M000294425

Comprehensive Treatment of Chronic Pain by Medical, Interventional, and Integrative Approaches

Timothy R. Deer
Editor-in-chief

Michael S. Leong
Associate Editor-in-chief

Asokumar Buvanendran • Vitaly Gordin
Philip S. Kim • Sunil J. Panchal • Albert L. Ray
Associate Editors

Comprehensive Treatment of Chronic Pain by Medical, Interventional, and Integrative Approaches

the AMERICAN ACADEMY *of* PAIN MEDICINE
Textbook on Patient Management

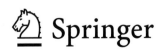 Springer

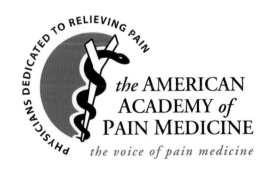

Editor-in-chief
Timothy R. Deer, M.D.
President and CEO
The Center for Pain Relief
Clinical Professor of Anesthesiology
West Virginia University School of Medicine
Charleston, WV, USA

Associate Editor-in-chief
Michael S. Leong, M.D.
Clinic Chief
Stanford Pain Medicine Center
Redwood City, CA, USA
Clinical Associate Professor
Department of Anesthesiology
Stanford University School of Medicine
Stanford, CA, USA

Associate Editors
Asokumar Buvanendran, M.D.
Professor
Department of Anesthesiology
Rush Medical College
Director
Orthopedic Anesthesia
Rush University Medical Center
Chicago, IL, USA

Vitaly Gordin, M.D.
Associate Professor
Associate Vice Chair of Pain Management
Department of Anesthesiology
Pennsylvania State University
College of Medicine
Director
Pain Medicine
Milton S. Hershey Medical Center
Hershey, PA, USA

Philip S. Kim, M.D.
Medical Director
Center for Interventional Pain & Spine,
Newark, DE and Bryn Mawr, PA, USA

Sunil J. Panchal, M.D.
President
National Institute of Pain
Tampa, FL, USA

Albert L. Ray, M.D.
Medical Director
The LITE Center
South Miami, FL, USA
Clinical Associate Professor
University of Miami Miller School of Medicine
Miami, FL, USA

ISBN 978-1-4614-1559-6   ISBN 978-1-4614-1560-2   (eBook)
DOI 10.1007/978-1-4614-1560-2
Springer New York Heidelberg Dordrecht London

Library of Congress Control Number: 2012954791

© American Academy of Pain Medicine 2013
This work is subject to copyright. All rights are reserved by the Publisher, whether the whole or part of the material is concerned, specifically the rights of translation, reprinting, reuse of illustrations, recitation, broadcasting, reproduction on microfilms or in any other physical way, and transmission or information storage and retrieval, electronic adaptation, computer software, or by similar or dissimilar methodology now known or hereafter developed. Exempted from this legal reservation are brief excerpts in connection with reviews or scholarly analysis or material supplied specifically for the purpose of being entered and executed on a computer system, for exclusive use by the purchaser of the work. Duplication of this publication or parts thereof is permitted only under the provisions of the Copyright Law of the Publisher's location, in its current version, and permission for use must always be obtained from Springer. Permissions for use may be obtained through RightsLink at the Copyright Clearance Center. Violations are liable to prosecution under the respective Copyright Law.
The use of general descriptive names, registered names, trademarks, service marks, etc. in this publication does not imply, even in the absence of a specific statement, that such names are exempt from the relevant protective laws and regulations and therefore free for general use.
While the advice and information in this book are believed to be true and accurate at the date of publication, neither the authors nor the editors nor the publisher can accept any legal responsibility for any errors or omissions that may be made. The publisher makes no warranty, express or implied, with respect to the material contained herein.

Printed on acid-free paper

Springer is part of Springer Science+Business Media (www.springer.com)

To my wonderful wife, Missy, and the blessings I have been given in my children Morgan, Taylor, Reed, and Bailie.
I also want to thank my team for their awesome, continued support: Chris Kim, Rick Bowman, Doug Stewart, Matt Ranson, Jeff Peterson, Michelle Miller, Wil Tolentino, and Brian Yee.

Timothy R. Deer, M.D.

To all of my mentors, colleagues, and patients who have taught me about pain medicine. I would also like to acknowledge the patience and love of my family, particularly my children, Isabelle and Adam, as well as Brad, PFP, and little Mia. I have discovered more about myself during my short career than I thought possible and hope to help many more people cope with pain in the exciting future.

Michael S. Leong, M.D.

To Maria, Yuri, and Jacob for their patience and understanding, and to my fellows for choosing the field of pain management.

Vitaly Gordin, M.D.

To my very supportive wife, Gowthy, and my wonderful kids: Dhanya and Arjun Asokumar.

Asokumar Buvanendran, M.D.

To my very supportive wife, Claire, and my wonderful kids: Alex, Keira, and Grant.

Philip S. Kim, M.D.

To my children, Neha, Anjali, and Naresh, for their patience, support, and understanding.

Sunil J. Panchal, M.D.

To my family and The LITE Center team, who have been patient and allowed me time to do this work.

Albert L. Ray, M.D.

Foreword

A brand new textbook is a testament to many things—an editor's vision, many authors' individual and collective expertise, the publisher's commitment, and all told, thousands of hours of hard work. This book encapsulates all of this, and with its compendium of up-to-date information covering the full spectrum of the field of pain medicine, it stands as an authoritative and highly practical reference for specialists and primary care clinicians alike. These attributes would be ample, in and of themselves, yet this important addition to the growing pain medicine library represents a rather novel attribute. It is a tangible embodiment of a professional medical society's fidelity to its avowed mission. With its commission of this text, under the editorial stewardship of highly dedicated and seasoned pain medicine specialists, the American Academy of Pain Medicine has made an important incremental step forward to realizing its ambitious mission, "to optimize the health of patients in pain and eliminate the major public health problem of pain by advancing the practice and specialty of pain medicine."

This last year, the Institute of Medicine (IOM) of the National Academies undertook the first comprehensive evaluation of the state of pain care in the United States. This seminal work culminated in a report and recommendations entitled "Relieving Pain in America: A Blueprint for Transforming Prevention, Care, Education, and Research." Clearly, as a nation, we have much work to do in order to meet the extraordinary public health needs revealed by the IOM committee. This comprehensive textbook is both timely and relevant as a resource for clinicians, educators, and researchers to ensure that the converging goals of the American Academy of Pain Medicine and the Institute of Medicine are realized. This book has been written; it is now all of ours to read and implement. Godspeed!

Salt Lake City, UT, USA   Perry G. Fine, M.D.

Foreword

The maturation of a medical specialty rests on both its ability to project its values, science, and mission into the medical academy and the salience of its mission to the public health. The arrival of the American Academy of Pain Medicine (AAPM)'s *Comprehensive Treatment of Chronic Pain by Medical, Interventional, and Integrative Approaches*: *the American Academy of Pain Medicine Textbook on Patient Management* is another accomplishment that signals AAPM's emergence as the premier medical organization solely dedicated to the development of pain medicine as a specialty in the service of patients in pain and the public health.

Allow me the privilege of brief comment on our progress leading to this accomplishment. The problem of pain as both a neurophysiological event and as human suffering has been a core dialectic of the physician-healer experience over the millennia, driving scientific and religious inquiry in all cultures and civilizations. The sentinel concepts and historical developments in pain medicine science and practice are well outlined in this and other volumes. Our history, like all of medicine's, is replete with examples of sociopolitical forces fostering environments in which individuals with vision and character initiated major advances in medical care. Thus the challenge of managing chronic pain and suffering born of injuries to troops in WWII galvanized John Bonica and other pioneers, representing several specialties, into action. They refused to consider that their duty to these soldiers, and by extension their brethren in chronic pain of all causes, was finished once pain was controlled after an acute injury or during a surgical procedure. They and other clinicians joined scientists in forming the IASP (International Association for the Study of Pain) in 1974, and the APS (American Pain Society) was ratified as its American chapter in 1978. Shortly thereafter, APS physicians with a primary interest in the development of pain management as a distinct medical practice began discussing the need for an organizational home for physicians dedicated to pain treatment; in 1984, they formally chartered AAPM. We soon obtained a seat in the AMA (American Medical Association). Since then, we have provided over two decades of leadership to the "House of Medicine," culminating in leadership of the AMA's Pain and Palliative Medicine Specialty Section Council that sponsored and conducted the first Pain Medicine Summit in 2009. The summit, whose participants represented all specialties caring for pain, made specific recommendations to improve pain education for all medical students and pain medicine training of residents in all specialties and to lengthen and strengthen the training of pain medicine specialists who would assume responsibility for the standards of pain education and care and help guide research.

Other organizational accomplishments have also marked our maturation as a specialty. AAPM developed a code of ethics for practice, delineated training and certification requirements, and formed a certifying body (American Board of Pain Medicine, ABPM) whose examination was based on the science and practice of our several parent specialties coalesced into one. We applied for specialty recognition in ABMS (American Board of Medical Specialties), and we continue to pursue this goal in coordination with other specialty organizations to assure the public and our medical colleagues of adequate training for pain medicine specialists. We have become a recognized and effective voice in medical policy. The AAPM, APS, and AHA (American Hospital Association) established the Pain Care Coalition (PCC), recently joined by the ASA (American Society of Anesthesiologists). Once again, by garnering sociopolitical support galvanized by concern for the care of our wounded warriors, the PCC was able to partner with the American Pain Foundation (APF) and other organizations to pass three new laws requiring the Veterans Administration and the military to report yearly on advances in pain management, training, and research and requiring the NIH (National Institute of Health) to examine its pain research portfolio and undertake the recently completed IOM report on pain.

AAPM has developed a robust scientific presence in medicine. We publish our own journal, *Pain Medicine*, which has grown from a small quarterly journal to a respected monthly publication that represents the full scope of pain medicine science and practice. Annually, we conduct the only medical conference that is dedicated to coverage of the full scope of pain medicine science and practice and present a robust and scientific poster session that represents our latest progress. Yet, year to year, we lament that the incredible clinical wisdom displayed at this conference, born out of years of specialty practice in our field, is lost between meetings. Now comes a remedy, our textbook—*Comprehensive Treatment of Chronic Pain by Medical, Interventional, and Integrative Approaches*.

Several years ago, Editor Tim Deer, who co-chaired an Annual Meeting Program Committee with Todd Sitzman, recognized the special nature of our annual conference and proposed that the AAPM engages the considerable expertise of our membership in producing a textbook specifically focused on the concepts and practice of our specialty. Under the visionary and vigorous leadership of Tim as Editor-in-Chief and his editorial group, *Comprehensive Treatment of Chronic Pain by Medical, Interventional, and Integrative Approaches* has arrived. Kudos to Tim, his Associate Editor-in-Chief Michael Leong, Associate Editors Asokumar Buvanendran, Vitaly Gordin, Philip Kim, Sunil Panchal, and Albert Ray for guiding our busy authors to the finish line. The expertise herein represents the best of our specialty and its practice. And finally, a specialty organization of physician volunteers needs a steady and resourceful professional staff to successfully complete its projects in the service of its mission. Ms. Susie Flynn, AAPM's Director of Education, worked behind-the-scenes with our capable Springer publishers and Tim and his editors to assure our book's timely publication. Truly, this many-faceted effort signals that the academy has achieved yet another developmental milestone as a medical organization inexorably destined to achieve specialty status in the American medical pantheon.

Philadelphia, PA, USA   Rollin M. Gallagher, M.D., MPH

Preface

In recent years, I have found that the need for guidance in treating those suffering from chronic pain has increased, as the burden for those patients has become a very difficult issue in daily life. Our task has been overwhelming at times, when we consider the lack of knowledge that many of us found when considering issues that are not part of our personal repertoire and training. We must be mentors of others and elevate our practice, while at the same time maintain our patient-centric target. Not only do we need to train and nurture the medical student, but also those in postgraduate training and those in private and academic practice who are long separated from their training. We are burdened with complex issues such as the cost of chronic pain, loss of functional individuals to society, abuse, addiction, and diversion of controlled substances, complicated and high-risk spinal procedures, the increase in successful but expensive technology, and the humanistic morose that are part of the heavy load that we must strive to summit.

In this maze of difficulties, we find ourselves branded as "interventionalist" and "non-interventionalist." In shaping this book, it was my goal to overcome these labels and give a diverse overview of the specialty. Separated into five sections, the contents of this book give balance to the disciplines that make up our field. There is a very complete overview of interventions, medication management, and the important areas of rehabilitation, psychological support, and the personal side of suffering. We have tried to give a thorough overview while striving to make this book practical for the physician who needs insight into the daily care of pain patients. This book was created as one of the many tools from the American Academy of Pain Medicine to shape the proper practice of those who strive to do the right things for the chronic pain patient focusing on ethics and medical necessity issues in each section. You will find that the authors, Associate Editor-in-chief, Associate Editors, and I have given rise to a project that will be all encompassing in its goals.

With this text, the American Academy of Pain Medicine has set down the gauntlet for the mission of educating our members, friends, and concerned parties regarding the intricacies of our specialty. I wish you the best as you read this material and offer you my grandest hope that it will change the lives of your patients for the better.

We must remember that chronic pain treatment, like that of diabetes and hypertension, needs ongoing effort and ongoing innovation to defeat the limits of our current abilities. These thoughts are critical when you consider the long standing words of Emily Dickinson…

"Pain has an element of blank; it cannot recollect when it began, or if there were a day when it was not. It has no future but itself, its infinite realms contain its past, enlightened to perceive new periods of pain."

Best of luck as we fight our battles together.

Charleston, WV, USA   Timothy R. Deer, M.D.

Contents

Contributors

Miriam Abbas Department of Neurosurgery, Regina General Hospital, Regina, SK, Canada

Nirmala R. Abraham, M.D. Sycamore Pain Management Center, Miamisburg, OH, USA

Hakan Alfredson, M.D., Ph.D. Sports Medicine Unit, University of Umea, Umea, Sweden

Marco Araujo, M.D., FACIP APM Green Bay Clinic, Green Bay, WI, USA

Charles E. Argoff, M.D. Department of Neurology, Albany Medical College, Albany, NY, USA

Comprehensive Pain Center, Albany Medical Center, Albany, NY, USA

Ignacio Badiola, M.D. Capitol Spine and Pain Centers, Fairfax, VA, USA

Ray M. Baker, M.D. Evergreen Spine and Musculoskeletal Program, Medical Director EvergreenHealth, Kirkland, WA, USA

John F. Barnes, PT, LMT, NCTMP Myofascial Release Treatment Centers and Seminars, Paoli, PA, USA

Brian Belnap, DO Department of Anesthesiology and Pain Medicine, University of California Davis Medical Center, Sacramento, CA, USA

Honorio T. Benzon, M.D. Department of Anesthesiology, Northwestern University Feinberg School of Medicine, Chicago, IL, USA

Cheryl D. Bernstein, M.D. University of Pittsburgh School of Medicine, Pittsburgh, PA, USA

Sharon Bishop, BScN, MHLTHSci Department of Neurosurgery, Regina General Hospital, Regina, SK, Canada

Cady Block, MS Department of Psychology, University of Alabama at Birmingham, Birmingham, AL, USA

Iwona Bonney, Ph.D. Department of Anesthesiology, Tufts Medical Center and Tufts University School of Medicine, Boston, MA, USA

Brandi A. Bottiger, M.D. Department of Anesthesiology, Duke University Hospital, Durham, NC, USA

Gary J. Brenner, M.D., Ph.D. Department of Anesthesia, Critical Care and Pain Medicine, Massachusetts General Hospital, Boston, MA, USA

Harvard Medical School, Boston, MA, USA

Christopher R. Brigham, M.D. Improvement Resources LLC, San Diego, CA, USA
American Board of Independent Medical Examiners, San Diego, CA, USA

AMA Guides Newsletter and Guides to Casebook, San Diego, CA, USA

Brian M. Bruel, M.D., MBA Department of Pain Medicine, The University of Texas MD Anderson Cancer Center, Houston, TX, USA

Daniel Bruns, PsyD Health Psychology Associates, Greeley, CO, USA

Chester Buckenmaier III, M.D. Department of Anesthesiology, Walter Reed National Medical Center, Rockville, MD, USA

Adam R. Burkey, M.D., MSCE Jefferson University, Medical Office Building, Phoenixville, PA, USA

Asokumar Buvanendran, M.D. Department of Anesthesiology, Rush Medical College, Chicago, IL, USA

Orthopedic Anesthesia, Rush University Medical Center, Chicago, IL, USA

Kevin D. Cairns, M.D., MPH Nova Southeastern University, Fort Lauderdale, FL, USA Broward General Medical Center, Fort Lauderdale, FL, USA

Marsha Campbell-Yeo, RN, MN, Ph.D. Candidate IWK Health Care, Maternal Newborn Program, Halifax, NS, Canada

Kenneth D. Candido, M.D. Department of Anesthesiology, Advocate Illinois Masonic Medical Center, Chicago, IL, USA

Daniel B. Carr, M.D., DABPM, FFPMANZCA (Hon) Departments of Public Health, Anesthesiology, Medicine, and Molecular Physiology and Pharmacology, Tufts University School of Medicine, Boston, MA, USA

Christopher J. Centeno, M.D. Physical Medicine and Rehabilitation, Pain Medicine, and Regenerative Medicine, Centeno-Schultz Clinic, Broomfield, CO, USA

George C. Chang Chien, DO Department of Physical Medicine and Rehabilitation, Rehabilitation Institute of Chicago, Northwestern Memorial Hospital, Chicago, IL, USA

Kiran K. Chekka, M.D. Department of Anesthesiology, Northwestern Memorial Hospital, Chicago, IL, USA

Leanne R. Cianfrini, Ph.D. Pain and Rehabilitation Institute, Birmingham, AL, USA

Robert I. Cohen, M.D., M.A. (Educ) Department of Anesthesia, Critical Care and Pain Medicine, Beth Israel Deaconess Medical Center, Boston, MA, USA

David Crane, M.D. Regenerative Medicine, Crane Clinic Sports Medicine, Chesterfield, MO, USA

Geralyn Datz, Ph.D. Forrest General Pain Management Program, Hattiesburg, MS, USA

Peter Davis, M.D. Departments of Anesthesiology and Pediatrics, University of Pittsburgh School of Medicine, Pittsburg, PA, USA

Department of Anesthesiology, Children's Hospital of Pittsburgh, Pittsburg, PA, USA

Miles R. Day, M.D., DABIPP, FIPP Department of Anesthesiology, Texas Tech University School of Medicine, Lubbock, TX, USA

International Pain Center, Texas Tech University Health Sciences Center, Lubbock, TX, USA

Timothy R. Deer, M.D. The Center for Pain Relief, Charleston, WV, USA

Department of Anesthesiology, West Virginia University School of Medicine, Charleston, WV, USA

Richard Derby, M.D. Spinal Diagnostics and Treatment Center, Daly City, CA, USA

Jagan Devarajan, M.D. Department of Anesthesiology, Cleveland Clinic, Cleveland, OH, USA

John Mark Disorbio, EdD Integrated Therapies, LLC, Lakewood, CO, USA

Daniel M. Doleys, Ph.D. Pain and Rehabilitation Institute, Birmingham, AL, USA

Kelly Donnelly, DO Department of Neurology, Albany Medical Center, Albany, NY, USA

Beth Dove, B.A. Dover Medical Communications, LLC, Salt Lake City, UT, USA

Allen R. Dyer, M.D., Ph.D. International Medical Corps, Washington, DC, USA

Jill Eckert, DO Pennsylvania State University College of Medicine, Hershey, PA, USA

Department of Anesthesiology, Pennsylvania State Milton S. Hershey Medical Center, Hershey, PA, USA

Jason S. Eldrige, M.D. Department of Anesthesiology and Pain Medicine, Rochester Methodist Hospital, Mayo Clinic, Rochester, MN, USA

Mitchell P. Engle, M.D. Department of Pain Medicine, University of Texas MD Anderson Cancer Center, Houston, TX, USA

Rachel Feinberg, PT, DPT Feinberg Medical Group, Palo Alto, CA, USA

Steven D. Feinberg, M.D. Feinberg Medical Group, Palo Alto, CA, USA

Stanford University School of Medicine, Stanford, CA, USA

American Pain Solutions, San Diego, CA, USA

Ananda Fernandes, MSN, Ph.D. Candidate Coimbra School of Nursing, Coimbra, Lisbon, Portugal

Scott M. Fishman, M.D. Division of Pain Medicine, Department of Anesthesiology and Pain Medicine, University of California, Davis School of Medicine, Sacramento, CA, USA

Kennth A. Follett, M.D., Ph.D. Department of Neurosurgery, University of Nebraska College of Medicine, Omaha, NE, USA

Robert D. Foreman, Ph.D. Department of Anesthesiology, University of Oklahoma Health Sciences Center, Oklahoma City, OK, USA

Department of Physiology, University of Oklahoma College of Medicine, Oklahoma City, OK, USA

Eduardo M. Fraifeld, M.D. Southside Pain Solutions, Danville, VA, USA

Michael C. Francis, M.D. St. Jude Medical, New Orleans, LA, USA
Integrative Pain Medicine Center, New Orleans, LA, USA

Raymond R. Gaeta, M.D. HELP Pain Medical Network, San Mateo, CA, USA

Rollin M. Gallagher, M.D., MPH Department of Psychiatry, Anesthesiology and Critical Care, University of Pennsylvania Perelman School of Medicine, Philadelphia, PA, USA

Pain Policy Research and Primary Care, Penn Pain Medicine Center, Philadelphia, PA, USA

Pain Management, Philadelphia Veterans Health System, Philadelphia, PA, USA

Robert J. Gatchell, Ph.D., ABPP Department of Psychology, College of Science, The University of Texas at Arlington, Arlington, TX, USA

Robert Gerwin, M.D. Department of Neurology, Johns Hopkins University School of Medicine, Baltimore, MD, USA

David M. Giampetro, M.D. Department of Anesthesiology, Pennsylvania State University College of Medicine, Hershey, PA, USA

Stuart Gitlow, M.D., MPH, MBA Department of Psychiatry, Mount Sinai School of Medicine, New York, NY, USA

Mark P. Gjolaj, M.D., MBA Stanford Pain Management Center, Redwood City, CA, USA

Division of Pain Medicine, Stanford University School of Medicine, Stanford, CA, USA

Joshua D. Goldner, M.D. Department of Anesthesiology, University Hospitals Case Medical Center, Cleveland, OH, USA

Stanley Golovac, M.D. Departments of Anesthesia, Pain Management, Surgery, Cape Canaveral Hospital, Cocoa Beach, FL, USA

Space Coast Pain Institute, Merritt Island, FL, USA

Claire Elaine Goodchild, B.Sc., M.Sc., Ph.D. Department of Psychology, Clinical Institute of Psychiatry, King's College London, London, UK

Vitaly Gordin, M.D. Department of Anesthesiology, Penn sylvania State Milton S. Hershey Medical Center, Hershey, PA, USA

Eric J. Grigsby, M.D. Napa Pain Institute, Queen of the Valley, St Helena Hospital, Napa, CA, USA

J. David Haddox, DDS, M.D., DABPM, MRO Tufts University School of Medicine, Boston, MA, USA

Department of Health Policy, Purdue Pharma L.P., Stamford, CT, USA

Julia Hallisy, DDS San Francisco, CA, USA

Ji-Sheng Han, M.D. Neuroscience Research Institute, Peking University, Beijing, China

Nathan J. Harrison, M.D. University of California, Davis Medical Center, Sacramento, CA, USA

Mandeville, LA, USA

Salim M. Hayek, M.D., Ph.D. Department of Anesthesiology, Case Western Reserve University, Division of Pain Medicine University Hospitals, Cleveland, OH, USA

James E. Heavner, DVM, Ph.D. Department of Anesthesiology, Texas Tech University School of Medicine, Lubbock, TX, USA

Department of Anesthesia, University Medical Center, Lubbock, TX, USA

Andrea G. Hohmann, Ph.D. Department of Psychological and Brain Sciences, Indiana University, Bloomington, IN, USA

Gary L. Horowitz, M.D. Department of Pathology, Beth Israel Deaconess Medical Center, Boston, MA, USA

Harvard Medical School, Boston, MA, USA

Marc A. Huntoon, M.D. Department of Anesthesiology, Mayo Clinic, Rochester, MN, USA

Piotr K. Janicki, M.D., Ph.D., DSci, DABA Department of Anesthesiology, Pennsylvania State Milton S. Hershey Medical Center, Hershey, PA, USA

Laboratory of Perioperative Geriatrics, Pennsylvania State University College of Medicine, Hershey, PA, USA

Valerie Johnson-Montieth, M.A., Ph.D. Candidate Department of Psychology, University of Texas at Arlington, Arlington, TX, USA

Celeste Johnston, RN, DEd School of Nursing, McGill University, Montreal, QC, Canada

Abdallah I. Kabbara, M.D. Department of Pain Management, St. John Medical Center, Westlake, OH, USA

Fnu Kailash, M.D. Department of Pain Management, Institute for Pain Diagnostics and Care, Ohio Valley General Hospital, McKees Rocks, PA, USA

Leonardo Kapural, M.D., Ph.D. Carolinas Pain Institute and Center for Clinical Research, Winston-Salem, NC, USA

Department of Anesthesiology, Wake Forest University School of Medicine, Winston-Salem, NC, USA

Jordan F. Karp, M.D. University of Pittsburg School of Medicine, Pittsburgh, PA, USA

Department of Psychiatry, University of Pittsburgh Medical Center, Pittsburgh, PA, USA

Manpreet Kaur, M.D. Department of Neurology, Albany Medical Center, Albany, NY, USA

John C. Keel, M.D. Spine Center, Beth Israel Deaconess Medical Center, Boston, MA, USA

Department of Orthopedics, Harvard Medical School, Boston, MA, USA

Barry Kerner, M.D., DABPM Silver Hill Hospital, New Canaan, CT, USA

Philip S. Kim, M.D. Center for Interventional Pain & Spine, Newark, DE and Bryn Mawr, PA, USA

Kenneth L. Kirsh, Ph.D. Department of Behavioral Medicine, The Pain Treatment Center of the Bluegrass, Lexington, KY, USA

Hendrick Klopper, M.D. Department of Neurosurgery, University of Nebraska Medical Center, Omaha, NE, USA

Timothy Y. Ko, M.D. LakeHealth Department of Anesthesiology, Division of Pain, Medicine, Pinnacle Interventional Pain and Spine Consultants, Concord Township, OH, USA

Lynn R. Kohan, M.D. Department of Anesthesiology, Pain Management Center, University of Virginia School of Medicine, Charlottesville, VA, USA

Krishna Kumar, M.B.B.S., MS, FRCSC Department of Neurosurgery, Regina General Hospital, Regina, SK, Canada

Tim J. Lamer, M.D. Department of Anesthesiology and Pain Clinic, Rochester Methodist Hospital, Mayo Clinic, Rochester, MN, USA

Mayo College of Medicine, Rochester, MN, USA

Melinda M. Lawrence, M.D. Department of Anesthesiology, University Hospitals Case Medical Center, Cleveland, OH, USA

Erin F. Lawson, M.D. Department of Anesthesiology, University of California, San Diego Medical Center, La Jolla, CA, USA

Michael S. Leong, M.D. Stanford Pain Medicine Center, Redwood City, CA, USA

Department of Anesthesiology, Stanford University School of Medicine, Stanford, CA, USA

Felix S. Linetsky, M.D. Department of Osteopathic Principles and Practice, Nova Southeastern University of Osteopathic Medicine, Clearwater, FL, USA

Sean Mackey, M.D., Ph.D. Department of Anesthesiology, Standford University, Palo Alto, CA, USA

Division of Pain Medicine, Stanford University School of Medicine, Stanford, CA, USA

Gagan Mahajan, M.D. Department of Anesthesiology and Pain Medicine, University of California, Davis School of Medicine, Sacramento, CA, USA

Jianren Mao, M.D., Ph.D. Department of Anesthesia, Harvard Medical School, Boston, MA, USA

Department of Anesthesia, Critical Care and Pain Medicine, Massachusetts General Hospital, Boston, MA, USA

Norman Marcus, M.D. Division of Muscle Pain Research, Departments of Anesthesiology and of Psychiatry, New York University Langone School of Medicine, New York, NY, USA

Marte A. Martinez, M.D. Department of Anesthesiology, University of Oklahoma Health Sciences Center, Oklahoma City, OK, USA

Gerald A. Matchett, M.D. Department of Anesthesiology and Management, University of Texas Southwestern School of Medicine, Dallas, TX, USA

Ali Mchaourab, M.D. Department of Anesthesiology, Cleveland Department of Veterans Affairs Medical Center, Cleveland, OH, USA

Porter McRoberts, M.D. Department of Interventional Spine and Pain Medicine, Holy Cross Hospital, Fort Lauderdale, FL, USA

Irina Melnik, M.D. Comprehensive Spine and Sports, Mill Valley, CA, USA
Spinal Diagnostics and Treatment Center, Daly City, CA, USA

Beth Mintzer, M.D., MS, CBE Department of Pain Management, Cleveland Clinic, Cleveland, OH, USA

Natalia E. Morone, M.D., MS University of Pittsburgh School of Medicine, Pittsburgh, PA, USA

Geriatric Research Education and Clinical Center, VA Pittsburgh Healthcare System, Pittsburgh, PA, USA

Garret K. Morris, M.D. Department of Anesthesiology, University of Rochester School of Medicine, Rochester, NY, USA

Beth B. Murinson, MS, M.D., Ph.D. Department of Neurology, Johns Hopkins University School of Medicine, Baltimore, MD, USA

Samer N. Narouze, M.D., M.Sc., DABPM, FIPP Department of Pain Management, Summa Western Reserve Hospital, Cuyahoga Falls, OH, USA

Department of Anesthesiology and Pain Management, Ohio University College of Osteopathic Medicine, Athens, OH, USA

Bruce D. Nicholson, M.D. Division of Pain Medicine, Department of Anesthesiology, Lehigh Valley Health Network, Allentown, PA, USA

Dermot More O'Ferrall, M.D. Advanced Pain Management, Greenfield, WI, USA

Chima O. Oluigbo, M.D. Department of Neurological Surgery, The Ohio State University Medical Center, Columbus, OH, USA

Denny Curtis Orme, DO, MPH Billings Anesthesiology PC, Billings, MT, USA

Jason Ough, M.D. Department of Pain Management/Anesthesiology, New York University Langone Medical Center, New York, NY, USA

Sunil J. Panchal, M.D. National Institute of Pain, Tampa, FL, USA

Steven D. Passik, Ph.D. Professor of Psychiatry and Anesthesiology, Vanderbilt University Medical Center, Psychosomatic Medicine, 1103 Oxford House, Nashville, TN 37232, USA

Jeffrey T. B. Peterson The Center for Pain Relief, Inc., Charleston, WV, USA

Jason E. Pope, M.D. Napa Pain Institute, Queen of the Valley, St Helena Hospital, Napa, CA, USA

Department of Anesthesiology, Vanderbilt University School of Medicine, Nashville, TN, USA

Lawrence R. Poree, M.D., MPH, Ph.D. Department of Anesthesia and Perioperative Care, University of California San Francisco, San Francisco, CA, USA

Pain Management, Pain Clinic of Monterey Bay, Aptos, CA, USA

Gabor Bela Racz, M.D., DABIPP, FIPP Department of Anesthesiology, Texas Tech University School of Medicine, Lubbock, TX, USA

International Pain Center, Texas Tech University Health Sciences Center, Lubbock, TX, USA

Maunak V. Rana, M.D. Department of Anesthesiology, Chicago Anesthesia Pain Specialists, Advocate Illinois Masonic Medical Center, Chicago, IL, USA

Department of Anesthesiology, University of Illinois at Chicago Medical Center, Chicago, IL, USA

Manon Ranger, RN, Ph.D. Candidate School of Nursing, McGill University, Montreal, QC, Canada

Louis J. Raso, M.D. Jupiter Interventional Pain Management Corp, Jupiter, FL, USA

Richard L. Rauck, M.D., FIPP Department of Anesthesiology, Wake Forest University School of Medicine, Carolinas Pain Institute, Winston-Salem, NC, USA

Albert L. Ray, M.D. The LITE Center, South Miami, FL, USA

University of Miami Miller School of Medicine, Miami, FL, USA

Selina Read, M.D. Department of Anesthesiology, Penn State College of Medicine, Penn State Milton S. Hershey Medical Center, Hershey, PA, USA

Ali R. Rezai, M.D. Department of Neurological Surgery, The Ohio State University Medical Center, Columbus, OH, USA

Center for Neuromodulation, The Ohio State University School of Medicine, Columbus, OH, USA

Ben A. Rich, JD, Ph.D. Department of Bioethics, University of California, Davis School of Medicine, Sacramento, CA, USA

Syed Rizvi, M.D. Department of Neurosurgery, Regina General Hospital, Regina, SK, Canada

William Rowe, M.A. American Pain Foundation, Baltimore, MD, USA

Ethan B. Russo, M.D. GW Pharmaceuticals, Vashon, WA, USA

Pharmaceutical Sciences, University of Montana, Missoula, MT, USA

Lloyd Saberski, M.D. Advanced Diagnostic Pain Treatment Centers, Yale-New
Haven Hospital, New Haven, CT, USA

Mehul Sekhadia, DO Northwestern University, Feinberg School of Medicine,
Chicago, IL, USA

Saloni Sharma, M.D. Pittsburgh, PA, USA

Naileshni Singh, M.D. Department of Anesthesiology, UC-Davis Medical Center,
Sacramento, CA, USA

Department of Anesthesiology, UC-Davis Medical Center,
Sacramento, CA, USA

Todd B. Sitzman, M.D., MPH Advanced Pain Therapy, PLLC, Hattiesburg, MS, USA

Konstantin V. Slavin, M.D., FAANS Department of Neurosurgery, University of Illinois
at Chicago School of Medicine, Chicago, IL, USA

Howard S. Smith, M.D., FACP, FAAPM, FACNP Department of Anesthesiology,
Albany Medical College, Albany Medical Center, Albany, NY, USA

Jeffrey P. Smith, M.D., MBA Department of Anesthesiology and Pain Management,
Texas Tech University School of Medicine, Lubbock, TX, USA

David Spiegel, M.D. Department of Psychiatry and Behavioral Sciences, Stanford
University School of Medicine, Stanford, CA, USA

Steven Stanos, DO Department of Physical Medicine and Rehabilitation, Center for
Pain Management, Rehabilitation Institute of Chicago, Chicago, IL, USA

Northwestern University Medical School, Feinberg School of Medicine, Chicago, IL, USA

Michael Stanton-Hicks, M.D., M.B.B.S., FRCA, ABPM, FIPP Department of Pain
Management, Cleveland Clinic, Clevland, OH, USA

Department of Anesthesiology, Cleveland Clinic Lerner College of Medicine,
Cleveland, OH, USA

Christopher A. Steel, M.D. Department of Anesthesiology, Pennsylvania State University
Milton S. Hershey Medical Center, Hershey, PA, USA

Richard L. Stieg, M.D., MHS Denver, CO, USA

Heidi J. Stokes Minneapolis, MN, USA

Mariel Szapiel, M.D. Department of Neurological Surgery, The Ohio State University
Medical Center, Columbus, OH, USA

South Denver Neurosurgery, Littleton, CO, USA

Alexander Taghva, M.D. Department of Neurological Surgery, Ohio State University
Medical Center, Columbus, OH, USA

Nicole K.Y. Tang, D. Phil (Oxon) Department of Primary Care Sciences,
Arthritis Research UK Primary Care Centre, Keele University, Staffordshire, UK

Kyle Tokarz, DO Department of Anesthesiology, Naval Medical Center, San Diego,
San Diego, CA, USA

Andrea Trescot, M.D. Algone Pain Center, St. Augustine, FL, USA

Rhonwyn Ullmann, MS The LITE Center, South Miami, FL, USA

Thuong D. Vo, M.D. Southern California Spine & Pain Institute, Westminster, CA, USA

Kevin E. Vorenkamp, M.D. Department of Anesthesiology, Pain Management Center, University of Virginia School of Medicine, Charlottesville, VA, USA

Yakov Vorobeychik, M.D., Ph.D. Department of Anesthesiology, Pennsylvania State University, Milton S. Hershey Medical Center, Hershey, PA, USA

Mark S. Wallace, M.D. Department of Anesthesiology, University of California, San Diego School of Medicine, La Jolla, CA, USA

Carol A. Warfield, M.D. Department of Anesthesia, Harvard Medical School, Boston, MA, USA

Prides Crossing, MA, USA

Thomas J. Weber, DO Chronic Pain Medicine Center, Wake Forest University Baptist Health, Carolinas Pain Institute, Winston-Salem, NC, USA

Lynn R. Webster, M.D. Lifetree Clinical Research and Pain Clinic, Salt Lake City, UT, USA

Debra K. Weiner, M.D. University of Pittsburgh College of Medicine, Pittsburgh, PA, USA

Geriatric Research Education and Clinical Center, VA Pittsburgh Healthcare System, Pittsburgh, PA, USA

Ashley J. Wiese, DVM, MS, DACVA Department of Anesthesiology, University of California, San Diego School of Medicine, La Jolla, CA, USA

Bryan S. Williams, M.D., MPH Comprehensive Pain Medicine, Kaiser Permanente, Mid Atlantic Permanente Medical Group, Rush University College of Medicine, Chicago, IL, USA

September Williams, M.D. Ninth Month Productions, San Francisco, CA, USA

Channing D. Willoughby, M.D. Department of Anesthesiology, Pennsylvania State University Milton S. Hershey Medical Center, Hershey, PA, USA

Linda L. Wolbers, M.D. MPH Pain Clinic of Monterey Bay, Aptos, CA, USA

Tony L. Yaksh, Ph.D. Department of Anesthesiology, University of California, San Diego School of Medicine, La Jolla, CA, USA

Thomas L. Yearwood, M.D., Ph.D. Pain Consultants ASC, LLC, Pascagoula, MS, USA

Marc D. Yelle, M.D., Ph.D. Department of Anesthesiology, Wake Forest Baptist Medical Center, Winston-Salem, NC, USA

Part I

Medical Approaches

Vitaly Gordin, M.D.

Introduction

It is my great pleasure to introduce the Medical Approaches part to our readers. While this part covers a variety of topics, ranging from the neurobiological basis of pharmacological agents' utility in treating chronic pain to innovative agents and drug delivery systems, this part could not possibly address all medication-related issues facing the practicing physician. Rather than attempt to cover the entire spectrum of topics, our goal was to provide our readers with a body of work that serves as a reference as to the most common classes of medications a health care provider might prescribe on a daily basis. In addition to the chapters on frequently prescribed agents, this part reviews the adverse effects of opioid analgesics, monitoring of opioid use and abuse, the emerging role of cannabinoids in the treatment of pain, emerging trends in pharmacogenomics, drug interactions and polypharmacy. Experts from both academia and private practice, by collaborating throughout this part, provide the reader with an opportunity to learn from different perspectives on subjects that deeply affect both realms of medical practice. I must recognize and thank my distinguished, dedicated colleagues for sharing their expertise through contributions to this part. Were it not for the encouragement and fortitude of Dr. Tim Deer, this project would not have come to fruition. Additional gratitude is due to Ms. Elektra McDermott and Ms. Shelley Reinhardt, both from Springer, who helped to bring this part as the final product to the finish line.

A Survey of Systems Involved in Nociceptive Processing

Tony L. Yaksh and Ashley J. Wiese

Key Points

- A pain state can be generated by high-intensity stimuli, injury and inflammation, and injury to the peripheral nerve.
- Acute stimuli activate small primary afferents through terminal transducer protein that lead to a frequency dependent activation of the second-order dorsal horn neurons which project contralaterally in the ventrolateral tract to (i) the somatosensory thalamus that project to the somatosensory cortex and (ii) into the medial thalamus to project into limbic forebrain.
- With tissue injury, there is the local release of active products that sensitize the peripheral terminal and initiate an ongoing discharge which by its persistency leads to a spinal sensitization that yields an enhanced response to any given stimulus.
- Nerve injury leads to initiation of an ongoing (ectopic) activity which arises from trophic changes generated by the nerve injury at the terminal (neuroma) and in the dorsal root ganglion of the injured axon.
- In addition to the afferent traffic, nerve injury leads to changes in dorsal horn sensory processing such that large afferent input can initiate a strong activation in spinal nociceptive neurons as a result of a loss of local dorsal horn inhibitory control.

T.L. Yaksh, Ph.D. (✉)
Department of Anesthesiology, Anesthesia Research Lab 0818,
UC San Diego, 9500 Gilman Dr (CTF-312), La Jolla, CA 92093, USA

University of California, San Diego School of Medicine,
La Jolla, CA, USA
e-mail: tyaksh@ucsd.edu

A.J. Wiese, DVM, MS, DACVA
Anesthesia Research Lab 0818, UC San Diego,
9500 Gilman Dr (CTF-312), La Jolla, CA 92093, USA

Department of Anesthesiology, University of California,
San Diego Medical Center, La Jolla, CA, USA
e-mail: ajwiese@ucsd.edu

Background

High-intensity afferent input, tissue injury and inflammation, and injury to the peripheral nerve will initiate pain states with characteristic psychophysical properties. As will be considered below, this information processing can be modified to change the content of the message generated by a given stimulus to enhance the pain state (e.g., produce hyperalgesia), normalize a hyperalgesic state, or produce a decrease in pain sensitivity (e.g., produce analgesia). Management of that pain state is addressed by the use of agents or interventions which though specific targets at the level of the sensory afferent, the spinal dorsal horn or at higher-order levels (supraspinal) modify the contents of the sensory message generated by that physical stimulus. The important advances in the development of pain therapeutics have reflected upon the role played by specific underlying mechanisms which regulate these events. The aim of this overview chapter is to provide a context for the more detailed discussion of analgesics and their actions, which occur in accompanying chapters.

Overview of the Psychophysics of Nociception

Acute Stimulation

Transient thermal or mechanical stimulus of an intensity as to *potentially* yield injury evokes an escape response and an autonomic reaction (increased blood pressure and heart rate). The functional phenotype typically has four characteristics. (i) The response magnitude or pain report covaries with stimulus intensity. (ii) Removal of the stimulus immediately terminates the sensation and/or attendant behaviors. (iii) The sensation/ behavior is referred specifically to the site of stimulation, for example, it is somatotopically delimited, typically to the dermatome to which the stimulus is applied and the response, for example, the stimulated paw is the paw that is withdrawn. (iv) Often with an acute stimulus (such as a thermal probe), there are two perceived components to the

Pain psychophysics

Acute high intensity stimulus

• Coincident with stimulus

• Localized pain referral

• Limited to area of stimulation

• Proportional to stimulus intensity

Tissue injuring stimulus

• Persists after removal of stimulus

• Referred to area of injury (1˚) and to area adjacent to injury (2˚)

• Initiated by moderately aversive (hyperalgesia) or otherwise innocuous lstimuli (allodynia)

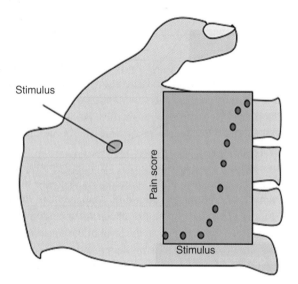

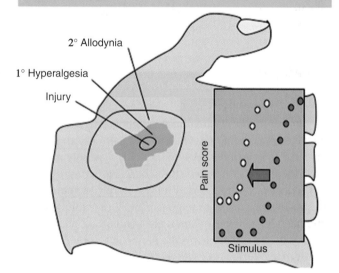

Fig. 1.1 Schematic displays the defining psychophysical properties that characterize the pain report after an acute high-intensity stimulus (*left*) and that after a local tissue injury (*right*). As indicated, in the inset plotting pain score vs. stimulus intensity, with the acute stimulus, the pain report for a given displays a threshold above which there is a monotonic increase in the magnitude of the reported pain state. After a tissue injury, there is an ongoing pain, and a stimulus applied to the injury site reveals that there is a greater pain report for a given stimulus (e.g., a primary hyperalgesia). In addition, it is appreciated that an innocuous mechanical stimuli applied to an adjacent uninjured area yields an enhanced response referred to secondary tactile allodynia

aversive sensation: an immediate sharp stinging sensation followed shortly by a dull throbbing sensation (Fig. 1.1).

Tissue Injury

The psychophysics of pain associated with a tissue injury and inflammation has several distinct psychophysical elements that distinguish it from the events initiated by an acute high-intensity stimulus (Fig. 1.1):

(i) With local tissue injury (such as burn, abrasion, or incision or the generation of a focal inflammatory state as in the joint), an acute sensation is generated by the injuring stimulus which is followed by an ongoing dull throbbing aching sensation which typically referred to the injury site—skin, soft tissue, or joint—and which evolves as the local inflammatory state progresses.

(ii) Application of a thermal or mechanical stimulus to the injury sited will initiate a pain state wherein the pain sensation is reported to be more intense than would be expected when that stimulus was applied to a non-injured site. That is to say, as shown in Fig. 1.1, the stimulus response curve is shifted up (e.g., an ongoing pain) and to the left. This lowered threshold of stimulus intensity required to elicit an aversive response to a stimuli applied to the injury site is referred to as primary hyperalgesia. Thus, modest flexion of an inflamed joint or moderate distention of the gastrointestinal (GI) track will lead to behavioral reports of pain.

(iii) Local injury and a low-intensity stimuli applied to regions adjacent to the injury may also produce a pain condition, and this is referred to as 2˚ hyperalgesia or allodynia. Thus, light touch may be reported as being aversive and is referred to as tactile allodynia.

These examples of "sensitization" secondary to local injury and inflammation are observed in all organ systems. Common examples would be sunburn (skin inflammation) leads to extreme sensitivity to warm water, inflammation of the pleura leads to pain secondary to respiration, and eyelid closure is painful secondary to corneal abrasion [1, 2].

In the case of inflammation of the viscera, the ongoing pain sensations are typically referred to specific somatic dermatomes. Thus, cardiac ischemia is referred to the left arm and shoulder, while inflammation of the bowel is associated with ongoing pain and hypersensitivity to light touch applied to the various quadrants of the abdomen. Such "referred" pain states reflect the convergence of somatic and visceral pain systems [3].

Nerve Injury

As described by Silas Weir Mitchell in 1864, frank trauma leads to two identifying elements: ongoing dysesthetic pain typically referred to the dermatome innervated by the injured nerve and prominent increase in the sensitivity to light touch applied to these regions. Injury to the nerve may be initiated by a wide variety of physical (extruded intervertebral disc compression section), toxic (chemotherapy), viral (postherpetic neuralgia: HIV), and metabolic (diabetes). In most of these syndromes, these two elements are expressed to varying degrees [4].

Encoding of Acute Nociception

As outlined in Fig. 1.2, the systems underlying these effects of acute high-intensity stimulation may be considered in terms of the afferents, the dorsal horn, and projection components. Under normal conditions, activity in sensory afferents is largely absent. However, peripheral mechanical and thermal stimuli will evoke intensity-dependent increases in firing rates of lightly myelinated (A∂) or unmyelinated (C) afferents. Based on differential blockade, these two fiber types, differing markedly in conduction velocity, are thought to underlie the acute sharp pain and subsequent dull throbbing sensation, respectively.

Transduction Channels and Afferent Terminal Activation

The transduction of the physical stimulus is mediated by specific channels which increase their conductance when certain stimulus properties are present. Channels vary in the range of temperatures which activate them, ranging from hot (such as the TRPV1) to cool to cold (TRPM1). The acute response properties of the afferent are thus defined by the collection of transducer channels that are expressed on its terminals. Activation of these channels increases inward sodium and calcium currents and progressive depolarization of the terminal (Fig. 1.2a) [5, 6].

Chemical Sensitivity of Temperature Channels

An important element regarding these channels is that while they are to varying degrees temperature sensitive, they also show sensitivity to specific chemicals. Thus, the TRPV1 responds to capsaicin, while the TRPM1 responds to menthol. Accordingly, when these agents are applied to the tongue, the sensation associated with their application corresponds with the sensation produced by the fibers which normally activate these fibers, hot and cool, respectively [7].

Action Potential Generation

Peripheral terminal depolarization leads to activation of the voltage-gated sodium channels which then leads to action potentials in the respective afferent. Subtypes of sodium channels (designated as NaV 1.1 through NaV 1.9 channels) have been identified.

These channels differ in terms of their activation properties as well as their pharmacology (e.g., tetrodotoxin sensitive or insensitive) and their distribution. Thus, some channels may be found principally on unmyelinated afferents (Nav 1.7) or distributed widely on all types of excitable membranes ranging from myocytes to brain neurons to a variety of afferents. Importantly, the frequency of afferent discharge is proportional to terminal depolarization which is proportional to stimulus intensity (Fig. 1.2b) [8, 9].

Encoding Properties of Primary Afferents

There are three important properties that define the encoding properties of any given class of primary afferents (Fig. 1.2b) [10]:

(i) Under resting conditions, the primary afferent, whether A or C, shows little or no spontaneous activity.

(ii) Primary afferents typically begin to respond to their respective stimulus modality (e.g., Aβ-tactile or C-thermal/mechanical/chemical) at some minimal intensity (e.g., threshold).

(iii) Above threshold, the frequency of firing evoked in the afferent axon will be proportional to stimulus intensity over a range of intensities. "Low-threshold" afferents will typically discharge at intensities that are considered to be nonnoxious. "High-threshold" or nociceptive

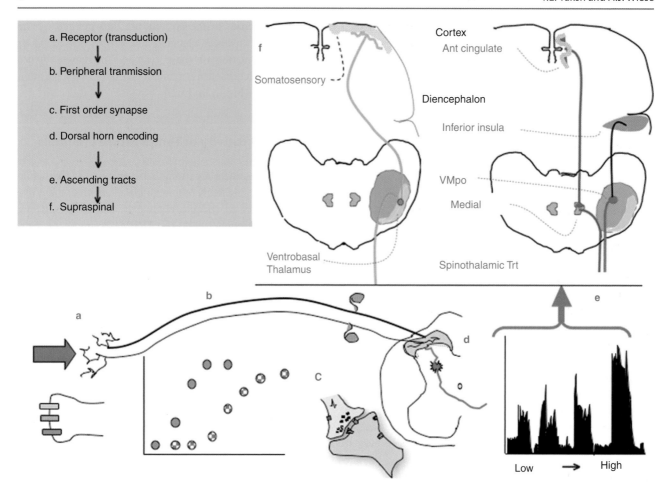

Fig. 1.2 This schematic provides an overview of the organization of events that initiate pain state after an acute high-intensity stimulus applied to the skin. (**a**) A physical stimulus activates channels such as the TRP channels on the terminal of small diameter afferents (*light line*). (**b**) There are two classes of afferents: large low-threshold afferents (Aβ: *dark line*) and small high-threshold afferents (A∂/C: *light line*). As the stimulus intensity increases, there is a monotonic increase in the discharge rate of each class of afferents with the low-threshold afferents showing an increase at low intensities, whereas the high-intensity afferents show an increase at higher intensities. The low and high threshold afferents project respectively into the deep and superficial dorsal horn. (**c**) The afferent input leads to depolarization of these spinal afferent terminals (**d**) which release excitatory transmitters yielding an (**e**) intensity-dependent depolarization of the second-order neuron. (Shown here is an example of the response of a neuron receiving convergent input from high and low threshold afferents.) Populations of these neurons project into the contralateral ventrolateral pathways to project to higher centers. (**f**) Broadly speaking, there are two classes of outflow. There are those which project into the somatosensory (ventrobasal) thalamus which then sends projection to the somatosensory cortex. A second type of projections goes to more medial thalamic regions and sends projection into areas of the old limbic forebrain (e.g., anterior cingulate/inferior insula)

afferents will discharge at intensities that are considered to be aversive in character.

Afferent Synaptic Transmission

Afferent action potentials invade the spinal terminal and depolarize these terminals. Such activation opens voltage-sensitive calcium channels which activate a variety of synaptic proteins which mediate the mobilization of synaptic vesicles and thereby initiate transmitter release.

Calcium Channels and Afferent Transmitter Release

There are a variety of voltage-sensitive calcium channels that regulate terminal transmitter release (referred to as CaV channels). These channels are distinguished on the basis of their voltage sensitivity, their location, and the agents which block them. The best known of these channels are the N-type calcium channel blocked by the therapeutic agent ziconotide. Block of this channel will block the release of many afferent terminal transmitters [11].

Table 1.1 Overview of classes of primary afferents characterized by common transmitter and cell markers

Fiber	Spinal termination	Cell marker		Channel/receptor		Transmitter	
		NF200	IB4	TRPV1 channel	Mu opioid receptor	Glutamate	Peptide (sP)
Aβ	III–VI	X				X	
A∂	II, III–V1	X				X	
C	I–II		X	X	X	X	X
C	II					X	

IB4 Isolectin B4, *NF200* Neurofilament 200

Spinal Afferent Terminal Transmitters

Sensory afferent uniformly releases excitatory transmitters. In terms of transmitters (Table 1.1), virtually all afferents contain and release the excitatory amino acid glutamate. Small afferent releases not only glutamate but also one or more of several peptides, such as substance P or calcitonin gene-related peptide (CGRP) (Fig. 1.2c). These transmitters in turn act postsynaptically upon eponymous receptors present on several of populations of dorsal horn neurons (Fig. 1.2d) [12]:

(i) Glutamate exerts the primary depolarizing effect through the activation of the AMPA receptor which leads to a short lasting increase in sodium conductance yielding a potent and short lasting depolarization of the membrane.

(ii) Substance P acts upon a G protein-coupled receptor that leads to a long slow depolarization of the membrane. Importantly, such receptors lead not only to a depolarization of the membrane, but to an increase in intracellular calcium, the glutamate by activating voltage-sensitive calcium channel and the NK1 by mobilizing intracellular calcium stores.

Laminar Organization of Spinal Dorsal Horn

The spinal dorsal horn is organized transversely in laminae (Rexed laminae), ranging from the most superficial dorsal horn marginal layer (lamina I), the substantia gelatinosa (lamina II), and the deeper nucleus proprius (laminae III–VI) [13].

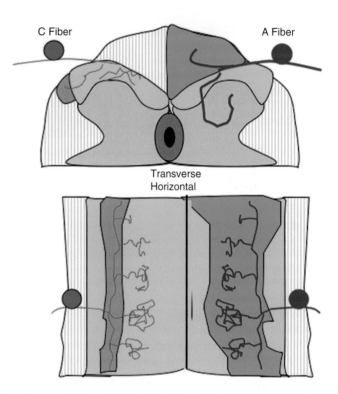

Fig. 1.3 Schematic presenting the spinal cord in transverse section (*top*) and horizontal (*bottom*) and showing: (i) (*left*) the ramification of C fibers in the superficial dorsal horn (laminae I and II) and collateralization into the tract of Lissauer and (ii) (*right*) the ramification of A fibers in the dorsal horn (terminating in the deep dorsal horn) and collateralization rostrocaudally into the dorsal columns and at each segment into the dorsal horn. The densest terminations are within the segment of entry. There are less dense collateralizations into the dorsal horns at the more distal spinal segments. This density of collateralization corresponds to the potency of the excitatory drive into these distal segments. Thus, distal segments may receive input from a given segment, but the input is not sufficiently robust to initiate activation of the neurons in the distal segment under normal circumstances

Primary Afferent Projections

There are several important principles reflecting the pattern of termination of afferent terminals in the dorsal horn (Fig. 1.3) [14]:

(i) Small afferents (A∂/C) terminate superficially in the lamina I (marginal layer) and lamina II. In contrast, the large afferents (Aβ) project deep into the dorsal horn and curve upwards to terminate just deep to lamina III.

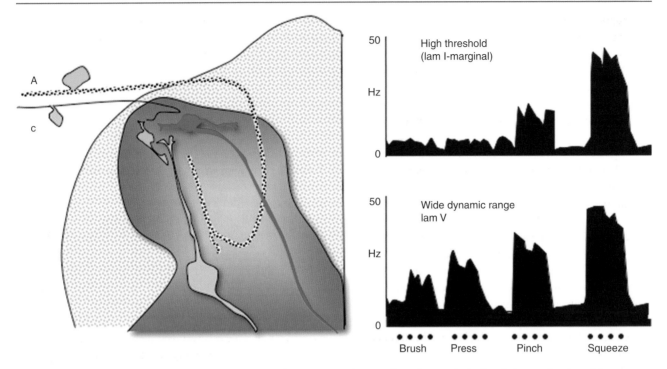

Fig. 1.4 Schematic displays (*left*) two principal classes of second-order neurons. As indicated, small afferents tend to terminate superficially (laminae I and II), while large afferents tend to project deep into the dorsal horn and terminate below lamina II. Accordingly, cells lying in lamina I (marginal layer) receive largely high-threshold input. Cells lying deeper (lamina V) received input from large afferents on their proximal dendrites and can receive excitatory input directly or through excitatory interneurons on their distal dendrites. (*right*) Single-unit recording from spinal dorsal horn, showing firing pattern (impulses/s) of a (*top*) high-threshold (nociceptive-specific marginal) neuron and (*bottom*) a horn wide-dynamic-range neuron, (WDR) located primarily in lamina V in response to graded intensities of mechanical stimulation (brush, pressure, pinch, squeeze) applied to the receptive fields of each cell. Both cells project supraspinally. Note the relationship between firing patterns and the response properties of the afferents with which each cell makes contact

(ii) Observing the spinal cord from the dorsal surface, it is noted that the central processes of the afferents collateralize, sending processes rostrally and caudally up to several segments into the dorsal columns (large afferents) or in the tract of Lissauer (small C-fiber afferents). Periodically, these collaterals send sprays into the dorsal horn at distal segments. Thus, neurons up to several segments distal to a given root entry zone of any given segment will receive afferent input from a given root (e.g., the L5 root will make synaptic contact with dorsal horn cells as far rostral as spinal segment L1). Importantly, the primary excitation occurs at the level of entry where the synaptic connections are strongest. At more distal segments, the degree of excitation from the proximal root is progressively reduced.

Dorsal Horn Neurons

Based on the organization of afferent termination, one can appreciate that superficial lamina I marginal neurons are primarily activated by small, high-threshold afferent input; hence they are "nociceptive specific." In contrast, the deeper lying cells have their cell bodies in lamina V and are hence called lamina V neurons but send their dendrites up into the superficial laminae. Interestingly, they receive input from Aβ (low-threshold) input on their ascending dendrites and C-fiber (high-threshold) input on their distal terminals (Fig. 1.4). Accordingly, these cells with their convergent input show activation at low intensities (mediated by the Aβ input) and increasing activation as the intensity rise (mediated by the C-fiber input). Accordingly, as shown in Fig. 1.2e, the cell shows increasing discharge rates over the range from very low to very high-threshold stimuli. Accordingly, these cells are referred to as wide-dynamic-range (WDR) neurons [15].

Dorsal Horn Projections

These lamina I and lamina V neurons then project via the ventrolateral tracts to higher centers and thence to cortical levels. Projections may occur ipsilaterally or contralaterally in the ventrolateral tracts. Ipsilaterally projecting axons typically project to terminate in the medial brainstem reticular nuclei. Cells receiving these projections then project to the thalamus. Contralateral axons project into several thalamic nuclei [13, 16].

Supraspinal Organization

The supraspinal projections can be broadly classified in two motifs (Fig. 1.2e) [13]:

(i) Dorsal horn, ventrobasal thalamic complex-somatosensory cortex. This is the classic somatosensory pathway. In these cases, the nervous system undertakes to maintain a specific intensity-, spatial-, and modality-linked encoding of the somatic stimulus, as summarized in Fig. 1.2. This pathway possesses the characteristics that relate to the psychophysical report of pain sensation in humans and the vigor of the escape response in animals. In the absence of tissue injury, removal of the stimulus leads to a rapid abatement of the afferent input and disappearance of the pain sensation. At all levels, the intensity of the message is reflected by the specific populations of axons which are activated and by the frequency of depolarization: the more intense the stimulation, the more frequent is the firing of the afferent; the greater is the dorsal horn transmitter release, the greater is the evoked discharge and the higher is the frequency of firing in the ascending pathway.

(ii) Dorsal horn-medial thalamus-limbic cortex. Here, there appears to be little precise anatomical mapping. Cells in this region project to regions such as the anterior cingulate cortex or inferior insula. The anterior cingulate is part of the older limbic cortex and is believed to be associated with emotional content.

The above subdivision reflects the orthogonal component of the pain experience, notably the "sensory-discriminative" components ("I hurt here on a scale of 1–10, 6") and the "affective-motivational" component of the pain pathway ("I have cancer, I am mortal") as proposed by Ronald Melzack and Kenneth Casey.

Encoding of Nociception After Tissue Injury

As reviewed above, with tissue injury, a distinct pattern of aversive sensations is observed. The psychophysical profile noted with injury or inflammation is composed of (i) an ongoing sensory experience that is described as dull throbbing aching ongoing pain, (ii) enhanced responsiveness to subsequent stimulation (e.g., hyperalgesia/tactile allodynia), and (iii) secondary pain referral (e.g., sensations which are aversive when applied to adjacent uninjured areas).

Peripheral Changes in Afferent Transmission Resulting from Tissue

As described in Fig. 1.1, in the event that a stimulus leads to a local injury, as in a tissue crush (trauma) or an incision, such stimuli may lead to the subsequent local elaboration of active products that directly activate the local terminals of afferents (that are otherwise silent) innervating the injury region and facilitating their discharge in response to otherwise submaximal stimuli. This then leads to an ongoing afferent barrage and enhanced response to any given stimulus (e.g., peripheral sensitization) (Fig. 1.5).

Origin of Ongoing Activity and Enhanced Terminal Responsiveness After Tissue Injury

The source of these active factors may be considered in terms of their source including the following (Fig. 1.5):

(i) Damaged cells which yield increased extracellular contents (potassium).

(ii) Products of plasma extravasation (clotting factors, cellular products such as platelets and erythrocytes which release products including amines (5HT), peptides (bradykinin), and various lipidic acids (prostaglandins)).

(iii) Innate immune cascade wherein given the chemoattractants present in the injury site, there will be a migration of inflammatory cells including neutrophils and macrophages. These contribute products such as myeloperoxidases, cytokines (TNF/IL1β), nerve growth factors (NGF), and serine proteases (trypsin).

(iv) Terminal of primary afferent C fibers activated by the local milieu will lead to a local release of sP and CGRP which respectively cause vasodilation (erythema) and capillary leakiness (e.g., tissue swelling).

Importantly, these products have several effects on terminal function that are dependent upon the presence of the eponymous receptors on those terminals (e.g., trypsin activates proteinase-activated receptors: PARs; TNF) and the concentrations of the ligand (Fig. 1.6) [17].

(i) Activate the sensory terminal, increase intracellular calcium, and initiate a conducted action potential.

(ii) Activate terminal kinases which serve to phosphorylate many membrane channels (e.g., sodium channels) and receptors (TRPV receptors) to increase their excitability. These actions are generally considered to result in spontaneous "afferent discharges" and to an enhanced responsiveness of the terminal to subsequent stimuli manifested by a left shift in the stimulus response curve for the sensory afferent. Overall, these properties are consistent with an ongoing pain stimulus and the ability of a given stimulus applied to that afferent in innervating the injured tissue to show a greater response (Fig. 1.2a).

It should be noted that these events are ubiquitous. This scenario has been demonstrated in numerous body systems, for example, cornea of the eye (sensitivity to light touch after abrasion), joint (pain of modest movement after inflammation of the knee), tooth pulp (sensory experience of cardiac-induced pressure changes in the tooth after inflammation of the pulp),

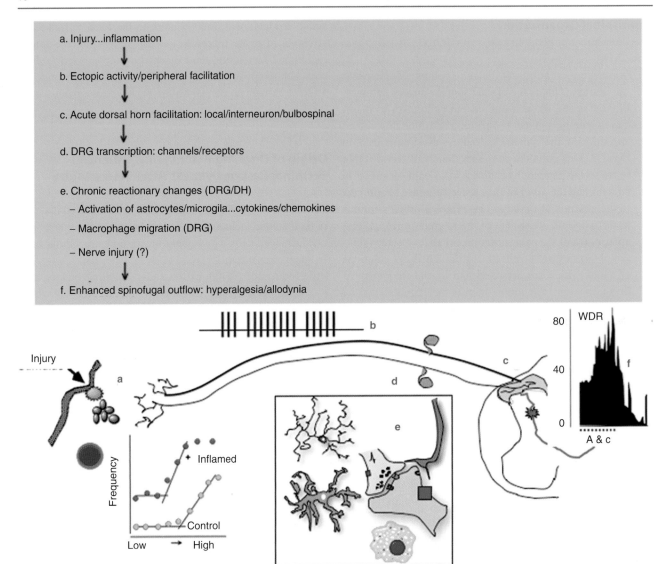

Fig. 1.5 This schematic provides an overview of the organization of events that initiate pain state after a tissue injuring stimulus of the skin. (**a**) Local tissue injury leads to the initiation of an innate immune response that yields the release of a variety of active factors. The factors acting through eponymous receptors on the terminals of C fibers lead to a activation of the C fiber and a state of sensitization. Accordingly, such products initiate an ongoing activity and an enhanced response to an otherwise innocuous stimulus. (**b**) The injury thus leads to an ongoing activity in small afferent. (**c**) The ongoing activity activates dorsal horn neurons and initiates a state of facilitation (windup). (**d**) The ongoing afferent traffic and injury products lead to a change in the tropic functions of the dorsal root ganglion leading to changes in protein synthesis and the expression of various receptors and channels which serve to enhance afferent responsiveness. (**e**) In the dorsal horn, the ongoing afferent drive initiates additional changes related to the activation of microglia and astrocytes as well as the invasion of typically nonneuronal cells including neutrophils and lymphocytes in the extreme. The net effect is to enhance the outflow initiated by any given stimulus, for example, hyperalgesia and allodynia. (**f**) With facilitation, the wide dynamic range neurons (WDR) are activated in response to stimuli that would normally not activate these neurons.[AW1]

and migraine (activation of the meningeal afferents which, like those in the tooth pulp, are not activated by normal mechanical movement or vascular pulsation). Indeed, think of any disease pathology described by the suffix "-itis" (Fig. 1.6).

Spinal Changes in Afferent Transmission Resulting from Tissue Injury

As reviewed above, acute activation of small afferents by extreme stimuli results in a spinal activation of dorsal horn neurons, the magnitude of which is proportional to the frequency (and identity) of the afferent input (Fig. 1.2e). Factors increasing that input-output relationship will cause a given stimulus to appear more intense (e.g., hyperalgesia). Conversely, factors reducing that function will cause a more intense stimulus to be encoded as less intense (e.g., analgesia). In the preceding section, it was appreciated that inflammation causes an enhanced response at the peripheral level. It is appreciated that there is also an enhanced response mediated in the spinal dorsal horn.

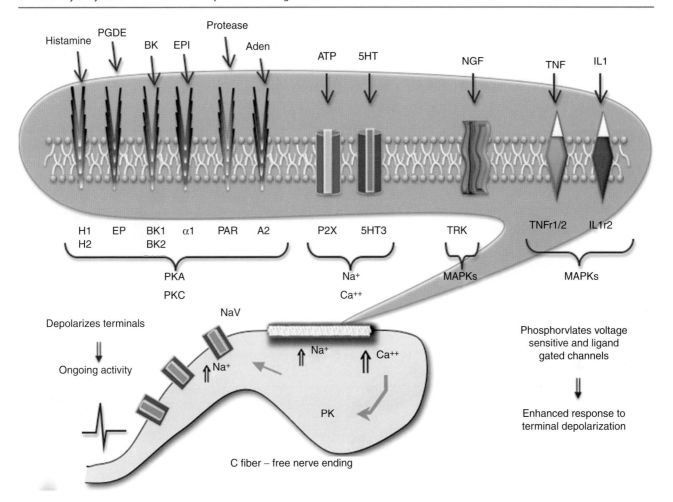

Fig. 1.6 This schematic provides an overview of the organization of events that initiate pain state after an injury to soft tissue. In the face of tissue injury, a variety of active products are released from local tissues, inflammatory cells, and the blood. These products exert a direct effect upon the small afferent terminal, free nerve endings, through specific receptors on the terminal. These receptors are coupled through a variety of second messengers which can lead to a local depolarization because of increased sodium and calcium influx. This leads to the activation of voltage-sensitive sodium channels (*NaV*) that initiate the regenerative action potential. In addition, the kinases and the increased intracellular calcium can initiate phosphorylation (*PK*) of channels and receptors, leading to an enhanced responsiveness of these channels and receptors. The net effect is to initiate an ongoing activity after the injuring stimulus has been removed and an increase in the discharge arising from any given stimulus

Central (Spinal) Facilitation

Animal research has demonstrated that repetitive afferent activation causes dorsal horn wide-dynamic-range (WDR) neurons to show evident signs of facilitation, labeled "windup" by Lorne Mendell and Patrick Wall (Fig. 1.4). This facilitation is characterized by following properties [18]:

 (i) High-frequency repetitive stimulation of C (but not A) fibers results in a progressively facilitated discharge of the WDR neurons.

(ii) The receptive field of the WDR neuron showing windup was significantly expanded acutely following the conditioning afferent stimulation, for example, stimulation of an adjacent dermatome which hitherto did not activate that cell, would now lead to activity in that neuron (Fig. 1.7).

Enhanced Response of WDR Neuron

The enhanced responsiveness of the cell was shown by intracellular recording to reflect a progressive and sustained (after termination of the stimulation) excitability of the neuron of the cell, rendering the membrane increasingly susceptible to even weak afferent inputs.

The enlarged receptive field can be explained by the ability of subliminal input coming from afferent input arising from an adjacent non-injured receptive field which was otherwise insufficient to activate a normally excitable cell.

Pharmacology of Central Facilitation

The enhanced excitability of dorsal horn neurons secondary to repetitive small afferent input reflects a series of complex

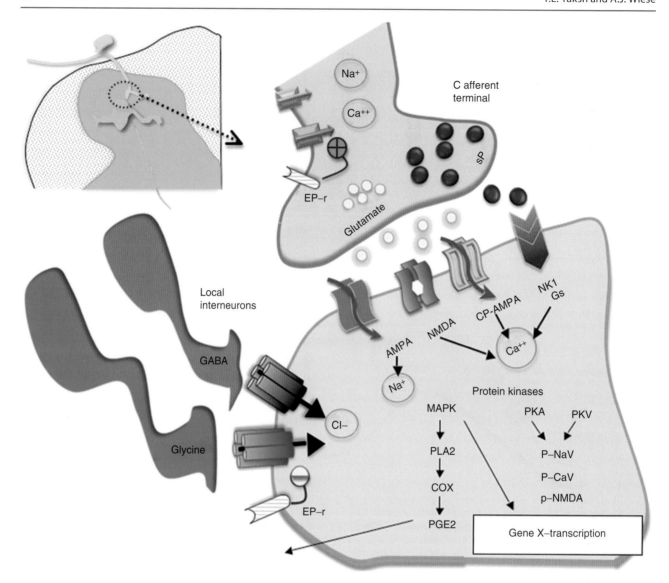

Fig. 1.7 This schematic provides an overview of the organization of the events transpiring at the level of the first-order synapse. (i) As indicated, the presynaptic effects of depolarization lead to opening of voltage-sensitive calcium and sodium channels with increases in intracellular sodium and calcium and mobilization and release of transmitters (*sP* and glutamate). (ii) These act upon eponymous receptors (see text), leading to depolarization and increase in intracellular calcium. (iii) Activation of kinases which phosphorylate a variety of channels and receptors activates intracellular enzyme cascades such as for PLA2 and

increasing gene transcription. (iv) Release of products such as prostanoids (*PGE2*) which can act upon the local membrane through their eponymous receptors (*EP-r*) where presynaptically they enhance the opening of voltage-sensitive calcium channels and postsynaptically reduce the activity of glycine receptors. (v). As indicated in addition, the first-order synapse is regulated by inhibitor interneurons such as those release GABA and glycine. These interneurons can be activated by afferent collaterals and by descending pathways to downregulate the excitability of this synapse

mechanistic motifs that have a diverse pharmacology which will be briefly reviewed below. These can be broadly considered in terms of those systems which are (i) postsynaptic to the primary afferent and (ii) mediated by local neuronal networks, extraspinal networks, and nonneuronal networks. Examples will be reviewed below (Fig. 1.8).

Primary Afferents

Small afferents release peptides (e.g., sP/CGRP) and excitatory amino acids (glutamate) which evoke excitation in second-order neurons through their eponymous receptors (Table 1.2; Fig. 1.7) [19–22].

(i) AMPA. Activation of the AMPA receptor leads to a short lasting but prominent increase in sodium conductance, yielding a robust, transient depolarization. Direct monosynaptic afferent-evoked excitation is largely mediated by the AMPA receptors, for example, AMPA receptor antagonists will block most acute excitatory input and produce an acute analgesia. A subtype of AMPA receptor is Ca permeable. For example, activation of these receptors leads to large increases in intracellular calcium.

(ii) NMDA. NMDA is a glutamate-activated ionophore that passes sodium and calcium. At normal resting membrane potential, the NMDA receptor is blocked by a

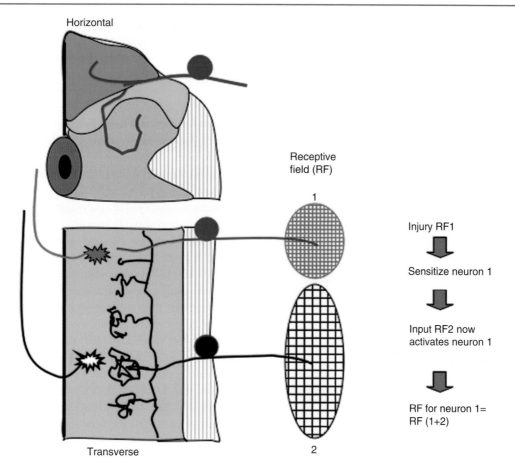

Fig. 1.8 Schematic presents the spinal cord in horizontal section (see Fig. 1.3). Receptive field of dorsal horn neuron depends upon the origin of its segmental input and the input from other segments, which can activate it. Thus, neuron 1 receives strong input from RF1 and very weak (ineffective) input from RF2. After injury in receptive field (*RF*) 1, neuron 1 becomes "sensitized." Collateral input from RF2 normally is unable to initiate sufficient excitatory activity to activate neuron 1, but after sensitization, RF2 input is sufficient. Now, the RF of neuron 1 is effectively RF1 + RF2. Thus, local injury can by a spinal mechanism leads acutely to increased receptive fields such that stimuli applied to a non-injured RF can contribute to the post-tissue injury sensation

Table 1.2 Summary of classes of spinal receptors postsynaptic to primary afferents

Transmitter	Receptor	Receptor type	Ion permeability
Glutamate	AMPA	Ionophore	Na
	AMPA-Ca permeable	Ionophore	Na, Ca
	NMDA	Ionophore	Na, Ca
sP	NK1	G protein cAMP dependent	None (Ca)
CGRP	CGRP1	G protein cAMP dependent	None (Ca)
BDNF	TRK B	Tyrosine kinase	–

sP substance P, *NMDA* N-methyl-D-aspartate, *BDNF* brain-derived neurotrophic factor, *NK1* neurokinin 1, *TRK B* tyrosine-related kinase B, *AMPA* α-amino-3-hydroxy-5-methyl-4-isoxazolepropionic acid

magnesium ion. In this condition, occupancy by glutamate will not activate the ionophore. If there is a modest depolarization of the membrane (as produced during repetitive stimulation secondary to the activation of AMPA (glutamate) and neurokinin 1 (NK1) (substance P) receptors), the Mg block is removed, permitting glutamate to now activate the NMDA receptor. When this happens, the NMDA channel permits the passage of Ca. Accordingly, block of the NMDA receptor has no effect upon acute activation but will prevent windup.

(iii) NK1 and CGRP. For sP and CGRP, excitation is through G protein-coupled receptors, neurokinin 1 (NK1) and CGRP, the effects of which are cAMP dependent and couple through the activation of phospholipase C. Activation of these receptors leads to slow, relatively long-lasting membrane depolarization accompanied by an increase in intracellular calcium. Agents which block the NK1 or CGRP receptor will produce minor effects upon the behavior evoked by acute excitation but will reduce the onset of the facilitated state and behaviorally defined hyperalgesia.

(iv) Growth factors. In addition to classic transmitters, growth factors such as brain-derived nerve growth factor (BDNF) is synthesized by small DRGs and released from spinal terminals, packaged in dense-cored vesicles, and transported within axons into terminals in the dorsal horn of the spinal cord. BDNF has potent sensitizing effect on spinal neurons mediated through TRK receptors.

As noted, with ongoing afferent drive, a progressive increase in excitation is noted. Aside from activation of the NMDA receptors, other components to this facilitatory process can be noted. These can be broadly considered in terms of those systems which are local to the neuronal networks in the dorsal horn, extraspinal networks, and nonneuronal networks. Several examples of each will be reviewed below.

Postsynaptic to the Primary Afferents

Repetitive activation of the primary afferent yields membrane depolarization and a significant increase in intracellular calcium. The increased intracellular calcium activates a series of intracellular cascades. Several examples are given below (Fig. 1.6):

(i) Activation of kinases. Persistent afferent input leads to a marked increase in intracellular Ca^{++} which leads to activation of a wide variety of phosphorylating enzymes, including protein kinase A and C, calcium calmodulin-dependent protein kinases, as well as mitogen-activated kinases (MAPKs) including p38 MAP kinase and ERK. Each of these kinases leads to a variety of downstream events which serve to increase the excitability of the neuron [23, 24].

(ii) Channel phosphorylation. The excitability of many channels is controlled by phosphorylation. Several examples may be cited. (1) PKA- and PKC-mediated phosphorylation of the NMDA ionophore leads to a facilitated removal of the Mg^{++} block and an increase in calcium current. (2) P38 leads MAPK activation to activation of phospholipase A2 (PLA2) which initiates the release of arachidonic acid and provides the substrate for cyclooxygenase (COX) to synthesize prostaglandins. In addition, this MAPK activates transcription factors such as NFKβ, which in turn activates synthesis of a variety of proteins, such as the inducible cyclooxygenase, COX2. Spinal P38 MAPK inhibitors thus reduce acutely initiated hyperalgesia and reduce the upregulation of COX2 otherwise produced by injury [23, 24].

(iii) Lipid cascades. A variety of phospholipases, cyclooxygenases, and lipoxygenases are constitutively expressed in the dorsal horn in both neuronal and nonneuronal cells. Lipid products including prostaglandins and other eicosanoids are synthesized and released after small afferent input. They serve to enhance the opening of voltage-sensitive calcium channels, augmenting afferent transmitter release. In addition, prostaglandins act postsynaptically to *reduce* glycine-mediated inhibition on second-order dorsal horn neurons. Such reduction in glycine or GABA interneuron activity leads to an increase in dorsal horn excitability (to be discussed further below). Spinal delivery of PGE will increase, while PLA2 or COX inhibitors will reduce, injury-induced hyperalgesia [25, 26].

(iv) Nitric oxide synthase (NOS). The neuronal and inducible forms of NOS are found in the spinal cord, and NO plays a facilitatory role, acting presynaptically through cGMP to enhance transmitter release. Spinal NOS inhibitors reduce post-tissue injury hyperalgesia [27].

Local Interneuronal Networks

The spinal dorsal horn has many local interneuronal circuits which are activated by primary afferent input:

(i) These interneurons may contain and release glutamate to act upon AMPA and NMDA receptors and are intrinsically excitatory. This polyneuronal chain can enhance the excitatory drive from a given afferent.

(ii) In addition, there are a wide variety of local interneurons which contain and release inhibitory amino acids such as GABA and glycine which act respectively on GABA A receptors and glycine receptors which are chloride ionophores that serve typically to downregulate the excitability of the membrane. These interneurons may project onto primary afferent terminals (presynaptic) and onto higher-order neurons (postsynaptic inhibition). The net excitatory outflow from the dorsal horn depends upon this local inhibitory regulation. Anything that increases that activity will diminish outflow, while events that inhibit the functionality of these inhibitory circuits will increase excitatory outflow.

As noted above, second-order deep dorsal horn neurons can receive excitatory input from large (Aβ) afferents. In spite of this afferent input onto dorsal horn neurons which are believed to play a role in nociceptive processing, this Aβ input will not typically evoke a pain state. However, after tissue injury such low-threshold mechanical stimuli may initiate a pain state (tactile allodynia). An element of this transition is believed to reflect a loss of local GABA or glycine inhibition. Thus, block of spinal GABA A and glycine receptors yields a markedly enhanced response of these WDR neurons to Aβ input and a behaviorally defined tactile allodynia. As noted above, repetitive small afferent input leads to a dorsal horn release of PGE2 which in turn reduces glycine-mediated opening of the glycine receptor and leads to a reduction in this local inhibition. The net effect is a corresponding increase in excitation evoked by low-threshold afferents.

Bulbospinal Systems

Serotonergic pathways (arising from the midline raphe nuclei of the medulla) project into the spinal dorsal horn. The effects of this bulbospinal projection are mediated by the presence of a variety of dorsal horn 5HT receptors. Some are inhibitory (5HT1a,b), and some are directly excitatory (5HT 2,3,7). The net effect is complexly defined by the nature of the neurons upon which the receptor is located. Inhibitory receptors on an excitatory neuron will lead to an

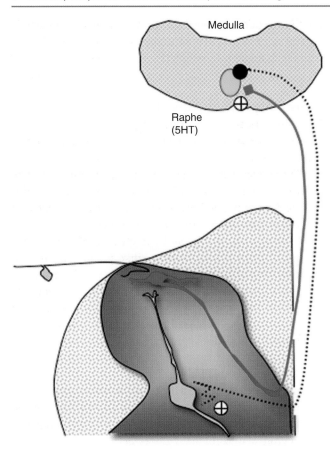

Medulla

Raphe
(5HT)

Fig. 1.9 Schematic shows bulbospinal 5HT arising from caudal raphe projects to the dorsal horn to synapse on 5HT3 cells and enhance excitability. This pathway may be activated by projections from lamina I neurons projecting to the raphe resulting in a spino-bulbo-spinal positive feedback loop

inhibition of excitation. Conversely, inhibition of an inhibition will lead to an excitation.

The most prominent effect however appears to be a net increase in excitability mediated by 5HT3 bearing dorsal horn neurons. A particularly interesting circuit involves the observation that lamina I (marginal) neurons project into the medullary brainstem to activate these bulbospinal serotonin neurons to activate deep dorsal horn neurons through the 5HT3 receptor. This spino-bulbo-spinal feedback pathway is believed to play an important role in afferent-driven spinal facilitation (Fig. 1.9) [28].

Nonneuronal Cells

Within the spinal parenchyma, there are a variety of nonneuronal cells. These include (i) astrocytes which arise from a multipotent neural stem cells, (ii) monocyte-derived cells (e.g., macrophages) which enter the nervous systems around parturition to become resident microglia, and (iii) circulating cells which enter the nervous systems during the course of peripheral injury and inflammation (neutrophils, lymphocytes, and macrophages). Classically, astrocytes were believed

to play a role in trophic systems function. The microglia were considered to be activated by CNS injury, and the circulating cells were part of the response to catastrophic injury and infection.

Current thinking now emphasizes the enormous constitutive contributions of these cells to the excitability of local neuronal circuits. While there are no direct synaptic linkages, neuraxial astrocytes and microglia can be activated by several linkages [29–32]:

(i) High-intensity afferent input leading to synaptic overflow of products such as glutamate, substance P, and BDNF.

(ii) Networks of astrocytes which may communicate over a distance by the spread of excitation through local nonsynaptic contacts ("gap" junctions) and by ATP acting on purine receptors on the glia.

(iii) Release of products from neurons. Microglia can be activated by release of chemokines (fractalkine) from the neuronal membrane. In addition to afferent input after tissue injury and inflammation, *circulating* cytokines (such as IL1β/TNF) can activate perivascular astrocytes/microglia.

(iv) Circulating products such as cytokines and lipids can activate these perivascular nonneuronal cells.

(v) Activation of spinal innate immune systems. It is appreciated that glial cells express a variety of toll-like receptors (TLRs). These TLRs are primitive recognition sites (first discovered in fruit flies) that can lead to glial activation. While these recognition sites have classically been considered relevant to recognizing membrane or molecular components of nonself entities such as viruses and bacteria, it is now appreciated that in the course of inflammation there are products that are released that can also activate these TLRs and their intracellular cascades. Activation of these receptors can initiate hyperalgesic states, while their blockade or knockout can minimize post-inflammatory hyperalgesia [33].

When activated, these glial cells can regulate synaptic excitability by (i) releasing excitatory products including ATP, free radicals, nitric oxide, lipid mediators, and cytokines and (ii) regulating extracellular parenchymal glutamate (by transporter-mediated uptake and release).

Preclinical work with spinal inhibitors of microglial activation such as minocycline (a second-generation tetracycline) and pentoxyfiline that have been reported to block indices of an acute or chronic glial activation and diminish hyperalgesic states has supported the role of nonneuronal cells in inflammation and injury-induced pain. These agents, while not clinically useful, suggest important directions in drug therapy development [34].

These events outlined above involving the nonneuronal cells are referred to broadly as "neuroinflammation." The work emphasizes that astrocytes and microglia are *constitutively* active and contributing to acute changes in spinal network excitability and can contribute to the enhanced response of the dorsal horn after peripheral tissue injury and inflammation.

Evolution of a Chronic Pain State After Acute Injury

In the preceding sections, we have focused on the events which occur after tissue injury and inflammation. After such tissue injury and inflammation, for example, as after trauma and surgery, pain typically resolves with a time course that is typically consistent with the resolution of the inflammation, a consequence which parallels the healing process. In a variable but significant fraction of patients, a failure to resolve the pain state in spite of healing may be noted. The persistency may be the result of an occult inflammation (e.g., failure to heal) or perhaps injury to the nerve which leads to events that are evidently unable to heal (see below). Alternatively, there is increasing evidence that in the face of persistent inflammation (as say in arthritis) that there may be fundamental changes in the functionality of the afferent/DRG to yield a state of persistent sensitization. For example, in the face of a persistent (weeks) inflammation in animal models, an allodynic state is noted that continues after the resolution of the inflammation. Importantly, the knockout of the TLR4 receptors has no effects upon the inflammation but prevents the evolution of the persistent tactile allodynia. This is an important area of ongoing research [35, 36].

Summary

Tissue injury and inflammation initiate a behavioral phenotype characterized by ongoing pain and the appearance of states where mildly aversive or innocuous stimuli lead to an enhanced pain state at the site of injury (primary) and adjacent to the site of injury (secondary). The mechanisms underlying these behavioral states reflect release of "active factors" at the injury site initiating afferent traffic and sensitizing the afferent terminal, yielding an enhanced response to a given stimulus. The ongoing afferent activity leads to a complex series of events in the dorsal horn representing local changes in membrane excitability, activation of local facilitatory circuits, blocking local inhibitory circuits, activation of spino-bulbo-spinal links, and engaging a complex "neuroinflammatory" process involving spinal nonneuronal cells.

Encoding of Nociception After Nerve Injury

The mechanisms underlying the spontaneous pain and the miscoding of low-threshold tactile input are not completely understood. However, the organizing concept is that these

events reflect (i) an increase in spontaneous activity the injured afferent and (ii) an exaggerated response of spinal neurons to low-threshold afferent input (Fig. 1.10).

Events Initiated by Nerve Injury

Injury leads to prominent changes at the site of nerve injury and in the DRG of the injured axon [8, 9, 37, 38]:

(i) Injury site: After acute injury of the peripheral afferent axon, there is an initial dying back (retrograde chromatolysis) until the axon begins to sprout, sending growth cones forward. Such axonal growth cone often fails to contact with the original target, and these sprouts show proliferation. Collections of these proliferated sprouts form neuromas.

(ii) DRG: Although the original injury is restricted to the peripheral nerve site, the distal injury has an enormous impact upon the dorsal root ganglion. Several events should be emphasized. (i) Markers of neuronal injury (such as ATF-3, an injury-evoked transcription factor) show a large-scale increase in expression in the DRG of the injured axons. (ii) There is an increased activation of the glial satellite cells (expressing GFAP) present. The DRG neurons are markedly enhanced. (iii) The DRG neurons show prominent increases in the expression of a variety of proteins such as those for sodium channels, calcium channels, and auxiliary calcium channel proteins (such as the alpha 2 delta subunit) and (iv) conversely decreases in the expression of other proteins such as those for certain potassium channels.

Origins of Spontaneous Pain State

As reviewed in the preceding sections, under normal conditions, the normal primary afferent axons show little of any spontaneous activity. After acute injury, the afferent axons display (i) an initial burst of afferent firing secondary to the injury, (ii) silence for intervals of hours to days, and (iii) development over time of spontaneous afferent traffic in both myelinated and unmyelinated axons.

Ongoing afferent input origin of ongoing pain. The ongoing afferent input is believed to provide the source of the afferent activity that leads to spontaneous ongoing sensation (Fig. 1.4). Evidence for this assertion that the ectopic afferent activity is in part responsible for the associated pain behavior is based on the observations that (i) parallel onset of pain and ectopic activity in neuroma and DRG, (ii) pain behavior blocked by application of TTX/local anesthetics to neuroma/DRGs, (iii) dorsal rhizotomy transiently reverse the pain behavior, and (iv) irritants applied to DRG initiate activity and importantly, evoke pain behavior [39].

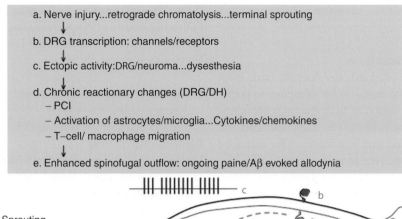

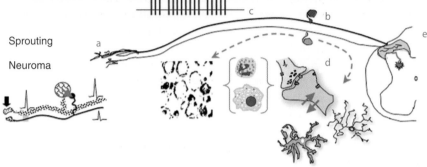

Fig. 1.10 This schematic provides an overview of the organization of events that initiate pain state after a peripheral nerve injury. (**a**) Nerve injury leads to retrograde chromatolysis and then sprouting to form local neuromas. (**b**) In addition to the changes in the terminals, there are trophic changes in the DRG leading to significant changes in the expression of a variety of channel and receptor proteins. (**c**) Over time, there is the appearance of ectopic activity in the injured axon. This activity arises from both the neuroma as well as the dorsal root ganglion. (**d, e**) In the dorsal horn, there are a series of reactive changes which lead to a reorganization of nociceptive processing. These changes include changes in the excitability of the second-order neurons, changes in the inhibitory control which normally regulates dorsal horn excitability, and then the activation of nonneuronal cells which contribute to the pro-excitatory nature of the nerve injury

Site of Origin of Spontaneous Afferent Traffic

Recording from the afferent axon has indicated that origin of the spontaneous activity in the injured afferent arises *both* from the neuroma and from the DRG of the injured axon (Fig. 1.4).

Mechanisms of Ongoing Activity

The generation of ongoing activity in the neuroma/DRG of the injured axon results from upregulation of excitable channels/receptors and appearance of excitatory substances in the DRG/neuroma.

Increased Sodium Channel Expression

Cloning shows that there are multiple populations of sodium channels, differing in their current activation properties and structure contributing to the action potential [8, 9].

Multiple sodium channels have been identified based on structure (NaV 1.1–NaV 1.9), whether they are tetrodotoxin sensitive (TTX), and their activation kinetics. Based on these designations, some subtypes are spatially limited in their distribution. Thus, NaV 1.8 and 1.9 are present in small primary afferents.

Importance of sodium channel subtypes in humans has been shown in identified loss- and gain-of-function mutations.

The SCN9A gene encodes the voltage-gated sodium channel NaV 1.7, a protein highly expressed in pain-sensing dorsal root ganglion neurons and sympathetic ganglion neurons. Mutations in SCN9A cause three human pain disorders:

(i) Loss of function: Loss-of-function mutations results in insensitivity to pain, no pain perception, and anosmia, but patients are otherwise normal.

(ii) Gain of function: Activating mutations cause severe episodic pain in paroxysmal extreme pain disorders with episodic burning pain in mandibular, ocular, and rectal areas as well as flushing, and primary erythermalgia, a peripheral pain disorder in which blood vessels are episodically blocked then become hyperemic with associated with severe burning pain.

Peripheral nerve injury increases the expression of many sodium channels in the DRG, and these channels are transported to the distal terminals. Increased channel increases ionic conductance and appears to increase spontaneous activity in the sprouting axon terminal. Note that systemic (IV/IP) lidocaine at concentrations which do *not* block conducted action potentials will block the "ectopic" discharges originating in DRG and neuroma. These concentrations are notable in that they will correspondingly block hyperpathia in the nerve jury pain state otherwise observed in humans and in animal models.

Decreased K Channel Expression

Many classes of types of gated K+channels have been described. Opening of K+channels yields membrane hyperpolarization and a reduced excitability. In the face of nerve injury, a reduced expression of such channels has been described, and it is hypothesized that this may contribute to the increased ectopic afferent activity observed after nerve injury [40].

Inflammatory Products

The sprouted terminals of the injured afferent axon display transduction properties that were not possessed by the original axon, including mechanical (e.g., compression) and chemical sensitivity. Thus, neuromas display sensitivity humoral factors, such as prostanoids, catecholamines, and cytokines (TNF). DRGs also respond to these products.

These products are released from local sources such as satellite cells in the DRG and Schwann cells in the periphery. The DRG is of particular interest as it lies outside the blood-brain barrier, for example, it can be influenced by circulating factors. This evolving sensitivity is of particular importance given that following local nerve injury, there is the release of a variety of cytokines, particularly TNF, which can thus directly activate the nerve and neuroma.

Following nerve injury, there is an important sprouting of postganglionic sympathetic efferents that can lead to the local release of catecholamines. This scenario is consistent with the observation that following nerve injury, the postganglionic axons can initiate excitation in the injured axon (see below). These events are believed to contribute to the development of spontaneous afferent traffic after peripheral nerve injury.

Origins of Evoke Hyperpathia

The observation that low-threshold tactile stimulation yields a pain states has been the subject of considerable interest. The psychophysical properties of this state emphasize that the pain results from activation of low-threshold mechanoreceptors (Aβ afferents). This ability of light touch evoking this anomalous pain state is *de facto* evidence that the peripheral nerve injury has led to a reorganization of central processing, that is, it is not a simple case of a peripheral sensitization of otherwise high-threshold afferents. In addition to these behavioral changes, the neuropathic pain condition may display other contrasting anomalies, including on occasion an ameliorating effect of sympathectomy of the afflicted limb and an attenuated responsiveness to spinal analgesics such as opiates. Several underlying mechanisms have been proposed to account for this seemingly anomalous linkage.

Dorsal Root Ganglion Cell Cross Talk

Following nerve injury, evidence suggests that "cross talk" develops between afferents in the DRG and in the neuroma. Here, action potentials in one axon generate depolarizing currents in an adjacent quiescent axon. Thus, activity arising in one axon (a large afferent) would drive activity on a second axon (small C fiber) [41].

Afferent Sprouting

Under normal circumstances, large myelinated (Aβ) afferents project into the spinal Rexed lamina III and deeper (see above). Small afferents (C fibers) tend to project into spinal laminae II and I, a region consisting mostly of nocisponsive neurons. Following peripheral nerve injury, it has been argued that the central terminals of these myelinated afferents (A fibers) sprout into lamina II of the spinal cord. With this synaptic reorganization, stimulation of low-threshold mechanoreceptors (Aβ fibers) could produce excitation of these neurons and be perceived as painful. The degree to which this sprouting occurs is a point of current discussion, and while it appears to occur, it is less prominent than originally reported.

Loss of Intrinsic GABAergic/Glycinergic Inhibitory Control

As reviewed above, GABA/glycinergic interneurons display a potent regulation of large afferent-evoked WDR excitation. The relevance of this intrinsic inhibition to pain processing is evidenced by the observation that spinal delivery of GABA A receptor or glycine receptor antagonists yields a powerful behaviorally defined tactile allodynia [42, 43].

In general, while there are changes in dorsal horn after nerve injury, the predominant evidence does not support a loss of dorsal horn inhibitory amino acids circuitry. Recent observations now suggest an important alternative. After nerve injury, spinal neurons regress to a neonatal phenotype in which GABA A activation becomes excitatory. As noted, the GABA A and glycine channels are chloride ionophores, wherein their activation (increasing Cl permeability) normally leads to a mild hyperpolarization of the postsynaptic membrane as Cl moves inside the cell. After injury, there is a loss of the Cl exporter (so-called KCC2), and there is an accumulation of Cl inside the cell. Now, increasing conductance leads to an extracellular movement of the Cl. This loss of negative charge causes the cell to mildly hypopolarize. This accordingly would turn an inhibitory regulation circuit for larger afferent to a facilitatory circuit for large afferent drive of the WDR neuron [44, 45].

Nonneuronal Cells and Nerve Injury

Nerve section or compression leads to activation of spinal microglia and astrocytes in spinal segments receiving input from injured nerves with a time course that parallels the changes in pain states. While the origin of this activation is not clear, it will lead to an increased spinal expression of COX/NOS/glutamate transporters/proteinases. The effects of such changes in spinal cord afferent processing have been previously reviewed above [46].

Sympathetic Dependency

Following peripheral nerve injury, an increased innervation by postganglionic sympathetic terminals of the neuroma and of the DRG of the injured axons is reliably noted. In the DRG, these postganglionic fibers form baskets of terminals around the ganglion cells. Several properties of this hyperinnervation are noteworthy [47, 48]:

(i) They invest ganglion cells of all sizes, but particularly large ganglion cells (so-called type A).

(ii) Postganglionic innervation occurs largely in the ipsilateral DRG but also occurs to a lesser degree in the contralateral DRG.

(iii) Activation of the preganglionic efferents (traveling in the ventral roots) will activate the sensory axon by an interaction at the site of injury or at the level of the DRG.

(iv) Activation is blocked by intravenous phentolamine, emphasizing an adrenergic effect.

Generalization to Many Nerve Injury Pain States

After nerve injury, there evolves an increase in ongoing dysesthesia and an enhanced response to low-threshold mechanical stimuli (allodynia). These effects are believed to reflect an increase in ectopic activity that arises from the neuromas well as the injured axon. The origin of the ectopic activity is believed to reflect an increased expression of sodium channel, decreased expression of K channels in the neuroma, and DRG leading to enhanced excitability. The allodynia is considered to reflect an alteration in the activation produced by large low-threshold afferents (Aβ). This alteration may result from cross talk between axons and/or a loss of inhibitory regulation.

It should be noted that the above review generically considers the "injured" axon. These changes reviewed above have been observed in animal models following chemotherapy, varicella zoster, extruded intervertebral disks (compressing the nerve root), and osteosarcoma. Accordingly, these changes described in preclinical models are believed to have a great likelihood of being relevant to the human condition.

Conclusions

In the preceding sections, we have provided an overview of the various systems that underlie the three heuristic subdivisions of acute, post-tissue injury and post-nerve injury pain states. An important concept is that in many clinical conditions, it is virtually certain that the clinical state is not one or the other, but rather a combination. Table 1.3 presents a superficial analysis of the types of mechanisms which may be involved in, for example, cancer pain. It is compelling to consider that such a patient may experience a pain state that reflects all three conditions between the events that arise from the tumor itself, the chemotherapy and the surgery (Tables 1.3 and 1.4).

The likelihood of multiple mechanisms mediating a particular pain state has an important ramification when it comes to the appropriateness of any particular analgesic therapy. Table 1.3 presents a summary of the basic mechanisms of actions of several classes of analgesic agents. Though not specifically discussed in this chapter (see elsewhere in this text), it is appreciated that they act to

Table 1.3 Summary of primary classes of analgesic therapeutics, mechanisms of action, and pain sites targeted by the agent as defined preclinical models [49–53]

Drug class	Mechanisms	Pain classification		
		Acute	Tissue injury	Nerve injury
Opiate (morphine)	Opiate receptors on high-threshold C fibers	X	X	x
NMDA antagonist (ketamine)	Blocks spinal glutamate-evoked facilitation	O	X	X
NSAID (ibuprofen)	Inhibits cyclooxygenase at injury site and in cord	O	X	O
Local anesthetic (IV lidocaine)	Sodium channel blocker	O	X	X
Anticonvulsant (gabapentin)	Reduces spontaneously active neuronal activity	O	X	X
Tricyclic antidepressant	Increase catecholamine levels	O	X	X
N-type calcium channel blocker (ziconotide)	Blocks spinal N-type calcium channel	O	X	X

Representative preclinical pain models include: Acute nociception: thermal-hot plate/tail flick; Tissue injury: intraplantar carrageenan-hyperalgesia, intraplantar formalin; Nerve injury: nerve ligation, nerve compression yielding tactile allodynia
X significant action, x minimal action, O no activity

Table 1.4 Summary of multiple mechanisms involved in the pain state of a cancer patient

Cancer	Acute Spinal neurons $A\partial/C$	Tissue injury Sensitization (peripheral, central)	Nerve injury Ectopic activity Spinal inhibition Sprouting
Tumor erosion (bone/tissue)		X	
Tumor release of factors	X	X	
Immune response (paraneoplastic)			X
Movement (incident pain)	X	X	
Tumor compression			X
Radiation			X
Chemotherapy			X
Surgery		X	X

$A\partial$ lightly myelinated, C unmyelinated

alter nociceptive transmission in a variety of ways. Opiates have a potent effect upon spinal transmission initiated by small primary afferents, whereas an NSAID largely has an effect when there is a facilitated state initiated by local inflammation. As reviewed above, there is in addition a central role for NSAIDs because of the constitutive expression of COX in the spinal dorsal horn and the role of prostaglandins in enhancing presynaptic transmitter release and diminish the inhibitory efficacy of the glycine receptor. In the face of multiple pain mechanisms, it can be appreciated that to minimize any pain state may well require addressing multiple therapeutic targets. Hence, it is not surprising that the profile of analgesic management of complex states, such as cancer, often shows 3–4 analgesic agents being employed.

References

1. Dougherty PM. Central sensitization and cutaneous hyperalgesia. Semin Pain Med. 2003;1:121–31.
2. Johanek L, Shim B, Meyer RA. Chapter 4 Primary hyperalgesia and nociceptor sensitization. Handb Clin Neurol. 2006;81:35–47.
3. Mayer EA, Gebhart GF. Basic and clinical aspects of visceral hyperalgesia. Gastroenterology. 1994;107:271–93.
4. Baron R. Neuropathic pain: a clinical perspective. Handb Exp Pharmacol. 2009;194:3–30.
5. Stucky CL, Dubin AE, Jeske NA, Malin SA, McKemy DD, Story GM. Roles of transient receptor potential channels in pain. Brain Res Rev. 2009;60:2–23.
6. Binshtok AM. Mechanisms of nociceptive transduction and transmission: a machinery for pain sensation and tools for selective analgesia. Int Rev Neurobiol. 2011;97:143–77.
7. Cortright DN, Szallasi A. TRP channels and pain. Curr Pharm Des. 2009;15(15):1736–49.
8. Dib-Hajj SD, Black JA, Waxman SG. Voltage-gated sodium channels: therapeutic targets for pain. Pain Med. 2009;10(7):1260–9.
9. Cohen CJ. Targeting voltage-gated sodium channels for treating neuropathic and inflammatory pain. Curr Pharm Biotechnol. 2011;12:1715–9.
10. Raja SN, Meyer RA, Campbell JN. Peripheral mechanisms of somatic pain. Anesthesiology. 1988;68:571–90.
11. Yaksh TL. Calcium channels as therapeutic targets in neuropathic pain. J Pain. 2006;7(1 Suppl 1):S13–30.
12. Ruscheweyh R, Forsthuber L, Schoffnegger D, Sandkühler J. Modification of classical neurochemical markers in identified primary afferent neurons with abeta-, adelta-, and C-fibers after chronic constriction injury in mice. J Comp Neurol. 2007;502:325–36.
13. Willis Jr WD. The somatosensory system, with emphasis on structures important for pain. Brain Res Rev. 2007;55:297–313.
14. Todd AJ, Spike RC. The localization of classical transmitters and neuropeptides within neurons in laminae I-III of the mammalian spinal dorsal horn. Prog Neurobiol. 1993;41:609–45.
15. Todd AJ. Neuronal circuitry for pain processing in the dorsal horn. Nat Rev Neurosci. 2010;11:823–36.
16. Ralston 3rd HJ. Pain and the primate thalamus. Prog Brain Res. 2005;149:1–10.
17. Reichling DB, Levine JD. Critical role of nociceptor plasticity in chronic pain. Trends Neurosci. 2009;32:611–8.
18. Herrero JF, Laird JM, López-García JA. Wind-up of spinal cord neurones and pain sensation: much ado about something? Prog Neurobiol. 2000;61:169–203.
19. Dickenson AH, Chapman V, Green GM. The pharmacology of excitatory and inhibitory amino acid-mediated events in the transmission and modulation of pain in the spinal cord. Gen Pharmacol. 1997;28:633–8.
20. Bleakman D, Alt A, Nisenbaum ES. Glutamate receptors and pain. Semin Cell Dev Biol. 2006;17:592–604.
21. Luo C, Seeburg PH, Sprengel R, Kuner R. Activity-dependent potentiation of calcium signals in spinal sensory networks in inflammatory pain states. Pain. 2008;140:358–67.
22. Latremoliere A, Woolf CJ. Central sensitization: a generator of pain hypersensitivity by central neural plasticity. J Pain. 2009;10:895–926.
23. Ji RR, Kawasaki Y, Zhuang ZY, Wen YR, Zhang YQ. Protein kinases as potential targets for the treatment of pathological pain. Handb Exp Pharmacol. 2007;177:359–89.
24. Velázquez KT, Mohammad H, Sweitzer SM. Protein kinase C in pain: involvement of multiple isoforms. Pharmacol Res. 2007;55:578–89.
25. Svensson CI, Yaksh TL. The spinal phospholipase-cyclooxygenase-prostanoid cascade in nociceptive processing. Annu Rev Pharmacol Toxicol. 2002;42:553–83.
26. Zeilhofer HU. The glycinergic control of spinal pain processing. Cell Mol Life Sci. 2005;62:2027–35.
27. Tang Q, Svensson CI, Fitzsimmons B, Webb M, Yaksh TL, Hua XY. Inhibition of spinal constitutive NOS-2 by 1400 W attenuates tissue injury and inflammation-induced hyperalgesia and spinal p38 activation. Eur J Neurosci. 2007;25:2964–72.
28. Suzuki R, Rygh LJ, Dickenson AH. Bad news from the brain: descending 5-HT pathways that control spinal pain processing. Trends Pharmacol Sci. 2004;25:613–7.
29. Milligan ED, Watkins LR. Pathological and protective roles of glia in chronic pain. Nat Rev Neurosci. 2009;10:23–36.
30. Ren K, Dubner R. Neuron-glia crosstalk gets serious: role in pain hypersensitivity. Curr Opin Anaesthesiol. 2008;21:570–9.

31. Abbadie C, Bhangoo S, De Koninck Y, Malcangio M, Melik-Parsadaniantz S, White FA. Chemokines and pain mechanisms. Brain Res Rev. 2009;60:125–34.

32. Clark AK, Staniland AA, Malcangio M. Fractalkine/CX3CR1 signalling in chronic pain and inflammation. Curr Pharm Biotechnol. 2011;12:1707–14.

33. Grace PM, Rolan PE, Hutchinson MR. Peripheral immune contributions to the maintenance of central glial activation underlying neuropathic pain. Brain Behav Immun. 2011;25:1322–32.

34. Ledeboer A, Sloane EM, Milligan ED, Frank MG, Mahony JH, Maier SF, Watkins LR. Minocycline attenuates mechanical allodynia and proinflammatory cytokine expression in rat models of pain facilitation. Pain. 2005;115:71–83.

35. Kehlet H, Jensen TS, Woolf CJ. Persistent postsurgical pain: risk factors and prevention. Lancet. 2006;367:1618–25.

36. Xu Q, Yaksh TL. A brief comparison of the pathophysiology of inflammatory versus neuropathic pain. Curr Opin Anaesthesiol. 2011;24:400–7.

37. Tuchman M, Barrett JA, Donevan S, Hedberg TG, Taylor CP. Central sensitization and Ca(V) α2δ ligands in chronic pain syndromes: pathologic processes and pharmacologic effect. J Pain. 2010;12:1241–9.

38. Bráz JM, Ackerman L, Basbaum AI. Sciatic nerve transection triggers release and intercellular transfer of a genetically expressed macromolecular tracer in dorsal root ganglia. J Comp Neurol. 2011;519:2648–57.

39. Zimmermann M. Pathobiology of neuropathic pain. Eur J Pharmacol. 2001;429:23–37.

40. Takeda M, Tsuboi Y, Kitagawa J, Nakagawa K, Iwata K, Matsumoto S. Potassium channels as a potential therapeutic target for trigeminal neuropathic and inflammatory pain. Mol Pain. 2011;7:5.

41. Devor M, Wall PD. Cross-excitation in dorsal root ganglia of nerve-injured and intact rats. J Neurophysiol. 1990;64(6):1733–46.

42. Yaksh TL. Behavioral and autonomic correlates of the tactile evoked allodynia produced by spinal glycine inhibition: effects of modulatory receptor systems and excitatory amino acid antagonists. Pain. 1989;37:111–23.

43. Sivilotti L, Woolf CJ. The contribution of GABAA and glycine receptors to central sensitization: disinhibition and touch-evoked allodynia in the spinal cord. J Neurophysiol. 1994;72:169–79.

44. Polgár E, Hughes DI, Riddell JS, Maxwell DJ, Puskár Z, Todd AJ. Selective loss of spinal GABAergic or glycinergic neurons is not necessary for development of thermal hyperalgesia in the chronic constriction injury model of neuropathic pain. Pain. 2003;104:229–39.

45. Price TJ, Cervero F, de Koninck Y. Role of cation-chloride-cotransporters (CCC) in pain and hyperalgesia. Curr Top Med Chem. 2005;5(6):547–55.

46. Cao H, Zhang YQ. Spinal glial activation contributes to pathological pain states. Neurosci Biobehav Rev. 2008;32(5):972–83.

47. McLachlan EM, Jänig W, Devor M, Michaelis M. Peripheral nerve injury triggers noradrenergic sprouting within dorsal-root ganglia. Nature. 1993;363:543–6.

48. Drummond PD. Involvement of the sympathetic nervous system in complex regional pain syndrome. Int J Low Extrem Wounds. 2004;3:35–42.

49. Borsook D, Becerra L. CNS animal fMRI in pain and analgesia. Neurosci Biobehav Rev. 2011;35:1125–43.

50. D'Souza WN, Ng GY, Youngblood BD, Tsuji W, Lehto SG. A review of current animal models of osteoarthritis pain. Curr Pharm Biotechnol. 2011;12:1596–612.

51. Mogil JS. Animal models of pain: progress and challenges. Nat Rev Neurosci. 2009;10:283–94.

52. Waszkielewicz AM, Gunia A, Słoczyńska K, Marona H. Evaluation of anticonvulsants for possible use in neuropathic pain. Curr Med Chem. 2011;18:4344–58.

53. Xu J, Brennan TJ. The pathophysiology of acute pain: animal models. Curr Opin Anaesthesiol. 2011;24:508–14.

Pharmacogenomics of Pain Management

2

Piotr K. Janicki

Key Points

- Individual pain variability and differences in the efficacy of analgesic drugs are genetically controlled.
- Drug-metabolizing enzymes represent a major target of current effort to identify associations between individuals' analgesic drug response and genetic profile.
- Genetic variants in other candidate genes influencing drug effector sites, such as those encoding receptors, transporters, and other molecules important for pain transmission represent another, less well-defined target.
- The pharmacogenomics-based approach to pain management represents a potential tool to improve the effectiveness and the side effect profile of therapy; however, well-designed prospective studies are needed to demonstrate superiority to conventional dosing regimes.

Introduction

Medicine has been continuously challenged, as well as stimulated, by the extraordinary variability in patient response to pharmacotherapy. The new age of identification of risk factors associated with pharmacotherapy using the methods of molecular medicine focuses on generating predictions regarding clinical outcome on the basis of each individual's unique DNA sequence. This new field has been coined *pharmacogenomics*.

P.K. Janicki, M.D., Ph.D., DSci, DABA
Department of Anesthesiology,
Pennsylvania State Milton S. Hershey Medical Center,
500 University Drive, Mailcode H187, Hershey, PA 17033, USA

Laboratory of Perioperative Genomics, Pennsylvania State University
College of Medicine, Hershey, PA, USA
e-mail: pjanicki@hmc.psu.edu

The goal of pharmacogenomics is to use information provided by advances in human genetics to identify patients at risk for significantly altered response during pharmacotherapy. The field of pharmacogenomics represents the major drive behind the introduction of the concept of *personalized medicine* in which the medical treatment is customized according to the individual patient genomic signature [1].

Background

Association of genome variability with increased or decreased pain, or modified effects of analgesics, has demonstrated that pain therapy is subject to pharmacogenomics [2–6].

There are two major components of pain management and pharmacogenomics (see Fig. 2.1). The use of genetic information from basic science and clinical studies to examine the impact of genetic variability on factors modulating the risk of developing pain, its clinical course, and intensity is called *functional pain genomics*. Functional pain genomics aims to discover the biologic function of particular genes and to uncover how a set of genes and their products work together in regulating the response to pain.

The second, more traditional, and better established component of pain related genomics is called *pharmacogenomics of pain management* and aims to characterize how genetic variations contribute to an individual's sensitivity and response to a variety of drugs important to pain management practice. Pharmacogenomics is traditionally divided into two parts describing genetic variants influencing pharmacokinetics and pharmacodynamics.

The molecular basis for the observed variability in patient response is defined by different forms of the detected genetic variants. These variants, consisting of the interindividual differences in the DNA sequences, produce the individual *phenotypes* of the human being. There are many different types of genetic variants (see Fig. 2.2). The most common (more than ten million types known so far) are single *nucleotide polymorphisms (or SNP)*, which represent a point mutation

T.R. Deer et al. (eds.), *Comprehensive Treatment of Chronic Pain by Medical, Interventional, and Integrative Approaches,*
DOI 10.1007/978-1-4614-1560-2_2, © American Academy of Pain Medicine 2013

23

Fig. 2.1 Framework of genetic
background influencing the
response to analgesic drugs

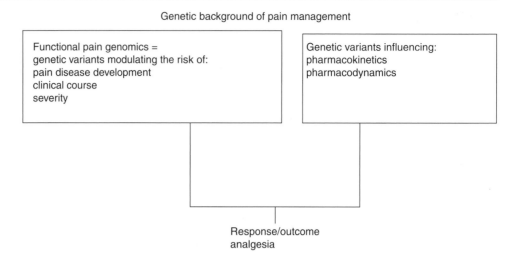

Fig. 2.2 Types of genetic
variants taking part in modifying
pain phenotype

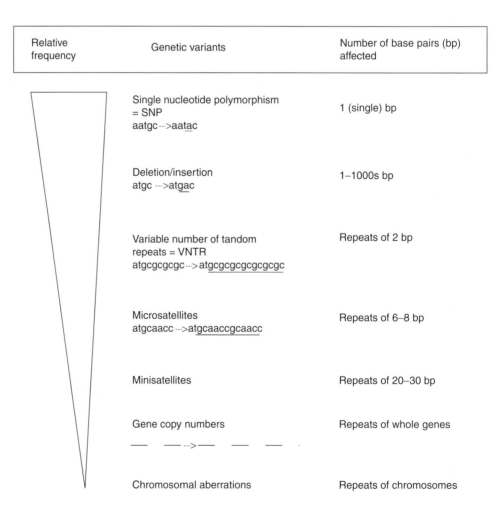

(change of one base) in the DNA fragments. Other allelic mutations include insertion or deletion of a single base (*indels*), multiple, continuous repeats of 2–4 bases (*variable number of tandem repeats or VNTR*); repeats of longer DNA fragments (*micro- and mini-satellites*); *copy number vari-* *ants* (CNV, deletion or multiplication of large, >1,000 bases fragments of chromosomes); and finally *chromosomal aber-* *rations*. The genetic variants may produce alterations in the protein's function through either changes in the protein expression or its structure.

Functional Genomics of Pain

Pain as a complex trait is expected to have a polygenic nature shaped by the environmental pressures. Identification of specific genetic elements of pain perception promises to be one of the key elements for creating novel and individualized pain treatments. It was demonstrated previously that both rare deleterious genetic variants and common genetic polymorphisms are mediators of human pain perception and clinical pain phenotypes [7, 8]. A higher or lower intensity of pain is very likely to require higher or lower doses of analgesics for efficient pain management. The genetic control of human pain perception and processing is therefore likely to modulate analgesic therapy.

The complete inability to sense pain in an otherwise healthy individual is a very rare phenotype. At present, five types of congenital insensitivity to pain (or HSAN=hereditary sensory and autonomic neuropathy) were identified which are caused by mutations in five different genes [9].

Recently, several new genomic mutations were identified which are described as "channelopathy-associated insensitivity to pain" [10] which are characterized by complete and selective inability to perceive any form of pain. It includes mutations in the alpha-subunit of sodium channel $Na_v1.7$ (SCN9A), causing the loss of function in this specific form of sodium channel [10, 11]. By contrast, mutations in SCN9A that leads to excessive channel activity trigger activation of pain signaling in humans and produce primary erythermalgia (more frequently used term is erythromelalgia), which is characterized by burning pain in response to exposure to mild warmth [12, 13]. Mutations in this gene also produce a rare condition referred to as "paroxysmal extreme pain disorder," which is characterized by rectal, ocular, and submandibular pain [14].

These syndromes probably have no importance in the everyday clinical pain management as they are very rare, and the affected people probably do not require pain therapy (with exception of erythromelalgia which causes severe pain that is considered a true pain-related emergency). However, defining the molecular causes for hereditary insensitivity to pain may serve as an important source of information to find new targets for analgesic drugs. This assumption was confirmed in the recently published study, in which the authors after investigating 27 common polymorphisms in the SCN9A gene found out that the minor A allele of the SNP rs6746030 was associated with an altered pain threshold and the effect was mediated through C-fiber activation [15]. They concluded that individuals experience differing amounts of pain, per nociceptive stimulus, on the basis of their SCN9A rs6746030 genotype.

Pain in the average population is controlled by fairly frequent genetic variants (allelic frequency > 10 %). Each of them, however, modifies the pain phenotype to only modest degree, and in the majority of cases, the evidence for their involvement in the efficacy of analgesics is either lacking or remains controversial [7, 8]. The involvement of common variants of the opioid receptors, kappa and mu, are discussed below in the part describing pharmacodynamic modifications of activity of opioid analgesics. A variant of third type of opioid receptor, delta, has been associated with lower thermal pain intensity with no association, so far, with the efficacy of opioid analgesics [16].

GTP cyclohydrolase (GCH1), recently implicated in shaping pain responses in humans, regulates production of tetrahydrobiopterin (BH4), an essential factor for the synthesis of dopamine, serotonin, and nitric acid. Tegeder et al. discovered a haplotype associated with reduction of experimental pain in normal volunteers and a favorable outcome with regard to long-term pain reduction that underwent pain (did you mean "a painful surgery"?) surgery [17]. In another study, Tegeder et al. showed that carriers of the particular GCH1 haplotype had higher pain threshold to mechanical and thermal pain following capsaicin sensitization [18]. However, Kim and Dionn and Lazarev et al. failed to replicate significant associations between the same GCH1 genomic variants and pain responses, both in assessment of experimental pain and postoperative pain after dental surgery, as well chronic pancreatic pain [19, 20]. Conversely, the most recent study confirmed again that the five previously identified GCH1 SNPs were profoundly affecting the ratings of pain induced by capsaicin in healthy human volunteers [21]. It was also suggested that the carriers of this particular GCH1 haplotype (which may be responsible for the decreased function of GCH1) display delayed need for pain therapy [2, 22].

Pharmacogenomics of Pain Therapy and Its Usefulness in Clinical Practice

Pharmacogenomics of pain management represents the most familiar area of practical pain genomics. It includes several examples of genomic variations, dramatically changing response to analgesic drugs through either change in their metabolism or receptor targets.

The current list of genetic polymorphisms which may affect the action of analgesic drugs is quite long and appears to be growing rapidly. The best known mechanisms involved in the altered effects of analgesics involve polymorphic changes in its metabolism. In this respect, three major mechanisms have been identified, involving genetic variations in the metabolic activation of the analgesics administered as an inactive or less active prodrug, variations in the metabolic degradation of the active components, and variations in its transmembrane transport.

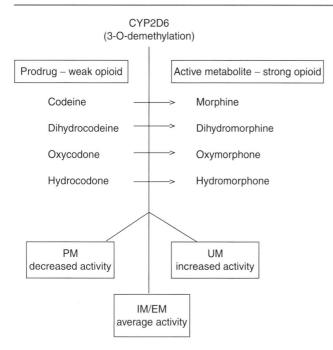

CYP2D6
(3-O-demethylation)

| Prodrug – weak opioid | | Active metabolite – strong opioid |

Codeine → Morphine

Dihydrocodeine → Dihydromorphine

Oxycodone → Oxymorphone

Hydrocodone → Hydromorphone

| PM decreased activity | | UM increased activity |

| IM/EM average activity |

Fig. 2.3 Opioid analgesics influenced by polymorphic CYP2D6 metabolism (3-O-demethylation)

Genetic Variations in the Prodrug Activation

The better known example involves polymorphisms in genes of the liver isoforms of the cytochrome P450 system (CYP) [23]. In particular, the most well-characterized *CYP2D6* polymorphism is responsible for the considerable variation in the metabolism (and clinical responses) of drugs from many therapeutic areas, including several analgesics (Fig. 2.3) [24–26]. More than 100 CYP2D6 alleles have been identified, ranging from nonsynonymous mutations to SNPs that either alter RNA splicing or produce deletions of the entire gene [27]. Of these, *3, *4, and *8 are nonfunctional, *9, *10, and *41 have reduced function, and *1,*2, *35, and *41 can be duplicated, resulting in greatly increased expression of functional CYP2D6. There are also interethnic differences in the frequencies of these variant alleles. Allele combinations determine phenotype: two nonfunctional = poor metabolizer (PM); at least one reduced functional = intermediate metabolizer (IM); at least one functional = extensive metabolizers (EM); and multiple copies of a functional and/or allele with promoter mutation = ultrarapid metabolizer (UM). The most recent update of CYP2D6 nomenclature and terminology could be found on home Web page of the Human Cytochrome P450 (CYP) Allele Nomenclature *at* http://www.cypalleles.ki.se/.

Codeine and other weak opioids are extensively metabolized by polymorphic CYP2D6 which regulates its O-demethylation to more potent metabolites (e.g., after a single oral dose of 30 mg codeine, 6 % is eventually transformed

to morphine). The clinical analgesic effect of codeine is mainly attributed to its conversion to morphine, which has a 200 times higher affinity and 50 times higher intrinsic activity at MOR than codeine itself [28]. Since CYP2D6 is genetically highly polymorphic, the effects of codeine are under pharmacogenetic control.

Genetically, altered effects of codeine may occur in subjects with either decreased, absent, or highly increased CYP2D6 activity when compared with the population average [29, 30]. Decreased or absent CYP2D6 activity in PMs causes production of only very low or absent amount of morphine after codeine administration. The ultrafast metabolizers (UM) produce on the other hand excessive amount of morphine after typical dose of codeine. Roughly, one out of seven Caucasians is at risk of either failure or toxicity of codeine therapy due to extremely low or high morphine formation, respectively. Recent case reports of codeine fatalities highlighted that the use of this weak opioid, particularly in young children, is associated with a substantial risk in those subjects displaying UM genotype [31–37]. The polymorphic variants in the CYP2D6 system are responsible for some but not all variability observed after codeine administration. The other causes for the observed high variability in codeine efficacy include both polymorphisms in other genes involved in opioid expression or trafficking, as well as nongenetic factors. In addition to differences in codeine metabolism between EM and PM, the differences between EM of various ethnicities have also been highlighted. The Chinese EM reported having a lower rate of codeine O-demethylation when compared with the Caucasian EM, because of the much higher frequency (50 %) of the *10 (reduced function) allele in the Chinese [27].

Other popular analgesic drug which depends on activation by the CYP2D6 includes *tramadol*. Tramadol is a mu-opioid receptor (MOR) agonist but has a lower affinity at MORs than its active metabolite O-desmethyltramadol. Tramadol itself has weak analgesic activity which becomes evident when CYP2D6 is blocked and also acts through non-opioid-dependent mechanisms which involve serotonin- and noradrenaline-mediated pain inhibition originating in brain stem. The analgesic activity of tramadol is strongly modulated by CYP2D6 activity. The analgesic activity on experimental pain is reduced in CYP2D6 PMs, a finding later confirmed in pain patients [38–42]. It is interesting to note that the pharmacokinetics of tramadol (which is administered as racemic substance containing equal amount of (−) and (+) optical isomers producing analgesia by a synergistic action of its two enantiomers and their metabolites) is enantioselective in CYP2D6 poor and extensive metabolizers, meaning that the production of either optical isomer differs depending on the metabolic status [41, 43, 44]. The clinical significance of this finding for pain management remains to be further explored.

As far as other CYP2D6 substrates with active analgesic metabolites are concerned (see Fig. 2.3), the evidence for variation in its analgesic with altered CYP2D6 function is less evident when compared with codeine or tramadol. These examples are either negative, such as for dihydrocodeine [45, 46], or explained at a nongenetic level, such as for oxycodone. In other cases, the evidence is based only on animal studies, such as hydrocodone, or restricted to single case reports for inadequate activity of oxycodone [3].

Tilidine (an opioid analgesic) is activated to active metabolite nortilidine, and *parecoxib* (an NSAID) is activated into valdecoxib by CYP3A system. This enzyme is phenotypically highly variable, but only a minor part of this variability can be attributed to genetics [2]. Individuals with at least one CYP3A5*1 allele copy produce fully active active copy of CYP3A5 enzyme; however, the majority of Caucasians have no active CYP3A5 due to a premature stop codon.

Genetic Variations in the Elimination of Analgesic Drugs

Many of the opioids contain hydroxyl group at position 6, and the potent opioids have a hydroxyl at position 3 of the 4,5-methoxymorphinan structure. The glucuronidation of morphine, codeine, buprenorphine, dihydrocodeine, dihydromorphine, hydromorphone, dihydromorphine, oxymorphone, as well as opioid receptor antagonists (naloxone and naltrexone) is mainly mediated by the uridine diphosphate (UDP) glucuronyltransferase (UGT)2B7 [3]. Similar to CYP genes, the UGT2B7 gene is also polymorphic, although less than 20 allelic variants have been identified. The main proportion of morphine is metabolized to morphine-6-glucuronide, M6G (approximately 70 %), and to lesser degree to morphine-3-glucuronide (M3G). Both metabolites are active, with effects opposite to each other, consisting in excitation and anti-analgesia for M3G and in typical opioid agonist effects for M6G. Despite the role of UGT2B7 in the formation of M6G and M3G, the clinical effect of the UGT2B7*2 (268Y) variant has only produced conflicting results so far. Different variants in the 5′ untranslated region of UGT2B7 are associated with reduced M6G/morphine ratios in patients. In addition, it was reported that UGT2B7 *2/*2 genotypes and CYP2D6 UM phenotypes were associated with severe neonatal toxicity after breast-feeding and oral ingestion of opioids. The above preliminary data indicate that the consequences of UGT variants were so far restricted to alterations of plasma concentrations, while none of the UGT variants alone have been associated with the altered efficacy of opioid analgesics [3, 4].

The increased enzyme activity associated with the CYP3A5*1 allele may cause accelerated elimination of CYP3A substrates, such as alfentanil, fentanyl, or sufentanil. However, positive associations of CYP3A polymorphisms with analgesic actions have not been reported so far. The CYP3A5 genotype did not affect the systemic or apparent oral clearance as well as the pharmacodynamics of alfentanil and levomethadone [47, 48].

In addition to CYP2D6 and CYP2A5, there is also clinical evidence about the involvement of other CYP systems in the metabolism of frequently used nonsteroid anti-inflammatory drugs (NSAIDs). Human CYP2C9 metabolizes numerous drugs (e.g., warfarin, oral sulfonylurea hypoglycemics, antiepileptics, and others) [49]. In addition, CYP2C9 polymorphism might play a significant role in the analgesic efficacy and toxicity of traditional NSAIDs, for example, diclofenac, ibuprofen, naproxen, tenoxicam, and piroxicam, as well as selective COX-2 inhibitors such as celecoxib and valdecoxib [50]. More than 33 variants and a series of subvariants have been identified for CYP2C9 to date. The two missense mutations, CYP2C9*2 (rs1799853) and CYPC9*3 (rs1057910), yield enzymes with decreased activity [51]. These alleles are mainly present in Caucasians, while their frequency is lower in African and Asian subjects. More than twofold reduced clearance after oral intake of celecoxib was observed in homozygous carriers of CYP2C9*3 compared with carriers of the wild-type genotype CYP2C9*1/*1 [52]. Similarly, ibuprofen-mediated inhibition of COX-1 and COX-2 is significantly decreased (by 50 %) in carriers of two CYP2C9*3 alleles [53]. Further investigations demonstrating the relevance of the CYP2C9*3 allele for naproxen, tenoxicam, piroxicam, and lornoxicam pharmacokinetics have been also published [4, 54]. Although CYP2C9 is the major determinant of clearance, it is necessary to also consider CYP2C8 genotype, as it contributes to some smaller extent in NSAIDs metabolism. In the study performed in healthy volunteers, it was demonstrated that metabolism of diclofenac was significantly slower in individuals carrying CYP2C8*3 (rs10509681) or CYP2C8*4 (rs1058930) allele than in those homozygous for the wild-type allele [55].

Whereas numerous clinical trials have demonstrated the impact of CYP2C9*3 on therapy with Coumadin, less information is available on the CYP2C9 genotype-related efficacy of NSAIDs in the pain management. Some publications focus, however, on the incidence and severity of adverse effects (e.g., gastrointestinal (GI) bleeding, effects on coagulation). It was that the combined presence of CYP2C8*3 and CYP2C9*2 was a relevant determinant in the risk of developing GI bleeding in patients receiving NSAIDs metabolized by CYP2C8/9 [56]. Similar results were also presented by Agundez et al. [57]. However, to date, the study results from other authors are conflicting, with several other trials reporting no association [58, 59]. More studies are clearly necessary to confirm the relevance of CYP2C8/9 genotype with increased incidence of GI bleeding.

Another typical adverse effect is the influence of classical NSAIDs on coagulation. The risk of altered coagulation was substantially increased in patients with either CYP2C9*3 and CYP2C9*3 (mentioned twice) genotypes taking Coumadin together with NSAIDs which are known CYP2C9 substrates [60].

Genetic Variations in the Transmembrane Transport of Analgesics

P-glycoprotein (P-gp) coded by the ATP-binding cassette subfamily (ABCB1)/multidrug resistance (MDR1) gene is mainly located in organs with excretory functions (e.g., liver, kidneys). It is also expressed at the blood-brain barrier where it forms an outward transporter. Therefore, functional impairment of P-gp-mediated drug transport may be expected to result in increased bioavailability of orally administered drugs, reduced renal clearance, or an increased brain concentration of its substrates. Some opioids are P-gp substrates. The ABCB1 3435 C>T variant (rs1045642) is associated with decreased dosage requirements in opioids that are P-gp substrates, as assessed in outpatients. Moreover, a diplotype consisting of three polymorphic positions in the ABCB1 gene (1236TT-rs1128503, 2677TT-rs2032582, and 3435TT) is associated with increased susceptibility to respiratory depression caused by fentanyl in Korean patients [61]. The results suggest that analysis of ABCB1 polymorphisms may have clinical relevance in the prevention of respiratory suppression by intravenous fentanyl or to anticipate its clinical effects. With the OPRM1 118 A>G variant (see below), the ABCB1 3435 C>T predicted the response to morphine in cancer patients with a sensitivity close to 100 % and a specificity of more than 70 % [62]. Trials in patients suffering from chronic and cancer pain had shown decreased opioid consumption in carriers of the 3435T allele [63, 64]. Finally, methadone analgesia may be subject to P-gp pharmacogenetic modulation. The pupillary effects of orally administered methadone are increased following the pharmacological blockade of P-gp by quinidine, and the methadone dosing for heroin substitution can be decreased in carriers of ABCB1 variants associated with decreased transporter expression, for example, ABCB1 2435 C>T and others [65, 66].

Pharmacodynamics of Pain Therapy

The alterations in effects of analgesics may also result from pharmacodynamic interferences, consisting of altered receptor binding, activation or signaling mechanisms, or of altered expression of the drug's target, such as opioid receptors or cyclooxygenases. Genetic factors have been found to act via any of these mechanisms.

Opioid Receptors

The mu-opioid receptor (MOR) is part of the family of several types of opioid receptors which are 7-transmembrane domain, G-protein-coupled receptors (GPCR), and inhibit cellular activity. MOR is clinically most relevant target of opioid analgesics. The OPRM1 gene coding for MOR in humans is highly polymorphic, with excess of 1,800 SNPs listed in the current edition (2010) of the NCBI SNP database (http://www.ncbi.nlm.nih.gov/snp). Coding mutations affecting the third intracellular loop of MOR (e.g., 779 G>A, 794 G>A, 802 T>C) result in reduced G-protein coupling, receptor signaling, and desensitization, leading to an expectation that opioids should be almost ineffective in patients carrying those polymorphisms. However, these polymorphisms are extremely rare (<0.1 % population) and are therefore restricted to very rare single cases.

Evidence for a function of OPRM1 variants with allelic frequencies >5 % is sparse, except for the 118 A>G polymorphism (rs1799971). This SNP causes an amino acid exchange of the aspartate with an asparagine at position 40 of extracellular part of MOR, deleting one of a putative glycosylation sites. This change can cause altered expression of MOR or its signaling [67–69]. The OPRM1 118 A>G polymorphism has an allele frequency of 8–17 % in Caucasians and considerably higher in Asians, with a frequency of 47 % reported from Japan. It is also worth noting that the frequency of homozygotes for the GG allele is by much higher in Asian population with only very rare (<1 %) occurrence in Caucasian population [70]. The data obtained so far with the OPRM1 118 A>G polymorphism have been controversial [71]. The molecular changes associated with SNP 118 A>G translate to a variety of clinical effects (predominantly decrease) of many opioids in experimental settings and clinical studies [72–81]. The consequences of the SNP 118 A>G have consistently been related to a decrease in opioid potency for pupil constriction (e.g., for morphine, M6G, methadone). For analgesia, the SNP decreases the concentration-dependent effects of alfentanil on experimental pain. Specifically, the variant decreases the effect of opioids on pain-related activation mainly in those regions of the brain that are processing the sensory dimension of pain including the primary and secondary somatosensory cortex and posterior insular cortex [82]. In clinical settings, greater postoperative requirements of alfentanil and morphine have been reported for carriers of the variant, and higher concentrations of alfentanil of M6G were needed to produce analgesia in experimental pain models [2, 48, 83–87]. It should be noted that other studies described only moderate to no significant effects of the OPRM1 118 A>G polymorphism on opioid requirements or pain relief. Several studies did not demonstrate any association between OPRM1 variant and analgesic needs [88–92]. Contradictory results were reported by Landau et al. who investigated the influence of OPRM1 118 A>G polymorphism on the analgesic effectiveness of fentanyl in females after its intrathecal administration during labor and delivery. The analgesic requirements in this study were increased in homozygous carriers of AA allele, the opposite effect compared with most other studies [93]. In the chronic pain patients, it was reported that in the high-quartile opioid utilization group, the homozygous carriers of the minor allele required significantly higher opioid doses than the carriers of the minor allele [91]. In another studies, GG homozygote patients were characterized by higher morphine consumption than carriers of the major AA allele [76, 94]. In summary, an influence of OPRM1 genetic variants on opioid requirements and degree of pain relief under opioid medication has been demonstrated in some studies; however, this could not be replicated in all subsequent investigations. Patients stratification; a low number of patients with the GG genotype (in particular in studies performed in Caucasian populations); presence of multiple, uncontrolled co-variables influencing the phenotype; and a clinically questionable reduction in opioid consumption are some major concerns. The requirements of high opioid doses may in part reflect an addiction component or a higher/faster rate of tolerance development in certain pain patients. It was reported that OPRM1 A118G polymorphism is a major determinant of striatal dopamine responses to alcohol. Social drinkers recruited based on OPRM1 genotype were challenged in separate sessions with alcohol and placebo under pharmacokinetically controlled conditions and examined for striatal dopamine release using positron emission tomography and [(11)C]-raclopride displacement. A striatal dopamine response to alcohol was restricted to carriers of the minor 118G allele. Based on the results of this study, it was concluded that OPRM1 A118G variation is a genetic determinant of dopamine responses to alcohol, a mechanism by which it likely modulates alcohol reward [95].

In addition, the most recent study seems to suggest that some of the effect of SNP A>G could be explained by the linkage disequilibrium with other functional SNPs located in the OPRM1 region [96]. For example, SNP rs563649 is located within a structurally conserved internal ribosome entry site in the 5′-UTR of a novel exon 13-containing OPRM1 isoforms (MOR-1K) and affects both mRNA levels and translation efficiency of these variants. Furthermore, rs563649 exhibits very strong linkage disequilibrium throughout the entire OPRM1 gene locus and thus affects the functional contribution of the corresponding haplotype that includes other functional OPRM1 SNPs. These results might provide evidence for an essential role for MOR-1K isoforms in nociceptive signaling and suggest that genetic variations in alternative OPRM1 isoforms may contribute to individual differences in opiate responses.

Catechol-O-Methyltransferase (COMT)

CMOT degrades catecholamine neurotransmitters such as norepinephrine, epinephrine, and dopamine. Increased dopamine concentrations suppress the production of endogenous opioid peptides. Opioid receptor expression is in turn upregulated, which has been observed with the Val158Met variant of COMT, coded by the COMT 772 G>A (rs4680) SNP in human postmortem brain tissue and in vivo by assessing radiolabeled 11C-carfentanil MOR binding [97, 98]. This variant leads to a low-function COMT enzyme that fails to degrade dopamine, which may cause a depletion of enkephalin. Patients with cancer carrying the Val158Met variant needed less morphine for pain relief than patients not carrying this variant. Finally, the variants exerts its opioid enforcing effects also in cross relation with the OPRM1 118 A>G variant [94, 97–101]. During the past decade, several new polymorphisms were identified in the COMT gene which contains at least five functional polymorphisms that impact its biological activity and associated phenotypes (including pain). The potentially complex interactions of functional variations in COMT imply that the overall functional state of the gene might not be easily deduced from genotype information alone, which presumably explains the inconsistency in the results from association studies that focus on the V158Met polymorphism [102, 103].

Melanocortin 1 Receptor (MC1R)

Nonfunctional variants of the MC1R which produces bright red hair and fair skin phenotype were associated with an increased analgesic response to kappa opioid receptors (KOR)-mediated opioid analgesia. Red-headed women required less of the KOR agonist drug – pentazocine – to reach a specific level of analgesia compared with all other groups [104, 105]. This study presented the first strong evidence for a gene-by-sex interaction in the area of pain genetics, because the authors also showed that red-headed men did not experience enhanced KOR analgesia.

Cyclooxygenases (COX)

Polymorphisms in the prostaglandin endoperoxidase synthase 2 gene (PTGS2) coding for COX-2 may modulate the development of inflammation and its response to treatment with inhibitors of COXs, especially those specific for COX-2 [106]. This has been proposed for the PTGS2-765 G>C SNP (rs20417), which was reported to be associated with more than a twofold decrease in COX-2 expression [107]. By altering a putative Sp1 binding site in the promoter region of PTGS2, this gene variant was found to decrease the promoter activity by 30 % [108]. However, the controversial results were reported so far in clinical studies with this polymorphisms and different COX-2 inhibitors. The inhibitory effect of celecoxib on COX-2 was not associated with the presence of this variant in volunteers [109];

conversely, significantly decreased analgesic effects of rofe-coxib were observed in the homozygous carriers of this variant [110].

Future Direction of Pharmacogenomics in Pain Treatment

The influence of different genetic variants on analgesic requirements and degree of pain relief has been demonstrated in some studies; however, there is relatively less information available about the interactions between these variants. Each of the genetic variants investigated up to now seems to contribute in a modest way to the modulation of analgesic response [111]. However, a global approach investigating multiple possible variables within one trial has not been performed. After more than a decade of identifying genetic associations, the current challenge is to intensify compilation of this information for precisely defined clinical settings for which improved pain treatment is possible.

The current knowledge about the impact of genetics in the pain management is based on the association studies. In contrast to traditional family or pedigree-based studies (linkage analysis), in this type of studies, two cohorts of unrelated patients (with and without the observed phenotype, i.e., changes in the efficacy of analgesics) are compared in respect to the frequency of different genetic variants (adjusted for other known risk factors and for environmental differences). Candidate-gene association studies are focused on selected genes which are thought to be relevant for a specific observed outcome.

The alternative to targeted association studies are genome-wide association studies (GWAS). In this type of studies, there is no a priori hypothesis about the gene candidates. Instead, the microarray-based genomic scans are performed throughout the whole genome in order to find all SNPs possibly associated with observed phenotypic changes in the cohorts of patients with investigated traits (and controls). The modern microarray platforms allow for the cost-effective, parallel analysis of approximately one million genomic variants in one sample (or pooled samples) and, using sophisticated computer strategy, enable finding the most relevant statistical associations between control and affected patients. The main advantage of GWAS is that it is an unbiased hypothesis-free approach. In contrast to other areas of medicine, the GWAS approach lags behind in pain genomics, but the next few years should bring about the results of several studies currently being performed in the area of pain medicine. One of the first pain pharmacogenomic studies using GWAS technology was recently published by Kim et al. and demonstrated association of minor allele variant in a zinc finger protein (ZNF429) gene with delayed onset of action of ketorolac in the oral surgery patients [112].

Table 2.1 List of the most common analgesic drugs and polymorphic genes for which some evidence exists that the pharmacokinetics and/or pharmacodynamics of these analgesic drugs are modulated by functional genetic variants

Analgesic drug	Genes
Opioid analgesics	
Codeine	CYP2D6, UGT2B7, ABCB1, OPRM1
Pentazocine	MC1R
Tramadol	CYP2D6
Morphine	UGT2B7, ABCB1, COMT, OPRM1, CGH1
Methadone	CYP2D6, UGT2B7, ABCB1, OPRM1
Tilidine	CYP3A
Dihydrocodeine, hydrocodone, oxycodone	CYP2D6, ABCB1, COMT, OPRM1
NSAIDs	
Ibuprofen	CYP2C9
Diclofenac	CYP2C9
Naproxen	CYP2C9
Valdecoxib	CYP2C9, PTGS2
Celecoxib	CYP2C9, PTGS2
Parecoxib	CYP3A, CYP2C9, PTGS2

Summary

In summary, genetics continues to make rapid progress in terms of technology and understanding, but there are still, as yet, no large randomized, multicenter controlled trials to support the use of widespread genetic screening to predict an individual's response to pain medication (Table 2.1) [113]. Despite intensive research, genetics-based personalized pain therapy has yet to emerge. Monogenetic heredity of pain conditions seems to be restricted to very rare and extreme phenotypes, whereas common phenotypes are very complex and multigenetic. Many common variants, of which only a fraction have been identified so far, produce only minor effects that are sometimes partly canceled out. For most clinical settings and analgesic drug effects, common genetic variants cannot yet be used to provide a relevant prediction of individual pain and analgesic responses. However, genetics has some potential practical uses: CYP2D6, MC1R, and potentially PTGS2 could provide guidance on the right choice of analgesics. We still have a way to go before genetic screening becomes a routine practice and much further still before the contribution of gene-environment interactions is fully realized. However, continued identification of genotypes which are predictive of efficacy of pain management may not only further our understanding of the pain mechanisms but also potentially help discover new potential molecular targets for pain therapy.

References

1. Eichelbaum M, Ingelman-Sundberg M, Evans WE. Pharmacogenomics and individualized drug therapy. Annu Rev Med. 2006;57:119–37.
2. Lotsch J, Geisslinger G, Tegeder I. Genetic modulation of the pharmacological treatment of pain. Pharmacol Ther. 2009;124:168–84.
3. Somogyi AA, Barratt DT, Coller JK. Pharmacogenetics of opioids. Clin Pharmacol Ther. 2007;81:429–44.
4. Stamer UM, Zhang L, Stuber F. Personalized therapy in pain management: where do we stand? Pharmacogenomics. 2010; 11:843–64.
5. Lacroix-Fralish ML, Mogil JS. Progress in genetic studies of pain and analgesia. Annu Rev Pharmacol Toxicol. 2009;49:97–121.
6. Landau R. One size does not fit all: genetic variability of mu-opioid receptor and postoperative morphine consumption. Anesthesiology. 2006;105:235–7.
7. Diatchenko L, Nackley AG, Tchivileva IE, Shabalina SA, Maixner W. Genetic architecture of human pain perception. Trends Genet. 2007;23:605–13.
8. Fillingim RB, Wallace MR, Herbstman DM, Ribeiro-Dasilva M, Staud R. Genetic contributions to pain: a review of findings in humans. Oral Dis. 2008;14:673–82.
9. Nagasako EM, Oaklander AL, Dworkin RH. Congenital insensitivity to pain: an update. Pain. 2003;101:213–9.
10. Cox JJ, Reimann F, Nicholas AK, et al. An SCN9A channelopathy causes congenital inability to experience pain. Nature. 2006; 444:894–8.
11. Goldberg YP, MacFarlane J, MacDonald ML, et al. Loss-of-function mutations in the Nav1.7 gene underlie congenital indifference to pain in multiple human populations. Clin Genet. 2007;71:311–9.
12. Waxman SG. Neurobiology: a channel sets the gain on pain. Nature. 2006;444:831–2.
13. Waxman SG, Dib-Hajj SD. Erythromelalgia: a hereditary pain syndrome enters the molecular era. Ann Neurol. 2005;57:785–8.
14. Fertleman CR, Baker MD, Parker KA, et al. SCN9A mutations in paroxysmal extreme pain disorder: allelic variants underlie distinct channel defects and phenotypes. Neuron. 2006;52:767–74.
15. Reimann F, Cox JJ, Belfer I, et al. Pain perception is altered by a nucleotide polymorphism in SCN9A. Proc Natl Acad Sci USA. 2010;107:5148–53.
16. Kim H, Mittal DP, Iadarola MJ, Dionne RA. Genetic predictors for acute experimental cold and heat pain sensitivity in humans. J Med Genet. 2006;43:e40.
17. Tegeder I, Costigan M, Griffin RS, et al. GTP cyclohydrolase and tetrahydrobiopterin regulate pain sensitivity and persistence. Nat Med. 2006;12:1269–77.
18. Tegeder I, Adolph J, Schmidt H, Woolf CJ, Geisslinger G, Lotsch J. Reduced hyperalgesia in homozygous carriers of a GTP cyclohydrolase 1 haplotype. Eur J Pain. 2008;12:1069–77.
19. Kim H, Dionne RA. Lack of influence of GTP cyclohydrolase gene (GCH1) variations on pain sensitivity in humans. Mol Pain. 2007;3:6.
20. Lazarev M, Lamb J, Barmada MM, et al. Does the pain-protective GTP cyclohydrolase haplotype significantly alter the pattern or severity of pain in humans with chronic pancreatitis? Mol Pain. 2008;4:58.
21. Campbell CM, Edwards RR, Carmona C, et al. Polymorphisms in the GTP cyclohydrolase gene (GCH1) are associated with ratings of capsaicin pain. Pain. 2009;141:114–8.
22. Lotsch J, Klepstad P, Doehring A, Dale O. A GTP cyclohydrolase 1 genetic variant delays cancer pain. Pain. 2010; 148:103–6.
23. Ingelman-Sundberg M, Sim SC, Gomez A, Rodriguez-Antona C. Influence of cytochrome P450 polymorphisms on drug therapies: pharmacogenetic, pharmacoepigenetic and clinical aspects. Pharmacol Ther. 2007;116:496–526.
24. Wang B, Yang LP, Zhang XZ, Huang SQ, Bartlam M, Zhou SF. New insights into the structural characteristics and functional relevance of the human cytochrome P450 2D6 enzyme. Drug Metab Rev. 2009;41:573–643.
25. Zhou SF. Polymorphism of human cytochrome P450 2D6 and its clinical significance: Part I. Clin Pharmacokinet. 2009;48:689–723.
26. Zhou SF, Liu JP, Lai XS. Substrate specificity, inhibitors and regulation of human cytochrome P450 2D6 and implications in drug development. Curr Med Chem. 2009;16:2661–805.
27. Zanger UM, Raimundo S, Eichelbaum M. Cytochrome P450 2D6: overview and update on pharmacology, genetics, biochemistry. Naunyn Schmiedebergs Arch Pharmacol. 2004;369:23–37.
28. Mignat C, Wille U, Ziegler A. Affinity profiles of morphine, codeine, dihydrocodeine and their glucuronides at opioid receptor subtypes. Life Sci. 1995;56:793–9.
29. Thorn CF, Klein TE, Altman RB. Codeine and morphine pathway. Pharmacogenet Genomics. 2009;19:556–8.
30. Zhou SF. Polymorphism of human cytochrome P450 2D6 and its clinical significance: part II. Clin Pharmacokinet. 2009; 48:761–804.
31. Ciszkowski C, Madadi P, Phillips MS, Lauwers AE, Koren G. Codeine, ultrarapid-metabolism genotype, and postoperative death. N Engl J Med. 2009;361:827–8.
32. Gasche Y, Daali Y, Fathi M, et al. Codeine intoxication associated with ultrarapid CYP2D6 metabolism. N Engl J Med. 2004;351:2827–31.
33. Koren G, Cairns J, Chitayat D, Gaedigk A, Leeder SJ. Pharmacogenetics of morphine poisoning in a breastfed neonate of a codeine-prescribed mother. Lancet. 2006;368:704.
34. Madadi P, Koren G. Pharmacogenetic insights into codeine analgesia: implications to pediatric codeine use. Pharmacogenomics. 2008;9:1267–84.
35. Madadi P, Koren G, Cairns J, et al. Safety of codeine during breast-feeding: fatal morphine poisoning in the breastfed neonate of a mother prescribed codeine. Can Fam Physician. 2007;53:33–5.
36. Madadi P, Ross CJ, Hayden MR, et al. Pharmacogenetics of neonatal opioid toxicity following maternal use of codeine during breast-feeding: a case-control study. Clin Pharmacol Ther. 2009;85:31–5.
37. Voronov P, Przybylo HJ, Jagannathan N. Apnea in a child after oral codeine: a genetic variant – an ultra-rapid metabolizer. Paediatr Anaesth. 2007;17:684–7.
38. Enggaard TP, Poulsen L, Arendt-Nielsen L, Brosen K, Ossig J, Sindrup SH. The analgesic effect of tramadol after intravenous injection in healthy volunteers in relation to CYP2D6. Anesth Analg. 2006;102:146–50.
39. Poulsen L, Arendt-Nielsen L, Brosen K, Sindrup SH. The hypoalgesic effect of tramadol in relation to CYP2D6. Clin Pharmacol Ther. 1996;60:636–44.
40. Stamer UM, Lehnen K, Hothker F, et al. Impact of CYP2D6 genotype on postoperative tramadol analgesia. Pain. 2003;105:231–8.
41. Stamer UM, Musshoff F, Kobilay M, Madea B, Hoeft A, Stuber F. Concentrations of tramadol and O-desmethyltramadol enantiomers in different CYP2D6 genotypes. Clin Pharmacol Ther. 2007;82:41–7.
42. Stamer UM, Stuber F, Muders T, Musshoff F. Respiratory depression with tramadol in a patient with renal impairment and CYP2D6 gene duplication. Anesth Analg. 2008;107:926–9.
43. Musshoff F, Madea B, Stuber F, Stamer UM. Enantiomeric determination of tramadol and O-desmethyltramadol by liquid chromatography- mass spectrometry and application to postoperative patients receiving tramadol. J Anal Toxicol. 2006;30:463–7.
44. Pedersen RS, Damkier P, Brosen K. Enantioselective pharmacokinetics of tramadol in CYP2D6 extensive and poor metabolizers. Eur J Clin Pharmacol. 2006;62:513–21.

45. Hufschmid E, Theurillat R, Wilder-Smith CH, Thormann W. Characterization of the genetic polymorphism of dihydrocodeine O-demethylation in man via analysis of urinary dihydrocodeine and dihydromorphine by micellar electrokinetic capillary chromatography. J Chromatogr B Biomed Appl. 1996;678:43–51.

46. Wilder-Smith CH, Hufschmid E, Thormann W. The visceral and somatic antinociceptive effects of dihydrocodeine and its metabolite, dihydromorphine. A cross-over study with extensive and quinidine-induced poor metabolizers. Br J Clin Pharmacol. 1998; 45:575–81.

47. Kharasch ED, Walker A, Isoherranen N, et al. Influence of CYP3A5 genotype on the pharmacokinetics and pharmacodynamics of the cytochrome P4503A probes alfentanil and midazolam. Clin Pharmacol Ther. 2007;82:410–26.

48. Lotsch J, Skarke C, Wieting J, et al. Modulation of the central nervous effects of levomethadone by genetic polymorphisms potentially affecting its metabolism, distribution, and drug action. Clin Pharmacol Ther. 2006;79:72–89.

49. Zhou SF, Zhou ZW, Huang M. Polymorphisms of human cytochrome P450 2C9 and the functional relevance. Toxicology. 2010;278:165–88. Epub 2009 Aug 26.

50. Rodrigues AD. Impact of CYP2C9 genotype on pharmacokinetics: are all cyclooxygenase inhibitors the same? Drug Metab Dispos. 2005;33:1567–75.

51. Kirchheiner J, Brockmoller J. Clinical consequences of cytochrome P450 2C9 polymorphisms. Clin Pharmacol Ther. 2005;77:1–16.

52. Kirchheiner J, Stormer E, Meisel C, Steinbach N, Roots I, Brockmoller J. Influence of CYP2C9 genetic polymorphisms on pharmacokinetics of celecoxib and its metabolites. Pharmacogenetics. 2003;13:473–80.

53. Kirchheiner J, Meineke I, Freytag G, Meisel C, Roots I, Brockmoller J. Enantiospecific effects of cytochrome P450 2C9 amino acid variants on ibuprofen pharmacokinetics and on the inhibition of cyclooxygenases 1 and 2. Clin Pharmacol Ther. 2002;72:62–75.

54. Bae JW, Kim JH, Choi CI, et al. Effect of CYP2C9*3 allele on the pharmacokinetics of naproxen in Korean subjects. Arch Pharm Res. 2009;32:269–73.

55. Dorado P, Cavaco I, Caceres MC, Piedade R, Ribeiro V, Llerena A. Relationship between CYP2C8 genotypes and diclofenac 5-hydroxylation in healthy Spanish volunteers. Eur J Clin Pharmacol. 2008;64:967–70.

56. Blanco G, Martinez C, Ladero JM, et al. Interaction of CYP2C8 and CYP2C9 genotypes modifies the risk for nonsteroidal anti-inflammatory drugs-related acute gastrointestinal bleeding. Pharmacogenet Genomics. 2008;18:37–43.

57. Agundez JA, Garcia-Martin E, Martinez C. Genetically based impairment in CYP2C8- and CYP2C9-dependent NSAID metabolism as a risk factor for gastrointestinal bleeding: is a combination of pharmacogenomics and metabolomics required to improve personalized medicine? Expert Opin Drug Metab Toxicol. 2009;5:607–20.

58. Ma J, Yang XY, Qiao L, Liang LQ, Chen MH. CYP2C9 polymorphism in non-steroidal anti-inflammatory drugs-induced gastropathy. J Dig Dis. 2008;9:79–83.

59. Vonkeman HE, van de Laar MA, van der Palen J, Brouwers JR, Vermes I. Allele variants of the cytochrome P450 2C9 genotype in white subjects from The Netherlands with serious gastroduodenal ulcers attributable to the use of NSAIDs. Clin Ther. 2006;28:1670–6.

60. Visser LE, van Schaik RH, van Vliet M, et al. Allelic variants of cytochrome P450 2C9 modify the interaction between nonsteroidal anti-inflammatory drugs and coumarin anticoagulants. Clin Pharmacol Ther. 2005;77:479–85.

61. Park HJ, Shinn HK, Ryu SH, Lee HS, Park CS, Kang JH. Genetic polymorphisms in the ABCB1 gene and the effects of fentanyl in Koreans. Clin Pharmacol Ther. 2007;81:539–46.

62. Zwisler ST, Enggaard TP, Noehr-Jensen L, et al. The antinociceptive effect and adverse drug reactions of oxycodone in human experimental pain in relation to genetic variations in the OPRM1 and ABCB1 genes. Fundam Clin Pharmacol. 2010;24:517–24. Epub 2009 Oct 21.

63. Campa D, Gioia A, Tomei A, Poli P, Barale R. Association of ABCB1/MDR1 and OPRM1 gene polymorphisms with morphine pain relief. Clin Pharmacol Ther. 2008;83:559–66.

64. Lotsch J, von Hentig N, Freynhagen R, et al. Cross-sectional analysis of the influence of currently known pharmacogenetic modulators on opioid therapy in outpatient pain centers. Pharmacogenet Genomics. 2009;19:429–36.

65. Coller JK, Barratt DT, Dahlen K, Loennechen MH, Somogyi AA. ABCB1 genetic variability and methadone dosage requirements in opioid-dependent individuals. Clin Pharmacol Ther. 2006;80:682–90.

66. Levran O, O'Hara K, Peles E, et al. ABCB1 (MDR1) genetic variants are associated with methadone doses required for effective treatment of heroin dependence. Hum Mol Genet. 2008; 17:2219–27.

67. Beyer A, Koch T, Schroder H, Schulz S, Hollt V. Effect of the A118G polymorphism on binding affinity, potency and agonist-mediated endocytosis, desensitization, and resensitization of the human mu-opioid receptor. J Neurochem. 2004;89:553–60.

68. Margas W, Zubkoff I, Schuler HG, Janicki PK, Ruiz-Velasco V. Modulation of Ca^{2+} channels by heterologously expressed wild-type and mutant human micro-opioid receptors (hMORs) containing the A118G single-nucleotide polymorphism. J Neurophysiol. 2007;97:1058–67.

69. Kroslak T, Laforge KS, Gianotti RJ, Ho A, Nielsen DA, Kreek MJ. The single nucleotide polymorphism A118G alters functional properties of the human mu opioid receptor. J Neurochem. 2007;103:77–87.

70. Tan EC, Lim EC, Teo YY, Lim Y, Law HY, Sia AT. Ethnicity and OPRM variant independently predict pain perception and patient-controlled analgesia usage for post-operative pain. Mol Pain. 2009;5:32.

71. Walter C, Lotsch J. Meta-analysis of the relevance of the OPRM1 118A>G genetic variant for pain treatment. Pain. 2009;146:270–5.

72. Bruehl S, Chung OY, Donahue BS, Burns JW. Anger regulation style, postoperative pain, and relationship to the A118G mu opioid receptor gene polymorphism: a preliminary study. J Behav Med. 2006;29:161–9.

73. Chou WY, Wang CH, Liu PH, Liu CC, Tseng CC, Jawan B. Human opioid receptor A118G polymorphism affects intravenous patient-controlled analgesia morphine consumption after total abdominal hysterectomy. Anesthesiology. 2006;105:334–7.

74. Chou WY, Yang LC, Lu HF, et al. Association of mu-opioid receptor gene polymorphism (A118G) with variations in morphine consumption for analgesia after total knee arthroplasty. Acta Anaesthesiol Scand. 2006;50:787–92.

75. Fillingim RB, Kaplan L, Staud R, et al. The A118G single nucleotide polymorphism of the mu-opioid receptor gene (OPRM1) is associated with pressure pain sensitivity in humans. J Pain. 2005;6:159–67.

76. Klepstad P, Rakvag TT, Kaasa S, et al. The 118 A>G polymorphism in the human micro-opioid receptor gene may increase morphine requirements in patients with pain caused by malignant disease. Acta Anaesthesiol Scand. 2004;48:1232–9.

77. Oertel BG, Schmidt R, Schneider A, Geisslinger G, Lotsch J. The mu-opioid receptor gene polymorphism 118A>G depletes alfentanil-induced analgesia and protects against respiratory depression in homozygous carriers. Pharmacogenet Genomics. 2006;16:625–36.

78. Sia AT, Lim Y, Lim EC, et al. A118G single nucleotide polymorphism of human mu-opioid receptor gene influences pain perception and patient-controlled intravenous morphine consumption after

intrathecal morphine for postcesarean analgesia. Anesthesiology. 2008;109:520–6.

79. Wand GS, McCaul M, Yang X, et al. The mu-opioid receptor gene polymorphism (A118G) alters HPA axis activation induced by opioid receptor blockade. Neuropsychopharmacology. 2002; 26:106–14.

80. Ginosar Y, Davidson EM, Meroz Y, Blotnick S, Shacham M, Caraco Y. Mu-opioid receptor (A118G) single-nucleotide polymorphism affects alfentanil requirements for extracorporeal shock wave lithotripsy: a pharmacokinetic-pharmacodynamic study. Br J Anaesth. 2009;103:420–7.

81. Wu WD, Wang Y, Fang YM, Zhou HY. Polymorphism of the micro-opioid receptor gene (OPRM1 118A>G) affects fentanyl-induced analgesia during anesthesia and recovery. Mol Diagn Ther. 2009;13:331–7.

82. Lotsch J, Stuck B, Hummel T. The human mu-opioid receptor gene polymorphism 118A>G decreases cortical activation in response to specific nociceptive stimulation. Behav Neurosci. 2006; 120:1218–24.

83. Lotsch J, Freynhagen R, Geisslinger G. Are polymorphisms in the mu-opioid receptor important for opioid therapy? Schmerz. 2005;19:378–82. 384–95.

84. Lotsch J, Geisslinger G. Relevance of frequent mu-opioid receptor polymorphisms for opioid activity in healthy volunteers. Pharmacogenomics J. 2006;6:200–10.

85. Lotsch J, Geisslinger G. Current evidence for a genetic modulation of the response to analgesics. Pain. 2006;121:1–5.

86. Lotsch J, Skarke C, Grosch S, Darimont J, Schmidt H, Geisslinger G. The polymorphism A118G of the human mu-opioid receptor gene decreases the pupil constrictory effect of morphine-6-glucuronide but not that of morphine. Pharmacogenetics. 2002;12:3–9.

87. Lotsch J, Zimmermann M, Darimont J, et al. Does the A118G polymorphism at the mu-opioid receptor gene protect against morphine-6-glucuronide toxicity? Anesthesiology. 2002;97:814–9.

88. Coulbault L, Beaussier M, Verstuyft C, et al. Environmental and genetic factors associated with morphine response in the postoperative period. Clin Pharmacol Ther. 2006;79:316–24.

89. Fukuda K, Hayashida M, Ide S, et al. Association between OPRM1 gene polymorphisms and fentanyl sensitivity in patients undergoing painful cosmetic surgery. Pain. 2009;147:194–201.

90. Huehne K, Leis S, Muenster T, et al. High post surgical opioid requirements in Crohn's disease are not due to a general change in pain sensitivity. Eur J Pain. 2009;13:1036–42.

91. Janicki PK, Schuler G, Francis D, et al. A genetic association study of the functional A118G polymorphism of the human mu-opioid receptor gene in patients with acute and chronic pain. Anesth Analg. 2006;103:1011–7.

92. Hayashida M, Nagashima M, Satoh Y, et al. Analgesic requirements after major abdominal surgery are associated with OPRM1 gene polymorphism genotype and haplotype. Pharmacogenomics. 2008;9:1605–16.

93. Landau R, Kern C, Columb MO, Smiley RM, Blouin JL. Genetic variability of the mu-opioid receptor influences intrathecal fentanyl analgesia requirements in laboring women. Pain. 2008;139:5–14.

94. Reyes-Gibby CC, Shete S, Rakvag T, et al. Exploring joint effects of genes and the clinical efficacy of morphine for cancer pain: OPRM1 and COMT gene. Pain. 2007;130:25–30.

95. Ramchandani VA, Umhau J, Pavon FJ, et al. A genetic determinant of the striatal dopamine response to alcohol in men. Mol Psychiatry. 2011;16:809–17. Epub 2010 May 18.

96. Shabalina SA, Zaykin DV, Gris P, et al. Expansion of the human mu-opioid receptor gene architecture: novel functional variants. Hum Mol Genet. 2009;18:1037–51.

97. Berthele A, Platzer S, Jochim B, et al. COMT Val108/158Met genotype affects the mu-opioid receptor system in the human brain: evidence from ligand-binding, G-protein activation and pre-proenkephalin mRNA expression. Neuroimage. 2005;28:185–93.

98. Zubieta JK, Heitzeg MM, Smith YR, et al. COMT val158met genotype affects mu-opioid neurotransmitter responses to a pain stressor. Science. 2003;299:1240–3.

99. Rakvag TT, Klepstad P, Baar C, et al. The Val158Met polymorphism of the human catechol-O-methyltransferase (COMT) gene may influence morphine requirements in cancer pain patients. Pain. 2005;116:73–8.

100. Rakvag TT, Ross JR, Sato H, Skorpen F, Kaasa S, Klepstad P. Genetic variation in the catechol-O-methyltransferase (COMT) gene and morphine requirements in cancer patients with pain. Mol Pain. 2008;4:64.

101. Ross JR, Riley J, Taegetmeyer AB, et al. Genetic variation and response to morphine in cancer patients: catechol-O-methyltransferase and multidrug resistance-1 gene polymorphisms are associated with central side effects. Cancer. 2008;112:1390–403.

102. Nackley AG, Shabalina SA, Lambert JE, et al. Low enzymatic activity haplotypes of the human catechol-O-methyltransferase gene: enrichment for marker SNPs. PLoS One. 2009;4:e5237.

103. Nackley AG, Shabalina SA, Tchivileva IE, et al. Human catechol-O-methyltransferase haplotypes modulate protein expression by altering mRNA secondary structure. Science. 2006;314:1930–3.

104. Mogil JS, Ritchie J, Smith SB, et al. Melanocortin-1 receptor gene variants affect pain and mu-opioid analgesia in mice and humans. J Med Genet. 2005;42:583–7.

105. Mogil JS, Wilson SG, Chesler EJ, et al. The melanocortin-1 receptor gene mediates female-specific mechanisms of analgesia in mice and humans. Proc Natl Acad Sci USA. 2003;100:4867–72.

106. Esser R, Berry C, Du Z, et al. Preclinical pharmacology of lumiracoxib: a novel selective inhibitor of cyclooxygenase-2. Br J Pharmacol. 2005;144:538–50.

107. Cipollone F, Patrono C. Cyclooxygenase-2 polymorphism: putting a brake on the inflammatory response to vascular injury? Arterioscler Thromb Vasc Biol. 2002;22:1516–8.

108. Papafili A, Hill MR, Brull DJ, et al. Common promoter variant in cyclooxygenase-2 represses gene expression: evidence of role in acute-phase inflammatory response. Arterioscler Thromb Vasc Biol. 2002;22:1631–6.

109. Skarke C, Reus M, Schmidt R, et al. The cyclooxygenase 2 genetic variant -765 G>C does not modulate the effects of celecoxib on prostaglandin E2 production. Clin Pharmacol Ther. 2006;80:621–32.

110. Lee YS, Kim H, Wu TX, Wang XM, Dionne RA. Genetically mediated interindividual variation in analgesic responses to cyclooxygenase inhibitory drugs. Clin Pharmacol Ther. 2006;79:407–18.

111. Lotsch J, Fluhr K, Neddermayer T, Doehring A, Geisslinger G. The consequence of concomitantly present functional genetic variants for the identification of functional genotype-phenotype associations in pain. Clin Pharmacol Ther. 2009;85:25–30.

112. Kim H, Ramsay E, Lee H, Wahl S, Dionne RA. Genome-wide association study of acute post-surgical pain in humans. Pharmacogenomics. 2009;10:171–9.

113. Lotsch J, Geisslinger G. A critical appraisal of human genotyping for pain therapy. Trends Pharmacol Sci. 2010;31:312–7.

Nonsteroidal Anti-inflammatory Drugs

3

Asokumar Buvanendran

Key Points

- NSAIDs are analgesic compounds with anti-inflammatory activity determined by their ability to decrease prostaglandin formation through inhibition of COX following tissue injury.
- There are two major isoforms of COX. COX-1 is largely constitutive and is responsible for the production of prostaglandins involved in homeostatic processes in the gastric protection, kidney, and platelet aggregation. COX-2 is an inducible form created in the presence of inflammation and is largely responsible for the production of prostaglandins involved in pain and inflammation. Selective COX-2 inhibitors are capable of producing the same analgesic effect of the nonselective NSAIDs but without affecting platelet function and gastropathy.
- Initiation of NSAIDs should occur with the patient education of side effects and should be prescribed with the lowest effective dose and for the shortest duration.
- Combination medications (opioid/NSAID) should occur with patient education of the contents of the combination medication.
- The NSAIDs are extremely effective as part of a multimodal perioperative analgesic regimen. Selective COX-2 inhibitors provide an additional advantage in the perioperative period of not affecting platelet coagulation profile.

Introduction

Nonsteroidal anti-inflammatory drugs (NSAIDs) are the most widely used analgesic medications in the world because of their ability to reduce pain and inflammation [1–3]. The NSAIDs are structurally diverse, but all have antipyretic, anti-inflammatory, and analgesic properties. The salicylates (aspirin-like medications) have been used to treat pain conditions for thousands of years [4]. Greater than 100 million prescriptions for NSAIDS are written by clinicians in the United States each year, and more than 30 million Americans use prescription or over-the-counter (OTC) NSAIDs regularly [5, 6]. This class of medications contains compounds that are often chemically diverse which are grouped together based on their therapeutic actions. Many of these NSAIDs used today are available as OTC products with greater than 14 million patients use NSAIDs for relief of symptoms associated with arthritis alone [7]. NSAIDs are the most widely prescribed drugs in the world with sales in the United States alone of nearly five billion dollars [3]. They have even demonstrated clear clinical utility in such severe pain states as osteoarthritis, rheumatoid arthritis, and metastatic spread of cancer to bone, usually supplementing rather than replacing the role of opioids [8, 9].

Often labeled as a NSAID, acetaminophen and NSAIDs have important differences such as acetaminophen's weak anti-inflammatory effects and its generally poor ability to inhibit COX in the presence of high concentrations of peroxides, as are found at sites of inflammation [10, 11] nor does it have an adverse effect on platelet function [12] or the gastric mucosa [11].

Mechanism of Action

The mechanism of action of the NSAIDs is inhibition of prostaglandin production from arachidonic acid by either reversible or irreversible acetylation of the cyclooxygenase (Fig. 3.1). Cyclooxygenase (COX) is present in at least two

A. Buvanendran, M.D.
Department of Anesthesiology, Rush Medical College, Chicago, IL, USA

Orthopedic Anesthesia, Rush University Medical Center, Chicago, IL, USA
e-mail: asokumar@aol.com

T.R. Deer et al. (eds.), *Comprehensive Treatment of Chronic Pain by Medical, Interventional, and Integrative Approaches*,
DOI 10.1007/978-1-4614-1560-2_3, © American Academy of Pain Medicine 2013

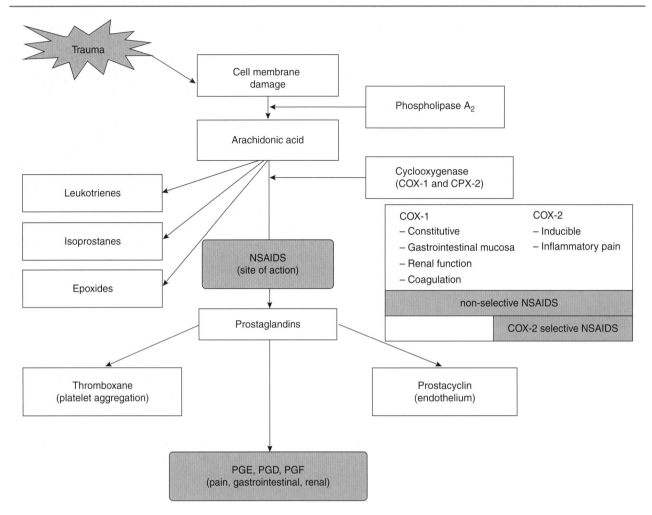

Fig. 3.1 Site of action of NSAIDs

isoforms (COX-1 and COX-2) and is dispersed throughout the body. The COX-1 isoform is constitutive, causing hemostasis, platelet aggregation, and the production of prostacyclin, which is gastric mucosal protective. The inhibition of COX-1 isoform may be responsible for the adverse effects related to the nonselective NSAIDs [13]. It is the COX-2 isoform that is induced by pro-inflammatory stimuli and cytokines causing fever, inflammation, and pain and thus the target for antipyresis, anti-inflammation, and analgesia by NSAIDs [4]. COX-1, as the constitutive isoform, is necessary for normal functions and is found in most cell types. COX-1 mediates the production of prostaglandins that are essential in the homeostatic processes in the stomach (gastric protection), kidney, and platelet aggregation. The COX-2 is generally considered to be an inducible enzyme, induced pathologic processes such as fever, pain, and inflammation. COX-2, despite being the inducible isoform, is expressed under normal conditions in a number of tissues, which probably include brain, testis, and kidney. In inflammatory states, COX-2 becomes expressed in macrophages and other cells

propagating the inflammatory process [14]. The pain associated with inflammation and prostaglandin production results from the production of prostanoids in the inflamed body tissues that sensitize nerve ending and leads to the sensation of pain [15].

Originally thought of as possessing solely peripheral inhibition of prostaglandin production, more recent research indicates that NSAIDs have peripheral and central mechanisms of action [2, 16, 17]. Peripherally, prostaglandins contribute to hyperalgesia by sensitizing nociceptive sensory nerve endings to other mediators (such as histamine and bradykinin) and by sensitizing nociceptors to respond to nonnociceptive stimuli (e.g., touch) [16, 18]. Peripheral inflammation induces a substantial increase in COX-2 [19] and prostaglandin synthase expression in the central nervous system. Centrally, prostaglandins are recognized to have direct actions at the level of the spinal cord enhancing nociception, notably the terminals of sensory neurons in the dorsal horn [20]. Both COX-1 and COX-2 are expressed constitutively in dorsal root ganglia and spinal dorsal and ventral gray matter, but inhibition of COX-2 and not COX-1 reduces hyperalgesia [21]. Additionally, the pro-inflammatory cytokine interleukin-1beta (IL-1β) plays a major role in inducing COX-2 in local inflammatory cells by activating the transcription factor NF-κB. In the central nervous system (CNS), IL-1β causes increased production of COX-2 and PGE_2, producing hyperalgesia, but this is not the result of neural activity arising from the sensory fibers innervating the inflamed tissue or of systemic IL-1β in the plasma [22]. Peripheral inflammation possibly produces other signal molecules that enter the circulation, crossing the blood-brain barrier, and act to elevate IL-1β, leading to COX-2 expression in neurons and nonneuronal cells in many different areas of the spinal cord [22, 23]. At present, evidence suggests that interleukin-6 (IL-6) triggers the formation of IL-1β in the CNS, which in turn causes increased production of COX-2 and PGE_2 [22].

There appear to be two forms of input from peripheral-inflamed tissue to the CNS. The first is mediated by electrical activity in sensitized nerve fibers innervating the inflamed area, which signals the location of the inflamed tissue as well as the onset, duration, and nature of any stimuli applied to this tissue [21]. This input is sensitive to peripherally acting COX-2 inhibitors and to neural blockade with local anesthetics [24]. The second is a humoral signal originating from the inflamed tissue, which acts to produce a widespread induction of COX-2 in the CNS.

Pharmacokinetics

NSAIDs are most often administered enterally, but intravenous, intramuscular, rectal, and topical preparations are available. NSAIDs are highly bound to plasma proteins, specifically to albumin (>90 %), and therefore, only a small portion of the circulating drug in plasma exists in the unbound (pharmacologically active) form. The volume of distribution of NSAIDs is low, ranging from 0.1 to 0.3 L/kg, suggesting minimal tissue binding [25]. Most NSAIDs are weak acids with pK_as < 6, and since weak acids will be 99 % ionized two pH units above their pK_a, these anti-inflammatory medications are present in the body mostly in the ionized form. In contrast, the coxibs are nonacidic which may play a role in the favorable tolerability profile.

Absorption

NSAID's pH profile facilitates absorption via the stomach, and the large surface area of the small intestine produces a major absorptive site for orally administered NSAIDs. Most of the NSAIDs are rapidly and completely absorbed from the gastrointestinal tract, with peak concentrations occurring within 1–4 h. The presence of food tends to delay absorption without affecting peak concentration [10]. Ketorolac is one of the few NSAIDs approved for parenteral administration, but most NSAIDs are not available in parenteral forms in the United States. Recently, injectable ibuprofen has been approved as an injectable formulation for pain and fever. Parenteral administration may have the advantage of decreased direct local toxicity in the gastrointestinal tract, but parenteral ketorolac tromethamine does not decrease the risk of adverse events associated with COX-1 inhibition. Topical NSAIDs possess the advantage of providing local action without systemic adverse effects. These medications, such as diclofenac epolamine transdermal patch (Flector®) and diclofenac sodium gel (Voltaren®) are formulated to traverse the skin to reach the adjacent joints and muscles and exert therapeutic activity.

Distribution

The majority of NSAIDs are weakly acidic, highly bound to plasma proteins (albumin), and lipophilic. The relatively low pH of most NSAIDs, in part, determines the distribution too because they are ionized at physiologic pHs. In areas with acidic extracellular pH values, NSAIDs may accumulate (inflamed tissue, gastrointestinal tract, kidneys) [24]. Additionally, the unbound drug is generally considered responsible for pharmacological effects, and the apparent volume of distribution (Vd/F), determined after oral administration, is usually 0.1–0.3 L/kg, which approximates plasma volume [25]. This high-protein binding places only a small portion in the active, unbound form. However, some NSAIDs (i.e., ibuprofen, naproxen, salicylate) have activity that is concentration-dependent because their plasma concentration approaches that of plasma albumin and the Vd/F increases with dose [24]. The high-protein binding (>90 %) of the NSAIDs has particular relevance in the state of hypoalbuminemia or decrease albumin concentrations (e.g., elderly, malnourished). A greater fraction of unbound NSAIDs are present in the plasma which may enhance efficacy, but also increase toxicity.

Elimination

The major metabolic pathway for elimination of NSAIDs is hepatic oxidation or conjugation. The half-lives of NSAIDs vary as active metabolites may be present or the metabolite is the active form when liberated from the prodrug. Also, the elimination of the NSAIDs may determine the dosing frequency as NSAID plasma elimination half-lives vary widely from 0.25 to 70 h [24]. Renal excretion of unmetabolized drug is a minor elimination pathway for most NSAIDs accounting for less than 10 % of the administered dose.

Specific Medications

Salicylates

Aspirin

Acetylsalicylic acid (ASA) is the most widely used analgesic, antipyretic, and anti-inflammatory agent in the world and remains the standard for which all other NSAIDs are compared. Aspirin inhibits the biosynthesis of prostaglandins by means of an irreversible acetylation and consequent inactivation of COX; thus, aspirin inactivates COX permanently. This is an important distinction among the NSAIDs because aspirin's duration action is related to the turnover rate of cyclooxygenases in different target tissues. The duration of action of other NSAIDs, which competitively inhibit the active sites of the COX enzymes, relates more directly to the time course of drug disposition [26]. Platelets are devoid of the ability to produce additional cyclooxygenase; thus, thromboxane synthesis is arrested.

Propionic Acid

Naproxen

Naproxen is a nonprescription NSAID, but a newly formulated controlled-release tablet is available (Naprelan®). It is fully absorbed after enteral administration and has a half-life of 14 h. Peak concentrations in plasma occur within 4–6 h. Naproxen has a volume of distribution of 0.16 L/kg. At therapeutic levels, naproxen is greater than 99 % albumin-bound. Naproxen is extensively metabolized to 6-0-desmethyl naproxen, and both parent and metabolites do not induce metabolizing enzymes. Most of the drug is excreted in the urine, primarily as unchanged naproxen. Naproxen has been used for the treatment of arthritis and other inflammatory diseases. Metabolites of naproxen are excreted almost entirely in the urine. About 30 % of the drug undergoes 6-demethylation, and most of this metabolite, as well as naproxen itself, is excreted as the glucuronide or other conjugates.

Ibuprofen

Ibuprofen is one of the most widely used NSAIDs after ASA, and N-acetyl-p-aminophenol (APAP) in OTC is used for the relief of symptoms of acute pain, fever, and inflammation. Ibuprofen is rapidly absorbed from the upper GI tract, with peak plasma levels achieved about 1–2 h after administration. Ibuprofen is highly bound to plasma proteins and has an estimated volume of distribution of 0.14 L/kg. Ibuprofen is primarily hepatically metabolized (90 %) with less than 10 % excreted unchanged in the urine and bile. and mild-to-moderate pain conditions [27]. Ibuprofen at a dose of 1,200–2,400 mg/day has a predominately analgesic effect for mild-to-moderate pain conditions, with dose of 3,200 mg/day only recommended under continued care of clinical professionals. Even at anti-inflammatory doses of more than 1,600 mg/day, renal side effects are almost exclusively encountered in patients with low intravascular volume and low cardiac output, particularly in the elderly [28]. The effectiveness of ibuprofen has been demonstrated in the treatment of headache and migraine, menstrual pain, and acute postoperative pain [29–31]. The recent injectable formulation will gain increased use for acute pain and fever.

Ketoprofen

The pharmacological properties of ketoprofen are similar to other propionic acid derivative, although the different formulations differ in their release characteristic. Not available in the United States, the optically pure (S) enantiomer (dexketoprofen) is available which is rapidly reabsorbed from the gastrointestinal tract, having a rapid onset of effects. Additionally, capsules release drug in the stomach, whereas the capsule pellets (extended release) are designed to resist dissolution in the low pH of gastric fluid but release drug at a controlled rate in the higher pH environment of the small intestine. Peak plasma levels achieved about 1–2 h after oral administration for the capsules and 6–7 h after administration of the capsule pellets. Ketoprofen has high plasma protein binding (98–99 %) and an estimated volume of distribution of 0.11 L/kg. Ketoprofen is conjugated with glucuronic acid in the liver, and the conjugate is excreted in the urine. The glucuronic acid moiety can be converted back to the parent compound. Thus, the metabolite serves as a potential reservoir for parent drug, and this may be important in persons with renal insufficiency. The extended release ketoprofen is not recommended for the treatment of acute pain because of the release characteristics. Individual patients may show a better response to 300 mg daily as compared to 200 mg, although in well-controlled clinical trials patients on 300 mg did not show greater mean effectiveness. The usual starting dose of ketoprofen is 50 or 75 mg with immediate release capsules every 6–8 h or 200 mg with extended release capsules once daily. The maximum dose is 300 mg daily of immediate release capsules or 200 mg daily of extended release capsules. Ketoprofen has shown statistical superiority over acetaminophen on the time-effect curves for pain relief and pain intensity difference in the treatment of moderate or severe postoperative pain and acute low back pain [32–34].

Oxaprozin

In contrast to the other propionic acid derivatives, oxaprozin peak plasma levels are not achieved until 3–6 h after an oral dose and its half-life of 40–60 h allows for once-daily administration [35]. Oxaprozin is highly bound to plasma proteins and has an estimated volume of distribution of 0.15 L/kg. Oxaprozin is primarily metabolized by the liver, and 65 % of the dose is excreted into the urine and 35 % in the feces as metabolites. Oxaprozin diffuses readily into inflamed synovial tissues after oral administration and is capable of inhibiting both anandamide hydrolase in neurons and NF-kappaB activation in inflammatory cells, which are crucial for synthesis of pro-inflammatory and histotoxic mediators in inflamed joints [36–38].

Acetic Acid

Diclofenac

Diclofenac has COX-2 selectivity, and the selective inhibitor of COX-2 lumiracoxib is an analog of diclofenac. Its potency against COX-2 is substantially greater than that of indomethacin, naproxen, or several other NSAIDs and is similar to celecoxib [10]. Diclofenac is rapidly absorbed after oral administration, but substantial first-pass metabolism of only about 50 % of diclofenac is available systemically. After oral administration, peak serum concentrations are attained within 2–3 h. Diclofenac is highly bound to plasma proteins and has an estimated volume of distribution of 0.12 L/kg. Diclofenac is excreted primarily in the urine (65 %) and 35 % as bile conjugates. Diclofenac is available in two enteral formulations, diclofenac sodium and diclofenac potassium. Diclofenac potassium is formulated to be released and absorbed in the stomach. Diclofenac sodium, usually distributed in enteric-coated tablets, resists dissolution in low-pH gastric environments, releasing instead in the duodenum [39]. Hepatotoxicity, elevated transaminases, may occur, and measurements of transaminases should be measured during therapy with diclofenac. Other formulations of diclofenac include topical gels (Voltaren® Gel) and transdermal patches (Flector® Patch). Additionally, diclofenac is available in a parenteral formulation for infusion (Voltarol® Ampoules), and more recently, a formulation for intravenous bolus has been developed (diclofenac sodium injection [DIC075V; Dyloject®]). Uniquely, diclofenac accumulates in synovial fluid after oral administration [40], which may explain why its duration of therapeutic effect is considerably longer than the plasma half-life of 1–2 h. Oral preparations have been shown to provide significant analgesia in the postoperative period for adults experiencing moderate or severe pain following a surgical procedure [41].

The transdermal application of diclofenac has also shown efficacy in the treatment of musculoskeletal disorders including ankle sprains, epicondylitis, and knee osteoarthritis [42, 43]. The advantage of the transdermal formulation is the lack of appreciable systemic absorption and accumulation of the medication at the site of application, thereby providing local pain relief. In comparison to enteral delivery, topical application of diclofenac provides analgesia by peripheral activity and not central mediation.

Etodolac

Etodolac has some degree of COX-2 selectivity conferring less gastric irritation compared with other NSAIDs [44]. The analgesic effect of full doses of etodolac is longer than that of aspirin, lasting up to 8 h. After oral administration, peak serum concentrations of 16 and 25 mg/L are attained within 2 h of administering 200 and 400 mg, respectively. Etodolac is highly bound to plasma proteins and has an estimated volume of distribution of 0.4 L/kg. Etodolac is excreted primarily in the urine, and 60 % of a dose is recovered within 24 h. Greater than 60 % of the metabolites are hydroxylated with glucuronic conjugation. The half-life of etodolac is approximately 7 h in healthy subjects. When compared with other NSAIDs, etodolac 300 and 400 mg daily has tended to be more effective than aspirin 3–4 g daily and was similar in efficacy to sulindac 400 mg daily [10]. Clinical doses of 200–300 mg twice a day for the relief of low back or shoulder pain have been equated to analgesia with naproxen 500 mg twice a day [45]. In postsurgical pain, etodolac 100–200 mg was approximately equivalent to aspirin 650 mg in providing pain relief, although etodolac had a longer duration of action [46].

Indomethacin

It is a nonselective COX inhibitor introduced in 1963, but has fallen out of favor with the advent of safer alternatives. Indomethacin is a more potent inhibitor of the cyclooxygenases than is aspirin, but patient intolerance generally limits its use to short-term dosing. Oral indomethacin has excellent bioavailability. Peak concentrations occur 1–2 h after dosing. Indomethacin is 90 % bound to plasma proteins and tissues. The concentration of the drug in the CSF is low, but its concentration in synovial fluid is equal to that in plasma within 5 h of administration [10]. Complaints associated with gastrointestinal irritation are common, including diarrhea, and ulcerative lesions are a contraindication to indomethacin use. Indomethacin has FDA approval for closure of persistent patent ductus arteriosus, but side effect profile limits other uses.

Ketorolac

Ketorolac Tromethamine is a NSAID with activity at COX-1 and COX-2 enzymes thus blocking prostaglandin production. After oral administration, peak serum concentrations are attained within 1–2 h. Ketorolac is highly bound to plasma proteins and has an estimated volume of distribution of

0.28 L/kg. Ketorolac is excreted primarily in the urine and has a half-life of approximately 5–6 h in healthy subjects. Administration of ketorolac is available for enteral, ophthalmic, and parenteral delivery and is the only parenteral NSAID currently available in the United States. Ketorolac has been utilized to treat mild-to-severe pain following major surgical procedures including general abdominal surgery, gynecologic surgery, orthopedic surgery, and dentistry. Multiple studies have investigated the analgesic potency of ketorolac, and in animal models, the analgesic potency has be estimated to be between 180 and 800 times that of aspirin [47, 48]. When compared to morphine, ketorolac 30 mg intramuscular (IM) has been shown to be equivalent to 12 mg morphine IM and 100 mg meperidine IM [49]. It was observed that the mean values for total body clearance of ketorolac were decreased by about 50 % and that the half-life was approximately doubled in patients with renal impairment compared with healthy control subjects [50], and it may precipitate or exacerbate renal failure in hypovolemic, elderly, or especially those with underlying renal dysfunction. Therefore, ketorolac is recommended for limited use (3–5 days). Recently, intranasal route of administration of ketorolac (Sprix™) has been approved by the FDA for acute pain. The CSF penetration of this compound via the nasal route should be superior.

Nabumetone

Nabumetone is a prodrug, which undergoes hepatic biotransformation to the active component, 6-methoxy-2-naphthylacetic acid (6MNA), that has some degree of COX-2 selectivity conferring less gastric irritation compared with other NSAIDs [51]. Nabumetone is highly bound to plasma proteins and has an estimated volume of distribution of 0.68 L/kg. Nabumetone is excreted primarily in the urine and has a half-life of approximately 20–24 h in healthy subjects enabling single-daily dosing. When compared with other NSAIDs, nabumetone has tended to show efficacy [52] and tolerability in the treatment of arthritis [53, 54].

Anthranilic Acid

Mefenamic Acid

Peak serum concentrations are attained within 2–4 h and a half-life of 3–4 h. Mefenamic acid has been associated with severe pancytopenia and many other side effects. Hence, therapy is not to be for more than 1 week [55].

Meloxicam

The enolic acid derivative shows nonselectivity, except for meloxicam which shows relative COX-2 selectivity. For example, meloxicam shows dose-dependent COX selectivity, where 7.5 mg is more selective for COX-2 while at 15 mg meloxicam becomes less selective [56]. After oral administration, peak serum concentrations are attained within 5–10 h after administration. Meloxicam is highly bound to plasma proteins and has an estimated half-life of approximately 15–20 h in healthy subjects.

COX-2 Inhibitors

COX-2 inhibitors (celecoxib, rofecoxib, and valdecoxib) were approved for use in the United States and Europe, but both rofecoxib and valdecoxib have now been withdrawn from the market due to their adverse event profile. Recently, parecoxib and etoricoxib have been approved in Europe. The newest drug in the class, lumiracoxib, is under consideration for approval in Europe. Upon administration, most of the coxibs are distributed widely throughout the body with celecoxib possessing an increased lipophilicity enabling transport into the CNS. Despite these subtle differences, all of the coxibs achieve sufficient brain concentrations to have a central analgesic effect [57] and all reduce prostaglandin formation in inflamed joints. The estimated half-lives of these medications vary (2–6 h for lumiracoxib, 6–12 h for celecoxib and valdecoxib, and 20–26 h for etoricoxib). Likewise, the relative degree of selectivity for COX-2 inhibition is lumiracoxib = etoricoxib > valdecoxib = rofecoxib >> celecoxib [10].

Celecoxib

Currently, celecoxib is the only selective COX-2 inhibitor available in the United States. After oral administration, peak serum concentrations of celecoxib are attained 2–3 h after administration. Celecoxib is highly bound to plasma proteins, is excreted primarily by hepatic metabolism, and has a half-life of approximately 11 h in healthy subjects. Celecoxib does not interfere with platelet aggregation; thus, perioperative administration can be conducted as part of a multimodal analgesic regimen without increased risk of bleeding. Additionally, NSAID-induced GI complications are one of the most common drug-related serious adverse events, but celecoxib preferentially inhibits the inducible COX-2 isoform and not the constitutive COX-1 isoform thus conferring some gastroprotective effect.

The efficacy and tolerability of celecoxib has been studied in multiple studies. Celecoxib has demonstrated effectiveness in both placebo and active-control (or comparator) clinical trials in patients with osteoarthritis, rheumatoid arthritis, and postoperative pain relief [58–60].

Etoricoxib

Etoricoxib is a second-generation, highly selective cyclooxygenase 2 (COX-2) inhibitor with anti-inflammatory and analgesic properties [61]. It shows dose-dependent inhibition of COX-2 across the therapeutic dose range, without inhibition of COX-1, does not inhibit gastric prostaglandin synthesis and has no effect on platelet function [62]. Etoricoxib shows 106-fold selectivity for COX-2 over COX-1 [63], compared with 7.6-fold selectivity observed with celecoxib [62, 63].

Acetaminophen

Acetaminophen (paracetamol – APAP) is an analgesic and antipyretic medication that produces its analgesic effect by inhibiting central prostaglandin synthesis with minimal inhibition of peripheral prostaglandin synthesis [10, 11]. After oral administration, peak serum concentrations are attained within 0.5–3 h. A small portion of acetaminophen is bound to plasma proteins (10–50 %) and has an estimated volume of distribution of 0.95 L/kg. Acetaminophen is eliminated from the body primarily by formation of glucuronide and sulfate conjugates in a dose-dependent manner. The half-life of acetaminophen is approximately 2–3 h in healthy subjects. As previously stated, acetaminophen and NSAIDs have important differences such as acetaminophen's weak anti-inflammatory effects and its generally poor ability to inhibit COX in the presence of high concentrations of peroxides, as are found at sites of inflammation [10, 11] nor does it have an adverse effect on platelet function [12] or the gastric mucosa [11]. It is absorbed rapidly, with peak plasma levels seen within 30 min to 1 h, and is metabolized in the liver by conjugation and hydroxylation to inactive metabolites and has duration of action of 4–6 h [64, 65]. Paracetamol is perhaps the safest and most cost-effective non-opioid analgesic when it is administered in analgesic doses [66]. Paracetamol is available in parenteral form as propacetamol, and 1 g of propacetamol provides 0.5 g paracetamol after hydrolysis [67]. Propacetamol is widely used in many countries other than the United States and has shown to reduce opioid consumption by about 35–45 % [68] in postoperative pain studies [68, 69] including after cardiac surgery [70].

Safety, Toxicity, and Adverse Effects

Although NSAIDs are the most widely used OTC medications, with a long history of use, research, and medication advancements, NSAIDs remain as a source of adverse effects. NSAIDs not only share therapeutic actions but also similar adverse effects that include GI ulceration and bleeding, disturbance of platelet function, sodium and water retention, nephrotoxicity, and hypersensitivity reactions [71]. The adverse effects range from minor (e.g., nausea, gastric irritation, dizziness) to major (e.g., allergic reaction, gastrointestinal, renal and coagulation derangements, and delay in bone healing) in acute use. Chronic use of these medications may increase minor or major adverse effects. The three most common adverse drug reactions to NSAIDs are gastrointestinal, dermatological, and neuropsychiatric, the last one oddly not being age related [55, 72].

Gastrointestinal

Gastrointestinal bleeding is one of the most frequently reported significant complications of NSAID use. The effects of NSAIDs on gastric mucosa have been estimated to occur in 30–40 % of users [73]. NSAIDs affect the GI tract with symptoms of gastric distress alone and through actual damage with ulceration. Dyspepsia has been shown to have an annual prevalence with NSAID use of about 15 % [55]. One review estimated 7,000 deaths and 70,000 hospitalizations per year in the USA among NSAID users. Among rheumatoid arthritis patients, an estimated 20,000 hospitalizations and 2,600 deaths per year are related to NSAID GI toxicity [55, 74]. Evidence of the association between NSAIDs and gastropathy accrued in the 1970s with the increased use of endoscopy and the introduction of several new NSAIDs [55, 75].

The risk of developing GI complications with the continued and long-term use of NSAIDs is now well recognized. Likewise, risk factors have been identified for the development of NSAID-induced gastropathy. Risk factors include history of GI complications, high-dose or multiple NSAIDs, advanced age, concomitant corticosteroid use, and alcohol use [76]. Administration of GI protective agents (H_2-receptor antagonist and proton pump inhibitors), may attenuate the complications associated with long-term NSAID use. Other strategies include the use of selective COX-2 inhibitors, such as celecoxib, which are less ulcerogenic compared with nonselective NSAIDs.

Renal

NSAIDs can decrease renal function and cause renal failure. Renal impairment has been reported to occur in as many as 18 % of patients using ibuprofen, whereas acute renal failure has been shown to occur in about 6 % of patients using NSAIDs in another study [55, 77, 78]. The proposed mechanism is reduction in prostaglandin production leading to reduced renal blood flow with subsequent medullary ischemia that may result from NSAID use in susceptible individuals [79]. Acute renal failure may occur with any COX-2-selective or nonselective NSAID [80]. The risk factors for NSAID-induced renal toxicity include chronic NSAID use, high-dose or multiple NSAIDs, volume depletion, congestive heart failure, vascular disease, hyperreninemia, shock, sepsis, systemic lupus erythematosus, hepatic disease, sodium depletion, nephrotic syndrome, diuresis, concomitant drug therapy (diuretics, ACE inhibitors, beta blockers, potassium supplements), and advanced age [81].

Hepatic

Hepatotoxicity seems to be a rare complication of most NSAIDs [82]. Hepatic-related side effects of NSAIDs have been reported to occur in 3 % of patients receiving the drugs [83]. In contrast, paracetamol has a recognized potential for hepatotoxicity and is thought to be responsible for at least 42 % of acute liver failure cases observed and has become the most common cause of acute liver failure in the United States [27]. Most of these cases were due to intentional or unintentional overdose with 79 % reported taking the analgesic specifically for pain and 38 % were taking two different preparations of the drug simultaneously [27]. Acetaminophen is almost entirely metabolized in the liver, and the minor metabolites are responsible for the hepatotoxicity seen in overdoses [84]. Mechanisms of acetaminophen hepatotoxicity include depletion of hepatocyte glutathione, accumulation of the toxic metabolite NAPQI, mitochondrial dysfunction, and alteration of innate immunity [85]. Risk factors include concomitant depression, chronic pain, alcohol or narcotic use, and/or take several preparations simultaneously [27]. The lowest dose of acetaminophen to cause hepatotoxicity is believed to be between 125 and 150 mg/kg [86, 87]. The threshold dose to cause hepatotoxicity is 10–15 g of acetaminophen for adults and 150 mg/kg for children [86, 88]. The most recognized dosing limit is 4 g/24 h in healthy adult patients. Clinicians should continually inquire medication usage as many patients are not aware that prescription narcotic–acetaminophen combinations contain acetaminophen and unintentionally combine these medications with OTC acetaminophen.

Cardiovascular

The inhibition of cyclooxygenase reduces the production of thromboxane and prostacyclin. Thromboxane functions as a vasoconstrictor and facilitates platelet aggregation. Thromboxane A_2 (TXA_2), produced by activated platelets, has prothrombotic properties, stimulating activation of new platelets as well as increasing platelet aggregation. Endothelium-derived prostacyclin (PGI_2) functions in concert with thromboxane, primarily inhibiting platelet activation, thus, preventing the formation of a hemostatic plug. Nonselective NSAIDs inhibit both the COX-1 and COX-2 thus reducing the production of thromboxane and prostacyclin. The nucleated endothelial cells are able to regenerate prostacyclin, but the anucleated platelets are incapable of regenerating this enzyme. The imbalance of thromboxane

and prostacyclin may lead a thrombogenic situation. Low-dose aspirin (81 mg/day) has been advocated as a platelet aggregation inhibitor, thus reducing thrombotic events related to platelet aggregation. Aspirin at larger doses 1.5–2 g/day has been described to result in a paradoxical thrombogenic effect [2, 89]. The analgesic effects of aspirin are usually at higher doses, possibly negating the antithrombotic effects of aspirin. Celecoxib is an anti-inflammatory agent that primarily inhibits COX-2, an inducible enzyme not expressed in platelets and thus does not interfere with platelet aggregation. A systematic review and meta-analysis assessing the risks of serious cardiovascular events with selective COX-2 inhibitors and nonselective NSAIDs indicates that rofecoxib was associated with a significant dose-related risk (relative risk, 2.19 [>25 mg daily]) of serious cardiovascular events during the first month of treatment although celecoxib was not associated with an elevated risk. Among the nonselective NSAIDs, diclofenac had the highest risk (relative risk, 1.40), ibuprofen (relative risk, 1.07) and piroxicam (relative risk, 1.06), and naproxen (relative risk, 0.97) [90].

Summary

NSAIDs are useful analgesics for many pain states, especially those involving inflammation. Acetaminophen provides comparable analgesic effects but lacks clinically useful anti-inflammatory activity. The COX-2 selective inhibitors are continuing its development to attenuate the GI and hematological side effects of traditional NSAIDs. Overall, NSAIDs have similar pharmacokinetic characteristics: they are rapidly and extensively absorbed after oral administration, tissue distribution is very limited, they are metabolized extensively in the liver with little dependence on renal elimination, and therefore, the choice of NSAID may be determined by the efficacy and side-effect profile. This chapter has provided an overview of the NSAIDs and acetaminophen, but there remains research to be conducted in newer and more efficacious NSAIDs, adverse effect preventative strategies.

References

1. De Ledinghen V, Heresbach D, Fourdan O, et al. Anti-inflammatory drugs and variceal bleeding: a case-control study. Gut. 999; 44(2):270–3.
2. Godal HC, Eika C, Dybdahl JH, et al. Aspirin and bleeding-time. Lancet. 1979;1(8128):1236.
3. Laine L. Approaches to nonsteroidal anti-inflammatory drug use in the high-risk patient. Gastroenterology. 2001;120(3):594–606.
4. Vane JR, Botting RM. Mechanism of action of nonsteroidal anti-inflammatory drugs. Am J Med. 1998;104(3A):2S–8. discussion 21S–22S.

5. Singh G. Gastrointestinal complications of prescription and over-the-counter nonsteroidal anti-inflammatory drugs: a view from the ARAMIS database. Arthritis, rheumatism, and aging medical information system. Am J Ther. 2000;7(2):115–21.

6. Jouzeau JY, Terlain B, Abid A, et al. Cyclo-oxygenase isoenzymes. How recent findings affect thinking about nonsteroidal anti-inflammatory drugs. Drugs. 1997;53(4):563–82.

7. Talley NJ, Evans JM, Fleming KC, et al. Nonsteroidal antiinflammatory drugs and dyspepsia in the elderly. Dig Dis Sci. 1995;40(6):1345–50.

8. Tannenbaum H, Bombardier C, Davis P, et al. An evidence-based approach to prescribing nonsteroidal antiinflammatory drugs. Third Canadian Consensus Conference. J Rheumatol. 2006; 33(1):140–57.

9. Eisenberg E, Berkey CS, Carr DB, et al. Efficacy and safety of nonsteroidal antiinflammatory drugs for cancer pain: a meta-analysis. J Clin Oncol. 1994;12(12):2756–65.

10. Burke Anne SE, FitzGerald Garret A. Chapter 26: Analgesic-antipyretic and antiinflammatory agents; pharmacotherapy of gout. In: Goodman & Gilman's the pharmacological basis of therapeutics. 2011. [11th: http://www.accessmedicine.com/content. aspx?aID=942390]. Accessed 11 Feb 2010.

11. Graham GG, Scott KF. Mechanism of action of paracetamol. Am J Ther. 2005;12(1):46–55.

12. Munsterhjelm E, Munsterhjelm NM, Niemi TT, et al. Dose-dependent inhibition of platelet function by acetaminophen in healthy volunteers. Anesthesiology. 2005;103(4):712–17.

13. Lanza FL. A review of gastric ulcer and gastroduodenal injury in normal volunteers receiving aspirin and other non-steroidal anti-inflammatory drugs. Scand J Gastroenterol Suppl. 1989; 163:24–31.

14. Seibert K, Zhang Y, Leahy K, et al. Pharmacological and biochemical demonstration of the role of cyclooxygenase 2 in inflammation and pain. Proc Natl Acad Sci USA. 1994;91(25):12013–17.

15. Gordon SM, Brahim JS, Rowan J, et al. Peripheral prostanoid levels and nonsteroidal anti-inflammatory drug analgesia: replicate clinical trials in a tissue injury model. Clin Pharmacol Ther. 2002;72(2):175–83.

16. McCormack K. The spinal actions of nonsteroidal anti-inflammatory drugs and the dissociation between their anti-inflammatory and analgesic effects. Drugs. 1994;47 Suppl 5:28–45; discussion 46–47.

17. Cashman JN. The mechanisms of action of NSAIDs in analgesia. Drugs. 1996;52 Suppl 5:13–23.

18. Bjorkman R. Central antinociceptive effects of non-steroidal anti-inflammatory drugs and paracetamol. Experimental studies in the rat. Acta Anaesthesiol Scand Suppl. 1995;103:1–44.

19. Kroin JS, Buvanendran A, McCarthy RJ, et al. Cyclooxygenase-2 inhibition potentiates morphine antinociception at the spinal level in a postoperative pain model. Reg Anesth Pain Med. 2002;27(5): 451–5.

20. Vasko MR. Prostaglandin-induced neuropeptide release from spinal cord. Prog Brain Res. 1995;104:367–80.

21. Svensson CI, Yaksh TL. The spinal phospholipase-cyclooxygenase-prostanoid cascade in nociceptive processing. Annu Rev Pharmacol Toxicol. 2002;42:553–83.

22. Samad TA, Moore KA, Sapirstein A, et al. Interleukin-1beta-mediated induction of Cox-2 in the CNS contributes to inflammatory pain hypersensitivity. Nature. 2001;410(6827):471–5.

23. Samad TA, Sapirstein A, Woolf CJ. Prostanoids and pain: unraveling mechanisms and revealing therapeutic targets. Trends Mol Med. 2002;8(8):390–6.

24. Brune K, Glatt M, Graf P. Mechanisms of action of anti-inflammatory drugs. Gen Pharmacol. 1976;7(1):27–33.

25. Davies NM, Skjodt NM. Choosing the right nonsteroidal anti-inflammatory drug for the right patient: a pharmacokinetic approach. Clin Pharmacokinet. 2000;38(5):377–92.

26. Munir MA, Enany N, Zhang JM. Nonopioid analgesics. Med Clin North Am. 2007;91(1):97–111.

27. Larson AM, Polson J, Fontana RJ, et al. Acetaminophen-induced acute liver failure: results of a United States multicenter, prospective study. Hepatology. 2005;42(6):1364–72.

28. Mann JF, Goerig M, Brune K, et al. Ibuprofen as an over-the-counter drug: is there a risk for renal injury? Clin Nephrol. 1993;39(1): 1–6.

29. Silver S, Gano D, Gerretsen P. Acute treatment of paediatric migraine: a meta-analysis of efficacy. J Paediatr Child Health. 2008;44(1–2):3–9.

30. Derry C, Derry S, Moore RA, et al. Single dose oral ibuprofen for acute postoperative pain in adults. Cochrane Database Syst Rev. 2009;3:CD001548.

31. Grimes DA, Hubacher D, Lopez LM, et al. Non-steroidal anti-inflammatory drugs for heavy bleeding or pain associated with intrauterine-device use. Cochrane Database Syst Rev. 2006;4: CD006034.

32. Olson NZ, Otero AM, Marrero I, et al. Onset of analgesia for liqui-gel ibuprofen 400 mg, acetaminophen 1000 mg, ketoprofen 25 mg, and placebo in the treatment of postoperative dental pain. J Clin Pharmacol. 2001;41(11):1238–47.

33. Barden J, Derry S, McQuay HJ, et al. Single dose oral ketoprofen and dexketoprofen for acute postoperative pain in adults. Cochrane Database Syst Rev. 2009;4:CD007355.

34. Moore RA, Barden J. Systematic review of dexketoprofen in acute and chronic pain. BMC Clin Pharmacol. 2008;8:11.

35. Davies NM. Clinical pharmacokinetics of oxaprozin. Clin Pharmacokinet. 1998;35(6):425–36.

36. Kean WF. Oxaprozin: kinetic and dynamic profile in the treatment of pain. Curr Med Res Opin. 2004;20(8):1275–7.

37. Kurowski M, Thabe H. The transsynovial distribution of oxaprozin. Agents Actions. 1989;27(3–4):458–60.

38. Dallegri F, Bertolotto M, Ottonello L. A review of the emerging profile of the anti-inflammatory drug oxaprozin. Expert Opin Pharmacother. 2005;6(5):777–85.

39. Olson NZ, Sunshine A, Zighelboim I, et al. Onset and duration of analgesia of diclofenac potassium in the treatment of postepisiotomy pain. Am J Ther. 1997;4(7–8):239–46.

40. Davies NM, Anderson KE. Clinical pharmacokinetics of diclofenac. Therapeutic insights and pitfalls. Clin Pharmacokinet. 1997;33(3): 184–213.

41. Derry P, Derry S, Moore RA, et al. Single dose oral diclofenac for acute postoperative pain in adults. Cochrane Database Syst Rev. 2009;2:CD004768.

42. Bruhlmann P, de Vathaire F, Dreiser RL, et al. Short-term treatment with topical diclofenac epolamine plaster in patients with symptomatic knee osteoarthritis: pooled analysis of two randomised clinical studies. Curr Med Res Opin. 2006;22(12):2429–38.

43. Petersen B, Rovati S. Diclofenac epolamine (Flector) patch: evidence for topical activity. Clin Drug Investig. 2009;29(1):1–9.

44. Warner TD, Giuliano F, Vojnovic I, et al. Nonsteroid drug selectivities for cyclo-oxygenase-1 rather than cyclo-oxygenase-2 are associated with human gastrointestinal toxicity: a full in vitro analysis. Proc Natl Acad Sci USA. 1999;96(13):7563–8.

45. Pena M. Etodolac: analgesic effects in musculoskeletal and postoperative pain. Rheumatol Int. 1990;10(Suppl):9–16.

46. Lynch S, Brogden RN. Etodolac. A preliminary review of its pharmacodynamic activity and therapeutic use. Drugs. 1986;31(4): 288–300.

47. Gillis JC, Brogden RN. Ketorolac. A reappraisal of its pharmacodynamic and pharmacokinetic properties and therapeutic use in pain management. Drugs. 1997;53(1):139–88.

48. Buckley MM, Brogden RN. Ketorolac. A review of its pharmacodynamic and pharmacokinetic properties, and therapeutic potential. Drugs. 1990;39(1):86–109.

49. Morley-Forster P, Newton PT, Cook MJ. Ketorolac and indomethacin are equally efficacious for the relief of minor postoperative pain. Can J Anaesth. 1993;40(12):1126–30.

50. Resman-Targoff BH. Ketorolac: a parenteral nonsteroidal antiinflammatory drug. DICP. 1990;24(11):1098–104.

51. Laneuville O, Breuer DK, Dewitt DL, et al. Differential inhibition of human prostaglandin endoperoxide H synthases-1 and -2 by non-steroidal anti-inflammatory drugs. J Pharmacol Exp Ther. 1994;271(2):927–34.

52. Lanier BG, Turner Jr RA, Collins RL, et al. Evaluation of nabumetone in the treatment of active adult rheumatoid arthritis. Am J Med. 1987;83(4B):40–3.

53. Appelrouth DJ, Baim S, Chang RW, et al. Comparison of the safety and efficacy of nabumetone and aspirin in the treatment of osteoarthritis in adults. Am J Med. 1987;83(4B):78–81.

54. Krug H, Broadwell LK, Berry M, et al. Tolerability and efficacy of nabumetone and naproxen in the treatment of rheumatoid arthritis. Clin Ther. 2000;22(1):40–52.

55. Katz JA. NSAIDs and COX-2-selective inhibitors. In: Benzon HT, Raja SN, Molloy RE, Liu SS, Fishman SM, editors. Essentials of pain medicine and regional anesthesia. 2nd ed. Philadelphia: Elsevier Churchill Livingstone; 2005. p. 141–58.

56. Patoia L, Santucci L, Furno P, et al. A 4-week, double-blind, parallel-group study to compare the gastrointestinal effects of meloxicam 7.5 mg, meloxicam 15 mg, piroxicam 20 mg and placebo by means of faecal blood loss, endoscopy and symptom evaluation in healthy volunteers. Br J Rheumatol. 1996;35 Suppl 1:61–7.

57. Buvanendran A, Kroin JS, Tuman KJ, et al. Cerebrospinal fluid and plasma pharmacokinetics of the cyclooxygenase 2 inhibitor rofecoxib in humans: single and multiple oral drug administration. Anesth Analg. 2005;100(5):1320–4, table of contents.

58. Derry S, Barden J, McQuay HJ, et al. Single dose oral celecoxib for acute postoperative pain in adults. Cochrane Database Syst Rev. 2008;4:CD004233.

59. Singh G, Fort JG, Goldstein JL, et al. Celecoxib versus naproxen and diclofenac in osteoarthritis patients: SUCCESS-I study. Am J Med. 2006;119(3):255–66.

60. Towheed TE, Maxwell L, Judd MG, et al. Acetaminophen for osteoarthritis. Cochrane Database Syst Rev. 2006;1:CD004257.

61. Takemoto JK, Reynolds JK, Remsberg CM, et al. Clinical pharmacokinetic and pharmacodynamic profile of etoricoxib. Clin Pharmacokinet. 2008;47(11):703–20.

62. Croom KF, Siddiqui MA. Etoricoxib: a review of its use in the symptomatic treatment of osteoarthritis, rheumatoid arthritis, ankylosing spondylitis and acute gouty arthritis. Drugs. 2009;69(11):1513–32.

63. Riendeau D, Percival MD, Brideau C, et al. Etoricoxib (MK-0663): preclinical profile and comparison with other agents that selectively inhibit cyclooxygenase-2. J Pharmacol Exp Ther. 2001;296(2):558–66.

64. Strassels SA, McNicol E, Suleman R. Postoperative pain management: a practical review, part 1. Am J Health Syst Pharm. 2005;62(18):1904–16.

65. Burke Anne SE, FitzGerald Garret A. Analgesic-antipyretic and antiinflammatory agents; pharmacotherapy of gout. 11th ed. New York: The McGraw-Hill Companies, Inc.; 2006.

66. White PF. The changing role of non-opioid analgesic techniques in the management of postoperative pain. Anesth Analg. 2005;101(5 Suppl):S5–22.

67. Flouvat B, Leneveu A, Fitoussi S, et al. Bioequivalence study comparing a new paracetamol solution for injection and propacetamol after single intravenous infusion in healthy subjects. Int J Clin Pharmacol Ther. 2004;42(1):50–7.

68. Delbos A, Boccard E. The morphine-sparing effect of propacetamol in orthopedic postoperative pain. J Pain Symptom Manage. 1995;10(4):279–86.

69. Sinatra RS, Jahr JS, Reynolds LW, et al. Efficacy and safety of single and repeated administration of 1 gram intravenous acetaminophen injection (paracetamol) for pain management after major orthopedic surgery. Anesthesiology. 2005;102(4):822–31.

70. Cattabriga I, Pacini D, Lamazza G, et al. Intravenous paracetamol as adjunctive treatment for postoperative pain after cardiac surgery: a double blind randomized controlled trial. Eur J Cardiothorac Surg. 2007;32(3):527–31.

71. Laffi G, La Villa G, Pinzani M, et al. Arachidonic acid derivatives and renal function in liver cirrhosis. Semin Nephrol. 1997;17(6):530–48.

72. Clark DW, Ghose K. Neuropsychiatric reactions to nonsteroidal anti-inflammatory drugs (NSAIDs). The New Zealand experience. Drug Saf. 1992;7(6):460–5.

73. Garcia Rodriguez LA. Nonsteroidal antiinflammatory drugs, ulcers and risk: a collaborative meta-analysis. Semin Arthritis Rheum. 1997;26(6 Suppl 1):16–20.

74. Fries JF. NSAID gastropathy: the second most deadly rheumatic disease? Epidemiology and risk appraisal. J Rheumatol Suppl. 1991;28:6–10.

75. Wallace JL. Nonsteroidal anti-inflammatory drugs and gastroenteropathy: the second hundred years. Gastroenterology. 1997;112(3):1000–16.

76. Fries JF, Williams CA, Bloch DA, et al. Nonsteroidal anti-inflammatory drug-associated gastropathy: incidence and risk factor models. Am J Med. 1991;91(3):213–22.

77. Murray MD, Brater DC. Adverse effects of nonsteroidal anti-inflammatory drugs on renal function. Ann Intern Med. 1990;112(8):559–60.

78. Corwin HL, Bonventre JV. Renal insufficiency associated with nonsteroidal anti-inflammatory agents. Am J Kidney Dis. 1984;4(2):147–52.

79. Nies AS. Renal effects of nonsteroidal anti-inflammatory drugs. Agents Actions Suppl. 1988;24:95–106.

80. Vonkeman HE, van de Laar MA. Nonsteroidal anti-inflammatory drugs: adverse effects and their prevention. Semin Arthritis Rheum. 2010;39(4):294–312.

81. Taber SS, Mueller BA. Drug-associated renal dysfunction. Crit Care Clin. 2006;22(2):357–74, viii.

82. Garcia Rodriguez LA, Perez Gutthann S, Walker AM, et al. The role of non-steroidal anti-inflammatory drugs in acute liver injury. BMJ. 1992;305(6858):865–8.

83. Rabinovitz M, Van Thiel DH. Hepatotoxicity of nonsteroidal anti-inflammatory drugs. Am J Gastroenterol. 1992;87(12):1696–704.

84. Stewart DM, Dillman RO, Kim HS, et al. Acetaminophen overdose: a growing health care hazard. Clin Toxicol. 1979;14(5):507–13.

85. Chun LJ, Tong MJ, Busuttil RW, et al. Acetaminophen hepatotoxicity and acute liver failure. J Clin Gastroenterol. 2009;43(4):342–9.

86. Makin AJ, Williams R. Acetaminophen-induced hepatotoxicity: predisposing factors and treatments. Adv Intern Med. 1997;42:453–83.

87. Dargan PI, Jones AL. Acetaminophen poisoning: an update for the intensivist. Crit Care. 2002;6(2):108–10.

88. Larson AM. Acetaminophen hepatotoxicity. Clin Liver Dis. 2007;11(3):525–48, vi.

89. Amezcua JL, O'Grady J, Salmon JA, et al. Prolonged paradoxical effect of aspirin on platelet behaviour and bleeding time in man. Thromb Res. 1979;16(1–2):69–79.

90. McGettigan P, Henry D. Cardiovascular risk and inhibition of cyclooxygenase: a systematic review of the observational studies of selective and nonselective inhibitors of cyclooxygenase 2. JAMA. 2006;296(13):1633–44.

The Role of Antidepressants in the Treatment of Chronic Pain

4

Beth B. Murinson

Key Points

- Selected antidepressants are effective against pain, and these include the tricyclic antidepressants: amitriptyline, desipramine, and imipramine as well as specific selective serotonin and noradrenergic reuptake inhibitors: duloxetine, venlafaxine, and milnacipran.
- Most antidepressants carry a black box warning regarding increased risk of suicidality. This is generally more common in young people including teens and young adults. It is important to remain vigilant for symptoms of suicidal ideation and to provide appropriate guidance and warnings.
- Tricyclic antidepressants are contraindicated in the immediate period following a myocardial infarction and should be used with caution in patients with known heart disease; they are however generally safe and well tolerated over sustained periods of treatment.
- Newer pain-active antidepressants, e.g., duloxetine, have relatively mild side effects and can be quite effective, but clinical trials have indicated that these agents have a lower "number needed to treat" (NNT), meaning that for an individual patient, the chance of experiencing a therapeutic response may be one in four or lower.
- Pain-active antidepressants are an important component of treating chronic pain. They are not "habit forming" and should be used where appropriate in the treatment for persistent pain-producing conditions reducing the requirements for long-term opioids.

B.B. Murinson, M.S., M.D., Ph.D.
Department of Neurology,
Johns Hopkins University School of Medicine,
Baltimore, MD, USA

Depearment of Neurology, Clinical, Technion Faculty
of Medicine, Haifa, Israel
e-mail: bethmurinson@hotmail.com

Introduction

A number of antidepressants are essential for the treatment of chronic pain; these are referred to as the "pain-active" antidepressants. As a group, these agents manifest noradrenergic modulation. They have a number of advantages in this context: well-documented efficacy, mechanism or mechanisms of action that are complimentary to other agents used for persistent pain, distinctive and unique side effect profiles, excellent long-term tolerability, and a spectrum of cost-range options. Because the onset of action for the pain-active antidepressants can take days to weeks, these drugs are generally not appropriate for acute pain treatment with notable exceptions [1]. It is because of their numerous advantages including efficacy and tolerability for long-term usage that antidepressants have become a staple of medical management of chronic pain (Table 4.1).

Some antidepressants have not consistently demonstrated clinical efficacy against pain [2]. These include the most commonly prescribed antidepressants: fluoxetine (Prozac) and escitalopram (Lexapro) [3]. Paroxetine (Paxil) has been suggested as an agent that may modulate important pain-signaling events in the dorsal root ganglion; however, clinical trials have been inconsistent in demonstrating efficacy against pain.

As a group, pain-active antidepressants can serve as alternative single-agent therapy or complement the actions of agents in other classes. However, antidepressants used for the treatment of chronic pain have specific advantages. Giannopoulos et al. [4] reported that compliance and mood were higher in those chronic pain patients treated with antidepressants compared to those treated with GBP (gabapentin); however the effect size was small. Overall, both treatments demonstrated efficacy against neuropathic pain in about half of those treated as measured by patient satisfaction (Table 4.1).

In this chapter, seven "pain-active antidepressants" are discussed. The chapter begins with the most recent entry to the field and then takes a step back in time to examine aspects of selected tricyclic antidepressants and finishes with the two newer pain-active antidepressants.

T.R. Deer et al. (eds.), *Comprehensive Treatment of Chronic Pain by Medical, Interventional, and Integrative Approaches*,
DOI 10.1007/978-1-4614-1560-2_4, © American Academy of Pain Medicine 2013

Table 4.1 Pain-active antidepressants

Drug (trade name)	Class	Available dosages	FDA-approved indication	Side effects, warnings[a,b]	Notes
Imipramine	TCA	75, 100, 125, or 150 mg	Depression	Dry mouth, constipation, tremor black, box warning[a]	Potentially alerting
Desipramine	TCA	10, 25, 50, 75, 100, or 150 mg	Depression	Tachycardia, avoid in those with history of dysrhythmias, black box warning[a]	Metabolite of imipramine Nonsedating
Amitriptyline (Elatrol) (Elavil?)	TCA	10, 25, 50, 75, 100, or 150 mg	Depression	Dental caries with prolonged use, hypersomnia, black box warning[a]	Heavily sedating
Nortriptyline (Pamelor)	TCA	10, 25, 50, and 75 mg	Depression	Constipation, urinary retention, black box warning[a]	Mildly sedating
Venlafaxine (Effexor)	SNRI	25, 37.5, 50, 75, or 100 mg; 37.5, 75, or 150 mg XR	Depression	Nausea, elevated blood pressure, nervousness, insomnia, black box warning[a]	Primarily serotonergic at low-dose Half-life: 4 h short half-life means extended release dosing necessary
Duloxetine (Cymbalta)	SNRI	20, 30, or 60 mg	Depression, GAD[c], diabetic peripheral neuropathic pain, fibromyalgia, chronic musculoskeletal pain	Hepatotoxicity, black box warning[a]	Higher affinity for 5HT than for NE Half-life: 12 h
Milnacipran (Savella)	SNRI	12.5, 25, 50, or 100 mg	Fibromyalgia	Nausea (10 %), headache (<10 %), black box warning[a]	Balanced NE/5HT Half-life: 8 h

[a]Black box warning for suicidality applies to all agents discussed here
[b]MAO inhibitors should not be prescribed with any of these agents
[c]GAD generalized anxiety disorder

Imipramine

Imipramine is a tricyclic antidepressant, the first to be synthesized and to undergo clinical testing. It was widely marketed as "Tofranil." Imipramine is available in tablets of the following dosages: 75, 100, 125, or 150 mg.

Imipramine carries the same black box warning as amitriptyline and nortriptyline [Imipramine]. It requires special monitoring for clinical worsening, suicidality, and behavior changes that are unusual. The proposed mechanism of action against depression is through the blockage of norepinephrine reuptake. The FDA has approved imipramine for the treatment of the symptoms of depression. It is noted that treatment effects may not be apparent for 1–3 weeks.

The absolute contraindications, as for the other tricyclics, include acute myocardial ischemia and recovery from such, current or recent use of MAO inhibitors, and hypersensitivity to the medication.

The package insert for imipramine notes the necessity for EKG screening prior to administering *larger than usual* doses of the medication. Although it has been recommended that a screening EKG be obtained prior to TCA treatment for all patients over age 40 [5], a recent study suggests that patients without known cardiovascular history in fact have a lower risk for MI during treatment with tricyclic antidepressants [6]. Clinical judgment is clearly appropriate. Abrupt

cessation of the medication should be avoided as headache, nausea, and malaise may ensue.

Imipramine is less potent than the other tricyclic antidepressants, and the recommended starting dose is 75 mg daily, with lower starting doses recommended for older adults and those younger. The medication is not recommended for use in children [Imipramine].

Imipramine was among the earliest antidepressants to demonstrate efficacy against neuropathic pain [7]. It has been shown in repeated clinical studies to have good efficacy against the symptoms of diabetic neuropathy; however, side effects may interfere with successful management [8, 9]. A recent Cochrane Database Review indicates that imipramine is efficacious against neuropathic pain with a NNT of 2.2 [10]. Among the earliest references to imipramine in the treatment of pain is the efficacy of amitriptyline and imipramine in the treatment of tension headache [11]. Amitriptyline was superior to all other therapies attempted in this early study.

Desipramine

Desipramine is a tricyclic antidepressant and a metabolite of imipramine. It is available in tablets of 10, 25, 50, 75, 100, or 150 mg dosage. Widely marketed as "Norpramin," it should not be confused with nortriptyline.

Relative to amitriptyline, desipramine is a more potent as a relative inhibitor of norepinephrine reuptake, compared with inhibition of serotonin reuptake. Relative to imipramine, it is noted that the onset of treatment effects with desipramine is more rapid and benefits may be observed as soon as 2–5 days following the initiation of treatment [Desipramine]. An additional potential benefit of desipramine is that it is relatively nonsedating and is well tolerated when taken twice daily. Thus, in those patients for whom pain is a more constant feature of their daily routine, desipramine may be an excellent choice. There are those patients who are very busy with work demands and for whom the residual sedating effects of amitriptyline, which may persist even with nighttime administration, preclude successful dose titration for pain relief. In these patients also, desipramine may represent a useful alternative. It was shown in one high-quality study to have efficacy against PHN, and it is observed to work well with gabapentin in clinical practice.

Desipramine is metabolized in the liver but largely excreted in the urine. There is a wide range in serum levels among individuals receiving the same dose. Serum levels are generally higher with fixed doses in the elderly, consistent with decreased renal function. Cimetidine impedes metabolism and raises serum levels, whereas tobacco, barbiturates, and alcohol resulted in induced metabolic losses. It is recommended that caution be exercised in considering coadministration of SSRIs with desipramine as metabolic interactions will result in increased concentrations of desipramine.

TCAs have idiosyncratic metabolism, and serum levels can vary widely potentially accounting for variations in clinical responses. Metabolism is markedly decreased in a small but significant percentage of patients. Partially due to a polymorphism in CYP2D6 metabolizing protein transcripts, variants result in higher than anticipated serum drug levels [12].

The contraindications for desipramine are similar to those for other tricyclics that are discussed here and include MAO inhibitor administration, recent myocardial ischemia, and allergy to the medication.

The black box warning for the tricyclic antidepressants pertains also to desipramine. Patients should be monitored during therapy, and caregivers should receive appropriate instructions regarding behavioral changes and the need to contact health providers with concerns.

"Extreme caution" is urged in considering use of this medication in those with cardiovascular disease, a family history of sudden death, difficulty with urination, glaucoma, thyroid disease, or seizure disorder. It is established that desipramine can lower the seizure threshold.

The usual adult dosage is noted as 100–200 mg daily with recommendations not to exceed 300 mg daily. The starting dose should be lower than the usual dosage. Dosage adjustment for adolescents and geriatric patients includes recommendations for doses of 25–100 mg daily.

Although desipramine does not carry FDA approval for the treatment of any pain condition, it has been investigated for such in clinical trials and may be used at the discretion of the prescribing physician. In 1990, desipramine was described as effective against pain in patients with postherpetic neuralgia. In this randomized, double-blind crossover trial, the average desipramine dose was 167 mg daily. Compared with placebo, desipramine provided significant pain relief beginning at week 3 of the active treatment [13]. A study of desipramine for the treatment of painful diabetic neuropathy found that somewhat higher doses were prescribed following titration (201 mg daily) and that significant pain relief was demonstrable following week 5 of the treatment period [14]. Comparison with amitriptyline and fluoxetine demonstrated that amitriptyline and desipramine were both efficacious in relieving the pain of diabetic neuropathy while fluoxetine was not significantly different from placebo. The mean titrated dose of desipramine was 111 mg daily which compared to 105 for amitriptyline [15]. Recent Cochrane Database Review indicates that desipramine is efficacious against neuropathic pain with a NNT of 2.6 [10]. The use of TCAs for acute pain management is not common practice; however, in a trial of preemptive analgesia for pain following dental surgery, desipramine was effective in reducing opioid requirements [1]. Other applications for acute or subacute pain have not been extensively studied.

Amitriptyline

Amitriptyline was approved by the FDA for the relief of symptoms of depression in 1961 and widely prescribed as "Elavil." It is metabolized to nortriptyline, another "pain-active" antidepressant described below. Although amitriptyline is not FDA approved for indications other than depression, it is used for a variety of conditions including diabetic neuropathy, fibromyalgia, migraine prophylaxis, neuropathic pain, postherpetic neuralgia, and tension headache [11].

Amitriptyline has multiple mechanisms of action that may be important for notable activity against neuropathic pain. These include both central (noradrenergic) and peripheral (sodium channel blocking) mechanisms.

Nortriptyline

Nortriptyline is a tricyclic antidepressant, widely prescribed as "Pamelor." It is a metabolite of amitriptyline but is relatively less sedating. Nortriptyline is FDA approved for the relief of symptoms of depression [Nortriptyline]. It has multiple potential mechanisms of action but clearly "interferes with the transport, release, and storage of catecholamines"

[Nortriptyline]. According to the package insert, preclinical trials of nortriptyline indicated that it has both "stimulant and depressant properties."

Nortriptyline carries the same black box warning as amitriptyline and imipramine. It requires special monitoring for clinical worsening, suicidality, and behavior changes that are unusual. The absolute contraindications, as for the other tricyclics, include acute myocardial ischemia and recovery from such, current or recent use of MAO inhibitors, and hypersensitivity to the medication. It has been written that nortriptyline carries significant cardiovascular dangers [5], but the study that supports this compared nortriptyline to a SSRI that was not pain-active, in patients who were post-MI and who were depressed. Relative to the SSRI used for the treatment of depression, nortriptyline did produce an increase in average heart rate (eight beats per minute) and did result in more patients discontinuing therapy for cardiac-related side effects (sinus tachycardia and ventricular ectopy) [16]. In follow-up studies of this effect, it was shown that these effects of nortriptyline relate to the vagolytic activity of nortriptyline relative to paroxetine [17], an aspect of this medication that may have a significant relationship to its mechanism of action against pain. There is little evidence to support the notion that nortriptyline is more pronounced in this effect than other pain-active antidepressants. One point of interest is that in recent preclinical studies screening a large compound library for efficacy against hypoxic injury, nortriptyline has in fact shown a neuroprotective effect in models of *cerebral* ischemia [18].

Caveats aside, nortriptyline is an important medication option in the management of persistent pain. For many pain specialists, it is the tricyclic of choice. In a clinical trial of postherpetic neuralgia, nortriptyline and desipramine showed similar efficacy to morphine [19]. In diabetic and postherpetic neuralgia, nortriptyline has been shown to be at least as effective as gabapentin in the treatment of these disorders [20]. It is accompanied by dry mouth in the majority of patients, but nortriptyline in combination with gabapentin provided additional incremental pain relief [20].

Contraindications for Imipramine, Desipramine, Amitriptyline, and Nortriptyline

Amitriptyline and other tricyclic antidepressants (nortriptyline, desipramine) are contraindicated for concomitant prescription with MAO inhibitors. MAO inhibitors block the metabolism of catecholamines, and in concert with agents which block the reuptake of amines from the synaptic cleft can produce a life-threatening syndrome of elevated temperature and seizures. It is recommended that tricyclics should not be started sooner than 14 days after discontinuation of

MAO inhibitors [Amitriptyline]. Amitriptyline and the tricyclic antidepressants are also contraindicated during the acute recovery phase following myocardial ischemia. One of the important side effects of tricyclic antidepressants and a serious problem in the setting of medication overdose is the prolongation of the Q-T interval. TCAs should be avoided in patients with conduction defects such as AV block [5]. Patients with hypersensitivity to amitriptyline or other tricyclic antidepressants should not receive this drug [Amitriptyline].

Although there is a strong contraindication for using tricyclic antidepressants in the acute period following MI, an important recent study indicates no hazard in using antidepressants for those who do not have an established history of cardiovascular disease [6]. The findings of this study suggest that those patients who complete at least 12 weeks of treatment with antidepressant medications have a reduced risk for MI and lower all causes of mortality.

Black Box Warnings for Imipramine, Desipramine, Amitriptyline, and Nortriptyline

Amitriptyline and all tricyclic antidepressants carry a black box warning indicating that patients receiving these medications may be at increased risk for suicide. The warning indicates that providers prescribing these medications should monitor patients for clinical worsening and suicidality. They are further instructed to advise caregivers and family members about the need for close observation and specifically to watch for signs of irritability, agitation, and worsening of depression.

Coadministration of tricyclic antidepressants with SSRIs may produce a metabolic interaction such that the resulting plasma levels are markedly and variably elevated. Caution, clinical experience, and clear-cut therapeutic rationale should dictate the use of these agents in combination.

Amitriptyline was noted from the earliest studies of pharmacological treatment of chronic pain to be highly effective against persistent pain and provide the added benefit of improved sleep [11]. Although early dosing regimens involved three-times daily dosing, daytime sedation is a frequent concomitant of this approach. Switching patients to single-dose administration at bedtime resolves many of the concerns with hypersomnia and has the added benefit of mitigating the effects of amitriptyline in producing orthostatic hypotension. The sedation of amitriptyline may ameliorate with time; however, the sedation when present can be profound so that patients should be instructed not to drive following the evening medication dose. Dry mouth is a prominent side effect of amitriptyline. This phenomenon goes beyond being a minor annoyance and can have a devastating effect by accelerating dental caries.

Diligent attention to professional dental care and enhanced attention to daily dental hygiene should be urged for patients receiving amitriptyline long-term.

The sedating effects of amitriptyline can be used to great advantage in patients with increased pain severity at night or in the evening. It is typical that patients with painful small fiber neuropathy will describe pain that is markedly worse once they get into bed for the evening or even once they put their feet up to rest. Patients with neuropathy will also describe difficulty tolerating sheets on the feet at night, a phenomenon that may represent mechanical allodynia, or may represent aberrant sensory processing that occurs with mild warming of the feet. In either case, a burning, occasionally searing pain is provoked by resting the feet under covers. The ordinary comfort that comes from climbing under warm blankets is completely replaced by spontaneous dysesthesias for these patients with early neuropathy. The elicitation of a night pain history is quickly accomplished with the question "At what time of day is your pain the worst?" The patient with night pain or with sleep disruption due to neuropathic pain may find that amitriptyline provides excellent therapeutic relief.

Amitriptyline is available in a wide range of doses including 10, 25, 50, 75, 100, or 150 mg tablets. The half-life is relatively short, but the therapeutic benefit can be obtained with once daily dosing over the longer treatment intervals. Amitriptyline is not appropriate for the treatment of acute pain.

Amitriptyline has not been shown to provide significant pain relief in the treatment of HIV-associated sensory neuropathy [21].

Amitriptyline at low dose (25 mg daily) has been found in meta-analysis to provide relief from symptoms of fibromyalgia including pain relief, sleep, and fatigue at the 6-week time point [22].

Amitriptyline has shown consistent efficacy against neuropathic pain as assessed by recent meta-analysis; the number needed to treat (NNT) is in the range of 3.1 [10].

Venlafaxine

Venlafaxine (marketed as Effexor) is an SNRI that has FDA approval for the treatment of depression [Venlafaxine]. It is available in tablets of 2, 37.5, 50, 75, or 100 mg and extended release capsules of 37.5, 75, or 150 mg XR. Among the major potential side effects are nausea, persistently elevated blood pressure, nervousness, and insomnia. Like all of the antidepressants, it carries a black box warning indicating that patients should be monitored for increased suicidality and unusual behavior changes that might herald suicide attempts or worsening depression. The drug has activity against serotonin and norepinephrine reuptake pumps but is primarily serotonergic at low dose. Venlafaxine has a short half-life of about 4 h. The short half-life means extended release dosing is generally necessary for efficacy.

Venlafaxine has been demonstrated in randomized controlled trials to be efficacious in the treatment of painful neuropathy [23]. In comparison to imipramine, it is indistinguishably effective; however, the NNT for venlafaxine, around 4.5, is higher than that of the TCAs [8, 9]. Although generally used in the context of treating established chronic pain, a recent randomized study has shown that venlafaxine provides pain relief in the first 10 days after mastectomy, superior even to gabapentin [24]. Venlafaxine, although having an NNT higher than the TCAs, is valuable medication in the armamentarium against neuropathic pain as it has a more targeted mechanism of action, and for many patients, the side effects are more tolerable.

Duloxetine

Duloxetine, trade name Cymbalta, is an SNRI that is FDA approved for the treatment of depression as well as diabetic peripheral neuropathic pain, fibromyalgia, and chronic musculoskeletal pain [Duloxetine]. In this respect, the medication has a significant advantage over the other pain-active antidepressants as it clearly has a stamp of approval from the FDA for a wide range of pain-associated conditions. One limitation of duloxetine that may frustrate its use in clinical practice is the observation that the NNT is estimated at 5.7. This could be expected to mean that a number of patients will try the treatment and not obtain clinically significant relief. The NNT for duloxetine compares with more favorable NNTs, less than 3, for the tricyclic antidepressants. Duloxetine is available in delayed release capsules of the following dosages: 20, 30, or 60 mg.

Like the other pain-active antidepressants, duloxetine carries a black box warning for the worsening of depression and the risk for increased suicidality. Patients should be monitored for suicidality. In some cases, patients with no prior experience of suicidal ideation will find the emergence of suicidal ideation to be deeply troubling. Immediate discontinuation is appropriate for patients who develop these intrusive and emotionally disturbing thoughts. Caregivers should also receive appropriate guidance to observe patients for irritability, aggression, and unusual behavior changes.

Contraindications for duloxetine include the prohibition against co-prescribing with MAO inhibitors due to the severe serotonin syndrome effects that result. There is also a contraindication for prescribing this medication to patients with untreated narrow-angle glaucoma.

Elevation of liver transaminases and fatal liver failure has been observed in patients taking duloxetine. These patients present with jaundice, abdominal pain, or elevated transaminases. Elevated transaminases resulted in the discontinuation of duloxetine in 0.3 % of patients in clinical trials, and in placebo-controlled trials, significant elevations of ALT occurred in an excess of 0.8 % of treated patients relative to placebo. For these reasons, duloxetine should not be prescribed to patients with "substantial alcohol use or evidence of chronic liver disease." Other potential side effects include nausea, somnolence, orthostatic hypotension, hyponatremia, and worsening of glycemic control in diabetes.

Duloxetine is metabolized by both CYP1A2 and CYP2D6, and drug interactions reflect this. Concomitant administration with desipramine resulted in increased desipramine concentrations. Drug interactions should be reviewed as appropriate for this medication.

Duloxetine is significantly more potent in blocking serotonin reuptake than norepinephrine. For this reason, at lower doses, serotonergic effects may dominate.

Duloxetine has been found to provide pain relief comparable to gabapentin and pregabalin in patients with diabetic peripheral neuropathy (meta-analysis) [25].

A recent Cochrane Database Review of duloxetine indicated efficacy for the treatment of both diabetic peripheral neuropathy and fibromyalgia at doses of 60 and 120 mg daily. The NNT to treat for these conditions was quite high however at 6 and 8, respectively. Despite the potential for side effects and adverse events, these events are relatively uncommon compared with side effect profiles of other pain-active antidepressants. In those patients who do respond to the pain-relieving effects, duloxetine is usually a well-tolerated medication that dramatically improves quality of life. For these reasons, duloxetine has become a valued treatment option for patients with neuropathic pain [26].

Milnacipran

Milnacipran is one of the newer SNRIs approved for the treatment of chronic pain conditions, specifically fibromyalgia. Distinctive from the other two SNRIs discussed here, it has nearly balanced efficacy against serotonin and norepinephrine reuptake [27]. Although milnacipran is Food and Drug Administration (FDA) approved for fibromyalgia and not for depression, it is used internationally for depression and there is literature to suggest that milnacipran has efficacy against depression that is comparable to imipramine [28]. It is generally well tolerated with most side effects being comparable to placebo. Exceptions to this are infrequent, occurring in fewer than 5 % of the patients studied in meta-analysis, but include dysuria, palpitations, hot flushes, anxiety, sweating, and vertigo.

Milnacipran is available as tablets of 12.5, 25, 50, or 100 mg. Rapidly absorbed, milnacipran has high bioavailability (85 %). The half-life of milnacipran is around 8 h which suggests that twice daily dosing may provide better efficacy. The prescribing information for milnacipran indicates that titration is recommended when starting this medication with an initial dose of 12.5 mg tapered upward over the course of a week to 50 mg twice daily. There is no significant inhibition or induction of metabolic enzymes, and for this reason, milnacipran has relatively few drug-drug interactions. It is excreted largely unmetabolized.

There are important absolute contraindications to prescribing this medication: concurrent irreversible MAO inhibitors such as selegiline may result in serotonergic crisis. Recent (within 14 days) use of MAO inhibitors is also contraindicated. Milnacipran is contraindicated in patients with untreated narrow-angle glaucoma. The medication is also not to be used concurrently with digitalis glycosides or with 5HT-1D agonists (triptans) as myocardial ischemia may result. Hepatotoxicity has been observed, and mild elevations in blood pressure and heart rate have been reported.

As with all of the antidepressants discussed in this chapter, Milnacipran carries a black box warning for increased risk of suicidality especially in children, adolescents, and young adults. Patients of all ages who are starting this medication are required to have appropriate monitoring and should be "observed closely for clinical worsening, suicidality or unusual changes in behavior."

Summary

Antidepressants are widely used in the treatment of neuropathic pain. Though the number of agents that are FDA approved for use in chronic pain states are very limited at this time, there is now good evidence from a wide range of clinical trials and meta-analysis studies that specific antidepressants are very effective in particular circumstances. Pain-associated conditions that may respond well to treatment with antidepressants include diabetic peripheral neuropathy, postherpetic neuralgia, fibromyalgia, tension headache, migraine prophylaxis, chronic musculoskeletal pain, and fibromyalgia. It is important to understand the particulars of each agent and its demonstrated efficacy from clinical trials to appropriately select therapies. Although the pain-active antidepressants offer significant advantages in terms of complementary mechanisms of action and long-term tolerability, it is important to prescribe these agents only when appropriate and with the recognition that increased suicidality, concomitant use of MAO inhibitors, cardiac disease, and allergies remain important impediments to broader, freer use of these agents. On a positive note, it is a monumental advance in the treatment of pain that so many diverse and generally effective agents are available today [29].

Electronic Sources for Prescribing Information

Duloxetine. Eli Lilly and Company. http://dailymed.nlm.nih.gov/dailymed/lookup.cfm?setid=2f7d4d67-10c1-4bf4-a7f2-c185fbad64ba. Accessed October 2, 2011.

Venlafaxine. Wyeth Pharmaceuticals Company. http://dailymed.nlm.nih.gov/dailymed/lookup.cfm?setid=53c3e7ac-1852-4d70-d2b6-4fca819acf26. Accessed September 28, 2011.

Milnacipran. Forrest Laboratories. http://dailymed.nlm.nih.gov/dailymed/lookup.cfm?setid=16a4a314-f97e-4e91-95e9-576a3773d284. Accessed October 2, 2011.

Amitriptyline. Sandoz Inc. http://dailymed.nlm.nih.gov/dailymed/lookup.cfm?setid=705a2bae-031d-4218-82fe-4346542c0baa. Accessed September 27, 2011.

Nortriptyline. Mallinckrodt Inc. http://dailymed.nlm.nih.gov/dailymed/lookup.cfm?setid=e17dc299-f52d-414d-ab6e-e809bd6f8acb. Accessed September 27, 2011.

Desipramine. Sanofi-Aventis Inc. http://dailymed.nlm.nih.gov/dailymed/lookup.cfm?setid=3e593725-3fc9-458e-907d-19d51d5a7f9c. Accessed October 2, 2011.

Imipramine. Sandoz Inc. http://dailymed.nlm.nih.gov/dailymed/lookup.cfm?setid=7d52c40c-bbcb-4698-9879-d40136301d31. Accessed October 2, 2011.

References

1. Levine JD, Gordon NC, Smith R, McBryde R. Desipramine enhances opiate postoperative analgesia. Pain. 1986;27(1):45–9.
2. Watson CP, Gilron I, Sawynok J, Lynch ME. Nontricyclic antidepressant analgesics and pain: are serotonin norepinephrine reuptake inhibitors (SNRIs) any better? Pain. 2011;152(10):2206–10.
3. Dharmshaktu P, Tayal V, Kalra BS. Efficacy of antidepressants as analgesics: a review. J Clin Pharmacol. 2011. doi:10.1177/0091270010394852.
4. Giannopoulos S, Kosmidou M, Sarmas I, Markoula S, Pelidou SH, Lagos G, Kyritsis AP. Patient compliance with SSRIs and gabapentin in painful diabetic neuropathy. Clin J Pain. 2007;23(3):267–9.
5. Dworkin RH, O'Connor AB, Backonja M, Farrar JT, Finnerup NB, Jensen TS, Kalso EA, Loeser JD, Miaskowski C, Nurmikko TJ, Portenoy RK, Rice AS, Stacey BR, Treede RD, Turk DC, Wallace MS. Pharmacologic management of neuropathic pain: evidence-based recommendations. Pain. 2007;132(3):237–51.
6. Scherrer JF, Garfield LD, Lustman PJ, Hauptman PJ, Chrusciel T, Zeringue A, Carney RM, Freedland KE, Bucholz KK, Owen R, Newcomer JW, True WR. Antidepressant drug compliance: reduced risk of MI and mortality in depressed patients. Am J Med. 2011;124(4):318–24.
7. Kvinesdale B, Molin J, Frøland A, Gram LF. Imipramine treatment of painful diabetic neuropathy. JAMA. 1984;251(13):1727–30.
8. Sindrup SH, Gram LF, Brøsen K, Eshøj O, Mogensen EF. The selective serotonin reuptake inhibitor paroxetine is effective in the treatment of diabetic neuropathy symptoms. Pain. 1990;42(2):135–44.
9. Sindrup SH, Ejlertsen B, Frøland A, Sindrup EH, Brøsen K, Gram LF. Imipramine treatment in diabetic neuropathy: relief of subjective symptoms without changes in peripheral and autonomic nerve function. Eur J Clin Pharmacol. 1989;37(2):151–3.
10. Saarto T, Wiffen PJ. Antidepressants for neuropathic pain. Cochrane Database Syst Rev. 2007;17(4):005454.
11. Lance JW, Curran DA. Treatment of chronic tension headache. Lancet. 1964;1(7345):1236–9.
12. Oscarson M. Pharmacogenetics of drug metabolising enzymes: importance for personalised medicine. Clin Chem Lab Med. 2003;41(4):573–80.
13. Kishore-Kumar R, Max MB, Schafer SC, Gaughan AM, Smoller B, Gracely RH, Dubner R. Desipramine relieves postherpetic neuralgia. Clin Pharmacol Ther. 1990;47(3):305–12.
14. Max MB, Kishore-Kumar R, Schafer SC, Meister B, Gracely RH, Smoller B, Dubner R. Efficacy of desipramine in painful diabetic neuropathy: a placebo-controlled trial. Pain. 1991;45(1):3–9; discussion 1–2.
15. Max MB, Lynch SA, Muir J, Shoaf SE, Smoller B, Dubner R. Effects of desipramine, amitriptyline, and fluoxetine on pain in diabetic neuropathy. N Engl J Med. 1992;326(19):1250–6.
16. Roose SP, Laghrissi-Thode F, Kennedy JS, Nelson JC, Bigger Jr JT, Pollock BG, Gaffney A, Narayan M, Finkel MS, McCafferty J, Gergel I. Comparison of paroxetine and nortriptyline in depressed patients with ischemic heart disease. JAMA. 1998;279(4):287–91.
17. Yeragani VK, Pesce V, Jayaraman A, Roose S. Major depression with ischemic heart disease: effects of paroxetine and nortriptyline on long-term heart rate variability measures. Biol Psychiatry. 2002;52(5):418–29.
18. Zhang WH, Wang H, Wang X, Narayanan MV, Stavrovskaya IG, Kristal BS, Friedlander RM. Nortriptyline protects mitochondria and reduces cerebral ischemia/hypoxia injury. Stroke. 2008;39(2):455–62.
19. Raja SN, Haythornthwaite JA, Pappagallo M, Clark MR, Travison TG, Sabeen S, Royall RM, Max MB. Opioids versus antidepressants in postherpetic neuralgia: a randomized, placebo-controlled trial. Neurology. 2002;59(7):1015–21.
20. Gilron I, Bailey JM, Tu D, Holden RR, Jackson AC, Houlden RL. Nortriptyline and gabapentin, alone and in combination for neuropathic pain: a double-blind, randomised controlled crossover trial. Lancet. 2009;374(9697):1252–61.
21. Phillips TJ, Cherry CL, Cox S, Marshall SJ, Rice AS. Pharmacological treatment of painful HIV-associated sensory neuropathy: a systematic review and meta-analysis of randomised controlled trials. PLoS One. 2010;5(12):e14433.
22. Nishishinya B, Urrútia G, Walitt B, Rodriguez A, Bonfill X, Alegre C, Darko G. Amitriptyline in the treatment of fibromyalgia: a systematic review of its efficacy. Rheumatology (Oxford). 2008;47(12):1741–6.
23. Rowbotham MC, Goli V, Kunz NR, Lei D. Venlafaxine extended release in the treatment of painful diabetic neuropathy: a double blind, placebo-controlled study. Pain. 2004;110:697–706.
24. Amr YM, Yousef AA. Evaluation of efficacy of the perioperative administration of venlafaxine or gabapentin on acute and chronic post-mastectomy pain. Clin J Pain. 2010;26:381–5.
25. Quilici S, Chancellor J, Löthgren M, Simon D, Said G, Le TK, Garcia-Cebrian A, Monz B. Meta-analysis of duloxetine vs. pregabalin and gabapentin in the treatment of diabetic peripheral neuropathic pain. BMC Neurol. 2009;9:6.
26. Lunn MP, Hughes RA, Wiffen PJ. Duloxetine for treating painful neuropathy or chronic pain. Cochrane Database Syst Rev. 2009;7(4):CD007115.
27. Stahl SM, Grady MM, Moret C, Briley M. SNRIs: their pharmacology, clinical efficacy, and tolerability in comparison with other classes of antidepressants. CNS Spectr. 2005;10(9):732–47.
28. Kasper S, Pletan Y, Solles A, Tournoux A. Comparative studies with milnacipran and tricyclic antidepressants in the treatment of patients with major depression: a summary of clinical trial results. Int Clin Psychopharmacol. 1996;11 Suppl 4:35–9.
29. Attal N, Cruccu G, Baron R, Haanpää M, Hansson P, Jensen TS, Nurmikko T, European Federation of Neurological Societies. EFNS guidelines on the pharmacological treatment of neuropathic pain: 2010 revision. Eur J Neurol. 2010;17(9):1113-e88. Epub 2010 Apr 9. Review.

Anticonvulsant Medications for Treatment of Neuropathic and "Functional" Pain

5

Bruce D. Nicholson

Key Points
- Anticonvulsant therapy is effective for the treatment of neuropathic pain.
- Efficacy is well demonstrated in selected neuropathic pain syndromes.
- Little evidence is available to support generalized use in treatment of neuropathic pain.
- Further research is required to evaluate the utility of anticonvulsant therapy in combination with other drugs.

Introduction

The broad definition of neuropathic pain as articulated by the International Association of Pain, "pain initiated or caused by a primary lesion or dysfunction of the nervous system," unfortunately has done little to guide the clinician when attempting to develop an effective treatment plan that may include an anticonvulsant medication. Current guidelines and indications for use of anticonvulsant therapy primarily utilize a lesion-based approach when recommending treatment for patients suffering from neuropathic pain. However, recent work by Baron and colleagues would suggest that selection of patients based on sensory symptoms and signs rather than strictly by disease etiology has potential benefits in identifying successful therapeutic outcomes [1].

Initial use of anticonvulsant drugs for the etiologic-based treatment of neuropathic pain dates back almost 50 years, with the sequential trials of carbamazepine for the treatment of trigeminal neuralgia [2–4]. From the mid-1960s until the mid-1990s, only a limited number of clinical trials utilizing anticonvulsants had been completed for the treatment of neuropathic pain. Subsequent to the introduction of gabapentin for the treatment of epilepsy in the mid-1990s, case reports of successful treatment of neuropathic pain began to appear in the medical literature [5, 6]. Several recent reviews of the literature along with meta-analysis of randomized controlled trials (RCT) now support the use of anticonvulsant therapy for first-line treatment of selected neuropathic pain syndromes [7–9]. More recently, fibromyalgia (functional pain) now widely considered to be a neuropathic pain syndrome manifested by widespread pain due to underlying changes in sensory processing has been effectively treated with anticonvulsant therapy [3].

The body of evidence supporting the use of anticonvulsant therapy for the treatment of neuropathic pain as a generalized category is rather limited. The vast majority of clinical trials involving anticonvulsant drugs have been narrowly focused on treatment of specific conditions such as painful peripheral diabetic neuropathy and postherpetic neuralgia [8, 10, 11]. To date, only one trial has been published supporting the use of anticonvulsant therapy for the treatment of neuropathic cancer pain [12]. Of considerable interest is that the literature is devoid of a single trial demonstrating efficacy of anticonvulsant therapy in one of the most common forms of neuropathic pain that being neuropathic low back pain. The following review of anticonvulsant drugs will focus on clinically relevant aspects for the practicing clinician.

Carbamazepine and Oxcarbazepine

Few neuropathic pain conditions are more effectively managed with anticonvulsant therapy than classic trigeminal neuralgia [13, 14]. Consensus guidelines remain clear that carbamazepine is the drug of first choice with initial efficacy of upwards to 80 % and long-term efficacy of 50 % at doses between 200 and 400 mg administered three times a day [14]. Carbamazepine exerts a use-dependent inhibition of sodium

B.D. Nicholson, M.D.
Division of Pain Medicine, Department of Anesthesiology,
Lehigh Valley Health Network,
1240 South Cedar Crest BLVD, Suite 307,
Allentown PA 18103, USA
e-mail: bruce.nicholson@lvhn.org

T.R. Deer et al. (eds.), *Comprehensive Treatment of Chronic Pain by Medical, Interventional, and Integrative Approaches*,
DOI 10.1007/978-1-4614-1560-2_5, © American Academy of Pain Medicine 2013

channels that leads to a reduction in the frequency of sustained repetitive firing of action potentials in neurons. The effect on pain suppression is hypothesized to occur through both central and peripheral mechanisms. Carbamazepine use in three placebo-controlled studies for treatment trigeminal neuralgia demonstrated a combined numbers needed to treat (NNT) for effectiveness of 1.7 [15].

In a single 2-week placebo-controlled trial involving only 30 participants, carbamazepine demonstrated an NNT of 2.3 for treatment of painful diabetic neuropathy (PDN) [16]. However, several other clinical trials involving various neuropathic pain conditions that include PDN and postherpetic neuralgia (PHN) have failed to demonstrate clinical benefit measured by improvement in pain scores [10].

Unfortunately, problematic issues that may significantly limit the use as well as long-term efficacy include hepatic enzyme induction effects of carbamazepine. This particularly vexing side effect frequently requires close monitoring of other drug activity such as warfarin. Ongoing monitoring of liver function and blood count is recommended as well. The second-generation anticonvulsant oxcarbazepine has a structurally similar sodium channel inhibitor effect as carbamazepine but with significantly fewer complicating side effects. In two relatively small randomized controlled trials, oxcarbazepine was found to be similar to carbamazepine in reduction of number of attacks in patients suffering with trigeminal neuralgia [14]. Titration dosing from 300 mg QD to maximum of 900 mg BID over 5 days is recommended in order to minimize side effects such as dizziness and sedation. One concerning serious side effect is hyponatremia, which may occur in approximately 3 % of individuals taking oxcarbazepine; therefore, monitoring of sodium levels is recommended [10, 15].

Gabapentin and Pregabalin

Gabapentin original synthesized in 1977 as a drug for the treatment of spasticity and subsequently introduced in the mid-1990s for the treatment of epilepsy has garnered over 3,200 citations in the medical literature, with over 1,200 citations in the area of pain [17]. Since 1995, gabapentin has gained approval for the treatment of postherpetic neuralgia in the USA and for the broader indication of peripheral neuropathic pain in many countries outside of the United States [18]. In 2003, a second-generation alpha-2-delta-binding drug pregabalin was introduced in the United States, and FDA approved it for the treatment of epilepsy, postherpetic neuralgia, and painful diabetic peripheral neuropathy and more recently for the treatment of fibromyalgia [19, 20].

Whereas gabapentin and pregabalin both bind to the presynaptic neuronal alpha-2-delta subunit of voltage-gated calcium channels, pregabalin's unique chemical structure confers several clinically important features that distinguish it from gabapentin. Both drugs share the similar characteristics when binding to the alpha-2-delta subunit of voltage-gated calcium channels which results in decreased expression and release of certain neurotransmitters that include substance P, glutamate, and calcitonin-related gene peptide all of which are considered important for induction and maintenance of neuropathic pain states. The suppression of the above-mentioned neuronal peptide activity occurs primarily after tissue or nerve injury has occurred. This unique upregulation of the alpha-2-delta subunit on voltage-gated calcium channels is thought to be required for drug activity, as there is minimal drug effect on activity of normal nerve transmission [21, 22].

Pharmacokinetic characteristic particular to pregabalin that may have clinical benefit over gabapentin includes the linear absorption of pregabalin, which increases proportionally with each dose, resulting in a uniformly linear dose-exposure response across patient populations. On the other hand, the pharmacokinetic profile of gabapentin is considered nonlinear, and bioavailability (approximately 60 % at a dose of 900 mg) is significantly lower and less predictable across patient populations. The amount of gabapentin absorbed is dose dependent, with the proportion of drug absorbed decreasing with increasing dose to the point where only a fraction of the dose is absorbed at relatively higher doses. In single-dose absorption studies, the amount of gabapentin absorbed decreases from 80 % at 100 mg to 27 % at 1,600 mg [18]. On the contrary, pregabalin absorption is independent of dose administered; it is constant and averages >90 % over the dose range of 10–300 mg in single-dose trials [19]. Consequently, this particular pharmacokinetic difference translates into minimal variations between patients in plasma concentrations for pregabalin with dose titration. Whether this has any clinically important, significance remains to be determined, as this has not been measured in any head-to-head trials between gabapentin and pregabalin.

Clinically important characteristics of both gabapentin and pregabalin that simplify the use of these drugs include minimal protein binding and minimal or little drug-drug interaction which importantly includes warfarin. As well, favorable elimination characteristics include minimal metabolism and no CYP 450 interaction for both gabapentin and pregabalin, allowing the clinician to prescribe either drug in a patient who may be taking multiple other medications that may be affected by hepatic enzyme induction. It is particularly important to note clinically that gabapentin and pregabalin do not have any effect on renal function, as quite often this is a misunderstood concept that results in the withdrawal of therapy in patients with renal impairment. However, it is important to take into consideration when dosing both drugs that approximately 95 % of ingested gabapentin and pregabalin is eliminated, unchanged through renal excretion. Therefore, with decreasing creatinine clearance (CC), the dose of drug administered may be decreased proportionally from full-recommended dosing levels when CC is above 60–30 % or less of the normal dose when CC is below 30 [18, 19].

Gabapentin Therapy

Fourteen studies detailing use of gabapentin included the following conditions: two studies in postherpetic neuralgia (PHN), seven studies in painful diabetic neuropathy (PDN), and one each in cancer related neuropathic pain, phantom limb pain, Guillain-Barré syndrome, spinal cord injury pain, and mixed neuropathic pain states [12, 17, 23, 24]. In 2002, gabapentin was the first medication to be granted FDA approval for the treatment of postherpetic neuralgia. RCT results demonstrated in 336 PHN patients that dosing between 1,800 and 3,600 mg/day resulted in a 33–35 % reduction in pain compared to a 7.7 % pain score reduction in the placebo group. Overall, 43.2 % of subjects treated with gabapentin categorized their pain as "much" or "moderately" improved at the end of the study, whereas only 12.1 % in the placebo group experienced any significant improvement [25]. Three trials considered of fair quality conducted over 6–8-week duration at dosing levels varying between 900 and 3,600 mg/day demonstrated mixed results in the same condition [9, 17]. The Cochrane database analysis supports the use of gabapentin for treatment of chronic neuropathic pain and suggests that the numbers needed to treat (NNT) for improvement in all trials with evaluable data is around 5.1. Clinically, it is important to understand that on average, only one in approximately every five patients who receive gabapentin for the treatment of neuropathic pain will report significant improvement [11].

Of clinical importance are the adverse events that occurred more frequently in the gabapentin group compared to those in receiving placebo in decreasing order included somnolence, dizziness, and peripheral edema. The former-mentioned side effect of somnolence may be clinically beneficial in patients suffering from sleep deprivation due to neuropathic pain. The usual starting dose of gabapentin may vary depending on patient tolerance to pharmacotherapy. Therefore, one may start at a very low dose of 100 mg TID of QID titrating to efficacy that is usually seen at an average total daily dose between 900 and 1,800 mg, with occasional dosing to 2,400 mg/day. As mentioned above, asymmetric dosing of gabapentin giving a larger dose of drug at bedtime (600–1,200 mg) to induce somnolence and a lower dose in the morning (300–600 mg) and afternoon (300–600 mg) may help mitigate the somnolence and dizziness side effect profile during the waking hours while improving the sleep-related comorbidity found in up to 80 % of patients suffering with chronic neuropathic pain [9, 26, 27].

Pregabalin Therapy

Pregabalin, a second-generation alpha-2-delta analogue, has demonstrated efficacy in the treatment of postherpetic neuralgia, painful diabetic neuropathy, and central neuropathic pain. In general, the 19 published clinical trials have demonstrated that total daily doses of 150, 300, 450, and 600 mg daily were effective in patients suffering with neuropathic pain. The NNT for at least 50 % pain relief at 600 mg daily dosing compared with placebo were 3.9 for postherpetic neuralgia in five studies, 5.0 for painful diabetic neuropathy in seven studies, and 5.6 for central neuropathic pain in two studies [8, 10, 11, 16].

Seven randomized controlled trials were completed, evaluating the efficacy of pregabalin for treatment of painful diabetic neuropathy (PDN). Dosing ranged between 150 mg/day and a maximum of 600 mg/day with duration of treatment varying from 5 to 13 weeks. Average onset to significant improvement in pain was somewhat related to dosing being 4 days at 600 mg/day and 5 days at 300 mg/day. The longest onset to pain relief occurred in the 150 mg/day treatment group occurring as long as 13 days after start of drug. Analysis of the various dosing schedules for the PDN trials revealed that TID dosing was effective at 150–450 mg/day; however, efficacy in BID dosing was only seen at a total daily dose of 600 mg/day (300 mg BID). Although efficacy was demonstrated across a dosing range of 150–600 mg/day, FDA approval is for total daily dosing of 150–300 mg divided and given TID [28–30].

Three randomized controlled trials varying between 8 and 13 weeks in duration have looked at the efficacy of pregabalin for the treatment of postherpetic neuralgia. Consistent improvement across all three trials was found at dosing strengths between 150 and 600 mg/day. The dosing interval of BID or TID did not seem to affect patient responses at any total dose between 150 and 600 mg/day [20, 31, 32]. Of clinical interest was the varying response in overall pain relief that was targeted at 50 % improvement, but varied depending on the study between 20 and 50 % for the participants.

Two clinical trials involving over 300 patients with central pain found that relatively high doses of pregabalin 600 mg/day were required to achieve even results of minor significance. NNT for 35 % improvement were around 3.5 (2.3–7) and for 50 % improvement around 5.6 (3.5–14), while the discontinuation rates due to lack of efficacy and side effects (all minor) were somewhere around 50 % of participants [8, 11].

Of clinical importance is that consistent across all neuropathic pain trials regardless of condition treated, there was a generalized tendency towards greater improvement in pain relief with increasing dose of drug to a maximum of 600 mg/day. In addition, when compared to placebo on several of the SF-36 subscales, pregabalin demonstrated general improvement [33].

As with gabapentin, the beneficial effect on sleep has been demonstrated with pregabalin therapy in patients suffering with neuropathic pain [31, 34].

In conclusion, when looking at the pregabalin clinical trial data, substantially greater benefit was found at doses between 300 and 600 mg/day administered either BID or TID for the treatment of postherpetic neuralgia and painful diabetic neuropathy and with less but still clinically relevant benefit in central neuropathic pain [33]. Regardless of the pregabalin dose, only a minority of patients will have attained substantial benefit with pregabalin >50 %; however, the majority will demonstrate moderate benefit of between 30 and 50 % reduction in pain [9, 11, 16].

Adverse Events Profile for Gabapentin and Pregabalin

The most common adverse events for both drugs reported in clinical trials by participants were dizziness (22–38 %), somnolence (15–28 %), and peripheral edema (10–15 %). Review of clinical trial side effect data suggest that overall, similar side effects are present for gabapentin but somewhat lower than with pregabalin for dizziness as well as for weight gain. Of importance for the practicing clinician is that the number needed to harm (NNH/safety) for adverse events leading to withdrawal from a clinical trial with gabapentin was 26.1, which suggests a rather high-safety profile [35, 36].

As with gabapentin, the most common side effects with pregabalin therapy included dizziness, reported in 27–46 % of participants with somnolence being reported in 15–25 % of participants. Side effects were most significant with pregabalin aggressive dose escalation to 600 mg daily. Overall, 18–28 % of participants in pregabalin clinical trials discontinued treatment due to adverse events [35].

The current guidelines for dosing of pregabalin recommend a starting dose of 50 mg TID for PDN and 75 mg BID for PHN. However, due to the side effect profile and pharmacokinetic of pregabalin, individualization of treatment is needed to maximize pain relief and minimize adverse events [28, 32]. In the pregabalin study by Stacey and colleagues that utilized flexible verses fixed dosing schedules (150–600 mg/day) in 269 patients with postherpetic neuralgia, flexible dose therapy was demonstrated to be slightly more effective for treatment of allodynia. More importantly, pregabalin was better tolerated at a higher average dosage of 396 mg/day versus 295 mg/day in the fixed dose group. As well, of clinical importance is the onset of measurable reductions in pain that occurred at 1.5 days in the fixed dose group and 3.5 days in the flexible dose group. Reduction in allodynia was present as early as 1 week after onset of therapy. Equally important was the finding that discontinuation rates due to adverse events were more frequent in the fixed dose therapy group [32].

Although weight gain approximately 2–3 kg is relatively unique to pregabalin and has been reported in 4–14 % of participants across multiple studies, few withdrawal-related issues from therapy were seen, that is, <3 % of participants. More importantly, glycemic control was not an issue in diabetic patients as demonstrated by no change in hemoglobin A-1-C levels. A rather unique reported finding was the euphoric effect experienced by approximately 5 % of participants in the generalized anxiety disorder clinical trials with pregabalin. This finding combined with limited evidence suggesting subjective drug "liking" in a study of pregabalin in recreational drug users led the US Drug Enforcement Administration to list pregabalin as a Schedule V drug [19]. However, to date, no current data would suggest that pregabalin presents a significant health-related issue related to drug abuse or misuse.

Combination Drug Therapy

The construct of utilizing drugs from different classes and with different mechanisms of action has long been advocated, although few trials have been published in support of this approach. Meta-analysis of current single-drug therapy trials utilizing anticonvulsants indicates that less than two-thirds of patients suffering with neuropathic pain obtain satisfactory relief [12]. Therefore, combination drug trials may potentially offer greater improvement in various outcome measures related to neuropathic pain syndromes, such as dose-limiting side effects related to therapy, that most likely play a significant role in the low-therapeutic efficacy rates with currently available single-drug treatment protocols.

Gilron and colleagues have demonstrated that when given in combination, gabapentin and nortriptyline seemed to be more efficacious than when given as a single entity for treatment of neuropathic pain. A total of 56 patients, 40 with PDN and 16 with PHN, were randomized in a double-blind, double-dummy crossover-designed study which suggested that combination therapy improved sleep and had a weak effect on SF-36 quality of life outcomes. Of particular interest is the finding that the average dose of each drug was lower in the combination therapy group compared to when monotherapy was utilized [37]. An earlier study by Gilron published in 1995 demonstrated that combination therapy of gabapentin and morphine was superior to gabapentin alone for treatment of neuropathic pain [38]. On the contrary, a recent randomized controlled trial of oxycodone and pregabalin in combination demonstrated no enhanced pain relief. Unfortunately, the trial design required a forced titration of pregabalin to 600 mg/day in the pregabalin/placebo group. This aggressive pregabalin titration approach was thought to result in the high success of pain reduction >50 %, leading to no significant difference compared to the combination of low-dose oxycodone 10 mg/day and pregabalin [27].

Fibromyalgia (Functional Pain)

Fibromyalgia, a chronic pain condition characterized by widespread pain and tenderness, is considered to result from dysfunctional central sensory processing [3]. It is estimated that somewhere around five million Americans suffer from fibromyalgia and manifest symptoms that include widespread allodynia and hyperalgesia clinically identified by anatomical tender points [9]. The central sensitization process underlying this amplified pain perception is thought to result from an imbalance of neurotransmitters involved in pain processing [3]. Several industry-sponsored studies involving over 3,300 participants have demonstrated the efficacy of pregabalin for treatment of symptoms related to fibromyalgia.

The efficacy of pregabalin was demonstrated in clinical trials that utilized the American College of Rheumatology criteria for diagnosis of fibromyalgia. The trials included one 14-week randomized double-blind placebo-controlled multicenter study and one 6-month randomized withdrawal design study. Pregabalin also was shown to be superior to placebo in four randomized double-blind placebo-controlled trials lasting between 8 and 14 weeks for two main efficacy outcome measures that included the visual analogue scale (VAS) for pain and the patient global impression of change (PGIC). The balance between efficacy and side effects has been measured in several short- and long-term open-label safety extension studies [39].

Recommendations from review of these studies would suggest that effective dosing for treatment of fibromyalgia is between a total daily dosage of 300 and 450 mg/day administered BID. The suggested starting dose should be 75 mg BID and increased within 1 week to 150 mg BID based on efficacy and tolerability; importantly, dosing at 150 mg/day was not shown to be superior to placebo. Further up-titration should be considered to a maximum dose of 225 mg BID (total 450 mg/day), again based on individual patient response and tolerability. Dosing above 450 mg/day is not recommended, as patient global impression of change was lower when dosing at 600 mg/day and may have been the result of an increased dose-related side effect burden [40, 41].

On average, individuals with fibromyalgia manifest widespread pain for greater than 3 months and suffer with their symptoms for at least 5 years prior to diagnosis [42, 43]. Therefore, of special interest is the single, 6-month randomized withdrawal study that demonstrated efficacy and durability of pregabalin for the treatment of fibromyalgia. This 6-month study was designed to evaluate the response and durability of pregabalin over placebo therapy in participants whom already had demonstrated at least a 50 % improvement in an open-label run in phase. At the end of study, 68% of the participants administered pregabalin had ongoing therapeutic effect of >30 % pain relief as well as improvement in PGIC scores [39]. The NNT with pregabalin is quite favorable being 3.5 in order to prevent one participant from losing efficacy for treatment of fibromyalgia-related pain symptoms.

In a 12-week randomized placebo-controlled trial, gabapentin at dosages between 1,200 and 2,400 mg/day demonstrated a 51 % response versus 31 % for placebo with improvement of pain. Measures included the Brief Pain Inventory and Fibromyalgia Impact Questionnaire, which demonstrated improvement in symptoms related to fibromyalgia. Of particular interest was that tender point pain thresholds were not improved [42].

Other Anticonvulsant Drugs

Lamotrigine, a sodium channel-blocking AED, has been trialed in several neuropathic pain conditions with conflicting results. In a double-blind, placebo-controlled crossover-design study of 14 patients with trigeminal neuralgia refractory to carbamazepine or phenytoin, lamotrigine was superior to placebo at 400 mg/day [10]. A 14-week long study in HIV painful neuropathy patients, with titration to 300 mg/day, demonstrated benefit compared to placebo [36, 44]. A small 8-week long study in central post-stroke pain patients with titration to 200 mg/day demonstrated pain relief benefit over placebo [45]. Unfortunately, significant side effects including rash, dizziness, and somnolence combined with a painfully slow titration schedule limit the utility of lamotrigine in clinical practice.

The seldom used anticonvulsant sodium valproate has been studied for the treatment of PDN and PHN. Divalproex sodium studied in a randomized placebo-controlled clinical trial has demonstrated benefit at dosing between 800 and 1,600 mg/day. Treatment-limiting side effects were significant and may include nausea (42 %), infection (39 %), alopecia (31 %), and tremor (28 %) as experienced in migraine trials [10].

Lacosamide, a recent addition second-generation voltage-gated sodium channel-blocking agent, has conflicting evidence of efficacy for treatment of painful diabetic neuropathy. After review of phase 2 and phase 3 trial results, both the FDA and the European Medicines Agency rejected the request for approval to treat painful diabetic neuropathy [7]. Various other first-generation drugs such as phenytoin and clonazepam and second-generation drugs including topiramate, tiagabine, and levetiracetam have either not been tested in randomized controlled trial or have been shown not to have benefit in reducing neuropathic pain as in the case of topiramate [9, 10, 12].

Conclusions

As a group, anticonvulsants can be recommended as initial therapy for the treatment of neuropathic pain with significant pain relief of 50 % in approximately 30 % of patients and 30 % relief in 50 % of patients [46]. However, it is important to emphasize that only three peripheral neuropathic pain syndromes including PDN, PHN, and HIV neuropathy have been utilized to validate efficacy and generalized use for the treatment of neuropathic pain. Anticonvulsants, similar to other therapeutic classes of drugs for the treatment of central neuropathic pain, have for the most part demonstrated minimal efficacy. The one exception to this generalization is the 80 % efficacy data for carbamazepine in the treatment of trigeminal neuralgia. The most widely used anticonvulsants gabapentin [47] and pregabalin have been studied extensively and have demonstrated at best moderate efficacy in treatment of peripheral neuropathic pain.

References

1. Baron R, Tolle T, et al. A cross-sectional cohort survey in 2100 patients with painful diabetic neuropathy and postherpetic neuralgia: differences in demographic data and sensory symptoms. Pain. 2009;146:34–40.
2. Blom S. Trigeminal neuralgia: its treatment with a new anticonvulsant drug (G32883). Lancet. 1962;1:829–40.
3. Branco JC. State of the art on fibromyalgia mechanism. Acta Reumatol Port. 2010;35(1):10–5.
4. Rockoff BW, Davis EH. Controlled sequential trials of carbamazepine in trigeminal neuralgia. Arch Neurol. 1966;15:129–36.
5. Mellick LB, Mellick GA. Successful treatment of reflex sympathetic dystrophy with gabapentin. Am J Emerg Med. 1995;13:96.
6. Rosner H, Rubin L, Kestenbaum A. Gabapentin adjuvant therapy in neuropathic pain states. Clin J Pain. 1996;12:56–8.
7. Doworkin R, O'Connor A, et al. Recommendations for the pharmacologic management of neuropathic pain: an overview and literature update. Mayo Clin Proc. 2010;85 Suppl 3:S3–14.
8. Finnerup NB, Sindrup S, Jensen T. The evidence for pharmacological treatment of neuropathic. Pain. 2010;150:573–81.
9. Wiffen P, Collins S, McQuay H, Carroll D, Jadad A, Moore A. Anticonvulsant drugs for acute and chronic pain. Cochrane Database Syst Rev. 2005;20(3):CD001133.
10. Spina E, Perugi G. Antiepileptic drugs: indications of than epilepsy. Epileptic Disord. 2004;6(2):57–75.
11. Finnerup NB, Otto M, et al. Algorithm for neuropathic pain treatment: an evidence based proposal. Pain. 2005;118:289–305.
12. Goodyear-Smith F, Joan Halliwell. Anticonvulsants for neuropathic pain gaps in evidence. Clin J Pain. 2009;25(6):528–36.
13. Campbell FG, Graham JG, Zilkha KJ. Clinical trial of carbamazepine (Tegretol) in trigeminal neuralgia. J Neurol Neurosurg Psychiatry. 1966;29:265–7.
14. Cruccu G, Gronseth G, Alksne J, Argoff C, Brainin M, Burchiel K, et al. AAN-EFNS guidelines on trigeminal neuralgia management. Eur J Neurol. 2008;15:1013–28.
15. Gronseth G, Cruccu G, Alksne J, Argoff C, Brainin M, Burchiel K, et al. Practice parameter: the diagnostic evaluation and treatment of trigeminal neuralgia (an evidence-based review): report of the quality standards subcommittee of the American Academy of Neurology and the European Federation of Neurological Societies. Neurology. 2008;71:1183–90.
16. Zin C, Nissen LM, et al. An update on the pharmacologic management of post herpetic neuralgia and painful diabetic neuropathy. CNS Drugs. 2008;22(5):417–25.
17. Gilron I. Gabapentin and pregabalin for chronic neuropathic and early postsurgical pain: current evidence and future directions. Curr Opin Anaesthesiol. 2007;20:456–72.
18. Neurontin® (gabapentin) [package insert]. New York: Pfizer Inc; 2004.
19. Lyrica™ (pregabalin) capsules [package insert]. New York: Pfizer Inc; 2005.
20. Moore RA, Straube S, Wiffen PJ, Derry S, McQuay HJ. Pregabalin for acute and chronic pain in adults. Cochrane Database Syst Rev. 2009;3 Article No.: CD007076. doi: 10.1002/14651858.CD007076.pub2.
21. Dooley DJ, Taylor CP, et al. Ca²⁺ channel alpha-2-delta ligands; novel modulators of neurotransmission. Trends Pharmacol Sci. 2007;28(2):7582.
22. Taylor CP. Mechanisms of analgesia by gabapentin and pregabalin-calcium channel alpha-2-delta ligands. Pain. 2009;145(1–2):259.
23. Backonja M, Beydoun A, Edwards KR, Schwartz SL, Fonseca V, Hes M, LaMoreaux L, Garofalo E. Gabapentin for the symptomatic treatment of painful neuropathy in patients with diabetes mellitus. JAMA. 1998;280:1831–6.
24. Bennett M, Simpson K. Gabapentin in the treatment of neuropathic pain. Palliat Med. 2004;18:5–11.
25. Rowbotham M, Harden N, Stacey B, Bernstein P, Magnus-Miller L. Gabapentin for the treatment of postherpetic neuralgia. JAMA. 1998;280:1837–42.
26. Serpell M, Neuropathic Pain Study Group. Gabapentin in neuropathic pain syndromes: a randomised, double-blind, placebo-controlled trial. Pain. 2002;99:557–66.
27. Zin C, Nissen L, et al. A Randomized controlled trial of oxycodone vs placebo in patients with postherpetic neuralgia and painful diabetic neuropathy treated with pregabalin. J Pain. 2009;11:1–10.
28. Freynhagen R, Strojek K, et al. Efficacy of pregabalin in neuropathic pain evaluated in a 12-week, randomized, double-blind, multicentre, placebo-controlled trial of flexible- and fixed-dose regimens. Pain. 2005;115:254–63.
29. Lesser H, Sharma U, et al. Pregabalin relieves symptoms of painful diabetic neuropathy: a randomized controlled trial. Neurology. 2004;63:2104–10.
30. Richter RW, Portenoy R, Sharma U, et al. Relief of painful diabetic peripheral neuropathy with pregabalin: a randomized, placebo-controlled trial. J Pain. 2005;6(4):253–60.
31. Sabatowski R, Galvez R, Cherry DA, et al. Pregabalin reduces pain and improves sleep and mood disturbances in patients with postherpetic neuralgia: results of a randomized, placebo-controlled clinical trial. Pain. 2004;109:26–35.
32. Stacey BR, Barrett JA, et al. Pregabalin for postherpetic neuralgia: placebo-controlled trial of fixed and flexible dosing regimens on allodynia and time to onset of pain relief. J Pain. 2008;9(11):1006–17.
33. Siddall PJ, Cousins MJ, et al. Pregabalin in central neuropathic pain associated with spinal cord injury: a placebo-controlled trial. Neurology. 2006;67:1792–800.
34. van Seventer R, Feister HA, et al. Efficacy and tolerability of twice-daily pregabalin for treating pain and related sleep interference in postherpetic neuralgia: a 13-week, randomized trial. Curr Med Res Opin. 2006;22(2):375–84.
35. Killian JM, Fromm GH. Carbamazepine in the treatment of neuralgia. Arch Neurol. 1968;19:129–36.

36. Simpson DM, McArthur JC, et al. Lamotrigine for HIV-associated painful sensory neuropathies: placebo-controlled trial. Neurology. 2003;60:1508–14.

37. Gilron I, Bailey J, et al. Nortriptyline and gabapentin, alone and in combination for neuropathic pain: a double-blind, randomized controlled crossover trial. Lancet. 2009;374:1252–61.

38. Gilron I, Bailey J, et al. Morphine, gabapentin, or their combination for neuropathic pain. N Engl J Med. 2005;352:1324–34.

39. Crofford LJ, Mease PJ, Simpson SL, et al. Fibromyalgia relapse evaluation and efficacy for durability of meaningful relief (FREEDOM): a 6-month, double-blind, placebo-controlled trial with pregabalin. Pain. 2008;136(3):419–31.

40. Arnold LM, Russell IJ, Diri EW, et al. A 14-week, randomized, double-blind, placebo-controlled, monotherapy trial of pregabalin in patients with fibromyalgia. J Pain. 2008;9:792–805.

41. Mease PJ, Russell IJ, Arnold LM, et al. A randomized, double-blind, placebo-controlled, phase III trial of pregabalin in the treatment of patients with fibromyalgia. J Rheumatol. 2008;35(3):502–14.

42. Arnold LM, Goldenberg DL, et al. Gabapentin in the treatment of fibromyalgia: a randomized, double-blind, placebo-controlled, multicenter trial. Arthritis Rheum. 2007;56:1336–44.

43. Wolfe F, Smythe H, et al. The American College of Rheumatology 1990 criteria for the classification of fibromyalgia. Arthritis Rheum. 1990;33(2):160–72.

44. Simpson DM, Olney R, et al. A placebo controlled trial of lamotrigine for painful HIV-associated neuropathy. Neurology. 2000;54:2115–9.

45. Vestergaard K, Andersen G, et al. Lamotrigine for central post-stroke pain: a randomized controlled trial. Neurology. 2001; 56:184–90.

46. Chou R, Norris S, Carson S, Chan BKS. Drug class review on drugs for neuropathic pain. 2007. http://www.ohsu.edu/drugeffectiveness/reports/final.cfm. Accessed 2007.

47. Rice AS, Maton S, Postherpetic Neuralgia Study Group. Gabapentin in postherpetic neuralgia: a randomised, double blind, placebo controlled study. Pain. 2001;94:215–24.

NMDA Receptor Antagonists in the Treatment of Pain

6

Yakov Vorobeychik, Channing D. Willoughby, and Jianren Mao

Key Points

- NMDA receptors play a pivotal role in a number of essential physiological functions including neuroplasticity. However, persistent and excessive stimulation of this receptor could be detrimental to the central nervous system, leading to neuronal degenerative changes and neurotoxicity. In this regard, NMDA receptors may play a significant role in the development and maintenance of persistent pathological pain.
- Preclinical evidence suggests that blockade of NMDA receptors would prevent the development of a persistent pain state and effectively reverse signs of a persistent pain. Therefore, NMDA receptor antagonists also would be expected to have a therapeutic role in treating persistent pain states in the clinical setting.
- Many clinical studies demonstrated that NMDA receptor antagonists could be efficacious in the treatment of chronic pain states, particularly neuropathic pain, as well as in the management of any non-neuropathic opioid-resistant pain due to developing opioid tolerance or opioid-induced hyperalgesia (OIH). Apparent opioid-sparing effects of these drugs also make them an attractive therapy in the acute pain setting. However, some other studies have failed to prove the clinical usefulness of these medications.
- The perioperative use of an NMDA receptor antagonist may lead to the reduction of postoperative pain from a surgical procedure that is more likely to involve central sensitization but may not provide significant pain reduction if the major component of postoperative pain is considered to be nociceptive.
- Side effects of NMDA receptor antagonists, when administered at therapeutic doses, are a primary limiting factor in their use in clinical practice today. Powerful direct competitive NMDA receptor blockers, as well as high-affinity noncompetitive antagonists, exhibit inadequate therapeutic margins for human use when evaluated in clinical trials. An obvious limitation in assessing the role of the NMDA receptor mechanism in clinical pain management has been the lack of highly selective NMDA receptor antagonists suitable for clinical use.
- It may be anticipated that chronic pain treatment can be improved through the use of NMDA receptor antagonists displaying minimal clinical side effects at therapeutic doses.

Y. Vorobeychik, M.D., Ph.D. (✉)
Department of Anesthesiology, Pennsylvania State University
Milton S. Hershey Medical Center,
500 University Drive, HU-32, P.O. Box 850,
Hershey, PA 17033, USA

Pennsylvania State University College of Medicine,
Hershey, PA, USA
e-mail: yvorbeychik@psu.edu

C.D. Willoughby, M.D.
Department of Anesthesiology, Pennsylvania State University Milton
S. Hershey Medical Center,
500 University Drive, HU-32,
P.O. Box 850, Hershey, PA 17033, USA
e-mail: channingwilloughby@gmail.com

J. Mao, M.D., Ph.D.
Department of Anesthesia, Harvard Medical School,
Boston, MA, USA

Department of Anesthesia, Critical Care and Pain Medicine,
Massachusetts General Hospital,
15 Parkman St, Boston, MA 02114, USA
e-mail: jmao@partners.org

T.R. Deer et al. (eds.), *Comprehensive Treatment of Chronic Pain by Medical, Interventional, and Integrative Approaches*,
DOI 10.1007/978-1-4614-1560-2_6, © American Academy of Pain Medicine 2013

Introduction

Over the past three decades, the central glutamatergic system, particularly the role of the N-methyl-D-aspartate (NMDA) receptor in the neural mechanisms of persistent pain, has been extensively investigated. Chronic pain can be sustained by way of a central sensitization process involving the NMDA receptor system. A considerable number of clinical trials have also been carried out to evaluate the potential application of such mechanisms in clinical pain management. Data from the preclinical studies have consistently supported a crucial role of the central glutamatergic system and NMDA receptors in the induction and maintenance of persistent pain resulting from pathological conditions such as inflammation and nerve injury. To date, clinical trials have resulted in mixed conclusions as to the overall effectiveness in treating persistent pain with NMDA receptor antagonists. Nonetheless, NMDA receptor antagonists have been demonstrated as an effective treatment option in the management of chronic pain, particularly for pain which has been refractory to other treatment modalities.

NMDA Receptors

The NMDA receptor is a subgroup of a large family of glutamate receptors that utilize excitatory amino acids such as glutamate and aspartate as the endogenous agonist. At least three major families of genes have been identified that encode NMDA receptor subunits, namely, NR1, NR2, and NR3 subunits [1]. Various combinations of NR1 and other NR subunits determine the property of NMDA receptor activity. The NR1 subunit is necessary for the NMDA receptor-coupled channel activity, and other subunits are likely to modulate the properties of such channel activities. Recent studies have examined the NR2B subunit of the NMDA receptor and its effect on modulation of pain, proposing that a positive feedback pathway of this subunit as an explanation for cortical sensitization of chronic pain [2, 3].

A unique characteristic of the NMDA receptor is that this receptor is both voltage- and ligand-gated, such that activation of this receptor requires not only an agonist binding but also cell membrane depolarization. As such, activation of NMDA receptors often involves simultaneous activation of other subtypes of glutamate receptors and/or neuropeptidergic receptors. The NMDA receptor-channel complex can be regulated at multiple sites including glutamate, glycine, and calcium channel sites.

NMDA receptors have been localized in both supraspinal and spinal regions from a number of species including mice, rats, and human subjects. There appears to be a minimal variation of NMDA receptor distributions among different species. At the supraspinal level, NMDA receptor binding has been found in hippocampus, cerebral cortex, thalamus, stria-

Table 6.1 Common NMDA receptor antagonists

Ketamine
Amantadine
Memantine
Phencyclidine
Dextromethorphan
Methadone[a]

[a]Commonly clinically utilized for opioid agonist properties

tum, cerebellum, and brain stem. At the spinal level, NMDA receptor binding has been demonstrated mainly within the substantia gelatinosa of the dorsal horn with limited, very low-level binding elsewhere in the spinal gray matter [1].

Since most studies show NMDA receptor binding or immunocytochemical labeling in the neuronal somata, the location of NMDA receptors generally is considered to be postsynaptic. However, presynaptic NMDA receptors also have been demonstrated within the terminals of primary afferent fibers using the combined electron microscopic and immunocytochemical technique. The presynaptic NMDA receptors also are likely to be auto-receptors [4]. It is likely that these receptors may have a role in regulating release of excitatory amino acids from presynaptic terminals. NMDA receptors play a pivotal role in a number of essential physiological functions including neuroplasticity. Neuroplasticity takes place in a variety of forms and contributes to such events as memory formation. It is the persistent and excessive stimulation of this receptor that could be detrimental to the central nervous system, leading to neuronal degenerative changes and neurotoxicity [1]. In this regard, NMDA receptors may play a significant role in the development and maintenance of persistent pathological pain following inflammation (inflammatory pain) and/or nerve injury (neuropathic pain).

NMDA Receptors and Pain Mechanisms

Preclinical Studies

Compelling evidence has emerged from preclinical studies that indicate a critical role of NMDA receptors in the neural mechanisms of persistent nociceptive states including neuropathy and inflammation (Table 6.1) [5–10]. These studies reveal several fundamental features of the NMDA receptor involvement in such pain states. First, NMDA receptors are involved in pain states induced by either partial or complete nerve injury or by persistent inflammation. Second, experimental pain states can be prevented and/or reversed by using either experimental (AP5, MK-801) or clinically available (ketamine, amantadine, dextromethorphan) NMDA receptor antagonists. Third, thermal hyperalgesia, mechanical allodynia, and, in some cases, spontaneous pain behaviors were reduced effectively with an NMDA receptor antagonist in experimental persistent pain states.

By and large, preclinical evidence regarding the role of NMDA receptors in persistent pain states is reproducible and reliable. Such preclinical evidence suggests that blockade of NMDA receptors would prevent the development of a persistent pain state in a clinical setting. Because NMDA receptor antagonists also effectively reverse signs of a persistent pain state in preclinical studies, an NMDA receptor antagonist also would be expected to have a therapeutic role in treating persistent pain states in the clinical setting. These are two key hypotheses (the preventive and therapeutic role of an NMDA receptor antagonist) that have been tested in many clinical trials carried out over the last several years.

Clinical Studies

Currently, clinically available NMDA receptor antagonists include ketamine, dextromethorphan, amantadine, and memantine. They bind to the channel site and are considered relatively low-affinity agents. The opioid analgesic methadone is also known to express NMDA receptor antagonistic properties. Unfortunately, direct competitive NMDA receptor blockers that bind to the site of glutamate (e.g., AP5), as well as high-affinity noncompetitive antagonists, all exhibit inadequate therapeutic margins for human use when evaluated in clinical trials [11–15].

The antagonism of NMDA activity and subsequent inhibition of central sensitization offers a valuable pain treatment approach. NMDA antagonists can be efficacious in the treatment of chronic pain states, particularly neuropathic pain, as well as in the management of any non-neuropathic opioid-resistant pain due to developing opioid tolerance or opioid-induced hyperalgesia (OIH). Apparent opioid-sparing effects of these drugs also make them an attractive therapy in the acute pain setting.

In patients with chronic pain states that have been refractory to more standard therapy, particularly neuropathic pain, NMDA receptor antagonists have been frequently utilized. Studies evaluating high-dose IV ketamine in the treatment of complex regional pain syndrome (CRPS) have demonstrated substantial decreases in pain scores and, in some instances, complete resolution of study subjects' pain [16, 17]. There is also some evidence that the use of ketamine at sub-anesthetic doses also improves a multitude of pain parameters in patients with CRPS [15, 18–20]. One particular case series of six patients with CRPS who underwent treatment with the NMDA receptor antagonist memantine for 6 months demonstrated improved pain scores and other markers of disease, including functional MRI changes [21].

In postherpetic neuralgia that has been refractory to more conventional treatment, intravenous ketamine has shown to be an effective therapy in decreasing initial visual analogue scale (VAS) pain scores and offering sustained pain relief 1 year following initial treatment [22]. Several studies have focused upon the use of ketamine in the treatment of phantom limb pain. One such study demonstrated ketamine to be superior to calcitonin in the treatment of persistent phantom limb pain [23]. Yet another study evaluating epidurally administered ketamine with local anesthetic demonstrated improved short-term analgesia and decreased mechanical sensitivity in patients suffering from phantom limb pain condition, further substantiating the role of NMDA receptor antagonism and its inhibition of central sensitization [24]. Memantine has also been evaluated for the treatment of phantom limb pain. While some findings were inconclusive, the overall trend suggests that memantine may serve as a useful adjuvant agent for this disorder [25–28].

NMDA receptor antagonists may play a particularly important role in cancer-related opioid- resistant pain treatment. Utilization of high doses of opioid analgesics may lead to the development of opioid unresponsiveness in oncology patients. OIH, pharmacodynamic, pharmacokinetic, and learned tolerance can all cause decreased opioid efficacy in this patient population [29]. Many studies published during the last decade showed that low to moderate doses of ketamine significantly improve analgesia in patients with opioid refractory cancer pain [30–34]. In dissonance, one systemic review demonstrated lack of suitable randomized trials and insufficient evidence to make recommendations for routine use of ketamine for cancer pain [35]. The most recent work by Kapural et al. failed to prove the use of ketamine as an effective way to lower long-term pain scores in patients taking high-dose opioids in the settings of neuropathic or nociceptive pain [16].

The role of OIH in clinical situations has been demonstrated in some chronic pain patients, many of who were taking "megadoses" of opioid [36–39]. It has been shown that the addition of an NMDA receptor antagonist for the management of patients who have failed to benefit from opioid rotation or other adjunctive treatments may lead to a more favorable clinical outcome. Several publications report the successful use of ketamine for OIH [40–42]. Methadone, with its D-isomer demonstrating NMDA receptor antagonism, is also mechanistically appealing for the treatment of OIH [43–46]. Dextromethorphan has been studied to assess its clinical utility in treating OIH or limiting tolerance with mixed results [47, 48].

Opioid-sparing effects of NMDA receptor antagonists is well established. The combination of NMDA antagonists with opioid and other non-opioid analgesics can act in synergism, providing an optimal multimodal approach to the management of pain. Ketamine has been demonstrated to provide opioid-sparing effects, facilitate postsurgical rehabilitation, and offer decreased postoperative pain in patients following total hip arthroplasty [49]. Likewise, low-dose ketamine administration has been shown to decrease postoperative morphine consumption and improve postoperative analgesia in patients undergoing major abdominal surgery [50]. Amantadine, most known for its antiviral and antiparkinsonian effects, has been shown to lower the morphine dose requirements and VAS pain scores in patients undergoing radical prostatectomy [51].

Discrepancies Between Preclinical and Clinical Studies

A considerable number of clinical studies (both controlled randomized studies and case observations) have been conducted to test the above hypotheses. Clinically available agents, all with the NMDA receptor antagonist properties, were commonly used in these studies. Unlike unequivocal results from the bench studies, however, clinical outcomes of pain relief using NMDA receptor antagonists have varied substantially among different studies.

The role of the NMDA receptor mechanism in persistent pain states is overwhelmingly supported by the data from a large number of preclinical studies, yet outcomes from clinical studies are far less certain. One obvious limitation in assessing the role of the NMDA receptor mechanism in clinical pain management has been the lack of highly selective NMDA receptor antagonists suitable for clinical use.

NMDA Receptor Antagonists and Preemptive Analgesia

The concept of preemptive analgesia suggests that postoperative pain intensity could be enhanced due to the process of central sensitization driven by repeated peripheral nociceptive input and mediated through the NMDA receptor. As such, blocking the establishment of central sensitization preoperatively with a clinically available NMDA receptor antagonist would be expected to prevent the development of postoperative pain hypersensitivity. This potentially beneficial effect would be reflected as diminished pain intensity, hence a lower pain score and/or a reduced consumption of analgesics (such as opioids) in surgical patients who receive perioperative treatment with a clinically available NMDA receptor antagonist. To date, nearly all of the clinical studies examining preemptive analgesia have been conducted along this line of experimental design. Several important issues on this topic deserve some discussion.

Is Postoperative Pain Primarily due to Central Sensitization?

This fundamental question needs to be better addressed for two important reasons. First, although NMDA receptors play a pivotal role in central sensitization, they are not primarily involved in the processing of nociceptive pain. Second, because NMDA receptors do not play a major role in the processing of nociceptive pain, an NMDA receptor antagonist by itself could not function as an effective analgesic.

Thus, the perioperative use of an NMDA receptor antagonist alone may not provide significant pain reduction if the major component of postoperative pain is considered to be nociceptive pain. By the same token, one would expect that the reduction of postoperative pain from a surgical procedure that is more likely to involve central sensitization, such as limb amputation, would be better achieved with the perioperative use of an NMDA receptor antagonist.

Is the Study Design Sufficiently Sensitive to Make a Distinction Between the Reduction of Nociceptive Pain and Decreased Pain Hypersensitivity?

It is conceivable that central sensitization would be contributory to postoperative pain if repeated intra- and postoperative nociceptive input is the driving force for the NMDA receptor-mediated cellular and molecular changes underlying the development of neuronal plasticity. In this regard, one might argue that regardless of the relative contribution of nociceptive pain and/or increased pain hypersensitivity, perioperative use of an NMDA receptor antagonist (hence the prevention of pain hypersensitivity) would lead to a reduction of pain scoring and/or sparing of postoperative analgesic use. The issue is whether the clinical trial design is sensitive enough to make such a distinction. Thus, an adequate power of analysis should be considered for clinical studies.

Adverse Effects

Side effects of NMDA receptor antagonists when administered at therapeutic doses are a primary limiting factor in their use in clinical practice today (Table 6.2). They may cause psycho-cognitive issues, sedation, respiratory depression, and cardiostimulatory derangements.

Table 6.2 Potential side effects of NMDA antagonists

Psychosocial	Confusion
	Hallucinations
	Delirium
	Anxiety
	Insomnia
Cardiovascular	Arrhythmias
	Hemodynamic instability
Respiratory	Apnea
Gastrointestinal	Nausea/vomiting
	Anorexia
Ocular	Diplopia
	Nystagmus
Musculoskeletal	Myoclonus

Alterations in body image and mood, feelings of unreality, floating sensation, hallucinations, restlessness, vivid dreams, dissociation, insomnia, fatigue, delirium, confusion, and drowsiness are among the cognitive adverse effects described in the literature [52]. Increased blood pressure and heart rate are the most common cardiovascular complications [40]. NMDA receptor antagonists were found to trigger a dose-dependent neurotoxic reaction in the cingulated and retrosplenial cortices of adult rats when administered as a short-term treatment [53]. Prolonged continuous infusion of intrathecal ketamine has been associated with spinal cord vacuolization [54]. However, most of the mentioned side effects have been reported with intravenous or subcutaneous administration of this NMDA receptor blocker. Oral ketamine produces few adverse effects [55]. Moreover, the incidence of side effects with ketamine's systemic use in combination with opioids is low and does not differ from controls treated with opioids only [56]. Specifically, hallucinations occur in 7.4 %, "pleasant dreams" in 18.3 %, nightmares in 4 %, and visual disturbance in 6.2 % of patients [57]. The overall rate of central nervous system adverse effects in patients receiving low-dose ketamine is about 10 % [58]. It is believed that ketamine may cause psychotomimetic effects by disinhibiting certain excitatory transmitter circuits in the human brain [59]. Some drugs such as benzodiazepines can restore the inhibition to this circuitry, providing a neuroprotective effect and reducing the rate of complications [60]. Therefore, concomitant use of benzodiazepines is recommended during ketamine infusion treatment [61]. Another class of medications, alpha-2 adrenergic agonists, may also protect against neurotoxic, psychotomimetic, and cardiostimulatory side effects of NMDA antagonists and, in the case of neuropathic pain, exert a synergistic analgesic effect [18, 62, 63]. Recent studies focusing upon the neramexane and memantine suggest that NMDA antagonists may be used at therapeutic doses without adverse side effects [64, 65].

Conclusion

In summary, NMDA receptors are likely to play a significant role in the central mechanisms of persistent pain. It is conceivable that the outcome of clinical use of NMDA receptor antagonists may vary significantly depending on pain condition, onset of treatment, dosing regimen, and pain assessment tools. NMDA receptor antagonists are more likely to be helpful in improving pain conditions such as neuropathic pain involving the mechanisms of central sensitization. Thus, it is important to recognize the limitation of using NMDA receptor antagonists in clinical pain management. Recent studies have indicated potential clinical benefits of using agents that target new NMDA receptor sites (e.g., NR2 subunit)

[2, 3, 66, 67]. It may be anticipated that chronic pain treatment can be improved through the use of NMDA receptor antagonists displaying minimal clinical side effects at therapeutic doses.

References

1. Mao J. NMDA and opioid receptors: their interactions in antinociception, tolerance, and neuroplasticity. Brain Res Rev. 1999;30:289–304.
2. Hu J, Wang Z, Guo YY, et al. A role of periaqueductal grey NR2B-containing NMDA receptor in mediating persistent inflammatory pain. Mol Pain. 2009;5:71.
3. Zhuo M. Plasticity of NMDA receptor NR2B subunit in memory and chronic pain. Mol Brain. 2009;2:4.
4. Liu J, Wang H, Sheng M, Jan LY, Jan YN, Basbaum AI. Evidence for presynaptic N-methyl-D-aspartate autoreceptors in the spinal cord dorsal horn. Proc Natl Acad Sci USA. 1994;91(18):8383–7.
5. Dickenson AH. A cure for wind-up: NMDA receptor antagonists as potential analgesics. Trends Pharmacol Sci. 1990;11:307–9.
6. Woolf CJ, Thompson SWN. The induction and maintenance of central sensitization is dependent on N-methyl-D-aspartic acid receptor activation: implications for the treatment of post-injury pain hypersensitivity states. Pain. 1991;44:293–9.
7. Woolf CJ, Mannion RJ. Neuropathic pain: aetiology, symptoms, mechanisms, and management. Lancet. 1999;353:1959–64.
8. Dubner R. Neuronal plasticity and pain following peripheral tissue inflammation or nerve injury. In: Bond M, Charlton E, Woolf CJ, editors. Proceedings of 5th world congress on pain. Pain research and clinical management, vol. 5. Amsterdam: Elsevier; 1991. p. 263–76.
9. Mao J, Price DD, Mayer DJ. Mechanisms of hyperalgesia and opiate tolerance: a current view of their possible interactions. Pain. 1995;62:259–74.
10. Chaplan SR, Malmberg AB, Yaksh TL. Efficacy of spinal NMDA receptor antagonism in formalin hyperalgesia and nerve injury evoked allodynia in the rat. J Pharmacol Exp Ther. 1997;280:829–38.
11. Yenari MA, Bell TE, Kotake AN, et al. Dose escalation safety and tolerance study of the competitive NMDA antagonist selfotel (CGS-19755) in neurosurgery patients. Clin Neuropharmacol. 1998;21(1):28–34.
12. Muir KW, Lees KR. Excitatory amino acid antagonists for acute stroke. Cochrane Database Syst Rev. 2003;3:CD001244.
13. Hoyte L, Barber PA, Buchan AM, et al. The rise and fall of NMDA antagonists for ischemic stroke. Curr Mol Med. 2004;4(2):131–6.
14. Wood PL. The NMDA receptor complex: a long and winding road to therapeutics. IDrugs. 2005;8(3):229–35.
15. Harbut RE, Correll GE. Successful treatment of a nine-year case of complex regional pain syndrome type-I (reflex sympathetic dystrophy) with intravenous ketamine-infusion therapy in a warfarin-anticoagulated adult female patient. Pain Med. 2002;3:147–55.
16. Kapural L, Kapural M, Bensitel T, et al. Opioid-sparing effect of intravenous outpatient ketamine infusions appears short-lived in chronic-pain patients with high opioid requirements. Pain Physician. 2010;13:389–94.
17. Goldberg ME, Torjman MC, Schwartzman RJ, et al. Pharmacodynamic profiles of ketamine (R)- and (S)- with 5-day inpatient infusion for the treatment of complex regional pain syndrome. Pain Physician. 2010;13:379–87.
18. Correll EC, Maleki J, Gracely EJ, et al. Subanesthetic ketamine infusion therapy: a retrospective analysis of a novel therapeutic approach to complex regional pain syndrome. Pain Med. 2004;5(3):263–75.

19. Schwartzman RJ, Alexander GM, Grothusen JR, et al. Outpatient intravenous ketamine for the treatment of complex regional pain syndrome: a double-blind placebo controlled study. Pain. 2009;147:107–15.

20. Nama S, Meenan DR, Fritz WT. The use of sub-anesthetic intravenous ketamine and adjuvant dexmedetomidine when treating acute pain from CRPS. Pain Physician. 2010;13:365–8.

21. Sinis N, Birbaumer N, Gustin S, et al. Memantine treatment of complex regional pain syndrome: a preliminary report of six cases. Clin J Pain. 2007;23:237–43.

22. Tsuneyoshi I, Gushiken T, Kanmura Y, Yoshimura N. Changes in pain intensity of post-herpetic neuralgia following intravenous injections of ketamine hydrochloride. J Anesth. 1999;13(1):53–5.

23. Urs E, Neff F, Sveticic G, et al. Chronic phantom limb pain: the effects of calcitonin, ketamine, and their combination on pain and sensory thresholds. Anesth Analg. 2008;106(4):1265–73.

24. Wilson JA, Nimmo AF, Fleetwood-Walker SM, et al. Randomized double blind trail of the effect of pre-emptive epidural ketamine on persistent pain after lower limb amputation. Pain. 2008;135:108–18.

25. Schley M, Topfner S, Wiech K, Schaller HE, Konrad CJ, Schmelz M, Birbaumer N. Continuous brachial plexus blockade in combination with the NMDA receptor antagonist memantine prevents phantom pain in acute traumatic upper limb amputees. Eur J Pain. 2007;11:299–308.

26. Nikolajsen L, Gottrup H, Kristensen AG, Jensen TS. Memantine (a N-methyl-d-aspartate receptor antagonist) in the treatment of neuropathic pain after amputation or surgery: a randomized, double-blinded, cross-over study. Anesth Analg. 2000;91:960–96.

27. Wiech K, Kiefer RT, Topfner S, Preissl H, Braun C, Unertl K, Flor H, Birbaumer N. A placebo-controlled randomized crossover trial of the N-methyl-d-aspartic acid receptor antagonist, memantine, in patients with chronic phantom limb pain. Anesth Analg. 2004; 98:408–13.

28. Maier C, Dertwinkel R, Mansourian N, Hosbach I, Schwenkreis P, Senne I, Skipka G, Zenz M, Tegenthoff M. Efficacy of the NMDA-receptor antagonist memantine in patients with chronic phantom limb pain–results of a randomized double-blinded, placebo-controlled trial. Pain. 2003;103:277–83.

29. Chang G, Chen L, Mao J. Opioid tolerance and hyperalgesia. Med Clin North Am. 2007;91(2):199–211.

30. Mercadante S, Arcuri E, Tirelli W, et al. Analgesic effect of intravenous ketamine in cancer patients on morphine therapy. J Pain Symptom Manage. 2000;20:246–52.

31. Good P, Tullio F, Jackson K, et al. Prospective audit of short-term concurrent ketamine, opioid and anti-inflammatory "triple-agent" therapy of episodes of acute on chronic pain. Intern Med J. 2005; 35:39–44.

32. Kannan TR, Saxena A, Bhatnagar S, et al. Oral ketamine as an adjuvant to oral morphine for neuropathic pain in cancer patients. J Pain Symptom Manage. 2002;23:60–5.

33. Fitzgibbon EJ, Viola R. Parenteral ketamine as an analgesic adjuvant for severe pain: development and retrospective audit of a protocol for a palliative care unit. J Palliat Med. 2005;8(1):49–57.

34. Lossignol DA, Obiols-Portis M, Body JJ. Successful use of ketamine for intractable cancer pain. Support Care Cancer. 2005;13(3):188–93.

35. Bell RF, Eccleston C, Kalso E. Ketamine as adjuvant to opioids for cancer pain. A qualitative systematic review. J Pain Symptom Manage. 2003;26:867–75.

36. Gardell LR, Wang R, Burgess SE, et al. Sustained morphine exposure induces a spinal dynorphin-dependent enhancement of excitatory transmitter release from primary afferent fibers. J Neurosci. 2002;22(15):6747–55.

37. Gardell LR, King T, Ossipov MH, et al. Opioid receptor-mediated hyperalgesia and antinociceptive tolerance induced by sustained opiate delivery. Neurosci Lett. 2006;396(1):44–9.

38. Mao J. Opioid-induced abnormal pain sensitivity: implications in clinical opioid therapy. Pain. 2002;100(3):213–7.

39. Chu LF, Angst MS, Clark D. Opioid induced hyperalgesia in humans: molecular mechanisms and clinical considerations. Clin J Pain. 2008;24(6):479–96.

40. Okon T. Ketamine: an introduction for the pain and palliative medicine physician. Pain Physician. 2007;10:493–500.

41. Joly V, Richebe P, Guignard B, et al. Remifentanil-induced postoperative hyperalgesia and its prevention with small-dose ketamine. Anesthesiology. 2005;103(1):147–55.

42. Singla A, Stojanovic MP, Chen L, et al. A differential diagnosis of hyperalgesia toxicity, and withdrawal from intrathecal morphine infusion. Anesth Analg. 2007;105(6):1816–9.

43. Vorobeychik Y, Chen L, Bush MC, et al. Improved opioid analgesic effect following opioid dose reduction. Pain Med. 2008;5(6): 724–7.

44. Axelrod DJ, Reville B. Using methadone to treat opioid-induced hyperalgesia and refractory pain. J Opioid Manag. 2007;3(2):113–4.

45. Mercadante S, Arcuri E. Hyperalgesia and opioid switching. Am J Hosp Palliat Care. 2005;22:291–4.

46. Chung KS, Carson S, Glassman D, et al. Successful treatment of hydromorphone induced neurotoxicity and hyperalgesia. Conn Med. 2004;68:547–9.

47. Galer BS, Lee D, Ma T, et al. Morphidex (morphine sulfate/dextromethorphan hydrobromide combination) in the treatment of chronic pain: three multicenter, randomized, double-blend, controlled clinical trials fail to demonstrate enhanced opioid analgesia or reduction in tolerance. Pain. 2005;115:284–95.

48. Katz NP. Morphidex (MS:DM) double-blind, multiple-dose studies in chronic pain patients. J Pain Symptom Manage. 2000;19:S42–9.

49. Remérand F, Le Tendre C, Baud A, et al. The early and delayed analgesic effects of ketamine after total hip arthroplasty: a prospective, randomized, controlled, double-blind study. Anesth Analg. 2009;109(6):1963–71.

50. Zakine J, Samarcq D, Lorne E, et al. Postoperative ketamine administration decreases morphine consumption in major abdominal surgery: a prospective, randomized, double blind, controlled study. Anesth Analg. 2008;106(6):1856–61.

51. Snijdelaar DG, Koren G, Katz J. Effects of perioperative amantadine on postoperative pain and morphine consumption in patients after radical prostatectomy. Anesthesiology. 2004;100:134–41.

52. Fisher K, Coderre TJ, Hagen NA. Targeting the N-methyl-D-aspartate receptor for chronic pain management: preclinical animal studies, recent clinical experience and future research directions. J Pain Symptom Manage. 2000;20(5):358–73.

53. Jevtovic-Todorovic V, Wozniak DF, Benshoff ND, et al. A comparative evaluation of neurotoxic properties of ketamine and nitrous oxide. Brain Res. 2001;895:246–7.

54. Stoltz M, Oehen HP, Gerber H. Histological findings after long-term infusion of intrathecal ketamine for chronic pain: a case report. J Pain Symptom Manage. 1999;18:223–8.

55. Fisher K, Hagen NA. Analgesic effect of oral ketamine in chronic neuropathic pain of spinal origin: a case report. J Pain Symptom Manage. 1999;18:61–6.

56. Visser E, Schug SA. The role of ketamine in pain management. Biomed Pharmacother. 2006;60(7):341–8.

57. Elia N, Tramer MR. Ketamine and postoperative pain – a quantitative systematic review of randomized trials. Pain. 2005; 113(1–2):61–70.

58. Subramaniam K, Subramaniam B, Steinbrook RA. Ketamine as adjuvant analgesic to opioids: a quantitative and qualitative systematic review. Anesth Analg. 2004;99(2):482–95.

59. Jevtovic-Todorovic V, Olney JW. Neuroprotective agents. In: Evers AS, Mayes M, editors. Anesthetic pharmacology, physiologic principles and clinical practice. Philadelphia: Churchill Livingstone; 2004. p. 557–72.

60. Farber NB, Kim SH, Dikranian K, et al. Receptor mechanisms and circuitry underlying NMDA antagonist neurotoxicity. Mol Psychiatry. 2002;7:32–43.

61. Prommer E. Ketamine to control pain. J Palliat Med. 2003; 6(3):443–6.

62. Kim SH, Price MT, Olney JW, et al. Excessive cerebrocortical release of acetylcholine induced by NMDA antagonists is reduced by GABAergic and alpha- adrenergic agonists. Mol Psychiatry. 1999;4:344–52.

63. Handa F, Tanaka M, Nishikawa T, et al. Effects of oral clonidine premedication on side effects of intravenous ketamine anesthesia: a randomized, double-blind placebo-controlled study. J Clin Anesth. 2000;12:19–24.

64. Chen S-R, Samoriski G, Pan H-L. Antinociceptive effects of chronic administration of uncompetitive NMDA receptor antagonists in a rat model of diabetic neuropathic pain. Neuropharmacology. 2009;57(2):121–6.

65. Hackworth RJ, Tokarz KA, Fowler IA, Wallace SC, Stedje-Larsen ET. Profound pain reduction after induction of memantine treatment in two patients with severe phantom limb pain. Anesth Analg. 2008;107(4):1377–9.

66. Chazot PL. The NMDA receptor NR2B subunit: a valid therapeutic target for multiple CNS pathologies. Curr Med Chem. 2004; 11:389–96.

67. Tao YX, Raja SN. Are synaptic MAGUK proteins involved in chronic pain? Trends Pharmacol Sci. 2004;25:397–400.

Role of Muscle Relaxants in the Treatment of Pain

7

Robert I. Cohen and Carol A. Warfield

Key Points

- Muscle relaxants are a diverse group of medications with limited indications which share few structural similarities and where known, few mechanisms of action.
- There are four different mechanisms by which muscle relaxants are thought to work. Baclofen is active at the GABA-B receptor, tizanidine at the alpha-2 receptor, cyclobenzaprine at small TLRs in spinal microglia, and flupirtine (available in Europe) activates a potassium "M-current" in Kv7 potassium channels.
- As a group, muscle relaxants have a high side effect profile and produce limited benefit.
- FDA indications include treatment of "musculoskeletal disorders" and treatment of "spasticity."
- When used in musculoskeletal disorders such as low back pain, benefit has been established compared with placebo. However, there are few head-to-head trials against active agents suggesting that this group should be utilized as the first-line treatment. At the same time, there is some evidence that these drugs should not be used long term for chronic back pain.
- While evidence of efficacy is poor compared with other classes of drugs, usage of these medications is high, especially among primary care physicians

(PCPs) and to a lesser degree by rheumatologists, psychiatrists, and neurologists.
- One of the most commonly prescribed agents, cyclobenzaprine is very closely related to the tricyclic antidepressants and it differs from amitriptyline by only one double bond.
- Carisoprodol is probably the most controversial member of this class which is metabolized by cytochrome P450-CYP2C19 to the barbiturate meprobamate.
- Baclofen is the mainstay for treatment of upper motor neuron syndromes leading to spasticity. Unacceptable sedation at therapeutically effective oral doses makes it desirable to administer this drug intrathecally which minimizes side effects.

R.I. Cohen, M.D., M.A. (Educ) (✉)
Department of Anesthesia, Critical Care and Pain Medicine,
Beth Israel Deaconess Medical Center,
330 Brookline Avenue, Boston, MA 02215, USA
e-mail: ricohen@bidmc.hardvard.edu

C.A. Warfield, M.D.
Department of Anesthesia, Critical Care and Pain Medicine,
Harvard Medical School,
Boston, MA, USA

P.O. Box 222, Prides Crossing, MA 01965, USA
e-mail: cwarfiel@bidmc.harvard.edu

Introduction

This chapter is about drugs approved to treat both spastic upper motor neuron conditions like cerebral palsy or multiple sclerosis and drugs that are used to relieve muscle spasm associated with musculoskeletal conditions such as acute non-radicular cervical or low back pain. Unlike other analgesic classes such as opioids and NSAIDS, the muscle relaxant drugs as a group share neither chemical structure nor mechanism of action. For example, two drugs approved to treat spasm, baclofen and tizanidine, work by different mechanisms. The former blocks GABA-B receptors and the latter is an alpha-2 agonist. Cyclobenzaprine, a drug approved for treating spasm-type pain in the low back, except for one double bond, is chemically identical to the tricyclic antidepressant amitriptyline.

If muscle relaxants are dissimilar in structure and mechanism of action, one thing they share as a class is a high side effect profile. Because the evidence for harm is strong and the evidence for benefit is weak, muscle relaxants should not be first-line drugs for musculoskeletal conditions like acute low back pain, and when used, the course should be brief unless

T.R. Deer et al. (eds.), *Comprehensive Treatment of Chronic Pain by Medical, Interventional, and Integrative Approaches*,
DOI 10.1007/978-1-4614-1560-2_7, © American Academy of Pain Medicine 2013

there is clear evidence that for a given individual, there is ongoing benefit and lack of significant side effects [1].

While these drugs are not recommended as first-line drugs, in practice, that is frequently how they are used. In a study based on insurance claims of 211,511 patients with low back pain, 69 % were treated with prescription medication with the tendency to prescribe muscle relaxants first; then, on subsequent visits, drugs tended to be prescribed in the following order: NSAIDs, antidepressants, and opioids, with opioids being the last to be prescribed [2].

While there may be a response to the publication of guidelines for best practice, the effect is not necessarily sustained. In 1994, the Agency for Healthcare Research and Quality (AHRQ) published evidence-based guidelines for best practice for low back pain that included recommendations similar to the WHO pain ladder for increased use of acetaminophen and NSAIDs and recommended against the use of muscle relaxant medications. Three years after release of the guidelines, Jackson et al. reviewed a database of ten million patient visits, half in the 3 years before the guidelines were issued and half following release [3]. They report that the AHRQ guidelines had a modest impact on practice, showing increased use of acetaminophen and NSAIDs and decreased use of muscle relaxants. As far as muscle relaxants are concerned, educational efforts have been disappointing due to a lack of sustained effect and repeated efforts at education would seem to be necessary.

Driven by an effort to reduce cost in addition to providing better care, California commissioned an expert physician panel to work with a California Medicaid provider covering more than 100,000 recipients. They identified five overused PCP behaviors, one of which was long-term treatment of back pain with muscle relaxants. Muscle relaxant use decreased significantly after an intervention carried out among 45 primary care physicians where their behaviors were discussed, educational material provided, and ongoing behavior monitored [4]. This is a recent study, and long-term follow-up data is not available to describe whether the educational and monitoring effort will continue and if the behavioral changes in physician prescribing will be sustained.

In the North Carolina Back Pain Project population, more than 1,600 patients with new onset of low back pain had a mean functional recovery in 16 days (8 days median) after their first physician visit. Within this group, half received prescriptions for muscle relaxants. Muscle relaxant use was characterized by younger age, higher proportion of female sex, greater likelihood of being on workers compensation, and an increased history of prior episodes of treatment for low back pain. In terms of return to baseline function, outcome was worse for patients receiving muscle relaxants; however, those who received muscle relaxants also tended to have the highest reported pain intensity and lowest baseline function due to pain interference [5]. A more recent study in the same state surveyed 5,357 households and determined that the rate of prescribing muscle relaxants for low back pain in elders was significantly lower than for younger age groups [6].

While it would seem that muscle relaxants must be very effective based on the extent to which they are prescribed, universally accepted evidence is scarce for muscle relaxants as effective treatment for low back pain. For example, in a recent review, although 17 of 137 studies on medical management of low back pain showed evidence of benefit for opioid and NSAID agents, no study on muscle relaxant treatment of low back pain met their standard for evidence of benefit [7]. Other studies have found muscle relaxants effective for treatment of acute nonspecific low back pain compared to placebo. In a meta-analysis that included 23 high-quality trials of muscle relaxants compared to placebo for low back pain, patients taking active drug were 50 % more likely to have a side effect such as drowsiness, dizziness, or dry mouth (relative risk 1.5). This study showed significant efficacy for acute pain but questioned it for chronic low back pain [8]. A recent review of agents targeting nociceptive and neuropathic pain components mentions that side effects of muscle relaxants outweigh their limited potential benefit as monotherapy for chronic low back pain [9].

Myofascial pain is a muscle pain phenomenon with taught bands (trigger points) that might benefit from muscle relaxants. However, a recent Cochrane review found only two small studies showing efficacy of cyclobenzaprine over clonazepam and placebo [10]. Another soft tissue pain syndrome, fibromyalgia, might also be thought to benefit from muscle relaxant drugs. However, in a recent review comparing medical management of fibromyalgia by various specialties, muscle relaxants were not as commonly used as other analgesic classes, and among muscle relaxants, cyclobenzaprine was the most commonly prescribed. That said, they were prescribed by 35 % of primary care physicians compared to 9, 4, and 3 % of rheumatologists, psychiatrists, and neurologists, respectively [11]. Monotherapy with pregabalin or duloxetine is most common, although 8 % of a recent study group of patients with fibromyalgia are receiving muscle relaxants [12].

Because muscle tension or spasm is brought to mind when discussing tension-type headache, one might find it logical to expect that tension-type headache would respond well to muscle relaxants. However, this has not proved to be the case, even for tizanidine [13]. Compared to migraine, tension-type headache has a higher age of onset, a more even female to male distribution, a greater overall cost, is usually bilateral, and has a pressing-tightening character [13]. Although this type of headache is described in terms of muscular symptoms, the use of muscle relaxants is not indicated for this condition [13].

Metaxalone
$C_{11}H_{15}NO_3$

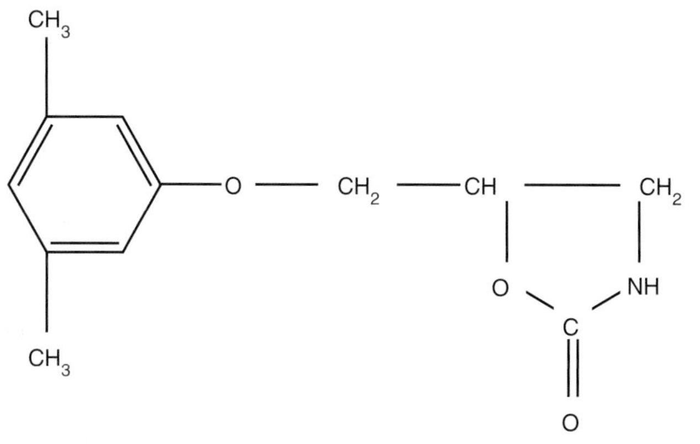

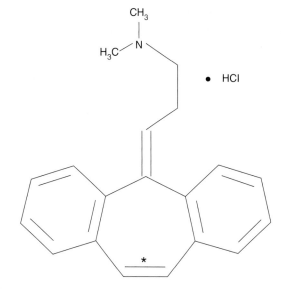

Fig. 7.1 Metaxalone was approved as a muscle relaxant in the 1960s when two small studies suggested benefit in degree of low back spasm over the painful area and decreased pain interference; however, there has been a dearth of recent studies establishing either a mechanism of action or efficacy

Fig. 7.2 Cyclobenzaprine is one of the most commonly prescribed muscle relaxants, and while the exact mechanism by which it produces a muscle relaxant effect is not known, it may produce inhibition of serotonergic descending systems

Metaxalone

Metaxalone was approved as a muscle relaxant in the 1960s when two small studies suggested benefit in degree of low back spasm over the painful area and decreased pain interference; however, there has been a dearth of recent studies establishing either a mechanism of action or efficacy (Fig. 7.1) [14]. A review of three muscle relaxants, including metaxalone, calls attention to the lack of understanding of the mechanism of action and lower standards for articles reporting on efficacy and safety when these drugs were brought to market in the 1960s and 1970s [14]. Proposed mechanisms for metaxalone included sedation or modulation of signals in polysynaptic fibers sensing passive stretch. Also reviewed were cyclobenzaprine and carisoprodol. Concern was raised for the abuse potential of the latter and thus suggested the former may be safer.

Cyclobenzaprine

Cyclobenzaprine is one of the most commonly prescribed muscle relaxants, and while the exact mechanism by which it produces a muscle relaxant effect is not known, it may produce inhibition of serotonergic descending systems (Fig. 7.2) [15].

Cyclobenzaprine is chemically related to amitriptyline from which it differs by only one double bond. Cyclobenzaprine metabolites also differ from amitriptyline metabolites by only one double bond. When doing forensic testing for the presence of these drugs and their metabolites, it may be necessary to use advanced techniques, such as high-performance liquid chromatography with ultraviolet detection or gas chromatography with nitrogen-phosphorus detection [16]. Laboratory technology involving high-performance liquid chromatography and tandem mass spectrometry is currently able to rapidly and quantitatively measure the following eight muscle relaxants in human blood: afloqualone, chlorphenesin carbamate, chlorzoxazone, dantrolene, eperisone, methocarbamol, pridinol, and tolperisone [17].

A meta-analysis of studies comparing cyclobenzaprine with placebo showed efficacy to be greatest on day 4 and then declining after the first week. NNT = 3, meaning three patients required treatment for one to show response [18]. In this now 10-year-old paper, a strong recommendation was made for comparing efficacy among active controls such as acetaminophen and NSAIDs which has since been done. A 2010 study shows efficacy for cyclobenzaprine 5 mg TID, but no benefit over an NSAID (ibuprofen 800 mg TID) during a 7-day treatment of acute cervical pain presenting at the emergency department of a large university hospital [19]. In this small study of 61 patients, although findings did not reach statistical significance, pain was more quickly relieved in patients receiving cyclobenzaprine, and the degree of pain intensity relief was greater for cyclobenzaprine compared to ibuprofen and was greatest with a combination of cyclobenzaprine and the NSAID. Cyclobenzaprine is commonly prescribed at a dose of 10 mg TID for muscle spasm with local pain and tenderness, is thought to increase range of motion, and is associated with a high incidence of side effects such as drowsiness and xerostomia. Interestingly, an industry-funded dose ranging study suggests 5 mg TID produces less side effect while maintaining efficacy [20].

Cylobenzaprine, like the related tricyclic antidepressants and also opioids, activates toll-like receptors (TLR) in spinal microglial cells [21]. Glial cell activation can have profound effects modulating pain and affect opioid-induced analgesia and tolerance. A mechanism by which tricyclic antidepressant class drugs including amitriptyline, imipramine, desipramine, cyclobenzaprine, carbamazepine, and oxcarbazepine can potentiate opioid analgesia has been demonstrated in mice [21]. These findings may explain how these drugs function as analgesics in chronic pain syndromes.

Carisoprodol

Regarding the non-tricyclic antidepressant muscle relaxants, one of the most controversial is carisoprodol (Fig. 7.3). Compared to placebo, it demonstrates efficacy for relief from acute muscle spasm and improved functional status at doses of 250 mg QID, although it is usually prescribed at 350 mg QID, a dose associated with a higher incidence of adverse effects [22]. Ralph et al. suggest carisoprodol would be a better drug if prescribed at the lower dose of 250 mg; however, the study was industry-sponsored, and authors disclosed they served on a speaker's bureau for the product [22].

Carisoprodol is metabolized to meprobamate, an anxiolytic and hypnotic with known abuse potential, which also has a longer half-life. Either drug at a sufficient dose can produce mental impairment. An extensive database on nonalcoholic impaired drivers maintained in Norway includes extensive testing of mental function matched with forensic blood testing for drugs including carisoprodol and meprobamate. Impaired drivers admitted to consuming doses of carisoprodol greater than 700 mg and high carisoprodol levels correlated with impairment. Interestingly, Bramness et al. also reported that regular users of carisoprodol did not demonstrate high levels of meprobamate. The study was not designed to identify the mechanism though it was suggested that these patients had developed tolerance for the impairment caused by this active metabolite, while occasional users of carisoprodol who had not yet developed tolerance tended to have higher levels of meprobamate [23]. Metabolism of carisoprodol to meprobamate occurs via the CYP2C19 variant of cytochrome P450 in the liver. If there is variation of the cytochrome P450-CYP2C19 gene, it would be expected to affect meprobamate levels and subsequent side effects. For example, an individual with two CYP2C19 alleles may make more meprobamate and may have increased potential risk for impairment while driving [24].

An extreme case of withdrawal occurred in a patient taking a very high dose of carisoprodol, more than 17 g/day. Some might conclude that if such large doses could be tolerated, carisoprodol may actually have a high therapeutic index. In this case, withdrawal delirium occurred in a patient with back pain due to trauma who purchased large doses of carisoprodol over the internet when her health insurance lapsed. She was noted to be taking very high doses, up to fifty 350 mg tablets per day. She was not overly sedated and

Carisoprodol
$C_{12}H_{24}N_2O_4$

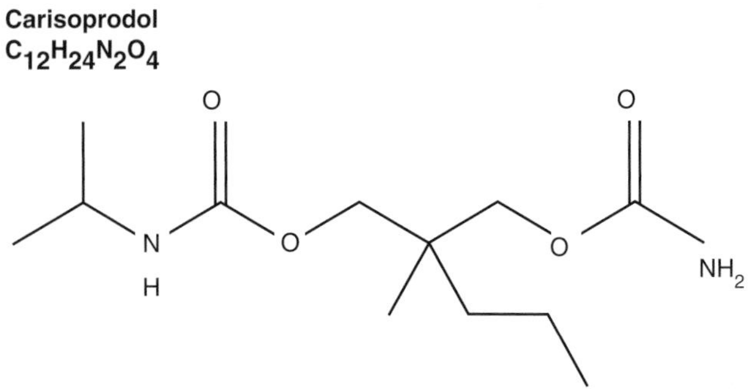

Fig. 7.3 Regarding the non-tricyclic antidepressant muscle relaxants, one of the most controversial is carisoprodol. Compared to placebo, it demonstrates efficacy for relief from acute muscle spasm and improved functional status at doses of 250 mg QID, although it is usually prescribed at 350 mg QID, a dose associated with a higher incidence of adverse effects

probably developed tolerance to the active metabolite, meprobamate. Seven days after deciding to stop, she lost orientation to person, place, and time and reported visual hallucinations, and postural and action tremors were noted on exam. Symptoms of delirium responded to treatment with 2 mg doses of lorazepam [25].

Concern for carisoprodol abuse since the Bramness study has led Norway to reclassify it as class-A (most restricted) led 39 of the United States to restrict its prescribing and led to a drive for the DEA to reclassify carisoprodol as a class-IV drug [26]. A case-control study was done in elderly patients identifying 8,164 cases and as many controls from a population of 1.5 million enrollees in a Medicare Advantage plan offered by a large HMO. Elderly patients receiving muscle relaxants were 1.4 times more likely to suffer a fracture injury, and the authors advised extreme caution be used prescribing muscle relaxants for older adults [27].

As our population ages, increased attention should be given to use and monitoring in elderly patients. Muscle relaxants are not recommended for patients over 65 years of age due to increased risk of injury due to side effects and should specifically to be avoided for elderly patients with bladder outflow obstruction and cognitive impairment [28].

However, while many reports as well as common wisdom advises against the use of muscle relaxants in the elderly, it has recently been suggested that skeletal muscle relaxants may be appropriate in this age group, especially if the patient does not have a high burden of disease and first-line medications were ineffective [29].

Baclofen

The muscle relaxants are a dichotomous group with indications for "skeletal muscle conditions" and for "spasticity" originating in the central nervous system, such as found in upper motor neuron disorders. Spasticity is an active muscle

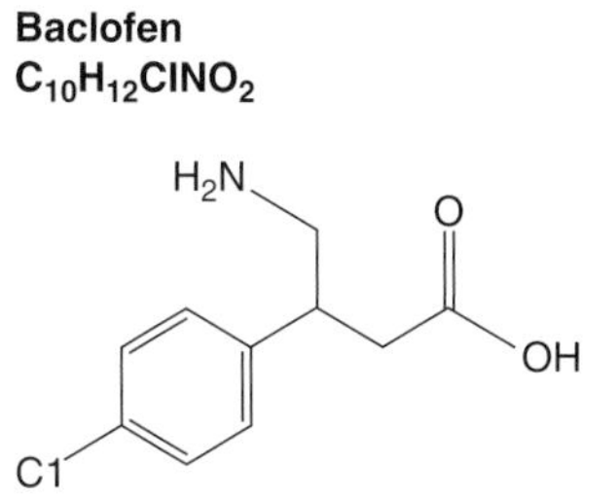

Baclofen
C$_{10}$H$_{12}$ClNO$_2$

Fig. 7.4 The traditional mainstay of treatment for upper motor neuron spasticity is baclofen, which has been used orally since the 1970s and, more recently, intrathecally

C$_{19}$H$_{21}$FN$_4$O$_6$
Mol. Wt.: 420.39

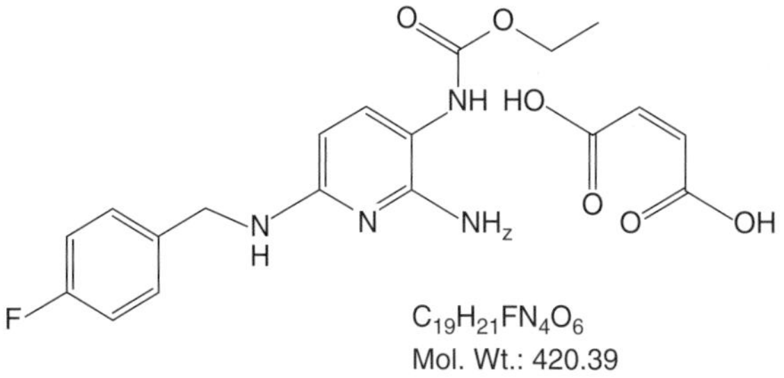

Fig. 7.5 Of the muscle relaxants not available in the United States, one that should be mentioned is flupirtine. Developed in Germany in the 1980s, flupirtine has been described as having many potential analgesic roles, and, equipotent to tramadol, it may also function as a muscle relaxant

process whereby loss of central modulation causes increased excitability of the stretch reflex such that there is a velocity-sensitive response to limb manipulation [30]. Spasticity results from upper motor neuron pathology with abnormal stretch reflexes that may be the result of changed muscle structure, development of new spinal level collaterals, and/or failure to adequately regulate supraspinal pathways resulting in increased spinal reflex responses [31].

The traditional mainstay of treatment for upper motor neuron spasticity is baclofen, which has been used orally since the 1970s and, more recently, intrathecally (Fig. 7.4). To assess the possible survival advantage of intrathecal baclofen for cerebral palsy patients, 359 patients from Minnesota with intrathecal baclofen pumps were compared with 349 matched controls that were selected from 27,962 Californians with CP who did not have pumps. Interestingly, the survival for those with intrathecal baclofen was somewhat better than their well-matched controls [32].

Whereas benzodiazepines work at GABA-A receptors, increasing chloride ion currents causing cell hyperpolarization and thus inhibiting action potentials, baclofen activates the GABA-B receptor [33]. Designed to mimic GABA, baclofen is basically a GABA molecule with a chlorinated phenol moiety, hence its chemical name p-chlorophenyl-GABA. The only available prescription medicine that activates GABA-B receptors, baclofen has been the drug of choice for the treatment of tetanus, stiff man syndrome, cerebral palsy, and multiple sclerosis. In addition to treatment of spasticity, GABA-B receptor activation may also have a role in treatment of pain, depression and anxiety, drug addiction, and absence epilepsy, and GABA-B receptor antagonism may have a role in treating cognitive impairment [33].

Baclofen as a visceral pain reliever has been studied in sensitized visceral pain models where it appears to have a central site of action in the dorsal horn of the spinal cord at GABA-B receptors and, in a dose response fashion, attenuates both pain behavior and expression of FOS (a nociceptive marker). However, in the dose range that produced the analgesic effect, marked sedation was also observed [34].

In addition to the side effects of its use, in its withdrawal, baclofen may produce respiratory failure, unstable hemody-

namics, seizures not responsive to usual treatment, and delirium. Interestingly, delirium is caused by both overdose and rapid withdrawal. If an intrathecal pump fails or needs to be removed due to infection, it is difficult using oral dosing to produce sufficient levels of baclofen in the CSF to prevent these catastrophic effects, and treatment with benzodiazepines, propofol, neuromuscular blocking agents, dantrolene, and tizanidine may be required in an ICU setting [35]. Baclofen and tizanidine withdrawal acutely produced extrapyramidal signs, delirium, and autonomic dysfunction that were eventually reversed when baclofen was restarted in a sufficient dose [36]. For a clear review of the differential diagnosis of baclofen withdrawal, the reader is referred to a recent case report with an excellent summary chart [37].

Other Muscle Relaxants

Of the muscle relaxants not available in the United States, one that should be mentioned is flupirtine (Fig. 7.5).

Developed in Germany in the 1980s, flupirtine has been described as having many potential analgesic roles, and, equipotent to tramadol, it may also function as a muscle relaxant. Flupirtine activates Kv7 potassium channels, produces an M-current, and dampens hyperexcitable neurons [38]. The Kv7 potassium channel is activated by muscarine and is receiving a great deal of attention recently. There is speculation that further work could lead to new treatments for Alzheimer's disease, seizure disorders, and chronic pain. The subtypes of Kv7 potassium channels regulate the potassium M-current activated by muscarine. Thus, muscarine (or other drugs acting at these sites) can lead to changes in potassium conductance with activation leading to hyperpolarization and blockade leading to increased neuronal activity. The M-current is a low-threshold, non-inactivating voltage-dependent potassium current at the Kv7 channel capable of limiting repetitive firing of neuronal action potentials [39]. Hyperexcitable states

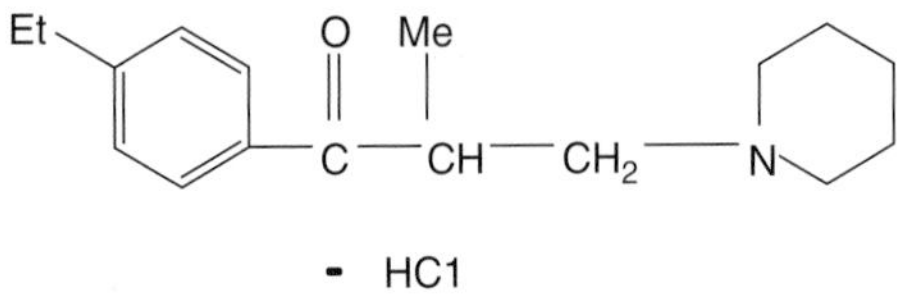

Fig. 7.6 Used to treat painful contracture and spasticity, eperisone inhibits gamma-efferent firing in the spinal cord and produces local vasodilatation and rarely has adverse CNS affects. It has good bioavailability, short onset time, and rapid elimination making it suitable for initial treatment of acute low back pain

Tizanidine HCl
$C_9H_8ClN_5S \cdot HCl$

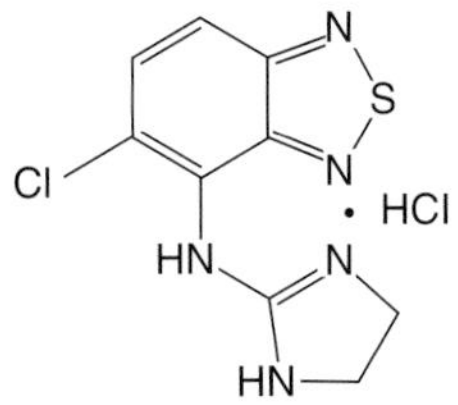

Fig. 7.7 Tizanidine is an alpha-2 agonist which has been shown to have beneficial results in the treatment of muscle spasm

such as seizure disorders and chronic pain, including muscle pain and spasm, may respond to channel activators, while blockers at Kv7 channels might increase neuronal activation and provide a treatment of Alzheimer's [39].

Used to treat painful contracture and spasticity, eperisone inhibits gamma-efferent firing in the spinal cord and produces local vasodilatation and rarely has adverse CNS effects (Fig. 7.6). It has good bioavailability, short onset time, and rapid elimination, making it suitable for initial treatment of acute low back pain [40].

While eperisone appears effective for treatment of muscle contracture and chronic low back pain, it is also touted to be free of sedative side effects [41]. Blood flow in low back muscles may increase with eperisone treatment over 4 weeks in comparison with placebo and active physical therapy protocols [42].

Tizanidine

Tizanidine is an alpha-2 agonist which has been shown to have beneficial results in the treatment of muscle spasm (Fig. 7.7). The reader is referred to a major review of the drug class muscle relaxants, Chou et al. [43]. This is an important work and will be given attention in the following paragraphs. The aim of the ambitious 237-page electronic book in the public domain, available at http://www.ncbi.nlm.nih.gov/pubmed/20496453, was to determine among nine muscle relaxants (baclofen, carisoprodol, chlorzoxazone, cyclobenzaprine, dantrolene, metaxalone, methocarbamol, orphenadrine, and tizanidine), whether one or more were superior in efficacy or safety for treatment of muscle spasticity mostly due to multiple sclerosis or for musculoskeletal conditions such as neck and low back pain compared with the others. Only tizanidine was found to have fair quality evidence for effectiveness in both spasticity and musculoskeletal conditions. Spasticity was evaluated in 59 trials; however, only 18 included an active control, which was sometimes another muscle relaxant. None of the 18 was considered high quality with each containing at least two methodological flaws. For example, there were nine trials comparing baclofen to tizanidine and eight comparing diazepam with tizanidine, baclofen, or dantrolene. Except for one trial comparing clonidine to baclofen, they reported no muscle relaxant trials where

the following common adjuvants were used as active controls: clonidine, gabapentin, and other benzodiazepines. There were 5 reviews and 52 trials reviewed for efficacy and safety for muscle relaxant use in musculoskeletal conditions (as opposed to spasticity). Twelve trials used a muscle relaxant as an active control against another muscle relaxant. No active control trials for efficacy or safety for musculoskeletal conditions were found for baclofen, dantrolene, metaxalone, or orphenadrine.

Based on nine head-to-head trials, Chou et al. report that tizanidine and baclofen have similar efficacy for the treatment of spasm including improvement in tone, clonus, and assessments of function and physician and patient preference [43].

Head-to-head trials of muscle relaxants used for musculoskeletal conditions are less common with only two showing carisoprodol or chlorzoxazone, both superior to the active control diazepam, and three showing cyclobenzaprine equivalent to it [43]. Although methodologies were flawed, Chou et al. report that compared to placebo, efficacy has been shown for cyclobenzaprine, carisoprodol, orphenadrine, and tizanidine, while evidence of efficacy is poor for baclofen, chlorzoxazone, dantrolene, methocarbamol, or metaxalone [43].

The Oregon Health & Science University group also reviewed relative risks of treatment including abuse, addiction, and other adverse effects. Used in treatment of spasticity, tizanidine and baclofen have different side effect profiles with the former associated with xerostomia and the latter with weakness [43]. Other muscle relaxants could not be compared head to head due to lack of good evidence. Major side effects included hepatic toxicity for dantrolene and tizanidine but not for baclofen, and quantitative comparisons could not be made for serious adverse events such as seizures, withdrawal reaction, and overdose. Frequent adverse events included somnolence, weakness, dizziness, and dry mouth. Abuse and addiction were not evaluated in these studies.

Diazepam

Benzodiazepines have been shown to reduce muscle spasm, especially in the postoperative period but their use is often limited by sedation (Fig. 7.8). This class of drugs is discussed elsewhere in the text.

Diazepam

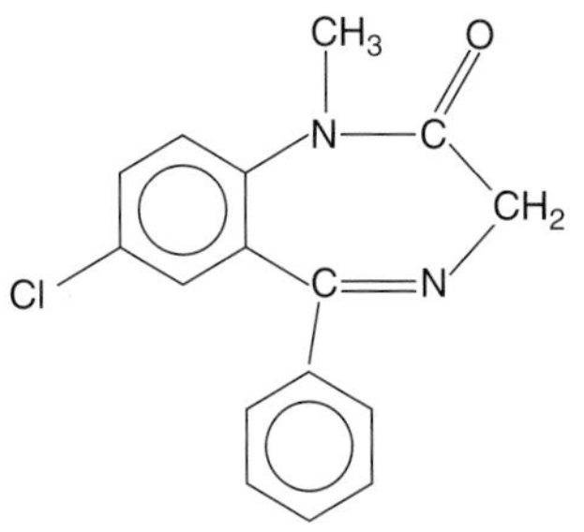

Fig. 7.8 Diazepam. Benzodiazepines have been shown to reduce muscle spasm, especially in the postoperative period but their use is often limited by sedation

Dantrolene
$C_{14}H_{10}N_4O_5$

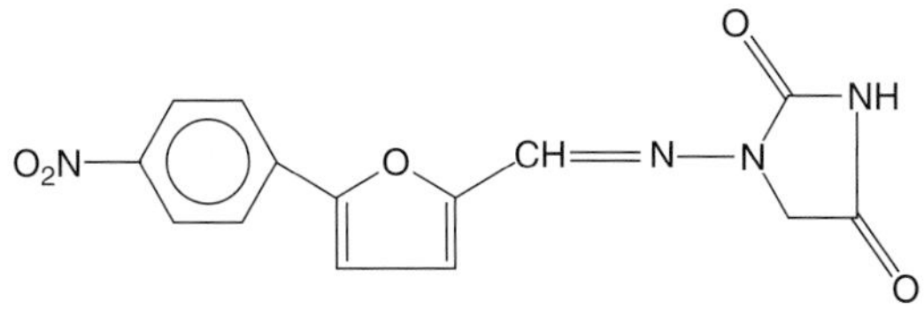

Fig. 7.9 Dantrolene appears to work by abolishing excitation/contraction coupling within muscle

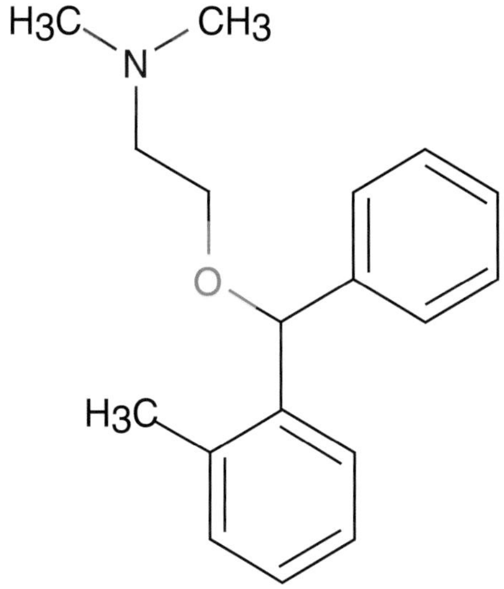

Fig. 7.10 While technically an anticholinergic of the antihistamine class and not a muscle relaxant drug, orphenadrine has been used to treat muscle spasm and pain, but its effectiveness in doing so has not been clearly proven

Quinine
$C_{20}H_{24}N_2O_2 \cdot \frac{1}{2}H_2O_4S \cdot H_2O$

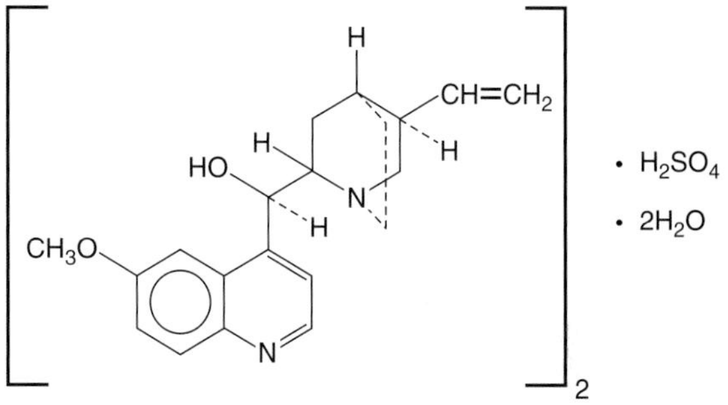

Fig. 7.11 Although not classified as a skeletal muscle relaxant, quinine has long been used to treat muscle cramps

Dantrolene

Dantrolene appears to work by abolishing excitation/contraction coupling within muscle (Fig. 7.9). While dantrolene has the capacity to reduce muscle spasm and spasticity, its use has been severely limited by its hepatic, cardiovascular, and pulmonary toxicity and by severe CNS side effects including visual disturbances, hallucinations, seizures, and depression. It remains useful as a treatment for malignant hyperthermia.

Orphenadrine

While technically an anticholinergic of the antihistamine class and not a muscle relaxant drug, orphenadrine has been used to treat muscle spasm and pain, but its effectiveness in doing so has not been clearly proven (Fig. 7.10).

Quinine

Although not classified as a skeletal muscle relaxant, quinine has long been used to treat muscle cramps (Fig. 7.11). An extensive Cochrane review summarizes 23 trials with 1,586 participants at daily doses between 200 and 500 mg and concludes there is evidence of moderate quality for reduction in intensity and frequency of cramping pain and that when used

for up to 60 days, although there is increase in side effects such as GI symptoms, the serious side effect rate is similar to placebo [44].

Botulinum Toxin

Finally, no discussion of muscle relaxants to treat musculoskeletal conditions and spasticity would be complete without mentioning botulinum toxin. Botulinum toxin type A, but not type B, is helpful for spasticity acting presynaptically at the myoneural junction by inhibiting acetylcholine vesicle release leading to decreased contraction strength and is now considered first-line treatment for spasticity (Fig.7.12) [31]. Further details in the mechanism of action and application of botulinum toxin in treatment of disease are discussed elsewhere in this textbook.

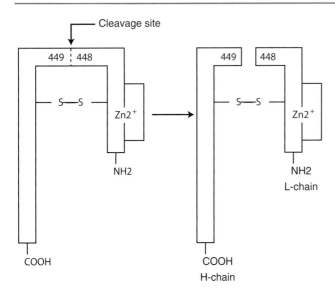

Fig. 7.12 Botulinum toxin type A, but not type B, is helpful for spasticity acting presynaptically at the myoneural junction by inhibiting acetylcholine vesicle release leading to decreased contraction strength and is now considered first-line treatment for spasticity

References

1. Chou R. Pharmacological management of low back pain. Drugs. 2010;70(4):387–402.
2. Ivanova JI, et al. Real-world practice patterns, health-care utilization, and costs in patients with low back pain: the long road to guideline-concordant care. Spine J. 2011;11:622–32.
3. Jackson JL, Browning R. Impact of national low back pain guidelines on clinical practice. South Med J. 2005;98(2):139–43.
4. Cammisa C, et al. Engaging physicians in change: results of a safety net quality improvement program to reduce overuse. Am J Med Qual. 2011;26(1):26–33.
5. Bernstein E, Carey TS, Garrett JM. The use of muscle relaxant medications in acute low back pain. Spine. 2004;29(12):1345–51.
6. Knauer SR, Freburger JK, Carey TS. Chronic low back pain among older adults: a population-based perspective. J Aging Health. 2010;22(8):1213–34.
7. Kuijpers T, et al. A systematic review on the effectiveness of pharmacological interventions for chronic non-specific low-back pain. Eur Spine J. 2011;20(1):40–50.
8. van Tulder MW, et al. Muscle relaxants for non-specific low back pain. Cochrane Database Syst Rev. 2003;2:CD004252.
9. Morlion B. Pharmacotherapy of low back pain: targeting nociceptive and neuropathic pain components. Curr Med Res Opin. 2011;27(1):11–33.
10. Kim CS, et al. Teaching internal medicine residents quality improvement and patient safety: a lean thinking approach. Am J Med Qual. 2010;25(3):211–7.
11. McNett M, et al. Treatment patterns among physician specialties in the management of fibromyalgia: results of a cross-sectional study in the United States. Curr Med Res Opin. 2011;27(3):673–83.
12. Dussias P, Kalali AH, Staud RM. Treatment of fibromyalgia. Psychiatry. 2010;7(5):15–8.
13. Bendtsen L, et al. EFNS guideline on the treatment of tension-type headache – report of an EFNS task force. Eur J Neurol. 2010;17(11):1318–25.

14. Toth PP, Urtis J. Commonly used muscle relaxant therapies for acute low back pain- a review of carisoprodol, cyclobenzaprine hydrochloride, and metaxalone. Clin Ther. 2004;26(9):1355–67.
15. Kobayashi H, Hasegawa Y, Ono H. Cyclobenzaprine, a centrally acting muscle relaxant, acts on descending serotonergic systems. Eur J Pharmacol. 1996;311(1):29–35.
16. Lofland JH, Szarlej S, Buttaro T, Shermock S, Jalali S. Cyclobenzaprine hydrochloride is a commonly prescribed centrally acting muscle relaxant which is structurally similar TCAs and differs amitriptyline one double bond. Clin J Pain. 2001;17(1):103–4.
17. Ogawa T, et al. High-throughput and simultaneous analysis of eight central-acting muscle relaxants in human plasma by ultra-performance liquid chromatography-tandem mass spectrometry in the positive and negative ionization modes. Anal Bioanal Chem. 2011;400(7):1959–65.
18. Browning R, Jackson JL, O'Malley PG. Cyclobenzaprine and back pain: a meta-analysis. Arch Intern Med. 2001;161(13):1613–20.
19. Khwaja SM, Minnerop M, Singer AJ. Comparison of ibuprofen, cyclobenzaprine or both in patients with acute cervical strain- a randomized controlled trial. CJEM. 2010;12(1):39–44.
20. Borenstein DG, Korn S. Efficacy of a low-dose regimen of cyclobenzaprine hydrochloride in acute skeletal muscle spasm- results of two placebo-controlled trials. Clin Ther. 2003;25(4):1056–73.
21. Hutchinson MR, et al. Evidence that tricyclic small molecules may possess toll-like receptor and myeloid differentiation protein 2 activity. Neuroscience. 2010;168(2):551–63.
22. Ralph L, et al. Double-blind, placebo-controlled trial of carisoprodol 250-mg tablets in the treatment of acute lower-back spasm. Curr Med Res Opin. 2008;24(2):551–8.
23. Bramness JG, Skurtveit S, Morland J. Impairment due to intake of carisoprodol. Drug Alcohol Depend. 2004;74(3):311–8.
24. Musshoff F, Stamer UM, Madea B. Pharmacogenetics and forensic toxicology. Forensic Sci Int. 2010;203(1–3):53–62.
25. Ni K, Cary M, Zarkowski P. Carisoprodol withdrawal induced delirium – a case study. Neuropsychiatr Dis Treat. 2007;3(5):679–82.
26. Fass JA. Carisoprodol legal status and patterns of abuse. Ann Pharmacother. 2010;44(12):1962–7.
27. Golden AG, et al. Risk for fractures with centrally acting muscle relaxants: an analysis of a national Medicare advantage claims database. Ann Pharmacother. 2010;44(9):1369–75.
28. Fick DM. Updating the beers criteria for potentially inappropriate medication use in older adults: results of a US consensus panel of experts. Arch Intern Med. 2003;163(22):2716–24.
29. Billups SJ, Delate T, Hoover B. Injury in an elderly population before and after initiating a skeletal muscle relaxant. Ann Pharmacother. 2011;45(4):485–91.
30. Nielsen JB, Crone C, Hultborn H. The spinal pathophysiology of spasticity – from a basic science point of view. Acta Physiol. 2007;189(2):171–80.
31. Simon O, Yelnik A. Managing spasticity with drugs. Eur J Phys Rehabil Med. 2010;46(3):401–10.
32. Krach LE, et al. Survival of individuals with cerebral palsy receiving continuous intrathecal baclofen treatment: a matched-cohort study. Dev Med Child Neurol. 2010;52(7):672–6.
33. Bowery NG. GABAB receptor: a site of therapeutic benefit. Curr Opin Pharmacol. 2006;6(1):37–43.
34. Liu LS, Shenoy M, Pasricha PJ. The analgesic effects of the GABA(B) receptor agonist, baclofen, in a rodent model of functional dyspepsia. Neurogastroenterol Motil. 2011;23(4):356–61.
35. Ross JC, et al. Acute intrathecal baclofen withdrawal: a brief review of treatment options. Neurocrit Care. 2011;14(1):103–8.
36. Karol DE, Muzyk AJ, Preud'homme XA. A case of delirium, motor disturbances, and autonomic dysfunction due to baclofen and tizanidine withdrawal: a review of the literature. Gen Hosp Psychiatry. 2011;33(1):84.e1–2.

37. Ross JC, et al. Acute intrathecal baclofen withdrawal: a brief review of treatment options. Neurocrit Care. 2010;14(1):103–8.

38. Devulder J. Flupirtine in pain management: pharmacological properties and clinical use. CNS Drugs. 2010;24(10):867–81.

39. Miceli F, et al. Molecular pharmacology and therapeutic potential of neuronal Kv7-modulating drugs. Curr Opin Pharmacol. 2008;8(1):65–74.

40. Melilli B, et al. Human pharmacokinetics of the muscle relaxant, eperisone hydrochloride by liquid chromatography-electrospray tandem mass spectrometry. Eur J Drug Metab Pharmacokinet. 2011;36(2):71–8.

41. Pham JC, et al. ReCASTing the RCA: an improved model for performing root cause analyses. Am J Med Qual. 2010;25(3):186–91.

42. Dull DL, Fox L. Perception of intimidation in a perioperative setting. Am J Med Qual. 2010;25(2):87–94.

43. Chou R, Peterson K. Drug class review on skeletal muscle relaxants: final report. Portland: Oregon Health & Science University; 2005.

44. El-Tawil S, et al. Quinine for muscle cramps. Cochrane Database Syst Rev. 2010;(12):CD005044.

Topical Analgesics

Charles E. Argoff, Manpreet Kaur,
and Kelly Donnelly

Key Points
- Topical analgesics differ from systemic analgesics especially because the systemic concentration of the analgesic is likely to be low compared to systemic analgesics.
- Do not confuse topical analgesics with transdermal analgesics that use the skin as a means for the analgesic to achieve a systemic concentration.
- Even though the site of action of a topical analgesic may be within the peripheral nervous system, there may be central nervous system effects of the topical analgesic.
- Topical analgesics are often more tolerable than systemic analgesics.
- There is significant evidence for the potential clinical benefit of topical analgesics for a broad range of chronic pain conditions including various neuropathic as well as non-neuropathic states.

Introduction

Topical analgesics differ from systemic analgesics by exhibiting analgesia without significant systemic absorption as compared to systemic analgesics, which require systemic absorption for their analgesic activity. Topical analgesics are frequently confused with transdermal agents; however, they differ from transdermal analgesics (e.g., transdermal fentanyl patch) because systemic absorption of a transdermal agent is required for clinical benefit. There is a variety of mechanism of actions of specific topical analgesics. Topical analgesics have been studied in acute pain as well as in various types of chronic pain including both non-neuropathic and neuropathic pain types. The results of many of these studies are described in this chapter. New data that suggest that topical analgesics which were assumed almost by definition, to act peripherally, may affect central pain processing are also discussed.

Background and Scientific Foundation

Pain, by definition, does not occur without the activation of relevant brain areas, and indeed, this fact has certainly been clearly established over the past few decades. At the same time, scientific advances have pointed to a significant role of the peripheral nervous system (PNS) in initiating and maintaining acute and chronic painful conditions; thus, it is not surprising that even though topical analgesics are believed to exert their principle analgesic activity peripherally, multiple chronic pain syndromes have been shown to be responsive to certain topical analgesics. In addition, while there are certain painful conditions such as central poststroke pain or spinal cord injury pain in which almost exclusively, the mechanisms of the pain lie entirely within the brain and/or central nervous system (CNS), other pain syndromes including those which we commonly encounter as clinicians including postherpetic neuralgia (PHN), chronic low back pain (CLBP), and osteoarthritis (OA) ultimately likely result from both peripheral as well as CNS mechanisms. The designation of a medication as a topical analgesic has been made when the analgesic is applied locally and directly to the painful areas and whose primary site of action is local to the site of analgesic application. The term "topical analgesic" should not be confused with the term "transdermal analgesic" which in contrast to a topical analgesic requires a systemic analgesic concentration to be effective. Be aware that not infrequently

C.E. Argoff, M.D. (✉)
Neurology/Comprehensive Pain Center, Albany Medical College,
4 Loudon Lane North, Loudonville, NY 12211, USA

Comprehensive Pain Center, Albany Medical Center,
Albany, NY, USA
e-mail: cargoff@nycap.rr.com

M. Kaur, M.D. • K. Donnelly, DO
Department of Neurology, Albany Medical Center,
47 New Scotland Avenue, Albany, NY 12208, USA
e-mail: kaurm@mail.amc.edu; donnelk1@mail.amc.edu

in the authors' experiences, analgesics have been inappropriately considered as "topical" agents even when formal pharmacological studies to demonstrate a lack of systemic activity and/or systemic drug concentration had not been completed.

Nociception, the activation of specialized nerve endings by mechanical, thermal, and/or chemical stimuli, is not equivalent to pain, yet interfering with nociception can possibly result in a person experiencing less pain. Consequently, even though the mechanism of action of a topical analgesic may largely be within the peripheral nervous system and thus on nociceptive mechanisms, this peripheral effect may actually lead to a reduction of central pain mechanisms and thus pain as well. Put another way, since the pain experience requires the brain receiving and processing pain-related information, if less such information from the PNS presents to the CNS for central processing, it is certainly possible that fewer central mechanisms will be activated and thus less pain experienced. This chapter reviews the use of topical analgesics in the treatment of various painful conditions and provides an update to previously published similar reviews [1–3].

The clinical effectiveness of any analgesic or, for that matter, any medication may be diminished by that medication's adverse effect profile, toxicities, and drug-drug interaction. The risk and severity of significant adverse effects and drug-drug interactions are less than for the same medication given systemically [4]. This may be especially important when considering what type of nonsteroidal anti-inflammatory (NSAID) agent to use for a given patient as will be discussed further below. Localized drug effects such as rash or unpleasant skin sensations have been described but are not generally experienced [5]. Additionally, since the use of a topical analgesic does not result in a significant systemic concentration of the analgesic, the use of a topical analgesic does not produce significant systemic accumulation of the specific analgesic. Of the FDA-approved topical analgesics, the 5 % lidocaine patch (Lidoderm®) has been one of the most extensively studied. It might help to illustrate some of the above principles by focusing briefly on this preparation. The tolerability and safety of daily, 24 h/day, use of four lidocaine 5 % patches has been specifically studied. The results demonstrate that there were no significant systemic side effects experienced and plasma lidocaine levels remained below those that have been associated with cardiac abnormalities. Similar safety and tolerability was noted regardless of whether or not the subject used the patch for 12- or 24-h daily [6]. In a separate investigation, patients with a history of chronic low back pain were treated safely with four lidocaine 5 % patches every 24 h for extended periods [5]. No significant dermal reactions were experienced in either of these reports [6, 7].

In addition to the potential for dermal sensitivity, other adverse effects may be associated with the use of specific topical analgesic that is, in general, specific to the particular chemical entity in the preparation. For example, upon application of topical capsaicin, severe burning at the site of application may occur in the overwhelming majority of treated patients. This effect may in fact lead to a reduced effectiveness of this type of topical analgesic because although this drug when applied topically in its currently available forms does not result in significant systemic accumulation or in any life-threatening outcomes, and even though the incidence of burning may decrease with repeated use, the frequent occurrence of this side effect may negatively impact upon patient compliance and, as a result, may potentially hinder the patient's ability to benefit from it [8]. However, as will be discussed below, the 8 % capsaicin patch (Qutenza®), now FDA approved for the treatment of PHN, was generally well tolerated in the clinical trials completed, leading to its approval.

The fact that drug-drug interactions may be minimized when using topical analgesics may be of enormous importance for a patient who must use systemic medications concurrently for additional medical conditions. This is a point that has been emphasized in recent guidelines for the pharmacotherapeutic management of persistent pain in older adults [9]. Consider, for example, an 82-year-old person who suffers from hypertension, coronary artery disease, and type 2 diabetes mellitus. Consider that this person requires analgesic treatment for his knee OA. He is using a total of six other medications for his other chronic medical conditions. Assuming that comparable or even better pain relief is experienced, the use of a topical medication in this setting may offer several advantages over a systemic agent due to the lack of drug-drug interactions [10]. The use of a topical analgesic in place of or in addition to a systemic analgesic may have an additional advantage in that the use of a topical analgesic does not typically require dose titration, making these relatively simple medications to use.

Not all "topical" analgesics are prescribed as commercially available, FDA-approved agents. When prescribing a topical analgesic, one must distinguish between those which are FDA (or other similar agency in non-US countries) approved, commercially available, and with consistent manufacturing standards/quality control and those that may be manufactured on an individualized basis by a specialized compounding pharmacy. Many of the "topical" analgesics currently in use are not commercially available products, and for many years, health-care providers have ordered other so-called topical agents from compounding pharmacies. Often the preparations prescribed are combinations of medications put into a single product. This chapter will only review the use of those topical agents which are commercially available or for which there is clear evidence that they were manufactured in a dependable manner. To the best of our knowledge, for many compounding pharmacies, no matter the good intentions of the prescriber or pharmacy, there is no proof of quality control or consistency from one batch to another as would be required for an FDA-approved product. The reader might nevertheless appreciate that compounded, noncommercially available agents are prescribed as topical agents quite often, likely in an attempt to help a patient for whom other perhaps FDA-approved measures have not yielded effective results. For example, in a survey of members of the American Society of Regional Anesthesia and Pain Medicine, 27 % of the survey responders indicated that they prescribed such an agent, and 47 % of the responders reported that they felt that their patient responded positively to the prescribed agent(s) [11].

There appears to be increasing interest in the commercial development of new topical analgesics. As will be discussed below in more detail, recently, three topical NSAIDs and one high-concentration capsaicin preparation have been FDA approved, and in addition, opioids, local anesthetics, antidepressants, glutamate receptor antagonists, alpha-adrenergic receptor agonists, adenosine, cannabinoids, cholinergic receptor agonists, gabapentinoids, prostanoids, bradykinin, ATP, biogenic amines, and nerve growth factor are each being considered as potential topical analgesics [12].

Not surprisingly, the mechanism of action of each topical analgesic depends upon the specific analgesic. For example, the mechanism of action of capsaicin-containing topical analgesics appears through their agonist activity at the transient receptor potential vanilloid receptor 1 (TRPV1) on A-delta and C-fibers [13, 14]. This results in the release of substance P as well as calcitonin gene-related peptide (CGRP). With the older preparations, therapeutic responses to capsaicin were generally achieved only with repeated topical application; however, as will be summarized below, the more recently FDA-approved 8 % capsaicin patch has been shown to provide analgesic benefit for up to 12 weeks following a single 1-h application [15]. It has been suggested that reduced peripheral as well as central excitability with resulting less pain through reduced afferent input is the outcome of the depletion of substance P in C-fibers [8, 13, 15]. Histopathological examination results of human nerve biopsies as well as animal experiments have suggested that application of capsaicin may lead to nerve fiber degeneration in the skin underneath the site of application. This neurodegenerative effect of capsaicin has been hypothesized to be one of its mechanisms of pain relief [16]. In contrast, the mechanism of action of a topical NSAID is probably related to the inhibition of prostaglandin synthesis and associated anti-inflammatory effect; however, because the anti-inflammatory effect is not always proportional to the amount of pain relief experienced, additional mechanisms of action might also be important to consider [17]. The combination of different topical therapies may be synergistic, and as an example, the antinociceptive effects of topical morphine have been shown to be enhanced by a topical cannabinoid in a recent study in rats in which the radiant tail-flick test was utilized [18].

No similar human studies have thus far been published. The analgesic action of local anesthetic agents based upon currently available data appears to be related to the ability of these agents to suppress the activity of peripheral sodium channels within sensory afferents and subsequent pain transmission; however, other mechanisms of action are under investigation. Reduced expression of messenger ribonucleic acid (mRNA) for specific sodium channel subtypes following local anesthetic use has been reported as well [1, 5]. Several local anesthetic-containing analgesics which may be considered topical agents are currently commercially available. Although use of the 5 % lidocaine patch is associated with an *analgesic* effect without creating *anesthetic* skin, in contrast, the use of EMLA® cream (eutectic mixture of local anesthetics, 2.5 % lidocaine/2.5 % prilocaine) or the FDA-approved Synera™ patch (lidocaine 70 mg/tetracaine 70 mg) may create both analgesia as well as anesthesia when applied topically. In certain clinical settings, for example, venipuncture, lumbar puncture, intramuscular injections, and circumcision, this property of EMLA® or Synera™may actually be desirable. In other clinical situations, it might not be [5]. Choosing which topical analgesic to use clearly depends upon the clinical setting in which the medication is being used. A mechanism of action of the lidocaine 5 % patch as a topical agent which is unrelated to the active medication is that the patch itself may reduce the allodynia experienced by those afflicted by neuropathic pain states such as PHN through the patch's ability to protect the skin [1].

The development of tricyclic antidepressants as topical analgesics is novel and is under investigation. These agents as a group are known to have multiple mechanisms of action including sodium channel blockade; the potential clinical benefit of their ability to block sodium channels when topically applied is being actively investigated at this time [19, 20]. In fact, in the United States, there is currently one commercially available topical antidepressant, Zonalon® (doxepin hydrochloride) cream. While it is indicated for use by the FDA for the short-term treatment of adult patients with pruritis associated with atopic dermatitis or lichen simplex chronicus, there have been sporadic anecdotal reports of use of this agent in an "off-label" manner as a topical analgesic [21]. Other topical agents including topical opioids, glutamate receptor antagonists, and cannabinoids have potential as topical analgesics as well. Certain studies of some of these agents will be commented upon further below.

Clinical Examples

What follows is a summary of the clinical uses of topical agents based upon the painful disorder for which they are being used and/or for some FDA approved.

Neuropathic Pain

Without a doubt, clinical trial data provide varying levels of evidence for the use of certain topical analgesics in the treatment of neuropathic pain, and various published reviews of the treatment of neuropathic pain have emphasized the role of these agents [22–24].

Local Anesthetics

The lidocaine 5 % patch is FDA approved for the treatment of PHN. In fact, this agent was the first medication approved by the FDA for PHN. Clinical trials of PHN patients which led to the FDA approval demonstrated that use of the lidocaine 5 % patch by patients compared to use of placebo patches resulted in statistically significant more pain reduction and was in addition safe and well-tolerated [25, 26]. After the FDA approval of this drug for PHN, an open-label study was completed that was designed to examine the effect, if any, of the lidocaine 5 % patch on various quality of life measures. A total of 332 patients with PHN were studied, and a validated pain assessment tool, the Brief Pain Inventory (BPI), utilized. As many as three lidocaine 5 % patches, 12 h each day, were utilized by enrolled patients; the BPI was completed daily over 4 weeks. There were 204/332 (67 %) of the patients reported reduced pain intensity following repeated lidocaine 5 % patch application by the end of the first week of the study. Pain intensity reduction was noted by the second week of patch use in over 40 % of the remaining patients. Seventy percent of enrolled patients experienced notable improvement by the study's conclusion [27]. In a separate randomized open-label study in which use of the 5 % lidocaine patch was compared to the use of pregabalin (Lyrica®) for PHN, the 5 % lidocaine patch was determined to be at least as effective as pregabalin for pain relief in PHN patients with a favorable safety profile. Furthermore, in this study, for patients who were unresponsive to either the lidocaine 5 % patch or pregabalin as monotherapy, combining the use of these agents provided additional efficacy and was well tolerated by such patients [28].

Patients with neuropathic pain states other than PHN have also been treated with the lidocaine 5 % patch in various studies. In Europe, a randomized, double-blind, placebo-controlled trial studied the efficacy of the lidocaine 5 % patch in the treatment of "focal" neuropathic pain syndromes such as mononeuropathies, intercostal neuralgia, and ilioinguinal neuralgia. Trial results suggested that when the lidocaine 5 % patch is added to other pharmacotherapeutic regimens, the 5 % lidocaine patch can reduce ongoing pain as well as allodynia as quickly as in the first 8 h of use but also over a period of 7 days [29]. The results of another smaller open-label study of 16 patients with various chronic neuropathic pain conditions (post-thoracotomy pain, complex regional pain syndrome, postamputation pain, painful diabetic

neuropathy, meralgia paresthetica, postmastectomy pain, neuroma-related pain) demonstrated that the lidocaine 5 % patch provided pain relief without significant side effects in 81 % of these patients [30]. It is worthy to note that according to the study's authors, patients enrolled in this study, prior to the use of the lidocaine 5 % patch, had experienced suboptimal outcomes with numerous other agents commonly prescribed for the treatment of neuropathic pain. Several other noncontrolled studies of patients with painful diabetic neuropathy who were treated with the lidocaine 5 % patch have been completed. These studies allowed patients to use as many as four lidocaine 5 % patches for as long as 18 h/ day. Considered together as a group, these studies reported pain reduction for the majority of patients and good tolerability of this medication [31–34]. In a 3-week single center, open-label study of the lidocaine 5 % patch in patients with painful idiopathic sensory polyneuropathy, noted over the treatment period, significant improvements in both pain and quality of life measures were noted [35].

Changes in the quality of the pain of patients with PHN treated with the lidocaine 5 % patch compared to placebo were examined in a multicenter, randomized, vehicle-controlled study of 150 PHN patients who were treated with either actual or placebo lidocaine 5 % patches (up to three lidocaine 5 % or vehicle patches for 12 h each day). The use of the lidocaine 5 % patch but not the vehicle patch was associated with reduced intensity of certain neuropathic pain qualities utilizing the Neuropathic Pain Scale (NPS). The results additionally demonstrated that some of the qualities of neuropathic pain (deep, sharp, and burning) which were reduced had previously been assumed not to be related to peripheral but to central nervous system mechanisms. The authors of this study proposed that their results suggested that peripheral mechanisms of neuropathic pain might also indeed play a role in the development of these neuropathic pain qualities [36]. Also of great interest are the results of a functional brain MRI study of patients with PHN who were treated with the 5 % lidocaine patch for various time periods. Depending upon the length of application, brain activity for the spontaneous pain of PHN appeared to be modulated by treatment with this medication, again suggesting that a peripherally acting agent may have an impact on central pain mechanisms [37].

EMLA® cream is another local anesthetic preparation (the eutectic mixture of 2.5 % lidocaine and 2.5 % prilocaine). It is indicated as a topical anesthetic for use on normal intact skin for analgesia, but it is not FDA approved for any specific neuropathic pain disorder. Regardless, it is worth noting that several studies of the use of the eutectic preparation of 2.5 % lidocaine and 2.5 % prilocaine cream in the treatment of PHN have been completed. In a randomized, controlled study of PHN patients, treatment with the eutectic preparation of 2.5 % lidocaine and 2.5 % prilocaine cream did not result in significant differences between the treated and placebo groups [38]. In two studies, each of which was uncontrolled and thus less rigorously designed, the results were more encouraging suggesting that use of the eutectic preparation of 2.5 % lidocaine and 2.5 % prilocaine cream might relieve the pain associated with PHN [39, 40].

Capsaicin

There has been great interest in using capsaicin in a number of neuropathic pain disorders such as diabetic neuropathy, painful HIV neuropathy, PHN, and postmastectomy pain, but past available strengths of capsaicin (0.025 % and 0.075 %) had yielded disappointing results with the treatment being poorly tolerated, regimens poorly adhered to, and not enough pain relief experienced [41]. In contrast, examining the results of a higher-strength capsaicin preparation, notable analgesia had been reported by patients with painful HIV neuropathy receiving a 7.5 % topical capsaicin cream. The patients, to be able to tolerate this medication, required concurrent treatment with epidural anesthesia [42]. At the 2004 Annual Scientific Meeting of the American Academy of Neurology, two open-label studies, one in patients with PHN and one in patients with painful HIV-associated distal symmetrical polyneuropathy, reported notable pain relief for the majority of patients following the single application of a high-concentration (8 %) capsaicin patch. The duration of pain relief lasted as long as 48 weeks (PHN) [15, 43]. A review of the published randomized trials involving the use of topical capsaicin in the treatment of either neuropathic or musculoskeletal pain syndromes concluded that "although topically applied capsaicin has moderate to poor efficacy in the treatment of chronic musculoskeletal or neuropathic pain, it may be useful as an adjunct or sole therapy for a small number of patients who are unresponsive to, or intolerant of, other treatments" [44]. Recently, the 8 % capsaicin patch (Qutenza®) has received FDA approval for the treatment of PHN. In studies leading to its FDA approval, it was shown to be more effective in reducing pain intensity than an active, lower concentration capsaicin product that served as placebo, and it was generally well tolerated. It has also been studied in other neuropathic pain states such as painful HIV neuropathy with favorable outcome as well [45–49].

A novel study comparing the analgesic effect of a topical preparation containing either 3.3 % doxepin alone or 3.3 % doxepin combined with 0.075 % capsaicin to placebo in patients with various different chronic neuropathic pain problems demonstrated that each treatment resulted in equal degrees of analgesia and each was superior to placebo [50].

Other Agents

There has been interest in the use of topical tricyclic antidepressants in the treatment of neuropathic pain with clinical trials completed. In each two such studies, the preparation tested was a combination of amitriptyline 2 % and ketamine 1 %. The results of one of these, a double-blind, randomized, placebo-controlled study involving 92 patients with diabetic neuropathy, PHN, postsurgical, or posttraumatic neuropathic pain, were no difference in pain relief among the four treatment groups (placebo, amitriptyline 2 % alone, ketamine 1 % alone, or combination amitriptyline 2 %/ketamine 1 %) [51]. In a separate open-label study by the same group, 28 patients with neuropathic pain for 6–12 months were treated with the combination topical analgesic amitriptyline 2 %/ketamine 1 %. The investigators reported that on average, patients experienced 34 % pain reduction [52]. In another open-label study by the same group, the benefit of a combination of topical amitriptyline and ketamine for neuropathic pain also demonstrated encouraging results; however, no controlled study has yet been published [53]. Noncontrolled studies of topical ketamine, one in patients with PHN and one in patients with complex regional pain syndrome type 1, have suggested that topical ketamine may be an effective topical analgesic; however, serum ketamine levels were not measured in either study [54]. There is one report that suggests that the topical application of geranium oil may provide temporary relief from PHN [55].

Case Example: A 35-year-old female with complex regional pain syndrome type 2 following a traumatic injury to her left peroneal nerve presents to your office for evaluation and treatment. She is married with two children and is currently working part-time as an accountant. She is utilizing several medications and complains of severe, burning pain and hypersensitivity to anything that touches her left leg and foot, with a visual analogue scale score of 6/10. The pain is continuous but worst at night. She has achieved 30 % pain relief taking both duloxetine and pregabalin at maximally tolerated doses. She has failed a trial of both spinal as well as peripheral nerve stimulation and had previously benefitted only temporarily from sympathetic nerve blocks. Should this person be treated as well with a topical analgesic, even in an "off-label" manner? If so, which and what evidence do we use in making this decision? We think it would be reasonable to attempt such treatment providing the patient was fully informed of the "off-label" use, the potential benefits and risk of the prescribed agent, and the evidence for its use and of course the patient was to be properly monitored.

Soft Tissue Injuries and Osteoarthritis

Soft tissue injuries and osteoarthritis are each an example of musculoskeletal pain states. The use of topical analgesics for these heterogeneous conditions has been actively studied, and in fact, since 2007, the FDA has approved three topical NSAIDs. The diclofenac sodium gel 1 % (Voltaren gel 1 %) was FDA approved for use in treating pain associated with OA in joints that can be managed with topical treatment such as the knees and hands. The diclofenac epolamine topical patch (Flector® patch) has been FDA approved for the topical treatment of acute pain due to minor strains, sprains, and contusions. The diclofenac sodium topical solution (Pennsaid) has been FDA approved for the treatment of the signs and symptoms of OA of the knee [56]. Additional information about these more recently FDA-approved agents as well as other topical therapies for these conditions is reviewed below.

NSAIDs

Outside of the US, other topical NSAIDs have been studied. The use of a topical ketoprofen patch (100 mg) was superior to placebo in reducing pain after 1 week of treatment in a 14-day randomized, placebo-controlled study of 163 patients with an ankle sprain [57]. A similar ketoprofen preparation has been studied in patients with tendonitis in a randomized, double-blind, placebo-controlled study. Results were positive in favor of the active treatment, and the treatment was in general, except for skin irritation, well tolerated [58]. In a child with Sever's disease, a common cause of heel pain in athletic children, ketoprofen gel has been used as adjunctive therapy to physical therapy with reported benefit [59]. In a randomized, controlled study of a diclofenac patch in 120 individuals experiencing acute pain following a "blunt" injury, use of the patch was well tolerated as well as significantly better than placebo in reducing the pain associated with this injury [60]. In two separate studies (one open-label and one multicenter, randomized, controlled study), each completed by different investigators, of pain associated with acute sports injuries, a diclofenac patch was found to be effective in providing pain relief and well tolerated. On average, patients experienced 60 % pain relief in the open-label study [61, 62]. An open-label study of patients with "soft tissue pain" concluded that topical flurbiprofen was associated with greater pain reduction than oral diclofenac with fewer adverse effects reported [63]. In another controlled study, the use of topical ibuprofen cream in the management of acute ankle sprains was found to be superior to placebo in reducing pain [64]. In a controlled study of ketoprofen gel in the management of acute soft tissue pain, the gel was found to be more effective than placebo in providing pain relief [65]. A topical formulation of 5 % ibuprofen gel was examined in a placebo-controlled study in patients with painful soft tissue injuries. Patients received either the 5 % ibuprofen gel ($n=40$) or placebo gel ($n=41$) for a maximum of 7 days. Pain intensity levels as well as limitations of physical activity were assessed daily. A significant difference ($p<0.001$) in pain reduction as well as improvement in physical activities for those patients who received the active gel compared to placebo recipients was noted [66]. An additional study of a similar population of patients

completed by the same investigators resulted in similar outcomes [67]. A recent Cochrane Database review has concluded that topical NSAIDs can provide good levels of pain relief without the systemic adverse effects of oral NSAIDs for the treatment of acute musculoskeletal pain [68].

There has also been interest in studying the use of topical analgesics in the treatment of osteoarthritis in addition to soft tissue injuries, and in fact, multiple recent reviews of this subject have been recently published [69–72]. A diclofenac patch has been studied in a randomized, double-blind, controlled study in patients with osteoarthritis of the knee, and the results have demonstrated that this patch may be safe and effective for this condition [73]. A randomized, controlled study comparing the use of topical diclofenac solution to oral diclofenac for the treatment of osteoarthritis of the knee concluded that use of this topical diclofenac solution in patients with osteoarthritis of the knee produced symptom relief which was equivalent to oral diclofenac while resulting in significantly reduced incidence of diclofenac-related gastrointestinal complaints [74]. A recently published long-term study with this preparation has confirmed the safety of this preparation during the study period [75]. In a study of patients with pain in the temporomandibular joint, a group of patients received diclofenac solution applied topically several times daily, and a second group received oral diclofenac. No significant difference was demonstrated with respect to pain relief between the two groups; however, there were significantly fewer gastrointestinal side effects experienced by the patients receiving the diclofenac topical solution [76]. Other topical NSAID trials include a placebo-controlled trial that has demonstrated the efficacy of topical diclofenac gel 1.16 % for patients with osteoarthritis of the knee and a randomized, controlled study demonstrating benefit from the application of a topical diclofenac solution compared to placebo after 6 weeks of treatment for patients with painful osteoarthritis of the knee [77, 78]. More than one meta-analysis of this topic has been completed. A meta-analysis examining the use of topical NSAIDs in the treatment of osteoarthritis concluded that there was evidence that topical NSAIDs are superior to placebo during the first 2 weeks of treatment only. This meta-analysis concluded as well that available evidence suggested that topical NSAIDs were inferior to oral NSAIDs during the first week of treatment [79]. Another meta-analysis examining the evidence for the use of topical NSAIDs for chronic musculoskeletal pain also concluded that topical NSAIDs are effective and safe in treating chronic musculoskeletal conditions for 2 weeks [80]. Yet another meta-analysis of the use of topical NSAIDs for osteoarthritis suggested that of the four studies which had been completed in which a topical NSAID was compared to placebo or vehicle lasting 4 weeks or more for patients with osteoarthritis of the knee, pain relief did occur for a longer duration than placebo, but not all preparations had uniform results [81].

One should recognize that topical salicylates are used by patients in nonprescription preparations. A meta-analysis examining the effects of topical salicylates in acute and chronic pain concluded that based on the sparse data available that use of topically applied rubefacients containing salicylates based upon available trials of musculoskeletal and arthritic pain resulted in moderate to poor efficacy. The authors emphasized that efficacy estimates for rubefacients were at present unreliable due to a lack of appropriate clinical trials [82]. A randomized, controlled study completed in Germany with another topical NSAID, eltenac, examined its effect compared to placebo in 237 patients with osteoarthritis of the knee. Demonstrated efficacy and safety of the use of topical eltenac in the treatment of osteoarthritis of the knee compared to placebo were concluded by the authors [83]. In a separate study, topical eltenac gel was compared to oral diclofenac and placebo in patients with osteoarthritis of the knee. While both therapies were found to be superior to placebo with respect to analgesia, as reported in the meta-analysis above, the incidence of gastrointestinal side effects was notably lower in the group treated with topical eltenac gel compared to those treated with oral diclofenac [84]. Multiple other additional studies have demonstrated that topical diclofenac may be effective in reducing the pain associated with various types of degenerative joint disease [85–87].

Other topical agents have been studied in these conditions as well. No benefit of 0.025 % capsaicin cream over vehicle (not active) cream in a randomized, double-blind study of 30 patients with pain in the temporomandibular joint has been noted [88]. A topical cream containing glucosamine sulfate, chondroitin sulfate, and camphor for osteoarthritis of the knee showed a significant reduction of pain in the treatment group after 8 weeks compared to the placebo group in a randomized, controlled study [89].

A recently published case series reported the potential benefit of "topical" morphine in the management of chronic osteoarthritis-related pain; however, since the report emphasized that morphine or its metabolites were identifiable in the urine of treated patients, it is unclear how truly "topical" this preparation was [90].

Case Report: Consider a 67-year-old female with osteoarthritis of both knees and severe hypertension and esophageal reflux, who may be considered to be an inappropriate candidate for an oral NSAID, who has had little to no response to opiates, injection therapy, and /or physical therapy and is not a candidate for knee replacement. Might she be a candidate for a topical analgesic?

Low Back and Myofascial Pain

Far fewer studies regarding the use of topical analgesics for low back pain or myofascial pain have been published. The results of a double-blind, placebo-controlled study comparing topical capsaicin to placebo in 154 patients with chronic low back pain indicated that 60.8 % of capsaicin-treated patients compared with 42.1 % of placebo patients experienced 30 % pain relief after 3 weeks of treatment ($p < 0.02$) [91]. Other studies have been published in abstract form only – two are novel since they both involve the use of a local anesthetic in conditions not typically thought of as response to such and will be considered here. A multicenter, open-label study involving treatment of 120 patients with acute (<6 weeks), subacute (<3 months), short-term chronic (3–12 months), or long-term chronic (>12 months) low back pain with the 5 % lidocaine patch was completed. During the 6-week study period, participants applied four lidocaine 5 % patches to areas of maximal low back pain every 24 h. Initial evaluation suggests that the majority of patients experience moderate or greater degree of pain relief. Significant positive changes in quality of life indicators on this scale have been noted as well as demonstrated by the use of the NPS in this study [7]. An open-label study of patients with chronic myofascial pain was presented at the 2002 Scientific Meeting of the American Pain Society; 16 patients with chronic myofascial pain were treated with the lidocaine 5 % patch. After 28 days of treatment, statistically significant improvements were noted for average pain, general activity level, ability to walk, ability to work, relationships, sleep, and overall enjoyment of life in approximately 50 % of the patients studied [91].

Other Uses of Topical Analgesics

Although only small numbers of patients have been studied, it is interesting to note other conditions in which topical analgesics have been used. Topical analgesic of various types including opiates may be helpful in reducing pain associated with pressure ulcers or dressing changes [92–97]. A topical analgesic may help to treat postoperative pain and reduce the need for systemic analgesics. Controlled studies have demonstrated the benefit of the eutectic mixture of local anesthetics, 2.5 % lidocaine/2.5 % prilocaine cream in the reduction of pain associated with circumcision and venipuncture as well as for the pain associated with breast cancer surgery [5, 98]. More than one study has suggested that either ketamine or morphine may be used topically for mucositis-associated pain following chemotherapy or radiation therapy in patients with head and neck carcinomas [99, 100]. Topical opiates have been reported to reduce pain for two children with epidermolysis bullosa who were treated successfully with topical opiates [101]. An interesting report notes that the analgesic effect of menthol, an ingredient common to many over-the-counter analgesic preparations, may in part be as the result of activation of kappa-opioid receptors [102]. Burn pain has been reported to be treated effectively with a topical loperamide preparation [103]. Two randomized, controlled studies – one involving postoperative pain (diclofenac patch) and one involving wound pain treatment (capsicum plaster topically applied at acupuncture sites) – have been published as well [104, 105]. Central neuropathic itch has been treated successfully with the lidocaine 5 % patch according to a single case report [106]. Two other novel approaches to studying topical analgesia are worth mentioning. The results of an enriched enrollment study in which an open-label initial study led to the randomization of responders in a placebo-controlled study of the use of either a 4 % amitriptyline/2 % ketamine cream, 2 % amitriptyline/1 % ketamine cream, or placebo for patients with PHN demonstrated that after 3 weeks of treatment, the average daily pain intensity was lowest in patients receiving the higher concentration combination cream compared to the lower concentration combination or placebo ($p = 0.026$ high-concentration cream vs. placebo). Plasma levels of either drug were detected in fewer than 10 % of those patients receiving active treatment [107]. An open-label study of the use of a 0.25 % capsaicin topical agent in a lidocaine-containing vehicle in 25 patients with painful diabetic polyneuropathy and seven patients with PHN demonstrated pain relief in the majority of patients who were studied [108, 109].

Future Directions and Summary

The use of topical analgesics should be considered for a variety of painful conditions. The number of FDA-approved topical agents has grown recently. Off-label use of available therapies requires careful consideration of the potential risks as well benefits and deserves further study. Since topical analgesic use is generally associated with a better side effect profile than orally, transdermally, parenterally, or intrathecally administered analgesics, this should be considered when developing a pharmacologic treatment regimen for an individual patient. Further large, well-designed studies including comparative trials with nontopical analgesics are needed to further understand the role of topical analgesics in the management of acute and chronic pain.

References

1. Argoff CE. New analgesics for neuropathic pain: the lidocaine patch. Clin J Pain. 2000;16 Suppl 2:S62–5.
2. Argoff CE. Topical treatments for pain. Curr Pain Headache Rep. 2004;8:261–7.
3. Argoff CE, Khan KR. Chapter 17: Topical analgesics for neuropathic pain. In: Rice A, Howard R, Justins D, Miaskowski C, editors. Clinical pain management. 2nd ed. London: Hodder Arnold. 2008.
4. Argoff CE. Targeted topical peripheral analgesics in the management of pain. Curr Pain Headache Rep. 2002;7(1):34–8.
5. Galer BS. Topical medications. In: Loeser JD, editor. Bonica's management of pain. Philadelphia: Lippincott-Williams & Wilkins; 2001. p. 1736–41.
6. Gammaitoni AR, Alvarez NA. 24-hour application of the lidocaine patch 5% for 3 consecutive days is safe and well tolerated in healthy adult men and women. Abstract PO6.20. In: Presented at the 54th Annual American Academy of Neurology Meeting, Denver, 13–20 Apr 2002.
7. Argoff C, Nicholson B, Moskowitz M, et al. Effectiveness of lidocaine patch 5% (Lidoderm®) in the treatment of low back pain. In: Presented at the 10th world congress on pain, San Diego, 17–22 Aug 2002.
8. Watson CPN. Topical capsaicin as an adjuvant analgesic. J Pain Symptom Manage. 1994;9:425–33.
9. American Geriatrics Society Panel on Pharmacological Management of Persistent Pain in Older Adults. Pharmacological management of persistent pain in older persons. J Am Geriatr Soc. 2009;57(8):1331–46.
10. Gammaitoni AR, Davis MW. Pharmacokinetics and tolerability of lidocaine 5% patch with extended dosing. Ann Pharmacother. 2002;36:236–40.
11. Ness TJ, Jones L, Smith H. Use of compounded topical analgesics – results of an internet survey. Reg Anesth Pain Med. 2002;27(3):309–12.
12. Sawynok J. Topical and peripherally acting analgesics. Pharmacol Rev. 2003;55:1–20.
13. Robbins W. Clinical applications of capsaicinoids. Clin J Pain. 2000;16 Suppl 2:S86–9.
14. Bley KR. Recent developments in transient receptor potential vanilloid receptor 1 agonist-based therapies. Expert Opin Investig Drugs. 2004;13(11):1445–56. Review.
15. Backonja M, Malan P, Brady S, et al. One-hour high concentration capsaicin applications provide durable pain relief in initial and repeat treatment of postherpetic neuralgia. In: Presented at the 2004 Annual Scientific Meeting of the American Academy of Neurology, San Francisco, 2004.
16. Rowbotham MC. Topical analgesic agents. In: Fields HL, Liebeskind JC, editors. Pharmacologic approaches to the treatment of chronic pain: new concepts and critical issues. Seattle: IASP Press; 1994. p. 211–27.
17. Cashman JN. The mechanism of action of NSAIDs in analgesia. Drugs. 1996;52 suppl 5:13–23.
18. Yesilyurt O, Dogrul A, Gul H, et al. Topical cannabinoid enhances topical morphine antinociception. Pain. 2003;105(1–2):303–8.
19. Sawynok J, Esser MJ, Reid AR. Antidepressants as analgesics: an overview of central and peripheral mechanisms of action. J Psychiatry Neurosci. 2001;26(1):21–9.
20. Gerner P, Kao G, Srinivasa V, et al. Topical amitriptyline in health volunteers. Reg Anesth Pain Med. 2003;28(4):289–93.
21. Physicians desk reference. 55th edn. Montvale: Medical Economics Company; 2002.
22. Sawynok J. Topical analgesics in neuropathic pain. Curr Pharm Des. 2005;11(23):2995–3004.
23. Attal N, Crucci G, Haanpaa M, et al. EFNS guidelines on pharmacological treatment of neuropathic pain. Eur J Neurol. 2006;13(11):1153–69.
24. Rowbotham MC. Pharmacologic management of complex regional pain syndrome. Clin J Pain. 2006;22(5):425–9.
25. Rowbotham MC, Davies PS, Verkempinck C, et al. Lidocaine patch: double-blind controlled study of a new treatment method for post-herpetic neuralgia. Pain. 1996;65:39–44.
26. Galer BS, Rowbotham MC, Perander J, et al. Topical lidocaine patch relieves post-herpetic neuralgia more effectively than vehicle patch: results of an enriched enrollment study. Pain. 1999;80:533–8.

27. Katz NP, Davis MW, Dworkin RH. Topical lidocaine patch produces a significant improvement in mean pain scores and pain relief in treated PHN patients: results of a multicenter open-label trial. J Pain. 2001;2:9–18.

28. Rehm S, Binder A, Baron R. Post-herpetic neuralgia: 5% lidocaine medicated plaster, pregabalin or a combination of both? A randomized, open clinical effectiveness study. Curr Med Res Opin. 2010;26(7):1607–19.

29. Meier T, Wasner G, Faust M, et al. Efficacy of lidocaine patch 5% in the treatment of focal peripheral neuropathic pain syndromes: a randomized, double-blind, placebo-controlled study. Pain. 2003;106: 151–8.

30. Devers A, Galer BS. Topical lidocaine patch relieves a variety of neuropathic pain conditions: an open-label study. Clin J Pain. 2000;16(3):205–8.

31. Data on file. Chadds Ford: Endo Pharmaceuticals, Inc.

32. Hart-Gouleau S, Gammaitoni A, Galer BS, et al. Open-label study of the effectiveness and safety of the lidocaine patch 5 % (Lidoderm®) in patients with painful diabetic neuropathy. In: Presented at the 10th world congress on pain, San Diego, 17–22 Aug 2002.

33. Galer BS, Jensen MP. Development and preliminary validation of a pain measure specific to neuropathic pain: the neuropathic pain scale. Neurology. 1997;48:332–8.

34. Barbano RL, Herrmann DN, Hart-Gouleau S, et al. Effectiveness, tolerability and impact on quality of life of lidocaine patch 5% in diabetic polyneuropathy. Arch Neurol. 2004;61(6):914–8.

35. Herrmann DN, Barbano RL, Hart-Gouleau S, et al. An open-label study of the lidocaine patch 5% in painful polyneuropathy. Pain Med. 2005;6(5):379–84.

36. Galer BS, Jensen MP, Ma T, et al. The lidocaine patch 5% effectively treats all neuropathic pain qualities: results of a randomized, double-blind, vehicle-controlled, 3-week efficacy study with use of the neuropathic pain scale. Clin J Pain. 2002;18:297–301.

37. Geha PY, Baliki MN, Chialvo DR, et al. Brain activity for spontaneous pain of post herpetic neuralgia and its modulation by lidocaine patch therapy. Pain. 2007;128(1–2):88–100.

38. Lycka BA, Watson CP, Nevin K, et al. EMLA® cream for the treatment of pain caused by post-herpetic neuralgia: a double-blind, placebo-controlled study. In: Proceedings of the annual meeting of the American Pain Society, 1996:A111(abstract).

39. Attal N, Brasseur L, Chauvin M, et al. Effects of single and repeated applications of a eutectic mixture of local anesthetics (EMLA®) cream on spontaneous and evoked pain in post-herpetic neuralgia. Pain. 1999;81:203–9.

40. Litman SJ, Vitkun SA, Poppers PJ. Use of EMLA® cream in the treatment of post-herpetic neuralgia. J Clin Anesth. 1996;8:54–7.

41. Rains C, Bryson HM. Topical capsaicin: a review of its pharmacological properties and therapeutic potential in post-herpetic neuralgia, diabetic neuropathy, and osteoarthritis. Drugs Aging. 1995;7:317–28.

42. Robbins WR, Staats PS, Levine J, et al. Treatment of intractable pain with topical large-dose capsaicin: preliminary report. Anesth Analg. 1998;86:579–83.

43. Simpson D, Brown S, Sampson J, et al. A single application of high-concentration capsaicin leads to 12 weeks of pain relief in HIV-associated distal symmetrical polyneuropathy: results of an open label trail. In: Presented at the 2004 Annual Scientific Meeting of the American Academy of Neurology, San Francisco, 2004.

44. Mason L, Moore RA, Derry S, et al. Systematic review of topical capsaicin for the treatment of chronic pain. BMJ. 2004;328(7446):991–6.

45. Backonja MM, Malan TP, Vanhove GF, et al. NGX-4010, a high concentration patch, for the treatment of post herpetic neuralgia: a randomized, double-blind, controlled study with an open-label extension. Pain Med. 2010;11(4):600–8.

46. Backonja M, Wallace MS, Blonsky ER, et al. NGX-4010, a high-concentration capsaicin patch, for the treatment of post herpetic neuralgia: a randomised, double-blind study. LancetNeurol. 2008;7(12): 1106–12.

47. Wallace M, Pappagallo M. Qutenza®: a capsaicin 8% patch for the management of post herpetic neuralgia. Expert Rev Neurother. 2011;11(1):15–27.

48. Simpson DM, Brown S, Tobias J, et al. Controlled trial of high-concentration capsaicin patch for treatment of painful HIV neuropathy. Neurology. 2008;70(24):2305–13.

49. Phillips TJ, Cherry CL, Cox S, et al. Pharmacological treatment of painful HIV-associated sensory neuropathy: a systematic review and meta-analysis of randomised controlled trials. PLoS One. 2010;5(12):e14422. Epub2010 Dec 28.

50. McCleane G. Topical application of doxepin hydrochloride, capsaicin and a combination of both produces analgesia in chronic neuropathic pain: a randomized, double-blind, placebo-controlled study. Br J Clin Pharmacol. 2000;49(6):574–9.

51. Lynch ME, Clark AJ, Sawynok J, et al. Topical 2% amitriptyline and 1% ketamine in neuropathic pain syndromes: a randomized, double-blind, placebo-controlled trial. Anesthesiology. 2005;103(1):140–6.

52. Lynch ME, Clark AJ, Sawynok J, et al. Topical amitriptyline and ketamine in neuropathic pain syndromes: an open-label study. J Pain. 2005;6(10):644–9.

53. Lynch ME, Clark AJ, Sawynok J. A pilot study examining topical amitriptyline, ketamine, and a combination of both in the treatment of neuropathic pain. Clin J Pain. 2003;19(5):323–8.

54. Quan D, Wellish M, Gilden DH. Topical ketamine treatment of postherpetic neuralgia. Neurology. 2003;60(8):1391–2.

55. Greenway FL, Frome BM, Engels TM, et al. Temporary relief of postherpetic neuralgia pain with topical geranium oil. Am J Med. 2003;115(7):586–7.

56. Barthel HR, Axford-Gatley RA. Topical non-steroidal anti-inflammatory drugs for osteoarthritis. Postgrad Med. 2010;122(6): 98–106.

57. Mazieres B, Rouanet S, Velicy J, et al. Topical ketoprofen patch (100 mg) for the treatment of ankle sprain: a randomized, double-blind, placebo-controlled study. Am J Sports Med. 2005;33(4):515–23.

58. Mazieres B, Rouanet S, Guillon Y, et al. Topical ketoprofen patch in the treatment of tendonitis: a randomized, double blind, placebo controlled study. J Rheumatol. 2005;32(8):1563–70.

59. White RL. Ketoprofen gel as an adjunct to physical therapy management of a child with Sever disease. Phys Ther. 2006;86(3):424–33.

60. Predel HG, Koll R, Pabst H, et al. Diclofenac patch for topical treatment of acute impact injuries: a randomized, double blind, placebo controlled, multicenter study. Br J Sports Med. 2004;38(3):318–23.

61. Galer BS, Rowbotham MC, Perander J, et al. Topical diclofenac patch significantly reduces pain associated with minor sports injuries: results of a randomized, double-blind, placebo-controlled, multicenter study. J Pain Symptom Manage. 2000;19:287–94.

62. Jenoure P, Segesser B, Luhti U, et al. A trial with diclofenac HEP plaster as topical treatment in minor sports injuries. Drugs Exp Clin Res. 1993;19:125–31.

63. Marten M. Efficacy and tolerability of a topical NSAID patch (local action transcutaneous flurbiprofen) and oral diclofenac in the treatment of soft-tissue rheumatism. Clin Rheumatol. 1997;16:25–31.

64. Campbell J, Dunn T. Evaluation of topical ibuprofen cream in the treatment of acute ankle sprains. J Accid Emerg Med. 1994;11:178–82.

65. Airaksinen O, Venalainen J, Pietilainen T. Ketoprofen 2.5% gel versus placebo gel in the treatment of acute soft tissue injuries. Int J Clin Pharmacol Ther Toxicol. 1993;31:561–3.

66. Machen J, Whitefield M. Efficacy of a proprietary ibuprofen gel in soft tissue injuries: a randomized, double-blind, placebo-controlled study. Int J Clin Pract. 2002;56(2):102–6.

67. Whitefield M, O'Kane CJ, Anderson S. Comparative efficacy of a proprietary topical ibuprofen gel and oral ibuprofen in acute soft tissue injuries: a randomized, double-blind study. J Clin Pharm Ther. 2002;27(6):409–17.

68. Massey T, Derry S, Moore RA, et al. Topical NSAIDs for acute pain in adults. Cochrane Database Syst Rev. 2010;6:CD007402.

69. Brewer AR, McCarberg B, Argoff CE. Update on the use of topical NSAIDs for the treatment of soft tissue and musculoskeletal pain: a review of recent data and current treatment options. Phys Sportsmed. 2010;38(2):62–70.

70. Stanos SP. Topical agents for the management of musculoskeletal pain. J Pain Symptom Manage. 2007;33(3):342–55.

71. Harovtiunian S, Drennan DA, Lipman AG. Topical NSAID therapy for musculoskeletal pain. Pain Med. 2010;11(4):535–49.

72. Baraf HS, Gloth FM, Barthel HR, et al. Safety and efficacy of topical diclofenac sodium gel for knee osteoarthritis in elderly and younger patients; pooled data from three randomized, double-blind, parallel-group, placebo-controlled, multicenter trials. Drugs Aging. 2011;28(1):27–40.

73. Bruhlmann P, Michel BA. Topical diclofenac patch in patients with knee osteoarthritis: a randomized, double-blind, controlled clinical trial. Clin Exp Rheumatol. 2003;21(2):193–8.

74. Tugwell PS, Wells GA, Shainhouse JZ. Equivalence study of a topical diclofenac solution (pennsaid) compared with oral diclofenac in symptomatic treatment of osteoarthritis of the knee: a randomized, controlled trial. J Rheumatol. 2004;31(10):2002–12.

75. Shainhouse JZ, Grierson LM, Naseer Z. A long-term open label study to confirm the safety of topical diclofenac solution containing dimethyl sulfoxide in the treatment of the osteoarthritic knee. Am J Ther. 2010;17(6):566–76.

76. Di Rienzo BL, Di Rienzo BA, D'Emilia E, et al. Topical versus systemic diclofenac in the treatment of temporo-mandibular joint dysfunction symptoms. Acta Otorhinolaryngol Ital. 2004;24(5):279–83.

77. Niethard FU, Gold MS, Solomon GS, et al. Efficacy of topical diclofenac diethylamine gel in osteoarthritis of the knee. J Rheumatol. 2005;32(12):2384–92.

78. Baer PA, Thomas LM, Shainhouse Z. Treatment of osteoarthritis of the knee with a topical diclofenac solution: a randomized, controlled, 6 week trial (ISRCTN53366886). BMC Musculoskelet Disord. 2005;6:44.

79. Lin J, Zhang W, Jones A, et al. Efficacy of topical non-steroidal anti-inflammatory drugs in the treatment of osteoarthritis: meta-analysis of randomized controlled trials. BMJ. 2004;329(7461):324–8.

80. Mason L, Moore RA, Edwards JE, et al. Topical NSAIDS for chronic musculoskeletal pain: a systematic review and meta-analysis. BMC Musculoskelet Disord. 2004;5:28.

81. Biswal S, Medhi B, Pandhi P. Longterm efficacy of topical non-steroidal anti-inflammatory drugs in knee osteoarthritis: metaanalysis of randomized placebo-controlled clinical trials. J Rheumatol. 2006;33(9):1841–4.

82. Mason L, Moore RA, Edwards JE, et al. Systematic review of topical rubefacients containing salicylates for the treatment of acute and chronic pain. BMJ. 2004;328:995.

83. Ottillinger B, Gomor B, Michel BA, et al. Efficacy and safety of eltenac gel in the treatment of knee osteoarthritis. Osteoarthritis Cartilage. 2001;9(3):273–80.

84. Sandelin J, Harilainen A, Crone H, et al. Local NSAID gel (eltenac) in the treatment of osteoarthritis of the knee. A double-blind study comparing eltenac with oral diclofenac and placebo gel. Scand J Rheumatol. 1997;26:287–92.

85. Dreiser RL, Tisne-Camus M. DHEP plasters as a topical treatment of knee osteoarthritis: a double-blind placebo-controlled study. Drugs Exp Clin Res. 1993;19:107–15.

86. Galeazzi M, Marcolongo R. A placebo-controlled study of the efficacy and tolerability of a nonsteroidal anti-inflammatory drug, DHEP plaster in inflammatory peri- and extra-articular rheumatological diseases. Drugs Exp Clin Res. 1993;19:107–15.

87. Gallachia G, Marcolongo R. Pharmacokinetics of diclofenac hydroxyethylpyrrolidine (DHEP) plasters in patients with monolateral knee joint effusion. Drugs Exp Clin Res. 1993;19:95–7.

88. Winocur E, Gavish A, Halachmi M, et al. Topical application of capsaicin for the treatment of localized pain in the temporomandibular joint area. J Orofac Pain. 2000;14(1):31–6.

89. Cohen M, Wolfe R, Mai T, et al. A randomized, double blind placebo-controlled trial of a topical crème containing glucosamine sulfate, chondroitin sulfate and camphor for osteoarthritis of the knee. J Rheumatol. 2003;30(3):523–8.

90. Wilken M, Ineck JR, Rule AM. Chronic arthritis pain management with topical morphine:case series. J Pain Palliat Care Pharmacother. 2005;19(4):39–44.

91. Keitel W, Frerick H, Kuhn U, et al. Capsicum pain plaster in chronic non-specific low back pain. Arzneimittelforschung. 2001;51:896–903.

92. Lipman AG, Dalpiaz AS, London SP. Topical lidocaine patch therapy for myofascial pain. Abstract 782. In: Presented at the Annual Scientific Meeting of the American Pain Society, Baltimore, 14–17 Mar 2002.

93. Briggs M, Nelson EA. Topical agents or dressings for pain in venous leg ulcers. Cochrane Database Syst Rev. 2003;1:CD001177.

94. Flock P. Pilot study to determine the effectiveness of diamorphine gel to control pressure ulcer pain. J Pain Symptom Manage. 2003;25(6):547–54.

95. Zeppetella G, Ribeiro PJ. Analgesic efficacy of morphine applied topically to painful ulcers. J Pain Symptom Manage. 2003;25(6):555–8.

96. Gallagher RE, Arndt DR, Hunt KL. Analgesic effects of topical methadone: a report of four cases. Clin J Pain. 2005;21(2):190–2.

97. Vernassiere C, Cornet C, Trechot P, et al. Study to determine the efficacy of topical morphine on painful chronic skin ulcers. J Wound Care. 2005;14(6):289–93.

98. Ashfield T. The use of topical opioids to relieve pressure ulcer pain. Nurs Stand. 2005;19(45):90–2.

99. Fassoulaki A, Sarantopoulos C, Melemeni A, et al. EMLA reduces acute and chronic pain after breast surgery for cancer. Reg Anesth Pain Med. 2000;25(4):35–355.

100. Cerchietti LC, Navigante AH, Bonomi MR, et al. Effect of topical morphine for mucositis-associated pain following concomitant chemoradiotherapy for head and neck carcinoma. Cancer. 2002;95(10):2230–6.

101. Slatkin NE, Rhiner M. Topical ketamine in the treatment of mucositis pain. Pain Med. 2003;4(3):298–303.

102. Watterson G, Howard R, Goldman A. Peripheral opiates in inflammatory pain. Arch Dis Child. 2004;89(7):679–81.

103. Galeotti N, DeCesare Mannelli L, Mazzanti G, et al. Menthol: a natural analgesic compound. Neurosci Lett. 2002;322(3):145–8.

104. Ray SB. Loperamide: a potential topical analgesic for the treatment of burn pain. J Burn Care Res. 2006;27(1):121–2.

105. Alessandri F, Lijoi D, Mistrangelo E, et al. Topical diclofenac patch for postoperative wound pain in laparoscopic gynecologic surgery: a randomized study. J Minim Invasive Gynecol. 2006;13(3):195–200.

106. Kim KS, Nam YM. The analgesic effects of capsicum plaster at the Zusanli point after abdominal hysterectomy. Anesth Analg. 2006;103(3):709–13.

107. Sandroni P. Central neuropathic itch: a new treatment option? Neurology. 2002;59:778–9.

108. Lockhart E. Topical combination of amitriptyline and ketamine for post herpetic neuralgia. J Pain. 2004;3 suppl 1:82.

109. Bernstein J, Phillips S, Group T. A new topical medication for the adjunctive relief of painful diabetic neuropathy and postherpetic neuralgia. J Pain. 2004;5(3 suppl 1):82.

Sleep Aids

Howard S. Smith

Key Points

- Insomnia relates to complaints of inadequate sleep (e.g., problems falling asleep, problems with staying asleep [sleep duration], and/or quality of sleep) and may need treatment especially if it is associated with significant patient distress and/or daytime sleepiness.
- Treatment for insomnia may require nonpharmacologic approaches as well as pharmacologic approaches.
- Medications that are FDA approved for the treatment of insomnia include benzodiazepines, "Z-drugs," and melatonin receptor agonists.
- "Z-drugs" (e.g., zaleplon, zolpidem, zopiclone, eszopiclone) may have less potential for rebound insomnia and withdrawal symptoms than benzodiazepines, but they still have a significant potential for abuse.

Introduction

Sleep is one of the most universal biological processes in existence. Depriving an organism of sleep altogether can be extremely detrimental and may even lead to death [1]. Sleep is therefore considered necessary for life, but why this is so remains unclear. Sleep is subdivided into rapid eye movement (REM) sleep, which is characterized by high-frequency electroencephalogram (EEG) recordings and muscle atonia [2], and non-REM (slow-wave) sleep, characterized by low-frequency EEG recordings and body rest [3].

While the cholinergic and monoaminergic systems act to promote wakefulness in conjunction with the orexins, there are other neuronal groups that act to promote sleep. The primary population of sleep-promoting neurons is located in the preoptic area, specifically the ventrolateral preoptic area of the hypothalamus (VLPO). Thus, multiple mediators can be targeted in efforts to combat insomnia and/or promote sleep/sedation (e.g., acetylcholine, norepinephrine, gamma-aminobutyric acid, histamine, serotonin, adenosine dopamine, melatonin, orexin).

Insomnia is a condition of perceived inadequate sleep, with patients typically presenting with difficulty falling asleep, difficulty maintaining sleep, or poor quality sleep [4]. To manage insomnia successfully, pharmacological treatments for insomnia may be required to reduce sleep latency, increase sleep maintenance, and improve sleep quality. In addition, such treatments should enable normal wakening with no subsequent impairment of daytime function and minimal risk of dependence.

Sivertsen et al. studied insomnia symptoms and the use of health-care services and medications and concluded that insomnia symptoms represent a significant public health concern, being independently associated with substantially elevated use of health-care services, medications, and alcohol overuse [5].

Kyle and colleagues concluded from the relatively small literature that insomnia impacts on diverse areas of health-related quality of life (HRQoL), and that both pharmacological and nonpharmacological interventions can produce, to varying degrees, improvements in domains spanning physical, social, and emotional functioning [6].

Insomnia Assessment

The following questions can serve as the initial assessment regarding sleep [7]: What time do you normally go to bed at night and wake up in the morning? Do you often have trouble falling asleep at night? About how many times do you wake

H.S. Smith, M.D., FACP, FAAPM, FACNP
Department of Anesthesiology, Albany Medical College,
Albany Medical Center, 47 New Scotland Avenue,
Albany, NY 12159, USA
e-mail: smithh@mail.amc.edu

up at night? If you do wake up during the night, do you usually have trouble falling back asleep? Does your bed partner say (or are you aware) that you frequently snore, gasp for air, or stop breathing—kick, thrash about, eat, punch, or scream during sleep? Are you sleepy or tired during much of the day? Do you unintentionally doze off during the day? Do you usually take one or more naps during the day?

The ISI, developed by Morin, is a seven-item Likert-type self-rating scale designed to assess the subjective perception of the severity of insomnia [8].The scale contains items that measure the symptoms and associated features and impacts of insomnia, including difficulty falling asleep, difficulty maintaining sleep, early morning awakening, satisfaction with sleep, concerns about insomnia, and functional impacts of insomnia.

Treatment for Insomnia

The treatment for insomnia may involve pharmacologic as well as nonpharmacologic approaches.

Nonpharmacologic Approaches to Insomnia

Sleep Hygiene and Sleep Education

Sleep hygiene refers to the general rules of behavioral practices and environmental factors that are consistent with good quality sleep. When defined broadly, it includes guidelines for general health practices (e.g., diet, exercise, substance use), environmental factors (e.g., light, temperature, noise), as well as sleep-related behavioral practices (e.g., regularity of sleep schedule, pre-sleep activities, efforts to try to sleep) [9]. The International Classification of Sleep Disorders even includes the diagnostic category "inadequate sleep hygiene," which is designated for the sleep disruption associated with poor sleep hygiene practices [10]. In addition, poor sleep-related habits leading to conditioned arousal in bed are considered to be one of the major etiological factors of psychophysiological insomnia [10]. Poor sleep hygiene practices have been considered to be a contributing factor to insomnia [9].

Previous studies have shown that sleep hygiene alone is not a sufficient treatment for insomnia [11–14]. Interventions aimed to reduce physiological or cognitive arousal (e.g., relaxation training, cognitive restructuring) and stimulus control instructions to reduce conditioned arousal with bedtime cues may be indicated to generate better results.

Behaviors and habits that may impair sleep include the following [7]: frequent daytime napping, spending too much time in bed, insufficient daytime activities, late-evening exercises, insufficient bright-light exposure, excess caffeine, evening alcohol consumption, smoking in the evening, late,

heavy dinner, watching television or engaging in other stimulating activities at night, anxiety and anticipation of poor sleep, clock watching, and environmental factors, such as the room being too warm, too noisy, or too bright; pets on the bed or in the bedroom; and active or noisy bed partners.

The following are helpful instructions for using stimulus control and practicing good sleep hygiene [7]: develop a sleep ritual, such as maintaining a 30-min relaxation period before bedtime or taking a hot bath 90 min before bedtime; make sure the bedroom is restful and comfortable; go to bed only if you feel sleepy; avoid heavy exercise within 2 h of bedtime; avoid sleep-fragmenting substances, such as caffeine, nicotine, and alcohol; avoid activities in the bedroom that keep you awake. Use the bedroom only for sleep and sex; do not watch television from bed or work in bed; sleep only in your bedroom; if you cannot fall asleep, leave the bedroom and return only when sleepy; maintain stable bedtimes and rising times. Arise at the same time each morning, regardless of the amount of sleep obtained that night, and avoid daytime napping. If you do nap during the day, limit it to 30 min and do not nap, if possible, after 2 p.m.

Relaxation Therapy

The goal of relaxation therapy is to guide individuals to a calm, steady state when they wish to go to sleep. The methods used include progressive muscle relaxation (tensing and then relaxing each muscle group), guided imagery, diaphragmatic breathing, meditation, and biofeedback [15].

Cognitive Behavioral Therapy

Vitiello et al. performed randomized controlled trial of cognitive behavioral therapy for insomnia (CBT-I) in patients with osteoarthritis and comorbid insomnia [16]. CBT-I subjects reported significantly improved sleep and significantly reduced pain after treatment. Control subjects reported no significant improvements. One-year follow-up found maintenance of improved sleep and reduced pain for both the CBT-I group alone and among subjects who crossed over from control to CBT-I, suggesting that improving sleep, per se, in patients with osteoarthritis may result in decreased pain [16].

Sivertsen and colleagues performed a randomized double-blind placebo-controlled trial examining short- and long-term clinical efficacies of cognitive behavioral therapy (CBT) and pharmacological treatment in older adults experiencing chronic primary insomnia [17]. Participants receiving CBT improved their sleep efficiency from 81.4 % at pretreatment to 90.1 % at 6-month follow-up compared with a decrease from 82.3 to 81.9 % in the zopiclone group, suggesting that interventions based on CBT may be superior to zopiclone treatment both in short- and long-term management of insomnia in older adults [17]. This agrees with the findings of Dolan et al. [18] and of a similar study which found

Table 9.1 Conclusions from the Agency for Healthcare Research and Quality Evidence Report/technology assessment regarding the manifestations and management of chronic insomnia [23]

Evidence exists to support that:
Chronic insomnia is associated with older age.
Benzodiazepines and nonbenzodiazepines are effective in the management of chronic insomnia. However, benzodiazepines, nonbenzodiazepines, and antidepressants pose a risk of harm.
Benzodiazepines have a greater risk of harm than nonbenzodiazepines.
Melatonin is effective in the management of chronic insomnia in subsets of the chronic insomnia population, and there is no evidence that melatonin poses a risk of harm.
Relaxation therapy and cognitive behavioral therapy are effective in the management of chronic insomnia in subsets of the chronic insomnia population.

temazepam equal to CBT in the short term but inferior to CBT in the long term [19]. Three meta-analyses [12, 14, 20] have concluded that 70–80 % of middle-aged adults with insomnia benefit from interventions based on CBT. Irwin et al. performed a meta-analysis and concluded that behavioral interventions were more effective in middle-aged adults versus older adults in improving both total sleep time and sleep efficiency [20]. Morin et al. conducted a prospective, randomized controlled trial involving 2-stage therapy for 160 adults with persistent insomnia [21]. Participants received CBT alone or CBT plus 10 mg/day (taken at bedtime) of zolpidem for an initial 6-week acute therapy, followed by extended 6-month therapy. The best long-term outcome was obtained with patients treated with combined therapy initially, followed by CBT alone, as evidenced by higher remission rates at the 6-month follow-up compared with patients who continued to take zolpidem during extended therapy [21].

Acupuncture

Cao and colleagues performed a systematic review of randomized controlled trials (RCTs) of acupuncture for treatment of insomnia [22]. They found that acupuncture appears to be effective in treatment of insomnia; however, further large, rigorous designed trials are warranted [22].

Pharmacologic Approaches to Insomnia

In 2005, the Agency for Healthcare Research and Quality released its Evidence Report/Technology Assessment (see Table 9.1) [23]. Several nutritional or herbal products are sold for the treatment of insomnia (e.g., valerian root, melatonin, hops, chamomile, St. John's wort). Only valerian and melatonin have demonstrated some benefit in promoting sleep. Melatonin, however, can cause sleep disruption, daytime fatigue, headaches, and dizziness at higher doses, while valerian root can cause residual daytime sedation and, in rare instances, hepatotoxicity [24].

Common drug classes used to treat insomnia, but not FDA approved for that use, include antihistamines (e.g., diphenhydramine), antidepressants (e.g., amitriptyline, doxepin, trazodone), atypical antipsychotics (quetiapine), and sedatives (e.g., chloral hydrate). These drug classes are used due to their sedative properties.

FDA-Approved Pharmacologic Therapies for Management of Insomnia

The FDA-approved therapies for the management of insomnia are classified as sedative-hypnotic agents. These sedative hypnotics can be categorized into three groups: benzodiazepines, nonbenzodiazepine selective GABA agonists, and melatonin receptor agonists (see Table 9.2).

Benzodiazepines

The first benzodiazepine, chlordiazepoxide (discovered serendipitously by Leo Sternbach in 1955), is a fusion of a benzene ring and a diazepine ring. Benzodiazepines such as chlordiazepoxide (Librium) and diazepam (Valium) were first developed as sedatives in the 1960s and rapidly gained popularity essentially replacing barbiturates as the sedatives of choice for "sleeping pills" [25]. Benzodiazepines could be acting on receptors directly within the VLPO to promote sleep, or they could be acting more globally to facilitate inhibitory GABA transmission [26]. The $\alpha 1$ subunit of the GABAA receptor is especially important for benzodiazepine-induced sedation. Mice with mutations in the $\alpha 1$ subunit are insensitive to the sedative effects of the traditional benzodiazepine diazepam but maintain sensitivity to its anxiolytic, myorelaxant, and motor-impairing functions, indicating that the sedating effects of benzodiazepines are primarily mediated by actions on the $\alpha 1$ subunit [27].

Nonbenzodiazepine Selective GABA Agonists

The $GABA_A$ receptor is a pentameric molecule composed of a combination of one or more specific subunit types. Although 19 different subunits are known to exist, the majority of $GABA_A$ receptors in the central nervous system consist of $\alpha_{(1-6)}$, $\beta_{(1-3)}$, and $\gamma_{(1-3)}$ subunits [28]. The interaction of benzodiazepines with multiple $GABA_A$ receptor subunits containing $\alpha_{(1-3,5)}$ is thought to elicit the variety of effects seen with these agents such as anxiolysis, amnesia, muscle relaxation, sedation, and anticonvulsant activity [28]. The theoretical advantage of having a selective α_1 subunit agonist of the GABA receptor is that sedating effects are achieved while avoiding other effects thought to be mediated by the other α subunits to which benzodiazepines bind.

In contrast to benzodiazepines, the nonbenzodiazepine sedative hypnotics (i.e., zolpidem, eszopiclone, zopiclone, zaleplon) are more selective for the $GABA_A$ receptors with

Table 9.2 Food and Drug Administration–approved drugs for insomnia

Drugs	Adult dose (mg)	Half-life (h)	Onset (min)	Peak effect (h)
BzRAs				
Estazolam	(1, 2)	10–24	15–60	0.5–1.6
(*ProSom*^{TM})	0.5–2			
Flurazepam	(15, 30)	47–100	15–20	3–6
(*Dalmane*^{TM})	15–30			
Quazepam	(15)	P: 25–41	15–60	15–3
(*Doral*^{TM})	7.5–15 (max. 30)	AM: 40–114 (2-oxoquazepam-[2 h] *N*-desalkyl-2-oxoquazepam [40–114 h])		
Temazepam	(17.5, 15, 22.5, 30)	6–16	15–60	1.5–3
(*Restoril*^{TM})	7.5–30			
Triazolam	(0.125, 0.25)	1.5–5.5	15–30	1.7–5
(*Halcion*^{TM})	0.125–0.25 (max. 0.5)			
Non–BzRAs				
Eszopiclone	(1, 2, 3)	6	30	1
(*Lunesta*^{TM})	1–2 (max. 3)	(9 in elderly)		
Zaleplon	(5, 10)	1	Rapid	1
(*Sonata*^{TM}, *Starnoc*^{TM})	5–10 (max. 20)			
Zopiclone	(5, 7.5)	~5–6	30	1–2
(*Imovane*^{TM})	5–15	(5–10 in elderly)		
Zolpidem tartrate IR	(5, 10)	~2.5	15–30	1–3
(*Ambien*^{TM})	5–20			
Zolpidem tartarate ER	(6.25, 12.5)	~3	30	1.5–4
(*Ambien CR*^{TM})	6.25–12.5			
Melatonin receptor agonist				
Ramelton	(8)	P: 0.5–2.6	30	0.5–1.5
(*Rozerem*^{TM})	8½h before bedtime	AM: 2–5 (M-II)		

Abbreviations: *P* parent drug, *AM* active metabolite, *BzRAs* benzodiazepines, *Non-BzRAs* nonbenzodiazepines, *IR* immediate release, *ER* extended release, *CR* controlled release, *( )* dosage forms

the α_1-receptor subunit [29]. Indiplon is a novel pyrazolopyrimidine, nonbenzodiazepine γ-aminobutyric acid (GABA) agonist with a high affinity and selectivity for the α1 subunit associated with sedation for the treatment of insomnia [29]. Petroski and colleagues [30] showed indiplon to be at least nine times more selective for α_1 as compared to α_2, α_3, and α_5 subunits [30]; a greater degree of selectivity for α_1, over the α_2 and α_3 subunits, was greater for indiplon as compared to zolpidem, zopiclone, and zaleplon.

"Z-DRUGS"

Initial nonbenzodiazepine selective GABA agonists are often referred to as the "Z-drugs" because they include zolpidem (Ambien), zaleplon (Sonata), zopiclone (Imovane), and eszopiclone (Lunesta). Zaleplon and zolpidem have much higher efficacy at benzodiazepine receptors containing the α1 subunit compared with other types of α subunits, whereas traditional benzodiazepines (e.g., triazolam) lack this specificity [31].

Zaleplon

It appears that zaleplon binds preferentially to alpha 1-containing GABAA receptors [32] and may be considered alpha

1-selective, and so zaleplon's effects are likely mediated via the alpha 1 receptor and are predominantly sedative in nature [30]. Zaleplon has a short T_{max} and the shortest $t_{\frac{1}{2}}$ of the current Z-drugs (see Table 9.2), explaining its fast onset and the fastest offset of action. Zolpidem IR has a longer $t_{\frac{1}{2}}$ than zaleplon, resulting in a longer duration of action. Zolpidem CR consists of a two-layer tablet: The outer layer dissolves quickly, while the second layer dissolves slowly to maintain plasma zolpidem concentrations above those seen for the IR formulation, particularly at 3–6 h post-dose [33].

Zolpidem

Zolpidem was the first subtype-selective GABAA receptor agonist and has the highest affinity at the alpha 1 subtype of all the nonbenzodiazepine GABAA receptor modulators. Zolpidem will activate alpha 2 and alpha 3 receptors, though at considerably higher concentrations than those that activate the alpha 1 subtype.

Zopiclone

Zopiclone shows relatively high binding affinity for the alpha 1 over the alpha 3 receptor subtype [34], and zopiclone also binds to the alpha 5 receptor with high affinity [35]. Sivertsen et al. examined polysomnographic parameters and sleep apnea and periodic limb movement disorder (PLMD) in chronic users of zopiclone compared with aged-matched drug-free patients with insomnia versus "good sleepers" [36]. Forty-one percent of the patients treated pharmacologically for insomnia also had sleep apnea. There were no differences between the zopiclone and insomnia group on any of the polysomnography parameters, and a similar pattern was found for data based on sleep diaries [36]. This study suggests that the sleep of chronic users of zopiclone is no better than that of drug-free patients with insomnia [36].

Zopiclone is a racemic mixture of (S)- and (R)-isomers, with stereoselective PK profiles [37, 38] and clinical outcomes [39]. Racemic zopiclone has the longest T_{max} of the Z-drugs, and plasma concentrations of the more active enantiomer, (S)-zopiclone, remain below the sleep-inducing threshold (of 10 ng/ml) for more than half an hour after administration [40]. Racemic zopiclone has a longer $t_{1/2}$ than either zaleplon or zolpidem, suggesting a longer duration of action. However, this means that (S)-zopiclone plasma concentrations may not fall below the sleep-inducing threshold until more than 9 h after racemic zopiclone dosing. An additional consideration is the duration of effects of zopiclone's active metabolite, (S)-desmethylzopiclone (SDMZ), and the less active enantiomer, (R)-zopiclone. Measurable plasma concentrations of both SDMZ and (R)-zopiclone are present 8 h after zopiclone dosing and could contribute to unwanted next-day residual effects [41].

Eszopiclone

Eszopiclone is the pure (S)-enantiomer of racemic zopiclone [42] and was licensed in the USA in December 2004. Although eszopiclone is the isolated (S)-enantiomer of zopiclone, this study revealed notable differences in the pharmacodynamic effects of eszopiclone compared with racemic (R, S)-zopiclone. The pattern of eszopiclone binding at alpha 1, alpha 2, alpha 3, and alpha 5 subtypes is similar (although not identical) to that of zopiclone, but the binding affinities of eszopiclone are all higher than those seen with zopiclone. Eszopiclone's potency is greatest at alpha 5 receptors, followed by alpha 2 and alpha 3 receptors, but it is still a very potent drug at the alpha 1 receptor subtype with an EC50 of the same order of magnitude as zaleplon and zopiclone. Eszopiclone is particularly efficacious at alpha 2 and 3 receptors, with the highest efficacy of the nonbenzodiazepine GABAA modulators when examined in the same study [35].

Melatonin Receptor Agonists (MRAs)

Melatonin is an endogenous neuromodulator synthesized by the pineal gland, and its secretion is regulated by the supra-chiasmatic nucleus (SCN), the circadian pacemaker of the brain [43]. The SCN receives light signals from the retina, which are transmitted to the dorsal medial hypothalamus (DMH), which acts as a relay center for signals to regions involved in sleep and wake maintenance [e.g., VLPO, locus coeruleus (LC)]. Melatonin acts largely through MT1 receptors in the SCN to suppress firing of SCN neurons, thereby disinhibiting the sleep-promoting neurons in the VLPO [43]. Secretion of melatonin is low during the day and high at night, and the onset of melatonin secretion coincides with the onset of nightly sleepiness. Exogenous melatonin crosses the blood–brain barrier, and various over-the-counter melatonin preparations are used to treat insomnia, jet lag, shift-work-related sleepiness, and delayed phase syndrome, with various degrees of effectiveness [44]. Melatonin, ramelteon (Rozerem), and agomelatine (Valdoxan) are all agonists for melatonin 1 (MT1) and melatonin 2 (MT2) receptors [43]. Ramelteon has an affinity for both receptors that is 3–16 times greater than melatonin, and it has a longer half-life. Agomelatine also has a high affinity for melatonin receptors, in addition to acting as an antagonist at serotonin 5-HT2C receptors to decrease anxiety as well as promote sleep. Both MT1 and MT2 play a role in sleep induction; MT1 activation suppresses firing of SCN neurons, and MT2 receptors are involved in entraining circadian rhythms.

The administration of melatonin (MEL) during the daytime, i.e., out of the phase of its endogenous secretion, can facilitate sleep [45]; however, if the treatment goal is to maintain daytime sleep for ~8 h, then fast-release oral MEL with its short elimination half-life (~40 min) may be more appropriate [46]. Aeschbach et al. show in healthy subjects that transdermal delivery of MEL during the daytime can elevate plasma MEL and reduce waking after sleep onset, by promoting sleep in the latter part of an 8-h sleep opportunity [46].

Antihistamines

Antihistaminergics exert their sedative effects by antagonizing the H1 receptors in the brain. The H1 antagonist cyproheptadine (Periactin) is effective at increasing slow-wave sleep and REM sleep in rats [47], whereas the H1 antagonists diphenhydramine (Benadryl) and chlorpheniramine (Chlor-Trimeton) decrease sleep latency but have no effect on amount of sleep. In humans, diphenhydramine initially increases subjective sleepiness and reduces latency to sleep compared with placebo, but after 4 days of administration, this effect is abolished, indicating tolerance to its effects [48].

Antidepressants/Atypical Antipsychotics

The effects of antidepressants on sleep are diverse, even within a class of medications. Sedation and drowsiness are common side effects of the TCAs (e.g., desipramine (Norpramin), imipramine (Tofranil), and amitriptyline (Elavil)). Amitriptyline increases drowsiness and shortens sleep latency compared with placebo, whereas imipramine actually increases sleep latency and decreases total sleep time. MAOIs and SSRIs (e.g., fluoxetine (Prozac), sertraline (Zoloft), and citalopram (Celexa)) can cause insomnia and decreased sleep efficiency. The TCAs which seem to be utilized most commonly to help combat insomnia include amitriptyline and doxepin. Notably, all these classes of antidepressants suppress REM sleep to some degree and have significant anticholinergic effects while doxepin has significant antihistaminergic effects. Cyclobenzaprine (an agent traditionally viewed as a muscle relaxant but structurally very similar to amitriptyline) has been used to help combat insomnia by some clinicians.

Trazodone (Desyrel) is an antidepressant that is also commonly prescribed for insomnia [49]. Trazodone acts as both a weak serotonin (5-HT) reuptake inhibitor and as an antagonist at 5-HT_{2A} and 5-HT_{2C}, α_1-adrenergic, and histamine H_1 receptors [50]. Trazodone has been shown to suppress REM sleep; however, its effects on sleep latency, sleep duration, and number of wakenings are controversial.

Schwartz et al. attempted to compare the effectiveness and tolerability of two hypnotic agents, trazodone (Desyrel) (50–100 mg) and zaleplon (Sonata) (10–20 mg), on psychiatric inpatients with insomnia. Schwartz and colleagues suggested that in their pilot study, it appeared that trazodone may be a better agent to promote longer, deeper subjective quality sleep for psychiatric inpatients with insomnia in terms of effectiveness. However, tolerability was much better with zaleplon as daytime residual side effects were less [51]. Meta-chlorophenylpiperazine (mCPP) is a synthetic drug that was identified for the first time in 2004 in Sweden as an illicit recreational drug and is also a metabolite of trazodone [52]. mCPP has stimulant and hallucinogenic effects similar to those of 3,4-methylenedioxymethamphetamine (MDMA) and has the potential to lead to the development of serotonergic syndrome when interacting with certain agents [53].

Cankurtaran and colleagues compared the effectiveness of mirtazapine and imipramine on multiple distressing symptoms (e.g., pain, nausea) and other symptoms, e.g., sleep disturbances and also depressive and anxiety symptoms [54]. For initial, middle, and late insomnia, only the mirtazapine group showed improvements, suggesting that mirtazapine is effective for helping to resolve insomnia [54].

If antidepressants are used to address insomnia, sedating ones should be preferred over activating agents such as serotonin reuptake inhibitors. In general, drugs lacking strong cholinergic activity should be preferred over agents with strong cholinergic activity (e.g., amitriptyline). Drugs blocking serotonin 5-HT2A or 5-HT2C receptors should be preferred over those whose sedative property is caused largely by histamine receptor blockade (e.g., doxepin). However, sometimes these "nonpreferred" agents (which tend to be very sedating) appear to address insomnia the best. The dose should be as low as possible (e.g., as an initial dose: doxepin 25 mg, mirtazapine

15 mg, trazodone 50 mg, trimipramine 25 mg) [55]. Regarding the lack of substantial data allowing for evidence-based recommendations, we are facing a clear need for well-designed, long-term, comparative studies to further define the role of antidepressants versus other agents in the management of insomnia. Atypical antipsychotic agents which have been utilized (largely because of their sedative effects) in patients that also have chronic insomnia with relatively little data include olanzapine, quetiapine, and clozapine [56].

Alpha 2-Delta Ligands

The use of gabapentin has been evaluated for sleep on healthy persons, patients with seizure, or alcoholic patients [57–60]. All of these studies, though not on persons with primary insomnia, showed generally beneficial effects of sleep and increased slow-wave sleep. Lo and colleagues studied 18 patients with primary insomnia who received gabapentin treatment for at least 4 weeks [61]. All patients received polysomnography, a biochemical blood test, and neuropsychological tests before and after the treatment period. They found that gabapentin enhances slow-wave sleep in patients with primary insomnia [61]. It also improves sleep quality by elevating sleep efficiency and decreasing spontaneous arousal. The results suggest that gabapentin may be beneficial in the treatment of primary insomnia [61]. Hindmarch and colleagues assessed the effects of pregabalin compared with alprazolam and placebo on aspects of sleep in healthy volunteers using a randomized, double-blind, placebo- and active-controlled, 3-way crossover study design [62]. Although there were no differences between the active treatments, both pregabalin and alprazolam reduced rapid eye movement sleep as a proportion of the total sleep period compared with placebo. Pregabalin also significantly reduced the number of awakenings of more than 1 min in duration [62]. Leeds Sleep Evaluation Questionnaire ratings of the ease of getting to sleep and the perceived quality of sleep were significantly improved following both active treatments, and ratings of behavior following awakening were significantly impaired by both drug treatments [62].

Sympatholytics

Sedation and fatigue are among the most common side effects in patients taking βAR antagonists, α1AR antagonists, and clonidine, an agonist for α2AR inhibitor autoreceptors that attenuates NE release. Interestingly, prazosin is used to alleviate nightmares in posttraumatic stress disorder patients [63], potentially by acting as a dual anxiolytic and sedative. Twenty-two veterans with posttraumatic stress disorder (PTSD) were assessed for trauma-related nightmares and nonnightmare distressed awakenings (NNDA) before and after treatment with the alpha-1 adrenoreceptor antagonist prazosin at an average bedtime dose of 9.6 mg/day. Ratings combining frequency and intensity dimensions of trauma-related nightmares decreased from 3.6 to 2.2, NNDA

Fig. 9.1 Insomnia relief ladder

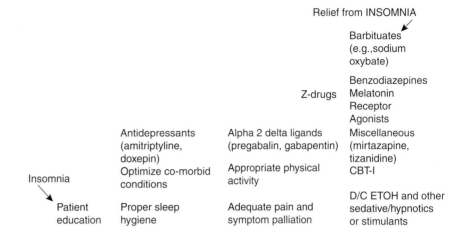

from 5.2 to 2.1, and sleep difficulty from 7.2 to 4.1 per week [64]. Tizanidine (an alpha 2 agonist traditionally viewed as a muscle relaxant/antispasticity agent) has been used by some clinicians to help combat insomnia.

Barbiturates

Gamma-hydroxybutyrate (GHB) is not a barbiturate; it is a euphoric, prosocial, and sleep-inducing drug that binds with high affinity to its own GHB receptor site and also more weakly to GABA (B) receptors [65]. GHB is only available from one pharmacy and has been used for patients with severe intractable sleep disturbances who also have fibromyalgia.

In addition to its established efficacy for the treatment of cataplexy and EDS, nightly sodium oxybate administration significantly reduces measures of sleep disruption and significantly increases slow-wave sleep in patients with narcolepsy [66].

Potential Future Sleep Aids

Accumulating evidence supports a role for 5-HT2A antagonism in the treatment of sleep maintenance insomnias [67]. Indeed, several selective 5-HT2A inverse agonists have entered clinical development for the treatment of insomnia; these include eplivanserin, volinanserin, pruvanserin, and nelotanserin [68].

In healthy human volunteers, nelotanserin was rapidly absorbed after oral administration and achieved maximum concentrations 1 h later. All doses (up to 40 mg) of nelotanserin significantly improved measures of sleep consolidation, including decreases in the number of stage shifts, number of awakenings after sleep onset, microarousal index, and number of sleep bouts, concomitant with increases in sleep bout duration [69].

EVT 201 is considered a partial $GABA_A$ receptor agonist because it produces a lower maximal potentiation of $GABA_A$ receptors than a full agonist [70]. It has an elimination half-life of 3–4 h and an active metabolite with similar affinity

and elimination characteristics but lower intrinsic activity [71]. Compared to placebo, EVT 201 1.5 and 2.5 mg increased total sleep time (TST), reduced wake after sleep onset, and reduced latency to persistent sleep [72].

Orexin Receptor Modulators

Almorexant (ACT-078573) is an orally active dual orexin receptor antagonist that is being developed for the treatment of primary insomnia [73]. Hoever and colleagues enrolled 70 healthy male subjects in a double-blind, placebo- and active-controlled study [74]. Population pharmacokinetic/pharmacodynamic modeling suggested that doses of ~500 mg almorexant and 10 mg zolpidem are equivalent with respect to subjectively assessed alertness [74].

Conclusion

The approach to insomnia/sleep disturbances is challenging and like the approach to patients with pain involves a multidimensional assessment with a history and physical examination as well as perhaps with other testing to develop a working diagnosis. Treatment approaches should begin with nonpharmacologic approaches and if necessary also involve pharmacologic approaches. An interdisciplinary team and sleep medicine specialist should be involved in complex and poorly responsive cases. A step-ladder approach may be helpful to health-care providers unfamiliar with sleep disturbance issues (Fig. 9.1) [75].

References

1. Rechtschaffen A, Bergmann BM, Everson CA, et al. Sleep deprivation in the rat. X. Integration and discussion of the findings. Sleep. 1989;12:68–87.
2. Remy P, Doder M, Lees A, et al. Depression in Parkinson's disease: loss of dopamine and noradrenaline innervation in the limbic system. Brain. 2005;128:1314–22.

3. Stenberg D. Neuroanatomy and neurochemistry of sleep. Cell Mol Life Sci. 2007;64:1187–204.

4. Roth T. Insomnia: definition, prevalence, etiology, and consequences. J Clin Sleep Med. 2007;3:S7–10.

5. Sivertsen B, Krokstad S, Mykletun A, Overland S. Insomnia symptoms and use of health care services and medications: the HUNT-2 study. Behav Sleep Med. 2009;7:210–22.

6. Kyle SD, Morgan K, Espie CA. Insomnia and health-related quality of life. Sleep Med Rev. 2010;14:69–82.

7. Joshi S. Non-pharmacological therapy for insomnia in the elderly. Clin Geriatr Med. 2008;24:107–19.

8. Morin CM. Insomnia: psychological assessment and management. New York: Guildford Press; 1993.

9. Yang CM, Lin SC, Hsu SC, Cheng CP. Maladaptive sleep hygiene practices in good sleepers and patients with insomnia. J Health Psychol. 2010;15:147–55.

10. AmericanAcademy of SleepMedicine. International classification of sleep disorders: diagnostic and coding manual. 2nd ed. Westchester: American Academy of Sleep Medicine; 2005.

11. Morin CM, Bootzin RR, Buysse DJ, et al. Psychological and behavioral treatment of insomnia: update of the recent evidence (1998–2004). Sleep. 2006;29:1398–414.

12. Morin CM, Culbert JP, Schwartz SM. Nonpharmacological interventions for insomnia: a meta-analysis of treatment efficacy. Am J Psychiatry. 1994;151:1172–80.

13. Morin CM, Hauri PJ, Espie CA, et al. Nonpharmacologic treatment of chronic insomnia. An American Academy of Sleep Medicine review. Sleep. 1999;22:1134–56.

14. Murtagh DR, Greenwood KM. Identifying effective psychological treatments for insomnia: a meta-analysis. J Consult Clin Psychol. 1995;63:79–89.

15. Manber R, Kuo TF. Cognitive-behavioral therapies for insomnia. In: Lee-Chiong TL, Sateia MJ, Carskadon MA, editors. Sleep medicine. Philadelphia: Hanley & Belfus; 2002. p. 177–85.

16. Vitiello MV, Rybarczyk B, Von Korff M, Stepanski E. Cognitive behavioral therapy for insomnia improves sleep and decreases pain in older adults with co-morbid insomnia and osteoarthritis. J Clin Sleep Med. 2009;5:355–62.

17. Sivertsen B, Omvik S, Pallesen S, et al. Cognitive behavioral therapy vs zopiclone for treatment of chronic primary insomnia in older adults: a randomized controlled trial. JAMA. 2006;295:2851–8.

18. Dolan DC, Taylor DJ, Bramoweth AD, Rosenthal LD. Cognitive-behavioral therapy of insomnia: a clinical case series study of patients with co-morbid disorders and using hypnotic medications. Behav Res Ther. 2010;48:321–7.

19. Morin CM, Colecchi C, Stone J, et al. Behavioral and pharmacological therapies for late-life insomnia: a randomized controlled trial. JAMA. 1999;281:991–9.

20. Irwin MR, Cole JC, Nicassio PM. Comparative meta-analysis of behavioral interventions for insomnia and their efficacy in middle-aged adults and in older adults 55+ years of age. Health Psychol. 2006;25:3–14.

21. Morin CM, Vallières A, Guay B, et al. Cognitive behavioral therapy, singly and combined with medication, for persistent insomnia: a randomized controlled trial. JAMA. 2009;301:2005–15.

22. Cao H, Pan X, Li H, Liu J. Acupuncture for treatment of insomnia: a systematic review of randomized controlled trials. J Altern Complement Med. 2009;15:1171–86.

23. Buscemi N, Vandermeer B, Friesen C, et al. Manifestations and management of chronic insomnia in adults. AHRQ publication no. 05-E021-2. 2008. Available at: www.ahrq.gov/downloads/pub/evidence/pdf/insomnia/insomnia.pdf. Accessed 27 May 2008.

24. Ramakrishnan K, Scheid DC. Treatment options for insomnia. Am Fam Physician. 2007;76:517–26.

25. Wafford KA, Ebert B. Emerging anti-insomnia drugs: tackling sleeplessness and the quality of wake time. Nat Rev Drug Discov. 2008;7:530–40.

26. Mitchell HA, Weinshenker D. Good night and good luck: norepinephrine in sleep pharmacology. Biochem Pharmacol. 2010;79:801–9.

27. Rudolph U, Crestani F, Benke D, et al. Benzodiazepine actions mediated by specific gamma-aminobutyric acid(A) receptor subtypes. Nature. 1999;401:796–800.

28. Möhler H, Fritschy JM, Rudolph U. A new benzodiazepine pharmacology. J Pharmacol Exp Ther. 2002;300(1):2–8.

29. Foster AC, Pelleymounter MA, Cullen MJ, et al. In vivo pharmacological characterization of indiplon, a novel pyrazolopyrimidine sedative hypnotic. J Pharmacol Exp Ther. 2004;311:547–59.

30. Petroski RE, Pomeroy JE, Das R, et al. Indiplon, is a high-affinity positive allosteric modulator with selectivity for α1 subunit-containing $GABA_A$ receptors. J Pharmacol Exp Ther. 2006;317: 369–77.

31. Sanger DJ. The pharmacology and mechanisms of action of new generation, non-benzodiazepine hypnotic agents. CNS Drugs. 2004;18:9–15.

32. Wegner F, Deuther-Conrad W, Scheunemann M, et al. GABAA receptor pharmacology of fluorinated derivatives of the novel sedative-hypnotic pyrazolopyrimidine indiplon. Eur J Pharmacol. 2008; 580:1–11.

33. Weinling E, McDougall S, Andre F, et al. Pharmacokinetic profile of a new modified release formulation of zolpidem designed to improve sleep maintenance. Fundam Clin Pharmacol. 2006;20: 397–403.

34. Sanna E, Busonero F, Talani G, et al. Comparison of the effects of zaleplon, zolpidem, and triazolam at various GABAA receptor subtypes. Eur J Pharmacol. 2002;451:103–10.

35. Brunello N, Cooper J, Bettica P, et al. Differential pharmacological profiles of the GABAA receptor modulators zolpidem, zopiclone, eszopiclone, and (S)-desmethylzopiclone. In: Abstract Presented at the World Psychiatric Association International Congress (WPA), Florence; 2009.

36. Sivertsen B, Omvik S, Pallesen S, et al. Sleep and sleep disorders in chronic users of zopiclone and drug-free insomniacs. J Clin Sleep Med. 2009;5:349–54.

37. Fernandez C, Maradeix V, Gimenez F, et al. Pharmacokinetics of zopiclone and its enantiomers in Caucasian young healthy volunteers. Drug Metab Dispos. 1993;21:1125–8.

38. Fernandez C, Alet P, Davrinche C, et al. Stereoselective distribution and stereoconversion of zopiclone enantiomers in plasma and brain tissues in rats. J Pharm Pharmacol. 2002;54:335–40.

39. McMahon LR, Jerussi TP, France CP. Stereoselective discriminative stimulus effects of zopiclone in rhesus monkeys. Psychopharmacology (Berlin). 2003;165:222–8.

40. Fernandez C, Martin C, Gimenez F, Farinotti R. Clinical pharmacokinetics of zopiclone. Clin Pharmacokinet. 1995;29:431–41.

41. Carlson JN, Haskew R, Wacker J, et al. Sedative and anxiolytic effects of zopiclone's enantiomers and metabolite. Eur J Pharmacol. 2001;415:181–9.

42. Najib J. Eszopiclone, a nonbenzodiazepine sedative-hypnotic agent for the treatment of transient and chronic insomnia. Clin Therapy. 2006;28:491–516.

43. Pandi-Perumal SR, Srinivasan V, Spence DW, Cardinali DP. Role of the melatonin system in the control of sleep: therapeutic implications. CNS Drugs. 2007;21:995–1018.

44. Reiter RJ, Tan DX, Manchester LC, et al. Medical implications of melatonin: receptor-mediated and receptor-independent actions. Adv Med Sci. 2007;52:11–28.

45. Wyatt JK, Dijk DJ, Ritz-De Cecco A, et al. Sleep facilitating effect of exogenous melatonin in healthy young men and women is circadian-phase dependent. Sleep. 2006;29:609–18.

46. Aeschbach D, Lockye Jr B, Dijk D-J, et al. Use of transdermal melatonin delivery to improve sleep maintenance during daytime. Clin Pharmacol Ther. 2009;864:378–82.

47. Tokunaga S, Takeda Y, Shinomiya K, et al. Effects of some H1-antagonists on the sleep–wake cycle in sleep-disturbed rats. J Pharmacol Sci. 2007;103:201–6.

48. Richardson GS, Roehrs TA, Rosenthal L, et al. Tolerance to daytime sedative effects of H1 antihistamines. J Clin Psychopharmacol. 2002;22:511–5.

49. Mendelson WB. A review of the evidence for the efficacy and safety of trazodone in insomnia. J Clin Psychiatry. 2005;66:469–76.

50. Morin AK, Jarvis CI, Lynch AM. Therapeutic options for sleep maintenance and sleep-onset insomnia. Pharmacotherapy. 2007;27:89–110.

51. Schwartz T, Nihalani N, Virk S, et al. A comparison of the effectiveness of two hypnotic agents for the treatment of insomnia. Int J Psychiatr Nurs Res. 2004;10:1146–50.

52. Ellenhorn MJ, Schonwald S, Ordog J, et al. Ellenhorn's medical toxicology: diagnosis and treatment of human poisoning. 8th ed. Baltimore: Williams and Wilkins; 2006.

53. m-chlorophénylpipérazine nouvelle identification. Observatoire Francxais des Drogues et des Toxicomanies web site. 2006. Available at: http://www.drogues.gouv.fr/IMG/pdf/note_mCPP. pdf. Accessed 14 Mar 2006.

54. Cankurtaran ES, Ozalp E, Soygur H, et al. Mirtazapine improves sleep and lowers anxiety and depression in cancer patients: superiority over imipramine. Support Care Cancer. 2008;16:1291–8.

55. Wiegand MH. Antidepressants for the treatment of insomnia: a suitable approach? Drugs. 2008;68:2411–7.

56. Miller DD. Atypical antipsychotics: sleep, sedation, and efficacy. J Clin Psychiatry. 2004;6:3–7.

57. Foldvary-Schaefer N, De Leon Sanchez I, Karafa M, et al. Gabapentin increases slow-wave sleep in normal adults. Epilepsia. 2002;43:1493–7.

58. Ehrenberg B. Importance of sleep restoration in co-morbid disease: effect of anticonvulsants. Neurology. 2000;54:S33–7.

59. Karam-Hage M, Brower KJ. Gabapentin treatment for insomnia associated with alcohol dependence [comment]. Am J Psychiatry. 2000;157:151.

60. Bazil CW, Battista J, Basner RC. Gabapentin improves sleep in the presence of alcohol. J Clin Sleep Med. 2005;1:284–7.

61. Lo HS, Yang CM, Lo HG, et al. Treatment effects of gabapentin for primary insomnia. Clin Neuropharmacol. 2010;33:84–90.

62. Hindmarch I, Dawson J, Stanley N. A double-blind study in healthy volunteers to assess the effects on sleep of pregabalin compared with alprazolam and placebo. Sleep. 2005;28:187–93.

63. Dierks MR, Jordan JK, Sheehan AH. Prazosin treatment of nightmares related to posttraumatic stress disorder. Ann Pharmacother. 2007;41:1013–7.

64. Thompson CE, Taylor FB, McFall ME, et al. Nonnightmare distressed awakenings in veterans with posttraumatic stress disorder: response to prazosin. J Trauma Stress. 2008;21:417–20.

65. van Nieuwenhuijzen PS, McGregor IS, Hunt GE. The distribution of gamma-hydroxybutyrate-induced Fos expression in rat brain: comparison with baclofen. Neuroscience. 2009;158:441–55.

66. Black J, Pardi D, Hornfeldt CS, Inhaber N. The nightly administration of sodium oxybate results in significant reduction in the nocturnal sleep disruption of patients with narcolepsy. Sleep Med. 2009;10:829–35.

67. Monti JM, Jantos H. Effects of the serotonin 5-HT2A/2C receptor agonist DOI and of the selective 5-HT2A or 5-HT2C receptor antagonists EMD 281014 and SB-243213, respectively, on sleep and waking in the rat. Eur J Pharmacol. 2006;553:163–70.

68. Teegarden BR, Al Shamma H, Xiong Y. 5-HT2A inverse-agonists for the treatment of insomnia. Curr Top Med Chem. 2008;8: 969–76.

69. Al-Shamma HA, Anderson C, Chuang E, et al. Nelotanserin, a novel selective human 5-hydroxytryptamine2A inverse agonist for the treatment of insomnia. J Pharmacol Exp Ther. 2010;332: 281–90.

70. Kemp JA, Baur R, Sigel E. EVT 201: a high affinity, partial positive allosteric modulator of GABAA receptors with preference for the a1-subtype. Sleep. 2008;31:A34.

71. Boyle J, Stanley N, Hunneyball I, et al. A placebo controlled, randomised, double-blind, 5 way cross-over study of 4 doses of EVT 201 on subjective sleep quality and morning after performance in a traffic noise model of sleep disturbance. Sleep. 2007;30:A262.

72. Walsh JK, Salkeld L, Knowles LJ, et al. Treatment of elderly primary insomnia patients with EVT 201 improves sleep initiation, sleep maintenance, and daytime sleepiness. Sleep Med. 2010;11:23–30.

73. Neubauer DN. Almorexant, a dual orexin receptor antagonist for the treatment of insomnia. Curr Opin Investig Drugs. 2010;11:101–10.

74. Hoever P, de Haas S, Winkler J, et al. Orexin receptor antagonism, a new sleep-promoting paradigm: an ascending single-dose study with almorexant. Clin Pharmacol Ther. 2010;87:593–600.

75. Smith HS, Barkin RL, Barkin SJ, et al. Personalized pharmacotherapy for treatment approaches focused at primary insomnia. AM J Ther. 2011 May;18(3):227–40.

Clinical Use of Opioids

10

Andrea Trescot

Key Points
- Opioids are extremely useful but potentially dangerous broad-spectrum analgesics.
- Understanding the pharmacology and metabolism of opioids may help predict effectiveness and potential side effects of opioids.
- Opioid use may differ when used for specific indications, such as cancer pain, acute versus chronic pain, and pediatric or geriatric population.

Introduction

Opioids are compounds that work at specific receptors in the brain to provide analgesia. Originally extracted from the sap of the poppy plant, opioids may be naturally occurring, semisynthetic, or synthetic, and their clinical activity is a function of their affinity for the opioid receptors in the brain. Opioids are useful for a wide variety of painful conditions, including acute pain, cancer pain, and chronic pain, as well as cough suppression and air hunger. However, opioid use is associated with a significant risk of addiction potential, which limits their use and contributes to the current "opioid phobia." In this chapter, we will discuss the history, pharmacology, clinical uses, and future directions.

History

Opioids have been used for their euphoric and analgesic properties for thousands of years. Records show that around 3400 BC [1], the opium poppy was cultivated in lower Mesopotamia by the Sumerians who referred to it as *Hul Gil*, the "joy plant." In 1817, a German pharmacist, Friedrich Wilhelm Adam Serturner, isolated morphine from opium [2]. After ingesting the crystals, Serturner discovered that the compound induced a dreamlike state; thus, he named the compound "morphium" after Morpheus, the Greek god of dreams [3]. Joseph Louis Gay-Lussac coined the term "morphine" later when he translated Serturner's article from German to French [4]. Morphine is only one of 24 alkaloids found within the resin of the opium poppy plant (*Papaver somniferum*) and comprises approximately 10 % of the total opium extract.

Opioid Receptors

"Opiates" are naturally occurring compounds derived from the poppy. The term "opioid" is now used broadly to describe any compound that exerts activity at an opioid receptor [5]. The opioid receptors were first discovered in 1972 [6], and the first endogenous opioid, or "endorphin," was identified in 1975 [7]. Multiple opioid receptors have now been identified, including *Mu*, *Kappa*, and *Delta* [8]. *Mu* receptors are found primarily in the brainstem, ventricles, and medial thalamus, and activation of these receptors can result in supraspinal analgesia, respiratory depression, euphoria, sedation, decreased gastrointestinal motility, and physical dependence. *Kappa* receptors are found in the limbic system, brainstem, and spinal cord and are felt to be responsible for spinal analgesia, sedation, dyspnea, dependence, dysphoria, and respiratory depression. *Delta* receptors are located largely in the brain itself and are thought to be responsible for psychomimetic and dysphoric effects.

A. Trescot, M.D.
Algone Pain Center,
4 Oceanside Circle, St. Augustine, FL 32080, USA
e-mail: drtrescot@gmail.com

T.R. Deer et al. (eds.), *Comprehensive Treatment of Chronic Pain by Medical, Interventional, and Integrative Approaches*,
DOI 10.1007/978-1-4614-1560-2_10, © American Academy of Pain Medicine 2013

Fig. 10.1 Intracellular opioid
actions (With permission from
Trescot et al. [5])

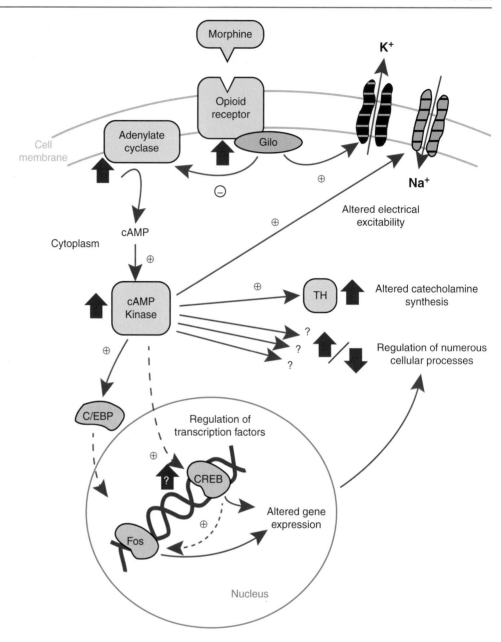

These opioid receptors are G-linked proteins within the membranes of cells; when activated, the receptor releases a protein, which migrates within the cell, activating Na/K channels or influencing enzymes within the cell or influencing nuclear gene transcription (Fig. 10.1) [9]. Presynaptic opioid receptors inhibit neurotransmitter release of compounds such as acetylcholine, norepinephrine, serotonin, and substance P. The inhibition of an inhibitory neuron may then result in excitation (Fig. 10.2) [9].

The dopaminergic system in the ventral tegmental area (VTA) is the site of the natural reward centers of the brain, and GABA neurons usually inhibit these dopaminergic systems. Opioids inhibit the presynaptic receptors on these GABA neurons, which increases the release of dopamine,

which is intensely pleasurable. These are the same areas of the brain associated with other drugs of abuse such as alcohol, nicotine, and benzodiazepines (Fig. 10.3) [10].

Opioid Genetics

Each opioid receptor has a different activity, as well as a different receptor affinity (which is genetically controlled). For example, OPRM1, the gene that encodes the mu receptor, is polymorphic, and approximately 20–30 % of the population has heterozygous changes in the alleles, associated with altered sensitivities to pain [11]. Different opioids also have different relative affinity for each receptor, so that the same opioid may have very different effects on different people, and the same person might have different effects from different opioids.

There is now considerable evidence suggesting genetic variability in the ability of individuals to metabolize and respond to drugs. All opioid drugs are substantially metabolized, mainly by the cytochrome P450 system as well as to a lesser degree the UDP-glucuronosyltransferase system (UGTs). Activity of these enzymes depends on whether patient is homozygous for nonfunctioning alleles (poor metabolizer or PM), has at least one functioning allele (extensive metabolizer or EM), or has multiple copies of a functional allele (ultrarapid metabolizer UM) [12].

As a result, the morphine dose needed for postoperative pain relief after similar surgery may vary fivefold between individuals, and the dose needed at a defined stage of cancer pain varies threefold [13]. As another example, CYP 450 2D6 is a critical enzyme involved in the metabolism of a variety of opioids described below; activity of this enzyme is highly variable, and there may be as much as a 10,000-fold difference among individuals [14]. Approximately 8–10 % of Caucasians but up to 50 % of people of Asian descent have an inactive form of this enzyme [15]. As discussed below, hydrocodone is metabolized to hydromorphone via CYP 2D6; in one study [16], the metabolism of hydrocodone to hydromorphone was eight times faster in EMs than in PMs. Medications may also interfere with enzyme activity; in this same study, quinidine, a potent CYP2D6 inhibitor, reduced the excretion of hydromorphone, resulting in plasma levels five times higher in EMs than PMs.

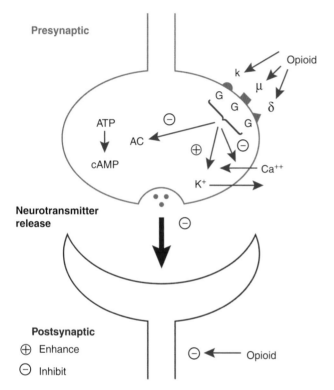

Fig. 10.2 Opioid receptors, pre- and postsynaptic (With permission from Trescot et al. [5])

Opioid Side Effects

Opioids are well known to cause a variety of side effects, most commonly nausea and vomiting, constipation, sedation, and respiratory depression [17]. These side effects can be significant, and some patients avoid opioids even in the face of significant pain, in an effort to limit such side effects, which may act as a significant barrier to adequate pain relief [18].

Constipation

Constipation is the most common adverse effect from opioids, occurring in 40–95 % of patients treated with opioids [19], and is caused by opioid receptor stimulation in the gut.

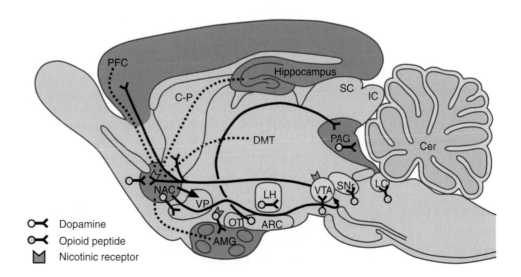

Fig. 10.3 Opioid activity sites (With permission from Trescot et al. [5])

The subsequent decrease in GI motility results in increased fecal fluid absorption, resulting in hard, dry stools. It is essential that prophylactic treatment be instituted on the initiation of opioid treatment since this, of all the side effects of opioids, does not resolve over time.

Nausea

Nausea has been reported to occur in up to 25 % of patients treated with opioids [20]. Mechanism for this nausea may include direct stimulation of the chemotactic trigger zone (CTZ), reduced gastrointestinal motility leading to gastric distention, and increased vestibular sensitivity [21].

Pruritus

Two to ten percent of patients on opioids will develop pruritus [18], which results from a direct release of histamine and not usually an antigen/antibody reaction. It is therefore better considered an adverse reaction than an allergic reaction and is usually treated symptomatically with antihistamines such as diphenhydramine.

Sedation and Cognitive Dysfunction

The incidence of sedation can vary from 20 to 60 % [22]; it is usually associated with an initiation or increase in opioids and is usually transient. Cognitive dysfunction can be confounded by the presence of infection, dehydration, metabolic abnormalities, or advanced disease [23].

Respiratory Depression

A significant proportion of patients taking long-term opioids develop central apnea during sleep. Teichtahl and colleagues [24] examined ten patients in a methadone maintenance program and performed a clinical assessment and overnight polysomnography. They found that all ten patients had evidence of central sleep apnea, with six patients having a central apnea index (CAI) [the number of central apnea events per hour] [25] greater than 5, and four patients with a CAI greater than 10. In a larger follow-up study of 50 patients taking long-term methadone, 30 % of the patients had a CAI greater than 5, and 20 % had a CAI greater than 10 [26].

Endocrine Effects

Endorphins appear to be primarily involved in the regulation of gonadotropins and ACTH release [27]. Amenorrhea developed in 52 % female patients on opioids for chronic pain [28], while the testosterone levels were subnormal in 74 % of males on sustained-release oral opioids [29]. These effects are more profound with IV or intrathecal opioids than oral opioids [30].

Immunologic Effects

Acute and chronic opioid administration can cause inhibitory effects on antibody and cellular immune responses, natural killer cell activity, cytokine expression, and phagocytic activity. Chronic administration of opioids decreases the proliferative capacity of macrophage progenitor cells and lymphocytes [31].

Relationship Between Side Effects and Sex or Ethnicity

Several studies suggest that sex and ethnic differences exist to explain the differences seen in side effect profiles. Women have, for instance, been found to be more sensitive to the respiratory effects of morphine [32] and more often have nausea and emesis with opioids [33]. Varying levels of opioid metabolites due to genetic differences in CYP 450 isoenzymes and glucuronidation between ethnic groups [34] may explain the variety of responses seen to similar doses of medications (see section "Opioid Metabolism").

Opioid Metabolism

Many of the positive effects, as well as the side effects of opioids, can be traced to their metabolites, and knowledge of these metabolites may help to explain many of the puzzling clinical scenarios seen by the practicing physician.

Morphine

Morphine is metabolized by glucuronidation, producing morphine-6-glucuronide (M6G) and morphine-3-glucuronide (M3G) in a ratio of 6:1. M6G is believed to be responsible for some additional analgesic effects of morphine [35]. M3G, on the other hand, is believed to potentially lead to hyperalgesia [36], with increased pain, agitation, and myoclonus. Morphine is also metabolized in small amounts to codeine and hydromorphone. For instance, in one study, hydromorphone was present in 66 % of morphine consumers without aberrant drug behavior [37]; this usually occurs with doses higher than 100 mg/day.

Codeine

It is believed that the analgesic activity from codeine occurs from metabolism of codeine to morphine by CYP2D6. Because of the great heterogeneity in the CYP2D6 enzyme, with both fast metabolizers and slow metabolizers, codeine may not be an effective drug in all populations. Recently, the FDA has issued a Public Health Advisory [38] regarding a serious side effect in nursing infants whose mothers are apparent CYP2D6 ultrarapid metabolizers, who, while taking codeine, had rapid and higher levels of morphine in the breast milk, with subsequent potentially fatal neonate respiratory depression.

Although codeine is often referred to as a "weak" analgesic, in a cancer pain study comparing 25 mg of hydrocodone (a "strong" analgesic) to 150 mg of codeine (a "weak" analgesic), 58 % of the codeine patients obtained relief compared to 57 % of the hydrocodone patients [39].

Hydrocodone

Hydrocodone is similar in structure to codeine and is a weak mu receptor agonist, but the CYP2D6 enzyme demethylates it into hydromorphone, which has much stronger mu binding [16]. Like codeine, it has been proposed that hydrocodone is a prodrug. In other words, patients who are CYP2D6 deficient, or patients who are on CYP2D6 inhibitors, may not produce the hydromorphone metabolites and may have less than expected analgesia.

Oxycodone

Oxycodone has activity at multiple opiate receptors including the kappa receptor, which gives it a unique anti-sedative effect ("perky Percocet"). It undergoes extensive hepatic metabolism by glucuronidation to noroxycodone (which has less than 1 % of the analgesia potency of oxycodone) and by CYP2D6 to oxymorphone [40]. Because oxycodone is dependent on the CYP2D6 pathway for clearance, it is possible that drug–drug interactions can occur with 2D6 inhibitors.

Oxymorphone

Although oxycodone has activity at multiple receptors, its metabolite oxymorphone is a pure mu agonist. Oxymorphone is about ten times more potent than morphine. It has limited protein binding and is not affected by CYP2D6 or CYP3A4, which decreases the risk of drug–drug interactions [41]. Oxymorphone has a reduced histamine effect and may be of use in patients who complain of headache or itching with other opioids [42].

Hydromorphone

Hydromorphone is a hydrogenated ketone of morphine [43]. Like morphine, it acts primarily on mu opioid receptors and to a lesser degree on delta receptors. While hydromorphone is 7–10 times more potent than morphine in single-dose studies [44], the oral and parenteral steady-state equivalence is 1:5, while the equivalence of chronic infusions may be as little as 1:3.5 [45]. It is highly water-soluble, which allows for very concentrated formulations, and in patients with renal failure, it may be preferred over morphine. Hydromorphone is metabolized primarily to hydromorphone-3-glucuronide (H3G), which, similar to the corresponding M3G, is not only devoid of analgesic activity but also evokes a range of dose-dependent excited behaviors including allodynia, myoclonus, and seizures in animal models [46].

Methadone

Methadone is a synthetic mu opioid receptor agonist medication. It is a racemic mixture of two enantiomers; the R form is more potent, with a tenfold higher affinity for opioid receptors (which accounts for virtually all of its analgesic effect), while S-methadone is the NMDA antagonist. The inherent NMDA antagonistic effects make it potentially useful in severe neuropathic and "opioid-resistant" pain states. The S isomer also inhibits reuptake of serotonin and norepinephrine, which should be recognized when using methadone in combination with SSRIs and TCAs. Although it has traditionally been used to treat heroin addicts, its flexibility in dosing, use in neuropathic pain, and cheap price have led to a recent increase in its use. Unfortunately, a lack of awareness of its metabolism and potential drug interactions, as well as its long half-life, has led to a dramatic increase in the deaths associated with this medication.

Methadone is unrelated to standard opioids, leading to its usefulness in patients with "true" morphine allergies. Methadone is metabolized in the liver and intestines and excreted almost exclusively in feces, an advantage in patients with renal insufficiency or failure.

The metabolism of methadone is always variable. Methadone is metabolized by CYP3A4 primarily and CYP2D6 secondarily; CYP2D6 preferentially metabolizes the R-methadone, while CYP3A4 and CYP1A2 metabolize both enantiomers. CYP1B2 is possibly involved, and a newly proposed enzyme CYP2B6 may be emerging as an important intermediary metabolic transformation [47]. CYP3A4 expression can vary up to 30-fold, and there can be genetic polymorphism of CYP2D6, ranging from poor to rapid metabolism. The initiation of methadone therapy can induce the CYP3A4 enzyme for 5–7 days, leading to low blood levels initially, but unexpectedly high levels may follow about a week later if the medication has been rapidly titrated upward. A wide variety of substances can also induce or inhibit these enzymes [48]. The potential differences in enzymatic metabolic conversion of methadone may explain the inconsistency of observed half-life.

Methadone has no active metabolites and therefore may result in less hyperalgesia, myoclonus, and neurotoxicity than morphine. It may be unique in its lack of profound euphoria, but its analgesic action (4–8 h) is significantly shorter than its elimination half-life (up to 150 h), and patient self-directed redosing and a long half-life may lead to the potential of respiratory depression and death.

Methadone also has the potential to cause cardiac arrhythmias, specifically prolonged QTc intervals and/or torsade de pointes under certain circumstances. Congenital QT prolongation, high methadone levels (usually over 60 mg/day), and conditions that increase QT prolongation (such as hypokalemia and hypomagnesemia) or IV methadone, because it contains chlorobutanol, which prolongs QTc intervals [49], may increase that risk [50]. Combining methadone with a CYP3A4 inhibitor such as ciprofloxin [51] potentially can increase that risk. It is recommended that a switch to methadone from another opioid be accompanied by a large (50–90 %) decrease in the calculated equipotent dose (Table 10.1) [53]. It cannot be too strongly emphasized that the dosing of methadone can be potentially lethal and must be done with knowledge and caution.

Fentanyl

Fentanyl is approximately 80 times more potent than morphine, is highly lipophilic, and binds strongly to plasma proteins. Fentanyl undergoes extensive metabolism in the liver. Fentanyl is metabolized by CYP3A4 to inactive and non-

Table 10.1 Oral morphine to methadone conversion

Oral morphine dose (mg)	MS: methadone ratio
30–90	4:1
90–300	8:1
300–800	12:1
800–1,000	15:1
>1,000	20:1

Ripamonti et al. [52]

toxic metabolites [54]; however, CYP3A4 inhibitors may lead to increased fentanyl blood levels. The transdermal formulation has a onset of action lag time of 6–12 h after application and typically reaches steady state in 3–6 days. When a patch is removed, a subcutaneous reservoir remains, and drug clearance may take up to 24 h.

Conversion Tables

The usual recommendation for calculating the equipotent dose of different opioids involves calculating the 24-h dose as "morphine equivalents" (see Table 10.2). However, Hanks and Fallon [54] instead suggest relating the starting doses to 4-h doses of morphine rather than 24-h doses. For example, in patients receiving 5–20 mg oral morphine every 4 h (or the equivalent in controlled-release morphine), start with 25 mcg/h fentanyl patches every 72 h; patients on 25–35 mg oral morphine every 4 h, 50 mcg/h of fentanyl; patients on 40–50 mg oral morphine every 4 h, 75 mcg/h fentanyl; and patients on 55–65 mg oral morphine every 4 h, 100 mcg/h fentanyl. They feel that the controversies over appropriate morphine to fentanyl potency ratio calculations miss the point that fentanyl transdermally behaves differently and cannot be equated with oral routes when calculating relative potency.

Tramadol

A unique analgesic, tramadol, is an atypical synthetic analogue of codeine [56]. The M1 derivative (O-demethyl tramadol) produced by CYP2D6 has a higher affinity for the mu receptor than the parent compound (as much as six times). Tramadol is a racemic mixture of two enantiomers—one form is a selective mu agonist and inhibits serotonin reuptake, while the other mainly inhibits norepinephrine reuptake [57]. Maximum dose is 400 mg/day, and toxic doses cause CNS excitation and seizures. Because it requires CYP2D6 metabolism for maximal analgesic effect, coadministration of CYP2D6 inhibitors such as fluoxetine, paroxetine, and sertraline is contraindicated. In addition, because tramadol has

Table 10.2 Opioid conversions

Drug	Initial po dose	PO:IV	PO MS:PO drug	PO drug: PO MS
Morphine	2.5–15 mg	3:1	1:1	1:1
Hydromorphone	1, 2, or 4 mg	4:1	1:0.25	1:4
Oxycodone	5 or 10 mg	N/A	1:0.66	1:1.5
Oxymorphone	2.5, 5, or 10 mg	10:1	1:0.33	1:3
Methadone	2.5 or 5 mg	2:1	[a]	[a]
TD fentanyl	25 mcg/h[b]	TD=IV/h	[b]	[b]

Modified from NHHPCO [55]
[a]See Table 10.1
[b]See section "Fentanyl"

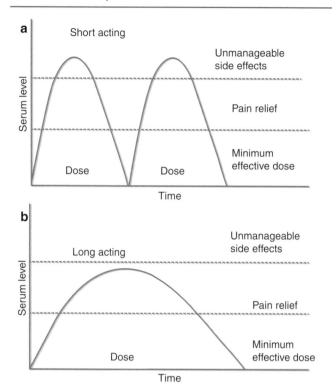

Fig. 10.4 Serum drug level following administration of (**a**) short-acting and (**b**) long-acting opioids (Modified from McCarberg and Barkin [59])

serotonin activity, SSRIs are relatively contraindicated because of the potential of a serotonin syndrome.

Although considered a "weak" opioid, it can have significant analgesic qualities (perhaps because of its dual opioid and SNRI action). In a study of 118 patients with moderate to severe cancer pain comparing 25 mg of hydrocodone to 200 mg of tramadol, 62 % of the tramadol patients obtained relief, compared to 57 % of the hydrocodone patients [58].

Opioid Routes of Administration

Oral

Major advances in the pharmacotherapy of chronic pain have led to the development of extended-release opioid delivery systems, thereby allowing less frequent dosing than the classic short-acting formulas. It is the patterns in serum drug levels that define the difference between short-acting opioids (SAO) and long-acting opioids (LAO); with SAOs, serum opioid levels rise rapidly following administration and then decline rapidly, while LAO administration allows for less fluctuation in serum opioid levels and an extended period within the therapeutic range (Fig. 10.4) [59]. The assumption that plasma levels of opioids correspond to analgesia has led to the additional concept of minimum effective concentration (MEC), the plasma level of an opioid below which there is ineffective analgesia.

There are many proposed advantages of the long-acting opioid formulas compared to the short-acting formulas. Because of the longer duration of action, there is a lessening of the frequency and severity of end-of-dose pain [60]. Furthermore, it has been suggested that less frequent dosing leads to increased compliance and improved efficacy [61]. Sustained analgesia and uninterrupted sleep are other potential advantages of the extended-release formulation compared to the short-acting variety. However, in a recent systematic review of long-acting versus short-acting opioids, Rauck [62] noted that, while it was clear that long-acting opioids achieved more stable drug levels, there was no clear evidence from appropriately designed comparative trials to make a case for the use of one type of formulation over the other on the basis of clinical efficacy.

Transmucosal

Oral transmucosal fentanyl citrate (OTFC) has become a mainstay in the treatment of breakthrough pain because it provides faster absorption of the lipophilic fentanyl than any other oral opioid formulation [63]. This "fentanyl lollipop" consists of medication on the end of a stick, which is applied to the buccal membrane. A newer formulation of fentanyl, the fentanyl buccal tablet (FBT), was designed to provide an even faster relief. Additional delivery systems for intranasal and inhaled fentanyl are being developed [64].

Intravenous

Intravenous delivery of opioids allows for rapid and reliable delivery of medicine, but veins for administration are not always available. In general, the IV dose is approximately 1/3 of the oral dose, since IV medications do not have a first-pass effect. Opioids can be delivered intermittently or continuously; patient-controlled analgesia (PCA) is now available for outpatient use so that small doses of opioids are delivered when the patient pushes a button, with or without a continuous infusion of opioid.

Subcutaneous

Subcutaneous opioid injections can be an option for the patient unable to tolerate oral medications but without IV access. The medication is administered through a butterfly needle and can be given intermittently or continuously. Onset is slower and lower peak effect than IV, but this may be a better option for acute or escalating pain than transdermal fentanyl, which has an even slower onset and prolonged effect [65]. Subcutaneous infusions up to 10 cc/h can be usually absorbed, but patients are usually more comfortable with 2–3 cc/h.

Rectal

The rectal mucosa absorbs many medications easily, including most opioids, and the blood flow from the rectum bypasses the liver so that rectal morphine results in blood levels that are almost 90 % of the oral dose [66]. A double-blind, double-dummy, crossover study in 1995 compared oral versus rectal morphine, which was shown to be effective, easy to manage, and inexpensive, with a rapid onset of action [67].

Transdermal

The skin is the largest organ in the body, with a surface area of 1–2 m², which makes it appealing as a drug absorption modality. However, the skin functions as a barrier to the elements, and those same properties limit its effectiveness as a drug delivery site. Medications must have a small molecular weight with high lipid solubility to pass across the skin barrier, and fentanyl is one of the most effective opioids for transdermal delivery [68]. Although all opioids have similar side effects (see section "Opioid Side Effects"), transdermal fentanyl appears to have less constipation but did show skin reactions in 1–3 % of the 153 cancer pain patients studied [69].

Intrathecal/Epidural

Oral and parenteral opioids work by dulling the brain so that it does not recognize the pain signals as easily. Intrathecal and epidural opioids attach to opioid receptors at the spinal level, blocking pain signals from reaching the brain. The medications are more potent in the spinal column; as an example, 300 mg of morphine by mouth is felt to be equivalent to 5 mg in the epidural space or 1 mg in the spinal fluid (intrathecal space). These dramatically lower doses result in less sedation and mental clouding. Single dose administration of intrathecal opioids has been used for acute pain, such as postoperative pain. Continuous infusions for cancer pain and chronic noncancer pain utilized implanted subcutaneous pumps connected to intrathecal catheters. However, because these systems require specialist's placement and care, they are often not considered until very late in the course of the cancer, and hematologic abnormalities such as chemotherapy-induced thrombocytopenia may severely limit the ability to safely access the spinal canal. Although intrathecal opioid pain relief can be dramatic, procedural complications remain high, including infection, pump failures, drug errors, and post-dural puncture headaches [70].

Pruritus is seen more commonly with neural axial opioids than systemic opioids, with an incidence between 30 and 100 %, and is effectively reversed by opioid antagonists.

Although respiratory depression is the dreaded complication of intrathecal opioids, its incidence is low (0.09–0.4 %) [71].

Opioid Conversion

Equianalgesic tables, like the one below (Table 10.2), can guide physicians to *estimate* the new opioid optimal dose for a patient that has started to develop tolerance to their current opioid dose. These tables provide only broad guidelines for selecting the dose of an opioid because of large individual pharmacokinetic and even larger pharmacodynamic differences in opioid pharmacology. Different pain syndromes, such as osteoarticular diseases, neuropathic pain, or oncologic pain states, may demonstrate very different and unpredictable clinical responses [72]. The majority of patients need a lower dosing of the new opioid than the dose theoretically calculated with an equianalgesic table [73]. Because of an incomplete cross-tolerance, it is recommended to reduce the calculated dose by 33 % (methadone should be decreased as much as 90%) [74]. For safety reasons, the new opioid should be initiated at a low dose that, if necessary, can be gradually increased to achieve adequate analgesia [75].

Opioid in Acute Pain

Opioids have typically been used in the treatment of acute pain, such as broken bones or postsurgical pain. In the emergency department, there has been a concern that opioids would mask the physical findings for surgical problems such as acute appendicitis. Yuan and colleagues [76] prospectively evaluated 102 patients with acute appendicitis who received either morphine or normal saline IV. In the morphine group, the abdominal pain was significantly relieved, and the patient's cooperation was improved while the physical exam was unaffected, supporting the premise that morphine did not obscure the physical signs.

Unfortunately, standard doses of opioids may not work effectively for acute pain; 621 consecutive ED patients were treated with titrated boluses of IV morphine [77]. The mean total dose of morphine was 10.5 mg with a range of 2–46 mg. The authors noted that sedation could not be arbitrarily attributed to the occurrence of an adequate level of analgesia because, among patients in whom morphine titration was discontinued because of sedation, 25 % still exhibit a level of pain above 50 (0–100).

Opioids in Cancer Pain

There are many causes of cancer pain, some caused by the cancer itself, and others caused by the effects of the cancer. Recently, a large study of almost 2,000 outpatient oncology patients [78] showed that 53 % of the patients had pain only due to their cancer and/or treatment, 25.3 % had noncancer pain, and 21.7 % had both cancer and noncancer pain. However, less than 25 % received a prescription for a strong opioid, only 7 % had a coanalgesic prescribed for pain, and approximately 20 % received no analgesic prescription. This suggests that oncologists are not adequately addressing pain needs.

Noncancer Pain in Cancer Pain Patients

Although often blamed on the cancer, patients with cancer can also suffer from the same pain conditions seen in noncancer pain patients. Thus, the lung cancer patient with pain going down the arm may have tumor involvement of the brachial plexus but may also have a herniated cervical disc or suprascapular nerve entrapment. In addition, there are multiple cancer-related pain issues, such as chemotherapy-induced peripheral neuropathy or postherpetic neuralgia, that may need to be addressed with opioids.

Noncancer Pain

Although originally considered contraindicated for chronic noncancer pain, opioids are now being used much more frequently for a variety of chronic painful conditions, such as post-laminectomy syndrome, peripheral neuropathy, and postherpetic neuralgia. The American Society of Interventional Pain Physicians (ASIPP) reviewed chronic opioid use in noncancer pain [79] and concluded that opioids are commonly prescribed for chronic noncancer pain and may be effective for short-term pain relief. However, evidence of long-term effectiveness for 6 months or longer is variable, with evidence ranging from moderate for transdermal fentanyl and sustained-release morphine to limited for oxycodone and indeterminate for hydrocodone and methadone.

Opioid Tolerance Versus Hyperalgia

When opioids become less effective over time, increased pain may represent tolerance, a pharmacodynamic desensitization induced by high opioid doses [80]. One method of addressing this increase in pain is the use of adjuvant medications. The cancer patient with neuropathic pain, for instance, from tumor invasion of a nerve plexus, would not be expected to respond well to opioids but might benefit from the addition of an anticonvulsant. Another option is opioid rotation (see below), a therapeutic maneuver aiming in improving analgesic response and/or reducing adverse effects, including change to a different medication using the same administration route, maintaining the current medication but altering administration route, or both.

Decreased response to opioids may also be due to pharmacokinetic and drug delivery factors, such as poor absorption or vascular compromise. However, most concerning is the concept of opioid-induced hyperalgesia, a reduced opioid responsiveness resulting in increased pain despite (or perhaps because of) escalating doses of opioids. Opioid-induced hyperalgesia might be considered in a patient who has no evidence of disease progression, who is on clinically reasonable doses of opioids, and whose pain escalates as opioid doses are increased [81]. A reduction of opioids and the addition of a low-dose N-methyl-D-aspartate (NMDA) receptor antagonist may provide a favorable clinical outcome in those patients who have failed to benefit from opioid rotation and other adjunctive pain treatments.

Opioid Rotation

Pain patients may not respond to increasing doses of opioids because they develop adverse effects before achieving an acceptable analgesia, or the analgesic response is poor despite a rapid dose escalation. Opioid switching may significantly improve the balance between analgesia and adverse effects. According to available data, opioid switching results in clinical improvement in more than 50 % of patients with chronic pain with poor response to one opioid [82].

Addiction

We currently have no satisfactory definition or criteria for addiction in patients receiving therapeutic opioids [83]. However, the rise of prescription opioid abuse has focused attention on the need for prevention in all exposed populations. The 2006 National Survey on Drug Use and Health found that 5.2 million Americans age 12 or older misused prescription analgesics, an increase from 4.7 million in 2005 [84]. Furthermore, analgesic use was the drug category with the most new initiates. Screening patients to determine their risk for drug abuse prior to beginning opioid therapy is considered good practice. Even more vital is the monitoring of patients to ensure compliance, including urine drug monitoring and surveillance of non-sanctioned opioid use via national prescription registers, a process that was associated with a 50 % reduction in opioid abuse in 500 patients receiving controlled substances [85].

Future Directions

Opioids of lower addictive potential, such as tamper-resistant extended-release opioids, are coming on the market, in an effort to expand the use of opioids while decreasing the addiction and diversion potential. Opioid abuse screening tools (such as the Opioid Risk Tool) and fMRIs to look at brain areas associated with addiction and pain perception may also help identify those patients at risk for opioid abuse while maintaining access for those patients in whom opioids are appropriate management for their painful condition.

Conclusion

Opioids are broad-spectrum analgesics, with multiple effects and side effects. When used wisely and with appropriate caution and knowledge of metabolism and interactions, opioids can offer significant relief from soul-draining pain.

Recommended Links

American Academy of Pain Medicine code of ethics
http://www.painmed.org/pract_mngmnt/ethics.html
ASIPP opioid guidelines
http://www.asipp.org/Guidelines.htm
American Pain Foundation
http://www.painfoundation.org/

References

1. Breasted JG. Ancient records of Egypt. University of Chicago Oriental Institute Publications, vol. III. Chicago: University of Chicago Press; 1930. p. 217.
2. Schwarz S, Huxtable R. The isolation of morphine. Mol Interv. 2001;1(4):189–91.
3. The role of chemistry in history. 2010. http://itech.dickinson.edu/chemistry/?cat=107. Accessed 15 Mar 2010.
4. Jurna I. Serturner and morphine – a historical vignette. Schmerz. 2003;17(4):280–3.
5. Trescot A, Datta S, Lee M, Hansen H. Opioid pharmacology. Pain Physician. 2008;11(opioid special issue):S133–53.
6. Pert CB, Snyder SH. Opiate receptor: its demonstration in nervous tissue. Science. 1973;179:1011–4.
7. Hughes J, Smith T, Kosterlitz H, Fothergill L, Morgan B, Morris H. Identification of two related pentapeptides from the brain with potent opiate agonist activity. Nature. 1975;258:577–80.
8. Fukuda K. Intravenous opioid anesthetics. In: Miller RD, editor. Miller's anesthesia. 6th ed. Philadelphia: Elsevier; 2005.
9. Chahl LA. Opioids – mechanism of action. Aust Prescr. 1996;19:63–5.
10. Nestler EJ. Molecular basis of long-term plasticity underlying addiction. Nat Rev Neurosci. 2001;2:119–28.
11. Fillingim RB, Kaplan L, Staud R, et al. The A118G single nucleotide polymorphism of the μ-opioid receptor gene (OPRM1) is associated with pressure pain sensitivity in humans. J Pain. 2005;6(3):159–67.
12. Smith HS. Variations in opioid responsiveness. Pain Physician. 2008;11:237–48.
13. Klepstad P, Kaasa S, Skauge M, Borchgrevink PC. Pain intensity and side effects during titration of morphine in cancer patients using a fixed schedule dose escalation. Acta Anaesthesiol Scand. 2000;44(6):656–64.
14. Bertilsson L, Dahl ML, Ekqvist B, Jerling M, Lierena A. Genetic regulation of the disposition of psychotropic drugs. In: Meltzer HY, Nerozzi D, editors. Current practices and future developments in the pharmacotherapy of mental disorders. Amsterdam: Elsevier; 1991. p. 73–80.
15. Stamer UM, Stuber F. Genetic factors in pain and its treatment. Curr Opin Anaesthesiol. 2007;20(5):478–84.
16. Otton SV, Schadel M, Cheung SW, Kaplan HL, Busto UE, Sellers EM. CYP2D6 phenotype determines the metabolic conversion of hydrocodone to hydromorphone. Clin Pharmacol Ther. 1993;54(5):463–72.
17. Benyamin R, Trescot AM, Datta S, et al. Opioid complications and side effects. Pain Physician. 2008;11(opioid special issue):S105–20.
18. McNicol E, Horowicz-Mehler N, Fisk RA, et al. Management of opioid side effects in cancer-related and chronic noncancer pain: a systematic review. J Pain. 2003;4:231–56.
19. Swegle JM, Logemann C. Opioid-induced adverse effects. Am Fam Physician. 2006;74(8):1347–52.
20. Meuser T, Pietruck C, Radbruch L, Stute P, Lehmann KA, Grond S. Symptoms during cancer pain treatment following WHO-guidelines: a longitudinal follow-up study of symptom prevalence, severity and etiology. Pain Med. 2001;93:247–57.
21. Flake ZA, Scalley RG, Bailey AG. Practical selection of antiemetics. Am Fam Physician. 2004;69:1169–74.
22. Cherny N, Ripamonti C, Pereira J, et al. Strategies to manage the adverse effects of oral morphine: an evidence-based report. J Clin Oncol. 2001;19:2542–54.
23. Cherny NI. The management of cancer pain. CA Cancer J Clin. 2000;50:70–116.
24. Teichtahl H, Prodromidis A, Miller B, et al. Sleep-disordered breathing in stable methadone programme patients: a pilot study. Addiction. 2001;96(3):395–403.
25. Downey R, Gold PM. Obstructive sleep apnea. 2010. http://emedicine.medscape.com/article/295807-print. Accessed Apr 2010.
26. Wang D, Teichtahl H, Drummer O, et al. Central sleep apnea in stable methadone maintenance treatment patients. Chest. 2005;128(3):1348–56.
27. Howlett TA, Rees LH. Endogenous opioid peptides and hypothalamopituitary function. Annu Rev Physiol. 1986;48:527–36.
28. Daniell HW. Opioid endocrinopathy in women consuming prescribed sustained action opioids for control of nonmalignant pain. J Pain. 2008;9:28–36.
29. Daniell HW. Hypogonadism in men consuming sustained-action oral opioids. J Pain. 2002;3:377–84.
30. Merza Z. Chronic use of opioids and the endocrine system. Horm Metab Res. 2010;42(9):621–6.
31. Roy S, Loh HH. Effects of opioids on the immune system. Neurochem Res. 1996;21(11):1375–86.
32. Zacny JP. Morphine responses in humans: a retrospective analysis of sex differences. Drug Alcohol Depend. 2001;63:23–8.
33. Zun LS, Downey LV, Gossman W, Rosenbaumdagger J, Sussman G. Gender differences in narcotic-induced emesis in the ED. Am J Emerg Med. 2002;20(3):151–4.
34. Cepeda MS, Farrar JT, Roa JH, et al. Ethnicity influences morphine pharmacokinetics and pharmacodynamics. Clin Pharmacol Ther. 2001;70(4):351–61.
35. Lotsch J, Geisslinger G. Morphine-6-glucuronide: an analgesic of the future? Clin Pharmacokinet. 2001;40:485–99.
36. Smith MT. Neuroexcitatory effects of morphine and hydromorphone: evidence implicating the 3-glucuronide metabolites. Clin Exp Pharmacol Physiol. 2000;27:524–8.
37. Wasan AD, Michna E, Janfaza D, Greenfield S, Teter CJ, Jamison RN. Interpreting urine drug tests: prevalence of morphine metabolism to hydromorphone in chronic pain patients treated with morphine. Pain Med. 2008;9:918–23.

38. MedWatch safety labeling change. 2010. www.fda.gov/medwatch/safety/2007/safety07.htm#Codeine. Accessed Jan 2010.

39. Rodriguez RF, Castillo JM, del Pilar Castillo M, et al. Codeine/acetaminophen and hydrocodone/acetaminophen combination tablets for the management of chronic cancer pain in adults: a 23-day, prospective, double-blind, randomized, parallel-group study. Clin Ther. 2007;29(4):581–7.

40. Poyhia R, Seppala T, Olkkola KT, Kalso E. The pharmacokinetics and metabolism of oxycodone after intramuscular and oral administration to healthy subjects. Br J Clin Pharmacol. 1992;33:617–21.

41. Sloan PA, Barkin RL. Oxymorphone and oxymorphone extended release: a pharmacotherapeutic review. J Opioid Manag. 2008;4(3):131–44.

42. Foley KM, Abernathy A. Management of cancer pain. In: Devita VT, Lawrence TS, Rosenberg SA, editors. Devita, Hellman & Rosenberg's cancer: principles & practice of oncology. 8th ed. Philadelphia: Lippincott Williams & Wilkins; 2008.

43. Murray A, Hagen NA. Hydrocodone. J Pain Symptom Manage. 2005;29:S57–66.

44. Vallner JJ, Stewart J, Kotzan JA, Kirsten EB, Honigberg IL. Pharmacokinetics and bioavailability of hydromorphone following intravenous and oral administration to human subjects. J Clin Pharmacol. 1981;214:152–6.

45. Davis MP, McPherson ML. Tabling hydromorphone: do we have it right? J Palliat Med. 2010;13(4):365–6.

46. Wright AW, Mather LE, Smith MT. Hydromorphone-3-glucuronide: a more potent neuro-excitant than its structural analogue, morphine-3-glucuronide. Life Sci. 2001;69(4):409–20.

47. Lynch ME. A review of the use of methadone for the treatment of chronic noncancer pain. Pain Res Manag. 2005;10:133–44.

48. Leavitt SB. Addiction treatment forums: methadone – drug interactions. 2009. www.atforum.com/SiteRoot/pages/rxmethadone/methadonedruginteractions.shtml. Accessed 2009.

49. Kornick CA, Kilborn MJ, Santiago-Palma J, et al. QTc interval prolongation associated with intravenous methadone. Pain. 2003;105(3):499–506.

50. Krantz MJ, Lewkowiez L, Hays H, Woodroffe MA, Robertson AD, Mehler PS. Torsade de pointes associated with very high dose methadone. Ann Intern Med. 2002;137:501–4.

51. Herrlin K, Segerdahl M, Gustafsson LL, Kalso E. Methadone, ciprofloxacin, and adverse drug reactions. Lancet. 2000;356:2069–70.

52. Ripamonti C, Conno FD, Groff L, et al. Equianalgesic dose/ratio between methadone and other opioid agonists in cancer pain: comparison of two clinical experiences. Ann Oncol. 1998;9(1):79–83.

53. Gazelle G, Fine PG. Methadone for the treatment of pain. J Palliat Med. 2003;6:621–2.

54. Hanks G, Cherny N, Fallon M. Opioid analgesic therapy. In: Doyle D, Hanks G, Cherny N, et al (eds) Oxford Textbook of Palliative Medicine (3rd ed). Oxford University Press, 2004; pp. 318–21.

55. New Hampshire Hospice and Palliative Care Organization. 2010. http://www.nhhpco.org/opioid.htm. Accessed Apr 2010.

56. Grond S, Sablotzki A. Clinical pharmacology of tramadol. Clin Pharmacokinet. 2004;43:879–923.

57. Raffa RB, Friderichs E, Reimann W. et al opioid and nonopioid components independently contribute to the mechanism of action of tramadol, an "atypical" opioid analgesic. J Pharmacol Exp Ther. 1992;260:275–85.

58. Rodriguez RF, Castillo JM, Castillo MP, et al. Hydrocodone/acetaminophen and tramadol chlorhydrate combination tablets for the management of chronic cancer pain: a double-blind comparative trial. Clin J Pain. 2008;24(1):1–4.

59. McCarberg B, Barkin R. Long-acting opioids for chronic pain; pharmacotherapeutic opportunities to enhance compliance, quality of life, and analgesia. Am J Ther. 2001;8:181–6.

60. Kaplan R, Parris WC, Citron ML, et al. Comparison of controlled-release and immediate-release oxycodone tablets AVINZA and chronic noncancer pain – 263 inpatients with cancer pain. J Clin Oncol. 1998;16:3230–7.

61. American Pain Society. Principles of analgesic use in the treatment of acute pain and cancer pain. Glenview: American Pain Society; 2003.

62. Rauck RL. What is the case for prescribing long-acting opioids over short-acting opioids for patients with chronic pain? A critical review. Pain Pract. 2009;9(6):468–79.

63. Coluzzi PH, Shwartzberg L, Conroy Jr JD, Charapata S, Gay M, Busch MA, et al. Breakthrough cancer pain: a randomized trial comparing oral transmucosal fentanyl citrate (OTFC®) and morphine sulfate immediate release (MSIR®). Pain. 2001;91:123–30.

64. Mercadante S, Radbruch L, Popper L, Korsholm L, Davies A. Efficacy of intranasal fentanyl spray (INFS) versus oral transmucosal fentanyl citrate (OTFC) for breakthrough cancer pain: open-label crossover trial. Eur J Pain. 2009;13:S198.

65. Ripamonti C, Fagnoni E, Campa T, et al. Is the use of transdermal fentanyl inappropriate according to the WHO guidelines and the EAPC recommendations? A study of cancer patients in Italy. Support Care Cancer. 2006;14:400–7.

66. McCaffery M, Martin L, Ferrell BR. Analgesic administration via rectum or stoma. J ET Nurs. 1992;19:114–21.

67. DeConno F, Ripamonti C, Saita L, MacEachern T, Hanson J, Bruera E. Role of rectal route in treating cancer pain: a randomized crossover clinical trial of oral versus rectal morphine administration in opioid-naive cancer patients with pain. J Clin Oncol. 1995;13(4):1004–8.

68. Jeal W, Benfield P. Transdermal fentanyl. A review of its pharmacological properties and therapeutic efficacy in pain control. Drugs. 1997;53(1):109–38.

69. Muijsers RB, Wagstaff AJ. Transdermal fentanyl: an updated review of its pharmacological properties and therapeutic efficacy in chronic cancer pain control. Drugs. 2001;61(15):2289–307.

70. Rathmell JP, Lair TR, Nauman B. The role of intrathecal drugs in the treatment of acute pain. Anesth Analg. 2005;101:S30–43.

71. Gustafsson LL, Schildt B, Jacobsen K. Adverse effects of extradural and intrathecal opiates: report of a nation-wide survey in Sweden. Br J Anaesth. 1982;54:479–86.

72. Galer BS, Coyle N, Pasternak GW, Portenoy RK. Individual variability in the response to different opioids: report of five cases. Pain. 1992;49:87–91.

73. Brant JM. Opioid equianalgesic conversion: the right dose. Clin J Oncol Nurs. 2001;5:163–5.

74. Vissers KC, Besse K, Hans G, Devulder J, Morlion B. Opioid rotation in the management of chronic pain: where is the evidence? Pain Pract. 2010;10(2):85–93.

75. Hanks GW, Conno F, Cherny N, et al. Morphine and alternative opioids in cancer pain: the EAPC recommendations. Br J Cancer. 2001;84:587–93.

76. Yuan Y, Chen JY, Guo H, et al. Relief of abdominal pain by morphine without altering physical signs in acute appendicitis. Chin Med J (Engl). 2010;123(2):142–5.

77. Lvovschi V, Aubrun F, Bonnet P, et al. Intravenous morphine titration to treat severe pain in the ED. Am J Emerg Med. 2008;26:676–82.

78. Valeberg BT, Rustoen T, Bjordal K, Hanestad BR, Paul S, Miaskowski C. Self-reported prevalence, etiology, and characteristics of pain in oncology outpatients. Eur J Pain. 2008;12(5):582–90.

79. Trescot AM, Boswell MV, Atluri SL, et al. Opioid guidelines in the management of chronic non-cancer pain. Pain Physician. 2006;9(1):1–39.

80. Chang G, Chen L, Mao J. Opioid tolerance and hyperalgesia. Med Clin North Am. 2007;91:199–211.

81. Vorobeychik Y, Chen L, Bush MC, Mao J. Improved opioid analgesic effect following opioid dose reduction. Pain Med. 2008;9(6):724–7.

82. Mercadante S, Bruera E. Opioid switching: a systematic and critical review. Cancer Treat Rev. 2006;32:304–15.

83. Ballantyne J. Opioid analgesia: perspective on right use and utility. Pain Physician. 2007;10:479–91.

84. Substance Abuse and Mental Health Services Administration. Results from the 2006 national survey on drug use and health. National findings. Office of Applied Studies, NSDUH Series: H-32, DHHS Publication No. SMA 07-4293. Rockville. 2007.

85. Manchikanti L, Manchukonda R, Damron KS, Brandon D, McManus CD, Cash K. Does adherence monitoring reduce controlled substance abuse in chronic pain patients? Pain Physician. 2006;9(1):57–60.

Opioid Adverse Effects and Opioid-Induced Hypogonadism

Saloni Sharma and David M. Giampetro

Key Points

- Recognize that opioids are known to have potentially serious adverse effects
- Review major adverse effects including nausea and vomiting, constipation, neuroendocrine effects, immune effects, respiratory depression, central nervous system effects, and pruritis
- Consider the risks and benefits of continued opioid therapy in light of adverse effects
- Become familiar with common treatment options for opioid-related adverse effects

Nausea and Vomiting

Nausea and vomiting are well-known side effects of opioid use. When used for treatment of chronic nonmalignant pain, nausea has been reported to occur in 21–32 % of patients with vomiting reported in 10 % [1, 2]. Opioid-induced nausea and vomiting often occurs with initiation of an opioid or with recent dose escalation. The majority of patients develop a tolerance to this over several days or weeks. These effects can occur via centrally and peripherally stimulated pathways. Activation of the emesis center in the medulla is the primary mechanism for opioid-induced nausea and vomiting. The emesis center is stimulated by input from gastrointestinal (GI) receptors, the cerebral cortex, the vestibular system, and the chemoreceptor trigger zone in the area postrema of the medulla. It also sends efferent information to the GI system (see Fig. 11.1).

S. Sharma, B.A., M.D. (✉)
Rehabilitation & Pain Specialists, 107 Gamma Drive, Suite 220,
Pittsburgh, PA 15238, USA
e-mail: salsharma@hotmail.com

D.M. Giampetro, M.D.
Department of Anesthesiology,
Pennsylvania State University College of Medicine,
500 University Blvd, Hershey, PA 17033, USA
e-mail: dgiampetro@psu.edu

Since tolerance to opioid-induced nausea and vomiting usually develops within days, prolonged treatment, if any, is usually not needed. Often, decreasing the opioid dose with a slower titration to escalating doses, changing the route of administration, or opioid rotation are sufficient strategies to manage this side effect. If possible, identifying an individual's trigger of opioid-induced nausea and/or vomiting can allow one to tailor etiology-specific treatment. If symptoms occur with movement or ambulation, the vestibular system may be involved and treatment with antihistamines or anticholinergics such as scopolamine may be of benefit. If symptoms are associated with meals, gastrointestinal causes may be triggering nausea and vomiting and the patient may benefit from multiple smaller volume meals as well as treatment with a motility agent such as metoclopramide [3].

If a clear mechanism cannot be identified, treatment is often determined based on a patient's comorbidities and other symptoms such as constipation. The potential for side effects from the treating medication must also be considered. Other potentially therapeutic drugs include prokinetic drugs, antipsychotics and related drugs, antihistamines, serotonin antagonists, anticholinergics, benzodiazepines, and steroids (see Table 11.1). Prokinetic agents such as metoclopramide improve gastric motility and decrease GI transit times and, therefore, may be beneficial to patients with nausea and constipation [4]. Antipsychotics work within the chemoreceptor trigger zone to block dopamine receptors and have been found to be effective for the treatment of opioid-associated nausea and vomiting in cancer patients [5]. Antihistamines act on the emesis center and vestibular system [3, 6]. Serotonin antagonists act by blocking serotonin release in the GI tract and the chemoreceptor trigger zone [6]. Anticholinergics act on the emesis center and GI tract [6]. Benzodiazepines act on the vestibular system and chemoreceptor trigger zone. The mechanism of steroids in reducing nausea and vomiting is not clear [6]. Peripherally acting mu-receptor antagonists have been shown to decrease gastric transit time and diminish opioid-related nausea and vomiting [7, 8] but have not been extensively used for this purpose.

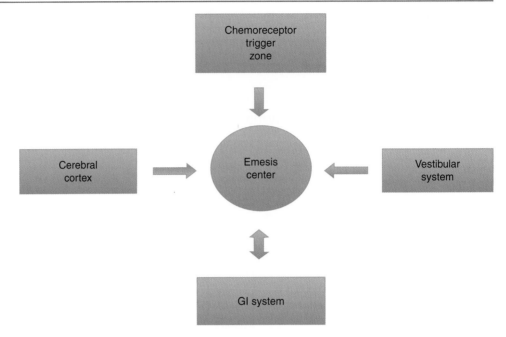

Fig. 11.1 Causes of opioid-induced nausea and/or vomiting

Table 11.1 Medications for treatment of opioid-induced nausea and/or vomiting[a] [3, 6, 7]

Motility drugs	Metoclopramide
Antipsychotics and related drugs	Haloperidol, droperidol, prochlorperazine, promethazine, chlorpromazine, methotrimeprazine
Antihistamines	Meclizine, cyclizine, hydroxyzine, diphenhydramine
Serotonin antagonists	Ondansetron, granisetron, dolasetron
Anticholinergics	Scopolamine
Benzodiazepines	Lorazepam
Steroids	Prednisone, dexamethasone
Potentially, peripherally acting mu-receptor antagonist	Methylnaltrexone, alvimopan

[a]An example(s) of each type of medication is listed and is not meant to be a comprehensive list

Medications may be delivered in a non-oral form if nausea and vomiting impair oral intake or if oral intake is limited for other reasons. A combination of antiemetics from different classes may be needed in resistant cases. All of these medications may result in side effects of their own, and the risks and benefits of initiating these therapies as opposed to decreasing the opioid dose, changing the route of administration, changing the type of opioid, or discontinuing opioid therapy must be considered.

Additionally, some have recommended use of alternative therapies including cannabinoids and acupressure [9]. Cannabinoids have been primarily studied for the treatment of nausea and vomiting related to chemotherapy. The results of the studies in this setting have shown some efficacy in patients who have failed treatment with other antiemetics but often resulted in a high rate of therapy discontinuation

secondary to adverse side effects [10]. Cannabinoids are not commonly used in the setting of opioid-induced nausea and vomiting and are not recommended for routine use in this setting. Acupuncture techniques including acupressure and electro-acutherapy treatments with use of acupuncture point Pericardium 6 have been found to be effective in the treatment of postoperative nausea and vomiting [11] as well as in a multitude of other settings including chemotherapy-induced nausea and vomiting [12]. Other alternative approaches include use of meditation and guided imagery to treat the anticipation of nausea and vomiting and have been studied in patients with cancer [13]. There is not a large amount of data supporting use of these treatments for opioid-induced nausea and vomiting, but they may be beneficial.

Most importantly, if an opioid has not recently been started or opioid dose recently escalated, or if there are other systemic signs and symptoms, other etiologies of nausea and/or vomiting must be considered (see Table 11.2).

Constipation

Constipation is a common side effect of opioid therapy. Constipation related to opioid use has been reported to occur in 15–90 % of patients [15]. Constipation as defined by the Rome III Diagnostic Criteria includes at least two of the following: less than three defecations per week, straining, lumpy or hard stools, feeling of incomplete evacuation or anorectal obstruction, and manual attempts to ease defecation [16].

There are multiple potential mechanisms for opioid-induced constipation, and it is widely known to be mediated via opioid receptors in the GI tract and central nervous system

Table 11.2 Differential diagnosis nausea and vomiting[a] [14]

Gastrointestinal (GI)	*Functional* (e.g., irritable bowel syndrome, dyspepsia, gastroparesis)
	Obstruction (e.g., adhesions, malignancy, hernia, stenosis)
	Organic (e.g., appendicitis, cholecystitis, hepatitis, peptic ulcers)
Infectious	(e.g., Food-borne toxins, urinary tract infection)
Medications/toxins	(e.g., Nonsteroidal anti-inflammatories, radiation)
Metabolic	(e.g., Adrenal disorder, pregnancy, uremia)
Miscellaneous	(e.g., Nephrolithiasis, pain, psychiatric)
Central nervous system	*Increased intracranial pressure, migraine, seizure disorder, head injury, vestibular*

[a]This is a summary and is not intended to include all potential causes

Table 11.3 Mechanisms of opioid-induced constipation [3, 15]

| 1. ↓ Peristalsis → ↓ GI motility → ↑ transit time → ↑ fluid absorption → ↓ fluid in stool |
| 2. ↑ Segment contractions that are ineffective in propelling stool forward |
| 3. ↑ Sphincter tone |
| 4. ↓ Mucosal secretions |

(see Table 11.3). Binding of opioid receptors, specifically mu, kappa, and delta receptors, within the enteric nervous system of the GI tract alters GI motility and contributes to constipation [17–19] as well as to nausea and vomiting. Once bound, the release of GI neurotransmitters is inhibited disrupting the appropriate intestinal contractions needed for GI motility, and mucosal secretions are decreased [15].

Constipation is thought to be dose-related, and unfortunately, tolerance to opioid-induced constipation does not typically occur [7]. Therefore, this side effect usually necessitates treatment. Lifestyle and dietary modifications including increasing physical activity, drinking more fluids, ingesting larger amounts of fiber, and creating a meal and toileting schedule may be trialed [20]. Typically, first-line treatment includes use of a stool softener such as sodium docusate and often is not effective as a sole treatment [21]. A stimulant laxative such as senna is typically added to use of stool softener. If constipation persists, addition of osmotic or bulk-forming laxatives, nonabsorbable solution, or enema may be therapeutic (see Table 11.4). Recently, peripherally acting mu-receptor antagonists have been found effective in treating peripheral causes of constipation. Methylnaltrexone is approved for treatment of opioid-induced constipation in patients receiving palliative care, and alvimopan is approved for aiding GI function after bowel resection [8].

As with most opioid side effects, one may consider decreasing opioid dose, opioid rotation, changing the route of administration, or discontinuing opioid therapy. There is

Table 11.4 Medications to treat opioid-induced constipation[a] [3, 4, 15, 19, 22]

Stool softeners	Sodium docusate
Stimulants	Senna, bisacodyl
Osmotic laxatives	Sorbitol, lactulose, magnesium, polyethylene glycol
Bulk laxatives	Wheat bran, psyllium seed, polycarbophil
Lubricant	Mineral oil
Peripherally, acting mu-receptor antagonist	Methylnaltrexone, alvimopan

[a]An example(s) of each type of medication is listed and is not meant to be a comprehensive list or suggests a preferred medication

Table 11.5 Differential framework for constipation[a] [26]

Functional	Dietary reasons, motility problem
Structural	Anorectal disorders, colonic strictures, or mass lesions
Endocrine and metabolic	Diabetes mellitus, hypercalcemia, hypothyroidism
Neurogenic	Cerebrovascular events, multiple sclerosis
Smooth muscle and connective tissue disorders	Amyloidosis, scleroderma
Psychogenic	Anxiety, depression, somatization
Drugs	Narcotics, anticholinergics, antidepressants

[a]This is a summary and is not intended to include all potential causes

literature reporting diminished rates of constipation with use of buprenorphine or transdermal fentanyl, but there is also literature refuting this in regard to transdermal fentanyl [23–25]. If opioid therapy has not recently been initiated or opioid dose increased, or if there are other symptoms, one must consider other causes of constipation (see Table 11.5).

Neuroendocrine Effects Including Hypogonadism

Opioids are known to alter the functioning of the hypothalamus-pituitary-adrenal axis in both acute and chronic settings. The hypothalamus has numerous functions including controlling the secretion of gonadotropin-releasing hormone (GrH), which stimulates the pituitary gland to secrete luteinizing hormone (LH) and follicle-stimulating hormone (FSH). These hormones, then, act on the testes and ovaries to result in the secretion of testosterone and estradiol. The release of GrH, LH, and FSH are regulated by negative feedback from testosterone and estradiol (see Fig. 11.2).

Chronic opioid therapy leads to suppression of the hypothalamus and pituitary [27–30]. This results in diminished GrH secretion contributing to a decreased release of LH and FSH as well as decreased testosterone and estradiol. Studies

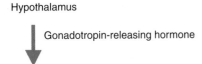

Hypothalamus

    Gonadotropin-releasing hormone

Pituitary

    Follicle-stimulating hormone and luteinizing hormone

Ovarises/testes

Estradiol/testosterone

Fig. 11.2 The hypothalamus-pituitary axis

Table 11.7 Differential diagnosis of hypogonadism in males[a] [35]

Pituitary tumors, pituitary insufficiency, hemochromatosis
Hyperprolactinemia
Transient hypogonadism due to serious illness or stress
Aging, metabolic syndrome
Autoimmune syndromes, acquired immunodeficiency syndrome
Fertile eunuch syndrome, mumps, orchitis
Cryptorchidism, vanishing testes syndrome, testicular trauma
Radiation treatment or chemotherapy
Sertoli cell only syndrome
Genetic syndromes:
Klinefelter's syndrome, 47 XYY syndrome, dysgenetic testes
Androgen receptor defects, testicular feminization, Reifenstein's syndrome
5 Alpha-reductase deficiency, myotonic dystrophy, Kallmann's syndrome

[a]This is a summary and is not intended to include all potential causes

Table 11.6 Symptoms of hypogonadism

In females	Amenorrhea, oligomenorrhea
In males	Erectile dysfunction
In both sexes	Decreased libido, decreased fertility, decreased muscle mass, osteopenia, osteoporosis, compression fractures, fatigue, decreased ability to concentrate, depression, anxiety

support the finding of opioid receptors in the hypothalamus and pituitary as well as the gonads [27, 28, 30–33]. Therefore, opioid-induced hypogonadism is thought to be mediated via central effects on the hypothalamus and pituitary and via direct gonadal effects.

Opioids also have been shown to alter neuroendocrine function by increasing thyroid-stimulating hormone and prolactin while decreasing oxytocin [34]. Additionally, studies have shown opioids may impact the autonomic nervous system and result in altered glycemic control and insulin release [34].

Opioid suppression of the hypothalamus, pituitary, and gonads can result in hypogonadism in both males and females potentially leading to fatigue, depression, anxiety, decreased libido, infertility, decreased muscle mass, osteopenia, osteoporosis, and compression fractures in either sex (see Table 11.6) [29, 35]. In females, there may be amenorrhea and oligomenorrhea and, in males, erectile dysfunction. Daniell reported that 87% of men receiving opioids noted a decreased libido or significant erectile dysfunction after initiating use of opioids [27]. This study was followed by a study treating men with opioid-induced androgen deficiency

with testosterone and revealed that testosterone treatment resulted in improved sexual function, decreased depression, and improved mood [36].

Patients receiving chronic opioid therapy with symptoms of hypogonadism should be monitored for abnormalities in sex hormones. Laboratory analysis should include free and total testosterone and estradiol in women. It has also been recommended that LH and dehydroepiandrosterone, an adrenal precursor to the primary sex hormones, be tested as well [37, 38]. If diagnosed with hypogonadism secondary to opioids, it has been suggested that the risks and benefits of continued opioid therapy be considered versus discontinuation of opioids, a trial of alternative opioid, or hormonal supplementation [37]. In current practice, sex hormones are often monitored if the patient has complaints consistent with hypogonadism as outlined above while receiving chronic opioid therapy. Hormonal supplementation may be beyond the scope of some pain management practitioners and require coordinated care through the patient's primary care physician or with referral to endocrinology. Nonetheless, sex hormone levels should be monitored in all symptomatic patients and potentially in all patients receiving chronic opioid therapy. In addition to monitoring of free testosterone, estradiol, and other hormones, measuring bone density may also be valuable [29]. The American Association of Clinical Endocrinologists recommends ordering bone density studies for all patients with hypogonadism [35]. Furthermore, depending on the patient's history, other causes of hypogonadism should be considered as well (see Tables 11.7 and 11.8). Many of these would likely have presented earlier in life or with additional symptoms. Detailed evaluation of these conditions may be left to an endocrinologist or other specialist.

Table 11.8 Differential diagnosis of hypogonadism in females[a] [39, 40]

Reproductive organ dysfunction	Congenital, Asherman's syndrome, Turner's syndrome, premature ovarian failure including secondary to autoimmune causes, polycystic ovarian syndrome, ovarian tumors
Pituitary disorders	Tumor, hemochromatosis, sarcoidosis, traumatic brain injury
Hypothalamic dysfunction	Kallmann's syndrome, radiation
Prolactin secreting tumors	
Hypercortisolism	
Thyroid disorders	

[a]This is a summary and is not intended to include all potential causes

Immune Effects

Opioids, especially morphine, are known to adversely affect the immune system. Morphine has been shown to inhibit phagocytosis as early as 1898 [41]. Numerous subsequent studies have verified this including early animal research by Kraft and Leitch in 1921 demonstrating a decreased resistance to streptococcal septicemia in animals treated with morphine [42].

This immunosuppression occurs via both central and direct cellular mechanisms. Centrally, opioids can lead to the release of corticosteroids via the hypothalamic-pituitary-adrenal axis [43], leading to suppression of immune system function with chronic use of opioids [44]. Acute exposure to morphine and related drugs is also believed to influence the immune system via activation of the sympathetic nervous system [43, 44]. The released catecholamines, including norepinephrine, bind to leukocytes to alter immune function [45]. Opioids can also directly affect immune cells via opioid receptors present on immune cells [43]. Studies suggest that opioids bind to immune cell opioid receptors resulting in a diminished ability of immune cells to produce lymphocytes and macrophage precursors [43]. Further studies reveal that immune cells possess mu-opioid receptors and are activated by morphine, which is the most immunosuppressive opioid [44].

Morphine has been the most extensively researched opioid, in both animals and humans, regarding its potentially immunosuppressive effect. In animal studies and studies of opioid abusers in which confounding factors were controlled, chronic morphine use has been shown to result in an increased risk in opportunistic infections including pneumonia, HIV, and tuberculosis [46]. In addition to morphine, fentanyl has also been studied and found to suppress immune function including natural killer cell function [47]. The immunosuppressive effects are prolonged with increased doses of fentanyl [48]. The immunomodulatory effect of other opioids has also been studied but to a lesser extent than morphine and fentanyl. Codeine has been found to suppress the immune system but to a lesser degree than morphine [49]. Both hydromorphone and oxycodone have not been found to suppress the immune system [49]. Interestingly, naloxone and naltrexone have been found to increase immune responses [49]. These findings have not been widely studied. Buprenorphine has not been found to exert a significant immunosuppressive effect when monitoring immune functioning [50, 51]. Therefore, current data suggests that morphine and fentanyl have immunosuppressive effects although the significance with short-term or long-term administration is not clear. Furthermore, buprenorphine, hydromorphone, and oxycodone have not been found to depress the immune system although there is somewhat limited data in regard to this finding.

There has been debate about the clinical significance of opioid-induced immunosuppression. Opioid-induced immune dysfunction including an increased risk for opportunistic infections may have implications for patients who already have alterations in their immune system or are already immunocompromised including cancer patients. Some practitioners suggest use of opioids without immunosuppressive properties at all times [52] while others feel there is not enough clinical data to change clinical practice at this point [53]. Currently, there is no clear recommendation in regard to individualized opioid selection based on a patient's comorbidities and consideration of opioid immunosuppressive effects. A consensus statement published in 2008 generally suggests use of buprenorphine over morphine or fentanyl for chronic opioid use in light of immunosuppressive effects [54]. Beyond this, no other formal recommendations are available, and further research must be done to elucidate the clinical significance of opioid immunosuppression and develop prescribing guidelines for the application of this knowledge.

Respiratory Depression

Respiratory depression is an established and potentially life-threatening event related to opioid use. It has been defined in relation to respiratory rate as well as oxygen saturation with severe respiratory depression considered to be a respiratory rate less than 8–10 breaths/min [55]. Opioids depress brainstem respiratory centers in a dose-dependent manner. Respiratory depression typically occurs in opioid-naive patients or patients suddenly receiving doses greater than their typical doses. As the depression becomes more significant, it is often accompanied by confusion and sedation. Opioid-naive patients and patients receiving gradually increasing doses of opioids usually develop a tolerance to this side effect quickly [3, 56]. Additionally, hypoventilation

Table 11.9 Causes of hypoventilation resulting in respiratory acidosis[a] [60]

Pulmonary	Airway (laryngospasm)
	Parenchymal (pneumonia, chronic obstructive pulmonary disease)
Nonpulmonary	Drugs (e.g., narcotics, benzodiazepines)
	Flail chest (spinal cord injury, cardiopulmonary arrest)
	Sleep apnea
	Neuromuscular and chest wall disease (Guillain-Barre syndrome)

[a]This is a summary and is not intended to be comprehensive

results in increased levels of carbon dioxide stimulating chemoreceptors centrally to increase the respiratory rate and arterial oxygen level [57].

Naloxone is an opioid receptor antagonist that may be used to treat opioid-related respiratory depression. Such treatment should be done in an emergent or inpatient setting with appropriate monitoring. Furthermore, one must recognize, especially, with respiratory depression related to a long-acting opioid, that multiple doses of naloxone may be required as the onset of action is 1–3 min with a duration of only 45 min depending on the naloxone dose [3, 58]. Methadone, a long-acting opioid, may result in prolonged respiratory depression requiring a continuous infusion of naloxone or frequent doses secondary to its average elimination half-life being 22 h [59]. One must assess other causes of respiratory depression, especially, if opioid therapy has not recently been initiated or dose escalated or if there are other symptoms (see Table 11.9).

Central Nervous System Effects

Opioids can have various effects on the central nervous system (CNS) including sedation, psychomotor slowing, delirium, hallucinations, muscle rigidity, myoclonus, and sleep disturbances. Opioid-induced sedation and cognitive effects typically occur with the initiation of an opioid or with dose escalation [56, 61]. Cognitive effects are usually transient and last 1–2 weeks [62, 63]. If patients do not develop tolerance to the sedative effects, they may be treated with CNS stimulants such as methylphenidate or modafinil or with acetylcholinesterase inhibitors such as donepezil [3]. Studies have demonstrated that driving ability is not impaired with use of a stable and chronic dose of opioid medication [64–66].

Pruritis

Pruritis has been reported to occur in 2–10 % patients taking oral morphine [67]. It is most commonly associated with morphine use and thought to occur via histamine release [7]. The likelihood of opioid-associated pruritis is increased with epidural or intrathecal opioids [68, 69]. Antihistamines are commonly used to treat pruritis. Use of antihistamines may compound potential sedation.

Other medications including mixed opioid receptor agonist-antagonists, serotonin 5-HT$_3$ receptor antagonists, opioid antagonists, propofol, NSAIDs, and dopamine receptor antagonists have been found to reduce opioid-related pruritis [70, 71]. Specifically, methylnaltrexone, naloxone, naltrexone, and nalbuphine have demonstrated efficacy in reducing pruritis [72, 73]. Acupuncture has also been shown to be helpful in reducing morphine-related pruritis [74]. As with other side effects, opioid rotation, dose reduction, or use of non-opioid therapy may be considered.

Conclusion

Opioid-related adverse effects are well known and studied. The risks and benefits of opioid treatments must be weighed against these. The development of adverse effects requires consideration of decreasing the opioid dose, changing the route of administration, changing the type of opioid, or discontinuing opioid therapy. If medications are used to treat these adverse effects, one must also recognize that these medications may result in side effects of their own. Novel approaches and medications as well as combination medications of opioids and other drugs that minimize side effects are continually being developed.

References

1. More RA, McQuay HJ. Prevalence of opioid adverse events in chronic non-malignant pain: systematic review of randomised trials of oral opioids. Arthritis Res Ther. 2005;7(5):R1046–51.
2. Kalso E, Allan L, Dellemijn PLI, Faura CC, Ilias WK, Jensen TS, Perrot S, Plaghki LH, Zenz M. Recommendations for using opioids in chronic non-cancer pain. Eur J Pain. 2003;7(5):381–6.
3. O'Mahony S, Coyle N, Payne R. Current management of opioid related side effects. Oncology. 2001;15(1):61–74.
4. Herndon CM, Jackson 2nd KC, Hallin PA. Management of opioid-induced gastrointestinal effects in patients receiving palliative care. Pharmacotherapy. 2002;22(2):240–50.
5. Okamoto Y, Tsuneto S, Matsuda Y, et al. A retrospective chart review of the antiemetic effectiveness of risperidone in refractory opioid-induced nausea and vomiting in advanced cancer patients. J Pain Symptom Manage. 2007;34:217–22.
6. Porreca F, Ossipov MH. Nausea and vomiting side effects with opioid analgesics during treatment of chronic pain: mechanisms, implications, and management options. Pain Med. 2009;10(4):654–62.

7. Swegle JM, Logemann C. Management of common opioid-induced adverse effects. Am Fam Physician. 2006;74:1347–54.

8. Moss J, Rosow CE. Development of peripheral opioid antagonists' new insights into opioid effects. Mayo Clin Proc. 2008;83(10):1116–30.

9. Harris JD. Management of expected and unexpected opioid-related side effects. Clin J Pain. 2008;24 Suppl 10:S8–13.

10. Voth EA, Schwartz RH. Medicinal applications of delta-9-tetrahy-drocannabinol and marijuana. Ann Intern Med. 1997;126(10):791–8.

11. Lee A, Fan LT. Stimulation of the wrist acupuncture point P6 for preventing postoperative nausea and vomiting. Cochrane Database Syst Rev. 2010;(2):CD003281.

12. Bao T. Use of acupuncture in the control of chemotherapy-induced nausea and vomiting. J Natl Compr Canc Netw. 2009;7(5):606–12.

13. Mansky PJ, Wallerstedt DB. Complementary medicine in palliative care and cancer symptom management. Cancer J. 2006;12(5):425–31.

14. Scorza K, Williams A, Phillips D, Shaw J. Evaluation of nausea and vomiting. Am Fam Physician. 2007;76(1):76–84.

15. Panchal SJ, Müller-Schwefe P, Wurzelmann JI. Opioid-induced bowel dysfunction: prevalence, pathophysiology and burden. Int J Clin Pract. 2007;61(7):1181–7.

16. Longstreth GF, Thompson WG, Chey WD, Houghton LA, Mearin F, Spiller RC. Functional bowel disorders. Gastroenterology. 2006;130:1480–91.

17. Fox-Threlkeld JE, Daniel EE, Christinck F, Hruby VJ, Cipris S, Woskowska Z. Identification of mechanisms and sites of actions of mu and delta opioid receptor activation in the canine intestine. J Pharmacol Exp Ther. 1994;268(2):689–700.

18. Holzer P. Opioids and opioid receptors in the enteric nervous system: from a problem in opioid analgesia to a possible new prokinetic therapy in humans. Neurosci Lett. 2004;361(1–3):192–5.

19. De Schepper HU, Cremonini F, Park MI, Camilleri M. Opioids and the gut: pharmacology and current clinical experience. Neurogastroenterol Motil. 2004;16(4):383–94.

20. Canty SL. Constipation as a side effect of opioids. Oncol Nurs Forum. 1994;21:739–45.

21. Michael AA, Arthur GL, Daniel C, Carla R. Principles of analgesic use in the treatment of acute pain and cancer pain. 5th ed. Glenview: American Pain Society; 2003.

22. Clemens KE, Klaschik E. Management of constipation in palliative care patients. Curr Opin Support Palliat Care. 2008;2(1):22–7.

23. Likar R. Transdermal buprenorphine in the management of persistent pain – safety aspects. Ther Clin Risk Manag. 2006;2:115–25.

24. Bach V, Kamp-Jensen M, Jensen N-H, Eriksen J. Buprenorphine and sustained release morphine – effects and side effects in chronic use. Pain Clin. 1991;4:87–93.

25. Allan L, Hays H, Jensen NH, de Waroux BL, Bolt M, Donald R, Kalso E. Randomised crossover trial of transdermal fentanyl and sustained release oral morphine for treating chronic non-cancer pain. BMJ. 2001;322(7295):1154–8.

26. Arce DA, Ermocilla CA, Costa H. Evaluation of constipation. Am Fam Physician. 2002;65(11):2283–90.

27. Daniell HW. Hypogonadism in men consuming sustained-action opioids. J Pain. 2002;3(5):377–84.

28. Cicero TJ. Effects of exogenous and endogenous opiates on the hypothalamic–pituitary–gonadal axis in the male. Fed Proc. 1980;39(8):2551–4.

29. Daniell HW. Opioid endocrinopathy in women consuming prescribed sustained-action opioids for control of nonmalignant pain. J Pain. 2008;9(1):28–36.

30. Genazzani AR, Genazzani AD, Volpogni C, et al. Opioid control of gonadotropin secretion in humans. Hum Reprod. 1993;8 suppl 2:151–3.

31. Jordan D, Tafani JA, Ries C, Zajac JM, Simonnet G, Martin D, Kopp N, Allard M. Evidence for multiple opioid receptors in the human posterior pituitary. J Neuroendocrinol. 1996;8(11):883–7.

32. Cicero TJ, Bell RD, Wiest WG, et al. Function of the male sex organs in heroin and methadone users. N Engl J Med. 1975;292:882–7.

33. Kaminski T. The involvement of protein kinases in signalling of opioid agonist FK 33-824 in porcine granulosa cells. Anim Reprod Sci. 2006;91:107–22.

34. Vuong C, Van Uum SH, O'Dell LE, Lutfy K, Friedman TC. The effects of opioids and opioid analogs on animal and human endocrine systems. Endocr Rev. 2010;31(1):98–132.

35. AACE Hypogonadism Task Force. American association of clinical endocrinologists medical guidelines for clinical practice for the evaluation and treatment of hypogonadism in adult male patients-2002 update. Endocr Pract. 2002;8(6):439–56.

36. Daniell HW, Lentz R, Mazer NA. Open-label pilot study of testosterone patch therapy in men with opioid induced androgen deficiency (OPIAD). J Pain. 2006;7:200–10.

37. Katz N, Mazer NA. The impact of opioids on the endocrine system. Clin J Pain. 2009;25(2):170–5.

38. Daniell HW. DHEAS deficiency during consumption of sustained-action prescribed opioids: evidence for opioid- induced inhibition of adrenal androgen production. J Pain. 2006;7:901–7.

39. Rothman MS, Wierman ME. Female hypogonadism: evaluation of the hypothalamic-pituitary-ovarian axis. Pituitary. 2008;11:163–9.

40. Makhsida N, Shah J, Yan G, Fisch H, Shabsigh R. Hypogonadism and metabolic syndrome: implications for testosterone therapy. J Urol. 2005;174(3):827–34.

41. Cantacuzene. Annales de L'Institut Pasteur. 1898; xli:273.

42. Kraft A, Leitch NM. The action of drugs in infection I. The influence of morphine in experimental septicemia. J Pharmacol Exp Ther. 1921;5:3877–84.

43. Roy S, Loh HH. Effects of opioids on the immune system. Neurochem Res. 1996;21(11):1375–86.

44. Mellon RD, Bayer BM. Evidence for central opioid receptors in the immunomodulatory effects of morphine: review of potential mechanism(s) of action. J Neuroimmunol. 1998;83(1–2):19–28.

45. Peterson PK, Molitor TW, Chao CC. Mechanisms of morphine-induced immunomodulation. Biochem Pharmacol. 1993;46:343–8.

46. Roy S, Wang J, Kelschenbach J, Koodie L, Martin J. Modulation of immune function by morphine: implications for susceptibility to infection. J Neuroimmune Pharmacol. 2006;1:77–89.

47. Shavit Y, Ben-Eliyahu S, Zeidel A, Beilin B. Effects of fentanyl on natural killer cell activity and on resistance to tumor metastasis in rats dose and timing study. Neuroimmunomodulation. 2004;11(4):255–60.

48. Beilin B, Shavit Y, Hart J, Mordashov B, Cohn S, Notti I, Bessler H. Effects of anesthesia based on large versus small doses of fentanyl on natural killer cell cytotoxicity in the perioperative period. Anesth Analg. 1996;82(3):492–7.

49. Sacerdote P, Manfredi B, Mantegazza P, Panerai AE. Antinociceptive and immunosuppressive effects of opiate drugs: a structure-related activity study. Br J Pharmacol. 1997;121(4):834–40.

50. Martucci C, Panerai AE, Sacerdote P. Chronic fentanyl or buprenorphine infusion in the mouse: similar analgesic profile but different effects on immune responses. Pain. 2004;110(1–2):385–92.

51. Sacerdote P. Opioids and the immune system. Palliat Med. 2006; 20 Suppl 1:s9–15.

52. Budd K. Pain management: is opioid immunosuppression a clinical problem? Biomed Pharmacother. 2006;60(7):310–7.

53. Sacerdote P. Opioid-induced immunosuppression. Curr Opin Support Palliat Care. 2008;2(1):14–8.

54. Pergolizzi J, Böger RH, Budd K, Dahan A, Erdine S, Hans G, Kress HG, Langford R, Likar R, Raffa RB, Sacerdote P. Opioids and the management of chronic severe pain in the elderly: consensus statement of an international expert panel with focus on the six clinically most often used World Health Organization Step III opioids (buprenorphine, fentanyl, hydromorphone, methadone, morphine, oxycodone). Pain Pract. 2008;8(4):287–313.

55. Dahan A, Aarts L, Smith TW. Incidence, reversal, and prevention of opioid-induced respiratory depression. Anesthesiology. 2010; 112:226–38.

56. McNicol E, Horowicz-Mehler N, Fisk RA, Bennett K, Gialeli-Goudas M, Chew PW, Lau J, Carr D. Management of opioid side effects in cancer-related and chronic noncancer pain: a systematic review. J Pain. 2003;4(5):231–56.

57. Mueller RA, Lundberg DB, Breese GR, Hedner J, Hedner T, Jonason J. The neuropharmacy of respiratory control. Pharmacol Rev. 1982;34:255–85.

58. Olofsen E, van Dorp E, Teppema L, Aarts L, Smith TW, Dahan A, Sarton E. Naloxone reversal of morphine- and morphine-6-glucuronide-induced respiratory depression in healthy volunteers: a mechanism-based pharmacokinetic-pharmacodynamic modeling study. Anesthesiology. 2010;112(6):1417–27.

59. Eap CB, Buclin T, Baumann P. Interindividual variability of the clinical pharmacokinetics of methadone: implications for the treatment of opioid dependence. Clin Pharmacokinet. 2002;41(14):1153–93.

60. Lerma EV, Berns JS, Nissenson AR. Current diagnosis & treatment: nephrology & hypertension. New York: The McGraw-Hill Companies; 2009. p. 58.

61. Christo PJ. Opioid effectiveness and side effects in chronic pain. Anesthesiol Clin North America. 2003;21(4):699–713.

62. Reissig JE, Rybarczyk AM. Pharmacologic treatment of opioid-induced sedation in chronic pain. Ann Pharmacother. 2005;39:727–31.

63. Bruera E, Macmillan K, Hanson J, MacDonald RN. The cognitive effects of the administration of narcotic analgesics in patients with cancer pain. Pain. 1989;39(1):13–6.

64. Byas-Smith MG, Chapman SL, Reed B, Cotsonis G. The effect of opioids on driving and psychomotor performance in patients with chronic pain. Clin J Pain. 2005;21(4):345–52.

65. Fishbain DA, Cutler RB, Rosomoff HL, Rosomoff RS. Can patients taking opioids drive safely? A structured evidence-based review. J Pain Palliat Care Pharmacother. 2002;16(1):9–28.

66. Fishbain DA, Cutler RB, Rosomoff HL, Rosomoff RS. Are opioid-dependent/tolerant patients impaired in driving-related skills? A structured evidence-based review. J Pain Symptom Manage. 2003;25(6):559–77.

67. Cherny N, Ripamonti C, Pereira J, Davis C, Fallon M, McQuay H, Mercadante S, Pasternak G, Ventafridda V, Expert Working Group of the European Association of Palliative Care Network. Strategies to manage the adverse effects of oral morphine: an evidence-based report. J Clin Oncol. 2001;19(9):2542–54.

68. Ballantyne JC, Loach AB, Carr DB. Itching after epidural and spinal opiates. Pain. 1988;33(2):149–60.

69. Chaney MA. Side effects of intrathecal and epidural opioids. Can J Anaesth. 1995;42(10):891–903.

70. Ganesh A, Maxwell LG. Pathophysiology and management of opioid-induced pruritus. Drugs. 2007;67(16):2323–33.

71. Szarvas S, Harmon D, Murphy D. Neuraxial opioid-induced pruritus: a review. J Clin Anesth. 2003;15(3):234–9.

72. Diego L, Atayee R, Helmons P, von Gunten CF. Methylnaltrexone: a novel approach for the management of opioid-induced constipation in patients with advanced illness. Expert Rev Gastroenterol Hepatol. 2009;3(5):473–85.

73. Kjellberg F, Tramèr MR. Pharmacological control of opioid-induced pruritus: a quantitative systematic review of randomized trials. Eur J Anaesthesiol. 2001;18(6):346–57.

74. Jiang YH, Jiang W, Jiang LM, Lin GX, Yang H, Tan Y, Xiong WW. Clinical efficacy of acupuncture on the morphine-related side effects in patients undergoing spinal-epidural anesthesia and analgesia. Chin J Integr Med. 2001;16(1):71–4.

Acute Management of the Opioid-Dependent Patient

Brandi A. Bottiger, Denny Curtis Orme, and Vitaly Gordin

Key Points

- Opioid-dependent patients are at substantial risk in postoperative period for being labeled as drug seeking and therefore have their pain inadequately controlled.
- When appropriate, use of regional anesthesia and adjuvant analgesics can have a beneficial effect on postoperative pain control and decrease the total dose of opioid analgesics.
- Perioperative period is an inappropriate setting for opioid tapering.
- Adequate pain control in opioid-dependent patient will decrease the psychological and physiologic burden of poorly controlled pain. It will improve surgical outcomes, decrease hospital stay, and prevent unnecessary admission after outpatient surgery.

Introduction

Seventy million patients are afflicted by and treated for chronic pain in the United States and treated more frequently with long-term opioids, particularly morphine, oxycodone, and

B.A. Bottiger, M.D. (✉)
Department of Anesthesiology, Duke University Hospital,
Box 3094 2301 Erwin Rd, Durham, NC 27705, USA
e-mail: brandi.bottiger@dm.duke.edu

D.C. Orme, DO, MPH
Billings Anesthesiology PC,
PO Box 1155, Billings, MT 59103, USA
e-mail: dennyxorme@hotmail.com

V. Gordin
Department of Anesthesiology,
Penn State Milton S. Hershey Medical Center,
500 University Drive, Hershey, PA 17033, USA

Department of Anesthesiology,
Pennsylvania State University College of Medicine,
Hershey, PA, USA
e-mail: vgordin@hmc.psu.edu

methadone in the treatment of non-cancer pain [1]. Many of these patients will arrive for surgical procedures and pain management will be a major part of their hospital stay [2–4]. According to various sources, approximately 40 % of all surgical patients still experience moderate to severe pain and almost a quarter of them experience inadequate pain relief [5, 6]. Allowing patients to suffer from poorly controlled pain not only may be considered a breach of human rights [3, 7, 8] but may result in emotional and cognitive problems negatively impacting postoperative rehabilitation and quality of life.

Unfortunately, there are only a small number of reports discussing the treatment of acute pain in patients with substance abuse disorders, opioid tolerance, and physical dependence, and even less discussion on opioid-dependent patients specifically [2–4, 7, 8].

Acute pain management of opioid-dependent patients is challenging not only for the primary team but also for anesthesiologists and pain specialists. Improving perioperative pain control in these patients may result in shortening of the hospital stay [9, 10], improving patient satisfaction and rehabilitation rate, and decreasing admissions for pain control from same day surgery units. In this chapter, we will review factors responsible for opioid tolerance, physical dependence, and addiction, and provide perioperative pain management strategies.

In the perioperative period, acute surgical pain must be treated in addition to the patient's underlying chronic pain, which may or may not be adequately controlled. An opioid-tolerant patient can consume up to three times the amount of opioid analgesics than an opioid-naïve patient [11]. This can be alarming for many practitioners, and inadequate pain control may result in unnecessary suffering. Fear of the adverse effects of opioid analgesics may prevent the practitioner from adequately treating an opioid-tolerant patient. Conversely attempts to treat pain with opioid analgesics alone may put patients at increased risk for adverse events such as respiratory depression and over-sedation. The ideal focus should be on preventative pain control using a multifaceted approach, rather than controlling pain postoperatively only.

Key concepts for consideration when managing a chronic pain patient include (1) understanding the adverse consequences of acute pain; (2) exploring basic concepts as they relate to definitions of substance abuse, dependence, tolerance, and addiction; (3) differentiating opioid dependency from addiction; (4) performing preoperative and postoperative assessments; and (5) developing multifaceted, balanced pain management plan.

Consequences of Acute Pain

The consequences of pain during surgical stimulation are well known to the anesthesiologist. The intraoperative pain response can be difficult to manage and often leads to large sympathetic responses. Neuroendocrine activation along the hypothalamo-adrenal axis leads to release of not only catecholamines but also ACTH, aldosterone, angiotensin, and antidiuretic hormone (ADH) as well as cortisol and glucagon [12, 13]. This results in an overall catabolic state promoting hyperglycemia, water retention, and release of proinflammatory mediators [14].

Catecholamine release, as well as direct effects of aldosterone, cortisol, ADH, and angiotensin, has direct effect on the cardiovascular system [15]. Increased cardiac work is a direct result of increased heart rate, preload, afterload, and oxygen consumption. These changes can lead to myocardial ischemia, congestive heart failure, or lung injury in predisposed patients. Regarding the pulmonary system, increased extracellular lung water contributes to ventilation-perfusion abnormalities. Patients undergoing upper abdominal or thoracic surgery with significant pain often exhibit splinting, decreased lung compliance, and hypoventilation, resulting in atelectasis [14, 16]. In high-risk patients, there may be a reduction in functional residual capacity up to 50 %. These sequelae could have detrimental effects particularly to the patient with preexisting pulmonary disease, advanced age, or obesity [17].

Importantly, the body's response to pain and surgical stress may result in a hypercoagulable state via alteration in blood viscosity, platelet function, fibrinolysis, and coagulation pathways [18–20]. Coupling this with catecholamine release and immobilization of the patient, the risk of a thromboembolic event significantly increases. Both cellular and immune function is impaired [21–23], and with the additional problem of hyperglycemia, the patient is predisposed for wound infection and poor wound healing. Further, catecholamines may further result in increased intestinal secretions and increased smooth muscle sphincter tone in the gastrointestinal and urinary tracts, resulting in decreased bowel motility and urinary retention, respectively [24, 25]. These sequelae of the physiologic response to pain may result in prolonged hospitalization and potentially detrimental complications.

Lastly, intense painful stimuli can result in gene expression changes that influence pain perception and impulse formation in as little as 1 h, perhaps influencing the development of chronic pain [26]. The concept of preemptive and balanced analgesia becomes essential to reduce this pain response, particularly in patients who have been previously sensitized [27, 28].

Basic Concepts and Definitions

During a preoperative history and physical examination, basic concepts and terms describing substance abuse, physical and psychological dependency, and addiction should be correctly applied to describe a patient characteristic or behavior.

Substance use disorder or substance dependence has been described as a maladaptive pattern of substance use, leading to clinically significant impairment or distress, as manifested by three or more of the following described in Table 12.1. The opioid-dependent patient may be legitimately and responsibly using opioids and labeled with a substance use disorder. However, he/she may be misdiagnosed with psychological dependence or addiction (see pseudoaddiction below). Physiologic dependence must be distinguished from psychological dependence if possible and described appropriately; misdiagnosis of psychological dependence or addiction may negatively impact the patient on a personal level and inhibit future care, as well as result in undertreatment of pain. Definitions of the major terms should be reviewed in Table 12.2 and are briefly described below [6].

Psychological dependence is described as a psychological need for specific substance to obtain positive effects or to avoid negative consequences. *Addiction* refers to the aberrant use of substance, including loss of control, compulsive use, preoccupation, and continued use despite harm. Opioid abuse or addiction is more common with polydrug abuse, or dependence on other substances, such as alcohol, marijuana, or nicotine. It is important, if possible, to distinguish the chronic pain patient from the opioid-abusing patient (Table 12.3) [6]. Unfortunately, to cloud the issue, there is significant opioid addiction within the chronic pain population, approximating 3–19 % [29]. This prevalence may be underestimated because these patients have a background of emotional and psychological instability, and develop a conditioning behavior resulting from relief of increasing pain intensity experienced from opioid use [30, 31].

There is another group of patients who have well-documented chronic pain and resemble opioid abusers because of their often obsessive drug-seeking behavior. These patients may have visited many physicians but are under-medicated, seeking adequate pain relief. This phenomenon was termed *pseudoaddiction* [32]. However, unlike patients with true addiction, the pseudoaddicted patient will obtain pain relief if the dose of opioid is increased and the behavior will be eliminated.

Table 12.1 Criteria for substance dependence

A maladaptive pattern of substance use, leading to clinically significant impairment or distress, as manifested by three (or more) of the following, occurring at any time in the 12-month period:
1. Tolerance, as defined by either of the following:
(a) A need for markedly increased amounts of the substance to achieve intoxication or desired effect
(b) Markedly diminished effect with continued use of the same amount of the substance
2. Withdrawal, as manifested by either of the following:
(a) The characteristic withdrawal syndrome for the substance (refer to criteria A and B of the criteria sets for withdrawal from the specific substances)
(b) The same (or a closely related) substance is taken to avoid or relieve withdrawal symptoms
3. The substance is often taken in larger amounts or for a longer period than was intended
4. There is a persistent desire or unsuccessful efforts to cut down or control substance abuse
5. A great deal of time is spent in activities to obtain the substance, use the substance, or recover from its effects
6. Important social, occupational, or recreational activities are given up or reduced because of substance use
7. The substance use is continued despite knowledge of having a persistent or recurrent physical or psychological problems that is likely to have been caused or exacerbated by the substance
With physiologic dependence: evidence of tolerance or withdrawal (i.e., either item 1 or item 2 is present)
Without physiologic dependence: no evidence of tolerance or withdrawal (i.e., neither item 1 nor item 2 is present)
Criteria for opioid withdrawal
(A) Either of the following:
1. Cessation of (or reduction in) opioid use that has been heavy and prolonged (several weeks or longer)
2. Administration of an opioid antagonist after a period of opioid use
(B) Three (or more) of the following, developing within minutes to several days after criterion A:
1. Dysphoric mood
2. Nausea or vomiting
3. Muscle aches
4. Lacrimation or rhinorrhea
5. Pupillary dilation, piloerection, or sweating
6. Diarrhea
7. Yawning
8. Fever
9. Insomnia

Reproduced with permission from Mitra and Sinatra [6]

Physiologic dependence is described as an alteration in physiologic response to a drug resulting from opioid binding to receptors, leading to withdrawal syndrome if drug is stopped. This can be seen both in patients in whom opioids are legitimately prescribed and in those abusing opioids. In general, the higher the daily dose is, the greater the degree of physiologic dependence and tolerance [33–35].

The opioid *withdrawal* syndrome is described as increased sympathetic and parasympathetic responses mediated via the myenteric plexus, brainstem vagal, and hypothalamic nuclei. These responses include hypertension, tachycardia, diaphoresis, abdominal cramping, and diarrhea. Quitting "cold turkey" is related to the abrupt withdrawal of opioids causing piloerection of the skin. Behavioral responses such as shaking, yawning, and leg jerking occur as well [33, 36, 37]. Rarely life threatening, these symptoms are extremely unpleasant and may be missed in the perioperative period [37]. The time course of withdrawal varies depending on the opioid being used; however, that for intermediate acting agents (e.g., morphine, heroine), it is listed in Table 12.4 [33,

38]. Abrupt halt of short-acting agents such as fentanyl or meperidine may result in withdrawal as early as 2–6 h after stopping the drug and have symptoms lasting only 4–5 days. In contrast, withdrawal from long-acting agents like methadone occurs 24–48 h after use and may last up to 6–7 weeks.

Opioid tolerance is a pharmacologic adaptation occurring when patients require increasing amounts of drug for same effect, shifting the dose-response curve to the right. Tolerance develops to the analgesic, euphoric, sedative, respiratory depression, and nauseating effects but not to miosis and constipation [33, 36, 37]. Duration of exposure, daily dose requirement, and receptor association/disassociation kinetics are predictive of the degree of opioid tolerance. Opioid agonists binding to the same receptor show asymmetric cross-tolerance depending on their intrinsic efficacy [33]. The number of receptors that need to be occupied to create an analgesic effect is inversely proportional to the intrinsic efficacy. In other words, a potent agonist with high efficacy binds to a small number of

Table 12.2 Commonly used terms in substance dependence

Addiction	Commonly used term meaning the aberrant use of a specific psychoactive substance in a manner characterized by loss of control, compulsive use, preoccupation, and continued use despite harm; pejorative term, replaced in the "DSM-IV" in a nonpejorative way by the term *substance use disorder* (SUD) with psychological and physical dependence
Dependence	1. Psychological dependence: need for a specific psychoactive substance either for its positive effects or to avoid negative psychological or physical effects associated with its withdrawal
	2. Physical dependence: a physiologic state of adaptation to a specific psychoactive substance characterized by the emergence of a withdrawal syndrome during abstinence, which may be relieved in total or in part by re-administration of the substance
	3. One category of psychoactive substance use disorder
Chemical dependence	A generic term relating to psychological and/or physical dependence on one or more psychoactive substances
Substance use disorders	Term of DSM-IV comprising two main groups:
	1. Substance dependence disorder and substance abuse disorder
	2. Substance-induced disorders (e.g., intoxication, withdrawal, delirium, psychotic disorders)
Tolerance	A state in which an increased dosage of psychoactive substance is needed to produce a desired effect; cross-tolerance: induced by repeated administration of one psychoactive substance that is manifested toward another substance to which the individual has not been recently exposed
Withdrawal syndrome	The onset of a predictable constellation of signs and symptoms after the abrupt discontinuation of or a rapid decrease in dosage of a psychoactive substance
Polydrug dependence	Concomitant use of two or more psychoactive substances in quantities and frequencies that cause individually significant physiologic, psychological, and/or sociological distress or impairment (polysubstance abuser)
Recovery	A process of overcoming both physical and psychological dependence on a psychoactive substance with a commitment to sobriety
Abstinence	Non-use of any psychoactive substance
Maintenance	Prevention of craving behavior and withdrawal symptoms of opioids by long-acting opioids (e.g., methadone, buprenorphine)
Substance abuse	Use of a psychoactive substance in a manner outside of sociocultural conventions

Reproduced with permission from Mitra and Sinatra [6]

Table 12.3 Distinguishing the chronic pain patient from the opioid-abusing patient

Chronic pain patient	Opioid-abusing patient
Using opioids as prescribed, follows treatment plan	Out of control with opioid use, does not follow treatment plan
Use of opioid improves quality of life	Opioids impair quality of life
Aware and concerned about side effects	Unconcerned about side effects
Will save previous medications, prescriptions	"Loses" prescriptions, runs out of medication early, makes excuses

Table 12.4 Typical withdrawal symptoms associated of opioid withdrawal, by stage

Stage 1 (1–36 h)
Anxiety
Craving for drug
Lacrimation
Rhinorrhea
Yawning
Stage II (12–72 h)
Diaphoresis
Piloerection
Anorexia
Mydriasis
Irritability
Mild-moderate sleep disturbance
Tremor
Stage III (24–72 h)
Abdominal pain
Muscle spasms
Nausea, vomiting, diarrhea
Severe insomnia
Violent yawning

receptors to achieve analgesia (e.g., sufentanil). The patient treated with this agent will develop tolerance more slowly than a patient treated with opioids having low intrinsic efficacy binding to a large number of receptors (e.g., morphine) [34, 39–42]. Briefly, acquired opioid tolerance can be classified into pharmacokinetic tolerance, learned tolerance, and pharmacodynamic tolerance. The pharmacokinetic tolerance refers to enzyme induction and subsequent acceleration of opioid metabolism [43, 44]. Learned tolerance refers to decreased drug affect due to learned compensatory mechanisms (i.e., can walk a straight line while intoxicated) [45, 46]. Pharmacodynamic tolerance refers to neuroadaptive changes that take place after long-term exposure to the drug [6]. The molecular mechanisms of

these adaptations are complex and result in long-term persistent neural adaptations, involving increased levels of cAMP, spinal dynorphin, glutamine, and activation of

NMDA receptors [47–50]. These changes ultimately result in receptor desensitization, decreased receptor density, and alterations in receptor coupling to G proteins and signal transduction pathways [33, 46, 48, 51, 67].

Vignette #1

An example of a particularly difficult patient is the patient with history of opioid addiction presenting for an elective ventral abdominal hernia repair. In this example, the patient is taking an antidepressant for depression, oxyContin for chronic abdominal pain, and gabapentin for neuropathic symptoms. The preoperative appointment should be utilized to discuss clarify expectations and create a management strategy for post operative pain.

Issues relative to undergoing the procedure include the necessity to continue her current medications and then plan for treatment of acute surgical pain from tissue trauma. A prudent approach for this patient should start with preoperative assessment and discussion with the surgeon, anesthesiologist, psychiatrist, and social work to clarify expectations. Placement of an epidural, if feasible, would be useful in perioperative pain control. In addition to general anesthesia, adjuncts may include intravenous infusions of dexmedetomidine or other alpha 2 agonist to reduce sympathetic outflow and an NMDA antagonist. In the acute postoperative period, adequate dosing of the epidural would provide analgesia with breakthrough intravenous opioids, perhaps via patient-controlled analgesia (PCA). This may avoid acute withdrawal and treat breakthrough pain. As early as possible, the home dose of opioids should be reinstated with adequate short-acting breakthrough pain medication to cover surgical pain. This is one possible regimen to obtain pain control and subsequent early discharge.

Types and Mechanisms of Pain

Although chronic back pain is by far the most common cause of chronic pain, peripheral neuropathy, cancer, abdominal disorders, or musculoskeletal disorders such as rheumatoid arthritis and fibromyalgia are common. Many patients are afflicted with multiple disorders, which can cause different types of pain, e.g., somatic and/or neuropathic, and may benefit from targeted non-opioid modalities or a multimodal approach.

Pain begins with the stimulation of specialized nerve endings called nociceptors, which exist throughout the body on sensory nerves. Nociceptive pain accounts for both visceral (related to internal organs) and somatic (related to bones, joints, muscles) pains involved with surgery. Nociceptors respond to direct stimulation as well as to mediators such as

prostaglandins, bradykinins, histamine, and serotonin, which are released at the site of tissue injury [26, 52, 53]. These act via nerve endings to cause pain impulse formation as well as amplifying further signals caused by direct stimulation [54].

Slow conduction takes place in the visceral unmyelinated C fibers which join somatic nerves and are responsible for referred pain. After entry into the dorsal horn, pain and temperature fibers cross the midline and ascend via the lateral spinothalamic tract. At this level, substance P is the primary mediator. Ascending fibers terminate primarily in the brainstem and thalamus, which then relay the information to the cerebral cortex. Here, the impulse is perceived and localized, and further signals to the limbic system are responsible for the emotional response to pain.

Descending pain fibers from the cerebral cortex and midbrain modulate the afferent nerve stimuli that transmit pain signals to the central nervous system. Enkephalin, norepinephrine, serotonin, and gamma aminobutyric acid (GABA) have been shown to modulate and inhibit the frequency and intensity of nociceptive impulses, thereby attenuating the pain response [28]. Endogenous opioids and endorphins are released from the central nervous system, bind to mu, delta, and kappa opioid receptors, and prevent presynaptic release of neurotransmitters, including substance P. They aslo inhibit the perception and response to painful stimuli.

Both ascending and descending pain pathways can be summarized in Fig. 12.1. Inflammatory pain acts via upregulation of nociceptors and recruiting nonstimulated or dormant receptors [52, 55–57]. Proinflammatory mediators such as IL-1, IL-6, and TNF alpha interferons decrease the threshold for impulse generation and raise the intensity of the impulse as well as the rate of impulse discharge. Further, inflammation perpetuates itself by neurogenic inflammation in which substance P is released and acts peripherally to induce more inflammation, vascular permeability, and ongoing tissue injury [26, 53].

Neuropathic pain occurs secondary to direct injury of peripheral or central nervous structures, or as a result of compression or tumor invasion. Opioid receptors (mu, kappa, and sigma) exist in the periphery, spinal cord, and central nervous system, as well as inflammatory and immunologic cells [59]. Most receptors are concentrated in the central nervous system, with the highest concentration in the dorsal horn of the spinal cord, periaqueductal gray matter, and rostral ventromedial medulla of the brainstem. Opioids are a mainstay for postoperative and intraoperative analgesia because of their potency. They act by binding to presynaptic receptors and preventing the release of substance P and impulse transmission. The mu receptor is responsible for spinal and supraspinal analgesia as well as having the undesirable side effects of respiratory depression, bowel dysmotility, urinary retention, and pruritus. Kappa, while providing supraspinal and spinal analgesia,

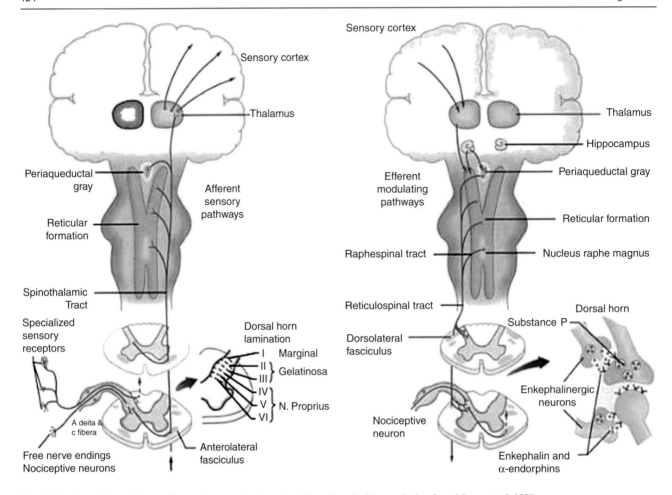

Fig. 12.1 Ascending and descending pathways of nociception (Reproduced with permission from Macres et al. [55])

also mediates miosis, sedation, and dysphagia. Lastly, the delta receptor mediates spinal and supraspinal analgesia only. A majority of opioids utilized in the perioperative period are mu agonists, having different degree of affinity for mu subtypes. Thus, a "new" opioid may have a different selectivity for the individual mu receptor subtype, explaining "incomplete cross-tolerance" [42]. As a class, opioids do not have a ceiling effect and escalating doses will stop pain once enough opioid is given [54]. The characteristics, pharmacokinetics, and pharmacodynamics of each drug are discussed in other chapters.

Opioid-Induced Hyperalgesia

The chronic pain patient may present perioperatively with an amplified pain response or hyperesthesia. They may also present with allodynia, or pain elicited by a normally non-painful stimulus. Compared to narcotic-naïve patients, opioid-dependent patients have relative pain intolerance and significantly increased sensitivity during cold, pressor, and thermal testing [58, 59]. This is referred to as

drug-induced hyperalgesia and is thought to result after continuous opioid receptor occupation. This occurs regardless of route of administration, dosing, and administration schedules [60, 61].

Both central and peripheral neural processes are influenced by the neuronal and humoral inputs caused by nociception [35, 62]. Generally, both types of hyperalgesia share underlying mechanisms mediated by glutamate via the N-methyl-D-aspartate (NMDA) receptor [63, 64]. Because of their amplified pain response, these patients might have extreme difficulty coping with sudden acute pain [11, 58, 65].

Treatment of the Chronic Pain Patient in the Perioperative Period

There are few controlled studies to guide the anesthesiologist in optimizing anesthetic and analgesic care in these patients although the prevalence of opioid dependency continues to increase [2–4, 11, 66]. Scientific literature in this area is mostly case reports and expert opinion. Although these have not been tested specifically, below are guidelines that may serve to improve analgesia and patient satisfaction based on the information we have.

The patient should take their daily maintenance opioid dose before induction of any anesthetic if possible. Most sustained release opioids provide 12 h or more of analgesic effect and should maintain baseline requirements during the preoperative and intraoperative period, particularly for an ambulatory surgery. If the patient forgets or is instructed not to take his or her baseline medication, they should be loaded with an equivalent loading dose of intravenous narcotic at induction or during the procedure. Transdermal fentanyl patches should be maintained. The patient may safely change the patch on their scheduled date if it happens to be the scheduled surgery date without the need for intravenous fentanyl. However, if removed >6–12 h prior this, it can be replaced with an equivalent intravenous maintenance rate. Replacing the patch may take 6–12 h to take full effect and intravenous fentanyl may be weaned after that time [67, 68]. Implanted intrathecal or epidural narcotic infusions are generally continued. If the baseline narcotic requirement is not maintained, withdrawal symptoms may be experienced, as demonstrated by some case reports [34]. While there are many computerized programs and online calculators available to convert various types of oral narcotic dosages to different available types of narcotics via intravenous and intramuscular routes, a narcotic conversion chart may be a useful place to start when calculating baseline opioid requirements (Table 12.5).

Some intravenous or intramuscular doses of morphine or hydromorphone may be titrated down from oral doses because parenteral administration bypasses first pass metabolism, having 2–3 times the bioavailability of oral dosing [70–72]. However, newer formulations such as oxycodone and oxymorphone have high oral bioavailability, approaching 83 % [70, 73, 74]. When providing these doses, close monitoring of patient the baseline oral dose can be approximated by nearly similar doses of intravenous awareness, oxygenation, heart rate, respiratory rate, and pupil diameter should be undertaken to avoid both under- and overmedication.

In an ambulatory surgery setting, patients may benefit from intraoperative boluses of fentanyl and sufentanil. After stabilization in the recovery area, they should be started on early oral opioids and might require doses higher than baseline, depending on the invasiveness of the procedure [75, 76]. Doses may need to be increased 30–100 % in comparison to opioid-naïve patients [3, 8, 76]. In a nonambulatory surgery setting, where a patient may be unable to take oral medications postoperatively, judicious doses of morphine, hydromorphone, or fentanyl can be provided to cover both baseline and postsurgical pain. Some anesthesiologists may prefer to titrate opioids preoperatively or "preemptively"

while maintaining active communication with the patient and monitoring vital signs. Others prefer to give half the estimated dose before the induction of anesthesia and the remainder as the case progresses [76].

Patient-Controlled Analgesia (PCA)

Lastly, use of an intravenous patient-controlled analgesia (PCA) to control postoperative pain has been shown to be useful in this population. These can be set to fulfill a patient's basal pain requirements as well as add a patient-controlled dose to provide acute pain relief [77, 78]. Due to receptor downregulation and opioid tolerance, higher than normal doses of morphine or hydromorphone may be required. Basal requirements can be met by converting the oral or transdermal daily dose to intravenous equivalent and starting a basal infusion or adding 1–2 boluses per hour to maintain baseline opioid requirements [77]. Although some studies first were concerned that individuals may self-administer excessive amounts of opioid [4, 75, 76], it is now widely accepted that PCA can be offered to selected patients provided that pain intensity, opioid consumption, and side effects are monitored [79].

Methadone has also been advocated for use in patients who have inadequate pain control despite treatment with high doses of morphine [80]. Methadone may have the ability of activating a different mu receptor subtype to which morphine tolerance has not developed as well as having the added benefits of alpha 2 agonist properties and NMDA receptor antagonism [59, 81, 82]. However, initial dosing of methadone should be started cautiously due to the prolonged half-life in some patients and potentially unclear dose conversion when compared to higher total dosages of morphine equivalents.

Postoperative Oral Narcotic Regimens

When a postoperative oral narcotic regimen is chosen, baseline requirements should be supplemented with additional 20–50 % above baseline to accommodate pain associated with surgical injury [76]. These should be slowly titrated down over 5–7 days to presurgical amounts, thereby reducing the risk of withdrawal. If the procedure reduces chronic pain (e.g., cordotomy, spine surgery, neurolysis) then the baseline dose may be reduced by 25–50 % the first postoperative day and then tapered 25 % every 24–48 h, as tolerated. Of course, during this time, the signs and symptoms of withdrawal should be closely monitored. Weaning of opioids and the prevention of withdrawal reaction can be facilitated by adding an alpha 2 agonist such as clonidine.

Table 12.5 Equianalgesic dosing of opioids for pain management

Drug[a]	Equianalgesic doses (mg)		Approximate equianalgesic 24-h dose (assumes around-the-clock dosing)[b]		Usual starting dose (adults) (doses not equianalgesic)	
	Parenteral	Oral	Parenteral	Oral/other	Parenteral	Oral/other
Morphine (immediate-release tablets, oral solution)	10	30	3–4 mg q 4 h	10 mg q 4 h	2–5 mg q 3–4 h	5–15 mg q 3–4 h
Controlled-release morphine (e.g., MS Contin, Kadian)	NA	30	NA	30 mg q 12 h (Kadian may be given as 60 mg q 24 h)	NA	15 mg q 8–12 h (Kadian may be started at 10–20 mg q 24 h)[g]
Extended-release morphine (Avinza [USA], Embeda [with naltrexone USA])	NA	30	NA	60 mg q 24 h	NA	Avinza: 30 mg q 24 h Embeda: 20 mg q 24 h
Hydromorphone (Dilaudid)	1.5–2	7.5–8	0.5–0.8 mg q 4 h	2–4 mg q 4 h	See footnotes c,d	See footnote c
Extended-release hydromorphone (Exalgo, Jurnista [Canada])	NA	See footnote e	NA	See footnote e	NA	See footnotes f,g
Oxycodone (e.g., Roxicodone [USA], OxyIR [Canada], also in Percocet, others)	NA	20–30	NA	5–10 mg q 4 h	NA	5 mg q 3–4 h
Controlled-release oxycodone (OxyContin)	NA	20–30	NA	20–30 mg q 12 h	NA	10 mg q 12 h
Oxymorphone (Opana [USA])	1	10	0.3–0.4 mg q 4 h	5 mg q 6 h	0.5 mg q 4–6 h	10 mg q 4–6 h
Extended-release oxymorphone (Opana ER [USA])[h]	NA	10	NA	10 mg q 12 h	NA	5 mg q 12 h
Hydrocodone (in Lortab [USA], Vicodin [USA], others)	NA	30–45	NA	10–15 mg q 4 h	NA	2.5–10 mg q 3–6 h
Codeine	100–130	200	30–50 mg q 4 h	60 mg q 4 h	10 mg q 3–4 h	15–30 mg q 3–4 h

Methadone (Dolophine [USA], Metadol [Canada])	Variable	Variable	The conversion ratio of methadone is highly variable depending on factors such as patient tolerance, morphine dose, and length of dosing (short term versus chronic dosing). Because the analgesic duration of action is shorter than the half-life, toxicity due to drug accumulation can occur within 3–5 days (see our detail document "Opioid Dosing")
Fentanyl	0.1	NA	All non-injectable fentanyl products are for opioid-tolerant patients only. Do not convert mcg for mcg among fentanyl products (i.e., patch, transmucosal [Actiq (USA)], buccal [Fentora (USA)], buccal soluble film [Onsolis]). See specific product labeling for dosing
Meperidine (Demerol)	75	300	Should be used for acute dosing only (short duration of action (2.5–3.5 h)) and neurotoxic metabolite, normeperidine [1]. Avoid in renal insufficiency and use caution in hepatic impairment and in the elderly (potential for toxicity due to accumulation of normeperidine). Seizures, myoclonus, tremor, confusion, and delirium may occur

An equianalgesic dose calculator is available at http://www.hopweb.org

From Therapeutic Research Center [69]

Project leaders in preparation of this detail document: Melanie Cupp, Pharm.D., BCPS (May 2010 update), Jennifer Obenrader, Pharm.D (original author 2004)

NA not available

Equianalgesic doses contained in this chart are approximate and should be used only as a guideline. Dosing must be titrated to individual response. There is often incomplete cross-tolerance among these drugs. It is, therefore, typically necessary to begin with a dose lower (e.g., 25–50 % lower) than the equianalgesic dose when changing drugs and then titrate to an effective response. Dosing adjustments for renal or hepatic insufficiency and other conditions that affect drug metabolism and kinetics may also be necessary. Most of the above opioids are available as generics. Exceptions (with example cost from drugstore.com) include Kadian ($4.81/30 mg cap), Avinza ($4.47/30 mg cap), Opana, Opana ER ($4.40/10 mg tab), Embeda ($4.60/20 mg cap), and Exalgo ($10/8 mg [AWP]). As a comparison, generic morphine controlled release = $1.63/30 mg tab

a Tramadol (e.g., Ultram [USA], Ralivia [Canada], potency is about one-tenth that of morphine, similar to codeine. The maximum daily dose of tramadol is 300–400 mg, depending on the product. Also check product information regarding appropriate dosing in elderly or in renal or hepatic dysfunction

b Examples of doses seen in clinical practice, taking into account available dosage strengths

c Product labeling for hydromorphone recommends a starting dose of 1 mg to 2 mg IV every 4–6 h or 2–4 mg orally every 4–6 h. Some institutions use even lower doses of hydromorphone (e.g., 0.2–0.5 mg every 2 h as needed). One regimen starts opioid-naïve patients at 0.2 mg IV every 2 h as needed for mild or moderate pain, with the option in moderate pain to give an extra 0.2 mg after 15 min if relief is inadequate after the first 0.2-mg dose. For severe pain, 0.5 mg IV every 2 h as needed is used initially. In adults <65 years of age, the 0.5-mg dose can be repeated in 15 min if relief is inadequate, for a maximum of 1 mg in 2 h

d Dilaudid Canadian monograph recommends parenteral starting dose of 2 mg. See footnote "c" for additional information and precautions

e Per the product labeling, convert to Exalgo 12 mg from oral codeine 200 mg, hydrocodone 30 mg, morphine 60 mg, oxycodone 30 mg, and oxymorphone 20 mg. The Jurnista product monograph recommends a 5:1 oral morphine to oral hydromorphone conversion ratio

f No initial dose for Exalgo. For opioid-tolerant patients only. Initial Jurnista dose (opioid naïve or <40 mg daily oral morphine equivalents) is 4–8 mg q 24 h

g Labeling for some products (MS Contin [USA], Kadian, Jurnista) suggests beginning treatment with an immediate-release formulation

h Per the product labeling, oral oxymorphone 10 mg ER is approximately equivalent to hydrocodone 20 mg or oxycodone 20 mg

Use of Mixed Agonists/Antagonists

Buprenorphine is a mixed partial opioid agonist/antagonist approximately 30 times more potent than morphine, with less respiratory depression than pure mu agonists [83]. Buprenorphine may be delivered via oral, intravenous, intramuscular, sublingual, or epidural routes. Although it may be used in the management of acute pain, it may be encountered in the patient receiving chronic treatment for past narcotic addiction. Like other chronic opioid use, long-term use of buprenorphine will result in physical dependence, but withdrawal symptoms will be less severe when compared with full mu agonists. Side effects to be wary of include constipation, headache, nausea, vomiting, sweating, dizziness, as well as respiratory depression, and changes in blood pressure and heart rate [84–87].

One approach to the patient taking chronic buprenorphine [88] is described below. Firstly, the prescribing physician should be contacted and be made aware of the surgery. If buprenorphine is being taken, the patient should continue as long as pain is controlled, and non-narcotic adjuncts should be provided for home use. If pain is uncontrolled preoperatively and surgery is elective, consider delaying the surgery until the prescribing physician can transition to short-acting opioids for 5 days. If surgery is emergent and pain is uncontrolled, buprenorphine should be discontinued and a PCA should be started if possible, realizing that patient requirements will be high due to opioid tolerance. Non-narcotic adjuncts with regional or neuraxial anesthesia should be considered. If they have been off buprenorphine for more than 5 days and pain is uncontrolled, the patient should be treated with pure opioid receptor agonists such as morphine, and the physician prescribing buprenorphine should be made aware of the switch. Buprenorphine can then be restarted by that physician after postoperative pain returns to baseline.

Use of Adjuvant Analgesics

Non-narcotic adjuvants are valuable resources in the treatment of acute pain. Each adjuvant works via a different mechanism to provide analgesia and diminished sensation of pain. All come with varying side effect profiles and efficacies. It is important to recognize these available options, and if begun preemptively, these medications can have opioid-sparing effect in the perioperative period. Effective perioperative analgesia with a combination of agents results in reducing perioperative morbidity, shortens hospital stays, and improves patient satisfaction [89–92].

Firstly, anxiolytics in the preoperative period may help the patient cooperate without fear or anxiety as well as reduce intraoperative anesthesia and postoperative analgesia requirements. The use of anxiolytic pretreatment may further lead to decrease in postoperative pain scores and postoperative anxiety [93, 94].

Local anesthetics bind to receptors in the sodium channel and block sodium influx, arresting depolarization, thereby interrupting afferent nerve conduction. Local anesthesia or peripheral nerve blockade is useful to provide incisional pain relief in the immediate perioperative period [95]. Although lidocaine patches have only been FDA approved for use in postherpetic neuralgia [94], they can also be used to decrease the incisional pain. The patches can be cut according to the size of a painful area; the manufacturer recommends leaving the patch on for 12 h and then off for 12 h. Some texts discuss the use of lidocaine patches 2–3 in. from the incision to help with incisional pain [14]. This allows lidocaine to diffuse into the dermis and epidermis, producing analgesia without numbness of the skin, with minimal systemic absorption [94]. Other medications such as tramadol, morphine, and ketorolac injected subcutaneously at the incision site have been used to decrease oral analgesic consumption [96, 97].

The use of non-opioid analgesic adjuvants may also reduce the amount of narcotic required. Acetaminophen is a commonly used agent that can be clinically useful in reducing postoperative opioid consumption and reduces inflammation via COX-2 and COX-3 inhibition. Doses less than 3 g over 24 h make hepatotoxicity unlikely in the patient without hepatic dysfunction, and it has an excellent safety profile. Intraoperative and postoperative opioid consumption is reduced via the use of nonsteroidal anti-inflammatory drugs (NSAIDs) as well. Postoperative opioid consumption may be reduced up to 50 % [98–101] and is particularly useful in same day surgeries [102]. These include the salicylates, propionic acids, acetic acids, oxylates, and fenamates. Although most NSAIDs are orally delivered, ketorolac is unique in that it can be delivered intramuscularly or intravenously in the perioperative period.

In general, NSAIDs inhibit the conversion of arachidonic acid to prostaglandins, bradykinins, and phospholipids via the cyclooxygenase enzyme. Cyclooxygenase (COX) inhibition increases leukotriene production, leading to rare asthmatic and anaphylactic reactions [103, 104]. COX-1 specifically influences platelet function, gastric mucosal protection, and hemostasis, while COX-2 affects inflammatory cascade and pain specifically [104]. The inhibition of COX-1 enzyme can thereby result in platelet inhibition, increased risk of gastric ulcers and gastrointestinal bleeding, as well as renal dysfunction. Initial enthusiasm regarding selective cyclooxygenase COX-2 inhibition has been quenched in recent years, as these have been associated with adverse cardiovascular events such as myocardial infarction and cerebrovascular accident [89, 105–110]. Despite this controversy, some authors still recommend its use in the acute setting as these agents are readily available, easy to administer, and effective [94].

Use of ketamine intraoperatively as an induction agent (1–2 mg/kg IV) or low-dose ketamine (0.5 mg/kg IV) postoperatively has been shown to reduce opioid dose requirements and provide analgesia via direct interaction with kappa opioid receptors [111] but more importantly via NMDA antagonism, inhibiting monoaminergic pain pathways [112, 113]. It also has mild local anesthetic properties, interacting with voltage-gated sodium channels. Ketamine is unique in that it does not cause respiratory depression while providing anesthesia and analgesia; however, it may be associated with increased salivation, emergence delerium, sympathetic stimulation, tachycardia, and hypertension at induction doses.

Clonidine and dexmedetomidine have also been shown to reduce total opioid requirements without respiratory depression via alpha 2 agonism and reduction of sympathetic outflow [46]. Clonidine is typically applied in a 0.1–0.2-mg/h transdermal patch or via oral routes. Dexmedetomidine is an alpha 2 receptor agonist, with less effect on alpha 1 receptors than clonidine, and may be used in the perioperative period in doses approximating 0.5 mg/kg/h via intravenous route. However, both may have side effects including sedation, dry mouth, hypotension, and bradycardia; abrupt discontinuation of clonidine may result in reflex hypertension and tachycardia.

Although it has not been studied in the chronic pain patient in the perioperative period, gabapentin has been shown to be particularly useful in patients with neuropathic pain. It has been shown to reduce postoperative morphine requirements in patients undergoing radical mastectomy and enhances morphine analgesia in healthy volunteers [114, 115]. It is renally excreted and has a few known drug interactions and can cause sedation. Although pregabalin works via a similar mechanism, this has not been studied as extensively. Both agents have been found to be effective in reducing nociception-induced hyperalgesia [35] and should be considered in a preemptive multimodal pain management plan. Ongoing study is necessary in the area of the opioid-tolerant patient.

Patients may also be chronically on antidepressants for chronic pain management, such as serotonin, norepinephrine reuptake inhibitors (SNRIs), and tricyclic antidepressants or (TCAs). These should be continued during the perioperative period, although the anesthesiologist should be aware of the profound response to pressor administration, particularly indirect agents such as ephedrine. TCAs also have anticholinergic effects and may cause somnolence.

Magnesium is thought to work as an NMDA antagonist and may be an adjuvant to consider in a comprehensive pain strategy. Its use is still an area of controversy and research. Some studies have shown a reduction of total intraoperative opioid requirements after an intravenous dose of 50 mg/kg [116, 117], while others showed reduction in postoperative opioid consumption after spinal anesthetics [118]. Evidence provided by a recent systematic review [119] demonstrated that magnesium is an inexpensive, available treatment for hypomagnesemia and shivering, and may or may not reduce postoperative opioid requirements. There are little to no recommendations from this review provided specifically to the chronic pain population.

Lastly, dextromethorphan, a commonly used antitussive, is also a low-affinity NMDA antagonist and may be used as an adjunct. More therapies are being actively developed to reduce opioid tolerance via NMDA receptors and production of nitric oxide synthase [114]. Recent studies have shown increasing levels of nitric oxide via transdermal nitroglycerin decreases the postoperative opioid requirements in cancer patients [120]. There may be some role for M5 muscarinic acetycholine receptors in mediating reward and withdrawal symptoms related to opioid use [121].

Neuraxial Analgesia for Postoperative Pain

Administration of opioids via the neuraxial rouge may be more efficacious than parenteral or oral opioids [40, 122]. Intrathecal and epidural doses are approximately 100 and 10 times more efficacious peroperatively than parenteral administration [24]. This increased efficacy may be due to downregulation of spinal opioid receptors. There have only been a few studies in opioid-dependent patients, on this route of administration and should be further explored.

Continuous epidural catheters are most appropriate in orthopedic, abdominal, pelvic, and thoracic procedures and in the treatment of blunt chest injury. When placed prior to induction of anesthesia, intraoperative and postoperative anesthetic requirements are reduced [123–127]. Ileus as well as postoperative nausea and vomiting, postoperative pulmonary complications, myocardial infarction, and thromboembolism are all reduced with epidural anesthesia [128].

If epidural anesthesia is chosen, serious complications can occur including inadvertent intravascular or intrathecal injection, epidural abscess, and epidural hematoma [129]. These risks should be assessed preoperatively and discussed with the patient.

Peripheral Nerve Blockade for Postoperative Pain

If possible and applicable for a given surgery, peripheral nerve blockade (PNB) should be considered in developing a comprehensive pain management plan for a chronic pain patient, particularly in extremity surgery. Advantages include reduction in parenteral and oral opioid requirements both intraoperative and several hours postoperatively with a "single-shot" technique, and some centers have trialed discharging patients home with an indwelling catheter for up to 48 h via disposable pumps. The goal is to minimize pain perception while reducing the need for oral or parental opioids beyond baseline requirements [4, 76].

Conclusions

In the opioid-dependent patient, preventing not only the withdrawal symptoms but also the adverse physiologic, emotional, and long-term effects of surgical pain are vital in humane perioperative pain treatment. There is a significant risk of both overdosing and underdosing narcotics in this patient population. Patients must be assessed preoperatively to determine the most appropriate plan of action for pain control. In developing a balanced analgesic plan, pain must be treated with the least amount of the most specific drug with a goal of treating stimulation, modulation, inflammation, and psychology of pain. Using a multimodal approach appropriately may reduce the amount of opioid consumed and thereby reduce the number of dose related side effects.

Vignette #2

A 33-year-old male presents for operative treatment of an ankle fracture 1 month after a severe motorcycle injury where he suffered injuries to both lower extremities. Since the accident, he has undergone multiple procedures including exploratory laparotomy, pelvic reconstruction, and femur and tibia surgeries. In the last month, he has become severely opioid tolerant and feels his pain has been vastly undertreated. This patient presents a significant challenge in the attempt to provide adequate pain control perioperatively. Even though he was in excellent health prior to his injury, over the last month, his increasing narcotic requirement and psychological impairment have led to uncontrolled pain.

The need for thorough counseling and discussion of expectations are highly important. In this patient, a balanced approach with preemptive analgesia will lead to a higher satisfaction rate and less risk of narcotic overdose and side effects of medications. The preoperative placement of popliteal and saphenous peripheral nerve blockade with local anesthesia and clonidine provides complete blockade of ongoing pain from the operative extremity. Intraoperatively, intermittent ketamine and intravenous narcotics with the peripheral nerve blockade provide analgesia. Intravenous magnesium could be considered intraoperatively. Upon emergence, patient-controlled analgesia with a basal rate to compensate for his preoperative requirements could be

instated as well. Oral home medications reinstituted as soon as possible to allow for an easy transition to discharge.

References

1. Bell JR. Australian trends in opioid prescribing for chronic non-cancer pain, 1986–1996. Med J Aust. 1997;167:26–9.
2. Jage J, Bey T. Postoperative analgesia in patients with substance use disorders. Acute Pain. 2000;3:140–55.
3. May JA, White HC, Leonard-White A, Warltier DC, Pagel PS. The patient recovering from alcohol or drug addiction: special issues for the anesthesiologist. Anesth Analg. 2001;92:160–1.
4. Hord AH, Sinatra RS. Postoperative analgesia in the opioid dependent patient. In: Hord AH, Ginsberg B, Preble LM, editors. Acute pain: mechanisms and management. St Louis: Mosby Yearbook; 1992. p. 390–8.
5. Dolin SJ, Cashman JN, Bland JM. Effectiveness of acute postoperative pain management: evidence from published data. Br J Anaesth. 2002;89:409–23.
6. Mitra S, Sinatra RS. Perioperative management of acute pain in the opioid dependent patient. Anesthesiology. 2004;101:212–27.
7. Streitzer J. Pain management in the opioid dependent patient. Curr Psychiatr Rep. 2001;3:489–96.
8. Collett BJ. Chronic opioid therapy for non cancer pain. Br J Anaesth. 2001;87:133–43.
9. Miaskowski C, Crews J, Ready LB, et al. Anesthesia-based pain services improve the quality of postoperative pain management. Pain. 1999;80:23–9.
10. Finlay RJ, Keeri-Szanto M, Boyd D. New analgesic agents and techniques shorten port-operative hospital stay. Pain. 1984;19:S397.
11. Rapp SE, Ready LB, Nessly ML. Acute pain management in patients with prior opioid consumption: a case-controlled retrospective review. Pain. 1995;61:195–201.
12. Weissman C. The metabolic response to stress: an overview and update. Anesthesiology. 1990;73:308.
13. Hagen C, Brandt MR, Kehlet H. Prolactin, LH, FSH, GH, and cortisol response to surgery and the effect of epidural analgesia. Acta Endocrinol Copenh. 1980;94:151.
14. Lubenow T, Ivankovich A, Barkin R. Management of acute postoperative pain. In: Barash P, Cullen B, Stoelting R, editors. Clinical anesthesia. 5th ed. Philadelphia: Lippincott, Williams & Wilkins; 2006. p. 1413.
15. Lee D, Kimura S, DeQuattro V. Noradrenergic activity and silent ischemia in hypertensive patients with stable angina: effect of metoprolol. Lancet. 1989;1:403.
16. Rademaker BM, Ringers J, Oddom JA, et al. Pulmonary function and stress response after laparoscopic cholecystectomy: comparison with subcostal incision and influence of thoracic epidural anesthesia. Anesth Analg. 1992;75:381.
17. Rawal N, Sjostrand U, Christoffersson E, et al. Comparison of intramuscular and epidural morphine for postoperative analgesia in the grossly obese; influence on postoperative ambulation and pulmonary function. Anesth Analg. 1984;63:583.
18. Tuman K, McCarthy R, March R, et al. Effects of epidural anesthesia and analgesia on coagulation and outcome after major vascular surgery. Anesth Analg. 1991;73:696.
19. Rosenfeld B, Beattie C, Christopherson R, et al. The effects of different anesthetic regimens on fibrinolysis and the development of postoperative anesthetic regimens on fibrinolysis and the development of postoperative arterial thrombosis. Anesthesiology. 1993;79:435.
20. Breslow MJ, Parker S, Frank S, et al. Determinants of catecholamine and cortisol responses to lower-extremity revascularization. Anesthesiology. 1993;79:1202.

21. Saol M. Effects of anesthesia and surgery on the immune response. Acta Anaesthesiol Scand. 1992;36:201.

22. Toft P, Svendsen P, Tonnesen E. Redistribution of lymphocytes after major surgical stress. Acta Anaesthesiol Scand. 1993;37:245.

23. Davis JM, Albert JD, Tracy KJ. Increased neutrophil mobilization and decreased chemotaxis during cortisol and epinephrine infusions. J Trauma. 1991;31:725.

24. Cousins M. Acute and postoperative pain. In: Wall P, Melzack R, editors. Textbook of pain. New York: Churchill Livingstone; 1999. p. 357–85.

25. Nimmo WS. Effect of anaesthesia on gastric motility and emptying. Br J Anaesth. 1984;56:29–36.

26. Carr DB, Goudas LC. Acute pain. Lancet. 1999;353:2051–8.

27. Wu CL, et al. Gene therapy for the management of pain: part I: methods and strategies. Anesthesiology. 2001;94:1119–32.

28. Wallace KG. The pathophysiology of pain. Crit Care Nurs Q. 1992;15:1–13.

29. Fishbain DA, Rosomoff HL, Rosomoff RS. Drug abuse, dependence, and addiction in chronic pain patients. Clin J Pain. 1992;8:77–85.

30. Savage SR. Addiction in the treatment of pain: significance, recognition and treatment. J Pain Symptom Manage. 1993;8:265–78.

31. Strain EC. Assessment and treatment of comorbid psychiatric disorders in opioid-dependent patients. Clin J Pain. 2002;18(suppl):S14–27.

32. Weissman DE, Haddox JD. Opioid pseudoaddiction: an iatrogenic syndrome. Pain. 1989;36:363–6.

33. Gustin HB, Akil H. Opioid analgesics. In: Hardman JG, Limbird LE, editors. Goodman and Gilman's the pharmacological basis of therapeutics. New York: McGraw-Hill; 2001. p. 569–619.

34. de Leon-Casasola OA, Lema MJ. Epidural sufentanil for acute pain control in a patient with extreme opioid dependency. Anesthesiology. 1992;76:853–6.

35. Wilder-Smith OH, Arendt-Nielsen L. Postoperative hyperalgesia: its clinical importance and relevance. Anesthesiology. 2006;104: 601–7.

36. Stoelting RK, Hillier SC. Chapter 6: nonbarbituate intravenous anesthetic drugs. In: Pharmacology & physiology in anesthetic practice. Philadelphia: Lippincott Williams & Wilkins; 2006. p. 167–75.

37. Stoelting RK, Miller RD. Opioids. Basics of anesthesia. 5th ed. Philadelphia: Churchill -Livingstone Elsevier; 2007. p. 113–21.

38. Kosten T, O'Connor PG. Management of drug and alcohol withdrawal. N Engl J Med. 2003;348:1786.

39. Sosnowski M, Yaksh TL. Differential cross-tolerance between intrathecal morphine and sufentanil in the rat. Anesthesiology. 1990;73:1141–7.

40. de Leon-Casasola OA, Lema MJ. Epidural bupivacaine/sufentanil therapy for postoperative pain control in patients tolerant to opioid and unresponsive to epidural bupivacaine/morphine. Anesthesiology. 1994;80:303–9.

41. Saeki S, Yaksh TL. Suppression of nociceptive responses by spinal mu opioid agonists: effects of stimulus intensity and agonist efficacy. Anesth Analg. 1993;77:265–74.

42. Dupen A, Shen D, Ersek M. Mechanisms of opioid induced tolerance and hyperalgesia. Pain Manag Nurs. 2007;8:113–21.

43. Howard LA, Sellers EM, Tyndale RF. The role of pharmacogenetically variable cytochrome P450 enzymes in drug abuse and dependence. Pharmacogenomics. 2002;3:85–99.

44. Liu J-G, Anand KJS. Protein kinases modulate the cellular adaptations associated with opioid tolerance and dependence. Brain Res Rev. 2001;38:1–19.

45. Liu S, Wu C. The effect of analgesic technique on postoperative patient-reported outcomes including analgesia: a systematic review. Pain Med. 2007;105:789–807.

46. O'Brien CP. Drug addiction and drug abuse. In: Hardman JG, Limbird LE, editors. Goodman and Gilman's the pharmacological basis of therapeutics. New York: McGraw-Hill; 2001. p. 621–42.

47. Nestler EJ, Aghajanian GK. Molecular and cellular basis of addiction. Science. 1997;278:58–63.

48. Nestler EJ. Molecular basis of long-term plasticity underlying addiction. Nat Rev Neurosci. 2001;2:119–28.

49. Nestler EJ. Molecular neurobiology of addiction. Am J Addict. 2001;10:201–17.

50. Mao J. Opioid-induced abnormal pain sensitivity: implications in clinical opioid therapy. Pain. 2002;100:213–7.

51. Kieffer BL, Evans CJ. Opioid tolerance: in search of the holy grail. Cell. 2002;108:587–90.

52. Caterina MJ, Julius D. The vanilloid receptor: a molecular gateway to the pain pathway. Annu Rev Neurosci. 2001;24:487–517.

53. Desborough JP. The stress response to trauma and surgery. Br J Anaesth. 2000;85:109–17.

54. Cohen M, Schecter WP. Perioperative pain control: a strategy for management. Surg Clin North Am. 2005;85:1243–57.

55. Macres S, Moore P, Fishman S. Acute pain management. In: Barash P, Cullen B, Stoelting R, Calahan M, Stock C, editors. Clinical anesthesiology. 6th ed. Philadelphia: Lippincott, Williams & Wilkins; 2009. p. 1474.

56. Schaible HG, Richter F. Pathophysiology of pain. Langenbecks Arch Surg. 2004;389:237–43.

57. Winkelstein BA. Mechanisms of central sensitization, neuroimmunology & injury biomechanics in persistent pain: implications for musculoskeletal disorders. J Electromyogr Kinesiol. 2004;14: 87–93.

58. Compton MA. Cold-pressor pain tolerance in opiate and cocaine abusers: correlates of drug type and use status. J Pain Symptom Manage. 1994;9:462–73.

59. Doverty M, Somogyi AA, White JM, Bochner F, Ali R, Ling W. Hyperalgesic responses in methadone maintenance patients. Pain. 2001;90:91–6.

60. Angst MS, Clark JD. Opioid-induced hyperalgesia: a qualitative systematic review. Anesthesiology. 2006;104:570–87.

61. Ossipov MH, Lai J, King T, Vanderah TW, Porreca F. Underlying mechanisms of pronociceptive consequences of prolonged morphine exposure. Biopolymers. 2005;80:319–24.

62. Wilder-Smith OH, Tassonyi E, Crul BJ, Arendt-Nielsen L. Quantitative sensory testing and human surgery: effects of analgesic management on postoperative neuroplasticity. Anesthesiology. 2003;98:1214–22.

63. Koppert W, Sittl R, Scheuber K, Alsheimer M, Schmelz M, Schuttler J. Differential modulation of remifentanil-induced analgesia and postinfusion hyperalgesia by S-ketamine and clonidine in humans. Anesthesiology. 2003;99:152–9.

64. Simonnet G, Rivat C. Opioid-induced hyperalgesia: abnormal or normal pain? Neuroreport. 2003;14:1–7.

65. Laulin JP, Celerier E, Larcher A, LeMoal M, Simonet G. Opiate tolerance to daily heroin administration: an apparent phenomenon associated with enhanced pain sensitivity. Neuroscience. 1999;89:631–6.

66. Compton P, Charuvastra VC, Kintaudi K, Ling W. Pain responses in methadone-maintained opioid abusers. J Pain Symptom Manage. 2000;20:237–45.

67. Caplan RA, Ready B, Oden RV, Matsen FA, Nessly ML, Olsson GL. Transdermal fentanyl for postoperative pain management. JAMA. 1989;261:1036–9.

68. Sevarino FB, Ning T, Sinatra RS, Hord AH, Ginsberg B, Preble LM. Transdermal fentanyl for acute pain management. In: Acute pain: mechanisms and management. St. Louis: Mosby Yearbook; 1992. p. 364–9.

69. Melanie C, Jennifer O. Therapeutic Research Center. Equianalgesic dosing of opioids for pain management. Canadian Pharm Lett. 2010;26(7):260712.

70. Foley RM. Opioids II: opioid analgesics in clinical pain management. In: Herz AAH, Simon EJ, editors. Handbook of experimental pharmacology. New York: Springer-Verlag; 1993. p. 697–743.

71. Pereira J, Lawlor P, Vigano A, Dorgan M, Bruera E. Equianalgesic dose ratios for opioids: a critical review and proposals for long-term dosing. J Pain Symptom Manage. 2001;22:672–87.

72. Steindler EM. ASAM addiction terminology. In: Graham AW, Schultz TK, editors. Principles of addiction medicine. 2nd ed. Chevy Chase: American Society of Addiction Medicine; 1998. p. 1301–4.

73. Ginsberg B, Sinatra RS, Adler LJ, Crews JC, Hord AH, Laurito CE, Ashburn MA. Conversion to oral controlled-release oxycodone from intravenous opioid analgesic in the postoperative setting. Pain Med. 2003;4:31–8.

74. Poyhia R, Vainio A, Kaiko E. A review of oxycodone's clinical pharmacokinetics and pharmacodynamics. J Pain Symptom Manage. 1993;8:63–7.

75. Pasero CL, Compton P. Pain management in addicted patients. Am J Nurs. 1997;4:17–9.

76. Saberski L. Postoperative pain management for the patient with chronic pain. In: Sinatra RS Hord AH, Ginsberg B, Preble LM, editors. Acute pain: mechanisms and management. St. Louis: Mosby Yearbook; 1992. p. 422–31.

77. Parker RK, Holtman B, White PF. Patient-controlled analgesia: does a concurrent opioid infusion improve pain management after surgery? JAMA. 1992;266:1947–52.

78. Macintyre PE. Safety and efficacy of patient-controlled analgesia. Br J Anaesth. 2001;87:36–46.

79. Hudcova J. Patient controlled opioid analgesia versus conventional opioid analgesia for postoperative pain. Cochrane Database Syst Rev. 2006;4:CD003348.

80. Sartain JB, Mitchell SJ. Successful use of oral methadone after failure of intravenous morphine and ketamine. Anaesth Intensive Care. 2002;30:487–9.

81. Morley JS, Makin MK. The use of methadone in cancer pain poorly responsive to other opioids. Pain Rev. 1998;5:51–8.

82. Davis AM, Inturrisi CE. d-Methadone blocks morphine tolerance and nmethyl-D-aspartate-induced hyperalgesia. J Pharmacol Exp Ther. 1999;289:1048–53.

83. Johnson RE, Jaffe JH, Fudala PJ. A controlled trial of buprenorphine treatment for opioid dependence. JAMA. 1992;287:2750–5.

84. Pickworth WB, Johnson RE, Holicky BA, Cone EJ. Subjective and physiologic effects of intravenous buprenorphine in humans. Clin Pharmacol Ther. 1993;53:570–6.

85. Lange WR, Fudala PJ, Dax EM, Johnson RE. Safety and side-effects of buprenorphine in the clinical management of heroin addiction. Drug Alcohol Depend. 1990;26:19–28.

86. Ling W, Wesson DR, Charuvastra C, Klett CJ. A controlled trial comparing buprenorphine and methadone maintenance in opioid dependence. Arch Gen Psychiatry. 1996;53:401–7.

87. Ling W, Charuvastra C, Collins JF, et al. Buprenorphine maintenance treatment of opiate dependence: a multicenter, randomized clinical trial. Addiction. 1998;93:475–86.

88. Brummett C. Perioperative management of buprenorphine. Department of Anesthesiology, Division of Pain Medicine, University of Michigan, 2008.

89. Barratt SM, et al. Multimodal analgesia and intravenous nutrition preserves total body protein following major upper gastrointestinal surgery. Reg Anesth Pain Med. 2002;27:15–22.

90. Basse L, et al. Accelerated postoperative recovery programme after colonic resection improves physical performance, pulmonary function and body composition. Br J Surg. 2002;89:446–53.

91. Brodner G, et al. Acute pain management: analysis, implications and consequences after prospective experience with 6349 surgical patients. Eur J Anaesthesiol. 2000;17:566–75.

92. Brodner G, et al. Multimodal perioperative management combining thoracic epidural analgesia, forced mobilization, and oral nutrition reduces hormonal and metabolic stress and improves convalescence after major urologic surgery. Anesth Analg. 2001;92:1594–600.

93. Kain ZN, Sevarino F, Pincus S, et al. Attenuation of the preoperative stress response with midazolam: effects on postoperative outcomes. Anesthesiology. 2000;93:141–7.

94. Olorunto WA, Galandiuk S. Managing the spectrum of surgical pain: acute management of the chronic pain patient. J Am Coll Surg. 2006;202:169–75.

95. Morrison JEJ, Jacobs VR. Reduction or elimination of postoperative pain medication after mastectomy through use of a temporarily placed local anesthetic pump vs control group. Zentralbl Gynakol. 2003;125:17–22.

96. Altunkaya H, Ozer Y, Kargi E, et al. The postoperative analgesic effect of tramadol when used as subcutaneous local anesthetic. Anesth Analg. 2004;99:1461–4.

97. Connelly NR, Reuben SS, Albert M, Page D. Use of preincisional ketorolac in hernia patients: intravenous versus surgical site. Reg Anesth. 1997;22:229–32.

98. Souter AJ, Fredman B, White PF. Controversies in the perioperative use of nonsterodial antiinflammatory drugs. Anesth Analg. 1994;79:1178–90.

99. Reuben SS, Connelly NR. Postoperative analgesic effects of celecoxib or rofecoxib after spinal fusion surgery. Anesth Analg. 2000;91:1221–5.

100. Katz WA. Cyclooxygenase-2-selective inhibitors in the management of acute and perioperative pain. Cleve Clin J Med. 2002;69:SI65–75.

101. Mercadante S, Sapio M, Caligara M, Serrata R, Dardanoni G, Barresi L. Opioid-sparing effect of diclofenac in cancer pain. J Pain Symptom Manage. 1997;14:15–20.

102. Rawal N. Analgesia for day-case surgery. Br J Anaesth. 2001;87: 73–87.

103. Schecter WP, et al. Pain control in outpatient surgery. J Am Coll Surg. 2002;195:95–104.

104. Zuckerman LF. Nonopioid and opioid analgesics. In: Ashburn MRL, editor. The management of pain. New York: Churchill Livingstone; 1998. p. 111–40.

105. Lefkowith JB. Cyclooxygenase-2 specificity and its clinical implications. Am J Med. 1999;106:43S–50.

106. Bresalier RS, et al. Cardiovascular events associated with rofecoxib in a colorectal adenoma chemoprevention trial. N Engl J Med. 2005;352:1092–102.

107. Drazen JM. COX-2 inhibitors: a lesson in unexpected problems. N Engl J Med. 2005;352:1131–2.

108. Nussmeier NA, et al. Complications of the COX-2 inhibitors parecoxib and valdecoxib after cardiac surgery. N Engl J Med. 2005; 352:1081–91.

109. Seibert K, et al. COX-2 inhibitors is there cause for concern? Nat Med. 1999;5:621–2.

110. Solomon DH, et al. Relationship between selective cyclooxygenase-2 inhibitors and acute myocardial infarction in older adults. Circulation. 2004;109:2068–73.

111. Hurstveit O, Maurset A, Oye I. Interaction of the chiral forms of ketamine with opioid, phencyclidine, and muscarinic receptors. Pharmacol Toxicol. 1995;77:355–9.

112. Connor DFJ, Muir A. Balanced analgesia for the management of pain associated with multiple fractured ribs in an opioid addict. Anaesth Intensive Care. 1998;26:459–60.

113. Clark JL, Kalan GE. Effective treatment of severe cancer pain of the head using low-dose ketamine in an opioid-tolerant patient. J Pain Symptom Manag. 1995;10:310–4.

114. Barton SF, Langeland FF, Snabes MC, LeComte D, Kuss ME, Dhadda SS, Hubbard RC. Efficacy and safety of intravenous parecoxib sodium in relieving acute postoperative pain following gynecologic laparotomy surgery. Anesthesiology. 2002;97:306–14.

115. Eckhardt K, Ammon S, Hofmann U, Riebe A, Gugeler N, Mikus G. Gabapentin enhances the analgesic effect of morphine in healthy volunteers. Anesth Analg. 2000;91:185–91.

116. Koinig H, Wallner T, Marhofer P, Andel KH, Mayer N. Magnesium sulfate reduces intra- and postoperative analgesic requirements. Anesth Analg. 1998;87:206–10.

117. Ryu JH, Kang MH, Park KS, Do SH. Effects of magnesium sulphate on intraoperative anaesthetic requirements and postoperative analgesia in gynaecology patients receiving total intravenous anaesthesia. Br J Anaesth. 2008;100:397–403.

118. Hwang JY, Na HS, Jeon YT, Ro YJ, Kim CS, Do SH. IV infusion of magnesium sulphate during spinal anaesthesia improves postoperative analgesia. Br J Anaesth. 2010;104:89–93.

119. Lysakowsky C, Dumont L, Czarnetzki C, Tramer MR. Magnesium as an adjuvant to postoperative analgesia: a systematic review of randomized trials. Anesth Analg. 2007;104:1532–9.

120. Lauretti GR, Perez MV, Reis MP, Pereira NL. Double-blind evaluation of transdermal nitroglycerine as adjuvant to oral morphine for cancer pain management. J Clin Anesth. 2002;14:83–6.

121. Basile AS, Fedorova I, Zapata A, Liu X, Shippenberg T, Duttaroy A, Yamada M, Wess J. Deletion of the M5 muscarinic acetylcholine receptor attenuates morphine reinforcement and withdrawal but not morphine analgesia. Proc Natl Acad Sci U S A. 2002;99:11452–7.

122. Harrison DH, Sinatra RS, Morgese L, Chung JH. Epidural narcotic and patient-controlled analgesia for post-cesarean section pain relief. Anesthesiology. 1988;68:454–7.

123. Fernandez MI, et al. Does a thoracic epidural confer any additional benefit following videoassisted thoracoscopic pleurectomy for primary spontaneous pneumothorax? Eur J Cardiothorac Surg. 2005;27:671–4.

124. Holte K, Kehlet H. Epidural analgesia and risk of anastomotic leakage. Reg Anesth Pain Med. 2001;26:111–7.

125. Holte K, Kehlet H. Effect of postoperative epidural analgesia on surgical outcome. Minerva Anestesiol. 2002;68:157–61.

126. Subramaniam B, Pawar DK, Kashyap L. Pre-emptive analgesia with epidural morphine or morphine and bupivacaine. Anaesth Intensive Care. 2000;28:392–8.

127. Wu CT, et al. Pre-incisional epidural ketamine, morphine and bupivacaine combined with epidural and general anaesthesia provides pre-emptive analgesia for upper abdominal surgery. Acta Anaesthesiol Scand. 2000;44:63–8.

128. Carli F, Mayo N, Klubien K, et al. Epidural analgesia enhances functional exercise capacity and health-related quality of life after colonic surgery: results of a randomized trial. Anesthesiology. 2002;97:540–9.

129. Cullen DJ, Bogdanov E, Htut N. Spinal epidural hematoma occurrence in the absence of known risk factors: a case series. J Clin Anesth. 2004;16:376–81.

Opioids and the Law

Selina Read and Jill Eckert

Key Points

- Opioids have been used for medicinal purposes since as early as 3000 B.C.; problems such as abuse and addiction have also been reported alongside.
- Understanding the definitions, incidence, and cost of chronic pain is important for anyone who will be prescribing these medications.
- The clinician must become familiar with both state and federal laws pertaining to opioid prescribing. Not adhering to both state and federal laws can put the prescriber at risk.
- Clinicians who prescribe opioids must be well versed in detecting abuse and be able to find avenues for treatment of both the abuse alongside with the chronic pain issue.
- Prescription monitoring programs have become a valuable tool in preventing diversion of controlled substances.

Introduction

As physicians, one of the most important aspects of our job is the alleviation of pain, both acute and chronic. Opioids have been an integral part of easing pain for thousands of years and continue to play an important role in the medical

S. Read, M.D. (✉)
Department of Anesthesiology,
Penn State College of Medicine, Penn State Milton S. Hershey Medical Center, 500 University Drive, H187,
Hershey, PA 17033, USA
e-mail: sread@hmc.psu.edu

J. Eckert, DO
Pennsylvania State University College of Medicine,
Hershey, PA, USA

Department of Anesthesiology,
Pennsylvania State Milton S. Hershey Medical Center,
P.O. Box 850, Hershey, PA 17033, USA
e-mail: jeckert@psu.edu

landscape today. The downside of these often powerful medications is the possibility of those taking them to become addicted and divert them away from the intended use.

History of Opioids and the Law

The earliest use of opioids dates back several thousand years, where in 3000 B.C. residents of Sumer, what is modern-day Iraq, used opium for both its medicinal and recreational characteristics. Hippocrates, one of the most important Greek physicians of his time, used opium to cure several ailments ranging from headache to depression. Other ancient Greeks and Romans used opium to relieve aches and pains. They also used opium for entertainment, enjoying the euphoric effects. Opium made its way to Europe and China sometime in the tenth century when Arab traders brought it from the Middle East. This efflux into Europe brought with it many of the problems we face today, namely, addiction. As early as the sixteenth century, manuscripts can be found discussing addiction and tolerance. It may be China that experienced the most problems with abuse in the seventeenth century when tobacco was outlawed, and the population began smoking opium as an alternative. There are no records of any of these ancient civilizations trying to pass laws to decrease or ban the use of opioids; however, many records indicate that abuse was prevalent and caused problems in society.

It wasn't until the nineteenth century when chemist Friedrich Sertürner isolated the active ingredient in opium that this plant found its birth in modern medicine. Sertürner named this isolated chemical morphine, after the Greek god of dreams, Morpheus. The safety of morphine was marginal as evidenced by untreatable respiratory depression which caused several deaths. Many companies began the search for a "safer, nonaddictive" opioid. Chemical modification of morphine began at the end of the nineteenth century when German chemists added two acetyl groups to the drug, forming heroin. This modification allowed the opioid to dissolve faster through the blood-brain barrier, making it twice as potent. Interestingly, this German company, known as Bayer, marketed heroin as a cough suppressant. Unfortunately, heroin had the same addictive properties and dangers as morphine, and the search continued into the twentieth century where meperidine and methadone were added to the physician's arsenal. An important discovery by Wejilard and Erikson in the middle of the twentieth century was nalorphine, the first opioid antagonist, providing clinicians the ability to reverse the dangerous effects of opioids [1].

As opioid use became more widespread, the United States government started placing heavy taxes on the medications, in an attempt to prevent unintended usage. The International Opium Convention of 1912 committed governments to restrict trade of these substances to medical and scientific purposes only. In 1924, the US banned all nonmedical use of opioids along with creating the Permanent Central Opium Board, which became the agency in charge of determining whether there was too much or too little opioid production around the world. The US government passed the federal Controlled Substance Act in 1970 which scheduled opioids according to their abuse potential. This act prohibited the use of opioids by any individuals not under a physician's care and assured the safety of the medications being prescribed. Then, in 1990, the International Narcotics Control Board, which was initially formed in 1961 to unite all the international agencies under one umbrella, determined that opioids are not sufficiently available for legitimate medical purposes and called for governments to take corrective actions to repair the problem [2].

Important Definitions

When discussing opioids, certain terminology must be understood to apply the prescribing laws, treating pain in patients with addiction/dependence and understanding a clinician's practice. Furthermore, not understanding or mislabeling definitions may actually hinder effective pain treatment, leading to unnecessary suffering.

In 1999, the American Academy of Pain Medicine, the American Pain Society, and the American Society of Addiction Medicine formed the Liaison Committee on Pain and Addiction (LCPA), allowing collaboration between these groups to develop consensus definitions regarding terminology. Prior to this, most clinicians would use the World Health Organization's definitions along with the DSM and ICD-10 classifications; however, consensus was needed because practitioners need a way to communicate in the same language, along with easily understood definitions to implement into their practice [3].

Addiction is defined as a primary, chronic, neurobiologic disease with genetic, psychosocial, and environmental factors influencing its development and manifestations. It is characterized by behaviors that include one or more of the

following: impaired control over drug use, compulsive use, or continued use despite harm and craving.

Physical dependence is defined as a state of adaptation that is manifested by a drug class that causes specific withdrawal syndrome that can be produced by abrupt cessation, rapid dose reduction, decreasing blood level of the drug, and/or administration of antagonist.

Tolerance is defined as a state of adaptation in which exposure to a drug induces change that results in a diminution of one or more of the drug's effects over time.

Clearly, both addiction and physical dependence can occur in the same patient; however, it is important to realize that physical dependence does not equal addiction. It is essential to understand that even though these are universally understood definitions, often state and federal governments have their own defined terminology. Whenever prescribing opioids, the prescriber should review not only the above definitions but also those set forth by their respective governing agencies they are prescribing under.

Incidence of Pain and Its Cost

It is expected that a patient will have pain following acute injury such as trauma or surgery; this pain is generally easily treated with current therapies, including opioids for short periods of time. Chronic pain presents a different set of problems due to the length of time needed for treatment, and the increasing dosage of medications that occurs with tolerance.

Chronic pain is defined as pain that persists beyond the usual course of an acute disease or pain that is not amenable to routine pain control methods. The prevalence of chronic pain ranges from 2 to 40 % in the adult population [4]. A survey in 1999 found that almost half of American households had at least one family member who suffers from chronic pain. The same survey found that one third of chronic pain sufferers did not feel they could function in society due to their pain; a majority of them felt that the pain was so horrible that they sometimes wanted to die [5]. More recently, a study from 2011 found that at least 116 million American adults suffer from pain, more than those affected by heart disease, cancer, and diabetes combined [6].

All of this adds up to billions of dollars in costs each year, $635 billion to be exact [6]. It is projected that the healthcare costs of patients with chronic pain may exceed the cost for treating patients with coronary artery disease, cancer, and AIDS combined [4].

How Common Is Abuse?

The statistics regarding abuse of prescription drugs is startling. In 2004, an estimated 19 million Americans, or 8 % of the population, admitted to abusing illicit drugs in the past year, and more than half of the public has tried an illicit drug during their lifetime [4]. The National Co-morbidity Study suggests that up to 14 % of Americans will develop alcohol addiction, and up to 7.5 % will develop addiction to illicit drugs over their lifetime [3]. According to the DEA, more than 6 million Americans are abusing prescription drugs – more than the number abusing cocaine, heroin, hallucinogens, and inhalants, combined. In the past 20 years, more people began abusing prescription pain medications (2.4 million) compared with marijuana (2.1 million) or cocaine (1.0 million) [4].

There are many types of prescription drugs abused, including opioid analgesics, tranquilizers, stimulants, and sedatives. About 75 % of the abuse is in the opioid analgesic class, with OxyContin, hydrocodone, Vicodin, morphine, and Dilaudid being the most commonly abused [4].

Although the true extent of prescription drug abuse is unknown, 10 % of patients receiving treatment for illicit drugs abuse prescription drugs only. The number abusing prescription medications is staggering, and the figures are climbing each year. Between 1992 and 2003, the United States population increased by 14 %; however, prescription drug abuse increased 94 %. During this time, the abuse rate for 12–17-year-olds increased 212 %, and it is known that those teens who abuse prescription drugs are more likely to abuse other illicit drugs such as alcohol, marijuana, cocaine, and heroin [4].

Demographics regarding abuse are varied, with the two extremes of age appearing to be the most susceptible. In 2004, the number of adolescents abusing tobacco, alcohol, marijuana, cocaine, and heroin appeared to be decreasing; however; this may be linked to an increase in the rate of prescription drug use. Monitoring the future, which is an epidemiological and etiological research project based at the University of Michigan, reported that OxyContin use among 12th graders increased almost 40 % over the previous 3 years. At the other extreme of age is the elderly who often are taking multiple prescriptions, which may lead to abuse or unintentional misuse [4].

Abuse is frequent in patients being treated for a chronic pain conditions, 15 % are concomitantly abusing prescription drugs, while 35 % are abusing illicit drugs. The direct cost of medical care is staggering in a pain clinic for those who abuse opioids, costing approximately $15,000 a year, compared with $1,800 for those on opioid therapy not abusing the prescriptions [4].

Possible Causes for Increased Abuse

It's not completely clear why there is such a significant rise in abuse rates. Some postulate it's due to increased supply, rising street values, and perceived safety of prescription medications in the general public [4].

Increased supply and demand can certainly play a large role in the ability of abusers to obtain controlled substances due to the simple fact that more medications being prescribed lend to more being available. The estimated number of prescriptions filled for controlled substances has been increasing dramatically since the early 1990s. Approximately 222 million controlled substance prescriptions were filled in 1994, compared with 354 million in 2003. This represents a 154 % increase in prescription filled for controlled substances contrasted with only a 57 % increase in all other prescription medications [4].

The street value for controlled substances is staggering; these medications sell for much more than most illicit drugs. Just a few examples will help the reader understand. The cost of 100 OxyContin 80-mg tablets to insurance is $1,081; the estimated street value for this same amount is $8,000. The pharmacy cost for 100 4-mg Dilaudid tablets is $88 where the street value is $10,000 [4]. Drug dealers will do almost anything to obtain prescriptions for these controlled substances because there is a large profit margin to be made.

The public may believe that prescribed medications are safer than the similar illicit drugs that may be found on the street. Most feel that if a doctor prescribes the medication, it must be safe. Furthermore, the acquisition of licit drugs poses much less of a threat, compared with purchasing a similar drug on the street.

Sequelae of Abuse

The increased incidence of prescription drug abuse has led to many socioeconomic problems. One of the most serious is an increase in the number of deaths due to unintentional overdose. According to the Centers for Disease Control and Prevention, the number of fatal poisonings due to prescription drugs increased 25 % from 1985 to 1995. The number of overdoses due to prescription opioids now surpasses both cocaine and heroin overdoses combined. Paulozzi et al. [5] hypothesized that this increase in fatal poisonings was linked to an increase in opioid prescriptions by physicians. They found that at the end of the 1980s, pain specialists began to argue that the risk of addiction should not prevent opioid analgesics from being prescribed for nonmalignant pain. This increased utilization of opioids for pain was linked to an increase in the sales of opioids and, not surprisingly, the number of deaths due to prescription opioids [5]. However, it is not completely clear that there is a cause and effect relationship. More information and further studies will need to be completed before definitive conclusions can be formed.

Abuse puts a significant strain on society, costing nearly $200 billion dollars a year. This cost comes from medical costs from misuse, crime involved supporting diversion/addiction, loss of productivity and wages, and cost of law enforcement. The illicit drug market was estimated at $322 billion dollars a year [5].

How Will This Affect Your Practice?

In the United States and around the world, pain goes untreated and undertreated every day. This inadequate treatment has been attributed to a lack of knowledge of pain management options, inadequate understanding of addiction, or fears of investigation and sanction by federal, state, and local regulatory agencies [4].

In response to this, multiple advocacy groups and professional organizations have been formed, with the goal of improving pain management. The Joint Committee on Accreditation of Healthcare Organizations labeled pain as the fifth vital sign and suggested hospitals use some form of pain assessment in all patients, allowing for more prompt and thorough treatment [3].

Nearly 90 % of patients being treated in a pain management setting are receiving opioid therapy, with many actually being treated with more than one type of opioid [4]. In order to protect yourself and your patient's well-being, it is vital to understand the laws governing prescribing of these medications. It's also essential to understand addiction, or have a specialist's advice, to help diagnose and adequately treat patients.

Federal Law

In 1973, the DEA was established to serve as the primary federal agency responsible for the enforcement of the Controlled Substances Act, which sets forth the federal law regarding both licit and illicit controlled substances. The Practitioner's Manual is designed to explain the basic federal requirements for prescribing, administering, and dispensing controlled substances to professionals, including physicians, mid-level providers, dentists, and veterinarians. The authors are explicit in explaining that the manual and the laws that guided its writing are not intended to hinder the practitioner's ability to treat pain, but to safeguard society against diversion [7].

In the United States, the Controlled Substances Act (CSA) placed controlled substances into five schedules. Substances are placed into their respective category based on whether they have an accepted medical use and the probability of causing dependence when abused. Schedule I drugs have no accepted medical use, with a very high potential for abuse. Some examples from this class are heroin, lysergic acid diethylamide, marijuana, and peyote. Schedule II substances have a high potential for abuse with severe psychological or physical dependence. Some examples include morphine, codeine, hydromorphone, fentanyl, and meperidine. Schedule III substances have a potential for abuse that is less than schedule II, including narcotics which contain less than 15 mg of hydrocodone and products that contain less than 90 mg of codeine per unit dosage. Schedule IV substances have a lower potential for abuse compared with schedule III and include partial agonist opioids, benzodiazepines, and long-acting barbiturates. Schedule V substances have the lowest potential for abuse and include most of the antitussive, antidiarrheal, and less potent analgesic medications.

In order to prescribe scheduled substances, a practitioner must be registered with the DEA or be considered exempt from the registration process. This registration grants the practitioner authority to handle and prescribe controlled substances and must be renewed every 3 years. In accordance with federal law, the practitioner may only engage in those activities that are authorized under state law for the jurisdiction in which the practice is located. When the state and federal laws conflict, the practitioner must abide by the more stringent aspects of both federal and state laws, in many cases the state laws being stricter. The certificate of registration must be maintained at the registered location in an easily retrievable location should official inspection be needed, and if operating in several states, the practitioner must register with the DEA for each of those states.

Practitioners who are agents or employees of a hospital may use a hospital DEA number to prescribe or administer controlled substances when acting in the usual course of business or employment. Examples include residents, staff physicians, and mid-level practitioners. In order to use the hospital DEA number, the employee must be authorized to do so by the state which they practice, verified by the hospital and acting within the scope of their employment. In 2004, the DEA, in conjunction with the Centers for Medicare and Medicaid Services, instituted an identification number that should be used for all noncontrolled substance prescriptions called the National Provider Identification (NPI). This was formed as a way to allow recognition of prescribers on noncontrolled substances without use of the DEA number, preventing its weakening and overuse.

In order to comply with federal law, a prescription for a controlled substance must be prescribed for a legitimate medical purpose by a practitioner acting in the usual course of professional practice. This prescription must include the drug's name, strength, dosage form, quantity prescribed, directions for use, and number of refills. In addition, all prescriptions must have a signature along with the date the medication was prescribed. Different scheduled medications have different prescribing limitations by the federal (and state) governments. Schedule II substances have no specific federal limitations on quantity and must be written, but cannot be given any refills. In 2007, the DEA passed an amendment that allows schedule II substances to be prescribed for up to 90 days by allowing sequential prescriptions that are written on the same day but, may be filled one at a time, each at 30-day intervals. Schedule III–V substances may be refilled up to five times within 6 months after the initial prescription was issued.

The CSA outlines safeguards that help protect the physician by decreasing diversion. Keeping blank prescriptions in a safe place where they cannot be stolen and limiting the number of prescription pads in use was recommended. Writing out the actual amount prescribed in words in addition to writing the number to help prevent alterations. Never sign out blank prescriptions and use tamper-resistant pads that cannot be photocopied. Each practitioner must maintain meticulous inventories and records of controlled substances. The DEA's Office of Diversion periodically issues informational brochures meant to help decrease the risk of diversion. One such brochure entitled "Don't be Scammed by a Drug Abuser" lists common characteristics of drug abusers. These include:

- Unusual behavior in the waiting room
- Assertive and often demanding personalities
- Strange physical appearance
- Unusual knowledge of controlled substances
- Requesting a specific controlled drug with reluctance to try any other medication
- Cutaneous signs of drug abuse

Patients with abuse problems may demand to be seen right away, request appointments at the end of the business day, call or come in after regular hours, state that they are just "passing through" seeing family members, state that a prescription has been lost or stolen, or pressure the physician by eliciting sympathy or guilt [8]. Any of these signs should tip the physician that the patient may be seeking controlled substances for reasons outside of legitimate pain relief.

When prescribing controlled substances, the practitioner must understand the federal definition of addiction. This definition requires either (a) habitual use that endangers the public morals, health, safety, or welfare or (b) addiction to the use of drugs to the point of loss of self-control over the addiction or (c) the use of narcotic drugs. This definition leaves much up to the practitioner, and some argue that it fails to distinguish psychological from physical dependence, the latter often occurring in chronic pain patients over time [9]. It is important to look for addiction in your practice because frequently when regulatory action is undertaken, it is against the physician, not the patient. The patient will often be given a "deal" that allows escape from prosecution in exchange for testimony against the prescriber. It would then be up to the prescriber to prove that he/she was acting within the established standard of practice [9]. This is not meant to scare the reader, but to elaborate on the importance of proper prescribing and record keeping.

The federal government amended the Controlled Substance Act in 1974 with the Narcotic Addiction Treatment Act and again in 2000 with the Drug Addiction Treatment Act to provide laws guiding the use of controlled substances in the medical treatment of addiction. These laws established "the approval and licensing of practitioners involved in the treatment of opioid addiction, as well as improving the quality and delivery of treatment to that segment of society." It is very clear that a physician cannot prescribe schedule II maintenance or detoxification treatment, such as methadone, without a separate DEA registration. A practitioner who wants to prescribe schedule III–V medications approved for addiction, such as buprenorphine, may do so if they request a waiver form and fulfill requirements under the Center for Substance Abuse Treatment Program. If there is any question, more information can be found on the DEA's Office of Diversion Control website [7]. It's essential to delineate this from tapering a patient after long-term opioid therapy, which is permitted under federal law. It is therefore up to the practitioner to actively watch for symptoms of addiction and for proper referral of the patient to a proper detoxification clinic if warranted [9].

State Laws

Individual states have different laws for prescriptions of controlled substances. It is extremely important that before prescribing controlled substances, you are familiar with the laws in the state you will be prescribing. Some states have laws which may raise concerns by limiting the amounts of opioids that can be prescribed, requiring special government issues prescriptions, restricting access to patients in pain who have a history of substance abuse, and requiring that opioids be a treatment of last resort [10]. It is impractical in the scope of this chapter to discuss all of the laws of each state. In 1997, the Federation of State Medical Boards undertook an initiative to develop model guidelines to encourage state medical boards and other health-care agencies to adopt unified policies encouraging adequate treatment of pain. The *Model Guidelines for the Use of Controlled Substances for the Treatment of Pain* is now widely distributed and many agencies throughout the health-care world endorse its use.

The first section of the model describes a patient's right to obtain adequate and effective pain relief, which allows for improved quality of life, along with reduction of morbidity and the costs associated with insufficient treatment. Inadequate treatment may result from the physician's lack of knowledge about pain management, fears of investigation, or sanction. The FSMB considers inadequate treatment a departure from the standard of practice; if complaints are filed, it may result in formal investigations. This imparts the importance of a clinician maintaining current knowledge of pain management and treatment modalities. However, they should also remain current with the state and federal laws that pertain to the prescribing of controlled substances. The laws of the state aim to protect public health and safety since improper prescribing of controlled substances may lead to abuse. Accordingly, the FSMB expects physicians to place safeguards to help reduce this potential [2].

The second section gives a basic outline of how a physician should evaluate a patient's pain. The components are:

1. Evaluation of the patient – a thorough medical history and physical exam
2. Treatment plan
3. Informed consent and agreement for treatment
4. Periodic review
5. Consultation
6. Medical records
7. Compliance with controlled substances laws and regulations

Many physicians spend a great deal of time in medical school and residency learning how to accurately obtain a medical history and physical exam. This is the core of what makes us diagnosticians, and it is not surprising that this is an important component of evaluating a patient's pain. This can sometimes be difficult though because we can define in words how the patient's pain feels to them, but we can never truly understand how the pain is affecting them. In Responsible Opioid Prescribing, Dr. Fishman describes this as the physician's paradox, stating: "perhaps one reason that physicians are reluctant to aggressively treat pain has to do with the often frustrating fact that we can't prove that someone is in pain." Pain is an "untreatable hypothesis," and it can be quite difficult to measure a patient's pain, even in the twenty-first century where we have the ability to order complex medical tests and imaging [10]. The FSMB tries to ensure adequate documentation by requiring that the medical record contains the following: nature and intensity of the pain, current and past treatments for pain, underlying or coexisting disease or conditions, the effect of pain on the physical and psychological function, and a history of substance abuse. In addition, the physician should document the presence of one or more recognized indications for or against the use of a controlled substance [2].

A written treatment plan is the second requirement by the FSMB. This will outline objectives that can be used to determine if treatment is a success, i.e., whether the patient benefits from treatment as evidenced by improved physical and psychosocial function. It will also outline whether additional diagnostic evaluation is planned. They recommend that the physician adjust drug therapy to the individual patient and make use of other treatment modalities, such as physical therapy and psychiatric services, when warranted.

Informed consent and agreement for treatment is an essential component of a treatment plan. The FSMB requires that the physician discuss with the patient, or the patient's legal guardian, all of the risks and benefits of using controlled substances. The patient should understand that it is important to only receive controlled substances from one physician and if possible only one pharmacy. If the patient is considered a high risk for abuse, or to protect the patient-physician relationship, a written contract can be formed between the prescriber and patient, defining in writing guidelines what is expected in order to continue the treatment [2]. This type of contract can be called by many different names; most common are "patient agreements," "pain contracts," or "patient care contract." These contracts often stipulate that the patient has urine/serum medication levels when requested, protecting both the patient and prescriber. These contracts offer several advantages, including allowing the patient to participate in the decision-making process, serving as an informed consent, helping to remind the patient of the specific goals of treatment, and preventing any misunderstandings or distortions of understanding [10].

Periodic review of a patient's progress and symptom management during treatment is essential in order to document continued improvements in the patient's condition. The FSMB recommends the clinician to monitor the patient's response to treatment by determining how the pain has changed, both subjective and objective, if the patient has improved quality of life after treatment and if the treatment plan should be altered. The physician should be willing to consult with other clinicians if additional information is needed to adequately treat a specific patient with special attention being given to patients who are at increased risk for abuse or diversion.

Medical records have become an important component of a physician's daily activities, protecting the physician by outlining the thought process behind the treatments undertaken for a patient. The FSMB urges the physician to keep complete and accurate records, something that can be easily neglected in today's busy practice. They recommend having several vital components in your medical record:

1. A complete medical history and comprehensive physical exam
2. Diagnostic, therapeutic, and laboratory results
3. Evaluation and consultations
4. Treatment objectives
5. Discussion of risks and benefits
6. Informed consent
7. Treatments
8. Medications (including date, type, dosage, and quantity prescribed)
9. Instructions and agreements
10. Periodic review

Many states control a practitioner's ability to prescribe opioids for pain with each state being very different. It is essential to know your own states laws. The Texas Medical Practice Act states that physicians cannot prescribe opioids for any patient that has been known to be a habitual user of narcotic drugs. In New York, prescribers are required to report "addicts" to the Commissioner of Public health. In Rhode Island, a practitioner must report the name and ailment of any patient who is being treated with a schedule II substance for more than 3 months. New Jersey limits dispensing of schedule II substances to a 30-day prescription that should not be greater than 120 dosage units [2].

Fear of governmental action has been cited as a possible barrier to proper treatment of pain. A study of medical boards' actions against physicians who prescribe opioids for patients in pain found that the fear is exaggerated compared to the actual risk. In 2006, researchers studied DEA actions for the 2003–2004 year against physicians. They found that of the 963,385 physicians holding DEA licenses, 557 were investigated for possible criminal activity. Three hundred twenty-four physicians lost their DEA number, 116 had the investigation discontinued, and 43 physicians were arrested. A variety of violations resulted in arrest such as prescriptions in exchange for sex, money, and personal use; prescriptions written over the internet without proper medical examination; and prescriptions written without a proper DEA license [11]. These studies suggest that federal agencies do not typically investigate physicians who are prescribing controlled substances appropriately. Although 116 of the 557 investigations resulted in cessation of the investigation, it's unlikely that these physicians were investigated without cause. The small number of investigations resulting in no action proves that the agencies are not out to penalize physicians treating pain. A physician can likely avoid investigation by adhering to proper prescribing laws and keeping meticulous records regarding patients on opioid therapy.

It's worth mentioning again that the practitioner must abide by the more stringent laws, whether that be state or federal. Furthermore, it is the practitioner's responsibility to be familiar with laws at all levels before prescribing opioids.

Assessing the Risk for Abuse

How does a physician adequately screen for patients that may be at risk for addiction or drug abuse? This is certainly not an easy task, and no conclusive answers have come to light. It would go against all of our training and our oath to first do no harm if we assume that all patients will abuse the controlled substances we prescribe, and therefore we should not treat patient's pain adequately. Physicians should remain vigilant and maintain a modicum of suspicion. Often, this may force the prescriber to ask questions the patient may not want to answer. When prescribing controlled substances, it is always essential to determine if abuse is a possibility. Unfortunately, there have not been any conclusive studies allowing us to develop stringent guidelines on which patients are likely to abuse and divert prescribed medications; however, treating everyone with the same diagnostic tests and psychological screens may allow the physician to remain objective with every patient [10].

Guidelines allowing us to determine which patients receiving controlled substances are at risk for abuse are still in their infancy; however, there are certainly risk factors that place a patient at increased risk. Patients with a personal history of substance abuse or a family history of substance abuse are at a much higher risk of misusing the controlled substance they are prescribed compared with patients who do not have these histories. Furthermore, the risk for abuse is higher in younger patients, in those with a history of sexual abuse, mental disease, psychological stress, poor social support, and unclear cause of pain. Additionally, tobacco abuse increases the risk [12].

It seems the most important risk factor for misuse of a prescribed substance is a personal history of substance abuse. Individuals who abuse one substance are seven times more likely to abuse another substance. This makes perfect sense; however, the clinician may need to do some detective work to discover whether a patient has a substance abuse history, because often patients are not forthcoming with this information. This risk increases in patients who have recently abused illicit or licit drugs and may be the highest in those who have abused the prescription medication they are being prescribed. Ives et al. found patients with a history of alcohol, cocaine, or opioid misuse along with those convicted of a DUI or drug offense had a higher rate of abuse when prescribed opioids for chronic pain [13]. The second most important risk factor for abuse is a family history of abuse tendencies. This contributes to increased risk of abuse due to genetic factors that have yet to be elucidated, along with the social ramifications that surround having family members abusing substances. Family attitudes toward misuse of prescription medications can foster a liberal and tolerant environment [12].

Risk factors help determine which patients are in danger of abuse, allowing the clinician to place patients on a hierarchy of potential abuse: high risk, moderate risk, and lower risk of abuse. Depending on which rung the patient is placed will influence how the clinician assesses and monitors the patient.

Assessment through screening tools plays a very important role in determining if a patient is at risk for abusing prescription medications. Unless you are fortunate and have an addiction specialist as part of the pain management care team, a tool will be needed to evaluate patient's risk of abuse. This evaluation should be brief, have easily interpreted results, and must be validated in patients who are suffering from pain. Most screening tools are designed to find patients at risk for abuse, not diagnose substance abuse. If a patient is found to be at risk through the screening tools, they should have a formal evaluation with a professional trained in diagnosing substance abuse disorders. There are several different screening tools available; some are geared more toward alcohol abuse while others for illicit drugs. Likely the most useful in the clinic will be combined screens which allow the clinician to determine if the patient is at risk for substance abuse for a variety of drugs. A new generation of screening tools has recently been developed specifically tailored to determine if a patient is at risk for opioid misuses [12]. Of course, these tests are not perfect; no test designed thus far has 100 % sensitivity and specificity nor are they able to conclude if a patient is not being forthcoming. They do allow for screening and can help prevent abuse in those with high risk by allowing the clinician to monitor that group of patients more closely. It is important to stress that even if a patient is at high risk for abuse, that patient still has the right to obtain adequate treatment of his pain.

Monitoring patients treated with opioids for chronic pain conditions is a very important step in helping detect abuse during treatment. There are several different guides available, and deciding which to use is a personal preference. The American Academy of Pain Medicine and the American Pain Society set forth five recommended steps of opioid prescribing. The first step is a thorough patient evaluation which should occur at the initial patient visit. Subsequent visits do not need to be as extensive; however, the clinician should be reassessing the patients risk for abuse and how effective the prescribed medications are in treating the patient's pain. Every patient should have an individualized plan tailored to their needs and medical history. Often having the patient actively involved in formulating this plan will solidify what is expected from the relationship. The clinician should obtain consultations when deemed necessary. These can include but are not limited to consultation with psychologists, psychiatrists, physical therapists, and addiction specialists. Finally, appropriate documentation cannot be overemphasized [12]. In addition to the above-mentioned steps, drug screening may be an important tool in detecting abuse. Maintaining doctor-patient trust is important; however, research indicates that relying on a patient's word regarding drug abuse is unwise. Drug screening both for illicit substance use and levels of prescribed medications should be viewed as another diagnostic test similar to blood glucose levels in diabetics. Periodic testing may be used as a deterrent to inappropriate drug use, provide a way to monitor the patient's response to treatment by obtaining levels of prescribed medications, and allowing the clinician to support their medical decisions. At a minimum, clinicians should test patients at the beginning of their therapy and again if any question arises whether the patient could be abusing an illicit substance or misusing the prescribed medicine [12].

The clinician should be aware of pseudoaddiction, a syndrome of abnormal behavior that develops due to inadequate treatment of pain developing tolerance. The three characteristic phases of pseudoaddiction include inadequate treatment with analgesics to meet the primary pain stimuli, escalation of analgesic demands by the patient associated with behavioral changes to convince others of the pain's severity, and crisis of mistrust between the patient and health-care team. This can easily be confused with addictive behaviors and may lead the prescriber to conclude the patient is addicted, instead of in need of higher doses or stronger pain medications [11].

Treating Pain in Patients with Addiction

It is estimated that up to 20–25 % of hospitalized patients have an addictive disorder. Most hospitalized patients will require some form of opioid therapy during their admission, including those with an addictive disorder [3]. In addition, patients in a chronic pain clinic are thought to have addictive disorders with a frequency of around 15 %. These patients can be difficult to manage since the risk of further addiction and diversion is more likely. In 2009, the American Pain Society and American Academy of Pain Medicine formed clinical guidelines for chronic opioid therapy. They recommend a higher level of monitoring and care for high-risk patients: those with a history of drug abuse, psychiatric issues, or serious aberrant drug-related behaviors. These patients will need to have more frequent visits and strict monitoring parameters along with possible consultation with addiction specialists. Furthermore, constant reevaluation should occur to determine if the patient is benefiting from chronic opioid therapy. If drug aberrant behavior occurs, the physician may need to discontinue the opioid therapy completely [14].

Terminating a physician-patient relationship is something that may become necessary when a patient does not adhere to the contract put forth by the provider. No physician should tolerate deviant behavior. Instead, a "zero tolerance" policy should be instituted. It is important that the patient fully understands the reasons that they are being discharged from the practice, and it is advisable to do so in both verbal and written formats. You may want to consider having a witness in the face-to-face conversations. Abandonment must be avoided, and if a physician has no experience with termination of a patient, consultation with professionals such as a bioethics committee or a professional consultant (such as addiction specialists) may help guide them through the process [10].

Prescription Monitoring Programs

Multiple states are adopting prescription monitoring programs, or PMPs, as a way to further prevent diversion of controlled substances. With the advent of computer pharmacy systems and the transition from paper to electronic prescriptions gaining popularity, it has become easier to monitor controlled substance prescribing. The main purpose of PMPs is to reduce diversion. Its objectives typically include not only monitoring but also education, early intervention, and investigative/enforcement arms. It is the goal of a PMP to be as unobtrusive as possible and not hinder the patient-physician relationship. PMPs can benefit the physician immensely when there is a question about prescribing habits (is it of another physician or medication use of the patient? Please clarify), because they allow information to be quickly and efficiently obtained. Additionally, they allow handling of complaints and avoidance of unnecessary investigations [15].

It is important to discuss the legal implications of prescription monitoring programs. To be considered effective, a monitoring system must reduce the abuse of controlled substances, but it also must not interfere with patient privacy or legitimate prescription of controlled substances. Patients are free to obtain prescriptions from any physician and have those prescriptions filled at any pharmacy. Most of the time, physicians and pharmacies do not share the information on what prescriptions are being filled and by whom, which can allow for diversion to easily occur.

Generally, when a state develops a monitoring program, they implement legislation which mandates pharmacies report through electronic databases the dispensing of certain or all controlled substances. The information required to report may vary between states, but the patient's name, physician prescribing the medication, name of the controlled substance, dose, and number dispensed are typically obtained. Once the data is obtained, the agency will do evaluation of the data and determine if certain physicians, pharmacists, or patients are associated with excessive substance prescribing or use. This report also allows physicians and pharmacists to determine if their patients are obtaining medications from other sources [15]. When properly used, the PMPs do their job well; however, there are a few glitches that are still being worked out. One is the accuracy of the data obtained. Some pharmacies provide incomplete or inconsistent data of prescriptions. Furthermore, although infrequent, identity theft occurs in patients on chronic opioid therapy. Both of these inconsistencies could lead to unnecessary investigations. It is important for those involved in gathering and interpreting the data to be looking closely when a question arises about prescribing or obtaining those substances. It should be thoroughly investigated not through the PMP databases alone but uses all other sources available [16].

In 2007, the president signed into law the Food and Drug Administration Amendments Act of 2007 (FDAAA) which authorized the FDA to require pharmaceutical companies to submit proposed risk evaluation and mitigation strategies (REMS) for medications which would ensure the benefits of a drug outweigh the risks. This law applied to both new medications and those already in use. In 2009, the FDA formed a multidisciplinary opioid REMS steering committee which was tasked with reducing the "epidemic" of prescription drug abuse in the United States. The committee revamped education programs for patients taking opioids, while recommending pharmaceutical companies making these medications to be part of this education by distributing information that was written in "consumer friendly language." The FDA also focused on physician education through multiple programs. Additionally, expansion of state prescription monitoring programs and increasing law enforcement to reduce of the number of "pill mills" and doctor shopping was initiated to decrease the excessive amount of opioid medications reaching the public. In 2012, other risk reduction measures such as doctor training and patient counseling are expected to become part of the REMS. These will be required for various "high-risk" medications such as hydromorphone, oxycodone, morphine, methadone, transdermal fentanyl, and oxymorphone [17].

Conclusion

Treatment of pain, both acute and chronic, is a vital part of any physician's practice. There are millions of patients who suffer from pain without getting appropriate treatment. However, the medications we use for this treatment can be fraught with problems such as abuse and addiction. It's important that any physician prescribing these medications distinguish between the signs of addiction and the treatments. Furthermore, a thorough understanding of both the federal and state laws is paramount to proper prescribing.

References

1. Brownstein MJ. A brief history of opiates, opioid peptides, and opioid receptors. Proc Natl Acad Sci. 1993;90:5391–3.
2. Shapiro RS. Legal basis for the control of analgesic drugs. J Pain Symptom Manage. 1994;9(3):153–9.
3. Savage SR, Covington EC, Joranson DE, Heit H, Gilson A. Definitions related to the medical use of opioids: evolution towards universal agreement. J Pain Symptom Manage. 2003;26(1):655–67.
4. Manchikanti L. Prescription drug abuse: what is being done to address this new drug epidemic? Testimony before the subcommittee on criminal justice, drug policy and human resources. Pain Physician. 2006;9(4):287–321.
5. Paulozzi LJ, Budnitz D, Xi Y. Increasing deaths from opioid analgesics in the United States. Pharmacoepidemiol Drug Saf. 2006;15:618–27.
6. Relieving pain in America: a blueprint for transforming prevention, care, education, and research. Washington, DC: National Academies; 2011.
7. Rannazzisi JT, Caverly MW. Practitioner's manual: an informational outline of the controlled substances act. Drug Enforcement Agency. 2006.
8. Publications – don't be scammed by a drug abuser. DEA diversion control program: welcome. 2010. http://www.deadiversion.usdoj.gov/pubs/brochures/drugabuser.htm. 24 Feb. 2010.

9. Clark W, Sees K. Opioids, chronic pain, and the law. J Pain Symptom Manage. 1993;8(5):297–305.
10. Fishman S. Responsible opioid prescribing: a physician's guide. Washington, DC: Waterford Life Sciences; 2009.
11. Jung B, Reidenberg M. The risk of action by the drug enforcement administration against physicians prescribing opioids for pain. Pain Med. 2006;7(4):353–7.
12. Webster LR, Dove B. Avoiding opioid abuse while managing pain: a guide for practitioners. North Branch: Sunrise River; 2007.
13. Ives TJ, Chelminski PR, Hammett-Stabler CA, Malone RM, Perhac SJ, Potisek NM, Shilliday BB, DeWalt DA, Pignone MP. Predictors of opioid misuse in patients with chronic pain: a prospective cohort study. BMC Health Serv Res. 2006;6:46.
14. Chou R, Fanciullo GJ, Fine PG, Adler JA, Ballantyne JC, Davies P, Donovan MI, Fishbain DA, Foley KM, Fundin J, Gilson AM, Kelter A, Mauskop A, O'Connor PG, Passik SD, Pasternak GW, Portenoy RK, Rich BA, Roberts RG, Todd KH, Miaskowski C. Clinical guidelines for the use of chronic opioid therapy in chronic noncancer pain. J Pain. 2009;10(2):113–30.
15. Joranson DE, Carrow GM, Ryan KM, Schaefer L, Gilson AM, Good P, Eadie J, Peine S, Dahl JL. Pain management and prescription monitoring. J Pain Symptom Manage. 2002;23(3):231–8.
16. Brushwood DB. Maximizing the value of electronic prescription monitoring programs. J Law Med Ethics. 2003;31:41–54.
17. FDA Acts to Reduce Harm from Opioid Drugs. U S food and drug administration home page. 2011. http://www.fda.gov/ForConsumers/ConsumerUpdates/ucm251830.htm. N.p., 1 Apr 2011. 27 May 2011.

Methadone for Chronic Pain

Naileshni Singh, Scott M. Fishman, and Kyle Tokarz

Key Points

- Methadone has pharmacological properties that make it unique among opioids including agonist action at mu and delta opioid receptors and antagonist action at NMDA receptors.
- Methadone's lipid solubility, long elimination half-life, high protein binding, and metabolism by the hepatic P450 system make predicting its pharmacokinetics difficult.
- Methadone has known efficacy for a variety of pain syndromes and clinical settings; however, its unstable metabolism, difficulty in predicting equianalgesic dosing, and other adverse effects raise its risk potential and mitigate its usefulness.
- Clinicians prescribing methadone must become familiar with its unique pharmacology and risk profile, including cardiac toxicity and data on rising rates of methadone-related deaths, in order to responsibly weigh risks and benefits of methadone before prescribing.

N. Singh, M.D. (✉)
Department of Anesthesiology, UC-Davis Medical Center,
4860 Y Street, Suite 3020, Sacramento, CA 95817, USA

University of California, Davis School of Medicine,
Sacramento, CA, USA
e-mail: naileshni.singh@ucdmc.ucdavis.edu

S.M. Fishman, M.D.
Division of Pain Medicine,
Department of Anesthesiology and Pain Medicine,
University of California, Davis School of Medicine,
4860 Y Street, Suite 3020, Sacramento, CA 95817, USA
e-mail: smfishman@ucdavis.edu

K. Tokarz, DO
Department of Anesthesiology, Naval Medical Center, San Diego,
2736 West Canyon Ave, San Diego, CA 92123, USA
e-mail: kyle.tokarz@med.navy.mil

Introduction

Methadone use for pain relief has surged over the past two decades. In this time, its special pharmacology has been elucidated which has led to speculation about special properties as well as far greater risks than with other opioid medications. Recently, increasing reports of methadone-related unintended deaths have spurred greater concern about this unique drug. Methadone has many advantages that are now well opposed by many posing serious risks for patients in pain. Advantages include cost, ease of use, and multiple opioid and non-opioid receptor actions. However, risks include metabolic instability related to unique P450 system hepatic clearance that poses drug-drug interactions that differ from other opioids, high protein binding, variable urine clearance, and the potential for cardiac arrhythmia. Thus, this drug that saw a renaissance over the past two decades has now been revealed as more dangerous than previously thought and widely noted to require heightened knowledge and risk management for safe use.

Pharmacology

Methadone, chemically known as 6-dimethylamino-4,4-diphenyl-3-heptanone, is an opioid commonly used in a variety of clinical settings (Fig. 14.1). The pharmacokinetics and unique receptor profile make it distinct from the other commonly used opioids such as morphine or hydromorphone. Methadone was originally created in 1938 in Germany as an alternative to morphine. Following World War II, the drug was manufactured in the United States, but its potential for analgesia was not well appreciated. The first use for methadone was for maintenance of heroin and opioid addiction during the 1950s as a once per day therapy. The use of methadone increased within the last several decades among many medical specialties including primary care and oncology. Also known as Dolophine or Methadose, methadone is now one of the most commonly used opioid analgesic therapies in the United States.

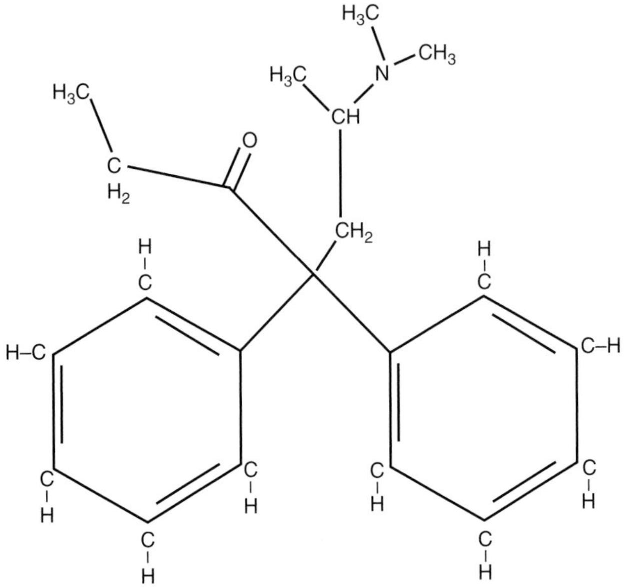

Fig. 14.1 Molecular structure of methadone

Methadone's activity at opioid sub-receptors is unique. Like morphine, methadone has agonist affinity for both the mu and delta opioid receptors. However, in animal studies, methadone has proportionately less mu receptor binding than morphine which may explain its more tolerable side effect profile. It is theorized that when compared to morphine which sensitizes the mu receptor, methadone's pharmacology may desensitize the mu receptor. This, coupled with affinity for the delta mu receptor, may lead some to use methadone to prevent dependence and tolerance. In comparison to other opioids, methadone has action on the serotoninergic and NMDA receptors. Animal and in vitro studies of the NMDA receptor suggest its possible role in neuropathic pain, as well as in tolerance and dependence of opioids. Theoretically, methadone's NMDA antagonist properties may make it better suited than other opioids for neuropathic pain syndromes. How the reuptake inhibition of serotonin and norepinephrine impacts its analgesic effects is currently unclear. Norepinephrine reuptake inhibition has specifically been a target for analgesic drug design in recent years. A medication with a broad ensemble of receptor affinities may have many medical uses. However, rising concerns about potential adverse effects may substantially temper such views.

Methadone has a basic pH and is available as a racemic mixture of enantiomers with different pharmacokinetic properties. The enantiomers, S-methadone (D-isomer) and R-methadone (L-isomer), can be reconstituted from a powder form into oral, rectal, intramuscular, and parenteral formulations. R-methadone acts largely at the mu opioid receptor site, while S-methadone antagonizes the NMDA receptor and inhibits the reuptake of 5-hydroxytryptamine (serotonin) and norepinephrine. The R isomer is thought to be less cardiotoxic compared to the racemic mixture. The potency of the R enantiomer at the mu opioid receptor is also greater than the S enantiomer.

Methadone has unique pharmacokinetic properties within the opioid class. The drug's high lipophilicity causes it to be stored in fat and released slowly into the plasma to reach a steady state. Elderly people who have higher body fat content may accumulate higher methadone doses and need less frequent dosing. In addition, methadone has a large volume of distribution, ranging from 1.71 to 5.34 l/kg in chronic pain patients and even higher in those with opioid addiction. Methadone is 80 to 90 % protein bound which has repercussions for its duration of action and circulating blood levels. The main binding protein is alpha-1-acid glycoprotein (AAG), an acute phase reactant whose levels can differ in disease states [1]. This fluctuation can predispose to serious variability of circulating methadone levels.

The oral bioavailability of methadone is high, ranging from 40 to 99 %, but is dependent on intestinal transporters. For the oral formulation, time to peak concentration is 2.5 to 4 hours, with a terminal half-life between 24 to 60 hours. The half-life is related to the chronicity of administration with the lower range in chronic methadone therapy versus the upper range in acute dosing. Oral absorption further depends on gastric pH and motility. Rectal bioavailability is similar to parenteral bioavailability with a quick onset of action within 15 to 45 minutes. Methadone, given rectally, is rapidly absorbed through mucosa and has duration of action of up to 10 h. Methadone's plasma concentrations by the intramuscular route will depend on the site of the injection. For example, when compared to administration in the gluteal region, the deltoid muscle offers an increase in peak plasma concentration and improved pain control. Methadone may be used subcutaneously or absorbed through the buccal mucosa due to high lipid solubility.

Methadone's metabolism is largely dependent on the hepatic metabolism. It undergoes N-demethylation in the liver by the P450 CYP enzymes to 2-ethyl-1,5-dimethyl-3,3-diphenylpyrrolinium (EDDP). The main metabolizers are thought to be CYP3A4, CYP2B6, and CYP2C19, while the CYP2B6 enzyme primarily generates EDDP. Other lesser CYP enzymes have varying roles in methadone's metabolism, but of note, certain enzymes may preferentially metabolize the S versus the R enantiomer. Further complicating metabolism is the fact that the type I CYP enzyme system exhibits genetic and ethnic variability in expression, which affects methadone's duration of action between individuals and groups. CYP3A4 is itself unique in being an autoinducible enzyme which brings about methadone's own metabolism over time.

The P450 system can be affected by induction or inhibition by a variety of substrates that are common and medically important. For example, various medications in the treatment of HIV such as ritonavir may prolong methadone action by inhibition of the CYP3A4 and CYP2B6 systems. Many antiepileptic, antibiotic, and antidepressant medications taken concomitantly can influence methadone levels by either inhibition or induction of enzymes. Drug-drug interactions with methadone may make management of complex patients on polypharmacy regimens challenging. In addition, pregnancy does not relate to a state of high gastric pH, elevated AAG; and urine pH < 6.0 can cause methadone to be metabolized faster or decrease its levels. Opioid transporters in the blood-brain barrier also regulate the access of methadone to sites of action. These variables make predicting methadone metabolism and subsequent blood plasma levels difficult.

Methadone use in pregnancy is not uncommon as it has long been recommended for substance abuse treatment and withdrawal prevention. Parturients have a decrease in half-life and an increase in clearance of methadone. Fetuses born to mothers on chronic methadone therapy should be assessed for respiratory depression even though placental transfer and breast milk exposure are thought to be low. Fetal abstinence syndrome has been described in newborns of mothers who were on methadone maintenance therapy. Infant mortality is higher in babies exposed to methadone in utero than for the general parturient population [2]. Methadone has been shown to prolong the QTc interval in human newborns. In addition, the use of opioids in early stages of pregnancy has been linked to birth defects of the cardiovascular system [3].

Methadone is often used in patients with complex medical problems for whom it seems to have certain advantages. The lack of active metabolites is one aspect of methadone's pharmacology that may make it beneficial in some frail patients. Use of methadone in liver disease has been described sparingly. Theoretically, methadone can accumulate in disease states that alter metabolism by the hepatic cytochrome P450 system. Patients in methadone maintenance treatment programs often have a history of intravenous drug use and subsequent chronic hepatitis. Regardless, methadone has been successfully used in patients with chronic hepatitis and cirrhosis.

Elimination of methadone is biphasic, following both an alpha (8 to 12 h) and beta (30 to 60 h) phase (Fig. 14.2). The alpha phase typically corresponds to the analgesic period that is far shorter than the terminal half-life. This alpha phase correlates with the analgesic phase and serves as the rational for 3–4 times a day dosing in chronic pain. The long beta phase prevents withdrawal symptoms but provides for little analgesia. This slow clearance allows for once a day dosing in maintenance therapy programs but dictates careful upward titration [4]. The use of methadone as a breakthrough medication is limited due to the long elimination phase and terminal half-life. Methadone taken in repetitive doses to achieve euphoric effects will often cause accumulation of the drug

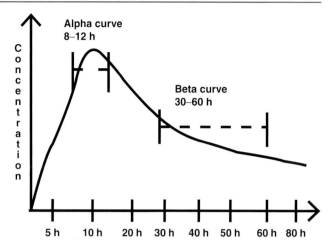

Fig. 14.2 Elimination curve for methadone depicting alpha (8 to 12 h) and beta phase (30 to 60 h)

resulting in subsequent adverse events due to long-lasting pharmacokinetics.

Methadone elimination is largely fecal with some contribution from the renal system. For this reason, it is largely safe for use in renal failure and is insignificantly dialyzed due to high lipid solubility. Patients with renal failure will excrete a vast majority of methadone in the feces. Acidic urine, with a pH < 6, causes more excretion of the unionized total methadone dose. While medications that may alkanize the urine allow methadone to accumulate. Methadone, however, has no neurotoxic metabolites that may accumulate in kidney disease as compared to morphine. This theoretically makes methadone a more tolerable medication in patients with a low glomerular filtration rate.

Clinical Issues

Side effects of methadone are not unlike those of shorter-acting opioids. There is still a serious risk of respiratory depression, sedation, constipation, and pruritis. Many studies attest to methadone having a comparable rate of side effects when compared to morphine. But unique to methadone is the tendency to prolong the QT interval corrected (QTc) for heart rate and predisposition to tachyarrhythmias such as ventricular fibrillation and torsades de pointes. Arrhythmias were originally described in the methadone maintenance population who were presenting with sudden death within weeks of starting the program or after dose escalation. Structural heart disease is often not found among these decedents. The mechanism is thought to be blockade of the cardiac ether-a-go-go-related gene (hERG) coding potassium channel that prevents repolarization during phase III of the cardiac action potential. This channel is the delayed rectifier potassium ion (Ikr) whose blockade causes bradycardia and predisposes to

Table 14.1 ACP recommendations for methadone use and QTc interval screening

Recommendation 1: Disclosure	Clinicians should inform patients of arrhythmia risk
Recommendation 2: history	Clinicians should ask patients about a history of cardiac disease
Recommendation 3: Screening	Obtain a baseline EKG to measure the QTc interval and a follow up 30 days after starting treatment, and then annually
Recommendation 4: Risk stratification	If the QTc interval is greater than 450 ms, then discuss risks of treatment with patients. If the QTc > 500 ms, consider stopping treatment
Recommendation 5: Drug Interactions	Be aware of methadone's interactions with other drugs that may encourage QTc prolongation or methadone accumulation

Adapted from the American College of Physician (2009) [7]

torsades [5]. Methadone, like other opioids, is a negative chronotrope which further slows the heart rate. Several risk factors have been identified for prolongation of the QTc in methadone patients including high dose, concomitant use of other QTc prolonging medications, antidepressants, antibiotics, electrolyte disturbances, congenital long QTc syndrome, structural heart disease, liver or renal disease, and alcohol and benzodiazepine use. Chronic pain patients may be on a variety of medicines that are otherwise potentially cardiotoxic such as tricyclic antidepressants, which theoretically may offer additive toxicity.

How tissue or blood concentrations of methadone exactly cause sudden cardiac death remains unclear. Prolongation of the QTc interval has been seen in patients on low-dose methadone. Unfortunately, in deaths related to methadone, serum blood levels have overlapped those of deaths that were not attributed to methadone, illustrating that a lethal level is difficult to determine [6]. This confusing interaction may be related to methadone's variable pharmacokinetics and the fact that blood concentrations are poor indicators of the potential for toxicity. Several medical organizations such as the American College of Physicians (ACP) recommend discussion of the risks with patients and baseline electrocardiograms prior to treatment initiation. Per ACP recommendations, patients with borderline QTc intervals between 450 and 500 ms should have frequent electrocardiograms during methadone treatment [7]. Cessation of treatment should be considered in patients with QTc intervals greater than 500 ms (Table 14.1). Other authors do not recommend frequent EKGs but do argue for vigilance on the part of the prescribing physician.

In 2006, the Federal Drug Administration issued a warning regarding methadone's potential for prolongation of the QTc interval along with modified dosage instructions. This resulted in a 2006 manufacturer's black box warning regarding the possibility for fatal cardiac arrhythmias. The warning included starting opioid-naïve patients on 2.5 to 10 mg every 8 to 12 h for a maximum daily dose of 30 mg/day. Many patients on methadone therapy are on substantially more medication than recommended with these guidelines.

Respiratory depression in a patient population with a high incidence of sleep apnea is another concerning issue when prescribing medications such as methadone. The rate of sleep apnea is high in methadone maintenance programs, while the overall prevalence is elevated in chronic pain patients. Opioids in general may worsen both obstructive and central sleep apnea by acting on central opioid receptors in the medulla and hypothalamus that regulate breathing and sleep. The dose of opioid agonists and their actions on hypoxic and hypercapnic respiratory drive is another contributing factor. NMDA receptors may also play a key role in multiple areas of the sleep regulatory centers. Combining methadone with other respiratory depressants, such as benzodiazepines, may synergistically contribute to morbidity and even unintended deaths in such a high-risk population. Multiple studies have identified benzodiazepines and other sedating medications in patients who died while on methadone therapy. Whether this is related to sleep apnea, respiratory depression, or cardiac toxicity or as a combination of all three factors or other factors is unknown.

As the popularity of methadone has increased in recent years, so has methadone-related adverse events. Prescribing of methadone increased by almost 400 %, from 1997 to 2002 in the United States [8]. Methadone has become an attractive alternative to other opioids due to the perception that it has low addiction potential combined with its relatively low cost. Increased attention to early and aggressive treatment of cancer pain and increased use of long-acting opioids in patients with noncancer-related pain has likely contributed to escalated prescribing. Due to this methadone has since added to the national epidemic of prescription opioid abuse, misuse, diversion, and addiction. By 2006, the Research Abuse, Diversion and Addiction-Related Surveillance (RADARS) noted methadone to be the second most abused or misused opioid in the United States. Of concern is methadone's particular side effect profile and prolonged duration of action.

Methadone-related deaths have been analyzed in a variety of patient populations to ascertain cause. The National Vital Statistics System (of the United States) noted a 16 % increase in methadone-related deaths between 1999 and 2005, especially among those aged 35 to 54 years old. Of all prescribed opioids and illegal drugs, methadone has had the highest rate of increase in related deaths in recent years. For example, between 2001 and 2006, the state of Florida reported more methadone-related deaths than heroin, and West Virginia saw an increase in unintended overdose deaths during 2007, even in those with valid methadone prescriptions. The U.S. Centers for Disease Control and Prevention (CDC) issued a warning that methadone is implicated in nearly 33% of all prescription opioid deaths [11]. Causes of death in methadone-related scenarios are difficult to assess as many were also taking concomitant drugs, such as illicit substances or benzodiazepines, that could increase the risk of fatal adverse events.

Despite the stated risks, methadone use is widespread. Methadone is often a second- or third-line opioid for chronic pain syndromes in which side effects of other opioids therapies cannot be tolerated or when a less expensive medication is desired. In many settings, methadone has been shown to be as efficacious as long-acting morphine or fentanyl transdermal systems [9]. Additionally, methadone has been used successfully in a variety of pain syndromes including neuropathic and cancer-related pain. Along with oral administration, methadone has been effectively used in patient-controlled analgesia (PCA) delivery systems. Rarely, the medication may be added to intrathecal therapy or used in the IV formulation for intractable pain or intraoperative use. Methadone's high oral availability may be useful in those with "short gut" or "dumping syndrome" who have impaired absorption of medications that depend on the gastrointestinal track. Patients with gastrostomy tubes may benefit from the elixir formulation, while those who are NPO may access the drug through rectal or intramuscular routes. The multiple available formulations and routes of delivery make methadone ideal for end-of-life patients who may have difficulty swallowing or poor intravenous access. Crushing of methadone tablets does not produce a shorter-acting agent, so the potential for abuse from this particular action is theoretically low. Nonetheless, methadone is abused.

Rotation to methadone from another opioid-based therapy can be complicated. Reports of equianalgesic dosing conversion ratios are inconsistent, but typically there is greater potency when patients are being switched from higher dose regimens of other opioids to methadone. Essentially, the more opioid an individual is exposed to prior to starting methadone, the more potent methadone is, mg/mg. For example, studies have recommended ratios between 1 and 4:1 for doses of oral morphine equivalents of less than 100 mg/day, 5:1 for doses greater than 500 mg/day, and up to 20:1 for doses greater than 1,000 mg/day. Conversion from methadone to morphine is equally as challenging; reported ratios have been up to methadone 1:10 of morphine [10]. The wide variation is thought to be related to individual differences in metabolism, pharmacokinetics, and cross tolerance between opioids. Many now consider methadone conversion to be so inexact as to recommend that practitioners start at the lowest dose and slowly titrate upwards to the effective dose. If the traditional rule of five half-lives is followed, then titration would be no faster than every 5 to 7 days.

Since methadone was initially used for the treatment of addiction, remnants of stigma surrounding its use for chronic or cancer-related pain may remain. Patients may be wary of being on a medication associated with drug addiction. Although practitioners from a variety of medical fields prescribe methadone, rarely is it a first choice medication and many physicians remain hesitant. Recent methadone-related deaths and the emergence of buprenorphine as an alternative long-acting opioid may also deter prescribing among physicians.

The cost of methadone is often substantially less compared to other common opioid therapies. The pharmacoeconomic benefit may be another reason to prescribe methadone over other medications and treatments. The drug is usually far less expensive than other opioids formulations. It should be noted that different formulations may have varying costs. For example, the liquid form is more expensive than the oral form. The oral formulation however remains the commonest form of methadone used often providing for a relative financial advantage.

Conclusions

Although methadone remains an effective analgesia, new information about its adverse event profile must give prescribers pause in evaluating the risk benefit ratio. QTc prolongation is one particular risk that must be kept in mind along with other adverse events such as respiratory depression. Other prescribed and nonprescribed medications, alcohol, and illicit substances concomitantly taken while on methadone therapy may be a confounding factor in assessing risk. Methadone continues to be a compelling choice for some clinicians due to its comparable efficacy to other opioids, attractive multiple pharmacologic actions, low cost, lack of active metabolites, and multiple available formulations. However, the growing body of evidence supporting much greater risks associated with methadone than previously appreciated should temper enthusiasm and heighten risk management required in using methadone for pain. Moreover, clinicians who choose to prescribe methadone must become familiar with its special properties and adverse effects and possess the risk management skills necessary for its safe use.

References

1. Fredheim OM, Moksnes K, Borchgrevink PC, Kaasa S, Dale O. Clinical pharmacology of methadone for pain. Acta Anaesthesiol Scand. 2008;52(7):879–89.
2. Burns L, Conroy E, Mattick RP. Infant mortality among women on a methadone program during pregnancy. Drug Alcohol Rev. 2010;29(5):551–6.
3. Broussard CS, Rasmussen SA, Reefhuis J, et al. Maternal treatment with opioid analgesics and risk for birth defects. Am J Obstet Gynecol. 2011;204(4):314.e1–11.
4. Fishman SM, Wilsey B, Mahajan G, Molina P. Methadone reincarnated: novel clinical applications with related concerns. Pain Med. 2002;3(4):339–48.

5. George S, Moreira K, Fapohunda M. Methadone and the heart: what the clinician needs to know. Curr Drug Abuse Rev. 2008;1(3): 297–302.

6. Gagajewski A, Apple FS. Methadone-related deaths in Hennepin county, Minnesota: 1992–2002. J Forensic Sci. 2003;48(3): 668–71.

7. Krantz MJ, Martin J, Stimmel B, Mehta D, Haigney MC. QTc interval screening in methadone treatment. Ann Intern Med. 2009; 150(6):387–95.

8. Paulozzi LJ, Ryan GW. Opioid analgesics and rates of fatal drug poisoning in the United States. Am J Prev Med. 2006;31(6): 506–11.

9. Mercadante S, Porzio G, Ferrera P, et al. Sustained-release oral morphine versus transdermal fentanyl and oral methadone in cancer pain management. Eur J Pain. 2008;12(8):1040–6.

10. Weschules DJ, Bain KT. A systematic review of opioid conversion ratios used with methadone for the treatment of pain. Pain Med. 2008;9(5):595–612.

11. Center for Disease Control & Prevention Prescription Painkiller Overdoses: Methadone. 2012. http://www.cdc.gov/Features/VitalSigns/ MethadoneOverdoses/index.html

Toxicology Screening for Opioids

15

Gary L. Horowitz

Key Points
- Screening immunoassays for opiates generate clinically significant false-negative and false-positive results.
- Urine is the specimen of choice for detecting opioids: concentrations are much higher, and opioids can be detected for much longer.
- The patterns and relative concentrations of opioids detected have clinical significance.

Introduction

Monitoring compliance in the field of pain medicine is critically important. The medications that are used are powerful, and the potential for abuse is high. Some patients do not take the prescribed medications in favor of diversion or trafficking [1, 2], and some patients may abuse opioids other than those prescribed. Further complicating matters is that laboratory testing for opioids, though it seems straightforward, can be confusing. Physicians rarely receive adequate training in test ordering and interpretation. Laboratory methods vary tremendously; in addition, laboratorians are rarely consulted and, when they are, may be ill-equipped to answer clinically important questions.

Among the issues covered in this chapter will be the clinical importance of the methods used to detect opioids, the reasons that urine is the preferred sample type, and some of the subtleties related to opioid concentrations and metabolites.

G.L. Horowitz, M.D.
Department of Pathology, Beth Israel Deaconess Medical Center, 330 Brookline Avenue, Boston, MA 02215, USA

Harvard Medical School,
Boston, MA, USA
e-mail: ghorowit@bidmc.harvard.edu

Background

The first question that confronts physicians when contemplating monitoring opioid compliance is what tests to order. Most clinical laboratories offer an "opiate screening assay," but it is often not clear which drugs such screens detect and which drugs they fail to detect. It would be logical, but wrong, to conclude that such screening methods detect all opioids; indeed, very few, if any, can detect all opioids [3]. Furthermore, even if a screening assay is positive, one cannot tell, from the screening assay alone, which opioid was detected, resulting in potentially very misleading, and unfortunate, consequences.

Screening methods were developed principally to help evaluate emergency room patients quickly in order to implement appropriate clinical care rapidly [4]. Traditional analytical methods require combinations of chromatography and mass spectroscopy to generate definitive results. Only specialized laboratories are able to offer such testing, and it often takes several hours to complete an analysis. A major advantage of these methods, though, is that they allow for the identification, and quantitation, of individual drugs (and, frequently, their metabolites).

In contrast, screening immunoassays can be performed by virtually any laboratory, from a physician's office laboratory to a community hospital to an academic medical center. They can be run by ordinary laboratory technologists, on conventional automated equipment used for other routine chemistry tests (such as glucose, creatinine, CK, ALT), and cost remarkably little to perform. When analyses of their clinical performance in the emergency department are compiled, screening immunoassays stand up quite well [5].

Nonetheless, applied to the field of pain medicine, as they so often are, a different picture emerges. In the emergency room, the physician may not care whether a patient is taking morphine versus hydromorphone; he simply needs to know whether there are opioids in the patient's system. For a pain medicine physician, though, the distinction is critical. If she has prescribed hydromorphone, she wants to know whether

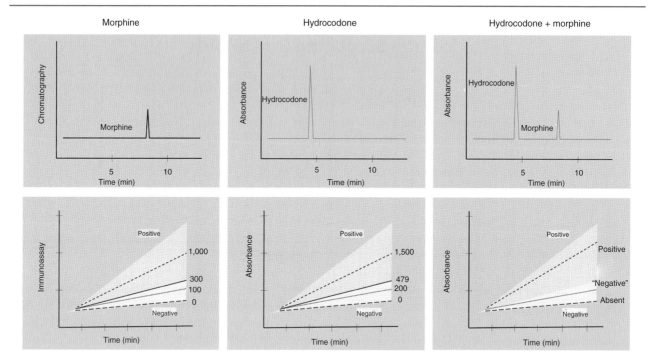

Fig. 15.1 In the top row, the three schematics for gas chromatography show that samples containing morphine, hydrocodone, and a combination of the two can be distinguished from one another because the time it takes the compounds to elute from the system differ. In contrast, in the bottom row, the three schematics show that an immunoassay cannot distinguish among these samples. In each case, the region shaded more darkly represents a positive result; the region shaded less darkly, a negative result. In the leftmost figure, a sample with a mor-phine concentration of 300 ng/mL is right at the threshold for a positive result; a sample with a morphine concentration of 1000 ng/ml, positive. In the middle figure, because of hydrocodone's reduced cross-reactivity, a hydrocodone concentration of 479 ng/mL is reguired to reach the positive thresold for the assay. In the right-hand figure, a sample containing both drugs would test positive, but one cannot know whether it represents only morphine, only hydrocodone, or a combination of the two

hydromorphone is present, but she also would like to know if any other opioids are present. With screening immunoassays, one can only say that an opioid is (probably) present. (As we will see later, one cannot be 100 % sure until the result is confirmed by another method based on a different principle.)

In other words, for pain management, screening immunoassays are not sufficient. They can be used, but one needs to ensure that they will detect all the drugs of interest, at relevant concentrations, and that all positive results will be confirmed by a second method.

Scientific Foundation

Methods: Screening Versus Gas Chromatography/Mass Spectroscopy

With chromatographic methods (most commonly, gas chromatography), individual drugs are typically identified by their "retention time," the time it takes them to travel through the system [6]. As reflected in Fig. 15.1, individual opioid drugs each elute from the system at characteristic times. Thus, hydrocodone and morphine elute at roughly 4

and 8 min, respectively. However, it is possible that another drug (or indeed substance of any kind), totally unrelated to hydrocodone (or morphine), could be present in the peak at 4 (or 8) min.

To be absolutely sure that another compound has not "co-eluted" at a given time, the compound(s) eluting at each time is (are) subjected to a second analysis, typically mass spectroscopy. In this technique, each compound presumptively identified by its retention time is ionized, and the resulting fragments, characteristic for the compound, are identified by their mass/charge ratios [7]. A typical mass spectrum for morphine is depicted in Fig. 15.2. If a compound other than morphine eluted at the same time by gas chromatography, it would have an entirely different mass spectrum.

Based on the retention time as well as the mass spectrum, the drug's identity can be assured. As will be seen in the examples later, this is a fundamental principle in clinical toxicology – one must identify each compound by two methods, each of which is based on a distinct analytical principle. It is possible that other compounds could co-elute and/or that other compounds might have the same (or similar) fragmentation patterns, but it is virtually impossible that another molecule would share both characteristics. These

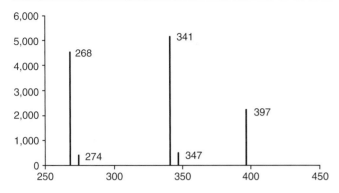

Fig. 15.2 Mass spectrum for morphine. After ionization, morphine is broken down into characteristic fragments, whose relative abundances are plotted against their mass/charge ratios. In this assay, the fragment with a mass/charge ratio of 341 is most abundant, followed by fragments with ratios of 268 and then 397; fragments with ratios of 274 and 347 are much less common. The pattern is unique for morphine

methods are the gold standards for identification, but they both are labor-intensive, demand significant expertise, and require expensive capital equipment.

It is relatively straightforward for the laboratory to determine whether its method can detect a given drug and the smallest concentration it can reliably detect. Thus, the laboratory should be able to provide its users with this data relatively easily. In addition, the laboratory should indicate which drugs are not in its repertoire, and it presumably would be able to offer advice on alternative ways to detect them. The laboratory report should explicitly indicate every individual drug for which the sample was tested, along with the detection limit. Thus, if the "opioid panel" does not explicitly indicate that testing for methadone (or tramadol, or buprenorphine, or fentanyl) was done, then the correct inference is that the test was not done. In most cases, none of these drugs is part of a typical opioid panel [8]. Too often, physicians infer that if a drug is not specifically mentioned, then it was not present.

As noted earlier, opiate screening immunoassays (which include techniques such as EMIT [9], FPIA [10], KIMS [11], CEDIA [12], etc.) can be, and are, performed by virtually any clinical laboratory, often in connection with an emergency toxicology program. Space does not permit a discussion of all the different methods here, but it may help to describe one method, one that is familiar to the author. The salient clinical performance characteristics are very similar for other methods.

In the EMIT assay [13], a small aliquot of a patient's sample is added to a cuvette in which an antibody and an enzyme-labeled drug are present. The drug from the patient and the enzyme-labeled drug compete for the limited sites on the antibody molecules. When the enzyme-labeled drug molecule binds to the antibody, the enzyme activity is inhibited. The more drug present in the patient sample, the less of the enzyme-labeled drug is bound to the antibody (i.e., this is a competitive immunoassay), and therefore, the more enzyme activity remains in the cuvette [14]. Substrate for the enzyme is added, and the enzyme activity is measured spectrophotometrically as the slope of the line relating absorbance to time, as depicted in Fig. 15.1. If the slope of the line is greater than that of the calibrator (in this case, 300 ng/mL morphine), the result is considered positive; if it is lower, then the result is negative.

As shown in Fig. 15.1, though, the enzyme activity for hydrocodone and the enzyme activity for morphine cannot be distinguished from each other. Each drug with which the antibody reacts will cause an increase in enzyme activity, but it is the same enzyme, and therefore there is nothing unique about the reaction. Thus, one cannot tell from this test which drug is present. In addition, one cannot know if there is one drug, or more than one drug, present. Moreover, one cannot know how much of any given drug is present because the cross-reactivities of the antibody with each drug are not 100 % (see later). In contrast to the case with gas chromatography (even when it is not paired with mass spectroscopy), then, one cannot determine from opiate screening immunoassays which opioids are present nor how much of any drug is present. As a result, it is important, at least in the field of pain management, that positive screening immunoassays be subjected to further analysis to identify which opioids are present.

Another important limitation of opiate screening immunoassays is that a number of important opioids are not detected. Although each assay has its own characteristics, opioids typically not detected include methadone, meperidine, oxycodone, tramadol, buprenorphine, and fentanyl [7]. At this point, it might be worthwhile pointing out that, although people tend to use the terms "opiate" and "opioid" interchangeably, there is a distinction. "Opioids" is the term used to describe all drugs with morphine-like actions; "opiates" are those opioids derived from opium, a group that includes morphine and codeine. Thus, it is perhaps not coincidental that the screening immunoassays are referred to as "opiate immunoassays" rather than "opioid immunoassays"; they are particularly adept at detecting the drugs with structures similar to morphine (see later) [15, 16].

Figure 15.3 provides a flow chart suggesting one way to utilize screening immunoassays effectively in connection with pain management programs; the flow chart needs to be customized to the specific assays available from each laboratory.

Specimen of Choice

Physicians often wonder why laboratories prefer to do opioid measurements on urine, a preference that gives rise to other

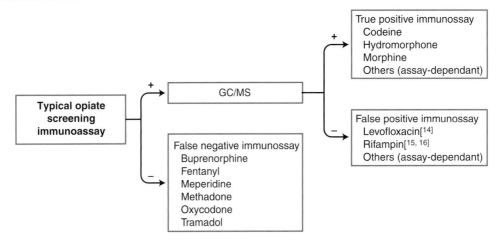

Fig. 15.3 Flow chart for using opiate immunoassays effectively. When using opiate immunoassays as the first step in screening urine samples, it is important to realize that several opioids may not be detected (buprenorphine, fentanyl, meperidine, methadone, oxycodone, and tramadol). Also, all positive results should be confirmed by a second method, such as gas chromatography/mass spectroscopy. If a specific opioid cannot be confirmed, then the original immunoassay result must be considered a false positive. As with all the examples in this chapter, the chart must be customized for each laboratory methods

Table 15.1 Urine versus serum morphine concentrations

Route (amount)	Serum peak (time)	Other serum (time)	Urine peak (time)	Other urine (time)
Intravenous [18] (0.125 mg/kg, ~9 mg)	440 (0.5 min)	20 (2 h)		
Intramuscular [18] (0.125 mg/kg, ~9 mg)	70 (15 min)	20 (4 h)		
By mouth [18] (30-mg tablet)	20 (4 h)			
By mouth [19] (7.5 mg from poppy seeds)	100 (2 h)	6 (24 h)	1,568 (3 h)	720 (24 h)

All concentrations are in ng/mL

problems (e.g., sample collection and adulteration). When a blood sample is drawn, one is reasonably certain that one knows the identity of the patient from whom it came and that it has not been adulterated in any way, not to mention that one can always get a blood sample from a patient.

There are many reasons for the analytic preference for urine. Drugs are typically concentrated manyfold in the urine, and drugs are present in the urine in relatively high concentrations for many hours [17]. Even in the best case scenario, where one knows exactly which opioid was ingested and when the ingestion occurred, so that one can predict reasonably well when the blood peak concentration will occur, the peak value is manyfold less than the typical urine concentration. For morphine, as shown in Table 15.1, a 0.125 mg/kg intravenous injection will result in a peak concentration in blood of 440 ng/mL after 1 min, which will rapidly decline to just 20 ng/mL at 2 h [18] (and less than that at later times). In contrast, in a study where the peak serum concentration was 100 ng/ml (4.4 fold lower than that just mentioned), the urine concentration averaged 1, 568 ng/mL at 3 h and 720 ng/mL at 24 h [19]. The lesson is clear – if one is trying to detect morphine (or other opioids), it will be easiest to detect it in the urine.

Another reason that most clinical laboratories prefer urine samples is that the assays they use (screening immunoassays) are FDA-approved for use with urine samples only. Laboratories are permitted to run these assays on urine after doing relatively straightforward validation studies. In order to run these same assays on blood, however, laboratories are required to undertake much more extensive validation studies, studies that few laboratories have the resources to do.

Nonetheless, there are a few caveats about using urine samples that are important to keep in mind. As mentioned earlier, specimen collection can be problematic. In the absence of a discrete witnessed voiding, it is possible for patients to substitute pristine urine samples for their own, and it is also possible for patients to add adulterants to a sample of their own urine, adulterants which can interfere with some testing methods [20, 21]. Even with a valid sample from the correct patient, massive hydration, or skipping a drug for several days, can render the concentration so low that it becomes undetectable by some methods [2, 21]. In other words, it is difficult to document conclusively that a patient has not used a drug.

Concentration/Metabolites

As mentioned earlier, with screening immunoassays, it is never clear which opioids are causing the positive reaction; a positive reaction looks the same no matter which opioid caused it. In truth, it is even a little more complicated. Although each assay is calibrated to turn positive at 300 ng/mL of morphine, other opioids show different amounts of cross-reactivity (Table 15.2) [22]. This is true whether one considers a given manufacturer's assay (columns) or whether one looks at a given opioid across manufacturers (rows). For example, for assay 1, hydrocodone will turn positive at a concentration of 100 ng/mL, but oxycodone will not turn

positive until the concentration reaches 1,000 ng/mL; for assay 2, the corresponding figures are 479 and 23,156 ng/mL; and for assay 3, 364 and 5,388 ng/mL. Does this mean a sample with a concentration of 250 ng/mL of hydrocodone will be reported as positive by assay 1 and negative by assays 2 and 3? Absolutely!

As mentioned earlier (and reflected in Table 15.2 for meperidine and oxycodone), none of the opiate screening immunoassays can be relied upon to detect buprenorphine, fentanyl, meperidine, methadone, or oxycodone. This is not entirely unexpected: these opioids have very different chemical structures, so one might predict that antibodies raised to morphine might not "recognize" them (Fig. 15.4).

There is yet another layer of complexity with opiate screening immunoassays. For emergency toxicology purposes, it may be important to prevent false positives by setting the positive threshold at 300 ng/mL, at which concentration morphine is present in potentially clinically significant amounts. But for pain management physicians, the real question is whether it is there at all. Put differently, as just described, a patient whose urine has a hydrocodone concentration of 250 ng/mL will be reported as negative for opiates by assays 2 and 3, but a patient whose urine has a morphine concentration of 200 ng/mL will be reported as negative by all three assays! To make matters even worse, some laboratories are now using as their positive threshold for opiate screening immunoassays a concentration of 2,000 ng/mL [4, 23].

Table 15.2 Immunoassay cross-reactivities

	Assay 1	Assay 2	Assay 3
Morphine	300	300	300
Codeine	50	225	247
Hydrocodone	100	479	364
Hydromorphone	100	620	498
Meperidine	250,000	30,508	>50,000
Oxycodone	1,000	23,166	5,388

Extracted from Magnani [22]
Shown above are the lowest concentrations of selected opioids that will cause a positive immunoassay result with three different commercial assays
All concentrations are in ng/mL

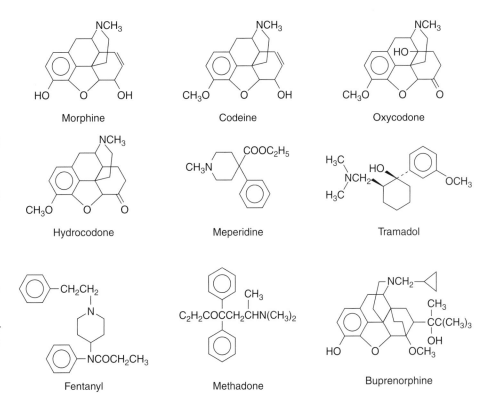

Fig. 15.4 Chemical structures of common opioids. The antibodies used in immunoassays are designed to detect morphine. One might predict that these antibodies would cross-react with codeine and hydrocodone, as their structures are so similar. By the same token, it is not surprising that these antibodies typically do not cross-react with meperidine, tramadol, fentanyl, methadone, and buprenorphine, whose structures are so different. Although, at first blush, oxycodone looks very similar to morphine, the presence of the (relatively large) hydroxyl (–OH) group in the center of the diagram must be sufficient to limit the cross-reactivity because few opiate immunoassays detect oxycodone (All structures were adapted from Magnani [22])

Table 15.3 Laboratory facts about opioid tests (applicable only at hospital XYZ)

Opioid	In-house (rapid TAT) opiate screening immunoassay		Gas chromatography/mass spectroscopy		Metabolites	Typical window of detection (days)
	Detected	Detection limit ng/mL	Included in GC panel?	Detection limit ng/mL		
Buprenorphine	No		No (order as individual test)	5	Norbuprenorphine	0.5–1
Codeine	Yes (not specifically identified)	224	Yes	50	Morphine (minor metabolite)	1–2
Fentanyl	No		No (order as individual test)	0.5	Norfentanyl	1 (3 for metabolite)
Hydrocodone	Probably (not specifically identified)	1,100	Yes	50	Hydromorphone dihydrocodeine	1–2
Hydromorphone	Probably (not specifically identified)	1,425	Yes	50	–	1–2
Meperidine	No		Yes	50	Normeperidine	0.5–1
Methadone	No (order methadone immunoassay)		No (order as individual test)	100	–	3–11
Morphine	Yes (not specifically identified)	300	Yes	50	–	1–2
Oxycodone	No		Yes	50	Oxymorphone noroxycodone	1–1.5 (3 for controlled release)
Tramadol	No		No (order as individual test)	500	–	0.5–1.5

Some information taken from White and Black [24]
Note that opiate immunoassay will not specifically identify any drug
Note that GC/MS detection limits are consistently much lower and that individual drugs are identified

In summary, there are many ways that opiate screening immunoassays may report as negative samples that have concentrations of opioids that would be of interest to the pain management physician: very poor cross-reactivity; thresholds set at levels more appropriate for emergency toxicology; and samples from patients who, by avoiding banned drugs for a few days or by overhydrating themselves, have succeeded in lowering their urine opioid concentrations to very low levels.

When testing is done by gas chromatography/mass spectroscopy, in addition to the specific drug(s) present, you can (and should) consider the expected patterns of metabolism [18]. Assuming your laboratory provides specific data on all the relevant compounds, you should not be surprised to see oxymorphone in the urine of patients on oxycodone therapy since it is a known metabolite. Similarly, since hydromorphone is a metabolite of hydrocodone, it would not be unexpected to find both opioids in a patient taking hydrocodone. In contrast, a patient taking oxymorphone should not have oxycodone in his urine, and a patient taking hydromorphone should not have hydrocodone in his urine because metabolism does not proceed in the reverse direction in either case. These relationships can be confusing, so Table 15.3 is a shortened version of a table the author prepared for use in his institution. As with all the previous examples, much of the data contained therein needs to be customized by each laboratory to take into account the specific assays in use locally.

Clinical Examples

Concrete examples can be very helpful in understanding the principles just described. Each of the examples that follow is based on a real case; indeed, many of them represent relatively common occurrences.

Since most physicians will use laboratories with screening immunoassays, the examples that follow assume that the initial testing is done in that manner. In some of the cases, the initial assay did not prompt an automatic confirmation by another method, which is often the case in practice (though, as described earlier, it should never be the case in pain management).

Clinical Example #1: I Really Am Taking My Oxycodone (False Negative)

A urine sample from a patient on oxycodone therapy is reported as negative for opiates by screening immunoassay. When you talk with your patient about the results and her apparent noncompliance, she is insistent that she has been taking her medication as prescribed.

You call the laboratory and discover that their opiate screening immunoassay, like most such assays, does not cross-react with oxycodone. In order to reliably detect oxycodone, the laboratory recommends using a different test (gas chromatography or an immunoassay specific for oxycodone). Applied to your patient's original sample, these methods indicate that oxycodone is indeed present.

Clinical Example #2: Methadone Does Not Cause a Positive Opiate Immunoassay

A urine sample from a patient on methadone therapy is reported as positive for opiates by screening immunoassay from your laboratory. In this case, no confirmatory testing was done. In addition, you ordered a methadone immunoassay on the sample, which was also reported as positive.

When you discuss these findings with the patient, he explains that his methadone is responsible for the positive reaction and that the test proves he is taking his medication as prescribed.

Because of its structure, which is very different from morphine (Fig. 15.4), methadone is not detected by opiate screening immunoassays. Indeed, this is the reason that a separate immunoassay is needed for its detection [8, 24, 25].

To prove that the positive opiate screening immunoassay result was not related to methadone, the specimen was referred for confirmatory testing by gas chromatography/mass spectroscopy, which came back positive for morphine.

Clinical Example #3: A True Positive Unrelated to Drug Use

A urine sample from a patient on oxycodone therapy is reported as positive for opiates by screening immunoassay from your laboratory. As requested, the laboratory refers the sample for confirmatory testing, which comes back positive for morphine by gas chromatography/mass spectrometry. There is no indication on the report that oxycodone is present.

If oxycodone is not mentioned, do not assume that it is not present. Good laboratories will report present or absent for each drug tested, often along with their detection limits. In this case, oxycodone was not part of the testing laboratory's opioid panel. One would have to request it specifically in order to have it done.

Fortunately, specific immunoassays are becoming available that make testing for oxycodone as easy as it is to test for methadone [26].

As to the morphine, the patient denied using morphine. A careful history taken after the fact revealed that she had consumed a large number of poppy seed crackers a few hours

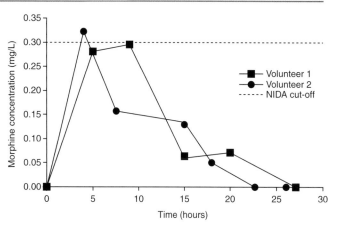

Fig. 15.5 Morphine concentration in urine after eating poppy seed crackers. At several time intervals after eating poppy seed crackers, two volunteers submitted urine samples to determine the morphine concentrations by gas chromatography/mass spectroscopy. As noted, samples from both individuals in the 5–10-h range had values that approached or exceeded the positive threshold (0.30 mg/L (300 ng/mL) (With permission from McCutcheon and Wood [27])

before submitting her urine sample. Although many people believe that poppy seeds cause a false-positive reaction for morphine, poppy seeds in fact contain genuine morphine. It has been well documented that ingestion of realistic numbers of crackers containing poppy seeds can cause true positive results for morphine (Fig. 15.5) [27].

Clinical Example #4: I Really Am Taking My Morphine (False Negative)

A urine sample from a patient on morphine therapy is reported as negative for opiates by screening immunoassay. Although the laboratory does refer samples that test positive for confirmation, this sample underwent no further testing.

When you discuss the apparent lack of compliance with your patient, she maintains that she has been taking the drug regularly. You call the laboratory to discuss the test results, and you discover that the patient's sample showed more reactivity than most negative samples (Fig. 15.1) but less than that required to be called positive. You ask that the sample be referred for more definitive testing. Gas chromatography/mass spectroscopy confirms that morphine is present at a concentration of 200 ng/mL. Most patients on morphine therapy will have urine concentrations far above the 300 ng/mL threshold. But it is possible for urine from patients who skip doses (sometimes a sign of bingeing) [2] or from patients who overhydrate themselves [21] to have lower levels. As a result, it is important to note that screening immunoassays are usually calibrated to turn positive at 300 ng/mL of morphine and that lower levels will be called negative.

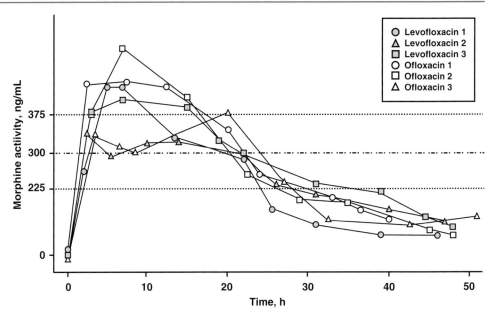

Fig. 15.6 False-positive opiate immunoassays following antibiotic ingestion. At several time intervals after single doses of levofloxacin or ofloxacin, three volunteers submitted urine samples for opiate screening by immunoassay. In every case, these urine samples tested positive for a prolonged period (roughly 24 h) (With permission from Baden et al. [14])

Clinical Example #5: I Really Am Taking My Hydromorphone (False Negative)

A urine sample from a patient on hydromorphone is reported as negative for opiates by screening immunoassay. When you call the laboratory for clarification, they assure you that their assay can detect the drug (in contrast to methadone and oxycodone). You insist that the sample be sent for a specific assay for hydromorphone, which comes back positive for hydromorphone at a concentration of 350 ng/mL.

Remember that opiate screening immunoassays are calibrated to turn positive at 300 ng/mL of morphine. Because of differences in cross-reactivity, it typically requires higher concentrations of hydrocodone to show this amount of reactivity (Table 15.2). Your patient's sample had 350 ng/mL and was therefore screen negative, but the drug was clearly present.

Clinical Example #6: It's Just Pneumonia (False Positive)

A patient on chronic methadone therapy has been compliant for many years. As his pain medicine consultant, you test him regularly for opiates as well as methadone (separate assay). His methadone test is always positive, and until this most recent test, his opiate screening immunoassay has been negative, just as you expect.

You share the positive opiate screening immunoassay test results with him, telling him how disappointed you are, but

he assures you that he has not taken any opioids other than methadone. You arrange to have the sample retested by gas chromatography/mass spectroscopy to identify the specific opiate involved, but no opioid could be identified by the more definitive technique. The opiate screening immunoassay must have been a false positive.

After sharing the good news with the patient, you review his history in more detail, and you uncover the fact that the week before he submitted his urine sample for testing, his primary care physician had started him on a course of levofloxacin for community-acquired pneumonia. Checking the literature, you discover quinolones have been reported to cause false-positive results with opiate screening immunoassays (Fig. 15.6) [14].

Clinical Example #7: When Two Opioids Are Present

A urine sample from a patient on hydromorphone tests positive for opiates by screening immunoassay. Your laboratory has a policy that all samples with positive screening tests be confirmed by gas chromatography/mass spectroscopy. This sample turns out to contain not only hydromorphone but also morphine.

In the absence of the gas chromatography/mass spectroscopy analysis, you would not have been aware of the noncompliance problem (i.e., that this patient is ingesting morphine as well as hydromorphone). With immunoassay screening, you do not know which, or how many, opioids are present in a sample.

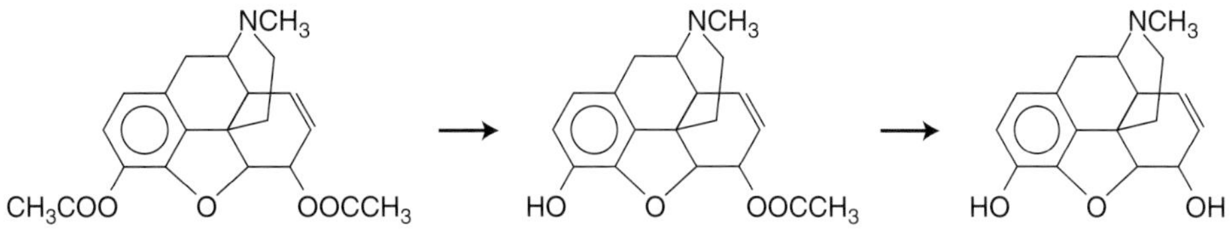

Heroin (diacetylmorphine) — $T_{½}$ ~ 10 min

6-MAM (6-monoacetylmorphine) — $T_{½}$ ~ 40 min

Morphine — $T_{½}$ ~ 3 h

Fig. 15.7 Metabolic pathways relating heroin and morphine. Heroin (diacetyl morphine) is rapidly broken down to 6-monoacetylmorphine (6-MAM), which is then converted to morphine. The half-lives of the three compounds are roughly 10, 40, and 180 min. Thus, if a patient uses heroin, one may only find morphine in the urine; if one does find 6-MAM in addition to morphine, though, it is proof that heroin was the source of the morphine (Adapted from Baselt [18])

Clinical Example #8: Understanding Metabolites #1

A patient on morphine therapy tests positive for opiates by screening immunoassay, and the confirmatory tests always show the presence of morphine only. On his most recent sample, the screening immunoassay is positive again, but the gas chromatography/mass spectroscopy report indicates the presence of a low concentration of hydromorphone (Dilaudid®).

You suspect that the patient has begun using hydromorphone illicitly. When you discuss your suspicion with him, he maintains that he has not used any opioids other than the morphine you prescribe for him.

Further investigation reveals that hydromorphone may be a minor metabolite of morphine and that the results from this sample do not conclusively prove that the patient ingested hydromorphone in addition to his prescribed morphine [28].

Clinical Example #9: Understanding Metabolites #2

A urine sample from a patient on oxycodone was referred to a laboratory for analysis by gas chromatography/mass spectroscopy. The report shows results for both oxycodone (positive) and oxymorphone (absent). Since you know that oxymorphone is a metabolite of oxycodone, you worry that the patient is not taking her oxycodone regularly, diverting the majority of her prescription, and crushing a tablet into her urine sample in order to test positive and remain under your care.

Even though oxymorphone is indeed a metabolite of oxycodone, whether or not it should be detected in urine samples is controversial [29, 30]. Possible explanations include the fact that some patients may not metabolize oxycodone efficiently and that the detection limits of some assays may not be sufficiently low enough. In any case, if pill crushing is a concern, one might decide to revert to a witnessed collection procedure [1].

Clinical Example #10: Understanding Metabolites #3

A patient on morphine therapy always tests positive for opiates by screening immunoassay, and the confirmatory tests always show the presence of morphine only. On his most recent sample, the screening immunoassay is positive again, but the gas chromatography/mass spectroscopy report indicates the presence of 6-monoacetylmorphine (6-MAM) as well as morphine.

You call the laboratory to find out what that means. As indicated in Fig. 15.7, heroin (diacetylmorphine) is metabolized to 6-MAM, which is then metabolized to morphine. The half-lives of heroin and 6-MAM are short (9 and 38 min, respectively), so they do not persist for long in patient samples. If 6-MAM is detected, it is proof that heroin has been taken [31]; morphine is not metabolized to 6-MAM. Its absence does not prove that heroin was not ingested; because of its short half-life, it is present in urine samples for a relatively short time. This patient may have been using heroin all along, but it was only on this sample that traces of the heroin metabolite (and morphine precursor) were found.

Recommendations

Know your laboratory! Compile a list of all the drugs you want to be able to detect in your patients and review it with your lab. Together, put together a set of test orders that will detect all the drugs you want. Common error includes thinking that methadone and oxycodone will be detected by opiate screening immunoassays; they will not!

Insist that all drugs detected by opiate screening immunoassay be confirmed by a second method so as to absolutely eliminate false positives.

Use urine as the preferred specimen to be sure you get the highest concentrations, but be aware of specimen integrity issues.

Concentrations, at least relative concentrations, as well as patterns of drugs detected can be helpful.

References

1. Braithwaite RA, Jarvie DR, Minty PS, et al. Screening for drugs of abuse (I): opiates, amphetamines and cocaine. Ann Clin Biochem. 1995;32:123–53.
2. Gourlay D, Heit HA, Caplan YH. Urine drug testing in primary care. Dispelling the myths & designing strategies. Monograph for California Academy of family Physicians. 2002. http://www.alaskaafp.org/udt.pdf. Accessed on 24 Aug 2012.
3. Hammett-Stabler CA, Pesce AJ, Cannon DJ. Urine drug screening in the medical setting. Clin Chim Acta. 2002;315:125–35.
4. Wu AHB, McKay C, Broussard LA, et al. Laboratory medicine practice guidelines: recommendations for the use of laboratory tests to support poisoned patients who present to the emergency department. Clin Chem. 2003;49:357–9.
5. Bailey DN. Results of limited versus comprehensive toxicology screening in a university medical center. Am J Clin Pathol. 1996;105:572–5.
6. Annesley TM, Rockwood AL, Sherman NE. Chromatography. In: Burtis CA, Ashwood ER, Bruns DE, editors. Tietz fundamentals of clinical chemistry. 6th ed. St. Louis: Saunders Elsevier; 2008. p. 112–27.
7. Annesley TM, Rockwood AL, Sherman NE. Mass spectrometry. In: Burtis CA, Ashwood ER, Bruns DE, editors. Tietz fundamentals of clinical chemistry. 6th ed. St. Louis: Saunders Elsevier; 2008. p. 128–39.
8. Heit HA, Gourlay D. Urine drug testing in pain medicine. J Pain Symptom Manage. 2004;27:260–7.
9. Rubenstein KE, Schneider RS, Ullman EF. "Homogeneous" enzyme immunoassay: new immunochemical technique. Biochem Biophys Res Commun. 1972;47:846–51.
10. Caplan YH, Levine B, Goldberger B. Fluorescence polarization immunoassay evaluated for screening amphetamine and methamphetamine in urine. Clin Chem. 1987;33:1200–2.
11. Adler FL, Liu CT. Detection of morphine by hemagglutination-inhibition. J Immunol. 1971;106:1684–5.
12. Henderson DR, Friedman SB, Harris JD, et al. CEDIA, a new homogeneous immunoassay system. Clin Chem. 1986;32:1637–41.
13. Kricka LJ. Principles of immunochemical techniques. In: Burtis CA, Ashwood ER, Bruns DE, editors. Tietz fundamentals of clinical chemistry. 6th ed. St. Louis: Saunders Elsevier; 2008. p. 155–70.
14. Baden LR, Horowitz G, Jacoby H, Eliopoulos GM. Quinolones and false-positive urine screening for opiates by immunoassay technology. JAMA. 2001;286:3115–9.
15. van As H, Stolk LM. Rifampicin cross-reacts with opiate immunoassay. J Anal Toxicol. 1999;23:71.
16. Daher R, Haidar JH, Al-Amin H. Rifampin interference with opiate immunoassays. Clin Chem. 2002;48:203–4.
17. Wolff K, Farrell M, Marsden J, et al. A review of biological indicators of illicit drug use, practical considerations and clinical usefulness. Addiction. 1999;94:1279–98.
18. Baselt RC. Disposition of toxic drugs and chemicals in man. 7th ed. Foster City: Biomedical Publications; 2004. p. 759–63.
19. Hayes LW, Krasselt WG, Mueggler PA. Concentrations of morphine and codeine in serum and urine after ingestion of poppy seeds. Clin Chem. 1987;33:806–8.
20. Cook JD, Caplan YH, LoDico CP, Bush DM. The characterization of human urine for specimen validity determination in workplace drug testing: a review. J Anal Toxicol. 2000;24:579–88.
21. Wu AHB. Urine adulteration before testing for drugs of abuse. In: Shaw LM, Kwong TC, editors. The clinical toxicology laboratory. Washington D.C.: AACC Press; 2001. p. 157–72.
22. Magnani B. Concentrations of compounds that produce positive results. In: Shaw LM, Kwong TC, editors. The clinical toxicology laboratory. Washington D.C.: AACC Press; 2001. p. 491–2.
23. Lee PR, Shahala DE. Changes to the cutoff levels for opiates for federal workplace drug testing programs. Substance abuse and mental health services administration. Fed Regist. 1995;60:575–85.
24. White RM, Black ML. Pain management. Washington D.C.: AACC Press; 2007.
25. Simpson D, Braithwaite RA, Jarvie DR, et al. Screening for drugs of abuse (II): cannabinoids, lysergic acid diethylamide, buprenorphine, methadone, barbiturates, benzodiazepines, and other drugs. Ann Clin Biochem. 1997;34:460–510.
26. Backer RC, Monforte JR, Poklis A. Evaluation of the DRI® oxycodone immunoassay for the detection of oxycodone in urine. J Anal Toxicol. 2005;29:675–7.
27. McCutcheon JR, Wood PG. Snack crackers yield opiate-positive urine. Clin Chem. 1995;41:769–70.
28. Reisfeld GM, Chronister CW, Goldberger BA, Bertholf RL. Unexpected urine drug testing results in a hospice patient on high-dose morphine therapy. Clin Chem. 2009;55:1765–9.
29. Smith HS. Opioid metabolism. Mayo Clin Proc. 2009;84:613–24.
30. Schneider J, Miller A. Oxycodone to oxymorphone metabolism. Pract Pain Manag. 2009;7:71–3.
31. von Euler M, Villen T, Svensson J-O, Stahle L. Interpretation of the presence of 6-monoacetylmorphine in the absence of morphine-3-glucoruronide in urine samples: evidence of heroin abuse. Ther Drug Monit. 2003;25:645–8.

Monitoring Drug Use and Abuse: The Evolution of a Paradigm

Steven D. Passik and Kenneth L. Kirsh

Key Points
- If a prescriber decides that a patient is a candidate for an opioid trial, the equally important decision of how opioid therapy is to be delivered in an individualized fashion must also be made.
- An opioid trial should be preceded by a risk assessment, and opioid therapy should be delivered in a fashion matched to the risk level of the individual.
- Once a trial is initiated and an initial risk assessment is completed, the job of monitoring and evaluating is not over; prescribers need to perform ongoing checkups and evaluations, including documentation in the domains of the 4 A's: analgesia, activities of daily living, adverse side effects, and potentially aberrant drug-taking behaviors.
- Many tools can be used in this initial and ongoing effort, including urine screening, use of prescription monitoring program reports, and creating a visit schedule tailored to the individual.

Introduction

Contrary to reports in the popular media that tend to focus solely on the recent problems of prescription drug abuse, our country faces two, not one, worrisome public health crises. The first is the problem of poorly treated chronic pain, and the second is the problem of prescription drug abuse. Pain

S.D. Passik, Ph.D. (✉)
Psychiatry and Anesthesiology,
Vanderbilt University Medical Center, Psychosomatic Medicine,
1103 Oxford House, Nashville, TN 37232, USA
e-mail: passiks@mskcc.org

K.L. Kirsh, Ph.D.
Department of Behavioral Medicine,
The Pain Treatment Center of the Bluegrass,
2416 Regency Road, Lexington, KY 40503, USA
e-mail: doctorken@windstream.net

clinicians do not have the luxury of focusing on only one of these two and instead have to attempt to find a balance in their practice that allows them to treat pain with controlled substances as needed and take reasonable steps to prevent drug abuse and diversion.

Affecting approximately 75 million Americans, poorly treated chronic pain causes losses of productivity that amount to more than 60 billion dollars per year while undermining quality of life for patients and families [1–4]. Indeed, chronic pain affects physical, psychological, and social well-being, and patients frequently experience sleep disturbance, depression, and anxiety [5]. Thus, despite advances in the knowledge of pain pathophysiology, understanding of treatments, and development of multidisciplinary approaches to pain management, pain care is still inadequate, and the problem is only expected to grow as the population continues to age.

Understanding Undertreatment

Why is pain still so poorly treated? The treatment of pain is complicated and often requires a multidisciplinary approach, which is becoming increasingly difficult to provide with poor reimbursement from managed care organizations. In addition, chronic pain is not usually associated with sympathetic arousal, and, therefore, the objective signs of physiological stress are often absent. Patients with chronic pain may not appear to be in physical pain, sometimes leading to skepticism by observers, which is particularly true when past histories of substance problems or the potential use of opioid medications are involved. Finally, with increasing regulatory scrutiny and the growth of prescription drug abuse, there has been a trend for clinicians to shy away from using opioids, and this fear reflects that the treatment of pain has become all the more controversial and undesirable [6, 7].

In truth, at the beginning of what became a massive expansion of opioid prescribing, there was a marked tendency to trivialize the risk of drug abuse and addiction, and we are now "playing catch-up." A new paradigm has emerged, one that attempts to incorporate the principles of addiction medicine into pain management, in a manner and fashion that is appropriate to each individual patient. Several instruments have been created to help with screening and ongoing documentation and management of pain patients being considered for or treated with opioid therapy. This does not answer all of the needs, however, and a novel set of guidelines and criteria are proposed that clinicians can use to determine whether they should apply routine or more intensive monitoring and documentation, given the risk level of the patient in question and within the guideposts of peer prescribing.

The Interface of Pain and Drug Abuse

Poorly treated chronic pain persists despite a massive increase of opioid prescribing in the country. Almost every class of analgesics has had substantial increases in prescribing during the last 3 years, with hydrocodone compounds being the most widely prescribed medication in the United States [8]. With the wider availability of opioids has also come a much larger concern about public abuse. From 2002 to 2005, there were 190 million prescriptions for opioids in the United States resulting in 9.4 billion doses [9]. In 2005, for the first time, opioids displaced marijuana to become the new illicit drug of choice [10]. A year later, the National Survey on Drug Use and Health data showed a minimum of 430 million abused doses [11]. Thus, clinicians are placed in a difficult position wherein they acknowledge on one hand that opioids are effective, but are faced with the potential that they might be contributing to drug abuse and diversion on the other. Unlike any other medication class, opioid prescribing requires documentation of informed consent or a treatment agreement.

With the dilemma of treating pain while avoiding abuse and diversion, it is crucial that proper assessments be performed to take reasonable steps to guard against abuse and diversion and to assure that patients are being treated safely and effectively – with gains not only in terms of pain relief but also in terms of stabilization or improvement in their functional status. While clearly a chronic pain assessment should include a detailed assessment of the pain itself, including intensity, quality, location, and radiation of pain, identification of factors that increase and decrease the pain should be elicited as well as a review of the effectiveness of various interventions that have been tried to relieve the pain, and of course, the impact of pain on sleep, mood, level of stress, and function in work, relationships, and recreational activities should be assessed, since improvement in these areas may be a goal of pain treatment and a measure of the efficacy of interventions. To aid in this endeavor, a number of general screening instruments, such as the Brief Pain Inventory, already exist for the clinical setting [12–14].

While these tools are useful for a good generalized assessment, we have been sorely in need of screening instruments designed specifically for identifying patients who are more likely to misuse their opioid medications. To answer this, many researchers have recently flooded the literature with a wide variety of assessment tools to examine potential risk when prescribing opioid analgesics. A few of the more promising measures are discussed below.

Tools for Predicting Risk of Misuse and Abuse in Pain Patients

Most of the recent research has focused on screening tools that can be used to prescreen patients to determine level of risk when considering opioids as part of the treatment regimen. Safe opioid prescribing demands proper risk stratification and the accommodation of that risk into a treatment plan. In addition, we must always keep in mind that a spectrum of nonadherence exists and that this spectrum is distinct for pain patients versus those who use these medications for nonmedical purposes. Nonmedical users can be seen as self-treating personal issues, purely as recreational users, or as having a more severe and consistent substance use disorder or addiction. On the other hand, pain patients are more complex, and their behaviors might range from strict adherence to chemically coping to a frank addiction. Thus, scores indicating increased risk on the following tools do not necessarily indicate addiction, but might be uncovering some of the grey areas of noncompliance.

Screener and Opioid Assessment for Patients With Pain

The Screener and Opioid Assessment for Patients with Pain (SOAPP) is a self-report measure with 14 items utilizing a 5-point scale (0=never, to 4=very often) and can be completed by patients while they are in the waiting room. Scores from each item are summed to create a total score, with a cutoff score of 8 or greater suggesting as the cut point to determine risk [15, 16]. The SOAPP has undergone a number of iterations, and the relatively low cutoff score of 8 or greater was chosen partially to account for the underreporting of behaviors. The SOAPP is an accurate tool for assessing abuse potential in patients considered for opioid therapy and has good psychometric properties, although the data available to date are correlational and not causal in nature. In addition, few demographic and medical data were recorded in the validation of the SOAPP, raising the chance for differences to exist in the cutoff scores among different subpopulations. Despite this, the SOAPP has an active research program behind it and will likely emerge as a clinically relevant tool for years to come.

Opioid Risk Tool

The Opioid Risk Tool (ORT) is made up of 5 yes-or-no self-report items, covering issues such as family and personal history of substance abuse, age, history of preadolescent sexual abuse, and psychological disease [17]. A self-report version is available so that patients can complete it in the waiting room. Alternately, the clinician form can be completed during the patient visit and can be done briefly as part of the patient intake. Positive endorsements are given a score based on patient gender (i.e., a family history of alcoholism equates to a score of 3 for male patients and 1 for female patients), and then, the scores are summed for a total score. Scores of 0–3 are associated with low risk, 4–7 with moderate risk, and 8 or more with high risk for addiction. The ORT was tested on 185 consecutive patients and displayed excellent discriminatory ability in both men and women for identifying patients who will go on to abuse their medications or develop an addiction, with observed c statistic values of 0.82 and 0.85, respectively. The ORT is useful due to its brevity and ease of scoring, but the face-valid nature of the ORT brings up the issue of susceptibility to deception. For many, this will be an acceptable risk tool, but may not be sufficient for all.

Pain Assessment and Documentation Tool

To initiate follow-up once a patient has been started on opioid therapy, it is important to consider four major domains. These domains have been labeled the "4 A's" (analgesia, activities of daily living, adverse effects, and aberrant drug-related behaviors) for teaching purposes [18]. The last "A," aberrant drug-taking behaviors, is perhaps the most salient when considering whether a patient should remain a candidate for opioid therapy. In short, aberrant drug-taking behaviors is a term encompassing a range of behaviors that may or may not be indicative of addiction in a patient, but definitely account for behaviors that need to be addressed and corrected. Examples of aberrant drug-taking behaviors less indicative of addiction can include increase in medication dose without authorization, requesting frequent early renewals, and appearing unkempt. More egregious aberrant drug-taking behaviors include doctor shopping, changing route of administration of medications, and forging prescriptions.

In application, Passik and colleagues [19, 20] set out to field test a short form that could be used as a charting note. The Pain Assessment and Documentation Tool (PADT) is a simple charting device based on the 4 A's that focuses on key outcomes and provides a consistent way to document progress in pain management therapy over time. The PADT is a two-sided chart note that can be easily included in the patient's medical record. It is designed to be intuitive, pragmatic, and adaptable to clinical situations. With regard to time burden, it took clinicians between 10 and 20 min to complete the original tool, and the revised PADT is substantially shorter and only requires a few minutes to complete. The PADT does not provide strict scoring criteria, as it is meant as a charting tool, but evidence from the trials suggests that four or more aberrant behaviors in a 6-month period predicts abuse and possibly true addiction.

Prescribing Outside the Bounds of Typical Practice

Should the prescriber decide that a patient appears to be an acceptable risk for opioid therapy based off one or more of the above screening tools along with clinical judgment, another set of criteria should come into play. Medicine is a peer-practiced art and science and thus requires that some thought be given to what other physicians are doing in their own practices. Where possible, some form of consensus should be established as standards of care while still acknowledging that a great deal of variability exists between physician philosophies and patients' responses and analgesic requirements.

The concept of monitoring opioid prescribing proposes that prescribing patterns can be viewed as either in the normal range of peer-related prescribing or outside of these norms. Prescribing in a normal range refers to the prescribing of opioids in a usual and customary fashion similar to that of their colleagues. Conversely, prescribing outside this zone refers to prescribing opioids in a manner which deviates from the usual prescribing habits of the majority of physicians writing opioid prescriptions. It is important to realize that there is nothing inherently wrong with prescribing outside these loose norms and there may be excellent reasons to do so. However, this concept may be helpful as a mechanism to alert certain prescribers to the fact that they are no longer in line with the usual prescribing practice of the majority of their colleagues, and so may decide to increase the degree, amount, or rigor of documentation.

It may be extremely appropriate to prescribe outside the bounds of typical practice long term for many decades on any given individual patient. The purpose of this label is not to highlight a prescriber as doing something wrong or aberrant, but to help notify prescribers that they are prescribing outside typical bounds for a given patient to ensure that they are aware of this so that they can choose to act (only if appropriate) or do nothing. Although experienced experts in pain medicine may know when they are doing this, novices and health-care providers from other disciplines of medicine may not.

Factors That Define Prescribing Outside the Scope of Normal Practice

Five factors may be important in defining whether a clinician is prescribing outside the scope of normal practice. Some of the factors have clear cut points, while others do not. The first thing to consider is the type of pain complaint; is it controversial or less common when considering opioid therapy (e.g., headaches)? Another thing is whether or not the patient has active psychiatric or substance abuse issues. While not all psychiatric disorders will be complicating factors, things such as depression, bipolar disorder, impulse control disorders, and substance use disorders will complicate care and may indicate prescribing outside the scope of normal practice. A third factor to consider is whether the patient has a significant amount of contact with nonmedical users of opioids. While difficult to determine at times, physicians learning of this social influence need to consider whether this pushes prescribing into a different category. The fourth factor is patient age. While exceptions definitely exist, problems of abuse and addiction are usually associated with younger adults, and this age group does increase risk of outside the box prescribing. Finally, the amount of opioid prescribed is the final factor to consider.

Of all the factors mentioned above, opioid dose is perhaps the most clear-cut (i.e., can be backed by prescribing statistics) but also the most controversial. The doses used in controlled studies are generally in the moderate range (up to 180 mg of morphine or a morphine equivalent per day), although a few patients received higher doses [21–23]. Daily doses above 180 mg of morphine or a morphine equivalent duration involving patients with chronic noncancer pain have not been validated in clinical trials of significant size and thus may be considered the high watermark for appropriate prescribing among peer physicians as reported in the literature (see Table 16.1) [21, 24–26].

Prescribing outside the scope of normal practice for any particular individual patient should not necessarily spark efforts to alter one's prescribing. Although no specific action is necessary when prescribing in this realm, actions which prescribers may choose to take include (a) consultation or referral to a pain specialist, (b) close reevaluation of the patient's clinical situation (e.g., repeat comprehensive history and physical examination and consideration for further medical work-up), (c) careful review of how the prescribing became outside the scope of normal practice and over what period of time, (d) investigation into the patient's home and social environment as well as their contacts with nonmedical users and where their pain medications are stored (e.g., whether they are secured in a locked space and who may have access), or (e) increase the degree of documentation and/or patient monitoring. Certain prescribers such as pain specialists who care for complex challenging patients with persistent pain may appropriately prescribe beyond normal bounds quite often.

Table 16.1 Listing of factors that may lead to opioid prescribing outside the scope of normal practice

#	Factor which may lead to increased medication dosing
1	Progression of the patient's painful condition
2	Development of a new painful condition
3	Aberrant drug-taking behavior
4	Chemical coping (or using medications to treat life stress while not rising to the level of an addiction)
5	Development of opioid tolerance/hyperalgesia
6	Pharmacokinetic phenomena (e.g., ultrarapid metabolizers) [26]
7	Increased spiritual/emotional or socioeconomic suffering
8	"Prescriber style" (e.g., aggressive opioid titration, perhaps with intent to entirely eliminate pain)
9	Pharmodynamic phenomena (e.g., decreased efficiency of the signaling processes of the opioid receptor) [26]
10	Pseudotolerance (e.g., increased physical activity, drug interactions) – a situation in which opioid dose escalation occurs and appears consistent with pharmacological tolerance but, after a thoughtful evaluation, is better explained by a variety of other variables [25]
11	Pseudoaddiction – drug-seeking behavior for the appropriate purpose of pain relief, rather than abuse or substance misuse [24]. It is characterized by a demand for more medication for analgesic purposes, as well as by behaviors that appear similar to those seen in addicted patients (e.g., anger, hostility). Pseudoaddiction can be differentiated from drug misuse by increasing the dose by an appropriate amount and determining whether the complaints abate

If after careful consideration of the individual patient's situation or discussion with a pain specialist a prescriber chooses to attempt to reduce dosing to more modest levels, potential therapeutic options which may be helpful include the opioid rotation, the addition of other medications (e.g., anti-inflammatory agents, adjuvants such as antidepressants and antiepileptic drugs), the addition of behavioral medicine treatment approaches, the addition of physical medicine treatment approaches, the addition of interventional treatment approaches, the addition of neuromodulation treatment approaches, a change to opioid administration intraspinally (with or without additional agents) [27], and/or the addition of complementary and alternative medicine treatment approaches.

Applying a Risk Management Package

Opioid abuse can have harmful consequences, such as stigmatization, opiophobia, and the undertreatment of pain [28]. Hence, it is important that the practice of opioid prescribing strikes a balance between the extremes of widespread opioid use and opioid avoidance, wherein risk stratification is used for patient selection and the principles of addiction medicine are applied during ongoing treatment. Exposure to drugs does not create drug addicts. Rather, only vulnerable individuals who are exposed to drugs have a risk of addiction. Only individuals exposed to alcohol or opioids, who have the genetic, social, and/or psychological predisposition to addiction, actually develop a problem. There is no problem inherent to the chemical nature of opioids; rather, the growing problem of prescription drug abuse is due to the increasing use of prescription drugs among individuals not screened for risk of drug abuse. The recent problems associated with oxycodone have stemmed from the prescription of the opioid to individuals who were not assessed for their risk of drug abuse and then were treated in the context of a low-risk drug treatment paradigm. The sustained-release preparation of oxycodone approved by the Food and Drug Administration (FDA) in 1995 was thought to have much lower abuse potential, leading to the unsubstantiated belief that the risk of opioid addiction was obviated with this slower-release oxycodone [6]. Truly, abuse deterrence is only tested and proven on the streets once the product is made available.

Opioid risk management techniques must be implemented to understand the risk of drug abuse of an individual in order to better guide the decision of whether or not opioids should be used for pain control and, if so, how best to deliver the analgesic and to tailor therapy accordingly. The assessment is directed at determining whether an individual will likely take their medication as prescribed and derive better function from the ~30–60 % pain relief that the opioids provide or whether the opioid will be used as a coping mechanism for other issues and will not lead to psychosocial gains. If the individual has a penchant for recreational drug use, prescription of opioids could lead to the abuse and or diversion of the analgesics and, at worst, addiction. Several patient factors have been found to be predictive of a patient's risk for opioid misuse or abuse. A mental health disorder is a moderately strong predictor of opioid abuse, while a history of illicit drug and alcohol abuse or legal problems is also predictive of future aberrant drug behaviors according to a survey of 145 patients being treated for chronic pain and a systematic review of the literature [29, 30]. Tobacco use is highly prevalent among substance misusers, and the Screening Instrument for Substance Abuse Potential (SISAP) and the Screener and Opioid Assessment for Patients with Pain (SOAPP) include tobacco use as a factor in determining risk [16, 31]. While smoking has been found to increase the desire to abuse drugs in an addict population ($N = 160$), alternatively, smoking can be used as a form of substance replacement in those trying to abstain from drug use [32, 33]. Furthermore, individuals who have chronic pain smoke at higher rates than the general population [34]. Cigarette use has been correlated with nonspecific low back pain, fibromyalgia, and headache disorders [35–37].

All patients being considered for opioid therapy need an individualized risk assessment. Patients considered for opioid therapy to treat chronic pain need to be assessed for risk of addiction with a validated tool; there have been many devices developed to assess addiction risk in order to help clinicians make better informed decisions regarding treatment for their patients [38]. As described above, the ORT and SOAPP are good choices for many clinics [15–17]. However, whatever tool may be chosen, it is important to approach this with patient from a standpoint that there are no right or wrong answers and that this is an important step in determining a treatment plan.

Delivering opioid therapy at a lower risk begins with learning how to document cases well. Chart reviews of primary care patients in pain management indicate that oftentimes the notes are not complete enough to support continuing opioid treatment. Typical notations such as "pain stable; renew hydrocodone #240" need to be modified to include the 4 A's of pain treatment outcomes discussed above in reference to the PADT [18–20]. This approach helps to broaden the focus of opioid effects beyond analgesia to other important aspects such as physical functioning. An example of a good chart note is, "Mr. Jones is taking hydrocodone for his chronic low back pain. His pain has reduced from severe to moderate and he is now able to attend church with his wife and help with household chores. Constipation had been noted, but he is responding to a bowel regimen; there is no evidence of aberrant drug-related behaviors." This documentation, along with a pain-focused physical examination and corroboration from a source other than self-report such as a significant other, caregiver, urine toxicology screen, or prescription monitoring report, is enough to thoroughly support pain management with opioids.

Addiction is a disorder characterized by craving, continued use despite harm, and compulsive and out-of-control behaviors. Behaviors that are common and sometimes ambiguous can be clearly associated with addiction when they continually reoccur. Fleming demonstrated in a primary care patient population that patients who self-report four or more aberrant drug behaviors over a lifetime are more likely to have a current substance use disorder [39]. Therefore, it is important to document the occurrence of even less predictive aberrant drug behaviors, because additively, they may indicate an addiction problem. Toward this end, there is a tool available called the Addiction Behaviors Checklist that has been designed and validated to longitudinally track behaviors potentially suggestive of addiction in patients taking long-term opioid therapy for chronic pain [40]. In the meantime, the available data suggests that patients should be given a second chance when one of these behaviors less predictive of addiction is noted; only when the problem reoccurs over a 6–12 month period should opioid therapy discontinuation or a referral be considered. Some individuals with chronic pain are treatable by primary care physicians, while others may require comanagement with a specialist or complete management by a clinician with addiction medicine training.

Aberrant behaviors can be due to several different etiologies, such as pseudoaddiction, in which poorly treated pain causes patients desperate for relief to appear as if they are addicted to their medication. Although pseudoaddiction was a concept first reported in the literature as a case study two decades ago, it has *not* been empirically validated, and it has been overextended. Moreover, sometimes in the face of circumstances that could be due to pseudoaddiction, dosages are escalated to unsafe levels. Instead, in cases where patients exhibit aberrant behaviors and complain of unrelieved pain, alternative approaches to pain control can be pursued instead of continued dose escalation [24, 41]. For example, for a patient who is seemingly unable to take their oxycodone as prescribed due to unrelieved pain, they can instead be prescribed a drug with a lower street value, such as sustained-release morphine. In addition, the patient could be given a urine toxicology screen and scheduled for an appointment with a psychologist in order to address the behavioral problems in opioid drug taking. Pseudoaddiction is a behavioral syndrome that needs to be addressed along with improving pain control. On the other hand, other individuals exhibit aberrant drug-taking behaviors when self-medicating to address a psychiatric issue, while still others may be selling their opioid medications. Individuals involved in drug diversion will be negative for opioids in a urine toxicology screen and will have no medicine to show when called in early for a pill count.

Tolerance and physiological dependence are *not* signs of addiction in an individual exposed to opioids for medical purposes. Although there are many behaviors that can be indicative of a developing drug addiction, such as stealing another patient's drugs or injecting an oral opioid formulation, most of these obvious signs are not reported by patients [42]. Meanwhile, other types of behaviors, such as early dosing, drug hoarding, and increasing the dose without physician's consent, are less predictive of addiction and very common. Opioid drug studies indicate that approximately 15–20 % of patients exhibit multiple behaviors possibly indicative of addiction. Therefore, with higher risk patients who are prone to engaging in aberrant behaviors, other systems of monitoring should be incorporated within their pain management program.

Once opioid treatment has begun, prescription monitoring program data can be an invaluable way to identify patients who are "doctor shopping"; however, this type of data varies in accessibility and quality from state to state, with many states now having operational prescription drug monitoring programs [43]. Still, a high-quality national database is yet needed to monitor opioid prescriptions in order to identify patients who doctor-shop across state lines. Prescribers who do not have the availability of a statewide program to track controlled substance prescriptions should at minimum develop a system to minimize duplicate prescriptions within their group practice.

Compliance monitoring with urine toxicology screens is also needed to corroborate patient claims due to the well-recognized unreliability of self-reported information [44]. The results of this drug testing can indicate whether the patient is taking their opioid medications as prescribed, whether they are obtaining controlled substances from another source, and whether they are concurrently taking illicit drugs. Urine toxicology screens are used for long-term monitoring in order to reduce the risk of a potentially serious adverse event, such as addiction or medication misuse, but are not intended to police patients. With chronic pain management, as with other chronic conditions such as heart disease and cancer, the ongoing consequences of treatment must be monitored to ensure safety. Observations of only patient behaviors are often not enough information to clearly indicate the presence or absence of drug misuse or abuse. Even pain and addiction specialists fail to identify a problem in one in five patients as indicated by surprise urine testing that showed drug use outside of the prescribed opioid and dose [44]. New technology developed for urine screening provides results in <5 min for 12 illicit or controlled substances at the point of care. The Federation of State Medical Board furnishes a strong foundation for support of the reimbursement of urine toxicology screening costs. Their model policy strongly recommends urine toxicology screens in patients who are considered high risk for nonadherence to taking their medications as prescribed and as an occasional screening tool to corroborate patient reports.

Due to the high prevalence of procurement of opioids from a family or friend, even adherent patients should be educated about drug storage and inventorying; "self-treaters" often have the misconception that sharing prescription medications is safe. Indeed, education regarding drug storage and sharing is another aspect of due diligence needed in comprehensive opioid risk management. Opioids should be locked away. New devices are being developed that allow the patient only to have access to medications on a schedule programmed by the clinician and, if tampered with, sends a notification email to the prescriber. When prescribing a pain reliever for a high-risk patient, it may be best not to initiate therapy with an opioid with a high abuse rate. Furthermore, highly structured approaches to therapy should be implemented for these patients. This type of strategy was assessed in a primary care population at a Veterans Affairs hospital in 335 patients who were referred due to aberrant drug behaviors [45]. Once enrolled in the "opioid renewal clinic," they signed an opioid treatment agreement, underwent frequent doctor visits, prescribed limited amounts of opioids on a short-term basis (either weekly or bi-weekly), and were given random urine toxicology screens and pill counts. When needed, the patients were given counseling and comanagement with addiction services. With this type of structured care intervention, 45 % of patients stopped abusing their opioids and pharmacy cost savings were noted [45]. Another study of 500 patients enrolled in an adherence monitoring program with similar structured care elements noted a 50 % reduction in the incidence of opioid abuse [46]. For actively drug-abusing patients with severe pain resulting in functional interference, a methadone-based program combined with adherence, motivational, and cognitive-behavioral therapies has been applied with positive outcomes [47]. A National Institute on Drug Abuse study of these interventions for 40 opioid-abusing patients with pain found significant reductions in positive tests for nonprescribed opioids and reductions in illicit drugs, along with positive tests for methadone after 6 months of treatment.

Conclusion and Future Directions

While the psychometrics of various screening tools still require further evaluation and the in/out of the box concept needs further refinement, we must remember that good pain management should lead to some decreases in pain perception for the patient combined with a corresponding increase in ability to function. By reviewing these tools and proposed novel guidelines for in/out of the box prescribing and adopting them into practice as appropriate, the physician will take a significant step in providing effective pain management for their pain patient while minimizing risk of opioid misuse.

References

1. ABC News/USA Today/Stanford University Medical Center Poll: Pain. Broad experience with pain sparks a search for relief. 2011. Available at: http://www.abcnews.go.com/images/Politics/979a1T heFightAgainstPain.pdf. Accessed 11 Jan 2011.
2. American Pain Foundation. Annual report. 2006. http://www.painfoundation.org/About/2006AnnualReport.pdf. Accessed 10 May 2010.
3. McCarberg BH, Billington R. Consequences of neuropathic pain: quality-of-life issues and associated costs. Am J Manag Care. 2006;12(9 Suppl):S263–8.
4. Stewart WF, Ricci JA, Chee E, Morganstein D, Lipton R. Lost productive time and cost due to common pain conditions in the US workforce. JAMA. 2003;290:2443–54.
5. Argoff CE. The coexistence of neuropathic pain, sleep, and psychiatric disorders: a novel treatment approach. Clin J Pain. 2007;23(1):15–22.
6. Cicero TJ, Inciardi JA, Munoz A. Trends in abuse of Oxycontin and other opioid analgesics in the United States: 2002–2004. J Pain. 2005;6(10):662–72.
7. Lipman AG. Does the DEA truly seek balance in pain medicine? J Pain Palliat Care Pharmacother. 2005;19(1):7–9.
8. Volkow ND. Scientific research on prescription drug abuse, before the Subcommittee on Crime and Drugs, Committee on the Judiciary and the Caucus on International Narcotics Control United States Senate. 2008. Available at: http://www.drugabuse.gov/Testimony/3-12-08Testimony.html. Accessed 10 May 2010.
9. SAMHSA. The NSDUH report: patterns and trends in nonmedical prescription pain reliever use: 2002 to 2005. Substance Abuse and Mental Health Services Administration, Department of Health and Human Services; 2007.
10. SAMHSA. Office of Applied Studies of the Substance Abuse and Mental Health Services Administration. Results from the 2005 National Survey on Drug Use and Health: National Findings. Department of Health and Human Services. Publication No. SMA 06–4194. Available at: http://www.oas.samhsa.gov/NSDUH/2k5NSDUH/2k5results.htm. Accessed 10 May 2010.
11. SAMHSA. Office of Applied Studies of the Substance Abuse and Mental Health Services Administration. Results from the 2006 National Survey on Drug Use and Health: National Findings. Department of Health and Human Services. Available at: http://www.oas.samhsa.gov/nsduh/2k6nsduh/2k6Results.pdf. Accessed 10 May 2010.
12. Cleveland CS, Ryan KM. Pain assessment: global use of the brief pain inventory. Ann Acad Med Singapore. 1994;23(2):129–38.
13. Kroenke K, Spitzer RL, Williams JB. The PHQ-9: validity of a brief depression severity measure. J Gen Intern Med. 2001;16(9):606–13.
14. Stratford PW, Binkley J, Solomon P, Finch E, Gill C, Moreland J. Defining the minimum level of detectable change for the Roland-Morris questionnaire. Phys Ther. 1996;76(4):359–65.
15. Akbik H, Butler SF, Budman SH, et al. Validation and clinical application of the screener and opioid assessment for patients with pain (SOAPP). J Pain Symptom Manage. 2006;32:287–93.
16. Butler SF, Budman SH, Fernandez K, Jamison RN. Validation of a screener and opioid assessment measure for patients with chronic pain. Pain. 2004;112:65–75.
17. Webster LR, Webster RM. Predicting aberrant behaviors in opioid-treated patients: preliminary validation of the opioid risk tool. Pain Med. 2005;6:432–42.
18. Passik SD, Weinreb HJ. Managing chronic nonmalignant pain: overcoming obstacles to the use of opioids. Adv Ther. 2000;17:70–83.
19. Passik SD, Kirsh KL, Whitcomb LA, Portenoy RK, Katz N, Kleinman L, Dodd S, Schein J. A new tool to assess and document pain outcomes in chronic pain patients receiving opioid therapy. Clin Ther. 2004;26(4):552–61.
20. Passik SD, Kirsh KL, Whitcomb LA, Schein JR, Kaplan M, Dodd S, Kleinman L, Katz NP, Portenoy RK. Monitoring outcomes during long-term opioid therapy for non-cancer pain: results with the pain assessment and documentation tool. J Opioid Manag. 2005;1(5):257–66.
21. Ballantyne JC, Mao J. Opioid therapy for chronic pain. N Engl J Med. 2003;349:1943–53.
22. Haythornthwaite JA, Menefee LA, Quatrano-Piacentini AL, Pappagallo M. Outcome of chronic opioid therapy for non-cancer pain. J Pain Symptom Manage. 1998;15:185–94.
23. Raja SN, Haythornthwaite JA, Pappagallo M, Clark MR, Travison TG, Sabeen S, Royall RM, Max MB. Opioids versus antidepressants in postherpetic neuralgia. A randomized, placebo-controlled trial. Neurology. 2002;59:1015–21.
24. Weissman DE, Haddox JD. Opioid pseudoaddiction – an iatrogenic syndrome. Pain. 1989;36:363–6.
25. Pappagallo M. The concept of pseudotolerance to opioids. J Pharm Care Pain Symptom Control. 1998;6:95–8.
26. Smith HS. Variations in opioid responsiveness. Pain Physician. 2008;11:237–48.
27. Smith HS, Deer T, Staats P, Singh V, Sehgal N, Cordner H. Intrathecal drug delivery: a focused review. Pain Physician. 2008;11:S89–104.
28. Zacny J, Bigelow G, Compton P, et al. College on problems of drug dependence taskforce on prescription opioid non-medical use and abuse: position statement. Drug Alcohol Depend. 2003;69(3):215–32.
29. Edlund MJ, Steffick D, Hudson T, et al. Risk factors for clinically recognized opioid abuse and dependence among veterans using opioids for chronic non-cancer pain. Pain. 2007;129(3):355–62.
30. Michna E, Ross EL, Hynes WL, et al. Predicting aberrant drug behavior in patients treated for chronic pain: importance of abuse history. J Pain Symptom Manage. 2004;28(3):250–8.

31. Coambs RB, Jarry JL, Santhiapillai AC, et al. The SISAP: a new screening instrument for identifying potential opioid abusers in the management of chronic malignant pain within general medical practice. Pain Res Manag. 1996;1(3):155–62.

32. Rohsenow DJ, Colby SM, Martin RA, et al. Nicotine and other substance interaction expectancies questionnaire: relationship of expectancies to substance use. Addict Behav. 2005;30(4):629–41.

33. Conner BT, Stein JA, Longshore D, et al. Associations between drug abuse treatment and cigarette use: evidence of substance replacement. Exp Clin Psychopharmacol. 1999;7(1):64–71.

34. Hahn EJ, Rayens MK, Kirsh KL, et al. Brief report: pain and readiness to quit smoking cigarettes. Nicotine Tob Res. 2006;8(3):473–80.

35. Jamison RN, Stetson BA, Parris WC. The relationship between cigarette smoking and chronic low back pain. Addict Behav. 1991;16(3–4):103–10.

36. Yunus MB, Arslan S, Aldag JC. Relationship between fibromyalgia features and smoking. Scand J Rheumatol. 2002;31(5):301–5.

37. Payne TJ, Stetson B, Stevens VM, et al. The impact of cigarette smoking on headache activity in headache patients. Headache. 1991;31(5):329–32.

38. Passik SD, Kirsh KL, Casper D. Addiction-related assessment tools and pain management: instruments for screening, treatment planning, and monitoring compliance. Pain Med. 2008;9(S2):S145–66.

39. Fleming MF, Davis J, Passik SD. Reported lifetime aberrant drug-taking behaviors are predictive of current substance use and mental health problems in primary care patients. Pain Med. 2008;9(8): 1098–106.

40. Wu SM, Compton P, Bolus R, et al. The addiction behaviors checklist: validation of a new clinician-based measure of inappropriate opioid use in chronic pain. J Pain Symptom Manage. 2006;32(4): 342–51.

41. Passik SD, Webster L, Kirsh KL. Pseudoaddiction revisited: a commentary on clinical and historical considerations. Pain Manag. 2011;1(3):239–48.

42. Passik SD, Portenoy RK, Ricketts PL. Substance abuse issues in cancer patients. Part 1: prevalence and diagnosis. Oncology (Williston Park). 1998;12(4):517–21, 524.

43. Office of Diversion Control. State prescription drug monitoring programs. http://www.deadiversion.usdoj.gov/faq/rx_monitor.htm.

44. Katz N, Fanciullo GJ. Role of urine toxicology testing in the management of chronic opioid therapy. Clin J Pain. 2002;18(4 suppl):S76–82.

45. Wiedemer NL, Harden PS, Arndt IO, et al. The opioid renewal clinic: a primary care, managed approach to opioid therapy in chronic pain patients at risk for substance abuse. Pain Med. 2007;8(7):573–84.

46. Manchikanti L, Manchukonda R, Damron KS, et al. Does adherence monitoring reduce controlled substance abuse in chronic pain patients? Pain Physician. 2006;9(1):57–60.

47. Bethea A, Acosta M, Haller D. Role of the therapeutic alliance in the treatment of pain patients who abuse prescription opioids. "PROJECT PAIN." NIDA (Grant #R01DA1369). In: Paper presented at: College on problems of drug dependence, Scottsdale, 17–22 June 2006.

Polypharmacy and Drug Interaction

17

Christopher A. Steel and Jill Eckert

Key Points

- When prescribing multiple drugs, consider the following:
  - The desired effect of each drug being administered, the clinical goal, or end point for each
  - Side effect profile of each of the drugs being administered and how they may be potentiated by an additional drug
  - Each of the drug effects on the metabolism of other drugs being administered
  - Impact of systemic illness such as renal or hepatic failure on specific drug levels
  - Likely risks of toxicity and which signs or symptoms to monitor for closely

Introduction

In days past, a basic understanding of a drug's mechanism of action was sufficient for the purpose of prescribing a medication to treat the vast majority of patients and their conditions. Those days are long gone with 48 % of Medicare beneficiaries over the age of 65 having three or more chronic medical conditions and 21 % having five or more of these conditions [1]. It has been estimated that the likelihood of a drug interaction in a patient taking only two different medications is only

6 %, whereas when the number of medication increases to ten, the likelihood of drug interaction increases to 100 % [2]. With this virtual certainty of frequently dealing with drug interaction, a physician must have a solid understanding of polypharmacy along with drug interactions.

Background

Not only has the increase in prescription medication influenced the need for understanding drug interactions; recent research has identified which specific enzymes are inhibited or induced by drugs and which drugs are substrates for these enzymes. This knowledge allows physicians to anticipate an added drug's likely pharmacokinetic response when administered to a patient already taking a variety of medications.

Pain physicians use a variety of medications and must therefore have a vast armamentarium of different drug groups and individual drugs. They must possess knowledge of not only what the drug does to target sites in the body (pharmacodynamics) but also how the body metabolizes and eliminates the drug (pharmacokinetics). Combining this information with reported adverse events and known side effects, a physician can dramatically reduce the chances of prescribing or administering a medication which will result in an adverse drug interaction. This chapter will discuss some of the more pertinent potential interactions; please refer to specific prescribing information for a specific medication to obtain a complete list of interactions and side effects.

Anticonvulsants

Anticonvulsant drugs exert their effect on pain via multiple pathways. Those felt to contribute greatly in the treatment of chronic pain include calcium channel blockade, depressed glutamate transmission, sodium channel blockade, and gamma-aminobutyric acid (GABA) potentiation [3].

C.A. Steel, M.D. (✉)
Department of Anesthesiology, Pennsylvania State University
Milton S. Hershey Medical Center, 500 University Drive,
P.O. Box 850, Hershey, PA 17033, USA
e-mail: chris_a_steel@yahoo.com

J. Eckert, DO
Department of Anesthesiology, Pennsylvania State University
Milton S. Hershey Medical Center, 500 University Drive,
P.O. Box 850, Hershey, PA 17033, USA
Pennsylvania State University College of Medicine,
Hershey, PA, USA
e-mail: jeckert@psu.edu

Anticonvulsant drugs are classified in two main groups: first generation and second generation. The first-generation drugs include benzodiazepines, carbamazepine, ethosuximide, phenobarbital, phenytoin, primidone, and valproic acid. The second generation consists of felbamate, gabapentin, lamotrigine, oxcarbazepine, pregabalin, tiagabine, topiramate, vigabatrin, and zonisamide. Of the above drugs, only those commonly used for the treatment of chronic pain will be discussed in detail.

First-generation drugs unfortunately exhibit high toxicity along with multiple drug interactions. This group has continued to be utilized due to its proven efficacy and low cost [4, 5]. To safely use this group of drugs, a practitioner must understand the pharmacodynamics including the mechanism of action of each drug, pharmacokinetics, and adverse effects to fully appreciate the implications of its use on the other medications being used by a patient.

Phenytoin

The effect of this medication is mediated via slowing of the recovery rate of the voltage-activated sodium channels even at low levels of this drug. At higher levels, potentiation of GABA and decreased glutamate transmission can be detected [3, 6]. Phenytoin is approximately 90 % bound by plasma proteins which allows small changes in albumin levels or competition with other drugs to greatly affect the free phenytoin level. The plasma half-life of phenytoin increases as the plasma concentration increases.

The drug interactions are due to the metabolism of phenytoin by certain liver enzymes and the induction of certain liver enzymes. Phenytoin is known to increase (or induce) the metabolism of drugs which are metabolized by CYP2C and CYP3A enzymes, and this maximum induction takes place 1–2 weeks after initiation of the drug [7]. This causes a decrease in the level of many drug groups including antiepileptic drugs (AEDs) and antidepressants. Oral contraceptive pills are known to be unreliable when phenytoin started. Notably, there is a decrease in the ethinylestradiol component of birth control when phenytoin is implemented, requiring at least 50 mcg ethinylestradiol in the patient's oral contraceptive and a warning to report any abnormal bleeding patterns [8]. Phenytoin is a substrate for CYP2C9, considering warfarin is also a substrate for this enzyme; addition of phenytoin to a stable warfarin regimen has led to significant bleeding problems.

The drug level of phenytoin can be increased or decreased when certain drugs are used with it simultaneously. Fluoxetine inhibits CYP2C19 enzyme for which phenytoin is a substrate, so the phenytoin level increases when fluoxetine is added to the regimen. Valproic acid is an inhibitor of the CYP2C9 enzyme which metabolizes phenytoin, so addition of valproic acid may increase the level of phenytoin. However, valproic acid also displaces phenytoin from albumin, so addition of valproic acid to a stable phenytoin regimen may increase, decrease, or not alter the phenytoin level [7]. The drug level of phenytoin is increased when these following drugs are coadministered: oxcarbazepine and topiramate [7–9]. Levetiracetam has been shown to cause no change in phenytoin levels [10]. The drug levels of phenytoin and carbamazepine are usually both decreased when they are used together [7].

Considering phenytoin is metabolized by the liver, hepatic disease can increase plasma phenytoin levels, and dose must be adjusted accordingly. It is known to only be 5 % excreted in the kidneys, so renal disease will not require dosing changes [11]. Toxic side effects include sedation, anorexia, nausea, megaloblastic anemia, gingival hyperplasia, osteomalacia, and hirsutism. Allergic reactions are thought to be responsible for serious skin, liver, and bone marrow effects. It is recommended to monitor complete blood count (CBC), electroencephalogram (EEG), liver function tests (LFTs), mean corpuscular volume (MCV), serum albumin level, and serum phenytoin level [11].

Valproic Acid

Valproic acid has been shown to block voltage-dependent sodium channels and to increase GABA levels, which are effective for the treatment of neuropathic pain. Calcium channels may also be blocked by this drug, but it requires a much higher drug level [12, 13].

Valproic acid is metabolized via hepatic glucuronidation and oxidation by CYP2A6, CYP2C9, and CYP2C19 and UGT [11, 14]. It is known to inhibit UGT and CYP2C9, thereby increasing the levels of phenytoin if it was being used, due to phenytoin's metabolism by CYP2C9. Valproic acid is also 90 % bound to albumin, which displaces other AEDs such as carbamazepine and phenytoin when used concurrently [7]. Cotherapy with valproic acid and topiramate causes a 17 % decrease in topiramate plasma concentrations and a 13 % increase in topiramate clearance [9]. Valproic acid does not, however, affect the use of birth control like other first-generation anticonvulsants due to its lack of action on the CYP3A enzyme [7].

Valproic acid is also affected by the use of other drugs. Felbamate inhibits the beta-oxidation pathway, thereby inhibiting the metabolism of valproic acid [7]. Topiramate is known to induce beta-oxidation and therefore decreases stable valproic acid levels by 11 % and increases its clearance, though the change is thought not to be clinically significant [9]. Carbamazepine and phenytoin both induce CYP2 enzymes which are responsible for valproic acid's metabolism, so both of these drugs will decrease stable valproic acid levels if added to a regimen [9].

Drug clearance can be affected by up to 50 % in hepatic dysfunction and with the possible change in serum albumin that can occur with severe liver disease; valproic acid levels should be dosed accordingly and followed closely [11]. It is 30–50 % excreted by the kidneys in the form of glucuronide conjugate and 3 % unchanged. Considering the significant changes that occur in protein binding in renal failure, valproic acid levels must be monitored closely. Common side effects noted with the use of valproic acid include nausea, sedation, peripheral edema, ataxia, diplopia, and nystagmus. In severe sedation, a physician must consider valproate-associated hyperammonemic encephalopathy (VHE) which has been reported [15, 16]. Some physicians follow blood tests due to reported thrombocytopenia and blood dyscrasias which occur in 0.4 % of patients [17, 18]. Other recommended monitoring tests include CBC including platelets, LFTs, serum ammonia levels, and serum valproic acid levels [11].

Carbamazepine

Carbamazepine has been implicated to work on a number of receptors and via number of mechanisms including sodium channels, calcium channels, potassium channels, adenosine receptors, release of serotonin, increase dopaminergic transmission, inhibition of glutamate release, interaction with peripheral-type benzodiazepine receptors, and decrease of basal and stimulated cAMP levels [19]. Pain relief has been attributed to disruption of synaptic transmission in the trigeminal nucleus [11]. Carbamazepine is known to induce metabolism not only of other drugs but also of itself, doubling its plasma clearance over the first few weeks of administration. This is due to the fact that it induces CYP3A4, which is one of the enzymes for which it is a substrate for (the other enzymes are CYP1A2, CYP2C8, and CYP2C9) [14]. As exhibited by phenytoin, carbamazepine decreases the levels of many other drugs. Carbamazepine also induces the enzyme which breaks down tricyclic antidepressants (TCAs), causing a decrease in TCA plasma concentration and an increase in metabolite concentration [7]. With the induction of CYP3A4, acetaminophen and codeine, which are broken down by this enzyme, have decreased levels due to their increased breakdown when used in coordination with carbamazepine [20]. Carbamazepine has a similar effect on oral contraceptives as was described with phenytoin [8]. It also can intensify the anticoagulant effect of warfarin as exhibited by phenytoin [21].

The interaction between carbamazepine and phenytoin is unpredictable as discussed earlier. Fluoxetine coadministration increases the level of carbamazepine. Also, the addition of valproic acid to a carbamazepine regimen can cause either no change or an increase in carbamazepine levels [7].

Stevens-Johnson syndrome (SJS) and another form of SJS known as toxic epidermal necrolysis only occur in 1–6 in 10,000 new carbamazepine users in this country, but can be up to ten times more prevalent in patients with Asian ancestry. These patients should undergo a test for HLA-B*1502 prior to starting this drug, and if the patient has this allelic variant, they should not start this medication [18]. Carbamazepine has a number of other side effects including severe hematologic disorders, antidiuretic effect, hepatic failure, hyperlipidemia, vertigo, drowsiness, and ataxia [6, 18, 22]. The latter being an important matter to consider in the elderly [12]. Blood dyscrasias are serious side effects and occur in 2.1 % of patients, causing most physicians to monitor blood tests on a weekly basis for the first 4–6 weeks [17]. Other significant labs to monitor include CBC, LFTs, serum carbamazepine level, and cholesterol profile [11, 18, 22, 23].

Second-Generation Anticonvulsants

Oxcarbazepine

Oxcarbazepine has been shown to inhibit sodium channels, potassium channels, calcium channels, and adenosine receptors and exhibit a dopaminergic effect. The other mechanisms of carbamazepine such as effects on peripheral-type benzodiazepine receptors, serotonergic effect, and the decrease in cAMP system have not yet been shown in oxcarbazepine. The main effect of both of the above agents, however, is their inhibition of the voltage-dependent sodium channels [19]. Oxcarbazepine is eliminated via glucuronide conjugation via glucuronyl transferases primarily and secondarily by renal excretion [21]. It is metabolized via CYP3A4 and shows mild inhibition of CYP2C19 [14]. Compared to carbamazepine, it has less metabolism via P450, no production of epoxide metabolite, and less protein binding, therefore leading most to believe it is more tolerable and has fewer drug interactions [24].

Oxcarbazepine induces the metabolism of oral contraceptives and requires the same precautions noted as with phenytoin. Doses of up to 900 mg/day have been shown not to affect the anticoagulant effect of warfarin, unlike carbamazepine [21]. Oxcarbazepine does increase stable phenytoin levels when added.

Approximately, 95 % of the drug is excreted by the kidneys, so requires dose decrease in renal failure, but no significant changes are need in hepatic failure [11]. Common side effects include dizziness, headache, diplopia, ataxia, nausea, and vomiting, which are less frequent and severe compared to carbamazepine. However, there is an increased risk of hyponatremia compared to carbamazepine [24]. Though side effects are noted, this drug does not require monitoring of laboratory tests compared to first-generation antiepileptics [11, 18].

Gabapentin

Gabapentin is structurally related to GABA, but does not directly interact with GABA receptors, though $GABA_B$ may be activated. It has shown to block hydroxy-5-methyl-4-isoxazolepropionic acid (AMPA) receptor-mediated transmission, enhance N-methyl-D-aspartate (NMDA) current at GABA interneurons, activate adenosine triphosphate-sensitive potassium channels, and modulate voltage-dependent calcium channels. It thereby inhibits the release of glutamate, aspartate, substance P, and calcitonin gene-related peptide (CGRP) [13, 25]. It is minimally metabolized and therefore excreted unchanged in the urine. Due to its renal excretion and lack of induction of hepatic enzymes, it has significantly fewer drug interactions. In the setting of renal failure with a creatinine clearance less than 60 ml/min, the dose of the medication will need to be reduced, and reduction should continue as renal function worsens [18]. It has been shown to act synergistically with NSAIDs and morphine, and that morphine can increase its area under the curve (AUC) [26, 27]. Side effects include somnolence, dizziness, peripheral edema, headache, and nausea, no interference with oral contraceptives [21].

Pregabalin

Pregabalin is a similar structure and is thought to have a similar mechanism of action as compared to gabapentin [28]. The main difference between pregabalin and gabapentin is that pregabalin has a uniform absorption from the GI tract whereas gabapentin demonstrates a decrease in absorption with escalating dosages [28]. In the setting of renal failure, the area under the curve (AUC) and half-life are increased, so it is recommended to decrease the dose by 50 % for creatinine clearance less than 60 ml/min [29]. Side effects are similar to gabapentin which include dizziness, somnolence, and peripheral edema. Due to the lack of metabolism and low protein binding, there are no significant drug interactions noted with the use of pregabalin [28]. No interference with oral contraceptives is also noted from pregabalin [21].

Topiramate

Topiramate inhibits sodium and calcium currents, blocks glutamate receptor at AMPA, and enhances GABA-mediated chloride channels [13]. Topiramate is approximately 15 % bound to plasma protein. It shows minimal CYP2C19 inhibition [14]. Adding either phenytoin or carbamazepine to a topiramate regimen can decrease the level of topiramate by approximately 40–50 %, whereas adding valproic acid to a topiramate regimen will decrease the topiramate level by only approximately 15 %. When topiramate is used with phenytoin, the phenytoin level is increased up to 25 % [7, 30]. Topiramate induces the metabolism of oral contraceptives, and similar precautions used with phenytoin should be employed [21].

Side effects of topiramate include psychomotor slowing, fatigue, and sedation. An observed increase in the rate of kidney stone formation was noted and found to be due to an increase in urinary bicarbonate excretion and urine pH along with a lower amount of citrate in the urine and the serum bicarbonate level. Also, metabolic acidosis, acute myopia, and oligohydrosis with hyperthermia have been rarely reported [18]. Considering this drug is excreted in the kidneys, the dose is usually decreased by 50 % in the setting of moderate to severe renal failure [11]. No specific recommendations have been made for prescribing in the setting of hepatic impairment [18]. For these reasons, serum electrolytes must be monitored, and the risk of kidney stone must be explained to patients [31].

Zonisamide

Zonisamide blocks sodium and calcium channels and also may inhibit monoamine release and metabolism. It also inhibits carbonic anhydrase [11, 13]. No interference with oral contraceptives is noted [21]. Zonisamide is a substrate for CYP3A4, UGT, and CYP2C19. It is not to inhibit or induce any CYP450 enzymes [11]. Therefore, its levels are significantly decreased with the concurrent use of phenytoin and carbamazepine, whereas the addition of valproic acid does not change the level of zonisamide. Phenytoin levels are increased by 16 % with the addition of zonisamide, and the carbamazepine levels have been variable in different studies with the addition of zonisamide [30].

In the setting of hepatic disease, zonisamide dose must be decreased due to its metabolism by the P450 system. In the setting of renal failure, there is an increase in the risk of metabolic acidosis which is thought to be due to the loss of bicarbonate via the inhibition of carbonic anhydrase. The dose is decreased in mild to moderate renal failure and should not be used with GFR < 50 ml/min [18]. Side effects include increased hepatic enzymes, azotemia, sedation, dizziness, metabolic acidosis, anorexia, and renal stones. It is recommended to monitor CBC, LFTs, serum bicarbonate, serum blood urea nitrogen (BUN) and serum creatinine, and urinalysis [11].

Levetiracetam

Levetiracetam is felt to bind to a specific site on the synaptic plasma membrane, though the exact mechanism of action is unknown [13]. It is not dependent on the CYP450 system for metabolism and is 66 % excreted unchanged in the urine and

27 % as inactive metabolites [11, 30]. Levetiracetam does not have any significant impact on other drug level, and no other drugs cause changes in levetiracetam levels [30]. There is no known interference with oral contraceptives [21].

Liver disease has little effect on this drug unless severe failure is present, in which the renal component will likely exert the greatest impact on the drug. In the setting of renal failure, the drug dose will need to be reduced accordingly [11]. Side effects include somnolence, dizziness, and fatigue. Serum BUN and serum creatinine are monitored due to extensive drug excretion [11].

Antidepressants

Selective Serotonin Reuptake Inhibitors (SSRIs)

The mechanism of action of SSRIs, as their name implies, is by blocking the reuptake of serotonin. The increased level of serotonin has been helpful in treating depression and OCD, in addition to other off-label uses. Side effects include sedation and sexual dysfunction [32]. Some specific agents do have significant drug interactions which must be considered.

Several SSRIs have been shown to increase warfarin levels due to inhibition of CYP2C9 and CYP3A4 and carbamazepine levels via inhibition of CYP3A4 [14, 20, 33]. The adverse effect of serotonin syndrome should lead practitioners to avoid combining MAOIs and SSRIs. One should also allow a 7-day washout period before starting MAOIs, and a 14-day washout period should be permitted prior to initiation of SSRI therapy after MAOIs have been used. Serotonin syndrome can occur when combined with triptans (naratriptan, rizatriptan, sumatriptan, and zolmitriptan) [34]. When combined with tramadol, there is an increased potential for seizures, and serotonin syndrome should be monitored [25]. SSRIs which inhibit CYP2D6 increase the concentration of TCAs when combined, and anticholinergic excess can occur [14, 34]. For SSRIs, no laboratory monitoring is absolutely required, though the inquiring into the presence of side effects will aid clinicians in determining when laboratory tests may be applicable [35].

Fluoxetine
Fluoxetine is metabolized by CYP2C9, CYP2C19, CYP2D6, and CYP3A4. It primarily inhibits enzyme CYP2D6, but also to lesser extent inhibits CYP2A1, CYP3A4, and CYP2C19 [20, 33]. It is known to significantly increase TCA levels when used in combination, which is ascribed to CYP2D6 inhibition. It can also increase the phenytoin level by almost twofold, which requires following phenytoin levels when implementing fluoxetine [33].

In the setting of the hepatic failure, the dose of this drug will need to be reduced, in contrast to renal failure which will not require a dose adjustment. Common side effects include somnolence, gastrointestinal dysfunction, headache, and sexual dysfunction. Rarely, hyponatremia occurs typically due to syndrome of inappropriate antidiuretic hormone secretion (SIADH) [36]. Weight loss, sexual dysfunction, hypothyroidism, hepatic disease, decreased bone growth, suicidal ideation, hyperglycemia, and impaired platelet aggregation have also been described [11, 18, 37, 38]. Therefore, monitoring has been recommended to include CBC with differential, LFTs, and thyroid function tests (TFTs), only if symptoms warrant these tests [11, 35, 39].

Sertraline
Sertraline is metabolized by CYP2B6, CYP2C9, CYP2C19, CYP2D6, and CYP3A4 and primarily inhibits CYP2D6, CYP1A2, CYP2C9, and CYP3A4. It has less of an impact on drug interactions compared to fluoxetine and paroxetine [14, 20, 33].

In patients with hepatic disease, sertraline doses will need to be decreased, as opposed to in the setting of renal failure, when the dose does not need to be changed. Side effects include hyponatremia, sexual dysfunction, and impaired platelet aggregation. Rarely, hypothyroidism and elevated liver transaminases are caused, and therefore, LFTs are monitored and baseline thyroid function tests (TFTs) are obtained [11, 23]. For this reason, monitoring has been recommended to include electrolytes, TFTs and LFTs, which should be obtained if signs or symptoms suggest derangements in these tests [11, 18, 23, 35].

Paroxetine
Paroxetine is metabolized by CYP2D6 and is the most potent SSRI for inhibition of enzyme CYP2D6, but is also known to inhibit CYP1A2 and CYP3A4 [14, 20, 33]. This leads to a dramatic increase in TCA levels when used in combination [20]. Specifically, desipramine plasma levels were increased 400 % by the addition of paroxetine [33]. Clinically, significant bleeding has been noted in patients who were taking warfarin when paroxetine was added, so monitoring INR would be prudent [33].

In mild to moderate renal failure and in hepatic failure, paroxetine plasma concentration is increased two times its normal value, whereas in severe renal failure, it can be up to four times the normal value. For this reason, dose adjustment for these dysfunctions is recommended [11, 18, 23]. Side effects including headache, somnolence, sexual dysfunction, and weight loss. Rarely, hypothyroidism, hepatic disease, and renal impairment occur, so it is recommended to monitor LFTs, TFTs, and serum BUN and creatinine, if signs and symptoms suggest possible derangements in these values [11, 23, 35].

Fluvoxamine
Fluvoxamine is metabolized by CYP1A2 and CYP2D6 and known to inhibit CYP1A2, CYP2C19, CYP3A4, and CYP2D6 [14, 20]. Of all the SSRIs, it is the most potent inhibitor of CYP

1A2 and likely CYP2C19. Due to its CYP enzyme inhibition, it has been shown to dramatically increase TCA levels. It can also increase warfarin levels, so INR levels should be monitored when this drug is added to chronic warfarin therapy [33].

In the setting of severe hepatic failure, the half-life is increased from 15 to 24 h, and dose frequency should be adjusted accordingly. There is no significant change in the half-life, and drug level in the setting of renal failure and dose and frequency of medication should not necessarily be changed. Side effects include headache, nausea, and sexual dysfunction. Rarely, hypothyroidism and elevated liver transaminases are caused, and therefore, LFTs are monitored and baseline TFTs are obtained, if signs and symptoms warrant these tests [11, 23, 35].

Citalopram

Citalopram is metabolized via CYP2C19 and CYP2D6 and possible CYP3A4 and is a weak inhibitor of CYP2D6, though this exerts less of an effect than other SSRIs [20, 40]. It has not shown to cause the same decrease in metabolism of TCAs, as seen with other SSRIs, but its breakdown products may decrease TCA metabolism [20]. In the setting of hepatic failure, clearance is decreased and the half-life is increased, so adjusting the dose accordingly may be warranted. In the setting of mild to moderate renal failure, no dose change will be needed, but in severe renal failure, a close monitoring and dose adjustment may be warranted [11, 23]. Side effects include somnolence, nausea, diaphoresis, and sexual dysfunction, which is less prominent than seen with some other SSRIs, along with the change of elevated liver enzymes and hypothyroidism. Therefore, signs and symptoms may prompt a clinician to perform lab tests such as LFTs and TFTs.

Escitalopram

Escitalopram is metabolized by CYP2C19, CYP2D6, and CYP3A4 and is a mild inhibitor of CYP2D6.

In the setting of hepatic failure, clearance is decreased and half-life is increased, so adjusting the dose accordingly may be warranted. In the setting of mild to moderate renal failure, no dose change will be needed, but in severe renal failure, a close monitoring and dose adjustment may be warranted [11, 23]. Side effects include headache, nausea, and sexual dysfunction. More rare side effects such as hypothyroidism, bleeding disorder, and elevated LFTs should prompt a clinician to obtain labs such as LFTs or TFTs if deemed clinically necessary [11, 23, 35].

Serotonin-Norepinephrine Reuptake Inhibitors (SNRIs)

Milnacipran

Milnacipran blocks the reuptake of norepinephrine and serotonin with preference given to the former. It is only 13 % protein bound. It minimally interacts with the P450 system and has little inhibition or induction on these enzymes. Severe reactions such as autonomic changes, muscle rigidity, and neuroleptic malignant syndrome can occur when MAO inhibitors are combined with milnacipran. Serotonin syndrome can occur when milnacipran is combined with SSRIs and other SNRIs. In the setting of severe hepatic failure, the half-life is increased by 55 % and area under the curve (AUC) increased by 31 %, therefore requiring a slight decrease in dosing in these patients. In the setting of severe renal failure, the half-life is increased by 122 %, and the AUC is increased 199 %, requiring significant dose reductions. Side effects include headache, hot flashes, and nausea.

Venlafaxine

Venlafaxine blocks the reuptake of serotonin, norepinephrine, and dopamine. This drug was created in attempt to provide the benefits of TCAs without the adverse side effects. It has been shown to have great efficacy in many chronic pain disorders while providing a more tolerable side effect profile as compared to TCAs and SSRIs [41]. It is metabolized by CYP2D6, and inhibition of this enzyme is mild compared to other agents. Combined with its low protein binding of 25–30 %, it has shown much fewer drug interactions than many of the TCAs and SSRIs. The adverse effect of serotonin syndrome should be avoided via observation of washout periods after discontinuation of MAOIs or starting of MAOIs described in the SSRI section [42]. Serotonin syndrome due to the combination of venlafaxine and MAOIs has been reported leading to death [43].

In the setting of renal failure, the dose should be reduced 25 %, and if the patient is undergoing hemodialysis, the dose should be reduced 50 %. This is because in renal failure, the clearance is decreased by 24 %, and the half-life is increased 50 %. In dialysis, in one study of six patients on maintenance hemodialysis, a 4-h dialysis treatment removed only about 5 % of a single 50 mg dose of venlafaxine [44]. In the setting of hepatic failure, the dose should be reduced by 50 % since the half-life is increased by 30 %, and the clearance is decreased by 50 %. Side effects include headache, nausea, insomnia, somnolence, gastrointestinal distress, and inhibition of sexual function [11, 23, 41]. Elevation of blood pressure and cholesterol is a potential side effect of this medication [11, 35].

Duloxetine

Duloxetine is a balanced inhibitor of serotonin and norepinephrine reuptake. The resultant increase in these levels is felt to play a significant role in treating neuropathic pain along with treating depression [41]. Duloxetine is metabolized by CYP1A2 and CYP2D6 and inhibits CYP2D6 [14]. Side effects include nausea, headache, sexual dysfunction, dry mouth, and insomnia. Since 1 % of these patients develop an elevated ALT, consider checking LFTs after initiation [11, 35]. Duloxetine should not be prescribed to patients with preexisting liver disease due to the risk of exacerbating this condition. In the setting of mild to moderate renal failure with a creatinine clearance of greater than 30 ml/min, there should be no adjustments made to this medication; however, it should not be administered to patients with creatinine clearance less than 30 ml/min [18].

Tricyclic Antidepressants (TCAs)

Tricyclic antidepressants are composed of secondary amines and tertiary amines. Secondary amines include desipramine and nortriptyline, and tertiary amines include amitriptyline, clomipramine, and imipramine, among others. The major difference between the groups is the increase in norepinephrine reuptake inhibition seen in the secondary amines versus their tertiary amine counterparts [45].

TCAs inhibit the reuptake of 5-HT and norepinephrine and exert postsynaptic antagonism of the H1, alpha-1, muscarinic, and 5-HT2a receptors, all to varying degrees [46]. The most potent property is that of H1 antagonism, which is intuitive, considering TCAs were developed from antihistamines in the 1950s [46].

Secondary amines are metabolized primarily by CYP2D6 followed to a lesser extent by CYP2C19 and CYP1A2 and is not affected by CYP 3A4 in nortriptyline [47]. Tertiary amines are metabolized by CYP2C19, CYP1A2, CYP3A4, and CYP2D6. The inhibition of CYP2C19 is significant. They have a moderate effect on CYP1A2 and CYP3A4 and a clinically insignificant effect on CYP2D6 [46]. TCA levels are known to be increased when combined with SSRIs [34]. When combined with MAOIs, they have been reported to cause serotonin syndrome and death [43]. Side effects stem from anticholinergic muscarinic (dry mouth, xerostomia, sinus tachycardia, and urinary retention), alpha-2 blockade (postural hypotension), dopaminergic blockade (extrapyramidal side effects and neuroleptic malignant syndrome), and histamine blockade (sedation) [48]. TCAs are known to cause various ECG changes including tachycardia; ventricular tachycardia; ventricular fibrillation; supraventricular tachycardia; sinus arrest; QRS, PR, and QT prolongation; AV block; and bundle branch block. With this in mind, it is recommended to obtain a baseline ECG prior to starting these medications. For long-term monitoring, if the patient fails to respond or shows signs or symptoms of TCA toxicity, some recommend obtaining TCA level to rule out toxic levels or to help guide therapy [35, 49, 50]. In the setting of renal or hepatic failure, TCAs should be used with caution, with little literature to guide their use currently in these patient settings [51].

Monoamine Oxidase Inhibitors (MAOIs)

Monoamine oxidase is an enzyme which metabolizes 5-HT, histamine, dopamine, norepinephrine, and epinephrine. MAOIs inhibit this enzyme which causes an increase in the level of these substances [52]. First created were hydrazine derivative MAOIs, but due to liver toxicity, bleeding, and hypertensive crises, non-hydrazine derivatives were created. Unfortunately, non-hydrazine MAOIs still were implicated in hypertensive crises, though the liver problems were avoided. The hypertension eventually was coined as the "cheese reaction" caused by combination of MAOIs with tyramine-containing foods including fermented cheese. Individual reversible and irreversible MAO A and MAO B inhibitors were designed, along with multiple nonselective inhibitors [52].

Side effects of MAOIs include orthostatic hypotension, weight gain, drowsiness, and dizziness.

When combined with SSRIs, they have been documented to causes serotonin syndrome and death [43].

Opioids

Opioids exert action via the opioid receptors by acting as opioid agonists. Most opioids exert their effects via the OP1 (delta), OP2 (kappa), and OP3 (mu). This group of medications all exhibit similar side effects including but not limited to constipation, nausea/vomiting, dizziness, respiratory depression, hypotension, urticaria, urinary retention, and drowsiness. Long-term use can lead to physical dependence, hyperalgesia, hormonal abnormalities, and impairment of the immune system [53, 54]. If compliance becomes an issue or the patient experiences signs or symptoms indicative of toxicity, the clinician should test for the specifically prescribed opioid level [55].

Codeine

The major metabolite of codeine is codeine-6-glucuronide which is produced via glucuronidation by UGT2B7. Two minor metabolites are morphine and norcodeine which are formed by O-demethylation by CYP2D6 and N-demethylation by CYP3A4, respectively. Usually, less than 10 % of codeine is converted into morphine, but in the presence of a CYP2D6 or CYP3A4 inhibitor or CYP2D6 genetic polymorphism, the residual morphine level may be higher or lower [56]. Baseline creatinine levels have been recommended to obtain prior to long-term therapy [51].

Morphine

Morphine predominantly exerts its effect on the opioid receptors via the mu-opioid receptors [57]. Morphine is metabolized via glucuronidation by UGT2B7 into morphine-6-glucuronide and morphine-3-glucuronide. The former possesses 2–3 times more analgesic properties than morphine, while the latter does not bind to opioid receptors [58, 59]. In the setting of hepatic or renal failure, morphine dose should be decreased and monitored closely for signs or symptoms of toxicity. Baseline creatinine levels have been recommended to obtain prior to long-term therapy [51].

Fentanyl

Fentanyl is a mu-agonist with a high lipid solubility and low molecular weight, which makes it very attractive for the use of transdermal formulations. Unfortunately, the absorption has been shown to decrease after 48–72 in cachectic patients when compared to normal patients, making it less attractive for patients in this condition [60]. Fentanyl is metabolized by CYP3A4 into norfentanyl, which has no analgesic activity itself [59, 61]. In the setting of hepatic or renal failure, fentanyl dose should be decreased and monitored closely for signs or symptoms of toxicity [18]. In patients who are taking a CYP3A4 inducer or inhibitor, they could have a higher or lower metabolism of fentanyl and require an increase or decrease in frequency of dosing, respectively.

Oxycodone

Oxycodone exerts an agonist effect on the mu-, kappa-, and delta-opioid receptors, causing inhibition on adenylyl cyclase, hyperpolarization of neurons, and decreased excitability. It is known to work via the kappa receptor, more than the mu and delta receptors. Morphine, on the other hand, has more of an effect on the mu receptors than oxycodone, and it is less metabolized and therefore has less bioavailability. O-demethylation by CYP2D6 occurs which converts oxycodone to oxymorphone (a potent analgesic) which is excreted by the kidneys [57, 62]. N-demethylation of oxycodone to noroxycodone (a weak analgesic) takes place via CYP3A5 and CYP3A4, and noroxycodone is then excreted via the kidneys [63]. In the setting of renal and hepatic impairment, the dose should be reduced and patient monitored closely [18]. Baseline creatinine levels have been recommended to obtain prior to long-term therapy [51].

Methadone

Methadone is an opioid agonist with a predominant effect on the mu-opioid receptor [64]. Methadone is also known to block the NMDA receptor which may aid in blocking the windup mechanism thought to be responsible for chronic pain [65]. Methadone is a racemic mixture of R- and S-methadone. R-methadone has a 10–50-fold greater affinity for the mu and delta-opioid receptors when compared to S-methadone. Methadone has a half-life of approximately 22 h, which only produces 6 h of analgesia on initiation of drug, but increases to 8–12 h of analgesia after repeated dosing [66]. R-methadone is predominantly metabolized by CYP3A4, and also metabolized by CYP2C8 and CYP2D6 to a lesser extent. S-methadone is metabolized by CYP3A4 and CYP2C8 equally and to a lesser extent by CYP2D6. The breakdown product of methadone is EDDP (2-ethylidene-1,5-dimethyl-3,3-diphenylpyrrolidine), although at least six others have been identified, and all are inactive [67]. Methadone has been shown to prolong the QT interval even in small doses and to a greater extent in higher doses even resulting in torsades de pointes. For this reason, a baseline ECG should be taken prior to methadone induction and again after a stabilized dose is reached. If the corrected QT interval (QT_c) is increased by 40 ms above baseline or the total QT_c is 500 ms or greater, the patient would be considered to be at risk for torsades de pointes, and the dose should be reduced or discontinued. Also if the patient is prone to electrolyte abnormalities, electrolytes should be checked more frequently due to risk of electrolyte abnormalities further prolonging the QT_c [68]. In addition to prolongation of QT interval, other side effects include respiratory depression, sedation, and anxiety. In the setting of renal or hepatic failure, the dose should be decreased and patient monitored closely for signs and symptoms of toxicity [18].

Opioid Combinations

Tramadol

Tramadol is a mu-opioid receptor agonist and a norepinephrine and serotonin reuptake inhibitor. Considering it has a similar mechanism of action to MAOIs, when it is combined with MAOIs or other antidepressants, serotonin syndrome has been reported, and possible fatalities due to this interaction have been reported [43, 69]. Considering tramadol is 60 % metabolized via hepatic metabolism via CYP2D6, CYP2B6, and CYP3A4 and excreted via renal excretion, in the setting of liver of renal failure, tramadol doses should be decreased by approximately 50 % [11, 62, 69]. Enzyme inducers of CYP2D6 (carbamazepine) cause approximately a 50 % decrease in tramadol levels [70].

Tramadol should be avoided in patients with codeine or other opioid allergy due to the risk of anaphylacticreaction from cross-reactivity. Side effects include dizziness, nausea, headache, seizures, and constipation [11, 18].

Agonist/Antagonist

Buprenorphine

Buprenorphine is a mixed agonist antagonist, with partial agonism of the mu-opioid receptor and antagonism of the kappa-opioid receptor. At low doses, the mu-agonist effect predominates, allowing pain control with a potency of 25–40 times that of morphine. In contrast to morphine, however, at higher doses, there is a ceiling effect due to the antagonistic properties. This is advantageous to avoid respiratory depression, yet the medication may be lacking in treatment of severe pain [71]. This drug is 96 % protein bound and is metabolized to its active metabolite norbuprenorphine via multiple enzymes including CYP3A4, CYP2C8, CYP2C9, CYP2C18, and CYP2C19. Of all of these enzymes, CYP3A4 is responsible for 65 % of the metabolite, and CYP2C8 creates 30 % of the metabolite [62, 72]. In the setting of renal failure, buprenorphine levels are not significantly affected. However, in the setting of hepatic failure, the risk of increased LFTs has been noted and warrants obtaining baseline LFTs and periodic monitoring of LFTs [73].

Side effects including headache, insomnia, anxiety, nausea, weakness, sedation with rare instances of hypotension, and respiratory depression. The risk of increased LFTs has been noted and warrants obtaining baseline LFTs and periodic monitoring of LFTs.

Muscle Relaxants

Baclofen

Baclofen works directly on the spinal cord by blocking afferent pathways traveling from the brain to the skeletal muscles. Considering baclofen is an analog of gamma-aminobutyric acid (GABA), it also may have GABA-like effects in decreasing the release of excitatory neurotransmitters such as aspartate and glutamate. Baclofen is only 15 % metabolized in the liver, and 70–85 % is excreted unchanged in the urine, and it is poorly dialyzable. For these reasons, hepatic failure should not significantly affect dosing, whereas in renal failure or dialysis dependence, the dose should be reduced [11, 23, 74]. Side effects include drowsiness, ataxia, insomnia, slurred speech, seizures, and weakness, which can also be signs of toxicity [23].

Cyclobenzaprine

Cyclobenzaprine is close in chemical structure to amitriptyline and has some similar effects of TCAs like anticholinergic activity. It is felt to relieve muscle spasms via some central action and not directly at the neuromuscular junction. Cyclobenzaprine is a substrate for CYP3A4 and CYP1A2 and to a lesser extent CYP2D6. It is then excreted as inactive metabolites by the kidneys. Even in mild hepatic impairment, the AUC can be increased by up to 100 %, requiring dose reduction. Dosing in the elderly should also be reduced and titrated slowly. Side effects include drowsiness, headache, dizziness, and xerostomia [11, 18, 23].

Tizanidine

Tizanidine is an alpha-2 agonist which has antinociceptive and antispasmotic properties. It is metabolized via the enzyme CYP1A2. Therefore, inhibitors of CYP1A2 can lead to toxic levels of tizanidine. Of clinical significance is fluvoxamine which is contraindicated with tizanidine due to its being shown to increase the plasma level of tizanidine 12-fold. Other CYP1A2 inhibitors including but not limited to oral contraceptives and ciprofloxacin are discouraged in their use with tizanidine [75]. In the setting of hepatic impairment, this drug should be avoided if possible, or significant drug reduction should be used. In the setting of renal dysfunction, the dose should be decreased. Side effects include hypotension, somnolence, and weakness. Occasionally, hepatic dysfunction has been reported. It is recommended to obtain baseline LFTs and BUN/creatinine, along with periodic LFTs, BUN/creatinine, and blood pressure measurements [18, 51].

Clonidine

Clonidine is an alpha-2 agonist which exerts its effects on peripheral nerves, spinal cord, and brain stem. It is used as an alternative in the setting of refractory neuropathic pain. It can also be administered in a variety of ways including transdermal, intrathecal, epidural, perineural, intravenous, and per os [51]. Fifty percent of clonidine undergoes hepatic metabolism via CYP2D6, and other minor hepatic enzymes, and much of the remainder is excreted unchanged in the urine [76, 77]. With this in mind, in the setting of renal or hepatic failure, the dose should be decreased [18]. Side effects include drowsiness, hypotension, rebound hypertension, xerostomia, skin rash, decreased intraocular pressure, and decreased retinal blood flow. Blood pressure should be monitored, and the patient should receive periodic eye exams [18, 78].

Metaxalone

Metaxalone is a skeletal muscle relaxant which acts centrally without working directly on the skeletal muscles but instead possesses sedative properties which indirectly relax the muscles [23]. It is metabolized by CYP1A2, CYP2D6, CYP2E1, and CYP3A4 and to a lesser extent by CYP2C8, CYP2C9, and CYP2C19. In the setting of hepatic failure, LFTs should be followed and dose should be decreased. In patients with renal disease, the dose should also be decreased. Side effects include drowsiness, dizziness, headache, nausea, GI irritability, seizure exacerbation, and increased liver transaminases [11, 18, 23].

Carisoprodol

Carisoprodol is a skeletal muscle relaxant which acts centrally without working directly on the skeletal muscles but instead possesses sedative properties which indirectly relax the muscles [79]. It is broken down by CYP2C19 into its major active metabolite meprobamate. Meprobamate is equipotent with carisoprodol and has a significantly longer half-life compared to its parent compound carisoprodol. Since CYP2C19 exhibits genetic polymorphisms, different races may metabolize carisoprodrol at different rate, which should be considered. In the setting of hepatic and renal failure, the dosage should be reduced. Obtaining baseline BUN/creatinine may aid in identifying underlying renal dysfunction [23]. The main side effect is drowsiness though its dose poses the risk of abuse, which must be considered prior to prescribing this medication [79]. Other side effects include GI irritability, nausea, seizures, pancytopenia, and adverse skin reactions [51].

The Future of Polypharmacy

The future of limiting polypharmacy and drug interaction lies in pharmacogenomics. Of the P450 enzymes, 40 % of the metabolic function takes place by polymorphic enzymes CYP2A6, CYP2C9, CYP2C19, and CYP2D6 [80]. Unfortunately, these polymorphisms lead to interpatient variability, which makes prescribing and administering certain drugs an inexact science at its best. This contributes highly to the reported two million hospitalized patients annually who have severe adverse drug reactions [81].

In December of 2004, the FDA approved AmpliChip CYP450 test. This test uses microarrays to determine if a patient possesses a genetic polymorphism for CYP2D6 or CYP2C19. It will provide information whether a patient is a slow metabolizer versus an ultrarapid metabolizer [82]. This will undoubtedly aid clinicians in dosing and avoid many adverse drug reactions. Future research will give clinicians similar tests to accurately predict drug levels in the setting of polypharmacy and individual genetic polymorphisms.

References

1. Boyd C, et al. Clinical practice guidelines and quality of care for older patients with multiple comorbid diseases, implications for pay for performance. JAMA. 2005;294(6):716–24.
2. Lin P. Drug interactions and polypharmacy in the elderly. Can Alzheimer Dis Rev. 2003;10–4.
3. Gilron I. The role of anticonvulsant drugs in postoperative pain management: a bench-to-bedside perspective. Can J Anaesth. 2006;53:562–71.
4. Misra UK, Kalita J, Rathore C. Phenytoin and carbamazepine cross reactivity: report of a case and review of literature. Postgrad Med J. 2003;79:703–4.
5. Wadzinski J, Franks R, Roane D, Bayard M. Valproate-associated hyperammonemic encephalopathy. J Am Board Fam Med. 2007; 20:499–502.
6. McNamara J. Pharmacotherapies of the epilepsies. Goodman & Gilman's the pharmacological basis of therapeutics. 11th ed. USA: McGraw Hill; 2006.
7. Anderson G. A mechanistic approach to antiepileptic drug interactions. Ann Pharmacother. 1998;32:554–63.
8. Crawford P. Interactions between antiepileptic drugs and hormonal contraception. CNS Drugs. 2002;16(4):263–72.
9. Garnett WR. Clinical pharmacology of topiramate: a review. Epilepsia. 2000;41:S61–5.
10. Browne TR, Szabo GK, Leppik IE, Josephs E, Paz J, Baltes E, Jensen CM. Absence of pharmacokinetic drug interaction of levetiracetam with phenytoin in patients with epilepsy determined by new technique. J Clin Pharmacol. 2000;40:590.
11. Elsevier Health. MD consult web site. Drugs. 2010. Available at: http://www.mdconsult.com/das/pharm/lookup/134025550-4?type=alldrugs. Accessed June 2010.
12. Jensen T. Anticonvulsants in neuropathic pain: rationale and clinical evidence. Eur J Pain. 2002;6:A61–8.
13. Kwan P, Sills GJ, Brodie MJ. The mechanisms of action of commonly used antiepileptic drugs. Pharmacol Ther. 2001;90:21–34.
14. Kutscher EC, Alexander B. A review of the drug interactions with psychiatric medicines for the pharmacy practitioner. J Pharm Pract. 2007;20(4):327–33.
15. Wadzinski J, Franks R, Roane D, Bayard M. Valproate-associated hyperammonemic encephalopathy. JABFM. 2007;20(5):499–502.
16. Mattson RH, Cramer JA, Williamson PD, Novelly RA. Valproic acid in epilepsy: clinical and pharmacological effects. Ann Neurol. 1978;3:20–5.
17. Tohen M, Castillo J, Baldessarini RJ, Zarate Jr C, Kando JC. Blood dyscrasias with carbamazepine and valproate: a pharmacoepidemiological study of 2,228 patients at risk. Am J Psychiatry. 1995; 152(3):413–8.
18. Lexi-Comp Online™, Pediatric Lexi-Drugs Online™, Hudson, Ohio: Lexi-Comp, Inc. 2007; 2010.
19. Ambrosio A, Soares-da-Silva P, Carvalho CM, Carvalho AP. Mechanisms of action of carbamazepine and its derivatives, oxcarbazepine, BIA 2-093, and BIA 2-024. Neurochem Res. 2002; 27:121–30.
20. Baker GB, Fang J, Sinha S, Coutis RT. Metabolic drug interactions with selective serotonin reuptake inhibitor (SSRI) antidepressants. Neurosci Biobehav Rev. 1998;22(2):325–33.
21. Perucca E. Clinically relevant drug interactions with antiepileptic drugs. Br J Clin Pharmacol. 2005;61:246–55.

22. Kumar P, et al. Effect of anticonvulsant drugs on lipid profile in epileptic patients. Int J Neurol. 2004;3(1).

23. Basow DS, editor. UpToDate web site. 2010. Available at: http://utdol.com/online/content/search.do. Accessed June 2010.

24. Kalis MM, Huff NA. Oxcarbazepine, an antiepileptic agent. Clin Ther. 2001;23(5):680–700.

25. Kong VKF, Irwin MG. Gabapentin: a multimodal perioperative drug? Br J Anesth. 2007;99(6):775–86.

26. Hurley R, et al. Gabapentin and pregabalin can interact synergistically with naproxen to produce anti-hyperalgesia. Anesthesiology. 2002;97(5):1263–73.

27. Gilron I, et al. Morphine, gabapentin, or their combination for neuropathic pain. N Engl J Med. 2005;352:1324–34.

28. Stacey BR, Swift JN. Pregabalin for neuropathic pain based recent clinical trials. Curr Pain Headache Rep. 2006;10:179–84.

29. Randinitis EJ, et al. Pharmacokinetics of pregabalin in subjects with various degrees of renal function. J Clin Pharmacol. 2003; 43:277–83.

30. Hachad H, Ragueneau-Majlessi I, Levy RH. New antiepileptic drugs: review on drug interactions. Ther Drug Monit. 2002;24: 91–103.

31. Welsh BJ, Graybeal D, Moe OW, et al. Biochemical and stone-risk profiles with topiramate treatment. Am J Kidney Dis. 2006;48(4): 555–63.

32. Remick RA. Diagnosis and management of depression in primary care: a clinical update and review. CMAJ. 2002;167(11):1253–60.

33. Elliot R. Pharmacokinetic drug interactions of new antidepressants: a review of the effects on the metabolism of other drugs. Mayo Clin Proc. 1997;72:835–47.

34. Ament PW, Bertolino JG, Liszewski JL. Clinically significant drug interactions. Am Fam Physician. 2000;61:1745–54.

35. Carlat D. Laboratory monitoring when prescribing psychotropics. Carlat Psychiatry Rep. 2007;5(8):1, 3, 6, 8.

36. Liu BA, Mittmann N, Knowles SR, Shear NH. Hyponatremia and the syndrome of inappropriate secretion of antidiuretic hormone associated with the use of selective serotonin reuptake inhibitors: review of spontaneous reports. CMAJ. 1996;155:519–27.

37. Christodoulou C, et al. Extrapyramidal side effects and suicidal ideation under fluoxetine treatment: a case report. Ann Gen Psychiatry. 2010;9(5):1–3.

38. Warden S, et al. Inhibition of the serotonin (5-hydroxytryptamine) transporter reduces bone growth accrual during growth. Endocrinology. 2005;146:685–93.

39. The Merck Manual. Unbound Medicine, Inc.; 2010.

40. Herrlin K, et al. Metabolism of citalopram enantiomers in CYP2C19/CYP2D6 phenotyped panels of healthy Swedes. Br J Clin Pharmacol. 2003;56:415–21.

41. Lyengar S, Webster AA, Hemrick-Luecke SK, Xu JY, Simmons RMA. Efficacy of duloxetine, a potent and balanced serotonin-norepinephrine reuptake inhibitor in persistent pain models in rats. JPET. 2004;311(2):576–84.

42. Barkin RL, Fawcett J. The management challenges of chronic pain: the role of antidepressants. Am J Ther. 2000;7:31–47.

43. Gillman PK. Monoamine oxidase inhibitors, opioid analgesics and serotonin toxicity. Br J Anaesth. 2005;95:434–41.

44. Troy SM, Schultz RW, Parker VD, Chiang ST, Blum RA. The effect of renal disease on the disposition of venlafaxine. Clin Pharmacol Ther. 1994;56:14–21.

45. Petroianu G, Schmitt A. First line symptomatic therapy for painful diabetic neuropathy: a tricyclic antidepressant or gabapentin? Int J Diab Metab. 2002;10:1–13.

46. Gillman PK. Tricyclic antidepressant pharmacology and therapeutic drug interactions updated. Br J Pharmacol. 2007;151:737–48.

47. Oleson OV, Linnet K. Hydroxylation and demethylation of the tricyclic antidepressant nortriptyline by cDNA-expressed human cytochrome P-450 isozymes. Drug Metab Dispos. 1997;25(6):740–4.

48. Barkin RL, Barkin D. Pharmacologic management of acute and chronic pain: focus on drug interactions and patient specific pharmacotherapeutic selection. South Med J. 2001;94(8):756–70.

49. Harrigan R, Brady W. ECG abnormalities in tricyclic antidepressant ingestion. Am J Emerg Med. 1999;17:387–93.

50. Wiechers I, Smith F, Stern T. A guide to the judicious use of laboratory tests and diagnostic procedures in psychiatric practice. Psychiatric Times. 2010.

51. Eisenach JC, De Kock M, Klimscha W. Alpha sub 2 -adrenergic agonists for regional anesthesia: a clinical review of clonidine (1984–1995). Anesthesiology. 1996;85(3):655–74.

52. Youdim MBH, Edmondson D, Tipton KF. The therapeutic potential of monoamine oxidase inhibitors. Nat Rev. 2006;7:295–309.

53. Furlan AD, Sandoval JA, Mailis-Gagnon A, Tunks E. Opioid for chronic noncancer pain: a meta-analysis of effectiveness and side effects. CMAJ. 2006;174(11):1589–94.

54. Ballantyne JC, Mao J. Opioid therapy for chronic pain. N Engl J Med. 2003;349:1943–53.

55. White S, Wong S. Standards of laboratory practice: analgesic drug monitoring. Clin Chem. 1998;45(5):1110–23.

56. Caraco Y, Tateishi T, Guengerich FP, Wood AJJ. Microsomal codeine n-demethylation: cosegregation with cytochrome P4503A4 activity. Drug Metab Dispos. 1996;24(7):761–4.

57. Gallego AO, Baron MG, Arranz EE. Oxycodone: a pharmacological and clinical review. Clin Transl Oncol. 2007;9:298–307.

58. Coffman BL, King CD, Rios GR, Tephly TR. The glucuronidation of opioid, other xenobiotics, and androgens by human UGT2B7Y(268) and UGT2B7H(268). Drug Metab Dispos. 1998;26(1):73–7.

59. Miser AW, Narang PK, Dothage JA, Young RC, Sindelar W, Miser JS. Transdermal fentanyl for pain control in patients with cancer. Pain. 1989;39:15–21.

60. Heiskanen T, Matzke S, Haakana S, Gergov M, Vuori E, Kalso E. Transdermal fentanyl in cachectic cancer patients. Pain. 2009;144:218–22.

61. Feierman DE, Lasker JM. Metabolism of fentanyl, a synthetic opioid analgesic, by human liver microsomes. Drug Metab Dispos. 1996;24(9):932–9.

62. Pergolizzi J, et al. Opioids and the management of chronic severe pain in the elderly: consensus statement of an international expert panel with focus on the six clinically most often used world health organization step III opioids (buprenorphine, fentanyl, hydromorphone, methadone, morphine, oxycodone). Pain Pract. 2008;8(4): 287–313.

63. Lalovic B, Phillips B, Risler LL, Howald W, Shen DD. Quantitative contribution of CYP2D6 and CYP3A to oxycodone metabolism in human liver and intestinal microsomes. Drug Metab Dispos. 2004;32(4):447–54.

64. Ripamonti C, Zecca E, Bruera E. An update on the clinical use of methadone for cancer pain. Pain. 1997;70:109–15.

65. Andersen S, Dickenson AH, Kohn M, Reeve A, Rahman W, Ebert B. The opioid ketobemidone has a NMDA blocking effect. Pain. 1996;67:369–74.

66. Toombs J, Kral L. Methadone treatments for pain states. Am Fam Physician. 2005;71:1353–8.

67. Wang J, DeVane CL. Involvement of CYP3A4, CYP2C8, and CYP2D6 in the metabolism of (R)- and (S)-methadone in vitro. Pain. 2003;31(6):742–7.

68. Martell BA, Arnsten JH, Ray B, et al. The impact of methadone induction on cardiac conduction in opiate users. Ann Intern Med. 2003;139(2):154–5.

69. Klotz U. Tramadol – the impact of its pharmacokinetic and pharmacodynamic properties on the clinical management of pain. Arzneim Forsch Drug Res. 2003;53(10):681–7.

70. Grond S, Sablotzki A. Clinical pharmacology of tramadol. Clin Pharmacokinet. 2004;43(13):879–923.

71. Sporer KA. Buprenorphine: a primer for emergency physicians. Ann Emerg Med. 2004;43:580–4.

72. Picard N, Cresteil T, Djebli N, Marquet P. In vitro metabolism study of buprenorphine: evidence for new metabolic pathways. Drug Metab Dispos. 2005;33:689–95.

73. Taikato M, et al. What every psychiatrist should know about buprenorphine in substance misuse. Psychiatr Bull. 2005;29:225–7.

74. Addolorato G, et al. Effectiveness and safety of baclofen for maintenance of alcohol abstinence in alcohol-dependent patients with liver cirrhosis: randomized, double-blind controlled study. Lancet. 2007;370:1915–22.

75. Granfors MT, et al. Fluvoxamine drastically increases concentrations and effects of tizanidine: a potentially hazardous interaction. Clin Pharmacol Ther. 2004;75:331–41.

76. Abraham BK, Adithan C. Genetic polymorphism of CYP2D6. Indian J Pharmacol. 2001;33:147–69.

77. Elliot JA. α_2-Agonists. In: Smith HS, editor. Current therapy in pain. Philadelphia: Saunders; 2009. p. 476–9. Print.

78. Weigert G, Resch H, Luksch A, et al. Intravenous administration of clonidine reduces intraocular pressure and alters ocular blood flow. Br J Ophthalmol. 2007;91:1354–8.

79. Toth P, Urtis J. Commonly used muscle relaxant therapies for acute low back pain: a review of carisoprodol, cyclobenzaprine hydrochloride, and metaxalone. Clin Ther. 2004;26(9):1355–67.

80. Ingelman-Sundberg M, Oscarson M, McLellan R. Polymorphic human cytochrome P450 enzymes: an opportunity for individualized drug treatment. Trends Pharmacol Sci. 1999;20(8):342–9.

81. Phillips K, et al. Potential role of pharmacogenomics in reducing adverse drug reactions: a systematic review. JAMA. 2001;286(18):2270–9.

82. AmpliChip CYP450 test package insert. Roche Molecular Systems, Inc.; 2009.

Role of Cannabinoids in Pain Management

18

Ethan B. Russo and Andrea G. Hohmann

Key Points

- Cannabinoids are pharmacological agents of endogenous (endocannabinoids), botanical (phytocannabinoids), or synthetic origin.
- Cannabinoids alleviate pain through a variety of receptor and non-receptor mechanisms including direct analgesic and anti-inflammatory effects, modulatory actions on neurotransmitters, and interactions with endogenous and administered opioids.
- Cannabinoid agents are currently available in various countries for pain treatment, and even cannabinoids of botanical origin may be approvable by FDA, although this is distinctly unlikely for smoked cannabis.
- An impressive body of literature supports cannabinoid analgesia, and recently, this has been supplemented by an increasing number of phase I–III clinical trials.

Introduction

Plants and Pain

It is a curious fact that we owe a great deal of our insight into pharmacological treatment of pain to the plant world [1]. Willow bark from *Salix* spp. led to development of aspirin and eventual elucidation of the analgesic effects of prostaglandins and their role in inflammation. The opium poppy (*Papaver somniferum*) provided the prototypic narcotic analgesic morphine, the first alkaloid discovered, and stimulated the much later discovery of the endorphin and enkephalin systems. Similarly, the pharmacological properties of cannabis (*Cannabis sativa*) prompted the isolation of Δ^9-tetrahydrocannabinol (THC), the major psychoactive ingredient in cannabis, in 1964 [2]. It is this breakthrough that subsequently prompted the more recent discovery of the body's own cannabis-like system, the endocannabinoid system (ECS), which modulates pain under physiological conditions. Pro-nociceptive mechanisms of the endovanilloid system were similarly revealed by phytochemistry of capsaicin, the pungent ingredient in hot chile peppers (*Capsicum annuum* etc.), which activates transient receptor potential vanilloid receptor-1 (TRPV1). Additional plant products such as the mints and mustards activate other TRP channels to produce their physiological effects.

The Endocannabinoid System

There are three recognized types of cannabinoids: (1) the phytocannabinoids [3] derived from the cannabis plant, (2) synthetic cannabinoids (e.g., ajulemic acid, nabilone, CP55940, WIN55, 212-2) based upon the chemical structure of THC or other ligands which bind cannabinoid receptors, and (3) the endogenous cannabinoids or endocannabinoids. Endocannabinoids are natural chemicals such as anandamide (AEA) and 2-arachidonoylglycerol (2-AG) found in animals whose basic functions are "relax, eat, sleep, forget, and protect" [4]. The endocannabinoid system encompasses the endocannabinoids themselves, their biosynthetic and catabolic enzymes, and their corresponding receptors [5]. AEA is hydrolyzed by the enzyme fatty-acid amide hydrolase (FAAH) into breakdown products arachidonic acid and ethanolamine [6]. By contrast, 2-AG is hydrolyzed primarily by the enzyme monoacylglycerol lipase (MGL) into breakdown products arachidonic acid and glycerol [7] and to a lesser extent by the enzymes ABHD6 and ABHD12. FAAH, a

E.B. Russo, M.D. (✉)
GW Pharmaceuticals,
20402 81st Avenue SW, Vashon, WA 98070, USA

Pharmaceutical Sciences, University of Montana,
Missoula, MT, USA
e-mail: ethanrusso@comcast.net

A.G. Hohmann, Ph.D.
Department of Psychological and Brain Sciences, Indiana University,
101 East 10th Street, Bloomington, IN 47405, USA
e-mail: hohmanna@indiana.edu

T.R. Deer et al. (eds.), *Comprehensive Treatment of Chronic Pain by Medical, Interventional, and Integrative Approaches*,
DOI 10.1007/978-1-4614-1560-2_18, © American Academy of Pain Medicine 2013

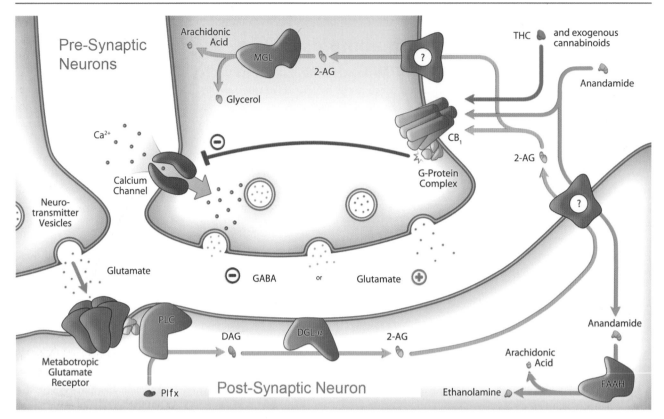

Fig. 18.1 Putative mechanism of endocannabinoid-mediated retrograde signaling in the nervous system. Activation of metabotropic glutamate receptors (*mGluR*) by glutamate triggers the activation of the phospholipase C (*PLC*)-diacylglycerol lipase (*DGL*) pathway to generate the endocannabinoid 2-arachidonoylglycerol (*2-AG*). First, the 2-AG precursor diacylglycerol (*DAG*) is formed from PLC-mediated hydrolysis of membrane phospholipid precursors (*PIPx*). DAG is then hydrolyzed by the enzyme DGL-α to generate 2-AG. 2-AG is released from the postsynaptic neuron and acts as a retrograde signaling molecule. Endocannabinoids activate presynaptic CB_1 receptors which reside on terminals of glutamatergic and GABAergic neurons. Activation of CB_1 by 2-AG, anandamide, or exogenous cannabinoids (e.g., tetrahydrocannabinol, *THC*) inhibits calcium influx in the presynaptic terminal, thereby inhibiting release of the primary neurotransmitter (i.e., glutamate or GABA) from the synaptic vesicle. Endocannabinoids are then rapidly deactivated by transport into cells (via a putative endocannabinoid transporter) followed by intracellular hydrolysis. 2-AG is metabolized by the enzyme monoacylglycerol lipase (*MGL*), whereas anandamide is metabolized by a distinct enzyme, fatty-acid amide hydrolase (*FAAH*). Note that MGL co-localizes with CB_1 in the presynaptic terminal, whereas FAAH is localized to postsynaptic sites. The existence of an endocannabinoid transporter remains controversial. Pharmacological inhibitors of either endocannabinoid deactivation (e.g., FAAH and MGL inhibitors) or transport (i.e., uptake inhibitors) have been developed to exploit the therapeutic potential of the endocannabinoid signaling system in the treatment of pain (Figure by authors with kind assistance of James Brodie, GW Pharmaceuticals)

postsynaptic enzyme, may control anandamide levels near sites of synthesis, whereas MGL, a presynaptic enzyme [8], may terminate 2-AG signaling following CB_1 receptor activation. These enzymes also represent therapeutic targets because inhibition of endocannabinoid deactivation will increase levels of endocannabinoids at sites with ongoing synthesis and release [9]. The pathways controlling formation of AEA remain poorly understood. However, 2-AG is believed to be formed from membrane phospholipid precursors through the sequential activation of two distinct enzymes, phospholipase C and diacylglycerol lipase-α. First, PLC catalyzes formation of the 2-AG precursor diacylglycerol (DAG) from membrane phosphoinositides. Then, DAG is hydrolyzed by the enzyme diacylglycerol lipase-α (DGL-α) to generate 2-AG [199].

There are currently two well-defined cannabinoid receptors, although additional candidate cannabinoid receptors have also been postulated. CB_1, a seven transmembrane spanning G-protein-coupled receptor inhibiting cyclic AMP release, was identified in 1988 [10]. CB_1 is the primary neuromodulatory receptor accounting for psychopharmacological effects of THC and most of its analgesic effects [11]. Endocannabinoids are produced on demand in postsynaptic cells and engage presynaptic CB_1 receptors through a retrograde mechanism [12]. Activation of presynaptic CB_1 receptors then acts as a synaptic circuit breaker to inhibit neurotransmitter release (either excitatory or inhibitory) from the presynaptic neuron (*vide infra*) (Fig. 18.1). CB_2 was identified in 1992, and while thought of primarily as a peripheral immunomodulatory receptor, it also has important effects on pain. The role of CB_2 in modulating persistent inflammatory and neuropathic pain [13] has been recently reviewed [14, 15]. Activation of CB_2 suppresses neuropathic pain mechanisms through nonneuronal (i.e., microglia and astrocytes) and neuronal mechanisms that may involve interferon-gamma [16]. THC, the prototypical classical cannabinoid, is a weak partial agonist at both CB_1 and CB_2 receptors. Transgenic mice lacking cannabinoid receptors (CB_1, CB_2, GPR55), enzymes controlling endocannabinoid breakdown (FAAH, MGL, ABHD6), and endocannabinoid synthesis (DGL-α, DGL-β) have been generated [17]. These knockouts have helped elucidate the role of the endocannabinoid system in controlling nociceptive processing and facilitated development of inhibitors of endocannabinoid breakdown (FAAH, MGL) as novel classes of analgesics.

A Brief Scientific History of Cannabis and Pain

Centuries of Citations

Cannabis has been utilized in one form or another for treatment of pain for longer than written history [18–21]. Although this documentation has been a major preoccupation of the lead author [22–25], and such information can provide provocative direction to inform modern research on treatment of pain and other conditions, it does not represent evidence of form, content, or degree that is commonly acceptable to governmental regulatory bodies with respect to pharmaceutical development.

Anecdotes Versus Modern Proof of Concept

While thousands of compelling stories of efficacy of cannabis in pain treatment certainly underline the importance of properly harnessing cannabinoid mechanisms therapeutically [26, 27], prescription analgesics in the United States necessitate Food and Drug Administration (FDA) approval. This requires a rigorous development program proving consistency, quality, efficacy, and safety as defined by basic scientific studies and randomized controlled trials (RCT) [28] and generally adhering to recent IMMPACT recommendations [29], provoking our next question.

Can a Botanical Agent Become a Prescription Medicine?

Most modern physicians fail to recognize that pharmacognosy (study of medicinal plants) has led directly or indirectly to an estimated 25 % of modern pharmaceuticals [30]. While the plethora of available herbal agents yield an indecipherable cacophony to most clinicians and consumers alike, it is certainly possible to standardize botanical agents and facilitate their recommendation based on sound science [31]. Botanical medicines can even fulfill the rigorous dictates of the FDA and attain prescription drug status via a clear roadmap in the form of a blueprint document [32], henceforth termed the *Botanical Guidance*: http://www.fda.gov/downloads/Drugs/ GuidanceComplianceRegulatoryInformation/Guidances/ ucm070491.pdf. To be successful and clinically valuable, botanicals, including cannabis-based medicines, must demonstrate the same quality, clinical analgesic benefit, and appropriately safe adverse event profile as available new chemical entities (NCE) [28].

The Biochemical and Neurophysiological Basis of Pain Control by Cannabinoids

Neuropathic Pain

Thorough reviews of therapeutic effects of cannabinoids in preclinical and clinical domains have recently been published [33, 34]. In essence, the endocannabinoid system (ECS) is active throughout the CNS and PNS in modulating pain at spinal, supraspinal, and peripheral levels. Endocannabinoids are produced on demand in the CNS to dampen sensitivity to pain [35]. The endocannabinoid system is operative in such key integrative pain centers as the periaqueductal grey matter [36, 37], the ventroposterolateral nucleus of the thalamus [38], and the spinal cord [39, 40]. Endocannabinoids are endogenous mediators of stress-induced analgesia and fear-conditioned analgesia and suppress pain-related phenomena such as windup [41] and allodynia [42]. In the periphery and PNS [13], the ECS has key effects in suppressing both hyperalgesia and allodynia via CB_1 [43] and CB_2 mechanisms (Fig. 18.2). Indeed, pathological pain states have been postulated to arise, at least in part, from a dysregulation of the endocannabinoid system.

Antinociceptive and Anti-inflammatory Pain Mechanisms

Beyond the mechanisms previously mentioned, the ECS plays a critical role in peripheral pain, inflammation, and hyperalgesia [43] through both CB_1 and CB_2 mechanisms. CB_1 and CB_2 mechanisms are also implicated in regulation of contact dermatitis and pruritus [44]. A role for spinal CB_2 mechanisms, mediated by microglia and/or astrocytes, is also revealed under conditions of inflammation [45]. Both THC and cannabidiol (CBD), a non-euphoriant phytocannabinoid common in certain cannabis strains, are potent anti-inflammatory antioxidants with activity exceeding that of

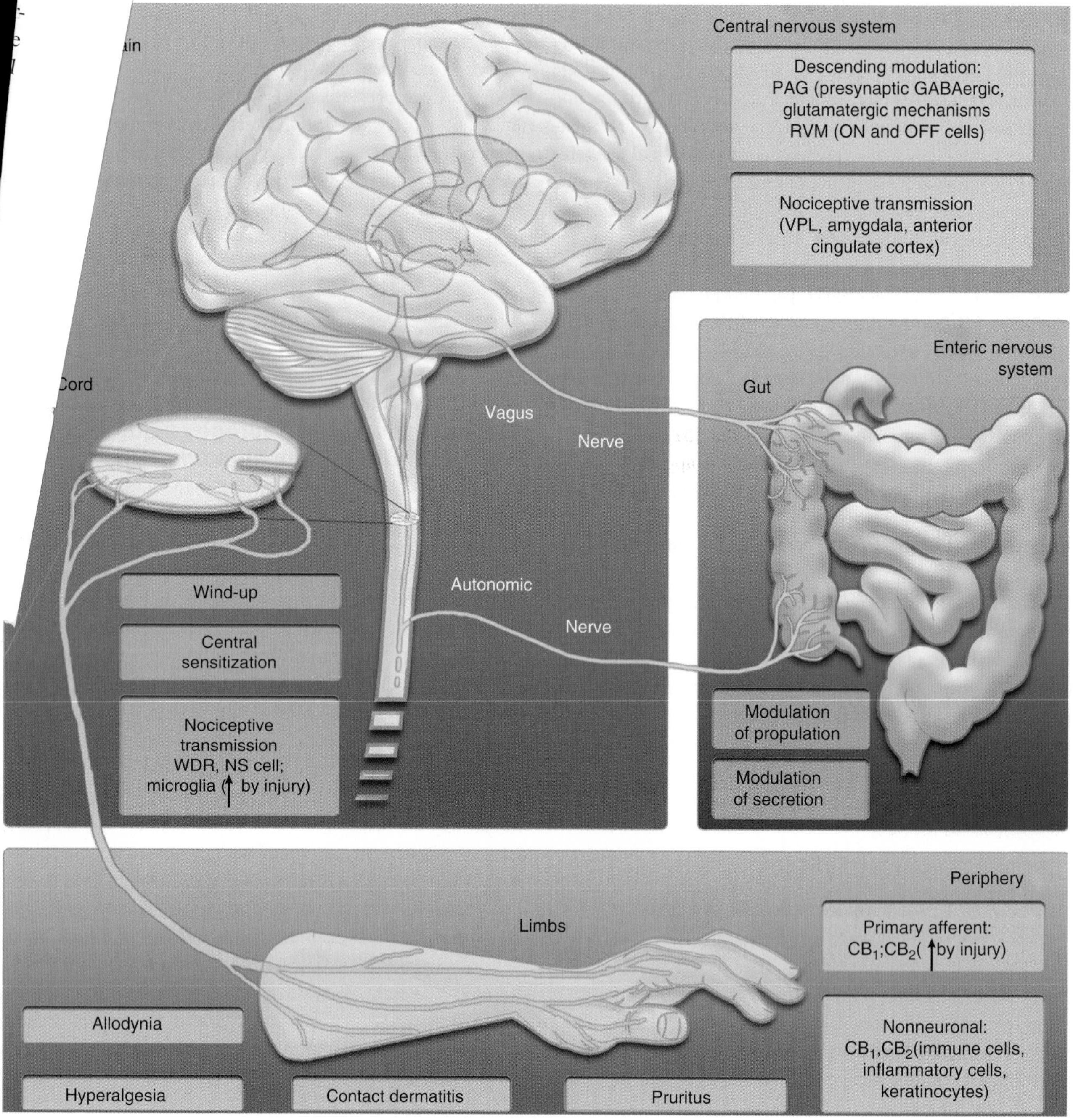

Fig. 18.2 Cannabinoids suppress pain and other pathophysiological (e.g., contact dermatitis, pruritis) and physiological (e.g., gastrointestinal transit and secretion) processes through multiple mechanisms involving CB_1 and CB_2 receptors. Peripheral, spinal, and supraspinal sites of cannabinoid actions are shown. In the periphery, cannabinoids act through both neuronal and nonneuronal mechanisms to control inflammation, allodynia, and hyperalgesia. CB_1 and CB_2 have been localized to both primary afferents and nonneuronal cells (e.g., keratinocytes, microglia), and expression can be regulated by injury. In the spinal cord, cannabinoids suppress nociceptive transmission, windup, and central sensitization by modulating activity in the ascending pain pathway of the spinothalamic tract, including responses of wide dynamic range (*WDR*) and nociceptive specific (*NS*) cells. Similar processes are observed at rostral levels of the neuraxis (e.g., ventroposterolateral nucleus of the thalamus, amygdala, anterior cingulate cortex). Cannabinoids also actively modulate pain through descending mechanisms. In the periaqueductal gray, cannabinoids act through presynaptic glutamatergic and GABAergic mechanisms to control nociception. In the rostral ventromedial medulla, cannabinoids suppress activity in ON cells and inhibit the firing pause of OFF cells, in response to noxious stimulation to produce antinociception (Figure by authors with kind assistance of James Brodie, GW Pharmaceuticals)

vitamins C and E via non-cannabinoid mechanisms [46]. THC inhibits prostaglandin E-2 synthesis [47] and stimulates lipooxygenase [48]. Neither THC nor CBD affects COX-1 or COX-2 at relevant pharmacological dosages [49].

While THC is inactive at vanilloid receptors, CBD, like AEA, is a $TRPV_1$ agonist. Like capsaicin, CBD is capable of inhibiting fatty-acid amide hydrolase (FAAH), the enzyme which hydrolyzes AEA and other fatty-acid amides that do not bind to cannabinoid receptors. CBD additionally inhibits AEA reuptake [50] though not potently. Thus, CBD acts as an endocannabinoid modulator [51], a mechanism that various pharmaceutical firms hope to emulate with new chemical entities (NCEs). CBD inhibits hepatic metabolism of THC to 11-hydroxy-THC, which is possibly more psychoactive, and prolongs its half-life, reducing its psychoactivity and attenuating attendant anxiety and tachycardia [51]; antagonizes psychotic symptoms [52]; and attenuates appetitive effects of THC [53] as well as its effects on short-term memory [54]. CBD also inhibits tumor necrosis factor-alpha (TNF-α) in a rodent model of rheumatoid arthritis [55]. Recently, CBD has been demonstrated to enhance adenosine receptor A2A signaling via inhibition of the adenosine transporter [56].

Recently, GPR18 has been proposed as a putative CBD receptor whose function relates to cellular migration [57]. Antagonism of GPR18 (by agents such as CBD) may be efficacious in treating pain of endometriosis, among other conditions, especially considering that such pain may be endocannabinoid-mediated [58]. Cannabinoids are also very active in various gastrointestinal and visceral sites mediating pain responses [59, 60].

Cannabinoid Interactions with Other Neurotransmitters Pertinent to Pain

As alluded to above, the ECS modulates neurotransmitter release via retrograde inhibition. This is particularly important in NMDA-glutamatergic mechanisms that become hyperresponsive in chronic pain states. Cannabinoids specifically inhibit glutamate release in the hippocampus [61]. THC reduces NMDA responses by 30–40 % [46]. Secondary and tertiary hyperalgesia mediated by NMDA [62] and by calcitonin gene-related peptide [40] may well be targets of cannabinoid therapy in disorders such as migraine, fibromyalgia, and idiopathic bowel syndrome wherein these mechanisms seem to operate pathophysiologically [63], prompting the hypothesis of a "clinical endocannabinoid deficiency." Endocannabinoid modulators may therefore restore homeostasis, leading to normalization of function in these pathophysiological conditions. THC also has numerous effects on serotonergic systems germane to migraine [64], increasing its production in the cerebrum while decreasing reuptake [65]. In fact, the ECS seems to modulate the trigeminovascular system of migraine pathogenesis at vascular and neurochemical levels [66–68].

Cannabinoid-Opioid Interactions

Although endocannabinoids do not bind to opioid receptors, the ECS may nonetheless work in parallel with the endogenous opioid system with numerous areas of overlap and interaction. Pertinent mechanisms include stimulation of beta-endorphin by THC [69] as well as its ability to demonstrate experimental opiate sparing [70], prevent opioid tolerance and withdrawal [71], and rekindle opioid analgesia after loss of effect [72]. Adjunctive treatments that combine opioids with cannabinoids may enhance the analgesic effects of either agent. Such strategies may permit lower doses of analgesics to be employed for therapeutic benefit in a manner that minimizes incidence or severity of adverse side effects.

Clinical Trials, Utility, and Pitfalls of Cannabinoids in Pain

Evidence for Synthetic Cannabinoids

Oral dronabinol (THC) has been available as the synthetic Marinol® since 1985 and is indicated for nausea associated with chemotherapy and appetite stimulation in HIV/AIDS. Issues with its cost, titration difficulties, delayed onset, and propensity to induce intoxicating and dysphoric effects have limited clinical application [73]. It was employed in two open-label studies of chronic neuropathic pain in case studies in 7 [74] and 8 patients [75], but no significant benefit was evident and side effects led to prominent dropout rates (average doses 15–16.6 mg THC). Dronabinol produced benefit in pain in multiple sclerosis [76], but none was evident in postoperative pain (Table 18.1) [77]. Dronabinol was reported to relieve pruritus in three case-report subjects with cholestatic jaundice [78]. Dronabinol was assessed in 30 chronic noncancer pain patients on opioids in double-blind crossover single-day sessions vs. placebo with improvement [79], followed by a 4-week open-label trial with continued improvement (Table 18.1). Associated adverse events were prominent. Methodological issues included lack of prescreening for cannabinoids, 4 placebo subjects with positive THC assays, and 58 % of subjects correctly guessing Marinol dose on test day. An open-label comparison in polyneuropathy examined nabilone patients with 6 obtaining 22.6 % mean pain relief after 3 months, and 5 achieving 28.6 % relief after 6 months, comparable to conventional agents [80]. A pilot study of Marinol in seven spinal cord injury patients with neuropathic pain saw two withdraw, and the remainder appreciate no greater efficacy than with diphenhydramine [81].

Table 18.1 Randomized controlled trials of cannabinoids in pain

Agent	N=	Indication	Duration/type	Outcomes/reference
Ajulemic acid	21	Neuropathic pain	7 day crossover	Visual analogue pain scales improved over placebo ($p=0.02$)/Karst et al. [92]
Cannabis, smoked	50	HIV neuropathy	5 days/DB	Decreased daily pain ($p=0.03$) and hyperalgesia ($p=0.05$), 52 % with >30 % pain reduction vs. placebo ($p=0.04$)/Abrams et al. [94]
Cannabis, smoked	23	Chronic neuropathic pain	5 days/DB	Decreased pain vs. placebo only at 9.4 % THC level ($p=0.023$)/Ware et al. [98]
Cannabis, smoked	38	Neuropathic pain	Single dose/DBC	NSD in pain except at highest cannabis dose ($p=0.02$), with prominent psychoactive effects/Wilsey et al. [95]
Cannabis, smoked	34	HIV neuropathy	5 days /DB	DDS improved over placebo ($p=0.016$), 46 % vs. 18 % improved >30 %, 2 cases toxic psychosis/Ellis et al. [97]
Cannabis, vaporized	21	Chronic pain on opioids	5 days/DB	27 % decrement in pain/Abrams et al. [118]
Cannador	419	Pain due to spasm in MS	15 weeks	Improvement over placebo in subjective pain associated with spasm ($p=0.003$)/Zajicek et al. [120]
Cannador	65	Postherpetic neuralgia	4 weeks	No benefit observed/Ernst et al. [122]
Cannador	30	Postoperative pain	Single doses, daily	Decreasing pain intensity with increased dose ($p=0.01$)/Holdcroft et al. [123]
Marinol	24	Neuropathic pain in MS	15–21 days/DBC	Median numerical pain ($p=0.02$), median pain relief improved ($p=0.035$) over placebo/Svendsen et al. [76]
Marinol	40	Postoperative pain	Single dose/DB	No benefit observed over placebo/Buggy et al. [77]
Marinol	30	Chronic pain	3 doses, 1 day/DBC	Total pain relief improved with 10 mg ($p<0.05$) and 20 mg ($p<0.01$) with opioids, AE prominent/Narang et al. [79]
Nabilone	41	Postoperative pain	3 doses in 24 h/DB	NSD morphine consumption. Increased pain at rest and on movement with nabilone 1 or 2 mg/Beaulieu [85]
Nabilone	31	Fibromyalgia	2 weeks/DBC	Compared to amitriptyline, nabilone improved sleep, decrease wakefulness, had no effect on pain, and increased AE/Ware et al. [90]
Nabilone	96	Neuropathic pain	14 weeks/DBC vs. dihydrocodeine	Dihydrocodeine more effective with fewer AE/Frank et al. [88]
Nabilone	13	Spasticity pain	9 weeks/DBC	NRS decreased 2 points for nabilone ($p<0.05$)/Wissel et al. [87]
Nabilone	40	Fibromyalgia	4 weeks/DBC	VAS decreased in pain, Fibromyalgia Impact Questionnaire, and anxiety over placebo (all, $p<0.02$)/Skrabek et al. [89]
Sativex	20	Neurogenic pain	Series of 2-week N-of-1 crossover blocks	Improvement with Tetranabinex and Sativex on VAS pain vs. placebo ($p<0.05$), symptom control best with Sativex ($p<0.0001$)/Wade et al. [132]
Sativex	24	Chronic intractable pain	12 weeks, series of N-of-1 crossover blocks	VAS pain improved over placebo ($p<0.001$) especially in MS ($p<0.0042$)/Notcutt et al. [133]
Sativex	48	Brachial plexus avulsion	6 weeks in 3 two-week crossover blocks	Benefits noted in Box Scale-11 pain scores with Tetranabinex ($p=0.002$) and Sativex ($p=0.005$) over placebo/Berman et al. [134]
Sativex	66	Central neuropathic pain in MS	5 weeks	Numerical Rating Scale (NRS) analgesia improved over placebo ($p=0.009$)/Rog et al. [135]

(continued)

Table 18.1 (continued)

Agent	N=	Indication	Duration/type	Outcomes/reference
Sativex	125	Peripheral neuropathic pain	5 weeks	Improvements in NRS pain levels ($p=0.004$), dynamic allodynia ($p=0.042$), and punctuate allodynia ($p=0.021$) vs. placebo/Nurmikko et al. [136]
Sativex	56	Rheumatoid arthritis	Nocturnal dosing for 5 weeks	Improvements over placebo morning pain on movement ($p=0.044$), morning pain at rest ($p=0.018$), DAS-28 ($p=0.002$), and SF-MPQ pain at present ($p=0.016$)/Blake et al. [138]
Sativex	117	Pain after spinal injury	10 days	NSD in NRS pain scores, but improved Brief Pain Inventory ($p=0.032$), and Patients' Global Impression of Change ($p=0.001$) (unpublished)
Sativex	177	Intractable cancer pain	2 weeks	Improvements in NRS analgesia vs. placebo ($p=0.0142$), Tetranabinex NSD/Johnson et al. [139]
Sativex	135	Intractable lower urinary tract symptoms in MS	8 weeks	Improved bladder severity symptoms including pain over placebo ($p=0.001$) [200]
Sativex	360	Intractable cancer pain	5 weeks/DB	CRA of lower and middle-dose cohorts improved over placebo ($p=0.006$)/ [201]

Nabilone, or Cesamet®, is a semisynthetic analogue of THC that is about tenfold more potent, and longer lasting [82]. It is indicated as an antiemetic in chemotherapy in the USA. Prior case reports in neuropathic pain [83] and other pain disorders [84] have been published. Sedation and dysphoria are prominent associated adverse events. An RCT of nabilone in 41 postoperative subjects dosed TID actually resulted in increased pain scores (Table 18.1) [85]. An uncontrolled study of 82 cancer patients on nabilone noted improved pain scores [86], but retention rates were limited. Nabilone improved pain ($p<0.05$) vs. placebo in patients with mixed spasticity syndromes in a small double-blind trial (Table 18.1) [87], but was without benefits in other parameters. In a double-blind crossover comparison of nabilone to dihydrocodeine (schedule II opioid) in chronic neuropathic pain (Table 18.1) [88], both drugs produced marginal benefit, but with dihydrocodeine proving clearly superior in efficacy and modestly superior in side-effect profile. In an RCT in 40 patients of nabilone vs. placebo over 4 weeks, it showed significant decreases in VAS of pain and anxiety (Table 18.1) [89]. A more recent study of nabilone vs. amitriptyline in fibromyalgia yielded benefits on sleep, but not pain, mood, or quality of life (Table 18.1) [90]. An open-label trial of nabilone vs. gabapentin found them comparable in pain and other symptom relief in peripheral neuropathic pain [91].

Ajulemic acid (CT3), another synthetic THC analogue in development, was utilized in a phase II RCT in peripheral neuropathic pain in 21 subjects with apparent improvement (Table 18.1) [92]. Whether or not ajulemic acid is psychoactive is the subject of some controversy [93].

Evidence for Smoked or Vaporized Cannabis

Few randomized controlled clinical trials (RCTs) of pain with smoked cannabis have been undertaken to date [94–97]. One of these [96] examined cannabis effects on experimental pain in normal volunteers.

Abrams et al. [94] studied inpatient adults with painful HIV neuropathy in 25 subjects in double-blind fashion to receive either smoked cannabis as 3.56 % THC cigarettes or placebo cigarettes three times daily for 5 days (Table 18.1). The smoked cannabis group had a 34 % reduction in daily pain vs. 17 % in the placebo group ($p=0.03$). The cannabis cohort also had a 52 % of subjects report a >30 % reduction in pain scores over the 5 days vs. 24 % in the placebo group ($p=0.04$) (Table 18.1). The authors rated cannabis as "well tolerated" due to an absence of serious adverse events (AE) leading to withdrawal, but all subjects were cannabis experienced. Symptoms of possible intoxication in the cannabis group including anxiety (25 %), sedation (54 %), disorientation (16 %), paranoia (13 %), confusion (17 %), dizziness (15 %), and nausea (11 %) were all statistically significantly more common than in the placebo group. Despite these findings, the authors stated that the values do not represent any serious safety concern in this short-term study. No discussion in the article addressed issues of the relative efficacy of blinding in the trial.

Wilsey et al. [95] examined neuropathic pain in 38 subjects in a double-blind crossover study comparing 7 % THC cannabis, 3.5 % THC cannabis, and placebo cigarettes via a complex cumulative dosing scheme with each dosage given once, in random order, with at least 3 day intervals separating sessions (Table 18.1). A total of 9 puffs maximum were allowed over several hours per session. Authors stated, "Psychoactive effects were minimal and well-tolerated, but neuropsychological impairment was problematic, particularly with the higher concentration of study medication." Again, only cannabis-experienced subjects were allowed entry. No withdrawals due to AE were reported, but 1 subject was removed due to elevated blood pressure. No significant differences were noted in pain relief in the two cannabis potency groups, but a significant separation of pain reduction from placebo ($p=0.02$) was not evident until a cumulative 9 puffs at 240 min elapsed time. Pain unpleasantness was also reduced in both active treatment groups ($p<0.01$). Subjectively, an "any drug effect" demonstrated a visual analogue scale (VAS) of 60/100 in the high-dose group, but even the low-dose group registered more of a "good drug effect" than placebo ($p<0.001$). "Bad drug effect" was also evident. "Feeling high" and "feeling stoned" were greatest in the high-dose sessions ($p<0.001$), while both high- and low-dose differentiated significantly from placebo ($p<0.05$). Of greater concern, both groups rated impairment as 30/100 on VAS vs. placebo ($p=0.003$). Sedation also demarcated both groups from placebo ($p<0.01$), as did confusion ($p=0.03$), and hunger ($p<0.001$). Anxiety was not considered a prominent feature in this cannabis-experienced population. This study distinguished itself from some others in its inclusion of specific objective neuropsychological measures and demonstrated neurocognitive impairment in attention, learning, and memory, most noteworthy with 7 % THC cannabis. No commentary on blinding efficacy was included.

Ellis et al. [97] examined HIV-associated neuropathic pain in a double-blind trial of placebo vs. 1–8 % THC cannabis administered four times daily over 5 days with a 2-week washout (Table 18.1). Subjects were started at 4 % THC and then titrated upward or downward in four smoking sessions dependent upon their symptom relief and tolerance of the dose. In this study, 96 % of subjects were cannabis-experienced, and 28 out of 34 subjects completed the trial. The primary outcome measure (Descriptor Differential Scale, DDS) was improved in the active group over placebo ($p=0.016$), with >30 % relief noted in 46 % of cannabis subjects vs. 18 % of placebo. While most adverse events (AE) were considered mild and self-limited, two subjects had to leave the trial due to toxicity. One cannabis-naïve subject was withdrawn due to "an acute cannabis-induced psychosis" at what proved to be his first actual cannabis exposure. The other subject suffered intractable cough. Pain reduction was greater in the cannabis-treated group ($p=0.016$) among completers, as was the proportion of subjects attaining >30 % pain reduction (46 % vs. 18 %, $p=0.043$). Blinding was assessed in this study; whereas placebo patients were inaccurate at guessing the investigational product, 93 % of those

receiving cannabis guessed correctly. On safety issues, the authors stated that the frequency of some nontreatment-limiting side effects was greater for cannabis than placebo. These included concentration difficulties, fatigue, sleepiness or sedation, increased duration of sleep, reduced salivation, and thirst.

A Canadian study [98] examined single 25-mg inhalations of various cannabis potencies (0–9.4 % THC) three times daily for 5 days per cycle in 23 subjects with chronic neuropathic pain (Table 18.1). Patients were said to be cannabis-free for 1 year, but were required to have some experience of the drug. Only the highest potency demarcated from placebo on decrements in average daily pain score (5.4 vs. 6.1, $p=0.023$). The most frequent AE in the high-dose group were headache, dry eyes, burning sensation, dizziness, numbness, and cough, but with "high" or "euphoria" reported only once in each cannabis potency group.

The current studies of smoked cannabis are noteworthy for their extremely short-term exposure and would be of uncertain relevance in a regulatory environment. The IMMPACT recommendations on chronic neuropathic pain clinical trials that are currently favored by the FDA [29] generally suggest randomized controlled clinical trials of 12-week duration as a prerequisite to demonstrate efficacy and safety. While one might assume that the degree of pain improvement demonstrated in these trials could be maintained over this longer interval, it is only reasonable to assume that cumulative adverse events would also increase to at least some degree. The combined studies represent only a total of 1,106 patient-days of cannabis exposure (Abrams: 125, Wilsey: 76, Ellis: 560, Ware 345) or 3 patient-years of experience. In contrast, over 6,000 patient-years of data have been analyzed for Sativex between clinical trials, prescription, and named-patient supplies, with vastly lower AE rates (data on file, GW Pharmaceuticals) [28, 99]. Certainly, the cognitive effects noted in California-smoked cannabis studies figure among many factors that would call the efficacy of blinding into question for investigations employing such an approach. However, it is also important to emphasize that unwanted side effects are not unique to cannabinoids. In a prospective evaluation of specific chronic polyneuropathy syndromes and their response to pharmacological therapies, the presence of intolerable side effects did not differ in groups receiving gabapentinoids, tricyclic antidepressants, anticonvulsants, cannabinoids (including nabilone, Sativex), and topical agents [80]. Moreover, no serious adverse events were related to any of the medications.

The current studies were performed in a very select subset of patients who almost invariably have had prior experience of cannabis. Their applicability to cannabis-naïve populations is, thus, quite unclear. At best, the observed benefits might possibly accrue to some, but it is eminently likely that candidates for such therapy might refuse it on any number of grounds: not wishing to smoke, concern with respect to intoxication, etc. Sequelae of smoking in therapeutic outcomes have had little discussion in these brief RCTs [28]. Cannabis smoking poses substantial risk of chronic cough and bronchitic symptoms [100], if not obvious emphysematous degeneration [101] or increase in aerodigestive cancers [102]. Even such smoked cannabis proponents as Lester Grinspoon has acknowledged are the only well-confirmed deleterious physical effect of marihuana is harm to the pulmonary system [103]. However, population-based studies of cannabis trials have failed to show any evidence for increased risk of respiratory symptoms/chronic obstructive pulmonary disease [100] or lung cancer [102] associated with smoking cannabis.

A very detailed analysis and comparison of mainstream and sidestream smoke for cannabis vs. tobacco smoke was performed in Canada [104]. Of note, cannabis smoke contained ammonia (NH_3) at a level of 720 µg per 775 mg cigarette, a figure 20-fold higher than that found in tobacco smoke. It was hypothesized that this finding was likely attributable to nitrate fertilizers. Formaldehyde and acetaldehyde were generally lower in cannabis smoke than in tobacco, but butyraldehyde was higher. Polycyclic aromatic hydrocarbon (PAH) contents were qualitatively similar in the comparisons, but total yield was lower for cannabis mainstream smoke, but higher than tobacco for sidestream smoke. Additionally, NO, NO_x, hydrogen cyanide, and aromatic amines concentrations were 3–5 times higher in cannabis smoke than that from tobacco. Possible mutagenic and carcinogenic potential of these various compounds were mentioned. More recently, experimental analysis of cannabis smoke with resultant acetaldehyde production has posited its genotoxic potential to be attributable to reactions that produce DNA adducts [105].

Vaporizers for cannabis have been offered as a harm reduction technique that would theoretically eliminate products of combustion and associated adverse events. The Institute of Medicine (IOM) examined cannabis issues in 1999 [106], and among their conclusions was the following (p. 4): "Recommendation 2: Clinical trials of cannabinoid drugs for symptom management should be conducted with the goal of developing rapid-onset, reliable, and safe delivery systems." One proposed technique is vaporization, whereby cannabis is heated to a temperature that volatilizes THC and other components with the goal of reducing or eliminating by-products of combustion, including potentially carcinogenic polycyclic aromatic hydrocarbons, benzene, acetaldehyde, carbon monoxide, toluene, naphthaline, phenol, toluene, hydrogen cyanide, and ammonia. Space limitations permit only a cursory review of available literature [107–115].

A pilot study of the Volcano vaporizer vs. smoking was performed in the USA in 2007 in 18 active cannabis consumers, with only 48 h of presumed abstinence [116]. NIDA 900-mg cannabis cigarettes were employed (1.7, 3.4, and 6.8 % THC) with each divided in two, so that one-half would be smoked or vaporized in a series of double-blind sessions. The Volcano vaporizer produced comparable or slightly higher THC plasma concentrations than smoking. Measured CO in exhaled vapor sessions diminished very slightly, while it increased after smoking ($p < 0.001$). Self-reported visual analogue scales of the associated high were virtually identical in vaporization vs. smoking sessions and increased with higher potency material. A contention was advanced that the absence of CO increase after vaporization can be equated to "little or no exposure to gaseous combustion toxins." Given that no measures of PAH or other components were undertaken, the assertion is questionable. It was also stated that there were no reported adverse events. Some 12 subjects preferred the Volcano, 2 chose smoking, and 2 had no preference as to technique, making the vaporizer "an acceptable system" and providing "a safer way to deliver THC."

A recent [202, 117] examined interactions of 3.2 % THC NIDA cannabis vaporized in the Volcano in conjunction with opioid treatment in a 5-day inpatient trial in 21 patients with chronic pain (Table 18.1). All subjects were prior cannabis smokers. Overall, pain scores were reduced from 39.6 to 29.1 on a VAS, a 27 % reduction, by day 5. Pain scores in subjects on morphine fell from 34.8 to 24.1, while in subjects taking oxycodone, scores dropped from 43.8 to 33.6.

The clinical studies performed with vaporizers to date have been very small pilot studies conducted over very limited timeframes (i.e., for a maximum of 5 days). Thus, these studies cannot contribute in any meaningful fashion toward possible FDA approval of vaporized cannabis as a delivery technique, device, or drug under existing policies dictated by the *Botanical Guidance* [32]. It is likewise quite unlikely that the current AE profile of smoked or vaporized cannabis would meet FDA requirements. The fact that all the vaporization trials to date have been undertaken only in cannabis-experienced subjects does not imply that results would generalize to larger patient populations. Moreover, there is certainly no reason to expect AE profiles to be better in cannabis-naïve patients. Additionally, existing standardization of cannabis product and delivery via vaporization seem far off the required marks. Although vaporizers represent an alternate delivery method devoid of the illegality associated with smoked cannabis, the presence of toxic ingredients such as PAH, ammonia, and acetaldehyde in cannabis vapor are unlikely to be acceptable to FDA in any significant amounts. Existing vaporizers still lack portability or convenience [28]. A large Internet survey revealed that only 2.2 % of cannabis users employed vaporization as their primary cannabis intake method [118]. While studies to date have established that lower temperature vaporization in the Volcano, but not necessarily other devices, can reduce the relative amounts of noxious by-products of combustion, it has yet to be demonstrated that they are totally eliminated. Until or unless this goal is achieved, along with requisite benchmarks of herbal cannabis quality, safety, and efficacy in properly designed randomized clinical trials, vaporization remains an unproven technology for therapeutic cannabinoid administration.

Evidence for Cannabis-Based Medicines

Cannador is a cannabis extract in oral capsules, with differing THC:CBD ratios [51]. Cannador was utilized in a phase III RCT of spasticity in multiple sclerosis (CAMS) (Table 18.1) [119]. While no improvement was evident in the Ashworth Scale, reduction was seen in spasm-associated pain. Both THC and Cannador improved pain scores in follow-up [120]. Cannador was also employed for postherpetic neuralgia in 65 patients, but without success (Table 18.1) [121, 122]. Slight pain reduction was observed in 30 subjects with postoperative pain (CANPOP) not receiving opiates, but psychoactive side effects were notable (Table 18.1).

Sativex® is a whole-cannabis-based extract delivered as an oromucosal spray that combines a CB_1 and CB_2 partial agonist (THC) with a cannabinoid system modulator (CBD), minor cannabinoids, and terpenoids plus ethanol and propylene glycol excipients and peppermint flavoring [51, 123]. It is approved in Canada for spasticity in MS and under a Notice of Compliance with Conditions for central neuropathic pain in multiple sclerosis and treatment of cancer pain unresponsive to opioids. Sativex is also approved in MS in the UK, Spain, and New Zealand, for spasticity in multiple sclerosis, with further approvals expected soon in some 22 countries around the world. Sativex is highly standardized and is formulated from two *Cannabis sativa* chemovars predominating in THC and CBD, respectively [124]. Each 100 μl pump-action oromucosal spray of Sativex yields 2.7 mg of THC and 2.5 mg of CBD plus additional components. Pharmacokinetic data are available [125–127]. Sativex effects begin within an interval allowing dose titration. A very favorable adverse event profile has been observed in the development program [27, 128]. Most patients stabilize at 8–10 sprays per day after 7–10 days, attaining symptomatic control without undue psychoactive sequelae. Sativex was added to optimized drug regimens in subjects with uncontrolled pain in every RCT (Table 18.1). An Investigational New Drug (IND) application to study Sativex in advanced clinical trials in the USA was approved by the FDA in January 2006 in patients with intractable cancer pain. One phase IIB dose-ranging study has already been completed [201]. Available clinical trials with Sativex have been independently assessed [129, 130].

In a phase II study of 20 patients with neurogenic symptoms [131], significant improvement was seen with both Tetranabinex (high-THC extract without CBD) and Sativex on pain, with Sativex displaying better symptom control ($p < 0.0001$), with less intoxication (Table 18.1).

In a phase II study of intractable chronic pain in 24 patients [132], Sativex again produced the best results compared to Tetranabinex ($p < 0.001$), especially in MS ($p < 0.0042$) (Table 18.1).

In a phase III study of brachial plexus avulsion ($N = 48$) [133], pain reduction with Tetranabinex and Sativex was about equal (Table 18.1).

In an RCT of 66 MS subjects, mean Numerical Rating Scale (NRS) analgesia favored Sativex over placebo (Table 18.1) [134].

In a phase III trial ($N = 125$) of peripheral neuropathic pain with allodynia [135], Sativex notably alleviated pain levels and dynamic and punctate allodynia (Table 18.1).

In a safety-extension study in 160 subjects with various symptoms of MS [136], 137 patients showed sustained improvements over a year or more in pain and other symptoms [99] without development of any tolerance requiring dose escalation or withdrawal effects in those who voluntarily discontinued treatment suddenly. Analgesia was quickly reestablished upon Sativex resumption.

In a phase II RCT in 56 rheumatoid arthritis sufferers over 5 weeks with Sativex [137], medicine was limited to only 6 evening sprays (16.2 mg THC + 15 mg CBD). By study end, morning pain on movement, morning pain at rest, DAS-28 measure of disease activity, and SF-MPQ pain all favored Sativex (Table 18.1).

In a phase III RCT in intractable cancer pain on opioids ($N = 177$), Sativex, Tetranabinex THC-predominant extract, and placebo were compared [138] demonstrating strongly statistically significant improvements in analgesia for Sativex only (Table 18.1). This suggests that the CBD component in Sativex was necessary for benefit.

In a 2-week study of spinal cord injury pain, NRS of pain was not statistically different from placebo, probably due to the short duration of the trial, but secondary endpoints were positive (Table 18.1). Additionally, an RCT of intractable lower urinary tract symptoms in MS also demonstrated pain reduction (Table 18.1).

The open-label study of various polyneuropathy patients included Sativex patients with 3 obtaining 21.56 % mean pain relief after 3 months (2/3 > 30 %), and 4 achieving 27.6 % relief after 6 months (2/4 > 30 %), comparable to conventional agents [80].

A recently completed RCT of Sativex in intractable cancer pain unresponsive to opioids over 5 weeks was performed in 360 subjects (Table 18.1). Results of a Continuous Response Analysis (CRA) showed improvements over placebo in the low-dose ($p = 0.08$) and middle-dose cohorts ($p = 0.038$) or combined ($p = 0.006$). Pain NRS improved over placebo in the low-dose ($p = 0.006$) and combined cohorts ($p = 0.019$).

Sleep has improved markedly in almost all Sativex RCTs in chronic pain based on symptom reduction, not a hypnotic effect [139].

The adverse event (AE) profile of Sativex has been quite benign with bad taste, oral stinging, dry mouth, dizziness, nausea, or fatigue most common, but not usually prompting discontinuation [128]. Most psychoactive sequelae are early and transient and have been notably lowered by more recent application of a slower, less aggressive titration schedule. While no direct comparative studies have been performed with Sativex and other agents, AE rates were comparable or greater with Marinol than with Sativex employing THC dosages some 2.5 times higher, likely due to the presence of accompanying CBD [28, 51]. Similarly, Sativex displayed a superior AE profile compared to smoked cannabis based on safety-extension studies of Sativex [28, 99], as compared to chronic use of cannabis with standardized government-supplied material in Canada for chronic pain [140] and the Netherlands for various indications [141, 142] over a period of several months or more. All AEs are more frequent with smoked cannabis, except for nausea and dizziness, both early and usually transiently reported with Sativex [27, 28, 128]. A recent meta-analysis suggested that serious AEs associated with cannabinoid-based medications did not differ from placebo and thus could not be attributable to cannabinoid use, further reinforcing the low toxicity associated with activation of cannabinoid systems.

Cannabinoid Pitfalls: Are They Surmountable?

The dangers of COX-1 and COX-2 inhibition by nonsteroidal anti-inflammatory drugs (NSAIDS) of various design (e.g., gastrointestinal ulceration and bleeding vs. coronary and cerebrovascular accidents, respectively) [143, 144] are unlikely to be mimicked by either THC or CBD, which produce no such activity at therapeutic dosages [49].

Natural cannabinoids require polar solvents and may be associated with delayed and sometimes erratic absorption after oral administration. Smoking of cannabis invariably produces rapid spikes in serum THC levels; cannabis smoking attains peak levels of serum THC above 140 ng/ml [145, 146], which, while desirable to the recreational user, has no necessity or advantage for treatment of chronic pain [28]. In contrast, comparable amounts of THC derived from oromucosal Sativex remained below 2 ng/ml with much lower propensity toward psychoactive sequelae [28, 125], with subjective intoxication levels on visual analogue scales that are indistinguishable from placebo, in the single digits out of 100 [100]. It is clear from RCTs that such psychoactivity is not a necessary accompaniment to pain control. In contrast, intoxication has continued to be prominent with oral THC [73].

In comparison to the questionable clinical trial blinding with smoked and vaporized cannabis discussed above, all indications are that such study blinding has been demonstrably effective with Sativex [147, 148] by utilizing a placebo spray with identical taste and color. Some 50 % of Sativex subjects in RCTs have had prior cannabis exposure, but results of two studies suggest that both groups exhibited comparable results in both treatment efficacy and side effect profile [134, 135].

Controversy continues to swirl around the issue of the potential dangers of cannabis use medicinally, particularly its drug abuse liability (DAL). Cannabis and cannabinoids are currently DEA schedule I substances and are forbidden in the USA (save for Marinol in schedule III and nabilone in schedule II) [73]. This is noteworthy in itself because the very same chemical compound, THC, appears simultaneously in schedule I (as THC), schedule II (as nabilone), and schedule III (as Marinol). DAL is assessed on the basis of five elements: intoxication, reinforcement, tolerance, withdrawal, and dependency plus the drug's overall observed rates of abuse and diversion. Drugs that are smoked or injected are commonly rated as more reinforcing due to more rapid delivery to the brain [149]. Sativex has intermediate onset. It is claimed that CBD in Sativex reduces the psychoactivity of THC [28]. RCT AE profiles do not indicate euphoria or other possible reinforcing psychoactive indicia as common problems with its use [99]. Similarly, acute THC effects such as tachycardia, hypothermia, orthostatic hypotension, dry mouth, ocular injection, and intraocular pressure decreases undergo prominent tachyphylaxis with regular usage [150]. Despite that observation, Sativex has not demonstrated dose tolerance to its therapeutic benefits on prolonged administration, and efficacy has been maintained for up to several years in pain conditions [99].

The existence or severity of a cannabis withdrawal syndrome remains under debate [151, 152]. In contrast to reported withdrawal sequelae in recreational users [153], 24 subjects with MS who volunteered to discontinue Sativex after a year or more suffered no withdrawal symptoms meeting Budney criteria. While symptoms such as pain recurred after some 7–10 days without Sativex, symptom control was rapidly reattained upon resumption [99].

Finally, no known abuse or diversion incidents have been reported with Sativex to date (March 2011). Formal DAL studies of Sativex vs. Marinol and placebo have been completed and demonstrate lower scores on drug liking and similar measures at comparable doses [155].

Cognitive effects of cannabis also remain at issue [155, 156], but less data are available in therapeutic applications. Studies of Sativex in neuropathic pain with allodynia have revealed no changes vs. placebo on Sativex in portions of the Halstead-Reitan Battery [135], or in central neuropathic pain in MS [134], where 80 % of tests showed no significant differences. In a recent RCT of Sativex vs. placebo in MS patients, no cognitive differences of note were observed

[157]. Similarly, chronic Sativex use has not produced observable mood disorders.

Controversies have also arisen regarding the possible association of cannabis abuse and onset of psychosis [156]. However, an etiological relationship is not supported by epidemiological data [158–161], but may well be affected by dose levels and duration, if pertinent. One may speculate that lower serum levels of Sativex combined with antipsychotic properties of CBD [52, 162, 163] might attenuate such concerns. Few cases of related symptoms have been reported in SAFEX studies of Sativex.

Immune function becomes impaired in experimental animals at cannabinoid doses 50–100 times necessary to produce psychoactive effects [164]. In four patients smoking cannabis medicinally for more than 20 years, no changes were evident in leukocyte, CD4, or CD8 cell counts [155]. MS patients on Cannador demonstrated no immune changes of note [165] nor were changes evident in subjects smoking cannabis in a brief trial in HIV patients [166]. Sativex RCTs have demonstrated no hematological or immune dysfunction.

No effects of THC extract, CBD extract, or Sativex were evident on the hepatic cytochrome P450 complex [167] or on human CYP450 [168]. Similarly, while Sativex might be expected to have additive sedative effects with other drugs or alcohol, no significant drug-drug interactions of any type have been observed in the entire development program to date.

No studies have demonstrated significant problems in relation to cannabis affecting driving skills at plasma levels below 5 ng/ml of THC [169]. Four oromucosal sprays of Sativex (exceeding the average single dose employed in therapy) produced serum levels well below this threshold [28]. As with other cannabinoids in therapy, it is recommended that patients not drive nor use dangerous equipment until accustomed to the effects of the drug.

Future Directions: An Array of Biosynthetic and Phytocannabinoid Analgesics

Inhibition of Endocannabinoid Transport and Degradation: A Solution?

It is essential that any cannabinoid analgesic strike a compromise between therapeutic and adverse effects that may both be mediated via CB_1 mechanisms [34]. Mechanisms to avoid psychoactive sequelae could include peripherally active synthetic cannabinoids that do not cross the blood-brain barrier or drugs that boost AEA levels by inhibiting fatty-acid amide hydrolase (FAAH) [170] or that of 2-AG by inhibiting monoacylcerol lipase (MGL). CBD also has this effect [50] and certainly seems to increase the therapeutic index of THC [51].

In preclinical studies, drugs inhibiting endocannabinoid hydrolysis [171, 172] and peripherally acting agonists [173] all

show promise for suppressing neuropathic pain. AZ11713908, a peripherally restricted mixed cannabinoid agonist, reduces mechanical allodynia with efficacy comparable to the brain penetrant mixed cannabinoid agonist WIN55,212-2 [173]. An irreversible inhibitor of the 2-AG hydrolyzing enzyme MGL suppresses nerve injury-induced mechanical allodynia through a CB_1 mechanism, although these anti-allodynic effects undergo tolerance following repeated administration [172]. URB937, a brain impermeant inhibitor of FAAH, has recently been shown to elevate anandamide outside the brain and suppress neuropathic and inflammatory pain behavior without producing tolerance or unwanted CNS side effects [171]. These observations raise the possibility that peripherally restricted endocannabinoid modulators may show therapeutic potential as analgesics with limited side-effect profiles.

The Phytocannabinoid and Terpenoid Pipeline

Additional phytocannabinoids show promise in treatment of chronic pain [123, 163, 174]. Cannabichromene (CBC), another prominent phytocannabinoid, also displays anti-inflammatory [175] and analgesic properties, though less potently than THC [176]. CBC, like CBD, is a weak inhibitor of AEA reuptake [177]. CBC is additionally a potent TRPA1 agonist [178]. Cannabigerol (CBG), another phytocannabinoid, displays weak binding at both CB_1 and CB_2 [179, 180] but is a more potent GABA reuptake inhibitor than either THC or CBD [181]. CBG is a stronger analgesic, anti-erythema, and lipooxygenase agent than THC [182]. CBG likewise inhibits AEA uptake and is a TRPV1 agonist [177], a TRPA1 agonist, and a TRPM8 antagonist [178]. CBG is also a phospholipase A2 modulator that reduces PGE-2 release in synovial cells [183]. Tetrahydrocannabivarin, a phytocannabinoid present in southern African strains, displays weak CB_1 antagonism [184] and a variety of anticonvulsant activities [185] that might prove useful in chronic neuropathic pain treatment. THCV also reduced inflammation and attendant pain in mouse experiments [187]. Most North American [187] and European [188, 189] cannabis strains have been bred to favor THC over a virtual absence of other phytocannabinoid components, but the latter are currently available in abundance via selective breeding [124, 190].

Aromatic terpenoid components of cannabis also demonstrate pain reducing activity [123, 163]. Myrcene displays an opioid-type analgesic effect blocked by naloxone [191] and reduces inflammation via PGE-2 [192]. β-Caryophyllene displays anti-inflammatory activity on par with phenylbutazone via PGE-1 [193], but contrasts by displaying gastric cytoprotective activity [194]. Surprisingly, β-caryophyllene has proven to be a phytocannabinoid in its own right as a selective CB_2 agonist [195]. α-Pinene inhibits PGE-1 [196], and linalool acts as a local anesthetic [197].

Summary

Basic science and clinical trials support the theoretical and practical basis of cannabinoid agents as analgesics for chronic pain. Their unique pharmacological profiles with multimodality effects and generally favorable efficacy and safety profiles render cannabinoid-based medicines promising agents for adjunctive treatment, particularly for neuropathic pain. It is our expectation that the coming years will mark the advent of numerous approved cannabinoids with varying mechanisms of action and delivery techniques that should offer the clinician useful new tools for treating pain.

References

1. Di Marzo V, Bisogno T, De Petrocellis L. Endocannabinoids and related compounds: walking back and forth between plant natural products and animal physiology. Chem Biol. 2007;14(7):741–56.
2. Gaoni Y, Mechoulam R. Isolation, structure and partial synthesis of an active constituent of hashish. J Am Chem Soc. 1964;86:1646–7.
3. Pate D. Chemical ecology of cannabis. J Int Hemp Assoc. 1994;2:32–7.
4. Di Marzo V, Melck D, Bisogno T, De Petrocellis L. Endocannabinoids: endogenous cannabinoid receptor ligands with neuromodulatory action. Trends Neurosci. 1998;21(12):521–8.
5. Pacher P, Batkai S, Kunos G. The endocannabinoid system as an emerging target of pharmacotherapy. Pharmacol Rev. 2006;58(3):389–462.
6. Cravatt BF, Giang DK, Mayfield SP, Boger DL, Lerner RA, Gilula NB. Molecular characterization of an enzyme that degrades neuromodulatory fatty-acid amides. Nature. 1996;384(6604):83–7.
7. Dinh TP, Freund TF, Piomelli D. A role for monoglyceride lipase in 2-arachidonoylglycerol inactivation. Chem Phys Lipids. 2002;121(1–2):149–58.
8. Gulyas AI, Cravatt BF, Bracey MH, et al. Segregation of two endocannabinoid-hydrolyzing enzymes into pre- and postsynaptic compartments in the rat hippocampus, cerebellum and amygdala. Eur J Neurosci. 2004;20(2):441–58.
9. Mangieri RA, Piomelli D. Enhancement of endocannabinoid signaling and the pharmacotherapy of depression. Pharmacol Res. 2007;56(5):360–6.
10. Howlett AC, Johnson MR, Melvin LS, Milne GM. Nonclassical cannabinoid analgetics inhibit adenylate cyclase: development of a cannabinoid receptor model. Mol Pharmacol. 1988;33(3):297–302.
11. Zimmer A, Zimmer AM, Hohmann AG, Herkenham M, Bonner TI. Increased mortality, hypoactivity, and hypoalgesia in cannabinoid CB1 receptor knockout mice. Proc Natl Acad Sci USA. 1999;96(10):5780–5.
12. Wilson RI, Nicoll RA. Endogenous cannabinoids mediate retrograde signalling at hippocampal synapses. Nature. 2001;410(6828):588–92.
13. Ibrahim MM, Porreca F, Lai J, et al. CB2 cannabinoid receptor activation produces antinociception by stimulating peripheral release of endogenous opioids. Proc Natl Acad Sci USA. 2005;102(8):3093–8.
14. Guindon J, Hohmann AG. Cannabinoid CB2 receptors: a therapeutic target for the treatment of inflammatory and neuropathic pain. Br J Pharmacol. 2008;153(2):319–34.
15. Pacher P, Mechoulam R. Is lipid signaling through cannabinoid 2 receptors part of a protective system? Prog Lipid Res. 2011;50:193–211.
16. Racz I, Nadal X, Alferink J, et al. Interferon-gamma is a critical modulator of CB(2) cannabinoid receptor signaling during neuropathic pain. J Neurosci. 2008;28(46):12136–45.
17. Guindon J, Hohmann AG. The endocannabinoid system and pain. CNS Neurol Disord Drug Targets. 2009;8(6):403–21.
18. Fankhauser M. History of cannabis in Western medicine. In: Grotenhermen F, Russo EB, editors. Cannabis and cannabinoids: pharmacology, toxicology and therapeutic potential. Binghamton: Haworth Press; 2002. p. 37–51.
19. Russo EB. History of cannabis as medicine. In: Guy GW, Whittle BA, Robson P, editors. Medicinal uses of cannabis and cannabinoids. London: Pharmaceutical Press; 2004. p. 1–16.
20. Russo EB. History of cannabis and its preparations in saga, science and sobriquet. Chem Biodivers. 2007;4(8):2624–48.
21. Mechoulam R. The pharmacohistory of Cannabis sativa. In: Mechoulam R, editor. Cannabinoids as therapeutic agents. Boca Raton: CRC Press; 1986. p. 1–19.
22. Russo E. Cannabis treatments in obstetrics and gynecology: a historical review. J Cannabis Ther. 2002;2(3–4):5–35.
23. Russo EB. Hemp for headache: an in-depth historical and scientific review of cannabis in migraine treatment. J Cannabis Ther. 2001;1(2):21–92.
24. Russo EB. The role of cannabis and cannabinoids in pain management. In: Cole BE, Boswell M, editors. Weiner's pain management: a practical guide for clinicians. 7th ed. Boca Raton: CRC Press; 2006. p. 823–44.
25. Russo EB. Cannabis in India: ancient lore and modern medicine. In: Mechoulam R, editor. Cannabinoids as therapeutics. Basel: Birkhäuser Verlag; 2005. p. 1–22.
26. ABC News, USA Today, Stanford Medical Center Poll. Broad experience with pain sparks search for relief. 9 May 2005.
27. Russo EB. Cannabinoids in the management of difficult to treat pain. Ther Clin Risk Manag. 2008;4(1):245–59.
28. Russo EB. The solution to the medicinal cannabis problem. In: Schatman ME, editor. Ethical issues in chronic pain management. Boca Raton: Taylor & Francis; 2006. p. 165–94.
29. Dworkin RH, Turk DC, Farrar JT, et al. Core outcome measures for chronic pain clinical trials: IMMPACT recommendations. Pain. 2005;113(1–2):9–19.
30. Tyler VE. Phytomedicines in Western Europe: potential impact on herbal medicine in the United States. In: Kinghorn AD, Balandrin MF, editors. Human medicinal agents from plants (ACS symposium, No. 534). Washington, D.C.: American Chemical Society; 1993. p. 25–37.
31. Russo EB. Handbook of psychotropic herbs: a scientific analysis of herbal remedies for psychiatric conditions. Binghamton: Haworth Press; 2001.
32. Food and Drug Administration. Guidance for industry: botanical drug products. In: Services UDoHaH, editor. US Government; 2004. p. 48. http://www.fda.gov/downloads/Drugs/GuidanceCompliance RegulatoryInformation/Guidances/ucm070491.pdf.
33. Walker JM, Hohmann AG. Cannabinoid mechanisms of pain suppression. Handb Exp Pharmacol. 2005;168:509–54.
34. Rahn EJ, Hohmann AG. Cannabinoids as pharmacotherapies for neuropathic pain: from the bench to the bedside. Neurotherapeutics. 2009;6(4):713–37.
35. Richardson JD, Aanonsen L, Hargreaves KM. SR 141716A, a cannabinoid receptor antagonist, produces hyperalgesia in untreated mice. Eur J Pharmacol. 1997;319(2–3):R3–4.
36. Walker JM, Huang SM, Strangman NM, Tsou K, Sanudo-Pena MC. Pain modulation by the release of the endogenous cannabinoid anandamide. Proc Natl Acad Sci. 1999;96(21):12198–203.
37. Walker JM, Hohmann AG, Martin WJ, Strangman NM, Huang SM, Tsou K. The neurobiology of cannabinoid analgesia. Life Sci. 1999;65(6–7):665–73.
38. Martin WJ, Hohmann AG, Walker JM. Suppression of noxious stimulus-evoked activity in the ventral posterolateral nucleus of the

thalamus by a cannabinoid agonist: correlation between electrophysiological and antinociceptive effects. J Neurosci. 1996;16: 6601–11.

39. Hohmann AG, Martin WJ, Tsou K, Walker JM. Inhibition of noxious stimulus-evoked activity of spinal cord dorsal horn neurons by the cannabinoid WIN 55,212-2. Life Sci. 1995;56(23–24):2111–8.

40. Richardson JD, Aanonsen L, Hargreaves KM. Antihyperalgesic effects of spinal cannabinoids. Eur J Pharmacol. 1998;345(2):145–53.

41. Strangman NM, Walker JM. Cannabinoid WIN 55,212-2 inhibits the activity-dependent facilitation of spinal nociceptive responses. J Neurophysiol. 1999;82(1):472–7.

42. Rahn EJ, Makriyannis A, Hohmann AG. Activation of cannabinoid CB(1) and CB(2) receptors suppresses neuropathic nociception evoked by the chemotherapeutic agent vincristine in rats. Br J Pharmacol. 2007;152:765–77.

43. Richardson JD, Kilo S, Hargreaves KM. Cannabinoids reduce hyperalgesia and inflammation via interaction with peripheral CB1 receptors. Pain. 1998;75(1):111–9.

44. Karsak M, Gaffal E, Date R, et al. Attenuation of allergic contact dermatitis through the endocannabinoid system. Science. 2007;316(5830):1494–7.

45. Luongo L, Palazzo E, Tambaro S, et al. 1-(2′,4′-Dichlorophenyl)-6-methyl-N-cyclohexylamine-1,4-dihydroindeno[1,2-c]pyrazole-3-carboxamide, a novel CB2 agonist, alleviates neuropathic pain through functional microglial changes in mice. Neurobiol Dis. 2010;37(1):177–85.

46. Hampson AJ, Grimaldi M, Axelrod J, Wink D. Cannabidiol and (-) Delta9-tetrahydrocannabinol are neuroprotective antioxidants. Proc Natl Acad Sci USA. 1998;95(14):8268–73.

47. Burstein S, Levin E, Varanelli C. Prostaglandins and cannabis. II. Inhibition of biosynthesis by the naturally occurring cannabinoids. Biochem Pharmacol. 1973;22(22):2905–10.

48. Fimiani C, Liberty T, Aquirre AJ, Amin I, Ali N, Stefano GB. Opiate, cannabinoid, and eicosanoid signaling converges on common intracellular pathways nitric oxide coupling. Prostaglandins Other Lipid Mediat. 1999;57(1):23–34.

49. Stott CG, Guy GW, Wright S, Whittle BA. The effects of cannabis extracts Tetranabinex & Nabidiolex on human cyclo-oxygenase (COX) activity. Paper presented at: Symposium on the Cannabinoids, Clearwater, June 2005.

50. Bisogno T, Hanus L, De Petrocellis L, et al. Molecular targets for cannabidiol and its synthetic analogues: effect on vanilloid VR1 receptors and on the cellular uptake and enzymatic hydrolysis of anandamide. Br J Pharmacol. 2001;134(4):845–52.

51. Russo EB, Guy GW. A tale of two cannabinoids: the therapeutic rationale for combining tetrahydrocannabinol and cannabidiol. Med Hypotheses. 2006;66(2):234–46.

52. Morgan CJ, Curran HV. Effects of cannabidiol on schizophrenia-like symptoms in people who use cannabis. Br J Psychiatry. 2008;192(4):306–7.

53. Morgan CJ, Freeman TP, Schafer GL, Curran HV. Cannabidiol attenuates the appetitive effects of delta 9-tetrahydrocannabinol in humans smoking their chosen cannabis. Neuropsychopharmacology. 2010;35(9):1879–85.

54. Morgan CJ, Schafer G, Freeman TP, Curran HV. Impact of cannabidiol on the acute memory and psychotomimetic effects of smoked cannabis: naturalistic study. Br J Psychiatry. 2010;197(4):285–90.

55. Malfait AM, Gallily R, Sumariwalla PF, et al. The nonpsychoactive cannabis constituent cannabidiol is an oral anti-arthritic therapeutic in murine collagen-induced arthritis. Proc Natl Acad Sci USA. 2000;97(17):9561–6.

56. Carrier EJ, Auchampach JA, Hillard CJ. Inhibition of an equilibrative nucleoside transporter by cannabidiol: a mechanism of cannabinoid immunosuppression. Proc Natl Acad Sci USA. 2006;103(20):7895–900.

57. McHugh D, Hu SS, Rimmerman N, et al. N-arachidonoyl glycine, an abundant endogenous lipid, potently drives directed cellular migration through GPR18, the putative abnormal cannabidiol receptor. BMC Neurosci. 2010;11:44.

58. Dmitrieva N, Nagabukuro H, Resuehr D, et al. Endocannabinoid involvement in endometriosis. Pain. 2010;151(3):703–10.

59. Izzo AA, Camilleri M. Emerging role of cannabinoids in gastrointestinal and liver diseases: basic and clinical aspects. Gut. 2008;57(8):1140–55.

60. Izzo AA, Sharkey KA. Cannabinoids and the gut: new developments and emerging concepts. Pharmacol Ther. 2010;126(1):21–38.

61. Shen M, Piser TM, Seybold VS, Thayer SA. Cannabinoid receptor agonists inhibit glutamatergic synaptic transmission in rat hippocampal cultures. J Neurosci. 1996;16(14):4322–34.

62. Nicolodi M, Volpe AR, Sicuteri F. Fibromyalgia and headache. Failure of serotonergic analgesia and N-methyl-D-aspartate-mediated neuronal plasticity: their common clues. Cephalalgia. 1998;18 Suppl 21:41–4.

63. Russo EB. Clinical endocannabinoid deficiency (CECD): Can this concept explain therapeutic benefits of cannabis in migraine, fibromyalgia, irritable bowel syndrome and other treatment-resistant conditions? Neuroendocrinol Lett. 2004;25(1–2):31–9.

64. Russo E. Cannabis for migraine treatment: the once and future prescription? An historical and scientific review. Pain. 1998;76(1–2):3–8.

65. Spadone C. Neurophysiologie du cannabis [neurophysiology of cannabis]. Encéphale. 1991;17(1):17–22.

66. Akerman S, Holland PR, Goadsby PJ. Cannabinoid (CB1) receptor activation inhibits trigeminovascular neurons. J Pharmacol Exp Ther. 2007;320(1):64–71.

67. Akerman S, Kaube H, Goadsby PJ. Anandamide is able to inhibit trigeminal neurons using an in vivo model of trigeminovascular-mediated nociception. J Pharmacol Exp Ther. 2003;309(1):56–63.

68. Akerman S, Kaube H, Goadsby PJ. Anandamide acts as a vasodilator of dural blood vessels in vivo by activating TRPV1 receptors. Br J Pharmacol. 2004;142:1354–60.

69. Manzanares J, Corchero J, Romero J, Fernandez-Ruiz JJ, Ramos JA, Fuentes JA. Chronic administration of cannabinoids regulates proenkephalin mRNA levels in selected regions of the rat brain. Brain Res Mol Brain Res. 1998;55(1):126–32.

70. Cichewicz DL, Martin ZL, Smith FL, Welch SP. Enhancement of mu opioid antinociception by oral delta9-tetrahydrocannabinol: dose-response analysis and receptor identification. J Pharmacol Exp Ther. 1999;289(2):859–67.

71. Cichewicz DL, Welch SP. Modulation of oral morphine antinociceptive tolerance and naloxone-precipitated withdrawal signs by oral delta 9-tetrahydrocannabinol. J Pharmacol Exp Ther. 2003;305(3):812–7.

72. Cichewicz DL, McCarthy EA. Antinociceptive synergy between delta(9)-tetrahydrocannabinol and opioids after oral administration. J Pharmacol Exp Ther. 2003;304(3):1010–5.

73. Calhoun SR, Galloway GP, Smith DE. Abuse potential of dronabinol (Marinol). J Psychoactive Drugs. 1998;30(2):187–96.

74. Clermont-Gnamien S, Atlani S, Attal N, Le Mercier F, Guirimand F, Brasseur L. Utilisation thérapeutique du delta-9-tétrahydrocannabinol (dronabinol) dans les douleurs neuropathiques réfractaires. The therapeutic use of D9-tetrahydrocannabinol (dronabinol) in refractory neuropathic pain. Presse Med. 2002;31(39 Pt 1):1840–5.

75. Attal N, Brasseur L, Guirimand D, Clermond-Gnamien S, Atlami S, Bouhassira D. Are oral cannabinoids safe and effective in refractory neuropathic pain? Eur J Pain. 2004;8(2):173–7.

76. Svendsen KB, Jensen TS, Bach FW. Does the cannabinoid dronabinol reduce central pain in multiple sclerosis? Randomised double blind placebo controlled crossover trial. BMJ. 2004;329(7460):253.

77. Buggy DJ, Toogood L, Maric S, Sharpe P, Lambert DG, Rowbotham DJ. Lack of analgesic efficacy of oral delta-9-tetrahydrocannabinol in postoperative pain. Pain. 2003;106(1–2):169–72.

78. Neff GW, O'Brien CB, Reddy KR, et al. Preliminary observation with dronabinol in patients with intractable pruritus secondary to cholestatic liver disease. Am J Gastroenterol. 2002;97(8): 2117–9.

79. Narang S, Gibson D, Wasan AD, et al. Efficacy of dronabinol as an adjuvant treatment for chronic pain patients on opioid therapy. J Pain. 2008;9(3):254–64.

80. Toth C, Au S. A prospective identification of neuropathic pain in specific chronic polyneuropathy syndromes and response to pharmacological therapy. Pain. 2008;138(3):657–66.

81. Rintala DH, Fiess RN, Tan G, Holmes SA, Bruel BM. Effect of dronabinol on central neuropathic pain after spinal cord injury: a pilot study. Am J Phys Med Rehabil. 2010;89(10):840–8.

82. Lemberger L, Rubin A, Wolen R, et al. Pharmacokinetics, metabolism and drug-abuse potential of nabilone. Cancer Treat Rev. 1982;9(Suppl B):17–23.

83. Notcutt W, Price M, Chapman G. Clinical experience with nabilone for chronic pain. Pharm Sci. 1997;3:551–5.

84. Berlach DM, Shir Y, Ware MA. Experience with the synthetic cannabinoid nabilone in chronic noncancer pain. Pain Med. 2006;7(1):25–9.

85. Beaulieu P. Effects of nabilone, a synthetic cannabinoid, on postoperative pain: Les effets de la nabilone, un cannabinoide synthetique, sur la douleur postoperatoire. Can J Anaesth. 2006;53(8):769–75.

86. Maida V. The synthetic cannabinoid nabilone improves pain and symptom management in cancer patietns. Breast Cancer Res Treat. 2007;103(Part 1):121–2.

87. Wissel J, Haydn T, Muller J, et al. Low dose treatment with the synthetic cannabinoid nabilone significantly reduces spasticity-related pain: a double-blind placebo-controlled cross-over trial. J Neurol. 2006;253(10):1337–41.

88. Frank B, Serpell MG, Hughes J, Matthews JN, Kapur D. Comparison of analgesic effects and patient tolerability of nabilone and dihydrocodeine for chronic neuropathic pain: randomised, crossover, double blind study. BMJ. 2008;336(7637):199–201.

89. Skrabek RQ, Galimova L, Ethans K, Perry D. Nabilone for the treatment of pain in fibromyalgia. J Pain. 2008;9(2):164–73.

90. Ware MA, Fitzcharles MA, Joseph L, Shir Y. The effects of nabilone on sleep in fibromyalgia: results of a randomized controlled trial. Anesth Analg. 2010;110(2):604–10.

91. Bestard JA, Toth CC. An open-label comparison of nabilone and gabapentin as adjuvant therapy or monotherapy in the management of neuropathic pain in patients with peripheral neuropathy. Pain Pract. 2011;11:353–68. Epub 2010 Nov 18.

92. Karst M, Salim K, Burstein S, Conrad I, Hoy L, Schneider U. Analgesic effect of the synthetic cannabinoid CT-3 on chronic neuropathic pain: a randomized controlled trial. JAMA. 2003;290(13):1757–62.

93. Dyson A, Peacock M, Chen A, et al. Antihyperalgesic properties of the cannabinoid CT-3 in chronic neuropathic and inflammatory pain states in the rat. Pain. 2005;116(1–2):129–37.

94. Abrams DI, Jay CA, Shade SB, et al. Cannabis in painful HIV-associated sensory neuropathy: a randomized placebo-controlled trial. Neurology. 2007;68(7):515–21.

95. Wilsey B, Marcotte T, Tsodikov A, et al. A randomized, placebo-controlled, crossover trial of cannabis cigarettes in neuropathic pain. J Pain. 2008;9(6):506–21.

96. Wallace M, Schulteis G, Atkinson JH, et al. Dose-dependent effects of smoked cannabis on capsaicin-induced pain and hyperalgesia in healthy volunteers. Anesthesiology. 2007;107(5):785–96.

97. Ellis RJ, Toperoff W, Vaida F, et al. Smoked medicinal cannabis for neuropathic pain in HIV: a randomized, crossover clinical trial. Neuropsychopharmacology. 2009;34(3):672–80.

98. Ware MA, Wang T, Shapiro S, et al. Smoked cannabis for chronic neuropathic pain: a randomized controlled trial. CMAJ. 2010;182(14):E694–701.

99. Wade DT, Makela PM, House H, Bateman C, Robson PJ. Long-term use of a cannabis-based medicine in the treatment of spasticity and other symptoms in multiple sclerosis. Mult Scler. 2006;12:639–45.

100. Tashkin DP. Smoked marijuana as a cause of lung injury. Monaldi Arch Chest Dis. 2005;63(2):93–100.

101. Tashkin DP, Simmons MS, Sherrill DL, Coulson AH. Heavy habitual marijuana smoking does not cause an accelerated decline in FEV1 with age. Am J Respir Crit Care Med. 1997;155(1):141–8.

102. Hashibe M, Morgenstern H, Cui Y, et al. Marijuana use and the risk of lung and upper aerodigestive tract cancers: results of a population-based case-control study. Cancer Epidemiol Biomarkers Prev. 2006;15(10):1829–34.

103. Grinspoon L, Bakalar JB. Marihuana, the forbidden medicine. Rev. and exp. edn. New Haven: Yale University Press; 1997.

104. Moir D, Rickert WS, Levasseur G, et al. A comparison of mainstream and sidestream marijuana and tobacco cigarette smoke produced under two machine smoking conditions. Chem Res Toxicol. 2008;21(2):494–502.

105. Singh R, Sandhu J, Kaur B, et al. Evaluation of the DNA damaging potential of cannabis cigarette smoke by the determination of acetaldehyde derived N2-ethyl-2′-deoxyguanosine adducts. Chem Res Toxicol. 2009;22(6):1181–8.

106. Joy JE, Watson SJ, Benson Jr JA. Marijuana and medicine: assessing the science base. Washington D.C.: Institute of Medicine; 1999.

107. Gieringer D. Marijuana waterpipe and vaporizer study. MAPS Bull. 1996;6(3):59–66.

108. Gieringer D. Cannabis "vaporization": a promising strategy for smoke harm reduction. J Cannabis Ther. 2001;1(3–4):153–70.

109. Storz M, Russo EB. An interview with Markus Storz. J Cannabis Ther. 2003;3(1):67–78.

110. Gieringer D, St. Laurent J, Goodrich S. Cannabis vaporizer combines efficient delivery of THC with effective suppression of pyrolytic compounds. J Cannabis Ther. 2004;4(1):7–27.

111. Hazekamp A, Ruhaak R, Zuurman L, van Gerven J, Verpoorte R. Evaluation of a vaporizing device (Volcano) for the pulmonary administration of tetrahydrocannabinol. J Pharm Sci. 2006;95(6):1308–17.

112. Van der Kooy F, Pomahacova B, Verpoorte R. Cannabis smoke condensate I: the effect of different preparation methods on tetrahydrocannabinol levels. Inhal Toxicol. 2008;20(9):801–4.

113. Bloor RN, Wang TS, Spanel P, Smith D. Ammonia release from heated 'street' cannabis leaf and its potential toxic effects on cannabis users. Addiction. 2008;103(10):1671–7.

114. Zuurman L, Roy C, Schoemaker RC, et al. Effect of intrapulmonary tetrahydrocannabinol administration in humans. J Psychopharmacol (Oxford, England). 2008;22(7):707–16.

115. Pomahacova B, Van der Kooy F, Verpoorte R. Cannabis smoke condensate III: the cannabinoid content of vaporised *Cannabis sativa*. Inhal Toxicol. 2009;21(13):1108–12.

116. Abrams DI, Vizoso HP, Shade SB, Jay C, Kelly ME, Benowitz NL. Vaporization as a smokeless cannabis delivery system: a pilot study. Clin Pharmacol Ther. 2007;82(5):572–8.

117. Abrams DI, Couey P, Shade SB, Kelly ME, Benowitz NL. Cannabinoid-opioid interaction in chronic pain. Clinical pharmacology and therapeutics. 2011;90(6):844–51.

118. Earleywine M, Barnwell SS. Decreased respiratory symptoms in cannabis users who vaporize. Harm Reduct J. 2007;4:11.

119. Zajicek J, Fox P, Sanders H, et al. Cannabinoids for treatment of spasticity and other symptoms related to multiple sclerosis (CAMS study): multicentre randomised placebo-controlled trial. Lancet. 2003;362(9395):1517–26.

120. Zajicek JP, Sanders HP, Wright DE, et al. Cannabinoids in multiple sclerosis (CAMS) study: safety and efficacy data for 12 months follow up. J Neurol Neurosurg Psychiatry. 2005;76(12):1664–9.

121. Ernst G, Denke C, Reif M, Schnelle M, Hagmeister H. Standardized cannabis extract in the treatment of postherpetic neuralgia: a randomized, double-blind, placebo-controlled cross-over study. Paper presented at: international association for cannabis as medicine, Leiden, 9 Sept 2005.

122. Holdcroft A, Maze M, Dore C, Tebbs S, Thompson S. A multi-center dose-escalation study of the analgesic and adverse effects

of an oral cannabis extract (Cannador) for postoperative pain management. Anesthesiology. 2006;104(5):1040–6.

123. McPartland JM, Russo EB. Cannabis and cannabis extracts: greater than the sum of their parts? J Cannabis Ther. 2001; 1(3–4):103–32.

124. de Meijer E. The breeding of cannabis cultivars for pharmaceutical end uses. In: Guy GW, Whittle BA, Robson P, editors. Medicinal uses of cannabis and cannabinoids. London: Pharmaceutical Press; 2004. p. 55–70.

125. Guy GW, Robson P. A phase I, double blind, three-way crossover study to assess the pharmacokinetic profile of cannabis based medicine extract (CBME) administered sublingually in variant cannabinoid ratios in normal healthy male volunteers (GWPK02125). J Cannabis Ther. 2003;3(4):121–52.

126. Karschner EL, Darwin WD, McMahon RP, et al. Subjective and physiological effects after controlled Sativex and oral THC administration. Clin Pharmacol Ther. 2011;89(3):400–7.

127. Karschner EL, Darwin WD, Goodwin RS, Wright S, Huestis MA. Plasma cannabinoid pharmacokinetics following controlled oral delta9-tetrahydrocannabinol and oromucosal cannabis extract administration. Clin Chem. 2011;57(1):66–75.

128. Russo EB, Etges T, Stott CG. Comprehensive adverse event profile of Sativex. 18th annual symposium on the cannabinoids. Vol Aviemore, Scotland: International Cannabinoid Research Society; 2008. p. 136.

129. Barnes MP. Sativex: clinical efficacy and tolerability in the treatment of symptoms of multiple sclerosis and neuropathic pain. Expert Opin Pharmacother. 2006;7(5):607–15.

130. Pérez J. Combined cannabinoid therapy via na oromucosal spray. Drugs Today. 2006;42(8):495–501.

131. Wade DT, Robson P, House H, Makela P, Aram J. A preliminary controlled study to determine whether whole-plant cannabis extracts can improve intractable neurogenic symptoms. Clin Rehabil. 2003;17:18–26.

132. Notcutt W, Price M, Miller R, et al. Initial experiences with medicinal extracts of cannabis for chronic pain: results from 34 "N of 1" studies. Anaesthesia. 2004;59:440–52.

133. Berman JS, Symonds C, Birch R. Efficacy of two cannabis based medicinal extracts for relief of central neuropathic pain from brachial plexus avulsion: results of a randomised controlled trial. Pain. 2004;112(3):299–306.

134. Rog DJ, Nurmiko T, Friede T, Young C. Randomized controlled trial of cannabis based medicine in central neuropathic pain due to multiple sclerosis. Neurology. 2005;65(6):812–9.

135. Nurmikko TJ, Serpell MG, Hoggart B, Toomey PJ, Morlion BJ, Haines D. Sativex successfully treats neuropathic pain characterised by allodynia: a randomised, double-blind, placebo-controlled clinical trial. Pain. 2007;133(1–3):210–20.

136. Wade DT, Makela P, Robson P, House H, Bateman C. Do cannabis-based medicinal extracts have general or specific effects on symptoms in multiple sclerosis? A double-blind, randomized, placebo-controlled study on 160 patients. Mult Scler. 2004;10(4):434–41.

137. Blake DR, Robson P, Ho M, Jubb RW, McCabe CS. Preliminary assessment of the efficacy, tolerability and safety of a cannabis-based medicine (Sativex) in the treatment of pain caused by rheumatoid arthritis. Rheumatology (Oxford). 2006;45(1):50–2.

138. Johnson JR, Burnell-Nugent M, Lossignol D, Ganae-Motan ED, Potts R, Fallon MT. Multicenter, double-blind, randomized, placebo-controlled, parallel-group study of the efficacy, safety, and tolerability of THC:CBD extract and THC extract in patients with intractable cancer-related pain. J Pain Symptom Manage. 2010;39(2):167–79.

139. Russo EB, Guy GW, Robson PJ. Cannabis, pain, and sleep: lessons from therapeutic clinical trials of Sativex, a cannabis-based medicine. Chem Biodivers. 2007;4(8):1729–43.

140. Lynch ME, Young J, Clark AJ. A case series of patients using medicinal marihuana for management of chronic pain under the Canadian Marihuana Medical Access Regulations. J Pain Symptom Manage. 2006;32(5):497–501.

141. Janse AFC, Breekveldt-Postma NS, Erkens JA, Herings RMC. Medicinal gebruik van cannabis: PHARMO instituut. Institute for Drug Outcomes Research; 2004.

142. Gorter RW, Butorac M, Cobian EP, van der Sluis W. Medical use of cannabis in the Netherlands. Neurology. 2005;64(5):917–9.

143. Fitzgerald GA. Coxibs and cardiovascular disease. N Engl J Med. 2004;10:6.

144. Topol EJ. Failing the public health – rofecoxib, Merck, and the FDA. N Engl J Med. 2004;10:6.

145. Grotenhermen F. Pharmacokinetics and pharmacodynamics of cannabinoids. Clin Pharmacokinet. 2003;42(4):327–60.

146. Huestis MA, Henningfield JE, Cone EJ. Blood cannabinoids. I. Absorption of THC and formation of 11-OH-THC and THCCOOH during and after smoking marijuana. J Anal Toxicol. 1992;16(5): 276–82.

147. Wright S. GWMS001 and GWMS0106: maintenance of blinding. London: GW Pharmaceuticals; 2005.

148. Clark P, Altman D. Assessment of blinding in phase III Sativex spasticity studies. GW Pharmaceuticals; 2006.

149. Samaha AN, Robinson TE. Why does the rapid delivery of drugs to the brain promote addiction? Trends Pharmacol Sci. 2005;26(2):82–7.

150. Jones RT, Benowitz N, Bachman J. Clinical studies of cannabis tolerance and dependence. Ann N Y Acad Sci. 1976;282:221–39.

151. Budney AJ, Hughes JR, Moore BA, Vandrey R. Review of the validity and significance of cannabis withdrawal syndrome. Am J Psychiatry. 2004;161(11):1967–77.

152. Smith NT. A review of the published literature into cannabis withdrawal symptoms in human users. Addiction. 2002;97(6): 621–32.

153. Solowij N, Stephens RS, Roffman RA, et al. Cognitive functioning of long-term heavy cannabis users seeking treatment. JAMA. 2002;287(9):1123–31.

154. Schoedel KA, Chen N, Hilliard A, et al. A randomized, double-blind, placebo-controlled, crossover study to evaluate the abuse potential of nabiximols oromucosal spray in subjects with a history of recreational cannabis use. Hum Psychopharmacol. 2011;26:224–36.

155. Russo EB, Mathre ML, Byrne A, et al. Chronic cannabis use in the Compassionate Use Investigational New Drug Program: an examination of benefits and adverse effects of legal clinical cannabis. J Cannabis Ther. 2002;2(1):3–57.

156. Fride E, Russo EB. Neuropsychiatry: schizophrenia, depression, and anxiety. In: Onaivi E, Sugiura T, Di Marzo V, editors. Endocannabinoids: the brain and body's marijuana and beyond. Boca Raton: Taylor & Francis; 2006. p. 371–82.

157. Aragona M, Onesti E, Tomassini V, et al. Psychopathological and cognitive effects of therapeutic cannabinoids in multiple sclerosis: a double-blind, placebo controlled, crossover study. Clin Neuropharmacol. 2009;32(1):41–7.

158. Degenhardt L, Hall W, Lynskey M. Testing hypotheses about the relationship between cannabis use and psychosis. Drug Alcohol Depend. 2003;71(1):37–48.

159. Macleod J, Davey Smith G, Hickman M. Does cannabis use cause schizophrenia? Lancet. 2006;367(9516):1055.

160. Macleod J, Hickman M. How ideology shapes the evidence and the policy: what do we know about cannabis use and what should we do? Addiction. 2010;105:1326–30.

161. Hickman M, Vickerman P, Macleod J, et al. If cannabis caused schizophrenia–how many cannabis users may need to be prevented in order to prevent one case of schizophrenia? England and Wales calculations. Addiction. 2009;104(11):1856–61.

162. Zuardi AW, Guimaraes FS. Cannabidiol as an anxiolytic and antipsychotic. In: Mathre ML, editor. Cannabis in medical practice: a legal, historical and pharmacological overview of the therapeutic use of marijuana. Jefferson: McFarland; 1997. p. 133–41.

163. Russo EB. Taming THC: potential cannabis synergy and phytocannabinoid-terpenoid entourage effects. Br J Pharmacol. 2011;163:1344–64.

164. Cabral G. Immune system. In: Grotenhermen F, Russo EB, editors. Cannabis and cannabinoids: pharmacology, toxicology and therapeutic potential. Binghamton: Haworth Press; 2001. p. 279–87.

165. Katona S, Kaminski E, Sanders H, Zajicek J. Cannabinoid influence on cytokine profile in multiple sclerosis. Clin Exp Immunol. 2005; 140(3):580–5.

166. Abrams DI, Hilton JF, Leiser RJ, et al. Short-term effects of cannabinoids in patients with HIV-1 infection. A randomized, placbo-controlled clinical trial. Ann Intern Med. 2003;139:258–66.

167. Stott CG, Guy GW, Wright S, Whittle BA. The effects of cannabis extracts Tetranabinex and Nabidiolex on human cytochrome P450-mediated metabolism. Paper presented at: Symposium on the Cannabinoids, Clearwater, 27 June 2005.

168. Stott CG, Ayerakwa L, Wright S, Guy G. Lack of human cytochrome P450 induction by Sativex. 17th annual symposium on the cannabinoids. Saint-Sauveur, Quebec: International Cannabinoid Research Society; 2007. p. 211.

169. Grotenhermen F, Leson G, Berghaus G, et al. Developing limits for driving under cannabis. Addiction. 2007;102(12):1910–7.

170. Hohmann AG, Suplita 2nd RL. Endocannabinoid mechanisms of pain modulation. AAPS J. 2006;8(4):E693–708.

171. Clapper JR, Moreno-Sanz G, Russo R, et al. Anandamide suppresses pain initiation through a peripheral endocannabinoid mechanism. Nat Neurosci. 2010;13:1265–70.

172. Schlosburg JE, Blankman JL, Long JZ, et al. Chronic monoacylglycerol lipase blockade causes functional antagonism of the endocannabinoid system. Nat Neurosci. 2010;13(9):1113–9.

173. Yu XH, Cao CQ, Martino G, et al. A peripherally restricted cannabinoid receptor agonist produces robust anti-nociceptive effects in rodent models of inflammatory and neuropathic pain. Pain. 2010;151(2):337–44.

174. Izzo AA, Borrelli F, Capasso R, Di Marzo V, Mechoulam R. Non-psychotropic plant cannabinoids: new therapeutic opportunities from an ancient herb. Trends Pharmacol Sci. 2009;30(10):515–27.

175. Wirth PW, Watson ES, ElSohly M, Turner CE, Murphy JC. Anti-inflammatory properties of cannabichromene. Life Sci. 1980; 26(23):1991–5.

176. Davis WM, Hatoum NS. Neurobehavioral actions of cannabichromene and interactions with delta 9-tetrahydrocannabinol. Gen Pharmacol. 1983;14(2):247–52.

177. Ligresti A, Moriello AS, Starowicz K, et al. Antitumor activity of plant cannabinoids with emphasis on the effect of cannabidiol on human breast carcinoma. J Pharmacol Exp Ther. 2006;318(3):1375–87.

178. De Petrocellis L, Starowicz K, Moriello AS, Vivese M, Orlando P, Di Marzo V. Regulation of transient receptor potential channels of melastatin type 8 (TRPM8): effect of cAMP, cannabinoid CB(1) receptors and endovanilloids. Exp Cell Res. 2007;313(9):1911–20.

179. Gauson LA, Stevenson LA, Thomas A, Baillie GL, Ross RA, Pertwee RG. Cannabigerol behaves as a partial agonist at both CB1 and CB2 receptors. 17th annual symposium on the cannabinoids. Vol Saint-Sauveur, Quebec: International Cannabinoid Research Society; 2007, p. 206.

180. Cascio MG, Gauson LA, Stevenson LA, Ross RA, Pertwee RG. Evidence that the plant cannabinoid cannabigerol is a highly potent alpha2-adrenoceptor agonist and moderately potent 5HT1A receptor antagonist. Br J Pharmacol. 2010;159(1):129–41.

181. Banerjee SP, Snyder SH, Mechoulam R. Cannabinoids: influence on neurotransmitter uptake in rat brain synaptosomes. J Pharmacol Exp Ther. 1975;194(1):74–81.

182. Evans FJ. Cannabinoids: the separation of central from peripheral effects on a structural basis. Planta Med. 1991;57(7):S60–7.

183. Evans AT, Formukong E, Evans FJ. Activation of phospholipase A2 by cannabinoids. Lack of correlation with CNS effects. FEBS Lett. 1987;211(2):119–22.

184. Pertwee RG. The diverse CB1 and CB2 receptor pharmacology of three plant cannabinoids: delta9-tetrahydrocannabinol, cannabidiol and delta9-tetrahydrocannabivarin. Br J Pharmacol. 2008; 153(2):199–215.

185. Hill AJ, Weston SE, Jones NA, et al. Delta-tetrahydrocannabivarin suppresses in vitro epileptiform and in vivo seizure activity in adult rats. Epilepsia. 2010;51(8):1522–32.

186. Bolognini D, Costa B, Maione S, et al. The plant cannabinoid delta9-tetrahydrocannabivarin can decrease signs of inflammation and inflammatory pain in mice. Br J Pharmacol. 2010; 160(3):677–87.

187. Mehmedic Z, Chandra S, Slade D, et al. Potency trends of delta(9)-THC and other cannabinoids in confiscated cannabis preparations from 1993 to 2008. J Forensic Sci. 2010;55:1209–17.

188. King LA, Carpentier C, Griffiths P. Cannabis potency in Europe. Addiction. 2005;100(7):884–6.

189. Potter DJ, Clark P, Brown MB. Potency of delta 9-THC and other cannabinoids in cannabis in England in 2005: implications for psychoactivity and pharmacology. J Forensic Sci. 2008;53(1): 90–4.

190. Potter D. Growth and morphology of medicinal cannabis. In: Guy GW, Whittle BA, Robson P, editors. Medicinal uses of cannabis and cannabinoids. London: Pharmaceutical Press; 2004. p. 17–54.

191. Rao VS, Menezes AM, Viana GS. Effect of myrcene on nociception in mice. J Pharm Pharmacol. 1990;42(12):877–8.

192. Lorenzetti BB, Souza GE, Sarti SJ, Santos Filho D, Ferreira SH. Myrcene mimics the peripheral analgesic activity of lemongrass tea. J Ethnopharmacol. 1991;34(1):43–8.

193. Basile AC, Sertie JA, Freitas PC, Zanini AC. Anti-inflammatory activity of oleoresin from Brazilian Copaifera. J Ethnopharmacol. 1988;22(1):101–9.

194. Tambe Y, Tsujiuchi H, Honda G, Ikeshiro Y, Tanaka S. Gastric cytoprotection of the non-steroidal anti-inflammatory sesquiterpene, beta-caryophyllene. Planta Med. 1996;62(5):469–70.

195. Gertsch J, Leonti M, Raduner S, et al. Beta-caryophyllene is a dietary cannabinoid. Proc Natl Acad Sci USA. 2008;105(26): 9099–104.

197. Gil ML, Jimenez J, Ocete MA, Zarzuelo A, Cabo MM. Comparative study of different essential oils of Bupleurum gibraltaricum Lamarck. Pharmazie. 1989;44(4):284–7.

198. Re L, Barocci S, Sonnino S, et al. Linalool modifies the nicotinic receptor-ion channel kinetics at the mouse neuromuscular junction. Pharmacol Res. 2000;42(2):177–82.

199. Gregg, L.C., Jung, K.M., Spradley, J.M., Nyilas, R., Suplita II, R.L., Zimmer, A., Watanabe, M., Mackie, K., Katona, I., Piomelli, D. and Hohmann, A.G. (2012) Activation of type-5 metabotropic glutamate receptors and diacylglycerol lipase-alpha initiates 2-arachidonoylglycerol formation and endocannabinoid-mediated analgesia in vivo. The Journal of Neuroscience, in press [DOI:10.1523/JNEUROSCI.0013-12.2012].

200. Kavia R, De Ridder D, Constantinescu C, Stott C, Fowler C. Randomized controlled trial of Sativex to treat detrusor overactivity in multiple sclerosis. Mult Scler. 2010;16(11):1349–59.

201. Portenoy RK, Ganae-Motan ED, Allende S, Yanagihara R, Shaiova L, Weinstein S, et al. Nabiximols for opioid-treated cancer patients with poorly-controlled chronic pain: a randomized, placebo-controlled, graded-dose trial. J Pain. 2012;13(5):438–49.

202. Abrams DI, Couey P, Shade SB, Kelly ME, Benowitz NL. Cannabinoid-opioid interaction in chronic pain. Clinical pharmacology and therapeutics. 2011;90(6):844–51.

The Future of Pain Pharmacotherapy

Iwona Bonney and Daniel B. Carr

Key Points
- Improve existing analgesics' safety profiles, dosing requirements, and convenience of administration routes (e.g., using controlled-release formulations and other novel delivery systems).
- Provide multimodal analgesia including combination products to achieve it safely and with few side effects.
- Design novel, condition-specific molecules whose structure is based upon understanding of pain mechanisms, neurotransmitters, and pathways involved in nociception.

Introduction

According to the American Academy of Pain Medicine (AAPM) and the Institute of Medicine [1], pain affects more Americans than cancer, diabetes, and cardiac disease combined. Current analgesics only provide modest relief, frequently carry black box warnings, and are susceptible to abuse. The ability of current medical science to treat pain effectively is limited by an incomplete understanding of the mechanisms of pain signaling in diverse individuals across different circumstances and the high prevalence of side effects after systemic or regional administration of available analgesics. Despite increasing interest in developing new analgesic

I. Bonney, Ph.D. (✉)
Department of Anesthesiology, Tufts Medical Center and Tufts University School of Medicine,
800 Washington Street, #298, Boston, MA 02111, USA
e-mail: ibonney@tuftsmedicalcenter.org

D.B. Carr, M.D., DABPM, FFPMANZCA (Hon)
Department of Public Health, Anesthesiology, Medicine, and Molecular Physiology and Pharmacology,
Tufts University School of Medicine,
136 Harrison Avenue, Boston, MA 02111, USA
e-mail: daniel.carr@tufts.edu

molecules by translating preclinical research on mechanisms of pain processing and harnessing innovative methods of drug delivery, the majority of new analgesic drug launches from 1990 to 2010 were reformulations of existing pharmaceuticals within well-established drug categories such as opioids and NSAIDs (nonsteroidal anti-inflammatory drugs). A distant second were novel drugs acting via well-known mechanisms [novel opioid molecules, norepinephrine reuptake inhibitors (NRI), serotonin-norepinephrine reuptake inhibitors (SNRI), and novel NSAIDs and coxibs]. Finally, there were those few novel molecules that acted via mechanisms not targeted by earlier approved drugs (Lyrica, Prialt, Sativex, Qutenza). At present and for the foreseeable future, drug development and discovery are likely to continue to involve these three approaches, supplemented by occasional leaps forward such as gene therapy to transfect neural cells with DNA that enables them to synthesize and secrete native or nonnative analgesic compounds. This chapter summarizes background knowledge on targets already exploited by existing analgesics including novel formulations of same, surveys other targets recently recognized as potentially worth addressing, and recounts the rapidly changing developmental status of the latter. We recognize that the fast pace of and frequent unexpected findings during clinical drug development will date many of our brief status reports, but this is unavoidable and in any event highlights the dynamic nature of translational research in analgesia. The chapter concludes with the question "Quo vadis?" ("Where are you going?") which we approach using current estimates of the number of "drugable" targets and our assessment of the progress made towards harnessing these therapeutically.

Pharmacological Background

A number of neurotransmitters of various chemical classes are released from afferent fibers, ascending and descending neurons, and interneurons upon peripheral nociceptive input. Neurotransmitters display a complex pattern of colocalization, comodulation, and corelease in primary afferent fibers and central nociceptive pathways [2]. All potentially relevant to analgesic pharmacology, these include substance P, gamma-aminobutyric acid (GABA), serotonin, norepinephrine, leu- and met-enkephalin, neurotensin, acetylcholine, dynorphin, cholecystokinin (CCK), vasocative intestinal peptide (VIP), calcitonin gene-related peptide (CGRP), somatostatin, adenosine, neuropeptide Y, glutamate, and prostaglandins. Also relevant are the enzymes involved in their generation or degradation, such as nitric oxide synthase, enkephalinases, and cholinesterases.

Changes in the magnitude and patterns of neurotransmitter release, along with diminished inhibitory interneuron function [3], contribute to altered nociceptor function after tissue damage, inflammation, or nerve injury. Those conditions can alter the threshold, excitability, and transmission properties of nociceptors, contributing to hyperalgesia and spontaneous pain. Hyperalgesia may be primary (in the immediate area of tissue injury, due to sensitization of local primary afferent nociceptors by locally released inflammatory mediators) and secondary (surrounding the area of injury that is centrally mediated) [4]. Hyperalgesia often coexists with allodynia (a painful response to normally innocuous stimulus).

Immune cells are also involved in pain, as they are activated peripherally and within the central nervous system by peripheral tissue damage, inflammation, or mechanical nerve lesions [5]. Immune cells enhance nociception through the release of cytokines or (e.g., for granulocytes and monocytes) promote analgesia by secreting β-endorphin and enkephalins [6]. For example, interleukin (IL-6) induces allodynia and hyperalgesia in dorsal horn neurons, IL-1β enhances the release of substance P in spinal cord and induces cyclooxygenase (COX)-2 expression, and tissue necrosis factor α (TNFα) may facilitate postsynaptic ion currents provoked by excitatory amino acids (EAA) [7]. Opioid peptide precursors, including pro-opiomelanocortin (POMC) and proenkephalin (PENK), have been detected in immune cells. POMC was found to be expressed by leukocytes, and pre-PENK mRNA was found in T and B cells, macrophages, and mast cells [8]. Opioid peptides are released from immune cells by stress or by secretagogues (CRH and/or IL-1) to bind to and activate opioid receptors located on peripheral terminals of sensory neurons [8]. Immune cells producing opioid peptides can migrate to inflamed tissue, where the peripheral actions of opioid peptides can contribute to potent, clinically relevant analgesia. The neurotrophin family includes nerve growth factor (NGF), brain-derived neurotrophic factor (BDNF), neurotrophins-3 (NT-3), and NT-4/5. NGF has been shown to play an important role in nociceptive function in adults [9]. Upregulation of NGF after inflammatory injury to the skin leads to increased levels of substance P and CGRP. NGF can also regulate the levels of

BDNF. BDNF levels in sensory neurons may be increased by exogenous administration of NGF or by endogenous NGF whose synthesis is increased after tissue injury. NGF is released from mast cells, macrophages, lymphocytes, fibroblasts, and keratinocytes following tissue injury and may contribute to the transition from acute to chronic pain, especially in inflammatory conditions. Recent studies suggest that within the spinal cord, BDNF functions as a retrograde modulator of presynaptic neurotransmitter release. BDNF rapidly and specifically enhances phosphorylation of the postsynaptic NMDA receptor, whose activation plays a pivotal role in the induction and maintenance of central sensitization [10].

Based on their involvement in nociceptive processing, the TRPV1 receptor and glycine receptor subtype α3 (GlyR α3) are viewed as promising targets for drug development. The vanilloid TRPV1 receptor is part of a family of transient receptor potential (TRP) channels densely expressed in small diameter primary afferent fibers. The TRPV1 receptor integrates noxious stimuli, including heat and acids, and endogenous pro-inflammatory substances [11]. The abnormal expression of TRPV1 in neurons that normally do not express TRPV1 has been linked to the development of inflammatory hyperalgesia and neuropathic pain [11, 12], as does the observation that TRPV1 −/− mice exhibit reduced hyperalgesia compared to wild-type mice.

Scientific Basis for Pharmacotherapy

As we shift from a biomedical to a patient-centered model, pain assessment and management have received growing attention. Individuals vary considerably in their reports of pain and their estimates of the efficacy of identical analgesics given at the same doses under seemingly identical circumstances.

Even allowing for interindividual differences, an important reality in pain care is that different mechanisms of nociception predominate in different conditions, resulting in different apparent rank efficacies of the same drugs across different models. Drugs such as NSAIDs and coxibs are anti-hyperalgesic, reducing the increased nociceptive input from damaged tissue or sensitized sensory neurons.

NSAIDs are the most widely prescribed drugs worldwide, but not all are equally effective. The potency and intrinsic efficacy of some NSAIDs is greater than others. Several of the newer NSAIDs have potency comparable to or greater than that of opioid analgesics and are therefore applied for postoperative pain management. With many NSAIDs, a higher dose provides a faster onset time, higher peak effect, and a longer duration. Most NSAIDs display a dose-response relationship for analgesia up to a certain ceiling. Patients' responses to NSAIDs vary considerably, and therapeutic failure to one drug does not preclude success with other within the same broad class. To achieve a greater analgesic response to a constant opioid dose, NSAIDs or acetaminophen analgesics are often used in combination; examples of common combinations with acetaminophen include hyodrocodone or oxycodone.

Acute moderate to severe pain generally requires an opioid analgesic to bring it under control, although pains of various etiologies and mechanisms are not equally opioid sensitive. Adjuvant drugs that boost opioid efficacy and minimize opioid side effects can be also beneficial. NSAIDs, acetaminophen, glucocorticoids, antidepressants, anxiolytic agents, and anticonvulsants have all been reported to act as analgesic adjuvants. Opioid analgesics can control nearly all types of pain. Systemic opioids induce analgesia by acting on different levels of central nervous system (spinal cord, limbic system, hypothalamus) via mu, delta, and kappa opioid receptors and in the periphery. Opioid analgesia is dose-dependent, and its side effects also increase with increasing doses. Common opioid side effects include sedation, drowsiness, dizziness, constipation, respiratory depression, nausea and vomiting, pruritus, and the development of tolerance and physical dependence.

In an effort to gain better control over acute and chronic pain, doctors involved in pain treatment often advance from single drug therapy to combination drugs [13]. The potential benefits of such multimodal therapy include improvement of analgesic efficacy through additive or synergistic interactions, reduction of side effects through dose reductions of each component, and slowing of opioid dose escalation. In combination therapies, an opioid is typically coadministered with another opioid (e.g., morphine with sufentanil or fentanyl), a local anesthetic (morphine or fentanyl and bupivacaine), clonidine, or NMDA antagonists such as ketamine [13].

A Brief Survey of Novel Analgesics

Oral delivery is the most popular route of administration due to its versatility, ease, and probably most importantly, high level of patient compliance. Providing patients with simplified, convenient oral medications that improve compliance has been a major driver of innovation in the oral drug delivery market. Oral products represent about 70 % of the value of pharmaceutical sales and 60 % of drug delivery market [14]. A review of recent Food and Drug Administration (FDA) approvals over the past years shows that new chemical entities (NCEs) have accounted for only 25 % of all products approved; the majority of approvals have been reformulations or combinations of previously approved products [15]. With a reformulation costing approximately $40 million and taking 4–5 years to develop compared to the average clinical

development cost of a next-generation product—in the region of $330 million—the potential for reformulation using oral controlled-release technologies has never been greater [16, 17]. Moreover, the entire developmental cost of an NCE has been estimated at between $1.3 and 1.7 billion [18].

Extended-release formulations deliver a portion of the total dose shortly after ingestion and the remainder over an extended time frame. Typically, oral drug delivery systems are developed as matrix or reservoir systems. Two of the most widely commercialized controlled-release technologies are the OROS (the osmotic controlled-release oral delivery system that uses osmotic pressure as the driving force to deliver drug) and SODAS (spheroidal oral drug absorption system) technologies. Avinza® (King and Pfizer) uses the proprietary SODAS® technology for morphine sulfate extended-release capsules. Avinza® is a long-acting opioid for patients with moderate to severe chronic pain who require around-the-clock pain relief for an extended period of time. Avinza® consists of two components: an immediate release component that rapidly achieves plateau morphine plasma concentrations and an extended-release component that maintains plasma concentrations throughout the 24-h dosing interval. Within the gastrointestinal tract, due to the permeability of the ammonio methacrylate copolymers of the beads, fluid enters the beads and solubilizes the drug that then diffuses out in a predetermined manner.

Other examples of extended-release oral formulations of opioid analgesics indicated for moderate to severe pain for tolerant patients requiring continuous, around-the-clock opioid therapy for extended period of time are hydromorphone hydrochloride (Exalgo®, Covidien) and oxymorphone hydrochloride (Opana® ER, Endo).

Another area of opportunity to improve opioid oral formulations is to create abuse-resistant delivery systems. At present, a record of 36 million Americans has abused prescription drugs at least once in their lifetime [19]. It is estimated that the market for abuse-resistant opioid formulations, driven by oxycodone and morphine anti-abuse formulations, will be $1.2 billion by 2017 [20]. Conversely, a concern evident in some FDA decisions not to approve abuse-resistant formulations is that it is still possible for patients to experience serious adverse events related to the opioid component of a properly taken abuse-resistant formulation that has not been tampered with.

King Pharmaceuticals Inc. and Pain Therapeutics, Inc. in 2010 resubmitted a New Drug Application (NDA) for Remoxy®. Remoxy, based on Durect's ORADUR® technology, offers a controlled-release formulation of oxycodone. The company presently markets EMBEDA™ capsules that contain pellets of morphine sulfate and naltrexone hydrochloride in a 100:4 ratio. The latter component may reduce the adverse outcomes associated with sudden ingestion of the opioid provided in this form.

Combination products of existing compounds have been developed to improve efficacy or reduce unwanted side effects. Examples include combination products of oxycodone with ibuprofen, hydrocodone with acetaminophen, or naproxen in combination with the proton pump inhibitor esomeprazole (Vimovo). Vimovo (naproxen and esomeprazole magnesium, AstraZeneca, and Pozen Inc.) has been approved by the US FDA on April 30, 2010, as a new drug combination. It is a delayed-release combination tablet for arthritis whose proton pump component decreases the risk of developing NSAID-associated gastric ulcers in patients prone to this complication.

There are a number of examples where observations of analgesic properties of medicines originally developed for other therapeutic indications led to their application for the treatment of pain. Historically, such agents include medications to treat depression or seizures.

Antiepileptic drugs (AEDs) affect various neurotransmitters, receptors, and ion channels to achieve their anticonvulsant activity that overlap with targets for controlling pain and other dysfunctions. Both conventional and newer AEDs may be used in patients suffering from migraine, essential tremor, spasticity, restless legs syndrome, and a number of psychiatric disorders (e.g., bipolar disease or schizophrenia). AEDs are widely used to treat neuropathic pain syndromes such as postherpetic neuralgia (PHN), painful diabetic neuropathy (PDN), central post-stroke pain syndrome, trigeminal neuralgia, and human immunodeficiency virus (HIV)-associated neuropathic pain.

Lyrica®(pregabalin,(S)-3-(aminomethyl)-5-methylhexanoic acid, Pfizer) is a second-generation anticonvulsant structurally similar to gabapentin. It is the S-enantiomer of racemic 3-isobutyl GABA. The binding affinity of pregabalin for the $Ca_v\alpha2\beta1$ subunit is six times greater than that of gabapentin, which allows pregabalin to be clinically effective at lower doses than gabapentin. Pregabalin is indicated for the treatment of neuropathic pain associated with diabetic peripheral neuropathy (DPN), PHN, and fibromyalgia and as an adjunctive therapy for adult patients with partial onset seizures. Pregabalin binds with high affinity to the alpha2-delta site (an auxiliary subunit of voltage-gated neuronal calcium channels) in the central nervous system. Results with genetically modified mice and with compounds structurally related to pregabalin (such as gabapentin) suggest that binding to the alpha2-delta subunit may be involved in pregabalin's antinociceptive and antiseizure effects in animals. In animal models of nerve damage, pregabalin has been shown to reduce calcium-dependent release of pronociceptive neurotransmitters in the spinal cord, possibly by disrupting alpha2-delta-containing calcium channel trafficking and/or reducing calcium currents. Additional preclinical evidence suggests that the antinociceptive activities of pregabalin may also be mediated through interactions with descending inhibitory noradrenergic and serotonergic pathways originating from the brainstem and descending to the spinal cord.

The L-type VGCC blocker, Topiramate (brand name Topamax) is another AED. Its off-label and investigational uses include the treatment of essential tremor, bulimia nervosa, obsessive-compulsive disorder, alcoholism, smoking cessation, idiopathic intracranial hypertension, neuropathic pain, cluster headache, and cocaine dependence.

Nucynta® (tapentadol, Ortho-McNeil-Janssen) combines two analgesic mechanisms: a mu-opioid agonist and norepinephrine reuptake inhibitor. It is indicated for the relief of moderate to severe acute pain in patients 18 years of age or older. In a recent phase III open-label study, tapentadol extended-release (ER) tablets were compared to an existing prescription pain medication, oxycodone controlled-release (CR) tablets [ClinicalTrials.gov Identifier: NCT00361504].

Tapentadol ER provided sustained relief of moderate to severe chronic knee or hip osteoarthritis pain or chronic low back pain for up to 1 year, with a lower overall incidence of gastrointestinal adverse events than oxycodone CR in patients with chronic knee or hip osteoarthritis pain or chronic low back pain [21].

Savella® (milnacipran hydrochloride) (Forest and Cypress) is a selective serotonin and norepinephrine reuptake inhibitor similar to some drugs used for the treatment for depression and other psychiatric disorders. It is FDA-approved for the treatment of fibromyalgia.

Cymbalta® (duloxetine HCL, delayed-release capsules, Lilly) is indicated for the treatment of major depressive disorder (MDD) and generalized anxiety disorder (GAD). The efficacy of Cymbalta was established, and it is now approved for the management of diabetic peripheral neuropathic pain (DNP), fibromyalgia, and chronic musculoskeletal pain.

Current active strategies for novel analgesic development target ion channels (sodium, calcium, TRP channels), enzymes, receptors (neurotrophins, cannabinoids), and cytokines involved in pain processing.

Voltage-gated sodium channels (VGSCs) are fundamental components to the induction and propagation of neuronal signals. There are at least nine different VGSC subtypes in the nervous system, the distribution of which in aggregate is widespread but distinct for various subtypes. Their expression on afferent neurons has made VGSCs attractive targets to decrease the flow of nociceptive signals to spinal cord. Nonselective inhibitors of VGSCs, such as local anesthetics, have been employed for a century, but the use and in particular the dosing of such agents is limited to undesirable and potentially lethal side effects. Thus, there has been interest in selective VGSC blockers with improved therapeutic indices, particularly $Na_v1.8$ and 1.9 channels. Promising results have been reported for the selective sodium $Na_v1.8$ channel blocker, A-803467, in animal models of both inflammatory and neuropathic pain. The effects were dose-dependent and reversible. Systemic administration of A-803467 decreased the mechanically evoked and spontaneous firing of spinal neurons in nerve-injured rats [22].

Voltage-gated calcium channels (VGCC) or their subunits are another family of molecules with therapeutic potential for chronic pain management. Based on their physiological and pharmacological properties, VGCC can be subdivided into low voltage-activated T type ($Ca_v3.1$, $Ca_v3.2$, $Ca_v3.3$) and high voltage-activated L ($Ca_v1.1$, through $Ca_v1.4$), N ($Ca_v2.2$.), P/Q ($Ca_v2.1$) and R ($Ca_v2.3$) types depending on the channel forming $Ca_v\alpha1$ subunits [23]. All five sub-classes are found in the central and peripheral nervous systems [23, 24]. Most neurons, including sensory neurons and spinal dorsal horn neurons, express multiple types of VGCC. Several types of VGCC are considered potential targets for analgesics based on their distribution, biophysical/patho-logical roles, and plasticity under pain-inducing conditions. Blocking the N-type VGCC at the levels of spinal cord and sensory neurons results in inhibition of stimulus-evoked release of algesic peptides, such as substance P and CGRP and the excitatory neurotransmitter, glutamate. Results from animal studies indicate that N-type VGCC are more directly involved in chronic nociception. Direct blockade of N-type VGCC by cone snail peptides (ω-conotoxins isolated from the marine fish-hunting cone snail, Conus magus) inhibits neuropathic and inflammatory pain but not acute pain, in animal models. In December 2004, the FDA approved ziconotide (a synthetic version of ω-conotoxin MVIIA) for intrathecal treatment of chronic severe pain refractory to other pain medications. ω-conotonix MVIIA is a 25-amino acid peptide. The analgesic effect of ziconotide (Prialt, Elan) is more potent and longer lasting than intrathecal morphine without tolerance or cross-tolerance to morphine analgesia. Ziconotide has been used in patients with severe chronic pain, including neuropathic pain secondary to cancer or AIDS, and in patients with recalcitrant spinal cord injury pain. The use of this drug is limited due to route of adminis-tration and undesirable side effects, including sedation, diz-ziness, nausea, emesis, headache, urinary retention, slurred speech, double or blurry vision, confusion, memory impair-ment, amnesia, anxiety, ataxia, and depression.

The ongoing search for safer and more effective N-type channel blockers continues. The compound Xen2174 (Xenome), a derivative of the χ-conopeptide from cone snail Conus marmoreus, is a peptide whose therapeutic properties were improved through structure-activity analyses to opti-mize its potency, efficacy, safety, stability, and ease of manu-facturing. It is a stable peptide with ability to noncompetitively inhibit norepinephrine transporter. A phase I, double-blind, randomized, single-IV dose escalation study on healthy vol-unteers demonstrated that Xen2174 was safe and well toler-ated. Phase I/II studies, designed as an open-label, single IT bolus, dose-escalating study on cancer patients suffering severe chronic pain, found it to be efficacious and well toler-ated with an acceptable side-effect profile across a wide range of dose levels. A randomized, placebo-controlled, single intrathecal injection study for acute postoperative pain using the bunionectomy model is currently underway.

The unique features of $Ca_v\alpha2\beta$ subunit of calcium chan-nel and recent findings have suggested that the $Ca_v\alpha2\beta_1$ sub-unit may play an important role in neuropathic pain development. The $Ca_v\alpha2\beta_1$ subunit is upregulated in the spi-nal dorsal horn and DRG after nerve injury in correlation with neuropathic pain behavior. The $Ca_v\alpha2\beta_1$ subunit is also the binding site for gabapentin. Both gabapentin and pregab-alin are structural derivatives of the inhibitory neurotransmit-ter GABA, but they do not bind to $GABA_A$, $GABA_B$, or benzodiazepine receptors or alter GABA regulation. Binding of gabapentin and pregabalin to the $Ca_v\alpha2\beta_1$ subunit of VGCC results in a reduction in the calcium-dependent release of multiple neurotransmitters leading to efficacy and tolerability for neuropathic pain management.

Gabapentin is approved by FDA for postherpetic neuralgia, neuropathic pain, and partial seizures. Several studies also suggest a clinical role for restless leg syndrome, general anxi-ety, and general neuropathic pain. Gabapentin is used as a first-line agent to treat neuropathic pain from central (stroke, spinal cord injury) or peripheral origin (peripheral neuropathy, radiculopathy). It has a short half-life and the administration needs to be frequent. A gabapentin extended-release (ER) has been developed. Gabapentic ER was formulated using poly-mer-based AcuForm technology (DepoMed). When taken with a meal, the tablet is retained in stomach for up to 8 h and the drug is gradually released over 10 h in the small intestine, its optimal site of absorption. A recent randomized, double-blind, placebo-controlled study evaluated gastric-retentive gabapentin in patients with chronic pain from postherpetic neuralgia, with statistically significant reductions in pain scores in the gabapentin ER twice-daily group. However, pain scores in the once-daily gabapentin group were not reduced more than those in the placebo group [25].

A novel prodrug of gabapentin, XP13512/GSK 1838262 (Horizant and GlaxoSmithKline) was recently developed for the treatment of restless legs syndrome (RLS), PHN, PDN, and migraine prophylaxis. This drug has significant absorp-tion in the large intestine, allowing an extended-release for-mulation. XP13512 improved symptoms in all patients and reduced pain associated with RLS significantly more than placebo. A later study included 222 patients with moderate to severe RLS and showed that XP13512 significantly improved the mean International RLS total score compared with pla-cebo at week 12. The most common treatment-related adverse events included somnolence and dizziness [26].

Transient receptor potential (TRP) channels are nonse-lective monovalent and divalent cation channels. TRPV channels are present in small unmyelinated and myelinated (C and A delta) fibers of primary afferent neurons, dorsal root, trigeminal ganglia, the dorsal horn of the spinal cord (lamina I and II), and spinal nucleus of the trigeminal tract.

The principal interest in TRP channels has focused on TRPV1 (vanilloid receptors) due to their role in nociceptive transmission, amplification, and sensitization. The search for perfect TRPV antagonist has yielded several drugs that underwent clinical trials. In phase II, clinical trials are SB-705498 (for migraine), NGD-8243/MK-2295 (for acute pain), and GRC (for acute pain); in phase I are AMG-517, AZD-1386, and ABT-102 (for chronic pain). During phase I clinical trials with AMG 517, a highly selective TRPV1 antagonist, it was found that TRPV1 blockade elicited marked, but reversible, and generally plasma concentration-dependent hyperthermia. AZD1386 was discontinued from development in 2010 due to liver enzyme elevations.

SB-705498 is a potent, selective, and orally bioavailable TRPV1 antagonist with efficacy in preclinical pain models. The compound was safe and well tolerated at single oral doses in a phase I study. A phase II trial used a randomized, placebo-controlled, single-blind crossover design to assess the effects of SB-705498 (400 mg) on heat-evoked pain and skin sensitization induced by capsaicin or UVB irradiation. Compared with placebo, SB-705498 reduced the area of capsaicin-evoked flare and raised the heat pain threshold on non-sensitized skin at the site of UVB-evoked inflammation [27].

Because they are not neural cells, microglia represent a relatively novel therapeutic target for analgesia. Activation of p38 mitogen-activated protein kinases (p38MAPK) and P2X4 in spinal cord microglia is essential for allodynia after nerve injury. The allodynia was reversed rapidly by pharmacological blockade of p38MAPK activation or inhibiting the expression of P2X4 receptors. Inhibitions of P2X4 expression, inhibiting the function of these receptors and/or p38MAPK in spinal microglia, are therefore potential therapeutic approaches. Losmapimod (GW856553X) is a selective p38MAPK inhibitor developed by GlaxoSmithKline. p38MAPK inhibition has been shown to produce antidepressant and antipsychotic effects in animal studies, with the mechanism thought to involve increased neurogenesis probably related to BDNF release. Losmapimod has completed phase II human clinical trials for the treatment of depression, although its safety and efficacy have yet to be proven in further trials.

There are several phase I study completed (a first-time-in-human randomized, single-blind placebo-controlled study to evaluate the safety, tolerability, pharmacokinetics, and pharmacodynamics of single escalating doses of GSK1482160, in male and female healthy subjects, and to make a preliminary assessment of the effect of food), phase II completed (a randomized, double-blind study to evaluate the safety and efficacy of the p38 kinase inhibitor, GW856553, in subjects with neuropathic pain from lumbosacral radiculopathy), or under way (a randomized, double-blind study to evaluate the safety and efficacy of the p38 kinase inhibitor, GW856553, in subjects with neuropathic pain from peripheral nerve injury) [28].

Tanezumab is a monoclonal antibody that inhibits the production of NGF. NGF stimulates nerve development, triggers pain, and is often present in inflamed tissues, such as arthritic joints. Treatment with tanezumab led to significant improvements in osteoarthritis knee pain in a phase II proof-of-concept study. Patients who received various doses of tanezumab had significant reductions in knee pain while walking. However, there were reports of progressively worsening osteoarthritis that emerged following completion of this study. These reports included 16 patients who had radiographic evidence of bone necrosis that required total joint replacement [29]. The investigators concluded that the efficacy profile for tanezumab was favorable but called for more safety data. In the fall of 2010, the FDA halted the tanezumab clinical development program. It was suggested that the pain relief conferred by tanezumab was so substantial that patients increased their physical activity enough to accelerate joint damage, ultimately causing them to need earlier joint replacement. The FDA also asked the company to stop phase II stage of testing of the drug to treat chronic low back and painful diabetic peripheral neuropathy; studies testing on the drug's efficacy in patients suffering from cancer pain and chronic pancreatitis are continuing.

Also, FDA in December 2010 asked Regeneron to stop testing REGN475, another fully human antibody that selectively targets NGF, fearing that acceleration of avascular necrosis of a joint may occur. Before that point, initial results from a randomized, double-blind, four-arm, placebo-controlled phase II trial in 217 patients with osteoarthritis of the knee were very promising. REGN475 demonstrated significant improvements at the two highest doses tested as compared to placebo in average walking pain scores over 8 weeks following a single intravenous infusion. Similarly, in the end of December 2010, the FDA put on hold phase II testing of fulranumab (Johnson & Johnson) over concerns that, as with other drugs in anti-NGF class, it may cause rapidly progressive osteoarthritis or osteonecrosis resulting in the need for earlier total joint replacement.

Abbott Laboratories have ongoing (but not actively recruiting participants) phase I studies of the monoclonal antibody PG110 (a randomized, double-blind, placebo-controlled, single ascending dose, phase I study to evaluate the safety, tolerability, and pharmacokinetics of PG110 (anti-NGF monoclonal antibody) in patients with pain attributed to osteoarthritis of the knee, NCT00941746) [30]. The status of the study is "ongoing, but not recruiting participants."

All but one study with Johnson & Johnson JNJ-42160443 (fulranumab) testing it in osteoarthritis pain, cancer-related pain, diabetic painful neuropathy, neuropathic pain (postherpetic neuralgia and post-traumatic neuralgia), and bladder pain have likewise been suspended. One phase II study, "a randomized, double-blind, placebo-controlled, dose-ranging, dose-loading study to evaluate the efficacy, safety, and tolerability of JNJ-42160443 as adjunctive therapy in subjects with inadequately controlled, moderate to severe, chronic low back pain" is ongoing but not recruiting participants [31].

Marijuana and cannabinoids are now available for medicinal purposes in many US states, although inconsistencies with Federal prohibitions have interfered widely with legal patient access of such agent. The main pharmacological effects of marijuana, as well as synthetic and endogenous cannabinoids, are mediated through G protein-coupled receptors (GPCRs), including CB-1 and CB-2 receptors. The CB-1 receptor is the major cannabinoid receptor in the central nervous system and has gained increasing interest as a target for drug discovery for treatment of nausea, cachexia, obesity, pain, spasticity, neurodegenerative diseases, and mood and substance abuse disorders. GW Pharmaceuticals conducted Sativex clinical trials in over 3,000 patients, including over 20 phase II and phase III trials worldwide including patients with multiple sclerosis, cancer pain, neuropathic pain, and rheumatoid arthritis. Sativex is delivered as an oromucosal spray in which each 100-µl spray contains 2.7 mg delta-9-tetrahydrocannabinol (THC) and 2.5 mg cannabidiol (CBD) extracted from farmed *Cannabis sativa* leaf and flower. Sativex includes, among its other indications, the improvement of symptoms in patients with moderate to severe spasticity due to multiple sclerosis (MS) who have not responded adequately to other anti-spasticity medication and who demonstrate clinically significant improvement in spasticity-related symptoms during an initial trial of therapy.

In 2010, GW Pharmaceuticals announced results of phase IIb dose-ranging trial evaluating the efficacy and safety of Sativex® in the treatment of pain in patients with advanced cancer, who experience inadequate analgesia during optimized chronic opioid therapy [32]. Sativex showed statistically significant differences from placebo in pain scores. In Europe, Sativex is approved in the UK and Spain as a treatment for multiple sclerosis spasticity. In Canada, Sativex is approved for the treatment for central neuropathic pain due to MS. In the USA, cancer pain represents the initial target indication for Sativex.

Sativex showed positive results in a phase II placebo-controlled trial in 56 patients with rheumatoid arthritis (RA). RA is the most common form of inflammatory arthritis and afflicts up to 3 % of the population of Western countries. In this 56 patient study, statistically significant improvements in favor of Sativex were found for pain on movement, pain at rest, quality of sleep, and DAS28 scores. The DAS28 is the present gold standard inflammation activity measure, and this result suggests an effect on the progression of the disease itself. Sativex is approved and marketed in the UK for the relief of spasticity in MS.

Sativex is approved and marketed in Canada for the relief of neuropathic pain in MS as well as for the relief of spasticity in MS. Other completed phase III clinical studies have tested the effectiveness of Sativex in peripheral neuropathic pain [33], diabetic neuropathy [34], and cancer pain [35]. There are active phase I and II studies being conducted in California of vaporized cannabis as an analgesic for PDN [36]. In Canada, an open phase III study is exploring the effect of Sativex in treatment of neuropathic pain caused by chemotherapy [37].

ILARIS (canakinumab; ACZ885; Novartis Pharmaceuticals; injection for subcutaneous use only) is an interleukin-1β monoclonal antibody initially approved in the USA in 2009 for the treatment of cryopyrin-associated periodic syndromes (CAPS), a group of rare inherited autoinflammatory conditions including familial cold autoinflammatory syndrome (FCAS) and Muckle-Wells syndrome (MWS) (initial US approval in 2009). Signs and symptoms include recurrent rash, fever/chills, joint pain, fatigue, and eye pain/redness. Currently, there are two open phase II, placebo-controlled trials in the USA and Europe assessing the ability of canakinumab to inhibit IL-1β activity for sustained time periods and thus favorably impact OA symptoms including pain, decreased function, and stiffness [38]. Another trial taking place in Ireland, Italy, and the UK assesses the safety and efficacy of ACZ885 in patients with active recurrent or chronic TNF receptor-associated periodic syndrome (TRAPS) [39].

Botox® (botulinum toxin A (BTX-A), Allergan) is currently available in approximately 75 countries for injection into muscles to treat upper limb spasticity in people 18 years and older, abnormal head position and neck pain of cervical dystonia (CD) in people 16 years and older, and certain eye muscle problems (strabismus) or eyelid spasm (blepharospasm) in people 12 years and older. As post-marketing experience has accumulated with these and other conditions such as headache, above and beyond its wide application for cosmetic purposes, clues have emerged that its beneficial effects upon pain are separable from those upon muscle contraction. French investigators have demonstrated the long-term efficacy of repeated applications of BTX-A in a small group of patients with post-traumatic or postherpetic neuralgia. These investigators are now seeking to confirm these findings in a larger randomized, placebo-controlled phase IV study [40]. Other studies are accruing patients with diabetic neuropathic foot pain, shoulder pain, male pelvic pain syndrome, back pain, and upper thoracic muscular pain.

In 2010, Pfizer Inc. acquired FoldRx and its portfolio of investigational compounds to treat diseases caused by protein misfolding, increasingly recognized as an important mechanism of many chronic degenerative diseases. The company's lead product candidate, tafamidis meglumine, is in registration as an oral, disease-modifying therapy for transthyretin (TTR) amyloid polyneuropathy (ATTR-PN), a progressively fatal genetic neurodegenerative disease, for which liver transplant is the only current treatment option. Tafamidis is a new chemical entity, first-in-class, oral, disease-modifying agent that stabilizes TTR and prevents dissociation of the tetramer, the rate-limiting step in TTR amyloidosis. Early results from FoldRx's randomized, controlled phase II/III clinical study show that once-daily oral treatment was safe and well tolerated, while halting disease progression and reducing the burden of disease after 18 months compared to placebo.

Telcagepant (formerly MK-0974, Merck) is a calcitonin gene-related peptide receptor (CRLR) antagonist under investigation for the acute treatment and prevention of migraine. Calcitonin gene-related peptide (CGRP) is an algesic peptide involved in nociceptive neurotransmission, as well as a strong vasodilator primarily found in nervous tissue. Since vasodilation in the brain is thought to be involved in the development of migraine and CGRP levels are increased during migraine attacks, this peptide was considered a potential target for new antimigraine drugs. It was equally efficacious as rizatriptan and zolmitriptan in two phase III clinical trials. A phase IIa clinical trial studying telcagepant for the prophylaxis of episodic migraine was stopped on March 26, 2009, due to significant elevations in serum transaminases. It is still possible that this safety concern may be addressed satisfactorily and, if so, that this drug will come to the market.

Alternative Delivery Routes

Intranasal and Inhalational Drug Delivery

Intranasal formulations are in wide use and are easy to administer. Potential benefits of intranasal drug delivery include rapid onset of action and improved compliance with unit dosage forms. Intranasal opioids, in the form of a dry powder or water or saline solution, are delivered using syringe, nasal spray or dropper, or nebulized inhaler. In addition to needle-free administration, the intranasal opioid route of administration (especially fentanyl) bypasses hepatic first-pass metabolism; because of the excellent perfusion of the nasal mucosa, there is rapid absorption and a prompt rise in plasma concentrations comparable to that seen with IV injection.

Intranasal morphine (Rylomine, Javelin now Hospira) is a patient-controlled nasal spray that provides rapid analgesic onset comparable to IV simply and noninvasively to control moderate to severe pain. The drug product combines morphine mesylate and chitosan, a natural polymer derived from the shells of crustaceans. Chitosan serves as a mucoadherent to facilitate and linearly dispense morphine absorption through the nasal mucosa. A single-spray unit dose delivers 7.5 mg of morphine mesylate in 0.1-ml metered dose. Early clinical trials in acute postoperative pain showed safety and efficacy comparable to those seen with equivalent doses of systemic morphine.

A similar approach to regularizing the intranasal absorption of an opioid, in this case fentanyl, has been approved in 2011 for Lazanda (Archimedes). In the case of Lazanda, fentanyl is coformulated with the pectin, which forms a gel when it contacts the nasal mucosa thus allowing the active ingredient to be delivered in a rapid but controlled manner. This drug product is indicated to treat episodes of breakthrough pain in patients with cancer.

Intranasal ketamine (Ereska, Javelin now Hospira) has been tested in metered, subanesthetic doses with the intention to offer an alternative to morphine for acute pain and potentially to treat cancer breakthrough pain in patients on chronic opioid therapy.

AeroLEF (aerosolized liposome-encapsulated fentanyl, YM BioSciences) is a proprietary formulation of free and liposome-encapsulated fentanyl intended to provide rapid and extended inhalational analgesia for patients with acute pain episodes. AeroLEF is in development for the treatment of moderate to severe pain, including cancer pain.

Fentanyl TAIFUN (Akela and Janssen) is a dry powder being developed for inhalational use to treat breakthrough pain. Following favorable results in an open-label phase II clinical trial, phase III testing is ongoing in patients with cancer pain during maintenance opioid therapy [41].

Mucoadhesive Drug Delivery

The BioErodible MucoAdhesive (BEMA) delivery system is designed to deliver either local or systemic levels of drugs across mucosal tissues. This delivery system offers rapid onset of action, avoidance of first-pass hepatic metabolism, and improved drug bioavailability compared with the oral route. The BEMA delivery system consists of a dime-sized disk with bioerodible layers that deliver drugs rapidly across a sequence of specified time intervals. One example of this technology is the BEMA Fentanyl mouth patch from BioDelivery Sciences International (Raleigh, NC), approved by FDA in 2009 as Onsolis to manage breakthrough cancer pain.

Rapinyl (Orexo and ProStrakan) is similar in concept, i.e., a fast-dissolving tablet of fentanyl under development for the treatment of breakthrough cancer pain.

Transdermal Drug Delivery

Poultices of medications, salves, and ointments have been applied since prehistory. A heat-assisted transdermal delivery system for fentanyl briefly under development in recent decades is reminiscent of the traditional Chinese practice of "cupping" in which smoldering herbs applied to the skin are covered with a glass of porcelain cup. Since the approval of Duragesic, the original "fentanyl patch" developed by Alza and Janssen in the 1980s, a steady increase of new delivery methods has taken place for both opioids (including heat-assisted transdermal delivery) and non-opioids.

Fentanyl transdermal system (Mylan Pharmaceuticals) has an innovative matrix design that, in contrast to Duragesic, employs neither metal nor a gel reservoir. Like Duragesic, it is indicated only for use in patients who are already tolerant to opioid therapy and for management of persistent, moderate to severe chronic pain that requires continuous opioid administration for an extended time and that cannot be managed by nonsteroidal analgesics, opioid combination products, or immediate release opioids.

The Flector® Patch (diclofenac epolamine topical patch) (King, now Pfizer) 1.3 % is used for the topical treatment of acute short-term pain due to minor strains, sprains, and contusions (bruises). Flector® Patch adheres to the affected area and delivers the efficacy of the NSAID diclofenac epolamine to the site of acute pain for 12 h of pain relief. Although the amount of systemic uptake of diclofenac is low compared with the traditional oral formulations, any of the typical NSAID and diclofenac adverse effects may occur. Therefore, as for all NSAIDs, it is recommended that the lowest strength of Flector be used for the shortest possible duration.

Future Directions: "Quo Vadis?"

The idea that there is single universal analgesic compound for pain treatment has been largely abandoned. Pain is a complex phenomenon with heterogeneous etiologies, mechanisms, and temporal characteristics. Consequently, treatment must be targeted not at the general symptom, pain, or its temporal properties, acute or chronic, but rather at the underlying neurobiological mechanisms. Recent comprehensive summaries of analgesic drugs under development attest to the ingenuity of scientists and clinical researchers in exploring many options for reformulation of existing molecules as well as creating new chemical entities [42]. Identification of key molecular targets involved in nociception and discovery and characterization of specific activators and inhibitors are not yet complete. Efforts to describe genetic influences upon pain, nociception, and the response to analgesics are likewise in the early stages. Still, it is relevant to the future of pain pharmacotherapy to step back and consider how far along we really are in the discovery process. The human genome, although large, is now fully sequenced and known to be finite. Together with comprehensive biological knowledge as to the range of possible drug targets (enzymes, receptors, ion channels, transporter proteins, etc.), it is now possible to estimate the total number of potential drug targets [43]. That number in turn is linked to, albeit not tightly, the total number of drugs that are likely to find a place in analgesic pharmacotherapy [44].

Figure 19.1 is the authors' attempt to convey that with increasing time, the number of available analgesic drugs will reach a plateau. One may ask what the scales should be for

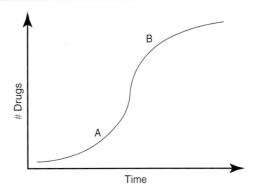

Fig. 19.1 A hypothetical graph of the number of available drugs as a function of time. The scales on the abscissa and ordinate are deliberately not specified (See text for discussion)

the abscissa and ordinate of this graph and whether we now are at point "A" or point "B." We would suggest "B" for the following reason: The relief of pain has been a continuous goal of humankind globally since prehistory [45]. Humans have swallowed, smoked, daubed on, or otherwise evaluated the analgesic properties and tolerability of nearly all substances within reach for tens of thousands of years. From this point of view, we would assert that the abscissa in Fig. 19.1 spans tens of thousands of years. It should come as no surprise that this prolonged, worldwide, high-throughput (if decentralized) screening for analgesic effectiveness has yielded agents that even today remain the foundation for analgesic pharmacotherapy: anti-inflammatories (e.g., willow bark), opioids (e.g., opium), and local anesthetics (e.g., cocaine). These drugs are supplemented by nondrug interventions first identified centuries or millennia ago such as heat, cold, splinting, and counter-stimulation with needles and/or electricity. Although the capacity of today's organized drug discovery processes dwarfs that of previous eras' empirical ad hoc observations, the former approach has proceeded for about a century while the latter has been in place for at least a hundredfold longer.

Summary/Conclusions

Despite efforts to maximize the utility of existing pain medicines, obvious shortfalls in the analgesic armamentarium persist. Analgesics based upon novel molecular and genetic mechanisms are being intensively explored to address the unmet needs of patients in pain [42]. The discovery and development of such medicines may require a surprising amount of effort and expense, however, to progress only slightly up the curve shown in Fig. 19.1. To some degree, this slowness to progress may reflect the many late-stage failures among recently developed analgesic compounds due to an unintended negative bias in the current FDA drug approval framework, such as overlooking subgroups of responders [46]. Further, on a global scale, many of the analgesic gaps between ideal and actual practice may be addressed simply by providing access to simple inexpensive agents such as anti-inflammatory drugs or opioids [47]. Nonetheless, even after taking these factors under consideration, it is safe to predict that in the wealthier nations, the search for new analgesics with an improved effect to side-effect profile and improved methods for the delivery of familiar agents will continue for some time to come.

Acknowledgment   Partial support for this work was provided by the Saltonstall Fund for Pain Research.

References

1. Institute of Medicine. Relieving pain in America: a blueprint for transforming prevention, care, education and research. Washington D.C.: The National Academies Press; 2011.
2. Coggeshall RE, Carlton SM. Receptor localization in the mammalian dorsal horn and primary afferent neurons. Brain Res Rev. 1997;24:28–66.
3. Traub RJ. The spinal contribution of the induction of central sensitization. Brain Res. 1997;778:34–42.
4. Dickenson AH. Spinal cord pharmacology of pain. Br J Anaesth. 1995;75:193–200.
5. Scholz J, Woolf CJ. Can we conquer pain? Nat Neurosci. 2002;5(Suppl):1062–7.
6. Rittner HL, Brack A, Machelska H, et al. Opioid peptide-expressing leukocytes: identification, recruitment, and simultaneously increasing inhibition of inflammatory pain. Anesthesiology. 2001;95:500–8.
7. Millan MJ. The induction of pain: an integrative review. Prog Neurobiol. 1999;57:1–164.
8. Machelska H, Stein C. Immune mechanisms in pain control. Anesth Analg. 2002;95:1002–8.
9. Shu X-Q, Mendell LM. Neurotrophins and hyperalgesia. Proc Natl Acad Sci U S A. 1999;96:7693–6.
10. Thompson SWN, Bennett DLH, Kerr BJ, Bradbury EJ, McMahon SB. Brain-derived neurotrophic factor is an endogenous modulator of nociceptive responses in the spinal cord. Proc Natl Acad Sci U S A. 1999;96:7714–8.
11. Cortright DN, Szallasi A. Biochemical pharmacology of the vanilloid receptor TRPV1: an update. Eur J Biochem. 2004;271:1814–9.
12. Rashid MH, Inoune M, Kondo S, Kawashima T, Bakoshi S, Ueda H. Novel expression of vanilloid receptor 1 on capsaicin-insensitive fibers accounts for the analgesic effect of capsaicin cream in neuropathic pain. J Pharmacol Exp Ther. 2003;304:940–8.
13. Walker SM, Goudas LC, Cousins MJ, Carr DB. Combination spinal analgesic chemotherapy: a systematic review. Anesth Analg. 2002;96:674–715.
14. Colombo P, Sonvico F, Colombo G, et al. Novel platforms for oral drug delivery. Pharm Res. 2009;26(3):601–11.
15. Drug and Biologic Approval Reports. United States Food and Drug Administration. 2011. FDA Web site www.fda.gov/. Accessed 10 Jan 2011.
16. Business Insights. Lifecycle management strategies: maximizing ROI through indication expansion, reformulation and Rx-to-OTC switching. Business Insights Report. 2006.
17. Grudzinskas C, Balster RL, Gorodetzky CW, et al. Impact of formulation on the abuse liability, safety and regulation of medications: the expert panel report. Drug Alcohol Depend. 2006;83(Supp 1):S77–82.
18. Collier R. Drug development cost estimates hard to swallow. CMAJ. 2009;180(3):279–80.
19. Associated Press. Scientists explore abuse-resistant painkillers. MSNBC Web site. 2007. Available at www.msnbc.msn.com/id/17581544/. Accessed 21 May 2009.
20. Commercial and Pipeline Insight: Opioids - Short acting and anti-abuse technologies set to fragment and grow the market. Datamonitor. March 2008. Abstract. http://www.marketresearch.com/Datamonitor-v72/Commercial-Pipeline-Insight-Opioids-Short-1728798/ Accessed 10 Feb 2011.
21. Wild JE, Grond S, Kuperwasser B, et al. Long-term safety and tolerability of tapentadol extended release for the management of chronic low back pain or osteoarthritis pain. Pain Pract. 2010;10:416–27.
22. McGaraughty S, Chu KC, Scanio MLC, Kort ME, Faltynek CR, Jarvis MF. A selective $Na_v1.8$ sodium channel blocker, A-803467 [5-(4-chlorophenyl-N-(3,5-dimethoxyphenyl)furan-2-carboxamide], attenuates spinal neuronal activity in neuropathic rats. J Pharmacol Exp Ther. 2008;324:1204–11.
23. Catterall WA. Structure and regulation of voltage-gated Ca2+ channels. Annu Rev Cell Dev Biol. 2000;16:521–55.
24. Ertel EA, Campbell KP, Harpold MM, et al. Nomenclature of voltage-gated calcium channels. Neuron. 2000;25:533–5.
25. Irving G, Jensen M, Cramer M, et al. Efficacy and tolerability of gastric-retentive gabapentin for the treatment of postherpetic neuralgia: results of double-blind, randomized, placebo-controlled clinical trial. Clin J Pain. 2009;25:185–92.
26. Kushida CA, Becker PM, Ellenbogen AL, Canafax DM, Barrett RW. Randomized, double-blind, placebo-controlled study of XP13512/GSK 1838262 in patients with RLS. Neurology. 2009;72:439–46.
27. Gunthorpe MJ, Chizh BA. Clinical development of TRPV1 antagonists: targeting a pivotal point in the pain pathway. Drug Discov Today. 2009;14(1–2):56–67.
28. A randomized, double blind study to evaluate the safety and efficacy of the p38 kinase inhibitor, GW856553, in subjects with neuropathic pain from peripheral nerve injury. GlaxoSmithKline GSK: Protocol Summaries: Compounds: Losmapimod. GSK Study ID112967. Study completed. http://www.gsk-clinicalstudyregister.com/protocol_comp_list.jsp;jsessionid=275F763F1C36638B02758F5A4C276956?compound=Losmapimod. Accessed 11 Feb 2011.
29. Lane NE, Schnitzer TJ, Birbara CA, et al. Tanezumab for the treatment of pain from osteoarthritis of the knee. N Engl J Med. 2010;363:1521–31.
30. Safety and tolerability of PG110 in patients with knee osteoarthritis pain. 2011. http://clinicaltrials.gov/ct2/show/NCT00941746. Study completed. Accessed 11 Feb 2011.
31. A dose-ranging study of the safety and effectiveness of JNJ-42160443 as add-on treatment in patients with low back pain. 2011. http://clinicaltrials.gov/ct2/show/NCT00973024. Study terminated. Accessed 11 Feb 2011.
32. A study of Sativex® for relieving persistent pain in patients with advancedcancer. 2011. http://clinicaltrials.gov/ct2/show/NCT01262651. Study currently active. Accessed 11 Feb 2011.
33. A study of Sativex® for pain relief of peripheral neuropathic pain, associated with allodynia. 2011. http://clinicaltrials.gov/ct2/show/NCT00710554. Study completed. Accessed 11 Feb 2011.
34. A study of Sativex® for pain relief due to diabetic neuropathy. 2011. http://clinicaltrials.gov/ct2/show/NCT00710424. Study completed. Accessed 11 Feb 2011.
35. Study to compare the safety and tolerability of Sativex® in patients with cancer related pain. 2011. http://clinicaltrials.gov/ct2/show/NCT00675948. Study completed. Accessed 11 Feb 2011.
36. Efficacy of inhaled cannabis in diabetic painful peripheral neuropathy. 2011. http://clinicaltrials.gov/ct2/show/NCT00781001. Study currently active. Accessed 11 Feb 2011.
37. A double blind placebo controlled crossover pilot trial of Sativex with open label extension for treatment of chemotherapy induced neuropathic pain. 2011. http://clinicaltrials.gov/ct2/show/NCT00872144. Study currently active. Accessed 11 Feb 2011.

38. A randomized, double blind, placebo and naproxen controlled, multi-center, study to determine the safety, tolerability, pharmacokinetics and effect on pain of a single intra-articular administration of canakinumab in patients with osteoarthritis in the knee. 2011. http://clinicaltrials.gov/ct2/show/NCT01160822. Study completed. Accessed 11 Feb 2011.

39. An open-label, multicenter, efficacy and safety study of 4-month canakinumab treatment with 6-month follow-up in patients with active recurrent or chronic TNF-receptor associated periodic syndrome (TRAPS). 2011. http://clinicaltrials.gov/ct2/show/NCT01242813. Study currently active. Accessed 11 Feb 2011.

40. Randomized double blind placebo controlled multicenter study of the efficacy and safety of repeated administrations of botulinum toxin type A (Botox) in the treatment of peripheral neuropathic pain. 2011. http://clinicaltrials.gov/ct2/show/NCT01251211. Study currently active. Accessed 11 Feb 2011.

41. The safety of fentanyl TAIFUN treatment after titrated dose administration and the current breakthrough pain treatment for breakthrough pain in cancer patients. 2011. http://clinicaltrials.gov/ct2/show/NCT00822614. Study currently active. Accessed 11 Feb 2011.

42. Sinatra RS, Jahr JS, Watkins-Pitchford JM, editors. The essence of analgesia and analgesics. New York: Cambridge University Press; 2011.

43. Overington JP, Al-Lazikani B, Hopkins AL. How many drug targets are there? Nat Rev Drug Discov. 2006;5:993–6.

44. Imming P, Sinning C, Meyer A. Drugs, their targets, and the nature and number of drug targets. Nat Rev Drug Discov. 2006;5:821–34.

45. Gallagher RM, Fishman SM. Pain medicine: history, emergence as a medical specialty, and evolution of the multidisciplinary approach. In: Cousins MJ, Bridenbaugh PO, Carr DB, Horlocker TT, editors. Cousins & Bridenbaugh's neural blockade in clinical anesthesia and management of pain. 4th ed. Philadelphia: Lippincott Williams & Wilkins; 2009. p. 631–43.

46. Dworkin RH, Turk DC. Accelerating the development of improved analgesic treatments: the ACTION public-private partnership. Pain Med. 2011;12:S109–17.

47. Brennan F, Carr DB, Cousins MJ. Pain management: a fundamental human right. Anesth Analg. 2007;105:205–21.

Part II

Interventional Approaches: Anatomy and Physiology of Pain

Asokumar Buvanendran, Sunil J. Panchal, and Philip S. Kim

Introduction

Interventional procedures are covered in three parts:
Part II reviews the anatomy and physiology of pain, as relevant to the practitioner
Part III details neural blockade and neurolysis blocks
Part IV provides guidance to the full range of neuromodulation techniques

As supported by this volume, comprehensive pain care is the optimal method to help patients progress to recovery. Interventional pain procedures are one part of the comprehensive approach. New procedures continue to be developed and established procedures continue to evolve as our understanding of the pathophysiology of pain grows. At the same time, the evidence base for interventional pain procedures is under intense scrutiny. The issue is a familiar one in the realm of interventional treatments. As with other surgical procedures, having a control group in a clinical study of interventions for patients with chronic pain presents significant ethical concerns.

The contributors to these parts and we share the belief that the decision to use a procedure solely on the basis of evidence misses the importance of the context of treatment. By the time a patient seeks out a pain medicine physician, he or she is looking for a practice that provides advanced and novel interventional treatments. The primary care physician has already started the patient on non-surgical approaches such as physical therapy and analgesics, and the interventional procedure acts as a therapeutic bridge between the patient's non-surgical management and psychological coping strategies, often significantly reducing the dose requirements of oral analgesics. From trigger point injections and epidural steroids, to radiofrequency ablation and implantable devices (for spinal cord stimulation, peripheral nerve stimulation, and intraspinal drug delivery), interventional procedures are among the most efficient ways of effecting change in pain reporting.

As the population of patients coping with pain grows older, maintenance on oral analgesics, particularly opioids for chronic non-cancer pain, becomes less of an option due to the development of comorbid medical conditions and the addition of other medications. Interventions for painful conditions, such as vertebral compression fractures, spondylosis, and spinal stenosis, can help older patients with acute pain and provide immediate and temporizing relief.

Given the fast evolutionary pace of technology, we expect that the chapter content in these parts will change significantly when the next edition of the book is published. In this inaugural edition, our aim is to provide you with up-to-the-minute expert guidance and practical tips for the current practice of simple and complex interventions for pain control. Furthermore, we hope to offer you a glimpse into the future, of therapies to come.

Neuroanatomy and Neurophysiology of Pain

20

Adam R. Burkey

Key Points

- All chronic pain, to a greater or lesser extent, alters nervous system physiology and is therefore neuropathic.
- Electrical neuromodulation may be employed against the peripheral and intraspinal nervous system in a variety of ways to "gate" the flow of pain information to consciousness.
- Modern functional imaging of the forebrain has confirmed and extended our understanding of pain neuroanatomy and may be an outcome measure for studies of pain in the future.
- In the future, research may be able to better match particular clinical characteristics to underlying pain physiology, understand how to act on autonomic and visceral pathways, and control glial and inflammatory activity to reduce neuropathic pain.

Introduction

The neuroanatomy and neurophysiology of pain can be discussed with regard to every level of the nervous system, from peripheral nerve to cerebral cortex. Rudimentary *nociception* is the physiologic perception of a potentially tissue-damaging stimulus and is the commonplace conception that holds when one claims that "something hurts." However, as we review here, "something hurting" for an extended period of time will induce changes in the nervous system that may be irreversible. For this reason, many experts believe that all chronic pain is, to some extent, *neuropathic*. This makes it

often impossible to merely remove the thorn from the lion's paw (treat a defined bodily source) and eliminate chronic pain, as much as patients wish we could. Pain as a subjective, even abstract, experience involving a complex array of emotions may occur independent of *any* discernable bodily tissue damage, such as the case of fibromyalgia. For this reason, most chronic pain treatments – whether with medications, cognitive therapies or interventional procedures – attempt to alter physiological pain processing in the peripheral nerve, spinal cord, or forebrain.

In the modern era, there have been three watershed moments in the scientific understanding of pain. The first was the "gate theory" of Melzack and Wall [1]. This theory held that circuitry existed in the spinal cord whereby an innocuous stimulus could block transmission of a noxious stimulus to the brain. This theory is still discussed and referenced by researchers who study pain processing in the spinal dorsal horn. The second was the delineation of a descending pathway from the brain stem to the spinal dorsal horn that could block ascending pain-related information, the so-called descending inhibitory system [2]. This opened the door for the study of mechanisms of analgesia, as it became clear that many analgesics, including morphine, utilized this endogenous circuitry to produce their effects. Thirdly, the advent of functional imaging in the early 1990s has yielded a wealth of information on how chronic pain is processed in the forebrain, defining potential sites of action for novel analgesics and providing more objective data than previously available on chronic pain outcomes and the mechanisms of action of therapeutic interventions.

Pain Neuroanatomy and Physiology

Peripheral and Spinal Neuroanatomy

Primary afferent (or sensory) neurons provide ongoing information about the external environment and the internal bodily milieu. Primary afferent nociceptors (PANs) detect chiefly temperature, trauma, and acidosis of tissues [3]. Their cell

20

A.R. Burkey, M.D., MSCE
Jefferson University,
Medical Office Building I, 824 Main Street, Suite 307,
Phoenixville, PA 19460, USA
e-mail: phxpain@aol.com

T.R. Deer et al. (eds.), *Comprehensive Treatment of Chronic Pain by Medical, Interventional, and Integrative Approaches*,
DOI 10.1007/978-1-4614-1560-2_20, © American Academy of Pain Medicine 2013

bodies reside in the "dorsal root ganglion" (DRG) which sits just outside the spinal cord. Their axons bifurcate within the ganglion, sending one branch out to innervate various tissues and the other to innervate the dorsal horn of the spinal cord. Most PANs have smaller cell bodies and thin lightly myelinated (Aδ) or unmyelinated (C) axons, the latter terminating as free nerve endings in various organs – skin, muscle, and visceral organs. The conduction velocities of PAN are slower than the large, heavily myelinated axons that act as motoneurons or mechanoreceptors that detect vibration or position sense.

Lightly myelinated Aδ nociceptors enter the spinal cord often in or near Lissauer's tract with terminations primarily in laminae I and IIo of the superficial dorsal horn [4]; some terminations can be found in deeper laminae III–V and X as well. A subset of Aδ nociceptors ramify rostrally and caudally through several spinal segments of Lissauer's tract before terminating. These neurons respond to different stimulus modalities (mechanical or thermal) and are thought to convey fast pricking or sharp pain.

Unmyelinated C fibers respond to a diversity of noxious mechanical, thermal, or chemical modalities. They are classified into two broad types: peptidergic and non-peptidergic [5]. Peptidergic C fibers carry TrkA, the high-affinity receptor for nerve growth factor, and contain peptides such as calcitonin gene-related peptide, substance P and/or galanin. The second type appears to lack peptide neurotransmitters, responds to glial cell line-derived neurotrophic factor, and can be identified using binding sites for the lectin IB4. Studies indicate that these two types of C fiber segregate differently in the dorsal horn. Non-peptidergic IB4-labeled C fibers gather in the central part of inner lamina II, while peptidergic fibers branch out through lamina I and outer lamina II, but with scattered terminals deeper (laminae III–V) [5].

Nearly all visceral afferents are small unmyelinated C fibers which express similar markers to somatic nociceptors, such as vanilloid receptor TRPV1 and tetrodotoxin-resistant sodium channels [6]. Visceral afferents terminate in laminae I, V–VII, and X of the spinal cord. Laminae I and V contribute fibers to the spinothalamic tract in the contralateral lateral-ventral portion of the cord; thus, visceral travels with somatic nociceptive information from both somatic C fibers (lamina I) and Aδ fibers (lamina V) rostrally [7, 8]. In addition, a second pathway for visceral pain information from medial lamina VII and lamina X propagates along the dorsal columns [9]. Viscerally innervated lamina X neurons are particularly numerous in the sacral spinal cord and important for pelvic and perineal pain transmission.

Peripheral and Spinal Physiology

Injury to peripheral nerves is believed to cause paroxysmal, spontaneous pain through changes in voltage-sensitive sodium channel expression that lead to ectopic action potentials in sensory neurons [10]. These Na(v) channels accumulate in neuromas and demyelinated areas of peripheral nerve in animal and human models. Four such channels are of particular interest given their restricted distribution in nociceptors and their experimental association with neuropathic pain: tetrodotoxin-sensitive Na(v) 1.3 and 1.7 and tetrodotoxin-resistant Na(v) 1.8 and 1.9 [11]. Demyelination and the more even distribution of sodium channels along axons after peripheral nerve injury can lead to difficulty with obtaining a peripheral block in response to local anesthetic agents.

A phenotypic switch has been observed after axotomy, whereby large Aβ fibers begin to express neuromediators that transmit nociceptive information, including substance P [12, 13]. Some investigators insist that a subset of Aβ fibers maintains extensive projections throughout the superficial dorsal horn which, after the phenotypic switch, could excite spinothalamic neurons [14]. There is a larger body of work to suggest ingrowth of large-diameter sensory afferents into the superficial dorsal horn when there has been loss of small-fiber inputs due to cell death [15]. Because large-diameter afferents transmit innocuous sensory information such as light touch, it is believed that a pathological change allowing them to excite the superficial dorsal horn – either through a phenotypic switch that provides them with pain-related neurotransmitters or pathological ingrowth into deafferented portions of superficial dorsal horn – underlies the phenomenon of mechanical allodynia.

Nociceptive afferents provided excitatory glutamatergic, and sometimes peptidergic (substance P), inputs to their respective spinal laminae that increase activity in spinothalamic projection neurons. Glutamate acts primarily on AMPA or NMDA receptors and substance P on the neurokinin-1 (NK1) receptor. Glutamatergic activity leads to increased intracellular calcium and changes in gene expression of these neurons, or, in some cases, neuronal cell death [16].

Two primary mechanisms reduce excitation in the dorsal horn. The first is presynaptic inhibition of neurotransmitter release from primary afferent terminals in the dorsal horn. Serotonergic, adrenergic, opioidergic, and dopaminergic receptors are present on nociceptive afferents whose activity will block calcium entry and vesicular release of glutamate or substance P. Secondly, dopaminergic D2, serotoninergic 5-HT1A, and GABAergic receptors on spinothalamic neurons will inhibit neuronal cell firing when those receptors are activated. The monoamines, serotonin, norepinephrine, and dopamine acting on pre- and postsynaptic receptors in the dorsal horn are released from the terminals of descending fibers from brain stem nuclei. As a sidenote, spinal *presynaptic* serotonergic 5-HT3, *postsynaptic* 5-HT2 and dopaminergic D1 receptors are all generally pro-nociceptive, in that activation of these receptors will either increase excitatory transmitter release and/or directly increase spinothalamic neuronal activity [17–19].

Intrinsic local inhibitory neurons containing GABA will reduce activity in spinothalamic neurons. About 30 % of neurons in superficial laminae I–III are inhibitory, all GABAergic of which some also contain glycine [4]. Most islet cells in the substantia gelatinosa contain GABA and receive excitatory input from C fibers; they provide monosynaptic, bicuculline-sensitive input to excitatory "central" neurons which also receive direct excitatory input from other C fibers. The "central" neurons, responding to convergent inputs from islet cells and C fibers, gate output from lamina I through the spinothalamic tract [20]. A recent study [21] detected large numbers of GABA-inhibitory interneurons postsynaptic to large, heavily myelinated dorsal root ganglia neurons (presumably Aβ fibers) in spinal laminae III–V, consistent with the gate theory of large-fiber inhibition of nociceptive transmission [1]. It has been shown that partial nerve injury will lead to loss of GABAergic inhibition in the superficial dorsal horn secondary to neuronal cell death [22, 23]; loss of this endogenous suppression of central sensitization is a key factor in the difficulty with treating neuropathic pain.

Inflammatory and immune mediators also maintain neuropathic pain. With peripheral nerve injury, mast cells, neutrophils, and macrophages will release immune mediators such as prostaglandin E2, histamine, and tumor necrosis factor-alpha [24]. Supportive glia and Schwann cells can also release nerve growth factor, interleukins, cytokines, chemokines, and ATP which excite axons under pathological conditions [25]. Central glial cells can modulate neuronal activity in other ways, i.e., by acting as ion buffers, and their role has lead to the term "gliopathic" pain [26].

Preganglionic sympathetic neurons, which reside in the intermediolateral cell column of the thoracic spinal cord to the upper second or third lumbar segments, are controlled by both spinal and supraspinal inputs. Particularly, they appear to be subject to tonic GABAergic inhibition which is lifted to quickly increase sympathetic outflow ("disinhibition") [27, 28]. Preganglionic sympathetic fibers exit through the ventral root of the spinal nerve and then connect to the paravertebral sympathetic chain via the "white ramus communicantes" to travel to the appropriate sympathetic ganglion to synapse with its postsynaptic neuron. Visceral afferents travel with the sympathetic nerves to that organ, and therefore, the clinician should consider the possibility of thoracic radiculopathy when confronted with poorly localized unilateral flank and abdominal or pelvic pain, especially if a separate thoracic dermatomal pain can be determined on careful interview.

Sympathetic nerve terminals have been observed to form basket structures around dorsal root ganglion cells after peripheral nerve lesions and can thereby activate these neurons [29, 30]. Nociceptive axons as well may exhibit adrenergic sensitivity in peripheral nerve. These anatomical observations may have relevance to mechanisms of sympathetically maintained pain and their responsiveness to blockade of sympathetic ganglia and dorsal column neuromodulation (see below).

Supraspinal Pain Neuroanatomy

Functional imaging methods have been a powerful complement to traditional anatomical methods in ascertaining the supraspinal networks involved in pain processing. The spinothalamic tract terminates in six distinct regions of the thalamus, mostly intralaminar and ventrolateral complex nuclei. Along the way, terminations from spinobulbar neurons, which travel with spinothalamic tract neurons, are found in the brain stem reticular formation, periaqueductal gray (PAG), parabrachial nucleus, and regions of catecholamine cell groups. It is also likely that the hypothalamus receives spinothalamic tract input either through a mono- or multisynaptic pathway.

The PAG and rostral ventromedial (RVM) nuclei of the brain stem are involved with descending pain inhibitory modulation already mentioned above [31]. The PAG controls spinal nociceptive activity through relays in the RVM and the dorsolateral pontine tegmentum. The RVM contains both serotonergic and non-serotonergic projection neurons that can increase or decrease nociceptive activity in the spinal dorsal horn. The dorsolateral pontine tegmentum sends noradrenergic fibers to the dorsal horn to reduce activity through alpha-2 receptor activation.

Ascending spinothalamic input from lamina I of the dorsal horn is relayed by the thalamus to four principal regions of the cerebral cortex: area 24c of the anterior cingulate gyrus, area 3a of the primary somatosensory cortex (SI), secondary somatosensory cortex on the parietal operculum (SII), and dorsal insular cortex. Not coincidentally, these four regions have shown activation in a consistent way across functional imaging studies, including PET and fMRI, using many different experimental paradigms [32, 33]. Ascending spinothalamic input from wide dynamic range neurons in lamina V is ultimately received in the SI and SII cortices. Of all the cerebral cortical areas activated by pain, the anterior cingulate cortex appears to be the most specific for pain itself. The insular cortex serves a more general role for visceral integration and monitoring bodily homeostasis [34]. Finally, nociceptive input to the parabrachial area may be relayed to the central nucleus of the amygdala, where a major lamina I pathway exists in rats [35]. This input could account in part for some of the emotional, "suffering," aspects of pain experience.

Clinical Applications

Neuromodulation

Virtually every level of the nervous system discussed above can be subjected to electrical neuromodulation with some benefit for chronic pain, particularly neuropathic pain. Here, we briefly list these targets with appropriate references for further review by the interventionalist.

Forebrain

Typically, the forebrain is modulated through superficial motor cortex stimulation or deep brain stimulation. To date, regions targeted for deep brain stimulation include the medial septal nuclei, sensory thalamus, and PAG. More commonly, superficial motor cortex stimulation is chosen for dense neuropathic pain conditions [36, 37]. Typical indications include central neuropathic pain, trigeminal neuralgia, phantom limb pain, and postherpetic neuralgia. Anatomic mapping is performed by identifying the central sulcus with electrophysiologic stimulation and monitoring. EMG and somatosensory-evoked potentials are used to match the motor cortex area with the pain pattern. The mechanism of action of motor cortex stimulation is unknown; it may have to do with the relationship of the motor cortex to suppression of activity in SI and SII somatosensory cortices.

Intraspinal Neuromodulation

The commonest location for placement of electrodes for pain relief is within the spinal canal. Dorsal column neuromodulation via epidural electrodes is an implantable, surgical treatment modality commonly used for chronic pain and vascular disorders [37, 38]. Several features of the neural target influence the efficacy of stimulation: a longitudinal rather than transverse orientation of the fibers relative to the electrode, the distance from the electrode to the fiber, and the fiber diameter itself [39]. Currently available devices activate heavily myelinated Aβ fibers, not the unmyelinated C fibers or lightly myelinated Aδ fibers. Every attempt should be made to align the electrode along the axis of the fibers being stimulated. Furthermore, neuromodulation will be more effective at levels of the spinal cord with less intervening CSF volume, such as at the lumbar and cervical enlargements, when leads are placed in the epidural space.

The ability of dorsal column neuromodulation to block neuropathic pain depends on endogenous mechanisms to reduce excitability in the dorsal horn. A substantive body of work implicates GABAergic mechanisms of analgesia for dorsal column neuromodulation [40]. Conversely, treatment failures for dorsal column neuromodulation may be attributable to loss of large-fiber function, transformation in the phenotype or connectivity of large fibers, or loss of GABAergic inhibitory networks in the dorsal horn.

For traditional neuromodulation, a Tuohy needle is placed into the epidural space after aseptic preparation of the skin several segments caudal to the final desired position. Using fluoroscopic guidance, the electrode is advanced into the midline position overlying the spinal segments to be stimulated. Trial stimulation is carried out using an external programmable pulse generator. The patient describes the location and type of paresthesia in relation to their pain. Sometimes, more than one electrode is required to cover all of the painful areas. A variety of paddle and alternately spaced quadric and octopolar leads are available to cover the necessary area of the dorsal columns; sometimes, staggered leads are placed one above the other in a linear fashion to cover a greater rostrocaudal number of segments.

With satisfactory stimulation obtained, the lead(s) are sutured into place for a trial period of up to 2 weeks. The needle is withdrawn without disturbing the electrode placement and anchored into place on skin with bandaging of a tension loop to decrease the likelihood of dislodgement. The externalized leads can be reprogrammed throughout the trial period to optimize capture of the painful territory. At any sign of superficial infection, they are removed. If successful, permanent leads can be placed in the dorsal epidural space and tunneled to a rechargeable, programmable battery pack.

Other intraspinal neural targets have been successfully utilized to provide relief from neuropathic pain. Electrodes may be placed laterally over the entering dorsal root entry zone, which includes the dorsal roots, Lissauer's tract, and the spinal dorsal horn; this technique has been referred to as "intraspinal nerve root stimulation" (INRS; Fig. 20.1). INRS benefits from a closer apposition of the electrode to the target fibers than in the dorsal columns. The electrodes are placed along the rostrocaudal axis of the spine and therefore are oriented in parallel to ramifying fibers in Lissauer's trace. Placement of an electrode along laterally over the entering dorsal roots uses the same approach as for midline dorsal column placement. Lateral fluoroscopic views should be used to ascertain that the electrode is not ventrally located in the epidural space but rather along the posterior border of the neural foraminae.

Selective nerve root stimulation (SNRS) involves targeting the dorsal root of the spinal nerve at the neural foramen through an intra- or extraspinal approach where the electrode lies in a parallel with the entering fibers. We include sacral nerve stimulation in this category. SNRS accomplishes the goal of capturing paresthesia in some difficult-to-treat lumbosacral segments where traditional methods fail. A cephalocaudal (retrograde) lateral epidural approach at L2/3 below the conus was developed to facilitate placement of the electrode "in line" with lumbosacral roots. Using this technique, a quadripolar electrode enters at midline and is rotated toward but not into the L4 foramen. The distal contact is commonly programmed as an anode and the three proximal contacts as cathodes. Appropriately positioned, one may capture the L4, 5 and S1 roots with a single lead. Retrograde cervicothoracic electrode placements have not been performed due to the risk of cord injury.

S2–4 roots can be captured by directing the quadrupole toward but not through the S2 foramen. For sacral neuromodulation, trial leads are commonly placed through the caudal sacral hiatus and advanced over the lumbosacral nerve roots of interest; if successful, a surgically implanted paddle

Fig. 20.1 Dual Octrode leads for INRS (a) The left, lateral lead (*arrow*) in this case overlies the entering fibers of C5, C6, and C7 for treatment of C6 dermatome central pain in an MS patient. The more medial lead guards the lateral lead to isolate stimulation over the dorsal root entry zone at C6. On the lateral view (**b**), the lateral lead is positioned immediately at the dorsal border of the neural foraminae. The more medial lead rises dorsally over the convexity of the spinal cord as it courses rostrally toward the dorsal columns [53]

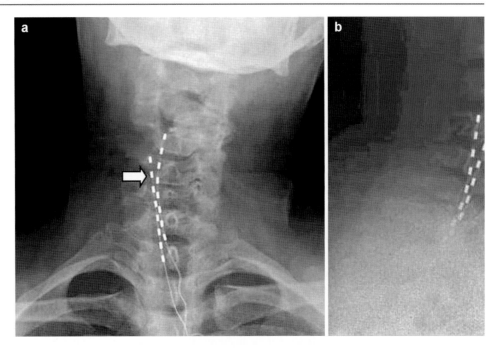

lead may be placed via laminotomy. Conditions treated with this approach include interstitial cystitis and perineal and rectal pain syndromes.

The DRG is another potential target for neuromodulation (Fig. 20.2). The DRG is reliably located intraspinally between the pedicles of the neural foramen. This structure has been targeted with radiofrequency energy to treat radicular neuropathic pain. It may be that a reversible treatment like neuromodulation is preferable to a destructive technique like radiofrequency. In the lumbosacral region, a retrograde approach is generally used and the electrode into the neural foramen. The difference between this target and SNRS is that the electrode is advanced farther into the foramen with this procedure, isolating a single dermatome and acting on the sensory cell bodies of the DRG. Although it may be more effective for this dermatome, it has less breadth of coverage than SNRS which can capture several nerve roots.

Peripheral Nervous System

Peripheral nerves may be individually stimulated or an electrical field generated through an electrode array placed subcutaneously [41]. In peripheral nerve stimulation, an attempt should be made to direct the electrode along the trajectory of the target nerve. Common peripheral nerves treated with neuromodulation include ilioinguinal nerves for post-herniorrhaphy pain, greater and lesser occipital nerves for occipital neuralgia, intercostal nerves for rib pain, and lower extremity nerves (saphenous, peroneal, tibial, sural) for foot pain. One may also use a combination of intraspinal and peripheral stimulation to treat, for instance, back and leg pain [42]. The lead is placed in proximity to the nerve rather than in contact to the nerve with most cases. In some cases,

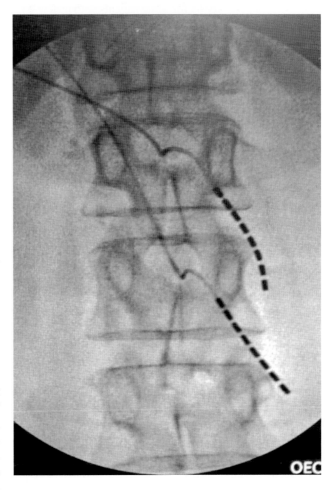

Fig. 20.2 DRG stimulation for postherpetic neuralgia. This patient had worsened symptoms with dorsal column neuromodulation. This arrangement of two leads stimulating the sensory neuronal perikarya at L1 and L2 provided 100 % relief with subthreshold stimulation (amplitude 0.5–0.8 mA with pulse width 120) (Photo courtesy of Dr. Christopher Vije, MD)

often because of lead migration or failure to capture with appropriate coverage, a paddle-type electrode is recommended for implantation.

In some cases it is not possible to isolate a single nerve branch that is responsible for the pain problem. Implantation of dual electrodes with appropriate spacing will generate a peripheral field that captures the pain problem. There is evidence that the two leads can cross talk to complete an electrical circuit and are thus creating a true field and not functioning independently [43]. This has been performed for a variety of conditions including lower back pain and abdominal pain [44].

Intrathecal Drug Delivery

Carefully selected patients may benefit from the implantation of an intrathecal drug-delivery system, typically an opioid with or without an adjunctive medication. These patients have failed more conservative options and have poor benefit and/or unacceptable side effects from oral medications. It is considered a good option for some patients with cancer pain who require large doses of opioid and suffer from severe constipation or sedation.

Typically, the catheter enters the intrathecal space at the lumbar level and is tunneled to a programmable, refillable pump usually in the lower quadrant of the abdomen. The catheter tip should be advanced to the optimal spinal level for the worst pain. For instance, back pain should have the catheter delivering medication at T10 or to the upper cervical spine for head and neck pain. These pumps are not without risk; beyond the immediate surgical risks of hematoma, cord injury, and infection, granulomas may form over time and require surgical intervention.

Pumps are typically filled with morphine, but the interventionalist may use other opioids such as hydromorphone or fentanyl. Common adjuncts to the opioid are clonidine or a local anesthetic such as bupivacaine. Clonidine takes advantage of the endogenous alpha-2 receptor mechanisms of spinal analgesia but can be complicated by hypotension or sedation. Intrathecal bupivacaine can cause numbness, edema, incoordination, or urinary retention; in other cases, it is difficult to deliver a clinically significant amount of bupivacaine, given that bupivacaine cannot be concentrated beyond 0.75 % and the low volumes required for intrathecal infusion.

Intrathecal opioid pumps produce their analgesia through an action on the mu-opioid receptors which are equally distributed on presynaptic fibers and postsynaptic neuronal cell bodies in the dorsal horn. Over time, typically several years, significant tolerance can develop. The loss of GABAergic inhibitory interneurons in the dorsal horn secondary to direct morphine neurotoxicity is thought to be one mechanism of tolerance development [45]. This is one factor that has prompted the development of alternative agents, such as ziconotide [46].

Ziconotide acts as a N-type voltage-dependent calcium channel. It blocks the release of glutamate and pro-nociceptive peptides in the dorsal horn. It has a narrow therapeutic window, with significant side effects of sedation, hallucinations, and dizziness. It has the benefit of no apparent development of tolerance or dependence, however. It is currently used for severe neuropathic pain refractory to other therapies.

Future Directions

Functional Imaging of Pain

PET and fMRI have disclosed activations in certain brain areas with chronic pain, including the anterior cingulate and insular gyri and the somatosensory cortices and thalamus. In some studies, standard MRI has shown reductions in gray matter volumes as a consequence not cause of the chronic pain of such common conditions as irritable bowel syndrome and chronic back pain [47–49]. In the case of chronic low back pain, effective treatment in one study showed reversal of the gray matter changes [50]. Should reliable protocols for common conditions such as back pain be developed, imaging studies could become outcome measures for interventional therapies.

Neuropathic Pain

Technological improvements in neuromodulation will continue to enhance their efficacy and improve our ability to treat certain pain states. Chief among these improvements, already on the horizon, is the development of small, self-contained stimulator devices that may be placed directly next to the nerve root or peripheral nerve, obviating the need for tunneling electrode leads to a battery pack. This will improve accessibility of the DRG and peripheral nerve targets, in particular, to neurostimulation.

The field of neuromodulation, like most other in medicine, would benefit from cohort studies of these different approaches used in different neuropathic pain states. Although the utility of dorsal column neuromodulation for failed back surgery syndrome/lumbosacral nerve root injury syndrome is well-established [37, 51, 52], to date, only anecdotal reports exist for the utility of this and alternate neuromodulatory strategies for other chronic neuropathic conditions. For instance, one case of central pain from multiple sclerosis was successfully treated by INRS [53]. Positive results from SNRS have been reported for lumbosacral nerve injury syndrome, ilioinguinal neuralgia, vulvodynia, interstitial cystitis, neuropathic extremity pain, and pelvic and rectal pain [54–59]. Subcutaneous peripheral nerve or field stimulation has been tried for neuropathic head and neck pain, occipital neuralgia, inguinal neuralgia, and chronic pelvic or abdominal pain [60–65].

"Sensory profiles" for neuropathic pain could enhance the study of alternate strategies and indications for neuromodulation. The concept proposes that a particular pattern of sensory description corresponds to a specific physiological change, even among patients with the same disease process. Thus, allodynia may represent a greater GABAergic inhibitory deficit in the dorsal horn; numbness, a significantly greater degree of deafferentation; spontaneous pain, a greater degree of Aδ fiber activity; and so on. Physiology in turn determines the efficacy of neuromodulation. These "sensory profiles" could then be used to stratify patients within a population to address the issue of nonresponders.

A case in point is postherpetic neuralgia, where dorsal column neuromodulation and peripheral field stimulation have both been reported effective in several patients [66, 67], yet is a condition where neurostimulation is not generally regarded as a useful modality [68, 69]. A descriptive study of 2,100 patients with either PHN or DPN demonstrated differences in hyperalgesia and allodynia between the two populations [70]; five patterns of sensory symptom description were detected within these two populations although differing in frequency within each. Distinct neuropathic signs and symptoms in PHN (i.e., paroxysmal vs. continuous pain) are generated by different patterns of abnormality among primary afferent neurons (Aβ- vs. Aδ- and C fibers). This type of research where clinical description is matched to underlying physiology may point the way forward, in identifying subtypes of neuropathic pain responsive (or not responsive) to different approaches to neuromodulation. This could greatly reduce the number of unnecessary trials and failed implants (see Fig. 20.2).

Visceral and Autonomic Systems

There exists a great deal of information on the utility of dorsal column neuromodulation for chronic stable angina and non-reconstructable lower extremity ischemia (Fig. 20.3) [38, 71, 72]. These indications are more widely used in Europe; practitioners in the USA have not managed to partner with vascular surgery, cardiology, and primary care in such a way as to be able to provide this treatment modality to the appropriate patients effectively. There is also burgeoning interest in the use of cervical spinal cord stimulation to increase cerebral perfusion in low-flow states, including enhancing chemotherapy delivery to brain tumors and improving cerebral oxygenation in patients poststroke [73, 74].

For chronic visceral pain such as pancreatitis, a guarded tripolar lead array is frequently used to drive stimulation deeper into the dorsal columns. Presumably, this allows activation of fibers in the midline visceral pain pathway which engages inhibitory mechanisms in deeper laminae VII and X where visceroceptive neurons reside. This existence of this pathway has led some to promote the efficacy of T10 midline

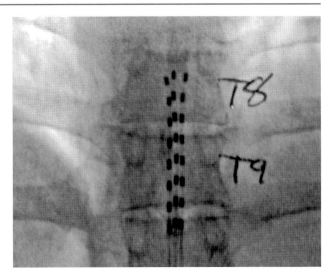

Fig. 20.3 Dorsal column tripole configuration. Using an Octrode lead on either side of a third Octrode allows one to "guard" the midline lead with positive charge. This drives the stimulation deeper into the dorsal columns and can prevent limb and thoracic dermatomal paresthesias. This arrangement has been used for chronic pancreatitis and axial low back pain

punctuate myelotomy for intractable cancer-related pelvic pain [75], which may be considered by the surgical interventionalist in their palliative care population.

Intrathecal Drug Delivery

Currently available technology would benefit greatly from novel analgesics to deliver intraspinally. Gabapentin, a well-established drug for the treatment of neuropathic pain, is one such candidate for intrathecal administration [76, 77]. Alternatively, it may be that adjuncts to morphine, such as baclofen, enhance its efficacy and reduce tolerance development [78]. An intriguing possibility in this regard would be medications to inhibit proinflammatory mediators in the spinal cord. Cytokine and chemokine activation appears not only to drive neuropathic pain itself, but to specifically reduce analgesia and promote tolerance development associated with opioids [79, 80].

Summary

Pain is a neurological condition that affects every level of the nervous system. The most reasonable target for therapy remains the peripheral nerve and spinal dorsal horn, as first proposed by the gate theory; at more rostral levels, pain-related activity is distributed among a "pain matrix" whose complexity makes it difficult to act upon. Imaging of this pain matrix, however, may become an objective surrogate marker for studies of pain and its treatment. Studies of neuromodulation for a variety of neuropathic pain states will benefit from correlation with clinical characteristics and physiology to reduce the number of failed implants. New medications, either alone or adjunctive to intrathecal opioids, will make infusion pumps a more attractive modality for pain control.

References

1. Melzack R, Wall PD. Pain mechanisms: a new theory. Science. 1965;150(699):971–9.
2. Basbaum AI, Fields HL. Endogenous pain control systems: brainstem spinal pathways and endorphin circuitry. Annu Rev Neurosci. 1984;7:309–38.
3. Levine JD, Fields HL, Basbaum AI. Peptides and the primary afferent nociceptor. J Neurosci. 1993;13(6):2273–86.
4. Todd AJ. Chapter 6 Anatomy and neurochemistry of the dorsal horn. Handb Clin Neurol. 2006;81:61–76.
5. Braz JM, et al. Parallel "pain" pathways arise from subpopulations of primary afferent nociceptor. Neuron. 2005;47(6):787–93.
6. Bielefeldt K, Christianson JA, Davis BM. Basic and clinical aspects of visceral sensation: transmission in the CNS. Neurogastroenterol Motil. 2005;17(4):488–99.
7. Traub RJ, Sengupta JN, Gebhart GF. Differential c-fos expression in the nucleus of the solitary tract and spinal cord following noxious gastric distention in the rat. Neuroscience. 1996;74(3):873–84.
8. Traub RJ, Stitt S, Gebhart GF. Attenuation of c-Fos expression in the rat lumbosacral spinal cord by morphine or tramadol following noxious colorectal distention. Brain Res. 1995;701 (1–2):175–82.
9. Palecek J, Paleckova V, Willis WD. Fos expression in spinothalamic and postsynaptic dorsal column neurons following noxious visceral and cutaneous stimuli. Pain. 2003;104(1–2):249–57.
10. Devor M. Sodium channels and mechanisms of neuropathic pain. J Pain. 2006;7(1 Suppl 1):S3–12.
11. Momin A, Wood JN. Sensory neuron voltage-gated sodium channels as analgesic drug targets. Curr Opin Neurobiol. 2008;18(4): 383–8.
12. Costigan M, et al. Replicate high-density rat genome oligonucleotide microarrays reveal hundreds of regulated genes in the dorsal root ganglion after peripheral nerve injury. BMC Neurosci. 2002;3(1):16.
13. Weissner W, et al. Time course of substance P expression in dorsal root ganglia following complete spinal nerve transection. J Comp Neurol. 2006;497(1):78–87.
14. Devor M. Ectopic discharge in Abeta afferents as a source of neuropathic pain. Exp Brain Res. 2009;196(1):115–28.
15. Nakamura S, Myers RR. Myelinated afferents sprout into lamina II of L3-5 dorsal horn following chronic constriction nerve injury in rats. Brain Res. 1999;818(2):285–90.
16. Whiteside GT, Munglani R. Cell death in the superficial dorsal horn in a model of neuropathic pain. J Neurosci Res. 2001;64(2): 168–73.
17. Yoshimura M, Furue H. Mechanisms for the anti-nociceptive actions of the descending noradrenergic and serotonergic systems in the spinal cord. J Pharmacol Sci. 2006;101(2):107–17.
18. Lu Y, Perl ER. Selective action of noradrenaline and serotonin on neurones of the spinal superficial dorsal horn in the rat. J Physiol. 2007;582(Pt 1):127–36.
19. Benarroch E. Descending monoaminergic pain modulation: bidirectional control and clinical relevance. Neurology. 2008;71(3): 217–21.
20. Lu Y, Perl ER. A specific inhibitory pathway between substantia gelatinosa neurons receiving direct C-fiber input. J Neurosci. 2003;23(25): 8752–8.
21. Braz JM, Basbaum AI. Triggering genetically-expressed transneuronal tracers by peripheral axotomy reveals convergent and segregated sensory neuron-spinal cord connectivity. Neuroscience. 2009;163(4):1220–32.
22. Moore KA, et al. Partial peripheral nerve injury promotes a selective loss of GABAergic inhibition in the superficial dorsal horn of the spinal cord. J Neurosci. 2002;22(15):6724–31.
23. Scholz J, et al. Blocking caspase activity prevents transsynaptic neuronal apoptosis and the loss of inhibition in lamina II of the dorsal horn after peripheral nerve injury. J Neurosci. 2005;25(32): 7317–23.
24. Rittner HL, Brack A, Stein C. Pro-algesic versus analgesic actions of immune cells. Curr Opin Anaesthesiol. 2003;16(5):527–33.
25. Moalem G, Tracey DJ. Immune and inflammatory mechanisms in neuropathic pain. Brain Res Rev. 2006;51(2):240–64.
26. Benarroch E. Central neuron-glia interactions and neuropathic pain: overview of recent concepts and clinical implications. Neurology. 2010;75(3):273–8.
27. Deuchars SA, et al. GABAergic neurons in the central region of the spinal cord: a novel substrate for sympathetic inhibition. J Neurosci. 2005;25(5):1063–70.
28. Wang L, et al. Tonic GABAergic inhibition of sympathetic preganglionic neurons: a novel substrate for sympathetic control. J Neurosci. 2008;28(47):12445–52.
29. McLachlan EM, et al. Peripheral nerve injury triggers noradrenergic sprouting within dorsal root ganglia. Nature. 1993;363(6429): 543–6.
30. Chung K, et al. Sympathetic sprouting in the dorsal root ganglia of the injured peripheral nerve in a rat neuropathic pain model. J Comp Neurol. 1996;376(2):241–52.
31. Ossipov MH, et al. Spinal and supraspinal mechanisms of neuropathic pain. Ann N Y Acad Sci. 2000;909:12–24.
32. Casey KL, Lorenz J, Minoshima S. Insights into the pathophysiology of neuropathic pain through functional brain imaging. Exp Neurol. 2003;184 Suppl 1:S80–8.
33. Garcia-Larrea L, et al. Functional imaging and neurophysiological assessment of spinal and brain therapeutic modulation in humans. Arch Med Res. 2000;31(3):248–57.
34. Craig AD. The functional anatomy of lamina I and its role in poststroke central pain. Prog Brain Res. 2000;129:137–51.
35. Al-Khater KM, Todd AJ. Collateral projections of neurons in laminae I, III, and IV of rat spinal cord to thalamus, periaqueductal gray matter, and lateral parabrachial area. J Comp Neurol. 2009;515(6): 629–46.
36. Canavero S, Bonicalzi V. Extradural cortical stimulation for central pain. Acta Neurochir Suppl. 2007;97(Pt 2):27–36.
37. Cruccu G, et al. EFNS guidelines on neurostimulation therapy for neuropathic pain. Eur J Neurol. 2007;14(9):952–70.
38. Ubbink DT, Vermeulen H. Spinal cord stimulation for non-reconstructable chronic critical leg ischaemia. Cochrane Database Syst Rev. 2005;20(3):CD04001.
39. Oakley JC, Prager JP. Spinal cord stimulation: mechanisms of action. Spine (Phila Pa 1976). 2002;27(22):2574–83.
40. Meyerson BA, Linderoth B. Mechanisms of spinal cord stimulation in neuropathic pain. Neurol Res. 2000;22(3):285–92.
41. Slavin KV. Peripheral nerve stimulation for neuropathic pain. Neurotherapeutics. 2008;5(1):100–6.
42. Lipov EG. 'Hybrid neurostimulator': simultaneous use of spinal cord and peripheral nerve field stimulation to treat low back and leg pain. Prog Neurol Surg. 2011;24:147–55.
43. Falco FJ, et al. Cross talk: a new method for peripheral nerve stimulation. An observational report with cadaveric verification. Pain Physician. 2009;12(6):965–83.

44. Verrills P, et al. Peripheral nerve field stimulation for chronic pain: 100 cases and review of the literature. Pain Med. 2011;3(10):1526–4637.
45. Mao J, et al. Neuronal apoptosis associated with morphine tolerance: evidence for an opioid-induced neurotoxic mechanism. J Neurosci. 2002;22(17):7650–61.
46. Staats PS, et al. Intrathecal ziconotide in the treatment of refractory pain in patients with cancer or AIDS: a randomized controlled trial. JAMA. 2004;291(1):63–70.
47. Blankstein U, et al. Altered brain structure in irritable bowel syndrome: potential contributions of pre-existing and disease-driven factors. Gastroenterology. 2010;138(5):1783–9.
48. May A. Chronic pain may change the structure of the brain. Pain. 2008;137(1):7–15.
49. Rodriguez-Raecke R, et al. Brain gray matter decrease in chronic pain is the consequence and not the cause of pain. J Neurosci. 2009;29(44):13746–50.
50. Seminowicz DA, et al. Effective treatment of chronic low back pain in humans reverses abnormal brain anatomy and function. J Neurosci. 2011;31(20):7540–50.
51. Kumar K, et al. Spinal cord stimulation versus conventional medical management for neuropathic pain: a multicentre randomised controlled trial in patients with failed back surgery syndrome. Pain. 2007;132(1–2):179–88. Epub 2007 Sep 12.
52. Turner JA, et al. Spinal cord stimulation for failed back surgery syndrome: outcomes in a workers' compensation setting. Pain. 2009;148(1):14–25.
53. Burkey AR, Abla-Yao S. Successful treatment of central pain in a multiple sclerosis patient with epidural stimulation of the dorsal root entry zone. Pain Med. 2010;11(1):127–32.
54. Alo KM, et al. Lumbar and sacral nerve root stimulation (NRS) in the treatment of chronic pain: a novel anatomic approach and neurostimulation technique. Neuromodulation. 1999;2:23–31.
55. Alo KM, McKay E. Sacral nerve root stimulation (SNRS) for the treatment of intractable pelvic pain and motor dysfunction: a case report. Neuromodulation. 2001;4:53–8.
56. Yearwood TL. Neuropathic extremity pain and spinal cord stimulation. Pain Med. 2006;7 Suppl 1:S97–102.
57. Haque R, Winfree CJ. Spinal nerve root stimulation. Neurosurg Focus. 2006;21(6):E4.
58. Stuart RM, Winfree CJ. Neurostimulation techniques for painful peripheral nerve disorders. Neurosurg Clin N Am. 2009;20(1):111–20, vii–viii.
59. Deer TR. Current and future trends in spinal cord stimulation for chronic pain. Curr Pain Headache Rep. 2001;5(6):503–9.
60. Tamimi MA, et al. Subcutaneous peripheral nerve stimulation treatment for chronic pelvic pain. Neuromodulation. 2008;11(4):277–81.
61. Weiner RL. Peripheral nerve neurostimulation. Neurosurg Clin N Am. 2003;14(3):401–8.
62. Weiner RL, Reed KL. Peripheral neurostimulation for control of intractable occipital neuralgia. Neuromodulation. 1999;2:217–21.
63. Oberoi J, Sampson C, Ross E. Head and neck peripheral stimulation for chronic pain: report of three cases. Neuromodulation. 2008;11(4):272–6.
64. Reverberi C, Bonezzi C, Demartini L. Peripheral subcutaneous neurostimulation in the management of neuropathic pain: five case reports. Neuromodulation. 2009;12(2):146–55.
65. Paicius RM, Bernstein CA, Lempert-Cohen C. Peripheral nerve field stimulation in chronic abdominal pain. Pain Physician. 2006;9(3):261–6.
66. Jang HD, et al. Analysis of failed spinal cord stimulation trials in the treatment of intractable chronic pain. J Korean Neurosurg Soc. 2008;43(2):85–9.
67. Kouroukli I, et al. Peripheral subcutaneous stimulation for the treatment of intractable postherpetic neuralgia: two case reports and literature review. Pain Pract. 2009;9(3):225–9.
68. Baron R. Mechanisms of postherpetic neuralgia–we are hot on the scent. Pain. 2008;140(3):395–6.
69. Truini A, et al. Pathophysiology of pain in postherpetic neuralgia: a clinical and neurophysiological study. Pain. 2008;140(3):405–10.
70. Baron R, et al. A cross-sectional cohort survey in 2100 patients with painful diabetic neuropathy and postherpetic neuralgia: differences in demographic data and sensory symptoms. Pain. 2009;146(1–2):34–40.
71. Wu M, Linderoth B, Foreman RD. Putative mechanisms behind effects of spinal cord stimulation on vascular diseases: a review of experimental studies. Auton Neurosci. 2008;138(1–2):9–23.
72. Deer TR. Spinal cord stimulation for the treatment of angina and peripheral vascular disease. Curr Pain Headache Rep. 2009;13(1):18–23.
73. Clavo B, et al. Modification of loco-regional microenvironment in brain tumors by spinal cord stimulation. Implications for radio-chemotherapy. J Neurooncol. 2011;12:12.
74. Robaina F, Clavo B. Spinal cord stimulation in the treatment of post-stroke patients: current state and future directions. Acta Neurochir Suppl. 2007;97(Pt 1):277–82.
75. Nauta HJ, et al. Punctate midline myelotomy for the relief of visceral cancer pain. J Neurosurg. 2000;92(2 Suppl):125–30.
76. Chu LC, et al. Chronic intrathecal infusion of gabapentin prevents nerve ligation-induced pain in rats. Br J Anaesth. 2011;106(5):699–705.
77. Takasusuki T, Yaksh TL. The effects of intrathecal and systemic gabapentin on spinal substance P release. Anesth Analg. 2011;112(4):971–6.
78. Saulino M. Simultaneous treatment of intractable pain and spasticity: observations of combined intrathecal baclofen-morphine therapy over a 10-year clinical experience. Eur J Phys Rehabil Med. 2011;28:28.
79. Hutchinson MR, et al. Proinflammatory cytokines oppose opioid-induced acute and chronic analgesia. Brain Behav Immun. 2008;22(8):1178–89.
80. Johnston IN, et al. A role for proinflammatory cytokines and fractalkine in analgesia, tolerance, and subsequent pain facilitation induced by chronic intrathecal morphine. J Neurosci. 2004;24(33):7353–65.

Spinal Targets for Interventional Pain Management

21

Lawrence R. Poree and Linda L. Wolbers

Key Points

- Interventional techniques that target specific nociceptive transmission sites can reduce pain without having the systemic impact that oral medication have on other organ systems.
- Convergence of nociceptive afferent signals in the spinal cord may explain the clinical observation that injury of different organs may produce the same pain sensations.
- Destruction of specific spinal neural targets with either neurolytic solutions or thermal probes provides long-term relief for a limited number of pain conditions.
- The primary pharmacological receptors that are targeted for intrathecal medication management of pain include opioid receptors, alpha-2 adrenergic receptors, sodium channel receptors, and calcium channel receptors.
- Electrical stimulation can provide effective analgesia by targeting various spinal targets including the spinal cord, nerve roots, and dorsal root ganglia.
- New minimally invasive percutaneous techniques have recently been developed to address some of the structural pathologies including spinal stenosis caused by ligamentum flavum hypertrophy.

L.R. Poree, M.D., MPH, Ph.D. (✉)
Department of Anesthesia and Perioperative Care,
University of California San Francisco,
San Francisco, CA, USA

Pain Management, Pain Clinic of Monterey Bay,
8057 Valencia Street, Ste A, Aptos, CA 95003, USA
e-mail: lporee@painclinicofmontereybay.com

L.L. Wolbers, M.D., MPH
Pain Clinic of Monterey Bay,
8057 Valencia Street, Ste A, Aptos, CA 95003, USA
e-mail: lwolbers@painclinicofmontereybay.com

Introduction

As noted in the previous chapter, the transmission of pain signals from the peripheral nervous system to the brain involves a variety of specialized neuronal and nonneuronal cells each with a host of specific receptors involved in the processing of these signals. The goal of this chapter is to briefly review the various image-guided interventional pain management techniques that target spinal structures aimed at reducing pain and improving patients' quality of life. Comprehensive medical management aims to accomplish these goals by utilizing systemic medications that target specific receptors throughout the peripheral and central nervous system. In many cases, this approach is successful with few untoward complications. However, in more severe pain conditions or higher doses of medications, patients may experience medication side effects and toxicities that limit the utility of a systemic approach. In contrast, interventional pain management techniques employ a variety of technologies to influence specific targets involved in nociceptive transmission while aiming to minimize the effects on systems not involved in the nociceptive process. For the purposes of this chapter, the interventional pain management techniques to be discussed will be limited to fluoroscopic procedures that target the structural and neural components in four distinctive spinal regions: the paraspinal region located immediately adjacent to the spine, the structural components of the spine including the bone and connective tissues, the intraforaminal region located within the spinal foramen, and the intraspinal region located within the spinal canal. Where appropriate, a distinction will be made between the epidural targets and intrathecal targets located within the intraspinal region. Knowledge of the spinal structures subject to interventional procedures is critical for all pain physicians, not just those who perform the interventions. For example, by understanding the spinal components involved in nociception and how they can be targeted, the clinician can explain not only how a patient with cholecystitis can present with clinical complaints of angina but also why

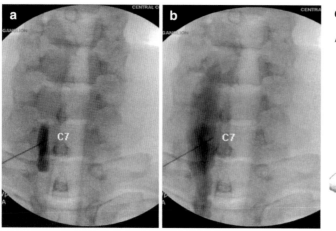
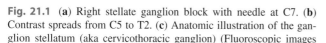
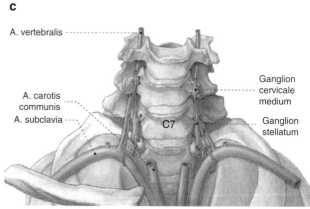

Fig. 21.1 (**a**) Right stellate ganglion block with needle at C7. (**b**) Contrast spreads from C5 to T2. (**c**) Anatomic illustration of the ganglion stellatum (aka cervicothoracic ganglion) (Fluoroscopic images courtesy of Lawrence Poree, MD Ph.D. Illustration courtesy of Rogier Trompert Medical Art. http://www.medical-art.nl; reprinted with permission from van Eijs et al. [5])

targeting the spinal cord may be beneficial [1, 2]. While this clinical observation was a mystery when first described over 100 years ago, animal studies characterized the convergent spinal pathways and processing centers responsible for this clinical observation [3, 4]. Armed with this knowledge, the interventionalist is able to target these centers with interventional techniques to disrupt the nociceptive processing at the spinal level. The techniques discussed here include both established as well as emerging technologies.

Paraspinal Targets for Interventional Pain Management

Chapter 20 described the role that the sympathetic nervous system plays in both the transmission and maintenance of pain. With efferent sympathetic fibers traversing along the paravertebral sympathetic chain adjacent to the cervical through sacral vertebral bodies, it is no surprise that these nerve bundles are a common target for neural blockade and ablation in patients diagnosed with sympathetically maintained pain. In addition, these same nerve bundles are often conduits of visceral nociceptive afferent fibers. Neural blockade with local anesthetic of nerve fibers in the cervical and lumbar sympathetic chain is a common therapeutic technique used in the treatment of complex regional pain syndrome (CRPS) of the upper and lower extremities, respectively. In a recent multicenter review of randomized clinical trials, sympathetic blockade for the treatment of CRPS was given a score of 2B+. This score indicates that one or more RCTs demonstrate effectiveness and that the treatment is recommended by the group [5]. In the cervical spine, the cervicothoracic ganglion (aka stellate ganglion) sympathetic blockade is performed by advancing a needle to the anterior tubercle of the C7 vertebral body under fluoroscopic guid-

ance. Injection of contrast confirms flow of the solution along the course of the cervical sympathetic chain in a craniocaudal direction and is followed by injecting 10 ml of local anesthetic (Fig. 21.1). Similarly, blockade of the lumbar sympathetic chain is performed by advancing a needle in the oblique fluoroscopic view to the anterior lateral surface of the L2 and/or L3 vertebral body under fluoroscopic guidance using a paramedian approach. Once proper needle placement is confirmed in the anterior-posterior and lateral views, 1 cc of contrast is injected and observed to spread in a craniocaudal direction and is followed by injecting 15 ml of local anesthetic (Fig. 21.2). In the thoracic spine, the sympathetic chain gives rise to the greater and lesser splanchnic nerves that provide sympathetic innervations of many visceral organs along with serving as a conduit for nociceptive afferents. As such, they are a favorite target for neural blockade and/or ablation in the treatment of visceral pain. For decades, the neural destruction of the celiac plexus with alcohol or phenol has been a mainstay in the treatment of pain associated with pancreatic cancer. While highly effective, this therapy is associated with significant risks, including inadvertent spread of neurolytic solution toward the nerve roots and lumbar plexus which may result in foot drop, paraplegia, sexual dysfunction, loss of anal and bladder sphincter tone, and dysesthesia [6]. To avoid these complications of chemical neurolysis, radiofrequency ablation is rapidly emerging as the preferred method for denervating the pancreas, especially in non-cancer patients [7]. The technique is accomplished by targeting the greater and lesser splanchnic nerves as they traverse along the lateral portion of the T11–T12 vertebral bodies (Fig. 21.3). Unlike the unpredictable flow of neurolytic solutions, RF lesions are limited to 1 mm lateral to the needle. Prior to lesioning, sensory stimulation at 50 Hz is performed up to 1 V to elicit stimulation in the epigastric region and motor stimulation at 2 Hz up to 3 V to rule out stimulation of

Fig. 21.2 Lumbar sympathetic block. (**a**) Needle placed on the anterolateral surface of the L3 vertebral body. (**b**) Contrast spreads from L2 to L4 (Fluoroscopic images courtesy of Lawrence Poree, M.D., Ph.D.)

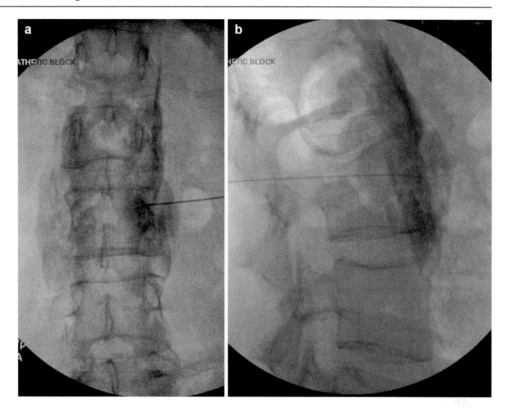

Fig. 21.3 15-mm active tip R-F (Racz-Finch) curved blunt needle for lesioning the splanchnics at T11–T12 placed over the splanchnic nerve dissected on a cadaver (With permission from Raj et al. [7])

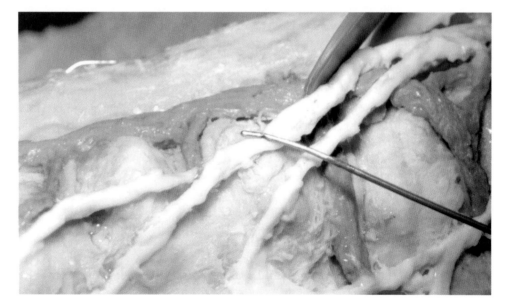

the intercostal nerves as noted by lack of contraction of the intercostal muscles. Once the location is confirmed both fluoroscopically in the A/P and lateral projections and with sensory and motor stimulation, the area is anesthetized with local anesthetic and then lesioned at 80 °C for 90 s. A second lesion is performed by turning the curved needle 180° to widen the lesion size. The primary complication of splanchnic nerve blocks/RF lesions is pneumothorax if the needle punctures the diaphragm [8].

Similarly, local anesthetic blocks and radiofrequency lesions of the lower portion of the sympathetic chain is targeted to treat pelvic and perineal pain. For bladder and uterine pain, the superior hypogastric plexus block is employed, whereas for perineal, rectal, and vaginal pain, the ganglion of impar is the target. The superior hypogastric plexus is located on the anterior lateral border of the lower third of the L5 vertebral body and accessed via an oblique fluoroscopic view of the anterior lateral surface of the L5 vertebra or an

Fig. 21.4 Illustration of spinal
innervation and targets for
neural blockade/neurolysis
including the sympathetic
ganglia, ramus communicans,
and ramus medialis (facet nerve)
(Illustration courtesy of Rogier
Trompert Medical Art. http://
www.medical-art.nl. Reprinted
with permission from
Kallewaard et al. [20])

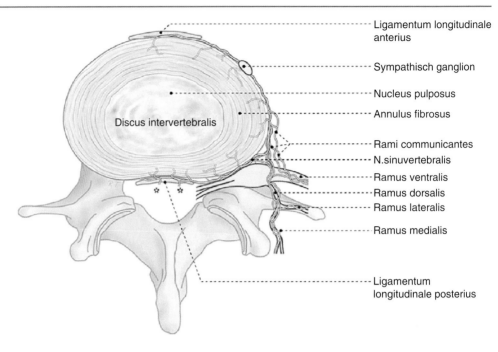

L5–S1 transdiscal approach [9, 10]. The ganglion of impar is accessed by passing a needle through the sacrococcygeal ligament [11, 12]. Neurolysis of these structures with alcohol or phenol is typically reserved for those with cancer pain; however, botulinum toxin has emerged as a novel tool to aid in providing sympathetic neurolysis beyond the duration of local anesthetic but without the long-term sequel of alcohol or phenol [13, 14].

In addition to the sympathetic chain, another anterior column target for neurolysis is the ramus communicans (Fig. 21.4) [15, 16]. These nerves contribute to nociceptive innervation of the intervertebral disc. Radiofrequency ablation of these nerves at two adjacent levels was first reported to provide pain relief in patients with single level of discogenic pain over 20 years ago, but only one randomized clinical trial has been published on the procedure in that time period [17]. These nerves can be accessed via a 20° oblique fluoroscopic view with a 2-gauge spinal or RF needle advanced to the vertebral body just anterior to the posterior edge. The proper location is identified when sensory stimulation produces a sensation in the back at less than 1.5 V and motor stimulation at twice the sensory stimulation fails to cause contractions of the leg muscles. Once the proper location is identified, a radiofrequency lesion is made at 80 °C for 60 s. One randomized clinical trial compared radiofrequency lesioning of the ramus communicans with a sham treatment. The RF-treated group had significantly lower VAS scores and improved SF-36 scores as compared to the sham-treated group 4 months after treatment [18]. Although there are few studies and only one RCT, the quality of evidence supporting this procedure secured it a level 2B+ positive recommendation using a

modified grading system [19, 20]. This procedure is also reportedly effective in the treatment of pain due to vertebral fractures as the ramus communicans also innervates the vertebral bodies. However, further studies are needed to make this a recommended procedure [21].

In the posterior column, the most common targets for paraspinal neurolysis are the medial branches of the spinal posterior rami (aka ramus medialis or facet nerves). These nerves branch off the spinal nerves as they exit the intervertebral foramen to innervate the facet joints (aka zygapophyseal joint). With aging and injury, the facet joint may become sclerotic and hypertrophied and contribute to chronic back pain. Denervating the joint by ablating the medial branch nerves relieves the pain and improves range of motion. The primary target for denervation is the medial branch nerve as it passes over the junction of the transverse process and pedicle in the lumbar spine and in the middle of the facet pillar in the cervical spine [22, 23]. Pain relief after a local anesthetic blockade of these nerves is the diagnostic criteria used to determine which spinal segments are contributing to a patient's back pain. Two of these nerves are lesioned for each painful facet joint as each joint is innervated by two separate medial branches. Radiofrequency neurolysis at 80° for 90 s is the most common technique for neurolysis although cryoneurolysis is also effective. Two recent analyses of the available literature using the Cochrane Musculoskeletal Review Group criteria for interventional techniques for randomized trials and the Agency for Healthcare Research and Quality (AHRQ) criteria for observational studies evaluated the efficacy of radiofreqency neurotomies of the medial branch nerves to treat facet joint pain and found that the available evidence supported recommending this procedure for the treatment of lumbar and cervical facet joint pain. This recommendation is based on quality of evidence reaching a level II-1 or II-2 when utilizing the grading criteria developed by the US Preventive Services Task Force [24, 25].

Percutaneous facet fusion, a new interventional pain management procedure, has recently been introduced as another technique to address facet joint pain. This fluoroscopically guided technique identifies the facet joint in an oblique view, and using a percutaneous portal system, a drill is advanced to the facet joint. A hole is made large enough to insert an 8-mm bone dowel into the joint which is allowed to fuse over the course of 6 weeks. This technique presumes that fusing the facet joint will relieve facet joint pain, but more clinical trials are needed to fully evaluate the effectiveness of this procedure as a stand-alone procedure for facet pain [26].

Spinal Bone and Connective Tissue Targets for Interventional Pain Management

As patients age, the bone and connective tissue components of the spine are subject to a wide array of degenerative processes that contribute to chronic pain, including but not limited to, vertebral fractures, disc herniations and ruptures, and hypertrophy and sclerosis of facets joints and ligamentum flavum. In the past 10–20 years, various minimally invasive image-guided interventional procedures have been developed to address each of these conditions with varying degrees of success.

Vertebral fractures, a condition common to patients with osteoporosis, can cause both acute and chronic pain. Two fluoroscopically driven procedures have emerged to address this condition, vertebroplasty and kyphoplasty. These vertebral augmentation procedures involve fluoroscopic placement of a needle into the fractured vertebral body and introduction of bone cement in an effort to stabilize the vertebral fracture and regain vertebral height and reduce pain [27]. A systematic review of the available studies from 1980 to 2008 graded the level of evidence using the North American Spine Society guidelines and concluded that there was good evidence to recommend vertebral augmentation in the treatment of vertebral fractures, although only one of the 74 studies was a randomized clinical trial. Subsequently, four additional randomized clinical trials were published that offered conflicting recommendations, two supporting and two not supporting vertebral augmentation for vertebral fractures. The two in support were both open-label trials randomized to kyphoplasty versus medical management in one study [28] and vertebroplasty versus medical management in the other [29] with both having an inclusion criteria of edema noted on MRI. Each study reported significant decreases in VAS scores 1 month posttreatment in the augmented groups versus the medical management groups. Less of a difference was noted at the 1-year point,

presumably due to fracture healing. In the kyphoplasty study, quality of life, mobility, and function also showed greater improvement in the surgical versus nonsurgical group. The two studies which did not support vertebral augmentation for vertebral fractures were sham versus vertebroplasty. All patients had radiographic evidence of vertebral fractures and back pain for less than a year, but not all had MRI evidence of edema [30, 31]. Each study reported trends of pain improvement in the vertebroplasty group at the 1-month time point that did not reach statistical significance. As each group continued to improve, there was no discernable difference between them in pain, physical functioning, or disability scores. The authors concluded that there was no significant difference between patients treated with vertebroplasty or a sham procedure. To help resolve these conflicting results, a more rigorous sham-controlled study was designed to include MRI evaluations by two independent radiologists, outcome measurements at 1 day, 1 week, 1,3,6, and12 months after treatment to include VAS, disability, and quality of life scores [32]. The results of this study are pending.

The intervertebral disc is another source of chronic spinal pain targeted by interventional procedures [33]. Derangements of the intervertebral disc can become a source of both acute and chronic back pain and is estimated to constitute up to 45 % of all cases of low back pain [19].

Herniated disc or extruded disc fragments can create pain as a result of a mass effect on neural structures including the spinal cord and exiting nerve roots. In addition, annular tears can allow leakage of the acidic nucleus pulposus leading to neural irritation of the sinuvertebral nerves that innervate the outer annulus as well as spinal nerves if the nucleus pulposus extends beyond the borders of the disc (Fig. 21.4). Diagnosis of this discogenic pain is most often determined by provocative discograms whereby 1–2 ml of contrast is injected into the disc and observed to reproduce concordant pain. The structural integrity of the disc is also evaluated by measuring intradiscal pressure to see if and at what pressure contrast may leak outside the normal boundaries of the nucleus pulposus up to a maximum of 100 psi, the normal pressure of a lumbar disc in the seated position (Fig. 21.5) [15, 19, 34]. Early interventional procedures attempted to treat discogenic pain with intradiscal injections of chymopapain, but anaphylaxis and clinical benefit less than that obtained with surgical discectomy lead to the abandonment of this chemonucleolysis technique [35]. In the intervening 20 years, a number of intradiscal procedures have been introduced utilizing a variety of lesioning, injection, and decompressive technologies, including intradiscal electrothermal therapy (IDET), annuloplasty and other radiofrequency lesioning techniques, injection of corticosteroids, ozone, hypertonic dextrose, and methylene blue, as well as nucleoplasty and other percutaneous disc decompression techniques [36–38]. A recent multicenter analytical review of the available studies of these

Fig. 21.5 (**a**) A/P fluoroscopic image of needles placed within lumbar disc. (**b**) Lateral view with injection of contrast, note posterior leakage of contrast at the L3–4 disc (Fluoroscopic images courtesy of Lawrence Poree, MD Ph.D)

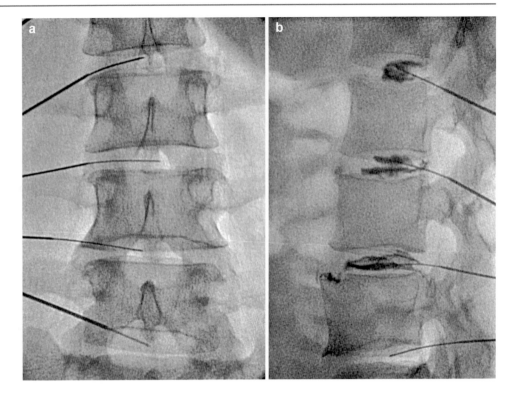

procedures made the following recommendation [19]: "Intradiscal corticosteroid injections and RF treatment of the discus are not advised for patients with discogenic low back pain. The current body of evidence does not provide sufficient proof to recommend intradiscal treatments, such as IDET and biacuplasty for chronic, nonspecific low back complaints originating from the discus intervertebralis. We are also of the opinion that at this time, the only place for intradiscal treatments for chronic low back pain is in a research setting. RF treatment of the ramus communicans is recommended." (See section above on paraspinal targets for a review of RF lesioning of the ramus communicans.) The authors went on to conclude "…provocative discography remains the gold standard for the determination of the diagnosis of discogenic pain."

Minimally invasive lumbar decompression (MILD) is another new interventional pain management technique that targets the hypertrophic ligamentum flavum in patients with lumbar spinal stenosis and neurogenic claudication [39]. As patients age, the ligamentum flavum hypertrophies in part due to replacement of the normal elastin with collagen in the posterior fibers of the ligamentum flavum [40]. Mechanical stress of the ligament causes an inflammatory response with infiltration of macrophages and fibroblast that in turn leads to scar formation. In addition, loss of disc height leads to buckling of the ligament and further narrows the spinal canal [41]. In later stages, calcification and ossification of the ligament develops and contributes even further to thickening and inflexibility of the ligamentum flavum [42]. Until recently, this condition was treated initially with epidural steroid

injections, and when this therapy no longer provided significant benefit, patients were treated with an open surgical decompression. The MILD procedure, performed with local anesthetic and minimal sedation, uses the placement of epidural contrast and fluoroscopy to outline the anterior border of the ligamentum flavum in a region where ligamentum flavum hypertrophy was identified on MRI images (Fig. 21.6). A small 5.1-mm trocar is advanced to the inferior lamina of interlaminar space to be treated. Removal of the trocar's stylet leaves a working portal through which instruments are passed and are used to remove osteophytes and the posterior fibers of the hypertrophied ligamentum flavum. Initial clinical trials revealed that this procedure showed statistically and clinically significant reduction of pain and improvement in the mobility as measured by VAS, ZCQ, SF-12v2, and ODI [43]. These improvements persisted at the 1-year follow-up [44]. A multicenter, randomized clinical trial is currently underway to compare the long-term benefits of the MILD procedure compared with epidural steroid treatments.

Intraforaminal Targets for Interventional Pain Management

Of course, the most important interventional pain management target within the vertebral foramen is the dorsal root ganglion (DRG). The primary sensory afferent neurons in the ganglion are the principle link between peripheral nociceptors and the processing centers of the central nervous system.

Fig. 21.6 (**a**) Axial MRI of lumbar spine showing spinal stenosis secondary to hypertrophy of the ligamentum flavum (LF). (**b**) Fluoroscopic image in contralateral oblique view showing epidurogram and failure of contrast to flow cephalad. (**c**) Tissue sculptor used to remove posterior portion of hypertrophic ligamentum flavum. (**d**) Epidurogram after decompression shows improvement in epidural flow (Images courtesy of Vertos Medical Aliso Viejo, CA)

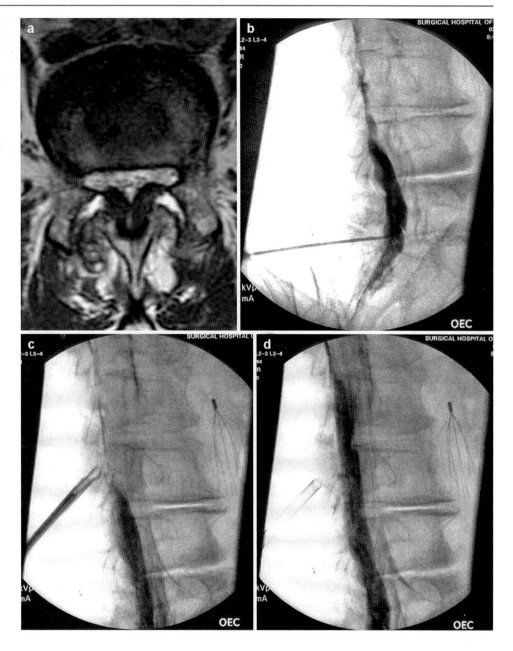

Injury of these nerves is common from mechanical trauma resulting from lateralized herniated disc or spondylolisthesis, chemical irritation from leakage of nucleus pulposus [45–48], and injury caused by infectious agents such as herpes zoster. All of these injuries can initiate a cascade of inflammatory mediators including cytokines that contribute to the development and maintenance of chronic pain [49]. Thus, it comes as no surprise that foraminal injection of glucocorticoids is a common target for interventional pain physicians [50, 51]. A recent analysis of the available literature using the Cochrane Musculoskeletal Review Group criteria for interventional techniques for randomized trials and the criteria developed by the Agency for Healthcare Research and Quality (AHRQ) criteria for observational studies evalu-

ated the efficacy of transforaminal epidural steroid injections and found that the available evidence supported recommending this procedure for the treatment of lumbar radiculitis. The quality of this evidence was ranked utilizing the US Preventive Services Task Force and found to reach a level II-1 for the short term and level II-2 for long-term management of lumbar nerve root and low back pain [52].

More recently, patients with acute lumbosacral radiculopathy due to intervertebral disc herniation have reportedly improved with transforaminal injections of clonidine [53]. The mechanism for this improvement remains uncertain; however, there may be multiple targets for intraforaminal clonidine. Chung and others observed that peripheral nerve injury leads to sympathetic nerve fiber spouting around the

DRG, and this observation was hypothesized to contribute to the development of sympathetically mediated neuropathic pain [54]. Thus, clonidine, an alpha-2 agonist with sympatholytic actions on sympathetic nerve endings, may reduce the effects of increased sympathetic innervation of the DRG after nerve injury. Another possibility is via direct anti-inflammatory action. Liu and Eisenach demonstrated decreased hyperexcitability in rodent-injured nerves after clonidine was applied perinurally and attributed this to inhibition of pro-inflammatory cytokines and prostaglandins [55]. A peripheral site of action for the antinociception activity of an alpha-2 agonist was also suggested by Poree et al. in an animal model of neuropathic pain. In this model, the antinociceptive actions of dexmedetomidine, an alpha-2 agonist, was antagonized by prior treatment with a peripherally restricted alpha2AR antagonist that does not cross the blood-brain barrier. The authors suggested the DRG as a possible peripheral site of action for dexmedetomidine after nerve injury [56].

The DRG has also been targeted for electrical and pulsed radiofrequency stimulation. Although high temperature lesioning radiofrequency energy is successfully employed to denervate medial branch nerves, this technique is avoided in the larger mixed nerves as it may lead to deafferentation pain and painful neuromas. Pulsed and low temperature radiofrequency treatments do not cause neural destruction but instead expose the nerves to a high voltage low to moderate temperature environment. In a prospective randomized double-blind study, 67 °C RF was reported to provide long-term relief of cervical brachial pain [57]. A recent retrospective chart review of 50 patients who received pulsed (42 °C) and moderate temperature (56 °C) radiofrequency treatment of the DRG for lumbar radiculitis reported that all patients received at least a 50 % improvement in their pain [58]. Another group reported that when low temperature (42 °C) pulsed RF was used alone, 30 % of the patients received greater than 50 % pain relief [59]. The observation that even low temperature electric fields applied to the DRG could provide long-lasting pain relief has prompted the recent development of an implantable DRG stimulation system to provide a continuous electric field around the DRG [60]. Excellent results from multiple prospective clinical trials have resulted in approval of DRG stimulation for the treatment of chronic pain in Europe and Australia with clinical trials currently underway in the USA (Fig. 21.7).

Intraspinal Targets for Interventional Pain Management

Targeting the intrathecal space with opioids and local anesthetic has been available for cancer pain management since it was first reported in 1899 [61]. However, widespread utilization of intraspinal (epidural and intrathecal) analgesics

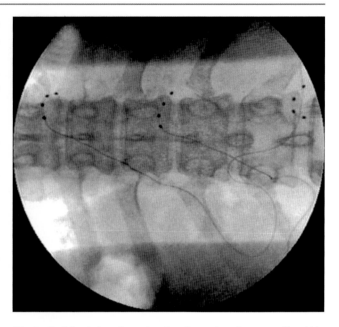

Fig. 21.7 Stimulating electrodes placed over dorsal root ganglia within the right T8–9, T10–11, and T12–L1 foramen. Stimulating electrodes placed over dorsal root ganglia within the right T8–9, T10–11, and T12–L1 foramen (Courtesy of Eric Grigsby MD, Napa Pain Institute, Napa, CA. and Jeff Kramer, Ph.D. Spinal Modulation, Menlo Park, CA [60]

outside of the operating room was not practical until the advent of long-term catheters and implantable pumps in the 1980s [62]. Dupen epidural catheters had an antimicrobial sleeve located at the skin exit site, thereby reducing the risk of infection and allowing for intraspinal delivery via an external pump for more than a year. While these catheters are no longer commercially available, they have been replaced by long-term epidural catheters attached to subcutaneous ports which provide even greater protection from infection [63]. For even longer-term intrathecal infusions and even greater protection against infection, implantable pumps have emerged as the preferred method for intrathecal delivery in the past 30 years. While these pumps are initially more expensive than externalized systems, they become cost neutral after 3 months and actually provide a cost savings thereafter as compared with externalized pumps [64, 65]. Most of the current systems are computer controlled, and some have the option for patient-controlled activation of programmed bolus doses [66]. The advantage of intrathecal management over systemic administration is one of inhibition of nociceptive transmission at the spinal level and reduced systemic toxicity. In a randomized clinical trial comparing intrathecal drug delivery systems (IDDS) to comprehensive medical management (CMM), cancer patients treated with IDDS had less medication-induced toxicity, greater pain control, and longer survival than did CMM patients [67]. Nonetheless, it is estimated that only 10–20 % of patients with cancer-related pain fail comprehensive medical management using the World Health Organization

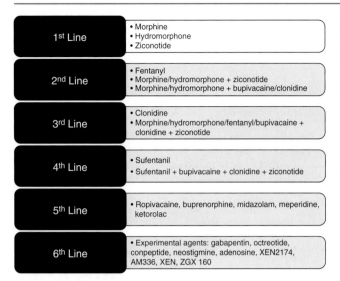

1st Line	• Morphine • Hydromorphone • Ziconotide
2nd Line	• Fentanyl • Morphine/hydromorphone + ziconotide • Morphine/hydromorphone + bupivacaine/clonidine
3rd Line	• Clonidine • Morphine/hydromorphone/fentanyl/bupivacaine + clonidine + ziconotide
4th Line	• Sufentanil • Sufentanil + bupivacaine + clonidine + ziconotide
5th Line	• Ropivacaine, buprenorphine, midazolam, meperidine, ketorolac

6th Line	• Experimental agents: gabapentin, octreotide,
	  conpeptide, neostigmine, adenosine, XEN2174,
	  AM336, XEN, ZGX 160

Fig. 21.8 Polyanalgesic algorithm for intrathecal therapy for cancer pain. With permission from Deer et al. [71])

guidelines and require more advanced pain management interventions such as IDDS [68]. Guidelines on appropriate selection of patients and intrathecal medication admixtures for patients with intractable cancer-related pain has recently been updated and includes the use of medications approved by the FDA for approved IDDS, medications that are by expert consensus, commonly used for IDDS therapy, and medications that are experimental and are recommended only as a means to provide greater analgesia in the final stages of life (Fig. 21.8) [70–72]. The common pharmacological targets for IDDS therapy include the mu-opioid receptors, calcium channels, sodium channels, and α-2 adrenergic receptors. Figure 21.9 shows the presynaptic and postsynaptic location of the receptors in the dorsal horn that forms the pharmacological basis of IDDS therapy, although, only morphine and ziconitide (aka SNX-111), a novel N-type voltage-sensitive calcium channel antagonist, are currently FDA-approved analgesics for IDDS therapy [70, 73–75]. As IDDS therapy gains greater acceptance for the treatment of intractable cancer pain, the appropriate position in a continuum of care for chronic non-cancer pain remains a source of debate. A recent review aimed at addressing this issue systematically evaluated the available literature using the Agency for Healthcare Research and Quality (AHRQ) criteria for observational studies and the Cochrane Musculoskeletal Review Group criteria for randomized trials. The level of evidence was determined using five levels of evidence, ranging from level I to III with three subcategories in level II, based on criteria developed by the US Preventive Services Task Force (USPSTF) [76]. The authors found 20 studies that met both the inclusions and exclusion criteria. Based on their analysis, they concluded that high-quality evidence supported a moderate recommendation for intrathecal

infusion systems for cancer-related pain and that moderate quality of evidence supported a limited to moderate recommendation for non-cancer-related pain.

In addition to pharmacological receptors, intraspinal neural structures are also targeted with electrical stimulation. Although the first spinal cord stimulator was implanted in 1967, the exact mechanism for electrical stimulation-induced analgesia remains elusive [77]. It is currently hypothesized that the analgesic effects of spinal cord stimulation are explained in part by the gate control theory proposed by Melzack and Wall whereby activation of large-diameter afferents activate segmental GABAergic interneurons [78, 79]. However, recent findings also suggest that supraspinal pathways are also involved in spinal cord stimulation analgesia [80]. Successful analgesia with spinal cord stimulation is dependent most upon proper placement of epidural electrodes over the spinal cord that are programmed to deliver the amplitude, frequency, and pulse width that successfully provides analgesia without untoward stimulation in areas that are not painful. The distance between electrodes being placed in an area that provides good analgesia ("sweet spot") and an area that does not can be as small as a few millimeters. Thus, successful stimulation can be lost if an electrode migrates even a few millimeters away from the ideal target. To circumvent this problem, most manufactures have devised more complex electrode arrays that allow for greater maneuverability of the electric field. While earlier systems employed as few as two or four electrode contacts per array, more recent spinal cord stimulation systems employ 16–20 contact arrays (Fig. 21.10b). In addition to spinal cord stimulation, intraspinal nerve roots can also be individually targeted (Fig. 21.10a). As with DRG stimulation discussed above, this technique is advantageous when the region of neuropathic pain has a small focal distribution and spinal cord stimulation activates areas outside the region of pain that is uncomfortable for the patient. This is especially true when the pain is due to injury to an isolated nerve [81, 82]. For example, Fig. 21.10c shows the electrode configuration in a patient receiving sacral nerve stimulation for persistent focal neuropathic pain in the pelvic floor after cystectomy and hysterectomy for chronic pelvic pain. Spinal cord stimulation failed to provide adequate analgesia whereas she continues to receive good analgesic benefit from sacral nerve stimulation 3 years after implantation.

In spite of over 40 years of clinical experience and success, routine implementation of spinal cord stimulation in clinical practice has been stifled, in part due to limited well-controlled clinical studies, a trend that has reversed in recent years. In a randomized prospective crossover design study comparing spinal cord stimulation versus reoperation for persistent leg pain after spinal decompression, North et al. found that patients initially randomized to SCS were significantly less likely to cross over than were those

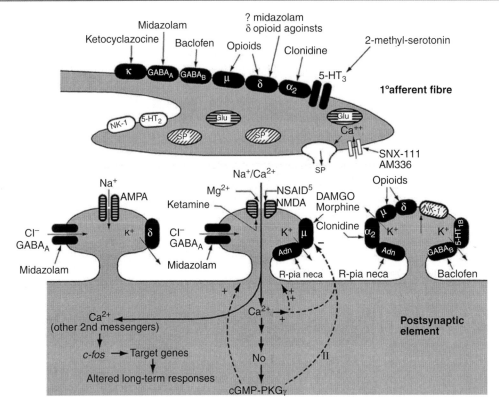

Fig. 21.9 Possible arrangement of pre- and postsynaptic receptors on structures in the dorsal horn of the spinal cord and potential sites of action of opioid and non-opioid spinal analgesics. Presynaptic release of the neurotransmitter glutamate (*Glu*) results in activation of the postsynaptic α-amino-3-hydroxy-5-methyl-4-isoxazolepropionic acid (*AMPA*) receptor, which controls a rapid-response sodium (*Na$^+$*) channel. Substance P (*SP*) interacts with the neurokinin (*NK-1*) receptor and results in activation of second messengers. With prolonged activation, the *N*-methyl-D-aspartate (*NMDA*) receptor is primed, Glu activates the receptor, the magnesium (*Mg^{2+}*) plug is removed, and the ion channel allows entry of Na$^+$ and calcium (*Ca^{2+}*) ions. The increase in intracellular Ca^{2+} then triggers a number of second-messenger cascades. Production of nitric oxide (*NO*) increases via the Ca^{2+}/calmodulin-dependent enzyme NO synthase. NO may diffuse out of the neuron to have a retrograde action on primary afferents and also activates guanylyl

cyclase, leading to increases in intracellular cyclic guanosine monophosphate (*cGMP*) and activation of cGMP-dependent protein kinases. Activation of the Ca^{2+}-dependent protein kinase C γ isoform (*PKCγ*) leads to phosphorylation of the NMDA receptor, which reduces the Mg^{2+} block (dotted line II) relating to the development of opioid tolerance. The increase in intracellular Ca^{2+} also results in the induction of proto-oncogenes such as c-*fos*, with a presumed action on target genes of altering long-term responses of the cell to further stimuli. κ, μ, and δ opioid receptors, *GABA* γ-aminobutyric acid, α$_2$ α$_2$ adrenoceptor, *5-HT* serotonin. Details of the potential analgesics are outlined in the text. *NSAID* nonsteroidal anti-inflammatory drug, *SNX-111* and *AM336* omega conopeptides that block neuronal Ca^{2+} channels. *DAMGO* [D-Ala^2,N-Me-Phe^4,Gly-ol^5]-enkephalin, *R-Pia* R-phenyl-isopropyl-adenosine, *Neca* N-ethylcarboxamide-adenosine (With permission from Walker et al. [69])

randomized to reoperation. Patients randomized to reoperation required increased opiate analgesics significantly more often than those randomized to SCS [83]. Kumar et al. followed shortly thereafter with a multicenter randomized prospective clinical study comparing spinal cord stimulation with conventional medical management (CMM) [84, 85]. This study found that compared with the CMM group, the SCS group experienced improved leg and back pain relief, quality of life, and functional capacity, as well as greater treatment satisfaction for over 2 years. More recently, a multicenter randomized study of SCS versus sham treatment demonstrated that spinal cord stimulation but not sham treatment decreased the frequency of angina attacks [86]. These pivotal studies have opened the door to even more investigations of SCS for an even greater number of disease states

including intractable angina, peripheral vascular disease, chronic pancreatitis, and chronic pelvic pain to name just a few [87–89]. As the clinical evidence grows in support of spinal cord stimulation for a wide range of chronic pain states, so does the resistance to approve this therapy by third-party payors due to concerns about initial cost. To address these concerns, Krames et al. proposed that spinal cord stimulation, as with other advanced therapies, be subject to a more comprehensive evaluation process whereby the initial cost is balanced with long-term health-care cost, safety, efficacy, and appropriateness of other therapies. They termed this new algorithm the SAFE (safety, appropriateness, fiscal neutrality, and effectiveness) principle [65, 90]. The authors went on to use this algorithm to assess when SCS should be used in the treatment of failed back surgery syndrome

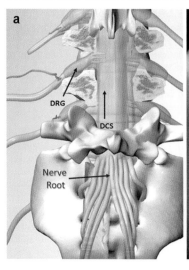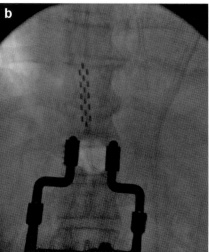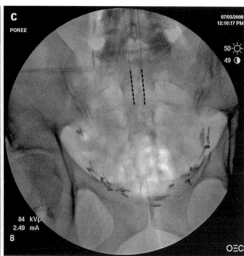

Fig. 21.10 (**a**) Illustration of intraspinal targets for electrical stimulation includes the dorsal columns (*DC*) of the spinal cord, the intraspinal nerve roots, and the dorsal root ganglia (*DRG*) (Courtesy of Jeff Kramer, Ph.D. Spinal Modulation, Menlo Park, CA) (**b**) Fluoroscopic image of intraoperative placement of 16 contact tripole paddle lead. Tripole configuration allows for greater maneuverability of the electric field. (**c**) Fluoroscopic image of retrograde placement of electrodes allows for stimulation of sacral nerve roots for patient with pelvic pain (Fluoroscopic images courtesy of Lawrence Poree MD PhD)

(FBSS). They concluded that SCS should be considered before submitting a patient to either long-term systemic opioid therapy or repeat spinal surgery for chronic pain resulting from FBSS [91].

As health-care costs continue to rise and advanced technologies rapidly emerge, employing the SAFE principle may provide a more rational approach to making individual as well as intuitional decisions regarding appropriate selection of therapies and allocation of resources.

References

1. Giamberardino MA, Costantini R, Affaitati G, et al. Viscero-visceral hyperalgesia: characterization in different clinical models. Pain. 2010;151:307–22.
2. Babcock RH. Chronic cholecystitis as a cause of myocardial incompetence; report of 13 cases. J Am Wed Assoc. 1909;52:1904–11.
3. Ammons WS, Blair RW, Foreman RD. Greater splanchnic excitation of primate T1-T5 spinothalamic neurons. J Neurophysiol. 1984;51(3):592–603.
4. Ammons WS, Blair RW, Foreman RD. Responses of primate T1–T5 spinothalamic neurons to gallbladder distension. AJP. 1984;247(6):R995–1002.
5. van Eijs F, Stanton-Hicks M, Van Zundert J, Faber CG, Lubenow TR, Mekhail N, van Kleef M, Huygen F. Evidence-based interventional pain medicine according to clinical diagnoses. 16. Complex regional pain syndrome. Pain Pract. 2011;11(1):70–87.
6. Alshab AK, Goldner JD, Panchal SJ. Complications of sympathetic blocks for visceral pain. Tech Reg Anesth Pain Manag. 2007;11:152–6.
7. Raj PP, Sahinler B, Lowe M. Radiofrequency lesioning of splanchnic nerves. Pain Pract. 2002;2(3):241–7.
8. Garcea G, Thomasset S, Berry DP, et al. Percutaneous splanchnic nerve radiofrequency ablation for chronic abdominal pain. ANZ J Surg. 2005;75:640–4.
9. Nabil D, Eissa AA. Evaluation of posteromedial transdiscal superior hypogastric block after failure of the classic approach. Clin J Pain. 2010;26(8):694–7.
10. Bosscher H. Blockade of the superior hypogastric plexus block for visceral pelvic pain. Pain Pract. 2001;1:162–70.
11. Toshniwal GR, Dureja GP, Prashanth SM. Transsacrococcygeal approach to ganglion impar block for management of chronic perineal pain: a prospective observational study. Pain Physician. 2007;10:661–6. ISSN 1533–3159.
12. Reig E, Abejón D, del Pozo C, Insausti J, Contreras R. Thermocoagulation of the ganglion impar or ganglion of Walther: description of a modified approach. Preliminary results in chronic, nononcological pain. Pain Pract. 2005;5:103–10.
13. Carroll I, Clark JD, Mackey S. Sympathetic block with botulinum toxin to treat complex regional pain syndrome. Ann Neurol. 2009;65:348–51.
14. Lim SJ, Park HJ, Lee SH, Moon DE. Ganglion impar block with botulinum toxin type a for chronic perineal pain. Korean J Pain. 2010;23(1):65–9.
15. Simopoulos TT, Malik AB, Sial KA, Elkersh M, Bajwa ZH. Radiofrequency lesioning of the L2 ramus communicans in managing discogenic low back pain. Pain Physician. 2005;8(1):61–5.
16. Schwarzer AC, Aprill CN, Derby R, Fortin J, Kine G, Bogduk N. The prevalence and clinical features of internal disc disruption in patients with chronic low back pain. Spine (Phila Pa 1976). 1995;20(17):1878–83.
17. Sluijter ME. Radiofrequency lesions of the communicating ramus in the treatment of low back pain. In: Raj PP, editor. Current management of pain. Philadelphia: Kluwer Academic publishers; 1989. p. 145–59.
18. Oh WS, Shim JC. A randomized controlled trial of radiofrequency denervation of the ramus communicans nerve for chronic discogenic low back pain. Clin J Pain. 2004;20(1):55–60.
19. Guyatt G, Gutterman D, Baumann MH, et al. Grading strength of recommendations and quality of evidence in clinical guidelines: report from an American college of chest physicians task force. Chest. 2006;129:174–81.
20. Kallewaard JW, Terheggen MA, Groen GJ, Sluijter ME, Derby R, Kapural L, Mekhail N, van Kleef M. Discogenic low back pain. Pain Pract. 2010;10(6):560–79.
21. Chandler G, Dalley G, Hemmer Jr J, et al. Gray ramus communicans nerve block. Novel treatment approach for painful osteoporotic vertebral compression fracture. South Med J. 2001;94:387–93.

22. Sluijter E, Mehta M. Treatment of chronic back and neck pain by percutaneous thermal lesions. In: Lipton S, Miles J, editors. Persistent pain: modern methods of treatment. London: Academic; 1981. p. 141–79.

23. Lord SM, McDonald GJ, Bogduk N. Percutaneous radiofrequency neurotomy of the cervical medial branches: a validated treatment for cervical zygapophysial joint pain. Neurosurg Q. 1988;8: 288–308.

24. Datta S, Lee M, Falco F, Bryce D, Hayek S. Systematic assessment of diagnostic accuracy and therapeutic utility of lumbar facet joint interventions. Pain Physician. 2009;12:437–60. ISSN 1533–3159.

25. Falco F, Erhart S, Wargo BW, et al. Systematic review of diagnostic utility and therapeutic effectiveness of cervical facet joint interventions. Pain Physician. 2009;12:323–44.

26. Beaubien BP, Mehbod AA, Kallemeier PM, Lew WD, Buttermann GR, Transfeldt EE, Wood KB. Posterior augmentation of an anterior lumbar interbody fusion: minimally invasive fixation versus pedicle screws in vitro. Spine (Phila Pa 1976). 2004;29(19): E406–12.

27. Boonen S, Wahl DA, Nauroy L, Brandi ML, Bouxsein ML, Goldhahn J, Lewiecki EM, Lyritis GP, Marsh D, Obrant K, Silverman S, Siris E, Akesson K; for the CSA Fracture Working Group of the International Osteoporosis Foundation. Balloon kyphoplasty and vertebroplasty in the management of vertebral compression fractures. Osteoporos Int. 2011;22:2915–34.

28. Wardlaw D, Cummings SR, Van Meirhaeghe J, Bastian L, Tillman JB, Ranstam J, Eastell R, Shabe P, Talmadge K, Boonen S. Efficacy and safety of balloon kyphoplasty compared with non-surgical care for vertebral compression fracture (FREE): a randomised controlled trial. Lancet. 2009;373(9668):1016–24.

29. Klazen CA, Lohle PN, de Vries J, Jansen FH, Tielbeek AV, Blonk MC, et al. Vertebroplasty versus conservative treatment in acute osteoporotic vertebral compression fractures (vertos II): an open-label randomised trial. Lancet. 2010;376(9746):1085–92.

30. Kallmes DF, Comstock BA, Heagerty PJ, et al. A randomized trial of vertebroplasty for osteoporotic spinal fractures. N Engl J Med. 2009;361:569–79.

31. Buchbinder R, Osborne RH, Ebeling PR, et al. A randomized trial of vertebroplasty for painful osteoporotic vertebral fractures. N Engl J Med. 2009;361:557–68.

32. Firanescu C, Lohle PN, de Vries J, Klazen CA, Juttmann JR, van Rooij WJ, VERTOS IV Study Group. A randomised sham controlled trial of vertebroplasty for painful acute osteoporotic vertebral fractures (VERTOS IV). Trials. 2011;12:93.

33. Manchikanti L, Singh V, Pampati V, Damron KS, Barnhill RC, Beyer C, Cash KA. Evaluation of the relative contributions of various structures in chronic low back pain. Pain Physician. 2001;4: 308–16.

34. Derby R, Howard MW, Grant JM, Lettice JJ, Van Peteghem PK, Ryan DP. The ability of pressure-controlled discography to predict surgical and nonsurgical outcomes. Spine. 1999;24:364–71; discussion 71–2.

35. Van Alphen HA, Braakman R, Bezemer PD, Broere G, Berfelo MW. Chemonucleolysis versus discectomy: a randomized multicenter trial. J Neurosurg. 1989;70:869–75.

36. Miller MR, Mathews RS, Reeves KD. Treatment of painful advanced internal lumbar disc derangement with intradiscal injection of hypertonic dextrose. Pain Physician. 2006;9(2):115–21.

37. Peng B, Pang X, Wub Y, Zhao C, Song X. A randomized placebo-controlled trial of intradiscal methylene blue injection for the treatment of chronic discogenic low back pain. Pain. 2010;149:124–9.

38. Henschke N, Kuijpers T, Rubinstein SM, van Middelkoop M, Ostelo R, Verhagen A, Koes BW, van Tulder MW. Injection therapy and denervation procedures for chronic low-back pain: a systematic review. Eur Spine J. 2010;19:1425–49.

39. DeerTR KL. New image-guided ultra-minimally invasive lumbar decompression method: the mild® procedure. Pain Physician. 2010;13:35–41.

40. Abbas J, Hamoud K, Masharawi YM, May H, et al. Ligamentum flavum thickness in normal and stenotic lumbar spines. Spine. 2010;35(12):1225–30.

41. Löhr M, Hampl JA, Lee JY, et al. Hypertrophy of the lumbar ligamentum flavum is associated with inflammation-related TGF-β expression. Acta Neurochir. 2011;153:134–41.

42. Kosaka H, Sairyo K, Biyani A, et al. Pathomechanism of loss of elasticity and hypertrophy of lumbar ligamentum flavum in elderly patients with lumbar spinal canal stenosis. Spine. 2007;32(25): 2805–11.

43. Chopko B, Caraway DL. MiDAS I (mild® decompression alternative to open surgery): a preliminary report of a prospective, multicenter clinical study. Pain Physician. 2010;13:369–78.

44. Mekhail N, Vallejo R, Coleman MH, Benyamin RM. Long-term results of percutaneous lumbar decompression mild(®) for spinal stenosis. Pain Pract. 2012;12:184–93. Epub 2012 Jan 16.

45. Levine JD, Lam D, Taiwo YO, et al. Hyperalgesic properties of 15 lipoxygenase products of arachidonic acid. Proc Natl Aca Sci U S A. 1986;83:5331–4.

46. Ozaktay AC, Kallakuri S, Cavanaugh JM. Phospholipase A2 sensitivity of the dorsal root ganglion. Spine. 1998;23:1296–306.

47. Franson R, Saal JS, Saal JA. Human disc phospholipase A2 is inflammatory. Spine. 1992;17(Suppl):S190–2.

48. Kang JD, Georgescu HI, McIntyre L, et al. Herniated lumbar intervertebral discs spontaneously produce matrix metalloproteinases, nitric oxide, interleukin-6, and prostaglandin E2. Spine. 1996;21: 271–7.

49. White FA, Jung H, Miller RJ. Chemokines and the pathophysiology of neuropathic pain. PNAS. 2007;104(51):20151–8.

50. Benny B, Azari P. The efficacy of lumbosacral transforaminal epidural steroid injections: a comprehensive literature review. J Back Musculoskelet Rehabil. 2011;24(2):67–76.

51. Roberts ST, Willick SE, Rho ME, Rittenberg JD. Efficacy of lumbosacral transforaminal epidural steroid injections: a systematic review. PMR. 2009;1(7):657–68.

52. Buenaventura RM, Datta S, Abdi S, Smith HS. Systematic review of therapeutic lumbar transforaminal epidural steroid injections. Pain Physician. 2009;12(1):233–51.

53. Burgher AH, Hoelzer BC, Schroeder DR, Wilson GA, Huntoon MA. Transforaminal epidural clonidine versus corticosteroid for acute lumbosacral radiculopathy due to intervertebral disc herniation. Spine (Phila Pa 1976). 2011;36(5):E293–300.

54. Chung K, Lee BH, Yoon YW, Chung JM. Sympathetic sprouting in the dorsal root ganglia of the injured peripheral nerve in a rat neuropathic pain model. J Comp Neurol. 1996;376(2):241–52.

55. Ririe DG, Liu B, Clayton B, Tong C, Eisenach JC. Electrophysiologic characteristics of large neurons in dorsal root ganglia during development and after hind paw incision in the rat. Anesthesiology. 2008;109(1):111–7.

56. Poree LR, Guo TZ, Kingery WS, Maze M. The analgesic potency of dexmedetomidine is enhanced after nerve injury: a possible role for peripheral alpha2-adrenoceptors. Anesth Analg. 1998;87(4): 941–8.

57. Van Kleef M, Liem L, Lousberg R, Barendse G, Kessels F, Sluijter M. Radiofrequency lesion adjacent to the dorsal root ganglion for cervical brachial pain: a prospective double blind randomized study. Neurosurgery. 1996;38:1127–32.

58. Nagda JV, Davis CV, Bajwa ZH, Simopoulos TT. Retrospective review of the efficacy and safety of repeated pulsed and continuous radiofrequency lesioning of the dorsal root ganglion/segmental nerve for lumbar radicular pain. Pain Physician. 2011;14:371–6. ISSN 1533–3159.

59. Van Boxem K, van Bilsen J, de Meij N, Herrler A, Kessels F, Van Zundert J, van Kleef M. Pulsed radiofrequency treatment adjacent to the lumbar dorsal root ganglion for the management of lumbosacral radicular syndrome: a clinical audit. Pain Med. 2011;12:1322–30. doi:10.1111/j.1526-4637.2011.01202.x.

60. Grigsby E, Deer T, Weiner R, Wilcosky B, Kramer J. Prospective, multicenter, Clinical Trial Studying Dorsal Root Ganglion Stimulation in the Treatment of Back Pain. North American Neuromodulation Society, 2010.

61. Barros S. Nothing new under the sun- a French (not Japanese) pioneer in the clinical use of intrathecal morphine history of spinal morphine. Int Congress Ser. 2002;1242:189–92.

62. Prager JP. Neuraxial medication delivery the development and maturity of a concept for treating chronic pain of spinal origin. Spine. 2002;27(22):2593–605.

63. de Jong PC, Kansen PJ. A comparison of epidural catheters with or without subcutaneous injection ports for treatment of cancer pain. Anesth Analg. 1994;78(1):94–100.

64. Bedder MD, Burchiel K, Larson A. Cost analysis of two implantable narcotic deliver systems. J Pain Symptom Manage. 1991; 6:368–73.

65. Krames E, Poree L, Deer T, Levy R. Implementing the SAFE principles for the development of pain medicine therapeutic algorithms that include neuromodulation techniques. Neuromodulation. 2009;12(2):104–13.

66. Ilias W, le Polain B, Buchser E, Demartini L, oPTiMa Study Group. Patient-controlled analgesia in chronic pain patients: experience with a new device designed to be used with implanted programmable pumps. Pain Pract. 2008;8(3):164–70.

67. Smith TJ, Staats PS, Deer T, Stearns LJ, Rauck RL, Boortz-Marx RL, et al. Randomized clinical trial of an implantable drug delivery system compared with comprehensive medical management for refractory cancer pain: impact on pain, drug-related toxicity, and survival. J Clin Oncol. 2002;20:4040–9.

68. Meuser T, Pietruck C, Radbruch L, Stute P, Lehmann KL, Grond S. Symptoms during cancer pain treatment following WHO-guidelines: a longitudinal follow-up study of symptom prevalence, severity and etiology. Pain. 2001;93:247–57.

69. Walker SM, Goudas LC, Cousins MJ, Carr DB. Combination spinal analgesic chemotherapy: a systematic review. Anesth Analg. 2002;95:674–715.

70. Stearns L, Boortz-Marx R, Du Pen S, Friehs G, Gordon M, Halyard M, Herbst L, Kiser J. Intrathecal drug delivery for the management of cancer pain a multidisciplinary consensus of best clinical practices. J Support Oncol. 2005;3:399–408.

71. Deer TR, Smith HS, Burton AW, Pope JE, Doleys DM, Levy RM, Staats PS, Wallace MS, Webster LR, Rauck RL, Cousins M. Comprehensive consensus based guidelines on intrathecal drug delivery systems in the treatment of pain caused by cancer pain. Pain Physician. 2011;14(3):E283–312.

72. Smith TJ, Staats PS, Deer T, Stearns LJ, Rauck RL, Boortz-Marx RL, Buchser E, Català E, Bryce DA, Coyne PJ, Pool GE, Implantable Drug Delivery Systems Study Group. Randomized clinical trial of an implantable drug delivery system compared with comprehensive medical management for refractory cancer pain: impact on pain, drug-related toxicity, and survival. J Clin Oncol. 2002;20:4040–9.

73. Deer T, Krames ES, Hassenbusch SJ, et al. Polyanalgesic consensus conference 2007: recommendations for the management of pain by intrathecal (intraspinal) drug delivery: report of an interdisciplinary expert panel. Neuromodulation. 2007;10:300–28.

74. Lawson EF, Wallace MS. Current developments in intraspinal agents for cancer and pain. Curr Pain Headache Rep. 2010;14(1):8–16.

75. Staats PS, Yearwood T, Charapata SG, Presley RW, Wallace MS, Byas-Smith M, Fisher R, Bryce DA, Mangieri EA, Luther RR, Mayo M, McGuire D, Ellis D. Intrathecal ziconotide in the treatment of refractory pain in patients with cancer or AIDS. JAMA. 2004;291:63–70.

76. Hayek SM, Deer TR, Pope JE, Panchal SJ, Patel V. Intrathecal therapy for cancer and non-cancer pain. Pain Physician. 2011;14:219–48.

77. Sealy CN, Mortimer JT, Reswick KB. Electrical inhibition of pain by stimulation of dorsal column: preliminary clinical reports. Anesth Analg. 1967;4:489–91.

78. Meizack K, Wall PD. Pain mechanism®: a new theory. Science. 1965;150:971–9.

79. Meyerson BA, Linderoth B. Mode of action of spinal cord stimulation in neuropathic pain. J Pain Symptom Manage. 2006;31: S6–12.

80. Linderoff B, Forman R. Physiology of spinal cord stimulation. Neuromodulation. 1999;2(3):150–64.

81. Ghazwani YQ, Elkelini MS, Hassouna MM. Efficacy of sacral neuromodulation in treatment of bladder pain syndrome: long-term follow-up. Neurourol Urodyn. 2011;30:1271–5.

82. McJunkin TL, Wuollet AL, Lynch PJ. Sacral nerve stimulation as a treatment modality for intractable neuropathic testicular pain. Pain Physician. 2009;12(6):991–5.

83. North RB, Kidd DH, Farrokhi R, Piantadosi SA. Spinal cord stimulation versus repeated lumbosacral spine surgery for chronic pain: a randomized, controlled trial. Neurosurgery. 2005;56:98–107.

84. Kumar K, Taylor R, Jacques L, et al. SCS versus conventional medical management for neuropathic pain: a multicentre randomised controlled trial in patients with failed back surgery syndrome. Pain. 2008;132:179–88.

85. Kumar K, Taylor R, Jacquies L, Eldabe SM, Eglio M, et al. The effects of spinal cord stimulation in neuropathic pain are sustained: a 24 month follow up of the prospective randomized controlled multicenter trial of the effectiveness of spinal cord stimulation. Neurosurgery. 2008;63(4):762–70.

86. Lanza GA, Grimaldi R, Greco S, Ghio S, Sarullo F, Zuin G, De Luca A, Allegri M, Di Pede F, Castagno D, Turco A, Sapio M, Pinato G, Cioni B, Trevi G, Crea F. Spinal cord stimulation for the treatment of refractory angina pectoris: a multicenter randomized single-blind study (the SCS-ITA trial). Pain. 2011;152(1):45–52.

87. Levy RM. Spinal cord stimulation for medically refractory angina pectoris: can the therapy be resuscitated? Neuromodulation. 2011;14(1):1–5.

88. North RB, Kumar K, Wallace MS, Henderson JM, Shipley JS, Hernandez JM, Jaax KN. Spinal cord stimulation versus re-operation in patientsWith failed back surgery syndrome: an international multicenter randomized controlled trial (EVIDENCE study). Neuromodulation. 2011;14:330–6.

89. Kapural L, Cywinski JB, Sparks DA. Spinal cord stimulation for visceral pain from chronic pancreatitis. Neuromodulation. 2011;14(5):423–7.

90. Krames E, Poree L, Deer T, Levy R. Rethinking algorithms of pain care: the use of the S.A.F.E. principles. Pain Med. 2009;10(1):1–5.

91. Krames ES, Monis S, Poree L, Deer T, Levy R. Using the SAFE principles when evaluating electrical stimulation therapies for the pain of failed back surgery syndrome. Neuromodulation. 2011;14(4): 299–311.

Functional Anatomy and Imaging of the Spine

22

John C. Keel and Gary J. Brenner

Key Points
- Spine pain concepts and standardized terminology
- Spine anatomical structures and functional unit concept, a basic foundation to take to clinic and fluoroscopy suite
- Basic spine imaging modalities and examples
- Awareness of references such as NASS, IASP, and ACR publications, writings of great anatomists, for example, Bogduk

Introduction

Painful disorders of the spine are among our most common medical complaints. Over a lifetime, 60–80 % of adults experience at least one significant episode of back pain [1, 2]. In a single year, 15–20 % will have back pain, and 2–5 % of the entire population will seek medical attention for back pain [2]. Low back pain has been estimated as the fifth leading cause of all medical visits and the second leading cause of symptom-related medical visits [3]. In the United States, the estimated annual cost of back pain is $20 billion to $50 billion [4]. In particular, low back pain is one of the most important factors in medical costs and disability.

J.C. Keel, M.D. (✉)
Spine Center, Beth Israel Deaconess Medical Center,
330 Brookline Avenue, Boston, MA 02215, USA

Department of Orthopedics, Harvard Medical School,
Boston, MA, USA
e-mail: jkeel@bidmc.harvard.edu

G.J. Brenner, M.D., Ph.D.
Department of Anesthesia, Critical Care and Pain Medicine,
Massachusetts General Hospital,
15 Parkman Street, Boston, MA 02114, USA

Harvard Medical School,
Boston, MA, USA
e-mail: gjbrenner@partners.org

Imaging of the spine is now nearly as ubiquitous as back pain itself. Imaging technology has become increasingly sensitive and detailed in its revelations, but improvements in images have outpaced our ability to interpret their significance, resulting in the conundrum of false-positive spine imaging [5]. Spine imaging is also expensive. A recent analysis of the Medical Expenditure Panel Survey (MEPS) from 1997 to 2005 showed that spine-related medical costs escalated significantly more than increases in general medical costs, and patients with spine problems accounted for a disproportionate share of expenditures. Spine imaging contributed to these costs without necessarily improving outcomes [6]. Several guidelines have been developed in hopes of ameliorating this trend, such as those of the American College of Radiology [7, 8].

This chapter introduces the essentials of spine anatomy and imaging. For the pain physician, mastery of spinal anatomy and imaging modalities is required to correlate clinical presentation with anatomic abnormalities and make a valid interpretation of the imaging.

Historical Background

The functional anatomy of the spine has been studied since antiquity. Imhotep, the founder of ancient Egyptian medicine, wrote about anatomy of the spine more than 4,500 years ago. The first description of spinal traction is in the Indian epic *Srimad Bhagwat Mahapuranam*, written between 3,500 and 1,800 B.C. Hippocrates (460–377 B.C.) described discs, ligaments, muscles, and curvatures of the spine and first described the effects of tuberculosis on the spine. He also devised the Hippocratic board and Hippocratic ladder to treat spinal deformities and performed spinal manipulation. Aristotle laid the philosophical foundation for kinesiology [9]. Galen (130–200 A.D.), the "father of sports medicine," wrote of the functional importance of spine anatomy and described spinal nerves in detail [10]. Vesalius (1514–1564), the "father of anatomy," made remarkably accurate observations about the spine [11] and described the spine as the "keel of the body [12]." The renowned medieval Persian physician, Ibn Sina (Avicenna), devoted eight chapters to the spine in *Al-Qanun fi al-Tibb (the Canons of Medicine)* [13]. Twentieth and twenty-first century spines experience great forces from automobiles and airplane ejection seats, and engineers collaborating with physicians have developed sophisticated models such as finite element analysis, in order to properly design equipment to protect the spine [14]. Technological advances and increased understanding of spine anatomy have led to more options for diagnosis and treatment of back pain, this major cause of human suffering.

Spine imaging is a most remarkable example of advancement in the diagnosis of painful spine disorders. In November 1895, Roentgen discovered X-rays, and within weeks, this powerful new tool was employed for medical use [15]. It is interesting for the pain physician to note that the first use of X-ray was really a form of fluoroscopy. In the 1930s, stratigraphy, planigraphy, and tomography techniques were developed, wherein the X-ray source and film are rotated in a precise way in order to obtain a picture of an internal structure, such as a vertebral fracture. Pneumoencephalography led to pneumomyelography in 1919, then Lipiodol myelography, using iodized poppy seed oil, in 1922. Pantopaque arrived in the 1940s, Conray in the 1960s, and the less toxic nonionic, water-soluble contrasts even later. Lindblom reported discography in 1948. Hounsfield invented computed tomography (CT) in 1973. MRI came into clinical use in 1984, after a long period of development [16].

Scientific Foundation and Relevance to Pain Care

The anatomic structures of the spine can be sources of somatic, inflammatory, neuropathic afferent, and peripheral deafferentation pain [17]. *Somatic pain* results from stimulation of nerve endings in bone, muscle, ligament, or joint. *Visceral pain* arises from stimulation of a body organ and can also be relevant to understanding back pain as visceral pain can both be referred to and radiate to the spine, for example, as in renal colic. *Inflammatory* pain results from pathology that, as the name suggests, involves inflammation; this can be either acute or chronic. Peripheral *neuropathic pain* results from stimulation of the axons or cell bodies of the peripheral nerve. *Central* or *deafferentation pain* can result from nerve root avulsion or injury to the spinal cord [18]. Furthermore, the spinal cord is a conduit for almost all pain, and so the spine is frequently the target of the pain physician's treatment modality, whether it is medication delivered orally, epidurally or intrathecally by catheter, or spinal cord stimulation [19].

Table 22.1 Bogduk's postulates

1. The structure must have a nerve supply
2. The structure should be capable of causing pain similar to what is clinically observed (e.g., when provoked in normal volunteers)
3. The structure should be susceptible to painful disease or injury; such disorders should be detectable by clinical, imaging, biomechanical, or post-mortem tests
4. The structure should be shown to be a source of pain in actual patients, using reliable and valid diagnostic tests

Table 22.2 Vertebral column structures with pain-fiber innervation

Structure

Innervation characteristics

1. *Fibrous capsules of facet joints*
   Plexus formations of unmyelinated nerve fibers, dense
2. *Ligaments: anterior longitudinal, posterior longitudinal, interspinous*
   Free nerve endings
3. *Periosteum*
   Plexus formations of unmyelinated nerve fibers, dense
4. *Fascia and tendons attached to periosteum*
   Plexus formations of unmyelinated nerve fibers, dense
5. *Dura mater*
   Plexus formations of unmyelinated nerve fibers, less dense
6. *Epidural adipose tissue*
   Plexus formations of unmyelinated nerve fibers, variably dense
7. *Adventitial walls of arteries and arterioles to facet joints and cancellous bone*
   Plexus formations of unmyelinated nerve fibers
8. *Walls of epidural and paravertebral veins*
   Plexus formations of unmyelinated nerve fibers, dense
9. *Walls of blood vessels to paravertebral muscles*
   Plexus formations of unmyelinated nerve fibers, dense
10. *Posterior anulus fibrosus of intervertebral disc*
    Free nerve endings at the superficial posterior anulus

Innervation characteristics (Modified from Wyke [20])
See Wyke et al. for references cited

In clinical practice, anatomic sources of pain have been referred to as *pain generators*. In order for an anatomic structure to be considered as a source of pain, several conditions should be present, as outlined in Table 22.1. Such criteria for the anatomic cause of back pain have come to be known as *Bogduk's postulates* and are analogous to Koch's postulates regarding bacterial cause of disease [17]. For example, several specific structures of the spine have long been known to have pain fibers. Table 22.2 summarizes pain fiber distribution in the vertebral column as described by Wyke in 1970 [20]. Understanding of the causes of spinal pain continues to develop.

The International Association for the Study of Pain (IASP) has published standardized definitions for spinal pain, based on perceived location of pain (Table 22.3) [11]. For example, lumbar spinal pain is pain felt to originate in

Table 22.3 Spinal pain defined by IASP

Cervical spinal or radicular pain syndromes
Thoracic spinal or radicular pain syndromes
Lumbar spinal or radicular pain syndromes
Sacral spinal or radicular pain syndromes
Coccygeal pain syndromes
Diffuse or generalized spinal pain
Low back pain of psychological origin with spinal referral

Table 22.4 Red flags of back pain that may prompt spine imaging

1. Recent significant trauma, or milder trauma, age >50
2. Unexplained weight loss
3. Unexplained fever
4. Immunosuppression
5. History of cancer
6. IV drug use
7. Prolonged use of corticosteroids, osteoporosis
8. Age >70
9. Focal neurologic deficit with progressive or disabling symptoms
10. Duration longer than 6 weeks

an area of the low back below the T12 spinous process, above the S1 spinous process, and medial to the lateral borders of the erector spinae muscles. Sacral spine pain is felt to originate in the sacrum below the S1 spinous process, above the sacrococcygeal joints, and medial to a line between the posterior superior and inferior iliac spines [11]. Pain perceived as being localized around the spine is termed *axial pain*. In contrast, radiculitis or referred pain is perceived more peripherally.

Pain originating from an area of the body with relatively low sensory innervation may be perceived in, or referred to, a different part of the body with greater sensory innervation from the same spinal root level. This *somatic referred pain* is due to *convergence* of high and low sensory inputs at the central nervous system level, such as spinal segmental level or thalamus [17, 21]. For example, low back pain is often perceived as spreading to the buttock. The low back is innervated by the lumbosacral dorsal rami, while the buttock is innervated by the ventral rami of the same spinal segmental levels. The quality of somatic referred pain is deep, constant aching that is diffuse and hard to localize. While it is more often an origin of referred pain, sometimes pain is referred to the lumbar spine. Pain can be referred to the lumbar spine from the lower thoracic spine, abdominal organs, or sacroiliac joints. Muscles may also refer pain to the spine [22].

Distinct from somatic referred pain, *radicular pain* is perceived as arising from a limb or other structure due to ectopic activation of sensory afferent fibers, typically at a spinal root level [21]. The classic quality of radicular pain is intermittent shooting or lancinating and is perceived as traveling down a limb in a narrow band, congruent with the quality of pain that has been produced by experimental stimulation of injured nerve roots [17]. However, in clinical practice, there is variation in pain referral from radiculitis; such pain patterns can be described as dermatomal, myotomal, sclerotomal, or even dynatomal [23–25]. *Radicular pain* is not equivalent to *radiculopathy*. Radiculopathy involves motor or sensory conduction block and does not cause pain by itself, but can accompany radicular or referred pain [17].

Evaluation of pain disorders begins with a careful history and evaluation, and this may often suggest that the anatomical source is the spine. The next step for the pain physician often involves a decision to pursue spine imaging or analysis of imaging that has already been ordered by referring physicians. As noted earlier, the utility of spine imaging is controversial. Low back pain with or without radiculopathy may be self-limited and may not require imaging. However, if *red flags* are present (Table 22.4), imaging of the spine may be warranted [7]. ACR guidelines for chronic neck pain are less clear, especially regarding whiplash. For chronic neck pain, patients with neurologic features may need MRI or CT regardless of X-ray findings, and patients without neurologic features generally do not require imaging beyond X-rays. If X-rays reveal bony or disc destruction, MRI or CT with contrast may be indicated [8]. More details on specific imaging modalities will follow below, and figures will provide examples.

Spine Anatomy and Function

Viewed as a whole, the typical adult spine has primary curvatures that are kyphotic in the thoracic, sacral, and coccygeal spine and secondary lordotic curvatures that develop after birth in the cervical and lumbar spine (Fig. 22.1). In the frontal plane there are typically no curvatures. A frontal curvature of more than 10° is scoliosis; thoracic kyphosis is typically limited to 30–35° and lumbar lordosis 50–60°.

A functional segmental unit of the spine consists of three joints that join adjacent vertebrae: anteriorly, the intervertebral disc (Fig. 22.2) and posteriorly, the two facet joints at that level [27, 28]. This functional unit was first described by Junghanns as a "mobile segment [29, 30]." The functional unit model applies to all mobile segments of the spine except at the atlantooccipital (C0–C1) and atlantoaxial (C1–C2) junctions, where there are no intervertebral discs. The muscles and nerves of the spine are intimately related to the functional unit. The following sections describe the specific anatomical structures of the spine, with an emphasis on function and pain.

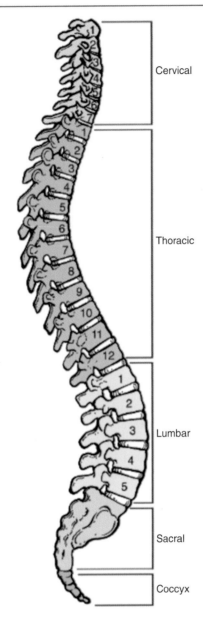

Fig. 22.1 Sagittal spine (Reprinted from Mathis [26])

Osteology

The vertebral column as a whole consists of 33 vertebrae: 7 cervical, 12 thoracic, 5 lumbar, 5 fused sacral, and 4 fused coccygeal [31]. Vertebrae are irregular, composite bones, consisting of a ventral body and a dorsal neural arch. The exception is the atlas, which has no vertebral body. The load-bearing system of the vertebral bones can be understood as a tripod: one vertebral body interface and two (paired) facet joint interfaces [32]. For example, lumbar vertebral bodies bear 80–90 % of the weight load, and lumbar pedicles and laminae function as struts, supporting the tripod "legs." Pedicles connect the anterior and posterior weight-bearing elements, spanning from the transverse process to the body.

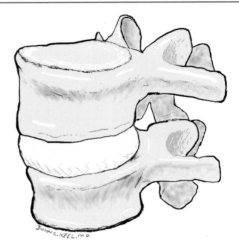

Fig. 22.2 Functional segmental unit

Transverse processes originate at the junction of the pedicle and the lamina, while the spinous process originates at the junction of right and left laminae. The functional significance of the transverse and spinous processes is to increase the moment arm of muscles attaching to these sites [17, 32]. The vertebral bodies have thin cortical bone and cancellous trabecular bone in vertical, oblique, and horizontal patterns [31]. This overlapping trabecular medullary structure provides great strength, but the relative lack of overlap in the anterior portion may predispose to compression fractures.

Cervical vertebrae (Fig. 22.3) bear the least weight, and their vertebral bodies are relatively narrow in AP dimension and have distinct uncinate processes at their superolateral borders, which articulate with the vertebral body above (uncovertebral joint). Vertebrae C1–C6 have bilateral foramen transversarium containing the vertebral artery (C7 has this foramen without the vertebral artery). As shown in the figure, the vertebral artery is very susceptible to injury in the anterolateral approach for cervical transforaminal injections (Fig. 22.4). The transverse processes have anterior and posterior projections for attachment of muscles, and the projections form a groove which contains the exiting spinal nerve. The cervical articular pillars are oblique to the horizontal plane and appear stacked as a column. The atlas, C1, has no vertebral body and has unique articular processes for occipital condyle and axis. The axis, C2, is most recognized by the odontoid process or dens. The occipital-atlantoaxial complex allows nodding and rotational movements: about 50 % of flexion-extension is at C0–C1, and 50 % of rotation is at C1–C2. C6 transverse process anterior tubercle is known as Chassaignac's tubercle (also known as carotid tubercle, an important landmark for stellate ganglion blocks). Vertebra C7 has a larger inferior body, a large spinous process (*vertebra prominens*), and steeply sloping articular pillars.

The defining features of the 12 thoracic vertebrae are the costotransverse and costovertebral articulations of the ribs

Fig. 22.3 Cervical vertebrae (Reprinted from Mathis et al. [33])

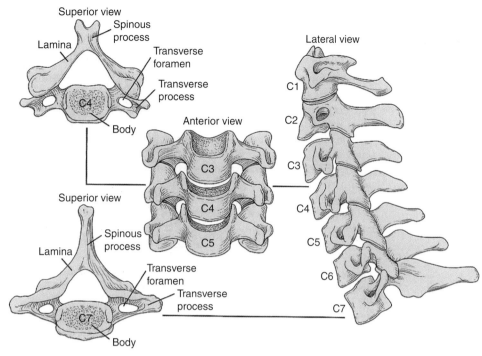

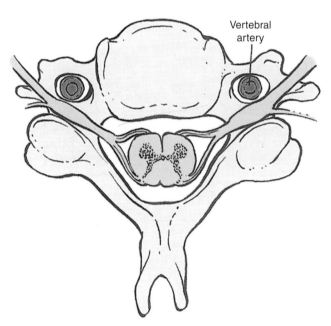

Fig. 22.4 Cervical vertebral artery (Reprinted from Mathis [26])

(Fig. 22.5). Thoracic facets are arranged in the coronal plane in a way that allows rotation and side bending.

Typical features of lumbar vertebrae are shown (Fig. 22.6). L5 is usually largest and more wedge-shaped when viewed laterally, which allows the superior aspect of L5 to be closer to horizontal [34]. The L5 disc is also wedge-shaped, allowing 16° average angle between the respective superior and inferior surfaces of S1 and L5 [35]. L5 has thick transverse processes but has the smallest lumbar spinous process. L1 has the shortest and L3 the longest transverse processes [36].

L5–S1 facets tend to be more flat, while other levels are more curved [31]. Because L5 is angled, more of its axial load is transmitted by its posterior elements, including the transverse processes and iliolumbar ligaments [37]. The lumbar vertebral bodies have indentations in the posterior aspects of superior and inferior rims, vestigial uncinate processes that may contribute to posterolateral disc protrusions [17]. The mamillary process is an attachment site for longissimus and rotator muscles. The accessory process is thought to be a vestigial costal process and is an attachment site for longissimus muscles. The mamilloaccessory ligament joins these two processes; this structure may be an obstacle in medial branch blocks or radiofrequency ablation.

The sacrum (Fig. 22.7) is formed of five fused vertebrae and vestigial costal elements. The sacrum articulates with the ilium. The sacrum has a central canal which is the terminal portion of the spinal canal. The ventral primary rami of S1–S4 exit via anterior foramina, and the posterior rami exit the posterior foramina. The center of mass is anterior to the vertebral column in 75 % of adults, typically 2 cm anterior to S2 [31]. The sacrum is tilted forward so that the most superior sacral end plate is 50–53° from horizontal [31, 38]. The coccyx is usually four vertebrae, with the first being larger and having cornua.

Arthrology

Movements of the functional unit of the spine include flexion, extension, side bending, and rotation. The zygapophyseal joints limit motion depending on their orientation and

Fig. 22.5 Thoracic vertebrae (Reprinted from Mathis et al. [33])

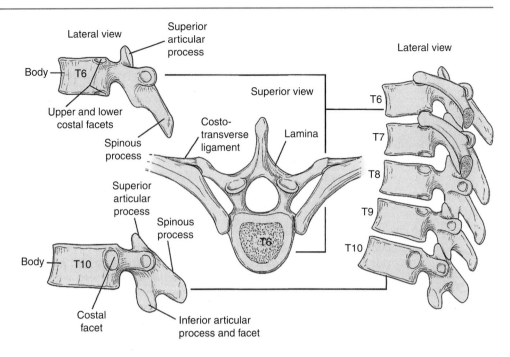

Fig. 22.6 Lumbar vertebrae (Reprinted from Mathis et al. [33])

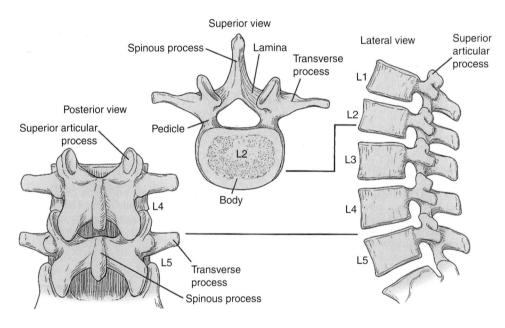

function to protect the intervertebral discs from rotational and translational strains [36]. The cervical spine has the greatest mobility. The thoracic spine is limited by the rib cage, as well as long, overlapping spinous processes. The lumbar spine is a relatively mobile section between the less mobile thoracic and sacral sections of the spine.

A facet joint is a diarthrodial joint formed from the *superior* articular process of the more *caudal* vertebra and the *inferior* articular process of the more *cephalad* vertebra. The facet joint capsule exists at the dorsal, superior, and inferior

margins and consists of the ligamentum flavum itself anteriorly [31]. The superior and inferior aspects of the joint capsule have loose pockets, subcapsular recesses that contain fat. Facet joints contain hyaline cartilage and *meniscoid* structures: fibroadipose meniscoids, adipose tissue pads, and connective tissue rims [17, 31, 39].

Facet joints have been known to cause pain since Goldwaithe's report in 1911 [40]. Ghormley coined the term "facet syndrome" to describe lumbosacral pain in 1933. Mooney and Robertson demonstrated referred pain from

Fig. 22.7 Sacrum (Reprinted from Mathis et al. [33])

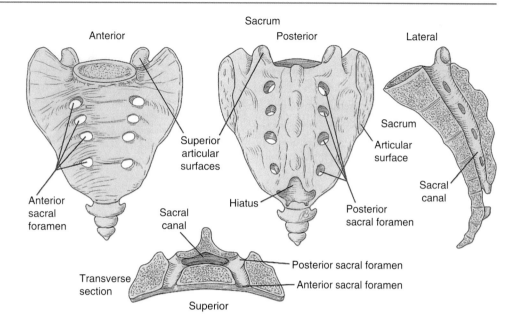

Fig. 22.8 Sacroiliac joint (Reprinted from Mathis et al. [33])

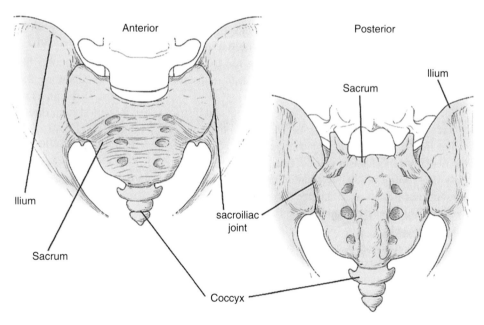

facet joints [41]. Lumbar facet joints bear about 20 % of the axial load and 40 % of the torsional and shear strength (as a pair). Recalling the tripod model, if the intervertebral disc is degenerated, the facets may bear up to 70 % of the axial load in that segment. They also bear more axial load with increased lumbar lordosis [27, 42]. Cervical and thoracic facet joints are also pain generators.

The sacroiliac joints consist of a C-shaped synovial portion and a syndesmosis portion (Fig. 22.8). The articular surface of the ilium is fibrocartilage, while the sacrum is hyaline cartilage that is much thicker [43]. Normal motion is slight, 2–3° in the transverse or longitudinal planes. *Nutation* (nod-

ding) is the rotation of the sacrum that causes forward tilting in relation to the ilium. *Counternutation* is the opposite movement, where the sacrum tilts posteriorly in relation to the ilium [27]. The sacroiliac joints can also be a source of pain.

Brief mention is warranted that other spine joints are sometimes considered pain generators: atlantooccipital, atlantoaxial, uncovertebral, costotransverse, and costovertebral, have all been described as sources of pain. A transitional lumbosacral junction may have an *assimilation joint*, wherein a large L5 transverse process articulates with the sacrum. A pars defect may form a pseudoarthrosis that can be painful.

Intervertebral Disc: A Special Joint

Mixter and Barr, respectively, from the neurosurgery and orthopedic surgery services of Massachusetts General Hospital, are often cited as the first to recognize the importance of intervertebral disc herniations, although Mixter and Barr themselves cite several prior reports [44]. Although the intervertebral disc has been compared to a diarthrodial joint, it is correctly classified as a symphysis, a major cartilaginous synarthrosis [45]. Adjacent vertebral levels are separated by an intervertebral disc (except at C0–C1 and C1–C2). The functions of the disc are to distribute force and allow movement between adjacent vertebral bodies and to hold the vertebral bodies together. The discs also comprise 20–25 % of the total length of the spine, separating the vertebrae, allowing nerve roots and vessels to travel between vertebrae [27].

The intervertebral disc is the largest avascular structure in the body [46]. Each disc contains superior and inferior cartilaginous end plates, anulus fibrosus, and nucleus pulposus. Nucleus pulposus is 70–90 % water, variable with age, and proteoglycans are the majority of the remainder. Type II collagen fibers join with proteoglycans, forming the matrix of the nucleus. Embedded in the proteoglycans, toward the end plate regions, are chondrocytes that synthesize the substance of the nucleus.

The nucleus pulposus functions to bear weight and distribute forces across vertebral segments. The healthy nucleus distributes load very evenly, in a manner as a fluid, according to Pascal's law, a mechanism that dissipates force and prevents injury [32]. With age, the glycosaminoglycan and water content of the nucleus decrease, and the fibrocartilaginous content increases. This transfers load bearing to the anulus and other structures.

The anulus fibrosus is the external ring of the disc and is formed by 10–20 sheets of parallel collagen fibers (lamellae), each sheet having fibers oriented in alternating directions 30–70° from vertical. The anulus is mostly water (60 %). Collagen is half of the remaining portion. The anulus can be divided into three zones: the outer zone is made of fibrocartilaginous Sharpey's fibers that attach to the vertebral body. The intermediate and inner zones are also fibrocartilage, but do not attach to the vertebral body. The posterolateral fibers of the lumbar anulus are most prone to injury and degeneration. While the posterocentral disc may be protected by attachments of posterior longitudinal ligament, there are no extrinsic ligament attachments to support the posterolateral disc [47]. The lumbar posterior anulus is thinner radially due to the eccentric location of the nucleus. It is also longitudinally thinner, due to the lordotic curve of the lumbar spine, which means that a given amount of displacement causes relatively greater strain on these shorter fibers.

Vertebral end plates are cartilaginous structures at the superior and inferior aspect of each vertebral body, between the

Table 22.5 Human studies on sensory innervation of intervertebral disc

Reference	Finding
Roofe [49]	Nerve fibers in disc and adjacent PLL
Malinsky [50]	Nerve endings in lateral outer 1/3 of annulus, encapsulated and non-encapsulated
Rabischong et al. [51]	Confirmed above
Yoshizawa et al. [52]	Confirmed above
	Also reported morphology similar to other known nociceptors
Bogduk [53]	Confirmed above
Palmgren et al. [54], Ashton et al. [55]	Immunohistochemical studies demonstrating sensory and autonomic fibers in the annulus

body and the disc. They are firmly attached to the disc by the collagenous fibers of the lamellae (intermediate and inner zones), which invest the fibrocartilaginous side of the end plate. Blood vessels on the surface of the vertebral bodies contact the hyaline side of the end plate, and nutrients diffuse through the end plate to the disc, a process of *imbibition* [48].

Several studies have confirmed nerve fibers in the outer portions of the anulus fibrosus, especially the posterolateral disc, likely rendering the disc capable of becoming a pain generator. Disc innervation may arise from sinuvertebral nerve, ventral rami direct branches, and rami communicans (Table 22.5) [17, 49–52, 54–57].

Pressure within the disc is affected by body position. The natural lordotic posture of the lumbar spine reduces vertical pressure on the disc. Direct vertical pressure increases fluid pressure within the disc. This can even lead to herniation of nucleus pulposus through defects in the end plate, known as Schmorl's nodes [first observed by Luschka [31]]. Fluid shifts in the disc also account for the 1–2 cm decrease in height that can be observed after a day of upright posture compared to the morning [58]. Disc pressure when standing is only 35 % of pressure when seated, while lifting greatly increases disc pressure and can be estimated at ten times the weight of the object lifted, as demonstrated in Nachemson's classic study [59].

Disc herniations can be classified as *protrusion, extrusion,* or *sequestration.* A protrusion has a base wider than the greatest extent of herniation (Fig. 22.9). Nucleus material extends into the epidural space in an extrusion, and the extent of herniation may exceed the width of the base (Fig. 22.10). In a sequestration, the nucleus material has been extruded as a fragment into the epidural space and has lost continuity with the disc. For further standardized terminology for description of location and type of disc herniations, the reader is referred to "Nomenclature and Classification of Lumbar Disc Pathology. Recommendations of the Combined Task Forces of the North American Spine Society, American Society of Spine Radiology, and American Society of Neuroradiology [47]."

Ligaments of the Spine

Ligaments of the spine are detailed in Tables 22.6, 22.7, and 22.8 [17, 32]. Of great practical interest to the pain physician is the ligamentum flavum, a paired structure, running from lumbar to cervical spine, composed of highly elastic fibers. There may be a narrow gap between the right and left halves [36]. It forms the posterior boundary of the epidural space as approached between vertebral lamina and may contribute to the boundary in the intervertebral foramen. On right and left, a ligamentum flavum attaches from the superior vertebral level to the adjacent level below. Laterally, fibers of ligamentum attach to the facet articular processes and form part of the joint capsule. Lateral fibers may attach to the pedicle. The lateral fibers of ligamentum contribute to the posterior boundary of the intervertebral foramen. In the lumbar spine, ligamentum flavum may be the strongest and most elastic of spinal ligaments and resists distraction and flexion. In the lumbar spine,

ligamentum flavum can be 2–3 mm thick [36]. The elasticity is important to prevent buckling of the ligament, which can compress neural structures. Buckling can occur if there is loss of intervertebral disc height. However, the ligamentum flavum is less robust in the cervical and upper thoracic spine, and its paper thinness and midline absence may affect cervical or thoracic interlaminar injections [60]. The interspinous and supraspinous ligaments are relatively weak and are often the first to be sprained [31, 61]. The iliolumbar ligament is a complex structure that begins as a muscle and becomes a ligament in the third decade and is only present in adults [31, 62].

The "false ligaments" are variably present and function more like membranes and may be encountered during injection procedures. In particular, the aforementioned mamilloaccessory ligament forms a foramen containing the medial branch nerve and is ossified in 10 % of cases [31, 53].

Muscles of the Spine

True back muscles are comprised of four groups of extensors, innervated by posterior rami (Table 22.9). In contrast, *appendicular* or limb muscles are also located in the back, more superficially. True back muscles are dorsal, deep to thoracolumbar fascia, multilayered, and redundant, with numerous attachments, whereas ventral muscles that flex the spine may effectively cross many vertebral levels with few direct attachments [32, 46]. For example, abdominal muscles are primary forward flexors (rectus abdominis, internal and external obliques). Psoas and iliacus are weak flexors of the spine and primarily flex the hip. The quadratus lumborum is considered a posterior abdominal muscle [63]. It does act as a lateral lumbar flexor, attaching to the transverse processes [64]. Also of interest are the suboccipital muscles, including

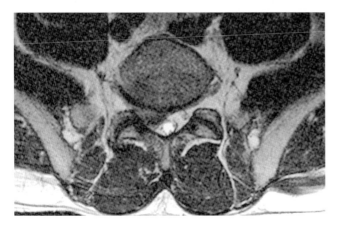

Fig. 22.9 Lumbar disc protrusion, rightward at L5–S1

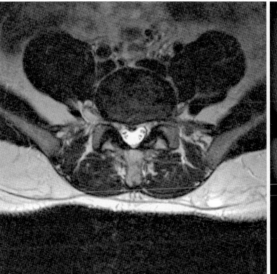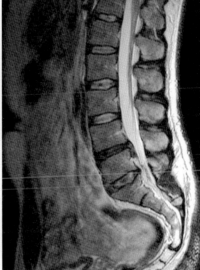

Fig. 22.10 Lumbar disc extrusion, central at L4–L5 with caudal subligamentous migration

Table 22.6 The ligaments of the spine

Ligament	Attachments	Function	Comments
Anterior longitudinal ligament	Cervical to sacral	Counters extension Stabilizes lordosis Restricts listhesis	Lumbar is most developed
Posterior longitudinal ligament	Cranium to sacrum	Resists flexion Reinforces posteromedial disc	Becomes tectorial ligament in cranium Can become ossified and cause stenosis
Ligamentum flavum	Cervical to lumbar Bifid	Resists distraction and flexion	See text
Interspinous	Adjacent spinous processes	Resists distraction and flexion	Lumbar is most developed Cervical may be absent
Supraspinous	Runs dorsally over spinous processes Terminates inferiorly at L4 in 73 %, L3 in 22 %, L5 in 5 %, is rarely at L5–S1	Resists distraction and flexion	
Iliolumbar	See separate table		
False ligaments	See separate table		

Table 22.7 The iliolumbar ligament

Portion	Origin	Insertion
Anterior	Anteroinferior border and tip of L5 transverse process	Ilium
Superior	Thickening of anterior and posterior quadratus lumborum fascia and anterosuperior L5 transverse process	Ilium
Posterior	Tip and posterior L5 transverse process	Ilium
Inferior	Lower L5 transverse process and L5 body	Superior and posterior iliac fossa
Vertical	Anteroinferior border of L5 transverse process	Iliopectineal line

Table 22.8 The false ligaments of the spine

Ligament	Attachments	Function	Comments
Intertransverse	Span adjacent pedicles	"Membranes"	Continue as middle layer of thoracodorsal fascia
Transforaminal	Variable	"Membranes"	May crowd spinal nerve
Mamilloaccessory	Mamillary and accessory processes	See text	See text

Table 22.9 True back muscles

Superficial to deep:	Individual muscles
Spinotransversales:	Splenius capitis
	Splenius cervicis
Erector spinae:	Iliocostalis
	Longissimus
	Spinalis
Transversospinal:	Semispinalis
	Multifidus
	Rotatores
Intersegmental:	Interspinalis
	Intertransversarius

Thoracolumbar Fascia

The anterior layer originates from anterior lumbar transverse processes and covers the quadratus lumborum. The middle layer originates from far lateral (tip) transverse processes, and the posterior layer arises from the midline. The posterior layer is an attachment site for latissimus dorsi and serratus posterior inferior. The thoracolumbar fascia layers join at the lateral border of erector spinae, where they become continuous with abdominal muscles (transversus abdominis and internal oblique). The posterior layer consists of deep fibers oriented caudo-laterally from the spinous processes and superficial fibers oriented rosto-laterally. This fiber arrangement, and continuity with abdominal muscles, allows abdominal muscle contraction to exert a force that resists spine flexion. The deep lamina of the posterior layer also functions as a series of accessory ligaments attaching the lumbar vertebrae to the ilium [65].

rectus capitis posterior minor and the suboccipital triangle formed by rectus capitis posterior major and obliquus capitis superior and inferior. For a complete description of specific pain referral patterns from individual muscles, the reader is referred to *Travell & Simons' Myofascial Pain and Dysfunction: The Trigger Point Manual* [22].

Spinal Canal and Foramina

The vertebral foramina are bounded by bone, including joints and ligaments. The superior boundary of the foramen is the inferior vertebral notch of the pedicle of the superior vertebra and part of the lateral-most ligamentum flavum. The inferior boundary is the superior vertebral notch of the pedicle of the inferior vertebral body. The anterior boundary includes the adjacent posterolateral vertebral bodies, that is, the inferior posterolateral part of the superior vertebral body and the superior posterolateral part of the inferior vertebral body, as well as the intervertebral disc. The anterior boundary also includes the lateral posterior longitudinal ligament and the anterior venous sinus. The posterior boundary is the pars interarticularis superiorly and facet joint inferiorly, as well as lateral ligamentum flavum. Therefore, two articulations form the boundaries of the foramen, the facet joint and the intervertebral body joint or disc; these allow the oval shape of the foramen to change with movement. The height of the disc also directly influences the size of the foramen. Proximally or medially, the foramen is bounded by dura. Especially in the lumbar spine, the foramen can be divided into three zones: the lateral recess, midzone, and exit zone [66]. The lateral recess contains the spinal nerve root that is descending to exit the next level.

In the lumbar spine, the intervertebral disc is located in the lower part of the anterior wall of the neural foramen. This is also true in the thoracic spine. However, in the cervical spine, the disc is in the middle of the anterior wall of the foramen. This relationship partly also determines which nerve is affected by disc herniations [32]. For example, a typical posterolateral disc herniation at L5–S1 will usually spare the L5 nerve root and is more likely to affect the most laterally placed nerve root in the spinal canal, which would be S1. In contrast, a C5–C6 herniation is likely to impact the exiting root, C6.

Nerve Supply to the Pain-Sensing Structures of the Spine

As the spinal nerve exits the neural foramen, it immediately divides into dorsal and ventral rami. Dorsal rami divide into medial, intermediate, and lateral branches. An exception is the L5 dorsal ramus which only divides into medial and intermediate branches. The typical medial branch nerve provides sensory innervation to two facet joints: (1) the inferior facet joint capsule that forms the posterior wall of its exiting foramen as well as (2) the superior facet joint at the next lower level. Thus, medial branch nerves are targets for treating pain from facet joints.

Table 22.10 Dorsal rami branches of lumbar spinal nerves

Lumbar dorsal rami of spinal nerve	Supplies motor innervation	Supplies sensory innervation
Medial branch	Multifidus muscle	Interspinous ligament
	Interspinalis muscle	Facet joints above and below
Intermediate branch L1–L4 only	Longissimus muscle	None
Lateral branch	Iliocostalis muscle	L1–L3: skin from iliac crest to greater trochanter

Medial branch nerve location is fairly consistent in relation to bony landmarks, which aids in targeting these nerves under fluoroscopic guidance. Medial branches of C3–C6 run across the center of the respective articular pillars, and C7 is high on the C7 superior articular process. The third occipital nerve alone innervates C2–C3 and runs directly across this joint, embedded in pericapsular fascia. Medial branches of T1–T3 and T9–T10 pass along the superolateral tip of the transverse process. Medial branches of T4–T8 pass posteriorly through the intertransverse space without contacting bone. Medial branch of T11 runs along the superior articular process of T12, and T12 medial branch follows the pattern of L1–L4. The lumbar medial branches of L1–L4 travel across the junction of the superior articular process and transverse process, then curve inferiorly and pass under the mamilloaccessory ligaments. The medial branch of L5 innervates the L5–S1 facet before it innervates the multifidus muscle. Lateral branches of dorsal rami supply longissimus, iliocostalis, and semispinalis muscles, as well as the skin over the medial two-thirds of the lumbosacral region (Table 22.10) [67].

The ventral ramus of the spinal nerve also gives rise to a somatic branch. The sympathetic trunk gives rise to the gray rami communicans. These join to form the sinuvertebral nerve, just outside the intervertebral foramen (recurrent meningeal nerve of Luschka). The sinuvertebral nerve courses medially into the foramen, dorsal to the posterior longitudinal ligament, where it sends ascending and descending branches to form a posterior plexus, providing innervation to structures adjacent to the spinal canal. These include the posterior longitudinal ligament, posterolateral disc (anulus fibrosus), ligamentum flavum, vertebral periosteum, dura, epidural fat, and local blood vessels.

An anterior nerve plexus also exists within the spinal canal, on the ventral aspect of the dura mater. It is formed by meningeal branches directly from the sinuvertebral nerve, branches from the posterior plexus, and perivascular branches. The ventral dura mater has nociceptive and autonomic innervation, whereas the posterolateral dura has little innervation. The dura has not been established as a typical pain generator [56]. A plexus of nerves is also formed along the anterior longitudinal ligament, from gray rami communicantes. These innervate the anterolateral vertebral bodies and discs. However, most of this innervation consists of autonomic fibers, and these structures have not been established as typical pain generators [56].

Spinal Cord, Nerve Roots, Ganglia

The conus medullaris is the terminal portion of the spinal cord. In the adult, this terminal portion is typically at L1–L2. In the lumbar spine, the lumbar and sacral nerve roots form the cauda equina, an intrathecal structure. Dura and arachnoid form the epineurium of the spinal nerve as the nerve exits the foramen.

The spinal nerve proper exists only within the intervertebral foramen, where it is formed as dorsal and ventral roots from the spinal cord converge. The dorsal roots contain sensory afferent fibers. The dorsal root ganglion containing the cell bodies of these fibers lies within the upper medial intervertebral foramen. The ventral roots contain efferent motor and a few sensory fibers. The ventral roots of T1–L2 contain preganglionic sympathetic efferent fibers. The dorsal and ventral roots leave the thecal sac one level superior to their foraminal exit level, and they travel in the radicular canal, within an extension of dural sheath. This dural sheath is attached by fibrous bands near its origin to the periosteum of the pedicle under which the nerve will exit. The nerve roots pass through the lateral recess of the foramen, formed by an osseous groove in the base of the pedicle. Just distal to the dorsal root ganglion, within the neural foramen, the dorsal and ventral roots merge to form the spinal nerve. A fibrous band anchors the spinal nerve to the superior and inferior pedicle as it exits the foramen. As the spinal nerve exits the neural foramen, it immediately divides into dorsal and ventral rami.

Vascular Structures of the Spine

Of particular interest are the blood vessels that can be encountered during interventional spine procedures. The vertebral artery, deep cervical, and ascending cervical arteries can be injured with devastating result in the cervical transforaminal approach [68–70]. Other chapters describe atlantooccipital and atlantoaxial injections, which can also lead to vertebral artery injury. The spinal segmental arteries travel proximally along the path of the spinal nerve, into the foramen, to supply the spinal cord. The presence of spinal segmental arteries is variable. A large conjoined spinal segmental artery, the artery of Adamkiewicz, may enter any level from T7 to L4, but in 80 %, it enters on the left between T9 and L1 [71]. A more recent study of 120 radiculomedullary arteries revealed all between T2 and L3, with 98 %

between T8 and L1, and 83 % on the left side, and often in the superior aspect of the foramen [72]. Spinal cord injury related to vascular insult is known to have occurred as low as S1 [73]. Vascular uptake has been reported in cervical interlaminar injections [74].

Spinal Cord Topology

The spinal cord is the conduit of pain of all types, so brief mention is made here of spinal cord topology. Other chapters will have more about receptor targets in the spinal cord. Targeting the spinal cord with treatment modalities can treat many types of pain, such as acute pain of labor, to the more chronic neuropathic and sympathetic pain syndromes. Melzack and Wall described the dorsal horn as the gate through which pain signals pass [75]. For example, spinal cord stimulation may work by stimulation of these dorsal columns, resulting in reduced activity of wide dynamic range neurons [76, 77]. Other chapters will describe spinal cord stimulation in more detail.

Spine Imaging

Choice of spine imaging involves consideration of several questions. How will information provided by imaging affect clinical decision making? What structure(s) needs to be visualized? Are there adverse effects or contraindications associated with obtaining the imaging? Are there "red flags" of a potential, more ominous condition, which might prompt more aggressive investigation? (Table 22.4) Described below are the most common imaging modalities encountered in the pain clinic, that is, X-rays, CT, MRI, and bone scans. The figures illustrate "fairly unremarkable" CT and MRI of the cervical and lumbar regions (Figs. 22.11, 22.12, and 22.13). Finally, several figures are used to illustrate important pain-related spine disorders (Figs. 22.14, 22.15, and 22.16). Other chapters will describe imaging modalities including fluoroscopy, provocative discography, and epiduroscopy. Relative sensitivities and specificities of patient history, X-ray, CT, and MRI are compared for spine conditions in Table 22.11 [79].

Radiographs, X-Rays

In patients with red flags suggestive of fracture, radiographs may be an acceptable, inexpensive initial choice. Fracture acuity typically cannot be judged by radiographs alone. Facet, sacroiliac, and intervertebral disc (disc space height and end plate changes) degenerative changes can be seen. Flexion-extension views may demonstrate instability at a

Fig. 22.11 Cervical CT and MRI. These images are relatively unremarkable studies from the same subject, comparing the appearance of the same structure on both CT and T2 MRI

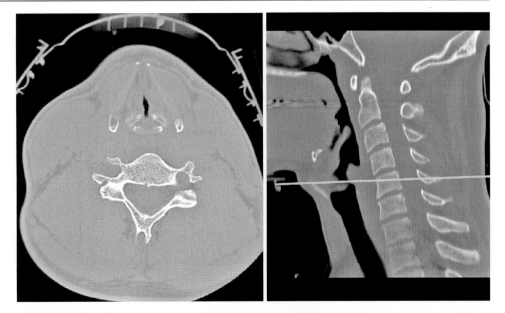

Fig. 22.12 Cervical CT and MRI. These images are relatively unremarkable studies from the same subject, comparing the appearance of the same structure on both CT and T2 MRI

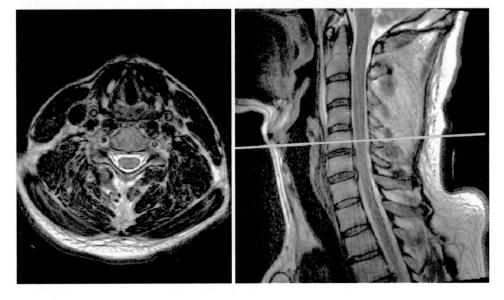

Fig. 22.13 Lumbar MRI. This unremarkable T2 MRI reveals normal disc hydration and height and no herniations or facet degeneration

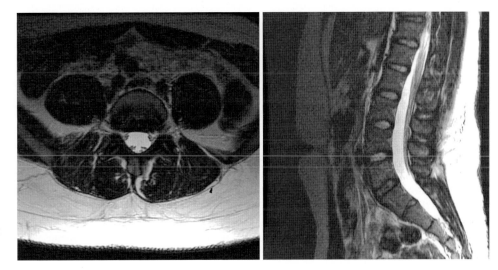

Fig. 22.14 Stenosis: L4–L5 disc degeneration, facet hypertrophy, ligamentum flavum hypertrophy, and central stenosis. There is also grade I anterolisthesis of L5 on S1

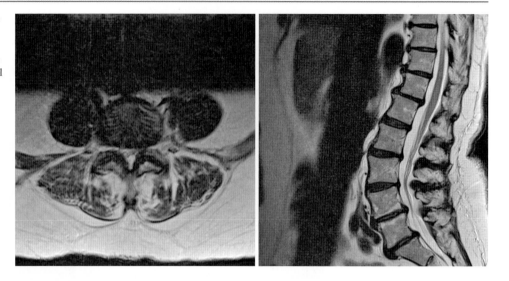

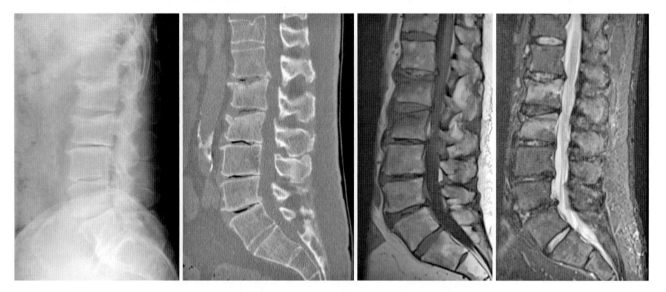

Fig. 22.15 Vertebral compression fractures. The same L1 and L2 compression fractures are seen on radiograph, CT, T1 MRI, and STIR MRI

Fig. 22.16 Osteomyelitis. T1 MRI with gadolinium contrast shows bright enhancement in L1, L2 and disc, with destruction of end plates, in a patient with osteomyelitis (Reprinted from Yang et al. [78])

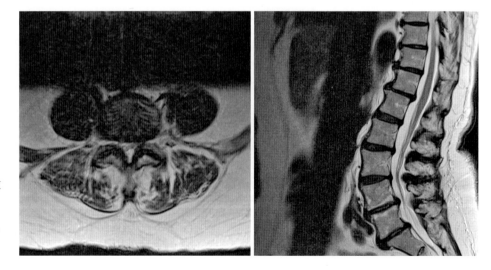

Table 22.11 Comparison of history, exam, radiography, CT, and MRI

Condition	History sensitivity/specificity	Radiograph sensitivity/specificity	CT sensitivity/specificity	MRI sensitivity/specificity
Cancer	No relief with bed rest >0.90, 0.46	0.60, 0.95–0.995		0.83–0.93, 0.90–0.97
Osteomyelitis	IVDA or infection 0.40, NA	0.82, 0.57		0.96, 0.92
Compression fracture	Age 50 or more 0.84, 0.61			
Herniated disc	Sciatica 0.95, 0.98		0.62–0.90, 0.70–0.87	0.6–1.0, 0.43–0.97
Stenosis	Age >65 0.77, 0.69		0.90, 0.80–0.96	0.9, 0.72–1.0

Modified from Jarvik and Deyo [79]

segment with listhesis. Pars defects may be seen readily on lateral and oblique views. Oblique views may also demonstrate encroachment of nerve pathways. Radiographs are often used to assess spinal curvatures. Radiographs demonstrate radiopaque implants such as fusion devices or spinal cord stimulators. Radiographs do carry risk of general and gonadal radiation exposure.

Computed Tomography

Computed tomography, or CT, uses X-rays to obtain images and is a superior modality when compared to MRI for observing bony cortex and trabeculae, but CT can also be used for soft tissue. For example, pre-procedure planning for kyphoplasty often includes CT to look for any fractures in the relatively anhydrous bony cortex, not visualized on MRI. CT can be a good imaging modality for patients with ferromagnetic implants that are not compatible with MRI. Modern helical multislice acquisition CT is very fast and thus does not require prolonged immobilization. Such CT acquisitions can be reconstructed to give images in multiple planes. Claustrophobia or morbid obesity is not typically problems preventing CT. Risks involve exposure to radiation (and may involve exposure to contrast, if used to detect abscess or tumor).

CT Myelography

Myelography carries risk as it is an invasive procedure involving lumbar puncture and injection of contrast, in addition to radiation exposure. Diagnosis is made by observing disruption of the contrast flow pattern. Therefore, the study does not give specific information about the cause of contrast flow alteration. Myelography may not visualize the lateral recesses. It may be useful in assessing the postoperative spine with metallic implants. CT myelogram outlines the cervical foramina with better resolution than MRI.

Magnetic Resonance Imaging

For most painful spine disorders, MRI is the best imaging modality to view soft tissue, discs, marrow, and nerves. MRI detects inflammation and edema and thus can detect acuity of spinal fractures. In MRI, the subject is placed in a very strong magnetic field, thereby aligning protons (hydrogen nuclei). The subject is then bombarded with various radio pulse sequences, and resonance of the hydrogen nuclei creates images. MRI "sees" proton density, which is essentially the amount of water in tissue. There are numerous types of sequence variations such as T1, T2, STIR (short tau inversion recovery), and various fat suppression techniques. Gadolinium contrast is bright on T1 images. The reader is directed to the ACR publication on contrast agents for more about the increasingly understood systemic risks of MRI contrast in the setting of renal disease (such as nephrogenic systemic fibrosis) [80]. There are no known risks from the MRI mechanism itself. MRI is contraindicated with certain metallic implants such as aneurysm clips or foreign bodies in the orbit. Claustrophobia is a common concern with MRI. Bony cortex does not show well on MRI.

Bone Scans, Scintigraphy, SPECT

This test involves injection of a radioactive substance such as Tc-methylene diphosphonate. Whole-body imaging is then performed via radiation detection. This method is useful in surveying the whole body for metabolically abnormal areas of skeleton. It has poor resolution and abnormal findings are nonspecific. The test takes many hours.

SPECT is a combined CT with single positron emission (SPE) tomography. The term "bone scan" is sometimes used to refer to SPECT. This modality increases the sensitivity and anatomic localization of spine and skeletal lesions. SPECT may have an increasing role in the imaging of spondylolysis [81].

Future Directions

Discogram

Discography, always controversial, is falling out of favor again, as it is well understood that confounds make this a flawed test, and risks, including now-established long-term risk of accelerated disc degeneration, are great compared with potential benefits [82]. Other chapters will provide more detail on discography.

Bone Mineral Density

Pain physicians are often medical spine experts and may be in the best position to initiate investigation and management of osteoporosis, the most common bone disease. In our facility, patients are screened, if not previously done, if a spine fracture is found or if they meet criteria established by the National Osteoporosis Foundation [83].

Ultrasound

Interest in ultrasound for intervention and diagnosis of musculoskeletal and pain conditions has exploded in the last few years [84, 85]. However, let us not forget so soon the widespread advocacy and abuse of diagnostic spine ultrasound in the 1990s [86, 87]. A prospective study found that paraspinal ultrasound is not accurate or reproducible in evaluating patients with cervical and lumbar back pain [87]. Several ultrasound-guided spine interventions have been described, including medial branch blocks, third occipital nerve blocks, and cervical epidural injections [88–92].

Conclusion

Forasmuch as we have previously set down almost everything which concerns the lumbar vertebrae and have no wish to prolong the description of them unnecessarily, we shall offer a brief summary…. Vesalius [93]

The spine holds great significance in the human experience, as a foundation for movement and strength, as a leading cause of suffering, and as an eternal symbol of each. This chapter has introduced concepts of spine anatomy and imaging. To gain an even more advanced understanding of functional anatomy, the reader is urged to refer to the cited literature and to explore the embryological development of the spine, as well as gain awareness of *kinesiology*, the all-encompassing study of human movement; *kinetics*, the study of the forces involved in the movements of the body; and *kinematics*, the study of the positions and motions of body structures [94, 95]. Through this knowledge, pain physicians become the doctors of the spine, best suited to understand and apply information from advanced imaging. One day, there may be an imaging test for pain itself, and doctors then will look back at our RF with amusement, much as we recall the hot poker of Hippocrates. If they still be physicians, they will remember: *primum non nocere*.

References

1. Borenstein D. Epidemiology, etiology, diagnostic evaluation, and treatment of low back pain. Curr Opin Rheumatol. 2001;13(2):128–34.
2. Rubin D. Epidemiology and risk factors for spine pain. Neurol Clin. 2007;25(2):353–71.
3. Hart L, Deyo R, Cherkin D. Physician office visits for low back pain: frequency, clinical evaluation, and treatment pattern from a US national survey. Spine. 1995;20(1):11–9.
4. Pai S, Sundaram L. Low back pain: an economic assessment in the United States. Orthop Clin North Am. 2004;35(1):1.
5. Boden S, et al. Abnormal magnetic-resonance scans of the lumbar spine in asymptomatic subjects. A prospective investigation. J Bone Joint Surg. 1990;72(3):403–8.
6. Martin B, et al. Expenditures and health status among adults with back and neck problems. JAMA. 2008;299(6):656–64.
7. Davis P, et al. Expert panel on neurologic imaging. ACR appropriateness criteria low back pain. 2008.
8. Daffner R, et al. Expert panel on musculoskeletal imaging. ACR appropriateness criteria chronic neck pain. 2010.
9. Naderi S, Andalkar N, Benzel E. History of spine biomechanics: part I–the pre-Greco-Roman, Greco-Roman, and medieval roots of spine biomechanics. Neurosurgery. 2007;60(2):382–90.
10. Marketos S, Skiadas P. Galen: a pioneer of spine research. Spine. 1999;24(22):2358.
11. Sanan A, Rengachary S. The history of spinal biomechanics. Neurosurgery. 1996;39(4):657–69.
12. Benini A, Bonar S. Andreas vesalius: 1514-1564. Spine. 1996;21(11):1388–93.
13. Naderi S, et al. Functional anatomy of the spine by Avicenna in his eleventh century treatise Al-Qanun fi al-Tibb (the canons of medicine). Neurosurgery. 2003;52(6):1449–53.
14. Naderi S, Andalkar N, Benzel E. History of spine biomechanics: part II–from the renaissance to the 20th century. Neurosurgery. 2007;60(2):392–403.
15. Spiegel P. The first clinical x ray made in America. AJR Am J Roentgenol. 1995;164:241–3.
16. Hesselink J. Spine imaging: history, achievements. Remaining frontiers. AJR. 1988;150:1223–9.
17. Bogduk N. Clinical anatomy of the lumbar spine and sacrum. 4th ed. Philadelphia: Elsevier Churchill Livingstone; 2005.
18. Backonja M. Defining neuropathic pain. Anesth Analg. 2003;97(3):785–90.
19. Mekhail N, et al. Clinical applications of neurostimulation: forty years later. Pain Pract. 2010;10(2):103–12.
20. Wyke B. The neurological basis of thoracic spinal pain. Rheumatol Phys Med. 1970;10:356–67.
21. Merskey H, Bogduk N, editors. Classification of chronic pain: descriptions of chronic pain syndromes and definitions of pain terms. Seattle: IASP Press; 1994.
22. Simons D, Travell J, Simons L. Travell & Simons' myofascial pain and dysfunction: the trigger point manual, vol. 2. Baltimore: Lippincott Williams & Wilkins; 1999.

23. Slipman C, et al. Symptom provocation of fluoroscopically guided cervical nerve root stimulation. Are dynatomal maps identical to dermatomal maps? Spine. 1998;23(20):2235–42.

24. Slipman C, et al. Clinical evidence of chemical radiculopathy. Pain Physician. 2002;5(3):260–5.

25. Huston C, Slipman C. Diagnostic selective nerve root blocks: indications and usefulness. Phys Med Rehabil Clin N Am. 2002;13:545–65.

26. Mathis J, editor. Image-guided spine interventions. New York, Berlin, Heidelberg: Springer; 2004.

27. Magee D. Orthopedic physical assessment. 4th ed. Philadelphia: Saunders; 2002.

28. White A, Panjabi M. Clinical biomechanics of the spine. Philadelphia: Lippincott; 1978.

29. Maigne R, Liberson W. Orthopedic medicine: a new approach to vertebral manipulations. Springfield: Charles C. Thomas; 1972.

30. Junghanns H. Der lumbosacralwinkel. Dtsch Z Chir. 1929;213:332.

31. Oliver J, Middleditch A. Functional anatomy of the spine. Oxford: Butterworth-Heinmann Ltd; 1991.

32. Schneck C. Functional and clinical anatomy of the spine. SPINE. 1995;9(3):525–58.

33. Mathis J, Deramond H, Belkoff S, editors. Percutaneous vertebroplasty and kyphoplasty. 2nd ed. New York: Springer; 2006.

34. Gilad I, Nisan M. Sagittal evaluation of elemental geometrical dimensions of human vertebrae. J Anat. 1985;143:115.

35. Schmorl G, Junghanns H. The human spine in health and disease. New York: Grune & Stratton; 1959.

36. Twomey L, Taylor J. Physical therapy of the low back. 2nd ed. Edinburgh: Churchill Livingstone; 1994.

37. Davis P. Human lower lumbar vertebrae: some mechanical and osteological considerations. J Anat. 1961;95:337–44.

38. Hellems H, Keates T. Measurement of the normal lumbosacral angle. Am J Roentgenol. 1971;113:642.

39. Bogduk N. The menisci of the lumbar zygapophyseal joints: a review of their anatomy and clinical significance. Spine. 1984;9(5):454–60.

40. Goldwaithe J. The lumbo-sacral articulation: an explanation of any cases of lumbago, sciatica and paraplegia. Boston Med Surg J. 1911;164:365–72.

41. Mooney V, Robertson J. The facet syndrome. Clin Orthop. 1976;115:149–56.

42. Yang K, King A. Mechanism of facet load transmission as a hypothesis for low-back pain. Spine. 1984;9(6):557–65.

43. Foley B, Buschbacher R. Sacroiliac joint pain: anatomy, biomechanics, diagnosis and treatment. Am J Phys Med Rehabil. 2006;85:997–1006.

44. Mixter W, Barr J. Rupture of the intervertebral disc with involvement of the spinal canal. N Engl J Med. 1934;211:210.

45. Grignon B, Roland J. Can the human intervertebral disc be compared to a diarthrodial joint? Surg Radiol Anat. 2000;22(2):101–5.

46. Mow V, Huiskes R. Basic orthpaedic biomechanics and mechanobiology. 3rd ed. Philadelphia: Lippincott Williams & Wilkins; 2005.

47. Fardon D, Milette P. Nomenclature and classification of lumbar disc pathology. Recommendations of the combined task forces of the North American Spine Society, American Society of Spine Radiology, and American Society of Neuroradiology. Spine. 2001;26(5):E93–113.

48. Benneker L, et al. 2004 Young investigator award winner: vertebral endplate marrow contact channel occlusions and intervertebral disc degeneration. Spine. 2005;30(2):167–73.

49. Roofe P. Innervation of anulus fibrosus and posterior longitudinal ligament. Arch Neurol Psychiatry. 1940;44:100–3.

50. Malinský J. The ontogenetic development of nerve terminations in the intervertebral discs of man. (Histology of intervertebral discs, 11th communication). Acta Anat. 1959;38:96–113.

51. Rabischong P, et al. The intervertebral disc. Anat Clin. 1978;1:55–64.

52. Yoshizawa H, et al. The neuropathology of intervertebral discs removed for low back pain. J Pathol. 1980;132:95–104.

53. Bogduk N. The lumbar mamillo-accessory ligament: its anatomical and neurosurgical significance. Spine. 1981;6(2):162–7.

54. Palmgren T, et al. An immunohistochemical study of nerve structures in the annulus fibrosus of human normal lumbar intervertebral discs. Spine. 1999;24:2075–9.

55. Ashton I, Roberts S, Jaffray D. Neuropeptides in the human intervertebral disc. J Orthop Res. 1994;12:186–92.

56. Slipman C, et al. Interventional spine: an algorithmic approach. Philadelphia: Saunders Elsevier; 2008.

57. Bogduk N, Tynan W, Wilson A. The nerve supply to the human lumbar intervertebral discs. J Anat. 1981;132:39–56.

58. Ledsome J, et al. Diurnal changes in lumbar intervertebral distance, measured using ultrasound. Spine. 1996;21(14):1671–5.

59. Nachemson A, Moriss J. In vivo measurements of intradiscal pressure: discometry, a method for the determination of pressure in the lower lumbar discs. J Bone Joint Surg. 1964;46:1077–92.

60. Lirk P, et al. Cervical and high thoracic ligamentum flavum frequently fails to fuse in the midline. Anesthesiology. 2003;99(6):1387–90.

61. Adams M, Hutton W, Stott J. The resistance to flexion of the lumbar intervertebral joint. Spine. 1980;5(3):245.

62. Leong J, et al. The biomechanical functions of the iliolumbar ligament in maintaining stability of the lumbosacral junction. Spine. 1987;12:669–74.

63. Windsor R, Falco F. Clinical orientation to spinal anatomy. Atlanta: O2 Communications; 2003.

64. Cailliett R. Low back pain syndrome. Philadelphia: F.A. Davis Company; 1981.

65. Bogduk N, MacIntosh J. The applied anatomy of the thoracolumbar fascia. Spine. 1984;9(2):164–70.

66. Lee C, Rauschning W, Glenn W. Lateral lumbar spinal canal stenosis: classification, pathologic anatomy and surgical decompression. Spine. 1988;13(3):313–20.

67. Bogduk N, editor. Practice guidelines: spinal diagnostic and treatment procedures. San Francisco: International Spine Intervention Society; 2004.

68. Baker R, et al. Cervical transforaminal injection of corticosteroids into a radicular artery: a possible mechanism for spinal cord injury. Pain. 2003;103(1–2):211–5.

69. Scanlon G, et al. Cervical transforaminal epidural steroid injections: more dangerous than we think? Spine. 2007;32(11):1249–56.

70. Huntoon M. Anatomy of the cervical intervertebral foramina: vulnerable arteries and ischemic neurologic injuries after transforaminal epidural injections. Pain. 2005;117(1–2):104–11.

71. Rathmell J. Atlas of image-guided intervention in regional anesthesia and pain medicine. Philadelphia: Lipincott; 2006.

72. Murthy N, Maus T, Behrns C. Intraforaminal location of the great anterior radiculomedullary artery (artery of adamkiewicz): a retrospective review. Pain Med. 2010;11:1756–64.

73. Houten J, Errico T. Paraplegia after lumbosacral nerve root block: report of three cases. Spine J. 2002;2(1):70–5.

74. Kaplan M, Cooke J, Collins J. Intravascular uptake during fluoroscopically guided cervical interlaminar steroid injection at C6-7: a case report. Arch Phys Med Rehabil. 2008;89(6):1206.

75. Melzack R, Wall P. Pain mechanisms: a new theory. Science. 1965;150:971–9.

76. Meyerson B, Linderoth B. Mechanisms of spinal cord stimulation in neuropathic pain. Neurol Res. 2000;22(3):285–92.

77. Prager J. What does the mechanism of spinal cord stimulation tell Us about complex regional pain syndrome? Pain Med. 2010;8(11):1278–83.

78. Yang S, et al. Identifying pathogens of spondylodiscitis: percutaneous endoscopy or CT-guided biopsy. Clin Orthop Relat Res. 2008;466:3086–92.

79. Jarvik J, Deyo R. Diagnostic evaluation of low back pain with emphasis on imaging. Ann Intern Med. 2002;137:586–97.

80. A.C.o.D.a.C. Media, editor. ACR manual on contrast media, Version 7 edn. American College of Radiology; 2010, p. 81.

81. Zukotynski K, et al. The value of SPECT in the detection of stress injury to the pars interarticularis in patients with low back pain. J Orthop Surg Res. 2010;5:13.

82. Carragee E, et al. 2009 ISSLS prize winner: does discography cause accelerated progression of degeneration changes in the lumbar disc: a ten-year matched cohort study. Spine. 2009;34(21):2338–45.

83. National Osteoporosis Foundation. Clinician's guide to prevention and treatment of osteoporosis. Washington D.C.: National Osteoporosis Foundation; 2010. Available at: http://www.nof.org/professionals/clinical-guidelines.

84. Smith J, Finnoff J. Diagnostic and interventional musculoskeletal ultrasound: part 1. Fundamentals. PMR. 2009;1(1):64–75.

85. Smith J, Finnoff J. Diagnostic and interventional musculoskeletal ultrasound: part 2. Clinical applications. PMR. 2009;1(2):162–77.

86. Ultrasound: not effective in diagnosing spinal injuries. ACR Bull, 1996.

87. Nazarian L, et al. Paraspinal ultrasonography: lack of accuracy in evaluating patients with cervical or lumbar back pain. J Ultrasound Med. 1998;17:117–22.

88. Greher M, et al. Ultrasound-guided lumbar facet nerve block. A sonoanatomic study of a new methodologic approach. Anesthesiology. 2004;100:1242–8.

89. Greher M, et al. Ultrasound-guided lumbar facet nerve block. Accuracy of a new technique confirmed by computed tomography. Anesthesiology. 2004;101:1195–200.

90. Shim J, et al. Ultrasound-guided lumbar medial branch block: a clinical study with fluoroscopy control. Reg Anesth Pain Med. 2006;31(5):451–4.

91. Eichenberger U, et al. Sonographic visualization and ultrasound-guided block of the third occipital nerve. Prospective for a new method to diagnose C2–C3 zygapophysial joint pain. Anesthesiology. 2006;104:303–8.

92. Kim S, et al. Sonographic estimation of needle depth for cervical epidural blocks. Anesth Analg. 2008;106(5):1542–7.

93. Vesalius A. On the fabric of the human body. A translation of De Humani Corporis Fabrica Libri Septem. San Francisco: Norman Publishing; 1998.

94. Rothstein J, Serge H, et al. The rehabilitation specialist's handbook. Philadelphia: F.A. Davis Company; 1998.

95. White A, Panjabi M. The basic kinematics of the human spine. A review of past and current knowledge. Spine. 1978;3(1):12–20.

Interventional Approaches: Neural Blockade and Neurolysis Blocks

Asokumar Buvanendran, Sunil J. Panchal, and Philip S. Kim

Introduction

Interventional procedures are covered in three parts:

Part II reviews the anatomy and physiology of pain, as relevant to the practitioner

Part III details neural blockade and neurolysis blocks

Part IV provides guidance to the full range of neuromodulation techniques

As supported by this volume, comprehensive pain care is the optimal method to help patients progress to recovery. Interventional pain procedures are one part of the comprehensive approach. New procedures continue to be developed and established procedures continue to evolve as our understanding of the pathophysiology of pain grows. At the same time, the evidence base for interventional pain procedures is under intense scrutiny. The issue is a familiar one in the realm of interventional treatments. As with other surgical procedures, having a control group in a clinical study of interventions for patients with chronic pain presents significant ethical concerns.

The contributors to these parts and we share the belief that the decision to use a procedure solely on the basis of evidence misses the importance of the context of treatment. By the time a patient seeks out a pain medicine physician, he or she is looking for a practice that provides advanced and novel interventional treatments. The primary care physician has already started the patient on non-surgical approaches such as physical therapy and analgesics, and the interventional procedure acts as a therapeutic bridge between the patient's non-surgical management and psychological coping strategies, often significantly reducing the dose requirements of oral analgesics. From trigger point injections and epidural steroids, to radiofrequency ablation and implantable devices (for spinal cord stimulation, peripheral nerve stimulation, and intraspinal drug delivery), interventional procedures are among the most efficient ways of effecting change in pain reporting.

As the population of patients coping with pain grows older, maintenance on oral analgesics, particularly opioids for chronic non-cancer pain, becomes less of an option due to the development of comorbid medical conditions and the addition of other medications. Interventions for painful conditions, such as vertebral compression fractures, spondylosis, and spinal stenosis, can help older patients with acute pain and provide immediate and temporizing relief.

Given the fast evolutionary pace of technology, we expect that the chapter content in these parts will change significantly when the next edition of the book is published. In this inaugural edition, our aim is to provide you with up-to-the-minute expert guidance and practical tips for the current practice of simple and complex interventions for pain control. Furthermore, we hope to offer you a glimpse into the future, of therapies to come.

Local Anesthetics

Michael S. Leong and B. Todd Sitzman

Key Points
- To describe local anesthetic pharmacology, types (amides, esters), and mechanism of action
- Typical dosages and local anesthetic used in clinical practice
- Common side effects from local anesthetics

Background

Local anesthetics in clinically appropriate concentrations will act on any part of the nervous system and on every type of nerve fiber to block conduction in a reversible manner without damage to nerve fibers or cells. This reversibility of action creates significant utility in diagnostic and therapeutic procedures. Local anesthetics (LAs) may abolish sensation in various parts of the body by topical application, injection in the vicinity of peripheral nerve endings and along major nerve trunks, or instillation within the epidural or subarachnoid space. The ensuing sensory block occurs locally and spreads to areas distal along the nerve pathway (Figs. 23.1 and 23.2).

Local anesthetics are composed of an acyl or aromatic group connected to an alkyl tertiary amine group by either an ester or amide bond. *Classification* into two groups is based on this bond which determines metabolic pathways. For the

M.S. Leong, M.D. (✉)
Stanford Pain Medicine Center,
450 Broadway Street, Redwood City, CA 94063, USA

Department of Anesthesiology,
Stanford University School of Medicine,
Stanford, CA, USA
e-mail: msleong@stanford.edu

B.T. Sitzman, M.D., MPH
Advanced Pain Therapy, PLLC,
7125 Highway 98, Hattiesburg, MS 39402, USA
e-mail: toddsitzman@msn.com

amino-ester LAs, there is relatively rapid breakdown by plasma cholinesterase to a common metabolite, para-aminobenzoic acid (PABA), with the exception of cocaine and articaine which have alternate metabolic pathways. Amino-amide LAs are metabolized by the cytochrome P450 system and conjugation as a route to elimination.

Thus, briefly, all local anesthetics have similar structures with an aromatic benzene ring and an amino group connected by a linkage. This linkage is either an amide or ester. All amide local anesthetics have an "I" in their generic name before "caine": lidocaine, bupivacaine, and ropivacaine. The other local anesthetics are esters: procaine and chloroprocaine. Local anesthetics block Na+ channels and stop nerve conduction of impulses.

Alkyl substitutions on LA increase the lipid solubility. The *potency* of LAs has been shown to be directly related to lipophilicity and is often expressed as the octanol-water partition coefficient.

All LAs are weak acids as quaternary amines and are positively charged. As tertiary amines, they are weak bases and uncharged. They must be in their lipophilic base form to access their site of action on the Na+ channel. The pKa of the LA and pH at the site of injection (usually physiologic pH of 7.4 but can be locally altered, e.g., in areas of infection) influence the amount of LA in base form and the *speed of onset* of block. The addition of bicarbonate to a solution to increase the pH and speed of onset can be done to epinephrine-containing LAs that are adjusted to an acidic pH for stability in commercial preparations. In general, the lower the pKa the LA has, the faster the onset. Other factors influencing the speed of onset include the concentration and amount of LA used and the anatomic location of injection or application.

LAs prevent generation and conduction of the nerve impulse by blocking voltage-gated Na+ channels within the cell membrane. This reduces or prevents the transient increase in Na+ permeability needed for depolarization and propagation of a nerve impulse. Not all nerve fibers are equally sensitive to block. A *differential sensitivity* to block

Fig. 23.1 Local anesthetics may abolish sensation in various parts of the body by topical application, injection in the vicinity of peripheral nerve endings and along major nerve trunks, or instillation within the epidural or subarachnoid space. The ensuing sensory block occurs locally and spreads to areas distal along the nerve pathway

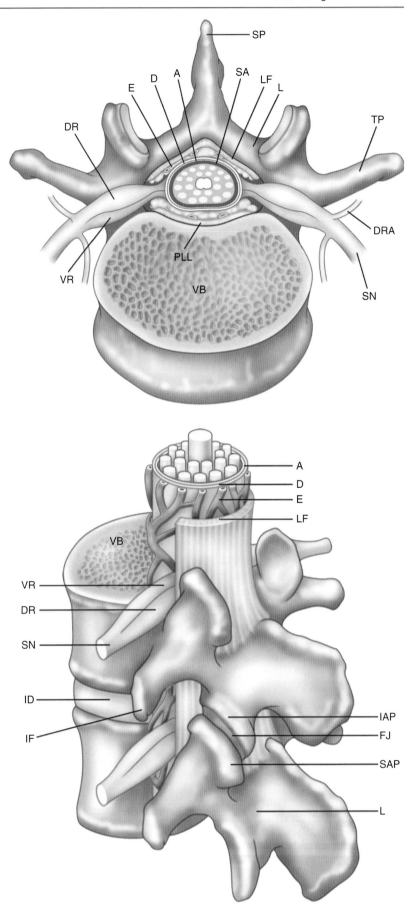

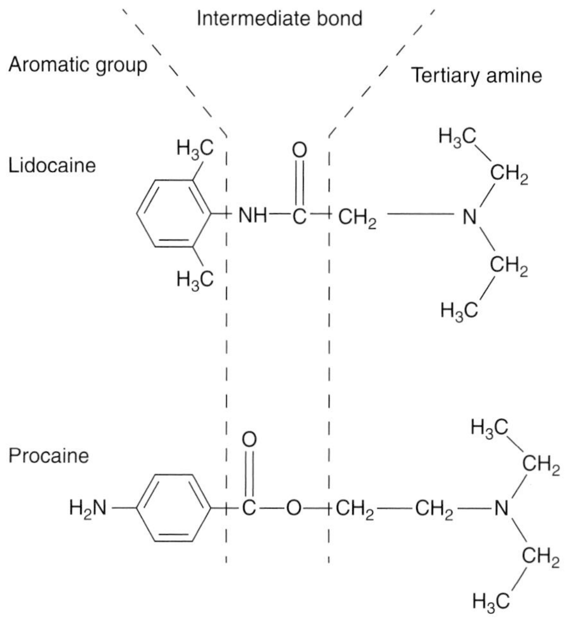

Fig. 23.2 Chemical composition and classification

is seen when the concentration of a LA is sufficient to block some nerve fiber types but not others. Clinically, small unmyelinated C fibers, autonomic fibers, and small myelinated A delta fibers (pain and temperature) are more sensitive than larger myelinated A gamma, A beta, and A alpha fibers (motor, proprioception, touch, and pressure). This differential sensitivity is of significant use in accomplishing pain or autonomic blockade without necessarily effecting motor block. LAs exhibit differences in their ability to provide differential sensitivity, and bupivacaine has been used for this capability since its introduction in 1963. More recently, ropivacaine is stated to be more motor sparing than bupivacaine with less cardiotoxicity at equipotent doses [1–3]. Interestingly, nearly the opposite differential sensitivity is seen with nerve in vitro studies. The reason for this is not known but thought to be due to phase block, which is the phenomenon that nerves that are frequently firing are more easily blocked, and anatomic considerations in nerve bundles.

A frequent consideration in the selection of a local anesthetic is *the duration of action*. There are multiple factors that determine duration of action. Increased lipid solubility of a particular agent generally increases its duration of action. As previously stated, the rate of metabolism can be a factor (e.g., amino-ester LAs). Generally, the speed of uptake and/or elimination from the site of deposition, which is also dependent on tissue perfusion, influences the duration of action. Perfusion of course is dependent on anatomic location (parauterine > intercostal > epidural > peripheral nerve > intrathecal) and sometimes is purposely manipulated by

the addition of vasoconstrictors to decrease perfusion and uptake and thus prolong block.

Mixtures of LAs to produce quick onset and/or a prolonged duration have been intermittently advocated. The results of this practice are varied, controversial, and depend on the location of utilization and the particular LAs used. There is some evidence to suggest that peripheral nerve block with bupivacaine/lidocaine or ropivacaine/lidocaine versus bupivacaine or ropivacaine alone provides a quicker onset but shorter duration of action [4]. Studies on epidural use suggest no significant difference when used in combination in terms of speed of onset or change in duration of action [5, 6]. Benefits in terms of reduced toxicity have not been elucidated. Toxicity is presumed to be additive when considering the maximum doses of more than one agent, see Table 23.1.

The important properties of LAs including potency, speed of onset, duration of action, differential block, and toxicity are dependent on the physiochemical properties of a LA as well as the way that it is used. The practitioner must become familiar with the LAs available, their individual properties, and utility. At this time, the most frequently used include lidocaine, bupivacaine, and ropivacaine.

Lidocaine is typically administered in 0.5–2 % concentrations or 5 % as a topical gel. The onset of action is approximately 5 min, with a 1–2-h duration without epinephrine. The maximal safe dose is 3 mg/kg or about 250 mg without epinephrine. With epinephrine, the safe dosage increases to 7 mg/kg or about 500 mg. Bicarbonating 0.5 % lidocaine will decrease initial pain of injection site pain.

Bupivacaine has a slower onset of action of 5–10 min but longer duration of action 3–6 h. Typical concentrations used are 0.25–0.75 % without epinephrine. A maximal safe dose is 150 mg without epinephrine. Bupivacaine is highly cardiotoxic, so ropivacaine, a chiral version of bupivacaine, is sometimes used in its place particularly for higher volume injections. Ropivacaine has concentrations from 0.2 to 1 % and a maximal safe dose of 300 mg, which is less cardiotoxic than bupivacaine.

One of the authors has received many calls from other physicians about patients with "lidocaine" allergies. Other than skin testing, the best option is avoid amide local anesthetics and use an ester: chloroprocaine.

2-chloroprocaine is a rapid-onset local anesthetic similar to lidocaine. It works within 5 min and has a duration of 30–60 min. Moreover, it is the most rapidly metabolized local anesthetic in use. Prior concerns existed over reports of spinal toxicity when administered into the epidural space. New formulations have had the prior EDTA removed which may have caused paraspinal spasms in the past [7]. Chloroprocaine may not be used if the patient reports an allergy to suntan lotion that contains benzocaine, a topical ester local anesthetic.

Table 23.1 Infiltration anesthesia

Drug	Plain solution			Epinephrine-containing solution	
	Concentration (%)	Max dose (mg)	Duration (min)	Max dose (mg)	Duration (min)
Short duration					
Procaine	1–2	500	20–30	600	30–45
Chloroprocaine	1–2	800	15–30	1,000	30
Moderate duration					
Lidocaine	0.5–1	300	30–60	500	120
Mepivacaine	0.5–1	300	45–90	500	120
Prilocaine	0.5–1	350	30–90	550	120
Long duration					
Bupivacaine	0.25–0.5	175	120–240	200	180–240
Ropivacaine	0.2–0.5	200	120–240	250	180–240

Adverse Reactions

Probably, the most common reactions are *autonomic responses* or anticipatory reactions to medical procedures. These include tachycardia, sweating, hypotension, and syncope. They are characteristically short-lived with resolution in minutes requiring no treatment or can be treated with muscarinic blockers or ephedrine.

Another common reaction is the response to vasoconstrictor additives, usually *epinephrine* which is either inadvertently injected intravascular or rapidly absorbed. Symptomatically, this produces tachycardia, hypertension, and anxiety or feelings of doom. If injected peri- or intra-arterial, it can produce distal ischemia from arterial spasm. This can produce serious complications from organ ischemia.

Local anesthetics can cause *local and systemic toxicity*. LAs used in highly concentrated solutions may be neurotoxic. Local toxicity can also occur with intraneural injections even with normal concentrations.

Systemic toxicity is estimated to occur with an incidence of 7–20/10,000 for peripheral nerve blocks and 4/10,000 for epidural blocks [8, 9]. Toxic levels usually occur due to excessive dose, intravascular injection or other reasons for unanticipated rapid absorption, predisposing medical conditions (e.g., seizure disorder), or difficulties with metabolism or elimination. Usually, systemic toxicity results first in central nervous system then cardiovascular effects, but this obviously depends on the rate of increase in blood concentration as well as the individual patient's comorbidities. CNS symptoms consist of metallic taste, perioral numbness, dizziness, muscle twitching, and ultimately generalized seizures. Toxic cardiovascular effects include arrhythmias, cardiac depression, vasodilation, hypotension, and cardiac arrest/collapse. The potent lipophilic LAs are more cardiotoxic, and resuscitation is known to be difficult using usual resuscitation efforts and medications [2]. The use of 20 % intralipid has been shown to be effective for resuscitation from bupivacaine-induced

cardiac toxicity [8–10]. The mechanism is uncertain but believed to be by extraction of the lipophilic LAs. There is evidence that it is more effective for bupivacaine and levobupivacaine than ropivacaine which is less lipophilic [10, 11], A published regimen consists of 20 % intralipid with a bolus of 1.2–2.0 ml/kg followed by infusion of 0.25–0.5 ml/kg. However, optimal dose has not been established [8].

Allergic reactions to LAs are relatively rare, constituting less than 1 % of adverse reactions [12, 13]. The majority of these allergic reactions are due to PABA from amino-ester LAs. PABA is a common metabolite of this class; there is near-complete cross-reactivity of allergy within this class of LA. Amino-amide LAs are exceedingly rarely responsible for allergic reactions, and because of their varying metabolic products, they do not have predictable allergic cross-reactivity. Paraben preservatives are structurally very similar to PABA and can show allergic cross-reactivity to amino-ester LAs. The commonest allergic reactions are delayed (24 h to a week) minor cutaneous rashes. These are generally self-limited and treated with antihistamines and topical corticosteroids. Of note is the possibility of allergic cross-reactivity to bisulfite preservatives in patients with known food allergies and to paraben preservatives in patients with sulfa antibiotic allergy.

Most local anesthetic allergies are to amide local anesthetic compounds, such as lidocaine or bupivacaine. Some patients also describe an allergy from a combination of the above agents mixed with epinephrine. Often, the epinephrine in the prior event was absorbed intravascularly causing an increase in heart rate.

An alternative to using amide local anesthetics are esters: chloroprocaine or procaine. The main question to ask is whether the patient had a "true" allergic reaction with skin rash, throat tightness, and difficulty breathing or swallowing. Moreover, if the patient has a rash to benzocaine, a common ester local anesthetic in suntan lotions, they may be allergic to esters. Typically, patients are allergic to one chemical structure of local anesthetic: amides or esters, so the other class may be dosed during procedures.

Intrathecal administration of LAs or *spinal block* can cause dense and widespread block. Spinal anesthetic techniques have been used for more than a century. Inadvertent placement of LA intrathecal can produce partial to complete spinal block depending on the amount and location of injection. A high-level or complete spinal block will result in respiratory compromise by diaphragmatic and accessory muscle paralysis and, in addition, total sympathectomy. Immediate resuscitation can be required, including respiratory and cardiovascular support. Intrathecal administration of some LAs (lidocaine, chloroprocaine) and additives (metabisulfite) are suspected of causing toxic effects ranging from transient neurological symptoms (TNS) to ascending or adhesive arachnoiditis and permanent neurologic injury. There is significant controversy around the toxic effects of intrathecal local anesthetics and additives regarding etiology and incidence of the reported complications [14].

References

1. Scott DB, Lee A, Fagan D, Bowler GM, Bloomfield P, Lundh R. Acute toxicity of ropivacaine compared with that of bupivacaine. Anesth Analg. 1989;69:563–9.
2. Zink W, Graf BM. The toxicity of local anesthetics: the place of ropivacaine and levobupivacaine. Curr Opin Anaesthesiol. 2008;21:645–50.
3. Leone S, Di Cianni S, Casati A, Fanelli G. Pharmacology, toxicology, and clinical use of new long acting local anesthetics, ropivacaine and levobupivacaine. Acta Biomed. 2008;79:92–105.
4. Cuvillon P, Nouvellon E, Ripart J, et al. A comparison of the pharmacodynamics and pharmacokinetics of bupivacaine, ropivacaine (with epinephrine) and their equal volume mixtures with lidocaine used for femoral and sciatic nerve blocks: a double-blind randomized study. Anesth Analg. 2009;108:641–9.
5. Seow LT, Lips FJ, Cousins MJ, Mather LE. Lidocaine and bupivacaine mixtures for epidural blockade. Anesthesiology. 1982;56:177–83.
6. Lucas DN, Ciccone GK, Yentis SM. Extending low-dose epidural analgesia for emergency Caesarean section. A comparison of three solutions. Anaesthesia. 1999;54:1173–7.
7. Corman SL, Skleda SJ. Use of lipid emulsion to reverse local anesthetic–induced toxicity. Ann Pharmacother. 2007;41:1873–7.
8. Corman SL, Skledar SJ. Use of lipid emulsion to reverse local anesthetic-induced toxicity. Ann Pharmacother. 2007;41:1873–7.
9. Mulroy MF. Systemic toxicity and cardiotoxicity from local anesthetics: incidence and preventive measures. Reg Anesth Pain Med. 2002;27:556–61.
10. Mazoit JX, Le Guen R, Beloeil H, Benhamou D. Binding of long-lasting local anesthetics to lipid emulsions. Anesthesiology. 2009;110:380–6.
11. Zausig YA, Zink W, Keil M, et al. Lipid emulsion improves recovery from bupivacaine-induced cardiac arrest, but not from ropivacaine- or mepivacaine-induced cardiac arrest. Anesth Analg. 2009; 109:1323–6.
12. Eggleston ST, Lush LW. Understanding allergic reactions to local anesthetics. Ann Pharmacother. 1996;30:851–7.
13. Phillips JF, Yates AB, Deshazo RD. Approach to patients with suspected hypersensitivity to local anesthetics. Am J Med Sci. 2007;334:190–6.
14. Drasner K. Chloroprocaine spinal anesthesia: back to the future? Anesth Analg. 2005;100:549–52.

Neurolytic Agents

Erin F. Lawson and Mark S. Wallace

Key Points

- Methods used to achieve neurolysis include surgical transection, cryoneurotomy, thermal radiofrequency, neuroselective toxins, and nonselective chemical ablation. None of these techniques completely destroy the nerve, and if the dorsal root ganglion is left intact, the nerve is capable of regeneration after which the pain will return.
- Nonselective neurolytic chemical agents including phenol, alcohol, and glycerol have potential for adverse outcomes. Classically, these agents are utilized in the setting of malignant pain when life expectancy is short. Imaging should be used when possible for these procedures. Heavy sedation of the patient should be avoided to allow patients to remain alert enough to report symptoms suggestive of any complication.
- Currently available neuroselective toxins include capsaicin and botulinum toxin.
- Capsaicin is a highly selective agonist for TRPV1 (vanilloid receptor 1 (VR1)). The prolonged exposure of small-diameter sensory neurons to small doses or short exposures to high doses of capsaicin result in a "desensitization" or "defunctionalization" of the nerve terminals.
- Exposure of nerve terminals to botulinum toxin has also been shown to result in rapid relief of pain. It is postulated that the botulinum toxin reduces peripheral and central release of neurotransmitters.

- Newer approaches such as pulsed radiofrequency ablation have widened the potential pool of patients for denervation due to decreased risk of permanent neurologic sequela.
- Sympathetic blocks are generally indicated for treatment of painful symptoms that are not confined to a dermatomal distribution, pain due to damage of peripheral nerve branches, pain caused or maintained by increased sympathetic tone, or pain due to circulatory disturbances.
- Intrathecal neurolysis provides a sensory block without a motor block. Positioning is of utmost importance. Thus, selection of neurolytic (hypobaric vs. hyperbaric) and patient cooperation is critical. Positioning is less critical with epidural neurolysis, which may be chosen to treat pain in the upper abdominal wall, thorax, or upper extremity.

Introduction

History

Neural blockade with neurolytic agents has been documented for the treatment of pain for over a century. In 1904, Schloesser was the first to report alcohol neurolysis for the treatment of trigeminal neuralgia [1, 2]. White, in 1935, applied alcohol neurolysis to the upper thoracic ganglia for the treatment of angina pain [3]. Doppler used phenol neurolysis to destroy presacral sympathetic nerves for treatment of pelvic pain in 1926 [3]. Mandl also studied phenol for cervical ganglion neurolysis in 1947 [3]. Today, the role of neurolytic agents is well established in the approach to cancer pain. Blocking neuronal transmission has the potential to relieve otherwise refractory cancer pain. However, all currently available neurolytic agents have potential for adverse outcomes making their use controversial in nonmalignant or nonterminal pain.

E.F. Lawson, M.D. (✉) • M.S. Wallace, M.D.
Department of Anesthesiology,
University of California, San Diego Medical Center,
9310 Campus Point Drive, Ste. A-106, La Jolla, CA 92037, USA
e-mail: erlawson@ucsd.edu, mswallace@ucsd.edu

T.R. Deer et al. (eds.), *Comprehensive Treatment of Chronic Pain by Medical, Interventional, and Integrative Approaches*,
DOI 10.1007/978-1-4614-1560-2_24, © American Academy of Pain Medicine 2013

Scientific Foundation

The specialty of pain medicine defines neurolysis as the selective, iatrogenic destruction of neural tissue to secure the relief of pain [4]. Methods used to achieve neurolysis include surgical transection, cryoneurotomy, thermal radiofrequency, neuroselective toxins, and nonselective chemical ablation. None of these techniques completely destroy the nerve, and if the dorsal root ganglion is left intact, the nerve is capable of regeneration after which the pain will return. This is an important point to convey to the patients as many will assume that if you destroy a nerve, the pain will cease forever. Of all the techniques, nonselective chemical ablation has the potential for the most side effects as the spread of the neurolytic agent is not controlled as with the other techniques where the control of the lesion is more precise. With the exception of neuroselective toxins, the ablative techniques are performed at the level of the axon after which a conduction block occurs. The chemical agents phenol, alcohol, and glycerol cause a dose-dependent, nonselective destruction of the nerve resulting in necrosis, death, Wallerian degeneration, and a complete conduction block in all fibers contained within the nerve [5]. When using neuroselective toxins, the agents are applied to the peripheral nerve terminals. For example, capsaicin is a highly selective agonist for TRPV1 (formerly known as vanilloid receptor 1 (VR1)), a ligand-gated, nonselective cation channel preferentially expressed on small-diameter sensory neurons, especially those nerve fibers that specialize in the detection of painful or noxious sensations [5, 6]. When capsaicin binds to the receptor, the TRPV1 calcium channel opens and calcium enters the intracellular space. The prolonged exposure of small-diameter sensory neurons to small doses or short exposures to high doses of capsaicin result in a "desensitization" or "defunctionalization" of the nerve terminals. The high concentration of intracellular calcium overwhelms the mitochondria, leading to dysfunction and nerve terminal death [7, 8]. Exposure of nerve terminals to botulinum toxin has also been shown to result in rapid relief of pain that cannot be explained by the muscle relaxation effect which takes days to take effect. It is postulated that the botulinum toxin is taken up by the free nerve endings where it cleaves the SNARE protein, SNAP-25. The peripheral release of neurotransmitters from the nerve terminal is dependent upon SNAP-25, and botulinum toxin reduces peripheral release of the neurotransmitter. Another mechanism is the transport of the toxin centrally where the SNARE proteins are cleaved resulting in the reduction of central release of neurotransmitters [9].

Patient Selection

Neurolytics are employed to produce long-lasting pain relief through disabling or destroying nerves. Due to potential for morbidity, neurolytics are selected after patients have failed noninvasive and less invasive therapy. Classically, these agents are utilized in the setting of malignant pain when life expectancy is short, which is the focus of this chapter. Pain is frequently inadequately controlled in cancer patients [10], leading to unnecessary suffering, physical debilitation, psychological deterioration, and avoidance of treatment. Cancer pain management has been identified as an international priority focus for improvement by the World Health Organization (WHO) [11]. While the WHO analgesic ladder usually establishes effective pain management for cancer patients with a less invasive approach, neurolytic procedures are required in 29 % of patients [12]. Although sometimes, more controversial, non-cancer patients with certain chronic pain conditions are also potential candidates for neurolysis. For example, some pain physicians do advocate for sympathetic neurolysis for patients with CRPS [13]. Newer approaches such as pulsed radiofrequency ablation have widened the potential pool of patients for denervation due to decreased risk of permanent neurologic sequela. For use of traditional nonselective neurolytic agents, however, a conservative approach continues to prevail. The use of chemical neurolytic blocks for chronic nonmalignant pain is controversial and not advocated by the authors of this chapter. Furthermore, it is critical that only experienced and skillful persons who are equipped to treat immediate effects perform these blocks [14]. Finally, radiographic guidance is recommended when appropriate.

Applications

Neurolysis is used to provide pain relief by interrupting pain transmission. It can therefore theoretically be applied anywhere along the sensory pathway. Peripheral nerves, sympathetic ganglia, and dorsal roots are all examples of potential targets for neurolysis. Peripheral nerve neurolysis is effective for painful symptoms limited to a single nerve distribution. Most peripheral nerves are mixed; therefore, peripheral neurolysis carries a high risk of motor block as well [13]. It is important to first perform a prognostic block with local anesthetic in order to assess efficacy. The local anesthetic block will determine appropriateness of location of block as well as provide the patient with an opportunity to evaluate the effect with a short-term block. If the patient is uncomfortable with the numb sensation or motor weakness, a neurolytic block is not indicated.

Sympathetic blocks are generally indicated for treatment of painful symptoms that are not confined to a dermatomal distribution, pain due to damage of peripheral nerve branches, pain caused or maintained by increased sympathetic tone, or pain due to circulatory disturbances. Stellate ganglion neurolysis is appropriate for upper extremity and possibly facial pain. Celiac plexus neurolysis is indicated for pain of the upper abdominal viscera. Lumbar plexus neurolysis targets

Table 24.1 Agents, dose, and location: the good and the bad

Agent	Strength	Unique property	Negative properties	Systemic toxicity
Alcohol	50–100 %	Hypobaric, fast onset	Painful on injection, risk of neuritis (peripheral nerves)	Disulfiram-like reaction
Phenol	4–15 %	Hyperbaric, painless, slow onset	Shorter-lived, affinity for vasculature	Convulsions, cardiovascular collapse
Glycerol	50 %	Historically applied to Gasserian ganglion for treatment of trigeminal neuralgia	Inability to control the spread	Severe headache or local dysesthesia
Capsaicin	8 %	Nociceptor-selective, topical	Painful application, only for localized neuropathic pain	
Ammonium salts	10 %	Sensory fiber-selective, motor intact, lack of postblock neuritis	Nausea and vomiting, headache and paresthesia	Nausea and vomiting, headache and paresthesia

pain in the lower extremity. Superior hypogastric plexus neurolysis targets lower abdominal or pelvic visceral pain. Finally, ganglion impar neurolysis treats sympathetically maintained perineal pain.

Intrathecal neurolysis or rhizolysis of the dorsal root will provide a sensory block without a motor block. Positioning is of utmost importance. Thus, selection of neurolytic (hypobaric vs. hyperbaric) and patient cooperation are critical. Epidural neurolysis may also be chosen to treat pain in the upper abdominal wall, thorax, or upper extremity. Positioning is less critical; thus, this approach may be an option when positioning for subarachnoid neurolysis is difficult.

Limitations

Following neurolysis, the nerves typically regenerate over time with return of pain. Nerves may regrow unpredictably and may form neuromas. In such cases, not only does pain return, but it is often worse than the initial pain experience. However, with terminal cancer pain, onset of this complication often exceeds the life expectancy of the patient. Therefore, the life expectancy of the patient should be considered when performing neurolytic procedures for pain management. Furthermore, neurolysis does not necessarily provide complete neuronal blockade. The neurolytic block often clinically provides less analgesia than the local anesthetic block [15].

Complications

Complications arise from all aspects of the procedure. Complications from the needle entry site include infection, bleeding, perforation of a viscus or organ, pneumothorax, unintentional subarachnoid or epidural injection, vascular laceration or injection, and peripheral nerve trauma. Complications from sympathectomy especially with celiac plexus block include hypotension that may be severe and

prolonged, diarrhea, and sexual dysfunction. These agents are nonselective; potentially catastrophic complications are possible. Complications from the neurolytic agent include motor block, paraplegia, neuropathic pain and dysesthesias, skin ulceration, soft tissue and muscle injury, phlebitis, thrombosis, and tissue ischemia [15]. Motor block is common and even expected with peripheral or neuraxial neurolysis due to the nonselective nature of most neurolytics. However, weakness and paraplegia may also occur during sympathetic blocks secondary to vascular injury. Bowel or urinary incontinence is possible following intrathecal neurolysis [16]. Although less devastating, neuralgias, hypesthesia, and anesthesia following neurolysis may be very distressing to patients expecting relief of suffering. These complications are more common following traditional neurolytic agents such as alcohol.

The Agents (Table 24.1)

Phenol

- Protein coagulation causes nonselective tissue destruction and initiates Wallerian degeneration in nerves [15].
- Intrathecal administration causes degeneration of large and small nerve fibers within the nerve roots but not the ganglia or spinal cord [17].
- It has affinity for vasculature and is toxic to vasculature [15]; therefore, use caution in vascular locations (celiac plexus).
- Neurolysis lasts for several months [18]; regeneration is more rapid than alcohol (14 weeks) [19]. Milder blockade (compared to alcohol).
- Concentrations <~2 % act as a local anesthetic and >5 % needed for neurolysis [18].
- Mixing possible with water or saline up to 6.67 %, mixing with glycerin for higher concentrations, and mixing with radiopaque dye possible.
- Not painful on injection.

- Hyperbaric compared to CSF (especially when mixed with glycerol); position patients with the painful side down during intrathecal injection in order to coat the dorsal roots.
- Phenol diffuses out of glycerin slowly; there is time for patient positioning after injection.
- Glycerin's high viscosity requires at least a 20-gauge needle for injection.

Alcohol

- Induces Wallerian degeneration in peripheral nerves [20].
- Subarachnoid application causes Wallerian degeneration, demyelination, and degeneration in the dorsal roots, posterior columns, and dorsolateral tract of Lissauer [16].
- Neuronal regeneration in peripheral nerves and spinal cord begins after 1–3 months [16].
- Concentrations up to 33 % destroy sensory nerves but spare motor nerves when applied peripherally.
- Concentrations >33 % may cause paralysis.
- Concentrations 50–100 % are used intrathecally.
- 40 % alcohol is equipotent to 5 % phenol.
- Available in the United States in a 95 % concentration in 5-ml vials.
- Rapidly spreads from the injection site
- Requires larger volumes (than phenol due to rapid spread)
- Easily absorbed into the bloodstream [21], peak blood alcohol levels after injection are usually below the legal limit for driving unless accidental intravascular injection has occurred.
- Hypobaric compared to CSF.
- When performing intrathecal neurolysis, the patient must be positioned with the painful side up in order to coat the appropriate dorsal roots.
- Alcohol is painful on injection.
- Give local anesthetic prior to application to peripheral nerves.
- Intrathecal application less painful than peripheral, with only transient mild burning.
- Toxic to vasculature, causes vasospasm and possibly thrombosis [15].
- Toxic to connective tissue, causes necrosis.
- Inject small volumes and flush the needle with sterile saline prior to withdrawal [19].

Glycerol

- The mechanism of action is unclear, but it appears to cause Wallerian degeneration [19].
- Historically most commonly used to treat trigeminal neuralgia but newer options including radiofrequency lesioning are replacing the use of glycerol.
- Rarely used to treat cancer pain.
- Concentration of 50 %.

Ammonium Compounds

- Not often used clinically.
- High incidence of nausea and vomiting, headache, and paresthesia [22].
- Ammonium sulfate is 10 % effective for intercostal neuralgia without painful post procedure neuritis [23].
- Intrafascicular injection has been shown to be less neurotoxic than phenol 5 % and to spare motor function in animal models [24, 25].

Hypertonic Solutions

- Serious complications including death secondary to hypertonic saline make them clinically undesirable [26].
- Hypertonic saline 10 % NaCl has been used in percutaneous epidural neuroplasty for the treatment of radiculopathy and low back pain.
- Intrathecal hypertonic saline (10–15 %) has been shown to decrease pain by 50 % in cancer patients for up to 3 months [27].

Vanilloids

- Capsaicin (active ingredient in hot chili peppers) and resiniferatoxin (RTX) are available for use.
- Desensitize unmyelinated C pain fibers.
- Activate the transient receptor potential vanilloid receptor 1 (TRPV1) on unmyelinated C fiber nociceptors; influx of calcium and sodium ions depolarize the nociceptive afferent terminals; release of stored neuropeptides causes initial pain signaling followed by desensitization [28].
- Early desensitization of nociceptors by conduction block.
- Delayed desensitization by downregulating TRPV1 receptors [29].
- TRPV1 receptors have been identified in visceral organs, spinal cord, and DRG [29].
- Selective for nociceptors.
- Speed of onset and duration of analgesia depends on dose, duration, and frequency of exposure [30].
- Effect is temporary, lasting hours to days, and requires frequent reapplication to maintain effect.
- Topical application several times daily.
- The topical application of low-dose capsaicin (<1 %); an effective adjunct to the treatment of postherpetic neuralgia, postmastectomy pain, and diabetic neuropathy [31].
- NGX-4010 (8 % capsaicin patch) provides pain relief for up to 12 weeks after one 60-min application [32].
- NGX-4010 is proven effective in the treatment of HIV-associated distal sensory polyneuropathy [33, 34] and postherpetic neuralgia [32].

- Intrathecal resiniferatoxin has been shown to reduce pain in a canine bone cancer model [35]. Phase I clinical trials in cancer patients will start soon.

Clostridial Neurotoxin

- Botulinum toxin is neurotoxic to cholinergic nerves by blocking acetylcholine release.
- Analgesic effect also secondary to inhibition of calcitonin gene-related peptide (CGRP) release from afferent nerve terminals [36], substance P from dorsal root ganglia, and glutamate in the dorsal horn [37].
- Botulinum toxin (BTX) has seven serotypes (A–G) which consist of a heavy chain bound to a light chain by a disulfide bond [38]. The heavy chain binds the nerve terminal and facilitates internalization of the light chain. The light chain internally inhibits neurotransmitter vesicle docking on the plasma membrane [38].
- Neurotransmitter vesicular docking is mediated by the soluble N-ethylmaleimide-sensitive factor attachment protein receptor (SNARE) complex which is the target for the BTX light chain.
- Normal nerve terminal function eventually recovers through restoration of the SNARE complex [37],
- Clinically, motor paresis develops within 5 days and lasts for several months.
- BTX is too large to penetrate the blood-brain barrier and is inactivated by retrograde axonal transport; therefore, there is no direct central nervous system effect [37]. Effective in treatment of painful muscle spasticity and myofacial pain, hyperhidrosis, hypersalivtion, and hyperlacrimation [38].
- In cancer patients, BTX has been shown to improve symptoms of radiation fibrosis syndrome [39] and neuropathic pain [40]. Currently approved for use in the United States are Onabotulinumtoxin A (Botox/Botox Cosmetic), Abobotulinumtoxin A (Dysport), and Rimabotulinumtoxin B (Myobloc).
- The dose equivalency is 20 U vs. 50 U vs. 2,000 U for Botox, Dysport, and Myobloc, respectively.
- BTX is injected into striated muscle in increments of units.
- Dosage units differ among the BTX products and are not comparable or convertible [41].
- BTX may be diluted in local anesthetic or sterile saline, and optimal dilutions have not been established for treatment of pain.
- Smaller effect or shorter duration of response seen over time due to development of antibodies against BTX [37].
- If antibodies are suspected, rotation to different serotype usually effective.
- Local complications include muscle atrophy, dysphagia, dysphonia, and ptosis.
- Systemic complications include dyspnea, respiratory compromise, weakness, and death. Systemic complications have mostly occurred in children treated for cerebral palsy-associated spasticity and have been reported between 1 day and several weeks following treatment [42].

Clinical Practice

The following clinical examples are the approaches the authors of this chapter have found most successful for neurolysis. These clinical descriptions are intended for example only and should be interpreted for use by experienced clinicians. We support the use of the following neurolytic agents for palliative pain control in patients with malignant pain. We urge caution when using these neurolytics in patients with non-cancer pain or those with normal life expectancy due to potential for permanent catastrophic complications. We endorse the use of imaging when possible for these procedures. We also recommend avoiding heavy sedation of the patient. Patients should remain alert enough to report symptoms suggestive of any complication.

While specific complication risks are mentioned below, complications may result from any aspect of neurolysis from technical procedural complications to agent-specific complications. Technical complications include infection, bleeding, perforation of a viscus or organ, pneumothorax, unintentional subarachnoid or epidural injection, vascular laceration or injection, and peripheral nerve trauma. Complications from the neurolytic agent include motor block, paraplegia, neuropathic pain and dysesthesias, skin ulceration, soft tissue and muscle injury, phlebitis, thrombosis, and tissue ischemia [15]. Although less devastating, neuralgias, hypesthesia, and anesthesia following neurolysis may be very distressing to patients expecting relief of suffering. These complications are more common following traditional neurolytic agents such as alcohol. Finally, neurolysis does not always provide complete neuronal blockade. The neurolytic block often clinically provides less analgesia than the local anesthetic block [15].

The strengths and volumes of neurolytic agents shown below are not supported by scientific literature but are based only on clinical experience. Absolute alcohol is available in the United States as ethanol 98 % and phenol 100 %. For lower concentrations for clinical use, phenol must be diluted with saline by a compounding pharmacy.

Subarachnoid Neurolysis

- Appropriate for well-localized, unilateral pain limited to a few dermatomes.
- Cervical subarachnoid neurolysis should be performed at the spinal segment level to be blocked because cervical

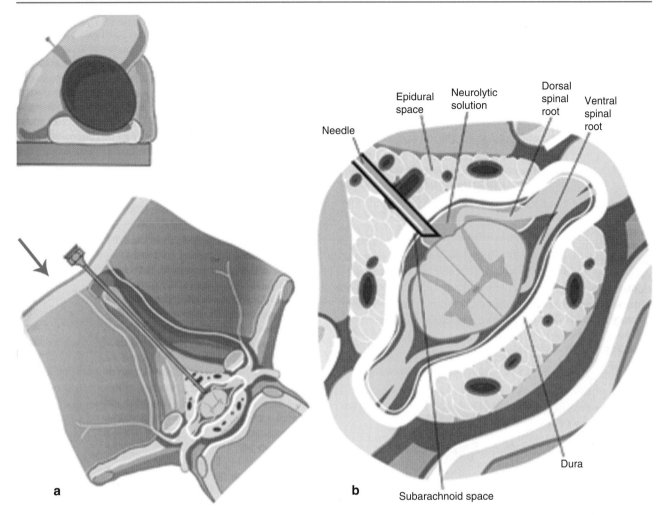

Fig. 24.1 Proper positioning of the patient with left-sided pain for intrathecal injection of alcohol (**a**) and close-up demonstration of proper needle entry into subarachnoid space (**b**). Note the 45° anterior tilt intended to bathe the posterior (sensory) nerve roots with hypobaric alcohol while sparing the anterior (motor) roots (With permissions from Waldman [44])

nerve roots pass horizontally from the cord through the intervertebral foramen [43].

- Upper thoracic subarachnoid neurolysis should be performed at the vertebral interspace of the dermatome to be blocked. Middle and lower thoracic subarachnoid neurolysis should be performed one or two segments above the vertebral interspace of the dermatome to be blocked due to the anatomic course of the thoracic nerve roots.
- Lumbar subarachnoid neurolysis should be performed at the T11–T12, and subarachnoid neurolysis for sacral dermatomes should be performed at the L1–L2 interspace.
- Intrathecal neurolysis or rhizolysis of the dorsal root will provide a sensory block without a motor block.
- Procedure
    - The patient should remain awake and alert throughout the procedure.
    - Sterile prep and drape.
    - Patient may be positioned sitting or lateral for initial needle positioning.

- A 20- or 22-gauge 3.5-in. spinal needle is advanced to intrathecal space at level of desired dermatome.
- After confirmation with (+) CSF, the patient is positioned for neurolytic injection.
- Alcohol is hypobaric; position patient with painful side up; positioning is critical as alcohol diffuses quickly and sets up quickly. Patient should be positioned laterally with 45 % forward tilt. Bilateral blocks with alcohol may be achieved with the patient in the prone position.
- Phenol is hyperbaric but diffuses out of glycerol slowly; therefore, positioning is less critical and may occur after injection. Patient should be positioned with painful side down with a 45 % posterior tilt.
- Absolute alcohol or phenol 6 % in glycerin, up to 1 ml is injected.
- Potential complications include painful setup (alcohol), coagulum with CSF (do not aspirate CSF prior to injection), bowel/bladder incontinence, lower extremity weakness, and motor block (Figs. 24.1 and 24.2).

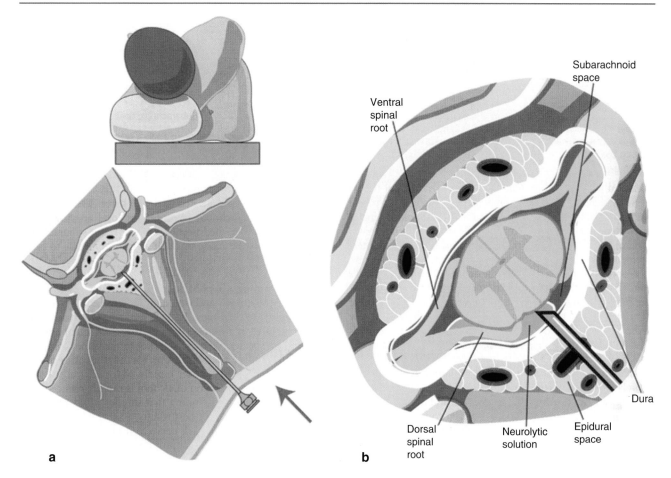

a

b

Fig. 24.2 Proper positioning of the patient with left-sided pain for intrathecal injection of phenol in glycerin (**a**) and close-up demonstration of proper need entry into the subarachnoid space (**b**). Note the 45° posterior tilt intended to bathe the posterior (sensory) nerve roots with hyperbaric phenol while sparing the anterior (motor) roots (From Waldman [45])

Epidural Neurolysis

- Appropriate for well-localized bilateral pain limited to a few dermatomes including pain in the upper abdominal wall, thorax, or upper extremity. Positioning is less critical; thus, this approach may be an option when positioning for subarachnoid neurolysis is difficult. Epidural neurolysis has less predictable spread than with intrathecal neurolysis.
- Procedure
  - The patient should remain awake and alert throughout the procedure.
  - The patient is positioned with painful side down in 45 % posterior tilt.
  - The patient is prepped and draped in a sterile manner.
  - Lidocaine 1 % local skin and subcutaneous tissue infiltration.
  - 17–18-gauge Tuohy epidural needle inserted into epidural space with loss of resistance technique. Epidural catheter threaded under fluoroscopic guidance to level of painful dermatomes to be treated.
  - Injection of small volume of contrast is performed to confirm epidural spread and rule out intrathecal or intravascular spread.
  - Absolute alcohol 8–10 ml; phenol 15 % in glycerol/75 % of LA volume 8–10 ml is injected.
  - The patient should ideally remain in this position 40 min following injection.
- Potential complications include motor block, numbness, neuritis, and deafferentation pain.

Peripheral Nerve Neurolysis

- Appropriate for pain localized to a single peripheral sensory nerve. Most peripheral nerves are mixed; therefore, peripheral neurolysis carries a high risk of motor block as well [13].
- Procedure: First, perform a prognostic block with local anesthetic in order to assess efficacy. The local anesthetic block will determine appropriateness of location of block as well as provide the patient with an opportunity to evaluate

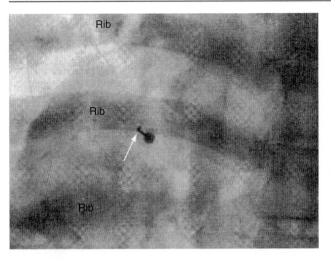

Fig. 24.3 Intercostal nerve block, anteroposterior view. The *arrow* indicates where the needle touches and stops below the rib (Raj Interventional Pain Management Image-Guided Procedures)

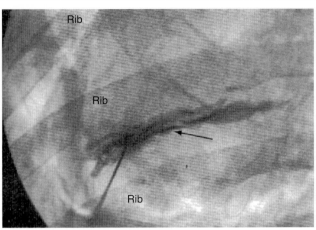

Fig. 24.4 Intercostal nerve block with contrast medium, anteroposterior view. The *arrow* indicates the spread of contrast in the intercostal groove (Raj Interventional Pain Management Image-Guided Procedures)

the effect with a short-term block. If the patient is uncomfortable with the numb sensation or motor weakness, a neurolytic block is not indicated.

- Ultrasound should be considered for nerve localization during the procedure.
- Procedure example: intercostal nerve neurolysis
  - The patient remained awake and alert throughout the procedure.
  - The patient is placed in the prone position.
  - The skin is prepped with chlorhexidine, and sterile drapes are applied.
  - The skin and soft tissues are anesthetized with lidocaine 1 %.
  - The injection is usually performed posteriorly at the angle of the rib just lateral to the paraspinous muscles [43].
  - A 20-gauge spinal needle is inserted percutaneously and advanced under fluoroscopic guidance using dorsal oblique, AP, and lateral projections.
  - The needle tip is advanced to contact bone at the dorsal caudal edge of the targeted rib. The needle is then advanced past the caudal and dorsal edge of the rib and stopped before reaching the ventral edge of the rib.
  - After negative aspiration for heme or air, contrast injection under live fluoroscopic guidance should spread longitudinally along the rib without evidence of intravascular spread.
  - 1–2 ml of 2 % lidocaine is injected to reduce the pain of the neurolytic agents. This is followed by absolute alcohol 1–2 ml, or phenol 6–12 % aqueous 1–2 ml is then injected.
- Potential complications include painful neuritis, motor weakness, and pneumothorax (Figs. 24.3 and 24.4).

Cranial Nerve Neurolysis

- Appropriate for pain localized to cranial nerves.
- Procedure example: Please see Sphenopalatine Ganglion Neurolysis described below
- CT guidance or use of digital subtraction fluoroscopy is recommended.
- 1 ml of 2 % lidocaine is injected followed by phenol 6–12 % aqueous 1 ml.
- Potential complications include painful neuritis and vascular injury with stroke.

Sphenopalatine Ganglion Neurolysis

- Appropriate for the treatment of intractable pain in the distribution of the maxillary nerve.
- Procedure
  - Position patient supine.
  - Sterile prep and drape of cheek on side where procedure is to be performed
  - The anterior view is taken with the C-arm, and the needle entry site is located under the zygoma in the coronoid notch. C-arm then rotated to a lateral view of the upper cervical spine and mandible. The patient's head is rotated until the rami of the mandible are superimposed one on the other. The C-arm is then rotated cephalad until the pterygopalatine fossa is visualized [46].
  - A 22-gauge 3.5-in. needle is advanced under fluoroscopic guidance until the needle tip is adjacent to the lateral nasal mucosa in the pterygopalatine fossa. The needle should never be advanced through resistance [46].

– Aspirate should be negative for heme and CSF.
– Inject 2 % lidocaine 1 ml followed by phenol 6–12 % 1 ml.
• Complications include hematoma if the maxillary artery or venous plexus is punctured; hypesthesia and numbness of the palate, maxilla, or posterior pharynx; meningitis; epistaxis; and trauma to the parotid gland or branches of the facial nerve (Figs. 24.5 and 24.6).

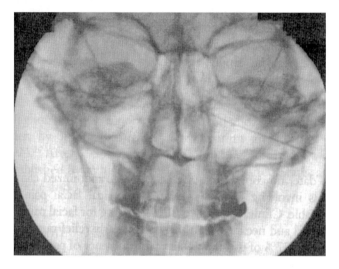

Fig. 24.5 The radiographic anteroposterior view of the face shows the needle tip at the lateral wall of the nose at the superomedial angle of the maxillary sinus (Raj Interventional Pain Management Image-Guided Procedures)

Thoracic Sympathetic Neurolysis

• Appropriate for the treatment of intractable pain of the upper two-thirds of the esophagus and pleuritic chest pain secondary to lung neoplasm [43]. The technical difficulty of multiple needle placements compared to effectiveness of epidural and subarachnoid neurolysis has limited the use of this procedure [43].
• Procedure
  – The patient should remain awake and alert throughout the procedure.
  – The patient is positioned prone with a pillow under the chest or optimal flexion of the thoracic spine.
  – Sterile prep and drape of the thorax.
  – The T2–T8 vertebral body levels may be approached based on location of pain. The selected vertebral body is "squared" under fluoroscopy. Rotate C-arm 20° oblique toward the ipsilateral side.
  – Local skin and soft tissue anesthesia with lidocaine 1 %.
  – A 20–22-gauge spinal needle is inserted percutaneously with tip directed to the lateral border of T2 above the third rib. Needle tip is advanced under fluoroscopic guidance to the lateral edge of the T2 vertebral body. The C-arm is then rotated laterally to view advancement of needle to the posterior third of the vertebral body while keeping needle tip in contact with the vertebral body edge.
  – After negative aspiration, contrast dye is injected under live fluoroscopy. Contrast should spread in a

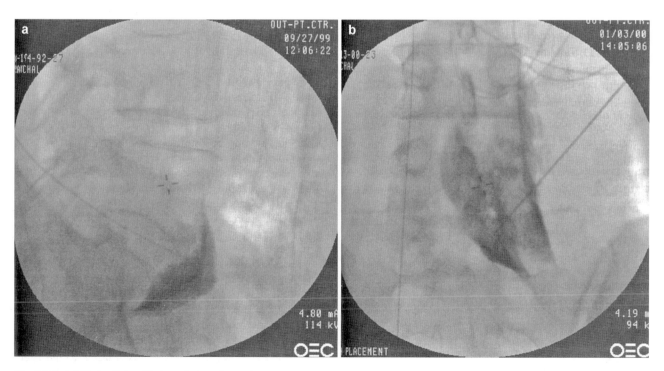

Fig. 24.6 (**a**) The radiographic lateral view shows the needle placed at the superior hypogastric plexus. (**b**) This image shows correct needle placement from the contralateral side. (Raj Interventional Pain Management Image-Guided Procedures)

cephalocaudal direction along the thoracic vertebral column without any evidence of intravascular uptake.

- Lidocaine 2 % 2.5 ml followed by phenol 10 % 2.5 ml is then injected.
- Complications include neuraxial injection, intravascular injection, nerve injury, pneumothorax, and intercostal neuralgia.

Celiac Plexus Neurolysis

- Appropriate for treatment of pain of upper abdominal viscera
- Procedure: posterior/retrocrural approaches
  - Fluoroscopic or CT guidance may be used.
  - The patient should remain awake and alert throughout the procedure.
  - The patient is positioned prone with a pillow under the abdomen.
  - Sterile prep and drape.
  - For fluoroscopically guided procedures, the L1 vertebral body is "squared" under fluoroscopic view, and then the C-arm is oblique to ipsilateral side to align the lateral tip of the transverse process with the edge of the L1 vertebral body. Needles are inserted bilaterally at the L1 vertebral body level.
  - The skin and soft tissues are anesthetized with lidocaine 1 %.

- A 20–22-gauge 15-cm spinal needle of adequate length for body habitus is inserted percutaneously with tip directed over the inferior one-third of the lateral L1 vertebral body.
- The needle is advanced under fluoroscopic guidance until contact is made with vertebral body. The C-arm is then rotated laterally to visualize the needle tip advance to appropriate location. The left needle tip is advanced 1.5–2 cm past the edge of the vertebral body, and right needle tip is advanced 3–4 cm past the edge of the vertebral body. Neurolytic agent is injected posterior and cephalic to the diaphragmatic crura [43].
- Aspiration should be negative for heme, CSF, urine, and thoracic duct fluid. Injection of contrast should demonstrate cephalocaudal spread without evidence of intravascular uptake. Injection of a test dose of injection solution is recommended.
- Lidocaine 2 % 10 ml (transcrural) or 5 ml (retrocrural or splanchnic) followed by alcohol 95 % (10 ml for transcrural approach, 5 ml each side for retrocrural or splanchnic approach) is injected.
- Side effects include diarrhea, hypotension, and sexual dysfunction.
- Complications include severe and prolonged hypotension, paraplegia, PTX, bowel injury, major vascular injury, bleeding, weakness, and paraplegia secondary to vascular injury (Figs. 24.7a, b).

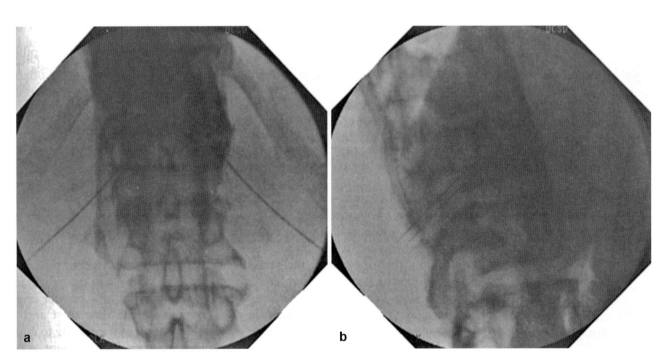

Fig. 24.7 Anteroposterior view (**a**) and lateral view (**b**) of correct needle locations for the retrocrural approach to the celiac plexus block. This technique requires bilateral needle placement, with the needle tip located at the anterolateral portion of L1 (Raj Textbook of Regional Anesthesia)

Superior Hypogastric Plexus Neurolysis

- Appropriate for the treatment of pelvic visceral pain
- Procedure
  - The patient should remain awake and alert throughout the procedure.
  - The patient is positioned prone with a pillow under the abdomen to reduce lumbar lordosis.
  - The lower back is sterilely prepped and draped.
  - The L5 vertebral body is identified under fluoroscopy.
  - Cranial tilt of the C-arm is utilized to align the top of the transverse process of L5 with the inferior border of the L5 vertebral body. The C-arm is then oblique ipsilaterally 20°. Needle entry site is 5–7 cm lateral to the midpoint of the L4–L5 interspinous space. Needles are advanced bilaterally.
  - Skin and soft tissues are infiltrated with lidocaine 1 %.
  - A 20–22-gauge 15-cm spinal needle is advanced percutaneously to pass just over the top of the L5 transverse process and target the anterior edge of the lower portion of the L5 vertebral body bilaterally.
  - After negative aspiration, injection of contrast should reveal cranial–caudal spread along the vertebral column without evidence of intravascular spread.
  - Lidocaine 2 % 4 ml followed by phenol 10 % 4 ml is injected on each side.
  - Potential complications include intravascular injection, neuraxial injection, discitis, urinary injury, bladder/bowel incontinence, weakness, and paraplegia secondary to vascular injury (Figs. 24.8 and 24.9a, b).

Ganglion Impar Neurolysis

- Appropriate for treatment of perineal pain or pain of rectum or anus.
- Procedure
  - The patient should remain awake and alert throughout the procedure.

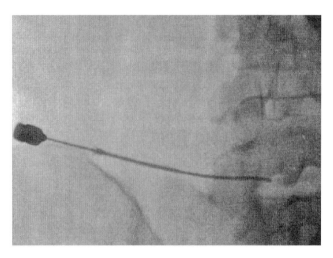

Fig. 24.8 Medial paraspinos approach: final position of the needle at L5 for hypogastric plexus block (posteroanterior view) (Raj Interventional Pain Management Image-Guided Procedures)

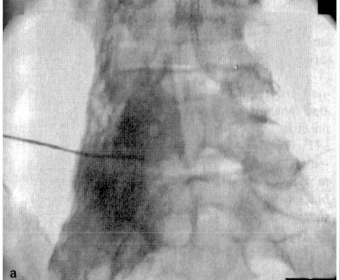
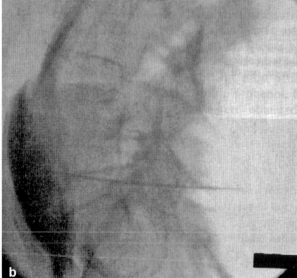

Fig. 24.9 (**a**) Posteroanterior view showing the dispersion of contrast Omnipaque (iohexol) solution to confirm the correct needle position. Note the solution spreading vertically hugging the spine. (**b**) Lateral view showing contrast solution spreading over the L5–S1 (Raj Interventional Pain Management Image-Guided Procedures)

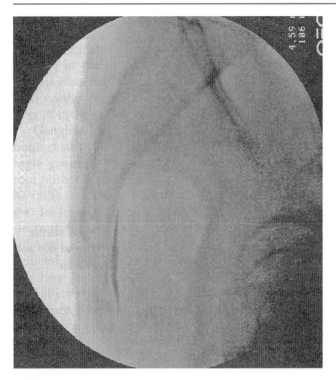

Fig. 24.10 Lateral fluoroscopic view that shows the needle tip in the perirectal space between rectum and the sacrum (Raj Interventional Pain Management Image-Guided Procedures)

– There are techniques described in the literature of patient positioning prone or in the lateral decubitus position. The prone positioning is discussed here.
– Patient is positioned prone with a pillow under the pelvis.
– Sterile prep and drape.
– Lidocaine 1 % is infiltrated into skin.
– Using AP and lateral fluoroscopic imaging, a 20-gauge 3.4-cm spinal needle is advanced through the sacro-coccygeal ligament just anterior to the anterior border of the sacrum.
– After negative aspiration, injection of contrast should reveal longitudinal spread along the anterior border of the sacrum without intravascular or rectal spread.
– Lidocaine 2 % 2 ml followed by phenol 10 % 2 ml is injected.
• Potential complications include rectal trauma or perforation, periosteal injection, epidural injection, or sacral root injury (Fig. 24.10).

High Dose Capsaicin

• FDA approved for the treatment of postherpetic neuralgia.
• A single 1-h treatment can provide up to 3 months of pain relief.
• Each patch contains 8 % capsaicin in a localized dermal delivery system.

• The patch is 14×20 cm (280 cm^2) and contains a total of 179 mg of capsaicin or 640 µg/cm^2. The patch can be cut to the size of the affected area.
  – Identify the area to be treated which includes areas of hypersensitivity and allodynia.
  – Use the patch only on dry, intact skin.
  – If necessary, clip (do not shave) the patient's hair to improve adherence of the patch.
  – Use only nitrile gloves when handling the patch and cleansing capsaicin residue from the skin. After handling the capsaicin patch, avoid contact with eyes or mucous membranes.
  – The patch is cut to the size of the painful area. Up to four patches can be used at once.
  – Prior to patch application, the area is gently washed with mild soap and water and dried thoroughly. This is to remove skin oils which will absorb the capsaicin (which is fat soluble) and reduce drug delivery.
  – The FDA-approved procedure is to pretreat with topical lidocaine. However, the studies showed that pretreatment with topical lidocaine did not reduce the pain of application. In general, the procedure is well tolerated with mild discomfort. In the author's experience, pretreatment with topical lidocaine has no effect on the pain of application, and it is not necessary [47]. If desired, pretreatment with oral oxycodone and Valium works well.
  – The patch is applied and left in place for 1 h. To ensure that the patch maintains contact with the treatment area, a dressing, such as rolled gauze, may be used.
  – Because aerosolization of capsaicin can occur upon rapid removal of the patches, remove the patches gently and slowly by rolling the adhesive side inward.
  – After removal, generously apply cleansing gel to the treatment area and leave for at least 1 min to remove any residual capsaicin. Remove the cleansing gel with a dry wipe and gently wash the area with mild soap and water.
  – Pain and erythema are the most common side effects of the treatment which rapidly resolves after removal. If pain is intolerable, application of local cooling or administration of appropriate analgesic medications are effective. In clinical trials, increases in blood pressure occurred during or shortly after exposure to the patch. Changes averaged less than 100 mmHg and appeared to be related to the amount of pain experienced with application.

Botulinum Toxin

• FDA approved for the treatment of migraine headaches.
• BTX is most effective for headaches and cervical and periscapular pain.

- Procedure
  - Myobloc comes premixed at 5,000 u/ml. Botox and Dysport should be diluted with either saline or local anesthetic at a concentration of 100 or 300 u/ml. Solutions are placed in a 1-ml tuberculin syringe.
  - Most common injections are into the following muscles:
    - Frontalis
    - Procerus
    - Orbicularis oculi
    - Temporalis
    - Masseter
    - Occipitalis
    - Cervical paraspinous
    - Trapezius
    - Levator scapulae
    - Supra- and infraspinatus
    - Rhomboids
    - Scalene muscles
    - Sternocleidomastoid
  - Injections are distributed through the different muscle groups depending on the painful area. Injections can be made on 0.025–0.05 ml increments. For migraines, the most common muscles injected are the frontalis, procerus, orbicularis, and temporalis. If the pain includes the cervico-occipital region, the upper cervical paraspinous and occipitalis muscles can be injected. Injections can also be inserted throughout the scalp. If scalp injections are performed, it is recommended that the patients wash their hair with chlorhexidine-based soap prior to treatment.
  - 100 U, 300 U, and 5,000 U of Botox, Dysport, and Myobloc are usually sufficient doses that can be spread throughout the muscle groups. However, some patients may require up to twice the dose.
  - Complications include ptosis if the injection is too close to the upper orbital rim. Even with properly placed injections in the frontal region, some patients may get a transient ptosis due to aberrancies in the muscles that provide upper eyelid tone. Injections in the cervical region can result in transient neck weakness.

Future Directions

Neurolysis for the treatment of refractory cancer pain continues to be an effective option. However, given the nonspecificity and complications associated with currently available agents, there is a need for further research in the area. Intrathecal resiniferatoxin holds the greatest promise due to the high specificity for the unmyelinated C fibers that transmit pain. However, a side effect of this therapy may be the inability to detect thermal pain which could lead to thermal injuries. Therefore, patients will require close observation and counseling on this risk. Topical 20 % capsaicin solution that is painted on the painful area is currently in clinical trials with postherpetic neuralgia. It was recently announced that the phase II trial met the primary end point and further trials are planned. This trial was performed without pretreatment with topical lidocaine, and the participants tolerated the procedure well confirming that pretreatment with lidocaine is not indicated. The application time is only 5 min which is considerably shorter than the 1-h application of the patch.

References

1. Apfelbaum R, Cole CD, Liu J. Historical perspectives on the diagnosis and treatment of: evolution therapies for TN. Neurosurg Focus. 2005;18(5):E4.
2. Stookey R. Trigeminal neuralgia: its history and treatment. Springfield: Charles C. Thomas; 1959.
3. Haxton HA. Chemical sympathetectomy. Br Med J. 1949;1:1026–8.
4. Govind J, Bogduk N. Neurolytic blockade for noncancer pain. In: Balantyne J, Fishman SM, Rathmell JP, editors. Bonica's management of pain. Philadelphia: Lippincott Willam and Wilkins; 2010. p. 1467–14845.
5. Caterina MJ, Schumacher M, Tominaga M, Rosen TA, Levine JD, Julius D. The capsaicin receptor: a heat-activated ion channel in the pain pathway. Nature. 1997;389:816–24.
6. Szallasi A, Blumberg PM. Vanilloid (capsaicin) receptors and mechanisms. Pharmacol Rev. 1999;51:159–211.
7. Nolano M, Simone DA, Wendelschafer-Crabb G, Johnson T, Hazen E, Kennedy WR. Topical capsaicin in humans: parallel loss of epidermal nerve fibers and pain sensation. Pain. 1999;81:135–45.
8. Sb M. The consequence of long-term topical capsaicin application in the rat. Pain. 1991;44:301–10.
9. McMahon HT, Foran P, Dolly JO, et al. Tetanus toxin and botulinum toxins type A and B inhibit glutamate, gamma-aminobutyric acid, aspartate, and metenkephalin release from synaptosomes: clues to the locus of action. J Biol Chem. 1992;267:21338–43.
10. Bonica J. The management of pain. In: Bonica J, editor. Cancer pain, vol. 1. 2nd ed. Philadelphia: Lea and Febiger; 1990.
11. WHO Expert Committee. Cancer pain relief and palliative care. In: W.H. Organization, editor. WHO technical report series. Geneva: WHO; 1990.
12. Ventafridda V, et al. A validation study of the WHO method for cancer pain relief. Cancer. 1987;59(4):850–6.
13. Raj PP. Current review of pain. In: Baumble C, editor. Current medicine. Philadelphia: Current Medicine; 1994.
14. A Jacox, DB Carr, R Payne. AHCPR Clinical Practice Guidelines, No.9 Management of cancer pain. Rockville: Agency for Health Care Policy and Research (AHCPR); 1994.
15. Benzon H, editor. Raj's practical management of pain. 4th ed. Philadelphia: Mosby Elsevier; 2008.
16. Gallager SM, Yonezawa T, Hay R, Derrick W. Subarachnoid alcohol block II: histologic changes in the central nervous system. Am J Pathol. 1961;38(6):679–93.
17. Smith M. Histological findings following intrathecal injections of phenol solutions for relief of pain. Br J Anaesth. 1964;36(7):387–406.
18. Gelber DAM, Jeffery DR, editors. Clinical evaluation and management of spasticity. Totowa: Humana Press Inc.; 2002.

19. Jain SAG, Rakesh. Neural blockade with neurolytic agents. In: Waldman SM, editor. Pain Management. Saunders; Philadelphia, PA. 2006.

20. Waldman SM, editor. Pain management. 1st ed. Philadelphia: Saunders Elsevier; 2007. p. 343–8.

21. Thompson GE, et al. Abdominal pain and alcohol celiac plexus nerve block. Anesth Analg. 1977;56(1):1–5.

22. Raj PP, Denson DD. Neurolytic agents. In: Raj PP, editor. Clinical practice of regional anesthesia. New York: Churchill Livingstone; 1991. p. 135–52.

23. Miller RD, Johnston RR, Hosobuchi Y. Treatment of intercostal neuralgia with 10 per cent ammonium sulfate. J Thorac Cardiovasc Surg. 1975;69(3):476–8.

24. Hertl MC, et al. Intrafascicular injection of ammonium sulfate and bupivacaine in peripheral nerves of neonatal and juvenile rats. Reg Anesth Pain Med. 1998;23(2):152–8.

25. Kobayashi J, et al. The effect of ammonium sulfate injection on peripheral nerve. J Reconstr Microsurg. 1997;13(6):389–96.

26. Lucas JT, Ducker TB, Perot Jr PL. Adverse reactions to intrathecal saline injection for control of pain. J Neurosurg. 1975;42(5):557–61.

27. Hitchcock E, Prandini MN. Hypertonic saline in management of intractable pain. Lancet. 1973;1(7798):310–2.

28. Wong GY, Gavva NR. Therapeutic potential of vanilloid receptor TRPV1 agonists and antagonists as analgesics: recent advances and setbacks. Brain Res Rev. 2009;60(1):267–77.

29. Yoshimura N, Chancellor MB. Physiology and pharmacology of the bladder and urethra. In: Wein, editor. Wein: Campbell-Walsh urology. Saunders, And Imprint of Elsevier; Philadelphia, PA. 2007.

30. Vyklicky L, et al. Calcium-dependent desensitization of vanilloid receptor TRPV1: a mechanism possibly involved in analgesia induced by topical application of capsaicin. Physiol Res. 2008;57 Suppl 3:S59–68.

31. Mason L, et al. Systematic review of topical capsaicin for the treatment of chronic pain. BMJ. 2004;328(7446):991.

32. Backonja M, Wallace MS, Blonsky E, Culter B, Malan P, Rauck R, Tobias J. NGX-4010, a high-concentration capsaicin patch, for the treatment of postherpetic neuralgia: a randomized, double-blind study. Lancet Neurol. 2008;7(12):1106–12.

33. Simpson DM, et al. An open-label pilot study of high-concentration capsaicin patch in painful HIV neuropathy. J Pain Symptom Manage. 2008;35(3):299–306.

34. Simpson KH, et al. Comparison of extradural buprenorphine and extradural morphine after caesarean section. Br J Anaesth. 1988;60(6):627–31.

35. Brown DC, et al. Physiologic and antinociceptive effects of intrathecal resiniferatoxin in a canine bone cancer model. Anesthesiology. 2005;103(5):1052–9.

36. Chuang YC, et al. Intravesical botulinum toxin a administration produces analgesia against acetic acid induced bladder pain responses in rats. J Urol. 2004;172(4 Pt 1):1529–32.

37. Dressler D, Saberi FA, Barbosa ER. Botulinum toxin: mechanisms of action. Arq Neuropsiquiatr. 2005;63(1):180–5.

38. Schiavo G, et al. Tetanus and botulinum-B neurotoxins block neurotransmitter release by proteolytic cleavage of synaptobrevin. Nature. 1992;359(6398):832–5.

39. Stubblefield MD, et al. The role of botulinum toxin type A in the radiation fibrosis syndrome: a preliminary report. Arch Phys Med Rehabil. 2008;89(3):417–21.

40. Luvisetto S, et al. Anti-allodynic efficacy of botulinum neurotoxin A in a model of neuropathic pain. Neuroscience. 2007;145(1): 1–4.

41. FDA. Information for healthcare professionals: OnabotulinumtoxinA (marketed as Botox/Botox Cosmetic), AbobotulinumtoxinA (Marketed as Dysport), and RimabotulinumtoxinB (marketed as Myoblock). In: U.S.D.o.H.a.H. Services, editor. http://www.fda.gov/Drugs/DrugSafety/PostmarketDrugSafetyInformationforPatientsandProviders/DrugSafetyInformationforHeathcareProfessionals/ucm174949.htm#.UBpVp-WBYTc.email FDA ALERT 08/2009.

42. FDA. Early communication about an ongoing safety review of botox and botox cosmetic (Botulinum toxin type A) and Myobloc (Botulinum toxin type B). In: U.S.D.o.H.a.H. Services, editor. http://www.fda.gov/Drugs/DrugSafety/PostmarketDrugSafetyInformationforPatientsandProviders/DrugSafetyInformationforHeathcareProfessionals/ucm143819.htm 4/2009.

43. Raj PP, editor. Textbook of regional anesthesia. Philadelphia: Churchhill Livingstone; An Imprint of Elsevier Science; 2002.

44. Waldman SD. Lumbar subarachnoid neurolytic block. In: Atlas of interventional pain management. 2nd ed. Philadelphia: Saunders; 2004. p. 529–30.

45. Waldman SD. Lumbar subarachnoid neurolytic block. In: Atlas of interventional pain management. 2nd ed. Philadelphia: Saunders; 2004. p. 531–2.

46. Lou L, Raj PP, Erdine S, Staats P, Waldman S, Racz G, Hammer M, Niv D, Ruiz-Lopez R, Heavner J, editors. Interventional pain management: image-guided procedures. 2nd ed. Philadelphia: Saunders Elsevier; 2008.

47. Lam VY, Wallace M, Schulteis G. Effects of lidocaine patch on intradermal capsaicin induced pain: a double-blind, controlled trial. J Pain. 2011;12(3):323–30.

Cryoanalgesia

25

Michael S. Leong, Philip S. Kim, and Lloyd Saberski

Key Points

Advantages

- Long history of analgesic treatment
- Treats nociceptive, neuropathic, and sympathetic maintained pain – coccydynia
- Produces Wallerian degeneration but leaves myelin sheath and endoneurium intact
- Anesthetic in treatment
- Low incidence of neuritis

Disadvantages

- Setup time for machine can be lengthy.
- Probe with introducer (up to 12 fr) can be large.
- Requires a separate nerve stimulator to test sensory and motor stimulation.
- Probe is not curved.

Future uses

- May be useful as office procedure for peripheral neuralgias
- Ultrasound guidance procedures with less sedation
- Randomization of cryoanalgesia with pulsed radio frequency

M.S. Leong, M.D.
Stanford Pain Medicine Center,
450 Broadway Street, Redwood City, CA 94063, USA

Department of Anesthesiology,
Stanford University School of Medicine,
Stanford, CA, USA
e-mail: msleong@stanford.edu

P.S. Kim, M.D.
Center for Interventional Pain & Spine,
Newark, DE and Bryn Mawr, PA, USA
e-mail: phshkim@yahoo.com

L. Saberski, M.D. (✉)
Advanced Diagnostic Pain Treatment Centers,
One Long Wharf, Ste 212, New Haven, CT 06511, USA
e-mail: lsaberski@ihurt.com

Introduction

Cryoanalgesia is an interventional pain therapy that seems less popular than newer techniques, such as pulsed radio-frequency ablation. Many studies show efficacy in multiple acute and chronic pain conditions. From a patient's perspective, cryoanalgesia or "freezing" of the nerves makes sense since they routinely use ice as a passive treatment modality. In this era of practice, with increasing emphasis on durability of treatment during repeated blocks as well as concern for long-term side effects (steroid effects, neuritis from continuous radio frequency, cryoanalgesia), the authors will present an introduction to this valuable pain management technique and suggest its integration into current clinical practice.

History

Cryoanalgesia is truly a cross-cultural pain treatment option through two millennia. Cryoanalgesia is a technique in which cold is applied to produce pain relief. The analgesic effect of cold has been known to humans for more than two millennia [1]. Hippocrates (460–377 B.C.) provided the first written record of the use of ice and snow packs applied before surgery as a local pain-relieving technique [2]. Early physicians, such as Avicenna of Persia (980–1070 A.D.) and Severino of Naples (1580–1656), recorded using cold for preoperative analgesia [3, 4]. In 1812, Napoleon's surgeon general, Baron Dominique Jean Larrey [5], recognized that the limbs of soldiers frozen in the Prussian snow could be amputated relatively painlessly. In 1751, Arnott [6] described using an ice-salt mixture to produce tumor regression and to obtain an anesthetic and hemostatic effect. Richardson introduced ether spray in 1766 to produce local analgesia by refrigeration; this was superseded in 1790 by ethyl chloride spray.

Modern interest in cryoanalgesia was sparked in 1961, after Cooper described a cryotherapy unit in which liquid nitrogen was circulated through a hollow metal probe that was vacuum insulated except at the tip. With this equipment, it was possible to control the temperature of the tip by interrupting the flow of liquid nitrogen at temperatures within the range of room temperature to −196 °C. Because the system was totally enclosed, cold could be applied to any part of the body accessible to the probe. The first clinical application of this technique was in neurosurgery for treatment of parkinsonism [7, 8]. In 1967, Amoils [9] developed a simpler handheld unit that used carbon dioxide or nitrous oxide. These devices were the prototypes for the current generation of cryoprobes used in cryoanalgesia. The coldest temperature applied today is approximately −70 °C.

Physics and Cellular Effects

Modern cryoneurolysis uses controlled cooling via the expansion of highly pressurized and compressed gas (nitrous oxide or carbon dioxide) through a narrow slit aperture. Cryoprobes are available in various sizes but with the same basic design: an inner and outer tube with outer insulation, except at the probe tip [9]. Gas under high pressure (650–800 psig) passes between the two tubes and is released through a small orifice into the chamber of the tip of the probe [10]. Compressed gas expands as it passes through the orifice, resulting in a rapid decrease in temperature at the probe tip (the Joule-Thomson effect). Absorption of heat from the surrounding tissues accompanies gas expansion and leads to the formation of an ice ball [10] by freezing of intracellular and extracellular water. Gas from the inner tube escapes and is scavenged through a ventilated outlet. The "closed-system" construction of the machine and probes allows for no gas to escape from the probe tip handle and the machine.

The rapid cooling at the tip results in temperatures of approximately −70 °C. Ice balls vary in size as a function of probe size, freeze time, tissue permeability to water, and presence of vascular "heat sinks." Modern cryoprobes develop ice balls approximately 3.5–5.5 mm in diameter.

Precise levels of gas flow are necessary for safe and effective cryoneurolysis. Inadequate gas flow will not result in tissue freezing, whereas excessive gas flow may result in freezing up to the stem of the probe with the potential for cold skin burns. Modern insulated cryoprobes and cryotherapy units have the ability for discriminative stimulation of sensory and motor nerves. Locating the precise "pain generator" with nerve stimulation is necessary because the size of the ice ball that can be generated may be large and can freeze other nontargeted tissues and nerves.

Histologically, the axons and myelin sheaths degenerate after cryolesioning (Wallerian degeneration), but the epineurium and perineurium remain intact, thus allowing subsequent nerve regeneration. The duration of the block is a function of the rate of axonal regeneration after cryolesioning, which is reported to be 1–3 mm/day [7]. Because axonal regrowth is constant, the return of sensory and motor activity is a function of the distance between the cryolesion and the end organ [1]. The absence of external damage to the nerve and the minimal inflammatory reaction to freezing ensure that regeneration is exact. The regenerating axons are unlikely to form painful neuromas. (Surgical and thermal lesions interrupt perineurium and epineurium.) Other neurolytic techniques (alcohol, phenol) potentially can produce painful residual neuromas because the epineurium and perineurium are disrupted, so regrowth is disordered.

A cryolesion provides a temporary anesthetic block. Clinically, a cryoblock lasts weeks to months. The result depends on numerous variables, including operator technique and clinical circumstances. The analgesia often lasts longer than the time required for axons to regenerate [11]. The reasons are still a matter of speculation, but it is obvious that cryoanalgesia is more than just a temporary disruption of axons. Possibly, sustained blockade of afferent input to the central nervous system (CNS) has an effect on CNS windup. One report suggested that cryolesions release sequestered tissue protein or facilitate changes in protein antigenic properties [7]. The result is an autoimmune response targeted at cryolesioned tissue. The first report of such a response was from Gander et al. [12] who showed tissue-specific autoantibodies after cryocoagulation of male rabbit accessory glands. This report was followed by a parallel clinical report of regression of metastatic deposits from prostatic adenocarcinoma after cryocoagulation of the primary tumor [13]. The significance for pain management is unclear; however, it does indicate that tumor growth and regression are affected by immune function. It is possible that immune mechanisms play a role in the analgesic response after cryoablation.

Indications and Contraindications

Cryoanalgesia can produce pain relief for weeks to months. Treatment does not permanently injure the nerves, and axonal regeneration is typical.

The median duration of pain relief is 2 weeks to 5 months [14, 15]. Cryoanalgesia is best suited for painful conditions that originate from small, well-localized lesions of peripheral nerves (e.g., neuromas, entrapment neuropathies, and postoperative pain) [11]. Longer than expected periods of analgesia has been reported and may result from the patient's ability to participate more fully in physical therapy or from an effect of prolonged analgesia on central processing of pain (preemptive analgesic effect). Sustained blockade of afferent impulses [16–19] with cryoanalgesia may reduce plasticity (windup) in the CNS and may decrease pain permanently [20].

Patient should be aware that the treatment entry site may be exposed to cryoanalgesia, especially if the probe or targeted region is superficial. Subsequently, numbness at the site of entry and possible skin depigmentation can occur if the ice ball frosts the skin.

Indications

- Focal peripheral nerves: neuromas, entrapment neuropathies
- Sympathetic maintained pain
- Postoperative pain

Contraindications

- Bleeding diathesis
- Local and systemic infection
- Patient consent

Pain Conditions

- Postoperative pain
- Post-herniorrhaphy (ilioinguinal nerve)
- Post-thoracotomy (intercostal nerves)
- Post-tonsillectomy (glossopharyngeal nerves)
- Chronic pain
- Facial pain syndromes
- Neuromas
- Intercostal neuralgia
- Facet arthropathy (cervical and lumbar)
- Interspinous ligaments
- Superior cluneal neuralgia
- Superior gluteal neuralgia
- Coccydynia
- Perineal pain
- Neuralgias of the groin (ilioinguinal, iliohypogastric, genitofemoral)
- Lower extremity neuralgias

Patient Preparation

The process of informed consent consists of discussing risk and benefits and specific contraindications to cryoneurolysis. Next, the cryoprobes are purged and machine checked. The patient is prepared under sterile conditions and is kept awake in order to determine location of pain generator by palpation and/or stimulation. Sensory and motor stimulations are then performed to identify the pain generator. Acceptable sensory stimulation thresholds are less than 0.4 mV. Motor stimulation should be 1.5 times greater than the sensory threshold.

Cryoneurolysis is then performed using 3–4-min freeze cycles with 30-s thaw periods in between. During the thaw period, sensory stimulation should be performed to check the success of the initial freeze. Two or three additional freezes are then performed with 30-s thaw periods in between.

Postoperative Pain Control

Post-thoracotomy Pain

Intraoperative intercostal cryoneurolysis was first reported by Nelson in 1974 [21]. The treatment of intercostal nerves on each side of the thoracotomy incision makes sense to lesion. Initial retrospective studies showed significant efficacy, even up to 3 months after treatment. Unfortunately, a randomized study comparing epidural analgesia and intercostal nerve cryoanalgesia by Ju in 2008 [22] suggested a troubling side effect of allodynia-like pain for the cryoanalgesia group. Mustola in 2011 [23] confirmed these findings for a smaller group. Subsequently, the authors do not recommend intraoperative cryoanalgesia for postoperative pain management.

Post-herniorrhaphy Pain

Cryoneurolysis after herniorrhaphy was first described by Wood et al. in 1979 [24]. A cryolesion of the ilioinguinal nerve reduced analgesic requirements during the postoperative period. The follow-up study in 1981 compared recovery from herniorrhaphy among three study groups: patients treated with oral analgesics, patients undergoing cryoanalgesia, and patients receiving paravertebral blockade (the last two treatments supplemented with oral analgesics as needed). The study indicated that the cryoanalgesia group not only had less pain in the postoperative period but also used less opioid, resumed a regular diet earlier, were mobilized faster, and returned to work sooner [25]. Despite these successes, the technique is not widely used. Given its effectiveness and freedom from side effects, it is ideal for ambulatory surgery. After repair of the internal ring, posterior wall of the inguinal canal, and internal oblique muscle, the ilioinguinal nerve on the surface of the muscle is identified and mobilized. The surgeon elevates the nerve above the muscle, and an assistant performs the cryoablation.

Chronic Pain Management Technique: Tips for Best Placement

Cryoanalgesia utilizes an introducer technique to place the tip of the probe in the closest proximity to the targeted nerve. The introducers are large-bored intravenous catheters, usually 14 or 16 ga but as large as 12 ga to accommodate the cryoprobe. The cryoprobe must be placed in a linear manner, and the tip cannot be curved due to the mechanism of the multiple treatment tubes carrying the nitrous oxide gas. The cryoprobe tip must be close enough to the targeted nerve to create a full ice ball and must extend far enough outside of the introducer catheter. Of course, regional anesthesia anatomy is imperative for the practitioner to place the cryoprobe appropriately and efficiently.

Several techniques are used to enhance precise placement of the cryoprobe, as follows:

1. Careful palpation with a small blunt instrument, such as a felt-tipped pen, can help to localize a soft tissue neuroma or another palpable pain generator.
2. An image intensifier (fluoroscopy) can identify bony landmarks.
3. Contrast medium improves definition of tissue planes, capsules, and spaces. (Nonionic contrast medium should be used in areas close to neural tissue.)
4. The nerve stimulator at the tip of the cryoprobe is used to produce a muscle twitch in a mixed nerve. The stimulator is set at 5 Hz for recruitment of motor fibers. The probe is closest to the nerve when the lowest output produces a twitch response. In general, twitches should occur at 0.5–1.5 V. Small sensory branches contain no motor component and do not twitch with electrical stimulation. These fibers are localized by using higher-frequency (100-Hz) stimulation, which produces overlapping dysesthesia in the distribution of the small sensory nerve. This procedure may reproduce the patient's pain. Use of low-output (<0.5–1.5 V) stimulation ensures closer placement of the cryoprobe to the nerve in question. The operator freezes the nerve for 2–3 min. Often, the patient has discomfort initially as cooling begins, but it should dissipate quickly. If significant pain persists beyond 30 s, the operator should investigate whether the ice ball is in the proper position. (If the ice ball is not sufficiently close to the nerve, and only partial freezing occurs, mostly of larger myelinated fibers, unchecked unmyelinated fiber input is left. This theoretically accounts for increased pain.) The brief cooling already may have altered nerve function, in which case, if positioning of the probe depends on feedback from the patient, it could be impeded. Before moving the probe, the operator must be sure to thaw the tip to prevent tissue damage from ice ball adherence to the tissues. In general, with closed procedures, two freeze cycles of 2 min each, followed by thaw cycles, are sufficient. In areas with a large vascular heat sink, longer periods of cryotherapy are necessary. Pain relief should be immediate and should be assessed subjectively and by physical examination while the patient is on the procedure table. All relevant clinical information should be recorded in the medical record.

A hard-copy radiograph should be obtained for most procedures when a fluoroscope is used.

Facial Neuralgias

Craniofacial nerves can be cryolesioned with a percutaneous or open technique [26, 27]. Entrapment neuropathies and neuromas are more responsive to local anesthetic and cryodenervations than neuropathies of medical causes. Meticulous diagnostic injection ensures the best outcome with cryoablation [15]. If the patient has a good analgesic response to a series of local anesthetic injections, cryodenervation is an option. The technique of cryodenervations of cranial and facial nerves is the same as that for other peripheral nerves. A nerve stimulator is used to localize the nerve. Because these areas are densely vascular, injecting a few milliliters of saline solution containing 1:100,000 epinephrine is recommended before inserting the cryoprobe introducer cannula. A post-procedural ice pack applied for 30 min reduces pain and swelling.

Irritative neuropathy of the *supraorbital nerve* often occurs at the supraorbital notch [27]. Vulnerable to blunt trauma, this nerve often is injured by deceleration against an automobile windshield. Commonly confused with migraine and frontal sinusitis, the pain of supraorbital neuralgia often manifests as a throbbing frontal headache. At times, many of the hallmarks of vascular headache are present, including blurred vision, nausea, and photophobia. This neuralgia often worsens over time, perhaps owing to scar formation around the nerve.

Neuropathic pain in the distribution of the supraorbital nerve can be addressed with an open or closed cryoablative procedure as long as appropriate conservative therapy has failed and the pain responds to a series of test local anesthetic injections. For an open procedure, the incision is buried beneath the eyebrow, so the patient has no obvious scar. For the percutaneous technique, the introducer catheter should be inserted at the eyebrow line to avoid damage to hair follicles.

The *infraorbital nerve* is the termination of the second division of the trigeminal nerve. Irritative neuropathy can occur at the infraorbital foramen secondary to blunt trauma or fracture of the zygoma with entrapment of the nerve in the bony callus. Commonly confused with maxillary sinusitis, the pain of infraorbital neuralgia most often is exacerbated by smiling and laughing. Referred pain to the teeth is common, and a history of dental pain and dental procedures is typical. Cryoablation can be accomplished by an open or closed technique. The closed technique can be performed from inside the mouth through the superior buccolabial fold. In both operations, the probe is advanced until it lies over the infraorbital foramen. The intraoral approach has cosmetic advantages only.

The *mandibular nerve* can be irritated at many locations along its path. It is often injured as the result of hypertrophy of the pterygoids secondary to chronic bruxism, but it also can be irritated if the vertical dimension of the oral cavity is reduced owing to tooth loss or altered dentition. Pain is often referred to the lower teeth, and patients frequently undergo dental evaluations and procedures.

Injury to the *mental nerve*, the terminal portion of the mandibular nerve, frequently occurs in edentulous patients. Pain can be reproduced easily with palpation.

The *auriculotemporal nerve* can be irritated at many sites, including immediately proximal to the parietal ridge at the attachment of the temporalis muscle and, less commonly, at the ramus of the mandible. Patients often present with temporal pain associated with retro-orbital pain. Pain often is referred to the teeth. Patients frequently awaken at night with temporal headache. The pain, described as throbbing, aching, and pounding, can be bilateral, and it is commonly associated with bruxism and functional abnormalities of the temporomandibular joint, maxilla, and mandible. The clinician must rule out other medical causes for this form of headache, including temporal arteritis, before considering treatments for auriculotemporal neuralgia. Posterior auricular neuralgia often follows blunt injury to the mastoid area. It is common in abused women and usually involves the left side owing to the preponderance of right-handed abusers. The clinical presentation consists of pain in the ear associated with a feeling of "fullness" and tenderness. This syndrome often is misdiagnosed as a chronic ear infection. The posterior auricular nerve runs along the posterior border of the sternocleidomastoid muscle, superficially and immediately posterior to the mastoid.

The *glossopharyngeal nerve* lies immediately subjacent to the tonsillar fossa. This painful condition can be treated by applying the cryoprobe for two cycles of 2 min each after local anesthetic injections have produced the appropriate responses. This is essentially a simple procedure, but it has distinct advantages over injection of this cranial nerve at the tip of the mastoid, where injection could block the vagus nerve in addition to the spinal accessory nerves [26].

Many other common peripheral nerve injuries are amenable to cryodenervation, including most cutaneous branches and the occipital, suprascapular, superficial radial, and anterior penetrating branches of the intercostal nerves. Applied carefully, the techniques outlined in this chapter help to achieve the safest and the best possible outcomes.

Intercostal Neuralgia

Percutaneous cryolesions of the intercostal nerves can be offered for various pain syndromes, including post-thoracotomy pain, traumatic intercostal neuralgia, rib fracture pain, and occasionally postherpetic neuropathy. For each of these conditions, a meticulous series of local anesthetic blocks are performed before consideration is given to cryoablation. The volume of local anesthetic should be kept to less than 3–4 ml to prevent tracking back into the epidural space. In addition, only two or three levels should be injected at any one time because systemic absorption could confound interpretation of the patient's response. Because the intercostal nerve runs with a large arterial and venous heat source, the use of two 4-min cryolesions at each level is suggested. The lesions should be made proximal to the pain at the inferior border of the rib. After the procedure, a chest film is obtained to check for pneumothorax. Effective blockade in some patients with postherpetic neuropathy suggests that this pain condition can have peripheral afferent input, as opposed to being strictly a central neuropathy.

A recent small retrospective study by Moore in 2010 [28] for CT-guided percutaneous cryoneurolysis for post-thoracotomy syndrome showed efficacy, but no allodynic syndrome was seen in the open-cryotherapy studies.

Neuromas

Cryoanalgesia seems the most effective when prior diagnostic blocks have mapped out a discrete pain generator. Initial test local anesthetic injections should contain 1 ml or less per site for the optimal benefit of cryoanalgesia. Either lidocaine or bupivacaine is typically injected with the patient's response and duration of analgesia recorded, sometimes longer than the duration of the local anesthetic. If the neuroma is successfully targeted, cryoanalgesia at this site could be a successful option.

Facet Arthropathy

Cryoanalgesia utilizes the same approach as typical facet and medial branch blocks also detailed in this textbook. Lumbar facet cryodenervations are performed at three levels similar to radio-frequency techniques. A 12 ga introducer catheter is introduced to the junction of the transverse process and the pedicle, the Scottie dog's eye. After sensory and motor testing via a nerve stimulator, two cryolesions are made, each for 2 min duration. Cervical facet cryodenervations are performed in the same manner as the initial diagnostic blocks, either in a prone or lateral manner.

Interspinous Ligament Pain

Interspinous ligament pain is common after a spine operation (lumbar, thoracic, or cervical). Pain impulses from interspinous ligaments are carried by the medial branch of the posterior ramus. Patients report severe movement-related spine pain, identified to the midline, which is worsened with hyperextension and relieved by small volumes of local anesthetic injected into the interspinous ligament. When cervical interspinous ligaments are involved, the patient frequently complains of posterior cervical headache. This headache often is mistaken for occipital neuralgia. Cryodenervation can be considered in local anesthetic responsive patients. The pain relief helps the patient to complete the necessary course of physical therapy.

Coccydynia

When coccygodynia has failed to respond to conservative therapy, including the patient's use of a donut pillow, NSAIDs, and local steroid injections, consideration can be given to coccygeal neural blockade as the coccygeal nerve exits from the sacral canal at the level of the cornu. Bilateral test injections should produce short-term analgesia before cryoablation is considered. For cryoablation of the coccygeal nerve, the probe must be inserted into the canal to make contact with the nerve. Accurate placement of the ice ball is facilitated by using the 100-Hz stimulator and gauging the patient's response. Care should be taken to prevent bending the relatively large cryoprobe while inserting it into the canal.

Perineal Pain

Pain over the dorsal surface of the scrotum, perineum, and anus that has not responded to conservative management at times can be managed effectively with cryodenervation from inside the sacral canal with bilateral S4 lesions. Test local anesthetic injections should produce a positive response before cryoablations are performed bilaterally at S4. Inserting the cryoprobe through the sacral hiatus up to the level of the fourth sacral foramen for placement of a series of cryolesions can provide good analgesia. Bladder dysfunction usually is not encountered, and analgesia lasts 6–8 weeks. Perineal pain is difficult to treat with intrathecal neurolytic agents without risking bladder and bowel dysfunction.

Ilioinguinal, iliohypogastric, and genitofemoral neuropathies often complicate herniorrhaphy, general abdominal surgery, and cesarean section. Patients present with sharp, lancinating to dull pain radiating into the lower abdomen or groin. The pain is exacerbated by lifting and defecating. If the patient is responsive to a series of low-volume test injections, consideration can be given to cryodenervation of the appropriate nerve. Significant care and time must be spent localizing the nerve with the sensory nerve stimulator. The patient may help to localize the pain generator by pointing with one finger to the point of maximum tenderness. These

nerves are difficult to localize percutaneously, and that difficulty has led to frequent misdiagnosis of the pain generator. In an effort to improve the accuracy of diagnosis, Rosser et al. [29] developed the *conscious pain mapping* technique. In a lightly sedated patient, a general surgeon working with a pain management specialist performs laparoscopic evaluation of the abdomen in an operating suite. The genitofemoral nerve, lateral femoral cutaneous nerve, and other structures are easily visualized. Blunt probing and patient feedback help to direct the physician to the area of pain. At times, objects such as ligatures and staples are found wrapped around the nerve, in which case they should be removed. If direct mechanical or electrical stimulation to the nerve reproduces the pain, cryoablation can be performed under direct vision. (Cryoablation is chosen as the appropriate test because the effect of bupivacaine does not outlast the discomfort of the perioperative period. The cryoblockade provides weeks to months of reliable analgesia and helps physicians and patients to determine whether that structure under surveillance carried the pain information.) Pain usually returns. A repeat cryoablation is possible when analgesia is long or an open surgical procedure with sectioning and burying can be performed.

Lower Extremity Pain

Many cutaneous nerve branches are responsive to cryodenervation. The clinician always must perform a complete physical examination, with careful touching of the painful area. After the primary pain generator is localized, a series of low-volume local anesthetic injections can be given. If the patient has a consistent response, cryodenervations, as outlined earlier, can be employed. Some common lower extremity nerve pain syndromes that are often amenable to cryodenervation are described next.

Neuralgia resulting from irritation of the *infrapatellar branch of the saphenous nerve* develops weeks to years after blunt injury to the tibial plateau or after knee replacement. The nerve is vulnerable as it passes superficial to the tibial collateral ligament, pierces the sartorius tendon and fascia lata, and runs inferior and medial to the tibial condyle. The clinical presentation consists of dull pain in the knee joint and achiness below the knee. Patients tend to adopt an antalgic gait. Pain with digital pressure is diagnostic. Patients are considered candidates for cryodenervation when they respond consistently to local anesthetic blocks. A 12-gauge intravenous catheter is used as the introducer to prevent cold injury to the skin. Because prodding with a felt-tipped pen alone is sufficient to localize the pain generator, the sensory nerve stimulator does not have to be used.

Neuralgia secondary to irritation of the *deep and superficial peroneal and intermediate dorsal cutaneous nerves* can be seen weeks to years after injury to the foot and ankle. These superficial sensory nerves pass through strong ligamentous structures and are vulnerable to stretch injury with inversion of the ankle, compression injury owing to edema, and penetrating trauma from bone fragments. The intermediate dorsal cutaneous nerve runs superficial and medial to the lateral malleolus, continues superficial to the inferior extensor retinaculum, and terminates in the fourth and fifth toes. This nerve is particularly vulnerable to injury after sprains of the lateral ankle. The clinical presentation consists of dull ankle pain that is worse with passive inversion of the ankle. Disproportionate swelling, vasomotor instability, and allodynia are remarkably common. Patients tend to adjust their gait to minimize weight bearing on the lateral aspect of the foot. Pain with digital pressure in the area between the lateral malleolus and extensor retinaculum is diagnostic.

Peroneal Nerve

Superficial and deep peroneal nerve injury often occurs in diabetic patients, who are vulnerable to compression injury from tight-fitting shoes, and is less common after blunt injury to the dorsum of the foot. The clinical presentation consists of dull pain in the great toe that is often worse after prolonged standing. Patients tend to adjust their gait to minimize weight bearing on the anterior portion of the foot. Pain with digital pressure in the area between the first and second metatarsal heads is often diagnostic.

Superior Gluteal Nerve

Neuralgia resulting from irritation of the superior gluteal branch of the sciatic nerve is common after injury to the lower back and hip sustained while lifting. After exiting the sciatic notch, the superior gluteal nerve passes caudal to the inferior border of the gluteus minimus and penetrates the gluteus medius. Vulnerable as it passes in the fascial plane between the gluteus medius and gluteus minimus musculature, the superior gluteal nerve is injured as a result of shearing between the gluteal muscles on forced external rotation of the leg and with extension of the hip under mechanical load. Rarely, it is injured by forced extension of the hip, an injury that may occur in a head-on automobile collision when the foot is pressed against the floorboards with the knee in extension as the patient braces for impact. The clinical presentation consists of sharp pain in the lower back, dull pain in the buttock, and vague pain to the popliteal fossa. Pain below the knee is unusual. Patients generally experience pain with prolonged sitting, leaning forward, or twisting to the contralateral side. Often, patients describe "giving way" of the leg. They usually sit with the weight on the contralateral buttock or cross their legs to minimize pressure on the involved side. With the patient in the prone position, the medial border of the ilium is palpated. The nerve is located 5 cm lateral and inferior to the attachment of the gluteus medius. The peripheral nerve stimulator is employed to ensure that motor units are not inadvertently blocked.

Future Directions

Cryotechnology offers potential analgesia for many different pain conditions both acute and chronic. Its effective and safe use on sensory and mixed nerves contrasts with radio-frequency technology, which has the potential to produce deafferentation pain syndromes particularly with continuous wave applied to peripheral nerves. The lack of controlled studies, the lack of uniform training, and the poor communication to referrers and patients have impeded widespread use of the technology. The application of ultrasound technology may expand the use of cryoanalgesia, with visualization helping the placement of the cryoprobe on larger nerves such as the intercostal nerves [30]. One area of interest could include a randomized study of cryotherapy compared to pulsed radio-frequency ablation for analgesia for peripheral neuropathies measuring efficacy and duration of effect. Given the long record for safety and the population's general acceptance of ice/cold-based therapies, cryoanalgesia could be revitalized for the future pain medicine providers.

References

1. Evans P. Cryo-analgesia: the application of low temperatures to nerves to produce anesthesia or analgesia. Anaesthesia. 1981;36:1003.
2. Hippocrates. Aphorisms, Heraclitus on the universe, vol. 4. London: Heinemann; 1931.
3. Gruner O. A treatise on the canon of medicine of Avicenna. London: Luzac; 1930.
4. Bartholini T. De nivis usu medico observationes variae, hafniae. Copenhagen: P. Haubold; 1661.
5. Larrey D. Surgical memoirs of the campaigns of Russia, Germany and France. Philadelphia: Carey and Lea; 1832.
6. Arnott J. On severe cold or congelation as a remedy of disease. London: Medical Gazette; 1748. p. 936.
7. Holden HB. Practical cryosurgery. London: Pitman; 1975. p. 2.
8. Cooper IS. Cryosurgery in modern medicine. J Neurol Sci. 1965;2:493.
9. Amoils SP. The Joule-Thomson cryoprobe. Arch Ophthalmol. 1978;78:201.
10. Evans P, Lloyd J, Green C. Cryo-analgesia: the response to alterations in freeze cycle temperature. Br J Anaesth. 1981;53:1121.
11. Peuria M, Krmpotic-Nemanic J, Markiewitz A. Tunnel syndromes. Boca Raton: CRC Press; 1991.
12. Gander MJ, Soanes WA, Smith V. Experimental prostate surgery. Invest Urol. 1964;1:610.

13. Soanes WA, Ablin RJ, Gander MJ. Remission of metastatic lesions following cryosurgery in prostatic cancer: immunologic considerations. J Urol. 1970;104:154.

14. Lloyd J, Barnard J, Glynn C. Cryo-analgesia: a new approach to pain relief. Lancet. 1976;2:932.

15. Barnard J, Lloyd J, Glynn C. Cryosurgery in the management of intractable facial pain. Br J Oral Surg. 1978;16:135.

16. Wall PD. The prevention of postoperative pain. Pain. 1988;33:289.

17. Armitage EN. Postoperative pain: prevention or relief? Br J Anaesth. 1989;63:136.

18. Cousins MJ. Acute pain and injury response: immediate and prolonged effects. Reg Anaesth. 1989;14:162.

19. McQuay HJ, Carroll D, Moore RA. Postoperative orthopedic pain: the effect of opiate premedication and local anesthetic blocks. Pain. 1988;33:291.

20. Woolf CJ, Wall PD. Morphine sensitive and insensitive actions of C-fibre input on the rat spinal cords. Neurosci Lett. 1986;64:221.

21. Nelson KM, Vincent RG, Bourke RS, Smith DE, Blakeley WR, Kaplan RJ, Pollay M. Intraoperative intercostal nerve freezing to prevent postthoracotomy pain. Ann Thorac Surg. 1974;18(3):280–5.

22. Ju H, Feng Y, Yang BX, Wang J. Comparison of epidural analgesia and intercostal nerve cryoanalgesia for post-thoracotomy pain control. Eur J Pain. 2008;12(3):378–84.

23. Mustola ST, Lempinen J, Saimanen E, Vilkko P. Efficacy of thoracic epidural analgesia with or without intercostal nerve cryoanalgesia for postthoracotomy pain. Ann Thorac Surg. 2011; 91(3):869–73.

24. Wood G, Lloyd J, Bullingham R, et al. Postoperative analgesia for day case herniorrhaphy patients: a comparison of cryo-analgesia, paravertebral blockade and oral analgesia. Anaesthesia. 1981; 36:603.

25. Wood G, Lloyd J, Evans P, et al. Cryo-analgesia and day case herniorrhaphy [letter]. Lancet. 1979;2:479.

26. Raj P. Practical management of pain. Chicago: Yearbook; 1986. p. 777.

27. Klein DS, Schmidt RE. Chronic headache resulting from postoperative supraorbital neuralgia. Anesth Analg. 1991;73:490.

28. Moore W, Kolnick D, Tan J, Yu HS. CT guided percutaneous cryoneurolysis for post thoracotomy pain syndrome: early experience and effectiveness. Acad Radiol. 2010;17(5):603–6. Epub 2010 Mar 15.

29. Rosser JC, Goodwin M, Gabriel NH, Saberski L. The use of minilaparoscopy for conscious pain mapping. Tech Reg Anesth Pain Manag. 2001;5(4):152–6.

30. Byas-Smith MG, Gulati A. Ultrasound-guided intercostal nerve cryoablation. Anesth Analg. 2006;103:1033–5.

Radiofrequency: Conventional and Pulsed

26

Maunak V. Rana

Key Points

- Radiofrequency uses an insulated needle with electrode and thermocouple to provide a precise controlled temperature lesion.
- The setup of a radiofrequency circuit [4–6] involves a generator to produce and drive the energy, a dispersive pad (grounding plate) to return energy to the generator, and an insulated introducer needle with an electrode and thermocouple to provide a precise, controlled temperature lesion.
- The exact mechanism of pulsed radiofrequency is unclear; however, pulsed radiofrequency is a *neuromodulatory* treatment option as opposed to the *ablative* conventional radiofrequency.
- Evidence exists for the routine use of CRF for treating pain due to trigeminal neuralgia and zygapophyseal joint pathology. Present data indicates that the benefit after pulsed radiofrequency may not be as long lasting when compared to conventional radiofrequency.
- Further investigations are warranted into the mechanism of PRF before disposing of this procedure as a viable technology.

Introduction

Radiofrequency technology, the manipulation of electrical energy to produce a desired clinical effect, has been utilized in various settings, including pain management, electrocar-

M.V. Rana, M.D.
Department of Anesthesiology, Chicago Anesthesia Pain Specialists,
Advocate Illinois Masonic Medical Center,
Chicago, IL, USA

University of Illinois at Chicago Medical Center,
Chicago, IL, USA

836 W. Wellington Avenue, 4815, Chicago, IL 60657, USA
e-mail: maunakr@gmail.com

diology [1], and oncology [2]. In the pain management universe, radiofrequency energy has been utilized for many indications; however, the treatment of cervical facet syndrome, lumbar facet syndrome, and sacroiliac discomfort [3–5] is the most common application for this technology. Pulsed radiofrequency (PRF) is a relatively recent [4] entity designed to provide the benefit of conventional radiofrequency (CRF) with a decrease in side-effect profile.

Physics of Radiofrequency

Before undertaking a discussion of radiofrequency, certain concepts of physics applicable to this technology must be reviewed to understand the technology. *Current* is the transfer of energy from an electrical source and is measured in hertz (Hz); *voltage* (volts) is the force that drives the current; *impedance* (ohms) is the resistance to the flow of current.

These concepts are represented by the following equation:

$$V = I \times R$$

where V is voltage, I is current, and R is impedance.

CRF involves controlled administration of alternating current electrical energy at 500 kHz (kilocycle/s) range. Current is utilized at the kilocycle Hz range, as alternating current (AC) at a lower frequency would be very painful in clinical use [6]. Direct current is not utilized in this radiofrequency technology as the frequency of this energy is zero and would lead to less precision during lesion formation.

The setup of a radiofrequency circuit [4–6] involves a generator to produce and drive the energy, a dispersive pad (grounding plate) to return energy to the generator, an insulated introducer needle to prevent dispersal of energy outside of the targeted area, and an electrode with a thermocouple to provide a precise area of therapy and temperature measurement.

The description of the electrical field that is responsible for the clinical effect of CRF is governed by Maxwell's equations on electromagnetism [4]. At the frequencies utilized in

RF technology, electrical and magnetic fields are generated; however, the magnetic field's effect is negligible [7]. The current density that is responsible for clinical effect is a function of the electrical conductivity of tissue [8]. Structures that readily conduct electrical energy such as nervous tissue and water will have higher current density than those structures with a lower conductivity (bone). Also, the coagulated tissue that is produced during CRF may serve to affect impedance as the resultant tissue may decrease the flow of energy into tissues.

As energy flows from the generator via electrical current to the electrode, ions in tissue electrolytes are activated and oscillated [6–8]. As a result of the kinetic energy produced by this Brownian motion, heat is dispersed from the ions and is measured by the thermocouple. Increasing the flow of current will increase the resultant temperature, known as ohmic or resistive heating of tissue, as measured at the thermocouple. In summary, the tissue heats up the electrode, and the electrode does not heat up the tissue.

Temperatures utilized typically range from 80 to 90 °C, although the minimum temperature to produce irreversible neuronal interruption is 44 °C [9]. Higher temperatures may lead to side effects including hematoma, smoke, and gas formation, along with adherence to tissues to the probe [9]. Nociceptive input is theoretically reduced as the therapy is aimed for sensory nerve fibers.

Utilizing a temperature-time controlled process, a lesion is produced with treatment. Precision in lesions developed with the introduction of a 22-G RF cannula, smaller than previous devices [10]. The size of the lesion is affected by factors including the diameter of the electrode, the active tip length, tissue characteristics, and vascular supply near the lesion site. The lesion size and tissue injury can be evaluated through the relation between the current divided by the electrode surface area known as the current density. For a given constant current, with a decrease in electrode surface area, a greater current density, tissue heating and resultant lesioning will occur.

Power [11] provided by the generator, along with lesion time, also affects lesion size. Lesion time has been found to be significant in increasing the size of the heat effect up to 40 s. The temperature at the thermocouple along with the cannula size is an important factor in the size of the lesion, as heat generated in the process believed to be responsible for the clinical effects of radiofrequency.

Due to the shape of the needle and the electrode, an oblate spheroid lesion is produced [6, 8, 9, 11]. A temperature-controlled system is preferred over a voltage-controlled system as lesion size and temperature achieved can more reliably result, leading to a more predictable lesion. Voltage-controlled lesioning may produce temperatures below or above target range, leading to lesions of variable efficacy [9].

Physics of Pulsed Radiofrequency

Pulsed radiofrequency differs from CRF in that pulsed radiofrequency does not lead to a neurodestructive process [3, 4]. This theoretical benefit is important for sensitive nerves such as peripheral nerves in the head and neck, dorsal root ganglia, trigeminal ganglia, and peripheral nerves in the abdominal and inguinal regions [12, 13], and the lower extremity.

During the developmental phases of what is now known to be pulsed radiofrequency, interest was sought for the possible beneficial role of the magnetic field in treatment. Cosman et al. [14] determined that the magnetic component was an incidental vector that would have negligible effects toward clinical benefit [7]. It was then proposed to deliver energy in waves or pulses with a short rest period between generator activation. This rest period would allow the dispersal of the heat that was generated (as in CRF). This interrupted treatment would theoretically deliver electrical energy to elicit a clinical response, but not lead to the side effects of denervation and its resultant complications. In the initial description by Sluijter et al. [14], the pulses were for 20 ms separated by 0.5 s. This separation allowed for a rest period whereby heat that is generated by oscillatory motion would be allowed to dissipate via vascular runoff. Still, this treatment should not be thought of as a "nonthermal" lesion as there is increased temperature at the thermocouple. Consequently, as the pulse duration is a fraction of total pulse time (pulse duration + interpulse duration), voltage utilized during PRF is higher without risking increased temperature change with the higher energy.

PRF technology, however, may also lead to lesion injury. Heavner et al. [15] however showed that when PRF is utilized (10 ms duration at 2 Hz), coagulation begins to occur in egg-white media at a temperature of 60 °C. Therefore, regardless of technology, PRF vs. CRF, increased temperature at the tip can lead to coagulation and tissue injury. In essence, PRF as is currently used is a *neuromodulatory* treatment option as opposed to the *ablative* CRF.

The exact mechanism of PRF's clinical benefit is unclear; initially, PRF was believed to play a role in causing neuronal plasticity with upregulating of c-Fos [16] in rat DRG. c-Fos is a proto-oncogene that is expressed in response to neuronal activity and may have a role in nociceptive transmission. Animals were exposed to RF at the C6 dorsal root ganglion, via CRF or PRF, at 38 °C for 120 s. Immunohistochemical assays for c-Fos were performed, and animals with PRF had an increased expression of the protein in laminae I and II of the spinal cord; this expression was not seen in animals exposed to CRF.

Additionally, c-Fos staining cells were found ipsilateral and contralateral to the side of PRF treatment. The implication of this finding is that PRF activates the dorsal horn laminae I and II neurons and could be a possible explanation for the clinical benefit of PRF, as both CRF and PRF animals were subject to the same temperature. This choice to have the temperatures of both CRF and PRF by the authors in the experimental design of this study leads to the possibility of deducing that a factor *intrinsic* to PRF not seen in CRF would lead to c-Fos expression.

This c-Fos selectivity for PRF-treated animals was subsequently refuted in a study by Van Zundert et al. [17] where sham, PRF, and continuous RF were applied adjacent to the cervical DRG of rats. All three groups had induction of c-Fos with staining that was noted 7 days after treatment study. Additional research is warranted regarding the genetic changes that may result and be responsible for the clinical effect of PRF.

Cahana et al. [18] evaluated in vitro neuronal preparations to determine tissue effects of CRF at 42 ° C versus PRF at 38 and 42 °C. The electrical energy required in CRF was less than that in PRF, yet CRF was found to be a destructive lesion in which heat was generated, with PRF specimens showing less tissue injury [18].

Cosman and Cosman [6] have opined that the heat produced with the pulsed energy may be responsible for the clinical benefit of PRF. This heat is subsequently removed during the rest phase, however. Additionally, they suggest that electroporation may be a factor in leading to the clinical effect of PRF. This concept is the alteration in electrical conductance and membrane permeability of a cell membrane in response to an applied electrical field, theoretically leading to analgesic benefit after PRF.

Hagiwara et al. [19] have opined that the analgesic action of PRF involves the action of the accessory adrenergic pain pathways. Hamann et al. [20] have looked at the possible mechanism of PRF and suggest that PRF targets neurons with small diameter axons by evaluating the role of activating transcription factor 3 (ATF-3), a marker of cellular stress, in rats. DRG application of PRF led to an increased presence of ATF-3 in neurons. The authors suggest that PRF can lead to increased cell stress in the absence of direct thermal lesioning. The role of this factor and others in regards to PRF is yet to be fully elucidated.

A proteomic study [21] has also been performed in rats to look at protein expression in animals treated with PRF. L5 dorsal root ganglia were exposed to PRF and sham therapy. Western blotting of samples showed increased levels of gamma-aminobutyric acid (GABA) and decreased 4-aminobutyrate aminotransferase (enzyme involved in production of GABA) in animals treated with PRF. GABA is a neurotransmitter regulating neuronal excitability. Further studies are warranted in exploring the role of PRF on GABA [22, 23].

Histological Effects of Radiofrequency

Animal studies have been performed evaluating the histological effects of CRF therapy. In a study involving CRF of goat (DRG), de Louw et al. [24] found that a temperature of 67 °C at the DRG can lead to hemorrhagic loss of myelinated fibers. This neural destruction is absent if the CRF is performed *adjacent* to the DRG. Consequently, the heat lesion leads to neuronal injury after a radiofrequency procedure. Animal research has led to the theory that CRF was a selective lesioning modality, preferentially targeting C and A-δ fibers occurred before affecting the larger myelinated A-α and A-β fibers. Other studies have contradicted this result, and CRF is now widely thought of as leading to heat-induced equal destruction of all nerve fibers. Dreyfuss et al. [25] showed that RF neurotomy is a nonselective treatment that affects and coagulates all nerves as a result of EMG studies [26].

Vatansever et al. [27] compared the effects on the sciatic nerve of male Wistar rats. Five groups were studied: no procedure, sham procedure, 40 °C CRF for 90 s, CRF 80 °C for 90 s, and PRF for 240 s. CRF 40 °C showed the presence of endoneurial edema in the subperineurial and perivascular areas of the nerve. Light microscopy specimen evaluation demonstrated transverse myelin fibers damaged along with separation of the axoplasma. This separation would lead to impaired nerve transmission. Electron microscopy also confirmed alteration of myelin configuration. Additionally, lamellous separation with protrusion of myelin and accumulation of neurofilaments was found, pointing to a diagnosis of neurodegeneration.

CRF 80 °C showed significant endoneurial edema and evidence of Wallerian degeneration. Electron microscopy showed evidence of neurodegeneration, including epineurial thickening, lamellous separation, intra-axonal vacuolization, increased intracellular endoplasmic reticulum, and Schwann cell damage.

PRF demonstrated changes similar to CRF 40, but the severity of lesions was less.

Podhajsky et al. [28] observed effects of 80 °C CRF and 42 °C PRF lesions on rat DRG and sciatic nerves for 2, 7, and 21 days after initial treatment and found similar results. Massive edema in specimens was seen on day 2 with 80 °C treatment. Wallerian degeneration and tissue coagulation were observed on the 7th day after treatment. With 42 °C, edema was also seen on the 2nd day of treatment, but *regressed* and *resolved* by the 7th day.

Animal studies were also performed in rabbits [29] to evaluate PRF vs. CRF current on the DRG. Animals were in a PRF, CRF, control, or sham grouping. No changes noted at 2 weeks after treatment under light microscopy. By electron microscopic sections, CRF-DRG specimens showed degenerative changes including evidence of cytoplasmic vacuoles, a large endoplasmic reticulum, mitochondrial degeneration, and the loss of nuclear membrane material. PRF did not show the intensity of these changes, with just the presence of large vacuoles throughout the cytoplasm.

Studies on the Efficacy of Radiofrequency

Trigeminal Neuralgia

CRF has been utilized for patients with trigeminal neuralgia, a devastating neuropathic pain state, often very difficult to treat. Radiofrequency has been shown to be the best option for complete pain relief when compared to other approaches including surgical treatments [30]. Kanpolat et al. [31] performed radiofrequency trigeminal rhizotomy on patients with trigeminal neuralgia, looking at 1,600 patients over a 25-year period. Excellent relief of pain symptoms was noted initially with a decrease of 57.7 % at 5-year follow-up. The number of patients with complete relief after a single procedure decreased to 52.3 % by the time a 10-year follow-up was performed. The study also provided side effects that may be present in patients undergoing an ablative procedure on the gasserian ganglion, highlighting the risks of corneal reflex changes, keratitis, masseter muscle dysfunction, cranial nerve II and VI paralysis, and anesthesia dolorosa. PRF has been evaluated against CRF [32], with the former not as effective as the latter in treating the pain of trigeminal neuralgia.

Cervical Zygapophyseal Joints

The "facets" are in actuality the zygapophyseal joints (z-joints) that are made of adjacent articular processes. The term facet describes the curved cartilaginous lining of the z-joints. The joints are involved in the range of motion of the cervical spine. The zygapophyseal joints in the cervical spine may be implicated in 54–60 % of patients with chronic neck pain [33]. Neural innervation of the joint is provided by medial branches of the spinal nerves with each joint is innervated by the adjacent two medial branches.

After successful block of the joint or the medial branches that supply the joints, radiofrequency treatment can be performed for longer-term benefit of painful symptoms. Cohen et al. [34] have evaluated in a multicenter analysis the factors that predict success for cervical radiofrequency denervation and noted the presence of pre-procedure paraspinal tenderness as the best prognostic sign. Lord et al. [35] evaluated patients with chronic z-joint pain after motor vehicle accident in a double-blinded randomized controlled trial, treated with CRF for analgesic relief. A positive result of 100 % pain relief with three diagnostic/therapeutic blocks with local anesthetic and steroid was required prior to inclusion in the study. Patients had a median time from initial relief to 50 % of pain returning at 263 days.

Sapir et al. [36] evaluated patients with cervical whiplash symptoms undergoing cervical neurolysis. There was a statistical significance in improvement in patients VAS scores regardless of litigation status by patients. Long-term follow-up and benefit was noted of the radiofrequency procedure in a paper by McDonald et al. [37]. The median duration in their study of 28 patients diagnosed as having cervical zygapophyseal joint pain was 219 days. In a Cochrane analysis, Niemisto et al. [38] evaluated the efficacy of cervical radiofrequency and found limited evidence for short-term benefit.

Other Painful Conditions of the Cervical Spine

Slappendel et al. [39] published a report of the results of a randomized, double-blinded multicenter trial on the effect of CRF of the cervical DRG to treat cervicobrachial pain. This study evaluated the difference in temperature between two groups: one population was treated with CRF at 67 °C and the other group at 40 °C. Both patient groups developed a decrease in VAS scores; however, the 40 °C group maintained their decrease at 3-month follow-up. Van Zundert et al. [40] have evaluated PRF in the treatment of cervical radicular pain adjacent to the cervical DRG and found the technique be satisfactory at reducing discomfort for a mean duration of 9 months.

The concept of cervicogenic headache is a controversial topic in pain management circles. Difference of opinion exists between physicians as to whether this entity deserves a diagnosis or not [41].

Multiple papers [41–43] have provided a description of this unilateral headache that is present in the occipital or neck region, radiating to the temporal and/or frontal aspect of the cranium. Stovner et al. [44] have evaluated the use of radiofrequency denervation of facet joints for cervicogenic headache via a double-blinded, sham-controlled randomized double-blinded study. Twelve patients with unilateral cervicogenic headache were evaluated with half randomized to receive C2–C6 neurotomy and the others to receive sham therapy. Patients were followed for 2 years, with improvement noted at 3 months in the treated group. The authors followed patients for 2 years after the initial treatment and found no significant benefit for the use of this technology. Haspeslagh et al. [45] compared the use of radiofrequency of the medial branches supplying the z-joints, the dorsal root ganglion against an injection of local anesthetic at the greater occipital nerve with subsequent application of transcutaneous electrical nerve stimulation. There was no evidence that cervical z-joint radiofrequency was superior to injection of the greater occipital nerve and TENS application. The results of this study may be questioned, however, because of the small sample size (15 patients) and a relatively large number of patient dropouts. Govind et al. [46] have evaluated radiofrequency denervation for headache pain by targeting the third occipital nerve a particularly tenacious nerve. Multiple lesions, larger electrode (greater than 22 G), were utilized for best clinical effect. Untoward side effects such as ataxia, paresthesia, numbness, and dysesthesia may result from this procedure.

Navani et al. [47] presented their report of the use of PRF in a patient with occipital neuralgia. The patient underwent PRF at the medial branches of C1 and C2 dorsal rami with three cycles of 42 °C for 120 s. The patient subsequently underwent another PRF treatment 4 months after initial therapy with improvement of symptoms. As with PRF in other cervical applications, the benefits of treatment as compared to CRF here are evident with less potential risk of neuritis pain induced by heat lesions. Further research is warranted for the use of PRF for this indication.

Thoracic

The thoracic zygapophyseal joints may be a source of discomfort in patients. These joints may be the source of thoracic spine and segmental discomfort in the thoracic region. Stolker et al. [48] evaluated thoracic facet joint CRF and reported benefit of neurolysis. Nearly half of patients were noted to be pain free after 2 months, 83 % of patients achieving greater than 50 % pain relief after 18–54-month follow-up. Cohen et al. [49] evaluated patients who were treated for post-thoracotomy pain with PRF of thoracic DRG vs. those patients treated with analgesics or PRF of the intercostal nerves and found that PRF of the DRG was superior.

Lumbar Pain

The lumbar z-joints are also paired, diarthrodial joints that are involved in the range of motion of the lumbar spine. Goldthwait [50] first presented the lumbosacral articulation as a source of low back pain in 1911. After a series of medial branch or z-joint injections, radiofrequency therapy may theoretically improve patient pain for a longer period than the duration of the agents utilized during injection therapies. Cohen et al. [51] also studied the predictors of success for a radiofrequency procedure in the lumbar region and again found paraspinal tenderness to be the most significant predictor of success. Additionally, the degree of pre-radiofrequency analgesia (percent improvement after block) had *no effect* on post-radiofrequency effect in patients who had at least 50 % pain relief with blocks.

Dreyfuss et al. [25] found that patients with the longest time of relief were those patients who had resultant multifidus muscle denervation based on EMG study after CRF. Nath et al. [52] evaluated patients receiving a positive facet joint injection block who subsequently underwent sham or CRF. Patients who were actively treated had a statistically significant improvement in back and leg pain with improved range of motion, indicating that the beneficial effects noted by patients were not due to placebo effect.

Gallagher et al. [53] evaluated radiofrequency for the z-joints as a treatment for low back pain in a double-blinded prospective study. The visual analog scale (VAS) was utilized to evaluate pain scores and relief after therapy. Patients receiving radiofrequency were compared to sham therapy with VAS was improved at 1 month and 6 months versus sham therapy. Van Kleef et al. [54] also demonstrated the benefit of radiofrequency by studying a group of 31 patients in a prospective double-blind randomized trial. Patients with lumbar facet degeneration after chronic low back pain who had benefit (50 % pain relief) with medial branch blocks underwent CRF vs. sham-treated patients. Test subjects were evaluated 8 weeks after the trial, then at present at 3, 6, and 12 months after initial therapy. There was statistically significant difference between the groups with CRF patients exhibiting lower analgesic requirements and improved disability status vs. patients receiving the sham therapy. The goal of DRG CRF is to perform a selective blockade of afferent nerve conduction with avoidance of damage to the ganglion. Geurts et al. [55] published a multicenter randomized control trial for evaluating lumbar DRG CRF in patients with chronic lumbosacral pain. Patients were evaluated with VAS and also the SF-36 quality of life pain measure. The results of this randomized double-blinded placebo-controlled study were that there was that CRF of lumbar DRG *should not* be routinely performed as benefit was not seen.

Radiofrequency ablation in the lumbar z-joint region did not have benefit in one study [56]. This placebo-controlled clinical trial resulted in negative recommendation for lumbar radiofrequency ablation. The criticism of this study is that there was a high inclusion rate of patients in this study. Slipman et al. [57] showed that radiofrequency ablation while leading to clinical improvement of pain was rated as having level III evidence based on evidence-based medicine criteria based on review of the literature. Manichikanti et al. [58] performed their own review of the literature that resulted in *strong* evidence for short-term relief of pain symptoms, but *moderate* evidence for lumbar radiofrequency for longer-term relief. Kornick et al. reported on complications [59] of lumbar radiofrequency noting that in 116 denervation procedures in 92 patients that no motor or sensory deficits were present in patients. This of course assumes that motor and sensory checks are performed by the operator before the lesioning procedure occurs.

Radiofrequency ablation has had effects for 6 months to a year [4]. In those patients who had repeat radiofrequency procedures, benefit may be achieved with the subsequent procedure. Schofferman and Kine [60] showed in a retrospective chart review of 20 patients who had an initial successful benefit with radiofrequency subsequently developed pain and then had a repeat radiofrequency procedure. Larger needle sizes (20-G electrode with a 10-mm active tip or a 16-G rhizotomy electrode) were utilized. Also, the CRF was 80 °C for 70 s. The mean duration of relief with the repeat RF was 11.6 months for a second RF procedure. Overall, improvement after repeat RF treatments was 10.6 months.

The first use of PRF was described by Sluijter in 1998 [14]. This prospective-controlled trial compared the results of utilizing the new technology with CRF at 42 °C. The authors concluded that PRF was superior to CRF at the parameters used due to a global perceived effect (GPE) that was higher in the former group.

Teixera has suggested the use of lumbar DRG PRF for surgical candidates with radicular pain. PRF DRG was recommended as an alternative to lumbar epidural injections as a treatment option, and 12/13 patients studied were able to avoid surgery for at least 1 year [61].

PRF has also been evaluated for use in patients having pain attributed to the z-joints in the lumbar region. Linder et al. performed a retrospective review [62] of patients undergoing PRF for low back pain. Patients in this study included those having back surgery and those with no history of prior surgical intervention. Prior to CRF, patients had analgesia with one diagnostic medial branch block. The authors found that PRF was beneficial in both patient populations, but more effective in patients who did not have prior back surgery. Mikeladzke et al. [63] evaluated the technology in patients with chronic z-joint pain and found that PRF was beneficial in providing pain relief lasting for almost 4 months.

Kroll et al. [64] performed a randomized double-blinded prospective study comparing CRF vs. PRF in the treatment of chronic z-joint pain. CRF was performed at 80 °C for 75 s and pulsed radiofrequency of 42 C with a pulse duration of 20 ms with a pulse rate of 2 Hz for 120 s. The VAS and the Oswestry Disability Questionnaire were utilized to gauge patient response to treatment at baseline and interval follow-up. There was no significant difference between CRF and PRF in long-term outcome. Additionally, there was greater improvement over time within CRF. A criticism of this study is the large dropout rate of 48 %.

Tekin et al. [65] evaluated the effects of CRF vs. PRF in 40 patients, with an additional 20 patients as control. The VAS and ODI were also utilized for evaluation at procedure, 6-month and 1-year follow-ups. While PRF and CRF patients had improvement in measured parameters, the maintenance of the decrease in VAS was greatest in patients who had CRF as opposed to patients with PRF. The result of therapy was longer lasting in the CRF group.

PRF has also been used in the lumbar region to treat discogenic pain [66]. High-voltage, long-duration PRF has been utilized to treat 8 patients. A 15-cm 20-G needle was placed in the nucleus pulposus for 20 min PRF at 2 × 20 ms at 60 V.

The study achieved 100 % improvement of pain on a VAS query. Further controlled studies are mandated for applicability in this domain.

Sacroiliac

The sacroiliac joint may be a common cause of back pain. Goldthwait and Osgood [67] proposed the SI joint to be an independent source of back pain. Estimates of the source of discomfort attributed to the SIJ range from 18 to 30 % [68, 69].

RF ablation of the sacroiliac joint has also been attempted with mixed results. Ferrante et al. [70] published the first description of an RF technique of this pain generator by describing a "leap frog" technique of overlapping bipolar lesions, less than 1 cm apart, along the length of a sacroiliac joint. Lesions were created at 90 °C for 90 s. The distance between lesions was questioned for this bipolar approach [71]. Cohen and others [72, 73] then presented a description of a lateral branch block radiofrequency.

Burnham and Yasui [74] have also described the use of a lateral branch approach for CRF of pain attributed to the SI joint. Nine subjects underwent strip RF lesions at the lateral dorsal foramina at S1–S3 along with monopolar lesions at the L5 dorsal ramus. Patients were then evaluated every 3 months up to a year. The results of this small-numbered, prospective cohort study indicated a decrease in analgesic requirements and back and leg pain.

Cooled RF has also been described [75, 76]. This is a technology devised to decrease the heating occurring at the electrode tip during CRF. The result is decreased impedance at the electrode tip, with a theoretical delivery of higher energy, with a larger lesion size than CRF.

Cooled RF was associated with a greater number of positive RF outcomes, likely because of the larger diameter lesion size associated with this technology compared to CRF. Kapural et al. [75] published a retrospective review of 47 procedures on 27 patients in which cooled RF was utilized for dorsal rami of L5 and S1–S3 lateral branches. Patients exhibited improvement in function (as measured by the Pain Disability Index-PDI) and VAS.

Pulsed RF has also been described in one study, with patients receiving PRF of the medial branches of L4 and L5 and the lateral branches of S1 and S2. The duration of pain relief in this study was 20 weeks [77].

Inguinal

PRF would show a theoretical advantage over CRF with the less risk of post-denervation discomfort. Studies [78–80] performed, however, are case series, and results should be evaluated, noting the small numbers of patients, as no control is present to minimize the concern of placebo effect. Rozen et al. [78] performed PRF on five patients with persistent inguinal pain after inguinal hernia surgery. Patients were treated with PRF at T12, L1, and L2 ganglia with noted improvement of their symptoms.

Radiofrequency Techniques

Cervical Medial Branch Anatomy

In normal human anatomy, here are eight cervical nerves but seven cervical vertebrae. To account for this discrepancy, the first seven nerve roots exit above the vertebral body whose number they share. That is, C4 nerve root exits the intervertebral foramen between C3 and C4 vertebral bodies. The first two cervical levels do not have dorsal primary rami innervating structures. Ventral primary rami are responsible for injection the atlanto-occipital and atlanto-axial joints. Two medial branches arise separately from the C3 dorsal ramus.

The superior and larger division is known as the third occipital nerve (TON). The TON travels dorsally and medially around the superior articular process of the C3 vertebra, crossing the C2–C3 zygapophyseal joint either just below or across the joint margin. Innervation of the C2–C3 facet joints comes from the TON and an articular branch of the dorsal ramus. Practically speaking, blocking the TON on the C3 articular process will denervate the C2–C3 joint.

The C3–C4 to C7–T1 joints are supplied by the medial branches of the cervical posterior rami at the same level and from the level above. These medial branches curve dorsally and medially, wrapping around the midportion, "waist", of the articular pillars. On lateral view, medial branches are in the middle of the trapezoid of the articular pillar. Of note, the C7 medial branch lies higher on the lateral projection of the C7 articular pillar. The medial branch of C8 crosses the root of the T1 transverse process. This branch hooks medially onto the lamina of T1 and sends branches to C7–T1 joint. The medial branches provide sensory input from nociceptors at each joint level.

Technique of Cervical MBB RF [81]

Monitors are attached for heart rate, blood pressure, and oxygen saturation. The patient is placed in the prone position on the fluoroscopy table with arms at sides and padding for the knees, abdomen, and chest. The patient's cervical spine should be flexed 10–15° (chin to chest position). The dispersive pad should be placed on the patient away from but as close to the site of the procedure. Traction of the arms toward the feet may be required to visualize the cervical facet pillars,

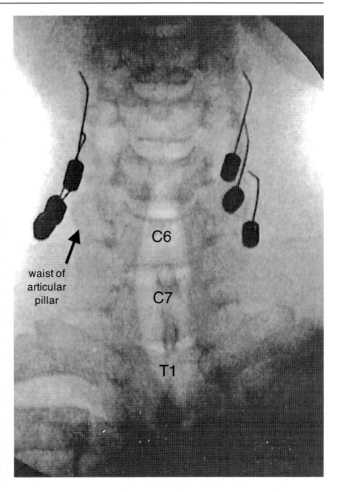

Fig. 26.1 Anterior-posterior view of needle placement for cervical z-joint medial branch radiofrequency procedure. Note the placement of the needles at the waist of the articular pillar. *C6* C6 vertebral body, *C7* C7 vertebral body, *T1* T1 vertebral body

particularly those patients with short necks. After proper positioning is performed, the patient may receive an anxiolytic. It is imperative that the operator is able to communicate with the patient and that the patient not is overly sedated. Using anterior-posterior fluoroscopic visualization, the relevant anatomic level is identified. The articular pillar should be seen, and the waist of the pillar should be identified (Figs. 26.1 and 26.2). The skin and subcutaneous tissues of this region should then be anesthetized with 1 % lidocaine. Care should be taken not to anesthetize the medial branch being tested, stimulated, and treated with CRF. Curved or straight tip may be utilized for the procedure.

Thereafter, a 20–22-G needle (50-mm, 5-mm active tip, author's suggestion) is inserted to access the previously anesthetized areas to contact the medial branch at the waist of the articular pillar. The long axis of the needle should be parallel to the course of the nerve targeted to provide the best lesion, as the lesion shape is an oblate spheroid around the active tip. All needles to be placed should be done so before stimulation

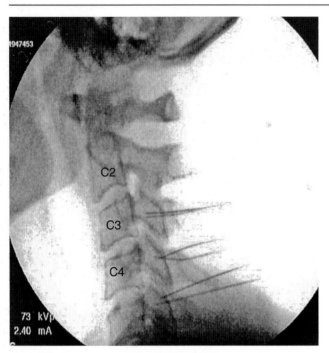

Fig. 26.2 Lateral view of needle placement for cervical z-joint medial branch radiofrequency procedure. Note the direction of the needles is parallel to the direction of the indicated nerves. *C2* C2 vertebral body, *C3* C3 vertebral body, *C4* C4 vertebral body

is tested to minimize patient discomfort. A thermocouple is then inserted into the needle, and sensory and motor nerve stimulation is performed.

Initially, sensory stimulation with 50-Hz current is performed to reproduce paresthesia localized to the site of discomfort at a delivered energy up to 1.0 V. If radicular stimulation is elicited, the needle should be repositioned as this may indicate dorsal root stimulation; a subsequent lesion at this location may then lead to motor or sensory dysfunction.

Next, 2-Hz motor stimulation should be performed to check that no motor recruitment other than localized neck muscle twitching is occurring. The upper threshold for motor stimulation should be 2.0 V. With a multilesioning system, stimulation would be checked at each site and then lesioning performed after successful testing occurs; in the situation of a generator that has single lesion capability, it is recommended that lesioning be performed immediately after checking stimulation at each level to decrease the likelihood of inaccurate lesioning.

Local anesthetic (0.5 ml) may be administered depending on operator preference: the discomfort of a heat lesion would be decreased by the local anesthetic. If the local anesthetic spreads beyond the needle at the lesion site, however, the risk of anesthetizing areas to be tested may occur, leading to motor/sensory stimulation that is inaccurate. Lesioning then

progresses at a temperature setting of 80 °C for 90 s for CRF and 42 °C for 120 s at PRF (author's technique).

Patients should be advised that they may note a multiphase response to CRF therapy: an initial phase with relief of symptoms lasting for a few days, followed by a 2–3-week period of discomfort that may result from the heat lesion. Thereafter, prolonged relief may result. This phase of discomfort may not be seen in a patient undergoing PRF as the temperature is kept at a nonlesioning level.

Patients are seen back in the clinic 3 weeks after an initial CRF procedure. The operator may provide an oral analgesic or muscle relaxant for the patient's discomfort.

Complications

Assuming that the patient had successful sensory and motor stimulation with the initial procedure, complications are expected to me at a minimum with radiofrequency procedures. Sterile technique is of utmost importance during interventional procedures involving spinal and paraspinal needle placement. The patient should have anticoagulants discontinued [82] prior to therapy for the requisite period prior to treatment. Also, patients should be afebrile with no evidence of infection prior to interventional techniques.

Patients may notice discomfort at the needle sites, which may be relieved with oral and topical analgesics, muscle relaxants, and conservative measures such as heat or ice packs. Myofascial pain may occur after CRF, which is treated by local anesthetic/steroid trigger point injections.

Thoracic Medial Branch Anatomy

The thoracic medial branches [83] have a typical course that has been verified by anatomical dissection. The medial branches cross the superior and lateral aspect of the transverse process, then curving inferiorly and medially across the transverse process, travelling to the multifidus muscle. Unlike the medial branch of the lumbar region, where the medial branch is targeted in a superomedial location on the transverse process, the target point would be along a superolateral to inferomedial line on the transverse process. This arrangement typically occurs from T1 to T4 and also from T9 to T10 levels; variation to this occurs at the T5–T8 levels where the nerve may be displaced in a superior location and may not cross the lateral aspect of the transverse process.

Technique of Thoracic MBB RF [48, 83]

The technique of thoracic MBB RF is similar to the description provided above of cervical RF. The fluoroscope tube is obliqued 10–15° toward the ipsilateral side to show the articulation of the transverse process and adjacent rib. The operator

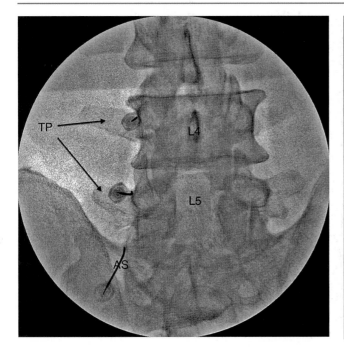

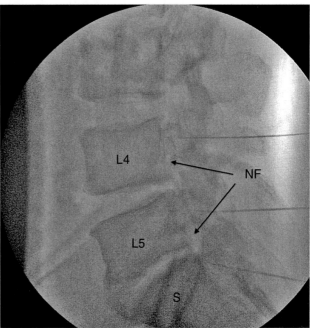

Fig. 26.3 Anterior-posterior radiograph of needle placement for lumbar medial branch RF procedure. *TP* transverse process of vertebral body, *AS* ala of sacrum, *L4* L4 vertebral body, *L5* L5 vertebral body

Fig. 26.4 Lateral view of needle placement for lumbar medial branch RF. Note location of needles in relation to relation to neural foramina. *L4* L4 vertebral body, *L5* L5 vertebral body, *S* sacrum *NF* neural foramina

should be cognizant of the location of the lungs in relation to the bony skeleton.

As described above, the target point of the medial branches is along the transverse process itself (Fig. 26.3). The skin and subcutaneous tissues of this region should then be anesthetized with 1 % lidocaine. Care should be taken not to anesthetize the medial branch being tested, stimulated, and treated with CRF. Curved or straight tip may be utilized for the procedure. Thereafter, a 20–22-G needle (100-mm, 10-mm active tip) is inserted to access the previously anesthetized areas to contact the medial branch at the transverse process.

Complications

In addition to the complications described in the cervical RF, the potential risk of pneumothorax exists due to accidental lung injury. Precision in evaluating perioperative fluoroscopy is required to note needle location vs. the lungs.

Myofascial pain may occur after CRF, which is treated by local anesthetic/steroid trigger point injections, being cautious of the risk of pneumothorax due to needle puncture of the pleura.

Lumbar Medial Branch Anatomy

In the lumbar region, the medial branch of the posterior ramus. The mamilo-accessory ligament is located in a groove on the base of the superior articular facet, adjacent to the base of the superior transverse process, the most reliable

location for a medial branch block. Each joint has dual segmental innervation, and each segmental nerve supplies two facet joints plus the soft tissues overlying them. There is considerable innervation overlap in the lower lumbar region. The L5 medial branch contributes an inferior segment at the ala of the sacrum. The posterior opening of the S1 nerve root in the sacrum runs cephalad to supply the L5–S1 joint.

Technique of Lumbar MBB RF

The technique of RF is similar to the technique described above. An intravenous is started in the patient. The natural lordotic curve of the lumbar spine should be minimized by placing a pillow underneath the abdomen; using anterior-posterior fluoroscopic guidance, the relevant anatomic level is identified. The procedure may be performed by identifying the juncture of the transverse process of the lumbar spine along with the articular process at the relevant level (Fig. 26.4). The L5 medial branch sends a contribution inferiorly which is addressed by placing a cannula at the ala of the sacrum.

Alternatively, the fluoroscope beam can be obliqued 15–20° to the ipsilateral side of the injection to visualize the "Scottie dog." The target point is the ear of the Scottie dog. Regardless of the technique being utilized, the long axis of the needle should be placed parallel to the direction of the target medial branch to maximize the resultant lesion with

CRF. Curved or straight tip may be utilized for the procedure. Thereafter, a 20–22-G needle (100-mm, 10-mm active tip, author's suggestion) is inserted to access the previously anesthetized areas to contact the target point. All needles to be placed should be done so before stimulation is tested to minimize patient discomfort. A thermocouple is then inserted into the needle, and sensory and motor nerve stimulation is performed. Initially, sensory stimulation with 50-Hz current is performed to reproduce paresthesia localized to the site of discomfort at a delivered energy up to 1.0 V. If radicular stimulation is elicited, the needle should be repositioned as this may indicate dorsal root stimulation; a subsequent lesion at this location may then lead to motor or sensory dysfunction. Next, 2-Hz motor stimulation should be performed to check that no motor recruitment other than localized multifidus muscle twitching is occurring. The upper threshold for motor stimulation should be 2.0 V.

Complications

The complications are as previously described above.

Conclusion

Radiofrequency technology has widespread use [84] in interventional pain management. Evidence exists for the routine use of CRF for treating pain due to trigeminal neuralgia and z-joint pathology. Pain physicians have traditionally utilized PRF as a way to provide the benefits of CRF minus the complication of post-denervation pain. The literature indicates that benefit after PRF may not be as long lasting when compared to CRF. Before disposing of PRF as a viable technology [85], however, further investigation into the mechanism of both CRF and PRF would be warranted and refinement of technique should occur. Failure to do so would deny patients a powerful neuromodulatory technique in the treatment of chronic painful conditions.

References

1. Morady F. Radiofrequency ablation as treatment for cardiac arrhythmias. New Engl J Med. 1999;340(7):534–44.
2. Curley S. Radiofrequency ablation of malignant liver tumors. Oncologist. 2001;6(1):14–23.
3. Bogduk N. Pulsed radiofrequency. Am Acad Pain Med. 2006; 7(5):396–407.
4. Sluijter M. Radiofrequency part I. Meggen: Flivo Press, SA; 2001.
5. Kline MT. Radiofrequency techniques in clinical practice. In: Waldman SA, Winnie AP, editors. Interventional pain management. 1st ed. Philadelphia: W.B. Saunders; 1996.
6. Cosman Jr ER, Cosman Sr ER. Electric and thermal field effects in tissue around radiofrequency electrodes. Pain Med. 2005; 6:405–24.
7. Cosman ER. A comment on the history of the pulsed radiofrequency technique for pain therapy. Anesthesiology. 2005; 103(6):312.
8. Cosman ER, Rittman WJ, Nashold BS, et al. Radiofrequency lesion generation and its effect on tissue impedance. Appl Neurophysiol. 1988;51:230–42.
9. Buijs EJ, van Wijk RMAW, Geurts JWM, et al. Radiofrequency lumbar facet denervation: a comparative study of the reproducibility of lesion size after 2 current radiofrequency techniques. Reg Anesth Pain Med. 2004;29(5):400–7.
10. Ahadian FM. Pulsed radiofrequency neurotomy: advances in pain medicine. Curr Pain Headache Rep. 2004;8:34–40.
11. Moringlane JR, Koch R, Schefer H, Ostertag CB. Experimental radiofrequency (RF) coagulation with computer-based on line monitoring of temperature and power. Acta Neurochir. 1989; 96:126–31.
12. Rohof OJJM. Radiofrequency treatment of peripheral nerves. Pain Pract. 2002;2:257–60.
13. Philip CN, Candido KD, Joseph NJ, Crystal GJ. Successful treatment of meralgia paresthetica with pulsed radiofrequency of the lateral femoral cutaneous nerve. Pain Physician. 2009; 12(5):881–5.
14. Sluijter ME, Cosman ER, Rittman WB, Van Kleef M. The effects of pulsed radiofrequency fields applied to the dorsal root ganglion—a preliminary report. Pain Clin. 1998;11:109–17.
15. Heavner JE, Boswell MV, Racz GB. A comparison of pulsed radiofrequency and continuous radiofrequency on thermocoagulation of egg white in vitro. Pain Physician. 2006;9:135–7.
16. Higuchi Y, Nashold BS, Sluijter M. Exposure of the dorsal root ganglion in rats to pulsed radiofrequency currents activates dorsal horn lamina I and II neurons. Neurosurgery. 2002;50(4): 850–6.
17. Van Zundert J, de Louw AJA, Joosten EAJ. Pulsed and continuous radiofrequency current adjacent to the cervical dorsal root ganglion of the rat induces late cellular activity in the dorsal horn. Anesthesiology. 2005;102:125–31.
18. Cahana A, Vutskits L, Muller D. Acute differential modulation of synaptic transmission and cell survival during exposure to pulsed and continuous radiofrequency energy. J Pain. 2003;4: 197–202.
19. Hagiwara S, Iwasaka H, Takeshima N, et al. Mechanisms of analgesic action of pulsed radiofrequency on adjuvant-induced pain in the rat: roles of descending adrenergic and serotonergic systems. Eur J Pain. 2009;13(3):249–52.
20. Hamann W, Abou-Sherif S, Thompson S, et al. Pulsed radiofrequency applied to dorsal root ganglia causes a selective increase in ATF3 in small neurons. Eur J Pain. 2006;10(2): 171–6.
21. Kim D, Lim YJ, Kim YC, Lee SC, Lee J, Kim SO. Comparative proteomic study of spinal cord after applying pulsed radiofrequency to dorsal root ganglion in the Rat. Anesth Pain Med. 2008; 3(2):86–93.
22. Brodkey JS, Miyazaki Y, Ervin FR, Mark H. Reversible heat lesions with radiofrequency current. A method of stereotactic localization. J Neurosurg. 1964;21:49–53.
23. Higuchi Y, Nashold B, Sluijter M, Cosman E, Pearlstein R. Exposure of the dorsal root ganglion in rats to pulsed radiofrequency currents activates dorsal horn lamina I and II neurons. Neurosurgery. 2002;50:850–6.
24. de Louw AJA, Vles HSH, Freling G, et al. The morphological effects of a radiofrequency lesion adjacent to the dorsal root ganglion. (RF-DRG)—an experimental study in the goat. Eur J Pain. 2001;5:169–74.
25. Dreyfuss P, Halbrook B, Pauza K, et al. Efficacy and validity of radiofrequency neurotomy for chronic lumbar zygapophyseal joint pain. Spine. 2000;25:1270–7.
26. Smith HP, McWhorter JM, Challa VR. Radiofrequency neurolysis in a clinical model: neuropathological correlation. J Neurosurg. 1981;55:246–53.

27. Vatansever D, Tekin I, Tuglu I, Erbuyun K, Ok G. A comparison of the neuroablative effects of conventional and pulsed radiofrequency techniques. Clin J Pain. 2008;24(8):717–24.

28. Podhajsky RJ, Sekiguchi Y, Kikuchi S, et al. The histologic effects of pulsed and continuous radiofrequency lesions at 42 C to rat dorsal root ganglion and sciatic nerve. Spine. 2005;1:1008–13.

29. Erdine S, Yucel A. Effects of pulsed versus conventional radiofrequency current on rabbit dorsal rot ganglion morphology. Eur J Pain. 2005;9:251–6.

30. Lopez BC, Hamlyn PJ, Zakrzewska JM. Systemic review of ablative neurosurgical techniques for the treatment of trigeminal neuralgia. Neurosurgery. 2004;54:973–82; discussion 82–3.

31. Kanpolat Y, Savas A, Bekar A, Berk C. Percutaneous controlled radiofrequency trigeminal rhizotomy for the treatment of idiopathic trigeminal neuralgia: 25-year experience with 1,600 patients. Neurosurgery. 2001;48:524–32; discussion 32–4.

32. Erdine S, Ozyalcin NS, Cimen A. Comparison of pulsed radiofrequency with conventional radiofrequency in the treatment of idiopathic trigeminal neuralgia. Eur J Pain. 2007;11(3):309–13.

33. Merskey H, Bogduk N. Classification of chronic pain: descriptions of chronic pain syndromes and definitions of pain terms. 2nd ed. Seattle: IASP Press; 1994.

34. Cohen SP, Bajwa ZH, Kraemer JJ, et al. Factors predicting success and failure for cervical facet radiofrequency denervation: a multicenter analysis. Reg Anesth Pain Med. 2007;32:495–503.

35. Lord SM, Barnsley L, Wallis B, McDonald GM, Bogduk N. Percutaneous radio-frequency neurotomy for chronic cervical zygapophyseal joint pain. N Engl J Med. 1996;335:1721–6.

36. Sapir D, Gorup JM. Radiofrequency medial branch neurotomy in litigant and nonlitigant patients with cervical whiplash. Spine. 2001;26:E268–73.

37. McDonald GJ, Lord SM, Bogduk N. Long-term follow-up of patients treated with cervical radiofrequency neurotomy for chronic neck pain. Neurosurgery. 1999;45(1):61–7; discussion 67–8.

38. Niemisto L, Kalso EA, Malmivaara A, Seitsalo S, Hurri H. Radiofrequency denervation for neck and back pain. A systematic review within the framework of the Cochrane collaboration back review group. Spine. 2003;28(16):1877–88.

39. Slappendel R, Crul BJ, Braak GJ, Geurts JW, Booij LH, Voerman VF, de Boo T. The efficacy of radiofrequency lesioning of the cervical spinal dorsal root ganglion in a double-blinded, randomized study: No difference between 40 degrees C and 67 degrees C treatments. Pain. 1997;73:159–63.

40. Lame IE, de Louw A, et al. Percutaneous pulsed radiofrequency treatment of the cervical dorsal root ganglion in the treatment of chronic cervical pain syndromes: a clinical audit. Neuromodulation. 2003;6:6–14.

41. Van Zundert J, Patijn J, Kessels A, et al. Pulsed radiofrequency adjacent to the cervical dorsal root ganglion in chronic cervical radicular pain: a double blind sham controlled randomized clinical trial. Pain. 2007;127:173–82.

42. Leone M, D'Amico D, Grazzi L, Attanasio A, Bussone G. Cervicogenic headache: a critical review of the current diagnostic criteria. Pain. 1998;78(1):1–5.

43. Headache Classification Subcommittee of the International Headache Society. The international classification of headache disorders: 2nd edition. Cephalalgia. 2004;24 Suppl 1:9–160.

44. Stovner LJ, Kolstad F, Heide G. Radiofrequency denervation of facet joints C2–C6 in cervicogenic headache: a randomized, double-blind, sham-controlled study. Cephalalgia. 2004;24:821–30.

45. Haspeslagh SR, Van Suijlekom HA, Lame IE, et al. Randomized controlled trial of cervical radiofrequency lesions as a treatment for cervicogenic headache. BMC Anesthesiol. 2006;6:1.

46. Govind J, King W, Bailey B, Bogduk N. Radiofrequency neurotomy for the treatment of third occipital headache. J Neurol Neurosurg Psychiatry. 2003;74:88–93.

47. Navani A, Mahajan G, Kreis P, et al. A case of pulsed radiofrequency lesioning for occipital neuralgia. Pain Med. 2006;7:453–6.

48. Stolker RJ, Vervest ACM, Groen GJ. Percutaneous facet denervation in chronic thoracic spinal pain. Acta Neurochir (Wien). 1993; 122:82–90.

49. Cohen SP, Sireci A, Wu CL, Larkin TM, Williams KA, Hurley RW. Pulsed radiofrequency of the dorsal root ganglia is superior to pharmacotherapy or pulsed radiofrequency of the intercostal nerves in the treatment of chronic postsurgical thoracic pain. Pain Physician. 2006;9:227–35.

50. Goldthwait JE. The lumbosacral articulation: an explanation of many cases of 'lumbago', 'sciatica', and 'paraplegia'. Boston Med Surg J. 1911;164:365–72.

51. Cohen SP, Hurley RW, Christo PJ, et al. Clinical predictors of success and failure for lumber facet radiofrequency denervation. Clin J Pain. 2007;23:45–52.

52. Nath S, Nath CA, Petterson K. Percutaneous lumbar zygapophyseal (facet) joint neurotomy using radiofrequency current, in the management of chronic Low back pain: a randomized double-blind trial. Spine. 2008;33(12):1291–7.

53. Gallagher J, Vadi PLP, Wesley JR. Radiofrequency facet joint denervation in the treatment of low back pain-a prospective controlled double-blind study in assess to efficacy. Pain Clin. 1994;7:193–8.

54. Van Kleef M, Barendse GAM, Kessels A, et al. Randomized trial of radiofrequency lumbar facet denervation for chronic low back pain. Spine. 1999;24:1937–42.

55. Geurts JW, van Wijk RM, Wynne HJ, et al. Radiofrequency lesioning of dorsal root ganglia for chronic lumbosacral radicular pain: a randomized, double-blind, controlled trial. Lancet. 2003; 361:21–6.

56. LeClaire R, Fortin L, Lambert R, Bergeron YM, Rossignol M. Radiofrequency facet joint denervation in the treatment of low back pain: a placebo-controlled clinical trial to assess efficacy. Spine. 2001;26:1411–6;discussion 7.

57. Slipman CW, Bhat AL, Gilchrist RV, et al. A critical review of the evidence for the use of zygapophysial injections and radiofrequency denervation in the treatment of low back pain. Spine J. 2003; 3:310–6.

58. Manchikanti L, Singh V, Vilims BD. Medial branch neurotomy in management of chronic spinal pain: systematic review of the evidence. Pain Physician. 2002;5:405–18.

59. Kornick C, Kramarich SS, Lamer TJ, Todd Sitzman B. Complications of lumbar radiofrequency denervation. Spine. 2004;29:1352–4.

60. Schofferman J, Kine G. Effectiveness of repeated radiofrequency neurotomy for lumbar facet pain. Spine. 2004;29:2471–3.

61. Teixeira A, Grandinson M, Sluijter ME. Pulsed radiofrequency for radicular pain due to herniated intervertebral disc: an initial report. Pain Pract. 2005;5:111–5.

62. Lindner R, Sluijter ME, Schleinzer W. Pulsed radiofrequency treatment of the lumbar medial branch for facet pain: a retrospective analysis. Pain Med. 2006;7:435–9.

63. Mikeladzke G, Espinal R, Finnegan R, Routon J, Martin D. Pulsed radiofrequency application in treatment of chronic zygapophyseal joint pain. Spine J. 2003;3:360–2.

64. Kroll HR, Kim D, Danic MJ, Sankey SS, Gariwala M, Brown M. A randomized, double-blind, prospective study comparing the efficacy of continuous versus pulsed radiofrequency in the treatment of lumbar facet syndrome. J Clin Anesth. 2008;20:534–7.

65. Tekin I, Mirzai H, Ok G, Erbuyun K, Vatansever D. A comparison of conventional and pulsed radiofrequency denervation in the treatment of chronic facet joint pain. Clin J Pain. 2007; 23:524–9.

66. Teixeira A, Sluijter ME. Intradiscal high-voltage, long duration pulsed radiofrequency for discogenic pain: a preliminary report. Pain Med. 2006;7(5):424–8.

67. Goldthwait JE, Osgood RB. A consideration of the pelvic articulations from an anatomical, pathological and clinical standpoint. Boston Med Surg J. 1905;152:593–601.

68. Schwarzer AC, Aprill CN, Bogduk N. The sacroiliac joint in chronic low back pain. Spine. 1995;20:31–7.

69. Maigne JY, Aivaliklis A, Pfefer F. Results of sacroiliac joint double blocks and value of sacroiliac pain provocation test in 54 patients with low back pain. Spine. 1996;21:1889–92.

70. Ferrante FM, King LF, Roche EA, et al. Radiofrequency sacroiliac joint denervation for sacroiliac syndrome. Reg Anesth Pain Med. 2001;26:137–42.

71. Pino CA, Hoeft MA, Hofsess C, et al. Morphologic analysis of bipolar radiofrequency lesions: implications for treatment of the sacroiliac joint. Reg Anesth Pain Med. 2005;30(4):335–8.

72. Cohen SP, Abdi S. Lateral branch blocks as a treatment for sacroiliac joint pain: a pilot study. Reg Anesth Pain Med. 2003; 28:113–9.

73. Cohen SP, Hurley RW, Buckenmaier 3rd CC, et al. Randomized, placebo-controlled study evaluating lateral branch radiofrequency denervation for sacroiliac joint pain. Anesthesiology. 2008; 109:279–88.

74. Burnham RS, Yasui Y. An alternate method of radiofrequency neurotomy of the sacroiliac joint: a pilot study of the effect of pain, function, and satisfaction. Reg Anesth Pain Med. 2007;32:12–9.

75. Kapural L, Nageeb F, Kapural M, Cata JP, et al. Cooled radiofrequency system for the treatment of chronic pain from sacroiliitis: the first case-series. Pain Pract. 2008;8(5):348–54.

76. Kapural L. Sacroiliac joint radiofrequency denervation: who benefits? Reg Anesth Pain Med. 2009;34(3):185–6.

77. Vallejo R, Benyamin RM, Kramer J, Stanton G, Joseph NJ. Pulsed radiofrequency denervation for the treatment of sacroiliac joint syndrome. Pain Med. 2006;7:429–34.

78. Rozen D, Ahn J. Pulsed radiofrequency for the treatment of ilioinguinal neuralgia after inguinal herniorrhaphy. Mt Sinai J Med. 2006;73:716–8.

79. Martin DC. Pulsed radiofrequency application for inguinal herniorrhaphy pain. Pain Physician. 2006;9:271.

80. Cohen SP, Foster A. Pulsed radiofrequency as a treatment for groin pain and orchialgia. Urology. 2003;61:645.

81. Faclier G, Kay J. Cervical facet radiofrequency neurotomy. Tech Reg Anesth Pain Manag. 2000;4(3):120–5.

82. Horlocker TT, Wedel DJ, Rowlingson JC, et al. Regional anesthesia in the patient receiving antithrombotic or thrombolytic therapy: American society of regional anesthesia and pain medicine evidence-based guidelines (third edition). Reg Anesth Pain Med. 2010;35:64–101.

83. Chua W, Bogduk N. The surgical anatomy of thoracic facet denervation. Acta Neurochir (Wien). 1995;136:140–4.

84. Van Boxem K, van Eerd M, Brinkhuize T. Radiofrequency and pulsed radiofrequency treatment of chronic pain syndromes: the available evidence. Pain Pract. 2008;8(5):385–93.

85. Richebe P, Rathmell JP, Brennan T. Immediate early genes after pulsed radiofrequency treatment; neurobiology in need of clinical trials. Anesthesiology. 2005;102:1–3.

Atlanto-Axial and Atlanto-Occipital Joints Injection in the Treatment of Headaches and Neck Pain

Samer N. Narouze

Key Points

- Atlanto-axial joint (AAJ) injection with local anaesthetic is used to make a definitive diagnosis of pain stemming from the AAJ. AAJ injection with local anaesthetic and steroids may be indicated in the management of AAJ pain.
- AAJ with local anaesthetic is usually considered first to predict the response to AAJ radiofrequency lesioning or arthrodesis in intractable cases.
- Atlanto-occipital joint (AOJ) injection is rarely performed.
- Spinal cord injury and syringomyelia are potential serious complications of AAJ and AOJ injections. Vertebral artery injection/injury has been reported with serious morbidity. Inadvertent puncture of the C2 dural sleeve with CSF leak or high spinal spread of the local anaesthetic may occur with AOJ injection.

occipital pain, and injection of local anaesthetic into the joint relieves the headache [1, 2].

Clinical presentations suggestive of pain originating from the lateral AAJ include occipital or suboccipital pain, focal tenderness over the suboccipital area or over the transverse process of C1, restricted painful rotation of C1 on C2, and pain provocation by passive rotation of C1.

These clinical presentations merely indicate that the lateral AAJ could be a possible source of occipital headache; however, they are not specific and therefore cannot be used alone to establish the diagnosis [3]. These clinical signs have a positive predictive value of only 60 % [1].

The pathology of lateral AAJ pain is usually osteoarthritis or post-traumatic in nature [4, 5]. However, the presence of osteoarthritic changes in imaging studies does not mean that the joint is necessarily painful; also the absence of abnormal findings does not preclude the joint from being painful, and the only means of establishing a definite diagnosis is a diagnostic block with intra-articular injection of local anaesthetic [1].

Introduction

Cervicogenic headache is referred pain from cervical structures innervated by the upper three cervical spinal nerves. The lateral atlanto-axial joint, which is innervated by the C2 ventral ramus, is a fairly common cause of cervicogenic headache. It may account for 16 % of patients with occipital headache [1]. In human volunteers, distending the lateral atlanto-axial joint (AAJ) with contrast agent produces

S.N. Narouze, M.D., Ph.D.
Department of Pain Management, Summa Western Reserve Hospital, 1900 23rd Street, Cuyahoga Falls, OH 44223, USA

Ohio University College of Osteopathic Medicine, Athens, OH, USA
e-mail: narouzs@hotmail.com

Indications

1. AAJ injection with local anaesthetic is used to make a definitive diagnosis of pain stemming from the AAJ.
2. AAJ injection with local anaesthetic and steroids may be indicated in the management of AAJ pain. Intra-articular steroids are effective in short-term pain relief originating from the lateral atlanto-axial joint [6, 7].
3. AAJ injection with local anaesthetic is usually considered first to predict the response to AAJ radiofrequency lesioning or arthrodesis in intractable cases. One report showed favourable long-term outcome after both pulsed and thermal radiofrequency lesioning of the AAJ [8]. In intractable cases, not responsive to more conservative management, arthrodesis of the lateral atlanto-axial joint may be indicated [9].

T.R. Deer et al. (eds.), *Comprehensive Treatment of Chronic Pain by Medical, Interventional, and Integrative Approaches*,
DOI 10.1007/978-1-4614-1560-2_27, © American Academy of Pain Medicine 2013

Fig. 27.1 Illustration showing the relevant anatomy of the atlanto-occipital and atlanto-axial joints

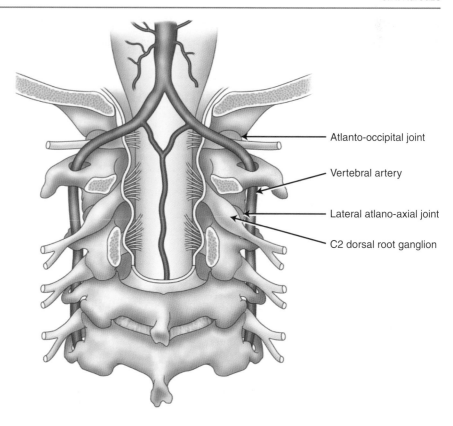

Atlanto-occipital joint

Vertebral artery

Lateral atlano-axial joint

C2 dorsal root ganglion

Anatomy of the Atlanto-Axial Joint (AAJ) and Atlanto-Occipital Joint (AOJ)

It is very crucial to be familiar with the anatomy of the AAJ and atlanto-occipital joint (AOJ) in relation to the surrounding vascular and neural structures (Fig. 27.1) to avoid serious complications. The vertebral artery is lateral to the AAJ as it courses through the C2 and C1 foramina. The vertebral artery then curves medially crossing the medial posterior aspect of the AOJ to go through the foramen magnum.

The C2 nerve root, dorsal root ganglion, and its surrounding dural sleeve cross the posterior aspect of the middle of the joint. Therefore, during AAJ injection, the needle should be directed towards the junction of the middle and lateral thirds of the posterior aspect of the joint. This will avoid injury to the C2 nerve root medially or the vertebral artery laterally (Fig. 27.1) [1, 7]. Conversely, the AOJ should be accessed posteriorly from the most superior lateral aspect to avoid injuring the vertebral artery medially.

Technique of AAJ Injections

With the patient placed in the prone position and a pillow under the chest to allow for slight neck flexion, the fluoroscopy C-arm is brought to the head of the table in an anteroposterior direction. Under fluoroscopic guidance, the C-arm is rotated in a cephalad-caudad direction to better visualize the lateral AAJ. The needle insertion site is marked on the skin overlying the lateral thirds of the AAJ. The skin is prepped and draped in the usual sterile fashion, and a skin wheel is raised with local anaesthetic at the insertion site. Then a 22–25-G 3½ inches blunt needle is advanced towards the posterolateral aspect of the inferior margin of the inferior articular process of the atlas (C1). This will avoid contact with the C2 nerve root and dorsal ganglion, which crosses the posterior aspect of the middle of the joint. It is "better" to seek and touch the bone to safely establish the correct depth. At this point, a lateral view is obtained. The needle is withdrawn slightly, directed towards the posterolateral aspect of the lateral atlanto-axial joint, and advanced for couple of millimetres. Usually a distinctive pop is felt signalling entering the joint cavity. Careful attention should be paid to avoid the vertebral artery that lies laterally to the lateral AAJ as it courses through the C1 and C2 foramina. After careful negative aspiration for blood or cerebrospinal fluid, 0.1–0.2 ml of water-soluble non-ionic contrast agent is injected to verify intra-articular placement of the tip of the needle.

Injection of the contrast agent is done under direct real-time fluoroscopy to check for inadvertent intra-arterial injection which is manifest by rapid clearance of the contrast agent. Anteroposterior and lateral views are obtained to insure that the contrast agent remained confined to the joint cavity without escape to the surrounding structures, especially

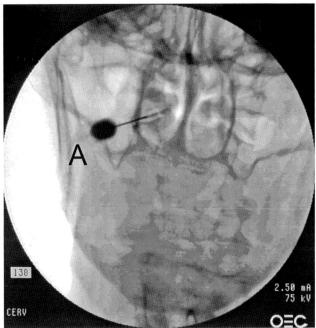

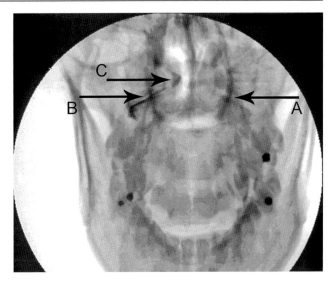

Fig. 27.4 Lateral atlanto-axial joint (AAJ) injection: *A* lateral atlanto-axial joint (AAJ). *B* contrast agent within the AAJ. *C* contrast spreading to the median atlanto-axial joint (Reproduced with permission from Ohio Pain and Headache Institute)

Fig. 27.2 Lateral atlanto-axial joint (AAJ) injection: AP view showing the needle (A) targeting the lateral third of the joint, and the contrast is contained within the joint space (Reproduced with permission from Ohio Pain and Headache Institute)

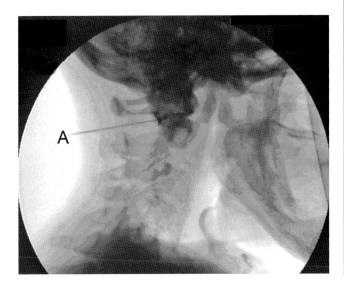

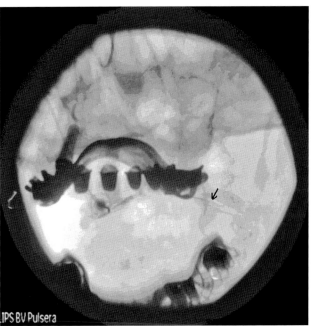

Fig. 27.3 Lateral atlanto-axial joint (AAJ) injection: lateral view showing the needle (A) and the contrast contained within the joint space (Reproduced with permission from Ohio Pain and Headache Institute)

Fig. 27.5 Lateral atlanto-axial joint (AAJ) injection: Needle inside the left AAJ with the contrast spreading to the right AAJ (*arrow*) (Reproduced with permission from Ohio Pain and Headache Institute)

the epidural space, or posteriorly to the C2 ganglion which will adversely affect the specificity of the block (Figs. 27.2 and 27.3). The anteroposterior view usually demonstrates the bilateral concavity of the joint with the contrast material inside the joint space (Fig. 27.2), and sometimes it shows that the lateral AAJ space communicates with that of the

median atlanto-axial joint (Fig. 27.4) and the contralateral AAJ (Fig. 27.5). After careful negative aspiration, 1.0 ml of a mixture of bupivacaine 0.5 % and 10 mg of triamcinolone is injected.

Every effort should be made to make the injection true intra-articular and not periarticular injection. Those procedures

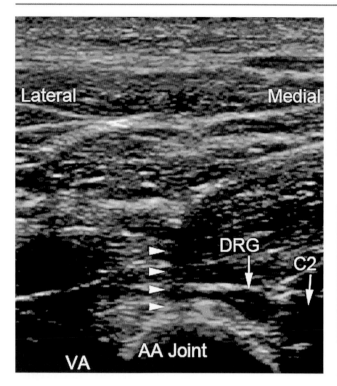

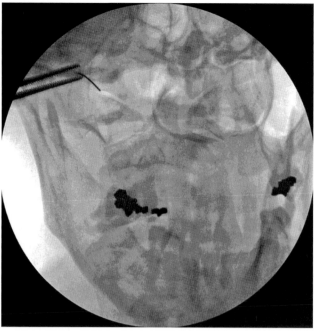

Fig. 27.7 Atlanto-occipital joint (AOJ) injection. AP view (Reproduced with permission from Ohio Pain and Headache Institute)

Fig. 27.6 Atlanto-axial joint (AAJ) injection. Short axis sonogram showing the needle targeting the AAJ (*arrowheads*). *C2* C2 nerve root, *DRG* dorsal root ganglion, *VA* vertebral artery (Reproduced with permission from Ohio Pain and Headache Institute)

which makes it vulnerable to injury while the needle is advanced towards the AOJ, especially with improper positioning of the patient.

are mainly utilized in the diagnosis of pain stemming from the joints, and periarticular injection is not target specific as the local anaesthetic may contaminate the C2 nerve root which crosses the posterior aspect of the AAJ. Intra-articular injection is more target specific as it selectively anesthetizes the joint [7].

Recently, ultrasound-assisted AAJ injection was reported. With real-time sonography, the vertebral artery can be identified laterally and the C2 dorsal root ganglion medially and accordingly; the needle can be advanced in-between (Fig. 27.6) [10].

Atlanto-Occipital Joint (AOJ) Injections

Indications

This procedure is rarely performed for few reasons. Isolated pain stemming from the atlanto-occipital joint (AOJ) is very rare, and usually the patient is presented with localized occipital pain that is aggravated mainly by head nodding. Activity modification and conservative management are usually all what is needed. Also the vertebral artery curves from lateral to medial crossing the posterior aspect of the C1 body

Technique of AOJ Injections

The positioning and approach is similar to that for AAJ injection. The patient needs to flex his head over the neck as much as possible (chin on chest) to open the suboccipital space posteriorly. The atlanto-occipital joint should be accessed posteriorly from the most superior lateral aspect to avoid the vertebral artery (Figs. 27.7 and 27.8).

More recently, ultrasound-assisted AOJ injection in conjunction with fluoroscopy was described. With real-time sonography, the vertebral artery is identified as it curves medially behind C1 body and accordingly can be avoided from the needle path, and then the procedure can be continued with fluoroscopy to confirm intra-articular placement of the needle (Fig. 27.9) [10].

Efficacy of AAJ and AOJ Injections

Narouze and colleagues [7] studied 115 patients with cervicogenic headache. Thirty-two patients had a clinical picture suggestive of atlanto-axial joint pain, and the diagnosis was

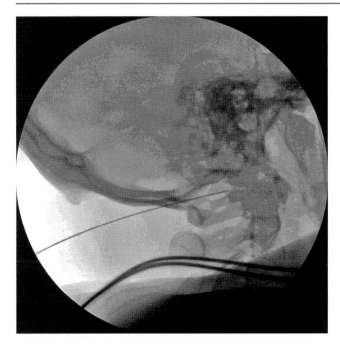

Fig. 27.8 Atlanto-occipital joint (AOJ) injection. Lateral view (Reproduced with permission from Ohio Pain and Headache Institute)

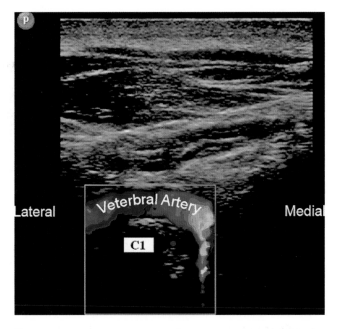

Fig. 27.9 Atlanto-occipital joint (AOJ) injection. Sonogram showing the vertebral artery as it curves medially posterior to C1 (Reproduced with permission from Ohio Pain and Headache Institute)

confirmed in 15 patients with complete abolition of the headache (pain score of zero) after AAJ injection. The prevalence of AAJ pain among patients with cervicogenic headache was 13 % (15/115 patients). At 1, 3, and 6 months after AAJ intra-articular steroid injection, the mean pain scores dropped from a baseline of 6.8 to 1.9, 3.6, and 3.7, respectively. The authors concluded that intra-articular steroid injection is effective in short-term relief of pain originating from the lateral AAJ. There is no data available to demonstrate the efficacy of AOJ intra-articular steroid injections.

Complications of AAJ and AOJ Injections

1. Spinal cord injury and syringomyelia are potential serious complications if the needle is directed further medially into the spinal canal [11].
2. Vertebral artery injection/injury was reported with serious morbidity. Injection of a contrast agent should be performed under real-time fluoroscopy, preferably with digital subtraction if available, prior to the injection of the local anaesthetic, as negative aspiration is unreliable [12]. Meticulous attention should be paid to avoid intravascular injection as vertebral artery anatomy may be variable. Recently, ultrasound-assisted AAJ and AOJ injections were reported in an effort to add more safety to the procedure as ultrasound can identify the relevant soft tissue structures nearby the joints (e.g. vertebral artery and C2 dorsal root ganglion) (Figs. 27.6 and 27.9) [10].
3. Inadvertent puncture of the C2 dural sleeve with CSF leak or high spinal spread of the local anaesthetic may occur with atlanto-axial joint injection if the needle is directed a few millimetres medially [11].

References

1. Aprill C, Axinn MJ, Bogduk N. Occipital headaches stemming from the lateral atlanto-axial (C1–2) joint. Cephalalgia. 2002;22(1):15–22.
2. Busch E, Wilson PR. Atlanto-occipital and atlanto-axial injections in the treatment of headache and neck pain. Reg Anesth. 1989;14 Suppl 2:45.
3. Bogduk N. The neck and headache. Neurol Clin. 2004; 22(1):151–71.
4. Ehni G, Benner B. Occipital neuralgia and the C1–2 arthrosis syndrome. J Neurosurg. 1984;61:961–5.
5. Schonstorm N, Twomey L, Taylor J. The lateral atlanto-axial joints and their synovial folds: an in vitro study of soft tissue injury and fractures. J Trauma. 1993;35:886–92.
6. Narouze SN, Casanova J. The efficacy of lateral atlanto-axial intra-articular steroid injection in the management of cervicogenic headache (abstract). Anesthesiology. 2004;101:A1005.
7. Narouze SN, Casanova J, Mekhail N. The longitudinal effectiveness of lateral atlanto-axial intra-articular steroid injection in the management of cervicogenic headache. Pain Med. 2007; 8:184–8.

8. Narouze SN, Gutenberg L. Radiofrequency denervation of the lateral atlantoaxial joint for the treatment of cervicogenic headache (abstract). Reg Anesth Pain Med. 2007;32:A-8.

9. Ghanayem AJ, Leventhal M, Bohlman HH. Osteoarthrosis of the atlantoaxial joints- long term follow up after treatment with arthrodesis. J Bone Joint Surg Am. 1996;78:1300–7.

10. Narouze S. Ultrasonography in pain medicine: future directions. Tech Reg Anesth Pain Manag. 2009;13(3):198–202.

11. Narouze S. Complications of head and neck procedures. Tech Reg Anesth Pain Manag. 2007;11:171–7.

12. Edlow BL, Wainger BJ, Frosch MP, Copen WA, Rathmell JP, Rost NS. Posterior circulation stroke after C1–C2 intraarticular facet steroid injection: evidence for diffuse microvascular injury. Anesthesiology. 2010;112:1532–5.

Sphenopalatine Ganglion Block

Michael S. Leong, Mark P. Gjolaj, and Raymond R. Gaeta

Key Points

- The sphenopalatine ganglion is the most cephalad region of input for the superior cervical sympathetic ganglion.
- Sphenopalatine blockade is indicated to treat headache (cluster, migraine), atypical facial pain and neuralgias, and possibly other sympathetic maintained conditions.
- There are three main techniques for performing sphenopalatine ganglion blockade, the simplest using cotton pledgets to the middle turbinates of the nasal sinuses, the most advanced with fluoroscopic-guided technique.
- Further clinical studies are required to demonstrate efficacy in neuropathic pain conditions other than cluster headache and facial neuralgias.

M.S. Leong, M.D. (✉)
Stanford Pain Medicine Center,
450 Broadway Street, Redwood City CA 94063, USA

Department of Anesthesiology,
Stanford University School of Medicine, Stanford, CA, USA
e-mail: msleong@stanford.edu

M.P. Gjolaj, M.D., M.B.A.
Stanford Pain Management Center,
450 Broadway Street, Redwood City CA 94063, USA

Department of Anesthesiology, Stanford Hospital and Clinics,
450 Broadway Street, Redwood City, CA 94063, USA

Division of Pain Medicine,
Stanford University School of Medicine, Stanford, CA, USA
e-mail: markmd@gmail.com

R.R. Gaeta, M.D.
HELP Pain Medical Network,
1900 O'Farrell Street, Ste 250, San Mateo, CA 94403, USA
e-mail: rgaeta@helppain.net

Introduction

A certain mystique surrounds the sphenopalatine ganglion as it seemingly rests in the middle of the head but is readily accessible for neural blockade. The sphenopalatine ganglion block is an older and relatively simple pain management block for treatment of headache (cluster and migraine) and facial neuralgias. This block was first described by Greenfield Sluder in 1908 for the treatment of nasal headaches [1]. Since it is localized to the back of the nasopharynx, it can be approached externally through the nares by using cotton pledgets soaked with local anesthetic to anesthetize this region. This simple approach has even been taught to headache sufferers to manage their own pain control at home [2]. Despite the ease of blockade, only recently has interest in the block been resurrected.

Anatomically, the sphenopalatine ganglion, also called pterygopalatine ganglion, is the superior most constellation of sensory (maxillary nerve), parasympathetic (greater petrosal nerve), and sympathetic (superior cervical ganglion) nervous system. The sensory branches of the palatine nerves pass through the ganglion from their origin as the sphenopalatine branches of the maxillary nerve. The parasympathetic portions arise from the nervus intermedius contribution of the greater petrosal nerve. These parasympathetic fibers are responsible for the secretory and vasodilatory functions of the various glands of the nasopharynx and lacrimal glands. The sympathetic fibers originate in the superior cervical plexus through the carotid plexus. The deep petrosal nerve then enters the ganglion to provide the sympathetic vasoconstriction function of the ganglion.

Alternative approaches to the sphenopalatine ganglion, intraoral and fluoroscopic radiofrequency ablation, have increased utilization of this procedure. Hence, a diagnostic and temporary sphenopalatine ganglion block via a nasopharynx approach in the pain management clinic can be used to predict whether further interventional fluoroscopic radiofrequency procedures should be attempted. In one study of the treatment of episodic cluster headache, 46 % of the 15 patients treated had a change in headache frequency for 18 months [3].

Literature Review

The main indications for the sphenopalatine ganglion block have traditionally been multiple headache conditions and facial neuralgias. Michael Sanders reported a 70-month follow-up study on 66 patients with cluster headaches, with 60.7 % of episodic patients having benefit and 30 % with chronic patients gaining benefit [4]. A more recent example of treatment of episodic cluster headache is Narouze's study above. Most recently, electrical stimulation of the sphenopalatine ganglion under fluoroscopic guidance seems effective for episodic cluster headaches [5]. Migraine, one of the most common headache syndromes, has been recognized as having cranial parasympathetic input to the trigeminovascular pain pathway, with intranasal lidocaine providing significant pain relief [6]. Similar to the cluster headache study above, electrical stimulation of acute migraine seems to be effective as well [7]. A case report by Shah and Racz demonstrated long-term relief of posttraumatic headache by sphenopalatine ganglion pulsed radiofrequency lesioning [8]. With regard to facial neuralgias, a case report of stereotactic radiosurgery has been used to treat sphenopalatine neuralgia [9]. Another case report reported treatment of trigeminal neuralgia [10]. A more extensive series for atypical facial and head pain using pulsed radiofrequency of the sphenopalatine ganglion in 30 patients showed 61 % having mild to moderate pain relief [11].

The sphenopalatine ganglion block has also been studied in other chronic pain conditions. Two case series have looked at its application to myofascial pain and fibromyalgia, with no differences between 4 % lidocaine and placebo [12–14]. Cancer pain due to carcinoma of the tongue and floor of the mouth has responded to sphenopalatine block [15]. Two cases of acute herpetic infection and even sinus arrest from postherpetic neuralgia have been treated with this block [16, 17]. One of the more intriguing case series involves two complex regional pain syndrome patients with lower extremity affected limbs [18]. Even after sympathetic blockade of the lower extremities had failed, sphenopalatine ganglion blocks with 4 % tetracaine provided 50 % pain reduction. Further clinical studies are required to demonstrate efficacy in neuropathic pain conditions other than cluster headache and facial neuralgias. Moreover, studies on block technique, full radiofrequency ablation versus pulsed and electrical stimulation, are also indicated.

Evidence-Based Assessment of Available Studies

Using the Guyatt grading strength of recommendations [19], most of the strongest studies were graded as 1C observational studies or case series: Sanders, Narouze, Ansarinia, Tepper, and Yarnitsky. These studies targeted episodic cluster headaches or migraine and had subject samples of five or more. In addition, Bayer's study of pulsed radiofrequency for treatment of atypical facial and head pain was also robust for an observational series – 30 subjects. Hence, the strongest recommendations for treatment so far include episodic cluster headaches, migraine headaches, atypical facial pain, and head pain.

The sphenopalatine ganglion block is a useful technique in the management of pain syndromes in the head region. Its application in the use of migraine is of particular interest in the future. More specific trials related to its treatment should be undertaken to clarify the exact indications and patient characteristics in which it would be useful. It is a safe technique with multiple approaches for both provocative testing and even therapeutic intervention with radiofrequency lesioning.

Intraoral Sphenopalatine Ganglion Block

This intraoral technique of blocking the sphenopalatine ganglion is also called the greater palatine foramen approach. It involves positioning the patient in a supine position, with the neck slightly extended using a pillow or foam wedge. The patient must have an appropriate oral aperture so that the practitioner can palpate the medial gum line of the third molar on the ipsilateral side. The foramen may be identified by a dimple on the medial aspect of the posterior hard palate [20]. A dental needle with a 120° angle is inserted into the foramen approximately 2.5 cm superiorly and slightly posterior [21]. The maxillary nerve is superior or cephalad to the sphenopalatine ganglion, so a facial paresthesia may be elicited if the placement is too deep. After negative aspiration for heme or cerebrospinal fluid, 2 mL of local anesthetic may be injected cautiously.

Sphenopalatine Ganglion Block via Anterior Approach

Access to the sphenopalatine ganglion is readily achieved through the nasal passages utilizing anesthetic-soaked pledgets and bayonet forceps or more easily with the use of cotton tip swabs. In either case, patency of the nares should be ascertained by having patients breathe alternatively through each of their nares, with the opposite side pressed closed. In addition, patients with nasal polyposis or a history of friable nasal mucosa should be approached with caution.

Classically, a nasal speculum to distend the nares allows the larger pledgets with a large surface area to be placed straight back into the nasal passages in the area of the sphenopalatine ganglion. Direct application of local anesthetic through the mucosa to the ganglion is thus achieved. The string attached to the pledget allows for easy recovery. Unfortunately, many patients may not tolerate the insertion of the pledgets, and thus, more significant sedation may be required.

An alternative which is well tolerated by many patients with very light or no sedation is the use of cotton tip swabs dipped in local anesthetic. Patience is required for the utilization of this technique with liberal amount of local anesthetics on the cotton tip swabs. After assuring patency, a liberal amount of lidocaine jelly can be applied to the nares prior to insertion of the cotton-tipped swabs. After a few minutes for the anesthetic to take effect, the cotton tip swabs should be advanced into the nares slowly in a twirling fashion. Generally, at the level of the turbinates, there may be slight resistance which can be overcome with gentle pressure, patience, and twirling of the cotton tip swab. As the nasal passages and the level of sphenopalatine ganglion are directly back from the midface, the angle of the cotton tip swab should almost be perpendicular to the face and advanced until the end of the nasopharynx is appreciated. With patience, 3–4 cotton tip swabs can be advanced into each nares. Additional local anesthetic can be dribbled onto the cotton tip swabs to provide more local anesthetic. Generally speaking, the cotton tip swabs may be left in place for 20–30 min after which they are removed.

Sphenopalatine Ganglion Block via Fluoroscopic Approach

Contraindications

- Absolute: local infection (skin or paranasal sinus); coagulopathy
- Relative: anatomic abnormalities of sinuses secondary to genetics, trauma, or surgery

Key Anatomic Landmarks

- Pterygopalatine fossa
- Zygomatic arch
- Maxillary nerve

Potential Side Effects

- Numbness at the root of the nose and potentially palate
- Lacrimation of the eye on ipsilateral side
- Reflex bradycardia for radiofrequency lesions
- Bleeding, infection, and epistaxis

Perioperative Medication and Conscious Sedation

Please refer to the current American Society of Anesthesiologist's (ASA) guidelines for conscious sedation [22] and/or Leong and Richeimer's "Conscious Sedation for Interventional Pain Procedures" in Lennard's Pain Procedures in Clinical Practice, 3 ed., Elsevier [23]. Standard monitors should also be applied during and post-procedure, including blood pressure monitoring, EKG, and pulse oximetry.

Procedure

Positioning
Most descriptions of the procedure advise the patient to be in a supine position with anterior-posterior view used initially to visualize the orbit and maxillary sinuses.

Imaging
The image intensifier should be placed in a lateral view and tilted cephalad until the pterygopalatine fossa is visualized. When the two pterygopalatine plates are superimposed, one will visualize an inverted flower "vase" just posterior to the posterior aspect of the maxillary sinus [24].

Needle Placement
The needle (typical – 22 gauge, 3.5 in spinal needle) is placed under the zygoma in the coronoid notch after local anesthetic skin infiltration. Using an AP view of the orbit and maxillary sinuses, the needle is advanced medial, cephalad, and slightly posterior into the pterygopalatine fossa. The needle should be positioned lateral to the lateral wall of the nose but medial to the maxillary sinus. When the needle enters the fossa, patients may experience a paresthesia from contact with the maxillary nerve [25]. One to two milliliters of local anesthetic (1–2 % lidocaine) is injected at this region prior to advancing the needle into the anterior superior corner of the fossa. If any resistance is encountered, needle positioning should be stopped and redirected to prevent advancing through the lateral wall of the nose.

It is important to place the needle into the sphenopalatine foramen, particularly when using radiofrequency ablation to prevent damage to the maxillary nerve. When

Table 28.1 Comparative costs of three nerve blocks

CPT code	Description	Medicare allowable – nonfacility	Medicare allowable – facility	Total
64505	Injection, anesthetic agent; spheno-palatine ganglion	$113.59	$92.39	$205.98
64510	Injection, anesthetic agent; stellate ganglion (cervical sympathetic)	$165.05	$75.59	$240.64
64400	Injection, anesthetic agent; trigeminal nerve, any division or branch	$129.45	$71.02	$200.47

positioned correctly, the patient will have a paresthesia at the root of the nose with nerve stimulation. If a paresthesia is felt in the upper teeth, the needle is placed too close to the maxillary nerve and needs to be redirected in a more caudal fashion [20].

Treatment

Local Anesthetic

One to two milliliters of lidocaine or bupivacaine with or without steroid may be placed at the sphenopalatine ganglion after negative aspiration for heme or CSF. A maximum of 5 mL of local anesthetic may be used for diagnostic block after negative aspiration. Numbness at the root of the nose as well as ipsilateral lacrimation may be a temporary result.

Radiofrequency

Lesioning can be performed using RFTC or pulsed EMF after a successful temporary block with local anesthetic. Typically a 20- or 20-ga, 10-cm, curved blunt-tipped RF needle is placed using a 5–10-mm active tip.

Confirmation of sensory paresthesia at the root of the nose should be elicited with approximately 0.5 V at 50 Hz. Again, if paresthesias are present in the upper teeth, the needle needs to be redirected caudally. Stimulation of the greater and less palatine nerves produces paresthesias of the hard palate. The needle is too lateral and anterior and needs to be redirected posteriorly and medially.

After best placement of the RF needle, RF lesioning is performed at 70–90 s at 80 °C. One to two lesions can be made after infiltration of 1–2 mL of local anesthetic. Pulsed RF does not require local anesthetic pretreatment since the lesioning is only at 42 °C for 120 s. Two to three lesions may be required for pulsed RF treatment.

As mentioned above, a reflex bradycardia may occur with RF and pulsed RF lesioning. A proposed mechanism suggests that a reflex similar to an oculocardiac reflex may be due to afferent transmission back to the dorsal vagal nucleus [26]. This reflex bradycardia stops with discontinuation of lesioning, but the patient may need atropine to complete the radiofrequency treatment.

Pharmacoeconomic Discussion of Sphenopalatine Blockade

Headache and facial pain produce both direct and indirect costs. Prescription drugs, physician office visits, emergency room visits, and inpatient hospitalizations represent the direct costs of an illness. For migraines alone, the national direct cost burden is estimated at $11 billion [Hawkins K. Value Health 2006;9:A85]. Indirect costs, due to missed workdays, short-term disability, and worker's compensation, make up over $13 billion annually, excluding presenteeism [27]. Presenteeism accounts for up to an additional $5 billion dollars annually of cost to employers in the United States [28].

In a large study of various pain disorders among the US workforce, headache was the most frequent cause of lost productive time over a 2-week period and caused the average affected individual to miss 3.5 h/week [29]. In the American Migraine Prevalence and Prevention (AMPP) study, the annual per person cost was $1,757 in episodic migraine and $7,750 in transformed migraine [30].

Approximately 15,000 new patients are diagnosed with trigeminal neuralgia each year in the United States alone [31]. An estimated 8,000 undergo surgery each year at an annual cost of greater than $100 million [32].

Sphenopalatine ganglion blockade represents a clinically and cost-effective intervention for facial pain and headaches. As shown in Table 28.1, the costs associated with sphenopalatine ganglion block match those of blocking one trigeminal nerve and are 20 % less than stellate ganglion block. When we consider the fact that patients can be instructed in performing the intranasal sphenopalatine ganglion block themselves, it becomes clear that it may be judged "the cheapest technique in the management of chronic pain" [33].

Summary

The sphenopalatine ganglion is located in the upper reaches of the nasopharynx and represents the most superior contribution of the superior sympathetic ganglion. Blockade of the sphenopalatine ganglion is easily achieved by a variety of techniques of increasing complexity, and it is deemed useful in the management of various pain syndromes of the head particularly migraine headache. Case series and observational studies have demonstrated its utility for treatment of painful syndromes, with the based designed study reaching 1C level of utility. While future studies should indeed be conducted to determine the exact indications and patient characteristics specific utility of the block, current practice provides a relatively safe and putatively effective treatment strategy for headache and facial pain. Local anesthetic blockade of the ganglion via the anterior nares approach is readily accomplished and serves as a therapeutic trial to determine whether more invasive and perhaps longer lasting treatment such as radiofrequency lesioning should be considered. The magnitude of patient suffering from migraine and facial pain and its societal implications with regard to economics and overall productivity should be a strong impetus to utilize sphenopalatine blockade via the multiple approaches until the definitive studies demonstrate the best algorithm for treatment.

References

1. Sluder G. The role of the sphenopalatine (or Meckel's) ganglion in nasal headaches. N Y Med J. 1908;87:989–90.
2. Saade E, Paige GB. Patient-administered sphenopalatine ganglion block. Reg Anesth. 1996;21(1):68–70.
3. Narouze S, Kapural L, Casanova J, Mekhail N. Sphenopalatine ganglion radiofrequency ablation for the management of chronic cluster headache. Headache. 2009;49(4):571–7. Epub 2008 Sep 9.
4. Sanders M, Zuurmond WW. Efficacy of sphenopalatine ganglion blockade in 66 patients suffering from cluster headache: a 12- to 70-month follow-up evaluation. J Neurosurg. 1997;87(6):876–80.
5. Ansarinia M, Rezai A, Tepper SJ, Steiner CP, Stump J, Stanton-Hicks M, Machado A, Narouze S. Electrical stimulation of sphenopalatine ganglion for acute treatment of cluster headaches. Headache. 2010;50(7):1164–74. Epub 2010 Apr 22.
6. Yarnitsky D, Goor-Aryeh I, Bajwa ZH, Ransil BI, Cutrer FM, Sottile A, Burstein R. 2003 Wolff Award: possible parasympathetic contributions to peripheral and central sensitization during migraine. Headache. 2003;43(7):704–14.
7. Tepper SJ, Rezai A, Narouze S, Steiner C, Mohajer P, Ansarinia M. Acute treatment of intractable migraine with sphenopalatine ganglion electrical stimulation. Headache. 2009;49(7):983–9. Epub 2009 May 26.
8. Shah RV, Racz GB. Long-term relief of posttraumatic headache by sphenopalatine ganglion pulsed radiofrequency lesioning: a case report. Arch Phys Med Rehabil. 2004;85(6):1013–6.
9. Pollock BE, Kondziolka D. Stereotactic radiosurgical treatment of sphenopalatine neuralgia. Case report. J Neurosurg. 1997;87(3):450–3.
10. Manahan AP, Malesker MA, Malone PM. Sphenopalatine ganglion block relieves symptoms of trigeminal neuralgia: a case report. Nebr Med J. 1996;81(9):306–9.
11. Bayer E, Racz GB, Miles D, Heavner J. Sphenopalatine ganglion pulsed radiofrequency treatment in 30 patients suffering from chronic face and head pain. Pain Pract. 2005;5(3):223–7.
12. Scudds RA, Janzen V, Delaney G, Heck C, McCain GA, Russell AL, Teasell RW, Varkey G, Woodbury MG. The use of topical 4 % lidocaine in spheno-palatine ganglion blocks for the treatment of chronic muscle pain syndromes: a randomized, controlled trial. Pain. 1995;62(1):69–77.
13. Janzen VD, Scudds R. Sphenopalatine blocks in the treatment of pain in fibromyalgia and myofascial pain syndrome. Laryngoscope. 1997;107(10):1420–2.
14. Ferrante FM, Kaufman AG, Dunbar SA, Cain CF, Cherukuri S. Sphenopalatine ganglion block for the treatment of myofascial pain of the head, neck, and shoulders. Reg Anesth Pain Med. 1998;23(1):30–6.
15. Prasanna A, Murthy PS. Sphenopalatine ganglion block and pain of cancer. J Pain Symptom Manage. 1993;8(3):125.
16. Prasanna A, Murthy PS. Combined stellate ganglion and sphenopalatine ganglion block in acute herpes infection. Clin J Pain. 1993;9(2):135–7.
17. Saberski L, Ahmad M, Wiske P. Sphenopalatine ganglion block for treatment of sinus arrest in postherpetic neuralgia. Headache. 1999;39(1):42–4.
18. Quevedo JP, Purgavie K, Platt H, Strax TE. Complex regional pain syndrome involving the lower extremity: a report of 2 cases of sphenopalatine block as a treatment option. Arch Phys Med Rehabil. 2005;86(2):335–7.
19. Guyatt G, Gutterman D, Baumann MH, Addrizzo-Harris D, Hylek EM, Phillips B, Raskob G, Lewis SZ, Schünemann H. Grading strength of recommendations and quality of evidence in clinical guidelines: report from an American college of chest physicians task force. Chest. 2006;129(1):174–81.
20. Day M. Sphenopalatine ganglion analgesia. Curr Rev Pain. 1999;3(5):342–7.
21. Waldman SD. Sphenopalatine ganglion block–80 years later. Reg Anesth. 1993;18(5):274–6.
22. American Society of Anesthesiologists (ASA) Guidelines for conscious sedation. American Society of Anesthesiologists. 2012. http://www.asahq.org/For-Healthcare-Professionals/Standards-Guidelines-and-Statements.aspx. Accessed 24 Jan 2012.
23. Leong M, Richeimer S. Conscious sedation for interventional pain procedures. In: Lennard TA, Walkowski SD, Singla AK, editors. Pain procedures in clinical practice. 3rd ed. Philadelphia: Elsevier; 2011.
24. Raj P, et al. Sphenopalatine galnglion block and neurolysis. In: Raj PP, Lou L, Erdine S, Staats PS, editors. Radiographic imaging for regional anesthesia and pain management. Philadelphia: Churchill Livingstone (Elsevier); 2003.
25. van Kleef M, Slujter M, van Zundert J. Radiofrequency treatment. In: Benzon H, Rathmell JP, Wu CL, Turk DC, Argoff CE, editors. Raj's practical management of pain. 4th ed. Philadelphia: Elsevier; 2008. p. 1063–78.
26. Konen A. Unexpected effects due to radiofrequency thermocoagulation of the sphenopalatine ganglion: Two case reports. Pain Dig. 2000;10:30–3.
27. Hawkins K, Wang S, Rupnow MF. Indirect cost burden of migraine in the United States. J Occup Environ Med. 2007;49:368–74.
28. Hu XH, Markson LE, Lipton RB, Stewart WF, Berger ML. Burden of migraine in the United States: disability and economic costs. Arch Intern Med. 1999;159(8):813–8.
29. Stewart WF, Ricci JA, Chee E, Morganstein D, Lipton RB. Lost productive time and cost due to common pain conditions in the US workforce. JAMA. 2003;290(18):2443–54.
30. Munakata J, Hazard E, Serrano D, et al. Economic burden of transformed migraine: results from the American Migraine Prevalence and Prevention (AMPP) Study. Headache. 2009;49(4):498–508.
31. Katusic S, Beard CM, Bergstralh E, et al. Incidence and clinical features of trigeminal neuralgia, Rochester, Minnesota, 1945–1984. Ann Neurol. 1990;27:89–95.
32. Pollock BE, Ecker RD. A prospective cost-effectiveness study of trigeminal neuralgia surgery. Clin J Pain. 2005;21(4):317–22.
33. Russell AL. Sphenopalatine block–the cheapest technique in the management of chronic pain. Clin J Pain. 1991;7(3):256–7.

Occipital Nerve Block

29

Garret K. Morris and Michael S. Leong

Key Points
- Anatomically, the greater occipital nerve is associated with the C2 dorsal root and ganglion and receives a contribution from the medial branch of the posterior division of the third cervical nerve.
- Occipital nerve blocks are a common component of the pain physician's armamentarium.
- Despite the relative frequency with which these blocks are performed, there is no standardized protocol, and considerable variation in technique exists.
- Occipital neuralgia, by definition, responds favorably.
- Cervicogenic and cluster headaches also appear to be prime candidates for the intervention.
- Migraineurs may obtain benefit, although the evidence is less substantial.
- Peripheral neuromodulation may be a viable option.
- Occipital nerve blocks are not predictive of the success of occipital peripheral nerve stimulation.

Introduction

Occipital nerve blocks have been performed for more than 50 years and are commonly employed in modern practice to treat pain not only in the distribution of the greater occipital nerve but also with increasing frequency in the treatment of myriad other painful conditions of the head and neck. Despite this prevalence, however, no formal, "standardized" protocol exists. Rather multiple, differing techniques for deposition of local anesthetic around the nerve have been described in the literature, making comparative analysis challenging. Regardless, evidence to date supports substantial analgesic benefit of the procedure, and future investigation may very well elucidate an even greater scope of implementation.

Anatomy

The origin of the greater occipital nerve can be traced back to the second cervical level, where an extradural convergence of root filaments forms the C2 dorsal root and ganglion, lateral to the atlantoaxial ligament and inferior to the obliquus capitis inferior. Here, the ganglion is confined to the intervertebral foramen: atlantoaxial joint ventrally, posteromedial arch of the atlas and lamina of the axis dorsally, posterior arch of the atlas rostrally, and lamina of the axis caudally. Following a horizontal course within the foramen, the second cervical nerve emerges and almost immediately divides, yielding the largest of all cervical posterior divisions and coursing below the obliquus capitis inferior and between the posterior arch of the atlas and the lamina of the axis. Here, the dorsal ramus splits into four braches, including a large medial branch known as the greater occipital nerve (GON) due to its size and anatomical course.

G.K. Morris, M.D. (✉)
Department of Anesthesiology,
University of Rochester School of Medicine,
601 Elmwood Avenue, Rochester, NY 14642, USA
e-mail: morris_garret@yahoo.com

M.S. Leong, M.D.
Stanford Pain Medicine Center,
450 Broadway Street, Redwood City, CA 94063, USA

Department of Anesthesiology,
Stanford University School of Medicine,
Stanford, CA, USA
e-mail: msleong@stanford.edu

Fig. 29.1 Schematic illustration depicting compression point 1, where the nerve exits from deep to the obliquus capitis, wrapping around as it moves cranially and superficially (With permission from Janis et al. [4])

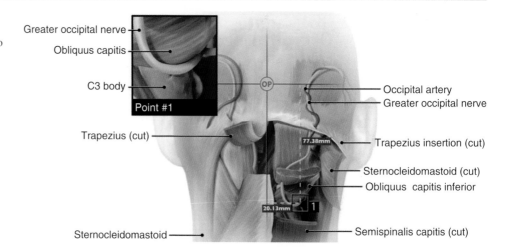

Fig. 29.2 Schematic illustration depicting compression point 2, the entrance of the nerve into the semispinalis muscle (With permission from Janis et al. [4])

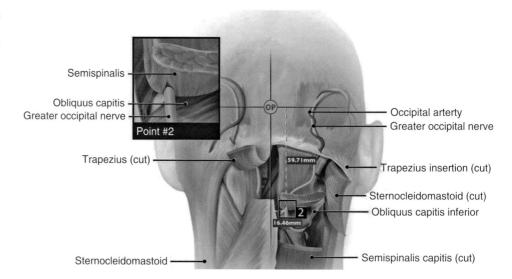

The subsequent path of the GON is critical to understanding the pathological states to which it is related. Following its emergence from the dorsal ramus, the GON quickly turns medially, coursing transversely and dorsally over the belly of the obliquus capitis inferior muscle and deep to the semispinalis capitis, splenius capitis, splenius cervicis, and trapezius. The nerve continues cephalad, penetrating the semispinalis capitis and trapezius and joining the occipital artery. In this area, the GON receives a contribution from the medial branch of the posterior division of the third cervical nerve, ascending parasagittally and obliquely to innervate the posterior occiput, vertex as far as the coronal suture, and as far laterally as the mastoid [1–5].

Over this complex anatomical path exist numerous locations with the potential to create entrapment neuropathies or compression injuries. From proximal to distal, these include (Figs. 29.1, 29.2, 29.3, 29.4, 29.5, and 29.6):

1. The space between the vertebral bones of C1 and C2
2. The atlantoaxial ligament as the dorsal ramus emerges

3. The deep to superficial turn around the inferiolateral border of the obliquus capitis inferior muscle and its tight investing fascia
4. The deep side of semispinalis capitis, where initial piercing can involve entrapment in either the muscle itself or surrounding fascia
5. The superficial side of semispinalis capitis, where completion of nerve piercing muscle and its fascia again poses risk
6. The deep side of the trapezius as the nerve enters the muscle
7. The tendinous insertion of the trapezius at the superior nuchal line
8. The neurovascular intertwining of the GON and the occipital artery

Traumatic extension injuries (i.e., whiplash) have also been proposed as potential causes, although a definitive mechanism by which such injury could occur has yet to be fully elucidated (Fig. 29.7) [7–9].

Fig. 29.3 Schematic illustration depicting compression point 3, where the greater occipital nerve exits from the semispinalis muscle (With permission from Janis et al. [4])

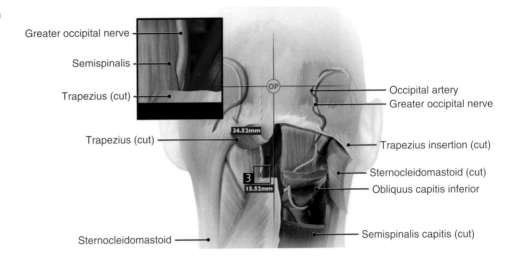

Greater occipital nerve
Semispinalis
Trapezius (cut)
Trapezius (cut)
34.52mm
3
15.52mm
Sternocleidomastoid
OP
Occipital artery
Greater occipital nerve
Trapezius insertion (cut)
Sternocleidomastoid (cut)
Obliquus capitis inferior
Semispinalis capitis (cut)

Fig. 29.4 Schematic illustration depicting compression point 4, where the nerve enters the trapezius (With permission from Janis et al. [4])

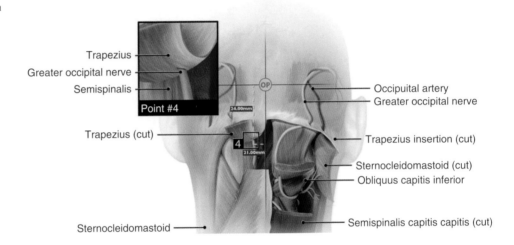

Trapezius
Greater occipital nerve
Semispinalis
Point #4
Trapezius (cut)
24.00mm
4
21.00mm
Sternocleidomastoid
OP
Occipuital artery
Greater occipital nerve
Trapezius insertion (cut)
Sternocleidomastoid (cut)
Obliquus capitis inferior
Semispinalis capitis capitis (cut)

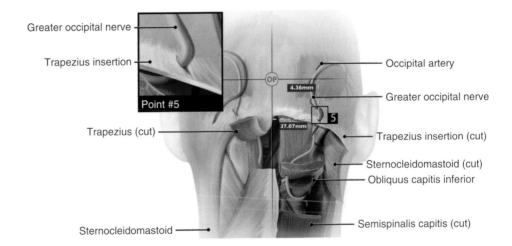

Greater occipital nerve
Trapezius insertion
Point #5
Trapezius (cut)
4.36mm
37.07mm
5
Sternocleidomastoid
OP
Occipital artery
Greater occipital nerve
Trapezius insertion (cut)
Sternocleidomastoid (cut)
Obliquus capitis inferior
Semispinalis capitis (cut)

Fig. 29.5 Schematic illustration depicting compression point 5, where the nerve enters the trapezius insertion (With permission from Janis et al. [4])

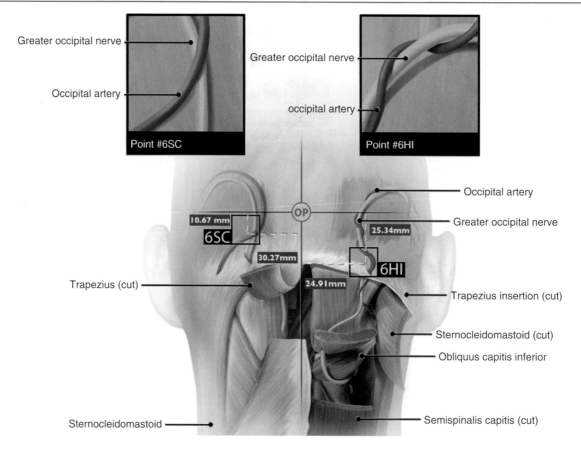

Fig. 29.6 Schematic illustration depicting compression point 6. Different types of greater occipital nerve–occipital artery relationships are shown. *SC* single cross, *HI* helical intertwining (With permission from Janis et al. [4])

Technique

As with all interventional procedures, a thorough and in-depth understanding of the relevant anatomy is an absolute a priori requirement to both successful neural blockade and minimization of potentially deleterious consequences. Unfortunately, despite the common frequency with which this block is internationally performed, there exists no standardized protocol for performing the procedure in either daily clinical practices or peer-reviewed medical literature.

Anatomical landmark identification [3, 10], point of maximal tenderness isolation [11], typical headache pain reproduction [11], ultrasonic Doppler flowmetry-assisted occipital artery localization [12], nerve stimulator guidance [13], and ultrasound image assistance [9] have all been employed in an effort to reproducibly identify the appropriate injection site. Nevertheless, the exact location for deposition of injectate varies widely in published studies in terms of both mediolateral and rostrocaudal orientation. All too often, no formal protocol is described at all, with authors simply stating that medications are injected in the "region of the greater occipital nerve" [14]. Clinically these discrepancies in localization may be serendipitously alleviated somewhat by the not inconsequential

injectate volumes employed, frequently five or even as many as 10 ml [15]. As such, any notion of specificity is rendered suspect at the very least and quite implausible at most, as in so doing yields procedures more akin to general field blocks than selective peripheral neural blockade.

Many authors employing landmark identification suggest palpation of the occipital artery, which frequently courses just lateral to the nerve. However, several pertinent issues may conspire to obscure such identification. One, anatomical variations to conventionally accepted neurovascular association are common. Two, the zone of palpation lies cephalad to typical hairlines, which may make palpation infeasible in the overly hirsute. Three, the occipital artery quite often lacks the vasodynamic bounding of more sizable vessels and thus may not be easily discernable, especially in patients of excess habitus. For these reasons, ultrasonic Doppler flowmetry may be employed to increase the likelihood of arterial localization, with purported increases in success rate and density of blockade, along with decreases in symptoms of vascular uptake as compared to more traditional approaches.

Although multiple techniques have been described, the clinical or statistical superiority of one method over competing

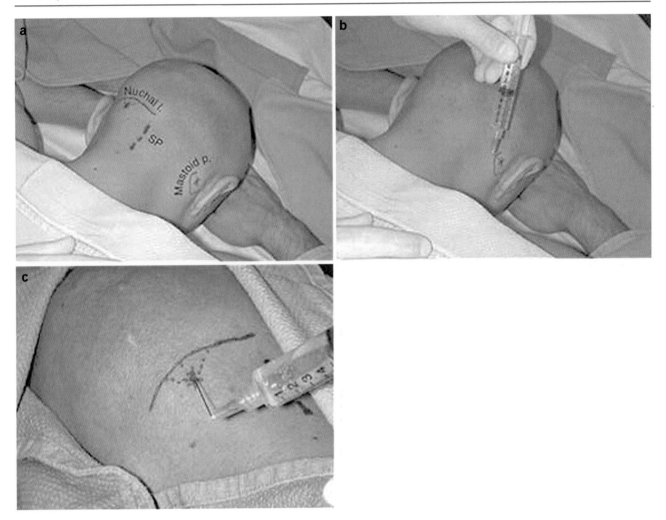

Fig. 29.7 (**a**) Surface anatomy of the occipital area. (SP spinous processe). (**b**) Lesser occipital nerve injection at the mastoid process. (**c**) Greater occipital nerve blockade at the superior nuchal ridge. Anatomic landmarks for greater and lesser occipital nerve block (From Chelly [6]. Copyright ©2009 Lippincott Williams & Wilkins)

approaches has never been validated. The practitioner, therefore, is left with myriad options from which to choose, depending on their personal experience, comfort level, and skill set. At the very least, it would appear that identification of the inion is a prerequisite to block performance, as is a topographical appreciation for the underlying subcutaneous and intermuscular course of the nerve.

Isolating a suitable location for injection is only one aspect of the procedure, however, which leads to the choice of injectate. Published study protocols have varied widely, including the use of both short- and long-acting local anesthetics, sometimes but not always including epinephrine, with or without a number of different steroids, plus or minus additives including but not limited to opioids and alpha-2 agonists. Botulinum toxin has also been employed with some success. Additionally, the chosen injectate volumes are far from uniform, with a single milliliter employed in some trials and as much as 10 ml in others.

What this implies, of course, is that there is either insufficient evidence at this stage to ascribe superiority of one medication regimen over another or, perhaps equally likely, there is simply no appreciable advantage to be elucidated. For instance, Naja et al. [16] injected 3 ml of a 10-ml mixture that included 3 ml of lidocaine 2 %, 3 ml of lidocaine 2 % with epinephrine 1:200,000, 2.5 ml of bupivacaine 0.5 %, 0.5 ml of fentanyl 50 mcg/ml, and 1 ml of clonidine 150 mcg/ml. The authors suggest that this mixture demonstrates superior longevity that exceeds the expected duration of action of the local anesthetic alone. However, Arner et al. [17], using 0.5 % bupivacaine alone, obtained analgesia that exceeded the expected duration of effect in 18/38 consecutive patients treated for peripheral neuralgia. Thus, the incremental improvements in dose response attributable to additives remain uncertain.

Lastly, there exists some evidence to substantiate the efficacy of frequently repeated injections over single interventions to achieve prolonged analgesia. Naja et al. [18] performed occipital nerve blocks repeatedly in 47 patients with cervicogenic headache and were able to achieve a 6-month period of pain relief in 96 %. Interestingly, the authors found that the number of blocks required to reach this end point could be predicted by adding one injection for every 3 years of headache history. Similarly, Caputi and Firetto [19] succeeded in obtaining a 50 % or greater reduction in the total pain index in 23/27 patients using repetitive local anesthetic-only blocks in the treatment of chronic migraineurs.

Indications

1. Occipital neuralgia
2. Cluster headache
3. Cervicogenic headache
4. Migraine
5. Cancer pain in the region [10]
6. Headache associated with muscular spasm or tension [10]
7. Anesthesia of posterior scalp [10]
8. Postconcussive headaches
9. Atypical orofacial pain [20]
10. Abnormal head movements, tinnitus, and dizziness associated with history of trauma [21]
11. Postdural puncture headache [13]
12. Rescue treatment for headaches proving recalcitrant to other measures
13. As an adjuvant to medication-overuse headache

Likely Ineffective

1. Tension headache
2. Hemicrania continua
3. Chronic paroxysmal hemicrania

Contraindications

1. Patient refusal
2. Bleeding diathesis
3. Local or systemic infection
4. Local neoplastic disease

Evidence-Based Review

In recent years, numerous studies have been published demonstrating the efficacy of GONB in multiple chronic pain and other conditions. Quite surprisingly, however, there are few randomized, double-blind, placebo-controlled trials, and the preponderance of evidence available is confounded by methodological discrepancies in diagnosis, technique, treatment, and outcome. Regardless, the available evidence does suggest that several conditions are likely to respond favorably to GONB. Perhaps this ambiguity in diagnostic response is more attributable to insufficient understanding of underlying pathophysiology and resultant overlap in ascribed diagnoses. Alternatively, the functional anatomical convergence of the occipital afferents and the trigeminal nerve complex in the proximal cervical spinal cord may render multiple distinct disease states susceptible to the same intervention. Evidence for this theory is supported by multiple findings. Goadsby et al. [22] showed that the cervical dorsal horn and trigeminal nucleus caudalis show increased metabolic activity during stimulation of the occipital nerve, suggesting that the second-order neurons overlap in their nociceptive processing. This finding was supported by the work of Piovesan et al. [23], who elicited pain in the distribution of the trigeminal nerve, including parasympathetic activation suggestive of trigeminal autonomic activation, during sterile water injection over the greater occipital nerve. More recently, Busch et al. [24, 25] have shown decreases in the nociceptive blink reflex area and increase in the reflex latency following occipital nerve blockade. The functional connectivity between cervicooccipital afferents and the trigeminal nerve complex would, as it appears, be central to the evidentiary link between GONB and its efficacy in the conditions described below. However, the response of primary headache disorders, in addition to occipital neuralgia, to GONB is felt by some to subvert the block's value as a diagnostic tool [26].

Cervicogenic Headache

Multiple studies have repeatedly shown positive responses to GONB in patients with cervicogenic headaches. Naja et al. [16] in a randomized, double-blind, placebo-controlled clinic trial investigated the efficacy of GONB and lesser occipital nerve block in patients with a diagnosis of cervicogenic headache. The facial nerve was also blocked in this study in patients with pain that extended into the orbital area. Using nerve stimulator guidance for localization, the authors injected 10 ml of a mixture containing 2 % lidocaine, 0.5 % bupivacaine, epinephrine, fentanyl, and clonidine to prolong duration of effect. The procedure reduced VAS and TPI scores by 50 % ($P=0.0001$), as well as reducing associated symptoms including duration and frequency of headache and analgesic consumption ($P<0.05$). In a prospective, open-label, case-series follow-up study that involved repeat injections as needed, the authors were able to achieve a 6-month period of pain relief in 96 % of the study participants in the setting of medication tapering. The study patients received an average of 5.3 injections, and the authors concluded that following the initial injection, patients would require one additional injection for each 3 years of headache history to achieve 6 months of relief. Multiple other unblinded studies have corroborated the findings of Naja et al. [27–29].

Cluster Headache

Cluster headache, like cervicogenic headache, has shown statistically significant improvement when treated by GONB in a number of studies. In a double-blind, randomized, placebo-controlled trial, Ambrosini et al. [30] randomized patients with cluster headache to receive 2 % lidocaine with either short- or long-acting betamethasone or normal saline. Headaches resolved in 85 % of patients, lasted for more than 4 weeks in 61 % and more than 4 months in 38 %. Retrospective analyses have also concluded that cluster headaches may respond to GONB. Afridi et al. [31] injected 3 ml of 2 % lidocaine plus 80 mg of methylprednisolone into a subgroup of patients with refractory cluster headache and found complete resolution in 53 % and partial resolution in an additional 16 %. The mean duration of benefit in this population from a single injection was 17 days. Likewise, Peres et al. [32] injected 14 cluster headache patients with 3 ml of 1 % lidocaine and 40 mg of triamcinolone, with 64 % of the study population rendered headache-free following injection and a mean duration of benefit of 13 days.

Occipital Neuralgia

According to the second edition of the International Headache Classification (ICHD-2), efficacy of GONB is, by definition, assumed. That is, in addition to the appropriate symptom complex and physical examination findings, pain must be, at least temporarily, alleviated by blockade of the occipital nerve. As such, prospective investigations determining response in patients presumed to have the diagnosis are rendered redundant. Retrospective analyses have been carried out, however. Anthony [14], using diagnostic criteria that included "unilateral occipital headache … with or without referral to the ipsilateral orbital or supraorbital areas, circumscribed tenderness over the GON … and hypoalgesia, hyperalgesia or dysaesthesiae in the area of distribution of the GON," found complete headache relief in 75 of 86 patients treated with GONB. The mean duration of relief in this study was 31 days when 160 mg of methylprednisolone was incorporated into the injectate. In another retrospective analysis performed by Tobin and Flitman [11], patients received GONBs if they had "significant headache pain … and if pressure on an ON reproduced their headache pain." In this group of patients, the authors achieved a 78 % success rate with local anesthetic and steroid and quite interestingly noted that systemic medication overuse increased the rate of failure threefold, more so in migraneurs than in patients diagnosed with occipital neuralgia.

Migraine Headaches

The evidence supporting GONB in migraneurs is not as compelling as it has been in other conditions (see above), but the procedure has been shown beneficial in some patients nonetheless. In a prospective, open-label, single-treatment-arm study, Weibelt et al. [33] decreased the number of headache days per month by at least 50 % in 78/150 patients, and 90/150 reported their symptoms to have subjectively improved. In a double-blind, controlled, crossover study, Piovesan et al. [34] found that GONB did not reduce the number or duration of migraine attacks, but did conclude that the intensity of headache symptoms was reduced 60 days following the injection. In a prospective, open-label, uncontrolled study, Caputi and Firetto [19] used GONB and supraorbital nerve blocks in on migraine patients whose physical examination was notable for tenderness to palpation over the respective nerves. The authors injected these areas until the tenderness had diminished to less than half its baseline value and noted that 5–10 injections would produce lasting and increasing benefit for as much as 6 months in 85 % of the patients studied. Afridi et al. [31] found benefit with GONB in patients with intractable migraine, obtaining complete or partial (>30 % improvement) response in 46 % of the injections, with a median duration of response of 30 days. Notably, the authors found no correlation between local anesthesia over the distribution of the GON and migrainous response. Gawel and Rothbart [35] retrospectively reviewed GONB with local anesthetic and steroid in their own migraine population and found that 54 % of patients with non-posttraumatic migraineurs felt "significantly better" for up to 6 months following the injection. The authors also noted that in patients with a diagnosis of posttraumatic migraine, the benefit was greater, with 72 % of patients reporting such benefit. The improved response rate in posttraumatic migraineurs has been substantiated by other studies, including Tobin and Flitman [11] who obtained 100 % efficacy (12/12) in postconcussive migraineurs.

Other Uses

The implications of convergence between the trigeminal nerve complex and occipital afferents suggest that the infiltration of medications around the GON may have applications well beyond typical occipital neuralgia. For instance, a recent prospective, randomized, single-blind, clinical study investigated the efficacy of nerve stimulator-guided GONB for the treatment of postdural puncture headache, with 68.4 % of the patients achieving complete relief after one to two blocks, with the remaining 31.6 % experiencing relief after three or four injections [13]. Given the side effect profile of epidural blood patches, this study raises the possibility of an equally effective treatment with far less risk, especially in the immunocompromised and/or anticoagulated postsurgical population.

Another potential avenue of pursuit in GONB involves the mitigation of withdrawal symptoms in patients being treated for chronic medication-overuse headaches. Afridi et al. [31] noted that in patients treated for migraine, there was no statistically significant association between block response and medication overuse. Data from Tobin and Flitman [11] is less supportive, but these authors still demonstrated a 56 % success rate even in those patients overusing abortive agents. In fact, the response rate in medication overusers was quite similar between the two studies, 20/31 (65 %) in Afridi et al. vs. 14/25 (56 %) in Tobin and Flitman's. Considering the difficulty with which many patients with medication-overuse headache wean from their pharmaceuticals, a procedure with the potential to moderate their course would certainly be advantageous.

Occipital Nerve Stimulation

Occipital nerve stimulation has become an increasingly popular modality for treating intractable headaches. In 1999, Weiner et al. [36] reported on a small group of patients with occipital neuralgia who had beneficial effects from subcutaneous neural stimulation. Since that initial report, use of occipital nerve stimulation has extended to more global headache diagnoses, such as migraine [1, 37, 38]. In the past, practitioners have used occipital nerve blocks to predict success with occipital nerve stimulation. However, recent studies show that occipital blocks are not useful for predicting success with occipital stimulation [39, 40]. Indeed, the most recent publication of the ONSTIM trial by Saper and others shows that response to occipital nerve block was not part of inclusion criteria [41].

Cautions

Despite the volume of scientific literature available supporting the use of GONB and the evidence for benefit in a number of clinical conditions, the results must be taken with caution. There are no uniform methods for GONB application, nor were the patient populations studied homogenous. Additionally, with rare exceptions, the bulk of data currently available was derived from uncontrolled investigations, confounding any conclusions that may be drawn. Determining whether the study findings are the result of the explicitly stated pathophysiological associations or more serendipitous interactions will require more focused investigation.

Another issue that clearly needs to be further delineated relates to the location of injection and the tissues through which the needle passes. Although advocated as primary block of the GON, it seems rather obvious that injections

performed more medially and caudally, where the GON exits the semispinalis capitis, are in fact also infiltrating local anesthetic into the paraspinal muscles. In effect, this represents a trigger-point injection in addition to any neural blockade that may be taking place and may be responsible, at least in part, for the finding by Afridi et al. [31] that anesthesia in the distribution of the greater occipital nerve did not correspond to degree of pain relief. This situation is made all the more ambiguous by the propensity of many practitioners to inject not according to any distinct anatomical location but rather in the area of greatest tenderness to palpation or reproduction of typical headache symptoms. Specifically, what is being "blocked" during such procedures is unclear, and as such, the mechanism of underlying pathophysiologic modification and subsequent clinical improvement remains uncertain.

Conclusions

Occipital nerve block has been, and will almost certainly remain, a frequently implemented tool in the pain physician's armamentarium. The procedure has proven effective for several conditions, including, by definition, occipital neuralgia, but also cervicogenic and cluster headaches. There also appears to be a role for treatment in migraineurs, although further investigation is needed. Despite the prevalence of the block, numerous technical variances obscure definitive conclusions.

References

1. Cohen DB, Oh MY, Whiting DM. Occipital neuralgia. In: Lozano AM, Gildenberg PL, Tasker RR, editors. Textbook of stereotactic and functional neurosurgery. Berlin: Springer; 2009. p. 2507–16.
2. Gray H. Anatomy of the human body. Philadelphia: Lea & Febiger; 1918.
3. Mosser SW, Guyuron B, Janis JE, Rohrich RJ. The anatomy of the greater occipital nerve: implications for the etiology of migraine headaches. Plast Reconstr Surg. 2004;113(2):693–7; discussion 698–700.
4. Janis JE, Hatef DA, Ducic I, Reece EM, Hamawy AH, Becker S, Guyuron B. The anatomy of the greater occipital nerve: part II. Compression point topography. Plast Reconstr Surg. 2010;126(5):1563–72.
5. Lu J, Ebraheim NA. Anatomic considerations of C2 nerve root ganglion. Spine. 1998;23(6):649–52.
6. Chelly JE. Peripheral nerve blocks: a color atlas. 3rd ed. Philadelphia: Lippincott Williams & Wilkins; 2009.
7. Hunter CR, Mayfield FH. Role of the upper cervical roots in the production of pain in the head. Am J Surg. 1949;48:743–52.
8. Bogduk N. Then anatomy of occipital neuralgia. Clin Exp Neurol. 1980;17:167–84.
9. Stechison MT, Mullin BB. Surgical treatment of greater occipital neuralgia: an appraisal of strategies. Acta Neurochir (Wein). 1994;131:236–40.
10. Benzon HT, Rathmell JP, Wu CL, Turk DC, Argoff CE. Raj's Practical management of pain. 4th ed. Mosby-Elsevier: Philadelphia; 2008.
11. Tobin JA, Flitman SS. Occipital nerve blocks: effect of symptomatic medication: overuse and headache type on failure rate. Headache. 2009;49(10):1479–85.

12. Na SH, Kim TW, Oh SY, Kweon TD, Yoon KB, Yoon DM. Ultrasonic Doppler flowmeter-guided occipital nerve block. Korean J Anesthesiol. 2010;59(6):394–7.

13. Naja Z, Al-Tannir M, El-Rajab M, Ziade F, Baraka A. Nerve stimulator-guided occipital nerve blockade for postdural puncture headache. Pain Pract. 2009;9(1):51–8.

14. Anthony M. Headache and the greater occipital nerve. Clin Neurol Neurosurg. 1992;94(4):297–301.

15. Fishman SM, Ballantyne JC, Rathmell JP, editors. Bonica's management of pain. 4th ed. Philadelphia: Wolters Kluwer/Lippincott, Williams and Wilkins; 2010.

16. Naja ZM, El-Rajab M, Al-Tannir MA, Ziade FM, Tawfik OM. Occipital nerve blockade for cervicogenic headache: a double-blind randomized controlled clinical trial. Pain Pract. 2006;6(2):89–95.

17. Arnér S, Lindblom U, Meyerson BA, Molander C. Prolonged relief of neuralgia after regional anesthetic blocks. A call for further experimental and systematic clinical studies. Pain. 1990;43(3):287–97.

18. Naja ZM, El-Rajab M, Al-Tannir MA, Ziade FM, Tawfik OM. Repetitive occipital nerve blockade for cervicogenic headache: expanded case report of 47 adults. Pain Pract. 2006;6(4):278–84.

19. Caputi CA, Firetto V. Therapeutic blockade of greater occipital and supraorbital nerves in migraine patients. Headache. 1997;37(3):174–9.

20. Sulfaro MA, Gobetti JP. Occipital neuralgia manifesting as orofacial pain. Oral Surg Oral Med Oral Pathol Oral Radiol Endod. 1995;80(6):751–5.

21. Matsushima JI, Sakai N, Uemi N, Ifukube T. Effects of greater occipital nerve block on tinnitus and dizziness. Int Tinnitus J. 1999;5(1):40–6.

22. Goadsby PJ, Knight YE, Hoskin KL. Stimulation of the greater occipital nerve increases metabolic activity in the trigeminal nucleus caudalis and cervical dorsal horn of the cat. Pain. 1997;73(1):23–8.

23. Piovesan EJ, Kowacs PA, Tatsui CE, Lange MC, Ribas LC, Werneck LC. Referred pain after painful stimulation of the greater occipital nerve in humans: evidence of convergence of cervical afferences of trigeminal nuclei. Cephalalgia. 2001;21(2):107–9.

24. Busch V, Jakob W, Juergens T, Schulte-Mattler W, Kaube H, May A. Functional connectivity between trigeminal and occipital nerves revealed by occipital nerve blockade and nociceptive blink reflexes. Cephalalgia. 2006;26(1):50–5.

25. Busch V, Jakob W, Juergens T, Schulte-Mattler W, Kaube H, May A. Occipital nerve blockade in chronic cluster headache patients and functional connectivity between trigeminal and occipital nerves. Cephalalgia. 2007;27(11):1206–14. Epub 2007 Sep 10.

26. Young WB. Blocking the greater occipital nerve: utility in headache management. Curr Pain Headache Rep. 2010;14(5):404–8.

27. Inan N, Ceyhan A, Inan L, Kavaklioglu O, Alptekin A, Unal N. C2/C3 nerve blocks and greater occipital nerve block in cervicogenic headache treatment. Funct Neurol. 2001;16(3):239–43.

28. Vincent M. Greater occipital nerve blockades in cervicogenic headache. Funct Neurol. 1998;13:78–9.

29. Bovim G, Sand T. Cervicogenic headache, migraine without aura and tension-type headache. Diagnostic blockade of the greater occipital and supra-orbital nerves. Pain. 1992;51:43–8.

30. Ambrosini A, Vandenheede M, Rossi P, Aloj F, Sauli E, Pierelli F, Schoenen J. Suboccipital injection with a mixture of rapid- and long-acting steroids in cluster headache: a double-blind placebo-controlled study. Pain. 2005;118(1–2):92–6.

31. Afridi SK, Shields KG, Bhola R, Goadsby PJ. Greater occipital nerve injection in primary headache syndromes–prolonged effects from a single injection. Pain. 2006;122(1–2):126–9. Epub 2006 Mar 9.

32. Peres MF, Stiles MA, Siow HC, Rozen TD, Young WB, Silberstein SD. Greater occipital nerve blockade for cluster headache. Cephalalgia. 2002;22(7):520–2.

33. Weibelt S, Andress-Rothrock D, King W, Rothrock J. Suboccipital nerve blocks for suppression of chronic migraine: safety, efficacy, and predictors of outcome. Headache. 2010;50(6):1041–4.

34. Piovesan EJ, Werneck LC, Kowacs PA, Tatsui CE, Lange MC, Vincent M. Anesthetic blockade of the greater occipital nerve in migraine prophylaxis [in Portuguese]. Arq Neuropsiquiatr. 2001;59(3-A):545–51.

35. Gawel MJ, Rothbart PJ. Occipital nerve block in the management of headache and cervical pain. Cephalalgia. 1992;12(1):9–13. Review.

36. Weiner RL, Reed KL. Peripheral neurostimulation for control of intractable occipital neuralgia. Neuromodulation. 1999;2(3):217–21.

37. Weiner RL. Occipital neurostimulation for treatment of intractable headache syndromes. Acta Neurochir Suppl. 2007;97(Pt 1):129–33. Review.

38. Paemeleire K, Bartsch T. Occipital nerve stimulation for headache disorders. Neurotherapeutics. 2010;7(2):213–9. Review.

39. Schwedt TJ, Dodick DW, Trentman TL, Zimmerman RS. Response to occipital nerve block is not useful in predicting efficacy of occipital nerve stimulation. Cephalalgia. 2007;27(3):271–4.

40. Schwedt TJ. Occipital nerve stimulation for medically intractable headache. Curr Pain Headache Rep. 2008;12(1):62–6. Review.

41. Saper JR, Dodick DW, Silberstein SD, McCarville S, Sun M, Goadsby PJ, ONSTIM Investigators. Occipital nerve stimulation for the treatment of intractable chronic migraine headache: ONSTIM feasibility study. Cephalalgia. 2011;31(3):271–85.

Neural Blockade for Trigeminal Neuralgia

30

Ali Mchaourab and Abdallah I. Kabbara

Key Points
- Review the history and epidemiology of trigeminal neuralgia.
- Highlight the clinical manifestations of trigeminal neuralgia.
- Review relevant anatomy of the trigeminal nerve and ganglion.
- Summarize the current treatment modalities and their effectiveness.
- Discuss neural blockade of the trigeminal nerve and ganglion and its application.
- Review potential complications of different invasive modalities.

Historical Background

The first case report of trigeminal neuralgia (TN) dates back to 1671, where it proved fatal to the unfortunate Johannes Laurentius Bausch, a physician. Later works by Nicolaus Andre, John Fothergill, and Charles Bell established "tic douloureux" as a disorder of the trigeminal nerve [1, 2]. In ancient times, facial pain was described by the Arabic physician Ibn Sina (980–1073). The description of interventional therapy dates back to 1677 when Locke applied sulfuric acid to the face of the Duchess of Northumberland to treat her facial pain [3]. The incidence of trigeminal neuralgia is estimated at 4–5 in 100,000 [4] with more prevalence in women (ratio of 1:1.5) [5]. It is the most common form of facial pain in people older than

50 years of age, and its highest incidence occurs in the ages between 50 and 70 years [3]. Described by Peter Jannetta as "the worst pain in the world," its presentation and management continues to present a challenge to modern-day medicine. In this chapter, the authors will review the current nonsurgical invasive modalities used to treat trigeminal neuralgia, placing an emphasis on proper diagnosis which is key for success.

The Clinical Syndrome

Clinical Manifestations

Trigeminal neuralgia pain is a neuropathic pain located in the distribution of the trigeminal nerve or cranial nerve V. It is classically described as sharp, stabbing, lancinating, electric shock-like, short lasting, intermittent and variable, and almost always unilateral. It is often so intense as to interfere with daily routines, speaking, or even eating. Pain can occur spontaneously, or can be triggered by movement or touching of the face or mouth. Therefore, patients typically avoid touching that area of their face, shaving, and chewing. Eating habits are affected, and often patients report weight loss. The fore mentioned avoidance is a valuable clue to diagnosis. In other facial pain syndromes, the opposite occurs: Patients tend to rub or massage the painful area of their face [6].

A typical attack lasts for seconds and is followed by a refractory period, a period of relief that lasts for seconds, minutes, or even hours. Any of the three branches of the trigeminal nerve may be affected. Typically, the neurologic examination is either normal or demonstrates a subtle decrease in sensation in the affected distribution, perhaps including suppression of the ipsilateral corneal reflex.

Differential Diagnosis

The etiology of trigeminal neuralgia is not fully understood. Abnormality of the trigeminal nerve myelin sheet has been

A. Mchaourab, M.D. (✉)
Department of Anesthesiology,
Cleveland Department of Veterans Affairs Medical Center,
10701 East Blvd, Cleveland, OH 44106, USA
e-mail: ali.mchaourab@va.gov

A.I. Kabbara, M.D.
Department of Pain Management, St. John Medical Center,
29000 Center Ridge Road, Westlake, OH 44145, USA
e-mail: drnopain@ymail.com

Table 30.1 Differential diagnosis of trigeminal neuralgia

Differential diagnosis of trigeminal neuralgia		
	Primary clinical characteristics	Mimicking characteristics
Glossopharyngeal neuralgia	Severe transient, stabbing or burning pain in the ear, base of the tongue, jaw, and tonsillar fossa	Pain in facial area; triggers can be chewing, swallowing, talking, or coughing
Geniculate neuralgia	Impairment of CN-VII sensory part; related to herpes zoster; pain is usually in the different ear structures	Pain may radiate from the ear to the face; has a burning dysesthetic quality
Herpetic and postherpetic neuralgia of the trigeminal nerve	Pain is steady and sustained, burning and aching. Often regresses in 2–3 weeks, months in patients older than 70 years of age	The steady pain is accompanied by shooting and sharp pain that radiates and is provoked by mechanical stimuli
Herpetic and postherpetic neuralgia of the cervical dorsal root ganglia	Steady pain in face, ear, and occiput	Facial pain, unilateral
Occipital neuralgia	Pain radiates following the greater occipital nerve distribution to the frontal region	Burning, unilateral pain that can radiate to the forehead, mimicking ophthalmic distribution of the trigeminal nerve
Atypical facial pain	Continuous aching or burning pain; unilateral or bilateral	Burning facial pain; may follow the nerve branches distribution; infrequently exacerbated by eating/talking
Rare disorders, that is, Raeder syndrome, trigeminal nerve neuritis from tumors, and other diseases	Usually Horner syndrome without anhidrosis	Sudden onset severe frontotemporal burning; often in periorbital or trigeminal distribution
Others: dental pathology, ear, nose, and throat; cluster or migraine headaches; temporomandibular joint syndrome	Variable presentations and patterns	Can mimic trigeminal neuralgia

described but not agreed upon [7]. Trigeminal neuralgia is divided into primary or idiopathic and secondary where a compressive etiology is identified such as a vascular structure or tumors, or a disease etiology such as multiple sclerosis. Establishing a diagnosis of trigeminal neuralgia is instrumental to a successful management strategy especially if surgical or invasive interventions are being considered. Pathognomonic criteria for diagnosis include paroxysmal pain that lasts from a fraction of a second to 2 min and pain characterized as intense, sharp, stabbing, and precipitated by trigger factors. Table 30.1 lists facial pain syndromes that could share some of the clinical manifestations of trigeminal neuralgia. The authors cannot stress enough the importance of establishing a firm diagnosis prior to proceeding to management, especially invasive modalities. A false-positive diagnosis will not only lead to failure of treatment but to possible non-indicated invasive treatments that carries potential morbidity and mortality (Table 30.1).

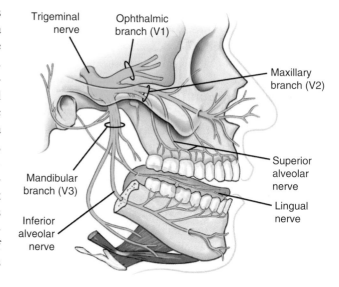

Fig. 30.1 The division of the three branches of the trigeminal nerve after exiting the middle cranial fossa (Copyright Elsevier)

The Gasserian Ganglion

Anatomy

Studying the gross and neuroanatomy of the trigeminal nerve is an essential task prior to neural blockade. The trigeminal nerve has both sensory and motor fibers. Visceral efferent fibers contribute to innervate some muscles of mastication and facial expression. Through its somatic afferent fibers, the trigeminal nerve transmits nociception, light touch, and temperature sensation from the skin of the face, teeth, anterior two thirds of the tongue, the nose, and oral cavity mucosa. Figure 30.1 shows the three branches of the trigeminal nerve (ophthalmic, maxillary, and mandibular).

The gasserian ganglion, also known as the trigeminal ganglion or the semilunar ganglion, sits in an invagination of the dura mater of the posterior cranial fossa, known as Meckel's cave (Fig. 30.1). Injection of local anesthetic in Meckel's cave, which contains cerebrospinal fluid, can potentially lead to total spinal anesthesia or spread to other cranial nerves. Its three sensory divisions, the ophthalmic (V1), maxillary (V2), and mandibular (V3), divide and exit anteriorly as shown in Fig. 30.1. The mandibular branch exiting through the foramen ovale has clinical applications as the reader will see in this chapter.

Blockade of the gasserian ganglion has been applied as surgical anesthetic for procedures of the head and neck in very limited instances. More commonly, it is used as a treatment for trigeminal neuralgia after failure of conservative therapy and also for cancer pain involving the face. Trigeminal ganglion neurolysis has been effective when oral therapy fails. The palliation of cancer-related pain arising from direct nerve involvement or surgical trauma has successfully been accomplished through blockade of the trigeminal ganglion or its divisions. Neurolysis of the trigeminal ganglion relieves cluster headaches refractory to oral therapy [8–12] and intractable atypical facial pain [13, 14].

Techniques for Gasserian Ganglion Blockade

To decrease the chances of adverse events, the use of radiological guidance such as computed tomography [15], fluoroscopy [16], or ultrasonography [17] along with a blunt-tipped curved needle is highly recommended. The blockade of the trigeminal ganglion has been performed without radiological guidance in the past but is not advisable. Those measures not only increase patient's safety but also improve the access to the main anatomical landmark, the foramen ovale.

The patient is placed in a supine position with the head slightly extended. Facial skin is sterilely prepped. It is recommended that conscious sedation be administered for patient comfort with blood pressure, pulse oximetry, and electrocardiogram monitoring. Fluoroscopic x-ray guidance is used. The skin entry site is usually located approximately 2–3 cm lateral to the commissural labialis (the corner of the mouth) in a mid-pupillary line. Localization of the foramen ovale is critical to the success of this block. The anteroposterior fluoroscopic view usually shows the petrous ridge through the orbit, and 1 cm medially, it also shows a dip in the petrous ridge. Rotation of the C-arm head obliquely away from the nose approximately 20–30° and approximately 30–35° in the caudo-cranial direction will bring the foramen into view just medial to the mandible and at the top of the petrous "pyramid." Lidocaine 1 % is applied to the skin and subcutaneous tissue over the shadow of the foramen ovale. For a diagnostic local anesthetic block, a 22-g B-bevel needle, 8–10 long, is used (for radiofrequency lesioning, an RFA 10-cm needle with a 2–5-mm active RFA tip is used). The needle is advanced through the entry point toward the fora-

men ovale, rotating the needle tip as needed to keep it on course initially downward and laterally, then medially aiming for the foramen ovale. To prevent intraoral entry, placement of one finger in the mouth could be done. When bone is encountered, the needle could be walked posteriorly along the skull into the foramen. A lateral view should be obtained, revealing the needle through the foramen ovale in a trajectory superior and toward the medial aspect of the external auditory meatus. A mandibular nerve paresthesia is commonly elicited. It is mandatory to test negative aspiration of cerebrospinal fluid (CSF) confirming that the needle did not penetrate the dura matter. The needle position is confirmed with injection of nonionic water-soluble contrast and negative aspiration of blood and CSF. For diagnostic local anesthetic blockade, small increments of local anesthetic (lidocaine 2 %, bupivacaine 0.5 %, or ropivacaine 0.5 %) are injected for a total of 1 ml. Monitoring the patient is essential to confirm that local anesthetic did not reach the CSF, putting the patient at risk of inadvertent spinal anesthetic and potential respiratory arrest. Figure 30.2 illustrates the trajectory of the needle in correct placement for the gasserian block.

Chemical Neurolysis

Currently, the most common agent used for neurolysis of the trigeminal ganglion is glycerol [18–24], knowing that phenol [25] and alcohol [26–28] have also been used in the past. A neurolytic solution up to 0.5 ml should be injected in small increments preferably of 0.1 ml to avoid inadvertent spread to structures of the brain stem. For the technique using glycerol, the needle is advanced into the trigeminal cistern and free CSF flow is confirmed. When using a hyperbaric neurolytic agent, the patient should sit with the head tipped forward for 2 h [29]. This maneuver ensures spread of the injectate to the maxillary and mandibular branches, sparing the ophthalmic branch. Acute unilateral total visual loss after gasserian phenol injection has been reported [30].

Radiofrequency Ablation

Conventional radiofrequency (RF) neurolysis is performed at temperatures ranging from 60° to 90° centigrade, for duration of 60–90 s. Knowing that the mandibular branch is the only branch carrying motor fibers, motor stimulation at 2 Hz within a range of 0.1–1.5 V will reproduce muscle contraction of the lower mandible. While performing lesioning for V1 or V2, motor stimulation at 2 Hz is not expected to show any muscular contraction. For confirmation of needle position, sensory stimulation at 50 Hz preferably below 0.6 V should precede any treatment. A correct needle position should reproduce a tingling-like sensation or paresthesia in the distribution of the targeted nerve branch. Adjustment of the needle position is performed to optimize desirable sensory patterns prior to any lesioning. Patient alertness and cooperation is of paramount importance: Patient feedback on

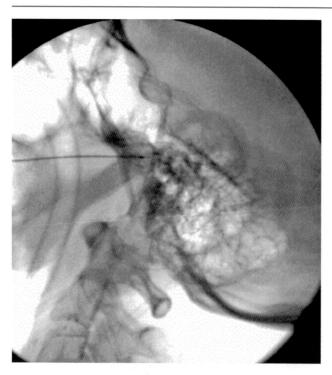

Fig. 30.2 Lateral fluoroscopic view showing trans-foramen ovale gasserian ganglion block: needle is in position and radio-opaque dye classic spread is shown

where the sensation is elicited will help the physician complete the desired block successfully (Fig. 30.2). Understanding the anatomy and how the rootlets of the trigeminal ganglion lay in a superomedial to inferolateral plane is very important: In case of a non-desirable motor response, the practitioner will adjust the needle from a lateral position to a more medial one. Confirmation of negative blood flow should be documented. Up to 0.5 ml of 0.5 % bupivacaine or 0.2 % ropivacaine should be injected prior to RF lesioning to alleviate procedure-related discomfort. If RF lesioning is performed on the 1st branch of the trigeminal nerve (V1), temperature should be limited to 60° to preserve the corneal reflex.

Pulsed radiofrequency [31–34] is another option for neurolysis usually done at 42 °C for 120 s. Even though Erdine et al. [35] could not confirm its effectiveness in this study, it is still being performed with variable results.

The Trigeminal Nerve Branches: Opthalmic, Maxillary, and Mandibular

Anatomy

The ophthalmic branch (V1) of the trigeminal branch is a purely sensory branch [36]. It enters the orbit via the superior orbital fissure. In turn, it divides into three branches, the frontal, nasociliary, and lacrimal nerves. The latter two pro-

vide innervations to nasal structures and the lacrimal gland, respectively. The supraorbital and the supratrochlear are terminal branches of the frontal nerve: They exit the orbit anteriorly and provide innervations to upper eyelid, forehead, and anterior scalp. As illustrated in the next paragraph, they are clinically most significant of the V1 branches.

The maxillary branch (V2) is also a pure sensory branch [37]. It exits the middle cranial fossa into the pterygopalatine fossa in a horizontal fashion through the foramen rotundum. Then, it passes through the inferior orbital fissure to the orbit before exiting to the face via the infraorbital foramen. That passage through the four facial compartments lead to the division of the many branches of V2 to four regional groups of branches. Understanding the exit of V2 from the middle cranial fossa to the face simplifies the understanding of its innervations of facial structures (Fig. 30.1). Table 30.2 summarizes the four groups and the facial areas they innervate.

The mandibular nerve is formed by the joining of the large sensory mandibular division of the trigeminal nerve and a small motor nerve root. They both cross the foramen ovale leaving the middle cranial fossa and forming the mandibular nerve [37]. This combined trunk then divides into a small anterior and larger posterior trunk (Fig. 30.1). Prior to this division, it gives off the nervus spinosus, innervating the dura matter and mucosal lining of the mastoid sinus, and the internal pterygoid, innervating the internal pterygoid and sending branches to the otic ganglion.

From the anterior trunk comes the buccinator nerve to innervate the skin and mucous membrane overlying the buccinator muscle. The anterior trunk also gives off three motor branches: the masseteric, deep temporal nerves, and the external pterygoid nerve. They provide motor innervations to the masseter muscle, temporalis muscle, and external pterygoid muscle, respectively.

The posterior trunk contains mostly sensory fibers. The following branches come off the posterior trunk: The auriculotemporal nerve provides sensory innervations to the following structures – the tympanic membrane, the lining of the acoustic meatus, the posterior temporomandibular joint, the parotid gland, the skin overlying the temporal region, and the skin anterior to the tragus and helix. The lingual nerve innervates the dorsum and lateral aspects of the anterior 2/3 of the tongue, the lateral mucous membrane, and the sublingual gland. The inferior alveolar nerve innervates the lower teeth and the mandible. Its terminal branch, the mental nerve, innervates the chin and the skin and mucous membrane of the lower lip.

Blockade of the Ophthalmic Branch

The most commonly blocked branches of V1 are the supraorbital and supratrochlear branches. To block the supraorbital

Table 30.2 The four regional groups of V2

The four regional groups of V2	V2 nerve branches	Facial areas innervated
1. Intracranial group	Middle meningeal nerve	The dura matter of the middle cranial fossa
2. Pterygopalatine group	Zygomatic nerve	The temporal and zygomatic region
	The sphenopalatine branches	The mucosa of the maxillary sinus, upper molars, upper gums, and the mucous membrane of the cheek
3. Infraorbital canal group	Anterosuperior alveolar branch	Incisors, canines, anterior wall of the maxillary antrum, floor of nasal cavity
	Middle superior branch	Premolars
4. Infraorbital facial group	Inferior palpebral branch	Conjunctiva and skin of lower eyelid
	External nasal branch	Side of the nose
	Superior labial branch	Skin of the upper lip and part of the oral mucosa

nerve, the patient is placed in a supine position. The landmark for this block, the supraorbital foramen, is palpated along the upper border of the orbit. After skin prepping, with precautions not to spill any disinfecting solution in the eye, a 25-gauge, 1.5-in.-long needle is introduced into the skin through the identified supraorbital foramen in a perpendicular plane to the skin. Some paresthesia is usually elicited; then, 3–4 ml of local anesthetic solution (lidocaine 1–2 %, bupivacaine 0.5 %, or ropivacaine 0.2 %) is injected in a fan-like fashion. Radiofrequency lesioning for the supraorbital nerve as a treatment for postherpetic neuralgia has been described. The technique for radiofrequency lesioning is similar to the local anesthetic block with the exception of using a RFA needle and confirmation of positive sensory response at 2-Hz stimulation in the somatic nerve distribution. To achieve a blockade of the supratrochlear branch of the ophthalmic division, simply direct the needle medially at the level of the supraorbital foramen and repeat similar steps as described above.

Blockade of the Maxillary and Mandibular Branches

The preferred approach for blockade of the maxillary (V2) and the mandibular (V3) branches of the trigeminal nerve is through the mandibular notch, also known as the coronoid notch. These blocks could be done without radiologic guidance. However, fluoroscopic guidance is highly recommended. Patient is placed in supine position, and the x-ray C arm is placed in a lateral view. The patient is asked to open and close his/her mouth few times if possible to facilitate palpation of the mandibular notch which could be marked. After skin sterilization, the skin is anesthetized with lidocaine 1 %. A 22-g B-bevel needle, 8–10 cm long is used (for radiofrequency lesioning, an RFA needle, 10 cm long, with a 2–5-mm active RFA tip is used). The needle is introduced under fluoroscopic guidance at the site already marked and advanced in a horizontal plane. Fluoroscopic guidance is used to direct the needle tip through the

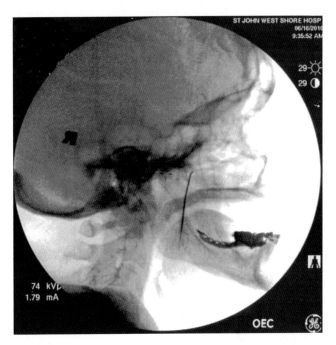

Fig. 30.3 Lateral fluoroscopic view showing needle though the coronoid notch in position for advancement

infratemporal fossa (Fig. 30.3). A small-angulation cephalad and slightly posterior will allow the needle to be in proximity to the lateral nasal mucosa taking extreme care not to pierce through it. The end point of the advancement of the needle is the lateral pterygoid plate. If the maxillary nerve is the final target, a slight superior and posterior angulation will elicit paresthesia into this nerve distribution (nose ridge, upper lip, gum, and face). If the mandibular nerve is targeted, a slight caudad and anterior angulation usually elicits paresthesia in its somatic distribution (lower mandible, lower lip, lower jaw, and tongue). If radiofrequency lesioning is planned, sensory testing at 50 Hz should be achieved preferably below 0.6 V in the nerve distribution prior to any treatment. Negative aspiration of blood and CSF should be demonstrated prior to any treatment. Figure 30.4 shows the advancement and final position of the needle. Figure 30.5 shows RF needle in position.

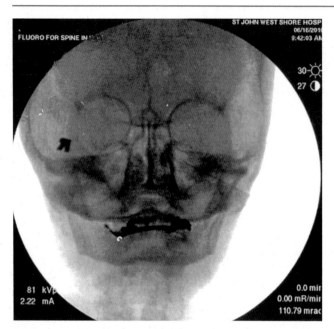

Fig. 30.4 Anteroposterior fluoroscopic view showing needle advancement for maxillary nerve block

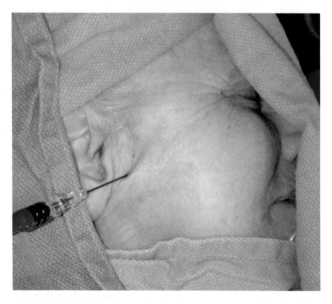

Fig. 30.5 Final needle placement for radiofrequency lesioning of the maxillary nerve

Efficacy and Safety

The efficacy and safety of radiofrequency (RF) lesioning for trigeminal neuralgia have been described in the literature. Review of current literature reveals one retrospective uncontrolled chart review [38] and four prospective uncontrolled clinical trials [39–42]. No randomized sham-controlled trials on the value of RF treatment of the trigeminal ganglion have been published. An initial complete pain relief was reported

in 83–99 % of patients treated with RF ablation in some studies [39, 40, 43–49]. Repeating the procedure has increased the long-term efficacy in three studies [38, 40, 42]. Kanpolat et al. [38] reviewed the records of 1,600 patients that received percutaneous radiofrequency rhizotomy as a treatment for trigeminal neuralgia. Even though initially up to 97.6 % reported acute pain relief at 5-year follow-up, only 57.7 % reported complete pain relief with a single procedure. This figure reaches 94.2 % for patients receiving multiple procedures. At 10- and 20-year follow-up, the percentage for single procedure was 52.3 % and 41 %, respectively, and for multiple procedures was 94.2 % and 100 %, respectively. The authors concluded that this technique is safe and effective.

Long-term safety from prospective uncontrolled and retrospective clinical studies up to 20 years was demonstrated. Taha and Tew [50] conducted a 15-year prospective study following 154 patients with trigeminal neuralgia treated with percutaneous stereotactic radiofrequency rhizotomy. Initial success was reported at 99 % after a single treatment. Similar results were confirmed in a prospective study by Scrivani et al. following 215 patients with trigeminal neuralgia for 15 years following rhizotomy. They found that patients had pain relief in 92 %. Table 30.3 summarizes the efficacy of RF lesioning for facial pain, trigeminal neuralgia, and headache.

Other retrospective comparative studies examined the safety and efficacy of RF lesioning compared with other established treatment modalities, such as microvascular decompression (MVD), balloon microcompression, glycerol rhizotomy, partial trigeminal rhizotomy, neurectomy, and alcohol block [50, 51]. Taha and Tew [50], in an extensive review, concluded that the highest rate of recurrence of pain is associated with glycerol rhizotomy. Trigeminal motor dysfunction is highest with balloon compression, while initial pain relief is best achieved with radiofrequency rhizotomy and MVD. Oturai et al. [51] sent questionnaires to 316 patients previously treated over 16 years for trigeminal neuralgia. They reported a success rate of 83 %, 51 %, and 42 %, respectively, after radiofrequency lesioning, neurectomy, and alcohol block. They concluded that radiofrequency lesioning has the highest success when compared to neurectomy and alcohol block. Table 30.4 summarizes studies conducted on the efficacy of glycerol neurolysis. The largest group of patients studied with glycerol neurolysis was reported by Saini [52]. After a single injection, 59 % and 8 % reported pain relief at 2 and 6 years, respectively. The best reported results with glycerol neurolysis were reported by Cappabianca, 93 % success within days of procedures [53].

There are fewer studies that address pulsed radiofrequency lesioning. One randomized controlled study indicates the superiority of conventional RF lesioning over pulsed RF lesioning for the management of idiopathic trigeminal neuralgia [35]. In a trial of 40 patients with trigeminal neuralgia

Table 30.3 Results of radiofrequency lesioning studies

Study	Technique	Results (%)	Number of patients	Comments
Kanpolat et al. [38]	RF	41–100	1,600	TN, 20-year follow-up
Taha et al. [39]	RF	99	154	TN, 15-year follow-up
Zakrzewska et al. [41]	RF	36–40 months pain-free	48	Chronic facial pain
Onofrio [43]	RF	86	140	Mainly TN
Tew et al. [44]	RF	93	>100	TN elderly
Sengupta and Stunden [45]	RF	92	39	TN
Piquer et al. [46]	RF	69	98	TN, 4.5-year follow-up
Maxwell [54]	RF	100	8	Migrainous neuralgia
Spincemaille et al. [47]	RF	85	53	TN, 2-year follow-up
Grunert et al. [55]	RF	92	250	TN
Choudhury et al. [56]	RF	78	40	TN
Moraci et al. [48]	RF	97	605	TN
Taha and Tew [11]	RF	100	7	Cluster HA
Yoon et al. [49]	RF	87	81	TN
Scrivani et al. [40]	RF	83–92	215	TN, 5-year follow-up

Table 30.4 Results of studies on gasserian neurolysis with glycerol

Study	Results (%)	Patient number	Comments
Dieckman et al. [57]	92	55	TN
Spaziante et al. [58]	94	50	TN
Saini [52]	59–8	552	Follow-up 2–6 years
Young [59]	86	162	TN
Burchiel [60]	80	60	TN
Waltz et al. [61]	80	200	TN
Van de Velde et al. [62]	76	20	TN
Ischia et al. [19]	92	112	TN
Borda et al. [63]	64	120	TN
Cappabianca et al. [53]	93	191	TN
Kondziolka et al. [64]	59	53	With MS 11-year follow-up
Linderoth and Hakanson [65]	90	23	Facial pain
Ekbom et al. [8]	57	7	Cluster HA
Pieper et al. [12]	83	18	Cluster HA

randomized to receive pulsed versus conventional RF lesioning of the trigeminal ganglia, Erdine et al. [35] confirmed the effectiveness of the conventional lesioning. Only 10 % of the pulsed RF group reported improvement. The authors concluded that pulsed RF lesioning was not an effective treatment for trigeminal neuralgia (Tables 30.3 and 30.4).

Complications and Side Effects

Complications are expected after neural blockade of the trigeminal nerve and the gasserian ganglion. Prior to any injection involving the trigeminal nerve, patient should be warned about potential common side effects including severe headache, dysesthesia, and significant facial or subscleral hematoma regardless of the technique used. Intravascular injection, more dangerously in the carotid artery, is a devastating complication. In an extensive review comparing results

and complications of percutaneous techniques performed as a treatment for trigeminal neuralgia, Taha and Tew reviewed 6,205 cases of RF ablation, 1,217 cases of glycerol injection, and 759 cases of balloon compression [50]. Facial numbness was the most common side effect reported varying between 60 % with glycerol and 98 % with RF. Anesthesia dolorosa was reported in less than 4 % [50, 66, 67]. The incidence of loss of the corneal reflex, ulceration, keratitis, and hypesthesia has all been reported [20, 43, 47, 60–63]. Dysesthesia occurs at the same rate independent of the technique and procedure. Acute unilateral total visual loss after Gasserian ganglion phenol injection has been reported [30]. Rhinorrhea after percutaneous radiofrequency lesioning is reported [68]. Masticatory muscle weakness was reported in many studies and was found to be reversible over time [50, 69–71]. Infection is always a potential complication with any of the techniques used. Due to the proximity to brain stem structures, a potential risk of meningitis is possible and had been reported in 24 out of 7,000 cases reviewed by Sweet [72]. Reactivation of a dormant herpetic infection is reported with the use of different techniques especially after trigeminal balloon compression [73]. Total spinal anesthesia, respiratory arrest, and fracture of the pterygomaxillary fissure are possible. Having mentioned how frequent and intractable some of these complications can be, it is recommended that only providers with adequate training and expertise perform these facial invasive procedures.

Neuro-Modulation for Trigeminal Neuralgia

With the emergence of neuro-modulation, we have witnessed a shift from neuro-destructive techniques to more neuro-modulatory ones. While deep brain and motor cortex stimulation have been used for treatment of trigeminal neuropathic pain and trigeminal neuralgia, the results are variable and the procedures are very invasive and complex. Attempts to place percutaneous neuro-modulatory electrodes at the gasserian ganglion using the trans-foramen ovale technique are being performed by trained neurosurgeons. However, technical limitations related to migration of electrodes have limited the success of such trials. While it is worthwhile mentioning because of its relatively less-invasive nature, the data on gasserian ganglion stimulation for trigeminal neuralgia is insufficient to recommend it use.

References

1. Lewy FH. The first authentic case of major trigeminal neuralgia and some comments on the history of the disease. Ann Med Hist. 1938;10:247–50.
2. Stookey B. Differential dorsal root section in the treatment of bilateral trigeminal neuralgia. J Neurosurg. 1955;12(5):501–15.
3. van Kleef M, van Genderen WE, Narouze S, Nurmikko TJ, van Zundert J, Geurts JW, Mekhail N. 1. Trigeminal neuralgia. Pain Pract. 2009;9:252–9.
4. Katusic S, Williams DB, Beard CM, Bergstralh EJ, Kurland LT. Epidemiology and clinical features of idiopathic trigeminal neuralgia and glossopharyngeal neuralgia: similarities and differences, Rochester, Minnesota, 1945–1984. Neuroepidemiology. 1991;10:276–81.
5. Rozen TD. Trigeminal neuralgia and glossopharyngeal neuralgia. Neurol Clin. 2004;22:185–206.
6. Dalessio DJ. Trigeminal neuralgia. A practical approach to treatment. Drugs. 1982;24:248–55.
7. Fisher A, Zakrzewska JM, Patsalos PN. Trigeminal neuralgia: current treatments and future developments. Expert Opin Emerg Drugs. 2003;8:123–43.
8. Ekbom K, Lindgren L, Nilsson BY, Hardebo JE, Waldenlind E. Retro-Gasserian glycerol injection in the treatment of chronic cluster headache. Cephalalgia. 1987;7:21–7.
9. Mathew NT, Hurt W. Percutaneous radiofrequency trigeminal gangliorhizolysis in intractable cluster headache. Headache. 1988;28:328–31.
10. Hassenbusch SJ, Kunkel RS, Kosmorsky GS, Covington EC, Pillay PK. Trigeminal cisternal injection of glycerol for treatment of chronic intractable cluster headaches. Neurosurgery. 1991;29:504–8.

11. Taha JM, Tew Jr JM. Long-term results of radiofrequency rhizotomy in the treatment of cluster headache. Headache. 1995;35:193–6.
12. Pieper DR, Dickerson J, Hassenbusch SJ. Percutaneous retrogasserian glycerol rhizolysis for treatment of chronic intractable cluster headaches: long-term results. Neurosurgery. 2000;46:363–8.
13. Stechison MT, Brogan M. Transfacial transpterygomaxillary access to foramen rotundum, sphenopalatine ganglion, and the maxillary nerve in the management of atypical facial pain. Skull Base Surg. 1994;4:15–20.
14. Sweet WH. Controlled thermocoagulation of trigeminal ganglion and rootlets for differential destruction of pain fibers: facial pain other than trigeminal neuralgia. Clin Neurosurg. 1976;23:96–102.
15. Koizuka S, Saito S, Sekimoto K, Tobe M, Obata H, Koyama Y. Percutaneous radio-frequency thermocoagulation of the Gasserian ganglion guided by high-speed real-time CT fluoroscopy. Neuroradiology. 2009;51:563–6.
16. Tator CH, Rowed DW. Fluoroscopy of foramen ovale as an aid to thermocoagulation of the Gasserian ganglion; technical note. J Neurosurg. 1976;44:254–7.
17. Tsui BC. Ultrasound imaging to localize foramina for superficial trigeminal nerve block. Can J Anaesth. 2009;56:704–6.
18. Elias M. Glycerol for trigeminal rhizolysis. Clin J Pain. 1997;13:272.
19. Ischia S, Luzzani A, Polati E. Retrogasserian glycerol injection: a retrospective study of 112 patients. Clin J Pain. 1990;6:291–6.
20. Fujimaki T, Fukushima T, Miyazaki S. Percutaneous retrogasserian glycerol injection in the management of trigeminal neuralgia: long-term follow-up results. J Neurosurg. 1990;73:212–6.
21. Orlandini G. Treatment of trigeminal neuralgia with retrogasserian glycerol injection. Preliminary results. Minerva Anestesiol. 1988;54:525–6.
22. Maksymowicz W. Treatment of trigeminal neuralgia by glycerol gangliolysis of the trigeminal ganglion. Neurol Neurochir Pol. 1987;21:45–8.
23. Igarashi S, Suzuki F, Iwasaki K, Koyama T, Umeda S. Glycerol injection method for trigeminal neuralgia. No Shinkei Geka. 1985;13:267–73.
24. Sindou M, Tatli M. Treatment of trigeminal neuralgia with glycerol injection at the Gasserian ganglion. Neurochirurgie. 2009;55:211–2.
25. Vasin NI. Methodology for and results of phenol blocks of the Gasserian ganglion in severe forms of facial pains. Vopr Neirokhir. 1973;37:16–22.
26. Longhi P, Graziussi G, Granata F. "Selective" percutaneous alcohol administration to the Gasserian ganglion in the treatment of trigeminal neuralgia. Riv Neurobiol. 1982;28:303–8.
27. Ecker A, Perl T. Selective Gasserian injection for tic douloureux. Technical advances and results. Acta Radiol Diagn (Stockh). 1969;9:38–48.
28. Fava E, Gentilli R. Taste sensitivity of the anterior two thirds of the tongue after alcohol block of the gasserian ganglion. Minerva Anestesiol. 1956;22:407–13.
29. Loar C. Peripheral nervous system pain. In: Raj P, editor. Pain medicine: a comprehensive review. 1st ed. St. Louis: Mosby; 1996. p. 453–60.
30. Aydemir O, Yilmaz T, Onal SA, Celiker U, Erol FS. Acute unilateral total visual loss after retrogasserian phenol injection for the treatment of trigeminal neuralgia: a case report. Orbit. 2006;25:23–6.
31. van Boxem K, van Eerd M, Brinkhuizen T, Patijn J, van Kleef M, van Zundert J. Radiofrequency and pulsed radiofrequency treatment of chronic pain syndromes: the available evidence. Pain Pract. 2008;8:385–93.
32. Nguyen M, Wilkes D. Pulsed radiofrequency V2 treatment and intranasal sphenopalatine ganglion block: a combination therapy for atypical trigeminal neuralgia. Pain Pract. 2010;10:370–4.

33. Orlandini G. Pulsed percutaneous radiofrequency treatment of the Gasserian ganglion for therapy of trigeminal neuralgia: technical notes, validity of the method and selection of the patients. Pain. 2004;108:297–8.

34. van Zundert J, Brabant S, Van de Kleft E, Vercruyssen A, Van Buyten JP. Pulsed radiofrequency treatment of the Gasserian ganglion in patients with idiopathic trigeminal neuralgia. Pain. 2003;104:449–52.

35. Erdine S, Ozyalcin NS, Cimen A, Celik M, Talu GK, Disci R. Comparison of pulsed radiofrequency with conventional radiofrequency in the treatment of idiopathic trigeminal neuralgia. Eur J Pain. 2007;11:309–13.

36. Neill RS. Head, neck and airway. In: Wildsmith JAW, editor. Principles and practice of regional anesthesia. New York: Churchill Livingston; 1987.

37. Hahn MB, Hahn MB, McQuillan PM. Trigeminal nerve block. In: Regional anesthesia. St-Louis: CV Mosby; 1996.

38. Kanpolat Y, Savas A, Bekar A, Berk C. Percutaneous controlled radiofrequency trigeminal rhizotomy for the treatment of idiopathic trigeminal neuralgia: 25-year experience with 1,600 patients. Neurosurgery. 2001;48:524–32.

39. Taha JM, Tew Jr JM. Buncher CR: a prospective 15-year follow up of 154 consecutive patients with trigeminal neuralgia treated by percutaneous stereotactic radiofrequency thermal rhizotomy. J Neurosurg. 1995;83:989–93.

40. Scrivani SJ, Keith DA, Mathews ES, Kaban LB. Percutaneous stereotactic differential radiofrequency thermal rhizotomy for the treatment of trigeminal neuralgia. J Oral Maxillofac Surg. 1999;57:104–11.

41. Zakrzewska JM, Jassim S, Bulman JS. A prospective, longitudinal study on patients with trigeminal neuralgia who underwent radiofrequency thermocoagulation of the Gasserian ganglion. Pain. 1999;79:51–8.

42. Mathews ES, Scrivani SJ. Percutaneous stereotactic radiofrequency thermal rhizotomy for the treatment of trigeminal neuralgia. Mt Sinai J Med. 2000;67:288–99.

43. Onofrio BM. Radiofrequency percutaneous Gasserian ganglion lesions. Results in 140 patients with trigeminal pain. J Neurosurg. 1975;42:132–9.

44. Tew Jr JM. Lockwood P, Mayfield FH: treatment of trigeminal neuralgia in the aged by a simplified surgical approach (percutaneous electrocoagulation). J Am Geriatr Soc. 1975;23:426–30.

45. Sengupta RP, Stunden RJ. Radiofrequency thermocoagulation of Gasserian ganglion and its rootlets for trigeminal neuralgia. Br Med J. 1977;1:142–3.

46. Piquer J, Joanes V, Roldan P, Barcia-Salorio JL, Masbout G. Long-term results of percutaneous gasserian ganglion lesions. Acta Neurochir Suppl (Wien). 1987;39:139–41.

47. Spincemaille GH, Dingemans W, Lodder J. Percutaneous radiofrequency Gasserian ganglion coagulation in the treatment of trigeminal neuralgia. Clin Neurol Neurosurg. 1985;87:91–4.

48. Moraci A, Buonaiuto C, Punzo A, Parlato C, Amalfi R. Trigeminal neuralgia treated by percutaneous thermocoagulation. Comparative analysis of percutaneous thermocoagulation and other surgical procedures. Neurochirurgia (Stuttg). 1992;35:48–53.

49. Yoon KB, Wiles JR, Miles JB, Nurmikko TJ. Long-term outcome of percutaneous thermocoagulation for trigeminal neuralgia. Anaesthesia. 1999;54:803–8.

50. Taha JM, Tew Jr JM. Comparison of surgical treatments for trigeminal neuralgia: reevaluation of radiofrequency rhizotomy. Neurosurgery. 1996;38:865–71.

51. Oturai AB, Jensen K, Eriksen J, Madsen FF. Neurosurgical treatment of trigeminal neuralgia. A comparative study of alcohol block, neurectomy and electrocoagulation. Ugeskr Laeger. 1998;160:3909–12.

52. Saini SS. Reterogasserian anhydrous glycerol injection therapy in trigeminal neuralgia: observations in 552 patients. J Neurol Neurosurg Psychiatry. 1987;50:1536–8.

53. Cappabianca P, Spaziante R, Graziussi G, Taglialatela G, Peca C, de Divitiis E. Percutaneous retrogasserian glycerol rhizolysis for treatment of trigeminal neuralgia Technique and results in 191 patients. J Neurosurg Sci. 1995;39:37–45.

54. Maxwell RE. Surgical control of chronic migrainous neuralgia by trigeminal ganglio-rhizolysis. J Neurosurg. 1982;57:459–66.

55. Grunert P, Pendl G, Ozturk E, Ungersbock K, Czech T. Results of electrocoagulation of Gasser's ganglion in 250 patients with idiopathic trigeminal neuralgia. Zentralbl Neurochir. 1988;49:196–201.

56. Choudhury BK, Pahari S, Acharyya A, Goswami A, Bhattacharyya MK. Percutaneous retrogasserian radiofrequency thermal rhizotomy for trigeminal neuralgia. J Indian Med Assoc. 1991;89: 294–6.

57. Dieckmann G, Veras G, Sogabe K. Retrogasserian glycerol injection or percutaneous stimulation in the treatment of typical and atypical trigeminal pain. Neurol Res. 1987;9:48–9.

58. Spaziante R, Cappabianca P, Peca C, De Divitiis E. Percutaneous retrogasserian glycerol rhizolysis. Observations and results about 50 cases. J Neurosurg Sci. 1987;31:121–8.

59. Young RF. Glycerol rhizolysis for treatment of trigeminal neuralgia. J Neurosurg. 1988;69:39–45.

60. Burchiel KJ. Percutaneous retrogasserian glycerol rhizolysis in the management of trigeminal neuralgia. J Neurosurg. 1988;69:361–6.

61. Waltz TA, Dalessio DJ, Copeland B, Abbott G. Percutaneous injection of glycerol for the treatment of trigeminal neuralgia. Clin J Pain. 1989;5:195–8.

62. Van de Velde V, Smeets P, Caemaert J, Van de Velde V. Transoval trigeminal cisternography and glycerol injection in trigeminal neuralgia. J Belge Radiol. 1989;72:83–7.

63. Borda L, Doczi T, Tarjanyi J. Treatment of trigeminal neuralgia with glycerin injected into Meckel's cavity. Orv Hetil. 1994;135:181–4.

64. Kondziolka D, Lunsford LD, Bissonette DJ. Long-term results after glycerol rhizotomy for multiple sclerosis-related trigeminal neuralgia. Can J Neurol Sci. 1994;21:137–40.

65. Linderoth B, Hakanson S. Paroxysmal facial pain in disseminated sclerosis treated by retrogasserian glycerol injection. Acta Neurol Scand. 1989;80:341–6.

66. Burchiel KJ, Steege TD, Howe JF, Loeser JD. Comparison of percutaneous radiofrequency gangliolysis and microvascular decompression for the surgical management of tic douloureux. Neurosurgery. 1981;9:111–9.

67. Broggi G, Franzini A, Lasio G, Giorgi C, Servello D. Long-term results of percutaneous retrogasserian thermorhizotomy for "essential" trigeminal neuralgia: considerations in 1000 consecutive patients. Neurosurgery. 1990;26:783–6.

68. Ugur HC, Savas A, Elhan A, Kanpolat Y. Unanticipated complication of percutaneous radiofrequency trigeminal rhizotomy: rhinorrhea: report of three cases and a cadaver study. Neurosurgery. 2004;54:1522–4.

69. Natarajan M. Percutaneous trigeminal ganglion balloon compression: experience in 40 patients. Neurol India. 2000;48:330–2.

70. Abdennebi B, Bouatta F, Chitti M, Bougatene B. Percutaneous balloon compression of the Gasserian ganglion in trigeminal neuralgia Long-term results in 150 cases. Acta Neurochir (Wien). 1995;136:72–4.

71. Lichtor T, Mullan JF. A 10-year follow-up review of percutaneous microcompression of the trigeminal ganglion. J Neurosurg. 1990;72:49–54.

72. Sweet WH. Complications of treating trigeminal neuralgia: an analysis of the literature and response to questionaire. In: Rovit RL, Murali R, Janetta PJ, editors. Trigeminal neuralgia. Baltimore: Williams & Wilkins; 1990. p. 251–79.

73. Simms HN, Dunn LT. Herpes zoster of the trigeminal nerve following microvascular decompression. Br J Neurosurg. 2006;20: 423–6.

Glossopharyngeal Nerve Block

31

Kenneth D. Candido and George C. Chang Chien

Key Points
- Glossopharyngeal neuralgia is characterized by unilateral paroxysmal pain in the oropharynx, nasopharynx, larynx, base of the tongue, tonsillar region, and lower jaw.
- Techniques for extraoral, intraoral, fluoroscopic, or ultrasound-assisted procedures have been described in the literature. Injections of local anesthetic and/or steroids or alcohol neurolysis and radiofrequency ablation are all options in management.
- Extraoral (peristyloid) technique is ideally performed under live fluoroscopy.
- The styloid process can be found equidistant between the mastoid process and the ipsilateral angle of the jaw.
- The advantages of the intraoral anterior tonsillar pillar method are that the ATP is easily identified and exposed and the tongue movement does not trigger the gag reflex.
- The posterior tonsillar pillar method becomes more difficult in patients with large tongues or small oral opening and may cause greater gag reflex.
- To test success of the glossopharyngeal nerve block (GNB), the operator can test for an obtunded gag reflex as a clinical indicator for analgesia.
- Patients need to be monitored for a minimum of 30 min following the block to verify that there has been no systemic response to the injected local anesthetic solution.

Introduction

The glossopharyngeal nerve (cranial nerve IX) is an important consideration as a pain generator or modulator in cases of recalcitrant pain of the face and neck. Although uncommon as an etiology of head and neck pain (0.57–1.3 % of cases of facial pain) [1–3], impingement or injury to the glossopharyngeal nerve can lead to glossopharyngeal neuralgia, a potentially life-threatening disease [4, 5]. Therefore, it is vital that the interventional pain management specialist learns to recognize disease of CN IX as well as to become facile with techniques of providing analgesia to this important structure.

Glossopharyngeal neuralgia, or Weisenburg-Sicard-Robineau syndrome, was first described by the American neurologist T.H. Weisenburg in 1910 in a case of facial pain misdiagnosed as tic douloureux (trigeminal neuralgia) secondary to a cerebellopontine tumor [6]. Although the French neurologists Jean-Athanase Sicard and Maurice Robineu also published cases in 1920 where they treated cases of atypical facial pain by dissection of the ninth cranial nerve [7], it was the British neurologist Wilfred Harris who coined the term "glossopharyngeal neuralgia" in 1921 [3, 4].

Glossopharyngeal neuralgia is characterized by unilateral paroxysmal pain in the oropharynx, nasopharynx, larynx, base of the tongue, tonsillar region, and lower jaw and can also radiate to the ipsilateral ear. These attacks are excruciatingly painful and typically described as sharp, stabbing, "shocks of electricity" that can last from seconds to minutes [2, 3, 8]. These painful attacks are triggered by

K.D. Candido, M.D. (✉)
Department of Anesthesiology,
Advocate Illinois Masonic Medical Center,
836 West Wellington Ave, Suite 4815,
Chicago, IL 60657, USA
e-mail: kdcandido@yahoo.com

G.C.C. Chien, DO
Department of Physical Medicine and Rehabilitation,
Rehabilitation Institute of Chicago,
Northwestern Memorial Hospital,
345 East Superior St,
Chicago, IL 60611, USA
e-mail: gchangchien@ric.org

T.R. Deer et al. (eds.), *Comprehensive Treatment of Chronic Pain by Medical, Interventional, and Integrative Approaches*,
DOI 10.1007/978-1-4614-1560-2_31, © American Academy of Pain Medicine 2013

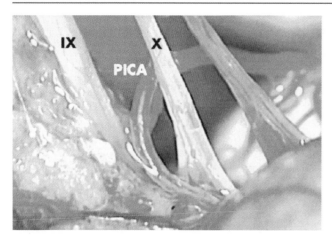

Fig. 31.1 Relationship of the glossopharyngeal nerve (*IX*) to the posterior inferior cerebellar artery (*PICA*) (Adapted from: Takaya [13])

Reported Causes of Glossopharyngeal Neuralgia (GPN)

- Trauma [21]
- Eagle's syndrome [23]
- Cerebellopontine angle tumors [4]
- Infection/parapharyngeal space lesions [20]
- Multiple sclerosis [24, 25]
- Posterior fossa arteriovenous malformation
- Arachnoiditis [26]
- Ossified styloid ligament
- Elongated styloid process
- Direct carotid puncture [4]
- Metastatic head and neck tumors [19]
- Chiari malformation [26]

Glossopharyngeal neuralgia may mimic trigeminal neuralgia. Both may present with facial/jaw pain worse elicited by the same mechanical and sensory mechanisms. Cases may be difficult to differentiate in patients with pain in the region of the tragus or deep to the angle of the jaw [2]. However, compared to trigeminal neuralgia, glossopharyngeal neuralgia is relatively rare [1–3]. A diagnostic interventional block may be useful in differentiating the two etiologies and indeed may be the only mechanism available to the interventional pain management physician to definitively establish CN IX as being responsible for the pain.

Anatomy

The glossopharyngeal nerve (cranial nerve IX) is a mixed function nerve with motor, sensory, and special sensory fibers. The rootlets originate in the upper part of the postolivary sulcus, between the olive and the inferior peduncle of the medulla oblongata, and exit the cranium with parasympathetic nerve fibers from the salivatory nucleus, the vagus and spinal accessory nerves (CN X and XI) via the jugular foramen. All three cranial nerves lie between the internal jugular vein and the internal carotid artery (Fig. 31.2).

The glossopharyngeal nerve has many distributive branches including the tympanic, carotid, pharyngeal, muscular, tonsillar, and lingual. The tympanic branch innervates the tympanic membrane. The carotid branch innervates the carotid sinus and carotid body. The pharyngeal branch carries sensory nerve from the walls of the pharynx. The tonsillar branch transmits sensory nerves from the tonsils. The lingual branch innervates the anterior surface of the epiglottis, the posterior third of the tongue, and the vallecula.

The motor component innervates the stylopharyngeus muscle, which elevates the pharynx during talking and swallowing. The sensory portion innervates the palatine tonsils, the posterior third of the tongue, and the mucous

stimulation to the oropharynx such as mechanical swallowing, yawning, coughing, laughing, chewing, and sensory stimulation such as cold, salty, acidic, or bitter foods [2, 3].

In 217 cases of glossopharyngeal neuralgia seen at the Mayo Clinic [9], 57 % of the cases were in patients greater than 50 years old, while 43 % were between the ages of 18 and 50. Twelve percent of these patients had bilateral involvement, but a bilateral frequency as high as 25 % has been reported [10]. Additionally, 12 % of the patients exhibited both glossopharyngeal and trigeminal neuralgia [9]. A greater prevalence in males has also been reported by some authors [2], while others have reported no difference in prevalence by gender.

Cardiovascular symptoms such as bradycardia, hypotension, and even cardiac arrest may accompany the attacks in 1–2 % of people with glossopharyngeal neuralgia [4, 5, 11]. It is believed that the close association between the glossopharyngeal nerve and the vagus nerve (CN X) underlies, in part, the etiology between glossopharyngeal neuralgia and these cardiac symptoms [12]. Seizures have also been associated with episodes of GPN [5, 13, 14].

Although most cases of glossopharyngeal neuralgia are categorized as "idiopathic," it is thought that the majority cases of glossopharyngeal neuralgia are caused by vascular compression of the glossopharyngeal nerve [11, 15].

Kawashima studied 14 cases of idiopathic GPN. In all of the cases, vascular compression on the glossopharyngeal nerve was found [16]. Most commonly, it is the posterior inferior cerebellar artery (PICA) (Fig. 31.1) followed by the anterior-inferior cerebral artery (AICA) that compresses the glossopharyngeal nerve [11, 16–18].

Other causes for GPN include tumors with local invasion [19], parapharyngeal abscess [20], trauma [21], multiple sclerosis [22], and carotid puncture [4].

Fig. 31.2 Base of the skull: the jugular foramen is where the glossopharyngeal, vagus, and accessory nerves exit the cranium (Photo courtesy of Kenneth D. Candido, M.D.)

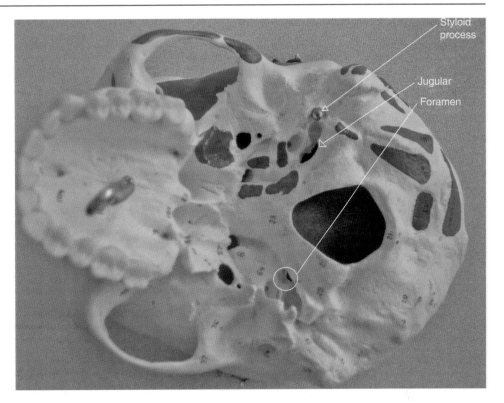

membranes of the oropharynx. Special sensory afferent fibers transmit information for taste from the posterior third of the tongue.

The carotid branch of CN IX, the carotid sinus nerve, innervates carotid body and carotid sinus. Therefore, damage to this branch has important implications for regulation of blood pressure, pulse, and respiration.

Indications for GPN Block or Neurolysis

- Glossopharyngeal neuralgia (GPN)
- Post-tonsillectomy pain control [27]
- Cancer pain [28–30]
- To reduce gag reflex for awake endotracheal intubation [31]
- Singultus (hiccups) [32]
- Carotid sinus syndrome [33]
- Patients that are poor candidates for microvascular decompression

Diagnosis

Imaging

High-resolution MRI [34, 35] or CT scan of the head may reveal tumor, bony erosion, multiple sclerosis plaques, abscess, or infection. Three-dimensional visualizations of the brain stem may identify, or MRA may show neurovascular compression or arteriovenous malformation. Visualization of the offending vessel was better in cases of compression from the PICA compared to the AICA [34].

Balloon Test Occlusion

Hasegawa et al. reported a case where magnetic resonance imaging suggested that the right vertebral artery (VA) was pressing on the glossopharyngeal nerve [36]. Balloon test occlusion of the VA was used to confirm the cause of the neuralgia. The neuralgia disappeared and reappeared with balloon inflation and deflation. Balloon test occlusion may be useful in the diagnosis of GPN and the selection of the most appropriate surgical treatment [36, 37].

Medical Treatment

Medical control treatment of GPN is similar to treatment for other forms of neuropathic pain, including trigeminal neuralgia. Antiepileptic drugs and tricyclic antidepressants alone or in combination have been studied with variable efficacy [38]. There is also a case report of GPN refractory to AEDs that responded well to opioids [39].

Antiepileptic drugs which have been used include carbamazepine, lamotrigine, diazepam, and gabapentin; tricyclic antidepressants used have included amitriptyline and nortriptyline [40–44].

Interventional Techniques

Techniques for extraoral, intraoral, fluoroscopic, or ultrasound-assisted procedures have been described in the literature. Injections of local anesthetic and/or steroids, or alcohol neurolysis [45] and radiofrequency ablation [46, 47] are all options in management of glossopharyngeal nerve dysfunction.

Although ultrasound-assisted intervention has been reported [48], the use of fluoroscopy also allows the advantage of real-time imaging of the contrast media, so that in cases in which the needle tip has penetrated either the carotid or jugular systems, this activity should be observable and intravascular injection subsequently preventable or at least minimized.

Patients need to be monitored for a minimum of 30 min following the block to verify that there has been no systemic response to the injected local anesthetic solution. Even taking these precautions and using fluoroscopic or ultrasound guidance does not completely eliminate the possibility of local anesthetic spillover onto the vagus nerve (with resultant ipsilateral vocal cord paralysis) or onto the spinal accessory nerve (weakness of the trapezius muscle).

To test success of the glossopharyngeal nerve block (GNB), the operator can test for an obtunded gag reflex as a clinical indicator for analgesia [27]. There is a strong relationship between extent of the obtunded gag reflex and the extent of post-tonsillectomy pain relief [27].

Extraoral (Peristyloid) Technique with Fluoroscopy

The patient is placed supine with the head rotated slightly opposite from the affected side. The styloid process is used to identify the course of the GPN. Once identification of the mastoid process and the ipsilateral angle of the mandible is performed, the styloid process can be found equidistant between these structures (Figs. 31.3a–d and 31.4a, b).

The skin overlying the styloid process should be prepped and draped in sterile fashion. A small skin wheal is made over the styloid process using a 25-gauge, 1.5-in. needle and 3–4 mL of 1 % plain lidocaine. Next, a 22-gauge, 1.5–2 in. blunt-tipped needle may be advanced perpendicular to the skin toward the process, aiming for its posterior aspect. The styloid process should be met at a depth approximating 1.5–4 cm. Once the styloid process is encountered, the needle is slightly withdrawn and "walked off" posteriorly. Aspiration should be performed to ensure that there is no blood or cerebrospinal fluid. Next, 1 mL of water-soluble, iodinated contrast media should be incrementally injected under live continuous fluoroscopy. Then, barring any intravascular spread, a short-acting, preservative-free (lidocaine, mepivacaine) and dilute

(1 % concentration) anesthetic with epinephrine 1:200,000 (5 μg/mL) in a volume of 3–5 mL should be incrementally injected in divided doses. Nonparticulate corticosteroid (dexamethasone, betamethasone) may be added to the injectate, although there is no literature support to a salubrious effect of adding an anti-inflammatory glucocorticoid medication.

Intraoral Technique (Figs. 31.5 and 31.6)

Anterior Tonsillar Pillar Method [31, 49, 50]

The patient is asked to open the mouth widely (Fig. 31.5). The operator may choose to anesthetize the tongue to facilitate the procedure. The tongue is swept to the opposite side with a tongue depressor, laryngoscope blade, or with gloved fingers. A 25-gauge, 3.5-in. spinal needle is inserted 0.5 cm deep, just lateral to the base of the anterior tonsillar pillar (ATP). Use of a spinal needle is advantageous for visualization of the tonsillar pillars by keeping the syringe out of the patient's mouth [51]. After careful aspiration for blood or cerebrospinal fluid, 2 mL of local anesthetic (LA) or LA plus nonparticulate steroid is injected. The advantages of this method are that the ATP is easily identified and exposed, and the tongue movement does not trigger the gag reflex (Fig. 31.6).

Posterior Tonsillar Pillar Method

The patient is asked to open the mouth widely. The tongue is depressed down with a laryngoscope blade (if done in the OR) or else with a tongue blade as described above. A 22-gauge, 3.5-in. spinal needle bent 1 cm from the distal end is directed laterally into the submucosa along the caudal aspect of the PTP (palatopharyngeal fold). After careful aspiration for blood and cerebrospinal fluid, 2 mL of local anesthetic and/or steroid is injected. The PTP method becomes more difficult in patients with large tongues or small oral opening and may cause greater gag reflex [52].

Potential Complications/Side Effects

Potential undesirable side effects of glossopharyngeal nerve block may include the following:

- Dysphagia secondary to weakness of the stylopharyngeus muscle [9]
- Upper airway obstruction/loss of protective reflexes secondary to bilateral nerve block [53]
- Ecchymoses/hematoma – trauma to internal carotid artery and/or internal carotid vein

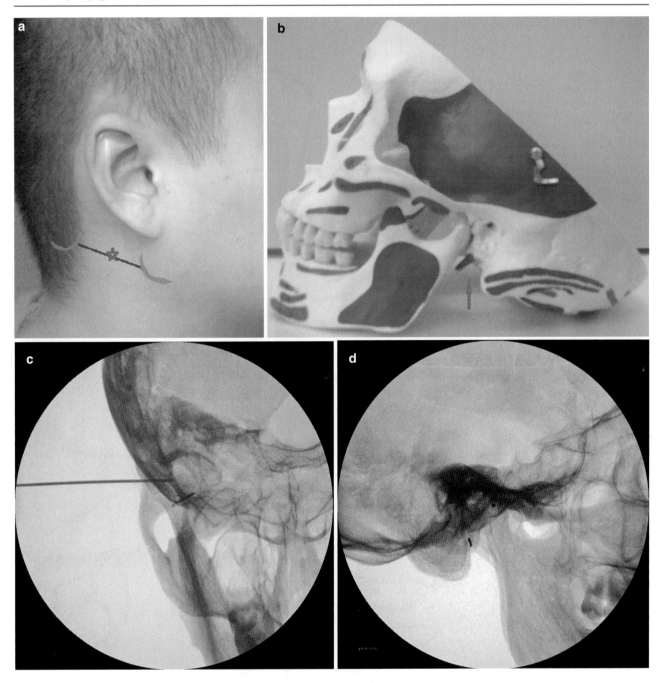

Fig. 31.3 (a, b) Surface anatomy: glossopharyngeal nerve block (Photo courtesy of George C. Chang Chien, D.O.). (c) AP fluoroscopic image of right GPN block (Photo courtesy of Steven D. Waldman, M.D., JD). (d) Lateral fluoroscopic image of right-sided GPN block (Photo courtesy of Steven D. Waldman, M.D., JD)

- Infection
- Trauma to the nerve
- Toxicity due intravascular injection of local anesthetic
- Tachycardia from vagus nerve block
- Hoarseness/dysphonia secondary to vagus nerve block and paralysis of the ipsilateral vocal cord
- Post-procedure dysesthesias or anesthesia dolorosa

- Cardiovascular complications resulting in acute onset hypotension with right bundle branch block secondary to dissection of the uppermost rootlets of the vagus nerve [54]
- Block of the hypoglossal nerve with resultant tongue weakness (CN XII)
- Trapezius muscle weakness secondary to inadvertent block of the spinal accessory nerve (CN XI)

Fig. 31.4 (**a**, **b**) Demonstrated is the relationship between the glossopharyngeal nerve and the styloid process. Ossification of the stylohyoid ligament (**a**) and elongation of the styloid process (**b**) can both cause compression of the glossopharyngeal nerve (Images courtesy of George C. Chang Chien, D.O.)

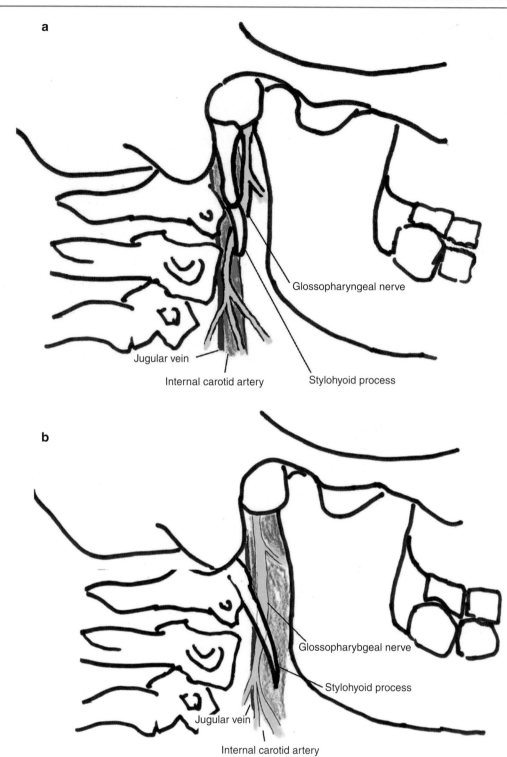

Fig. 31.5 Anatomy for intraoral GPN block (Photo courtesy of George C. Chang Chien, D.O.)

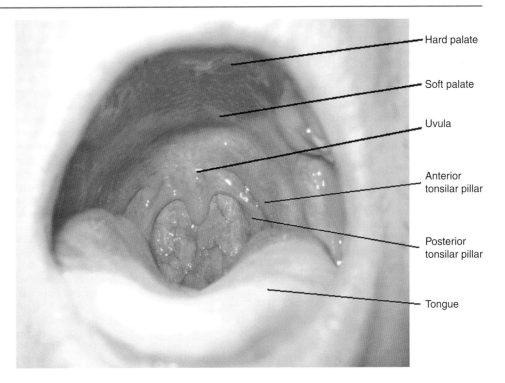

Hard palate

Soft palate

Uvula

Anterior tonsilar pillar

Posterior tonsilar pillar

Tongue

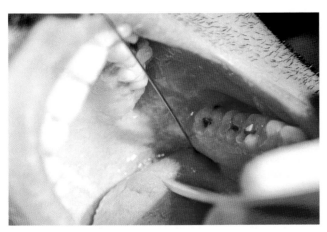

Fig. 31.6 Lateral tongue sweep prior to LA injection, needle in place (Photo courtesy of Kenneth D. Candido, M.D.)

Surgical Treatment

Surgical resection of the glossopharyngeal nerve performed for pain control was first described by Dandy in 1927 [8]. This remains an option in severe cases refractory to interventional pain management or microvascular decompression [55–58]. Two cases have been reported of successful pain treatment of GPN with use of the gamma knife [59].

Summary

In summary, facial pain continues to be a problem that is difficult to diagnose and even more difficult to treat [60]. The complicated neuroanatomical relationships between the glossopharyngeal nerve and other cranial structures, neural as well as osseous and ligamentous and vascular, create an imposing challenge for even seasoned interventional pain management physicians. The use of glossopharyngeal nerve block as part of a multidisciplinary and multimodal approach to pain control should be part of every pain physician's armamentarium.

References

1. Harris W. Persistent pain in lesions of the peripheral and central nervous system. Brain (Lond). 1921;44:557.
2. Chawla JC, Falconer MA. Glossopharyngeal and vagal neuralgia. Br Med J. 1967;3:529–31.
3. Fraioli B, Esposito V, Ferrante L, Trubiani L, Lunardi P. Microsurgical treatment of glossopharyngeal neuralgia: case reports. Neurosurgery. 1989;25:630–2.
4. Weinstein RE, Herec D, Friedman JH. Hypotension due to glossopharyngeal neuralgia. Arch Neurol. 1986;43:90–2.
5. Kong Y, Heyman A, Entman ML, McIntosh HD. Glossopharyngeal neuralgia associated with bradycardia, syncope, and seizures. Circulation. 1964;30:109–13.
6. Weisenburg TH. Cerebello-pontine tumor diagnosed for six years as a tic douloureux. The symptoms of irritation of the ninth and twelfth cranial nerves. J Am Med Assoc (Chic). 1910;54:1600–4.
7. Sicard R, Robineau J. Communications et presentations: I Algie velo-pharyngeal essentielle, traitement chirurgical. Rev Neurol. 1920;36:256.
8. Dandy WE. Glossopharyngeal neuralgia (tic douloureux). Arch Surg. 1927;15:I98.
9. Rushton JG, Stevens JC, Miller RH. Glossopharyngeal (vago-glossopharyngeal) neuralgia: a study of 217 cases. Arch Neurol. 1981;38:201–5.
10. Katusic S, Williams DB, Beard CM, Bergstralh E, Kurland LT. Incidence and clinical features of glossopharyngeal neuralgia, Rochester, Minnesota, 1945–1984. Neuroepidemiology. 1991;10:266–75.

11. Ferrante L, Artico M, Nardacci B, Fraioli B, Consentino F, Fortuna A. Glossopharyngeal neuralgia with cardiac syncope. Neurosurgery. 1995;36:58–63.

12. Karnosh LJ, Gardner WJ, Stowell A. Glossopharyngeal neuralgia: physiological consideration of the role of ninth and tenth cranial nerves–report of cases. Trans Am Neurol Assoc. 1947;72:205–7.

13. Takaya N, Sumiyoshi M, Nakata Y. Prolonged cardiac arrest caused by glossopharyngeal neuralgia. Heart. 2003;89:381.

14. Varrasi C, Strigaro G, Prandi P, Comi C, Mula M, Monaco F, Cantello RM. Complex pattern of convulsive syncope in glossopharyngeal neuralgia: video/EEG report and short review. Epilepsy Behav. 2011;20:407–9.

15. Soh KB. The glossopharyngeal nerve, glossopharyngeal neuralgia and the Eagle's syndrome–current concepts and management. Singapore Med J. 1999;40:659–65.

16. Kawashima M, Matsushima T, Inoue T, Mineta T, Masuoka J, Hirakawa N. Microvascular decompression for glossopharyngeal neuralgia through the transcondylar fossa (supracondylar transjugular tubercle) approach. Neurosurgery. 2010;66:275–80.

17. Resnick DK, Jannetta PJ, Bissonnette D, et al. Microvascular decompression for glossopharyngeal neuralgia. Neurosurgery. 1995;36:64–9.

18. Kondo A. Follow-up results of using microvascular decompression for treatment of glossopharyngeal neuralgia. J Neurosurg. 1998; 88:221–5.

19. Dykman TR, Montgomery Jr EB, Gerstenberger PD, Zeiger HE, Clutter WE, Cryer PE. Glossopharyngeal neuralgia with syncope secondary to tumor: treatment and pathophysiology. Am J Med. 1981;71:165–8.

20. Sobol SM, Wood BG, Conoyer JM. Glossopharyngeal neuralgia-asystole syndrome secondary to parapharyngeal space lesions. Otolaryngol Head Neck Surg. 1982;90:16–9.

21. Waga S, Kojima T. Glossopharyngeal neuralgia of traumatic origin. Surg Neurol. 1982;17:77–9.

22. Kahana E, Leibowitz U, Alter M. Brainstem and cranial nerve involvement in multiple sclerosis. Acta Neurol Scand. 1973; 49:269–79.

23. Shin JH, Herrera SR, Eboli P, Aydin S, Eskandar EH, Slavin KV. Entrapment of the glossopharyngeal nerve in patients with Eagle syndrome: surgical technique and outcomes in a series of 5 patients. J Neurosurg. 2009;111:1226–30.

24. Carrieri PB, Montella S, Petracca M. Glossopharyngeal neuralgia as onset of multiple sclerosis. Clin J Pain. 2009;25:737–9.

25. Fukuda H, Ishikawa M, Yamazoe N. Glossopharyngeal neuralgia caused by adhesive arachnoid. Acta Neurochir. 2002;144:1057–8.

26. Aicardi J. Disorders of the peripheral nerves. In: Aicardi J, editor. Diseases of the nervous system in childhood. London: MacKeith Press; 1998. p. 733.

27. Park HP. The effects of glossopharyngeal nerve block on postoperative pain relief after tonsillectomy: the importance of the extent of obtunded gag reflex as a clinical indicator. Anesth Analg. 2007;105:267–71.

28. Waldman SD. The role of neural blockade in the management of headaches and facial pain. Headache Dig. 1991;4:286–92.

29. Waldman SD, Waldman KA. The diagnosis and treatment of glossopharyngeal neuralgia. Am J Pain Manag. 1995;5:19–24.

30. Waldman SD. The role of neural blockade in the management of headaches and facial pain. Curr Rev Pain. 1997;1:346–52.

31. Benumof JL. Management of the difficult adult airway. Anesthesiology. 1991;75:1084–6.

32. Gallacher BP, Martin L. Treatment of refractory hiccups with glossopharyngeal nerve block. Anesth Analg. 1997;84:229.

33. Kodama K, Seo N, Murayama T, Yoshizawa Y, Terasako K, Yaginuma T. Glossopharyngeal nerve block for carotid sinus syndrome. Anesth Analg. 1992;75:1036–7.

34. Hiwatashi A, Matsushima T, Yoshiura T, Tanaka A, Noguchi T, Togao O, Yamashita K, Honda H. MRI of glossopharyngeal neuralgia caused by neurovascular compression. AJR Am J Roentgenol. 2008;191:578–81.

35. Gaul C, Hastreiter P, Duncker A, Naraghi R. Diagnosis and neurosurgical treatment of glossopharyngeal neuralgia: clinical findings and 3-D visualization of neurovascular compression in 19 consecutive patients. J Headache Pain. 2011;12:527–34.

36. Hasegawa S, Morioka M, Kai Y, Kuratsu J. Usefulness of balloon test occlusion in the diagnosis of glossopharyngeal neuralgia. Case report. Neurol Med Chir (Tokyo). 2008;48:163–6.

37. Matsushima T, Goto Y, Ishioka H, Mihara F, Fukui M. Possible role of an endovascular provocative test in the diagnosis of glossopharyngeal neuralgia as a vascular compression syndrome. Acta Neurochir (Wien). 1999;141:1229–32.

38. Dworkin R, Backonja M, Rowbotham MC, Allen R, Argoff C, Bennett G, Bushnell MC, Farrar JT, Galer BS, Haythornthwaite JA, Hewitt DJ, Loeser JD, Max MB, Saltarelli M, Schmader KE, Stein C, Thombson D, Turk DC, Wallace MS, Watkins LR, Weinstein SM. Advances in neuropathic pain: diagnosis, mechanisms, and treatment recommendations. Arch Neurol. 2003;60:1524–34.

39. Kouzaki Y, Takita T, Tawara S, Otsuka T, Hirano T, Uchino M. Opioid effectiveness for neuropathic pain in a patient with glossopharyngeal neuralgia. Rinsho Shinkeigaku. 2009;49:364–9.

40. Finnerup NB, Otto M, McQuay HK, Jensen TS, Sindrup SH. Algorithm for neuropathic pain treatment: an evidence based proposal. Pain. 2005;118:289–305.

41. Cheshire Jr WP. Defining the role for gabapentin in the treatment of trigeminal neuralgia: a retrospective study. J Pain. 2002;3:137–42.

42. Titlic M, Jukic I, Tonkic A, Grani P, Jukic J. Use of lamotrigine in glossopharyngeal neuralgia: a case report. Headache. 2006; 46:167–9.

43. Saviolo R, Fiascanaro G. Treatment of glossopharyngeal neuralgia by carbamazepine. Br Heart J. 1987;58:291–2.

44. Ekbom KA, Westerberg CE. Carbamazepine in glossopharyngeal neuralgia. Arch Neurol. 1966;14:595–6.

45. Funasaka S, Kodera K. Intraoral nerve block for glossopharyngeal neuralgia. Arch Otorhinolaryngol. 1977;215:311–5.

46. Isamat F, Ferran E, Acebes JJ. Selective percutaneous thermocoagulation rhizotomy in essential glossopharyngeal neuralgia. J Neurosurg. 1981;55:575–80.

47. Tew Jr JM. Treatment of pain of glossopharyngeal and vagus nerves by percutaneous rhizotomy. In: Youmans JR, editor. Neurological surgery. Philadelphia: W.B. Saunders Co; 1982. p. 3609–12.

48. Bedder MD, Lindsay D. Glossopharyngeal nerve block using ultrasound guidance: a case report of a new technique. Reg Anesth. 1989;14:304–7.

49. Isbir CA. Treatment of a patient with glossopharyngeal neuralgia by the anterior tonsillar pillar method. Case Rep Neurol. 2011;3:27–31.

50. Katz J. Glossopharyngeal nerve block. Atlas of regional anesthesia. Norwalk: Appleton and Lange; 1994. p. 54.

51. Saliba DL, McCutchen TA, Laxton MJ, Miller SA, Reynolds JE. Reliable block of the gag reflex in one minute or less. J Clin Anesth. 2009;21:463.

52. Nehthorn RW, Amayem A, Ganta R. Which method for intraoral glossopharyngeal nerve block is better? Letters to the Editor. Anesth Analg. 1995;81:1114.

53. Bean-Lijewski JD. Glossopharyngeal nerve block for pain relief after pediatric tonsillectomy: retrospective analysis and two cases of life-threatening upper airway obstruction from an interrupted trial. Anesth Analg. 1997;84:1232–8.

54. Nagashima C, Sakaguchi A, Kamisasa A, Kawanuma S. Cardiovascular complications on upper vagal rootlet section for glossopharyngeal neuralgia; case report. J Neurosurg. 1976;44:248–53.

55. Torigoe T, Kato I, Suzuki T, Kenmochi M, Takeyama I. Two cases with glossopharyngeal neuralgia treated by nerve reaction: oropharyngeal approach. Acta Otolaryngol Suppl. 1996;522:142–5.

56. Ceylan S, Karakuş A, Duru S, Baykal S, Koca O. Glossopharyngeal neuralgia: a study of 6 cases. J Neurosurg. 1997;20:196–200.

57. Ferroli P, Fioravanti A, Schiariti M, Tringali G, Franzini A, Calbucci F, Broggi G. Microvascular decompression for glossopharyngeal neuralgia: a long-term retrospectic review of the Milan-Blogna experience in 31 consecutive cases. Acta Neuochir. 2009;151: 1245–50.

58. Kandan SR. Neuralgia of the glossopharyngeal and vagal nerves: long-term outcome following surgical treatment and literature review. Br J Neurosurg. 2010;24(4):441–6.

59. Yomo S, Arkha Y, Donnet A, Régis J. Gamma knife surgery for glossopharyngeal neuralgia. J Neurosurg. 2009;110:559–63.

60. Koopman JS, Dieleman JP, Huygen FJ, de Mos M, Martin CG, Sturkenboom MC. Incidence of facial pain in the general population. Pain. 2009;147:122–7.

Cervical Plexus Block

Gerald A. Matchett and Sean Mackey

Abbreviations

CPB Cervical plexus block
SCM Sternocleidomastoid muscle
CEA Carotid endarterectomy

Key Points

- Cervical plexus block is safe and reliable for surgical anesthesia and analgesia.
- Superficial cervical plexus block has a lower complication rate than deep cervical plexus block.
- The most common complication of a cervical plexus block is phrenic nerve dysfunction.
- Superficial cervical plexus bock is sufficient for most surgical indications because of ready spread of local anesthetic within the fascial planes in the neck.
- Cervical plexus block may be useful in select patients with chronic pain disorders such as cervicogenic headache and cervicalgia arising from the cervical plexus.

Introduction

The purpose of this chapter is to provide an overview of the historical and current clinical use of the cervical plexus block (CPB). Historical interest in CPB dates to the 1840s, when reports described various topical therapies for cervical neuralgia arising from the cervical plexus [1]. Needle-based techniques were introduced in the early 1900s, and large case series describing CPB for open neck surgery soon followed [2, 3]. Numerous indications for CPB have been described for both acute and chronic pain (Table 32.1).

Anatomy of the Cervical Plexus

The cervical plexus is comprised of three loops that arise from the anterior rami of the cervical roots of C2–C4 (Fig. 32.1). The loops of the plexus lie anterior to the levator scapulae and scalenus medius muscles and posterior to the sternocleidomastoid (SCM) [4, 5]. Deep terminal branches of the plexus innervate deep muscular structures such as the scalenus medius, trapezius, levator scapulae, and SCM and communicate with the spinal accessory nerve. The superficial branches innervate the skin over the lateral head and neck via the occipital, anterior cutaneous, great auricular, and supraclavicular nerves (Fig. 32.2) [4, 5].

G.A. Matchett, M.D. (✉)
Department of Anesthesiology and Management,
University of Texas Southwestern School of Medicine,
5323 Harry Hines Blvd, Dallas, TX 75390-9068, USA
e-mail: gerald.matchett@utsouthwestern.edu

S. Mackey, M.D., Ph.D.
Department of Anesthesiology, Stanford University,
780 Welch Road #208, Palo Alto, CA 94304, USA

Division of Pain Medicine,
Stanford University School of Medicine,
Stanford, CA, USA
e-mail: smackey@standford.edu

Table 32.1 Indications for cervical plexus block

Atypical cervicogenic headache
Cervicalgia
Carotid surgery
Thyroid surgery
Parathyroid surgery
Lymph node biopsy in the neck
Surgery on the mastoid process
Central line placement (awake)
Other head and neck surgery

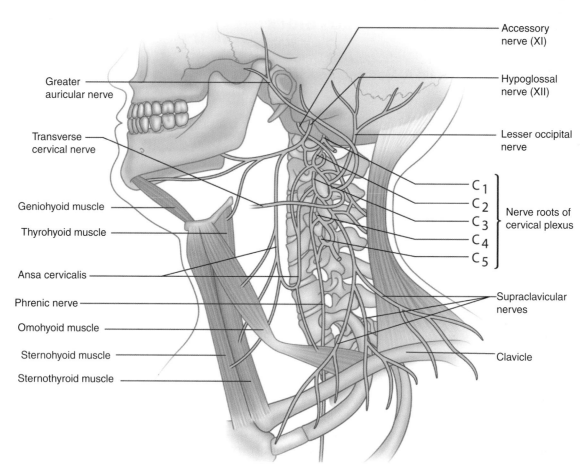

Fig. 32.1 Anatomy of the cervical plexus. Diagram of the cervical plexus as it emerges from the cervical roots of C2–4. Note the close relationship between the cervical plexus and the phrenic nerve, which is usually affected by a deep cervical plexus block

Techniques for Blocking the Cervical Plexus

Cervical plexus blocks are usually classified as "superficial" or "deep." Historically, a "superficial" block implied injection of local anesthetic into subcutaneous tissue without violating the fascial planes investing the SCM [6]. However, in current practice, a "superficial" block usually indicates administration of local anesthetic subcutaneously, around the SCM, and deep to fascial planes around the SCM [7, 8]. A "deep" block implies a plexus block at the level of the transverse processes of the cervical vertebrae [9]. Some have suggested the concept of an "intermediate" plexus block, defined by administration of local anesthetic subcutaneously and just deep to the investing fascial layers of the SCM [10]. However, as a practical matter, this definition overlaps considerably with what is currently known as a "superficial" block. In this chapter, we will use the term "superficial" to indicate an injection both in the skin and into layers just deep to the SCM as is commonly done today. A "deep" block refers to an injection at the level of the transverse processes

of the cervical spine. A "combined" cervical plexus block usually refers to the combination of a deep and superficial block.

Although the cervical plexus may be approached anteriorly, laterally, or posteriorly, the most common practice today is an anterolateral approach for both superficial and deep plexus blocks (Fig. 32.3a–f) [4, 9]. The superficial block is usually performed at the midpoint between the mastoid process and the sternal notch at the posterior edge of the sternocleidomastoid muscle (Fig. 32.3a–c). Local anesthetic is injected along the SCM, just deep to the SCM, and in the general direction of the terminal branches of the plexus [4].

Deep CPB is traditionally performed with three separate injections at the transverse process of C2–4 [4]. Historically, this block is performed using surface and bony landmarks, although our preference is to use fluoroscopic guidance with injection of iodinated contrast to help confirm needle placement. The bony landmark for this block is traditionally the C6 transverse process. This can be palpated, and C4–2 can be identified on a line drawn between C6 transverse process and the mastoid process (Fig. 32.3d–f). Alternately, a single

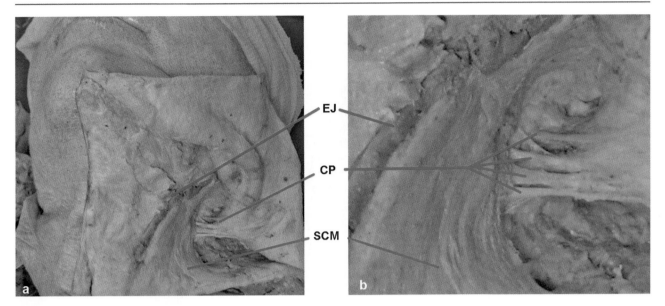

Fig. 32.2 Branches of the cervical plexus in situ. (**a**, **b**) Superficial cutaneous dissection of the left neck demonstrates the sternocleidomastoid (*SCM*), the external jugular vein (*EJ*), and the four branches of the cervical plexus (*CP*) emerging just posterior to the SCM. These branches are the great occipital, great auricular, transverse cervical, and supraclavicular nerves. In this dissection, the skin has been reflected posteriorly to the left (Courtesy of G. Matchett, made at the Gross Anatomy Lab at Stanford University School of Medicine)

injection at the transverse process of C3 or C4 may be used [9]. Needle placement for the deep block may be facilitated by surface landmarks, elicitation of paresthesias, elicitation of muscle twitches from levator scapulae [13], ultrasound [14, 15], or fluoroscopy [16]. Studies comparing single versus multiple injection techniques have reported similar outcomes [13, 17].

Local anesthetic spreads easily in the compartments of the neck after a superficial CPB. This has been demonstrated by cadaver study (Fig. 32.4) and clinical experience [7]. Likewise, after deep CPB, local anesthetic spreads easily, especially when large volumes are given (>20 mL) [18].

Indications: Surgical Anesthesia

The most common indication for CPB is surgical anesthesia. For example, the block may be used in addition to, or in place of, general anesthesia for carotid endarterectomy (CEA). Table 32.1 provides a list of common surgical indications.

Indications: Cervicalgia and Cervicogenic Headache

Historical interest in CPB arose out of a desire to treat cervicalgia arising from the cervical plexus [1]. A case series in 1955 reported the use of the block in 63 patients with atypical cervicogenic headache, 57 of who appeared to benefit from CPB [19]. Recent case series report similar findings. Goldberg et al. [16] described a 39-patient case series of deep cervical plexus block for atypical headaches that appeared to coincide predominately with a cervical or brachial plexus distraction-type injury. A majority of patients experienced a significant decrease in average pain scores immediately after the blocks, and a return to pre-block pain level took an average of 6.6 weeks [16]. Selective cervical plexus blocks may also be useful as an aid in diagnosis of atypical orofacial pain [20].

Choice of Local Anesthetic for Cervical Plexus Block

Bupivacaine and ropivacaine are commonly used for CPB, although nearly any local anesthetic can be used (Table 32.2). Pharmacokinetic studies have confirmed the safety of adding epinephrine to local anesthetic solutions for cervical plexus block [28–30]. This may help prolong the blockade and reduce serum concentration of local anesthetic [30]. Epinephrine may be associated with mild sympathomimetic effects on heart rate and blood pressure [29, 31].

Long-acting local anesthetics are usually used for CPB in order to ensure adequate duration of block (Table 32.2). Most comparative studies of one long-acting local anesthetic to another have reported similar clinical outcomes at equipotent doses [23, 32, 33]. Ropivacaine (0.75 or 1 %) was reported to be superior to mepivacaine (2 %) in the setting of deep cervical plexus block for CEA in one study [34]. Studies

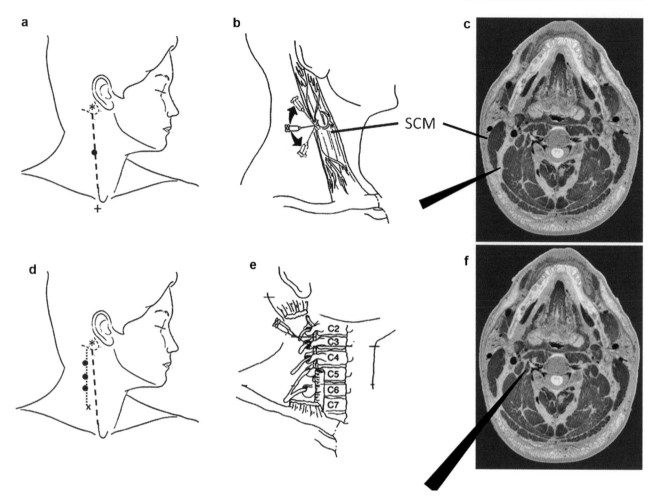

Fig. 32.3 Techniques for blocking the cervical plexus. (**a**) The superficial cervical plexus can be approached at the midline of the posterior border of the sternocleidomastoid (*SCM*) (*dashed line*). The SCM can be identified superiorly by the mastoid process (*) and inferiorly by the sternal notch (+). (**b**) Needle passage for a superficial block should be superior, inferior, and just deep to the sternocleidomastoid (*SCM*). (**c**) In transverse view at C4, the needle should pass just deep to the SCM. (**d**) The deep cervical plexus block can be performed by three individual injections at C2–4 or alternately can be performed by a single injection at C3 or C4. Typically, the location for the injections is noted by palpation of the C6 transverse process (*point x*). The transverse process of C2–4 can be identified superiorly to C6 on a line drawn between the mastoid process and the C6 transverse process (dot-

ted line). In an average adult, the transverse processes of C4–2 are approximately 2, 4, and 6 cm superiorly on the line connecting the mastoid process and C6. Once the transverse (superior tubercle) is contacted by the needle, the needle should be withdrawn 1–2 mm and local anesthetic injected following negative aspiration for blood. (**e**) Schematic diagram showing correct needle placement at C3. (**f**) Transverse section showing the transverse process of C4 (**a**, **d** – Reprinted with permission and adapted from Paul et al. [11]. © License from Wolters Kluwer Health License, 2009; **b**, **e** – Reprinted with permission and adapted from Stoneham and Knighton [12]. © License from Oxford University Press License, 2009; **c**, **f** – Reprinted with permission and adapted from the Visible Human Project of the National Library of Medicine – USA)

suggest that higher concentration local anesthetic solution (e.g., 0.75 % ropivacaine instead of 0.375 % ropivacaine) may be preferable for duration and density of block [27].

Reports have described other drugs such as clonidine [25] or corticosteroids [16] as part of CPB. The addition of clonidine (50 μg) to ropivacaine (150 mg) for superficial cervical plexus block was found to shorten the onset time and improve the quality of surgical anesthesia [25]. Steroids may be included for CPB in the setting of cervicalgia or cervicogenic headache [16].

Contraindications

Contraindications include patient refusal, marginal pulmonary status, severe coagulopathy, local infection, and severe anatomic distortion. Baseline pulmonary status is important to consider before a deep cervical plexus block. Deep blockade usually results in phrenic nerve paralysis with hemidiaphragmatic dysfunction, and this can potentially lead to respiratory distress in a patient with marginal baseline pulmonary function [4].

Fig. 32.4 Spread of local anesthetic with cervical plexus blocks. Superficial plexus block with methylene blue dye administered just deep to the sternocleidomastoid in a cadaver study. Following injection, methylene blue dye is widely distributed in the neck. 1-Ear, 2-mandible, 3-sterno-cleidomastoid muscle, 4-internal jugular vein, 5-subclavian artery, 6-omohyoid muscle (cut), 7-brachial nerve plexus, 8-trapezius muscle (cut). The inset picture denotes the orientation of the cadaver (Adapted and used with permission from Pandit et al. [7]. © License from Oxford University Press License, 2009)

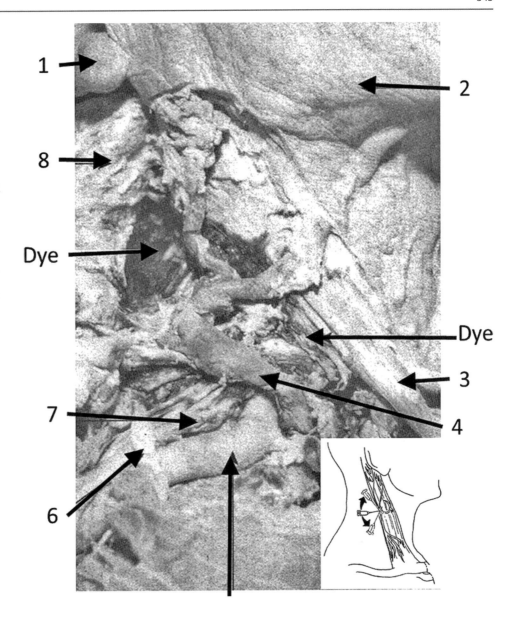

Complications

Blockade of the *superficial* cervical plexus is extremely safe and complications are very rare [35]. Most complications, serious or otherwise, occur with *deep* CPB [35]. A quantitative meta-analysis of 69 published reports covering more than 10,000 individual blocks found that deep CPB is significantly more likely to be associated with serious block-related complications and the need to convert to general anesthesia than superficial CPB (Fig. 32.5) [35].

The most common complication of deep CPB is phrenic nerve block which leads to hemidiaphragmatic dysfunction. This may occur in 55–100 % of patients who have a deep block [4, 36]. In patients with marginal pulmonary status, this may interfere with respiration and ventilation [36, 37].

Other common complications include the need for supplemental infiltration of local anesthetic (53 % of the time with carotid endarterectomy surgery) [38], and the need to convert from regional to general anesthesia (4.2 % of the time with carotid endarterectomy surgery) [39]. Table 32.3 provides a list of complications, most of which occur with deep blockade.

Bilateral Cervical Plexus Block

Bilateral regional anesthetic procedures in the neck should be approached with caution. Bilateral *superficial* CPB has been described for surgical anesthesia for thyroidectomy in several small randomized studies [42, 43, 44]. However, given

Table 32.2 Sample protocols for cervical plexus block

Local anesthetic	Dose	References
Superficial		
Bupivacaine	0.375 %, 1.4 mg/kg (average = 30 mL)	[21]
Bupivacaine	0.375 %, 20 mL	[22]
Levobupivacaine	0.5 %, 1 mg/kg	[23]
Levobupivacaine	0.5 %, 0.35 mL/kg	[24]
Ropivacaine	0.75 %, 20 mL + clonidine 50 mcg	[25]
Ropivacaine	1 %, 10 mL	[26]
Ropivacaine	0.75 %, 1.5 mg/kg	[23]
Ropivacaine	0.375–0.75 %, 20 mL	[27]
Deep		
Bupivacaine	0.25 %, 3–5 cc per level (C2–4)	[4]
Bupivacaine	0.375 %, 20 mL at C4	[9, 22]
Bupivacaine	0.25 %, 10 mL + 80 mg methylprednisolone (C2–4)	[16]
Lidocaine	2 % ± bicarbonate and epinephrine, (3–5 cc per level)	[4]
Mepivacaine	1.5 % ± bicarbonate and epinephrine, (3–5 cc per level)	[4]
Ropivacaine	0.5 %, 3–5 cc per level	[4]
Combined		
Bupivacaine	0.375 %, 1/3 of dose placed at C4 (deep), 2/3 of dose placed superficially, total dose = 1.4 mg/kg	[21]
Levobupivacaine	0.5 %, 0.2 mL/kg placed at C3, then 0.15 mL/kg placed superficially	[24]
Ropivacaine	0.375–0.75 %, 10 mL at C4 followed by 20 mL placed superficially	[27]

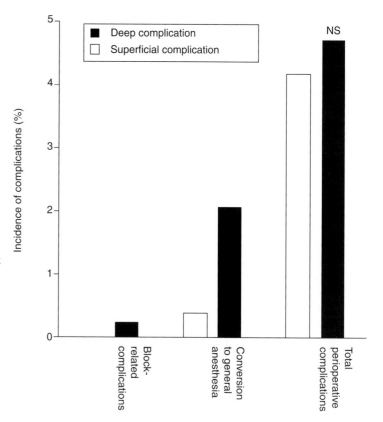

Fig. 32.5 Complications. In a large quantitative review of more than 10,000 patients who received cervical plexus block for carotid endarterectomy (CEA) surgery, the rate of serious, block-related complications for deep cervical plexus block was significantly greater than the rate of serious, block-related complications. Likewise, the rate of conversion to GA was significantly higher in the deep plexus block. The overall rate of serious complications associated with CEA surgery was the same in both groups. * indicates statistical significance, $p < 0.05$ for deep versus superficial comparison. *NS* not statistically significant (Reprinted and adapted with permission from Pandit et al. [35]. © License from Oxford University Press, 2009)

Table 32.3 Complications of cervical plexus block

Complication	Frequency	References
Common		
Phrenic nerve block or hemidiaphragmatic dysfunction	55–100 %	Occurs with deep CPB, occurs rarely with superficial CPB [4, 36]
Local anesthetic supplementation required during carotid endarterectomy	53 %	[38]
Blood aspirated during block placement	30 %	[38]
Block failure or conversion to general anesthesia for carotid endarterectomy	.039, 3, 4.2 %	[35, 39, 40]
Blockade of extraneous nerves such as cranial nerves	4.2 %	[40]
Uncommon		
Hematoma	0.6 %	[40]
Intravascular injection	0.6 %	[38]
Respiratory distress	0.1–0.3 %	[38, 41]
Seizure	0.3 %	[38]
Local anesthetic toxicity	0.2 %	[38]
Rare		
Infection	<<1%	
Intrathecal injection	<<1%	
Permanent nerve injury	<<1%	
Paralysis	<<1%	
Death	<<1%	

the relatively small amount of randomized data available, the absolute safety of this technique cannot be assured.

The safety of bilateral *deep* CPB is very uncertain. A small number of studies have reported the successful use of bilateral deep blocks for thyroid surgery, although this was done in the context of immediate induction of general anesthesia with definitive airway control [45, 46]. Given the likelihood of phrenic nerve paralysis with deep blockade, bilateral deep blocks should probably be avoided. In one small case series of bilateral combined (superficial and deep) cervical plexus block, 1/18 patients required conversion to general anesthesia because of respiratory distress (coughing) [47].

the higher complication rate of deep CPB compared to superficial CPB, there is a growing consensus that superficial cervical plexus block is preferable for most surgical indications, especially CEA. A recent quantitative meta-analysis of cervical plexus block supports the relative safety of superficial block over deep block (Fig. 32.5) [27].

The most plausible explanation for why superficial CPB is apparently as effective as deep CPB for surgical anesthesia relates to the ease of spread of local anesthetics. Local anesthetic solutions can spread easily through compartments in the neck after superficial (Fig. 32.4) [7] or deep [18] CPB. Superficial CPB is sufficient for most surgical indications, including carotid or thyroid surgery.

Superficial Versus Deep Cervical Plexus Block for Surgical Anesthesia

Several studies have compared superficial versus deep CPB in the context of surgical anesthesia. A prospective, randomized trial of superficial CPB versus combined CPB (both superficial and deep block) for parathyroidectomy reported equivalent outcomes between the two groups [24]. Notably, there was no discernable benefit from adding the deep block to the superficial block. This finding is consistent with earlier case series of parathyroidectomy under superficial cervical plexus block [48]. Similarly, at least two studies have compared superficial versus deep blocks for awake CEA and found no clear benefit from the deep block [21, 22]. Given

Outcome Data: Cervical Plexus Block Combined with General Anesthesia

Many surgical procedures may be performed with the combination of general anesthesia and CPB (Table 32.1). At least six recent prospective, randomized studies have examined the effect of combining a CPB with general anesthesia for thyroidectomy. Of these six studies, four reported a benefit of superficial cervical plexus block [42, 45, 46, 49]. These benefits included reduced intraoperative and/or postoperative analgesic use [45, 46, 49] and improved visual analog pain scores [42, 45, 46]. The other two studies reported essentially equivalent outcomes between patients with and without cervical plexus block for thyroidectomy done under general anesthesia [43, 44]. The combination of CPB with general anesthesia in CEA is associated with improved post-operative pain control and patient satisfaction [26].

Outcome Data: Cervical Plexus Block in Place of General Anesthesia

Many surgical procedures of the head and neck may be performed under regional anesthesia by CPB alone (Table 32.1). A case series published in 1934 reported a strong benefit of regional anesthesia with CPB over general anesthesia for thyroid surgery ($n = 125$) [3]. It seems likely that the benefit of regional anesthesia in this case series may have related to the relative danger of general anesthesia in the 1930s.

Recent studies have largely reported equivalent patient outcomes between surgeries performed with regional anesthesia alone via CPB versus surgeries under general anesthesia. The largest study to examine this question is the General Anesthesia versus Local Anesthesia for Carotid Endarterectomy (GALA) study [39]. In the GALA study, 3,526 patients scheduled for CEA were randomized to either general anesthesia (GA) or local anesthesia (LA) via CPB. The outcomes of this study included stroke, myocardial infarction, or death within 30 days after surgery. No difference in outcome between GA and LA was found, and the authors concluded that both techniques are appropriate. The 2009 Cochrane Database Review on the subject covering 4,335 patients echoes this conclusion [50].

Small studies have suggested improved hemodynamic stability during CEA with CPB than without [51, 52], and the GALA study reported similar findings in subgroup analyzes [39]. In the GALA study, more patients in the GA group required intermittent treatment for hypotension compared to the CPB group (43 % in the GA group vs. 17 % in the CPB group). Conversely, more patients in the CPB group required intermittent treatment for hypertension compared to the GA group (28 vs. 13 %). Of the two groups, hemodynamic manipulations were far more likely to be required in the GA group compared to the CPB group (72 vs. 54 %).

Conclusion

CPB is a safe and reliable plexus block that is widely used to provide surgical anesthesia and analgesia. CPB may also be useful in chronic pain disorders that arise from the cervical plexus. Both deep and superficial blocks are supported by current literature. Superficial block is safer than deep block, and superficial blockade is sufficient for most surgical indications because of ready spread of local anesthetic within the fascial planes in the neck.

Acknowledgment Thanks to Dr. John Gosling, Department Gross Anatomy, Stanford University, for assistance with Fig. 32.2.

References

1. Sandras M. Treatment of neuralgia according to their seat. BMJ Prov Med Surg J. 1849;s1–s3:191–4.
2. Carlton CH, Oxon MCH. Regional anaesthesia: an estimate of its place in practice. BMJ. 1925;1:648–51.
3. Graham JM, Wallace HL. Toxic goitre: a survey of 125 cases treated surgically. BMJ. 1934;2(3853): 845–9.
4. Hadzic A. Textbook of regional anesthesia and acute pain management. New York: McGraw-Hill Companies, Inc; 2007.
5. Loeser JD, Butler SH, Chapman CR Turk DC, editors. Bonica's management of pain. Philadelphia: Lippincott Williams & Wilkins; 2000.
6. Murphy TM. Somatic blockade of head and neck. Neural blockade in clinical anaesthesia and management of pain. Philadelphia: Lippincott Company; 1988.
7. Pandit JJ, Dutta D, Morris JF. Spread of injectate with superficial cervical plexus block in humans: an anatomical study. BJA. 2003;91(5):733–5.
8. Pandit JJ. Correct nomenclature of superficial cervical plexus blocks. BJA. 2004;91(5):733–5.
9. Winnie AP, Ramamurthy S, Durrani Z, Radonjic R. Interscalene cervical plexus block: a single-injection technique. Anesth Analg. 1975;54:370–5.
10. Telford RJ, Stoneham MD. Correct nomenclature of superficial cervical plexus blocks. BJA. 2003;91(5):733–5.
11. Paul R, Aradur A, Spencer F. Resection of an internal carotid artery aneurysm under regional anesthesia: posterior cervical block. Ann Surg. 1968;168(1):147–53.
12. Stoneham MD, Knighton JD. Regional anaesthesia for carotid endarterectomy. BJA. 1999;82(6):910–9.
13. Merle JC, Maxoit JX, Desgranges P, Abhay K, Rezaiguia S, Dhonneur G, Duvaldestin P. A comparison of two techniques for cervical plexus blockade: evaluation of efficacy and systemic toxicity. Anesth Analg. 1999;89:1366–70.
14. Sandeman DJ, Griffiths MJ, Lennox AF. Ultrasound guided deep cervical plexus block. Anaesth Intensive Care. 2006;34(2):240–4.
15. Roessel T, Wiessner D, Heller AR, Zimmermann T, Koch T, Litz R. High-resolution ultrasound-guided high interscalene plexus block for carotid endarterectomy. Reg Anesth Pain Med. 2007;32:247–53.
16. Goldberg ME, Schwartzman RJ, Domsky R, Sabina M, Torjman MC. Deep cervical plexus block for the treatment of cervicogenic headache. Pain Physician. 2008;11:849–54.
17. Gratz I, Deal E, Larijani GE, Domsky R, Goldberg ME. The number of injections does not influence absorption of bupivacaine after cervical plexus block for carotid endarterectomy. J Clin Anesth. 2005;17:263–6.
18. Dhonneur G, Saidi NE, Merle JC, Asfazadourian H, Ndoko SK, Bloc S. Demonstration of the spread of injectate with deep cervical plexus block: a case series. Reg Anesth Pain Med. 2007;32:116–9.
19. Pentecost PS, Adriani J. The use of cervical plexus block in the diagnosis and management of atypical cephalalgia of cervical origin. Anesthesiology. 1955;16(5):726–32.
20. Shinozaki T, Sakamoto E, Shiiba S, Ichikawa F, Arakawa Y, Makihara Y, Abe S, Ogawa A, Tsuboi E, Imamura Y. Cervical plexus block helps in diagnosis of orofacial pain originating from cervical structures. Tohoku J Exp Med. 2006;210:41–7.
21. Pandit JJ, Bree S, Dillon P, Elcock D, McLaren ID, Crider B. A comparison of superficial versus combined (superficial and deep) cervical plexus block for carotid endarterectomy: a prospective randomized study. Anesth Analg. 2000;91:781–6.
22. Stoneham MD, Doyle AR, Knighton JD, Dorje P, Stanley JC. Prospective, randomized comparison of deep or superficial cervical plexus block for carotid endarterectomy surgery. Anesthesiology. 1998;89(4):907–12.
23. Messina M, Magrin S, Bignami E, Maj G, Carozzo A, Minnella R, Landoni G, Zangrillo A. Prospective randomized, blind comparison of ropivacaine and levobupivacaine for superficial plexus anesthesia in carotid endarterectomy. Minerva Anestesiol. 2009;75:7–12.

24. Pintaric TS, Hocevar M, Jereb S, Casati A, Jankovic VN. A prospective, randomized comparison between combined (deep and superficial) and superficial cervical plexus block with levobupivacaine for minimally invasive parathyroidectomy. Anesth Analg. 2007;105:1160–3.

25. Danelli G, Nuzzi M, Salcuni PF, Caberti L, Berti M, Rossini E, Casati A, Fanelli G. Does clonidine 50 microg improve cervical plexus block obtained with ropivacaine 150 mg for carotid endarterectomy? A randomized, double-blinded study. J Clin Anesth. 2006;18:585–8.

26. Messner M, Albrecht S, Lang W, Sittl R, Dinkel M. The superficial cervical plexus block for postoperative pain therapy in carotid artery surgery. A prospective randomized controlled trial. Eur J Vasc Endovasc Surg. 2007;33:50–7.

27. Umbrain VJ, van Gorp VL, Schmedding E, Debing EE, von Kemp K, van den Brande PM, Camu F. Ropivacaine 3.75 mg/mL, 5 mg/mL or 7.5 mg/mL for cervical plexus block during carotid endarterectomy. Reg Anesth Pain Med. 2004;29(4):312–6.

28. Dawson AR, Dysart RH, Amerena JV, Braniff V, Davies MJ, Cronin KD, Mashford ML. Arterial lignocaine concentration following cervical plexus blockade for carotid endarterectomy. Anaesth Intensive Care. 1991;19(2):197–200.

29. McGlade DP, Murphy PM, Davies JM, Scott DA, Silbert BS. Comparative effects of plain and epinephrine-containing bupivacaine on the hemodynamic response to cervical plexus anesthesia in patients undergoing carotid endarterectomy. J Cardiothorac Vasc Anesth. 1996;10(5):593–7.

30. Harwood TN, Butterworth JF, Colonna DM, Samuel M. Plasma bupivacaine concentrations and effects of epinephrine after superficial cervical plexus blockade in patients undergoing carotid endarterectomy. J Cardiothoracic vasc Anesth. 1999;13(6):703–6.

31. Molnar RR, Davies MJ, Scott DA, Silbert BS, Mooney PH. Comparison of clonidine and epinephrine in lidocaine for cervical plexus block. Reg Anesth. 1997;22(2):137–42.

32. Junca A, Marret E, Goursot G, Mazoit X, Bonnet F. A comparison of ropivacaine and bupivacaine for cervical plexus block. Anesth Analg. 2001;92(3):720–4.

33. Cristalli A, Arlati S, Bettinelli L, Bracconaro G, Marconi G, Zerbi S. Regional anesthesia for carotid endarterectomy: a comparison between ropivacaine and levobupivacaine. Minerva Anestesiol. 2009;75:231–7.

34. Leoni A, Magrin S, Mascotto G, Rigamonti A, Galloli G, Muzzolon F, Fanelli G, Casati A. Cervical plexus anesthesia for carotid endarterectomy: comparison of ropivacaine and mepivacaine. Can J Anaesth. 2000;47(2):185–7.

35. Pandit JJ, Satya-Krishna R, Gration P. Superficial or deep cervical plexus block for carotid endarterectomy: a systematic review of complications. BJA. 2007;99(2):159–69.

36. Emery G, Handley G, Davies MJ, Mooney PH. Incidence of phrenic nerve block and hypercapnia in patients undergoing carotid endarterectomy under cervical plexus block. Anaesth Intensive Care. 1998;26(4):277–81.

37. Castresana MR, Masters RD, Castresana EJ, Stefsansson S, Shaker IJ, Neuman WH. Incidence and clinical significance of hemidiaphragmatic paresis in patients undergoing carotid endarterectomy during cervical plexus block anesthesia. J Neurosurg Anesthesiol. 1994;6(1):21–3.

38. Davies MJ, Silbert BS, Scott DA, Cook RJ, Mooney PH, Blyth C. Superficial and deep cervical plexus block for carotid artery surgery: a prospective study of 1000 blocks. Reg Anesth. 1997;22(5):442–6.

39. GALA Study Group. General anesthesia versus local anesthesia for carotid surgery (GALA): a multicentre, randomized controlled trial. Lancet. 2008;372:2132–42.

40. Hakl M, Michalek P, Sevcik P, Pavlikova J, Stern M. Regional anaesthesia for carotid endarterectomy: an audit over 10 years. BJA. 2007;99(3):415–20.

41. Peitzman AB, Webster MW, Loubeau JM, Grundy BL, Bahnson HT. Carotid endarterectomy under region (conductive) anesthesia. Ann Surg. 1982;196(1):59–64.

42. Dieudonne N, Gomola A, Bonnichon P, Ozier YM. Prevention of postoperative pain after thyroid surgery: a double-blind randomized study of bilateral superficial cervical plexus blocks. Anesth Analg. 2001;92:1538–42.

43. Herbland A, Cantini O, Reynier P, Valat P, Jougon J, Arimone Y, Janvier G. Bilateral superficial cervical plexus block with 0.75 % ropivacaine administered before or after surgery does not prevent postoperative pain after total thyroidectomy. Reg Anesth Pain Med. 2006;31(1):34–9.

44. Eti Z, Irmak P, Gulluoglu BM, Manukyan MN, Gogus FY. Does bilateral superficial cervical plexus block decrease analgesic requirement after thyroid surgery? Anesth Analg. 2006;102:1174–6.

45. Anuac S, Carlier M, Singelyn F, DeKock M. The analgesic efficacy of bilateral combined superficial and deep cervical plexus block administered before thyroid surgery under general anesthesia. Anesth Analg. 2002;95:746–50.

46. Suh YJ, Kim YS, In JH, Joo JD, Jeon YS, Kim HK. Comparison of analgesic efficacy between bilateral superficial and combined (superficial and deep) cervical plexus block administered before thyroid surgery. Eur J Anaesthesiol. 2009;26(12):1043–7.

47. Kulkarni RS, Braverman LE, Patwardhan NA. Bilateral cervical plexus block for thyroidectomy and parathyroidectomy in healthy and high risk patients. J Endocrinol Invest. 1996;19(11):714–8.

48. Carling T, Donovan P, Rinder C, Udelsman R. Minimally invasive parathyroidectomy using cervical block. Arch Surg. 2006;141:401–4.

49. Andrieu G, Amrouni H, Robin E, Carnaille B, Wattier JM, Pattou F, Vallet B, Lebuffe G. Analgesic efficacy of bilateral superficial cervical plexus block administered before thyroid surgery under general anaesthesia. BJA. 2007;99(4):561–6.

50. Rerkasem K, Rothwell PM. Local versus general anaesthesia for carotid endarterectomy. Cochrane Database Syst Rev. 2009;4: CD000126.

51. Hartsell PA, Calligaro KD, Syrek JR, Dougherty MJ, Raviola CA. Postoperative blood pressure changes associated with cervical block versus general anesthesia following carotid endarterectomy. Ann Vasc Surg. 1999;13:104–8.

52. Wallenborn J, Thieme V, Hertel-Gilch G, Grafe K, Richter O, Schaffranietz L. Effects of clonidine and superficial cervical plexus block on hemodynamic stability after carotid endarterectomy. J Cardiothorac Vasc Anesth. 2008;22(1):84–9.

Stellate Ganglion Blockade

33

Mehul Sekhadia, Kiran K. Chekka, and Honorio T. Benzon

Key Points

- Stellate ganglion blocks can be useful in the diagnosis and treatment of a variety of conditions; evidence is needed through randomized and controlled studies but is difficult to obtain.
- There are a variety of techniques available for both diagnostic blockade and neurolysis, but they should only be performed by those trained adequately to perform and monitor the outcomes of the blocks along with potential complications.
- The safety of stellate ganglion blocks and neurolysis is enhanced by the use of image guidance.
- The use of ultrasound is increasing and may increase efficacy, decrease complications, and reduce exposure to radiation.
- Regardless of technique, stellate ganglion block is a safe procedure when performed by properly trained physicians.

M. Sekhadia, DO (✉)
Feinberg School of Medicine, Northwestern University,
251 E. Huron, Feinberg Pavilion Suite 60611, Chicago,
IL 60611, USA
e-mail: msekhadi@nmff.org

K.K. Chekka, M.D.
Department of Anesthesiology, Northwestern Memorial Hospital,
675 N. St. Clair Street, Suite 20-100, Chicago, IL 60611, USA
e-mail: chekkamd@yahoo.com

H.T. Benzon, M.D.
Feinberg School of Medicine, Northwestern University,
251 E. Huron, Feinberg Pavilion Suite 60611, Chicago,
IL 60611, USA

Department of Anesthesiology, Feinberg School of Medicine,
Northwestern Memorial Hospital,
251 E. Huron, Feinberg Pavilion Suite 5-704, Chicago,
IL 60611, USA
e-mail: hbsenzon@nmff.org

Introduction

Physicians first began performing blocks of the sympathetic nervous system almost 100 years ago. In 1920, Jonnesco described the cervicothoracic block which Lawen [1] performed for the differential diagnosis of abdominal pain [1]. Kappis then used sympathetic blocks, including stellate blocks, for the treatment of several pain syndromes [2]. After World War I, a fair amount of research was done to elucidate the anatomy and function of the stellate ganglion, and soon after, the early techniques and indications for sympathetic blockade were developed. After World War II, these blocks became popular for the management of causalgia and reflex sympathetic dystrophies [2].

Sympathetic blocks can be used for diagnostic, prognostic, and therapeutic purposes. Diagnostic blocks are done to determine if acute or chronic pain is sympathetically mediated or independent. If a diagnostic block provides excellent relief of symptoms, then it is more likely that neurolysis or surgical sympathectomy would be beneficial [3]. Therapeutic blocks in series have been studied in the treatment of such syndromes such as complex regional pain syndromes [3, 4], phantom limb pain [1], postherpetic neuralgia [5, 6], ischemic pain [7], and cancer pain [8]. These blocks are usually an integral part of a comprehensive functional restoration program [4].

Once a block is performed, it is essential to verify that [1] the sympathetic chain was actually blocked and [2] that no other neural structures were blocked. The best practical model for monitoring blockade is by watching for a change in limb temperature without significant somatic sensory or motor blockade. While sympathetic blocks are performed for a plethora of reasons, there are only a few randomized, placebo-controlled, outcome studies to demonstrate their effectiveness [9]. Anecdotally, when the blocks provide pain relief, they can be profoundly effective in managing a patient's pain and facilitating participation in essential rehabilitation regimens. In this chapter, we intend to describe sympathetic anatomy and blockade technique, proper post-block monitoring, and the evidence which is there for sympathetic blockade.

Anatomy

There are three interconnected ganglia which make up the cervical sympathetic chain: the superior, middle, and inferior cervical ganglia. In 80 % of people, the lowest cervical ganglion fuses with the first thoracic ganglion and is commonly referred to as the stellate ganglion, so named because of the characteristic appearance [8, 10]. In the remaining 20 % of people, the first thoracic ganglion is named the stellate ganglion.

The cervical ganglia receive nerve fibers from two major contributors: (1) preganglionic fibers from the lateral gray column of the spinal cord and (2) myelinated preganglionic cell axons from the anterolateral horn of the spinal cord. These fibers originate in the upper thoracic segments, traverse the ventral rami, and then form the white rami communicantes, which enter into the thoracic ganglia and then traverse cephalad. The head and neck sympathetic innervations arise predominantly from T1 to T3, while the innervation of the upper extremity originates predominantly from T2 toT6. From these segments, the fibers climb cephalad through the sympathetic trunk into the cervicothoracic ganglion where they synapse. Then, the postganglionic fibers travel directly to the head and neck or to the brachial plexus to innervate the arm.

These postganglionic fibers control vasoconstrictor and sudomotor functions of the face and neck, secretory fibers to the salivary glands, dilator pupillae, and nonstriated muscle in the eyelid and orbitalis. As a consequence, blockade of these fibers results in ptosis, miosis, enophthalmos, and abolition of face and neck sweat response. Further, the stellate ganglion sends a gray ramus communicans to the seventh cervical, eighth cervical, and first thoracic nerves. There is also a cardiac branch and occasionally a vagal branch.

Most of the sympathetic innervation to the head and neck as well as the ipsilateral upper extremity can be blocked at the stellate ganglion. At this structure, preganglionic fibers synapse or traverse to a more cephalad ganglion and then send postganglionic fibers to the appropriate structures. Most preganglionic fibers which synapsed at a more caudad level still send their postganglionic fibers through the stellate ganglion. The first three intercostal nerves may also carry sympathetic innervation directly to the brachial plexus entirely bypassing the stellate ganglion. This anomalous pathway ("Kuntz's nerves") would not be blocked by a stellate ganglion blockade and maybe by an explanation for inadequate sympathetic blockade after an appropriately performed stellate block.

The cervical sympathetic chain lies just medial to the carotid space and is enclosed by the lateral aspect of the alar fascia which separates it from the retropharynx. Just posterior is the prevertebral musculature. This fascial plane is not entirely closed off from other tissue planes. Any medication deposited in this fascial plane may spread to the brachial plexus, spinal nerve roots, the prevertebral portion of the vertebral artery, and between the endothoracic fascia and the thoracic wall muscle at the T1–T2 level causing blockade of these structures and resultant side effects of stellate blockade. The stellate ganglion is consistently located anterior or just lateral to the longus colli muscle between the inferior margin of the seventh cervical transverse process and the first rib. At this level, the vertebral artery and vein are anterior (in the direct path of an anterior needle placement), and the C7 and T1 nerve roots are posterior to the ganglion.

By the C6 level, in over 90 % of patients, the vertebral artery is posterior to the sympathetic chain and shielded by bone. The variability in the size of the longus colli muscle can affect block success and complication rates and may explain ineffective neurolysis in a block responder [11].

Indications

Table 33.1 is a list of indications and contraindications for stellate ganglion block [1, 8]. This list includes diagnoses with variable amounts of research supporting their usage. Some indications are based on case reports or case series while others have legitimate outcome studies which are discussed later in this chapter.

Table 33.1 Indications and contraindications

CRPS I and II
Vascular insufficiency—Raynaud's, vasospasm, vascular disease
Accidental intra-arterial injection of drug
Postherpetic neuralgia and acute herpes zoster
Phantom pain
Frostbite
CRPS breast and postmastectomy pain
Quinine poisoning
Hyperhidrosis of upper extremity
Cardiac arrhythmias
Angina
Vascular headaches
Neuropathic pain syndromes including central pain
Cancer pain
Atypical facial pain and trigeminal neuralgia
Hot flashes
Contraindications
Coagulopathy (patients on warfarin or low-molecular-weight heparin, patients on aspirin or nonsteroidal anti-inflammatory agents are possible contraindications)
Contralateral pneumothorax (or contralateral phrenic palsy)
Systemic or local infection
Glaucoma
Bradycardia

Contradictions

See Table 33.1.

Techniques

There is huge range in stellate block success rates described in the literature (16–100 %) [12].

Seemingly, using some sort of guidance improves block success, but in practice, there continues to be debate on whether to use guidance and what sort of guidance should be used.

While CT guidance provides a very high success rate [13], there is the associated higher dose radiation and the typical inefficiencies and cost associated with CT which makes it less popular.

Ultrasound can be used to easily visualize superficial soft tissue structures including the stellate ganglion [14]. Also, the longus capitis muscle has been described as a possible landmark for cervical sympathetic block [15]. In this chapter, we describe the most commonly used surface landmark, ultrasound- and fluoroscopic-guided techniques. The techniques for CT-guided blocks are virtually identical to the fluoroscopic techniques.

Minimum requirements for stellate ganglion blocks:
- Informed consent
- IV access
- Standard resuscitative equipment
- ASA standard monitors
- Monitoring sympathetic blockade
- Fluoroscope (C-arm), ultrasound, or computed tomography
- 22- or 25-gauge needle, 2.5–3.5 in. long
- Local anesthetic—lidocaine versus bupivacaine
- Contrast—Omnipaque® or Isovue® (if using fluoroscopy)

Surface Landmark (Nonimage-Guided) Technique

The "blind" or non-guided techniques rely on the use of palpable surface landmarks to determine the site of injection. Typically, the patient is placed supine with slight neck extension using towels +/– a shoulder roll with the mouth open (an open mouth results in more relaxed neck musculature). The cricoid cartilage in the adult is a fairly accurate landmark to identify the C6 spinal level. Others have advocated using the skin crease caudad to the thyroid as a landmark to identify C6. Chassaignac's tubercle is identified with palpation at the C6 level. In most individuals, the tubercle is located approximately 3 cm cephalad to the sternoclavicular joint at the medial border of the sternocleidomastoid muscle. The carotid artery and trachea are gently retracted laterally. After intradermal local anesthetic injection with a 27-G needle, either 22- or 25-gauge Quincke or pencil-point needle is placed perpendicularly in an anterior-to-posterior fashion until the needle contacts bone at which point it is withdrawn 2 mm. After negative aspiration, 0.5–1 ml of 1 % lidocaine is injected slowly while the patient is awake and responsive to detect aberrant spread of the local anesthetic to surrounding structures. If negative, 5–8 ml of either 1 % lidocaine or 0.25 % bupivacaine is injected incrementally and frequent aspiration. The patient is then monitored for a minimum of 30 min to assess response to the blockade.

Fluoroscopic Technique

Positioning is unchanged from the blind procedure. The "C-arm" is then moved to achieve a posterior-anterior (PA) image. Then, using cephalad or caudad tilt, the end plates or C6 (or C7) are lined up. Either level can be utilized so long as the operator has thorough knowledge of the anatomy described in the previous section. The C7 level is preferred because of its closer proximity to the stellate ganglion, but the vertebral artery is uncovered at this level unlike at the C6 level where the vertebral artery travels posterior to Chassaignac's tubercle. To avoid the vertebral artery at C7, the needle should be placed more medial on the transverse process (see Fig. 33.1).

Local anesthetic is infiltrated with a 27-gauge needle intradermally at the site of injection as guided by the fluoroscope. Then, a 25-gauge by 1.5- or 2-in. needle is advanced coaxially to the anterior transverse process of the chosen level. Once contact is made, the needle is withdrawn 2 mm so that it is not in contact with periosteum and the stylet is removed. A lateral image can be taken to confirm that the needle is anterior to the vertebral body. A precontrast-flushed extension set is then connected to the needle, and after negative aspiration for blood, under live, real-time fluoroscopy or digital subtraction angiography, 1–5 ml of contrast is injected. The optimal spread of contrast should cover the C6–T2 levels to ensure blockade of the stellate ganglion (see Fig. 33.2). A test dose is then injected with 0.5–1 ml of 1 % lidocaine through the extension tubing (to minimize needle movement) assuring that the local anesthetic passes through the tubing. The patient is continuously assessed for possible intravascular or neuraxial spread which can result in seizure or high spinal.

If the test dose is negative, then approximately 5–10 ml of local anesthetic is injected incrementally. The greater the volume injected, the greater is the likelihood of spread to the recurrent laryngeal nerve, phrenic nerve, or brachial plexus. It is important to frequently aspirate during the injection and pause between boluses of injectate.

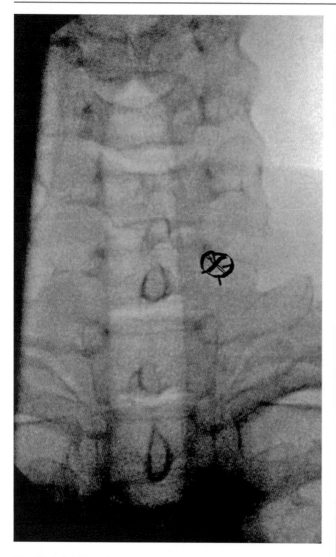

Fig. 33.1 Initial landmark (*x*) for the anterior approach to the stellate ganglion block

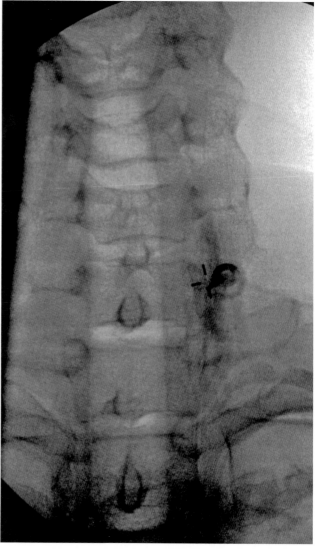

Fig. 33.2 Injection of contrast after needle placement demonstrating correct spread along the anterolateral borders of C5–T1

Other Fluoroscopic Approaches [16]

Patient preparation is unchanged with the patient placed in the supine position with established IV access. The head is then turned contralateral to the side to be blocked. The fluoroscope is used to identify the C5–C6 disk on AP view, and ipsilateral oblique rotation is added until the neural foramina are clearly demarcated. On this image, the target of the injection is the junction of the uncinate process and the vertebral body of C7. A 25-gauge needle is then passed coaxially with the fluoroscope beam until it reaches the target. As with all image-guided procedures, it is important to keep the needle coaxial and, in this case, avoid the needle going posterior into the foramina (direct entry into the thecal sac). Once contact with bone occurs, the stylet is removed and contrast is injected as described above in the previous section. The major reported advantage of this technique is

that only 3–5 ml of local anesthetic is needed to block the stellate ganglion as opposed to the other techniques described which use as much as 15–20 ml. Another advantage of the technique is that the needle is placed obliquely to allow for placement at C7 while avoiding the vertebral artery (which is anterior to the stellate ganglion) and the pleural dome in nonemphysematous patients (based on cadaver studies).

The authors outlined the following benefits [16]:
- Eliminating or pushing away vasculature and pressing on the potentially painful Chassaignac's tubercle
- Minimize the chance of intravascular injection
- Minimize esophageal perforation
- Minimize the chance of recurrent laryngeal nerve paralysis

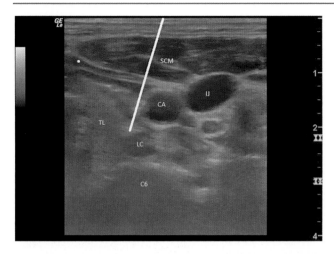

Fig. 33.3 Ultrasound-guided approach to stellate ganglion block done at C6 level. *TL* thyroid lobule, *LC* longus colli muscle, *CA* carotid artery, *IJ* internal jugular vein, *SCM* sternocleidomastoid muscle

- Reduce the volume of local anesthetic
- Easy to teach trainees

There is currently no prospective outcome data on this technique.

Ultrasound-Guided Approach

A newer ultrasound-guided technique for stellate ganglion blockade was first described by Kapral et al. (Fig. 33.3) [17]. Kapral et al. hypothesize a decrease in the incidence of retropharyngeal hematoma and increase the safety and efficacy of the block. Ultrasound allows direct visualization of the thyroid gland, vertebral artery, esophagus, pleura, nerve roots, longus colli muscle, and the correct fascial planes for nerve blockade along with real-time, direct visualization of local anesthetic spread [14, 18].

Positioning for the procedure is unchanged from the landmark-based technique. This block is considered an "expert" block by most ultrasonographers and should not be done by ultrasound beginners. A linear array, 3–12 MHz frequency probe (ideally with a small footprint) is placed transversely at the level of C6, just lateral to the trachea on the ipsilateral side. The carotid artery is easily visible with the use of ultrasound and can be a very good landmark. While some practitioners are performing exclusively ultrasound-guided blocks, many still use fluoroscopy to identify the C6 level, to verify what structures the needle is traversing, and to perform a live dye study. Sometimes, the ganglion itself can be visualized, but typically the goal is to use an in-plane approach and deposit medication in the fascial plane anterior to the longus colli muscle (which is almost always easily identified). Typically, small aliquots of 1–3 ml are injected under real-time visualization to verify a fill pattern in the appropriate fascial plane.

One validation study using the ultrasound approach showed that at the C6 level, the cervical sympathetic trunk lays entirely subfascially, and as a result, a subfascial injection via the lateral approach ensures reliable spread of solution to the stellate ganglion [14]. There are no randomized, prospective, outcome studies on using the ultrasound approach. One safety concern with ultrasound-guided injection is that there are no well-studied and validated contrast materials which can be used to insure that the injection is not intravascular. Still, one can use epinephrine to increase sensitivity, and others have reported a "wisping" in a visualized vessel when the injectate is intravascular.

Posterior Approach

Currently, the posterior approach is used principally when [1] a sympathectomy was not achieved using another technique or [2] when the block is being done as a diagnostic measure prior to percutaneous neurolysis (or rhizotomy) or surgical sympathectomy. Some advocate that this approach should be utilized for all upper extremity sympathectomies [19].

For this approach, the patient is in the prone position, and image guidance is an absolute necessity (usually fluoroscopy, but CT can be utilized). After IV placement and proper positioning, an AP image of T2 and T3 vertebrae is obtained. The C-arm is then rotated obliquely until the lateral margin of the transverse process is just overlapping the lateral margin of the vertebral body. Next, cephalocaudad tilt is used to square off the first rib. The target structure is the midpoint of the T2 or T3 vertebra. Pneumothorax is a significant concern which can be minimized by decreasing the degree of oblique angle. Practitioners often balance the concern for pneumothorax against the likelihood of a challenging or suboptimal needle placement as a result of decreased obliquity. As with anterior techniques, coaxial needle placement greatly reduces complications. Final needle position should be verified with a lateral image showing the needle at the midpoint of the vertebral body.

Next, 0.5–3 ml of contrast is injected under real-time imaging or digital subtraction angiography to observe for vascular uptake or extraneous spread. Local anesthetic of 5 ml is then injected in divided doses, and the patient is monitored for sympathetic blockade.

Comments

Variable injection volumes have been suggested from 5 to 20 ml [20]. Feigl et al. [20] cadaver study using the blind paratracheal approach at the C6 level showed that 5 ml of injectate almost always demonstrated spread over the C6–T2 levels without ventral or lateral spread. Injectate of 10–20 ml almost always spread to these spaces which in live humans can result in recurrent laryngeal nerve and phrenic nerve blockade. In another study, Hardy et al. [21] demonstrated that with 10 ml of local anesthetic injection, there is only a 10 % incidence of recurrent laryngeal nerve block, whereas with a 20 ml injection, the rate increases to 80 %. However, larger volumes may be needed to obtain complete blockade of T1 and T2 ganglia if injection is done at C6 compared to C7 [22].

Neurolysis

Percutaneous neurolysis can be simply performed using chemical (phenol or alcohol) neurolysis or radio-frequency (both pulsed and thermal) techniques. Radio-frequency techniques create small discrete lesions; chemical lesions are typically larger and less discrete. Both techniques have been utilized at the stellate ganglion. Usually if a diagnostic block consistently provides good but transient relief, neurolysis is a next potential therapeutic step. There are no randomized, placebo-controlled, prospective trials on the use of neurolytic agents for nonmalignant pain.

Chemical Neurolysis

Two to 3 ml of aqueous phenol (3–6 %) or alcohol (50–100 %) should be enough volume to neurolyse the ganglion without spread to adjacent structures [23]. Phenol is usually the agent of choice because of a decrease in incidence of neuritis post-procedure. Neurolysis can be performed using an anterior approach at C6 or C7 or using a posterior approach at T2 or T3 for upper extremity problems. Always inject a local anesthetic test before injecting the neurolytic to insure that no somatic sensory or motor nerves are destroyed.

Radio-Frequency Lesioning

Thermal radio-frequency (RF) lesioning produces discrete lesions whose size can be modulated with needle tip selection. Further, RF generators allow practitioners to perform nondestructive pulsed lesioning. Test dosing is not always necessary as stimulation can be used to verify that other neural structures are not at risk for neurolysis. Still local anesthetic is typically injected for patient comfort during lesioning.

RF lesioning is done at the C7 level because the probe must be in very close proximity to the structure being lesioned. Stimulation can be done while the patient is saying "EE" to see if there is any stimulation of the recurrent laryngeal nerve or phrenic nerve. A 22-gauge 50-mm cannula with a 5-mm active tip can be placed using an anterior approach with fluoroscopic guidance. Stimulation is performed at 2 Hz and up to 2.5 V (usual for motor stimulation) to assess prior to injection of local anesthetic and lesioning. The posterior approach at T2 and/or T3 will most likely avoid these two nerves [8, 24].

After placing the probes, the stylets are removed and sensory and motor testing is performed. Next, dense local anesthetic (i.e., 2 ml of 2 % lidocaine) is injected for thermal lesions. For pulsed lesions, the needle tip is withdrawn because the target should be in front of the needle, as opposed to parallel to the needle for thermal lesions. Sensory stimulation should be done (50 Hz) to determine the lowest threshold of stimulation, and motor stimulation should be done if doing a thermal lesion (2–5 Hz up to 3 V). Pulsed lesions are carried out at 42°, pulsed mode, 2×20 ms/s, 40–45 V (to titrate the temperature to 43°) for 120 s. With thermal lesioning, tip temperature is brought to 80 °C for 60–90 s [1, 8].

Complications

As with all interventional pain procedures, only those with proper training and experience should be performing these blocks. The potential complications for sympathetic blocks are real but if done properly, are rare. The risks with neurolysis are more severe (and potentially more permanent).

Stellate Ganglion Blockade and Neurolysis [8]

- Bleeding/hematoma
- Pneumothorax, hemothorax
- Vertebral artery injury or inadvertent injection
- Inadvertent injection into neuraxis
- Esophageal trauma
- Tracheal trauma
- Phrenic nerve injury
- Brachial plexus injury
- Recurrent laryngeal nerve injury
    - Neuritis—any nerve or plexus listed above
    - Postsympathectomy syndrome

Monitoring the Adequacy of Sympathetic Blockade

Stellate Block:
- Horner's syndrome (ptosis, miosis, enophthalmos, and anhidrosis)
- Guttman's sign (nasal stuffiness)
- Hyperemia of the tympanic membrane
- Warmth of face
- Increased temperature of the upper extremity by at least 1 °C

Successful stellate ganglion blockade results in Horner's syndrome (ptosis, miosis, and anhidrosis). Other signs include unilateral nasal stuffiness (Guttman's sign), hyperemia of the tympanic membrane, and warmth of the face.

The presence of Horner's syndrome signifies cephalic sympathetic blockade but does not verify upper extremity sympathetic blockade [25, 26]. If the block is used to treat the shoulder or upper limb, additional signs are needed to determine sympathetic blockade in the area. Complete block is reliably detected when a test of adrenergic fiber activity (thermography, plethysmography, laser Doppler flowmetry) is combined with a test of sympathetic cholinergic (sudomotor) fiber activity (sweat test, sympathogalvanic response).

Increase in skin temperature is the most practical and simple clinical sign of sympathetic blockade. Commonly, skin temperature is measured by using adhesive thermocouple probes that are placed distally on the extremity being monitored. For continuous skin temperature measurements, thermocouple devices are placed bilaterally. Infrared thermography can provide average sensitivity to skin temperature changes as minute as 0.1 °C. Another qualitative thermography technique is liquid crystal thermography, with reported sensitivity of about 0.8 °C. Different investigators considered different increases in skin temperature as signifying effective sympathetic blockade. After a stellate ganglion block, skin temperature increases of 1.5 °C [26], 3.8 °C [27], and 7.5 °C [13] have been considered as signifying successful sympathetic blockade. Hogan et al. [26] state that ipsilateral limb temperature should increase to a value greater than the contralateral temperature in the presence of successful sympathetic blockade. Stevens et al. found that a temperature increase that was 2 °C higher than the contralateral was attained with complete sympathectomy in most patients [28]. The magnitude of temperature increases after complete sympathetic blockade is largely dependent on the starting temperature [29]. With sympathectomy, skin temperature will nearly approximate core body temperature in the absence of peripheral vascular disease. Therefore, the upper limit of skin temperature in the fingers and toes is about 35–36 °C [30] in patients without significant organic peripheral vascular disease [29]. Patients whose baseline skin temperatures are low because of vasoconstriction (i.e., later stage CRPS patients) will attain a large temperature increase with complete sympathetic blockade. In a vasodilated patient (i.e., early stage CRPS), one cannot expect a large temperature increase.

Most other measures of sympathectomy are technically complex and usually infeasible in the typical clinical setting, but they are oftentimes used in research and academia. Laser Doppler flowmetry measures skin blood flow. A 50 % or greater increase in the skin blood flow is used to signify successful sympathetic block. Blood flow can also be accurately measured using plethysmographic methods such as venous-occlusion plethysmography. In this technique, a transducer is placed on the finger to measure the change of the finger volume over time. A tourniquet is inflated around the finger to a pressure which is greater than venous pressure but still allows arterial blood to enter the finger. The finger's rate of volume increase is measured using the volume transducer, and a plethysmographic trace is generated and then analyzed. First, a rapid increase is seen followed by a plateau phase which signifies that a sufficient amount of blood has entered the finger to equalize the venous pressure with tourniquet pressure. In the presence of sympathectomy, the upward slope is drastically increased due to a significant increase in the pulse wave. Kapural et al. found volume plethysmography better measured blood flow than skin surface temperature gradients than blood flow measurements by laser Doppler flowmetry [31].

Usually in a laboratory setting, the presence of complete sympathectomy can be verified by checking for abolition of sweat response and abolition of the sympathogalvanic response (SGR) [26, 28–35]. Today, ninhydrin and cobalt blue tests are most commonly used to verify abolition of sweating response. Benzon et al. have modified the preparation of the two sweat tests [34]. For the cobalt blue filter paper, 0.5 M $CoCl_2$ in 70 % ethanol is used, while 2 % ninhydrin in 70 % ethanol with 1 ml of 4 M acetate buffer (pH 5.5) per 100-ml solution is utilized for the ninhydrin filter paper. The solutions (cobalt blue or ninhydrin) are applied evenly on a Whatman no. 1 filter paper at 2 ml/100 cm^2. The papers are dried at room temperature and stored in a desiccator. Once setup is complete, cobalt blue paper or ninhydrin filter paper is clear taped to dry skin. If the patient still has the ability to sweat, cobalt blue paper will turn pink, and ninhydrin filter paper will have purple dots appear. The ability to sweat suggests that sympathectomy to the area tests was not complete.

Sympathogalvanic responses can be measured using the electrocardiogram, and the setup is simple. The right arm (RA) and left arm (LA) leads are placed on the limb being tested on the dorsum and palm (or sole). The other leads are placed contralaterally. Then, the patient is exposed to a stimulus such as deep breath, startling noise, or a pinprick. In healthy controls, either a monophasic up or down deflection or a biphasic response is seen. With partial sympathectomy, amplitude is diminished. With complete sympathectomy, a flat line trace is seen.

Benzon showed that sweat testing is more reliable than the SGR in predicting complete sympathetic blockade [34], but both had a sensitivity of 90 %. The specificity of the SGR was 56 % compared to 100 % for the sweat tests, resulting in stated accuracies of 74 and 95 %, respectively [34]. Whether or not a complete sympathectomy is achieved is really only clinically relevant when optimal (or complete) analgesia is not attained [35]. For example, patients can have full resolution of symptoms even with a partial sympathetic blockade. But if the patient has partial relief of symptoms, then the residual pain may be due to a somatic or central in etiology, or the remaining symptoms could be sympathetically mediated if only a partial sympathectomy was achieved [35].

Partial relief of symptoms occurs after the block due to a partial sympathectomy may be due to technique issues or to aberrant pathways (i.e., Kuntz's nerves) which were not blocked.

Studies

In this section, we present the data that is available for the efficacy of stellate ganglion blocks and rhizotomy.

In 2007, Day [36] reviewed 11 articles consisting of 4 case reports, 5 case series, 1 retrospective review [37], and 1 double-blind, placebo-controlled study. Using Guyatt's criteria, Day concluded that most evidence for stellate blocks was either 1B or 1C grade, including the randomized and blinded trial which had a very small sample size. There is one prospective comparison of RF ablation at T2 and T3 versus phenol/RF at T2 for severe Raynaud's phenomenon [38]. Fifty patients were randomized into the two groups and ablated, but no diagnostic blocks were done. Patients were followed for 3 months, and statistically significant improvement in visual analog pain scores, quality of life, and limb temperature were found in both arms. While the study was not placebo-controlled, it was concluded that both techniques showed efficacy in the treatment of Raynaud's disease [38].

Conclusions

Stellate ganglion block is an important tool in the arsenal of treating sympathetically mediated pain syndromes. The careful attention to patient selection, anatomical landmarks, and potential complications can lead to the successful use of this procedure.

References

1. Hansen HC, Trescot AM, Manchikanti L. Stellate ganglion block. In: Manchikanti L, Singh V, editors. Interventional techniques in chronic non-spinal pain. Paducah: ASIPP Publishing; 2009. p. 115–40.
2. Datta S, Pai UT, Manchikanti L. Lumbar sympathetic blocks. In: Manchikanti L, Singh V, editors. Interventional techniques in chronic non-spinal pain. Paducah: ASIPP Publishing; 2009. p. 141–67.
3. Stanton-Hicks M, Baron R, Boas R, et al. Complex regional pain syndromes: guidelines for therapy. Clin J Pain. 1998;14:155–66.
4. Stanton-Hicks M, Janig W, Hassenbusch S, et al. Reflex sympathetic dystrophy: changing concepts and taxonomy. Pain. 1995;63: 127–33.
5. Hashizume K. Herpes zoster and postherpetic neuralgia. Jpn J Clin Med. 2001;59:1738–42.
6. Peterson RC, Patel L, Cubert K, et al. Serial stellate ganglion blocks for intractable postherpetic itching in a pediatric patient: a case report. Pain Physician. 2009;12:629–32.
7. Cross F, Cotton L. Chemical lumbar sympathectomy for ischemic rest pain. A randomized, prospective controlled clinical trial. Am J Surg. 1985;150:341–5.
8. Elias M. Cervical sympathetic and stellate ganglion blocks. Pain Physician. 2000;3(3):294–304.
9. Cepeda MS, Carr DB, Lau J. Local anesthetic sympathetic blockade for complex regional pain syndrome. Cochrane Database Syst Rev. 2005;19:CD004598.
10. Marples IL, Atkin RE. Stellate ganglion block. Pain Rev. 2001;8:3–11.
11. Ates Y, Asik I, Ozgencil E. Evaluation of the longus colli muscle in relation to the stellate ganglion block. Reg Anesth Pain Med. 2009;34(3):219–23.
12. Schurmann M, Gradl G, Wizgal I, et al. Clinical and physiologic evaluation of stellate ganglion blockade for complex regional pain syndrome type I. Clin J Pain. 2001;17:94–100.
13. Erickson SJ, Hogan QH. CT-guided injection of the stellate ganglion: description of technique and efficacy of sympathetic blockade. Radiology. 1993;188:707–9.
14. Gofeld M, Bhatia A, Abbas S, et al. Development and validation of a new technique for ultrasound-guided stellate ganglion block. Reg Anesth Pain Med. 2009;34(5):475–9.
15. Usui Y, Kobayashi T, Kakinuma H. An anatomical basis for blocking of the deep cervical plexus and cervical sympathetic tract using an ultrasound-guided imaging technique. Anesth Analg. 2010;110:964–8.
16. Abdi S, Zhou Y, Patel N, et al. A new and easy technique to block the stellate ganglion. Pain Physician. 2004;7:327–31.
17. Kapral S, Krafft P, Gosch M, et al. Ultrasound imaging for stellate ganglion block: direct visualization of puncture site and local anesthetic spread. Reg Anesth. 1995;20:323–8.
18. Narouze S, Vydyanathan A, Patel N. Ultrasound-guided stellate ganglion block successfully prevented esophageal puncture. Pain Physician. 2007;10:747–52.
19. Wilkinson H. Neurosurgical procedures of the sympathetic nervous system. Pain Clin. 1995;1:43–50.
20. Feigl GC, Rosmarin W, Stelzl A, et al. Comparison of different injectate volumes for stellate ganglion block: an anatomic and radiologic study. Reg Anesth Pain Med. 2007;32(3):203–8.
21. Hardy PAJ, Wells JCD. Extent of sympathetic blockade after stellate ganglion block with bupivacaine. Pain. 1989;36:193–6.
22. Matsumoto S. Thermographic assessments of the sympathetic blockade by stellate ganglion block (1) comparison between C7-SGB and C6 SGB in 40 patients. Masui. 1991;40(4):562–9.
23. Racz G, editor. Techniques of neurolysis. Boston: Kluwer Academic Publications; 1989. p. 99–124.
24. Guerts JW, Stolker RJ. Percutaneous radiofrequency of the stellate ganglion in the treatment of pain in upper extremity reflex sympathetic dystrophy. Pain Clin. 1993;6:17–25.
25. Boas RA. Sympathetic blocks in clinical practice. In: Stanton-Hicks M, editor. International anesthesia clinics, regional anesthesia: advances in selected topics. 16th ed. Boston: Little Brown; 1978. p. 4.
26. Hogan QH, Taylor ML, Goldstein M, et al. Success rates in producing sympathetic blockade by paratracheal injection. Clin J Pain. 1994;10:139.
27. Carron H, Litwiller R. Stellate ganglion block. Anesth Analg. 1975;54:567.
28. Stevens RA, Stotz A, Kao TC, et al. The relative increase in skin temperature after stellate ganglion block is predictive of a complete sympathectomy of the hand. Reg Anesth Pain Med. 1998;23: 266–70.
29. Benzon HT, Avram MJ. Temperature increases after complete sympathetic blockade. Reg Anesth. 1986;11:27.

30. Coller FA, Maddock WG. The differentiation of spastic from organic vascular occlusion by the skin temperature response to high environmental temperature. Ann Surg. 1932;96:719.

31. Kapural L, Mekhail N. Assessment of sympathetic blocks. Tech Reg Anesth Pain Manag. 2001;5:82–7.

32. Malmqvist EL, Bengstsson M, Sorensen J. Efficacy of stellate ganglion block: a clinical study with bupivacaine. Reg Anesth. 1992;17:340.

33. Dhuner KG, Edshage S, Wihelm A. Ninhydrin test – an objective method for testing local anaesthetic drugs. Acta Anaesthesiol Scand. 1960;4:189.

34. Benzon HT, Cheng SC, Avram MJ, et al. Sign of complete sympathetic blockade: sweat test or sympathogalvanic response? Anesth Analg. 1985;64:415.

35. Benzon HT. Importance of documenting complete sympathetic denervation after sympathectomy. Anesth Analg. 1992;74:599.

36. Day M. Sympathetic blocks: the evidence. Pain Pract. 2008;8:98–109.

37. Forouzanfar T, van Kleef M, Weber WE. Radiofrequency lesions of the stellate ganglion in chronic pain syndromes: retrospective analysis of clinical efficacy in 86 patients. Clin J Pain. 2000;16:164–8.

38. Gabrhelik T, Michalek P, Adamus M, et al. Percutaneous upper thoracic radiofrequency sympathectomy in raynaud phenomenon: a comparison of T2/T3 procedure versus T2 lesion with phenol application. Reg Anesth Pain Med. 2009;34(5):425–9.

Epidural (Cervical, Thoracic, Lumbar, Caudal) Block/Injections

Nirmala R. Abraham, Ignacio Badiola, and Thuong D. Vo

Key Points
- Epidural steroid injections are relatively safe.
- Strict aseptic technique needs to be used.
- Fluoroscopic guidance is recommended.

Introduction

One of the first descriptions of access to the lumbar epidural space was described by Pages in 1921 [1]. Anesthesia through a caudal route had been reported much earlier, but his was the first to describe a method for accessing the lumbar epidural space. Since then, various epidural injection techniques have been developed, and there have been dramatic increases in their use, not only for acute and labor pain, but for chronic pain as well. The loss of resistance technique was described [2] as the "hanging drop" technique [3]. Soon after corticosteroids were introduced in the mid-twentieth century, physicians started using them in the epidural space.

The cervical, thoracic, and lumbar epidural spaces can be accessed using multiple approaches including interlaminar, transforaminal, and caudal approaches. All have the same purpose, which is to deliver higher concentrations of corticosteroid directly in the area of an inflamed nerve root. This is an alternative to the less targeted oral route, which leads to increased systemic side effects. All areas of the epidural space can be accessed including the cervical, thoracic, and lumbar regions.

N.R. Abraham, M.D. (✉)
Medical Director, Sycamore Pain Management Center,
4000 Miamisburg-Centerville Road, Suite 435,
Miamisburg, OH, USA
e-mail: nirmala.abraham@khnetwork.org

I. Badiola, M.D.
Capitol Spine and Pain Centers, Fairfax, VA, USA

T.D. Vo, M.D.
Southern California Spine & Pain Institute,
Westminster, CA, USA

Scientific Foundation

Epidural injections are believed to be effective due to targeted delivery of local anesthetic and/or corticosteroids to the space where spinal nerve roots travel on their way from the spinal cord to the body.

Corticosteroid molecules are highly protein-bound in plasma and enter the cell membrane by active transport after binding to surface proteins. Once inside the cell, they combine with glucocorticoid receptors, and the combined complex is taken into the nucleus by active transport. They upregulate production of anti-inflammatory proteins and repress the expression of pro-inflammatory proteins. Specifically, the enzyme phospholipase A2 which is involved in the formation of arachidonic acid is inhibited. Arachidonic acid is essential for the formation of inflammatory mediators. Glucocorticoids also suppress the expression of cyclooxygenase (COX-1 and COX-2), which adds to the anti-inflammatory effect. Overuse of corticosteroids may lead to many adverse effects including Cushing's syndrome, avascular necrosis, peptic ulcers, cataracts, immunosuppression, hyperglycemic syndromes and osteoporosis.

Anatomy of the Epidural Space

The epidural space starts at the point where the periosteal layer of the foramen magnum comes together with the dura. The inferior boundary is at the sacrococcygeal membrane, the anterior boundary is the posterior longitudinal ligament, the posterior boundary is the ligamentum flavum, and the lateral boundaries are the pedicles and the intervertebral foramina. The space contains fat, lymphatics, and venous plexus. The ligamentum flavum is thin in the cervical region and thickens as you move caudal [4]. In the cervical region, the distance between the ligamentum flavum and the dura is 1.5–2 mm at C7 (due to cervical enlargement) as opposed to the lumbar region where at L2, it is 5–6 mm.

Table 34.1 Common indications for cervical epidural injections

Cervical radiculopathy
Cervical degenerative disk disease
Cervical disk herniation
Cervical spinal stenosis
Cervical postlaminectomy (failed neck) surgery syndrome
Cervical vertebral compression fractures
Postherpetic neuralgia/herpes zoster
Complex regional pain syndrome (I and II)
Peripheral neuropathy (diabetic, chemotherapy induced, etc.)
Phantom limb pain
Cancer-related pain

Cervical Epidural Injections

There are two approaches to access the cervical epidural space: translaminar and transforaminal. There are no studies that have shown that one is better than the other; however, complications associated with each are significantly different [5]. A systematic review published in Pain Physician in 2009 looked at the efficacy of translaminar cervical epidural injections and concluded that they provide a significant effect on cervical radicular pain [6]. There are no major studies looking at the efficacy of transforaminal cervical epidural steroid injections.

Indications

This procedure has multiple indications for head, neck, shoulder, and upper extremity pain. Table 34.1 shows these indications.

Contraindications

Absolute: unwilling patient, localized infection over procedure area, current anticoagulant use (see current america society of regional anesthesia (ASRA) and pain medicine guidelines on anticoagulants), increased intracranial pressure (ICP), bleeding diathesis, and patient that cannot remain still during the procedure.

Relative: allergy to medications that will be injected (contrast, local anesthetic, steroid) pregnancy, immunosuppression, systemic infection, and anatomic changes that would prevent a safe procedure (congenital or surgical).

Cervical Epidural Transforaminal Epidural Injection Technique

Because of the risks associated with this procedure, only physicians who have training and experience in using fluoroscopy as well as precise injection techniques should perform this procedure. All patients should be fully monitored, and equipment to handle airway, local anesthetic toxicity, and cardiovascular emergencies should be readily available.

Although physicians may have different techniques, the primary aspects of all must include proper positioning of the patient in order to optimize visualization of the anatomy of the cervical spine at the target level(s). After discussing risks and benefits, answering questions, and obtaining written informed consent, an intravenous line is placed (for sedation or for emergency access). The patient is taken into the procedure suite and can be placed in the supine, oblique, or lateral position depending on physician preference. The area of the neck is prepped and draped in a sterile manner. The fluoroscopy beam is then adjusted to visualize the intervertebral foramen at its maximum diameter, usually an anterior oblique view. The anterior surface of the superior articular process of the inferior vertebrae (posterior aspect of foramen) is identified, and the entry point is marked. The skin and subcutaneous tissues are anesthetized with 1 % lidocaine. A 25-gauge needle is then directed toward the anterior portion of the superior articular process. It should always be directed toward this bony landmark, as going directly toward the foramen could result in a needle being placed too deep and into the spinal cord. Once the superior articular process is contacted, the depth of the needle should be noted. Repositioning of the needle should never exceed this noted depth by more than a few millimeters. The needle is then carefully adjusted so that it passes into the intervertebral foramen. The needle should always remain slightly anterior to the superior articular process. It should never be in the anterior portion of the intervertebral foramen as this may risk injection into the vertebral artery.

Once the needle is in the correct position, the fluoroscope is repositioned for a true anteroposterior (AP) view. This will allow the physician to see the depth of the needle. The correct depth is when the tip of the needle lies opposite the sagittal midline of the silhouettes of the articular pillars. If the needle contacts the existing nerve root, the patient will feel radicular pain. At this point, the needle should be slightly withdrawn and the procedure halted until the sensation disappears. If the sensation does disappear, the needle can be redirected back to its intended position, but avoiding the exact spot that caused the radicular pain. Fluoroscopy should be used to check in an oblique direction as well as an AP view to confirm needle position and depth. Only after this is done should anything be injected.

After negative aspiration is confirmed, less than 1 ml of contrast solution is injected under live fluoroscopy. It should enter the intervertebral foramen and outline the spinal nerve. It is of utmost importance to be sure there is no intra-arterial injection of contrast. Although this location of needle placement usually will not contain a radicular or a vertebral artery, these arteries can be atypically located. In case of an intra-arterial injection, the contrast will move and disappear during live fluoroscopy. If this is the case, one can redirect the needle until contrast is not seen entering an artery. However, it may be more prudent, given the severity of possible intra-articular injection through the punctured site, to abort the procedure. If contrast injection leads to rapid dilution of the contrast material, it may imply that there has been subarachnoid needle placement. In this case, abort the procedure and give enough time for the puncture to heal as injection even into another location may lead to entrance of medication into the subarachnoid space through the puncture hole created.

Once it has been confirmed by AP and oblique views that there has been correct needle placement, contrast injection has been negative for intra-arterial and subarachnoid injection, the contrast appropriately outlines the spinal nerve, and injection of contrast is negative for pain or paresthesia, the local anesthetic and steroid can be given. How much steroid depends on whether the pain is monoradicular or multiradicular. If monoradicular, betamethasone (3–6 mg), triamcinolone (20–40 mg), or dexamethasone (7.5–10 mg) can be used. If multiradicular, betamethasone (12 mg), triamcinolone (80 mg), or dexamethasone (15 mg) can be used.

Once the medication has been injected, the needle is removed with a saline or local anesthetic flush to clear the needle and track of steroid. The area that was prepped should be cleansed and a bandage placed over site of needle insertion. The patient should then be taken to a recovery area where they should be monitored for complications resulting from conscious sedation as well as complications from the procedure itself.

Cervical Translaminar Epidural Injection Technique

This procedure can be performed by either a loss of resistance technique or a hanging drop technique. One technique has not been shown to be better than the other; thus, the choice of technique is based on physician preference.

Loss of Resistance Technique

After discussing risks and benefits, answering questions, and obtaining written informed consent, an intravenous line is placed (for sedation or for emergency access). The cervical interlaminar technique can be performed in either a sitting, lateral, or prone position. Each position has its own advantages and disadvantages. Since most pain practitioners use fluoroscopy to perform cervical epidural injections, the prone or lateral position is utilized. The cervical spine should be flexed to maximize the opening of the intervertebral spaces.

Once the patient is appropriately positioned, the neck is prepped and draped in a sterile manner, and AP fluoroscopy is used to identify the interspace that will be entered. A 17- or 18-gauge Tuohy needle (3.5 in.) is suitable for most patients. The lamina of the inferior vertebra (i.e., the lamina of T1 if performing a C7–T1 injection) is noted on AP fluoroscopy. The skin and subcutaneous tissues overlying the area are then anesthetized with 1 % lidocaine. The epidural needle is then slowly advanced under intermittent fluoroscopy until contact is made with the lamina. The depth of the needle should be noted. Once the lamina has been contacted, the stylet is removed and a lubricated 5-ml glass syringe is connected to the needle. The syringe can be filled with air, sterile saline, or both. The needle is then walked off the lamina and into the epidural space. This should be performed using a two-handed technique with the hand holding the needle stabilized against the patient's neck to protect against needle movement if the patient moves. The syringe is slowly advanced while always maintaining continuous pressure against the plunger. Once the bevel passes into the epidural space, there is a sudden loss of resistance. The syringe is then removed from the needle, and 1 ml of contrast is injected. Epidural spread of the contrast should be noted. If subarachnoid spread (dilution) is noted, the procedure should be aborted as the puncture site may act as a gateway for local anesthetic and steroid to enter the subarachnoid space even if the injection is attempted in another intervertebral space.

Once needle location in the epidural space is confirmed, negative aspiration for blood and cerebrospinal fluid (CSF) must be confirmed; then, the medication can be injected. The needle is then withdrawn with a local anesthetic or saline flush to remove steroid from the needle and injection track.

The spread of medication in the epidural space is dependent on volume of injectate, dilation of the veins, anatomic differences in the epidural space, and age and height [7]. A number of local anesthetics can be used including lidocaine and bupivacaine. Generally, about 7 ml is enough volume to adequately cover the nerve roots with local anesthetic and steroid [8].

Hanging Drop Technique

The hanging drop technique is an alternative to the loss of resistance technique to signify entrance into the epidural space. The technique is similar to the loss of resistance technique initially as the Tuohy needle is advanced until lamina is contacted. At this point, instead of attaching a glass/plastic loss of resistance syringe, the needle is filled with saline until a bubble of fluid is visible at the hub. The needle is slowly advanced, and once the needle enters and passes through the ligamentum flavum, the drop of fluid is drawn in. This is thought to be due to the pressure in the epidural space being lower than atmospheric pressure. A lateral fluoroscopic view can be used to confirm proper positioning of the needle tip in the epidural space. The remainder of the procedure is similar to that described for a loss of resistance technique.

As an alternative to cervical transforaminal injections, a catheter can be used through the translaminar approach and directed to the nerve root as it comes off of the spinal cord. A smaller amount of medication can then be used. There is a much lower risk of injection into a vertebral artery or into a radicular artery while still accomplishing a selective nerve root block. No studies have been published comparing the efficacy of this approach versus a transforaminal approach.

Complications

Drug Related

Corticosteroids: mostly due to systemic absorption and are short-lived. It includes rash, nausea, pruritis, and hyperglycemia. More severe reactions include a Cushingoid response and adrenocortical failure.

Local anesthetics: rash, nausea, and accidental intrathecal injection with resultant spinal anesthesia. Systemic absorption can lead to seizures and refractory cardiac arrhythmias.

Procedure Related

Complications can be associated with both routes of access. These include postdural puncture headaches, infection, development of epidural hematoma (which could lead to quadriplegia), subarachnoid injection leading to a complete spinal block, and direct cervical spinal cord trauma. However, the incidences of these complications are lower in interlaminar injections if the procedure is carried out in a cooperative patient using fluoroscopy and contrast medium [9]. Multiple case reports of serious complications have been reported after cervical transforaminal injections, ranging from paraplegia to death. This is thought to be due to accidental injection of particulate steroid into a cervical radicular artery. This may lead to spinal cord infarction followed by impairment. As stated previously, no head-to-head comparisons have been done between interlaminar and transforaminal cervical epidural steroid injections. Given the positive results seen with the interlaminar approach and the serious complications associated with the transforaminal approach, it may be prudent to consider the former rather than the latter.

Thoracic Epidural Injections

This procedure is becoming more common in the chronic pain management arena. Similar to the cervical epidural procedure, the spinal cord can be injured during this procedure. It must also be remembered that the artery of Adamkiewicz can be located anywhere in the lower thoracic levels.

Indications

There are multiple uses for thoracic epidurals. One of the most common chronic pain uses is for treatment of postherpetic neuralgia. The thoracic dermatomes are the most common location for occurrence of postherpetic neuralgia. It has been shown that performing an epidural with local anesthetic during an acute herpes zoster outbreak may actually prevent PHN from developing [10].

Pain from metastatic disease to the thoracic spine can be treated with epidural analgesia. It is rare for there to be a disk herniation in the thoracic spinal cord, but this too will benefit from injection of local anesthetic and steroid into the epidural space. Other less common indications include pain from angina, pancreatic disease, or incisional neuralgia after thoracotomy or breast surgery.

Contraindications

Absolute: unwilling patient, localized infection over procedure area, current anticoagulant use, bleeding diathesis, increased ICP, and patient that cannot remain still during the procedure.

Relative: allergy to medications that will be injected (contrast, local anesthetic, steroid), pregnancy, immunosuppression, systemic infection, and anatomic changes that would prevent a safe procedure (congenital or surgical).

Thoracic Translaminar Epidural Injection Technique

After discussing the risks and benefits, answering questions, and obtaining written informed consent, the patient is brought into the procedure room and placed in a prone position. The skin overlying the thoracic region is then prepped and draped in a sterile manner.

The angulation of the thoracic spinous process differs at the cephalad and caudal portions of the thoracic levels. They are long and triangular when seen in a transverse section. They are directed obliquely downward and overlap each other between T5 and T8 [11]. This would make a midline approach to the epidural space very difficult if not unfeasible. The epidural space measures between 3 and 5 mm in width.

AP fluoroscopy can be used to identify the entry level. If the space is above T5 or below T8, a midline or paramedian approach can be used. Between T5 and T8, a paramedian approach must be used due to caudal angulation of the spinous process. The midline approach is performed in the same manner as lumbar level injections (see lumbar procedure in detail). It must be kept in mind that direct injury to the spinal cord is a risk at the thoracic and upper lumbar levels, unlike the lower lumbar levels.

For a paramedian approach, first, anesthetize the skin and subcutaneous tissues with 1 % lidocaine. Starting at 2 cm lateral to the spinous process, advance a 17- or 18-gauge Tuohy needle until contact is made with the lamina. Then, advance the needle 45° to the skin in a cephalad direction and a 30° angle to the midline. This is done with intermittent fluoroscopy to be sure the needle is in a correct path. A loss of resistance syringe is then attached. The needle is then angled cephalad, and for a right-handed practitioner, the left index finger and thumb is placed on the hub and rested on the patient's back. This will help stabilize the needle against inadvertent patient movement.

The loss of resistance technique can be done with continuous pressure on the syringe until there is loss of resistance. Another technique is to make small millimeter advances followed by tapping of the syringe plunger to confirm loss of resistance and entry into the epidural space. Once there is loss of resistance, lateral fluoroscopy can be utilized to confirm location of the needle tip in the epidural space. A false loss of resistance can occur in the subcutaneous tissue, though not commonly in the thoracic levels. It is also possible that a loss of resistance may not occur until the needle is in the subdural or subarachnoid space. Injection of contrast in the subdural space will give a "shifting lake" appearance, and injection in the subarachnoid space will lead to a myelographic pattern of contrast spread. Careful needle control as well as fluoroscopic images in the lateral view will minimize inaccurate needle placement.

Complications

Drug Related

Corticosteroids: mostly due to systemic absorption and are short-lived. It includes rash, nausea, pruritis, and hyperglycemia. More severe reactions include a Cushingoid response and adrenocortical failure.

Local anesthetics: rash, nausea, and accidental intrathecal injection with resultant spinal anesthesia. Systemic absorption can lead to seizures and refractory cardiac arrhythmias.

Procedure Related

Procedural complications include postdural puncture headache (from accidental dural puncture and CSF leak), vasovagal reaction, subdural infiltration, neural injury, and permanent injury to the spinal cord (if in the upper lumbar levels). Permanent spinal cord injury can be secondary to either direct needle trauma or disruption of blood supply to the spinal cord. The artery of Adamkiewicz is a major artery that supplies the lumbar region of the spinal cord. It enters the spinal canal in 80 % of people between T8 and L3 on the left [12]. Injury can be avoided by making sure the needle is not too lateral in the neural foramen on AP fluoroscopy [12].

Table 34.2 Common indications for lumbar epidural injections

Lumbar radiculopathy
Lumbar degenerative disk disease
Lumbar disk herniation
Lumbar spinal stenosis
Lumbar postlaminectomy (failed back) surgery syndrome
Lumbar vertebral compression fractures
Postherpetic neuralgia/herpes zoster
Complex regional pain syndrome (I and II)
Peripheral neuropathy (diabetic, chemotherapy induced, etc.)
Phantom limb pain
Cancer-related pain

Lumbar Epidural Injections

Given the high prevalence of back pain and radiculopathy, placing corticosteroid and local anesthetic into the lumbar epidural space is one of the most common procedures performed for chronic pain management. There are many structures in the lumbar region that can lead to pain, including the skin, muscle, fascia, facet joints, intervertebral disk, and the dura of the nerve root. Radicular pain may not always be secondary to nerve root compression by an intervertebral disk (i.e., many patients will have disk herniation by MRI, but not all will have radicular symptoms). Radicular pain can be due to partial axon damage, formation of a neuroma, intraneural edema, and impaired microcirculation [13].

A systematic review by Parr et al. [14] found positive correlations (Level II-2) between short-term pain relief of disk herniation or radiculitis with epidural corticosteroids. Evidence is lacking for long-term relief as well as short- and long-term relief of pain due to spinal stenosis and discogenic pain without radiculitis. This review was performed using studies that employed a blind injection technique (without fluoroscopy), and thus, may have limitations (i.e., incorrect subcutaneous placement of medication leading to false negatives).

Indications

There are many indications for lumbar epidural nerve block, with the most common being lumbar radiculopathy. Table 34.2 shows the more common indications.

Contraindications

Absolute: unwilling patient, localized infection over procedure area, current anticoagulant use, bleeding diathesis, increased ICP and patient that cannot remain still during the procedure.

Relative: allergy to medications that will be injected (contrast, local anesthetic, steroid), pregnancy, immunosuppression, systemic infection, and anatomical changes that would prevent a safe procedure (congenital or surgical).

Lumbar Transforaminal Epidural Injection Technique

After discussing the risks and benefits and obtaining written informed consent, the patient is taken to the fluoroscopy suite and placed in a prone position. The area of the lumbar spine is then prepped and draped in a sterile manner. AP fluoroscopy is used to identify the level to be injected. An oblique view is then obtained toward the side that will be injected. This is done until the superior articular process of the inferior level is in line with the 6 o'clock position of the pedicle of the superior level. Once the correct view has been obtained, the entry point is marked and the skin and subcutaneous tissues overlying the area are anesthetized with 1 % lidocaine. Using intermittent fluoroscopy, the needle is guided to the target point in small increments. The area in which it is appropriate to place the needle has the following boundaries on AP view: the upper border is a line that runs under the pedicle at the 6 o'clock position, the lateral boundary is a sagittal line that runs caudad from the lateral aspect of the pedicle to the segmental nerve, and the hypotenuse of this triangle connects the two lines and runs parallel to the lateral border of the nerve [15]. It is in this area where there is the least chance of hitting a segmental nerve or a vascular structure. Once the caudal aspect of the pedicle at the 6 o'clock position is encountered, the needle tip is turned caudad until it slips off the pedicle and into the neural foramen. Using a needle with the tip bent away from the bevel can make this step of the procedure easier to accomplish. Lateral fluoroscopy is then used to confirm that the needle is in the neural foramen. Occasionally, if the needle is placed too deep, the patient may experience a paresthesia due to accidental touching of the segmental nerve. The needle should be withdrawn and the paresthesia allowed to resolve. If the paresthesia does not resolve, the patient may be unable to tolerate the remainder of the procedure.

Once the needle is in the correct location, both AP and lateral fluoroscopy should be used to verify its position prior to injection. The AP view should show the needle just inferior to the 6 o'clock position of the superior level's pedicle. Lateral fluoroscopy should show the needle tip in the foramen below the pedicle and in the middle portion of the foramen. Once the needle position is confirmed and negative aspiration for blood or CSF has been observed, 1 ml of contrast is injected during live fluoroscopy in an AP view. The contrast should be seen outlining the nerve root and flowing into the epidural space. The medication can now be injected. The needle is removed with a local anesthetic or saline flush to clear the needle and injection track of steroid. The area that was prepped should be cleansed and a bandage placed over site of needle insertion. The patient should then be taken to a recovery area where they should be monitored for complications resulting from conscious sedation as well as complications from the procedure itself.

Lumbar Translaminar Epidural Injection Technique

After discussing the risks and benefits and obtaining written informed consent, the patient is taken to the fluoroscopy suite and placed in a prone position. A pillow or cushion can be placed under the abdomen to decrease lumbar lordosis and open up the intervertebral space. The area of the lumbar spine is then prepped and draped in a sterile manner. AP fluoroscopy is used to locate the target entry level. Cranial/caudal tilting can be done until the interspace is optimally visualized.

Once the site is chosen and the area is anesthetized, the needle is placed toward the side that the patient has pain (i.e., a patient with left lower extremity radiculopathy over the L4 dermatome should have the needle placed at the left-hand portion of the L4–L5 interspace). A 17- or 18-gauge Tuohy needle is directed under fluoroscopic guidance until the inferior lamina of the entry level is contacted. A loss of resistance syringe is then attached. The needle is then angled cephalad, and a two-handed technique is used to stabilize the needle and advance it slowly toward the epidural space.

The loss of resistance technique can be done with continuous pressure on the syringe until there is loss of resistance. Another technique is to make small millimeter advances followed by tapping of the syringe plunger to confirm loss of resistance and entry into the epidural space. Once there is loss of resistance, lateral fluoroscopy can be utilized to confirm location of the needle tip in the epidural space. A false loss of resistance can occur in the subcutaneous tissue. It is also possible that a loss of resistance may not occur until the needle is in the subdural or subarachnoid space. Injection of contrast in the subdural space will give a "shifting lake" appearance, and injection in the subarachnoid space will lead to a myelographic pattern of contrast spread. Careful needle control as well as fluoroscopic images in the lateral view will minimize inaccurate needle placement.

After confirming accurate needle placement, negative aspiration should be confirmed for blood and CSF, and 1–2 ml of contrast is then injected to visualize epidural spread. The contrast should have a smooth flow during injection. Once appropriate spread of contrast is confirmed, the medication can be injected. If the target level cannot be entered successfully, lower level can be chosen followed by placement of a catheter through the needle and advanced to intended level.

Injection of the medication may lead to transient paresthesia. It may or may not correspond to the same distribution where the patient has chronic pain. Caution must be exercised to avoid intraneural injection which would cause immediate and severe pain. If severe pain occurs on injection, the needle should be repositioned.

Complications

Drug Related

Corticosteroids: mostly due to systemic absorption and are short-lived. It includes rash, nausea, pruritis, and hyperglycemia. More severe reactions include a Cushingoid response and adrenocortical failure.

Local anesthetics: rash, nausea, accidental intrathecal injection with resultant spinal anesthesia. Systemic absorption can lead to seizures and refractory cardiac arrhythmias.

Procedure Related

Procedural complications include postdural puncture headache (from accidental dural puncture and CSF leak), vasovagal reaction, subdural infiltration, neural injury, and permanent injury to the spinal cord (if in the upper lumbar levels). Permanent spinal cord injury can be secondary to either direct needle trauma or disruption of blood supply to the spinal cord. The artery of Adamkiewicz is a major artery that supplies the lumbar region of the spinal cord. It enters the spinal canal in 80 % of people between T8 and L3 on the left [12]. Injury can be avoided by making sure the needle is not too lateral in the neural foramen on AP fluoroscopy [12].

Other complications associated with procedure are rare, but many case reports have been written. These include infectious processes like meningitis, abscess, and an epidural hematoma (a surgical emergency).

Caudal Epidural Injection

The caudal approach to the epidural space was performed years prior to the lumbar approaches. The first published report was done in 1901 [16]. It has been used for many purposes including obstetric and pediatric anesthesia. Table 34.3 describes some of the indications for a caudal block with emphasis on what is seen in a chronic pain clinic.

One of the primary uses for the caudal approach to the epidural space is in patients who have had lumbar surgery which could make lumbar approaches more difficult or even impossible. Severe degenerative changes may also warrant a caudal approach.

Indications

See Table 34.3.

Contraindications

Absolute: unwilling patient, localized infection over procedure area, current anticoagulant use, bleeding diathesis, increased ICP and patient that cannot remain still during the procedure.

Table 34.3 Common indications for caudal epidural injections

Lumbar radiculopathy
Lumbar degenerative disk disease
Lumbar spinal stenosis
Lumbar postlaminectomy (failed back) surgery syndrome
Postherpetic neuralgia/herpes zoster
Complex regional pain syndrome (I and II)
Peripheral neuropathy (diabetic, chemotherapy induced, etc.)
Phantom limb pain
Cancer-related pain
Sacral/coccygeal neuralgia
Interstitial neuritis
Pelvic pain
Penile/testicular pain

Relative: allergy to medications that will be injected (contrast, local anesthetic, steroid), pregnancy, immunosuppression, systemic infection, and anatomic changes that would prevent a safe procedure (congenital or surgical).

Caudal Epidural Injection Technique

After discussing risks and benefits, answering questions, and obtaining written informed consent, the patient is brought into the procedure room and placed in a prone position. A cushion can be placed under the lower abdomen which will decrease lumbar lordosis and help decrease the angle of the sacral hiatus. The skin overlying the lower lumbar and gluteal region is prepped and draped in a sterile manner. This procedure can be performed with or without fluoroscopy. Lateral fluoroscopy can be used to identify the sacral hiatus. Manual palpation can also be used to identify the sacral cornu at the entrance to the sacral hiatus. Once the sacral hiatus has been identified, the skin and subcutaneous tissues can be anesthetized. A 22- or 25-gauge needle can be used to enter the sacral canal. It does not need to be longer than 1.5 in. A 17- or 18-gauge Tuohy needle can be used if the plan is to thread a catheter to the lumbar region for more targeted block.

The needle is then inserted at a 45° angle until a "pop" is felt which signifies passage through the sacrococcygeal ligament and then angled caudal to avoid contact with the bone inside the sacral canal. The needle is then advanced about 1 cm, negative aspiration for blood is confirmed, and if using fluoroscopy, contrast can be injected to confirm placement of the needle in the canal. If fluoroscopy is not being used, air can be injected and palpation for crepitus can be performed. If there is resistance to injection of air or contrast, the needle can be rotated as the bevel may be against the bony wall of the sacral canal.

Once the needle is correctly placed, either a medication can be directly injected or a catheter can be placed and advanced to a higher level for a more targeted injection. The medication can then be injected slowly. The spread of medication depends on many factors including the volume and rate of injection. If a catheter is used, less volume can be used as the medication is deposited near the nerve roots, causing pain.

Once the medication has been injected, the needle is removed with a saline or local anesthetic flush to clear the needle and track of steroid. The area that was prepped should be cleansed and a bandage placed over site of needle insertion. The patient should then be taken to a recovery area where they should be monitored for complications resulting from conscious sedation as well as complications from the procedure itself.

Complications

Drug Related

Corticosteroids: mostly due to systemic absorption and are short-lived. It includes rash, nausea, pruritis, and hyperglycemia.

Local anesthetics: rash, nausea, and accidental intrathecal injection with resultant spinal anesthesia. Systemic absorption can lead to seizures and refractory cardiac arrhythmias.

Procedure Related

Procedural complications include postdural puncture headache (from accidental dural puncture and CSF leak), vasovagal reaction, subdural infiltration, and neural injury. Infection, although rare, can be a higher risk with this approach given the needles entry site closer to the anus when compared to lumbar approaches. This is very important consideration especially in immunocompromised patients.

Future Direction for Epidural Injections

Although studies have been performed on the effectiveness (both cost and therapeutic), many studies have been of low grade quality or of insufficient power to make meaningful determinations. There need to be more randomized controlled trials performed on each form of access to the epidural space. Comparison studies should also be performed to determine if access through one route is better than another (i.e., cervical translaminar vs cervical transforaminal).

Conclusion

There are multiple indications for performing epidural steroid injections in the cervical, thoracic, and lumbar regions. There are also many ways to access the epidural space. Each has its benefits and risks, and these must be considered when choosing which route to use in a given patient.

References

1. Pages E. Anesthesia metamerica. Rev Sanid Mil Madr. 1921;11:351.
2. Dogliotti AM. Segmental pudendal anesthesia. Am J Surg. 1933;20:107.
3. Guitierrez A. Valor De la Aspiracion Liquada En El Espacio Peridural En La Anestesia Peridural. Rev Circ. 1933;12:225.
4. Waldman SD. Pain management. 1st ed. Philadelphia: Saunders Elselvier; 2007. p. 1211–2.
5. Van Zundert J, Huntoon M, Patijn J, Lataster A, Mekhail N, Van Kleef M. Cervical radicular pain. Pain Pract. 2009;10:1–17.
6. Benyamin RM, Singh V, Parr AT, Conn A, Diwan S, Abdi S. Systematic review of the effectiveness of cervical epidurals in the management of chronic neck pain. Pain Physician. 2009;12:137–57.
7. Waldman SD. Pain management. 1st ed. Philadelphia: Saunders Elselvier; 2007. p. 1216.
8. Cronen MC, Waldman SD. Cervical steroid epidural nerve blocks in the palliation of pain secondary to tension-type headaches. J Pain Symptom Manage. 1990;5:379.
9. Abbasi A, Malhotra G, Malanga G, Elovic EP, Kahn S. Complications of interlaminar cervical epidural steroid injections: a review of the literature. Spine. 2007;32:2144–51.
10. Kumar V, Krone K, Mathieu A. Neuraxial and sympathetic blocks in herpes zoster and post herpetic neuralgia: an appraisal of current evidence. Reg Anesth Pain Med. 2004;29(15):454–61.
11. Waldman SD. Pain management. 1st ed. Philadelphia: Saunders Elselvier; 2007. p. 1244.
12. Waldman SD. Pain management. 1st ed. Philadelphia: Saunders Elselvier; 2007. p. 1291.
13. Waldman SD. Pain management. 1st ed. Philadelphia: Saunders Elselvier; 2007. p. 1281.
14. Parr A, Diwan S, Abdi S. Lumbar interlaminar epidural injections in managing chronic low back and lower extremity pain: a systematic review. Pain Physician. 2009;12:163–88.
15. Raj P, Lou L, Erdine S, Staats P, Waldman SD, Racz G, Hammer M, Niv D, Ruiz-Lopez R, Heavner J, editors. Interventional pain management image-guided procedures. 2nd ed. Philadelphia: Saunders Elselvier; 2008. p. 323–4.
16. Waldman SD. Pain management. 1st ed. Philadelphia: Saunders Elselvier; 2007. p. 1335.

Transforaminal Epidural Steroid Injections

35

Todd B. Sitzman

Key Points
- Epidural steroid injections are a clinical and cost-effective method for treating acute and chronic spinal pain.
- Transforaminal epidural injections are a more specific treatment than interlaminar epidural injections for radicular but not axial back pain.
- Many pain medicine specialists believe that cervical transforaminal epidural injections are contraindicated given the relatively high-risk benefit ratio; extra training is necessary to complete these procedures safely.

Introduction

Epidural steroid injections (ESIs) play a fundamental role in the treatment of acute and chronic spinal pain and have shown clinical and cost-effectiveness. This is especially true when used in well-selected patients as part of a conservative, nonsurgical rehabilitative program. While the epidural space can be targeted by interlaminar, transforaminal, or caudal approaches, this chapter will focus on transforaminal epidural steroid injections (TFESI) including anatomic considerations, patient selection, technique, and outcome. Complications and risk mitigation will be covered elsewhere.

Anatomic Considerations

Knowledge of spinal anatomy, specifically the epidural space, is of significant importance when deciding upon which approach to utilize for an ESI. The epidural space lies between the osseoligamentous structures of the vertebral canal and the dural membrane shielding the contents of the thecal sac: cerebrospinal fluid, nerve roots, and spinal cord. While the thecal sac extends from the foramen magnum to approximately the S2 level, the epidural space extends to the level of the sacral hiatus at S4 or S5.

The epidural space contains adipose tissue, loose areolar tissue, arteries, lymphatics, and a rich venous plexus network. Contiguous with the thecal sac along its entire spinal course, the epidural space is anatomically divided into posterior and anterior compartments. The pain medicine specialist must fully appreciate the anatomy of the epidural space and how it relates to the ESI technique being considered. The posterior epidural space, typically accessed using an *interlaminar* approach, is bordered anteriorly by the thecal sac and posteriorly by the ligamentum flavum and the laminae. The anterior epidural space, most often accessed by a *transforaminal* approach, is bordered anteriorly by the vertebral body, intervertebral disc, and posterior longitudinal ligament and posteriorly by the thecal sac. The sacral epidural space may be accessed inferiorly by a *caudal* approach via the sacral hiatus. There are relative advantages of using one ESI approach over another depending upon the targeted pain generator, anatomic considerations (e.g., previous spinal surgery, decreased interlaminar space), and medical conditions (e.g., anticoagulation status). Interlaminar and caudal ESI approaches are discussed in other chapters. This chapter will focus on the transforaminal ESI techniques, benefits, cautions, and a review of the literature regarding efficacy over non-transforaminal ESI techniques.

A misperception is that transforaminal ESIs have greater diagnostic and therapeutic specificity than interlaminar ESIs. The relative diagnostic "specificity" of a transforaminal ESI corresponds to radicular pain only – not for axial back pain. A smaller volume of injectate, local anesthetic and corticosteroid, used in the transforaminal ESI approach may be more selective for one spinal nerve level. However, the injectate also affects several additional neural structures including the sinuvertebral nerve and dorsal primary ramus and its branches.

T.B. Sitzman, M.D., MPH
Advanced Pain Therapy, PLLC,
7125 Highway 98, Hattiesburg, MS 39402, USA
e-mail: toddsitzman@msn.com

T.R. Deer et al. (eds.), *Comprehensive Treatment of Chronic Pain by Medical, Interventional, and Integrative Approaches*,
DOI 10.1007/978-1-4614-1560-2_35, © American Academy of Pain Medicine 2013

Patient Selection

Transforaminal ESIs can have a therapeutic role in the treatment of:

- Disc herniation
- Spinal nerve root compression
- Spinal nerve root irritation – traumatic
- Spinal nerve root inflammation – infectious, e.g., herpes zoster
- Spinal stenosis – foraminal or central canal

There may also be a diagnostic role for TFESIs in patients with radicular pain resulting from nerve root compression or in the planning for decompressive surgery [1, 2]. TFESIs may also benefit patients with radicular symptoms at the level of prior decompressive surgery. TFESIs avoid the potential for false-negative results and complications associated with an interlaminar approach at the site of previous surgery. In such cases, epidural fibrosis and adhesions may hinder the spread of epidural injectate from reaching the intended neural target, and scar tissue may increase the risk of dural puncture associated with interlaminar ESIs [1, 2].

Lumbar Transforaminal Approach

The patient is positioned in the prone position on the fluoroscopic table. An oblique view is obtained, aligning the pedicle of the superior vertebra with the superior articular process of the inferior vertebra. The target site is the 6 o'clock position of the pedicle. The skin over this target site is marked and prepped with an appropriate skin antiseptic. Using sterile technique throughout, the skin and subcutaneous tissues are anesthetized with 1 % lidocaine. A spinal needle is slowly advanced toward the target 6 o'clock position of the pedicle using intermittent fluoroscopic imaging. It is not necessary to advance the needle until bony contact, but imaging in multiple fluoroscopic planes (anterior-posterior, oblique, and lateral) is recommended to ensure proper needle tip position. The "safe triangle" for needle tip location, as visualized on an anterior-posterior fluoroscopic plane, corresponds to the following locations: *base* of the triangle is the inferior border of the pedicle, medial *side* of the triangle is the exiting spinal nerve, and lateral *side* of the triangle is lateral border of the vertebral body. The protection offered by the "safe triangle" relates to neural structures, not to vascular structures including the artery of Adamkiewicz.

Following negative aspiration for blood and cerebrospinal fluid, injection of 1 ml of radiocontrast agent under continuous fluoroscopic visualization should reveal contrast spread medially into the neural foramen and the epidural space. Once proper contrast flow has been determined, injection of local anesthetic and steroid admixture may be injected.

Thoracic Transforaminal Approach

In theory, the transforaminal approach to the thoracic epidural space is similar to the lumbar approach. However, there are anatomic differences that must be appreciated. The pedicles of the thoracic vertebrae are directed posterosuperiorly from the transverse process, and there are two costal articulations that are not present in the lumbar spine. In addition to zygapophysial joints, the head of each rib articulates with a superior costal facet at the posterolateral aspect of the vertebral body – located lateral to the base of the pedicle. A transverse costal facet is located at the lateral border of the transverse process. Visualized in the lateral fluoroscopic view, the relatively large neural foramina are bounded superiorly by the inferior undersurface of the pedicle and inferiorly by the superior articular process of the more caudal vertebra.

The patient is positioned in the prone position on the fluoroscopic table. An ipsilateral oblique view of approximately 20° is needed to visualize the pedicle. The target site is the 6 o'clock position of the pedicle. The skin over this target site is marked and prepped, and local anesthetic is infiltrated. A spinal needle is slowly advanced toward the target 6 o'clock position of the pedicle using intermittent fluoroscopic imaging. Fluoroscopic imaging in the oblique, anterior-posterior, and lateral planes is mandatory to ensure that the needle tip is in the superior aspect of the neural foramen, at the 6 o'clock position of the pedicle. Following negative aspiration for blood and cerebrospinal fluid, injection of 1 ml of radiocontrast agent under continuous fluoroscopic visualization should reveal contrast spread medially into the neural foramen and the epidural space. Once proper contrast flow has been determined, injection of local anesthetic and steroid admixture may be injected.

It is mandatory that radiocontrast injection occur under live fluoroscopy to visualize the possibility of vascular uptake. The *artery of Adamkiewicz* supplies the anterior spinal artery of the spinal cord and usually enters the superior aspect of a single neural foramen on the left from T9 through L4. Therefore, when performing left-sided TFESIs, it is recommended to advance the needle toward a more inferolateral position within the neural foramen than in the lumbar spine. Nevertheless, the location of the artery of Adamkiewicz is variable and can traverse the neural foramen bilaterally from T7 through S1. If fluoroscopic imaging reveals contrast flow anteriorly and at the midline, this usually represents trespass of the artery of Adamkiewicz. The needle should be withdrawn and the TFESI postponed while observing the patient for signs of anterior spinal artery ischemia. Additionally, only non-particulate corticosteroid should be administered with TFESIs to minimize the risk of embolic vascular occlusion of the anterior spinal artery should an intra-arterial injection occur.

Cervical Transforaminal Approach

The cervical epidural space is extremely vascular and is associated with an increased risk of unrecognized vascular injection. The potential for an intravascular injection, specifically arterial, with a subsequent catastrophic event, demands extreme vigilance when performing cervical TFESIs. In fact, many pain medicine specialists feel that there is no indication for a cervical TFESI given the relatively high-risk benefit ratio. Some practitioners would rather use an upper thoracic interlaminar epidural approach and place a radiopaque catheter up to the cervical treatment region for an inside out transforaminal injection.

Following informed consent, the patient is positioned in either a lateral decubitus position or a supine oblique position with a pillow or wedge placed under the ipsilateral shoulder to maintain this position. An oblique fluoroscopic view is obtained to reveal the target neural foramen. The actual needle target is the posteromedial aspect of the mid-superior articular process in the oblique view. This skin over this site is marked, prepped with antiseptic, and anesthetized with 1 % lidocaine. Using sterile technique throughout, the tip of a spinal needle (usually 22-guage) is slowly advanced until it contacts the superior articular process (SAP). Maintaining needle tip over the bony SAP minimizes the risk of inadvertent advancement through the neural foramen into the subarachnoid space – and the potential for cervical cord contact. Once the needle touches the SAP, it is gently walked ventromedially into the posterior aspect of the foramen. Care should be taken to maintain needle tip location in the mid-portion of the posterior neural foramen as the vertebral artery is usually located anteriorly and other vasculature is located superiorly.

After negative aspiration for blood and cerebrospinal fluid, injection of 0.5 ml of radiocontrast agent under continuous fluoroscopic visualization should reveal contrast spread and an outline of the proximal cervical nerve root. In the anterior-posterior view, the contrast agent should spread medially through the neural foramen into the lateral epidural space. Once proper contrast spread location is confirmed in multiple fluoroscopic planes, the local anesthetic and steroid admixture may be injected.

Complications

Transforaminal ESIs possess the potential for catastrophic complications. In general, these complications result from improper needle placement, infection, local anesthetic effect, or corticosteroid effect.

Needle placement complications include pain at the injection site, nerve root injury, puncture of the dural sac, spinal cord injury, epidural hematoma, and postdural puncture headache [3]. Infection risks may include skin or epidural abscess, meningitis, and osteomyelitis. Local anesthetic complications may include motor block or weakness, hypotension, cardiac arrhythmia, seizure, and allergic reaction. Lastly, corticosteroid effects may be more sensitive in some individuals than others. These adverse effects may include fluid retention, elevated blood pressure, hyperglycemia, suppression of the hypothalamic-pituitary-adrenal axis, Cushing syndrome, steroid myopathy, facial flushing, and allergic reaction.

While the complication rate of TFESIs is reported to relatively low, there is the potential for catastrophic events such as paraplegia, quadriplegia, stroke, and death. The mechanism of action is secondary to intra-arterial injection of particulate steroids into a radicular artery supplying the spinal cord, or with cervical TFESIs, direct trauma, or injection into a cervical radicular artery directly feeding into the anterior spinal artery. Intermittent fluoroscopic imaging may frequently miss intra-arterial uptake of contrast. As a result, not only is continuous fluoroscopic imaging of contrast spread mandatory when performing TFESIs at any spinal level, the use of digital subtraction fluoroscopy is highly advised for all cervical TFESIs.

References

1. Derby R, Kine G, Saal J, et al. Precision percutaneous blocking procedures for localizing spine pain: II. The lumbar neuraxial compartment. Pain Dig. 1993;3:175–83.
2. Dooley JF, McBroom RJ, Taguchi T, et al. Nerve root irritation in the diagnosis of radicular pain. Spine. 1988;13:79–83.
3. Verrills P, Nowesenitz G, Barnard A. Penetration of cervical radicular artery during a transforaminal epidural injection. Pain Med. 2010;11:229–31.

Facet Injections and Radiofrequency Denervation

36

Sunil J. Panchal

S.J. Panchal, M.D.
National Institute of Pain,
4911 Van Dyke Road, Tampa, FL 33558, USA
e-mail: sunilpanchal2000@yahoo.com

Key Points

- The facet joint (zygapophyseal) is a common cause of pain in both the cervical and lumbar spine and less frequently in the thoracic region.
- The innervation of these joints is well defined and varies based on the spinal region being evaluated.
- Lumbar facet arthropathy is characterized by low back pain, unilateral or bilateral, with or without radiation. The pain is described usually as a deep, dull ache; is difficult to localize; and frequently is referred into the buttock, groin, hip, or posterior thigh to the knee.
- Denervation of the medial branch can be accomplished by using either radiofrequency ablation or cryoneurolysis.
- The radiofrequency lesion generator has the following critical functions: (1) continuous online impedance measurement; (2) nerve stimulation; (3) monitoring of voltage, current, and wattage during radiofrequency lesioning; and (4) temperature monitoring. Electric impedance is measured to confirm the continuity of the electric circuit and to detect short circuits.
- Impedance is usually 300–500 in extradural tissue. The nerve stimulator is used to detect proximity to sensory or motor fibers of the segmental root. Stimulation at 50 Hz is used to detect sensory fibers; 2 Hz is used to detect motor fiber stimulation.

Introduction

Each spinal segment from C2 caudal possesses three joints: anteriorly, the disc and associated uncovertebral joint and posteriorly, the paired facet joints. For almost a century, the lumbar facet (zygapophyseal) joint has been considered a significant source of low back pain. Ghormley was the first to describe the facet syndrome, which he defined as a lumbosacral pain with or without radiculopathy, occurring most often after a sudden twisting or rotary strain of the lumbosacral region [1]. Hirsch et al. injected hypertonic saline in the region of the lumbar facet joints, which resulted in pain in the sacroiliac and gluteal regions with radiation to the greater trochanter [2]. Mooney and Robertson performed saline intra-articular facet injections that resulted in a similar pain referral pattern; however, they noted that the pain was relieved by intra-articular local anesthetic injection [3]. Similar findings were produced in the cervical spine, with cervical facet injection of hypertonic saline by Pawl, resulting in neck pain and headache [4].

While low back pain has typically been attributed to degenerative discs, surgical removal of the disc usually does not result in relief from axial back pain. A spinal fusion, which stops the motion of the facet joint, often is required for adequate control of back pain. The pathophysiology of low back pain is a complex issue, with various soft tissues and bony structures of the spine that should be considered as a possible pain generator, and commonly, there is contribution from more than one structure. Among these, the facet joint is involved more frequently.

Anatomy

Facet Joints

The facet joints are paired diarthrodial synovial joints formed by the inferior articular process of one vertebra and the superior articular process of the vertebra below [5]. They are present from the C1–C2 junction to the L5–S1 junction. A tough

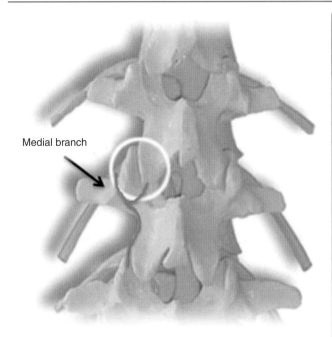

Medial branch

Fig. 36.1 Spine model where a lumbar facet joint is located within a white circle, and the course of a medial branch bifurcating after crossing the transverse process is shown to contribute to a dual innervation pattern

fibrous capsule is present on the posterolateral aspect of the joint. There is no fibrous capsule on the ventral aspect of the facet joint. Instead, the ligamentum flavum is located ventrally, in direct contact with the synovial membrane. Adipose tissue surrounding the spinal nerve is in direct contact with adipose tissue located in the superior recess of the facet joint, allowing direct spread of injectate from the joint to the epidural space and potentially to the spinal nerve [6, 7]. The capacity of the joint space averages only 1.0–2.0 mL in total volume. Communications between ipsilateral or contralateral facet joints do occur, often via defects in the pars interarticularis. These account for some of the spread of anesthetic that can occur during facet intra-articular injections.

Facet Innervation

Each spinal nerve root divides into a posterior and anterior ramus. The posterior ramus, also known as the sinuvertebral nerve of von Luschka, divides approximately 5 mm from its origin into medial, lateral, and intermediate branches. In turn, the medial branch divides into two branches that supply both the facet joint at the same level and the joint at the level below [8]. Therefore, each joint has a dual innervation supply (Fig. 36.1). The location of the medial branch and its divisions vary from the lumbar, cervical, and thoracic regions in relation to the bony structures. In the lumbar region, the medial branch is located in a groove at the base of the superior articular facet, where it crosses the transverse process

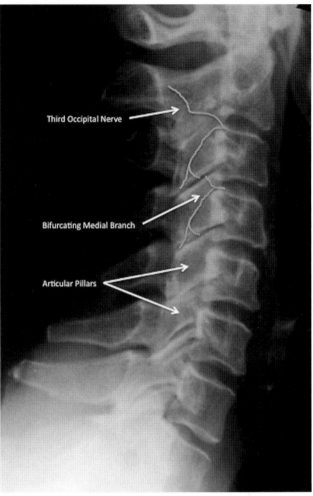

Third Occipital Nerve

Bifurcating Medial Branch

Articular Pillars

Fig. 36.2 Lateral radiograph of cervical spine identifying the articular pillars, demonstrating the bifurcation of the medial branch at C4 for a dual innervation pattern and the course of the third occipital nerve

posteriorly and inferiorly. It then divides, sending a branch medially and cephalad to the joint at the same level and a branch inferiorly to the joint below. The medial branch also supplies the multifidus and interspinalis muscles as well as the ligaments and periosteum of the neural arch [2]. Therefore, neural blockade of the medial branch is not specific for facet joint pain. There is some evidence of joint innervation from a third ascending branch, which originates directly from the mixed spinal nerve (Fig. 36.1) [5, 9, 10]. Innervation of the cervical facet region differs in that the medial branch predominantly supplies the facet joints, with minimal innervation of the posterior neck muscles [11]. The C3–C4 to C7–T1 facet joints are supplied by the medial branches from the same level and the level above [12, 13]. These branches wrap around the waist of each articular pillar bound to periosteum by investing fascia and the tendons of the semispinalis capitis [4]. The medial branch of C8 crosses facet innervation. The C3 medial branch divides earlier in its course into a deep, superficial (3rd occipital nerve) branch (Fig. 36.2). The deep C3 medial branch descends to innervate the C3–C4 facet joint; the superficial medial branch (3rd occipital nerve) traverses the lateral and dorsal surface of the C2–C3 facet joint before entering the joint capsule [11, 13, 14]. The atlantooccipital and lateral atlantoaxial joints receive innervation from the C1 and C2 ventral rami.

The thoracic facet joint innervation has a pattern similar to that of the lumbar region, except for findings from a study of four cadavers that demonstrated consistency of the medial branch course at the superolateral aspect of the transverse processes. The medial branches at these levels travel lateral from the foramen, cross the superior lateral border of the transverse process, and course medial to innervate the corresponding facet joint and level below. However at the T5–T8 levels, the inflection point of the nerve occurs at a point just superior to the superolateral corner of the transverse processes [15].

Pathophysiology

Intervertebral disc space narrowing occurs as the disc degenerates and loses hydration. The change in segment height can cause subluxation of the facet joints, resulting in abnormal stresses on the joint and nerve root impingement. Other sequelae, such as capsular irritation and local inflammation, may result in reflex spasm of the erector spinae muscles. As degeneration proceeds, abnormal motion leads to osteophyte production, further exacerbating the symptoms [16]. That the facet joint is a source of nociception has yet to be universally accepted. Opponents submit that local anesthetic blockade of the facet joint with subsequent pain relief lacks validity. This position is supported by observations of contrast injection spilling over into the epidural space or intervertebral foramen [7]. Pain elicited with hypertonic saline or relief with local anesthetic administration may be due to action on neural structures or on other pain-sensitive tissues. Proponents for the facet joint as a site of nociception point to the presence of substance P in facet capsule neurons [17]. In addition, most of the mechanosensitive somatosensory units in the facet joint are group-III high-threshold, slow-conduction units, which are thought to mediate nociception [18–20]. Chronic inflammation may lead to fluid accumulation and distension, stimulating the richly innervated synovial villi inside the capsule, resulting in pain.

Facet Block: Diagnostic or Therapeutic Tool?

Lumbar facet arthropathy is characterized by low back pain, unilateral or bilateral, with or without radiation. The pain is described usually as a deep, dull ache; is difficult to localize; and frequently is referred into the buttock, groin, hip, or posterior thigh to the knee. Fukui et al. described referral patterns for thoracic facet joints [21].

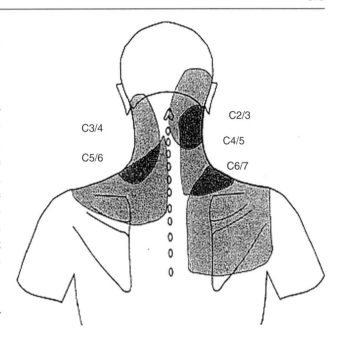

Fig. 36.3 The C3–C4 facet joint refers pain over the posterolateral cervical region, following the course of the levator scapulae. The lower cervical facet joints refer pain to the base of the neck and down to the scapulae

Some patients describe a sudden onset of pain, usually associated with twisting or bending. There is no exacerbation of the pain with Valsalva maneuver. In contrast to discogenic pain, sitting does not severely aggravate pain secondary to facet arthropathy. The cervical facet joints also cause pain described as deep and aching. Referral patterns vary, depending on which level is of concern. The C1–C2 facet joint may refer pain to the occipital and postauricular region [22]. The C2–C3 facet joint may cause pain referred to the occiput, ear, vertex, forehead, or eye [23, 24]. The C3–C4 facet joint refers pain over the posterolateral cervical region, following the course of the levator scapulae. The lower cervical facet joints refer pain to the base of the neck and down to the scapulae (Fig. 36.3) [23]. Physical examination often reveals tenderness over the facet joints and involves associated muscle spasm. The pain is exacerbated by extension or lateral bending as opposed to flexion as well as prolonged sitting. A few patients may exhibit mechanical hyperalgesia over the associated innervated skin. Whereas range of motion in all directions may be reduced, extension and rotation are most uncomfortable. Straight leg raise is usually negative. To make the diagnosis of a painful facet joint requires the typical history and physical findings already described in combination with diagnostic blocks. The use of facet block for diagnosis is hampered by certain pitfalls. There is a lack of a corresponding cutaneous innervation to the facet joint and thus an inability to determine when complete blockade has occurred. Injection into the joint often results in joint capsule rupture and spillage of local anesthetic into the epidural space or intervertebral foramen, which can interrupt nociceptive impulses from alternative sites [20, 25–27]. The medial branch nerve innervates muscles, ligaments, and periosteum in addition to the facet joints, again limiting specificity of the test. Facet blocks should be avoided in patients with systemic infection, infection at the site, or coagulopathies or in patients who refuse the procedure. Needle placement for facet injection as well as local anesthetic delivery can result in pain provocation. A provocative response that is concordant with the patient's ongoing complaints lends further support to the notion that the facet joint is the pain generator. Facet injections are commonly used for both therapeutic and diagnostic interventions. Intra-articular steroid injection often produces significant pain relief that outlasts the action of a local anesthetic [26, 28–30]. Although therapeutic benefit from steroid has been demonstrated, duration of outcomes is limited, similar to intra-articular steroids delivered to other joints [31–33]. Intra-articular block also does not correlate well with the success of radiofrequency denervation (only 64 %); therefore, medial branch block is the preferred procedure as a trial prior to facet denervation [34].

Technique

Lumbar and Thoracic Facet Blocks

For facet joint injection, the patient is positioned prone, with an abdominal cushion to reduce lumbar lordosis. Sterile preparation and draping of the back are performed. Intra-articular injection requires oblique fluoroscopic views. Best results are achieved at a 30–45° plane to "open" the joint. Either the table or the C-arm can be rotated for optimal viewing. The entry point through the skin then is identified and marked with the aid of a radiopaque instrument. The skin is infiltrated with 1 % lidocaine using a 25-gauge needle. A 22-gauge, 3.5-in. spinal needle then is introduced via the skin wheal and advanced into the joint using a trajectory parallel to the fluoroscopy beam. Local anesthetic alone or with steroid (0.25 % bupivacaine and 20 mg Depo-Medrol (methylprednisolone acetate)) is delivered in a volume of 1.0–1.5 mL. Volumes in excess of 2 mL will rupture the capsule and spill over into the epidural space (Fig. 36.4). For medial branch block, the patient is positioned prone, and the transverse process for each branch to be blocked is identified using fluoroscopy. Approximately 5 cm from the midline, a skin wheal is raised, and a 22-gauge, 3.5-in. spinal needle is advanced to the medial end of the transverse process, contacting the dorsal surface of the process near the superior edge. The L-5 medial branch is blocked at the groove between the ala of the sacrum and the superior articular process of the sacrum (Fig. 36.1). A total volume of 1.0 mL of 0.5 % bupivacaine is delivered at each site, and the patient is questioned for concordance compared with the original pattern of referred pain (Fig. 36.5). The technique is slightly altered for

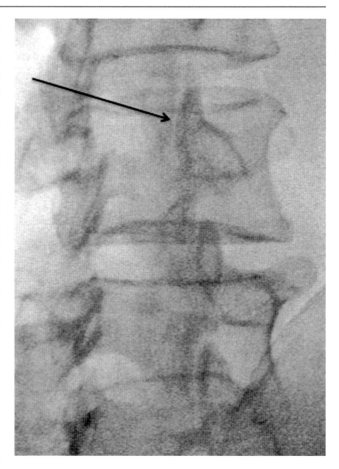

Fig. 36.4 "Scotty dog" view of facet joint at a 30° angle for intra-articular injection

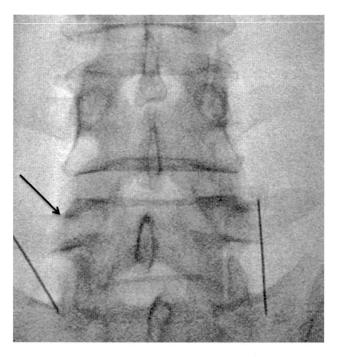

Fig. 36.5 AP view of lumbar facet medial branch block with needle at groove of sacral ala and arrow pointing to desired placement at superomedial aspect of the L5 transverse process

Fig. 36.6 With a lateral view of the cervical articular pillar, the intersection of lines connecting the opposite corners locates the centroid of the articular pillar where the medial branch typically will be found

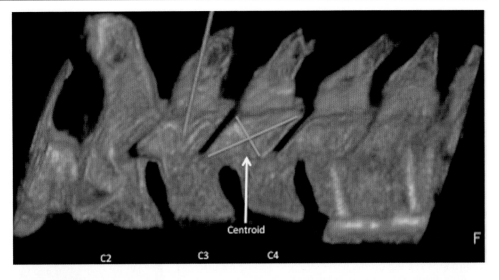

Fig. 36.7 Lateral view of 3-D reconstructed image demonstrating needle placement at the centroid of the C3 articular pillar

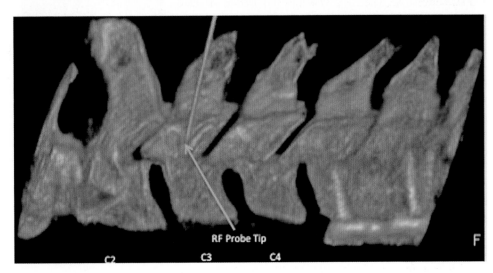

the thoracic levels, where the superolateral aspect of the transverse processes is the ideal site for placement.

Cervical Facet Block

The patient is ideally positioned prone to reduce potential injury to the vertebral arteries, but a lateral position has also been described. Sterile technique and needles are used as previously outlined. Needles are introduced 1–2 cm lateral to the waist of the articular pillar, guided by a posteroanterior view on fluoroscopy. The needle then is advanced to the centroid of the articular pillar as seen on a lateral view (Figs. 36.6 and 36.7). Again, 1.0 mL of local anesthetic is delivered. Intra-articular injection at the cervical level is not favored for several reasons. Cervical joint spaces are small and narrow. Further, the epidural space is immediately medial to the joint, and the vertebral artery is just lateral to the joint. Therefore, direct injection into cerebral circulation or blockade of cervical nerve roots is of great concern.

Facet Joint Denervation

Denervation of the medial branch can be accomplished by using either radiofrequency ablation or cryoneurolysis. This chapter will focus on the radiofrequency method in terms of its mechanism of action, followed by the results of long-term outcome studies.

Conventional Radiofrequency Ablation

The radiofrequency lesion generator has the following critical functions: (1) continuous online impedance measurement; (2) nerve stimulation; (3) monitoring of voltage, current, and wattage during radiofrequency lesioning; and (4) temperature monitoring. Electric impedance is measured to confirm the continuity of the electric circuit and to detect short circuits. Impedance is usually 300–500 Ω in extradural tissue. The nerve stimulator is used to detect proximity to sensory or motor fibers of the segmental root. Stimulation at

Table 36.1 Relationship of lesion size with tip sizes and temperatures

Authors	Electrode diameter (mm)	Exposed electrode tip length (mm)	Tip temperature (C)	Transverse lesion size (mm)	Test medium
Bogduk et al. [38]	186	5	80	2.2±0.4	Egg
	226	4	80	1.1±0.2	Egg
	226	4	90	1.6±0.2	Egg
Cosman et al. [36]	216	3	65	2–4	Egg
Guy, et al. [37]	216	2	60	3.7	Rabbit cortex
	216	2	70	5.5	Rabbit cortex
	216	2	80	7.2	Rabbit cortex
Vinas et al. [39]	206	4	80	4.9	Rabbit cortex

50 Hz is used to detect sensory fibers; 2 Hz is used to detect motor fiber stimulation. Ford et al. demonstrated that if the electrode is resting on the nerve, 0.25 V will be required to produce discharge, whereas 2 V will be required to produce discharge at a distance of 1 cm [35]. Therefore, monitoring voltage is important in determining proximity. Temperature monitoring occurs at the tip of the electrode only, with a thermocouple technique, producing a thermodionic voltage that is proportional to temperature. Bogduk et al. performed lesions in egg whites and meat and found that radiofrequency lesions do not extend distal to the electrode tip. Instead, lesions extended radially around the electrode tip in the shape of an oblate spheroid with a maximal effective radius of 2 mm using a 21-gauge electrode with a 3-mm exposed tip [38]. Table 36.1 demonstrates a survey of varying tip sizes and temperatures with the corresponding lesion size. The first signs of coagulation occur at 62 °C, but it is important to note that neural destruction begins at 45 °C. The maximal lesion size is attained once the "working" temperature is maintained for 20–40 s. Maintaining the temperature for longer periods did not result in any discernible increase in lesion size [39]. Although initial reports indicated selectivity for small fibers, Uematsu conclusively showed that radiofrequency at higher temperatures indiscriminately damages both small and large fibers [40]. Placement of the probes requires positioning of the active tip along the course of the medial branch as previously described (see Figs. 36.8 and 36.9).

Retrospective studies of lumbar facet RF denervation have demonstrated similar rates of success. Goupille et al. showed a 38.4 % success rate at 2-year follow-up, and North showed a 45 % success rate with a mean follow-up of 3.2 years [41–43]. North et al. went further, concluding that there was no difference in success for bilateral denervation for bilateral pain compared with unilateral denervation for unilateral pain [43]. Goupille et al. reported that patients who did not have prior spine surgery had better success with denervation, whereas North's group did not show any statistical difference between these groups (Table 36.2). Van Kleef et al. performed a lumbar facet RF denervation double-blinded

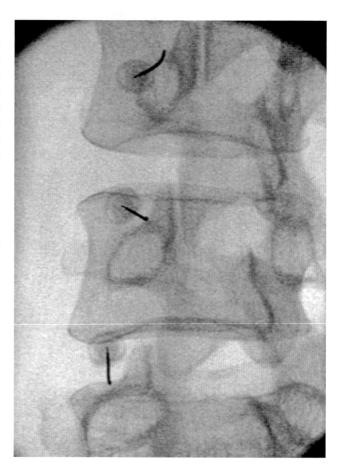

Fig. 36.8 Oblique view demonstrating placement of RF cannulae after contact with the "eye" of Scotty dog and slipped off the superior margin of the transverse processes

RCT in 31 patients with 80 C lesions at L3–L4, L4–L5, and L5–S1 with a sham control. At 8 weeks, mean VAS score was 4.8 for controls and 2.8 for the treated group. This was statistically significant for both differences in VAS but for Oswestry scores as well. In the treated group, 10/15 patients were successfully treated (at least 2-point reduction on VAS and greater than 50 % pain relief) at 8 weeks, and of these patients, seven were still a success at 12 months [44]. Nath et al. performed a sham-controlled RCT of lumbar facet RF

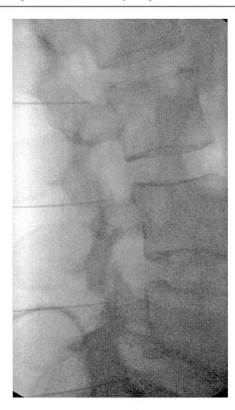

Fig. 36.9 Lateral view of placement of RF cannulae along the lumbar superior articular processes

denervation in 40 patients after at least 80 % pain relief was documented from controlled medial branch blocks. The RF group had multiple lesions performed at each level. At 6 months, the RF group had statistically significant improvement in VAS scores and with the patients' global assessment in comparison to the sham group. There was also significant improvement in secondary measures such as spine range of motion, quality of life measures, and physical exam findings posttreatment [45]. A 10-year prospective clinical audit of lumbar facet RF denervation in 209 patients was able to have 2-year follow-up data on 174 of the patients. Of these individuals, 119 (68.4 %) had good (>50 %) to excellent (>80 %) relief at 6 months. At 12 months, 81 patients still had good to excellent relief, and this was maintained in 36 patients at 24 months (Table 36.2).

Stolker et al. reported on 40 patients who underwent thoracic facet denervation with a mean follow-up of 31 months [47]. They found that 44 % were pain-free and 39 % had greater than 50 % relief. Stolker and coworkers also performed a cadaver study, with fluoroscopic guidance, in which radiofrequency denervations were performed bilaterally at T1–T12. They found that 61 % of the lesions hit neural tissue, but none hit the medial branch stem (the "target") [48]. The nerve stimulator should be used in an attempt to reproduce the patient's usual pain complaints and achieve better localization of the thoracic medial branch.

A randomized, double-blind trial of 24 patients with cervical facet pain after a motor-vehicle accident was performed to compare percutaneous radiofrequency denervation of multiple lesions at 80 °C with controls. Patients were selected for study after confirmation of cervical facet syndrome by use of double-blinded, placebo-controlled diagnostic local anesthetic blocks. Follow-up assessment was performed to determine the time until pain returned to 50 % of the preprocedural level. Radiofrequency patients had a median duration of relief of 263 days compared with 8 days in the control group [49]. In a separate study, psychological distress was measured by the McGill Pain Questionnaire and the SCL-90-R psychological questionnaire in patients with whiplash injury. A significant resolution of psychological distress was associated with pain relief from cervical facet radiofrequency denervation [50]. A prospective study was performed to assess for differences in outcomes of cervical facet RF denervation for treatment of whiplash symptoms based on litigation status. Patients with pain that persisted after 20 weeks were referred for RF treatment and followed for 1 year (N=46). There was significant improvement in pain immediately after treatment and at 1 year follow-up, but no statistical difference between litigants and nonlitigants. Pain scores for nonlitigants were reduced by 2.0 immediately and by 2.9 at 1 year and by 2.5 and 4.0, respectively, for litigants [51].

In regard to recurrence of pain and repeat treatment, two reports of small (20 and 24 patients) retrospective studies of repeat procedures after successful RF were identified for cervical and lumbar facet denervation. In both series, more than 80 % of patients had >50 % relief from repeat RF treatment, and mean duration of relief from subsequent RF treatments was comparable to the initial treatment [52, 53].

Pulsed Radiofrequency Ablation

Pulsed radiofrequency (PRF) treatments involve the application of short pulses of RF energy to neural tissue ranging from 5 to 50 ms with a frequency ranging from 1 to 10 Hz. The most common setting described is 2 Hz and 20 ms, with the goal of keeping the tissue temperature below the denaturation threshold of 45 °C. This method has been theorized to be non-ablative and provide relief by inducing intracellular changes, but has not been determined to have either of these benefits in a definitive manner [54–56]. In vitro studies suggest that PRF may change morphology of mitochondria, alter axonal structures, and has been demonstrated to reduce neuropathic pain behavior in the rat Chung model as well as sciatic nerve ligation study in rabbits [56, 57]. The clinical experience for utilization of PRF for lumbar facet pain has been positive, but does not appear to enjoy the same duration of effect as conventional RF. Tekin et al. performed a randomized trial of PRF vs. conventional RF, with similar

Table 36.2 Series showing lumbar facet RF denervation

Author, year	Technique	Study design	N	Length of follow-up	Outcomes	Key details
Goupille et al. 1993 [43]	Conventional RF	Retrospective	103 enrolled, 86 completed questionnaire	24 months	38.4 % had >50 % pain relief	Success rate was higher with no prior discectomy
North et al. 1994 [43]	Conventional RF	Retrospective	42	Mean follow-up of 3.2 years	45 % had >50 % pain relief	Assessment by disinterested 3rd party, no difference in success regardless of prior history of back surgery
Van Kleef et al. 1999 [44]	Conventional RF	Prospective, randomized double-blind, sham-controlled	31	12 months	Success = >50 % pain relief and ≥2-point decrease in VAS score Treated: 46.7 % at 6 months and at 12 months Sham: 18.8 % at 6 months and 12.5 % at 12 months	Excluded patients with prior history of back surgery
Nath et al. 2008 [45]	Conventional RF	Prospective, randomized double-blind, sham-controlled	40	6 months	Treated patients had mean decrease of VAS score by 1.9, only 0.4 decrease in the sham group	Treated patients had improved physical exam findings and statistically significant decrease in analgesic use
Gofeld et al. 2007 [46]	Conventional RF	Prospective, observational	209 treated, 174 completed 2-year assessment	24 months	Success = >50 % pain relief At 6 months, 68.4 % had success, 46.5 % at 12 months, 20.7 % at 24 months	83.2 % of patients with success reduced analgesic consumption

rates of improvement at 6 months, but only the RF group had maintained benefit at 1 year [58]. Van Zundert et al. randomized 23 patients to PRF vs. sham treatment, and had better results immediately, but not significantly different at 6 months [59].

Complications

Complications from facet block are infrequent and transient. A brief exacerbation of pain may occur and last a few days to a few weeks. Intrathecal injection has been reported, as well as one case of chemical meningitis [60]. Epidural blockade has occurred, and vertebral artery puncture and strokes have been described at the cervical level. Radiofrequency denervation resulted in postprocedure pain in 13 % of patients in one study; the pain resolved spontaneously over 2–6 weeks. No persistent motor or sensory deficits were reported.

Systematic Literature Reviews

A 2007 systematic review of facet joint interventions utilizing AHRQ criteria found that the evidence for pain relief with RF denervation is moderate for short- and long-term pain relief at the cervical and lumbar levels but was indeterminate for thoracic facets [61]. A 2009 systematic review of diagnostic utility and therapeutic effectiveness of cervical facet joint interventions by Falco et al. found level II-1 or II-2 evidence (controlled trials without randomization, and cohort or case control studies from more than one center) for RF neurotomy in the cervical spine using the US Preventive Services Task Force (USPSTF) quality ratings [62]. Using the same rating system, Datta and colleagues found level II-2 and level II-3 (cohort or case control studies from more than one center, and multiple time series with or without the intervention) evidence for lumbar radiofrequency neurotomy [63]. Van Boxem and colleagues in a review of evidence for continuous and pulsed RF note that RF at the cervical and lumbar level has produced the most solid evidence, and differences in outcome among RCTs can be attributed to differences in patient selection and/or inappropriate technique [64].

Conclusion

The facet joints are a common source of axial spine pain with well-described referral patterns, but methods for diagnosis remain underutilized. Specificity of local anesthetic injection is limited, but medial branch block is clearly preferred compared with intra-articular injection when attempting to prognosticate relief from denervation.

Local anesthetic injections as well as RF denervation are performed easily, are well tolerated by patients, and are extremely safe. Meaningful pain relief can be achieved in about 50 % of patients for a significant duration. Directions for future study include investigation of outcomes of thoracic facet RF denervation with a randomized controlled trial, and for patients with multiple areas of degenerative changes, outcomes of combined denervation treatments across targets are desirable.

References

1. Ghormley RK. Low back pain with special reference to the articular facet, with presentation of an operative procedure. JAMA. 1993;101:1773–7.
2. Hirsch C, Ingelmark B, Miller M. The anatomical basis for low back pain. Acta Orthop Scand. 1963;33:1.
3. Mooney V, Robertson I. The facet syndrome. CIin Orthop. 1976;115:149–56.
4. Pawl RP. Headache, cervical spondylosis, and anterior cervical fusion. Surg Annu. 1971;9:391–408.
5. Selby DK, Paris SV. Anatomy of facet joints and its clinical correlation with low back pain. Contemp Orthop. 1981;3:1097–103.
6. Xu GL, Hayerton VM, Carrera GF. Lumbar facet joint capsule: appearance at MR imaging and CT. Radiology. 1990;177:415–20.
7. McCormick CC, Taylor JR, Twang LT. Facet joint arthrography in lumbar spondylolysis: anatomic basis for spread of contrast medium. Radiology. 1989;171:193–6.
8. Bogduk N, Long D. The anatomy of the so-called "articular nerves" and their relationship to facet denervation in the treatment of low back pain. J Neurosurg. 1979;51:172–7.
9. Rashbaum RF. Radiofrequency facet denervation: a treatment alternative in refractory low back pain with or without leg pain. Orthop Clin North Am. 1983;14:569–75.
10. Schuster GD. The use of cryoanalgesia in the painful facet syndrome. J Neurol Orthop Surg. 1982;3:271–4.
11. Bogduk N. The clinical anatomy of the cervical dorsal rami. Spine. 1982;7:319–30.
12. Bogduk N, Marsland A. The cervical zygapophyseal joints as a source of neck pain. Spine. 1988;13:610–7.
13. Santavita S, Hopfner-Hallikainen D, Paukku P, et al. Atlantoaxial facet joint arthritis in the rheumatoid cervical spine: a panoramic zonography study. J Rheumatol. 1988;15:217–23.
14. Bovim G, Berg R, Gunnar Dale L. Cervicogenic headache: anesthetic blockades of cervical nerves and facet joint (C2/C3). Pain. 1992;49:315–20.
15. Chua WH, Bogduk N. The surgical anatomy of thoracic facet denervation. Acta Neurochir (Wien). 1995;136:140–4.
16. Wilde GP, Szypt ER, Mulholland RC. Unilateral lumbar facet joint hypertrophy causing nerve root irritation. Ann R Coll Surg Engl. 1988;70:307–10.
17. El-Bohy A, Cavanaugh JM, Getchell ML, et al. Localization of substance P and neurofilament immunoreactive fibers in the lumbar facet joint capsule and supraspinous ligament of the rabbit. Brain Res. 1988;460:379–82.
18. Yamashita T, Cavanaugh JM, El-Bohy AA, et al. Mechanosensitive afferent units in the lumbar facet joint. J Bone Joint Surg. 1990;72A:865–70.
19. Ashtar IK, Aston BA, Gibson SJ, et al. Morphological basis for back pain: the demonstration of nerve fibers and neuropeptides in the lumbar facet joint capsule but not in ligamentum flavum. J Orthop Res. 1992;10:72–8.

20. Yamashita I, Cavanaugh M, Ozaktay AC, et al. Effect of substance P on mechanosensitive units of tissue around and in the facet joint. J Orthop Res. 1993;11:205–14.

21. Fukui I, Ohseto K, Shiotani M. Patterns of pain induced by distending the thoracic zygapophyseal joints. Reg Anesth Pain Med. 1997;22:332–6.

22. Halla JT, Hardin JG. Atlantoaxial (C1–C2) facet joint osteoarthritis: a distinctive clinical syndrome. Arthritis Rheum. 1987;30: 577–82.

23. Aprill C, Dwyer A, Bogduk N. Cervical zygapophyseal joint pain patterns. II: a clinical evaluation. Spine. 1990;15:58–61.

24. Santavirta S, Konttinen Y, Lindquist C, Sandelin J. Occipital headache in rheumatoid cervical facet joint arthritis. Lancet. 1986;2:695.

25. Destouet JM, Gilul LA, Murphey WA, et al. Lumbar facet joint injection: indication, technique, clinical correlation, and preliminary results. Radiology. 1982;145:321–5.

26. Moran R, O'Connell D, Walsh MG. The diagnostic value of facet joint injections. Spine. 1988;13:1407–10.

27. Dory MA. Arthrography of the cervical facet joints. Radiology. 1983;148:379–82.

28. Carette S, Marcoux S, Truchon R, et al. A controlled trial of corticosteroid injection into facet joints for chronic low back pain. N Engl J Med. 1991;325:1002–7.

29. Lynch MC, Taylor JF. Facet joint injection for low back pain. J Bone Joint Surg Br. 1989;71:138–41.

30. Lilius G, Laassonen EM, Myllynen P, et al. Lumbar facet joint syndrome: a randomized clinical trial. Bone Joint Surg Br. 1989;71: 681–4.

31. Lau LS, Littlejohn GO, Miller MH. Clinical evaluation of intraarticular injections for lumbar facet joint pain. Med J Aust. 1985;143:563–5.

32. Marks RC, Houston T, Thulbourne T. Facet joint injection and facet nerve block: a randomized comparison in 86 patients with chronic low back pain. Pain. 1992;49:325–8.

33. Carrera GF. Lumbar facet joint injection in low back pain and sciatica: preliminary results. Radiology. 1980;137:665–7.

34. Lora J, Long D. So-called facet denervation in the management of intractable back pain. Spine. 1976;2:12l–6.

35. Ford DJ, et al. Comparison of insulated and uninsulated needles for locating peripheral nerves with a peripheral nerve stimulator. Anesth Analg. 1984;63:925–8.

36. Cosman ER, Rittman WJ, Nashold BS, et al. Radiofrequency lesion generation and its effect on tissue impedance. Appl Neurophysiol. 1988;51:230–42.

37. Guy G, et al. Surgical lesions of the brain stem. Neurochirurgie. 1989;35 Suppl 1:1–133.

38. Bogduk N, Macintosh J, Marsland A. Technical limitations to the efficacy of radiofrequency neurotomy for spinal pain. Neurosurgery. 1987;20:529–35.

39. Vinas FC, Zamorano L, Dujovny M, et al. In vivo and in vitro study of the lesions produced with a computerized radiofrequency system. Stereotact Funct Neurosurg. 1992;58:121–3.

40. Uematsu S. Percutaneous electrothermocoagulation of spinal nerve trunk, ganglion and rootlets. In: Schmidel HH, Sweet WS, editors. Current technique in operative neurosurgery. New York: Grune and Stratton; 1977. p. 469–90.

41. Silvers HR. Lumbar percutaneous facet rhizotomy. Spine. 1990;15: 36–40.

42. Goupille R, Cotty P, Fouquet B, et al. Denervation of the posterior lumbar vertebral apophyses by thermocoagulation in chronic low back pain: results of the treatment of 103 patients. Rev Rhum Ed Fr. 1993;60:791–6.

43. North RB, Han M, Zahurak M, et al. Radiofrequency lumbar facet denervation: analysis of prognostic factors. Pain. 1994;57:77–83.

44. Van Kleef M, Barendse GAM, Kessels A, et al. Randomized trial of radiofrequency lumbar facet denervation for chronic low back pain. Spine. 1999;24:1937–42.

45. Nath S, Nath CA, Pettersson K. Percutaneous lumbar zygapophysial (facet) joint neurotomy using radiofrequency current, in the management of chronic low back pain. Spine. 2008;33:1291–7.

46. Gofeld M, Jitendra J, Faclier G. Radiofrequency denervation of the lumbar zygapophysial joints: 10-year prospective clinical audit. Pain Physician. 2007;10:291–9.

47. Stolker RJ, Vervest AC, Groen GJ. Percutaneous facet denervation in chronic thoracic spinal pain. Acta Neurochir (Wien). 1993;122: 82–90.

48. Stolker RJ, Vervest AC, Groen GJ. Parameters in electrode positioning in thoracic percutaneous facet denervation: an anatomical study. Acta Neurochir (Wien). 1994;128:32–9.

49. Lord SM, Barnsley L, Wallis BJ, et al. Percutaneous radiofrequency neurotomy for chronic cervical zygapophyseal- joint pain. N Engl J Med. 1996;335:1721–6.

50. Wallis BJ, Lord SM, Bogduk N. Resolution of psychological distress of whiplash patients following treatment by radiofrequency neurotomy: a randomized, doubleblind, placebo-controlled trial. Pain. 1997;73:15–22.

51. Sapir DA, Gorup JM. Radiofrequency medial branch neurotomy in litigant and nonlitigant patients with cervical whiplash: a prospective study. Spine. 2001;26:E268–73.

52. Husted DS, Orton D, Schofferman J, et al. Effectiveness of repeated radiofrequency neurotomy for cervical facet joint pain. J Spinal Disord Tech. 2008;21(6):406–8.

53. Schofferman J, Kine G. Effectiveness of repeated radiofrequency neurotomy for lumbar facet pain. Spine. 2004;29(21):2471–3.

54. Erdine S, Yucel A, Cimen A, Aydin S, Sav A, Bilir A. Effects of pulsed versus conventional radiofrequency current on rabbit dorsal root ganglion morphology. Eur J Pain. 2005;9(3):251–6.

55. Erdine S, Bilir A, Cosman ER, Cosman Jr ER. Ultrastructural changes in axons following exposure to pulsed radiofrequency fields. Pain Pract. 2009;9(6):407–17.

56. Tun K, Cemil B, Gurcay AG, Kaptanoglu E, Sargon MF, Tekdemir I, Comert A, Kanpolat Y. Ultrastructural evaluation of pulsed radiofrequency and conventional radiofrequency lesions in rat sciatic nerve. Surg Neurol. 2009;72(5):496–500.

57. Aksu R, Ugur F, Bicer C, Menku A, Guler G, Madenoglu H, Canpolat DG, Boyaci A. The efficiency of pulsed radiofrequency application on L5 and l6 dorsal roots in rabbits developing neuropathic pain. Reg Anesth Pain Med. 2010;35(1):11–5.

58. Tekin I, Merzai H, Ok G, et al. A comparison of conventional and pulsed radiofrequency denervation in the treatment of chronic facet joint pain. Clin J Pain. 2007;23(6):524–9.

59. Van Zundert J, Patijn J, Kessels A, et al. Pulsed radiofrequency adjacent to the cervical root ganglion in chronic cervical radicular pain: a double-blind sham controlled randomized clinical trial. Pain. 2007;127(1–2):173–82.

60. Thomson SI, Lomax DM, Collett BJ. Chemical meningism after lumbar facet joint block with local anesthetic and steroids. Anaesthesia. 1997;46:563–4.

61. Boswell MV, Colson JD, Sehgal N, et al. A systematic review of therapeutic facet joint interventions in chronic spinal pain. Pain Physician. 2007;10:229–53.

62. Falco FJ, Erhart S, Wargo BW, et al. Systematic review of diagnostic utility and therapeutic effectiveness of cervical facet joint interventions. Pain Physician. 2009;12(2):323–44.

63. Datta S, Lee M, Falco FJ, et al. Systematic review of diagnostic utility and therapeutic utility of lumbar facet joint interventions. Pain Physician. 2009;12(2):437–60.

64. van Boxem K, van Eerd M, Brinkhuizen T, et al. Radiofrequency and pulsed radiofrequency treatment of chronic pain syndromes: the available evidence. Pain Pract. 2008;8(5):385–93.

Eduardo M. Fraifeld

Key Points
- Intercostal nerve blocks are relatively simple procedures that can prove effective in the properly selected patient.
- The anatomical knowledge required to do this procedure is straightforward.
- Despite the perceived simplicity of the procedure, the risks are serious and should be carefully considered prior to doing the block.
- The use of fluoroscopy is helpful in determining landmarks for needle placement.

And the Lord God caused a deep sleep to fall upon the man, and he slept; and He took one of his ribs, and closed up the place with flesh instead thereof. (Genesis 1:21)

Introduction

Intercostal nerve blocks (INBs) are relatively simple to perform and can provide excellent analgesia or anesthesia to the human torso. They provide relatively well-defined anatomical coverage, making them both an excellent diagnostic tool and a reliable therapeutic procedure. In addition, they are among the simplest of peripheral nerve blocks performed with a relatively low incidence of complications.

Many consider epidural anesthesia (see Chap. 34) the best method of providing analgesia to the torso; however, it requires greater technical skills and has potential side effects including undesired hypotension, urinary retention, and risks of nerve root or spinal cord injury. Furthermore,

the widespread use of anticoagulants often results in epidural techniques being contraindicated due to coagulopathy. Interpleural block (see Chap. 38) has similarly been suggested as a reliable method with the added advantage of a localized sympathetic block. However, its shorter lasting effect and resulting significantly higher plasma concentrations of local anesthetic [1] make it less optimal choice.

Increasingly, the literature is looking at paravertebral nerve blocks (PVNBs) as a better alternative to epidurals. One recent systematic review and meta-analysis of randomized trials comparing PVNB with epidural analgesia showed equivalent analgesia with better outcomes in PVNB [2] corroborating findings in previous studies [3–7].

Anatomy

The intercostal nerves originate from 12 paired thoracic nerve roots that are intimately associated with the thoracic ribs (see Figs. 37.1, 37.2 and 37.3). Knowledge of their anatomy and relation to surrounding structures is vital to successfully performing these procedures.

Ribs

- True ribs – first to seventh, connect directly to the sternum through costosternal cartilages.
- False ribs – eight to tenth, so-called because their cartilages do not reach the sternum directly but instead attach to the rib immediately above.
- Floating ribs – 11th and 12th, only reach to cover the back and do not have attachment to the sternum.
- Costochondral joints – the articulation between the rib and the cartilage connecting them to the sternum. They start at the first rib, just lateral to the sternum. As they go inferior, they become more lateral till the tenth rib; it is almost at the anterior axillary line.

E.M. Fraifeld, M.D.
Southside Pain Solutions,
P.O. Box 2639, Danville, VA 24541, USA
e-mail: efraifeld@me.com

T.R. Deer et al. (eds.), *Comprehensive Treatment of Chronic Pain by Medical, Interventional, and Integrative Approaches*,
DOI 10.1007/978-1-4614-1560-2_37, © American Academy of Pain Medicine 2013

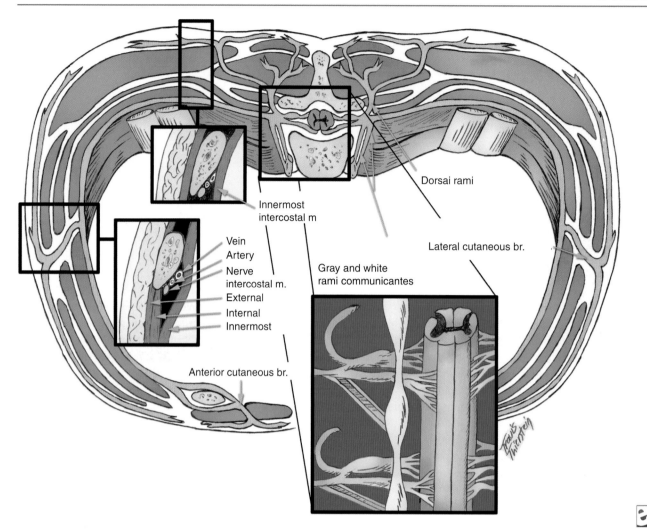

Fig. 37.1 Branches of thoracic spinal nerve roots (Reprinted with permission from eMedicine.com, 2010. Available at: http://emedicine.med-scape.com/article/1143675-overview)

Nerves

As the thoracic nerve roots emerge from the intervertebral foramen, they immediately split into the ventral rami that form the intercostal nerves and the posterior rami (see Fig. 37.1). Anterior branches form the gray and white rami communicantes of the thoracic sympathetic chain. The posterior rami innervate the zygapophyseal (facet) joints, muscles and skin of the thoracic midline, and paraspinous area of the back.

The intercostal veins, arteries, and nerves (VAN) travel for the most part in the costal grove, protected from direct trauma with the nerve being most inferior on the edge of the rib. After exiting the foramen, the intercostal nerves are near the middle of the intercostal space between the parietal pleura and the inner side of the intercostal muscles. As the nerve approaches the angle of the rib, the nerve then emerges between the internal intercostal muscle layer and the outer

portion of the innermost intercostal muscle to its location on the costal groove.

Small collateral nerve branches develop as the intercostal nerve progresses anteriorly, innervating the intercostal muscles and the ribs. At about the midaxillary line (MAL), the lateral cutaneous nerve arises. The lateral cutaneous nerve splits into posterior and anterior branches that innervate the skin of the chest wall from the scapular line to midclavicular line. The intercostal nerve continues anteriorly within the costal groove between the internal intercostal muscle layer and the outer portion of the innermost intercostal muscle, but as it progresses anteriorly, it once again emerges internal to the innermost intercostal muscle. As intercostal nerves approach the sternum, they emerge as the anterior cutaneous branches, innervating the anterior chest.

- Thoracic nerve roots – branch into the dorsal primary rami and the anterior rami which become the intercostal nerves.

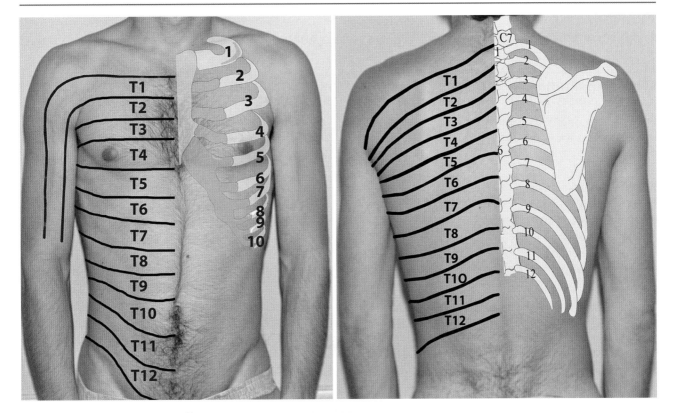

Figs. 37.2 and 37.3 Dermatomes of thoracic nerve roots and relation to ribs

- Dorsal primary rami – innervate the posterior midline and paraspinous muscles and skin.
- Intercostal nerves – innervate distinct band-like segments of muscles (myotomes) and skin (dermatomes).
- Collateral branches – arise from the intercostal nerves to innervate the intercostal muscles and ribs.
- Lateral cutaneous nerve branches – arise in the MAL and divide into anterior and posterior branches to innervate the skin of the majority of the torso.
- Anterior cutaneous nerves – divide into medial and lateral branches to innervate the skin of the anterior torso
- Cross innervation – as the nerves travel distally, they overlap so that even total loss of a single nerve root is unlikely to produce a noticeable sensory loss. To develop a complete sensory loss, usually you have to block two to three intercostal nerves.
- The optimal site for injection of the intercostal nerve is at the angle of the ribs where they are the thickest as noted in various studies [8–10]. This is about 15 cm from the spinous process [3, 4].

Special Considerations

1. First, intercostal nerve arises from the ventral ramus, but a portion of the ventral ramus goes on to join the brachial plexus.
2. Second, intercostal nerve also supplies a small branch of the ventral ramus to the brachial plexus.

Dermatomal Distribution

Dermatome distribution maps of intercostal nerves have long been published from a variety of sources and should always be viewed as approximations [11, 12]. In particular as noted above, a single intercostal nerve block seldom results in a total anesthesia of single dermatome due to cross innervation; however, dermatome charts can be used as a guide in selecting level of placement of intercostal nerve blocks (see Figs. 37.2 and 37.3).

Local Anesthetic

Local anesthetic choices are similar as in other nerve block procedures, the most common being lidocaine or bupivacaine. For single-shot INB, a volume of 3–5 mL is usually more than adequate per level injected. Total dose however should be monitored to reduce the risk of systemic toxicity. Alkalinization of the local anesthetic for intercostal nerve blocks has been found to be of little clinical benefit [13]. The use of epinephrine has been proposed as a possible increased safety factor by constricting local vessels and reducing uptake or by producing a tachycardia as a warning sign of accidental intravascular injection. However, other studies have called this into question and shown increased hemodynamic changes compared to other types of nerve blocks [14].

For continuous INB, an infusion of 0.25 % bupivacaine at 2 mL/h is usually adequate.

Clinical Applications

INB has been shown to be useful for a variety of anesthetic and analgesic uses in the distribution of the torso. Among these are:

1. Post-thoracotomy pain
2. Post-rib fracture pain
3. Cancer pain
4. Mastectomy and breast surgery pain
5. Shingles pain
6. Intercostal neuralgia
7. Costochondritis
8. Abdominal wall pain

Studies have shown that INB for post-thoracotomy pain offers advantages in preserving effort-dependent pulmonary function compared to opioid analgesia [15, 16].

The first three intercostals also innervate sensation portions of the upper arm and axilla, while the lower intercostals from T6 to T12 innervate the muscles of the upper abdomen and overlying skin [17]. Therefore, intercostal nerve blocks at the appropriate level can easily control symptoms in the affected region, allowing for decreased dependence on opioid analgesics. This can be useful in cases where one needs to avoid respiratory depressant or mental status changes.

Effective perioperative analgesia with continuous INB also has been demonstrated to reduce the incidence of chronic post-thoracotomy neuralgia [18]. While bupivacaine single-shot INB is reported to last longer than lidocaine, no significant difference has been reported in the outcome between infusions of lidocaine or bupivacaine for continuous infusions [19].

Trauma to an intercostal nerve by thoracotomy can lead to either pain or a sensory loss over the skin of the affected nerve or pain assisting in identifying the level injured. Similarly, trocar placement during laparoscopic procedures such a cholecystectomy can lead to similar problems. Numerous studies also have looked at use for a variety of conditions as noted above. Most studies are anecdotal, as noted in a recent case report on treatments for costochondritis [20].

Technical Tips

- Some studies have suggested that a short-beveled needle is likely to be safer and more accurate for INB [21].
- Continuous intercostal catheter analgesia is a more efficient way of performing INB, allowing a longer therapeutic effect. For most applications, an epidural catheter kit is the most convenient to use.

- Use of elastomeric infusion pumps has been shown to be a safe and effective adjunct in postoperative pain management after thoracotomy [22].

Paravertebral Nerve Block

The thoracic paravertebral space is a somewhat triangular space that is laterally continuous with the intercostal space [23, 24]. Anatomical borders are:

- Medial border – vertebral body, intervertebral disk, and spinal foramina
- Posterior border – transverse process, superior costotransverse ligaments, and ribs
- Anterior border – parietal pleura

Intercostal nerves, their collateral branches and posterior primary rami, and the thoracic sympathetic chain all pass through the paravertebral space, making it an ideal site for blockade of the various afferent nociceptive nerve impulses [25].

The mechanism of action of the PVNB is intercostal nerve block via the paravertebral spread of local anesthetic [26]. Spread of a mean of six dermatomes (range, five to seven) has been demonstrated by injection of methylene blue at thoracotomy and infusion of contrast medium in postoperative patients [26]. Techniques described have included blind placement [27, 28], by neurostimulator [29], by loss of resistance, by and ultrasound.

Clinically, PVNB is comparable with epidural block in respect to pain relief but without the well-known side effects of the epidural analgesia [30]. PVNB is therefore seen as a useful technique for pain control of breast, thorax, and abdomen, and many have considered it the technique of choice [31–33]. While one prospective study failed to that show a single-shot PVNB was superior to continuous wound infiltration [34], the technique of continuous catheter PVNB is gaining popularity. The ability to perform this effectively at bedside with ultrasound guidance [35] also simplifies the ability to perform this procedure in a greater variety of settings.

The effectiveness of PVNB injections with local anesthetic and steroids in acute herpes to prevent postherpetic neuralgia has been studied and been shown to be useful [36].

Complications

Complication rates for INB are low. They are reported to include:

1. Intravascular systemic injection with subsequent local anesthetic toxicity
2. Pleural puncture and pneumothorax
3. Hematoma
4. Neural injury

5. Infection

6. Total spinal anesthesia

Many studies have documented the higher plasma levels of local anesthetic concentrations after intercostal nerve block [37] relative to other nerve block locations. However, the incidence of local anesthetic toxicity is low.

Pneumothorax, one of the most commonly thought of complications, is actually also rare. One study in surgical patients looked at over 100,000 individual nerve blocks and found no severe systemic toxic reactions, and the incidence of pneumothorax was 0.073 % [38]. Another study in patients who received INB for rib fractures due to trauma showed a higher rate of 1.4 % [39], still a low rate considering the higher risk of pneumothorax in rib fractures.

Rare complications can include total spinal anesthesia. This may occur by inadvertent injection into a dural cuff extending outside the intervertebral foramen [40, 41]. This has been reported with paravertebral block injections and catheter placement [42], and similarly, neurolytic injections have led to total spinal cord injuries.

Procedure Description

Intercostal Nerve Block

- Standard monitors are applied.
- Patient is place in a comfortable prone position.
- Sedation with a combination of midazolam (0–3 mg) and fentanyl (0–150 μg).
- Identify the posterior spinous process by palpation and mark on skin.
- Draw a paramedian line at the lateral edge of the paraspinous muscles.
- Palpate for the inferior edge of each rib at this line and mark the skin at this site at the previously marked line.
- Inject local anesthetic into the skin at each one of the planned injection sites.
- Connect a 4-cm 25-gauge needle to a control syringe with the local anesthetic of choice.
- Use the nondominant hand and index and middle fingers to again palpate the inferior edge of the rib at the planned injection site (Fig. 37.4).
- Retract the skin over the rib.
- Holding the control syringe in the dominant hand, insert the needle in a slight cephalic direction towards the lower edge of the rib being palpated (Fig. 37.5).
- Carefully advance the needle until it contacts the rib.
- The nondominant hand will now release the skin and be used to steady the needle. This is of most importance to protect any movement by the patient resulting in unintentional lung puncture.

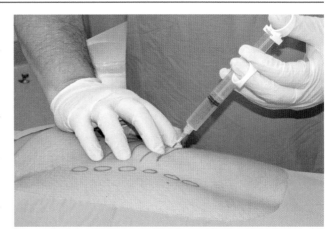

Fig. 37.4 Note the cephalic angle, initially aimed to the inferior rib edge

- Carefully walk the needle tip of the inferior edge of the rib and advance into the intercostal groove (about 2–4 mm) (Figs. 37.6 and 37.7).
- After negative aspiration for blood and air, 3–5 mL of local anesthetic solution is injected.

The procedure is repeated as outlined above at each planned level of injection. Intercostal nerves may also be injected along the midaxillary line if only an anterior block is desired such as a breast block.

Tips

- Palpation is best done by feeling for the intercostal spaces and sling fingers up to palpate lower edge of rib.
- Wetting fingertips and skin with the prepping solution allows fingers to slide over skin, making it easier to count ribs by palpation.
- In the obese patient, identification by palpation may be impossible and ultrasound guidance and fluoroscopy are both useful. At this time, there is inadequate data demonstrating the superiority of one method over the other.

Fluoroscopy Tips

- Read Chap. 4 regarding imaging for procedures and safety.
- For fluoroscopic guidance, follow directions as above. Tilt the fluoroscope in an ipsilateral direction slightly to get better visualization of the ribs and to move the hands and syringe from blocking the view (Fig. 37.8).
- Usage of microbore extension tubing can allow for more precise control of needle and remove obstruction of view caused by hand holding syringe.
- Contrast injection is helpful to rule out intravascular uptake and show filling into the costal grove and between the intercostal muscles (Fig. 37.9).
- With severely painful ribs, procedure can be more comfortably done in lateral position (Fig. 37.10) or alternately in sitting position with patient braced to prevent inadvertent movement.

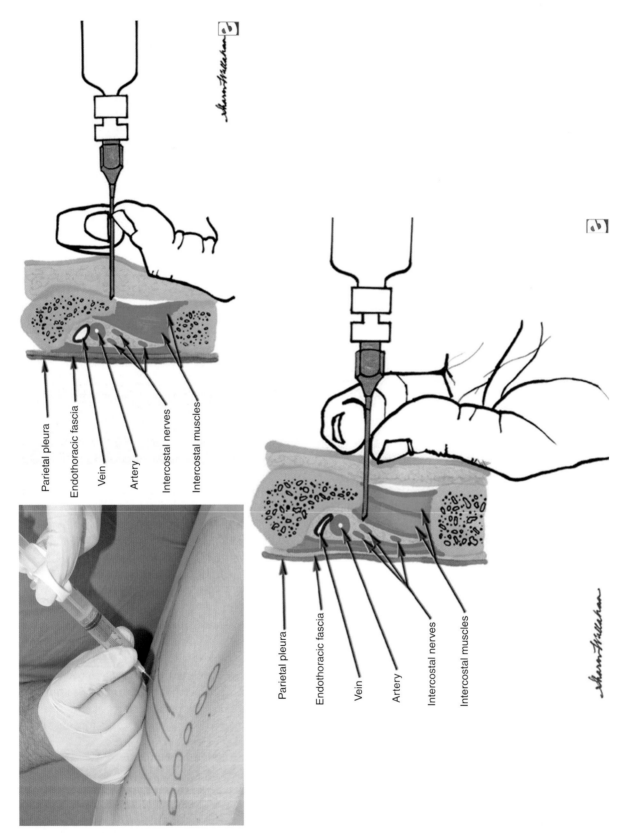

Figs. 37.5, 37.6, and 37.7 Bracing needle with hand firmly resting on patient will allow control of the needle and prevent accidental lung puncture if patient moves suddenly (Reprinted with permission from eMedicine.com, 2010. Available at: http://emedicine.medscape.com/article/1143675-overview)

Fig. 37.8 (*A*) Direction of fluoroscopy beam. (*B*) Direction of needle insertion

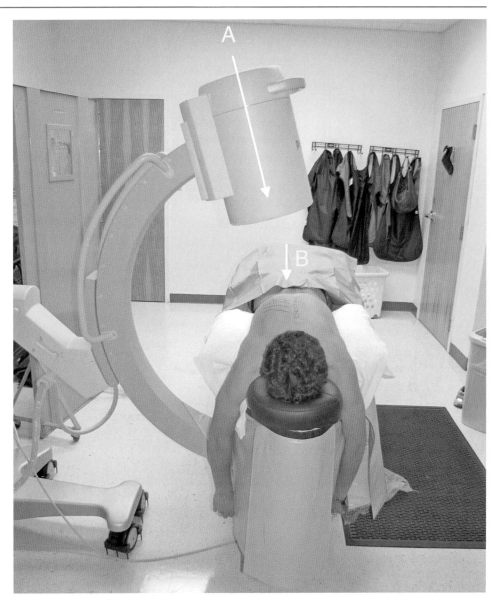

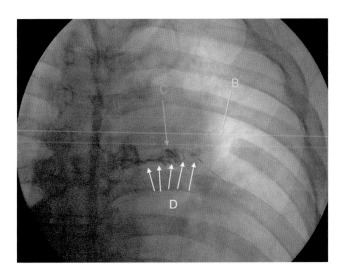

Paravertebral Nerve Block

- One to four steps as above.
- Mark skin entry point about 3 cm lateral to marks.
- Using a technique as above, insert the needle perpendicular to the skin.
- Advance the needle 2–4 cm, depending on body habitus, until the transverse process is contacted.

Fig. 37.9 (*A*) Surgical clip on intercostal artery. (*B*) Resected sixth rib from thoracotomy. (*C*) Needle placed for intercostal injection. (*D*) Contrast spread along intercostal groove and between intercostal inner muscles. Note that on medial side, contrast begins spread into paravertebral space

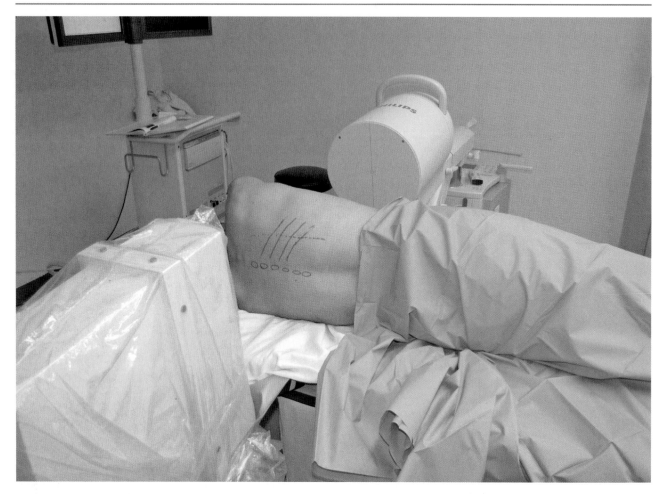

Fig. 37.10 Lateral placement for fluoroscopic intercostal nerve block. Can also be used with ultrasound

- The needle is then pulled back slightly and walked of the caudal edge of the transverse process.
- The needle is then advanced another 1.5–2 cm.
- After negative aspiration, 3–5 mL of local anesthetic is injected per level.
- Neurostimulator technique is performed with a 5-cm insulated needle in a similar fashion.
- Initially, stimulation of the paraspinous muscles is seen.
- On entering the paravertebral space, the needle is manipulated in an angular direction and by rotation of needle, not by in/out manipulation.
- Correct needle placement will result on stimulation at 0.4–0.6 mA of intercostal, low abdominal, inguinal, or cremaster contraction depending on the level being stimulated.
- Local anesthetic injection is then performed as above.

Paravertebral Nerve Block: Ultrasound Guided

Numerous reports have shown the value and possible increased safety of using ultrasound guidance [43].

- Standard monitors are applied.
- Patient is placed in a comfortable prone position.
- Sedation with a combination of midazolam (0–3 mg) and fentanyl (0–150 μg).
- Identify the posterior spinous process by palpation.
- Ultrasound scanning is done on the short axis lateral to the midline (Fig. 37.11).
  - Identify the ribs (Fig. 37.12).
  - Identify visceral and parietal pleura by having patient take deep breath.
  - Look for movement with respiration over each other.
- Rotate ultrasound so that it is on long axis to the rib midline (Fig. 37.13).
- Tilting probe side to side to get a sweeping view will help identify the muscles (Figs. 37.14 and 37.15).
- After identifying the location of entry, the skin is marked.
- Local anesthetic is infiltrated in the skin and subcutaneous tissue with Lidocaine 1 % using a 25-gauge needle.
- A 17-gauge Touhy needle is then inserted at the end of the ultrasound probe, in plane with the probe.
- The needle is advanced incrementally, aiming for the space between the internal intercostal muscle layer and

Fig. 37.11 Short axis view placement of linear ultrasound probe

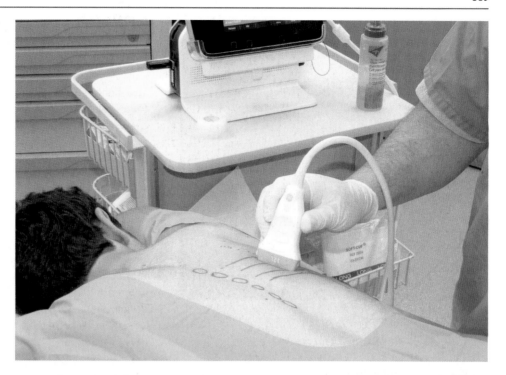

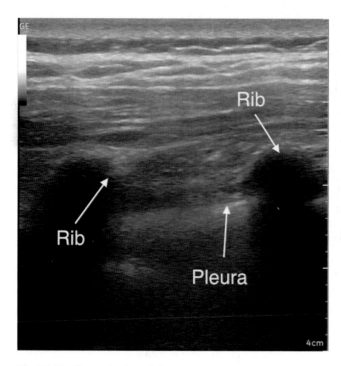

Fig. 37.12 Short axis view of ribs

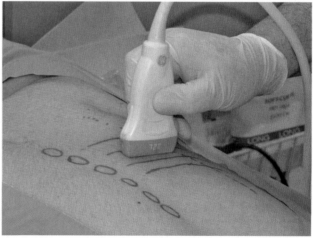

Fig. 37.13 Longitudinal placement of ultrasound for view of rib

the outer portion of the innermost intercostal muscle where the intercostal nerves reside.

- Small boluses of normal saline (1–2 mL) are injected as the needle is advanced between the muscle layers in order to dilate the space.
- Once the correct space is identified and slightly dilated, the syringe is disconnected from the needle hub.

- The patient is asked to breathe deeply looking for any airflow to rule out inadvertent pleural puncture.
- The syringe is reconnected. And aspiration is made for air or blood.
- After negative aspiration, 10 mL of local anesthetic is injected. A 19-gauge epidural catheter is advanced about 3–6 cm beyond the tip of the needle.
- The Touhy needle is removed over the catheter and taped to the skin.
- Reexamine the patient 15–30 min later and determine if the dermatome coverage of the block is adequate.

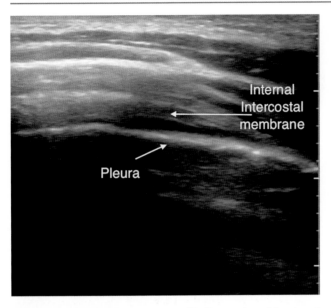

Fig. 37.14 Tilting ultrasound probe will allow a view of intercostal muscles and pleura

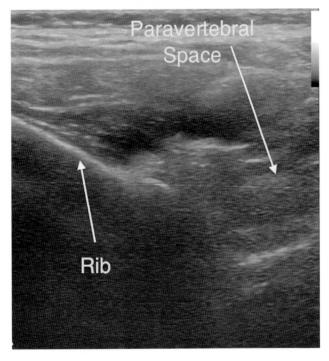

Fig. 37.15 More medical placement allows a view of edge of rib and paravertebral space

Tip: In obese patients, the movement of skin in relation to the intercostal nerve groove can be quite significant. Feeding some additional catheter into the adipose tissues as the needle is removed can reduce the incidence of catheter movement out of the proper space.

Infusion can then be started with the local anesthetic of choice.

Tips

- Have all equipments ready prior to starting procedure.
- Gently sweep side to side (during step 7a above) while on long axis view to not only identity muscle layers but to also identify tip of needle.
- Contrast injection and fluoroscopy can be used to confirm paravertebral spread of local anesthetic.

Future Directions

Future methods to prolong the effect of intercostal nerve blocks without increasing risks such as higher plasma concentrations of drugs will no doubt increase the usefulness of procedures such as intercostal nerve blocks in clinical practice. Studies on the injection of microcapsules of dexamethasone and bupivacaine are encouraging [44]. As the technology of 3-D echo continues to improve, it is likely to simplify this procedure and make bedside application even easier and safer.

References

1. van Kleef JW, Burn AGL, Vletter AA. Single-dose interpleural versus intercostal blockade: nerve block characteristics and plasma concentration profiles after administration of 0.5 % bupivacaine with epinephrine. Anesth Analg. 1990;70:484–8.
2. Davies RG, Myles PS, Graham JM. A comparison of the analgesic efficacy and side effects of paravertebral vs epidural blockade for thoracotomy – a systematic review and meta-analysis of randomized trials. Br J Anaesth. 2006;96(4):418–26.
3. Am K, et al. Prospective, randomized comparison of extrapleural versus epidural analgesia for postthoracotomy pain. Ann Thorac Surg. 1998;66:367–72.
4. Luketich JD, Sullivan EA, Ward J, Buenaventura PO, Landreneau RJ, Fernando HC. Thoracic epidural versus intercostal nerve catheter plus patient-controlled analgesia: a randomized study. Ann Thorac Surg. 2005;79:1845–50.
5. Joshi GP, Bonnet F, Wilkinson RC, Camu F, Fisher B, Rawal N, Schugg SA, Simanski C, Kehlet H. A systematic review of randomized trials evaluating regional techniques for postthoracotomy analgesia. Anesth Anal. 2008;107:1026–40.
6. Perttunen K, Nilsson E, Heinonen J, Hirvisalo EL, Salo JA, Kalso E. Extradural, paravertebral and intercostal nerve blocks for postthoracotomy pain. Br J Anaesth. 1995;75:541–7.
7. Detterbeck FC. Efficacy of methods of intercostal nerve blockade for pain after thoracotomy. Ann Thorac Surg. 2005;80:1550–9.
8. Moore DC, et al. Intercostal nerve block: a roentgenographic anatomy study of technique and absorption in humans. Anesth Analg. 1980;59(11):815–25.
9. Gross CM, editor. Gray's anatomy of the human body. 28th ed. Philadelphia: Lea & Febiger; 1996. p. 140–3, 983–7.
10. Nunn JF, Slavin G. Posterior intercostal nerve block for pain relief after cholecystectomy: anatomical basis and efficacy. Br J Anesthesiol. 1980;52:253–60.
11. Apok A, Gurusinghe NT, Mitchell JD, Emsley HCA. Dermatomes and dogma. Pract Neurol. 2001;11:100–5.
12. Greenberg SA. The history of dermatome mapping. Arch Neurol. 2003;60:126–32.
13. Swann DG, et al. The alkalinisation of bupivacaine for intercostal nerve blockade. Anaesthesia. 1991;46:174–6.

14. Cottrell WM, Schick LM, Perkins HM, Modell JH. Hemodynamic changes after intercostal nerve block with bupivacaine-epinephrine solution. Anesth Analg. 1978;57:492–5.

15. Faust RJ, Nauss LA. Post-thoracotomy intercostal block: comparison of its effects on pulmonary function with those of intramuscular meperidine. Anesth Analg. 1976;66:542–6.

16. Bridenbaugh PO, DuPen SL, Moore DC, Bridenbaugh LD, Thompson GE. Postoperative intercostal nerve block analgesia versus narcotic analgesia. Anesth Analg. 1973;52:81–5.

17. Moore KL, Dalley AF. Clinically oriented anatomy. 4th ed. Philadelphia: Lippincott Wiliams & Wilkins; 1999. p. 685–9.

18. Richardson J, Sabanathan S, Mearns AJ, Sides C, Goulden CP. Post-thoracotomy neuralgia. Pain Clin. 1994;7:87–97.

19. Watson DS, et al. Pain control after thoracotomy: bupivacaine versus lidocaine in continuous extrapleural intercostal nerve blockade. Ann Thorac Surg. 1999;67:825–8.

20. Freeston J, Karim Z, Lindsay K, Gough A. Can early diagnosis and management of costochondritis reduce acute chest pain admissions? J Rheumatol. 2004;31(11):2269–71.

21. Moore DC, Busch WH, Skurlock JE. Intercostal nerve block: a roentgenographic anatomic study of technique and absorption in humans. Anesth Analg. 1980;59:815–25.

22. Wheatley GH, et al. Improved pain management outcomes with continuous infusion of a local anesthetic after thoracotomy. J Thorac CV Surg. 2005;130:464–8.

23. Cowie B, McGlade D, Ivanusic J, Barrington MJ. Ultrasound-guided thoracic paravertebral blockade: a cadaveric study. Anesth Analg. 2010;110:1735–9.

24. Karmaker M. Ultrasound-guided thoracic paravertebral block. Tech Reg Anesth Pain Manag. 2009;13:142–9.

25. Sabanathan S, Mearns AJ, Bickford Smith PJ, et al. Efficacy of continuous extrapleural intercostal nerve block on post-thoracotomy pain and pulmonary mechanics. Br J Surg. 1990;77:221–5.

26. Eng J-B, Sabanathan S. Site of action of continuous extrapleural intercostal nerve block. Ann Thorac Surg. 1991;51:387.

27. Moore DC. Regional block. A handbook for use in the clinical practice of medicine and surgery. 4th ed. Springfield: Charles C. Thomas; 1965.

28. Katz J. Atlas of regional anesthesia. 2nd ed. Norwalk: Appleton & Lange; 1994.

29. Naja MZ, Ziade MF, Lönnqvist PA. Nerve-stimulator guided paravertebral blockade vs. general anaesthesia for breast surgery: a prospective randomized trial. Eur J Anaesth. 2003;20:897–903.

30. Richardson J, Sabanathan S, Eng J-B, et al. Comparison between continuous epidural morphine and extrapleural bupivacaine for relief of post thoracotomy pain. Ann Thorac Surg. 1993;55:377–80.

31. Coveney E, Weltz CR, Greengrass R, Iglehart JD, Leight GS, Steele SM, Lyerly HK. Use of paravertebral block anaesthesia in the surgical management of breast cancer. Experience in 156 cases. Ann Surg. 1998;227:496–501.

32. Klein SM, Bergh A, Steele SM, Georgiade GS, Greengrass RA. Thoracic paravertebral block for breast surgery. Anesth Analg. 2000;90:1402–5.

33. Wildling E. Single-injection paravertebral block compared to general anaesthesia in breast surgery. Acta Anaesthesiol Scand. 1999;43:770–4.

34. Sidiropoulou T, Buonmo O, Fabbi E, Silvi M, Kostopanagiotou G, Sabato A, Datri M. A prospective comparison of continuous wound infiltration with ropivacaine versus single-injection paravertebral block after modified radical mastectomy. Anesth Anal. 2008;106: 997–1001.

35. Ben-Ari A, Moreno M, Chelly J, Bigeleisen P. Ultrasound-guided paravertebral block using an intercostal approach. Anesth Analg. 2009;109:1691–4.

36. Ji G, Niu J, Shi Y, Hou L, Lu Y, Xiong L. The effectiveness of repetitive paravertebral injections with local anesthetics and steroids for the prevention of postherpetic neuralgia in patients with acute herpes zoster. Anesth Analg. 2009;109:1651–5.

37. Yokoyama M, Mizobuchi S, Nakatsuka H, Hirakawa M. Comparison of plasma lidocaine concentrations after injection of a fixed small volume in the stellate ganglion, the lumbar epidural space, or a single intercostal nerve. Anesth Analg. 1998;87:112–5.

38. Moore DC. Intercostal nerve block for postoperative somatic pain following surgery of thorax and upper abdomen. Br J Anaesth. 1975;47(suppl):284–6.

39. Shanti CM, Carlin AM, Tyburski JG. Incidence of pneumothorax from intercostal nerve block for analgesia in rib fractures. J Trauma. 2001;51:356–9.

40. Benumof JL, Semenza J. Total spinal anesthesia following intrathoracic intercostal nerve blocks. Anesthesiology. 1975;43:124–5.

41. Chaudhri BB, Macfie A, Kirk AJ. Inadvertent total spinal anesthesia after intercostal nerve block placement during lung resection. Ann Thorac Surg. 2009;88:283–4.

42. Gay GR, Evans JA. Total spinal anesthesia following lumbar paravertebral block: a potentially lethal complication. Anesth Analg. 1971;50:344–8.

43. Rianin SCO, Donnell BO, Cuffe T, Harmon DC, Fraher JP, Shorten G. Thoracic paravertebral block using real-time ultrasound guidance. Anesth Analg. 2010;110:248–51.

44. Kopacz DJ, et al. The dose response and effects of dexamethasone on bupivacaine microcapsules for intercostal blockade (T9 to T11) in healthy volunteers. Anesth Analg. 2003;96:576–82.

Intrapleural Catheters

38

Kevin E. Vorenkamp and Lynn R. Kohan

Key Points

- Reistad and Stromskag first described intrapleural analgesia in 1986.
- Intrapleural analgesia involves placing a catheter into the tissue plane within the chest wall (the intrapleural space) so that infusion of local anesthetic spreads to several nerves.
- The anatomy of the intrapleural space allows different types of nerve fibers to be anesthetized such as somatic, sympathetic, intercostal, and paravertebral nerves thereby increasing its overall utility in a variety of painful conditions.
- The main complication is the incidence of pneumothorax, which can range from 1 to 5 %.
- Intrapleural analgesia can be used in the management of pain for the upper extremity, chest wall, thoracic viscera, and upper abdominal viscera.
- Intrapleural catheter infusions offer an alternative technique that remains a viable option for a variety of pain states, especially if contraindications exist to other techniques.

Introduction

Reistad and Stromskag first described intrapleural analgesia in 1986 [1]. The "intrapleural" space refers to the space *inside* or *within* the pleural cavity, although the terms "interpleural" (referring to the same space *between* the visceral and parietal pleurae) and "subpleural" (referring to *below* the

parietal pleura) have also been used to describe the same space. Providing analgesia by infusing medications into the intrapleural space has been used in a variety of cases including but not limited to upper abdominal surgery, thoracic wall trauma, breast surgery, nephrostomy, esophagectomy, and thoracic surgery, in addition to chronic pain conditions such as chronic pancreatitis, complex regional pain syndrome (CRPS), and postherpetic neuralgia It is a relatively simple technique to learn with a low incidence of complications and few contraindications. It involves placing a catheter into the tissue plane within the chest wall (the intrapleural space) so that infusion of local anesthetic spreads to several intercostal or paravertebral nerves. The main complication is the incidence of pneumothorax, which can range from 1 to 5 % depending on the technique that is used to find the intrapleural space [2]. This complication combined with the risk for local anesthetic toxicity has limited its use; however, it can be used safely when performed with the proper technique.

History/Background

Mandl first described intrapleural injection in 1947 when he injected 6 % phenol into the intrapleural space of experimental animals without any evidence of pleural irritation or necrosis [3]. In 1978, interest in utilizing the intrapleural space for therapy resurfaced. At this time, Wallach injected tetracycline and lidocaine for malignant pleural effusions [4, 5]. The concept of intrapleural analgesia was first published in 1986 by Reistad and Stromskag as a way of treating pain after open cholecystectomy, kidney surgery, and breast surgery. Prior to that time, interest had focused on injecting multiple intercostal nerves. A cadaver study by Nunn and Slavin showed that local anesthetic of a single intercostal nerve gained access to other intercostal nerves in adjacent spaces above and below the injection site by means of both the intercostal and intrapleural spaces [6].

Kvalheim and Reistad demonstrated fluid spread by injecting local anesthetic and radiological contrast through a

K.E. Vorenkamp, M.D. (✉) • L.R. Kohan, M.D.
Department of Anesthesiology, Pain Management Center,
University of Virginia School of Medicine,
545 Ray. C. Hunt Drive, Suite 316, Charlottesville, VA 22908, USA
e-mail: kevin.vorenkamp@gmail.com; lynnkohan@gmail.com

T.R. Deer et al. (eds.), *Comprehensive Treatment of Chronic Pain by Medical, Interventional, and Integrative Approaches*,
DOI 10.1007/978-1-4614-1560-2_38, © American Academy of Pain Medicine 2013

Fig. 38.1 Anterior view
demonstrating the four parts
of the parietal pleura

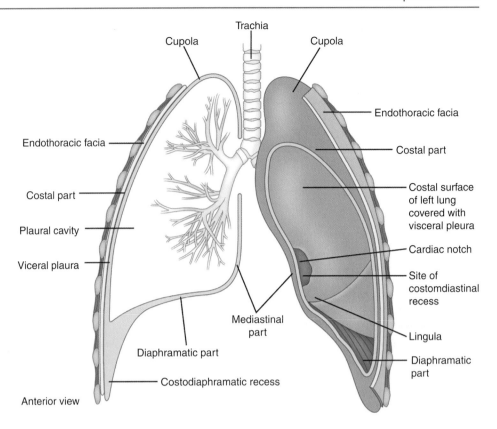

Anterior view

catheter that had been placed in the intercostal space. They found that, in addition to providing excellent analgesia, the contrast spread over the lung surface, leading them to conclude that the catheter was actually placed in the intrapleural space. They therefore decided to reproduce this type of analgesia by deliberately placing the catheter in the intrapleural space.

Anatomy

The visceral pleura surrounds the lungs. At the chest wall, diaphragm, and mediastinal borders of the lung, the pleura reflects back on itself to form the parietal pleura, which adheres to the chest wall. There are four parts of the parietal pleura: the mediastinal, which lines the mediastinum; diaphragmatic, which lines the diaphragm; costal, which lines the thoracic wall; and superiorly, the cupola (cervical), which extends superior to the first rib (Fig. 38.1).

The line where the costal pleura becomes diaphragmatic pleura is called the costodiaphragmatic reflection. The line where costal pleura becomes mediastinal pleura is called the costomediastinal reflection. The right pleural reflection passes across the sternoclavicular joint and proceeds near the midline of the sternum, inferiorly from the level of the second rib to the 6th costal cartilage, swings laterally to cross the 8th rib in the midclavicular line, the 10th rib in the midaxillary line, and the

12th rib posteriorly, near the midline. The left pleural reflection is similar except at the 4th costal cartilage; the line swings laterally to the left border of the sternum. At the left and right costodiaphragmatic reflection, the pleura extends caudally without intervening lung tissue. This caudal extension forms a potential space (in the pleural cavity), the costodiaphragmatic recess. At the costomediastinal reflection, on the left side, lung tissue does not extend up to the costomediastinal reflection because of the cardiac notch in the left lung, and another potential space, the costomediastinal recess, is formed.

As these lines of reflection are fixed, intrapleural analgesia can technically be instituted anywhere with those boundaries.

Anteriorly, laterally, and posteriorly, the parietal pleura is in close approximation to the intercostal nerves. The parietal pleura has abundant sensory innervation from the phrenic and intercostal nerves (Fig. 38.2). Superiorly, the lower roots of the brachial plexus pass a short distance over the cupola before reaching the first rib. Medially, the sympathetic chain, splanchnic, phrenic, and vagus nerves are also adjacent. Because the epidural and subarachnoid spaces are further away, they are generally not thought to be involved during an intrapleural injection. However, since these spaces are only separated from the parietal pleura by fat and loose connective tissue of the epidural and paravertebral spaces, there may be tracking of anesthetic solution if there is a breach of the parietal pleura.

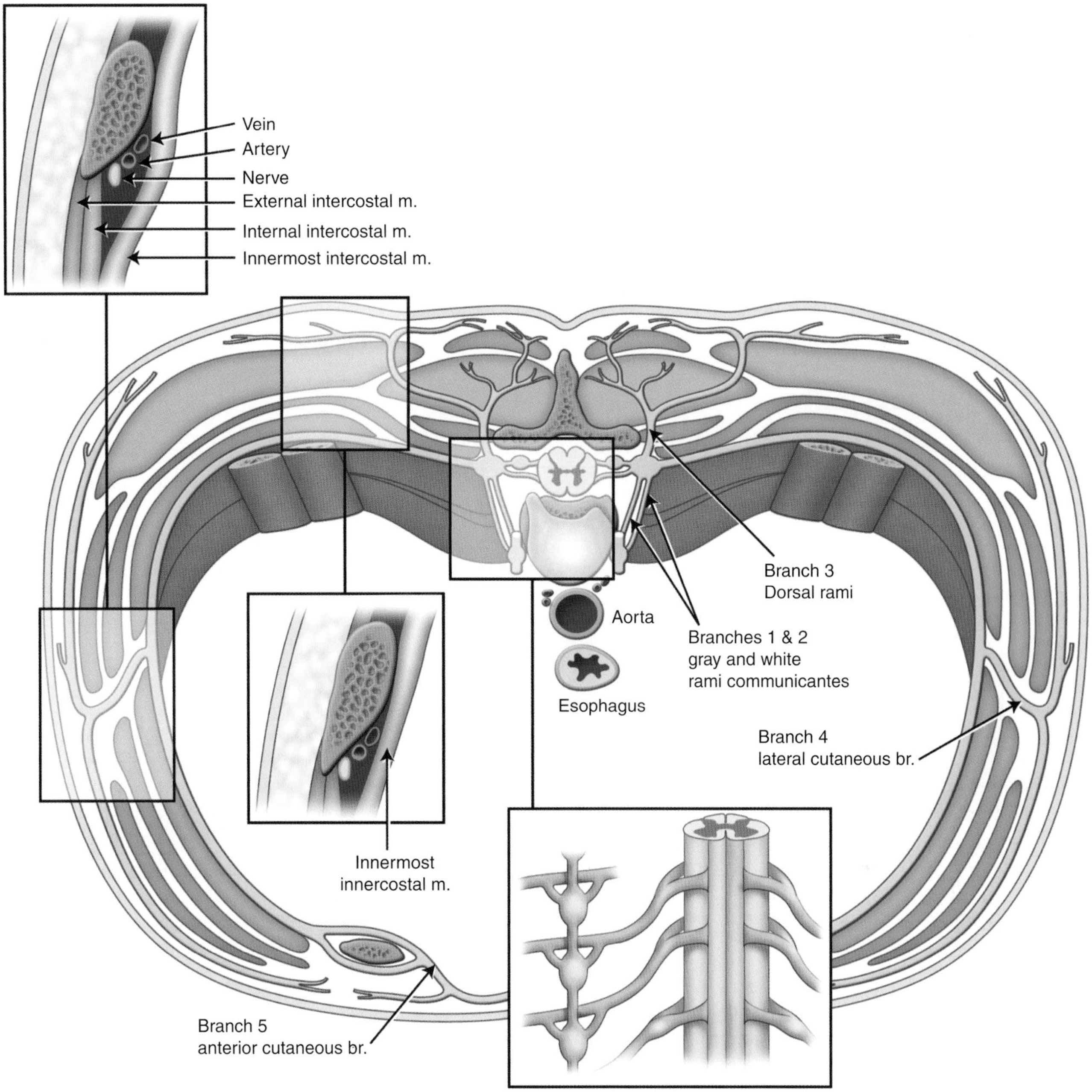

Fig. 38.2 Nerve supply of the thorax and intrapleural space

The visceral pleura is the innermost layer that is adherent to the substance of the lungs. It is continuous with the parietal pleura at the hilus of the lung. The intrapleural cavity is the potential space between the visceral and the parietal pleura. The space is 10–20 μm in width and has a static volume of 0.1–0.2 ml/kg. The micron-covered mesothelial surface of the parietal pleura facilitates the absorption of the local anesthetic and its diffusion into the intrapleural space. The pleura receives innervation from the phrenic and sympathetic nerves, and therefore, intrapleural administration of anesthetics may affect neural conduction on both types of nerves. Intrapleural analgesia can be accomplished by placing the anesthetic solution between the parietal and visceral pleurae, in this potential space (Fig. 38.3). Intrapleural analgesia can also be accomplished by placing a catheter deep to the internal intercostal muscle but superficial to the parietal pleura.

The intercostal space of the posterior chest wall has three layers: the external intercostal muscle; the posterior intercostal membrane, which is the aponeurosis of the internal intercostal muscle; and the intercostalis intimus muscle, which is a continuation of the transversus abdominis.

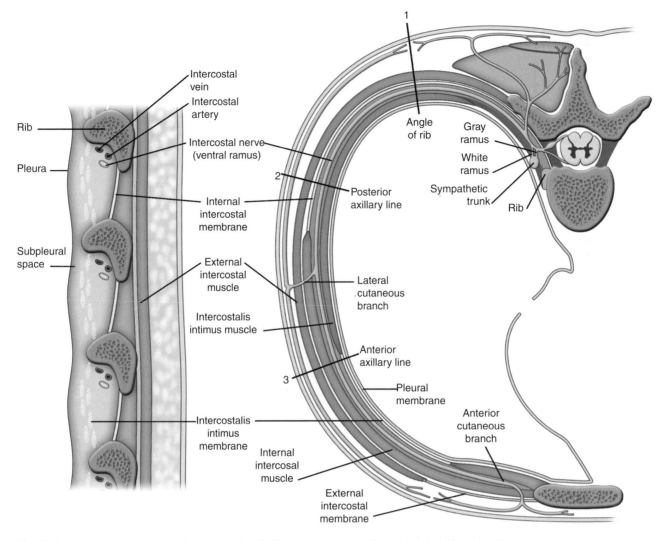

Fig. 38.3 Anatomy of the pleural cavity after (*left*) and before (*right*) injection of solution into the intrapleural space

The intercostal nerves lie in between the posterior intercostal membrane and the intercostalis intimus. The intercostal intimus is incomplete and allows fluid to pass freely into the intrapleural space, whereas the posterior intercostal membrane forms a complete barrier beneath the external intercostal muscle.

Therefore, as previously stated, intrapleural analgesia can be accomplished in one of two ways. A catheter can be placed either deep to the internal intercostal muscle but superficial to the parietal and the visceral layers of the pleura or the catheter can be placed between the parietal and the visceral layers of the pleura. The local anesthetic can thus spread to adjacent intercostal nerves and paravertebral nerves, but spread to the epidural or subarachnoid space does not usually occur. Local anesthetic that is placed in the intrapleural space will diffuse out to anesthetize the thoracic somatic and lower cervical and thoracic sympathetic nerves that lie close to the parietal pleura.

Indications

Intrapleural analgesia can be used in the management of pain for the upper extremity, chest wall, thoracic viscera, and upper abdominal viscera. It can also be used in more emergent pain states such as rib fractures, acute herpes zoster, and cancer pain. In addition, intrapleural analgesia has been found to be effective for percutaneous thoracostomy tubes, nephrostomy tubes, and biliary drainage tubes. It is also used in surgeries of the breast, chest wall, and flank. Additional pain states in which intrapleural analgesia can be used include postherpetic neuralgia, metastasis to the lung and liver, and post-thoracotomy pain (Table 38.1).

Gall Bladder and Liver Surgeries

There have been numerous studies examining the effectiveness of intrapleural analgesia in patients undergoing

Table 38.1 Indications for intrapleural analgesia

Type of surgery	Investigator	Evidence
Gall bladder	Tyagi et al. [7]	Supportive
	Shrestha et al. [8]	
	Dravid et al. [10]	
Gall bladder	Yaseen et al. [9]	Nonsupportive
Liver	Therasse et al. [11]	Supportive
Renal	Trivedi and Robalino [12]	Supportive
	Baude et al. [15]	
	Greif et al. [16]	
Breast	Colpaert et al. [17]	Supportive
	O'Donoghue et al. [18]	
CABG	Ogus and Selimoglu [19]	Supportive
Thoracotomy	Yildirim et al. [20]	Nonsupportive
	De Cosmo et al. [21]	
	Joshi et al. [22]	
Thoracotomy	Demmy et al. [23]	Supportive
Rib fractures	Wulf et al. [24]	Supportive
	Graziotti and Smith [25]	
	Knottenbelt et al. [26]	
Chronic pain	Reiestad et al. [27]	Supportive
	Reiestad et al. [28]	
	Perkins [29]	
	Dionne [30]	
	Fineman [31]	
	Lema et al. [32]	
	Main [33]	
	Myers and Lema [34]	
	Ahlburg et al. [35]	

cholecystectomies. Tyagi et al. studied the effects of intrapleural block in patients undergoing open cholecystectomy. He found that patients undergoing general anesthesia, with a preemptive intrapleural block, had lower mean systolic and diastolic blood pressures, improved hemodynamic stability, and utilized less isoflurane compared to a group who just received general anesthesia without an intrapleural block [7]. Another study on a patient undergoing open cholecystectomy found effective postoperative pain control for 24 h after receiving an intrapleural injection preop of 20 ml of 0.5 % bupivacaine in divided doses and postop an infusion of 0.125 % bupivacaine at a rate of 10 ml/h through a catheter [8]. In contrast, a study by Yaseen comparing the number of dermatomes blocked and time to regression of block between a group receiving an intrapleural block and a group receiving intercostal blocks found that the intercostal block group had more dermatomes blocked and had a more gradual regression of their block than did the group receiving an intrapleural block [9]. In contrast to open cholecystectomy, there has been less research investigating the use of intrapleural block following laparoscopic cholecystectomy. One such study found that intrapleural analgesia can be a very effective and safe method of pain control in patients undergoing laparoscopic cholecystectomy [10].

Liver

Intrapleural analgesia has also been found to be effective in cases involving percutaneous hepatobiliary drainage. A case study showed improved hemodynamic stability and lack of respiratory adverse effects in patients receiving intrapleural analgesia for percutaneous hepatobiliary drainage [11]. The same study also demonstrated lower pain intensity scores and less opioid requirement in patients receiving intrapleural analgesia during biliary drainage.

Renal

Intrapleural analgesia has also been found to be effective in patients undergoing percutaneous nephrostomy and nephrolithotomy. Studies in patients who received intrapleural analgesia have demonstrated adequate postop pain relief after percutaneous nephrostomy [12] and during extracorporeal shock wave lithotripsy [13, 14]. Two studies have found adequate pain relief without significant side effects in patients having undergone nephrectomies [15, 16].

Breast Surgeries

Intrapleural analgesia has been found to be effective in breast reconstructive surgeries. Colpaert found that in women undergoing latissimus dorsi flap reconstruction, patients who received intrapleural analgesia had lower morphine PCA requirements than patients who did not receive intrapleural analgesia. In addition, there were significantly lower levels of nausea and vomiting in the group having received the intrapleural analgesia [17]. Similar findings were reported by O'Donoghue who also found lower morphine requirements postop in patients who had received intrapleural analgesia both in the form of boluses and as a continuous infusion through the intrapleural catheter [18].

Coronary Artery Bypass Graft (CABG) Surgery

The role of intrapleural analgesia has also been investigated in regard to CABG. Ogus found that a group of patients, who had received boluses of 0.5 % bupivacaine every 6 h for 4 days after undergoing CABG, had shorter times to extubation, increased PaO_2 and decreased $PaCO_2$, and increased FEV1, FCV, VC, MVV, and FEF 25–75 %. In addition, they were found to have decreased postoperative opioid requirements and shorter ICU stays, although total hospital stay was unchanged [19].

Thoracotomy

The effectiveness of intrapleural analgesia in post-thoraco-tomy pain has shown mixed results. Overall, it appears that thoracic epidural analgesia or paravertebral blocks are more effective than intrapleural analgesia in relieving pain following thoracotomy. Yildirim compared intrapleural analgesia to thoracic epidural analgesia and found that those receiving thoracic epidural analgesia had better postop respiratory function, lower VAS pain scores, and better ABGs than those who received intrapleural analgesia [20]. Supporting this evidence, DeCosmo found that intrapleural analgesia was not as good as paravertebral blocks or thoracic epidural analgesia for patients with post-thoracotomy pain [21]. Similarly, Joshi found thoracic epidural analgesia or paravertebral blocks to be more effective than intercostal or intrapleural blocks in the management of thoracotomy patients. He concluded that intercostal blocks may be an alternative to thoracic epidural or paravertebral blocks in certain circumstances in which epidurals or paravertebral blocks were contraindicated but could not advocate intrapleural analgesia in such circumstances due to lack of effectiveness [22].

There has been a recent study which showed a possible role for intrapleural analgesia delivered via thoracostomy (chest) tube in patients undergoing non-rib-spreading thoracoscopy. Thirty patients with non-rib-spreading thoracoscopy were divided into three groups: those who did not receive any local anesthetic in the intrapleural block, those that received intermittent boluses of 30 ml of 0.25 % bupivacaine every 6 h, and those that received a continuous infusion of 0.25 % bupivacaine at 5 ml/h. He found that total VAS pain scores and fentanyl consumption were lower in the groups receiving intermittent boluses and continuous infusions than in the control group [23].

Rib Fractures

There have been many studies confirming the effectiveness of intrapleural analgesia in the treatment of multiple rib fractures [24–26]. Intrapleural analgesia may be particularly appealing in these cases as it may be difficult for the patient to assume a position enabling the placement of a thoracic epidural catheter. Additionally, if the patients already have a chest tube in place, a technique such that employed by Demmy could be utilized to avoid needle placement altogether [23].

Chronic Pain

Reistad et al. observed significant pain relief in upper extremity CRPS patients who had received five daily injections of

Table 38.2 Complications of intrapleural catheter placement and analgesia

Complications
Pneumothorax
Systemic local anesthetic toxicity
Catheter misplacement
Horner's syndrome
Phrenic nerve paralysis
Infection
Pleural effusion-serous or blood-stained
Intrabronchial injection
Ipsilateral bronchospasm
Cholestasis
Administrative error
Bronchopleural fistula
Direct myocardial depression

0.5 % bupivacaine through a catheter in the intrapleural space. Three of the seven patients were pain free for 4–10 months, while three of the other patients had minimal pain requiring no medications [27]. The same group later proved the effectiveness of intrapleural analgesia in the treatment of severe postherpetic neuralgia [28]. It has also been effective in the treatment of chronic ischemic pain of the upper limb [29] as well as various other pain states including tumors involving the brachial plexus [30], pain in the chest wall from metastatic bronchiogenic carcinoma [31], esophageal cancer [32], esophageal rupture [33], and chronic pain in terminally ill patients with pancreatic, renal cell, breast cancer, and lymphomas [34]. In addition, it has been found to be effective in patients with upper abdominal cancers and benign and neoplastic pancreatic pain [35, 36].

Contraindications and Complications

Overall, intrapleural catheter placement and infusion of local anesthetic into the intrapleural space is safe and well tolerated. One of the primary complications of the block may be pneumothorax, although other potential complications exist (Table 38.2). One of the potential advantages of intrapleural analgesia over other techniques (thoracic epidural analgesia, paravertebral) is that there are fewer contraindications, especially if the plan is to deliver intrapleural analgesia via a catheter through an existing thoracostomy tube (Table 38.3)

Technique

Spread of local anesthetic within the intrapleural space is determined by gravity and to a lesser extent the volume of anesthetic and location of the catheter. Intrapleural catheters are most commonly placed posteriorly with the patient in the lateral or semi-prone position. They have also been placed

Table 38.3 Contraindications to intrapleural analgesia

Absolute contraindications

Patient refusal

Allergy to local anesthetic

Extensive infection at block or catheter site

Relative contraindications

Emphysema

Bullous lung disease

Recent pulmonary infection or empyema

Pleural adhesions or pleurodesis

Hemothorax

Coagulopathy

Contralateral phrenic nerve paralysis

near the midaxillary line or anteriorly with the patient supine. The most important aspect of this technique is detection of negative intrapleural pressure. Therefore, the technique should be performed in awake patients either pre- or postoperatively or in patients under general anesthesia who are breathing spontaneously. Placement should be avoided during positive pressure ventilation, because the intrapleural pressure is no longer negative, thereby making this risk of pneumothorax or tension pneumothorax greater.

The technique used and thus the patient position should be based on the selection of nerves that are to be blocked. To treat sympathetically mediated pain of the upper extremity, the patient should be placed with the affected side up in order to block the lower cervical and upper thoracic sympathetic chains. After injecting the anesthetic solution, the patient should be placed in the head-down position in order to avoid block of the thoracic somatic nerves. In order to obtain a block of the thoracic somatic nerves including the thoracic spinal nerves and corresponding intercostal nerves, as well as the thoracic sympathetic chain, the patient is placed in the oblique position with the affected side down and the patient's back propped up against a pillow to encourage pooling of the anesthetic into the intrapleural gutter next to the thoracic spine. This will allow the anesthetic to maximally cover both the somatic and sympathetic nerves. If the patient cannot lie on the affected side secondary to rib fractures or other issues, the catheter can be placed with the patient in the sitting position or with the affected side up. After the injection, the patient can be placed supine and tilted away from the affected side to allow the flow of the anesthetic toward the intrapleural gutter next to the thoracic spine.

As described by Waldman [37], once the patient is in the appropriate position, the 8th rib is identified on the affected side. Next, the skin is marked at a site 10 cm from the origin of the rib. This area is prepped and draped in a sterile manner. The index and middle finger are then placed on the rib bracketing the side of needle insertion. This area is then anesthetized with local anesthetic, such as 1 % lidocaine. An 18-gauge, 9-cm-styletted Hustead or Touhy needle is then inserted through the previously anesthetized area. The needle is advanced perpendicular to the skin, aiming for the middle of the rib that is being bracketed by the ring and middle fingers. The needle usually hits bone at approximately ½ inch. Additional anesthetic is usually required at this point secondary to the sensitivity of the periosteum. After hitting bone, the needle is withdrawn slightly and walked off the superior margin of the rib, avoiding trauma to the neurovascular bundle that lies beneath the rib. In contrast to individual intercostal nerve blocks, where the entry point is at the inferior border of the rib, the entry point for intrapleural analgesia should be at the *superior* border of the rib to avoid trauma to the intercostal nerve and blood vessels by the large Touhy needle. As soon as bony contact is lost, the stylet is removed and the needle is attached to either a well-lubricated 5-ml syringe with a plunger containing air or 0.9 % preservative-free saline with the plunger removed. The needle and syringe are slowly advanced toward the intrapleural space. The needle is then "walked off" the superior edge of the rib. It should be advanced either just past the posterior intercostal membrane or between the parietal and the visceral pleural space. When the needle is positioned just past the posterior intercostal membrane, a "pop" is often felt. In contrast, when the needle is positioned between the parietal and visceral pleurae, a loss of resistance is encountered that is similar to that of epidural anesthesia. The pleural pressure remains negative throughout the respiratory cycle, whereas the pressure in the intercostal space oscillates from negative to positive at the end of inspiration and expiration, respectively. Spontaneous ventilation should be maintained during the procedure. Controlled ventilation increases the risk of tension pneumothorax during positive pressure ventilation. At this point, the plunger of the syringe, if utilizing the air method, will usually advance under its own response to the negative pressure of the intrapleural space. The syringe is then removed, and a catheter is advanced 6–8 cm into the intrapleural space. If utilizing the saline method, the column of saline in the syringe will fall once the intrapleural space has been identified. A catheter is then passed through the open-ended syringe barrel, through the saline and needle, and into the intrapleural space. The advantage of the saline technique is that no air is introduced or allowed to be entrained into the intrapleural space.

After careful aspiration for heme or air, the catheter is taped in place with sterile tape and the patient is placed in the appropriate position to allow block of the appropriate nerves. Twenty to 30 ml of local anesthetic can be injected in divided doses with negative aspiration between doses and with careful observation for signs of local anesthetic toxicity. If a higher concentration of local anesthetic is used, such as 0.5 % bupivacaine, then smaller volumes, such as 10–12 ml, can be used. Alternatively, a continuous infusion can be given via a pump. If long-term use is anticipated, the catheter should be tunneled to reduce the risk of infection. Plasma concentration of the local anesthetic peaks at 15–20 min after injection. Adding epinephrine to the solution slightly delays and reduces peak plasma concentration. For continuous infusion, a rate of 0.125 ml/kg/h is usually employed (10 ml/h for an 80-k patient).

The technique for tunneling the catheter can be performed as follows [37]. After the Touhy or Hustead needle has contacted bone at approximately ½ in., and with the needle still in place, a #15 blade scalpel is used to dissect all the subcutaneous connective tissue away from the needle. A small curved clamp can then be placed into the incision, and a small pocket is created overlying the superior part of the interspace that is made by blunt dissection. This technique will allow the catheter to lie in the subcutaneous space without kinking. After the pocket is made, the needle is removed, and a malleable tool is bent in the contour of the patient's chest wall. The tunneling device is then inserted in the subcutaneous pocket and guided laterally around the chest wall. The tunneling device is guided to the anterior chest wall. When it reaches its exit point, it is turned away from the patient so that the sharp tip is against the patient's skin. A scalpel is then used to cut down onto the tip. The tip of the tunneling device is then advanced through this exit incision and covered with a sterile dressing.

The styletted Touhy or Hustead needle is then reintroduced into the subcutaneous pocket and advanced until contact with the rib is made again. The needle is then slightly withdrawn and walked superiorly off the rib, again to avoid trauma to the neurovascular bundle. Once bony contact is made, the stylet is removed and the syringe attached. The needle is advanced until the tip penetrates the parietal pleura at which point a "pop" is usually felt. At this point, the plunger of the syringe will usually advance secondary to negative pressure of the intrapleural space. The syringe is removed, and a catheter is advanced 6–8 cm into the intrapleural space. The needle is then removed and withdrawn over the catheter. The catheter is aspirated. If no air or heme is identified, the distal end of the catheter is attached to the proximal end of the tunneling device. The tunneling device is then withdrawn from the exit incision, bringing the catheter with it into the subcutaneous tunnel. After the distal end of the catheter is drawn through the tunnel, the tunneling device is removed and the remaining catheter is withdrawn until the excess catheter falls into the subcutaneous pocket. An injection port is then attached to the distal end of the catheter. The port can then be injected with saline to ensure the integrity to the catheter. If the catheter injects easily without leakage, the midline incision can be closed. It can be closed with two layers of 4-0 nylon sutures. One must be careful to avoid damage to the catheter during closure of the incision. The catheter is then taped in place, and the patient

should be turned to the appropriate position in order to block the desired nerves.

Another technique was described for use during breast reconstructions [17]. In this study, the intrapleural space was identified using a variation of a technique described by Scott [38]. In this technique, the analgesia is given after the patient has been anesthetized under general anesthesia. The patient is positioned supine. The midaxillary line at the 4th or 5th intercostal space is identified. A 16G Touhy epidural needle is connected to a three-way tap, a fluid-giving set, and a bag of saline, which is suspended at least 60 cm above the patient. Under sterile conditions, the needle is inserted perpendicularly to the skin until the negative pressure of the intrapleural space is reached and saline starts running into the cavity. This is visible through the drip chamber in the infusion line. In this study, they used the three-way stop cock in order to facilitate consecutive bolus injection of local anesthetic and passage of a flexible epidural catheter for continuous infusion. While the catheter is being inserted, the proximal part of the needle is held downward to act as a water tap and avoid air entrapment. The procedure takes about 10 min.

An alternative approach in patient who has a chest tube in place is to infuse the local anesthetic through a catheter placed in the chest tube. For this technique, a 20-gauge epidural catheter with a flexible tip can be utilized. This catheter is inserted through the previously placed chest tube. The stiffness of this catheter allows for better advancement within the intrapleural space. The catheter can be inserted approximately 4–5 cm. After insertion, local anesthetic can be infused. It is important to clamp the chest tube temporarily (approximately 20 min) after infusion of the local anesthetic to prevent the local anesthetic from being removed to the suction of the chest tube.

Bupivacaine and lidocaine are two of the more commonly used agents for intrapleural analgesia. The most common agent appears to be 0.25 % or 0.5 % bupivacaine. These concentrations can either be delivered as a single injection or as a repeated bolus. Typical quantities include10–40 ml/injection. A single injection of 20 ml of 0.5 % bupivacaine with 5 mcg/ml of epinephrine has been found to reliably produce a cutaneous sensory block from T4 to T10 but has even been reported to produce cutaneous sensory block from T1–T12 [38]. The onset using this quantity and concentration of bupivacaine is usually within about 1–3 min. Complete pain relief has been achieved in about 30 min, and the analgesic duration is about 7 h. If a continuous infusion is to be used, lower concentrations from 0.125 to 0.375 % bupivacaine are typically chosen. The infusion is usually started after a bolus of 20 ml of 0.5 % bupivacaine [17].

Lidocaine 2 % with 1:200,000 epinephrine has not been found to produce consistent dermatomal analgesic levels.

Opioids can be added to the local anesthetic to improve pain control and to decrease the need to systemic narcotics.

Intrapleural opioids may act on opioid receptors in peripheral nerves.

Clonidine has also been used safely in the intrapleural space to increase the effectiveness with intrapleural analgesia.

Future Direction

More studies are needed to determine the overall clinical effectiveness of intrapleural catheters in various chronic pain conditions. Research should focus on alternatives to bupivacaine including NMDA receptor antagonists, steroids, or alpha-2 agonists as potential therapeutic options. In addition, ultrasound-guided intrapleural blocks may be a safer approach to lessen the risk on pneumothorax.

Summary/Conclusions

In summary, intrapleural analgesia is a relatively simple technique that can be used in a variety of situations for many diverse pain states. It has been proven to provide excellent analgesia over the chest wall and upper abdomen. It is generally a safe and easy procedure to perform, especially in cases where epidural analgesia may be difficult or contraindicated. The anatomy of the intrapleural space allows different types of nerve fibers to be anesthetized such as somatic, sympathetic, intercostal, and paravertebral nerves thereby increasing its overall utility in a variety of painful conditions. A variety of substances can be employed to achieve analgesia such as bupivacaine, ropivacaine, clonidine, or opioids. The technique rarely leads to systemic toxicity and has been shown to improve a variety of respiratory parameters in certain conditions [39]. At the current time, it appears that thoracic epidural analgesia and paravertebral blocks offer superior analgesia to intrapleural catheter infusion of local anesthetic for thoracotomy. However, intrapleural catheter infusions offer an alternative technique that remains a viable option for a variety of pain states, especially if contraindications exist to other techniques.

References

1. Reistad F, Stromskag KE. Intrapleural catheter in the management of postoperative pain: a preliminary report. Reg Anaesth. 1986;11:89–91.
2. Mandl F. Aqueous solution of phenol as substitute for alcohol in sympathetic block. J Int Coll Surg. 1950;13:566–72.
3. Stromskag KE, Minor B, et al. Side effects and complications related to intrapleural analgesia: an update. Acta Anaesthesiol Scand. 1990;34:473–7.
4. Wallach HW. Interpleural therapy with tetracycline and lidocaine for malignant pleural effusion. Chest. 1978;73:246.
5. Kvalheim L, Reiestad F. Interpleural catheter in the management of postoperative pain. Anesthesiology. 1984;61:A231.
6. Nunn JF, Slavin G. Posterior intercostal nerve block for pain relief after cholecystectomy. Anatomical basis and efficacy. Br J Anaesth. 1980;52:253–60.
7. Tyagi A, Sethi A, et al. Effect of preemptive intepleural block on the haemodynamic parameters during open cholecystectomy. J Anesthesiol Clin Pharmacol. 2007;23(1):47–52.
8. Shrestha BR, Tabadar S, et al. Interpleural catheter technique for perioperative pain management. Kathmandu Univ Med J. 2003;1(1):46–7.
9. Yaseen SS, Naqash I, et al. Interpleural block and intercostal block for postoperative pain relief following cholecystectomy: a comparative study. Indian J Anaesth. 1999;43(2):31–4.
10. Dravid RM, Mohroof R, et al. Interpleural block for day case laparoscopic cholecystectomy. J One Day Surg. 2006;16 Suppl 1:A2.
11. Therasse E, Choiniere M, et al. Percutaneous biliary drainage: clinical trial of analgesia with interpleural block. Radiology. 1997;205:663–8.
12. Trivedi N, Robalino J. Interpleural block: a new technique for regional anaesthesia during percutaneous nephrostomy and nephrolithotomy. Can J Anaesth. 1990;37(4 Pt 1):479–81.
13. Stromskag KE, Steen PA. Comparison of interpleural and epidural anesthesia for extracorporeal shock wave lithotripsy. Anaesth Analg. 1988;67:1181–3.
14. Reistad F, McIlvaine WB. Interpleural anesthesia for extracorporeal shock wave lithotripsy. Anaesth Analg. 1989;69:551–2.
15. Baude C, Long D, et al. Postoperative analgesia for nephrectomy. Cah Anesthesiol. 1991;39:533–6.
16. Greif R, Wasinger T, et al. Pleural bupivacaine for pain treatment after nephrectomy. Anesth Analg. 1999;89:440–3.
17. Colpaert SD, Smith PD, et al. Interpleural analgesia in breast reconstruction. Scand J Plast Reconstr Surg Hand Surg. 2008;42(1):32–7.
18. O'Donoghue J, Bahia H, et al. Intrapleural bupivacaine in latissimus dorsi breast reconstruction. Ann Plast Surg. 2008;61(3):252–5.
19. Ogus H, Selimoglu O. Effects of intrapleural analgesia on pulmonary function and postoperative pain in patients with chronic obstructive pulmonary disease undergoing coronary artery bypass graft surgery. J Cardiothorax Anaesth. 2007;21(6):816–9.
20. Yildirim V, Akay HT, et al. Interpleural versus epidural analgesia with ropivacaine for postthoracotomy pain and respiratory function. J Clin Anesth. 2007;19(7):506–11.
21. De Cosmo G, Aceto P, et al. Analgesia in thoracic surgery: a review. Minerva Anestesiol. 2009;75(6):393–400.
22. Joshi G, Bonnet F, et al. A systematic review of randomized trials evaluating regional techniques for postthoracotomy analgesia. Anesth Analg. 2008;107(3):1026–40.
23. Demmy T, Nwogu C, et al. Chest tube-delivered bupivacaine improves pain and decreases opioid use after thoracoscopy. Ann Thorac Surg. 2009;87:1040–7.
24. Wulf H, Jeckstrom W, et al. Intrapleural catheter analgesia in patients with multiple rib fractures. Anaesthetsist. 1991;40:19–24.
25. Graziotti P, Smith GB. Multiple fractures ribs and head injury-an indication for intercostal catheterisation and infusion of local anaesthetics. Anaesthesia. 1988;43:964–6.
26. Knottenbelt JD, James MF, et al. Intrapleural bupivacaine analgesia in hest trauma: a randomized double-blind controlled trial. Injury. 1991;22:114–6.
27. Reiestad F, McIlvaine WB, et al. Interpleural analgesia in treatment of upper extremity reflex sympathetic dystrophy. Anesth Analg. 1989;69:671–3.
28. Reistad F, McIlvaine WB, et al. Interpleural analgesia in the treatment of severe post-herpetic neuralgia. Reg Anesth. 1990;15:113.
29. Perkins G. Interpleural anaesthesia in the management of upper limb ischaemia. A report of three cases. Anaesth Intensive Care. 1991;19:575–8.

30. Dionne C. Tumour invasion of the brachia plexus: management of pain with interpleural analgesia. Can J Anaesth. 1992;39:520–1.

31. Fineman SP. Long-term post-thoracotomy cancer pain management with interpleural bupivacaine. Anesth Analg. 1989;68:694–7.

32. Lema MJ, Myers DP, et al. Pleural phenol therapy for the treatment of chronic oesophageal cancer pain. Reg Anaesth. 1992;17:166–70.

33. Main A. interpleural analgesia in the management of oesophageal perforation. Reg Anaesth. 1997;22:185–7.

34. Myers DP, Lema MJ. Interpleural analgesia for treatment of severe cancer pain in terminally ill patients. J Pain Symptom Manag. 1993;8:505–10.

35. Ahlburg P, Noreng M, et al. Treatment of pancreatic pain with interpleural bupivacaine: an open trial. Acta Anaesth Scand. 1990;34:156–7.

36. Reistad F, McIlvaine WB, et al. Successful treatment of chronic pancreatitis pain with intrapleural analgesia. Can J Anaesth. 1989;36:713–6.

37. Waldman S. Atlas of interventional pain management. 2nd ed. Philadelphia: Saunders; 2004.

38. Scott PV. Interpleural regional analgesia: detection of the interpleural space by saline infusion. Br J Anaesth. 1991;66:131–3.

39. Cheng J, Cata J. Interpleural analgesia. In: Smith H, editor. Current therapy in pain. Philadelphia: Saunders Elsevier; 2008. p. 92–5. http://books.google.com/books?id=U1ecpLvPiAIC&pg=PA92&lpg=PA92&dq=cheng+j+interpleural+analgesia&source=bl&ots=gLyNzHFvK6&sig=4Op4iNaSF0WHm-zqUovMEx2vD_g&hl=en&sa=X&ei=84WAUPaUKJTy8ATWjoHwAQ&ved=0CEsQ6AEwBQ#v=onepage&q=cheng%20j%20interpleural%20analgesia&f=false.

Epidural Lysis of Adhesions: Percutaneous and Endoscopic Techniques

39

Timothy Y. Ko and Salim M. Hayek

Key Points

- The purpose of using the lysis of adhesion technique is to bypass scar tissue and improve delivery of high concentrations of injected medications to the targeted area.
- The ideal patient would be one who may be suffering with more radicular symptoms from epidural fibrosis in close proximity to a nerve root.
- Identifying filling deficits that correlate well with patient's symptoms improves the likelihood of success.
- Minimizing the amount of adjustments to the catheter in the needle reduces the risk of equipment malfunction and risk to the patient.
- Resistance to the advancing catheter or epiduroscope should be respected as force may result in a complication.

Introduction

Epidural lysis of adhesions is an interventional technique that was initially described in 1989 [1]. It was designed to address refractory low back and leg pain due to epidural scarring by delivering high concentrations of injectable medication to targeted areas. These areas of scar tissue develop due to many reasons including postsurgical resection and chemical irritation from leaking nucleus pulposus. The contribution of epidural fibrosis to intractable low back pain and lumbosacral neuritis has been debated [2]. Kuslich and colleagues [3] performed an extensive evaluation on the origins of lumbar back pain throughout 193 operations under progressive local anesthesia delivered sequentially to different surgical planes. Back pain could be mostly reproduced by stimulation of the outer layer of the annulus fibrosis and the posterior longitudinal ligament. Sciatica could only be reproduced by stimulation of swollen, restricted, or compressed nerve roots. While epidural fibrosis itself was not painful, patients that had prior laminectomies were found to have perineural fibrosis that lead to painful and sensitive nerve roots [3]. The lysis of these adhesions has been reported to reduce pain in several prospective studies and systematic reviews [4–7].

The rate of lumbar spine surgery has grown exponentially in Western culture [8–10]. Studies like Weinstein and colleagues' Spine Patient Outcomes Research Trial (SPORT) have suggested a central role for spinal surgeries [11]. In their 4-year combined as-treated analysis, patients who underwent spine surgery for a herniated disk achieved greater improvement than the nonoperative cohort in all primary and secondary outcomes except work status. With this growth in surgical intervention, the number of failed back surgery syndrome has become an increasingly common diagnosis [12] for the interventional pain physician to treat. There is quite a range of treatment modalities for intractable back pain in patients who have had previous spine surgery. Conservative treatments include physical therapy, biofeedback, medication management, and epidural steroids. The use of epidural steroid injections for managing this syndrome is very common; unfortunately, only a moderate proportion of these patients have shown long-term and functional improvement in the failed back surgery population [13, 14]. Two recent studies do show some promise with the use of caudal epidural steroid injections in the failed back surgery and spinal stenosis populations [15, 16]. The purpose of using a lysis of adhesion technique is to bypass scar tissue and improve delivery of high concentrations of medications of injected drugs to the

T.Y. Ko, M.D. (✉)
LakeHealth Department of Anesthesiology, Division of Pain Medicine, Pinnacle Interventional Pain and Spine Consultants, 7580 Auburn Road, Suite 102, Concord Township, OH 44077, USA
e-mail: timothyko@pinnaclepainOH.com

S.M. Hayek, M.D., Ph.D.
Department of Anesthesiology, Case Western Reserve University, Division of Pain Medicine University Hospitals, 11100 Euclid Avenue, Cleveland, OH 44106, USA
e-mail: salim.hayek@uhhospitals.org

T.R. Deer et al. (eds.), *Comprehensive Treatment of Chronic Pain by Medical, Interventional, and Integrative Approaches,*
DOI 10.1007/978-1-4614-1560-2_39, © American Academy of Pain Medicine 2013

targeted area. The evidence for percutaneous lysis of epidural adhesions has been found to be moderate to strong in managing the pain for post-lumbar spine surgery syndrome [4, 13].

Indications for Epidural Lysis of Adhesions

Lysis of adhesions is a more advanced technique to provide relief of pain. Typically, it is preceded by more conservative treatments including physical therapy, transcutaneous electrical nerve stimulation, anti-inflammatories, muscle relaxants, membrane stabilizers, and traditional epidural corticosteroid injections. Once these have demonstrated failure, then consideration of this technique should be discussed with the patient. Ideally, this procedure was designed to aid in the management of pain related to failed back surgery syndrome, chemically sensitive disks, and other scenarios where epidural fibrosis and inflammation occur [17]. The ideal patient would be one who may be suffering with more radicular symptoms from epidural fibrosis in close proximity to a nerve root. The placement of the catheter or endoscope into this area allows for appropriate adhesiolysis and relief of pain. Indications for epidural lysis of adhesions according to the originator of this technique include post-laminectomy syndrome, disk disruption, metastatic carcinoma of the spine, multilevel degenerative arthritis, facet pain, spinal stenosis, and pain unresponsive to spinal cord stimulation and spinal opioids [18]. Caution should be used when selecting patients in order to improve overall outcome and reduction of complications.

Contraindications for Epidural Lysis of Adhesions

The usual absolute contraindications for interventional pain techniques exist and are as follows: sepsis, chronic infection, coagulopathy, local infection at site of the procedure, and patient refusal. Relative contraindications to consider include arachnoiditis or any other situation where there is significant disruption in the tissue planes in close proximity to the dura. There is an increased risk of inadvertent subdural administration of these medications that can lead to complications. One may consider referring appropriate candidates to practitioners with more experience in this technique.

Patient Preparation

The risks, benefits, and alternatives to the procedure should be explained in great detail to the prospective patient. An informed consent should be signed with the patient. The obvious benefits are pain relief and improved physical function. There is a possibility for reversal of some neurological symptoms. The usual risks include bleeding, infection, and reaction to any of the injected medications. Other risks include worsening of pain, no pain relief at all, damage to blood vessels, and dural puncture which may lead to a spinal headache.

A complete history and physical with well-documented neurological and/or urological findings should be documented before endeavoring with this technique. Appropriate imaging such as MRI, CT scans, and even CT myelograms are helpful, but epidural fibrosis is best diagnosed when performing an epidurogram with contrast and live fluoroscopy [19, 20]. Visualizing filling deficits that correlate well with patient's symptoms improves the likelihood of success.

Medications for Neuroplasty

There are many combinations of local anesthetic and corticosteroid preparations for this procedure. None have been found to be superior over the other; therefore, the final combination can be left to the individual practitioner to decide upon.

Hypertonic Saline

Hypertonic saline induces a shift of fluid from an intracellular to extracellular space across an osmotic gradient it generates. Traditionally, the applications for its use have been using the intravenous route in trauma, hyponatremia, and shock.

In the epidural space, this promotes an increase in fluid and possible improvement in flow of fluid around nerve roots and fibrosis. Other mechanisms of action include selective C fiber blockade of dorsal rootlets that may be related to elevated chloride ion concentrations [21]. Other work, on frog spinal neurons, showed some activity on GABA receptors that depresses the lateral column evoked ventral root response with the overall reduction in spinal cord water volumes [22]. Efficacy of the use of hypertonic saline alone in the epidural space has been determined in several studies [23, 24].

Complications with the use of epidural hypertonic saline are found mostly with inadvertent intrathecal injection. These complications include hypertension, tachycardia, and tachypnea with pulmonary edema [25]. Management of these sequelae is supportive in nature and would require intensive monitoring as they may be severe and life threatening. It is imperative for careful determination of epidural injection of contrast to avoid this potential complication. A dural puncture should postpone continuation of this procedure.

Hyaluronidase

Hyaluronidase is used for its ability to purportedly disrupt epidural adhesions. It catalyzes the hydrolysis of hyaluronic acid which is a major constituent in human tissue. This increases permeability in tissue planes and aids in the dispersement and delivery of medication. Hyaluronidase disrupts the proteoglycan ground substance in the adhesions of the epidural space and facilitates subsequent injections of local anesthetic and corticosteroids through the matrix. It does not affect collagen fibers [26]. Currently, there are animal-derived hyaluronidase available (Hydase TM – PrimaPharm Inc, Vitrase – ISTA Pharmaceuticals, and Amphadase – Amphastar Pharmaceuticals) as well as an FDA-approved (for subcutaneous administration) recombinant "human" hyaluronidase (Hylenex – Halozyme Therapeutics). Some potential risk arises as some patients may be allergic to these preparations, particularly the purified animal preparation which may have limited their use especially in the pediatric population [27, 28]. The use of human recombinant hyaluronidase is less likely to cause allergic reaction as it has up to 100 times greater purity than the reference standard, animal-derived formulation based on enzymatic activity [29, 30]. Reported allergic reactions include erythema at the site to urticaria and angioedema in those patients receiving human recombinant hyaluronidase (less than 0.1 %) [31].

The addition of hyaluronidase as part of the injected medications into the epidural space is controversial. Early studies comparing its use in adhesiolysis revealed a trend in the data toward reducing the need for additional treatments, but no evidence to support its exclusive use was found [7]. In fact, many subsequent studies and techniques were performed with only hypertonic saline [23, 24]. Subsequent systematic reviews also have not shown analgesic efficacy evidence from the addition of hyaluronidase [5, 32]. Emerging studies are showing some benefit of the addition of hyaluronidase to hypertonic saline, local anesthetics, and corticosteroids. Of note, all available studies have looked at hyaluronidase isolated from animal sources (bovine testes).

Yousef and colleagues [26] reported a prospective double-blinded, randomized study evaluating the addition of hyaluronidase to a typical caudal epidural steroid injection with hypertonic saline for patients with failed back surgery syndrome. They found that addition of hyaluronidase significantly reduced pain in long-term follow-up at 6 and 12 months compared to the hypertonic saline, local anesthetic, and corticosteroid group. Outcome measures included significant reduction of opioid and increased mobility in the lumbar spine [26]. Further study is needed in demonstrating a clear effect of hyaluronidase in lysis of epidural adhesions.

Technique

Two percutaneous methods will be described in the following sections. The first will be the Racz technique [33, 34]

performed over the course of 3 days, and the second will be a modified version proposed and studied by Manchikanti performed over the course of a single day. Numerous variations to these techniques have been proposed as well, including transforaminal approaches [34, 35].

The Racz Classical Technique

In the operating room:
1. The patient is placed into a prone position, and the general location of the sacral hiatus is prepared and draped in a sterile fashion. The appropriate amount of sedation can be administered based on physician and patient preference. The careful administration of midazolam and fentanyl is common practice, and the use of any stronger intravenous agents is usually unnecessary.
2. A local lidocaine anesthetic skin wheal is raised 1–2 cm inferior to the sacral hiatus. A small skin nick can be made with an 18-gauge needle to facilitate entrance of the larger epidural needle. A 15- or 16-gauge RK or Coudé epidural needle is placed into the sacral hiatus either using a midline approach or with an angle starting from the contralateral side of the suspected pathology. This initial angle allows for the final tip position to be biased toward the ipsilateral location of suspected fibrosis.
3. Fluoroscopy should be used first in a lateral approach to visualize the needle entry into the caudal space (Fig. 39.1). The needle can then be advanced in the anteroposterior view just below the S3 level to prevent accidental puncture of a low lying dura. Injection of a small amount of nonionic contrast can be used to ensure epidural location.
4. After negative aspiration for cerebrospinal fluid and blood, 5–10 ml of nonionic water soluble contrast (either Omnipaque 240 or Isovue 300) is injected smoothly under live fluoroscopy. An unremarkable epidurogram may have a "Christmas tree" pattern, the central canal making up the "trunk" of the tree and the nerve roots the "branches." An abnormal epidurogram will reveal filling deficits in areas of the presumed fibrosis (Fig. 39.2). This filling deficit should clinically correlate with the patient's symptoms before proceeding with the next step. There are some clinicians that perform the epidurogram after the catheter is in place by the suspected site of fibrosis (Fig. 39.3).
5. If the filling deficit correlates with symptoms, then a Racz Tun-L-Kath® or similar flexible catheter should be directed toward the area of filling deficits (Fig. 39.4). Placing a small bend to the tip of the catheter may improve the ability to steer toward these areas of filling deficits. A 30° bend in the first 1–2 cm of the catheter should be sufficient. Ventral placement of the catheter should be confirmed under lateral fluoroscopy.

Fig. 39.1 Lateral View: A 16 g Coude needle enters the caudal canal

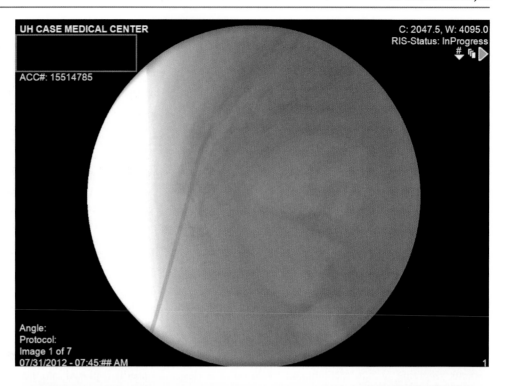

Fig. 39.2 Epidurogram: Injection of 2 ml of iohexol 240 with spread of contrast to L4/L5 junction with filling defect along right L5 nerve root

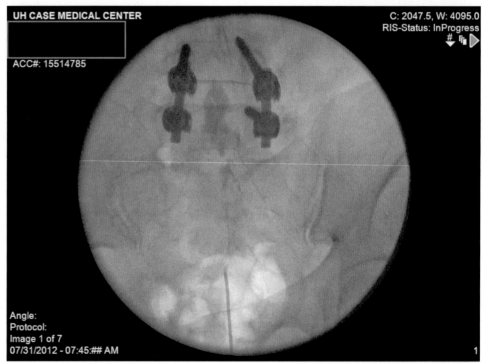

6. After correct placement, inject 10 ml of preservative-free normal saline with or without 1,500 units of hyaluronidase into the area surrounding the filling defect. Follow this with 2–3 ml more of contrast to visualize opening of the scarred area and spread of the injectate in the epidural space (Fig. 39.5).

7. Prepare a 10-ml syringe of 9 ml of 0.5 % lidocaine and 40 mg/ml of triamcinolone diacetate. Other common corticosteroid preparations include 40–80 mg methylprednisolone (Depo-Medrol®), 25–50 mg triamcinolone diacetate (Aristocort®), 40–80 mg triamcinolone acetonide (Kenalog®), and 6–12 mg betamethasone (Celestone Soluspan®) [36]. Administer a 3-ml test dose and wait for several minutes to confirm no signs of intrathecal injection. Resume the smooth injection of the rest of the syringe if the test dose reveals no untoward signs.

Fig. 39.3 Lateral View: The Racz catheter is advanced into the anterior epidural space until resistance is met

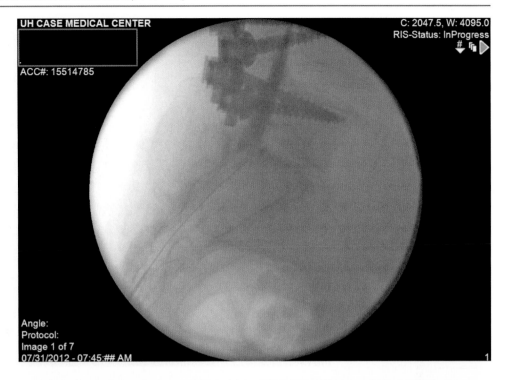

Fig. 39.4 AP View: The Racz catheter is seated more towards the filling defect on the right. The bevel is biased to the right side

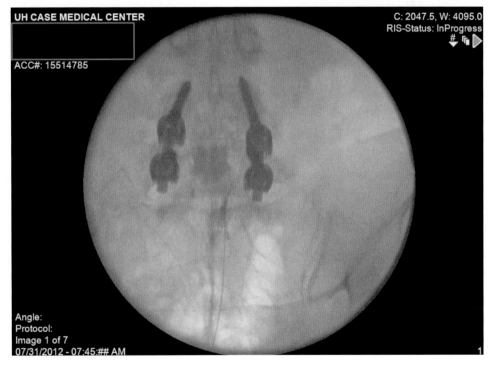

8. Remove the needle under live pulsed fluoroscopy and secure the catheter to the skin with tape. Place triple antibiotic ointment over the puncture site and place sterile dressings. Attach a bacteriostatic filter to the catheter.

In the postanesthesia care unit 20 min later:

1. Infuse 10 ml of 10 % hypertonic saline over the course of 30 min. If the patient complains of pain, add several ml of 0.5 % lidocaine, wait for 5 min, and then resume.

2. At the end of the infusion, flush the catheter with preservative-free normal saline.

On days 2 and 3:

1. Inject 10 ml of 0.5 % lidocaine, wait for 25–30 min, and then infuse 10 ml of 10 % hypertonic saline over 30 min.

2. Flush catheter with 2 ml of preservative-free NS.

3. Repeat above on day 3, remove catheter, and place sterile dressings.

Fig. 39.5 Repeat injection of local anesthetic with mechanical manipulation of catheter results in advancement of the catheter to top of L5 vertebral level

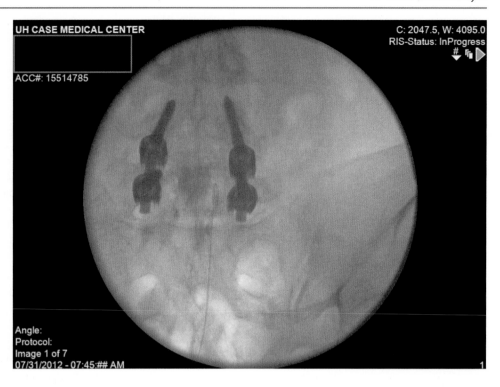

Modified Techniques [23] (Day 1)

The entrance into the caudal space is performed as described above. Adhesiolysis is carried out utilizing a Racz® catheter (EpiMed International, Inc.), with final positioning of the catheter on the side of the defect and the source of pain and an additional injection of contrast to identify successful adhesiolysis.

1. Following the completion of the adhesiolysis and repositioning of the catheter, an injection of 5 ml of lidocaine 1 % preservative-free with 6 mg of betamethasone phosphate acetate mixture should be injected.
2. After waiting 10–15 min, provided that there is no evidence of subarachnoid blockade, 6 ml 10 % sodium chloride solution in two divided doses of 3 ml over 10–15 min is administered. The catheter is then removed, and the patient may be discharged home when stable.

Endoscopic Lysis of Adhesions

The first in vivo exam of the spinal canal was performed by J. L. Pool in 1937 and was complicated by hemorrhage. Through persistence and refinement of his technique, he was able to document over 400 cases by 1942 with successful observation and identification of neuritis, herniated nucleus pulposus, hypertrophied ligamentum flavum, neoplasms, and arachnoid adhesions [37, 38].

Further improvements in endoscopy and fiber-optic light sources improved percutaneous placement. Ooi and

Morisaki from Japan were credited for these advancements throughout the 1960s and 1970s [37]. Shimoji and associates were the first to report the concomitant use of fiber-optic light sources and flexible fiber-optic catheters instead of rigid metal endoscopes. Fluoroscopy was used in conjunction with their technique which aided in identifying the spinal level in view. Significant anatomical findings including aseptic adhesive arachnoiditis and clumped nerve roots were also visualized with the use of this new technology [39]. Epiduroscopy may be useful in confirming a physiological basis for radiculitis when other diagnostic studies such as MRI are negative [37]. Direct visualization can be used to confirm clinical observations that may not otherwise be discovered by traditional tests. This would be a strong indication to use this technique over a percutaneous route if the practitioner has had appropriate training and experience.

Endoscopic Technique

The patient is placed into a prone position. Standard American Society of Anesthesiology recommendations for moderate sedation should be used. Prophylactic antibiotics should be administered prior to the start of the procedure.

1. After proper sterile preparation and draping, a skin wheal is raised over the sacral hiatus using 1–2 ml of 1 % lidocaine with a 25-gauge needle. A 16-gauge RK needle is then advanced into the hiatus under lateral and AP fluoroscopy.

2. An epidurogram is then performed with the injection of 10 ml of nonionic contrast dye.
3. A 0.9-mm guide wire is inserted through the needle, which is then advanced under fluoroscopic guidance to the level of suspected pathology and contrast filling defect. This is followed by a small incision with a #11 blade and advancement of a 9-French dilator with catheter (sheath) over the guide wire.
4. Once the catheter is advanced to the tip of the guide wire, the wire is removed. Following this, a 0.8-mm fiber-optic spinal endoscopic video-guided system is introduced into the catheter through the valve and is advanced until the tip is positioned at the distal end of the catheter, as determined by video and fluoroscopic images. The endoscope should be placed ventrolaterally toward the suspected side of the lesion.
5. In conjunction with gentle irrigation using normal saline, the catheter and fiber-optic endoscope are manipulated and rotated in multiple directions, with visualization of the nerve roots at various levels. Gentle irrigation is carried out by slow, controlled infusion. It is recommended that the infusion rate of saline irrigation should not exceed 30 ml/min and that the total infused volume should be less than 100 ml. (There will be retrograde flow that should not be counted toward the total volume) [37]. For prolonged cases with larger irrigation volumes, a continuous subarachnoid needle may be placed for continuous CSF pressure monitoring. Adhesiolysis and decompression are carried out by distension of the epidural space with normal saline and by mechanical means utilizing the fiber-optic endoscope. Visualization will be achieved only if the epidural space is kept distended by repeated injections of saline. Some structures that may be easily visualized include the dura mater.
6. Confirmation is accomplished with the injection of nonionic contrast material, and an epidurogram is performed on at least two occasions. Following completion of the procedure, generally, lidocaine 1 %, preservative-free, mixed with 6–12 mg of betamethasone acetate or 40–80 mg of methylprednisolone is injected after assuring that there is no evidence of subarachnoid leakage of contrast.
7. If pathology is determined to be at multiple levels, the procedure can be carried out at multiple levels, and the injectate should be injected in divided doses.

Complications

The usual risks of an invasive epidural procedure exist. The most commonly reported complications in percutaneous and endoscopic adhesiolysis include dural puncture, bleeding, infection, damage to blood vessels and nerves, unintentional dural puncture, inadvertent injection of medications, and catheter shearing [40].

Catheter shearing can occur as a result of frequent adjustment of the catheter against the needle. A Tuohy needle should not be used for this procedure as the back edge of the needle is a cutting surface and would shear the catheter [33]. Methods to minimize this include placement of the initial needle tip in the direction of the suspected lesion. This will minimize the amount of times the catheter will need to be adjusted and steered. Catheter shearing can present a problem of retained hardware. Removal of the catheter can require surgical intervention or the use of epidural endoscopy. Manchikanti described a case where this occurred, and the use of endoscopy alone was not sufficient, ultimately arthroscopy forceps where utilized to remove the catheter [41].

Other cases have been reported where fragments of the Racz catheter were sheared off and trapped in an L5-S1 foramen. Karaman and colleagues report on an incident where the catheter fragment was left in position in the epidural space. Careful monthly follow-up for a year revealed the patient to respond well to the neurolysis, and a decision was made to forgo an aggressive surgical resection to recover the very small fragment [42].

Until recently, there had been no published reports of serious side effects like arachnoiditis, paralysis, or bowel or bladder dysfunction. Justiz and colleagues describe the case of a 73-year-old woman who opted for endoscopic lysis of adhesions for severe scarring of the epidural space. Subsequently, the patient developed a neurogenic bladder with urinary retention. Three years later, she experienced resolution of the neurogenic bladder symptoms that coincided with the use of the antibiotic nitrofurantoin. Upon discontinuation of the antibiotic, the patient noted that she was unable to void spontaneously. With reinstitution of nitrofurantoin, the patient was once again able to void effectively and has been maintained on nitrofurantoin for >3 years [2].

Infection is a frequent concern when performing any neuraxial technique. Strict aseptic technique should be standard practice; however, infections still occur. Meningitis is a rare but reported complication of this particular procedure as well. Wagner and colleagues reported an incidence of severe meningitis with significant neurological sequelae after an epidural lysis of adhesions for unspecific low back pain. They cautioned that this procedure should be done under strict aseptic technique [43]. It is recommended to proceed with careful patient selection before embarking on this intervention to reduce overall complications.

The risk of damage to blood vessels is usually determined during administration of contrast. Venous uptake can be seen during live fluoroscopy and should prompt the interventionalist to adjust placement of the catheter accordingly especially if very little contrast remains in the epidural space after the injection. Arterial uptake should definitely prompt redirection of the catheter for fear of a thrombotic event if particulate steroid is injected. This seems to be a rare phenomenon either due to the elasticity of arterial walls in relation to the catheter or due to the overall prominence of venous vasculature in the caudal space.

Unintentional dural puncture can also be prevented using few precautions. The most important would be to avoid advancing the needle above the level of the S3 foramen as there is a chance of puncturing a low lying dura. The second manner would be to avoid advancing the catheter against resistance. Due to epidural fibrosis, the dural plane may become more distorted in relation to the epidural space. While the tips of the catheters are flexible, they are still able to puncture the dura given enough applied force. The injection of contrast will also be indicative of proper placement. If an inadvertent dural puncture occurs while performing a percutaneous adhesiolysis, the practitioner should consider canceling the procedure and reschedule for a future date.

During epiduroscopy, a dural puncture does not necessitate a mandatory cancelation of the case in the hands of expert practitioners. Shah and Heavner [44] reported two successful completions of endoscopic adhesiolysis and decompressive neuroplasty after inadvertent subarachnoid and subdural punctures with the endoscope. They were able to retract the endoscope and visualize the dural tears in each situation. The epidural catheter was then advanced into the epidural space and was confirmed under direct visualization and appropriate contrast flow identified epidural placement.

Complications may arise when direct visualization during epiduroscopy is compromised. The epidural space needs to be distended by repeated injection or infusion of saline to maximize the field of view. Careful monitoring of total volumes will prevent increased epidural pressures from developing. At times, the anatomical structures will be difficult to discern, and retraction of the endoscope may bring structures into view better. Easily recognized structures include dura mater, ligamentum flavum, epidural fat, fibrous connective tissue, and blood vessels. Spinal nerve roots may be difficult to identify. The concurrent use of fluoroscopic guidance can help identify the level being viewed on the screen and aid in orienting the interventionalist [37].

Complications may also arise when the cerebrospinal fluid pressure becomes elevated during epiduroscopy. The increase in epidural pressures is transmitted into the subarachnoid space to the optic nerve sheath, compressing the optic nerve and its vasculature. The vasculature compression ruptures retinal blood vessels, leading to retinal hemorrhage. In a review by Gill and colleagues, there have been only a dozen reported cases. The common finding was retinal hemorrhage with recovery occurring in 79.2 % of cases [45]. Bolus injections with or without epiduroscopy were considered the precipitating event. The volume varied between 20 and 120 ml of solution. To prevent this complication, it is recommended that the infusion rate of saline irrigation should not exceed 30 ml/min and that the total infused volume should be less than 100 ml [37]. For prolonged cases with larger irrigation volumes, a continuous subarachnoid needle may be placed for continuous CSF pressure monitoring.

Outcomes

There is some good evidence for short- and long-term relief with the use of percutaneous adhesiolysis. Unfortunately, there is still a paucity of literature in regard to the overall efficacy for this technique to solidify the role of adhesiolysis in the treatment algorithm of patients with intractable pain. Several randomized studies of this technique support its use in an interventionalist's armamentarium. Veihelmann et al. [46] evaluated 99 patients with chronic low back pain and sciatica (13 with prior back surgery). Nerve root compromise was confirmed by MRI and CT. A control group of 52 patients were treated with physical therapy. Forty-seven other patients underwent epidural neuroplasty with percutaneous adhesiolysis. The group undergoing neuroplasty had a catheter placed through the sacral hiatus to the level of the pathology after epidurogram. Postprocedure follow-up occurred at 3, 6, and 12 months. The outcome measures included the visual analog scale for the back and leg, Oswestry disability score, Gerbershagen score (explain briefly what it is), and analgesic score. An intent-to-treat analysis was performed. Among the adhesiolysis patients, there was a significant decrease in the VAS and Oswestry scores at 1, 3, 6, and 12 months. Twenty-eight patients undergoing adhesiolysis were able to decrease I Gerbershagen grade compared to 2 PT patients. The Gerbershagen score is commonly used in German pain clinic. It is a 4-axis operationally defined staging system for the chronicity of pain [47]. Epidural neuroplasty significantly reduced pain and functional disability in patients with chronic low back pain and sciatica caused by disk protrusion or failed back surgery syndrome in short-term (<6 months) and long-term (at 12 months) follow-up [46].

Another study by Manchikanti et al. [24] randomized 75 patients into three different treatment groups. Group I (25 patients) was a control group that received epidural catheterization but no adhesiolysis and injection of local anesthetic and steroid. Group II (25 patients) was treated with epidural adhesiolysis, followed by injection of normal saline, local anesthetic, and steroid. Group III (25 patients) consisted of adhesiolysis followed by injection of local anesthetic, hypertonic saline, and corticosteroid. Follow-up occurred at 3, 6, and 12 months. Outcome measures used included the VAS pain scale, Oswestry Disability Index 2.0, work status, opioid intake, range of motion measurements, and psychological evaluation by P-3. Significant improvement in these outcomes was found at 12-month follow-up. Seventy-two percent of patients in Group III (adhesiolysis and hypertonic saline neurolysis) and 60 % of patients in Group II (adhesiolysis only) compared to 0 % of Group I (control) demonstrated improvement. There was positive short-term (<6 months) and long-term relief (>6 months). In this study, adhesiolysis patients received good relief with or without hypertonic saline in neurolysis.

Heavner et al. [7] studied the efficacy and use of hypertonic saline and hyaluronidase in the percutaneous adhesiolysis. Eighty-three subjects with radiculopathy and low back pain were assigned to one of four epidural neuroplasty treatment groups: (a) hypertonic saline plus hyaluronidase, (b) hypertonic saline, (c) isotonic saline (0.9 % NaCl), or (d) isotonic saline plus hyaluronidase. Subjects in all treatment groups received epidural corticosteroids and local anesthetics. The results revealed 24 subjects did not complete the study. Most of the other 59 subjects receiving any of the four treatments as part of their pain management obtained significant relief immediately after treatment. Visual analog scale (VAS) scores for the area of maximal pain (VASmax; back or leg) were reduced in 25 % or more of subjects in all treatment groups at all posttreatment follow-up times (1, 3, 6, 9, and 12 months). A smaller fraction of subjects treated with hypertonic saline or hyaluronidase and hypertonic saline required more additional treatments than did subjects receiving the other treatments. The investigators were able to conclude that percutaneous epidural neuroplasty, as part of an overall pain management strategy, reduces pain (sometimes for over 1 year) in 25 % or more of subjects with radiculopathy and low back pain refractory to conventional therapies. The use of hypertonic saline may reduce the number of patients that require additional treatments.

There have been very few randomized double-blinded studies evaluating the efficacy of endoscopic neurolysis. Manchikanti and colleagues [48] did one such study in a prospective, randomized, double-blind trial to determine the outcome of spinal endoscopic adhesiolysis to reduce pain and improve function and psychological status in patients with chronic refractory low back and lower extremity pain. A total of 83 patients were evaluated, with 33 patients in Group I and 50 patients in Group II. Group I served as the control, with endoscopy into the sacral level without adhesiolysis, followed by injection of local anesthetic and steroid. Group II received spinal endoscopic adhesiolysis, followed by injection of local anesthetic and steroid. Among the 50 patients in the treatment group receiving spinal endoscopic adhesiolysis, significant improvement without adverse effects was shown in 80 % at 3 months, 56 % at 6 months, and 48 % at 12 months. The control group showed improvement in 33 % of the patients at 1 month and none thereafter. A significant number of patients obtained long-term (>12 months) relief with improvement in pain, functional status, and psychological status. This technique of spinal endoscopic adhesiolysis with targeted delivery of local anesthetic and steroid was found to be an effective treatment in a significant number of patients with chronic low back and lower extremity pain without major adverse effects.

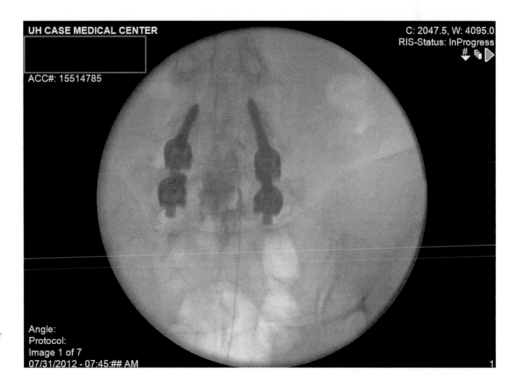

Fig. 39.6 Further catheter manipulation and contrast injection results in expansion of contrast spread to mid L4 vertebral level

Fig. 39.7 Final medication spread after depositing local anesthetic and steroids. Contrast has spread well into L4 and along the contour of the right L5 nerve root

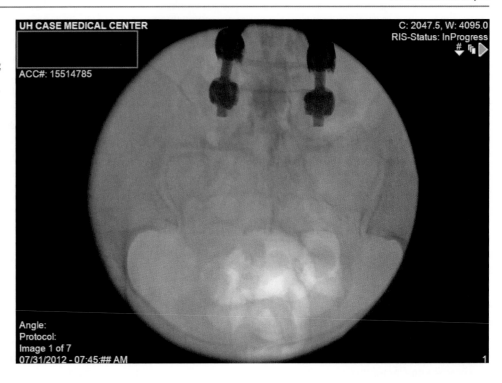

Summary

There has been an evolution of epidural neuroplasty over the last several decades [34]. Epidural adhesiolysis is a valuable technique in placing medications into areas of the epidural space that would otherwise be inaccessible by basic injections. There are many ways to perform adhesiolysis, and it is important for the practitioner to understand their limits before proceeding. Referral to a practitioner with more experience should be considered with more difficult cases. Careful selection of patients is important to avoid any untoward complications which are rare but serious. There is some evidence to support the use of this technique in an interventionalist's armamentarium to reduce suffering and pain particularly in patient with lumbar post-laminectomy syndrome, but more prospective randomized controlled studies are needed to solidify the role and value of epidural adhesiolysis.

References

1. Racz G, Holubec JT. Lysis of adhesions in the epidural space. In: Racz GB, editor. Techniques of neurolysis. Boston: Kluwer Academic Publishers; 1989. p. 57–72.
2. Justiz R, Taylor V, Day M. Neurogenic bladder: a complication after endoscopic adhesiolysis with return of bladder function while using nitrofurantoin. Anesth Analg. 2010;110(5):1496–8.
3. Kuslich SD, Ulstrom CL, Michael CJ. The tissue origin of low back pain and sciatica: a report of pain response to tissue stimulation during operations on the lumbar spine using local anesthesia. Orthop Clin North Am. 1991;22(2):181–7.
4. Trescot AM, Chopra P, Abdi S, Datta S, Schultz DM. Systematic review of effectiveness and complications of adhesiolysis in the management of chronic spinal pain: an update. Pain Physician. 2007;10(1):129–46.
5. Hayek SM, Helm S, Benyamin RM, Singh V, Bryce DA, Smith HS. Effectiveness of spinal endoscopic adhesiolysis in post lumbar surgery syndrome: a systematic review. Pain Physician. 2009;12(2):419–35.
6. Racz GB, Heavner JE, Trescot A. Percutaneous lysis of epidural adhesions – evidence for safety and efficacy. Pain Pract. 2008;8(4):277–86.
7. Heavner JE, Racz GB, Raj P. Percutaneous epidural neuroplasty: prospective evaluation of 0.9 % NaCl versus 10 % NaCl with or without hyaluronidase. Reg Anesth Pain Med. 1999;24(3):202–7.
8. Deyo RA, Mirza SK. Trends and variations in the use of spine surgery. Clin Orthop Relat Res. 2006;443:139–46.
9. Deyo RA, Nachemson A, Mirza SK. Spinal-fusion surgery – the case for restraint. N Engl J Med. 2004;350(7):722–6.
10. Lieberman IH. Disc bulge bubble: spine economics 101. Spine J. 2004;4(6):609–13.
11. Weinstein JN, Lurie JD, Tosteson TD, et al. Surgical versus nonoperative treatment for lumbar disc herniation: four-year results for the spine patient outcomes research trial (SPORT). Spine (Phila Pa 1976). 2008;33(25):2789–800.
12. Weinstein JN, Lurie JD, Olson PR, Bronner KK, Fisher ES. United States' trends and regional variations in lumbar spine surgery: 1992–2003. Spine (Phila Pa 1976). 2006;31(23):2707–14.
13. Boswell MV, Trescot AM, Datta S, et al. Interventional techniques: evidence-based practice guidelines in the management of chronic spinal pain. Pain Physician. 2007;10(1):7–111.
14. Abdi S, Datta S, Trescot AM, et al. Epidural steroids in the management of chronic spinal pain: a systematic review. Pain Physician. 2007;10(1):185–212.
15. Manchikanti L, Cash KA, McManus CD, Pampati V, Abdi S. Preliminary results of a randomized, equivalence trial of fluoroscopic caudal epidural injections in managing chronic low back pain: part 4 – spinal stenosis. Pain Physician. 2008;11(6):833–48.
16. Manchikanti L, Singh V, Cash KA, Pampati V, Datta S. Preliminary results of a randomized, equivalence trial of fluoroscopic caudal

epidural injections in managing chronic low back pain: part 3 – post surgery syndrome. Pain Physician. 2008;11(6):817–31.

17. Raj P, Lou L, Erdine S, Staats P, Waldman S. Decompressive neuroplasty. Radiographic Imagr Reg Anesth Pain Manag. 2003: 254–71.

18. Day M, Racz D. Technique of caudal neuroplasty. Pain Dig. 1999;9(4):255.

19. Devulder J, Bogaert L, Castille F, Moerman A, Rolly G. Relevance of epidurography and epidural adhesiolysis in chronic failed back surgery patients. Clin J Pain. 1995;11(2):147–50.

20. Manchikanti L, Bakhit CE, Pampati V. Role of epidurograpghy in caudal neuroplasty. Pain Dig. 1998;8:277.

21. King JS, Jewett DL, Sundberg HR. Differential blockade of cat dorsal root C fibers by various chloride solutions. J Neurosurg. 1972;36(5):569–83.

22. Lake DA, Barnes CD. Effects of changes in osmolality on spinal cord activity. Exp Neurol. 1980;68(3):555–67.

23. Manchikanti L, Pampati V, Fellows B, Rivera J, Beyer CD, Damron KS. Role of one day epidural adhesiolysis in management of chronic low back pain: a randomized clinical trial. Pain Physician. 2001;4(2):153–66.

24. Manchikanti L, Rivera JJ, Pampati V, et al. One day lumbar epidural adhesiolysis and hypertonic saline neurolysis in treatment of chronic low back pain: a randomized, double-blind trial. Pain Physician. 2004;7(2):177–86.

25. Lucas JT, Ducker TB, Perot Jr PL. Adverse reactions to intrathecal saline injection for control of pain. J Neurosurg. 1975;42(5):557–61.

26. Yousef AA, El-Deen AS, Al-Deeb AE. The role of adding hyaluronidase to fluoroscopically guided caudal steroid and hypertonic saline injection in patients with failed back surgery syndrome: a prospective, double-blinded, randomized study. Pain Pract. 2010;10:548–53.

27. Szepfalusi Z, Nentwich I, Dobner M, Pillwein K, Urbanek R. IgE-mediated allergic reaction to hyaluronidase in paediatric oncological patients. Eur J Pediatr. 1997;156(3):199–203.

28. Ebo DG, Goossens S, Opsomer F, Bridts CH, Stevens WJ. Flow-assisted diagnosis of anaphylaxis to hyaluronidase. Allergy. 2005;60(10):1333–4.

29. Yocum RC, Kennard D, Heiner LS. Assessment and implication of the allergic sensitivity to a single dose of recombinant human hyaluronidase injection: a double-blind, placebo-controlled clinical trial. J Infus Nurs. 2007;30(5):293–9.

30. Allen CH, Etzwiler LS, Miller MK, et al. Recombinant human hyaluronidase-enabled subcutaneous pediatric rehydration. Pediatrics. 2009;124(5):e858–67.

31. Hylenex. Highlights of Prescribing Information. Retrieved July 30, 2012 from http://www.hylenex.com/Theme/Hylenex/files/doc_downloads/LBL293-03.pdf. Accessed on Mar. 2012.

32. Epter RS, Helm 2nd S, Hayek SM, Benyamin RM, Smith HS, Abdi S. Systematic review of percutaneous adhesiolysis and management of chronic low back pain in post lumbar surgery syndrome. Pain Physician. 2009;12(2):361–78.

33. Day M, Racz GB. Lysis of epidural adhesions: the racz technique. In: Waldman S, editor. Pain management, vol. 2. 1st ed. Philadelphia: Saunders Elsevier; 2007.

34. Anderson SR, Racz GB, Heavner J. Evolution of epidural lysis of adhesions. Pain Physician. 2000;3(3):262–70.

35. Hammer M, Doleys DM, Chung OY. Transforaminal ventral epidural adhesiolysis. Pain Physician. 2001;4(3):273–9.

36. Manchikanti L. Role of neuraxial steroids in interventional pain management. Pain Physician. 2002;5(2):182–99.

37. Raj P, Lou L, Erdine S, Staats P, Waldman S. Epiduroscopy. Radiographic Imag Reg Anesth Pain Manag. 2003:272–81.

38. Pool J. Myeloscopy: intraspinal endoscopy. Surgery. 1942;11: 169–82.

39. Shimoji K, Fujioka H, Onodera M, et al. Observation of spinal canal and cisternae with the newly developed small-diameter, flexible fiberscopes. Anesthesiology. 1991;75(2):341–4.

40. Chopra P, Smith HS, Deer TR, Bowman RC. Role of adhesiolysis in the management of chronic spinal pain: a systematic review of effectiveness and complications. Pain Physician. 2005;8(1):87–100.

41. Manchikanti L, Bakhit CE. Removal of a torn Racz catheter from lumbar epidural space. Reg Anesth. 1997;22(6):579–81.

42. Karaman H, Ozturkmen Akay H, Turhanoglu S. Broken Racz catheter during application (case report). Agri. 2006;18(1):33–6.

43. Wagner KJ, Sprenger T, Pecho C, et al. Risks and complications of epidural neurolysis – a review with case report. Anasthesiol Intensivmed Notfallmed Schmerzther. 2006;41(4):213–22.

44. Shah RV, Heavner JE. Recognition of the subarachnoid and subdural compartments during epiduroscopy: two cases. Pain Pract. 2003;3(4):321–5.

45. Gill JB, Heavner JE. Visual impairment following epidural fluid injections and epiduroscopy: a review. Pain Med. 2005;6(5):367–74.

46. Veihelmann A, Devens C, Trouillier H, Birkenmaier C, Gerdesmeyer L, Refior HJ. Epidural neuroplasty versus physiotherapy to relieve pain in patients with sciatica: a prospective randomized blinded clinical trial. J Orthop Sci. 2006;11(4):365–9.

47. Pfingsten M, Schops P, Wille T, Terp L, Hildebrandt J. Classification of chronic pain. Quantification and grading with the Mainz pain staging system. Schmerz. 2000;14(1):10–7.

48. Manchikanti L, Boswell MV, Rivera JJ, et al. A randomized, controlled trial of spinal endoscopic adhesiolysis in chronic refractory low back and lower extremity pain. BMC Anesthesiol. 2005;5:10.

Thoracic and Lumbar Sympathetic Nerve Block and Neurolysis

Tim J. Lamer and Jason S. Eldrige

Key Points

- Preganglionic sympathetic neurons originate in the IML of T1–L2/3 and travel sequentially via the ventral root and then white rami communicantes to the paravertebral sympathetic chain or prevertebral ganglia. Postganglionic neurons originate in the sympathetic chain or prevertebral ganglia and then travel to (1) innervate end-organ structures or (2) follow a spinal nerve to the periphery via the postganglionic gray rami communicantes.
- Alcohol and phenol, in a variety of concentrations with various additives, are the two most commonly used neurolytic chemicals. Each has unique properties and side effects that warrant particular attention. Continuous radiofrequency involves the application of heat, generated by RF waves and typically held at 80 °C, to thermocoagulate nerve fibers.
- *Kuntz fibers*, arising from the upper thoracic sympathetic ganglia, may provide unrecognized sympathetic innervation to the upper extremity and be a contributory factor in stellate ganglion blocks which result in partial/incomplete sympathectomy.

T.J. Lamer, M.D. (✉)
Department of Anesthesiology and Pain Clinic, Rochester Methodist Hospital, Mayo Clinic,
1200 First Street S.W., Rochester, MN 55905, USA

Mayo College of Medicine,
Rochester, MN, USA
e-mail: lamer.tim@mayo.edu

J.S. Eldrige, M.D.
Department of Anesthesiology and Pain Clinic,
Rochester Methodist Hospital, Mayo Clinic,
1200 First Street S.W., Rochester, MN 55905, USA
e-mail: eldrige.jason@mayo.edu

Background and Historical Perspective

Sympathetic blockade of the thoracic and lumbar regions has been long described in the medical literature; initial techniques for a percutaneous thoracic block (paravertebral approach) were documented by Kappis in 1919 [1]. Earlier descriptions which postulated the role of the sympathetic system in the development and maintenance of neuropathic pain are detailed in the medical literature of the early 1900s. The sympathetic contribution to so-called causalgia was theorized in 1916 by Leriche, who argued that periarterial excision of sympathetic fibers may be of therapeutic benefit in relieving pain [2].

Over the next 20–30 years, various chemical and surgical techniques to denude, disrupt, ligate, or otherwise destroy the thoracic sympathetic innervation were devised. Most of these aforementioned methods were of limited therapeutic utility due to the inherent risks of open surgical techniques and the incomplete understanding of the complexities in relevant anatomy and physiology of the sympathetic system. One of the first percutaneous approaches to thoracic sympathetic blockade was accomplished by Leriche and Fontaine in 1925, who utilized a paravertebral technique [3]. Another noteworthy discovery, germane to the therapeutic success of stellate ganglionectomy for relieving upper extremity pain, was described by Albert Kuntz [2] in 1927. Kuntz noted that approximately 20 % of the population have sympathetic innervation to the upper extremity which does not pass through the stellate ganglion [4]. These so-called *nerves of Kuntz* (or *Kuntz fibers*) are composed of branches from the T2 and T3 thoracic sympathetic ganglia that route directly to the brachial plexus without passing through the sympathetic trunk proper. Contemporary clinical and cadaveric studies demonstrate that significant Kuntz Fibers occur more frequently than previously thought, with some studies claiming a 20–60 % incidence. As such, this *anatomic loophole* continues to be a scapegoat for failure to fully alleviate sympathetic-mediated symptoms after endothoracic surgical sympathectomy [4]. Additionally, the aforementioned discoveries have led to significant interest in procedures designed to ablate the T2 and T3 thoracic sympathetic ganglia [3–6].

Regardless, thorascopic sympathectomy (particularly endoscopic or video-assisted techniques) has enjoyed continued development and refinement over the last few decades. In addition, Wilkinson in 1979 was one of the first to illustrate a percutaneous approach to thoracic sympathetic structures for the purpose of chemical or radiofrequency neurolysis [6]. Fluoroscopic- and CT-guided percutaneous procedures are well described, but more recently, ultrasound technology has led to a revitalization of the procedure due to its presumed increased margin of safety while allowing similar diagnostic and therapeutic endpoints [7, 8].

The concept of lumbar sympathetic blockade was similar to the historical evolution of thoracic level sympathetics; the apparent first report in the literature was documented by Brunn and Mandl in 1924 using a paravertebral approach [9]. Similar to thoracic level interventions, lumbar sympathetic block was initially proposed as a therapy for vascular malperfusion (*Raynaud's disease*) and neuropathic "causalgia." The Second World War, primarily due to the frequency of lower extremity neuropathic injury, helped popularize interest in the lumbar sympathetic block [10]. Although several techniques of merit have been described, it is the original paravertebral approach of Kappis and Mandl described in the early 1920s that remains most popular [9]. Unlike the thoracic level, however, lumbar sympathetic blockade remains a commonly used interventional technique by pain practitioners worldwide.

Anatomic Considerations of the Sympathetic Nervous System

The sympathetic nervous system, a subset of the autonomic nervous system, subserves the body's need for rapid mobilization due to stress. As such, its chief role is one of initiation and maintenance of the familiar *fight-or-flight response*: characterized by peripheral extremity vasoconstriction, catecholamine surge, hastening of cardiopulmonary function, antagonism of intestinal activity, shunting of blood volume to large muscle groups, and many other functions. By clarifying the end function of this system in one's mind, the reader is better able to understand and even anticipate the anatomic connections required for sympathetic functionality to be established.

Alternatively known as the thoracolumbar nervous system, sympathetic nerves originate with cell bodies located in the intermediolateral horn (IML) of the T1 through L2–3 level of the spinal cord. These thoracolumbar cell bodies in the IML then give rise to preganglionic nerve fibers, which travel via the ventral root of the segmental spinal nerve and form white rami communicantes on their way to the paravertebral ganglia (i.e., sympathetic chain) or prevertebral gan-

glia (Fig. 40.1). When the preganglionic sympathetic nerve travels to the sympathetic chain (i.e., paravertebral ganglion), it has one of three choices for further course: synapse at the segmental paravertebral ganglion with a postsynaptic neuron, traveling up/down the sympathetic chain to synapse with a postsynaptic neuron at a remote level, or continue to pass through until synapsing with a postganglionic nerve in a prevertebral ganglion (Fig. 40.2) [11]. The postganglionic neuron then travels onward via the *gray rami communicantes* or prevertebral plexus to various final end-organ sites; typical postganglionic targets include the pupils, heart, blood vessels, sweat glands, and various visceral structures [2, 10–13]. It should be noted that *gray rami communicantes* (unmyelinated) allow for efferent connection between postganglionic sympathetic nerves to the segmental spinal nerve for vasomotor/sudomotor/pilomotor function, while *white rami communicantes* (myelinated) provide for efferent/afferent connections between preganglionic sympathetics (along with visceral afferents) and the central neuraxis (Fig. 40.2) [2, 10]. Consequently, the white rami communicantes form the sole pathway for neural traffic between the central nervous system and peripheral sympathetic system [10].

The sympathetic chain (paravertebral ganglia) extends from the top of the cervical spine down to the coccyx, traveling as two sympathetic trunks located along the anterolateral portion of the vertebral column. It is further subdivided into 23 sets of paired ganglia in the cervical [3], thoracic [12], lumbar [4], and sacral [4] regions, plus one single unpaired ganglion impar [2, 10–13]. Prevertebral ganglia, which provide neural intercession between the sympathetic chain and the postganglionic end-organ target, consist of specific ganglia and/or plexi located in the head, chest, abdomen, and pelvis. The major prevertebral sympathetic structures include the ciliary/otic/sphenopalatine/submaxillary ganglia, cardiac plexus, pulmonary plexus, celiac ganglia, superior and inferior mesenteric ganglia, and superior and inferior hypogastric plexuses [2, 10, 11].

The two anatomic areas most relevant to the discussion of this chapter are the cervicothoracic and lumbar ganglia regions. The cervicothoracic sympathetic region is principally composed of superior, middle, inferior, and stellate ganglia in the cervical region, along with 12 paired paravertebral ganglia in the thoracic region. The stellate ganglion, which is chiefly formed by the convalescence of inferior cervical and first thoracic ganglia elements, is of particular interest and lies ventrolaterally to the body of C7 with extension to the lateral portion of the T1 vertebral body [2, 11]. As mentioned previously, anatomic variants may include *Kuntz Fibers* which are postganglionic sympathetic branches from upper thoracic sympathetic ganglia (primarily T2 and T3) that may have direct neural connections to the brachial plexus external to the normal paravertebral (sympathetic chain) pathway.

Caudal to the stellate ganglion lies the *thoracic sympathetic chain*, which continues in a linear course along the

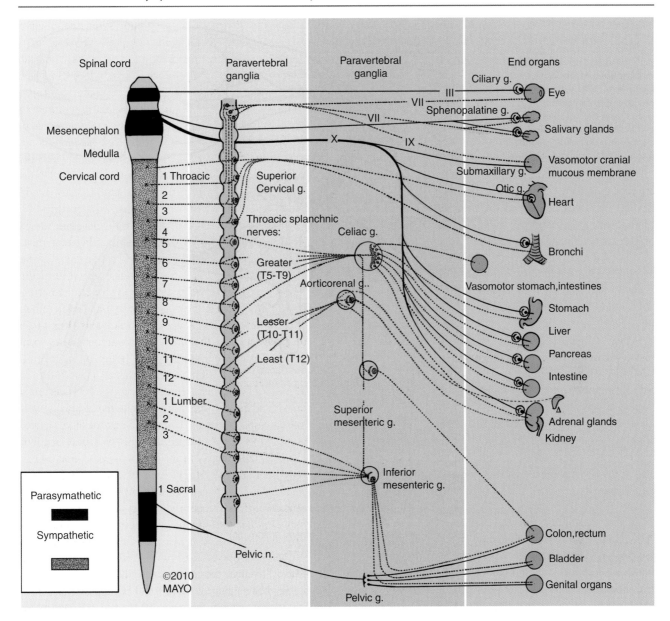

Fig. 40.1 Autonomic nervous system schematic, with special emphasis on common anatomic pathways of the sympathetic nervous system (With permission © Mayo Clinic, 2010)

dorsolateral aspect of the thoracic vertebral bodies; it is punctuated by paired segmental thoracic ganglia that lie just slightly caudad of the vertebral body midline (Fig. 40.3) [2, 9, 11]. The thoracic chain lies anterior to the head/neck of each rib in close approximation to the costovertebral interface and is bounded anterolaterally by the pleura of the lung [2, 11]. In the mid to lower thoracic regions, the sympathetic chain migrates to a more anterolateral position, relative to the vertebral bodies and lies at the anteromedial interface of the iliopsoas fascia as it further extends to the lumbar level. Typically, the lumbar sympathetic chain is found to have four discrete paired ganglia, but significant anatomic variation exists. Anatomic dissections have demonstrated a propensity for clustering of most significant lumbar sympathetic ganglia

at L3, which tends to be the classical target of percutaneous-based pain interventions [2]. More specific discussions regarding thoracic and lumbar sympathetic anatomy will follow in the interventional technique sections.

Methods of Neurolysis

Specific mention should be made of chemical neurolytic agents, since they are less commonly used and have unique properties that warrant particular attention. The most commonly used neurolytic chemicals are alcohol (33–100 %) and phenol (2–12 %, with or without glycerol additive). Alcohol is hypobaric relative to CSF, causes significant pain/

Fig. 40.2 Schematic of the central cord, exiting spinal nerve, and traditional anatomic path of the sympathetic nervous system that originates in the central lateral horn. Note that typical procedural targets include the lateral paravertebral chain (sympathetic trunk and ganglia) and/or the prevertebral ganglion/plexus (With permission © Mayo Clinic, 2010)

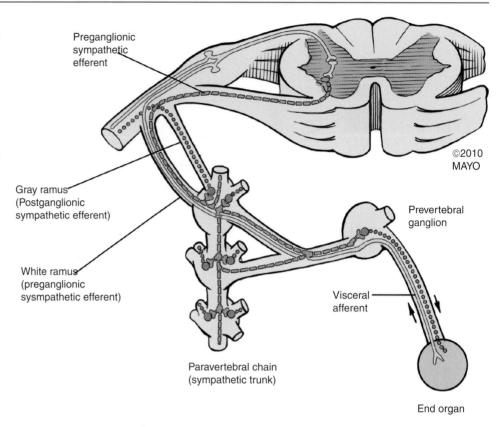

Preganglionic sympathetic efferent

©2010 MAYO

Gray ramus (Postganglionic sympathetic efferent)

Prevertebral ganglion

White ramus (preganglionic sysmpathetic efferent)

Visceral afferent

Paravertebral chain (sympathetic trunk)

End organ

Key

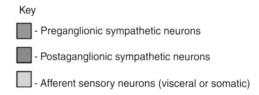

- Preganglionic sympathetic neurons

- Postaganglionic sympathetic neurons

- Afferent sensory neurons (visceral or somatic)

burning upon injection, and induces Wallerian degeneration from the direct neurodestructive effects of ethanol. Notably, alcohol may allow for selective neurolysis of small sensory fibers (sparing motor) when used in low concentrations less than 33 % [14]. Phenol is hyperbaric relative to CSF when glycerol 4–10 % is added, has local anesthetic properties that minimize discomfort when injected, and may enable selective neurolysis of sensory nerves when used in small concentrations (typically 2–3 %). Phenol imparts neurolysis due to denaturing of protein, which may explain its predilection to cause vascular injury (risk of spinal infarction with subarachnoid use, erodes Dacron graft material, etc.). While less likely than phenol to cause direct vascular injury, alcohol has been associated with increased risk of vascular spasm and subsequent ischemic blood flow [14]. Lastly, phenol has been linked with arrhythmia and cardiovascular collapse; the mechanism is not fully elucidated, but likely relates to phenol's sodium channel antagonist properties.

Continuous radiofrequency ablation (RFA) relies upon the application of heat, generated by continuous radiofrequency

(RF) waves, to cause thermocoagulation of nerve fibers. This technology heats adjacent tissue to 80 °C, typically for 90 s. Recognize that sensory testing at 50 Hz and 1 V and motor testing at 2 Hz and 3 V may help establish whether intercostal/somatic nerves are being stimulated. If one is unable to elicit somatic nerve (intercostal) stimulation at 2 Hz and up to 1.5 V, it is much less likely that thoracic sympathetic ganglion RFA will cause injury to the segmental somatic nerve [8]. Additionally, post-RF neuritis sometimes develops after lesioning; this is usually self-limited, spontaneously resolves, and may be treated with steroid administration (prophylactically or after neuritis develops).

Thoracic Sympathetic Block

Specific Anatomy and Physiology

The thoracic sympathetic nerves typically consist of 12 paired paravertebral ganglia that punctuate the sympathetic

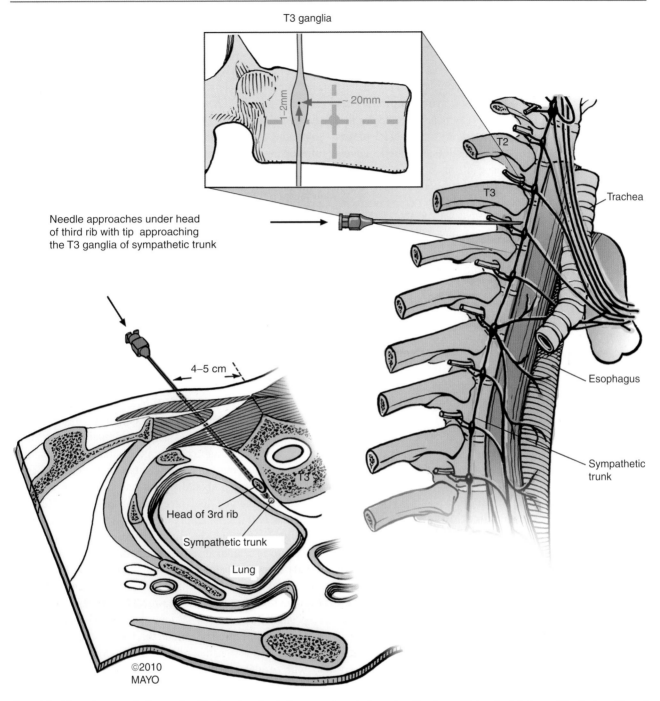

Fig. 40.3 Thoracic sympathetic ganglion block, using classic fluoroscopic technique, denoting the sagittal and axial views of the final position of the procedural needle tip (With permission © Mayo Clinic, 2010)

chain at each thoracic vertebral level. These thoracic level paravertebral trunks travel dorsolaterally relative to the vertebral body, just anterior to the transverse process and posterior to the pleura of the lung [2, 11–13]. The superior most thoracic ganglion (T1) typically fuses with the inferior cervical ganglion (C8) to form the stellate ganglion in the majority of patients [2, 11–13]. The upper thoracic sympathetic chain runs anterior and just lateral to the head of the rib, with the ganglia located slightly caudad to the inferior edge of the head of the rib (Fig. 40.3). As one progresses down the thoracic spine, the sympathetic chain gradually moves closer to the anterolateral position on the vertebral body assumed in the lumbar region. The thoracic sympathetic ganglia lie just inferior of the true vertical midpoint of the vertebral body, though the anteroposterior position moves more ventrally as one descends down the thoracic spine [8, 9]. To be sure, once at the T11 level, the low thoracic sympathetic chain has assumed a much more anterolateral position with individual ganglia located against the lateral surface of the vertebral body.

As mentioned previously, anatomic variants may include *Kuntz Fibers*, which are postganglionic sympathetic branches from the T2 and T3 (possibly T4) sympathetic ganglia that may have direct neural connections to the brachial plexus external to the normal paravertebral (sympathetic chain) pathway. The clinical relevance of this common anatomic pathway (10–20 % prevalence) is that a perfectly performed stellate ganglion block may not result in a complete sympathectomy for the entire upper extremity. *Kuntz fibers*, arising from the upper thoracic sympathetic ganglia, may provide unrecognized sympathetic innervation to the upper extremity [3, 6]. Consequently, it is possible to perform a successful stellate ganglion block that causes only a partial sympathectomy to the upper extremity due to unblocked *nerves of Kuntz*; this may appear clinically indistinguishable, in terms of asymmetric extremity temperature change, from a successful stellate blockade in patients without significant Kuntz Fibers. Thus, one must consider that sparing of Kuntz Fibers *may* be responsible for a stellate ganglion blocks that fail to relieve pain (regardless of evidence for successful sympathectomy). The primary clinical impetus for development of thoracic sympathetic blocks was an attempt to target these *Kuntz Fibers* at T2 and T3, though the techniques described can readily be applied throughout the thoracic spine.

Indications and Contraindications

Indications for thoracic level sympathetic block include hyperhidrosis, upper extremity vascular malperfusion (Raynaud's), and upper extremity or thoracic level sympathetically maintained neuropathic pain, along with visceral pain syndromes from the heart, lung, and/or esophagus. In general, because of the overlap in anatomic territory and existence of Kuntz fibers, one should consider upper thoracic level (T2 or T3) sympathetic blockade for any of the commonly accepted indications described for the stellate ganglion. Along with thoracic and upper abdominal visceral pain, consideration should be given for post-thoracotomy pain (particularly if sympathetic features are evident), postherpetic neuralgia, frostbite injuries to the upper extremity, and phantom breast pain [13].

Contraindications include the typical neuraxial *absolutes* of localized infection (skin or adjacent structures), systemic infection, and bleeding diathesis or coagulopathy. *Relative* contraindications relate primarily to the underlying function of adjacent anatomic structures, namely, pulmonary impairment and/or aneurysm of the great vessels (aorta or vena cava).

Complications and Expected Side Effects

Expected side effects from thoracic sympathectomy include ipsilateral Horner's syndrome, adjacent somatic nerve block, and cardiac accelerator fiber block. Unexpected, though entirely possible, complications include intrathecal, subdural, epidural, intravascular (intercostal, azygous, aorta) injections. Also possible, though very unlikely, is the danger of esophageal perforation if the needle is placed too anteriorly. The most feared of the complication is unintended puncture of the lung pleura and consequent development of pneumothorax. Pneumothorax may present with a delayed clinical presentation, which necessitates informing the patient of probable warning signs and when to seek medical attention. If using neurolytic techniques, damage to somatic nerves may occur from spread through the epidural, paravertebral, intervertebral foramen, or even intrathecal space (less likely); this may result in significant sensory and/or motor deficits that are not reversible.

Procedural Technique for Block Neurolysis

There are various descriptions of blocks and/or neurolysis to the thoracic sympathetic chain, but our discussion will focus on percutaneous approaches and intentionally omit reviews on surgically open and endoscopic techniques. One should also assume that real-time imaging, typically with ultrasound and/or fluoroscopy, should be utilized in order to optimize the safety, accuracy, and precision of these techniques. In particular, without the ability to visualize the lung, the risk of pneumothorax cannot be entirely eliminated. The technical procedure is similar throughout the thoracic spine, but the details described below are *most specific to the T2–3 levels* [7, 8, 11, 13]:

1. Plan to use a posterior approach, placing the patient prone.
2. If using fluoroscopy, orient the image intensifier in the true AP position, slightly oblique (15–20°, ipsilateral), with enough cephalad angulation to be in-plane with the neck of the rib at T2 or T3. This will allow coaxial placement of the procedural needle to a target point just anteroinferior to the head of the T2 or T3 rib (where the thoracic ganglion lies, see Fig. 40.3).
3. Initially, enter the skin approximately 2.5–5 cm lateral from true midline (depending upon degree of obliquity used) and coaxially advanced to the inferior edge of the rib or transverse process as applicable, depending upon degree of cephalad angulation used.
4. After touching bone, minimally redirect inferiorly until passing through the costotransverse ligament. The costotransverse ligament can be "felt" by a distinctive pop, or a loss or resistance technique can be utilized with a fluid or

Fig. 40.4 Paravertebral space schematic, denoting the position of thoracic somatic and sympathetic nerves/ganglia relative to the lung retroparietal space (With permission © Mayo Clinic, 2010)

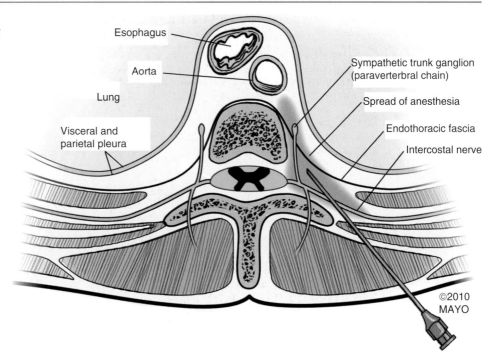

air-filled syringe. In either case, passage through this ligament heralds arrival at the retropleural space.

5. The needle should be closely approximated to the lateral edge of the adjacent vertebral body. The final needle tip position will be approximately just cephalad and posterior to the true midpoint along the dorsolateral aspect of the T2 or T3 vertebral body (Fig. 40.3).

6. Injection of contrast will demonstrate spread along the dorsolateral aspect of the thoracic vertebral column. If one breaches the parietal pleural, the lung dome will be outlined and the needle is too lateral (monitor patient for pneumothorax).

7. Proper sterile technique should be observed at all times, with appropriate monitoring established beforehand and local anesthetic infiltration taking place prior to the placement of the procedural needle. Aspiration should be negative for CSF, blood, and air before injecting local anesthetic, chemical neurolytic agents, or applying radiofrequency ablation. Care should be taken to verify no foraminal spread of contrast prior to neurolysis. Lastly, the use of local anesthetic test doses and/or digital subtraction angiography will help elucidate unintended vascular uptake prior to neurolytic procedures.

8. *Ultrasound procedural pearls*: With the recent renewed interest in perioperative paravertebral blocks, there are several techniques described utilizing real-time ultrasound. It has long been recognized anatomically that the sympathetic chain runs in the ventral region of the paravertebral compartment, such that intended somatic blockade of the segmental innervation often leads to ipsilateral sympathectomy. Ultrasound has the distinct advantage of

allowing in-plane visualization of needle placement, while also allowing direct visualization of costotransverse ligament, transverse processes, and the underlying lung pleura (Fig. 40.4). This likely translates into improved safety, in regard to pneumothorax risk specifically [7].

Efficacy (Measurable Endpoints for Success and Literature Review)

The single most effective measure for determining the successful sympathetic blockade is measurement of ipsilateral asymmetric temperature rise in the affected region [14]. This occurs because of the reflexive regional vasodilation that occurs once the concomitant sympathetic tone to that area is attenuated. Notably, with thoracic level blocks, it may be challenging to accurately record the cutaneous skin temperature; use of an infrared measuring device is often helpful. One should also observe asymmetric, ipsilateral sudomotor paralysis and anhidrosis (i.e., decreased sweat production). It is possible to observe an ipsilateral Horner's syndrome if the ascending cervical sympathetic chain is disrupted, though this is much less commonly observed, compared to stellate ganglion level blocks.

Unfortunately, there is a general paucity of robust medical evidence for efficacy in blocking thoracic sympathetic nerves (regarding pain indications). A recent review of the sympathetic block literature performed by Miles Day in 2008 demonstrated only two significant articles (one case report, one case review) related to percutaneous technique [13]. There are several other medical reports and case series available for

Fig. 40.5 Axial schematic of the typical needle trajectory for blocking the lumbar sympathetic ganglia at the L2 or L3 vertebral level (With permission © Mayo Clinic, 2010)

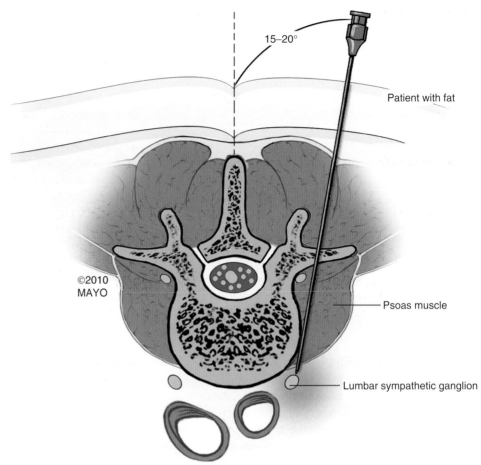

review in abstract form, but double-blind, randomized prospective trials continue to be lacking. The aforementioned review article by Day summarizes the evidence for percutaneous thoracic sympathetic block as being grade 1C–2C, defined as having low-medium quality evidence, where benefits may not clearly outweigh risks in all circumstances and the best clinical action may differ depending upon patient circumstance and societal values [13]. Consequently, there remains a significant need for larger studies, randomized trials, and long-term data.

Lumbar Sympathetic Block

Specific Anatomy and Physiology

The paired lumbar sympathetic trunks lie along the anterior lumbar vertebral bodies at the inferomedial margin of the psoas muscles (Figs. 40.1 and 40.5). The lumbar sympathetics send sympathetic efferent fibers to the lower extremities and lower abdominal and pelvic visceral organs. Some visceral afferent fibers from the lower abdominal and pelvic organs travel along the course of the sympathetic fibers and ultimately to the spinal cord via the

lumbar splanchnic nerves. Some anatomists have mentioned the existence of sympathetic fibers crossing the midline to the contralateral trunk, while others have failed to demonstrate this [15, 16]. These crossing fibers have been mentioned as a possible explanation for a seemingly technically successful sympathetic block failing to produce evidence of a sympathectomy.

Indications

Historically, lumbar sympathetic blocks (LSB) have been reported to treat a vast array of unrelated conditions including hyperhidrosis, postherpetic neuralgia, frostbite, phantom limb pain, and renal colic, to name a few [11]. Current indications for lumbar sympathetic block include complex regional pain syndrome (CRPS), peripheral vascular disease, with painful ischemic neuropathy, and some vascular pain syndromes. Despite the widespread use of LBS for the above indications, most of the literature support comes from anecdotal series and case reports rather than controlled trials.

The use of sympathectomy and sympathetic blocks for the treatment of CRPS was first described by Leriche and Fontaine in the 1930s [17]. The continuing use of sympathetic blocks for the diagnosis and treatment of CRPS and "sympathetically mediated" pain syndromes is based upon a large body of anecdotal reports, case series, and long-standing historical use. There are no high-quality RCTs in adults and only one RCT in a pediatric population [13, 18].

For lower extremity peripheral vascular disease (PVD), definitive management consists of surgical or minimally invasive bypass or angioplasty of the obstructed segments. Sympathetic blocks have a treatment role in those patients with symptomatic occlusive disease that is not amenable to surgery or in patients who are medically unsuitable for surgery.

A reasonable approach is to consider sympathetic neurolysis for patients who have failed medical therapy, who are not candidates for reconstruction or angioplasty, and who have ischemic pain and/or evidence of poor tissue perfusion. In most cases, it is advisable to first perform a diagnostic local anesthetic block to assess the degree of pain relief and demonstrate objective evidence of improved tissue perfusion.

Complication and Side Effects

Intravascular uptake or injection into the aorta, the vena cava, or the segmental radicular vessels can result in local anesthetic toxicity. These risks can be minimized by the usual block precautions of careful aspiration, use of a local anesthetic test does, and real-time fluoroscopic contrast injection. Needle trauma to the lumbar plexus nerves within the psoas muscle, the exiting nerve roots at the intervertebral foramen, or the radicular arteries can also occur and may result in temporary or permanent nerve injury.

Complications after neurolytic block are related to injection of the neurolytic agent near a somatic nerve or spread of the injected neurolytic agent from the area of the sympathetic trunks to a somatic nerve or nerve root. The use of fluoroscopy and small controlled volumes of injectant can help to minimize this complication. The genitofemoral nerve or L2 nerve roots are most commonly affected. This so-called post-neurolysis genitofemoral neuralgia has been reported in up to 5–10 % of cases and usually presents with neuropathic pain symptoms (burning, dysesthesia, allodynia) in the groin or anteromedial thigh [19].

Rare complications include organ puncture (kidney, ureter), intervertebral disk puncture, and retroperitoneal hematoma.

Procedural Technique

Over the years, numerous variations and techniques have been described to perform LSBs. Historically, most of the procedures involved needle entry at L2 or L3, approximately 6–7 cm from the midline, advancing the needle until it contacts the vertebral body and then "walking" the needle anteriorly off of the vertebral body until it slips off the body and through the anterior psoas muscle fascia, at which point the injectant is deposited [20].

Currently, image-guided LSB is the preferred technique. CT-guided techniques have been described, but there are few if any real advantages of this method over fluoroscopic guidance, and the increased expense and radiation exposure cannot be justified for most cases [21]. Ultrasound-guided techniques have been recently described, and, as techniques and equipment improve, this technique may become the preferred method in the future.

Currently, a fluoroscopic-guided approach is the preferred technique for most patients. The description that follows is suitable for the majority of patients encountered in clinical practice, though modifications may be needed for some patients depending on factors such as body habitus, spine surgery or spine deformity, etc.:

1. The patient is place prone, with a pillow under the pelvis and lower abdomen to straighten the lumbar lordosis.
2. Appropriate monitors are placed and sterile preparation and draping is performed.
3. Fluoroscopic guidance is then performed to identify and mark the surface landmarks and needle entry point(s). A single-needle technique should be performed at L2 or L3. Iliac vessels become more closely opposed to the vertebral bodies at the lower lumbar levels, increasing the likelihood of an intravascular injection.
4. The skin and deeper tissues are appropriately infiltrated with local anesthetic.
5. A 22-gauge needle with a curved tip works very well for this block. A 5–6-in. (12–15 cm) needle will suffice for the majority of patients.
6. Start with the fluoroscope at the midline posterior anterior position to identify the L2 or L3 vertebral bodies. Then, rotate the fluoroscopic beam approximately 15–20° from the sagittal plane (5–6 in. from midline in most patients) using this view. In this oblique view, the needle entry point should align with the anterior margin of the vertebral body approximately one-third of the distance caudal from the superior end plate of the vertebral body using a coaxial or "in-line" plane trajectory relative to the fluoroscope beam (Fig. 40.6). It is then advanced in 1-cm increments, using the curved needle tip to make adjustments in the trajectory to keep the needle tip coursing to the anterior margin of the vertebral body. Contact should be made at the anterior edge with the need curved medially. Then, the needle is curved 180° to point lateral and advanced to just slide past the vertebral body. Then, the fluoroscopic beam is turned to a lateral position and the tip advanced until it is even with the anterior margin of the vertebral body (Figs. 40.7, 40.8, 40.9, and 40.10).

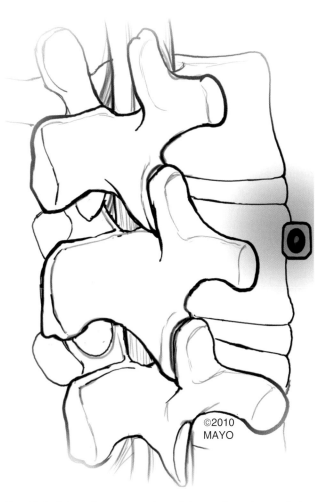

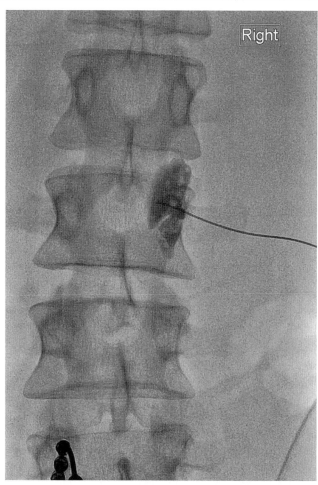

Fig. 40.6 Schematic representation of the needle trajectory during LSB in a coaxial or "in-line" plane relative to the fluoroscopy image intensifier (oblique view) (With permission © Mayo Clinic, 2010)

Fig. 40.7 Fluoroscopic image of right-sided lumbar sympathetic block, AP view

With experience, you should sense the needle tip pass or "pop" through the anterior psoas fascia.

7. Then, 1.0 ml of contrast is injected to be sure the needle tip is not in the psoas muscle and to verify that the solution layers are out in the anticipated location of the lumbar trunk (Figs. 40.7 and 40.8). Then, the fluoroscopic beam is turned to the posterior anterior orientation to again verify that the needle tip is in the correct location and that the contrast is not within the psoas muscle. If there is any question, another 1.0–2.0 ml of contrast can be injected. If there is a concern or question about vascular uptake, 1.0–2.0 ml of contrast should be injected using real-time injection, preferably with digital subtraction fluoroscopy.

8. Once the needle tip position is satisfactory, then inject 3–5 ml of local anesthetic.

9. For neurolytic injections, a smaller volume (1–2 ml) is recommended to decrease the possibility of posterior spread into the psoas muscle. This may reduce the likelihood of neuralgia.

10. In order to demonstrate a successful block pre- and post-procedure, measurements of distal extremity skin temperature or laser Doppler flowmetry should be preformed. Unless the patient has rather severe peripheral vascular disease (PVD), you should expect the skin temperature of the distal foot to rise to within approximately 3 °C of the core body temperature [22].

Efficacy

There is a paucity of well-designed randomized controlled trials (RCT) regarding the use of LSB for CRPS. In adults, a recent Cochrane review identified only one trial involving a very small number of patients, and the conclusion was that no consensus could be drawn concerning effectiveness [13, 23].

A recent double-blind, placebo-controlled trial of LSB in children with CRPS demonstrated significant pain reduction and improvement in sensory dysfunction compared to placebo and intravenous lidocaine [18]. Based upon the current literature, it is reasonable to continue to use local anesthetic

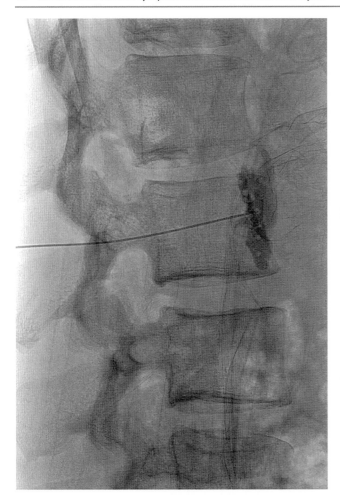

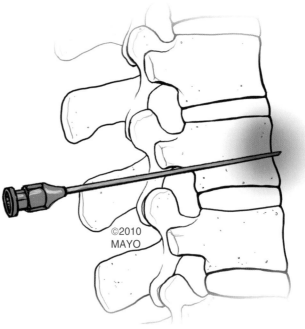

Fig. 40.9 Schematic representation of the final needle position for LSB, in the posterior anterior plane (With permission © Mayo Clinic, 2010)

Fig. 40.8 Fluoroscopic image of right-sided lumbar sympathetic block, lateral view

lumbar sympathetic blocks as part of a comprehensive treatment program in patients with early-stage CRPS that have not improved with less invasive conservative therapies.

There are several single center case series and two small RCTs that have examined the effectiveness of neurolytic LSB for patients with PVD [24–32]. In the RCTs, there was subjective symptomatic improvement (pain relief) but no significant improvement in objective testing such as ankle brachial pressure index (ABPI) and treadmill walking distance. Table 40.1 lists the clinical trials that have examined the results of chemical sympathectomy in patients with PVD. Based on the literature, it is reasonable to continue to consider lumbar sympathetic neurolysis to treat patients with painful lower extremity who have not responded to medical or surgical treatment or who are not candidates for surgery or angioplasty.

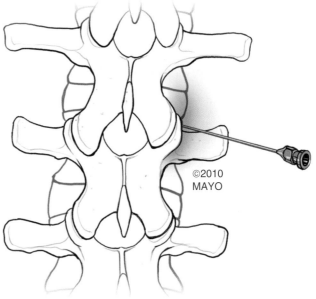

Fig. 40.10 Schematic representation of the final needle position for LSB in the lateral trajectory (With permission © Mayo Clinic, 2010)

Table 40.1 Summary review of research trials, which have studied the results of chemical sympathectomy in patients with peripheral vascular disease (PVD)

Sympathetic blocks for PVD				
Investigation	Patient number	Procedure[a]	Satisfactory response (%)	No response (%)
Hughes-David and Redman [28]	97	1	69	31
Strand [32]	167	3	56	44
Cousins et al. [24]	368	1,2	80	20
Haimovici et al. [27]	171	3	55	45
Froysaker [25]	32	3	5.5	94.5
Myers and Irvine [30]	26	3	69	31
Rosen et al. [31]	37	1	38	62
Fyfe et al. [26]	25	1	25	75
Mashiah et al. [29]	373	1	58.7	41.3

[a]1, Phenol sympathetic block; 2, Alcohol sympathetic block; 3, Local anesthetic sympathetic block

References

1. Kappis M. Sensibilitt und local ansthesie in chirurgischen gebiet der bauchhole mit besonderen bercksichtigung der splanchnichus-ansthesie. Bruns Beitr Klin Cher. 1919;15:161.
2. Finch P. Sympathetic neurolysis. In: Raj PP, editor. Textbook of regional anesthesia. Churchill Livingstone in cooperation with W B Saunders New York; 2002, p. 667–85.
3. Skabelund C, Racz G. Indications and technique of thoracic 2 and thoracic 3 neurolysis. Curr Rev Pain. 1999;3:400–5.
4. Marhold F, et al. Thoracoscopic and anatomic landmarks of Kuntz's nerve: implications for sympathetic surgery. Ann Thorac Surg. 2008;86:1653–8.
5. Ohseto K. Efficacy of thoracic sympathetic ganglion block and prediction of complications: clinical evaluation of the anterior paratracheal and posterior paravertebral approaches in 234 patients. J Anesth. 1992;6(3):316–31.
6. Wilkinson HA. Radiofrequency percutaneous upper-thoracic sympathectomy. Technique and review of indications. N Engl J Med. 1984;311(1):34–6.
7. Cowie B, et al. Ultrasound-guided thoracic paravertebral blockade: a cadaveric study. Anesth Analg. 2010;110(6):1735–9.
8. Stanton-Hicks M. Thoracic sympathetic block: a new approach. Tech Reg Anesth Pain Manag. 2001;5(3):94–8.
9. Raj PP, et al. Interventional pain management: image-guided procedures. Philadelphia: Saunders Elsevier; 2008.
10. Fishman SM, Ballantyne JC, Rathmell JP. Bonica's management of pain, in various chapters. Philadelphia: Lippincott Williams & Wilkins; 2009.
11. Lamer T. Sympathetic nerve blocks. In: Regional anesthesia and analgesia. Philadelphia: WB Saunders; 1996. p. 357–84.
12. Brown D. Atlas of regional anesthesia, in atlas of regional anesthesia. Philadelphia: Saunders Elsevier Publishing; 2006.
13. Day M. Sympathetic blocks: the evidence. Pain Pract. 2008;8(2): 98–109.
14. Loeser JD, Bonica JJ. Bonica's management of pain. 3rd ed. Philadelphia: Lippincott Williams & Wilkins; 2001. p. xxii, 2178 p.
15. Cowley RA, Yeager GH. Anatomic observations on the lumbar sympathetic nervous system. Surgery. 1949;25(6):880–90.
16. Gray H, Goss CM. Anatomy of the human body. 29th ed. Philadelphia: Lea & Febiger; 1973. p. xvii, 1466 p.
17. Leriche R. L'anesthesie isolee du ganglion etoile: sa technique, ses indications, ses resultats. Presse Med. 1934;42:849–50.
18. Meier PM, et al. Lumbar sympathetic blockade in children with complex regional pain syndromes: a double blind placebo-controlled crossover trial. Anesthesiology. 2009;111(2):372–80.
19. Kramis RC, Roberts WJ, Gillette RG. Post-sympathectomy neuralgia: hypotheses on peripheral and central neuronal mechanisms. Pain. 1996;64(1):1–9.
20. Cousins MJ, Bridenbaugh PO. Neural blockade in clinical anesthesia and management of pain. 2nd ed. Philadelphia: Lippincott; 1988. p. xix, 1171 p.
21. Heindel W, et al. CT-guided lumbar sympathectomy: results and analysis of factors influencing the outcome. Cardiovasc Intervent Radiol. 1998;21(4):319–23.
22. Tran KM, et al. Lumbar sympathetic block for sympathetically maintained pain: changes in cutaneous temperatures and pain perception. Anesth Analg. 2000;90(6):1396–401.
23. Cepeda MS, Carr DB, Lau J. Local anesthetic sympathetic blockade for complex regional pain syndrome. Cochrane Database Syst Rev. 2005;4:CD004598.
24. Cousins MJ, et al. Neurolytic lumbar sympathetic blockade: duration of denervation and relief of rest pain. Anaesth Intensive Care. 1979;7(2):121–35.
25. Froysaker T. Lumbar sympathectomy in impending gangrene and foot ulcer. Scand J Clin Lab Invest Suppl. 1973;128:71–2.
26. Fyfe T, Quin RO. Phenol sympathectomy in the treatment of intermittent claudication: a controlled clinical trial. Br J Surg. 1975;62(1):68–71.
27. Haimovici H, Steinman C, Karson IH. Evaluation of lumbar sympathectomy. Advanced occlusive arterial disease. Arch Surg. 1964;89:1089–95.
28. Hughes-Davies DI, Redman LR. Chemical lumbar sympathectomy. Anaesthesia. 1976;31(8):1068–75.
29. Mashiah A, et al. Phenol lumbar sympathetic block in diabetic lower limb ischemia. J Cardiovasc Risk. 1995;2(5):467–9.
30. Myers KA, Irvine WT. An objective study of lumbar sympathectomy-II. Skin ischaemia. Br Med J. 1966;1(5493):943–7.
31. Rosen RJ, et al. Percutaneous phenol sympathectomy in advanced vascular disease. AJR Am J Roentgenol. 1983;141(3):597–600.
32. Strand L. Lumbar sympathectomy in the treatment of peripheral obliterative arterial disease. An analysis of 167 patients. Acta Chir Scand. 1969;135(7):597–600.

Celiac Plexus, Splanchnic Nerve Block, and Neurolysis

Melinda M. Lawrence, Salim M. Hayek, and Joshua D. Goldner

Key Points

- Visceral abdominal pain secondary to upper gastro-intestinal malignancies and pancreatic disease can be very challenging to control.
- Optimization of pain may often require a multi-modal approach to obtain adequate analgesia.
- Numerous studies have shown that patients who suffer from viscerally mediated upper abdominal pain may experience great benefit from celiac plexus neurolysis. Regardless of the technique used, studies have shown that celiac plexus neurolysis has a long-lasting benefit in up to 70–90% of patients with pancreatic cancer.
- Neurolysis of the celiac plexus is a relatively safe procedure with commonly occurring mild side effects and uncommonly occurring serious adverse events.
- Celiac plexus neurolysis can be used as an alternative to or in conjunction with opioid analgesics for improvement in pain management and quality of life.

- It is important to keep in mind that celiac plexus blockade will only eliminate visceral-mediated pain but would not otherwise alter musculoskeletal or neuropathic components of pain; that should be clearly explained to the patient prior to entertaining the block.
- Intrathecal drug delivery is a valuable option in those who fail to have adequate relief from celiac plexus neurolysis or diagnostic block.

Introduction

In 1914, Max Kappis [1] performed the first celiac plexus block. Since the first reported celiac plexus block (CPB), there has been abundance of literature describing many indications, techniques, and complications associated with this procedure [1–9]. The celiac plexus innervates the gastrointestinal tract between the distal third of the esophagus and the transverse colon, including the liver, biliary tract, kidneys, spleen, adrenals, and mesentery. Due to the widespread visceral innervation of the gastrointestinal tract by the celiac plexus, blockade of these nerves is often used to treat viscerally mediated abdominal pain in patients with pancreatic cancer, upper abdominal malignancies, and chronic pancreatitis [2, 3]. Patients who undergo celiac plexus blockade have often failed to respond to conservative medical management, which may include nonsteroidal anti-inflammatories and opioids. Neurolytic celiac plexus blocks have been found to decrease post-procedural opioid consumption [4], improve pain control, improve mood, reduce pain interference with activity, and possibly increase life expectancy [5]. Typically, a diagnostic celiac plexus block is first performed, and if successful, it is then followed by a therapeutic neurolytic block with either ethanol or phenol for the purpose providing long-lasting relief. Physicians have reported performing this procedure with a wide variety of modalities including anatomical

M.M. Lawrence, M.D. (✉) • J.D. Goldner, M.D.
Department of Anesthesiology,
University Hospitals Case Medical Center,
11100 Euclid Ave., Cleveland, OH 44106, USA
e-mail: melinda.m.lawrence@gmail.com;
joshua.goldner@uhhospitals.org

S.M. Hayek, M.D., Ph.D
Department of Anesthesiology, Division of Pain Medicine,
Case Western Reserve University,
University Hospitals Case Medical Center,
11100 Euclid Ave., Cleveland, OH 44106, USA
e-mail: salim.hayek@uhhospitals.org

landmarks, radiography, computed tomography, fluoroscopy, bedside ultrasound, and endoscopic ultrasound [2, 6, 7].

Anatomy

Sympathetic innervation of the abdominal viscera originates in the anterolateral horn of the spinal cord. Preganglionic axons from T5 to T12 leave the spinal cord with the ventral spinal routes to join the white communicating rami en route to the sympathetic chain. These preganglionic sympathetic nerves are unique in that their axons do not synapse in the sympathetic chain; they pass through the chain and synapse at distal sites. Distal sites of synapse include the celiac, aorticorenal, and superior mesenteric ganglia [8]. The greater, lesser, and least splanchnic nerves provide the major preganglionic contribution to the celiac plexus and transmit the majority of nociceptive information from the viscera. The splanchnic nerves are contained in a narrow compartment made up by the vertebral body and the pleural laterally, the posterior mediastinum ventrally, and the pleural attachment to the vertebra dorsally. This compartment is bounded caudally by the crura of the diaphragm. The volume of this compartment is approximately 10 ml on each side.

The greater splanchnic nerve has its origin from the T5–10 spinal roots. The nerve travels along the thoracic paravertebral border through the crus of the diaphragm into the abdominal cavity, ending on the celiac ganglion of its respective side. The lesser splanchnic nerve arises from the T10–11 roots and passes with the greater nerve to end at the celiac ganglion. The least splanchnic nerve arises from the T11–12 spinal roots and passes through the diaphragm to the celiac ganglion [9].

Intrapatient anatomic variability of the celiac ganglia is significant, but the following generalizations can be drawn from anatomic studies of the celiac ganglia. The number of ganglia varies from 1 to 5 and range in diameter from 0.5 to 4.5 cm. The ganglia lie anterior and anterolateral to the aorta. The ganglia located on the left are uniformly more inferior than their right-sided counterparts by as much as a vertebral level, but both groups of ganglia lie below the level of the celiac artery. The ganglia usually lie approximately at the level of the first lumbar vertebra [9].

The celiac plexus is the largest prevertebral plexus and is composed of the right and left celiac ganglia, a dense network of parasympathetic and sympathetic efferent and afferent nerve fibers. The plexus is located in the epigastrium anterior to the crura of the diaphragm and the body of the first lumbar vertebra; it surrounds the celiac artery and the top of the superior mesenteric artery. The whole plexus is found posterior to the stomach and omental bursa. The right half of the plexus lies behind the upper part of the head of the pancreas, the small part of the duodenum, the lower end of the portal vein, and the inferior vena cava. The left half is covered by the pancreas and splenic vessels. The plexus is found to be anterior to the abdominal aorta. The phrenic arteries are superior and the renal vessels inferior to the plexus, while suprarenal vessels often pass through the plexus.

The celiac plexus occupies an area about 3 cm in length by 4 cm in width. In the transverse plane, it occupies the region between the two adrenal glands and extends beyond the lateral borders of the aorta on both sides. In the longitudinal plane, it occupies the area delineated by the celiac artery above and the renal arteries below. It is in front of the entire L1 vertebra and often the upper part of the L2 vertebra.

Techniques

Retrocrural

The retrocrural or posterior approach involves needle placement posterior and cephalad to the diaphragm. The patient is positioned prone, with the pillows placed under the abdomen to decrease lumbar lordosis. A 20- or 22-gauge needle that is 12–18 cm long is used for the procedure. Needle entry should be immediately caudal to the 12th rib and 7–8 cm lateral to the midline. Positioning of the needle toward the midline will depend on which nerves are to be blocked (splanchnic nerves vs. celiac plexus). To block the celiac plexus, one would direct the needle to the L1 spinous process, whereas the splanchnic nerves are blocked more cephalad toward the 11th or 12th thoracic spinous processes. The needle is inserted on left side at an angle of 45° and advanced following the direction of 12th rib medially until contact is made with the vertebral body of L1. The needle is then withdrawn a bit and redirected to pass by the vertebral body to a point 1–2 cm beyond anterior margin of the vertebral body or until aortic pulsation is felt. The procedure is repeated on the right side, and contrast medium is injected after negative aspiration under fluoroscopic guidance; at this time, a diagnostic block or neurolysis may be performed. The crus is the anatomical determinant of whether a block is a true celiac or splanchnic nerve block. If the needle tip is posterior to the crus, then the nerves blocked will be splanchnic. The crus attaches posteriorly at the T12 and L1 vertebral bodies; at these levels, the needle tip may be anterior or posterior to the crus. At T11, the needle tip will always be posterior to the crus and result in a splanchnic block [9].

Transcrural Approach

In the transcrural or anterocrural technique, the needle passes through the crus of diaphragm with the tip located anterior and caudad to the diaphragm just anterior to the aorta. The technique is similar to the retrocrural approach except that the needle is advanced 1–2 cm deeper. A loss of resistance should be felt once the crus of the diaphragm is pierced. The

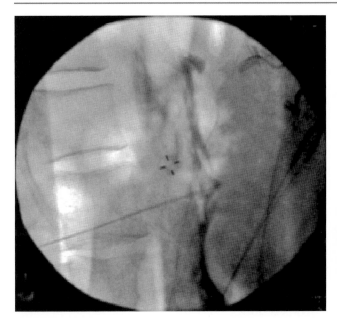

Fig. 41.1 Transaortic celiac plexus block. Lateral view

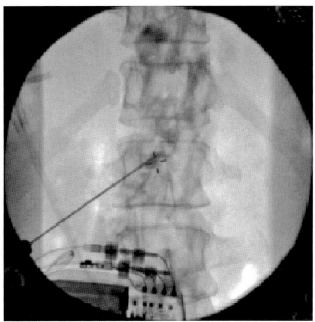

Fig. 41.2 Transaortic celiac plexus block. AP view

needle tips should be just anterolateral to the wall of the aorta bilaterally. With the one-needle method, the needle is inserted 5–6 cm off the midline on the right at the level of lower edge of L1 vertebral body and after passing it, advanced adjacent to the anterolateral wall of the aorta [9].

Transaortic Approach

The needle is placed immediately anterior to the aorta and is advanced slowly with frequent aspiration until the blood appears and the aorta is entered. The needle is then advanced until blood aspiration has stopped, and contrast is injected. Fluoroscopy confirms correct needle position in lateral projection; the needle tip projects just anterior to the edge of the lower third of the body of L1 and in posteroanterior projection; the needle lies in a plane between the left lateral edge of the body of L1 and spinous process (Fig. 41.1) [10].

Fluoroscopic imaging is one of the most commonly used methods of imaging for celiac plexus block [11]; however, there are many other imaging techniques that can be used, including computerized tomography-guided [12], injection by direct visualization [12], magnetic resonance imaging, and ultrasound-guided [13–15]. Ultrasound imaging can be used with a variety of techniques, including endoscopic [16, 17] and percutaneous [18].

In the literature, many approaches to celiac plexus blockade have been documented and include retrocrural, antecrural, transaortic, transcrural, transdiscal, and transabdominal. There are few studies on the different techniques used for celiac plexus neurolysis, and those that do exist demonstrate varying results. One study found no difference in pain scores with neurolysis between the retrocrural, transaortic, and

bilateral chemical splanchnicectomy groups [10]. In a non-randomized, prospective, case-controlled study of 59 patients [19], celiac plexus neurolysis was compared to videothoracoscopic splanchnicectomy. Stefaniak et al. [19] found that both techniques had similar efficacy in pain reduction and decreased daily opioid consumption. Celiac plexus neurolysis, however, was found to be associated with significantly improved physical, emotional, and social well-being with the added benefit of being less invasive [19]. As mentioned previously, in the meta-analysis by Eisenberg et al. [2], positive short-term outcomes from celiac plexus neurolysis, regardless of imaging modality used, were reported (Fig. 41.2).

Splanchnic

The patient is placed in the prone position with a pillow placed under the abdomen to decrease lumbar lordosis. The inferior margins of the 12th rib are identified and marked back to the T12 vertebral body. The spinous process of the L1 vertebral body is then identified and marked. A point approximately 2 in. slightly inferior and lateral to the spinous process of L1 is marked. Typically, 20-gauge, 12-cm needles are inserted bilaterally. The needles are initially oriented 45° toward the midline and about 35° cephalad. Once bony contact with the T12 vertebra is made and the depth noted, the needles are withdrawn to the subcutaneous tissue and redirected so that the needles may walk off the lateral surface of the T12 vertebral body. The needle tips should be at the junction of the anterior and lower third of the vertebral body in a lateral view. Contrast should be confined to the midline and concentrated near the T12 vertebral body in the fluoroscopic anteroposterior view.

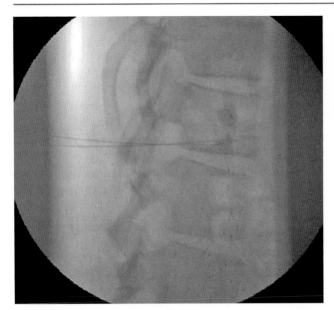

Fig. 41.3 Splanchnic nerve block. Lateral view

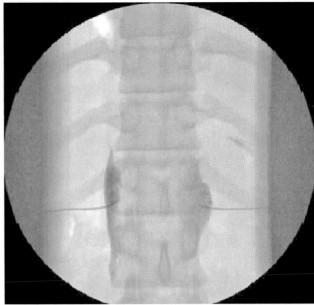

Fig. 41.4 Splanchnic nerve block. AP view

A smooth posterior contour can be observed that corresponds to the psoas fascia on the lateral view. The contrast should be observed to be entirely retrocrural. If there is precrural spread, the needles are withdrawn slightly back through the crura of the diaphragm (Fig. 41.3) [9].

The use of pulsed radio-frequency ablation of the splanchnic nerves has been described as an alternative to splanchnic neurolysis for the treatment of pancreatic and upper abdominal pain [20–22]. Raj et al. [21] reported that up to 40% of patients had excellent pain relief after a thoracic splanchnic nerve block, with only 15% of patients reporting poor results in a series of 107 patients with abdominal pain [21]. One study consisting of eight patients with chronic pancreatitis and two patients with chronic abdominal pain of an unknown etiology found that splanchnic radio-frequency ablation resulted in decreased pain scores, opiate usage, and hospital admissions for pain control [20]. Garcea et al. [20] also found patients to have improvement in their level of anxiety, daily activity, mood, and overall perception of health. One advantage of radio-frequency lesioning of splanchnic nerves is that the tissue that is damaged can be more precisely controlled, allowing the technique to be safer and perhaps more reliable than with the use of a neurolytic agent [21]. Radio-frequency lesioning also has the advantage of an immediate effect unlike neurolytic agents which could take anywhere from 7 to 10 days to achieve neurolysis (Fig. 41.4) [21].

Neurolytic Agents

Neurolytic celiac plexus blocks are commonly performed with 50–100% alcohol and 6–12% phenol. The mechanisms of action of alcohol include dehydration; extraction of phospholipids, cholesterol, and cerebrosides; and precipitation of mucoproteins and lipoproteins. These actions result in sclerosis and separation of the myelin sheath, edematous Schwann cells, and axons. The basal lamina of the Schwann cell tube is often spared, and the axon can regenerate along the previous course; if the ganglion is injected, it may produce cell destruction with no subsequent regeneration [23]. The mechanism of action of phenol depends on its concentration, protein denaturation occurs at concentrations less than 5%, and concentrations higher than 5% produce protein coagulation, nonspecific segmental demyelination, and orthograde degeneration [24, 25]. Axons of all sizes are affected and appear edematous, except posterior root ganglia which are unaffected by phenol. Some have suggested that phenol has a greater affinity for vascular than neuronal tissue [23, 26].

There are advantages and disadvantages to both alcohol and phenol as neurolytic agents. Alcohol is an irritant for soft tissue and is associated with a burning dysesthesia that warrants prior or simultaneous injection of local anesthetic. Alcohol spreads quickly from the injection site due to high solubility in the body. The higher solubility of alcohol can make it challenging to reach the targeted nerve; this also makes a larger volume of injectate necessary to increase the chance of neurolysis of the targeted tissue while also increasing the likelihood of damage to surrounding nerves. An advantage of not using a local anesthetic is that pain along the target nerve will confirm correct needle placement [23]. Phenol used in a concentration of 5–10% causes neurolysis by causing protein coagulation and necrosis when applied to nerves [24, 25]. Phenol is suspended in glycerol, and its high viscosity limits its spread. Phenol also has an advantage of being painless on injection. Just like alcohol, phenol has also been associated with the development of neuritis. However, there are many more case reports of persistent paraplegia following neurolysis with alcohol than with phenol. A study published by Abdalla and Schell [13] reviewed all of the previously reported cases (1974–1998) of temporary or permanent paralysis following neurolysis with alcohol or phenol. In that study, 10/11 cases involved alcohol as the neurolytic agent versus 1/11 in which phenol was used.

Complications may be related to spread of neurolytics to nearby structures, resulting in deafferentation pain of somatic nerves and neuritis. The intravascular spread of the neurolytic solution to the spinal cord may occur with any paraspinal block using neurolytics [13, 27–33]. Even with direct intraoperative visualization, administration of a neurolytic has been reported to lead to permanent paraplegia [13]. Alcohol results in pain upon injection and has been associated with neuritis following neurolysis. With a retrocrural approach, the spread of the neurolytic agent is limited by the diaphragm. Higher quantities of neurolytic agents are often used for the retrocrural approach, and the spread of the agent may cause increased risk of neurolysis to the somatic nerve roots with resulting paraplegia and/or neuritis [13].

Efficacy

The first double-blinded, randomized, controlled trial that studied the benefits of chemical splanchnicectomy in pancreatic cancer patients was done by Lillemoe et al. [5]. Chemical splanchnicectomy was performed with alcohol versus saline placebo at time of exploratory laparotomy for biopsy, staging, and possible palliative gastrointestinal bypass. In follow-up, mean pain scores were found to be lower in the alcohol group at 2, 4, and 6 months ($p < 0.05$). In this study, patients who underwent splanchnicectomy had a longer duration of pain relief (7.2 vs. 3 months of placebo, $p < 0.0001$) and needed lesser amounts of opioids compared to patients who received the placebo (46 and 68%, respectively, $p < 0.05$). Patients in both groups received rescue neurolytic celiac blocks, but time to rescue was significantly longer in those who underwent chemical intervention. In patients who did not have preoperative pain, chemical splanchnicectomy significantly reduced later pain scores and delayed or prevented onset of pain ($p < 0.05$).

Another double-blinded, randomized, control trial more recently conducted by Wong et al. [34] randomized 100 patients into two groups that received either a neurolytic celiac plexus block or analgesic therapy alone with a sham injection. This resulted in a greater reduction in pain intensity ($p = 0.01$) and showed improvement in quality of life ($p = 0.001$) in the first week after randomization in the neurolytic block group. In the first 6 weeks, fewer patients reported moderate to severe pain (rated as ≥5/10 on pain scale) in the neurolytic block group versus those in the systemic analgesic group (14 and 40%, respectively, $p = 0.005$). Although fewer patients in the neurolysis group required rescue blocks versus systemic analgesic group (6 and 20%, respectively), this finding was not statistically significant ($p = 0.07$). Overall, there was no significant difference between the groups for opioid consumption, frequency of adverse opioid effects, quality of life, and survival. However, pain relief was improved in the neurolysis group. In a randomized, double-blind study by Polati et al. [35], the efficacy of neurolytic CPB was compared with pharmacological therapy in the treatment of pain from pancreatic cancer. Twenty-four patients were divided into two groups: 12 patients underwent neurolytic CPB (group 1), and 12 were treated with pharmacological therapy (group 2). Immediate and long-term efficacy, mean analgesic consumption, mortality, and morbidity were evaluated at follow-up. Patients in group 1 reported significant pain relief compared with those in group 2 immediately after the block ($p < 0.05$), but long-term results did not differ between the groups. Overall, the mean analgesic consumption was lower in group 1. They also found a decrease in drug-related adverse effects including constipation (5/12 in group 1 vs. 12/12 in group 2), nausea, and/or vomiting (4/12 in group 1 vs. 12/12 in group 2) ($p < 0.05$).

A prospective study of 50 consecutive pancreatic cancer patients [35] assessed the efficacy of neurolytic celiac plexus blocks depending on primary tumor location. Patients with pancreatic head cancer experienced more pain relief (92% relief) from neurolysis when compared to those with pancreatic body/tail cancer (29% relief). Study results are likely secondary to more advanced tumors in those with body and tail tumors; in which case, neurolysis was ineffective for pain control [36].

Eisenberg et al. [2] performed a meta-analysis of the efficacy and safety of neurolytic celiac plexus blocks from 24 papers including two or more patients with abdominal cancers (total of 1,145 patients included). Good to excellent pain relief was reported in 878/989 patients at 2 weeks. Ninety percent of patients had partial to complete pain relief at 3-month postneurolysis and 70–90% percent had relief until death, even if beyond 3 months after neurolysis.

Although literature has clearly shown that there is a significant reduction in pain scores for most patients following neurolytic celiac plexus blocks, there have also been studies to support that celiac plexus neurolysis may also alter opioid consumption, quality of life, and overall patient survival. Survival in patients with pre-procedure pain was significantly increased by up to 15 months in the celiac plexus neurolysis group versus the placebo group in one study ($p = 0.0001$) [5]. Data also suggested that there may be improved mood and lower levels of disability; however, this was not statistically significant [5].

A more recent study also supports a significant positive effect on duration of life and mood scores following neurolytic celiac block [37]. This study found a correlation between a reduction in pain and increase in longevity. Overall, neurolytic block, when compared to medical management alone, improved pain, elevated mood, reduced pain interference with activity, and was associated with an increase in life expectancy [37].

Despite the commonality of decreased pain scores throughout the literature, not all studies were able to reproduce the results found by Lillemoe et al. [5] and Staats et al. [37]. Multiple studies were unable to find statistically significant differences between medically managed patients and patients who underwent neurolysis, when evaluating quality of life [6, 34, 38]. However, the results from Kawamata et al. [38] indicate celiac plexus blockade does not directly improve quality of life in patients with pancreatic cancer pain, but it may prevent deterioration in quality of life by the long-lasting analgesic effect, limitation of side effects, and reduction of morphine consumption, compared to treatment only with NSAIDs and morphine.

Conflicting results regarding reduction in opioid consumption have been found throughout the literature. Kawamata et al. [38] found a delayed but significant reduction in opioid requirement 4–7 weeks after neurolysis and that consumption continued to decrease over time. Another study found that celiac plexus neurolysis caused a significant but not complete decrease in opioid consumption; patients experienced a mean reduction of 40–80 mg/day of oral morphine [4]. A multicenter, randomized, control trial of 65 patients [39] with pancreatic and upper abdominal cancer found no difference in pain relief or opioid consumption between patients who underwent medical management versus celiac plexus neurolysis or thoracic splanchnicectomy.

Mercadante et al. [40] published a randomized trial of 20 patients, two groups of 10 patients each who were followed until death; pain scores and side effects of their treatment were recorded. Both groups received 1 week of pharmacotherapy, after which group A continued with NSAID-opioid management that followed the World Health Organization stepwise approach and group B who received neurolytic plexus blocks. Although there was a reduction in visual analogue scale pain scores in both groups, there was no statistical significant difference between the two. However, there was a significant decrease in opioid consumption in the celiac plexus neurolysis group; some effects were seen up to 7 weeks after neurolysis or until death.

A recent meta-analysis published in 2011 by Arcidiacono et al. [41] identified six randomized control trials, published between 1993 and 2008, which compared the percutaneous posterior bilateral block (five studies) or the intraoperative block (one study) with standard analgesic therapy for pancreatic and upper abdominal cancer pain. The mean difference for the visual analogue scale pain score at 4 weeks was significant ($p = 0.004$) for the experimental group celiac plexus block. The improvement in pain control coincided with a reduction in opioid consumption; the mean difference in the use of analgesic therapy in the two groups was much greater in the celiac plexus block group ($p < 0.00001$) versus those managed with standard pharmacologic therapy. Decreased opioid usage persisted until the death of the patient, with significantly lower opioid requirements in the CPB group ($p < 0.00001$). Although opioids were never completely stopped, their reduction translated into fewer side effects such as constipation, which was significantly higher in the control group ($p < 0.0001$) [41].

Complications

In general, celiac plexus blockade and neurolysis are considered relatively safe procedures. Adverse events are usually mild and transient, but serious complications including nerve damage, paraplegia, and aortic dissection may occur rarely. The most commonly reported adverse events are transient and include local pain (96%), hypotension (38%), and diarrhea (44%) [2]. A meta-analysis by Eisenberg [2] reports serious adverse events in only 13/628 or 2% of patients undergoing celiac plexus blockade. Serious events reported by Eisenberg et al. [2] included lower extremity weakness and paresthesia, epidural anesthesia and lumbar puncture, hematuria, pneumothorax, and shoulder, chest, and pleuritic pain. Davies [42] reported that paraplegia occurred in 1 of 683 patients undergoing celiac plexus blockade. This would be the most concerning risk for patients undergoing a neurolytic CPB. Hardy and Wells [43] found that during injection of the celiac plexus, the injected fluid typically spreads as high as midthoracic and cervical levels. A proposed etiology for development of paraplegia following neurolysis is the superior spread of injected alcohol or phenol causing spasm or thrombosis of the artery of Adamkiewicz [30, 31, 44]. The neurolytic-induced vasospasm of the artery of Adamkiewicz may occur secondary to compromised perfusion due to surrounding tissue edema or by direct contraction of the arterial muscle wall [45–47]. Paraplegia may also result from direct injection of neurolytic agents into the artery of Adamkiewicz or radicular artery [27, 29, 44, 48]. Even when CPB neurolysis has been performed under direct visualization by an open anterior approach, paraplegia has been a complication likely because of the close anatomical proximity of the celiac plexus to the artery of Adamkiewicz [49].

O'Toole and Schmulewitz [50] reported a complication rate of 1.8% after performing 220 endoscopic ultrasound-guided blocks on 158 patients. This study reported four complications, including asymptomatic hypotension after neurolysis, retroperitoneal abscess after celiac plexus block, and severe self-limited post-procedural pain in two patients after celiac plexus block [50]. Reports of retroperitoneal bleed and abscess [51], urinary retention [36], hiccoughing [52], bowel perforation, gastroparesis [53], hemorrhagic gastritis [54], loss of anal and bladder sphincter function [42], ejaculatory failure [55], anterior spinal artery syndrome and paraplegia [27, 30, 44], aortic dissection [56], and aortic pseudoaneurysm [57] have also been described.

Aortic dissection is one of the most concerning complications and has been reported to arise from the use of a transaortic approach to celiac plexus block [56, 58]. Loss of resistance technique may not prevent complications as one case report by Naviera et al. [58] described; they reported an atheromatous aortic plaque presenting as a loss of resistance and resulted in an aortic dissection. Reports have also documented needle aspiration of blood, cerebral spinal fluid, and urine prior to injection [59].

Celiac plexus block technique may be associated with increased incidence of complications depending on approach. In a prospective, randomized study of 61 patients with pancreatic cancer, Ischia et al. [10] compared the efficacy and incidence of complications associated with three approaches to celiac plexus neurolysis, including retrocrural, transaortic, and transcrural. Orthostatic hypotension occurred more often when the retrocrural (50%) or splanchnic (52%) technique was used than when the anterocrural approach (10%) was used. In contrast, transient diarrhea was more frequent with the anterocrural approach (65%) than with the splanchnic nerve block technique (5%) but not the retrocrural approach (25%). The incidence of dysesthesia, interscapular back pain, reactive pleurisy, hiccups, or hematuria was not statistically different among the three groups. Complications may be decreased with the use of blunt needles and appropriate imaging techniques [60].

Conclusions

Management of visceral abdominal pain that is often secondary to pancreatic and upper gastrointestinal malignancies can be very challenging. Optimization of pain may often require a multimodal approach to obtain adequate analgesia. Numerous studies have shown that patients who suffer from viscerally mediated upper abdominal pain may experience great benefit from celiac plexus neurolysis. Regardless of the technique used, studies have shown that celiac plexus neurolysis has a long-lasting benefit in up to 70–90% of patients with pancreatic cancer [2]. Neurolysis of the celiac plexus is a relatively safe procedure with commonly occurring mild side effects and uncommonly occurring serious adverse events. Celiac plexus neurolysis can be used as an alternative to or in conjunction with opioid analgesics for improvement in pain management and quality of life. However, it is important to keep in mind that celiac plexus blockade will only eliminate visceral-mediated pain but would not otherwise alter musculoskeletal or neuropathic components of pain; that should be clearly explained to the patient prior to entertaining the block.

References

1. Kappis M. Erfahrungen mit localanasthesie bie bauchoperationen. Verh Dtsch Gesellsch Chir. 1914;43:87–9.
2. Eisenberg E, Carr DB, Chalmers TC. Neurolytic celiac plexus block for treatment of cancer pain: a meta-analysis. Anesth Analg. 1995;80(2):290–5.
3. Brown DL. A retrospective analysis of neurolytic celiac plexus block for nonpancreatic intra-abdominal cancer pain. Reg Anesth. 1989;14(2):63–5.
4. Yan BM, Myers RP. Neurolytic celiac plexus block for pain control in unresectable pancreatic cancer. Am J Gastroenterol. 2007; 102(2):430–8.
5. Lillemoe KD, Cameron JL, Kaufman HS, et al. Chemical splanchnicectomy in patients with unresectable pancreatic cancer. A prospective randomized trial. Ann Surg. 1993;217(5):447–55.
6. Zhang CL, Zhang TJ, Guo YN, et al. Effect of neurolytic celiac plexus block guided computerized tomography on pancreatic cancer pain. Dig Dis Sci. 2008;53(3):856–60.
7. Bhatnagar S, Gupta D, Mishra S, Thulkar S, et al. Bedside ultrasound-guided celiac plexus neurolysis with bilateral paramedian needle entry technique can be an effective pain control technique inadvanced upper abdominal cancer pain. J Palliat Med. 2008; 11(9):1195–9.
8. Raj P. Practical management of pain. Missouri: Mosby Inc; 2000. p. 665–70.
9. Waldman SD. Splanchnic nerve block, pain review. Philadelphia: Saunders; 2009. p. 262–3.
10. Ischia S, Ischia A, Polati E, et al. Three posterior celiac plexus block techniques. A prospective, randomized study in 61 patients with pancreatic cancer pain. Anesthesiology. 1992;76(4):534–40.
11. Moore DC, Bush WH, Burnett LL. Celiac plexus block: a roentgenographic anatomic study of technique and spread of solution in patients and corpses. Anesth Analg. 1981;60(6):369–79.
12. Fitzgibbon DR, Schmiedl UP, Sinanan MN. Computed tomography guided neurolytic celiac plexus block with alcohol complicated by superior mesenteric venous thrombosis. Pain. 2001;92(1–2):307–10.
13. Abdalla EK, Schell SR. Paraplegia following intraoperative celiac plexus injection. J Gastrointest Surg. 1999;3(6):668–71.
14. Marcy PY, Magne N. Ultrasound guidance technique in celiac plexus block. J Radiol. 2000;81(12):1727–30.
15. Strong VE, Dalal KM, Malhotra VT, et al. Initial report of laparoscopic celiac plexus block for pain relief in patients with unresectable pancreatic cancer. J Am Coll Surg. 2006;203(1):129–31.
16. Abedi M, Zfass AM. Endoscopic ultrasound-guided (neurolytic) celiac plexus block. J Clin Gastroenterol. 2001;32(5):390–3.
17. Gress F, Schmitt C, Sherman S, et al. A prospective randomized comparison of endoscopic ultrasound and computed tomography guided celiac plexus block for managing chronic pancreatitis pain. Am J Gastroenterol. 1999;94:900–5.
18. Schonenberg P, BAstid C, Guedes J, et al. Percutaneous echography-guided alcohol block of the celiac plexus as treatment of painful syndromes of the upper abdomen, study of 21 cases. Schweiz Med Wochenschr. 1991;121(15):528–31.
19. Stefaniak T, Basinski A, Vingerhoets A, et al. A comparison of two invasive techniques in the management of intractable pain due to inoperable pancreatic cancer: neurolytic celiac plexus block and

videothoracoscopic splanchnicectomy. Eur J Surg Oncol. 2005; 31(7):768–73.

20. Garcea G, Thomasset S, Berry DP, et al. Percutaneous splanchnic nerve radiofrequency ablation for chronic abdominal pain. ANZ J Surg. 2005;75(8):640–4.

21. Raj PP, Sahinler B, Lowe M. Radiofrequency lesioning of splanchnic nerves. Pain Pract. 2002;2(3):241–7.

22. Brennan L, Fitzgerald J, McCrory C. The use of pulsed radiofrequency treatment for chronic benign pancreatitis pain. Pain Pract. 2009;9(2):135–40.

23. Georgescu V. Peripheral nerve blocks: a color atlas. Philadelphia: Lippincott; 2009. p. 409–15.

24. Worsey J, Ferson PF, Keenan RJ, et al. Thorascopic pancreatic denervation for pain control in irresectable pancreatic cancer. Br J Surg. 1993;80(8):1051–2.

25. Copping J, Willix R, Kraft R. Palliative chemical splanchnicectomy. Arch Surg. 1969;98(4):418–20.

26. Nour-Eldin F. Preliminary report: uptake of phenol by vascular and brain tissue. Microvasc Res. 1970;2(2):224–5.

27. Bacher T, Schiltenwolf M, Niethard FU, et al. The risk of paraplegia through medical treatment. Spinal Cord. 1999;37(3):172–82.

28. Houten JK, Errico TJ. Paraplegia after lumbosacral nerve root block, report of three cases. Spine J. 2002;2(1):70–5.

29. Glaser SE, Falco F. Paraplegia following a thoracolumbar transforaminal epidural steroid injection. Pain Physician. 2005; 8(3):309–14.

30. Hayakawa J, Kobyashi O, Murayama H. Paraplegia after intraoperative celiac plexus block. Anesth Analg. 1997;84(2):447–8.

31. Jabbal SS, Hunton J. Reversible paraplegia following coeliac plexus block. Anaesthesia. 1992;47(10):857–8.

32. Kumar A, Tripathi SS, Dhar D, et al. A case of reversible paraparesis following celiac plexus block. Reg Anesth Pain Med. 2001; 26(1):75–8.

33. De Cicco M, Matovic M, Bortolussi R, et al. Celiac plexus block: injectate spread and pain relief in patients with regional anatomic distortions. Anesthesiology. 2001;94(4):561–5.

34. Wong G, Schroeder DR, Carns PE, et al. Effect of neurolytic celiac plexus block on pain relief, quality of life, and survival in patients with unresectable pancreatic cancer: a randomized control trial. JAMA. 2004;291(9):1092–9.

35. Polati E, Finco G, Gottin L, et al. Prospective randomized double-blind trial of neurolytic coeliac plexus block in patients with pancreatic cancer. Br J Surg. 1998;85(2):199–201.

36. Rykowski JJ, Higlier M. Efficacy of neurolytic celiac plexus block in varying locations of pancreatic cancer. Anesthesiology. 2000; 92(2):347–54.

37. Staats PS, Hekmat H, Lilliemoe K, et al. The effects of alcohol celiac plexus block, pain, and mood on longevity in patients with unresectable pancreatic cancer: a double-blind, randomized, placebo controlled study. Pain Med. 2001;2(1):28–34.

38. Kawamata M, Ishitani K, Ishikawa K, et al. Comparison between celiac plexus block and morphine treatment on quality of life in patients with pancreatic cancer pain. Pain. 1996;64(3):597–602.

39. Johnson CD, Berry DP, Harris S, et al. An open randomized comparison of clinical effectiveness of protocol-driven opioid analgesia, celiac plexus block or thoracoscopic splanchnicectomy for pain management in patients with pancreatic and other abdominal malignancies. Pancreatology. 2009;9(6):755–63.

40. Mercadante S, Catala E, Arcuri E, et al. Celiac plexus block for pancreatic cancer pain: factors influencing pain, symptoms and quality of life. J Pain Symptom Manage. 2003;26(6):1140–7.

41. Arcidiacono PG, Calori G, Carrara S, et al. Celiac plexus block for pancreatic cancer pain in adults. Cochrane Database Syst Rev. 2011;16(3):CD007519.

42. Davies DD. Incidence of major complications of neurolytic coeliac plexus block. J R Soc Med. 1993;86(5):264–6.

43. Hardy PA, Wells JC. Coeliac plexus block and cephalad spread of injectate. Ann R Coll Surg Engl. 1989;71(1):48–9.

44. Woodham MJ, Hanna MH. Paraplegia after celiac plexus block. Anaesthesia. 1989;44(6):487–9.

45. Johnson ME, Sill JC, Brown DL, et al. The effect of the neurolytic agent ethanol on cytoplasmic calcium in arterial smooth muscle and endothelium. Reg Anesth. 1996;21(1):6–13.

46. Zafonte RD, Munin MC. Phenol and alcohol blocks for the treatment of spasticity. Phys Med Rehabil Clin N Am. 2001;12(4): 817–32, vii.

47. Mizisin AP, Kalichman MW, Myers RR, et al. Role of the blood-nerve barrier in experimental nerve edema. Toxicol Pathol. 1990;181(Pt 2):170–85.

48. Appelgren L, Nordborg C, Sjoberg M, et al. Spinal epidural metastasis: implications for spinal analgesia to treat "refractory" cancer pain. J Pain Symptom Manag. 1997;13(1):25–42.

49. Kinoshita H, Denda S, Shimoji K, et al. Paraplegia following coeliac plexus block by anterior approach under direct vision. Masui. 1996;45(10):1244–6.

50. O'Toole TM, Schmulewitz N. Complication rates of EUS-guided celiac plexus blockade and neurolysis: results of a large case series. Endoscopy. 2009;41(7):593–7.

51. Navarro-Martinez J, Montes A, Comps O, et al. Retroperitoneal abscess after neurolytic celiac plexus block from the anterior approach. Reg Anesth Pain Med. 2003;28(6):528–30.

52. Ischia S, Luzzani A, Ischia A, et al. A new approach to the neurolytic block of the coeliac plexus: the transaortic technique. Pain. 1983;16(4):333–41.

53. Iftikhar S, Loftus Jr EV. Gastroparesis after celiac plexus block. Am J Gastroenterol. 1998;93(11):2223–5.

54. Pello S, Miller A, Ku T, et al. Hemorrhagic gastritis and duodenitis following celiac plexus neurolysis. Pain Physician. 2009;12(6): 1001–3.

55. Shin SK, Kweon TD, Ha SH, et al. Ejaculatory failure after unilateral neurolytic celiac plexus block. Korean J Pain. 2010;23(4): 274–7.

56. Kaplan R, Schiff-Keren B, Alt E. Aortic dissection as a complication of celiac plexus block. Anesthesiology. 1995;83(3):632–5.

57. Sett SS, Taylor DC. Aortic pseudoaneurysm secondary to celiac plexus block. Ann Vasc Surg. 1991;5(1):88–91.

58. Naveira FA, Speight KL, Rauck RL. Atheromatous aortic plaque as a cause of resistance to needle passage during transaortic celiac plexus block. Anesth Analg. 1996;83(6):1327–9.

59. Saltzburg D, Foley KM. Management of pain in pancreatic cancer. Surg Clin North Am. 1989;69(3):629–49.

60. Heavner JE, Racz GB, Jenigiri B, et al. Sharp versus blunt needle: a comparative study of penetration of internal structures and bleeding in dogs. Pain Pract. 2003;3(3):226–31.

Superior Hypogastric Plexus, Ganglion Impar Blocks, and Neurolysis

42

Bryan S. Williams

Key Points

- Nearly 4% of women have ongoing chronic pelvic pain, and approximately 15–20% have had chronic pelvic pain of at least 1-year duration at some point in their lives (18–50).
- Many pelvic pain conditions can be attenuated by enteral or parenteral medications, along with psychosocial, physical therapy strategies. When conservative measures fail to provide adequate pain relief, interventional strategies can be employed.
- Patients with a history of vague, dull, burning, poorly localized pain of visceral origins (visceral pain) have been the patients thought to benefit from blockade of the superior hypogastric plexus or ganglion impar.
- Neuropathic pain usually manifests as allodynia and hyperalgesia and generates burning, lancinating pain, and paresthesias. The interruption of visceral pain transmission from the pelvis to the spinal cord can be accomplished by blocking the sympathetic pathway.
- The efficacy of local anesthetic blockade of the superior hypogastric and ganglion impar is based on the selective interruption of the sympathetic ganglia in those patients with sympathetically mediated pain. Patients without sympathetically mediated pain may not show attenuation in pain when a local anesthetic block is performed.

Introduction

Chronic pelvic pain (CPP) of malignant or nonmalignant origins can be attenuated by blockade of the superior hypogastric plexus (SHP) [1, 2] or the ganglion impar (GI) (ganglion of

B.S. Williams, M.D., MPH
Comprehensive Pain Medicine, Kaiser Permanente,
Mid Atlantic Permanente Medical Group,
Rush University College of Medicine,
1808 S. Miatican Ave #29, Chicago, IL 60616, USA
e-mail: bryan.williams@yahoo.com

Walther) [3]. Attempts to interrupt sympathetic pathways from the pelvis have been made since the late nineteenth century [4]. In 1921, Leriche performed a periarterial sympathectomy of the internal iliac arteries on a patient with "pelvic neuralgia," and later in the twentieth century. Plancarte et al. [2] showed excellent results from hypogastric plexus block in patients with chronic pelvic pain of malignant origins. The pelvis is innervated by an array of networking neural structures including sympathetic, parasympathetic, and somatic pathways. The SHP is the caudal, retroperitoneal, presacral confluence of the lumbar sympathetic chain. It is located anterior to the abdominal aorta at the L5–S1 intervertebral disk, with the common and internal iliac arteries and veins on either side. The SHP provides innervation to the descending and sigmoid colon, rectum, bladder, prostate, prostatic urethra, testes, seminal vesicles, vaginal fundus, uterus, and ovaries. The GI is the solitary, retroperitoneal termination of the left and right sympathetic chains located anterior to the sacrococcygeal junction. The ganglion of Walther provides innervation to the distal vagina, distal rectum, distal urethra, vulva, and perineum. Analgesia to the organs in the pelvis is possible because the afferent fibers innervating the pelvic structures travel with the sympathetic nerves, trunks ganglia, and rami. Patients with a history of vague, dull, burning, poorly localized pain of visceral origins (visceral pain) have been the patients thought to benefit from blockade of the SHP or GI. These patients include those with pelvic malignancies and nonmalignant origins (e.g., endometriosis).

Background

Malignant- and nonmalignant-associated chronic pelvic pain is a significant cause of pain. Chronic pelvic pain may be defined as noncyclic pain with duration of 6 or more months that localizes to the anatomic pelvis, the abdominal wall at or below the umbilicus, the lumbosacral back, or the buttocks and is of sufficient severity to cause functional disability or lead to medical care effects approximately 1 in 7 women [5]. CPP has been shown to be far more common in women as compared with men. Nearly 4% of women have ongoing CPP, and approximately 15–20% have had CPP of at least 1-year duration at some point in their lives (18–50) [5–7]. In one study of reproductive-aged women in primary care practices, the reported prevalence rate of pelvic pain was 39% [8]. Office visits to gynecologists have been estimated at 10% [9] resulting in 18% of all hysterectomies and up to 40% of all gynecologic laparoscopies performed by gynecologists [10]. This yields 881.5 billion dollars in health-care costs in the United States per year [5]. Malignant-related pain is equally significant with the overall prevalence of pain at 53% in patients of all stages combined and 58–69% in those with advanced cancer [11].

In males, an analogous condition chronic prostatitis/chronic pelvic pain syndrome (CP/CPPS) causes significant pain. Approximately 8.2% of men have prostatitis at some point in their lives. Estimates range from 2.2 to 16% in population-based studies [12–18]. Although prostatitis has been linked to pelvic pain, CP/CPPS has not been scientifically demonstrated to be primarily either a disease of the prostate or the result of an inflammatory process [15, 19]. The disease is named to recognize the limited understanding of the etiologies of this syndrome for most patients and the possibility that organs other than the prostate gland may be important in the cause of this syndrome [15, 20]. The new consensus definition recognizes genitourinary pain complaints as a primary component of this syndrome and includes several exclusion criteria, such as presence of active urethritis, urogenital cancer, urinary tract disease, urethral stricture, or neurological disease affecting the bladder [15]. Whether CPPS is a recognizable disease or not, blockade of the superior hypogastric plexus or ganglion impar may attenuate the pain complaint.

Scientific Foundation

Plancarte et al. [2] first described a percutaneous approach to blocking the superior hypogastric plexus and ganglion impar [3], and since many alternative descriptions have been published [21–26], pain may be nociceptive or neuropathic or mixed. The distention of visceral structures may present as vague, poorly localized, deep, crampy, and dull in nature, while somatic pain may present as well localized and often sharp. Neuropathic pain usually manifests as allodynia and hyperalgesia and generates burning, lancinating pain, and paresthesias. In particular with cancer-related pain, a neuropathic component may be present as pelvic masses invade neural structures. The interruption of visceral pain transmission from the pelvis to the spinal cord can be accomplished by blocking the sympathetic pathway. The blockade interrupts transmission of the pain signal from sympathetic pathways to the brain. In addition to local anesthetic blockade, neurolysis of the sympathetic axis has been employed to attenuate pain primarily in those suffering from malignant-related pain.

Table 42.1 Neurolytic agents

	Alcohol	Phenol
Mechanism of action	Dehydration, phospholipid extraction leading to Wallerian denaturation	Protein coagulation, segmental demyelination, and necrosis of all neural elements
Concentration (%)	50–100	5–10
Clinical onset	Fast	Slow
Clinical duration	Long	Short
Pain on injection	Yes	No

The efficacy of local anesthetic blockade of the SHP and GI is based on the selective interruption of the sympathetic ganglia in those patients with sympathetically mediated pain. Patients without sympathetically mediated pain may not show attenuation in pain when a local anesthetic block is performed. Since the ganglia may not purely be sympathetic, a ganglion/plexus block may not fully provide analgesia from pelvic-derived pain. The efficacy of superior hypogastric and ganglion impar local anesthetic blocks has been examined; although no randomized, placebo-controlled trials have been published, several publications report the efficacy of local anesthetic blocks and neurolytic procedures [27, 28]. High-quality studies are lacking and should be performed, but the use of local anesthetic sympathetic blockade serves a role in the treatment algorithm of visceral pain.

Neurolysis has traditionally been performed in malignant-related visceral pain. Local anesthetic blocks are performed prior to neurolysis as a prognostic measure, although successful temporary blockades do not guarantee the success of neurolysis [29]. The strongest evidence for neurolytic procedures is in those patients with pancreatic cancer [30, 31]. Plancarte et al. [2] present data that neurolysis of the superior hypogastric plexus produces a 70% VAS reduction. Chemical neurolysis with phenol (5–10%) or alcohol (50–100%) disrupts the transmission of pain signals by denaturing proteins and extracting fatty substance, causing Wallerian denaturation and necrosis of neural tissue. Alcohol may cause local pain on injection and neuritis. Phenol has some local anesthetic properties and, unlike alcohol, is not painful on injection. The effects of chemical neurolysis may persist between 3 and 6 months, although the response can vary depending on the extent of malignancy. Neurolysis is less commonly used for nonmalignant pain due to the risk of neuritis. The properties of the agents are presented in Table 42.1.

Patient Selection

These blocks may be associated with morbidity, and it is prudent to understand the indications, the relevant anatomy, and the appropriate patient selection. Patients with moderate to severe pain not controlled with oral analgesics and/or medication-related side effects are ideal candidates for interventional therapy.

Indications

- Acute intervention for acute pain
- Temporary treatment for chronic pain conditions until medication shows efficacy
- Pain affecting the pelvic visceral structures
    - *SHP*: descending and sigmoid colon, rectum, bladder, prostate, prostatic urethra, testes, seminal vesicles, vaginal fundus, uterus, and ovaries
    - *GI*: distal vagina, distal rectum, distal urethra, vulva, and perineum
- Malignant-related pain unresponsive to oral or parenteral medications (neurolysis)
- Excessive sedation or unacceptable side effects from oral or parenteral medications

Contraindications

- Patient refusal
- Coagulopathy
- Local/intra-abdominal infection and sepsis

Equipment

Superior Hypogastric Plexus Block

- Preparation kit, sterile gloves, surgical cap and mask, 18-gauge introducer needle, 22-gauge 5- or 7-in. spinal needle, extension tubing
- Fluoroscope
- Medications
    - Lidocaine 1%
    - Contrast media (e.g., iohexol)
    - Bupivacaine 0.5% or ropivacaine 0.5% and lidocaine 2%
    - Cefazolin 1 g (for intravenous infusion)

Ganglion Impar Block

- Preparation kit, sterile gloves, surgical cap and mask, 22-gauge 3.5-in. spinal needle, extension tubing
- Fluoroscope
- Medications
    - Lidocaine 1%

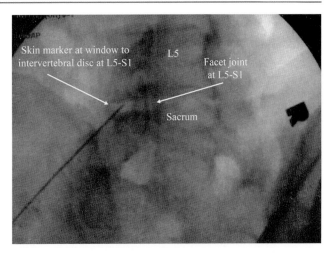

Fig. 42.1 Oblique radiographic view of entrance site

- Contrast media (e.g., iohexol)
- Bupivacaine 0.5% or ropivacaine 0.5% and lidocaine 2%

Neurolysis (Superior Hypogastric and Ganglion Impar)

- Preparation kit, sterile gloves, surgical cap and mask, 22-gauge 5- or 7-in. spinal needle (SHP) or 3.5-in. spinal needle (GI), extension tubing
- Fluoroscope
- Bupivacaine 0.5% or ropivacaine 0.5%
- 50–100% alcohol or 5–10% phenol

Technique

Superior Hypogastric Plexus Block (Transdiscal Approach)

Fluoroscopy guidance is recommended and is described. The patient is placed on the fluoroscopy table in the prone position. After sterile preparation and drape have been accomplished, an anterior-posterior (AP) fluoroscopic image of the lower lumbar spine is obtained, centered on the L5–S1 junction. The end plate of the sacrum is aligned, reducing parallax. The fluoroscope is angled obliquely 25–30° until the superior articular process of the sacrum is approximately one-third of the lateral portion of the disk and 25–30° cephalad, placing the L5–S1 intervertebral disk space into plane view. A site just lateral to the superior articular process "the window" is marked and anesthetized using 1% lidocaine (Fig. 42.1). An 18-gauge spinal introducer needle is inserted and advanced under coaxial technique and intermittent fluoroscopic guidance towards the L5–S1 intervertebral disk.

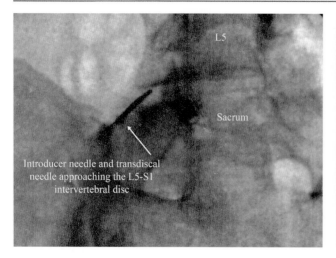

Fig. 42.2 Oblique radiographic view of transdiscal needle

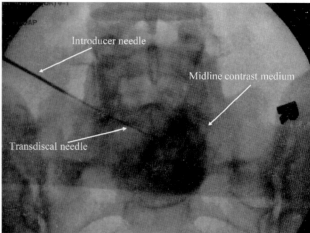

Fig. 42.4 AP radiographic view of transdiscal contrast medium

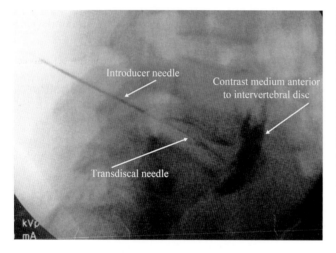

Fig. 42.3 Lateral radiographic view of transdiscal needle

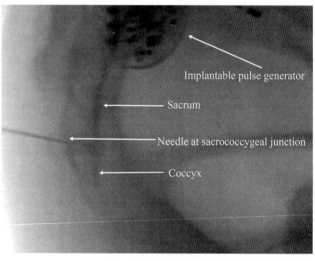

Fig. 42.5 Lateral radiographic view of transacrococcygeal approach

Following this, a 5-in. or 7-in. 22-gauge spinal needle is inserted through the 18-gauge introducer needle. The spinal needle is then advanced to enter the intervertebral disk (Fig. 42.2). The fluoroscope is rotated to lateral position, and the needle is advanced under intermittent fluoroscope until the needle is observed to be anterior to the L5–S1 disk. Then, 1–3 ml of contrast medium (Omnipaque 300 M) is injected anterior to the disk confirming correct needle placement (Fig. 42.3). An AP view is obtained confirming midline placement of the needle (Fig. 42.4). Following this, 8 ml of lidocaine 2%, 8 ml of bupivacaine 0.5% (16 ml total) is then injected with negative aspiration every 3 ml, utilizing intermittent fluoroscopy tracking the spread of the residual contrast anterior to the L5–S1 disk. Neurolysis is performed with phenol 5–10 ml of 5–10% or 5–10 ml of 50–100% alcohol. The needle is flushed with 2 ml of lidocaine 1% to prevent tracking of neurolytic agent and retracted from the subcutaneous tissue and skin.

Ganglion Impar Block (Transsacrococcygeal Approach)

Fluoroscopy guidance is recommended and is described. The patient is placed on the fluoroscopy table in the prone position. After sterile preparation and drape have been accomplished, an anterior-posterior fluoroscopic image of the sacrum is obtained. The ganglion impar block is approached by rotating the fluoroscope to the lateral position and anesthetizing the area overlying the sacrococcygeal junction. A 3.5-in. 22-gauge spinal needle is inserted and advanced under intermittent fluoroscopy towards and into the sacrococcygeal disk (Fig. 42.5). The needle is advanced until the needle is witnessed anterior to the sacrococcygeal disk. One to 3 ml of contrast medium (Omnipaque 300 M) is injected anterior to the disk, confirming correct needle placement. This may produce a "comma sign" in the lateral view (Fig. 42.6). An AP view is obtained confirming midline placement of the needle.

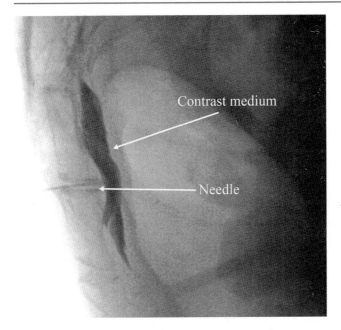

Fig. 42.6 Lateral radiographic view of contrast medium anterior to sacrum

Following this, 2 ml of lidocaine 2%, 2 ml of bupivacaine 0.5% (4 ml total) is then injected. Neurolysis is performed with phenol 1–3 ml of 5–10% or 1–3 ml of 50–100% alcohol. The needle is flushed with 2 ml of lidocaine 1% to prevent tracking of neurolytic agent and retracted from the subcutaneous tissue and skin.

Future Directions

Effective treatment of chronic pelvic pain remains limited. Many pelvic pain conditions can be attenuated by enteral and parenteral medications, along with psychosocial, physical therapy strategies. When conservative measures fail to provide adequate pain relief, interventional strategies should be employed. These strategies include hypogastric and ganglion impar block or neurolysis. Although a very limited number of studies have been published relating the efficacy of these interventional techniques, the prevalence and health-care costs associated with chronic pelvic pain warrant use of superior hypogastric plexus blocks, ganglion impar blocks, and neurolytic procedures in selective cases (e.g., malignant-related pain). Future work is required to confirm the findings of existing studies for nonmalignant pain and assist in developing a treatment strategy for pelvic pain patients.

Summary/Conclusions

Chronic pelvic pain causes significant disability and distress in men and women resulting in significant health-care causes. Specific causes and pathogenesis of CPP are poorly understood and difficult to identify, and treatment is often limited. When conservative therapy fails, sympathetic blocks and neurolysis can be efficacy and should be considered. These blocks can help reduce the requirement for oral analgesics while decreasing tolerance and side effects which develop with increasing doses and prolonged use of opioid medications. Whatever treatment is used, the approach and treatment of men and women with chronic pelvic pain should be multidisciplinary and targeted at different levels of the problem including symptomatic treatment of pain.

References

1. de Leon-Casasola OA, Kent E, Lema MJ. Neurolytic superior hypogastric plexus block for chronic pelvic pain associated with cancer. Pain. 1993;54(2):145–51.
2. Plancarte R, Amescua C, Patt RB, et al. Superior hypogastric plexus block for pelvic cancer pain. Anesthesiology. 1990;73(2):236–9.
3. Plancarte R, Amescua C, Patt RB, et al. Presacral blockade of the ganglion of Walther (ganglion impar). Anesthesiology. 1990; 73(3A):A751.
4. Jaboulay M. Le traitement de la nevralgie pelvienne par la paralysie du sympathique sacre. Lyon Med. 1899;90:467–46821.
5. Mathias SD, Kuppermann M, Liberman RF, et al. Chronic pelvic pain: prevalence, health-related quality of life, and economic correlates. Obstet Gynecol. 1996;87(3):321–7.
6. ACOG Practice Bulletin No. 51. Chronic pelvic pain. Obstet Gynecol. 2004;103(3):589–605.
7. Butrick CW. Chronic pelvic pain: how many surgeries are enough? Clin Obstet Gynecol. 2007;50(2):412–24.
8. Jamieson DJ, Steege JF. The prevalence of dysmenorrhea, dyspareunia, pelvic pain, and irritable bowel syndrome in primary care practices. Obstet Gynecol. 1996;87(1):55–8.
9. Reiter RC. A profile of women with chronic pelvic pain. Clin Obstet Gynecol. 1990;33(1):130–6.
10. Howard FM. The role of laparoscopy in chronic pelvic pain: promise and pitfalls. Obstet Gynecol Surv. 1993;48(6): 357–87.
11. van den Beuken-van Everdingen MH, de Rijke JM, Kessels AG, et al. Prevalence of pain in patients with cancer: a systematic review of the past 40 years. Ann Oncol. 2007;18(9):1437–49.
12. Collins M, Stafford RS, O'Leary MP, et al. How common is prostatitis? A national survey of physician visits. J Urol. 1998; 159(4):1224–8.
13. Krieger JN, Lee SW, Jeon J, et al. Epidemiology of prostatitis. Int J Antimicrob Agents. 2008;31 Suppl 1:S85–90.
14. Ku JH, Kim SW, Paick JS. Epidemiologic risk factors for chronic prostatitis. Int J Androl. 2005;28(6):317–27.
15. Murphy AB, Macejko A, Taylor A, et al. Chronic prostatitis: management strategies. Drugs. 2009;69(1):71–84.
16. Nickel JC, Downey J, Hunter D, et al. Prevalence of prostatitis-like symptoms in a population based study using the National Institutes of health chronic prostatitis symptom index. J Urol. 2001; 165(3):842–5.
17. Pontari MA. Chronic prostatitis/chronic pelvic pain syndrome in elderly men: toward better understanding and treatment. Drugs Aging. 2003;20(15):1111–25.
18. Roberts RO, Jacobson DJ, Girman CJ, et al. Prevalence of prostatitis-like symptoms in a community based cohort of older men. J Urol. 2002;168(6):2467–71.
19. Potts J, Payne RE. Prostatitis: infection, neuromuscular disorder, or pain syndrome? Proper patient classification is key. Cleve Clin J Med. 2007;74 Suppl 3:S63–71.

20. Ludwig M, Weidner W, Schroeder-Printzen I, et al. Transrectal prostatic sonography as a useful diagnostic means for patients with chronic prostatitis or prostatodynia. Br J Urol. 1994;73(6):664–8.

21. Datir A, Connell D. CT-guided injection for ganglion impar blockade: a radiological approach to the management of coccydynia. Clin Radiol. 2010;65(1):21–5.

22. Erdine S, Yucel A, Celik M, et al. Transdiscal approach for hypogastric plexus block. Reg Anesth Pain Med. 2003;28(4):304–30.

23. Kanazi GE, Perkins FM, Thakur R, et al. New technique for superior hypogastric plexus block. Reg Anesth Pain Med. 1999; 24(5):473–6.

24. Michalek P, Dutka J. Computed tomography-guided anterior approach to the superior hypogastric plexus for noncancer pelvic pain: a report of two cases. Clin J Pain. 2005;21(6):553–6.

25. Munir MA, Zhang J, Ahmad M. A modified needle-inside-needle technique for the ganglion impar block. Can J Anaesth. 2004;51(9):915–7.

26. Turker G, Basagan-Mogol E, Gurbet A, et al. A new technique for superior hypogastric plexus block: the posteromedian transdiscal approach. Tohoku J Exp Med. 2005;206(3):277–81.

27. Bosscher H. Blockade of the superior hypogastric plexus block for visceral pelvic pain. Pain Pract. 2001;1(2):162–70.

28. Day M. Sympathetic blocks: the evidence. Pain Pract. 2008; 8(2):98–109.

29. Practice guidelines for chronic pain management. A report by the American society of anesthesiologists task force on pain management, chronic pain section. Anesthesiology. 1997;86(4):995–1004.

30. Kawamata M, Ishitani K, Ishikawa K, et al. Comparison between celiac plexus block and morphine treatment on quality of life in patients with pancreatic cancer pain. Pain. 1996;64(3):597–602.

31. Mercadante S. Celiac plexus block versus analgesics in pancreatic cancer pain. Pain. 1993;52(2):187–92.

Peripheral Neurolysis

43

Beth Mintzer and Jagan Devarajan

Key Points

- Similar to central neuraxial neurolysis, neurolytic techniques can be utilized in peripheral nerves, sympathetic ganglia, and specific ganglia in order to alleviate pain arising from these structures.
- They are predominantly used for cancer pain management though they prove to be efficacious with minimal side effects for some benign conditions as well.
- Neurolysis can be performed by three means: physical (e.g., cryoprobe), chemical (e.g., phenol), and electrical (using high-frequency electrical current). All are aimed at interrupting the generation or propagation of action potentials along the corresponding neural structures.
- Alcohol (50–100 %) and phenol (6–10 %) are commonly used chemical neurolytic agents; glycerol (50–100 %) is exclusively used in Gasserian ganglion neurolysis.
- Cryoprobe works on Joule–Thomson effect, and pulsed radiofrequency acts by producing rapidly changing electrical field in a temperature-independent mechanism. It modulates the inflammatory response caused by the injury. It also initiates cascade of genetic events resulting in cellular prolifera-

tion which leads to decrease in pain and edema. It is presumed to cause less damage to nervous tissue.
- Trigeminal ganglion is located in apex part of petrous part of temporal bone in the middle cranial fossa, and one of the modalities of treatment of trigeminal neuralgia includes neurolysis with glycerol.
- The Gasserian ganglion can be targeted by many approaches: glycerol rhizolysis, application of radiofrequency thermocoagulation, balloon compression, and stereotactic radiosurgery using gamma knife.
- Radiofrequency thermocoagulation is associated with higher success rates, nevertheless, associated with greater incidence of complications.
- Sphenopalatine neurolysis is utilized in the treatment of sphenopalatine neuralgia and is performed by neurolysis infrazygomatic fluoroscopic-guided approach.
- Intercostal neurolysis serves in palliation of pain in the chest due to tumors involving breast, lung, and chest wall.
- Brachial plexus neurolysis is very seldom used due to fear of weakness and sensory disturbances.
- Celiac plexus neurolysis is indicated in refractory pain due to pancreatic adenocarcinoma and other intra-abdominal visceral malignancies.
- There are controversies surrounding the efficacy of block in improving quality of life and increase in life expectancy; nevertheless, it is consistently proven to provide superior analgesia compared to conservative management.
- Superior hypogastric plexus is commonly used to treat pain due to pelvic malignancies, though it has occasionally used in severe pain due to endometriosis.
- Neurolysis is one of the mainstays of treatment for Morton's neuroma due to compression of interdigital nerve and stump neuroma.
- Neurolysis of ganglion impar is occasionally used in pelvic pain.

B. Mintzer, M.D., M.S., CBE (✉)
Department of Pain Management, Anesthesia Institute, CCF,
9500 Euclid Av, C-25, Cleveland, OH 44195, USA
e-mail: minzteb@ccf.org

J. Devarajan, M.D.
Department of Pain Management, Anesthesia Institute, CCF,
9500 Euclid Av, C-25, Cleveland, OH 44195, USA

5936 Stumph Road Apt #205, Parma, OH 44130, USA
e-mail: drdjagan2000@yahoo.com

T.R. Deer et al. (eds.), *Comprehensive Treatment of Chronic Pain by Medical, Interventional, and Integrative Approaches*,
DOI 10.1007/978-1-4614-1560-2_43, © American Academy of Pain Medicine 2013

Introduction

The argument can be made that pain management is practiced best as a multidisciplinary specialty, and that interventional therapy is often required after conservative management and medication management have failed to provide adequate pain relief. Occasionally conventional therapeutic options fail because of the rapid progression of the disease such as in malignancy or in cases of uncontrolled proliferation of nerve fibers and unregulated transmission of nerve impulses. Very often, nontraditional methods of treatment need to be deployed to control a patient's pain. These methods include neurodestructive procedures. In general, neuroablative procedures are undertaken predominantly in malignant patients where pain control cannot be achieved with medications or in cases in which medications cause intolerable side effects.

Prevalence of pain among cancer patients is generally greater than 50 %, and as disease progresses, the incidence increases to 58–69 %, and its severity increases as well [1]. More often, these patients have a limited lifespan, and the provision of analgesia and improved quality of life will outweigh potential adverse effects arising from these interventional procedures. Various issues need to be considered before contemplating performance of these kinds of procedures, as the potential complications can be quite disabling. Often, in fact, they are permanent. Etiology of the pain, progression of the disease, expectations of the patients and their families, and availability of expertise should be analyzed thoroughly before the procedures. Despite their risks, neurolytic blocks nevertheless remain in the armamentarium of cancer pain management [2].

In the previous chapter, we discussed intrathecal and epidural neurolysis for intractable pain. In this chapter, we will discuss features of neurolysis at the level of ganglion, nerve roots, and peripheral nerves.

Substances Used for Neurolysis

There are three types of peripheral neurolysis reported in the literature. Chemical neurolysis is achieved by application of phenol, alcohol, or glycerol, or ammonium nitrate at the level of the peripheral nervous system. Physical neurolysis is by application of a cryoprobe to individual nerves. Electrical neuroablation is application of high-frequency electrical current resulting in disruption of transmission of nerve impulses.

The properties and side effects of different chemical agents used for neurolysis are discussed in the previous chapter. In brief, phenol is used in concentrations of 6–10 % and alcohol 50–100 %. Application of alcohol is painful; however, it is associated with longer duration of block (8–24 weeks). Phenol, on the other hand, is painless due to its local anesthetic properties but results in somewhat shorter duration of action (8–12 weeks). Glycerol is commonly used for trigeminal ganglion neurolysis. Glycerol is used only in trigeminal neurolysis, and the commonly administered concentration is 50–100 % [3].

Cryoanalgesia is based on the physical principle of Joule–Thomson effect [4]. Joule–Thomson effect results in rapid change in temperature when a gas is allowed to expand from a high pressure to low pressure in an adiabatic manner. The cooling is due to the fact that energy in the form of work is required to overcome the long-range attraction between gas molecules as they expand. A cryoprobe is a hollow tube with a smaller inner tube. Either N_2O or CO_2 is passed through the smaller tube at a pressure of 600–800 psi and is released into the larger tube where the pressure drops to 10–15 psi. The expansion decreases the temperature, resulting in the formation of an ice ball at the tip of the probe at a temperature of −70 °C. The probe may have nerve stimulator capability in order to localize the nerve better before freezing. Application of an ice ball on the surface of the nerve disrupts conduction of nerve impulses. Low temperature also causes severe vascular damage of vaso nervorum which causes severe endoneural edema. The long-term effect may also be explained by an autoimmune phenomenon with antibodies directed against the proteins released as a result of cryoablation. The degree of successful cryoablation depends on the temperature (how low) and duration of exposure to the cold. It also depends on the proximity of the probe to the nerve, the size of the probe and resultant ice ball formed, and the temperature of surrounding tissues. The use of a larger probe and accurate localization of the nerve with both ultrasound and nerve stimulator will improve the success rate.

The other approach is to apply high-frequency electrical current which would cause coagulation necrosis of the surrounding nerves [5]. This procedure is commonly referred to as radiofrequency ablation. The electrical energy is delivered in a circumferential manner around the needle tip. Pulsed radiofrequency has been used to treat pain arising from peripheral nerves and axial skeleton [6, 7]. In addition to heat production, exposure of nerve to radiofrequency electrical field causes changes in genetic expression of the nerves resulting in pain relief. Application of electrical current to the target in bursts of 20 ms followed by a quiescent period of 480 ms facilitates heat to be carried away.

Neurolysis

Peripheral Neurolysis Involving Ganglia

Trigeminal Neurolysis
Anatomy
The trigeminal ganglion is located within a fold of dura mater which is called Meckel's cave [8]. This fold of dura covers

the posterior two thirds of the ganglion. It is situated in the apex of the petrous portion of the temporal bone in the middle cranial fossa. It is bound medially by the cavernous sinus with the trochlear and optic nerves situated within it and superiorly by the inferior surface of temporal lobe and posteriorly by the brain stem. These boundaries reinforce the importance of placing the needle accurately in order to avoid serious side effects. Preganglionic fibers exit the brain stem and travel to synapse with second-order neurons in the Gasserian ganglion (GG) [9]. The GG is formed by three series of rootlets which originate from the ventral surface of brain stem at the midpontine level. The first rootlet is V1, the ophthalmic division, which passes through the superior orbital fissure and receives sensory afferents from the forehead and nose. The second is the maxillary division (V2), which consists of sensory afferents from the upper jaw and exits skull through the foramen rotundum, then entering the orbit through the inferior orbital fissure. The mandibular division (V3) passes through the foramen ovale and provides sensory supply to the lower jaw.

Indications

Though neurolysis of the trigeminal ganglion is predominantly used to treat persistent trigeminal neuralgia [10], this intervention has been used successfully to treat both cluster headache [11, 12] and atypical facial pain [13, 14]. It is also commonly utilized to treat refractory cancer pain [15] in the distribution of the V2 and V3 divisions of the trigeminal nerve.

Refractory trigeminal neuralgia can be treated by minimally invasive procedures percutaneously. These procedures can be neuroablative with destruction of the nerve or nonablative in which the nerve is decompressed without affecting nerve function.

Neuroablative procedures can be done at three levels [16]. They are done at the peripheral nerve, at the Gasserian ganglion, or at posterior fossa. The peripheral neurolysis is intended to destroy the sensory nerves innervating triggering zone for headache. The Gasserian ganglion can be targeted by many approaches: glycerol rhizolysis, application of radiofrequency thermocoagulation, balloon compression, and stereotactic radiosurgery using gamma knife. The posterior approach is intended to do partial rhizotomy surgery through gamma knife and microvascular decompression posterior fossa surgery. All techniques except surgical sensory rhizotomy are minimally invasive and require short hospital stay. Next trigeminal neurolysis at the level of the Gasserian ganglion is discussed in detail.

Approach to Gasserian Ganglion Through Foramen Ovale

It should be done under fluoroscopic guidance which aids in correct placement of the needle and decreases the incidence of adverse reactions. The use of a curved blunt-tipped needle is strongly recommended to facilitate access to the foramen and to decrease the incidence of complications.

Patient should be supine with the head slightly extended. The entry point is 2.5 cm lateral to the angle of mouth at midpupillary line. Sterile preparation and drape cannot be overemphasized. C-arm intensifier should be obliquely rotated contralaterally away from the nose 20–30°. C-arm is then rotated 30–35° in the cephalocaudal direction to bring foramen ovale into view. Fine adjustments are made to get the best possible view of the foramen ovale. The needle is advanced slowly after raising local anesthetic wheal at the skin entry site. The direction of the needle should be superior and towards the medial aspect of the external auditory meatus. After the needle contacts the bone, a lateral view should be utilized fluoroscopically to confirm the position of the needle, which is then advanced slowly through foramen ovale. If the tip of the needle does not enter the foramen ovale, the needle is usually redirected slightly posteriorly to negotiate through the foramen. Occasionally paresthesias in the distribution of the mandibular nerve may be elicited. After negative aspiration of blood and CSF, nonionic water-soluble contrast should be injected to confirm the needle position. Occasionally CSF can be seen at the needle tip, though this has not been shown to affect the outcome of the results. Absolute alcohol or phenol can be used to lyse the ganglion, but most commonly glycerol is used for neurolysis. The amount of glycerol required for neurolysis of the ganglia is usually 0.3–0.5 ml [17]. Local anesthetic test dose may be injected before neurolysis. Glycerol is usually injected in 0.1 ml increments in order to avoid spillage into surrounding intracranial structures. The patient is usually seated with his/her head tipped forward [18].

Currently, radiofrequency neuroablation is more frequently performed and is associated with higher success rates [19]. In conventional radiofrequency, the probe is heated to 60–90 °C and usually applied for 60–90 s. Local anesthetic must be injected in order to decrease the pain due to the high temperature. Electromagnetic field pulsed radiofrequency is another way to cause ablation of the trigeminal ganglion. The principle behind pulsed radiofrequency is that the nerve is considered to act as a capacitor and the high electric field created by EMF produces holes in the capacitor-like-acting nerve, thereby interrupting the transmission of signals. This lesioning is presumed to block sensory transmission selectively through A delta and C fibers. EMF lesioning is done at lower temperatures than conventional radiofrequency, and the working range of temperature is 42 °C and is applied for 120 s [20, 21].

Percutaneous microcompression of the trigeminal ganglion is performed by inserting a No. 4 Fogarty balloon catheter percutaneously through the foramen ovale and inflating it for a minute [22, 23]. Gamma knife surgery is the latest technique for trigeminal neurolysis and works by delivering cobalt-60 radiation to the root of the trigeminal nerve through stereotactic MRI approach [16, 24]. Selective neurolysis of the V2 and V3 divisions of the trigeminal nerve is possible for specific situations in patients with cancer-related pain [25].

These branches can be accessed below the zygomatic arch in the center of the coronoid notch by directing the needle in a perpendicular plane. The needle is advanced until the lateral pterygoid plate is encountered. If the needle is withdrawn and redirected superiorly and anteriorly, the maxillary nerve is encountered; if directed posteriorly and inferiorly, the mandibular nerve can be blocked. One to 2 ml of 6 % aqueous phenol is required to block the individual nerves.

The success rates of percutaneous glycerol rhizolysis (GR) and radiofrequency thermocoagulation (RFTC) are variable, and the studies in the literature are not uniform. Udipi et al. had shown 58.9 % success rate for GR and 84.6 % for RFTC which were not statistically significantly different from each other [26]. The recurrence rates were also not different between the two groups. Tew et al. [27] had reported a success rate of 93 % in a group of elderly patients who had undergone RFTC of the trigeminal ganglion. In the remaining 7 %, 5 % required repeat RFTC to which they responded well to treatment. In a study by Onofrio et al., all patients with classic trigeminal neuralgia responded well to RFTC, and those who were diagnosed with other types of neuralgia did not respond well [28]. Hundred percent pain relief was obtained in patients who suffered from chronic migrainous headaches [29]. The recurrence rate of headache has been reported to be 7 % in a follow-up period of 7 years. Recurrence rates in other studies were reported at 15 % [30] and 16 % [31], respectively. Glycerol rhizolysis has been shown to be successful in 92 % of patients by Dieckman et al. in 1–4 years of follow-up [32]. Spaziente has also obtained similar success rates in his patients [33].

However, Saini et al. in a large study involving 552 patients have shown a success rate of 68 % [34]. A cumulative 27.7 and 40.9 % relapsed in 1 and 2 years, respectively, after GR. Meta-analysis by Lopez had shown RFTC to have higher success rates compared to glycerol rhizolysis and stereotactic radiosurgery; nevertheless, it is associated with greatest number of complications [35]. The success rates in the literature in general are reported as 80–90 % in 1–2 years, and the relapse rate is 20–30 %. The success rates for GGGR are 80–90 % in patients who are diagnosed with cluster headaches [12, 36, 37].

Percutaneous microcompression (MC) of trigeminal neuralgia has been shown to be 93.2 % effective compared to improvement in 81.8 % of patients who underwent RFTC. However, the recurrence rates were 56 and 452.4 % following MDC and RFTC, respectively, and the recurrence occurred in a shorter period of time (6.5 months) compared to 18.5 months following RFTC [38].

Side Effects

Trigeminal neuralgia is associated with side effects which can be explained by the innervation of the trigeminal nerve. The trigeminal nerve serves as afferent pathway for corneal reflex; trigeminal ganglion blockade may result in loss of corneal reflex which can lead to hypesthesia, exposure keratitis, and corneal ulceration. Due to loss of innervation of masticatory muscles by the mandibular nerve, masticatory weakness can be observed. The incidence of numbness and paresthesia in the distribution of the trigeminal nerve is variable and ranges from 29 to 63 % [28, 39–41]. Anesthesia dolorosa can occur but the incidence is very low (0–1 %) [41–43]. Herpes simplex virus reactivation (incidence up to 10 %) has also been reported following GR [42].

Sphenopalatine Ganglion Neurolysis

Sphenopalatine ganglion (pterygopalatine ganglion or Meckel's, SPG) [44] is a major parasympathetic ganglion which is associated with branches of the maxillary nerve. It is located in the pterygopalatine fossa and consists of sensory, sympathetic, and parasympathetic roots. The boundaries of the pterygopalatine fossa are the posterior wall of maxillary sinus anteriorly, medial plate of pterygoid process posteriorly, the sphenoid sinus superiorly, and infratemporal fossa laterally. The ganglion is located on the posterior aspect of middle turbinate of the nose and lies very close to the lateral wall of the nose. Both maxillary artery and nerve are located within this region. Sensory branches arise from the maxillary nerve and are distributed along the nasal membranes, soft palate, and pharynx. The postganglionic sympathetic fibers which relay through the sphenopalatine ganglion are distributed to the lacrimal gland and nasal and palatine mucosa.

Indications for Neurolysis

The main indication for neurolysis is sphenopalatine neuralgia [45, 46], a painful condition of the head and neck where the patient experiences unilateral facial pain across the root of nose. This pain occasionally spreads retro-orbitally to the occiput and mastoid process. This painful syndrome related to irritation of the SPG can occur due to the existence of deformities such as a deviated nasal septum or nasal spur or a vasomotor phenomenon. Blockade of the sphenopalatine ganglia is occasionally used in the treatment of trigeminal neuralgia [47, 48] due to retrograde effect. It can also be used in the treatment of cluster headache, migraine, herpes zoster ophthalmicus, and atypical facial pain [49, 50] disorders.

Techniques

Neurolysis is performed by infrazygomatic fluoroscopic-guided approach [18]. A diagnostic block with local anesthetic is essential before proceeding with neurolysis.

Patient is positioned supine for the procedure.

The head is placed inside the C-arm and is passively rotated until rami of the mandible are superimposed. C-arm is tilted cephalad until pterygopalatine fossa is visualized. When the two pterygopalatine plates are superimposed, it will resemble a "vase." The needle insertion point is under the zygoma and anterior to the ramus of the mandible. The direction of the needle should be in a medial, cephalad, and slightly posterior direction towards the pterygopalatine fossa. The tip of the needle is advanced until it is adjacent to the lateral nasal mucosa. The needle tip is confirmed by an anteroposterior view. Extra care should be taken when advancing along the lateral nasal mucosa so as not to perforate it. If paresthesia in hard palate is felt, it indicates stimulation of the greater and lesser palatine nerves and requires redirection of needle posteriorly and medially. If paresthesia is felt on upper teeth due to stimulation of the maxillary nerve, the needle should be directed in a more caudal and medial direction. Contrast is injected to confirm the position of needle and to help predict the spread of neurolytic agent. It also is used to indicate vascular (or CSF) uptake so that the needle tip intravascular injection is avoided.

If spread is correct and there is no evidence of vascular uptake of contrast, then after negative aspiration neurolytic agent is injected in 0.1 ml increments. If radiofrequency lesioning is the preferred method of neuroablation, then it is performed twice at 67–80° for 70–90 s. Pulsed radiofrequency lesioning [46] is an alternative and is performed at 42 °C for 120 s and requires 2–3 lesions. A case report involving stereotactic radiosurgery has been reported to be successful for the treatment of sphenopalatine neuralgia [51].

Efficacy

RFTC of SPG has been found to be effective in relieving pain in patients with sphenopalatine neuralgia [46]. Duration of pain relief varied from 6 to 34 months. It has been shown to relieve intractable ear pain following herpes zoster ophthalmicus [52].

In cluster headache, the efficacy of sphenopalatine ganglion neurolysis was reported to be 60–70 % efficacious and 30 % in atypical headache [53]. Topical application of local anesthetic through the intranasal approach has been used to block the sphenopalatine ganglion. Local anesthetic soaked cotton-tipped applicator is inserted through the ipsilateral nose parallel to the zygomatic arch and advanced towards the back of the nasopharynx. To provide complete blockade, a second applicator can also be inserted superior and posterior to the first one. Sphenopalatine ganglion is located a few millimeters beneath lateral wall of nasal mucosa [54]. In a similar way, 88 % phenol has been applied to eight patients in an attempt to relieve sphenopalatine neuralgia [55]. This approach, however, is not generally recommended, as it has the potential of causing a perforation of the lateral nasal mucosa.

Side Effects

Hematoma formation is a potential complication due to the presence of a venous plexus in front of the pterygopalatine fossa. SPG blockade can cause sensory disturbances like numbness, hypesthesia, or dysesthesia in the region of the palate, maxilla, and posterior pharynx [46, 53]. The side effects are usually transient. The Konen reflex can occur [56], described as a bradycardia following blockade of SPG. It has a mechanism similar to that of the oculocardiac reflex. With recent introduction of pulsed radiofrequency, most side effects can be minimized.

Glossopharyngeal Nerve

Neurolysis of the glossopharyngeal nerve may be indicated in patients with refractory pain in the posterior third of the tongue and the oropharynx [25]. The nerve can be infiltrated by tumors of tonsils, tongue, and hypopharynx and can cause severe pain. This block may be diagnostic in Eagle's syndrome or glossopharyngeal neuralgia in which pain is distributed unilaterally across oropharynx, earlobe, and face. This pain syndrome is caused by compression of glossopharyngeal nerve due to presence of elongated styloid process or ossification of the stylohyoid ligament [57, 58].

The patient is kept in the supine or lateral decubitus position. The needle is inserted halfway between the angle of the mandible and the mastoid process. The styloid process is encountered at a depth of 3 cm, and the needle is withdrawn and redirected slightly posteriorly, just past the styloid process. Paresthesia can be elicited in the oropharynx, and 1 ml of 6 % phenol or absolute alcohol can be injected after negative aspiration. Pulsed radiofrequency can also be used for glossopharyngeal neuralgia which has been shown to be 50–75 % efficacious [59, 60]. Complications include deafferentation pain, neuritis, intravascular injection of neurolytic agent, and infection.

Blocks in Thorax

Intercostal nerve block can be utilized for palliation of pain in the chest due to tumors involving breast, lung, and chest wall. The pain can arise from the tumor itself or tumor-infiltrating nerves causing neuralgia [8]. Usually multiple intercostal nerve blocks are required to cover the region of pain.

It is very important to identify the dermatomes involved and the respective intercostal nerve which needs to be blocked. A diagnostic block with local anesthetic is absolutely necessary to predict the response.

Patients are positioned in the prone position for this procedure. The relevant intercostal nerve and the corresponding rib are identified with the aid of fluoroscopy or ultrasound. The intercostal nerve, along with its artery and nerve, runs along the inferior border of the rib. The puncture site is approximately 6 cm lateral to the midline. Usually a 22-gauge 50-mm needle is long enough to perform the block. The needle is advanced until it contacts the inferior border of the rib and then walked off the margin slightly. Radiocontrast dye is injected which can be seen to spread along the inferior border of the rib. Two to 3 ml of 6 % phenol is required to perform the block. Complications include hematoma, pneumothorax, neuritis, and intravascular injection. The most dangerous complication ever reported was occurrence of paraplegia which had happened to a patient with scoliosis who had undergone intercostal neurolysis with 7.5 % phenol [61]. It was postulated to be caused by diffusion of phenol through intervertebral foramen into spinal cord, damaging sensory and motor nerve roots. Usually somatic pain responds well to intercostal block.

For intractable visceral pain, interpleural phenol has been used in a case report. It was used to alleviate the suffering of a patient with pain due to esophageal cancer [62]. Ten milliliters of 6 % phenol mixed with bupivacaine produced 2 days of pain relief. This was followed by interpleural administration of 18 ml of 10 % phenol which produced substantial pain relief for 4 weeks until the patient's death. No postmortem histopathological changes were found which could be attributed to the effects of phenol.

Upper Extremity Neurolysis

Cancer pain in upper extremities is commonly due to Pancoast tumors and metastases or tumors involving the bone and soft tissues. Tumor invasion of the brachial plexus due to axillary metastases can cause intractable pain in the upper extremity. The brachial plexus originates from anterior primary rami of C5–T1 and provides innervation to the upper extremity. Brachial plexus neurolysis is performed very rarely as the incidence of side effects like numbness and paralysis is very high, and hence this procedure is usually restricted to terminally ill patients. Moreover, peripheral nerve stimulation and the availability of radiofrequency ablation make neurolysis fairly obsolete.

Neurolysis should be performed proximal to the nerves which act as pain generator. Most patients with involvement of neural structures may have preexisting sensory and motor weakness which should be carefully documented. This can also make identifying the nerve by nerve stimulator difficult; in these situations, identification with ultrasound can be very helpful.

To treat the pain secondary to Pancoast tumors, the interscalene approach to blockade of the brachial plexus is required. The brachial plexus can be identified by ultrasound, after which

diagnostic local anesthetic injection is helpful to determine the degree of pain relief which can be achieved. To perform neurolysis, 15–20 ml 6 % phenol can be injected slowly in increments. Side effects are intravascular injection, subarachnoid or epidural spread causing unwanted side effects, hematoma, pneumothorax, and involvement of phrenic nerve.

Involvement of the lumbosacral plexus by tumor causes pain in the lower extremities. This pain can be managed with central neuraxial neurolysis by selective blockade of sensory innervation. Transforaminal epidural phenol administration [63] to cause selective blockade of nerve root has been reported to alleviate pain successfully in the lower extremities due to leiomyosarcoma. Phenol was administered in two stages at three levels without any untoward side effects. Reportedly obturator nerve neurolysis successfully reduced adductor spasticity resulting from different pathological processes [64, 65].

The lytic effect lasted for a maximum of 3 months. It allowed for a decrease in VAS scores and improvement in range of motion and personal hygiene. Cryoanalgesia has been used to provide successful long lasting relief of adductor spasm and pain [66].

Details of the procedures for obturator nerve and transforaminal block are discussed elsewhere in the textbook.

Phenol neurolysis has also been used for certain conditions causing nonmalignant pain [67].

The pain was persisting even after opioids, NSAIDs, and adjuvants. The conditions where the neurolysis was effective were Tietze's syndrome, ilioinguinal nerve, medial branch neurolysis, lumbar sympathetic nerves, intercostal nerve, genitofemoral neuralgia, and meralgia paresthetica [67]. Neurolytic paravertebral block with phenol appears to have limited use [68]. There were no serious complications such as tissue necrosis or flaccid paralysis. Minor complications like local hematoma and pain occasionally occurs which usually resolve in 2 weeks. In 25 % of patients, a single injection is usually effective but in rest multiple setting was required. Concentration of phenol used was 4 %. Cryoablation has been reported to provide good pain relief in a patient with neuropathy of femoral component of genitofemoral nerve [69].

Neurolysis of Stump Neuroma

Phantom pain is quite common after limb amputation and the incidence could be as high as 72 % [70]. The incidence of stump pain is 50 % [71]. Development of stump neuroma is frequently associated with complex pathophysiology of development of both stump and phantom pain. Neuromas lead to reorganization of central neuronal circuits which cause structural and functional changes in somatosensory cortical areas corresponding to amputated limb.

Neurosclerosis of neuromas with phenol has been suggested as one of the treatment modalities for stump pain. Both blind- and ultrasound-guided administration of phenol have been shown to be effective. Complete pain relief was achieved in 26 % of patients, and rest of patients had more than 70 % decrease in VAS score [72, 73].

The success rate was much higher than even injecting under direct vision during surgery. An alternative is to apply cryoprobe to cause neurolysis in patients who had undergone amputation. The cryoprobes were applied under electrophysiological guidance. Sixty second freeze thaw cycles were applied using 2-mm cryoprobe [74]. The cycles were repeated until tenderness over the region of neuroma disappears to a maximum of five cycles. Nine out of ten patients experienced significant pain relief of more than 3 months.

Interdigital Nerve Compression of the Foot

The major cause of foot pain is interdigital nerve compression, commonly known as Morton's neuroma [75]. It causes numbness and burning in the toes, sensory disturbances, and a feeling of ball in the foot. This syndrome is due to entrapment of digital nerve between the metatarsal heads and beneath the intermetatarsal ligament. An intermetatarsal bursa can also compress the nerves causing symptoms. It can be managed by orthotic, pharmacological, or surgical methods. Application of alcohol or phenol is also a method to manage the condition in order to cause remission of symptoms.

Intermetatarsal space was accessed through dorsal approach, and 2.5 ml of 5 % phenol was injected after eliciting paresthesia, and the success rate was 80.3 %. Alcohol injection was also utilized; however, it required multiple injections, and 74 % of feet were improved after five settings of neurolysis treatment [76]. Complications included pain and erythema which usually resolve by 24 h.

Neurolysis in Abdomen

The ganglia which innervate abdominal and pelvic viscera include the celiac plexus, superior and inferior mesenteric plexuses, superior hypogastric plexus, and ganglion impar. Usually treatment with neurolysis of these ganglia is restricted to patients who have pain arising from malignancy. The celiac plexus provides sympathetic innervation to the liver, stomach, pancreas, gallbladder, spleen, kidneys, adrenal glands, small intestine, and a portion of the large intestine. Nociceptive afferents from bladder, prostate, rectum, uterus, ovaries, and vagina relay through the superior hypogastric plexus. The sympathetic chains terminate in the unpaired ganglion impar (ganglion of Walther) which carries visceral afferents from the distal rectum, anus, perineum, distal urethra, and vulva.

Celiac Plexus

It is a collection of 1–5 ganglia and contains fibers from the thoracic and lumbar sympathetic chains (sympathetic), vagus (parasympathetic), and the phrenic nerves (motor). The thoracic splanchnic nerves (greater, lesser, and least) arise from roots of T5–T12 paravertebral sympathetic ganglia and terminate in the celiac plexus.

Indications
Neurolytic block of the celiac plexus is used for both malignant [77] and nonmalignant pain. The most common and popular indication is pain arising from pancreatic adenocarcinoma [78, 79], although it has been used occasionally in chronic pancreatitis. It is reserved for patients whose pain cannot be controlled with opioids and/or who have developed intolerable side effects from opioids [80]. The optimal therapeutic effect is obtained if the procedure is performed early in the illness, and it has been postulated to prolong life expectancy [81] as well. However, later in the disease process, the incidence of complications arising from the block increases [82]. It can also be considered for treatment of visceral pain originating from malignancy involving stomach, liver, and pancreas.

Celiac plexus is located in the retroperitoneal region anterior to the crus of the diaphragm around the origin of celiac artery from the aorta. It is situated at the level of T12 and L1 vertebral bodies.

Procedure
Celiac plexus block can be performed percutaneously by fluoroscopic method (most common), directly during surgery, via CT guidance, and by endoscopic ultrasound. This block is most commonly performed by posterior percutaneous approach [83, 84]. Depending on the position of the needle tip, the procedure could be termed retrocrural [85] or precural [86].

Injection into the retrocrural space actually achieves blockade of the splanchnic nerves only (splanchnic nerve block), whereas precrural spread of the drug causes actual blockade of the entire celiac plexus. Retrocrural injection, however, also achieves spread of drug into the precrural space as well. According to the route of needle insertion, one can use a paravertebral (classic) approach or the transdiscal [85] or transaortic [87] route.

Although technique of celiac plexus block is described elsewhere in the textbook, we will describe the classic approach in which needle is inserted via paravertebral location with a posterolateral approach. In this technique, the needle is advanced until it contacts the lateral surface of the vertebral body. This approach requires bilateral injection of medication to achieve complete blockade of the plexus. In transaortic or transdiscal approach, a single injection is used. The efficacy of administration of drug via different approaches remains the same [87]. Transdiscal retrocrural approach is simpler and less invasive, though there exists the risk of infection of the intervertebral disk (diskitis).

The needle for CPB is inserted either under fluoroscopic or CT guidance [88, 89].

Loss of resistance to saline-containing antibiotics technique is used in transdiscal approach. Though CT-guided approach helps to place the needle more precisely, the efficacy is not different from that of fluoroscopy guidance. Contrast is often injected to confirm the needle tip position and rule out intravascular injection. A "butterfly-wing" shadow is seen in anteroposterior view in the transcrural approach, whereas a wedge-shaped appearance is seen in the retrocrural technique; 20–25 ml of 50–75 % alcohol is used for neurolysis (10 ml on each side if bilateral injections were planned). For splanchnic nerve block, needle is inserted at a higher level T10–T12 level. The anterior approach via CT guidance helps one avoid puncture of aorta (and lungs) and allows better visualization of structures. It can also be performed via an endoscopic ultrasound approach which allows simultaneous tissue sampling as well.

Expected and relatively common side effects include hypotension (38 %) and diarrhea (44 %) [90]. Rare complications also include infection, neuritis, pneumothorax (2 %), and renal, aortic, and intestinal injuries. Serious neurological complications like paraplegia is very rare but can occur, thought to be due to injury of the artery of Adamkiewicz. Spinal and epidural spread is possible though a rare complication [91–94]. Contrast injection before neurolytic administration helps reduce the incidence of many of these complications. When a semilateral diffusion of contrast medium is found, an additional inferior mesenteric plexus block can be performed using a transdiscal approach at the L2–L3 level. Though transdiscal approach is potentially associated with inflammation, degeneration, infection, and dislocation complications, no such complications have been reported [85, 86]. Acute alcoholic intoxication-like symptoms have been reported due to rapid absorption of alcohol from the surrounding venous plexus. Abdominal aortic dissection has been reported following celiac plexus block.

Efficacy

Meta-analysis of the studies involving celiac plexus neurolysis with 1,145 patients concluded that 89 % of patients had excellent pain relief for 2 weeks and 90 % had partial to complete pain relief for the duration of 3 months [95]. Patients with malignancy involving all upper abdominal structures manifest benefit in the same way as that of patients

with pancreatic adenocarcinoma. However, in a study by Wong et al. [96], celiac plexus neurolysis was associated with larger decrease pain scores in the first week compared to systemic opioids group; however, the consumption of opioids, side effects, and quality of life were not different between them. After 1 week, though percentage of patients who had severe pain was lower in neurolytic group, the quality of life was not improved by neurolysis.

Rykowski et al. in his study found better control of pain when the tumor is confined to pancreas. Neurolysis was more effective in patients with tumor involving head of pancreas [97]. Stefeniak et al. compared two methods of invasive celiac plexus neurolysis to control patient [98]. Percutaneous neurolytic group was associated with decreased pain and improved quality of life compared to control group. The follow-up period was up to 8 weeks. Staats et al. in a similar study had shown not only improvement of pain with neurolytic block but also was associated with elevated mood and improved life expectancy [81]. Elevated mood with neurolytic therapy will counter the depression causing decrease in immune function and antitumor activity. Vranken et al. in his small study involving 12 patients had also shown improved pain and quality of life with neurolytic celiac plexus block, but the effect was short lived [99]. Mercadante et al. [100] in a prospective controlled multicenter trial also had shown similar positive results with decreased opioid consumption and improved gastrointestinal adverse effects with neurolytic blocks. In the meta-analysis, Yan et al. found reduction in pain scores and opioid usage up to 8 weeks though there was no difference in the survival [95].

The predictors of poor pain relief are advanced age and prior surgery. There is no improvement in quality of life or survival in patients who had undergone EU-guided celiac plexus neurolysis. It did reduce the amount of morphine consumption and improved quality of pain relief.

The literature is not clear whether celiac plexus block improves quality of life and life expectancy; however, there is definite improvement in pain scores associated with reduction in opioid consumption for a variable duration of 2 weeks to 3 months.

Superior Hypogastric Plexus Block

Pain secondary to pelvic metastatic disease or de novo malignant tumors involving pelvic structures may be treated with superior hypogastric plexus blockade [101].

Superior hypogastric plexus is located in the retroperitoneal region bilaterally extending from the lower third of fifth lumbar body to the upper third of first sacral body. Nociceptive sympathetic fibers from pelvic viscera like prostate, bladder, uterus, ovaries, vagina, and rectum are carried through this superior hypogastric plexus. This plexus divides and forms into the inferior hypogastric plexus in front of S3 and after receives more parasympathetic innervations from S1–S3 [102].

Blockade of the superior hypogastric plexus is performed under fluoroscopy guidance with the patient in the prone position. The needle is inserted 5–7 cm lateral to the midline in the classic posterior approach. The tip of the needle is placed just anterolateral to the lower third of L5 and placement is confirmed in both anteroposterior and lateral views [103]. Ten milliliters of neurolytic agent is required to achieve complete blockade.

Superior hypogastric plexus neurolysis has been reported to provide excellent pain relief without major side effects in a patient with endometriosis which is unresponsive to medical treatment [104]. Superior hypogastric plexus blockade can also be performed from the anterior aspect of the patient via CT scan or ultrasound guidance [105]. CT-guided bilateral transdiscal approach [106] has been demonstrated to overcome anatomic obstacles to the block. It is an excellent choice in patients with intractable pain with genitourinary, rectal, and pelvic malignancies. This approach is particularly useful when challenges are encountered in doing classic posterior approach or when the sacral promontory [107] makes it impossible to place the needle at the correct location. The other obstacles occasionally encountered were osteophytes, surgically fused spines, orthopedic hardware, transverse process of L5, and an enlarged iliac crest. The risk of diskitis is possible but very rare, and disk rupture is a potential complication but never has been reported. Inferior hypogastric plexus can also be blocked by accessing it through the sacral foramen [102]. Superior hypogastric plexus block can also be done from anterior approach as well [108]. Complications include intravascular injection, neuraxial injection, diskitis, neuritis, and bladder and bowel dysfunction.

The success rate of the block was reported as 70 % in patients with pelvic pain associated with cancer [103]. In another study, the success rate was 72 % after repeated chemical neurolysis of the superior hypogastric plexus [109].

Ganglion Impar Block

The ganglion impar is located in the retroperitoneal region at the level of sacrococcygeal junction. It is an unpaired structure and marks the termination of the two sympathetic ganglia (chains). Neurolysis of this ganglion is useful in pelvic pain, but the published experience of neurolysis of this ganglion is limited.

For this procedure, the patient can be in either the prone or lateral decubitus position. A 20-gauge 1.5 needle is inserted through the sacrococcygeal in the midline and advanced until the tip of the needle is positioned posterior to rectum [110]. Care should be taken to avoid puncture of the

rectum. Contrast medium is injected to confirm the position and bilateral spread, and then, after negative aspiration, 4–6 ml of neurolytic agent may be injected in slow increments. Ultrasound can also be used to perform this block.

A modified technique has been described for thermocoagulation of ganglion impar where a two-needle technique is utilized. The first needle was placed through the sacrococcygeal ligament, the transsacrococcygeal needle, and the second one through a coccygeal disk, the transdiscal needle. A lateral view is shown in fluoroscopy which should include sacrum and coccyx. The tip of the needle should be placed 1–2 mm anterior to the sacrococcygeal ligament [111]. Complications include rectal puncture, caudal injection, and inadvertent intravascular administration.

Anesthesia Dolorosa (Deafferentation Pain)

Anesthesia dolorosa is described as pain in the distribution of an anesthetized area due to injury to the nerve. It has been reported more often after trigeminal rhizolysis though it could occur in other conditions associated with neurolysis and stereotactic surgery or any trauma causing nerve injury. The incidence is variable and reported to be between 0 and 5 % of patients who had Gasserian neurolysis.

Patients usually complain of altered sensation and pain in the injured area. The pain is often described as stabbing or burning or shooting and exacerbated with exposure to cold or rapid temperature changes [112].

There is no effective management of this condition. Shooting or lancinating pain can be managed with anticonvulsants, and burning pain can be treated with tricyclic antidepressants or serotonin reuptake inhibitors. If patient does not respond to above options, intravenous lidocaine or ketamine can be tried. Motor cortex stimulation is also used with intention of nonnociceptive sensory input replacing nociceptive pain [113].

Conclusion

Chemical neurolysis of peripheral nerves and sympathetic ganglia seems to be a relatively safe and cost-effective part of management of pain due to malignancy. Though there can be potentially dangerous complications, generally these are rare. Careful patient selection and counseling before blockade are important. The most commonly performed procedures are celiac plexus and superior hypogastric plexus neurolysis. The success rate (ability to achieve pain relief) of these procedures is >80 % for the first 3 months. These blocks are associated with good pain relief, reduction in the amount of opioid consumption, and hence reduction in side effects. Though they have also been shown to improve quality of life and survival, these benefits have not been conclusively established.

References

1. van den Beuken-van Everdingen MH, de Rijke JM, Kessels AG, Schouten HC, van Kleef M, Patijn J. Prevalence of pain in patients with cancer: a systematic review of the past 40 years. Ann Oncol. 2007;18:1437–49.

2. Burton AW, Hamid B. Current challenges in cancer pain management: does the WHO ladder approach still have relevance? Expert Rev Anticancer Ther. 2007;7:1501–2.

3. Jackson TP, Gaeta R. Neurolytic blocks revisited. Curr Pain Headache Rep. 2008;12:7–13.

4. Trescot AM. Cryoanalgesia in interventional pain management. Pain Physician. 2003;6:345–60.

5. Rohof OJ. Radiofrequency treatment of peripheral nerves. Pain Pract. 2002;2:257–60.

6. Ahadian FM. Pulsed radiofrequency neurotomy: advances in pain medicine. Curr Pain Headache Rep. 2004;8:34–40.

7. Cahana A, Van Zundert J, Macrea L, van Kleef M, Sluijter M. Pulsed radiofrequency: current clinical and biological literature available. Pain Med. 2006;7:411–23.

8. Cousins M, Bridenbaugh P. Clinical anesthesia and pain management. Cousins Lippincott. 1998. p. 489–514.

9. Raj P. Pain medicine: comprehensive review. Raj Mosby. 1996. p. 177–84.

10. Zakrzewska JM. Assessment and treatment of trigeminal neuralgia. Br J Hosp Med (Lond). 2010;71:490–4.

11. Mathew NT, Hurt W. Percutaneous radiofrequency trigeminal gangliorhizolysis in intractable cluster headache. Headache. 1988;28: 328–31.

12. Pieper DR, Dickerson J, Hassenbusch SJ. Percutaneous retrogasserian glycerol rhizolysis for treatment of chronic intractable cluster headaches: long-term results. Neurosurgery. 2000;46:363–8; discussion 368–70.

13. Sweet WH. Percutaneous methods for the treatment of trigeminal neuralgia and other faciocephalic pain; comparison with microvascular decompression. Semin Neurol. 1988;8:272–9.

14. Sweet WH. Controlled thermocoagulation of trigeminal ganglion and rootlets for differential destruction of pain fibers: facial pain other than trigeminal neuralgia. Clin Neurosurg. 1976;23:96–102.

15. Mehio AK, Shah SK. Alleviating head and neck pain. Otolaryngol Clin North Am. 2009;42:143–59, x.

16. Zakrzewska JM, Akram H. Neurosurgical interventions for the treatment of classical trigeminal neuralgia. Cochrane Database Syst Rev. 2011;9:CD007312.

17. Ischia S, Luzzani A, Polati E. Retrogasserian glycerol injection: a retrospective study of 112 patients. Clin J Pain. 1990;6:291–6.

18. Day M. Neurolysis of the trigeminal and sphenopalatine ganglions. Pain Pract. 2001;1:171–82.

19. Ischia S, Luzzani A, Polati E, Ischia A. Percutaneous controlled thermocoagulation in the treatment of trigeminal neuralgia. Clin J Pain. 1990;6:96–104.

20. Emril DR, Ho KY. Treatment of trigeminal neuralgia: role of radiofrequency ablation. J Pain Res. 2010;3:249–54.

21. Scholz MJ. A new option for trigeminal neuralgia. RN. 1997;60:70.

22. Mizuno M, Saito K, Takayasu M, Yoshida J. Percutaneous microcompression of the trigeminal ganglion for elderly patients with trigeminal neuralgia and patients with atypical trigeminal neuralgia. Neurol Med Chir (Tokyo). 2000;40:347–50; discussion 350–1.

23. Lee ST, Chen JF. Percutaneous trigeminal ganglion balloon compression for treatment of trigeminal neuralgia, part II: results related to compression duration. Surg Neurol. 2003;60:149–53; discussion 153–4.

24. Kondziolka D, Zorro O, Lobato-Polo J, Kano H, Flannery TJ, Flickinger JC, Lunsford LD. Gamma knife stereotactic radiosurgery for idiopathic trigeminal neuralgia. J Neurosurg. 2010;112: 758–65.

25. Koyyalagunta D, Burton AW. The role of chemical neurolysis in cancer pain. Curr Pain Headache Rep. 2010;14:261–7.

26. Udupi BP, Chouhan RS, Dash HH, Bithal PK, Prabhakar H. Comparative evaluation of percutaneous retrogasserian glycerol rhizolysis and radiofrequency thermocoagulation techniques in the management of trigeminal neuralgia. Neurosurgery. 2011. http://www.ncbi.nlm.nih.gov/pubmed/21866065.

27. Tew Jr JM, Lockwood P, Mayfield FH. Treatment of trigeminal neuralgia in the aged by a simplified surgical approach (percutaneous electrocoagulation). J Am Geriatr Soc. 1975;23:426–30.

28. Onofrio BM. Radiofrequency percutaneous Gasserian ganglion lesions. Results in 140 patients with trigeminal pain. J Neurosurg. 1975;42:132–9.

29. Maxwell RE. Surgical control of chronic migrainous neuralgia by trigeminal ganglio-rhizolysis. J Neurosurg. 1982;57:459–66.

30. Choudhury BK, Pahari S, Acharyya A, Goswami A, Bhattacharyya MK. Percutaneous retrogasserian radiofrequency thermal rhizotomy for trigeminal neuralgia. J Indian Med Assoc. 1991;89: 294–6.

31. Moraci A, Buonaiuto C, Punzo A, Parlato C, Amalfi R. Trigeminal neuralgia treated by percutaneous thermocoagulation. Comparative analysis of percutaneous thermocoagulation and other surgical procedures. Neurochirurgia (Stuttg). 1992;35:48–53.

32. Dieckmann G, Veras G, Sogabe K. Retrogasserian glycerol injection or percutaneous stimulation in the treatment of typical and atypical trigeminal pain. Neurol Res. 1987;9:48–9.

33. Spaziante R, Cappabianca P, Peca C, de Divitiis E. Percutaneous retrogasserian glycerol rhizolysis. Observations and results about 50 cases. J Neurosurg Sci. 1987;31:121–8.

34. Saini SS. Reterogasserian anhydrous glycerol injection therapy in trigeminal neuralgia: observations in 552 patients. J Neurol Neurosurg Psychiatry. 1987;50:1536–8.

35. Lopez BC, Hamlyn PJ, Zakrzewska JM. Systematic review of ablative neurosurgical techniques for the treatment of trigeminal neuralgia. Neurosurgery. 2004;54:973–82; discussion 982–3.

36. Ekbom K, Lindgren L, Nilsson BY, Hardebo JE, Waldenlind E. Retro-Gasserian glycerol injection in the treatment of chronic cluster headache. Cephalalgia. 1987;7:21–7.

37. Hassenbusch SJ, Kunkel RS, Kosmorsky GS, Covington EC, Pillay PK. Trigeminal cisternal injection of glycerol for treatment of chronic intractable cluster headaches. Neurosurgery. 1991;29: 504–8.

38. Meglio M, Cioni B, Moles A, Visocchi M. Microvascular decompression versus percutaneous procedures for typical trigeminal neuralgia: personal experience. Stereotact Funct Neurosurg. 1990; 54–55:76–9.

39. Spincemaille GH, Dingemans W, Lodder J. Percutaneous radiofrequency Gasserian ganglion coagulation in the treatment of trigeminal neuralgia. Clin Neurol Neurosurg. 1985;87:91–4.

40. Young RF. Glycerol rhizolysis for treatment of trigeminal neuralgia. J Neurosurg. 1988;69:39–45.

41. Waltz TA, Dalessio DJ, Copeland B, Abbott G. Percutaneous injection of glycerol for the treatment of trigeminal neuralgia. Clin J Pain. 1989;5:195–8.

42. Natarajan M. Percutaneous trigeminal ganglion balloon compression: experience in 40 patients. Neurol India. 2000;48:330–2.

43. Sahni KS, Pieper DR, Anderson R, Baldwin NG. Relation of hypesthesia to the outcome of glycerol rhizolysis for trigeminal neuralgia. J Neurosurg. 1990;72:55–8.

44. Waldman SD. Sphenopalatine ganglion block – 80 years later. Reg Anesth. 1993;18:274–6.

45. Brown CR. Sphenopalatine ganglion neuralgia. Pract Periodontics Aesthet Dent. 1997;9:99–100.

46. Salar G, Ori C, Iob I, Fiore D. Percutaneous thermocoagulation for sphenopalatine ganglion neuralgia. Acta Neurochir (Wien). 1987;84:24–8.

47. Gregoire A, Clair C, Delabrousse E, Aubry R, Boulahdour Z, Kastler B. CT guided neurolysis of the sphenopalatine ganglion for management of refractory trigeminal neuralgia. J Radiol. 2002;83:1082–4.

48. Manahan AP, Malesker MA, Malone PM. Sphenopalatine ganglion block relieves symptoms of trigeminal neuralgia: a case report. Nebr Med J. 1996;81:306–9.

49. Peterson JN, Schames J, Schames M, King E. Sphenopalatine ganglion block: a safe and easy method for the management of orofacial pain. Cranio. 1995;13:177–81.

50. Piagkou M, Demesticha T, Troupis T, Vlasis K, Skandalakis P, Makri A, Mazarakis A, Lappas D, Piagkos G, Johnson EO. The pterygopalatine ganglion and its role in various pain syndromes: from anatomy to clinical practice. Pain Pract. 2011. doi: 10.1111/j.1533-2500.2011.00507.x. http://www.ncbi.nlm.nih.gov/pubmed/21956040.

51. Pollock BE, Kondziolka D. Stereotactic radiosurgical treatment of sphenopalatine neuralgia. Case report. J Neurosurg. 1997; 87:450–3.

52. Prasanna A, Murthy PS. Combined stellate ganglion and sphenopalatine ganglion block in acute herpes infection. Clin J Pain. 1993;9:135–7.

53. Sanders M, Zuurmond WW. Efficacy of sphenopalatine ganglion blockade in 66 patients suffering from cluster headache: a 12- to 70-month follow-up evaluation. J Neurosurg. 1997;87:876–80.

54. Prasanna A, Murthy PS. Sphenopalatine ganglion block and pain of cancer. J Pain Symptom Manage. 1993;8:125.

55. Puig CM, Driscoll CL, Kern EB. Sluder's sphenopalatine ganglion neuralgia – treatment with 88 % phenol. Am J Rhinol. 1998;12:113–8.

56. Konen A. Unexpected effects due to radiofrequency thermocoagulation of the sphenopalatine ganglion: two case reports. Pain Dig. 2000;10:30–3.

57. Shin JH, Herrera SR, Eboli P, Aydin S, Eskandar EH, Slavin KV. Entrapment of the glossopharyngeal nerve in patients with Eagle syndrome: surgical technique and outcomes in a series of 5 patients. J Neurosurg. 2009;111:1226–30.

58. Soh KB. The glossopharyngeal nerve, glossopharyngeal neuralgia and the Eagle's syndrome–current concepts and management. Singapore Med J. 1999;40:659–65.

59. Abejon D, del Garcia Valle S, Nieto C, Delgado C, Gomez-Arnau JI. Pulsed radiofrequency treatment in idiopathic and secondary glossopharyngeal neuralgia: preliminary results in 2 cases. Rev Esp Anestesiol Reanim. 2005;52:109–14.

60. Arbit E, Krol G. Percutaneous radiofrequency neurolysis guided by computed tomography for the treatment of glossopharyngeal neuralgia. Neurosurgery. 1991;29:580–2.

61. Kowalewski R, Schurch B, Hodler J, Borgeat A. Persistent paraplegia after an aqueous 7.5 % phenol solution to the anterior motor root for intercostal neurolysis: a case report. Arch Phys Med Rehabil. 2002;83:283–5.

62. Lema MJ, Myers DP, De Leon-Casasola O, Penetrante R. Pleural phenol therapy for the treatment of chronic esophageal cancer pain. Reg Anesth. 1992;17:166–70.

63. Candido KD, Philip CN, Ghaly RF, Knezevic NN. Transforaminal 5 % phenol neurolysis for the treatment of intractable cancer pain. Anesth Analg. 2010;110:216–9.

64. Akkaya T, Unlu E, Alptekin A, Gumus HI, Umay E, Cakci A. Neurolytic phenol blockade of the obturator nerve for severe adductor spasticity. Acta Anaesthesiol Scand. 2010;54:79–85.

65. Yasar E, Tok F, Taskaynatan MA, Yilmaz B, Balaban B, Alaca R. The effects of phenol neurolysis of the obturator nerve on the distribution of buttock-seat interface pressure in spinal cord injury patients with hip adductor spasticity. Spinal Cord. 2010;48:828–31.

66. Kim PS, Ferrante FM. Cryoanalgesia: a novel treatment for hip adductor spasticity and obturator neuralgia. Anesthesiology. 1998;89:534–6.

67. Weksler N, Klein M, Gurevitch B, Rozentsveig V, Rudich Z, Brill S, Lottan M. Phenol neurolysis for severe chronic nonmalignant pain: is the old also obsolete? Pain Med. 2007;8:332–7.

68. Antila H, Kirvela O. Neurolytic thoracic paravertebral block in cancer pain. A clinical report. Acta Anaesthesiol Scand. 1998;42:581–5.

69. Campos NA, Chiles JH, Plunkett AR. Ultrasound-guided cryoablation of genitofemoral nerve for chronic inguinal pain. Pain Physician. 2009;12:997–1000.

70. Weeks SR, Anderson-Barnes VC, Tsao JW. Phantom limb pain: theories and therapies. Neurologist. 2010;16:277–86.

71. Flor H. Phantom-limb pain: characteristics, causes, and treatment. Lancet Neurol. 2002;1:182–9.

72. Gruber H, Kovacs P, Peer S, Frischhut B, Bodner G. Sonographically guided phenol injection in painful stump neuroma. AJR Am J Roentgenol. 2004;182:952–4.

73. Sivan M, Stoppard E. Sonographically guided phenol instillation of stump neuroma. AJR Am J Roentgenol. 2008;191:W208; author reply W209.

74. Neumann V, O'Connor RJ, Bush D. Cryoprobe treatment: an alternative to phenol injections for painful neuromas after amputation. AJR Am J Roentgenol. 2008;191:W313; author reply W314.

75. Magnan B, Marangon A, Frigo A, Bartolozzi P. Local phenol injection in the treatment of interdigital neuritis of the foot (Morton's neuroma). Chir Organi Mov. 2005;90:371–7.

76. Hyer CF, Mehl LR, Block AJ, Vancourt RB. Treatment of recalcitrant intermetatarsal neuroma with 4 % sclerosing alcohol injection: a pilot study. J Foot Ankle Surg. 2005;44:287–91.

77. Wyse JM, Carone M, Paquin SC, Usatii M, Sahai AV. Randomized, double-blind, controlled trial of early endoscopic ultrasound-guided celiac plexus neurolysis to prevent pain progression in patients with newly diagnosed, painful, inoperable pancreatic cancer. J Clin Oncol. 2011;29:3541–6.

78. Brogan S, Junkins S. Interventional therapies for the management of cancer pain. J Support Oncol. 2010;8:52–9.

79. Arcidiacono PG, Calori G, Carrara S, McNicol ED, Testoni PA. Celiac plexus block for pancreatic cancer pain in adults. Cochrane Database Syst Rev 2011;(3): CD007519.

80. de Oliveira R, dos Reis MP, Prado WA. The effects of early or late neurolytic sympathetic plexus block on the management of abdominal or pelvic cancer pain. Pain. 2004;110:400–8.

81. Staats PS, Hekmat H, Sauter P, Lillemoe K. The effects of alcohol celiac plexus block, pain, and mood on longevity in patients with unresectable pancreatic cancer: a double-blind, randomized, placebo-controlled study. Pain Med. 2001;2:28–34.

82. Ogawa S, Kanayama T, Yazaki S, Saito H, Ohshiima Y, Suzuki H. Mechanisms of pain relief following sympathetic ganglion block. Masui. 1982;31:927–32.

83. Boas RA. Sympathetic blocks in clinical practice. Int Anesthesiol Clin. 1978;16:149–82.

84. Moore DC, Bush WH, Burnett LL. Celiac plexus block: a roentgenographic, anatomic study of technique and spread of solution in patients and corpses. Anesth Analg. 1981;60:369–79.

85. Yamamuro M, Kusaka K, Kato M, Takahashi M. Celiac plexus block in cancer pain management. Tohoku J Exp Med. 2000;192: 1–18.

86. Ina H, Kitoh T, Kobayashi M, Imai S, Ofusa Y, Goto H. New technique for the neurolytic celiac plexus block: the transintervertebral disc approach. Anesthesiology. 1996;85:212–7.

87. Ischia S, Ischia A, Polati E, Finco G. Three posterior percutaneous celiac plexus block techniques. A prospective, randomized study in 61 patients with pancreatic cancer pain. Anesthesiology. 1992;76: 534–40.

88. Marra V, Debernardi F, Frigerio A, Menna S, Musso L, Di Virgilio MR. Neurolytic block of the celiac plexus and splanchnic nerves with computed tomography. The experience in 150 cases and an optimization of the technic. Radiol Med. 1999;98:183–8.

89. Zhang CL, Zhang TJ, Guo YN, Yang LQ, He MW, Shi JZ, Ni JX. Effect of neurolytic celiac plexus block guided by computerized tomography on pancreatic cancer pain. Dig Dis Sci. 2008;53:856–60.

90. Eisenberg E, Carr DB, Chalmers TC. Neurolytic celiac plexus block for treatment of cancer pain: a meta-analysis. Anesth Analg. 1995;80:290–5.

91. De Conno F, Caraceni A, Aldrighetti L, Magnani G, Ferla G, Comi G, Ventafridda V. Paraplegia following coeliac plexus block. Pain. 1993;55:383–5.

92. Kumar A, Tripathi SS, Dhar D, Bhattacharya A. A case of reversible paraparesis following celiac plexus block. Reg Anesth Pain Med. 2001;26:75–8.

93. Jabbal SS, Hunton J. Reversible paraplegia following coeliac plexus block. Anaesthesia. 1992;47:857–8.

94. Wong GY, Brown DL. Transient paraplegia following alcohol celiac plexus block. Reg Anesth. 1995;20:352–5.

95. Yan BM, Myers RP. Neurolytic celiac plexus block for pain control in unresectable pancreatic cancer. Am J Gastroenterol. 2007;102:430–8.

96. Wong GY, Schroeder DR, Carns PE, Wilson JL, Martin DP, Kinney MO, Mantilla CB, Warner DO. Effect of neurolytic celiac plexus block on pain relief, quality of life, and survival in patients with unresectable pancreatic cancer: a randomized controlled trial. JAMA. 2004;291:1092–9.

97. Rykowski JJ, Hilgier M. Efficacy of neurolytic celiac plexus block in varying locations of pancreatic cancer: influence on pain relief. Anesthesiology. 2000;92:347–54.

98. Stefaniak T, Basinski A, Vingerhoets A, Makarewicz W, Connor S, Kaska L, Stanek A, Kwiecinska B, Lachinski AJ, Sledzinski Z. A comparison of two invasive techniques in the management of intractable pain due to inoperable pancreatic cancer: neurolytic celiac plexus block and videothoracoscopic splanchnicectomy. Eur J Surg Oncol. 2005;31:768–73.

99. Vranken JH, Zuurmond WW, de Lange JJ. Increasing the efficacy of a celiac plexus block in patients with severe pancreatic cancer pain. J Pain Symptom Manage. 2001;22:966–77.

100. Mercadante S, Catala E, Arcuri E, Casuccio A. Celiac plexus block for pancreatic cancer pain: factors influencing pain, symptoms and quality of life. J Pain Symptom Manage. 2003;26: 1140–7.

101. Plancarte R, Amescua C, Patt RB, Aldrete JA. Superior hypogastric plexus block for pelvic cancer pain. Anesthesiology. 1990;73:236–9.

102. Schultz DM. Inferior hypogastric plexus blockade: a transsacral approach. Pain Physician. 2007;10:757–63.

103. Plancarte R, de Leon-Casasola OA, El-Helaly M, Allende S, Lema MJ. Neurolytic superior hypogastric plexus block for chronic pelvic pain associated with cancer. Reg Anesth. 1997;22:562–8.

104. Pollitt CI, Salota V, Leschinskiy D. Chemical neurolysis of the superior hypogastric plexus for chronic non-cancer pelvic pain. Int J Gynaecol Obstet. 2011;114:160–1.

105. Mishra S, Bhatnagar S, Gupta D, Thulkar S. Anterior ultrasound-guided superior hypogastric plexus neurolysis in pelvic cancer pain. Anaesth Intensive Care. 2008;36:732–5.

106. Dooley J, Beadles C, Ho KY, Sair F, Gray-Leithe L, Huh B. Computed tomography-guided bilateral transdiscal superior hypogastric plexus neurolysis. Pain Med. 2008;9:345–7.

107. Turker G, Basagan-Mogol E, Gurbet A, Ozturk C, Uckunkaya N, Sahin S. A new technique for superior hypogastric plexus block: the posteromedian transdiscal approach. Tohoku J Exp Med. 2005;206:277–81.

108. Kanazi GE, Perkins FM, Thakur R, Dotson E. New technique for superior hypogastric plexus block. Reg Anesth Pain Med. 1999;24:473–6.

109. Gamal G, Helaly M, Labib YM. Superior hypogastric block: transdiscal versus classic posterior approach in pelvic cancer pain. Clin J Pain. 2006;22:544–7.

110. Toshniwal GR, Dureja GP, Prashanth SM. Transsacrococcygeal approach to ganglion impar block for management of chronic perineal pain: a prospective observational study. Pain Physician. 2007;10:661–6.

111. Reig E, Abejon D, del Pozo C, Insausti J, Contreras R. Thermocoagulation of the ganglion impar or ganglion of Walther: description of a modified approach. Preliminary results in chronic, nononcological pain. Pain Pract. 2005;5:103–10.

112. Findler G, Feinsod M. Trigeminal somatosensory evoked responses in patients with facial anaesthesia dolorosa. Acta Neurochir (Wien). 1982;66:165–72.

113. Lazorthes Y, Sol JC, Fowo S, Roux FE, Verdie JC. Motor cortex stimulation for neuropathic pain. Acta Neurochir Suppl. 2007;97: 37–44.

Central Neuraxial Neurolysis

44

Beth Mintzer and Jagan Devarajan

Key Points
- Central neuraxial neurolysis is selective destruction of the sensory rootlets at the spinal cord to prevent transmission of nociception.
- Every effort is made to preserve motor, bladder, and bowel function.
- With the advent of continuous opioid delivery systems and the internalized intrathecal pump, this technique is needed less often and has fallen out of favor and use.
- This is a therapy offered to patients with pain due to malignancy who have limited life expectancy.
- The intrathecal (subarachnoid) route is preferred more often than the epidural route.
- Phenol (5 %) and absolute alcohol (33–100 %) are the commonly used therapeutic agents.
- Phenol is hyperbaric in relation to CSF and is required to be administered in patients positioned with the painful dermatome and sclerotome on the dependent side.
- Absolute alcohol is hypobaric relative to CSF and is injected with the painful segment on the nondependent side.
- Phenol injection is less painful and usually results in a shorter duration of effect compared to injection of alcohol, the latter of which causes burning pain and may provide up to 6 months pain relief in approximately 50 % of patients.

- Spread of phenol is better controlled than the spread of alcohol. After injection of alcohol, the patient needs to remain in the same position for a longer period of time (at least 30 min) than after phenol injection to diminish spread to other unintended regions of the spinal cord.
- Increased intracranial pressure and coagulopathy are contraindications to the performance of the procedure.
- The epidural route for neurolysis is occasionally chosen for patients with midline, bilateral, and extensive distribution of pain.
- Patient selection, informed consent, and follow-up care cannot be overemphasized.
- Complications of central neuraxial neurolysis include muscle weakness and bladder and bowel disturbances, which generally are transient and gradually improve over a period of 4–6 months. Permanent bladder dysfunction, however, occurs in 0.8 % of patients.
- Deafferentation pain and loss of sensory modalities in the involved dermatomes can be disturbing to a subgroup of patients.

B. Mintzer, M.D., MS, CBE (✉)
Department of Pain Management, Anesthesia Institute, CCF,
9500 Euclid Av, C-25, Cleveland, OH 44195, USA
e-mail: minzteb@ccf.org

J. Devarajan, M.D.
Department of Pain Management, Anesthesia Institute, CCF,
9500 Euclid Av, C-25, Cleveland, OH 44195, USA

5936 Stumph Road Apt #205, Parma, OH 44130, USA
e-mail: drdjagan2000@yahoo.com

Introduction

Central neuraxial neurolytic blockade is intended to destroy, selectively, sensory dorsal nerve roots and rootlets between the spinal cord and dorsal root ganglion (DRG) to prevent transmission of nociceptive impulses through the spinal cord [1]. Preservation of motor, bladder, and bowel function is the goal with optimal analgesia.

In the past two decades, this technique has fallen out of favor for several reasons. The development of intrathecal opioid delivery systems for the management of nonmalignant and malignant pain syndromes substantially decreased, to a large extent, the need for subarachnoid neurolysis. Moreover, fear of potential and disastrous complications of the procedure, accompanied by decreased experience with the technique, has rendered pain practitioners less than enthusiastic about the use of this intervention. Nevertheless, it is still an effective method of analgesia in cancer patients with terminal disease states. It remains more commonly performed in developing countries where access to opioids and dedicated follow-up care is limited [1].

It is a very effective method in those patients who have already undergone diversion procedures for bladder and bowel invasion. The greater susceptibility of the dorsal nerve rootlets compared to dorsal root ganglia and the separation of sensory and motor components in the spinal cord allow this technique to be used for selective disruption of nociceptive sensory pathways with preservation of motor function.

Patient selection plays a major role in the success of the procedure [2]. Application of selective neurolytic agent with the patient in the appropriate position cannot be overemphasized. It is important to understand that only a small subset of patients with pain due to malignancy is suitable for this procedure. It should also be emphasized that subarachnoid neurolysis is more effective in ameliorating somatic pain than visceral pain [3]. It is not found to be useful for neuropathic cancer pain. Despite these limitations, adverse effects can be minimized in experienced hands, and this is still a useful method of analgesia in selective patients.

History

Chemical neurolysis was developed to circumvent the adverse effects associated with surgical neurectomy performed for providing pain relief in earlier days. Neurolysis has been described as early as 1863 when Luton used the technique of subcutaneous injection of irritants to provide relief for sacral neuralgia. However, subarachnoid neurolysis was not performed until 1931 when Dogliotti performed subarachnoid neurolysis with alcohol to provide analgesia for intractable sciatica. Following this procedure, Suvansa used intrathecal carbolic acid for the treatment of tetanus [4]. Nevertheless, phenol was used for analgesic purposes only after 25 years. Maher from Liverpool reported the use of phenol for intractable pain in the trunk, pelvis, and legs, and he used phenol in combination with silver nitrate. Miller described usage of 10 % ammonium sulfate for intercostal neuralgia [5], and Korsten applied n-butyl p-aminobenzoate via the epidural route [6].

Pharmacology

Absolute alcohol and phenol are agents typically used for subarachnoid neurolysis and glycerol for blockade of the gasserian ganglion.

Phenol

Phenol is also known as carbolic acid. Chemically, it has a structure of C_6H_5OH where a hydroxyl group is substituted for a hydrogen atom in the benzene ring. It is available as a white crystalline solid. Therefore, it has to be prepared by the pharmacy as an injectate. Phenol is clear and less soluble in water than in alcohol or other organic compounds. It is mixed with distilled water, glycerin, or radiographic contrast dye for clinical use. Glycerin is required to dissolve the crystals when phenol is used at a concentration higher than 6.7 %. The phenol-glycerin mixture is made by dissolving 0.6–1 g of phenol crystals in 10 ml of dehydrated, sterilized glycerin to yield an effective concentration of 6–10 % [7]. Solution in glycerin is more viscous, requiring the use of large bore needles for administration. It is unstable at room temperature and needs refrigeration. If refrigerated, it can be stored up to a year as phenol itself is bactericidal and fungicidal [8]. When exposed to air, it undergoes oxidation and turns reddish in color. The major advantage of phenol is its very slow spread which limits its site of action to a very localized area.

Phenol is available in 4–12 % solution and is hyperbaric in relation to cerebrospinal fluid (CSF). The action of phenol is concentration-dependent, with concentrations of 1 % producing local anesthetic effect without any destruction of axons and 12 % producing maximal axonotomic effect which may cause spinal cord infarct, arachnoiditis, or meningitis [9]. An injection of 5 % solution produces more sensory blockade; a concentration greater than 5 % can affect motor function [10]. It is the preferred agent for use in the epidural space due to a differential blockade [10, 11]. Concentrations greater than 5 % cause protein denaturation, resulting in segmental and nonspecific demyelination [12] and Wallerian degeneration [13]. Phenol has a biphasic action: initially, it causes warmth and numbness due to its local anesthetic effect, followed by nonspecific degeneration of axons [14]. It thus allows one to assess the analgesic effect over 24 h which then helps to make decisions about repeated injection. Phenol produces a less intense block for shorter duration of effect compared to alcohol. It takes about 14 days for the degeneration of nerves and another 14 weeks for regeneration.

Lifschitz et al. have shown results of 1–2 months of pain relief in 52 % of patients and more than 2 months relief in 14 % of patients [15]. Phenol is metabolized rapidly through conjugation and oxidation in the liver. Its inactive metabolite is excreted in the urine. It is very unlikely to produce any systemic effects at doses clinically used for subarachnoid neurolysis (10 ml of 10 % solution). Doses exceeding 600–2,000 mg are neurotoxic to the central nervous system and can result in convulsions and stupor, followed by cardiovascular collapse [16]. Due to the systemic side effects, it is not advisable to use in vascular areas where systemic absorption can be very high [17].

Absolute Alcohol

Alcohol is used as an alternative to phenol for producing neurolysis. It is available in 1 or 5 ml ampules at a concentration of 100 %. Unlike phenol, it is associated with burning dysesthesia at the time of administration. The severity and duration of discomfort depend on the concentration of alcohol used. Local anesthetic may be used first to minimize the painful side effect. However, this burning sensation may be helpful to localize the dermatomal level of injection and action of the drug. It has a specific gravity of 0.789–0.807 and is hypobaric in relation to cerebrospinal fluid. Thus, the effect of alcohol is influenced by the position of the patient opposite to that of phenol. It is more soluble and hence spreads faster than phenol from the site of injection. It is also rapidly removed from the CSF by uptake and diffusion. Hence, a relatively large amount of solution is required to produce a given effect at a localized site of injection. Caution is necessary, however, as large volumes may result in surrounding tissue damage. Alcohol can produce arterial vasospasm in clinically effective concentrations and volumes, and hence, paraplegia is a risk during its administration by causing vasospasm of the artery of Adamkiewicz. This is similar to the risk of paraplegia during its use in celiac plexus block.

The mechanism of action of alcohol is by dehydration and extraction of cholesterol, phospholipids, cerebrosides and precipitation of mucoproteins. The nerve fibers and myelin sheath are sclerosed [18], resulting in demyelination and subsequent Wallerian degeneration [19]. Histopathology demonstrates patchy areas of demyelination in the posterior columns, Lissauer's tract, and dorsal roots [20]. These changes have also been observed in peripheral nerve injections and spinal nerve root injections. Alcohol has also been shown to be direct neurotoxic to posterior column of spinal cord. Alcohol produces inconsistent effects on sensory and motor discrimination; the lowest concentration of 33 % has been shown to produce satisfactory analgesia without motor compromise. The duration of effect of alcohol exceeds that of phenol and has been shown to last for more than 6 months in 50 % of patients who have undergone this procedure. CSF uptake with subsequent decrease in concentration takes up to 30 min to occur [21]; patients are required to remain in the same position used for administration of the alcohol for at least 30 min after injection.

The consensus is that the spread of hyperbaric phenol is better controlled compared to that of alcohol at the expense of decreased duration and potency of effect. If the patient cannot lie on the painful side, alcohol may be used preferentially.

Patient Selection

This may be the most important part of the entire procedure as it so strongly influences the success of the procedure. Great care should be exercised, as the adverse effects of the procedure can be severely disabling. This procedure is reserved for patients who have a short life expectancy of no more than 12 months and who have pain at a localized site not exceeding two to three dermatomes. Patients with diffuse and bilateral pain may not be suitable for this technique. Patients with bilateral pain may undergo the procedure two times, with the more painful side treated first, followed by ablation of pain on the other side at a later date. All other more conservative measures should be tried before resorting to this more destructive process. Patients should have undergone a thorough diagnostic workup including a detailed history and physical examination, laboratory tests, and imaging modalities, as appropriate. Evaluation for preexisting neurological deficits should be systematically performed and documented for medicolegal purposes. The diagnosis of the condition should be certain. One can consider performing a diagnostic injection with local anesthetic either before or at the time of the procedure. This may be especially helpful before phenol, as hyperbaric local anesthetic mimics the neurolytic agent fairly well. In contrast, it is difficult to get local anesthetic to have the same specific gravity as absolute alcohol, making it more difficult to perform a valid diagnostic block. Nevertheless, some practitioners routinely perform subarachnoid block with local anesthetic so that the patient may experience sensory blockade to decide that he/she can tolerate the "numbness." Strict selection criteria can be relaxed in those patients who have already developed bladder and bowel dysfunction and have undergone some kind of surgical drainage procedure such as an ostomy or conduit [10]. It should be remembered that the procedure is generally reserved for patients with pain from either somatic or visceral origin, and diagnosis of origin and type of pain should have been determined beyond doubt.

Contraindications

Anything which precludes performance of subarachnoid block contraindicates this procedure. Coagulopathy and presence of infection at the intended site of needle puncture prevent performance of this technique. Patients who are unable to understand and accept the potential adverse effects of the procedure and, generally, patients with neuropathic pain are not suitable candidates for this treatment modality. The presence of either primary or secondary tumor at the site of administration and elevated intracranial pressure are contraindications to the procedure. Subarachnoid neurolysis should generally not be utilized if six or more spinal segments are involved in the painful syndrome.

Preparation for Procedure

Informed Consent

It is paramount that patients understand the risks and adverse effects associated with the procedure. The possibilities of motor paresis, paralysis, and bladder and bowel dysfunction should be emphasized. They should have realistic expectations of analgesia from this procedure, i.e., improved comfort, decreased opioid requirements, and hence fewer side effects from opioids. They should be aware that this procedure probably will not completely eliminate the pain and will not control the primary source of pain. Numbness may result from the procedure, and the duration of effect varies between 1 and 6 months and may require that this procedure be repeated. Tumor may continue to grow and expand and produce pain in other sites.

Preparation

Neurolytic block should be performed at the level where the spinal cord receives the sensory rootlets from the affected dermatome(s). If there are any bony secondary metastases causing pain, the relevant sclerotome should be sought to target the block accurately at the site of pain.

It is essential to have a complete understanding of the affected dermatomes and the site of entrance of the specific dorsal nerve root in the vertebral column. Cervical nerve roots exit a level higher than their corresponding vertebrae and the remaining roots below their respective vertebral bodies. In the thoracic, lumbar, and sacral regions, nerve roots emerge from the spinal cord several segments above the level at which they exit through corresponding intervertebral foramina in the vertebral column due to differential growth of bony vertebral column and the spinal cord. Since the effects of alcohol are most pronounced at the level of the fine rootlets (i.e., fila radicularia), it is advisable to perform alcohol neurolysis at the level of origin of the nerve rootlets from the spinal cord.

A decision should be made whether hyperbaric phenol or hypobaric alcohol will be used during the procedure. If the patient cannot lie on the affected side, alcohol is a reasonable choice. The amount and concentration of the neurolytic agents administered determine the therapeutic and toxic effects of the drugs. Greater than recommended, therapeutic volumes can be used in the thoracic region, which is more distant from the brachial and lumbosacral plexuses. Similarly, upper limits of volume utilized can be liberal in terminally ill bedridden patients in whom mobility and continence are of less concern. It is also preferable to use smaller volumes and multiple needle approaches than one large volume and a single needle approach. Great care should be taken to minimize turbulence and barbotage during injection to prevent untoward aberrant spread of the agent and subsequent neurological injury.

Patients should be given instructions regarding the requirement to remain immobile during the procedure and for 30 min after the procedure, as movement from the original position can result in blockade and destruction of unin-

tended nerve roots without any therapeutic benefit. The patient may be expected to have some discomfort during needle placement and should expect to assume a potentially uncomfortable position immediately following the procedure. He/she should be prepared in advance to provide real-time feedback responses concerning the development of burning, warmth, numbness, or any unpleasant sensation, as well as pain relief experienced during and after the procedure. Assistance from one or more additional people is required to help the patient maintain his/her position and to assess and monitor vital signs during the procedure. Sedation needs to be kept to a minimum in order to obtain accurate feedback information and optimal cooperation from the patient. Observance of sterile precautions is mandatory and can be per usual protocol.

Alcohol Neurolysis

The patient should be positioned in lateral decubitus position with the painful side in a nondependent position. The patient is generally rolled 45° anteriorly (forward) to bring the dorsal nerve roots into a superior position, facing up (Fig. 44.1). The patient should be stabilized in this position with straps and bolsters and folded sheets to maximize comfort while maintaining

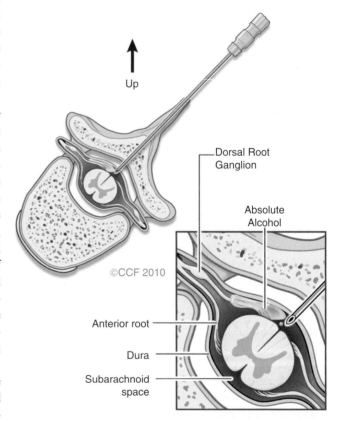

Fig. 44.1 Quieting dorsal nerve roots – alcohol and phenol

support. Fluoroscopy should be used to confirm the position of needle in the appropriate intervertebral space. A relatively large bore needle (22 G) should be used to ensure free flow of CSF and to minimize jet effects of injection. The bevel is oriented to the nondependent side to maximize the delivery of the alcohol toward targeted nerve roots which are positioned uppermost. Either a pencil point (e.g., Whitacre™) tip or cutting bevel (e.g., Quincke™) can be used for the procedure.

There are arguments for and against administration of a test dose. It is difficult to make local anesthetic as hypobaric as alcohol to determine accurately the behavior of the proposed alcohol injection. A small dose of lidocaine can be used to minimize the burning and unpleasant sensation associated with alcohol injection, but this will prevent the use of the symptoms of burning after alcohol injection as a valuable indicator of the particular segments which are going to be involved. Alcohol should be injected in 0.1-ml increments from a tuberculin syringe to ensure accuracy of volume administered. The patient should be asked to report the development of any burning sensation after each aliquot of injection and the location of such burning. The presence of a burning sensation at the painful area gives a strong indication that the injected drug has reached the corresponding site. The maximum injected volume required to produce the beneficial effect is usually 1 ml. If the patient indicates a burning sensation just cephalad or caudal to the original area of pain, the table can be tilted head up or down to modify the spread of neurolytic agent. However, if the unpleasant sensation is perceived distant from the painful areas, the spinal needle should be withdrawn and reinserted at a level below or above the initial site of injection as directed by the patient's perception of dysesthesia relative to the site of pain.

The needle should be flushed free of the alcohol or phenol with 0.2–0.3 ml of preservative-free normal saline or CSF before its withdrawal in order to avoid spilling of the drug in the subcutaneous tissue. Injection of 0.1–0.2 ml of neurolytic drug at a discordant site is associated with minimal demonstrable neurological damage. Constant communication and feedback from the patient is crucial to the success of the procedure and can greatly prevent unintentional neurologic deficits from occurring. If pain is present covering three or four segments, separate injections should be made at each level, observing the above precautions with each injection.

Phenol Neurolysis

As phenol is hyperbaric, the patient should be positioned with his/her painful side in a dependent position with slight posterior tilt to the torso so as to direct the solution to the posterior rootlets (Fig. 44.1). In patients with sacral pain, this procedure can be done in sitting position. Phenol is a viscous solution necessitating a larger bore needle to perform this procedure. Warming the phenol by immersing the ampoule in hot water prior to aspiration into the syringe reduces the viscosity and makes it easier to inject. The bevel of the needle should be directed inferiorly. Extreme care should be taken to minimize the likelihood of splashing phenol by creating a firm seal between the syringe and hub of the needle. Otherwise, due to the extreme viscous nature of the solution and subsequent increased pressure to inject the solution, the seal can break and the phenol solution can splash onto intact skin of the patient or even into the eyes of the clinician. Unlike alcohol, phenol does not produce any burning sensation during injection. It actually produces relatively mild warmth and tingling due to its local anesthetic properties. After the injection, the stylet should be replaced into the needle and the needle tip washed by the CSF to minimize the potential for sinus formation and backache due to the escape of residual drug as the needle is withdrawn.

Neurolysis is less common in the cervical region due to several factors. Compactness of the spinal cord and nerve roots make it difficult to perform a selective block. The compactness of neural elements in the cervical region makes selective neurolysis of sensory nerve roots more challenging to accomplish without causing unwanted adverse effects. Moreover, since the brachial plexus is in the cervical region, these adverse effects can be quite troublesome. In cases where the brachial plexus itself is involved in the pain syndrome, it may be a neuropathic rather than a somatic type of pain and therefore often resistant to successful treatment with subarachnoid neurolysis. Subarachnoid neurolysis for pain in the thoracic region is very effective but technically challenging compared to performance in the lumbosacral region due to the presence of the spinal cord. However, the consequences of motor dysfunction are less pronounced in the thoracic area, and paralyses of intercostal muscles usually are well tolerated. Intrathecal neurolysis in the lumbosacral region can be very effective for pain in the pelvic, perineal, rectal, and genital area, especially when it has been refractory to traditional therapeutic options.

A subarachnoid catheter technique has also been reported for use in neurolysis of selective thoracic posterior nerve roots for provision of analgesia in patients with lung cancer and pain [22]. The advantage of the catheter technique is simplicity and avoidance of multiple injections. A 19-G radiopaque catheter was inserted into the subarachnoid space through a 17-G Tuohy needle and was guided fluoroscopically cephalad to the spinal segment where analgesia was desired. After confirming the placement of the subarachnoid catheter, 0.4 ml of alcohol was injected at each level as the catheter was withdrawn slowly. Alcohol was injected at each level to produce the desired effect until a predetermined inferior level to be blocked was achieved.

Epidural Neurolytic Block

Despite the fact that epidural injection and catheter placement is a commonly performed technique, epidural neurolysis has been very disappointing in its results, probably because of reduced contact of neurolytic agent with the nerve roots due to the dural barrier. The potential for alcohol neuritis and disastrous complications of inadvertent intrathecal injection have made this technique less popular. This technique has been reported as early as 1940 for the treatment of pain due to general carcinomatosis. Nevertheless, there is less risk of bladder and bowel dysfunction with this approach. Solutions can be injected in an incremental fashion daily until the desired effect is obtained. CT scan or MRI should be performed prior to initiation of the procedure to rule out the presence of epidural tumor which could bleed during epidural needle placement. Uncontrolled bleeding, especially with tumor invasion and neovascularization, can lead to epidural or spinal hematoma.

Epidural neurolysis is more useful for midline and bilateral pain, as gravity plays little role in the spread of alcohol and phenol in the epidural space. Epidural administration is more preferable over the subarachnoid technique in patients with extensive topographic distribution of pain. Intracranial spread and meningeal irritation are uncommon. Overnight stay in the hospital may be required to titrate the injection to desired therapeutic effect given the need for multiple injections and titration to desired effect [23]. Use of at least a 20-G epidural catheter is required to allow for the injection of highly viscous phenol solutions in the epidural space. The suggested dosages are 0.5–5.0 ml, starting with the lower dosage. Confirmation of the site of injection and spread of medications with fluoroscopy and radiopaque contrast dye is highly desirable [24]. Fluoroscopy confirmation of the tip should be performed for every additional injection. Butamben has been successfully used via the epidural route for the treatment of both malignant and nonmalignant pain [25].

Although subdural neurolysis has been described in the older literature, particularly in the cervical region, due to technical difficulties and unpredictable distribution of drugs in the space, it is not used.

Efficacy

Patient selection and meticulous procedural technique are essential for the success of neuraxial neurolysis. Often, incomplete analgesia results, and therefore, patients should be informed realistically about reasonable expectations from the procedure. It is difficult to compare results of various studies, as the site of injection, choice of drug, presence and growth of tumor, and definition of pain relief vary between

different investigations. The success rate of subarachnoid neurolysis is slightly better with alcohol than of that with phenol, and complications are slightly higher with phenol than with alcohol [11, 15, 26, 27]. Table 44.1 illustrates the complications from two different types of neurolytic agents although there are no randomized studies. Phenol has been reported to give moderate to excellent pain relief in at least 50 % of the patients for at least a month.

Follow-up Care

Follow-up care is essential and obligatory following neuraxial neurolytic blockade. The aim of the post-procedural examination is to assess the efficacy of the block, taper systematically the dosage of systemic analgesic medications, and to address any adverse effects which may have occurred.

Functional pain scores and activity levels should be monitored. It can take up to a week for the patient to sense and appreciate the complete efficacy of the block. Hence, a 1-week follow-up is necessary to determine if there are any unblocked segments and to discuss the requirement of an additional procedure. Systemic opioid dose should be reduced gradually to avoid precipitation of any withdrawal symptoms. A suggested plan would be to reduce the dosage by a quarter to a third every week [28]. This reduction in opioid dosage may help minimize systemic opioid side effects and avoid sedation. This follow-up opportunity may also be utilized to identify adverse effects and institute appropriate rehabilitation as necessary.

Activities of daily living should be measured periodically as well. Frequent evaluation in follow-up also will assist the clinician to determine early the recurrence of pain and allow him/her to intervene in a timely fashion.

Complications

Complications depend upon the site of injection and the neurolytic agent used. Subarachnoid neurolysis is associated with potential major complications such as disability and loss of urinary and fecal continence. However, the majority

Table 44.1 Comparison of reported complications due to intrathecal phenol or intrathecal alcohol

Neurolytic agent	Phenol ($n=704$) (%)	Alcohol ($n=704$) (%)
Bladder dysfunction	9.0	3.5
Rectal sphincter dysfunction	2.0	0.0
Headache	3.0	0.0
Paresis	12.9	3.9
Dysesthesia	8.0	3.8

Modified from Charlton and Macrae [29]

of the complications are transient. The incidence and duration of complications vary. In a review of complications following subarachnoid neurolysis, Gerbershegan found that 51 % of complications resolved in a week, 21 % in a month, and 9 % in 4 months. However, 18 % of complications persisted even after 4 months [26].

The incidence of permanent paresis/paralysis and bladder dysfunction is 0.8 % each [26, 29]. One large case series reported a complication incidence of 14.3 % with 2.2 % [1] of those complications resulting in irreversible injury [1]. Neurolytic substances injected in the intrathecal space can cause aseptic meningitis. The most concerning event is the spread of the neurolytic agent to structures other than those intended as targets of the neurolytic agent. Neurolysis of sacral parasympathetic roots may cause bowel and bladder dysfunction.

Muscle weakness is more common with lumbosacral neurolysis, as the anterior and posterior nerve roots are in close proximity to each other below the level of L1. The motor dysfunction following neurolysis can be due to three different mechanisms: direct toxicity, arterial thrombosis causing spinal cord infarction, or arterial vasospasm. Direct toxicity can be caused by aberrant spread of neurolytic agent or via direct injection of the agent into the spinal cord [30, 31]. In a case series involving spinal cord injury following use of neurolytic agents, only one patient of 12 developed an injury due to direct toxicity [31]. Thrombosis of posterior spinal arteries causing infarction of the posterior spinal cord has been reported following phenol neurolysis [32]. Permanent paraplegia due to vasospasm of thoracic spinal arteries following alcohol injection has been reported in one case in which the symptoms were delayed by 1 day following the procedure [33]. The above mechanism was similar to that of paraplegia following celiac plexus neurolysis [34–36]. The mechanism of bladder and bowel disturbances is due to interruption of parasympathetic supply from anterior nerve roots of S2, S3, and S4 [29]. However, bladder disturbance has been shown to occur during blockade of thoracic segments as well.

Postdural puncture headache can occur following puncture of the dura by a large bore needle, though the incidence of persistent headache was lower than expected. Patt et al. reported a 6.1 % incidence of PDPHA (5 out of 82) when using ≥22-G needles. Two of these five headaches resolved spontaneously [28]. Epidural abscess, spinal hematoma, and aseptic meningitis are very rare potential complications. Systemic side effects can occur; these include malaise, nausea, headache, and dysesthesia, all of which may persist for as long as 2–3 weeks after the procedure. They occur more commonly with the injection of phenol at multiple levels due to the systemic effects of phenol. The other possible side effect can be loss of touch and position sensation due to involvement of the posterior columns; this sensory hypesthesia can be very disturbing for some patients.

Summary

1. Central neuraxial neurolytic block is a technique of providing analgesia for cancer patients that dates back to the 1930s. It is not frequently utilized for analgesia in the twenty-first century; nonetheless, it is a very effective mode of pain relief in a carefully selected patient population.
2. This procedure would be beneficial and worth considering in patients with a shortened life span, in patients with intractable pain not responding to conventional modes of analgesia, and in patients who have already lost bladder and bowel function or have undergone diversion procedures.
3. Patient selection and informed consent process play major roles in determining the overall success of the procedure.
4. Patients and/or families should be made aware of the limitations of efficacy of the technique and the potential for adverse effects.
5. Selection of appropriate neurolytic agent and proper positioning of the patient during the procedure cannot be emphasized enough.
6. Most of the adverse effects are transient, and the incidence of major adverse events, especially with respect to paralysis, is probably less than 1 %.

References

1. Ballantyne JC, Fishman SM, Rathmell JP. Bonica's management of pain. 4th ed. Philadelphia: Lippincott Williams & Wilkins; 2009.
2. Ferrer-Brechner T. Anesthetic techniques for the management of cancer pain. Cancer. 1989;63(11 Suppl):2343–7.
3. Candido K, Stevens RA. Intrathecal neurolytic blocks for the relief of cancer pain. Best Pract Res Clin Anaesthesiol. 2003; 17(3):407–28.
4. Suvansa S. Treatment of tetanus by intrathecal injection of carbolic acid. Lancet. 1931;1:1075, 1075–8.
5. Miller RD, Johnston RR, Hosobuchi Y. Treatment of intercostal neuralgia with 10 per cent ammonium sulfate. J Thorac Cardiovasc Surg. 1975;69(3):476–8.
6. Grouls RJ, Meert TF, Korsten HH, Hellebrekers LJ, Breimer DD. Epidural and intrathecal n-butyl-p-aminobenzoate solution in the rat. Comparison with bupivacaine. Anesthesiology. 1997;86(1): 181–7.
7. Ischia S, Luzzani A, Ischia A, Magon F, Toscano D. Subarachnoid neurolytic block (L5–S1) and unilateral percutaneous cervical cordotomy in the treatment of pain secondary to pelvic malignant disease. Pain. 1984;20(2):139–49.
8. Lipton S. Persistent pain: modern methods of treatment. New York: Grune & Stratton; 1977.
9. Iggo A, Walsh EG. Selective block of small fibres in the spinal roots by phenol. Brain. 1960;83:701–8.
10. Slatkin NE, Rhiner M. Phenol saddle blocks for intractable pain at end of life: report of four cases and literature review. Am J Hosp Palliat Care. 2003;20(1):62–6.
11. Maher RM. Relief of pain in incurable cancer. Lancet. 1955; 268(6853):18–20.

12. Hansebout RR, Cosgrove JB. Effects of intrathecal phenol in man. A histological study. Neurology. 1966;16(3):277–82.

13. Smith MC. Histological findings following intrathecal injections of phenol solutions for relief of pain. Br J Anaesth. 1964; 36:387–406.

14. Wood KM. The use of phenol as a neurolytic agent: a review. Pain. 1978;5(3):205–29.

15. Lifshitz S, Debacker LJ, Buchsbaum HJ. Subarachnoid phenol block for pain relief in gynecologic malignancy. Obstet Gynecol. 1976;48(3):316–20.

16. Totoki T, Kato T, Nomoto Y, Kurakazu M, Kanaseki T. Anterior spinal artery syndrome – a complication of cervical intrathecal phenol injection. Pain. 1979;6(1):99–104.

17. Raj PP. Clinical practice of regional anesthesia. New York: Churchill Livingstone; 2002.

18. Woolsey RM, Taylor JJ, Nagel JH. Acute effects of topical ethyl alcohol on the sciatic nerve of the mouse. Arch Phys Med Rehabil. 1972;53(9):410–4.

19. Rumsby MG, Finean JB. The action of organic solvents on the myelin sheath of peripheral nerve tissue. II. Short-chain aliphatic alcohols. J Neurochem. 1966;13(12):1509–11.

20. Gallager HS, Yonezawa T, Hay RC, Derrick WS. Subarachnoid alcohol block. II. Histologic changes in the central nervous system. Am J Pathol. 1961;38:679–93.

21. Matsuki M, Kato Y, Ichiyanagi K. Progressive changes in the concentration of ethyl alcohol in the human and canine subarachnoid spaces. Anesthesiology. 1972;36(6):617–21.

22. El-Sayed GG. A new catheter technique for thoracic subarachnoid neurolysis in advanced lung cancer patients. Pain Pract. 2007;7(1):27–30.

23. Korevaar WC. Transcatheter thoracic epidural neurolysis using ethyl alcohol. Anesthesiology. 1988;69(6):989–93.

24. Mehta M, Salmon N. Extradural block. Confirmation of the injection site by X-ray monitoring. Anaesthesia. 1985;40(10):1009–12.

25. Shulman M, Harris JE, Lubenow TR, Nath HA, Ivankovich AD. Comparison of epidural butamben to celiac plexus neurolytic block for the treatment of the pain of pancreatic cancer. Clin J Pain. 2000;16(4):304–9.

26. Gerbershagen HU. Neurolysis. Subarachnoid neurolytic blockade. Acta Anaesthesiol Belg. 1981;32(1):45–57.

27. Hay RC. Subarachnoid alcohol block in the control of intractable pain: report of results in 252 patients. Anesth Analg. 1962; 41:12–6.

28. Patt RB, Wu CL, Reddy S, Perkins FM, Isaacson S. The incidence of postdural puncture headache following intrathecal neurolysis with large caliber needles. Reg Anesth. 1994;19(2S):86.

29. Charlton JE, Macrae WA. In: Cousins MJ, Bridenbaugh PO, editors. Neural blockade in clinical anesthesia and management of pain. Complications of Neurolytic Neural Blockade. 2nd ed. Philadelphia: Lippincott; 1998.

30. Coles PG, Thompson GE. The role of neurolytic blocks in the treatment of cancer pain. Int Anesthesiol Clin. 1991;29(1):93–104.

31. Swerdlow M. Intrathecal neurolysis. Anaesthesia. 1978;33(8): 733–40.

32. Hughes JT. Thrombosis of the posterior spinal arteries. A complication of an intrathecal injection of phenol. Neurology. 1970;20(7):659–64.

33. McGarvey ML, Ferrante FM, Patel RS, Maljian JA, Stecker M. Irreversible spinal cord injury as a complication of subarachnoid ethanol neurolysis. Neurology. 2000;54(7):1522–4.

34. Wong GY, Brown DL. Transient paraplegia following alcohol celiac plexus block. Reg Anesth. 1995;20(4):352–5.

35. Hayakawa J, Kobayashi O, Murayama H. Paraplegia after intraoperative celiac plexus block. Anesth Analg. 1997;84(2):447–8.

36. Brown DL, Rorie DK. Altered reactivity of isolated segmental lumbar arteries of dogs following exposure to ethanol and phenol. Pain. 1994;56(2):139–43.

Provocative Discography

Irina Melnik, Richard Derby, and Ray M. Baker

Key Points

- Discography is an invasive diagnostic procedure not intended to be an initial screening examination due to associated potential risk to a patient.
- It is a confirmatory test, which can reveal the true source of pain and thus leads to precise and effective treatment as well as might help patients to avoid unnecessary surgical interventions.
- The value of the test is not only in providing morphologic characteristics of the disc structure and degrees of internal annular disc disrupture but also in providing unique clinical information by potentially evoking patients typical/concordant pain and confirming a specific level of the painful disc.
- As a provocative test, discography is liable to false-positive results, which can be potentially avoided by adherence to strict operational standards and interpretation criteria, including pain ≥7/10, pressure <50 psi a.o. , concordant pain, ≥ grade 3 annular tear, volume ≤3.5 mL, and the presence of a negative control disc.
- Technical challenges, potential complications, and interpretation mistakes can be avoided with proper selection of patients, including favorable psychological profiling, use of sterile technique, intravenous and intradiscal antibiotics, judicious use of sedation, and good technical training of a practitioner.
- Emerging alternative approaches including anesthetic discography and functional discography are gaining attention, as well as noninvasive MRI spectroscopy and other imaging tests, as an attempt to provide similar clinical information without putting patients at a potential short- or long-term risk.

I. Melnik, M.D.
Comprehensive Spine and Sports,
591 Redwood Highway, Suite 2300, Mill Valley, CA 94941, USA

Spinal Diagnostics and Treatment Center,
901 Campus Dr, Suite 310, Daly City, CA 94015, USA
e-mail: drmelnik@spinaldiagnostics.com

R. Derby, M.D. (✉)
Spinal Diagnostics and Treatment Center Medical Director,
901 Campus Dr, Suite 310, Daly City, CA 94015, USA
e-mail: rderby@spinaldiagnostics.com

R.M. Baker, M.D.
Evergreen Spine and Musculoskeletal Program,
Medical Director EvergreenHealth,
Kirkland, WA, USA
e-mail: rmbaker@ evergreenhealthcare.org

Introduction

Discography was introduced in the 1940s to diagnose herniation and internal annular disruption of the lumbar and subsequently cervical and thoracic intervertebral discs [1, 2]. While the development of CT and MRI scans unquestionably provide the physician with invaluable information, discography combined with a post-discography CT scan remains the most accurate method of detailing internal annular disruption and disc morphology [3]. Unlike noninvasive imaging tests, pressurizing the disc adds critical information if significant concordant pain is reproduced; and more importantly, a negative response to provocation discography assists in identifying negative discs for which surgery is not recommended. Theoretically, speed- and pressure-controlled injection of contrast media into the disc nucleus stimulates nerve endings via two mechanisms: a chemical stimulus from contact between contrast dye and sensitized nociceptors and a mechanical stimulus resulting from the fluid-distending stress simulating loading [4]. In the outer one-third of the normal disc, dissections and histochemical analysis reveal innervation by branches of the sinuvertebral nerves, the gray rami communicantes, and the ventral rami [5–8] which contain well-characterized nociceptive nerve fiber peptides such as substance P, VIP (vasoactive intestinal peptide), and CGRP (calcitonin-gene-related peptide) [9–11]. Distinct from normally aging discs, "pathologically painful" discs show a process of neo-innervation extending along annular fissures as well as to the inner annulus and nucleus pulposus which likely explains the pain of provocation discography [12–14].

Conceptually, provocation discography is an extension of the clinical examination, tantamount to palpating for tenderness [15]. In addition, post-discography CT findings suggest a firm correlation between a degree of a demonstrable annular disruption and reproduction of pain by disc stimulation [16, 17]. In a study by Vanharanta et al. greater than 75 % of painful discs on provocative discography (PD) had a grade 3 or greater annular tear. Provocation discography is particularly useful in challenging or inconclusive cases unresolved by MRI or myelography, such as in post-discectomy discs or recurrent disc herniations [18].

Provocative discography is an invasive diagnostic test, not intended to be an initial screening examination. Over the past decade, there have been debates challenging the validity and accuracy of discography, its long-term safety, and a need for alternative approaches such as functional anesthetic discography or innovative noninvasive biochemical imaging tests [19]. In this chapter, we discuss indications for provocative discography, technical considerations, and procedural descriptions as well as potential complications and future directions.

Indications and Contraindications

According to the position statement on discography by the North American Spine Society [3]:

> Discography is indicated in the evaluation of patients with unremitting spinal pain, with or without extremity pain, of greater than 4 months' duration, when the pain has been unresponsive to all appropriate methods of conservative therapy. Before discography, the patients should have undergone investigation with other modalities which have failed to explain the source of pain; such modalities should include, but not be limited to, either computed tomography (CT) scanning, magnetic resonance imaging (MRI) scanning and/or myelography.

The single purpose of discography is to obtain useful clinical information. The test endeavors to confirm or refute the hypothesis that a particular disc is a source of patient's familiar or accustomed pain. Since it is a provocation test, disc stimulation is liable to false-positive results; however, a recent meta-analysis of asymptomatic subjects demonstrated that a false-positive rate of less than 10 % can be obtained [20] if the discographer adheres to ISIS/IASP operational standards and interpretation criteria: pain $\geq 7/10$, pressure <50 psi a.o., concordant pain, $\geq$ grade 3

annular tear, volume ≤ 3.5 mL, and the presence of a negative control disc [21, 22].

Since abnormal disc morphology alone is not diagnostic, as shown on CT and MRI scans of subjects asymptomatic of low back pain [23], the prime indication for discography is to help to distinguish which disc is symptomatic. A parallel application is to identify asymptomatic discs. When a single disc is found to be symptomatic in the presence of adjacent asymptomatic discs, focused surgical therapy can be entertained. Patients with symptomatic or abnormal discs at multiple levels constitute a greater surgical challenge. Identification of asymptomatic discs which do not require intervention is also clinically invaluable.

Indications and Inclusion Criteria

- Failed conservative treatment for low back pain of probable spinal origin.
- Ongoing pain for greater than 4 months.
- Other common pain generators have been ruled out (e.g., facets, sacroiliac joints).
- Symptoms are clinically consistent with disc pain.
- Symptoms are severe enough to consider surgery or percutaneous interventions.
- Surgery is planned and the surgeon desires an assessment of the adjacent disc levels.
- The patient is capable of understanding the nature of the technique and can participate in the subjective interpretation.
- Both the patient and physician need to know the source of pain to guide further treatments.

Contraindications

- Unable or unwilling to consent to the procedure or to cooperate
- Inability to assess patient response during the procedure
- Coagulopathy (INR > 1.5 or platelets < 50,000/mm)
- Known localized or systemic infection
- Pregnancy (to prevent fetal radiation exposure)

Relative Contraindications to Discography

- Allergy to contrast medium, antibiotics, or local anesthetics
- Congenital, postsurgical, and anatomical derangements or psychological problems that can compromise safety and success of the procedure (including spinal cord compression and myelopathy in case of cervical and thoracic procedures)

Preprocedural Evaluation and Patient Preparation

Preprocedural Evaluation

A thorough patient evaluation as well as patient education about the nature of the procedure is critical to ensure optimal performance and the utility of the test. The evaluation should include history, physical examination, previous medical conditions, prior surgeries, medications, and allergies. Information about pain is recorded, including onset of symptoms, nature, frequency, and distribution of pain as well as its intensity in 0–10 pain scale. In most cases of lumbar discography and all cases of thoracic and cervical discography, an MRI or CT scan should be reviewed prior to discography. Furthermore, since false-positive rates may increase with severe somatization disorder, psychometric testing should be included such as DRAM (Distress and Risk Assessment Method) [24]. Prior to the procedure, patients have to understand the importance of reporting and recognizing whether the test reproduces their usual or so-called concordant pain and be able to distinguish this pain from other pain. Concordant pain is necessary to determine a positive response. For this reason, it is advisable to have a trained observer independently monitor patient pain responses while the operator concentrates on the technical aspects of the procedure.

Patient Preparation

Since the disc is a relatively avascular structure, there is an increased risk of discitis – a rare but serious potential complication of the discography procedure. The most common pathogens are *Escherichia coli*, *Staphylococcus aureus*, or *Staphylococcus epidermidis*. Intravenous (IV) antibiotic prophylaxis should be administered within 15–60 min before the procedure using cephazolin 1 g, gentamicin 80 mg, or ciprofloxacin 400 mg. For patients allergic to penicillin, clindamycin 900 mg is a possible alternative [25–27]. In addition, many discographers add 2–6 mg/mL of a cephalosporin antibiotic to the nonionic contrast solution [28]. The procedure should be performed under sterile conditions with double gloves. It is recommended to handle and touch any needle only with sterile gauze or instruments, not a gloved hand. Many injectionists scrub, gown, and glove as for an open surgical procedure. The C-arm image intensifier should also be draped.

As a provocative test, discography is at best uncomfortable and at worst very painful. For this reason, it is recommended that patients be judiciously sedated to manage anxiety, opiate withdrawal, and possible extraneous pain related to disc access. Patient response should be monitored with dosages titrated to establish a level of sedation permitting the patient to be conversant and responsive after needle placement. Short acting sedatives or analgesics are recommended, such as midazolam and fentanyl.

Technique of Lumbar Discography

Patient Position

Most lumbar discs can be safely and readily accessed using a postero-oblique, extrapedicular approach when patient lies in a prone oblique position on a fluoroscopy table. This technique, which has been described by Trosier [29] and modified by Aprill [30], prevents the potential complications associated with thecal puncture from a transdural approach [31]. Elevating the target side approximately 15° allows the fluoroscopy tube to remain in a more AP projection and reduces radiation scatter. If needed, a folded towel or soft wedge can be placed under the patient's flank to prevent side bending of the lumbar spine. A pillow or bolster can be placed under the patient's abdomen to slightly flex the spine and decrease the lumbar lordosis. Monitoring and light sedation are initiated. On the side selected for puncture, a wide area of the skin of the back is prepped and draped from the costal margin to the mid-buttock and from the midline to the flank. The puncture side should be opposite the patient's dominant pain to eliminate confusion between pain reproduced during contrast injection and the pain of penetrating the outer annulus fibrosus.

Disc Puncture

Prior to injection, a fluoroscopic examination of the spine is performed to confirm segmentation and to determine the appropriate level for needle placement. Using AP view, the beam should be parallel to the inferior vertebral endplate. After selecting the target disc using AP view, the fluoroscopic beam is axially rotated until the facet joint space is located midway between the anterior and posterior vertebral margins. In this view, the insertion point is 1 mm lateral to the lateral aspect of the superior articular process (SAP) and allows needles to be advanced parallel to the beam (Fig. 45.1).

Prior to needle placement, a skin wheal is made with lidocaine 1 % (~1 cc) using a 25-gauge 1.5-in. needle. To anesthetize the needle track, one can use a 25-gauge 3.5-in. needle advanced under to the level of the SAP. Excessive use of local anesthetic may obscure nerve root

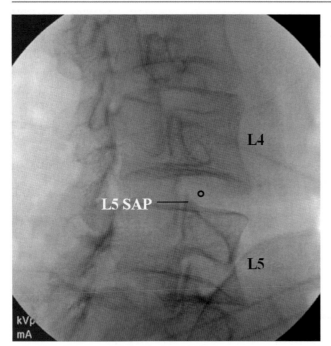

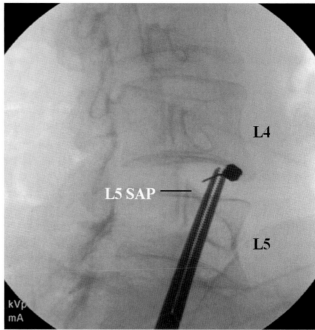

Fig. 45.1 In this view, the insertion point is 1 mm lateral to the lateral aspect of the superior articular process (*SAP*) and allows needles to be advanced parallel to the beam

Fig. 45.2 The introducer needle is advanced parallel to the fluoroscopic beam using an oblique fluoroscope view

impairment and could potentially anesthetize the sinuvertebral and ramus communicans nerves, thus altering the evoked pain response during disc stimulation and creating a false-negative response. A single- or double-needle technique may be used; however, both the North American Spine Society and the International Spinal Injection Society recommend a double-needle approach due to lower risk of disc infection (although single-needle techniques have proved adequate and safe since the use of prophylactic antibiotics) [3, 25, 32].

Puncture of L1–L5 Intervertebral Discs

In the double-needle technique, a styletted 25-gauge, 6-in. needle is placed into each disc through a 20-gauge 3.5-in. introducer needle under fluoroscopic guidance. To protect the discographer's hand from radiation exposure, forceps may be used to grasp the introducing needle. The introducer needle is advanced parallel to the fluoroscopic beam using an oblique fluoroscope view (Fig. 45.2). If bony obstruction is encountered, the physician must confirm whether the needle has contacted the SAP or the vertebral body. If necessary, the needle may be slightly withdrawn and its trajectory modified. The introducer needle can be either advanced just over the lateral edge of the SAP or advanced to the margin of the disc. After confirming introducer needle position with a lateral view, a 25-gauge, 6-in. discogram needle is slowly advanced into the center of the disc through the introducer needle while

monitoring the lateral view. A slight bend placed on the end of the discogram needle facilitates navigation. When the needle contacts the disc, position should be checked using AP and lateral views, with the ideal positioning of the needle on the line between midpoint of pedicles on AP view and posterior vertebral margin on lateral view (Fig. 45.3a, b).

Contact with the annulus fibrosus is characterized by the perception of firm resistance and frequently the patient experiencing a momentary sharp or sudden aching sensation in the back or the buttock. The needle is then advanced to the center of the disc. This requires confirmation both in AP and lateral views (Fig. 45.4a, b). If the needle tip is in the midline of the disc on the AP view but anterior on the lateral view, the needle entered the disc too far laterally. If the needle tip is centered on the AP view but posterior on the lateral image, the needle entered the disc too far medially.

Puncture of L5-S1 Intervertebral Disc

Disc access at the L5-S1 interspace can be more challenging because of an overlying iliac crest and broader interfacetal distance at that level. In this case, a curved, double-needle technique is recommended. The fluoroscopy tube is rotated only far enough to bring the facet joint space approximately 25 % of the distance between the anterior and posterior vertebral margins. The introducer needle is inserted between the S1 SAP and the iliac crest (Fig. 45.5). The discography needle is advanced under

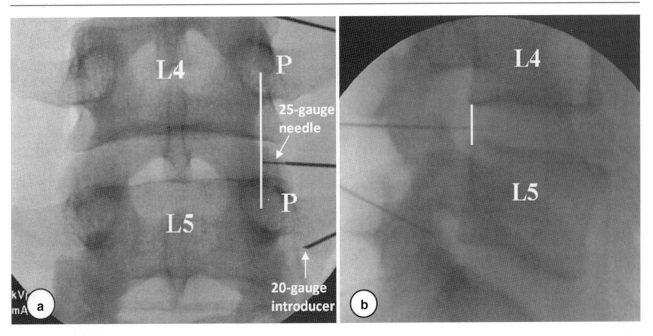

Fig. 45.3 (**a**, **b**) When the needle contacts the disc, position should be checked using AP and lateral views, with the ideal positioning of the needle on the line between midpoint of pedicles on AP view and posterior vertebral margin on lateral view

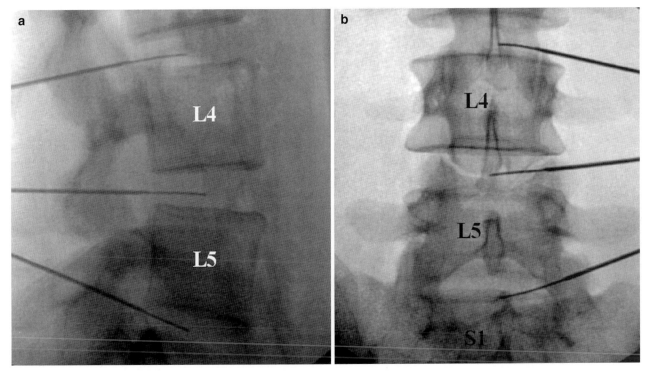

Fig. 45.4 (**a**, **b**) Contact with the annulus fibrosus is characterized by the perception of firm resistance and frequently the patient experiencing a momentary sharp or sudden aching sensation in the back or the buttock. The needle is then advanced to the center of the disc. This requires confirmation both in AP and lateral views

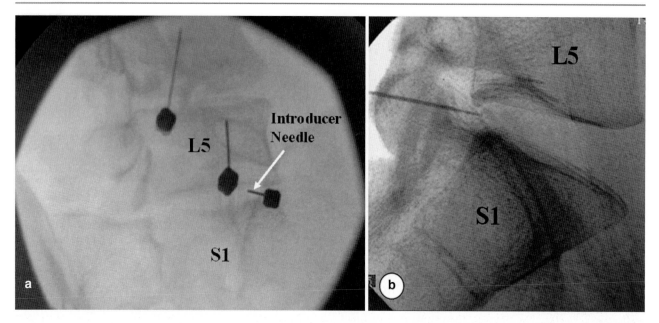

Fig. 45.5 (**a, b**) The fluoroscopy tube is rotated only far enough to bring the facet joint space approximately 25 % of the distance between the anterior and posterior vertebral margins. The introducer needle is inserted between the S1 SAP and the iliac crest

direct fluoroscopic vision, while the introducer needle is simultaneously retracted slightly. This unsheathes the discography needle, which should be turned so that the curve or bend bows the introducer needle in a medial and posterior direction through the "safe triangle." If the needle fails to track medially and posteriorly, it will not pass toward the center of the disc and may strike the ventral ramus, in which case the needle should be removed and its curvature accentuated. If the needle is blocked by the SAP, the inner needle is retracted into the introducer needle, and the pair is advanced to the lateral edge of the S1 SAP. The inner discography needle may then be directed toward the center of the disc. Ideally, the needle should be within 4–5 mm of the center on AP and lateral fluoroscopy (Fig. 45.6a, b).

Provocation Using Pressure Manometry

Provocation

Once the needle tip is in the center of nucleus pulposus, nonionic contrast medium mixed with antibiotic is injected into each disc at slow velocity, using preferably a controlled injection syringe with digital pressure readout. The disc is slowly pressurized by injecting 0.5 mL increments through a syringe attached to a pressure measuring device, while recording the opening pressure, the injection pressure, the location of contrast medium, and any pain response evoked. Injection continues until one of the following end points is reached: pain response ≥7/10, intradiscal pressure >50 psi a.o. above opening in a disc with a grade 3 annular tear or 80–100 psi a.o. with a normal-appearing nucleogram, or a total of 3.5 mL of contrast has been injected. Typical opening pressures are 5–25 psi a.o., depending on the degree of nuclear degeneration; if it exceeds 30 psi a.o., this usually indicates that the needle tip is lodged within the inner annulus and needs to be repositioned.

Imaging

AP and lateral images of all injected discs are saved as part of the permanent record. A variety of fluoroscopic patterns may occur in abnormal discs: cotton ball, lobular, irregular, fissured, and ruptured (Fig. 45.7a) [33]. The appearance of the normal nucleus following the injection of contrast medium is classic: the contrast medium assumes either a lobular pattern or a bilobed "hamburger" pattern (Fig. 45.7b). Contrast medium may extend into radial fissures of various lengths but remain contained within the disc (Figs. 45.7 and 45.8). Contrast may escape into the epidural spaces through a torn annulus or through a defect in the vertebral end plate [34]. In other cases, the disc can look completely fissured and disrupted. However, none of these patterns alone are indicative of whether the disc is

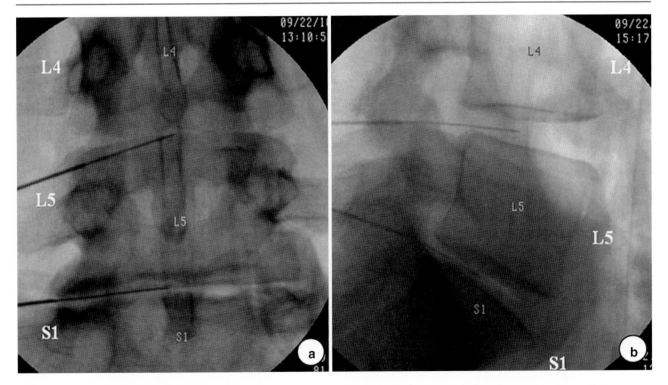

Fig. 45.6 (**a**, **b**) The inner needle may then be directed toward the center of the disc. Ideally, the needle should be within 4–5 mm of the center on AP and lateral fluoroscopy

painful; that can be ascertained only by the patient's subjective response to disc injection.

Post-discography axial CT scanning provides the most accurate depiction of internal disc architecture. The location of degeneration is described by dividing the disc into four quadrants [17] .If the contrast is confined to the nucleus, then no quadrant disruption is present; if the contrast is dispersed, then its location is described (e.g., single quadrant disruption, right posterior; two-quadrant disruption, left anterolateral and right posterior, etc.). The degree of radial and annular disruption is most commonly described [17, 35] using the modified Dallas discogram scale (Fig. 45.9) [32, 35–37]. Grade 0 describes contrast contained within the nucleus; grades 1–3 describe degree of fissuring extending to the inner, middle, and outer annulus, respectively; grade 4 describes a grade 3 annular fissure with a greater than 30° circumferential arc of contrast. A grade 5 annular tear indicates rupture or spread of contrast beyond the outer annulus (Fig. 45.8).

Interpretation

Discography is a provocational test which attempts to mimic physiologic disc loads and evoke the patient's pain by increasing intradiscal pressure with an injection of contrast medium. Increased intradiscal pressure is thought to stimulate annular nerve endings, sensitized nociceptors, and/or pathologically innervated annular fissures. The intensity of the provocation stimulus must be carefully controlled through the skilled operation of a manometer syringe or an automated manometer, permitting more precise comparisons between patient discs and between discographers. Most abnormal discs will be painful between 15 and 50 psi a.o. [38] and are termed "mechanically sensitive" based on a four-type classification introduced in the 1990s by Derby et al. in respect to annular sensitivity [39]. Discs which are painful at pressures <15 psi a.o. are termed low-pressure positive or "chemically sensitive" discs [39]; if discs are painful between 15 and 50 psi a.o., they are termed "mechanically sensitive" discs. Indeterminate discs are painful between 51 and 90 psi a.o., and normal discs are not painful on provocation. An operator using manual "thumb" disc pressurization to 100 psi a.o. reported to have higher false-positive rate in asymptomatic subjects than other operators [24, 40]. If a disc is painful at >50 psi a.o., the response must be reported as indeterminate, because it is difficult to distinguish between a pathologically painful disc and the pain evoked from simply mechanically stimulating a normal or subclinically

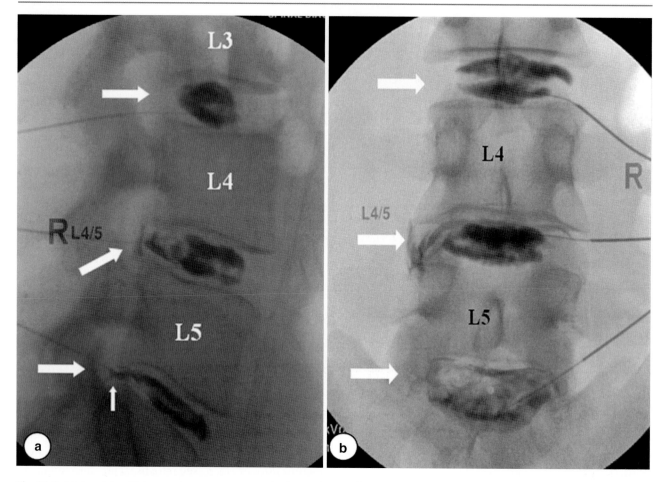

Fig. 45.7 (a) A variety of fluoroscopic patterns may occur in abnormal discs: cotton ball, lobular, irregular, fissured, and ruptured. (b) The appearance of the normal nucleus following the injection of contrast medium is classic: the contrast medium assumes a either a lobular pattern or a bilobed "hamburger" pattern

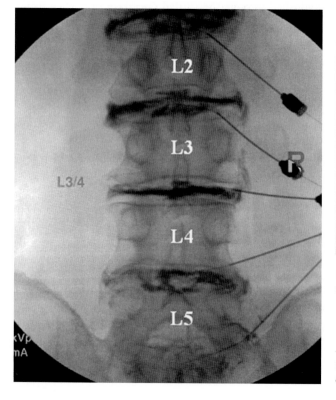

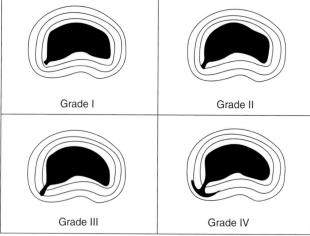

Fig. 45.9 The degree of radial and annular disruption is most commonly described [17, 35] using the modified Dallas discogram scale

Fig. 45.8 Contrast medium may extend into radial fissures of various degrees

Fig. 45.10 Pressure is applied with the index finger to the space between the trachea and the medial boarder of the sternocleidomastoid

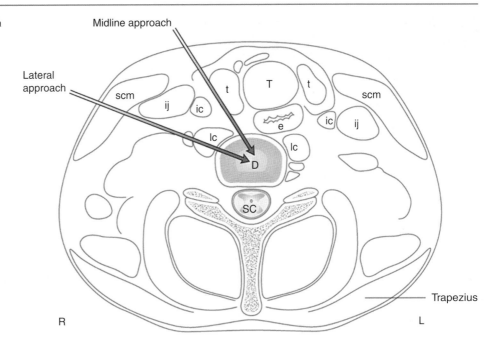

symptomatic disc. To limit false-positive responses, the most up-to-date discography standards are set at a pressure criteria of <50 psi a.o. to define a positive response [32, 41].

Injection speed is also a confounding factor and may account for inter-operator variability in results and increased false-positive responses. At high injection speeds, the true intradiscal pressure (dynamic pressure) is higher than the recorded static pressure [42]. The dynamic pressure, measured only in research settings, is the actual pressure which would be recorded with an intradiscal pressure sensor. Currently, the pressure is measured indirectly via a manometric syringe which records plateau static pressures, postinjection. The pain during activities of daily living is more closely correlated to dynamic peak pressure [39]. Static pressure is reflective of dynamic pressure when recorded by needle sensor and manometer only at slower injection speeds (<0.08 mL/s) [42].

Pain assessment during the disc provocation is the most important information obtained from discography. If the patient's pain intensity, location, and character are similar to or the same as the patient's clinical symptoms, the criteria for concordant pain are satisfied. A true positive pain response is ≥7/10, sustained for greater than 30–60 s; true discogenic pain is less likely to decrease rapidly. Pain which resolves within 10 s should be discounted. It is recommended to confirm all positive responses with manual repressurization with a small volume. If repressurization does not provoke concordant ≥7/10 pain at <50 psi a.o., then the response is considered indeterminate. Clinically, patients with discogenic pain tend to have increased pain postoperatively and an exacerbation of symptoms lasting 2–7 days.

Technique of Cervical Discography

Patient Position

The patient is placed supine on the fluoroscopy table with a cushion placed under his or her shoulders to slightly hyperextend the neck, which may help to improve a disc access. While the side to be punctured in lumbar discography is that opposite the patient's dominant pain, a right-sided approach is used for cervical discography because the esophagus lies to the left in the lower neck. The patient's neck is prepared and draped in a sterile fashion.

Disc Puncture

Midline Approach

The disc level to be studied is identified on the AP view of fluoroscopy. The tube is rotated in a cephalad-caudal direction to bring the end plates parallel to the beam. Pressure is applied with the index finger to the space between the trachea and the medial boarder of the sternocleidomastoid muscle (Fig. 45.10). Firm but gentle pressure will displace the great vessels laterally and the laryngeal structures and trachea medially. Below C4, the right common carotid artery and the internal carotid artery above C4 are palpated. The fingers are insinuated until they encounter the anterior surface of the vertebral column. Since the carotid artery is manually displaced to allow safe needle passage into the disc, and the carotid body may be compressed, administration of IV atropine is therefore suggested to minimize the possibility of vasovagal response [43, 44]. The needle entry point should be medial to the medial border of the sternocleidomastoid muscle, thus avoiding the pharynx

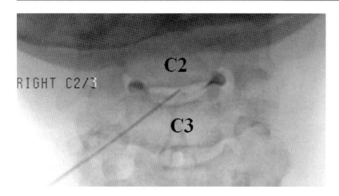

Fig. 45.11 The trachea is pushed medially by the fingernail of the index finger, and when the needle overlies the disc at 20–40° angle, the needle is introduced through the skin directed toward the anterior lateral aspect of the disc

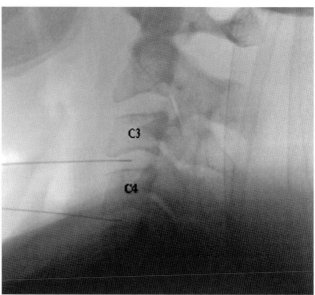

Fig. 45.12 Once the needle is passed several millimeters into the disc, the lateral view is used to guide further advancement, taking precaution to not pass the needle through the disc and into the epidural space or spinal cord

superiorly and the apex of the lungs inferiorly. A shorter 25-gauge 2.5-in. needle is recommended for easier and safer handling. With the point of the needle just medial to or under the index finger, both the needle and the index finger can be moved in unison. The trachea is pushed medially by the fingernail of the index finger, and when the needle overlies the disc at 20–40° angle, the needle is introduced through the skin directed toward the anterior lateral aspect of the disc (Fig. 45.11). Once the needle is passed several millimeters into the disc, the lateral view is recommended to guide further advancement, taking precaution to not pass the needle through the disc and into the epidural space or spinal cord (Fig. 45.12). In order to gauge the depth of penetration, the needle may be directed to and touch the anterior disc body just above or below the disc margin before the insertion into the center of the disc.

Lateral Approach

In this approach, after aligning the vertebral end plates of the target level, the fluoroscopic beam is axially rotated until the anterior margin of the uncinate process is moved approximately one-quarter of the distance between the anterior and posterior lateral vertebral margins. In this view, the target insertion point is 1–2 mm medial to the anterior margin of the uncinate process (Fig. 45.13). The skin entry point will be over the lateral neck muscles and posterior to the great vessels or trachea. Pressure displacement of the great vessels is difficult and usually not done. This region is highly vascular, and patients have to be observed for signs of hematoma. Before and during the injection of contrast, the needle position within the center of a disc and a spread of contrast material inside the disc have to be confirmed with both AP and lateral fluoroscopic images (Fig. 45.14a, b). At C7-T1, the medial approach is preferred to avoid puncturing the apex of the lung.

Provocation and Interpretation

The clinical utility of provocative discography for solving puzzling presentations of atypical pain resulting from cervical

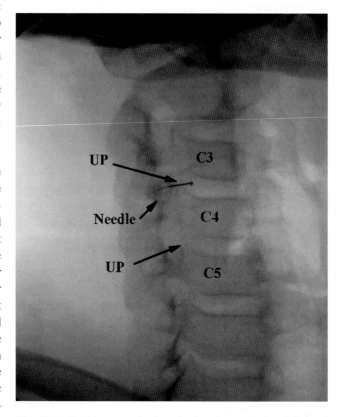

Fig. 45.13 In this approach, after aligning the vertebral end plates of the target level, the fluoroscopic beam is axially rotated until the anterior margin of the uncinate process (*UP*) is moved approximately one quarter of the distance between the anterior and posterior lateral vertebral margins. In this view, the target insertion point is 1–2 mm medial to the anterior margin of the uncinate process (*UP*)

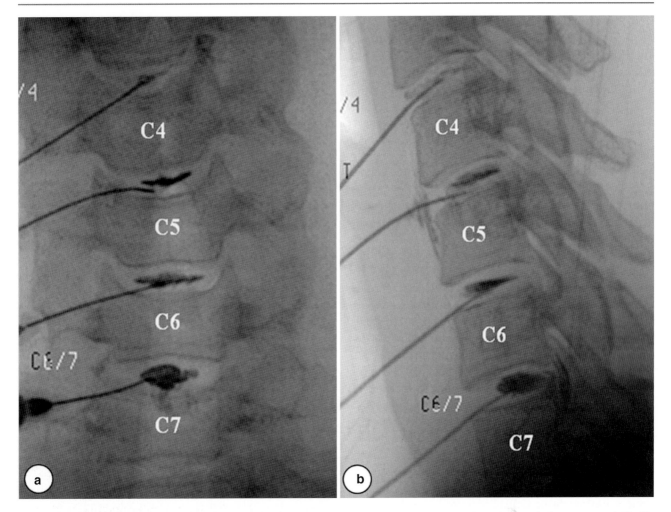

Fig. 45.14 (**a, b**) Before and during the injection of contrast, the needle position within the center of a disc and a spread of contrast material inside the disc have to be confirmed with both AP and lateral fluoroscopic images

discogenic lesions has been demonstrated. In a systematic review of the literature, Manchikanti showed a significant role for cervical discography in selecting surgical candidates and improving surgical outcomes, when strict criteria requiring a concordantly painful disc and two negative controlled discs, one above and one below the affected level, are utilized [45]. Normal cervical discs hold only 0.25–0.5 mL of fluid, and intradiscal injection of normal discs should not be painful. Schell et al. demonstrated an average pain response during disc stimulation in asymptomatic subjects as 2.2/10, whereas it was 5.2/10 in patients with neck pain. He showed that MRI cannot reliably identify the sources of neck pain and provocative discography results had better correlation between cervical discogenic pain and annular disc disruption compared to MRI [46, 47]. A 1–3-mL syringe with contrast media is attached to the needle. Manual syringe pressure is increased slowly until the intrinsic disc pressure is exceeded. Concordancy and pain intensity are recorded at 0.2 mL increments. A positive response requires provocation of significant

(>6–7/10) concordant pain during a confirmatory repeat injection of another 0.1–0.2 mL of contrast. Without an asymptomatic "control" disc, there is no evidence that the patient can discriminate between symptomatic and asymptomatic discs, especially in case of multiple concordant pain levels. It is observed that pressurization of the cervical discs will often cause separation of the end plates, and this movement may cause pain secondary to a symptomatic z-joint. It is recommended to rule out z-joint pain following an analgesic block protocol before performing cervical discography [48].

Technique of Thoracic Discography

Patient Positioning

The patient lies prone on the fluoroscopy table. Skin is prepared and draped in a sterile fashion. As a rule, the side to be punctured is that opposite the patient's dominant pain.

Disc Puncture

The current standard technique of thoracic discography was described by Schellhas et al. in 1994 [49]. After the selection of the target disc on AP view and the alignment of vertebral endplates, the fluoroscopic beam is then rotated ipsilaterally until the corner of the intervertebral disc space is visualized between the superior articular process (SAP) and the costovertebral joint (CVJ). Typically, this degree of ipsilateral rotation will superimpose the tip of the spinous process (SP) on the edge of the contralateral vertebral body. In this view, the insertion point is just lateral to the interpedicular line (Fig. 45.15) and approximately 3 cm lateral to the spinous process. Most discographers prefer a single-needle technique using 23–25-gauge, 3.5-in. needle. A slight bend placed on the end of the needle will facilitate changing directions by needle rotation. The trajectory of the needle is roughly parallel and behind the rib as it passes anterior to attach to the spine at the costovertebral joints. Aiming point is a round to square section of the posterior lateral disc that can be seen through a 1–3-mm opening between the SAP and the rib (Fig. 45.15). The needle should be advanced in short increments and the direction changed as necessary by needle rotation. If one stays medial to the costovertebral junction and just lateral to the SAP, there is no chance of penetrating the lung. It may be hard to visualize thoracic SAP; however, it always projects above the pedicle, which is easily visualized. Although passage of the needle behind the rib is usually uneventful, passage of the needle between the rib and SAP might be difficult due to the small aperture, requiring correctional rotations of the bent needle. Once the needle has passed anterior to the SAP using lateral fluoroscopic view, the needle bend is turned posteriorly to facilitate advancing the needle in a more posterior direction (Fig. 45.16a, b).

Provocation and Interpretation

Nonionic contrast medium is slowly injected into each disc in 0.2–0.3 mL increments under direct fluoroscopic observation, while recording pain response, including behavior, pain intensity, and concordance as well as morphologic abnormalities such as grade 1–3 annular tears or end plate defects. The normal thoracic nucleus usually looks like either a diffuse, elongated homogenous or lobulated pattern (Fig. 45.17). The end point is reached if the pain is >6/10, intradiscal pressure reaches a firm end point, or a total of 2.5 mL of contrast has been injected. CT-discography is often performed to define the exact location and size of annular fissures and protrusions. The most important information obtained is if there is a presence of concordant pain with evoked pain intensity >6/10 in the presence of at least one negative control disc.

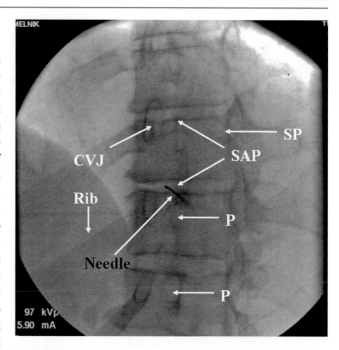

Fig. 45.15 Typically, this degree of ipsilateral rotation will superimpose the tip of the spinous process on the edge of the contralateral vertebral body. In this view, the insertion point is just lateral to the interpedicular line (P-pedicle) and approximately 3 cm lateral to the spinous process at the opening between the superior articular process (SAP) and the costovertebral joints (CVJ)

Postprocedural Care

After the procedure, patients are taken to the recovery room for vital signs and clinical status monitoring by nurses trained in spine injection management. The patient is checked immediately and 30 min postprocedure for any subcutaneous bleeding. Analgesic medications (oral, IV, or IM) are provided as needed. The patient is advised that he or she may experience an exacerbation of typical symptoms for 2–7 days and may experience postprocedure discomfort, including difficulty swallowing after cervical discography and lingering back pain after lumbar discography. The patient is instructed to contact the office if he or she develops fever, chills, or severe (or delayed) onset of pain. Patients are observed and discharged according to institutional protocol. Typically, the patient is discharged to the care of a responsible adult and instructed not to drive for the remainder of the day. Patients are contacted by phone 2–4 days postprocedure to screen for possible complications or adverse side effects.

Potential Risk and Complications

Lumbar Discography

Complications can result from the disc puncture itself, misadventures during needle placement, or medications

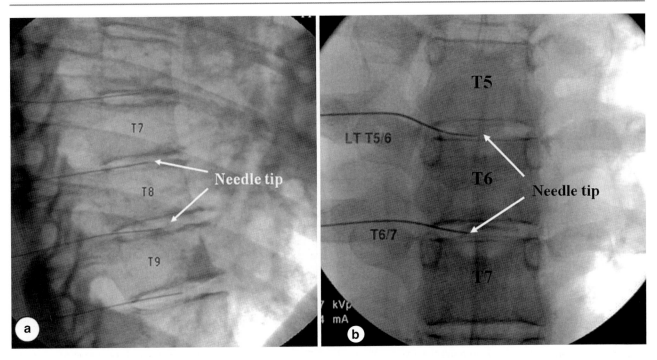

Fig. 45.16 (**a, b**) Once the needle has passed anterior to the SAP using lateral fluoroscopic view, the needle bend is turned posteriorly to facilitate advancing the needle in a more posterior direction

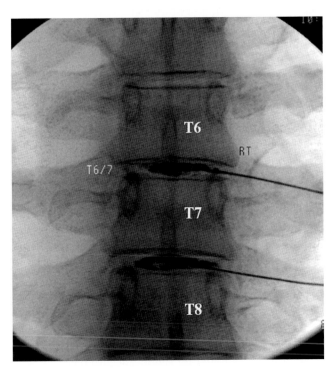

Fig. 45.17 The normal thoracic nucleus usually looks like either a diffuse, elongated homogenous or lobulated pattern

used during the procedure. Complications vary from minor (e.g., increased low back pain, nausea, headache) to major (discitis, seizures, permanent neurologic injury, and death)

[26, 50, 51]. Discitis is the most common serious complication of discography, reported to be less than 0.15 % per patient and 0.08 % per disc [3]. The incidence of discitis has been clearly diminished with the double- vs. single-needle technique [25]. Also, with careful preprocedure screening for infection (e.g., UTI or skin), aseptic skin preparation, styletted needles, and intravenous and intradiscal antibiotics, discitis is now very rare. However, even with prophylactic antibiotics, an epidural abscess after discography has been reported [52, 53].

Clinically, the patient with discitis presents with severe, unremitting, disabling axial pain beginning 5–21 days following the procedure, sometimes accompanied by fever and chills. Investigative tests may require blood work, including CBC, c-reactive protein (CRP), sedimentation rate (ESR), and blood cultures as well as a contrast-enhanced MRI and a disc biopsy. Empyema or abscess formation requires CT-guided drainage or surgical intervention [54–56]. Striking a ventral ramus is a potential hazard, but may be avoided by careful attention to correct technique. Other complications include spinal cord or nerve root injury, cord compression or myelopathy, urticaria, retroperitoneal hemorrhage, nausea, convulsions, headache, and, most commonly, increased pain [3]. An increase in the rate of disc degeneration over time following discography was also recently reported in a single small cohort study and requires further investigation [19]. Meanwhile, it is suggested to use smaller discography needles, gauges 25 or less.

Cervical Discography

Inadvertent passage of the needle through the cervical disc in the AP plane can cause spinal cord injury or post-thecal puncture cephalgia, which can be avoided by using a shorter needle, using a lateral view during needle advancement and conformation of needle depth penetration by touching the anterior vertebral margin prior to passage into the disc [46]. Penetration of viscera such as the pharynx and esophagus is not a problem per se, but increases the risk of infection such as epidural and retropharyngeal abscess and discitis [56–59]. The reported incidence of discitis is 0.1–0.5 % [58, 60]. Needle passage through the carotid artery may result in a hematoma which could potentially cause an airway obstruction, especially in patients with coagulation problems [46].

Thoracic Discography

The main complications include pneumothorax, discitis, and neural injury. Pneumothorax can complicate cervical, thoracic, or lumbar discography, but more frequent in the thoracic spine. A small traumatic pneumothorax after percutaneous needle procedures can be treated conservatively and usually does not require chest tube insertion [61].

Discussion

The single purpose and objective of disc stimulation is to identify a painful intervertebral disc. As in the case of palpation for tenderness, provocation does not reveal pathology or the cause of pain; it only indicates the structure that when stressed, reproduces the patient's pain. If an explicit, pathoanatomical diagnosis is to be made, such as internal disc disruption, the discography must be supplemented by post-discography CT in order to reveal the fissures characteristic of this condition. Another, not least important value of discography is in identification of "negative discs" in response to a disc stimulation, thus limiting the number of levels requiring surgical intervention or a need for interventional disc procedures altogether. However, the diagnostic power of discography remains controversial [62]. As a provocative test, it has been criticized to have a potentially high false-positive rate [24]. The reasons for that can occur due to technical errors, due to neurophysiological phenomena, or due to psychosocial factors [32].

Correct technical performance is paramount to the accuracy of the discography results and has been underestimated over the past decades, leading to questionable medical outcomes and important legal implications.

Discography without strict standards for pressure, volume, speed of injection controls, and limits is unsupportable. Dynamic and static pressures, volumes, and pain responses must be gathered and documented using a consistent and reproducible technique, preferably using a controlled injection syringe with digital pressure readout rather than manual pressurization [63]. It was shown that speed-sensitive dynamic pressure is more liable to provoke a positive pan response, thus requiring a slow injection rate (0.05–0.1 mL/s), which most accurately reflects the pressures transferred to the outer annulus [63]. Many of the reported false-positive responses occurred at pressures of 50 psi a.o. or greater. In addition, provocation response should not be accepted as a positive unless it can be confirmed by a repeat pressurization, and pain does not decrease more than 50 % over 30 s. Transient pain provocation may occur when an asymptomatic fissure opens or a thin membrane sealing the outer annulus ruptures during disc pressurization.

Central hyperalgesia also has to be taken into account as a physiological phenomenon when the perception of stimuli from a receptive field is facilitated by ongoing nociceptive activity arising from adjacent or nearby but separate receptive fields. In this regard, formal studies have shown that in patients with no history and no symptoms of back pain, but with a painful donor site on the iliac crest, disc stimulation can evoke back pain [40], producing false-positive response.

Concerns have been raised regarding psychological comorbidity and psychosocial factors as significant confounding factors in patients undergoing discography, questioning the results of discography in patients with chronic pain or somatization disorders other than back pain [40]. Evidence indicates that patients with chronic or chronic intermittent low back pain respond similarly to disc stimulation as do asymptomatic volunteers undergoing discography, as was shown by Derby in a prospective controlled study of patients with grade 3 disc tears [64]. Shin also confirmed that a majority of patients with grade 4 tears could distinguish between "positive" and "negative discs" by magnitude of pain response, causing doubt on the argument that a majority of patients with chronic pain undergoing discography would overreport pain [65].

In addition, a randomized controlled trial comparing discography results of 25 patients with and without somatization disorder found no significant difference in positive responses between groups [66]. There was also no difference in positive responses in patients with depression and/or general anxiety disorder. That calls into question the results of a limited Carragee study of six somatization patients, where only four of six were able to complete their discography test because of pain [24]. Derby et al. [67] reported DRAM scores of 81 patients undergoing discography: 15 % (12/81) were normal, 52 % (42/81) were at risk, and 33 % (27/81) were abnormal (distressed, depressive or somatic). The positive rates of discography were not statistically significant by subgroup ($p > 0.05$). In patients with chronic low back pain, no correlation was found between presenting DRAM score and discography result.

A recent meta-analysis of studies of asymptomatic subjects undergoing discography showed a high specificity of 0.94(95 % CI 0.89–0.98) and a relatively low false-positive rate of 6 % [20]. This critical examination of most studies in the literature since the 1960s showed that an acceptably low false-positive rate can be achieved when strict ISIS/IASP standards for a positive discography are utilized: pain ≥7/10, concordant pain, pressure <50 psi a.o., ≥grade 3 annular tear, volume limit ≤3.5 mL, and presence of a negative control disc.

In regard to post-discectomy subjects, it appeared that they have a slightly higher false-positive rate of 15 % per patient and 9.1 % per disc, as a group. Given our limited knowledge of discography in post-discectomy patients and the possibility that provocation may open previously healed granulation tissue along surgical planes, discographers have to consider pressure- and speed-controlled manometry and to use lower limits for pressure and volume when defining a positive value. Another recent concern raised by Carragee et al. [19] is a long-term risk that discography, as an invasive test, can potentially cause damage to punctured discs over time and result in accelerated disc degeneration. The authors showed a 21 % increase in the degree of disc degeneration using small gauge needles and an increase in the number of new disc herniations of all types in the discography vs. control group over 10 years. These results require attention and further investigation. It would be important to determine what proportion of those degenerative discs can be attributed to rather expected natural history of accelerated degeneration in this small cohort of patients with known cervical disc disease. Those patients might be already genetically predisposed to accelerated disc degeneration and multilevel spondylosis, compared to the normal population, as was shown in a well-designed twin study, when 74 % of degenerative findings at the lower lumbar levels were accounted for the heritability [68].

Even though the diagnostic power of discography remains controversial, it is a relatively safe and sensitive test for identifying painful discs, which may predict surgical outcomes. In a multicenter surgical and nonsurgical outcome study after pressure-controlled discography, Derby et al. [39] stated that precise prospective categorization of positive discographic diagnoses may predict treatment outcomes, surgical or otherwise, thereby greatly facilitating therapeutic decision-making.

Summary

Discography, when indicated and correctly performed, is a safe and sometimes powerful complement to the overall clinical context and is not intended to be a stand-alone test. Despite the controversy, this test can provide valuable information regarding the possible discogenic origin of pain and provide intricate details of inner disc morphology and annular disc disruption, when combined with a post-discography CT scan. It is not a screening procedure but rather a confirmatory one. Recent advances in discography technique, including use of pressure-controlled manometry and strict diagnostic criteria, helped to improved validity of this test significantly. In patients with chronic intractable neck or back pain but negative or indeterminate imaging findings who are being considered for surgical intervention, discography can help to localize the symptomatic level and potentially benefit the patients by surgical intervention or by avoiding it in case of "asymptomatic discs." Newer noninvasive imaging technologies like magnetic resonance spectroscopy, measuring biochemical markers of inflammation that could potentially correlate with "painful disc" on discography, are gradually emerging. They have the potential to replace more invasive disc stimulation tests in the near future, but to this day, discography remains the criterion of standard for the diagnosis of discogenic pain.

References

1. Lindblom K. Technique and results in myelography and disc puncture. Acta Radiol. 1950;34:321–30.
2. Lindblom K. Technique and results of diagnostic disc puncture and injection (discography) in the lumbar region. Acta Orthop Scand. 1951;20:315–26.
3. Guyer RD, Ohnmeiss DD. Lumbar discography. Position statement from the North American Spine Society Diagnostic and Therapeutic Committee. Spine. 1995;20:2048–59.
4. O'Neill C, Derby R. Percutaneous discectomy using nucleoplasty. In: International 21st course for percutaneous endoscopic spinal surgery and complementary techniques. Spital zolikerberg, Zurich; 2003.
5. Bogduk N, Tynan W, Wilson AS. The nerve supply to the human lumbar intervertebral discs. J Anat. 1981;132:39–56.
6. Yoshizawa H, O'Brien JP, Smith WT, Trumper M. The neuropathology of intervertebral discs removed for low-back pain. J Pathol. 1980;132:95–104.
7. Groen GJ, Baljet B, Drukker J. Nerves and nerve plexuses of the human vertebral column. Am J Anat. 1990;188:282–96.
8. Malinsky J. The ontogenetic development of nerve terminations in the intervertebral discs of man. (Histology of intervertebral discs, 11th communication). Acta Anat (Basel). 1959;38:96–113.
9. Weinstein J, Claverie W, Gibson S. The pain of discography. Spine (Phila Pa 1976). 1988;13:1344–8.
10. Korkala O, Gronblad M, Liesi P, Karaharju E. Immunohistochemical demonstration of nociceptors in the ligamentous structures of the lumbar spine. Spine. 1985;10:156–7.

11. Konttinen YT, et al. Neuroimmunohistochemical analysis of peri-discal nociceptive neural elements. Spine (Phila Pa 1976). 1990;15:383–6.

12. Peng B, et al. The pathogenesis of discogenic low back pain. J Bone Joint Surg. 2005;87:62–7.

13. Freemont AJ, et al. Nerve ingrowth into diseased intervertebral disc in chronic back pain. Lancet. 1997;350:178–81.

14. Coppes MH, Marani E, Thomeer RT, Groen GJ. Innervation of "painful" lumbar discs. Spine. 1997;22:2342–9; discussion 2349–50.

15. Bogduk N, Aprill C, Derby R, et al. Discography. In: Spine care: diagnosis and conservative treatment. St. Louis: Mosby; 1995. p. 219–36.

16. Moneta GB, et al. Reported pain during lumbar discography as a function of annular ruptures and disc degeneration. A re-analysis of 833 discograms. Spine (Phila Pa 1976). 1994;19:1968–74.

17. Vanharanta H, et al. The relationship of pain provocation to lumbar disc deterioration as seen by CT/discography. Spine. 1987;12:295–8.

18. Greenspan A, Amparo EG, Gorczyca DP, Montesano PX. Is there a role for diskography in the era of magnetic resonance imaging? Prospective correlation and quantitative analysis of computed tomography-diskography, magnetic resonance imaging, and surgical findings. J Spinal Disord. 1992;5:26–31.

19. Carragee EJ, et al. Does discography cause accelerated progression of degeneration changes in the lumbar disc: a ten-year matched cohort study. Spine (Phila Pa 1976). 2009;34:2338–45.

20. Wolfer LR, Derby R, Lee J-E, Lee S-H. Systematic review of lumbar provocation discography in asymptomatic subjects with a meta-analysis of false-positive rates. Pain Physician. 2008;11:513–38.

21. Bogduk N. Proposed discography standards. ISIS newsletter. Daly City: International Spinal Injection Society; 1994. p. 10–3.

22. Derby R. A second proposal for discography standards. ISIS newsletter. Daly City: International Spinal Injection Society; 1994. p. 108–22.

23. Jensen MC, et al. Magnetic resonance imaging of the lumbar spine in people without back pain. N Engl J Med. 1994;331:69–73.

24. Carragee EJ, et al. The rates of false-positive lumbar discography in select patients without low back symptoms. Spine. 2000;25:1373–80. discussion 1381.

25. Fraser RD, Osti OL, Vernon-Roberts B. Discitis after discography. J Bone Joint Surg Br. 1987;69:26–35.

26. Fraser RD, Osti OL, Vernon-Roberts B. Iatrogenic discitis: the role of intravenous antibiotics in prevention and treatment. An experimental study. Spine. 1989;14:1025–32.

27. Polk HC, Christmas AB. Prophylactic antibiotics in surgery and surgical wound infections. Am Surg. 2000;66:105–11.

28. Osti OL, Fraser RD, Vernon-Roberts B. Discitis after discography. The role of prophylactic antibiotics. J Bone Joint Surg Br. 1990;72:271–4.

29. Troiser O. Technique de la discographie extra-durale. J Radiol. 1982;63:571–8.

30. Aprill III C. Diagnostic disc injection. In: Frymoyer JW, editor. The adults spine: principles and practice. 2nd ed. Philadelphia: Lippincott-Raven; 1996.

31. Milette PC, Melanson D. A reappraisal of lumbar discography. J Can Assoc Radiol. 1982;33:176–82.

32. Bogduk N. Practice guidelines for spinal diagnostic and treatment procedures. San Francisco: International Spine Intervention Society; 2004.

33. Adams MA, Dolan P, Hutton WC. The stages of disc degeneration as revealed by discograms. J Bone Joint Surg Br. 1986;68:36–41.

34. Bogduk NC, April C, Derby R, et al. Discography. In: White A, editor. Spine care. Diagnosis and conservative treatment. St. Louis: Mosby Co; 1995. p. 219–36.

35. Derby R, Kim B-J, Chen Y, Seo K-S, Lee S-H. The relation between annular disruption on computed tomography scan and pressure-controlled diskography. Arch Phys Med Rehabil. 2005;86:1534–8.

36. Aprill C, Bogduk N. High-intensity zone: a diagnostic sign of painful lumbar disc on magnetic resonance imaging. Br J Radiol. 1992;65:361–9.

37. Sachs BL, et al. Dallas discogram description. A new classification of CT/discography in low-back disorders. Spine. 1987;12:287–94.

38. Derby R. Lumbar discometry. Sci Newsl Int Spine Injection Soc Newsl. 1993;1:8–17.

39. Derby R, et al. The ability of pressure-controlled discography to predict surgical and nonsurgical outcomes. Spine. 1999;24:364–71; discussion 371–62.

40. Carragee EJ, Tanner CM, Yang B, Brito JL, Truong T. False-positive findings on lumbar discography. Reliability of subjective concordance assessment during provocative disc injection. Spine. 1999;24:2542–7.

41. Derby R, Lee SH, Kim BJ. Discography. In: Slipman CW, Derby R, Simeone FA, Mayer TG, editors. Interventional spine: an algorithmic approach. Philadelphia: Saunders Elsevier; 2008. p. 291–302.

42. Seo K-S, et al. In vitro measurement of pressure differences using manometry at various injection speeds during discography. Spine J. 2007;7:68–73.

43. Singh V. The role of cervical discography in interventional pain management. Pain Physician. 2004;7:249–55.

44. Connor P, Darden BV. Cervical discography complications and clinical efficacy. Spine. 1993;18:2035.

45. Manchikanti L, et al. Systematic review of cervical discography as a diagnostic test for chronic spinal pain. Pain Physician. 2009;12:305–21.

46. Derby R, Melfi R, Talu G, Aprill C. Cervical discography: diagnostic value and complications. In: Curtis W, Slipman CW, Derby R, Simeone FA, Mayer TG, editors. Interventional spine: an algorithmic approach. New York: Saunders Publishers; 2007.

47. Schellhas KP, Smith MD, Gundry CR, Pollei SR. Cervical discogenic pain. Prospective correlation of magnetic resonance imaging and discography in asymptomatic subjects and pain sufferers. Spine. 1996;21:300–11.

48. Bogduk N, Aprill C. On the nature of neck pain, discography and cervical zygapophysial joint blocks. Pain. 1993;54:213–7.

49. Schellhas K, Pollei SR, Dorwart R. Thoracic discography. A safe and reliable technique. Spine. 1994;19:2103–9.

50. Thomas PS. Image-guided pain management. Philadelphia: Lippincott-Raven; 1997.

51. Vanharanta H, et al. Pain provocation and disc deterioration by age. A CT/discography study in a low-back pain population. Spine. 1989;14:420–3.

52. Tsuji N, Igarashi S, Koyama T. Spinal epidural abscess – report of 5 cases. No Shinkei Geka. 1987;15:1079–85.

53. Junila J, Niinimaki T, Tervonen O. Epidural abscess after lumbar discography. A case report. Spine. 1997;22:2191–3.

54. Baker AS, Ojemann RG, Swartz MN, Richardson EP. Spinal epidural abscess. N Engl J Med. 1975;293:463–8.

55. Ravicovitch MA, Spallone A. Spinal epidural abscesses. Surgical and parasurgical management. Eur Neurol. 1982;21:347–57.

56. Lownie SP, Ferguson GG. Spinal subdural empyema complicating cervical discography. Spine. 1989;14:1415–7.

57. Guyer RD, et al. Discitis after discography. Spine. 1988;13:1352–4.

58. Roosen K, Bettag W, Fiebach O. Complications of cervical discography(author's transl). ROFO Fortschr Geb Rontgenstr Nuklearmed. 1975;122:520–7.

59. Vogelsang H. Cervical intervertebral discitis after discography (author's transl). Neurochirurgia (Stuttg). 1973;16:80–3.

60. Brodsky AE, Binder WF. Lumbar discography. Its value in diagnosis and treatment of lumbar disc lesions. Spine. 1979;4:110–20.
61. Johnson G. Traumatic pneumothorax: is a chest drain always necessary? J Accid Emerg Med. 1996;13:173–4.
62. Carragee EJ. Prevalence and clinical features of internal disk disruption in patients with chronic low back pain. Spine. 1996;21:776–7.
63. Derby R, Guyer R, Lee SH, Seo KS, Chen Y. The rational use and limitations of provocative discography. International Spine Intervention Society 13th annual meeting in NY, ISIS Newsletter. 2004;5:6–20.
64. Derby R, et al. Comparison of discographic findings in asymptomatic subject discs and the negative discs of chronic LBP patients: can discography distinguish asymptomatic discs among morphologically abnormal discs? Spine J. 2005;5:389–94.
65. Shin D, Kim H, Jung J, Sin D, Lee J. Diagnostic relevance of pressure-controlled discography. J Korean Med Sci. 2006;21:911–6.
66. Manchikanti L, et al. Provocative discography in low back pain patients with or without somatization disorder: a randomized prospective evaluation. Pain Physician. 2001;4:227–39.
67. Derby R, et al. The influence of psychologic factors on diskography in patients with chronic axial low back pain. Arch Phys Med Rehabil. 2008;89:1300–4.
68. Derby R, Wolfer L, Summers J. Does discography cause accelerated progression of degeneration in the lumbar spine. SpineLine. 2010:Mar/Apr:26–30.

Brachial Plexus Block

46

Chester Buckenmaier III

Key Points

- Brachial plexus block is an ideal anesthetic for upper extremity surgery since plexus anatomy allows easy access by a variety of approaches.
- A detailed understanding of brachial plexus anatomy is essential for the safe and efficient application of all the approaches to brachial plexus block.
- As with all regional anesthetics, brachial plexus block should be performed in areas with standard monitors and emergency life support equipment.
- The existence of the brachial plexus "sheath" is supported by a preponderance of evidence as demonstrated in cadavers and with radiopaque injections.
- All approaches to the brachial plexus are suitable for continuous peripheral nerve block catheters.
- Brachial plexus block is particularly well suited for ultrasound technology though this technology does not preclude the need for the clinician to maintain a detailed understanding of anatomy.

History of the Brachial Plexus Block

The first brachial plexus block was performed less than a year following Carl Koller's discovery of the anesthetic properties of cocaine in 1884. William S. Halsted injected each of the roots of the brachial plexus with cocaine under direct visualization after surgical exposure. In some respects, the anesthetic method was as extensive as the surgical procedure [1]. In 1911, G. Hirschel described a percutaneous technique for brachial plexus blockade by injecting local anesthetic around

the axillary artery [2]. A century later, the science of brachial plexus block has become one of the most important anesthetic and analgesic techniques for the upper extremity.

The advantages of regional anesthesia include superior pain control, reductions in the surgical stress response, and preservation of immune function, among many others [3]. The numerous benefits of perioperative surgical stress attenuation using regional anesthesia were recently highlighted when breast cancer surgery patients were noted to have a reduced incidence of cancer recurrence or metastasis compared to patients who underwent breast cancer surgery under general anesthesia [4]. Brachial plexus block for upper extremity surgery has been suggested as an ideal anesthetic approach for most upper extremity surgery patients due to the profound analgesia provided, the anatomical realities of the plexus that allow relatively easy access by the anesthesiologist through a variety of approaches, and the excellent operating conditions afforded the surgeon [5]. As with all regional anesthetic techniques, a detailed understanding of brachial plexus anatomy, to include surrounding structures, is essential for the safe and efficient application of all the approaches to brachial plexus block.

Pearls of Brachial Plexus Block

As with any medical procedure, proper patient consent for the block procedure, conformation of side to be blocked, and documentation of the block is essential. Providers should counsel patients regarding the risks of regional anesthesia that include, but are not limited to, block failure, local anesthetic toxicity, and potential nerve injury. Additionally, patients should be informed that normal protective reflexes and proprioception for the blocked upper extremity will be diminished or absent for 24 h and they should therefore take special care of the blocked limb. All regional anesthetics should be performed in areas with standard monitors, oxygen, suction, airway, and emergency advanced cardiac life support equipment and medications. During local anesthetic injections, constant

C. Buckenmaier III, M.D.
Department of Anesthesiology,
Walter Reed National Medical Center, Defense and Veterans Center for Integrative Pain Management, 11300 Rockville Pike, Rockville, MD 20852, USA
e-mail: cbuckenmaier@dvcipm.org

T.R. Deer et al. (eds.), *Comprehensive Treatment of Chronic Pain by Medical, Interventional, and Integrative Approaches*,
DOI 10.1007/978-1-4614-1560-2_46, © American Academy of Pain Medicine 2013

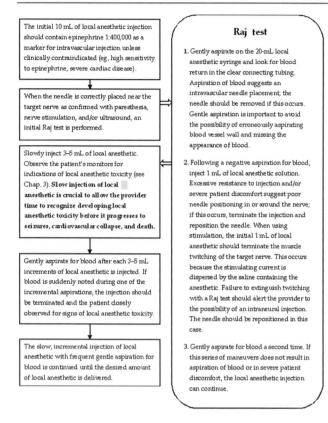

The initial 10 mL of local anesthetic injection should contain epinephrine 1:400,000 as a marker for intravascular injection unless clinically contraindicated (eg, high sensitivity to epinephrine, severe cardiac disease).

↓

When the needle is correctly placed near the target nerve as confirmed with paresthesia, nerve stimulation, and/or ultrasound, an initial Raj test is performed.

↓

Slowly inject 3–5 mL of local anesthetic. Observe the patient's monitors for indications of local anesthetic toxicity (see Chap. 3). **Slow injection of local anesthetic is crucial to allow the provider time to recognize developing local anesthetic toxicity before it progresses to seizures, cardiovascular collapse, and death.**

↓

Gently aspirate for blood after each 3–5 mL increments of local anesthetic is injected. If blood is suddenly noted during one of the incremental aspirations, the injection should be terminated and the patient closely observed for signs of local anesthetic toxicity.

↓

The slow, incremental injection of local anesthetic with frequent gentle aspiration for blood is continued until the desired amount of local anesthetic is delivered.

Raj test

1. Gently aspirate on the 20-mL local anesthetic syringe and look for blood return in the clear connecting tubing. Aspiration of blood suggests an intravascular needle placement; the needle should be removed if this occurs. Gentle aspiration is important to avoid the possibility of erroneously aspirating blood vessel wall and missing the appearance of blood.

2. Following a negative aspiration for blood, inject 1 mL of local anesthetic solution. Excessive resistance to injection and/or severe patient discomfort suggest poor needle positioning in or around the nerve; if this occurs, terminate the injection and reposition the needle. When using stimulation, the initial 1 mL of local anesthetic should terminate the muscle twitching of the target nerve. This occurs because the stimulating current is dispersed by the saline containing the anesthetic. Failure to extinguish twitching with a Raj test should alert the provider to the possibility of an intraneural injection. The needle should be repositioned in this case.

3. Gently aspirate for blood a second time. If this series of maneuvers does not result in aspiration of blood or in severe patient discomfort, the local anesthetic injection can continue.

Fig. 46.1 The preferred local anesthetic injection procedure used at Walter Reed Army Medical Center (With permission from Buckenmaier and Bleckner [71])

Table 46.1 Recommended techniques and conditions to minimize the risk of local anesthetic intravascular injection

Standard monitoring with audible oxygen saturation tone
Oxygen supplementation
Slow, incremental injection (5 mL, every 10–15 s)
Gentle aspiration for blood before injection and every 5 mL thereafter
Initial injection of local anesthetic test dose containing at least 5–15 μg epinephrine with observation for heart rate change >10 beats/min, blood pressure changes >15 mmHg, or lead II – wave amplitude decrease by 25 %
Pretreatment with benzodiazepines to increase the seizure threshold to local anesthetic toxicity
Patient either aware or sedated but still able to maintain meaningful communication with the physician
Resuscitation equipment and medications readily available at all times
If seizures occur, patient care includes airway maintenance, supplemental oxygen, and termination of the seizure with propofol (25–50 mg) or thiopental (50 mg)
Local anesthetic toxicity that leads to cardiovascular collapse should immediately be managed with prompt institution of advanced cardiac life support (ACLS) protocols

With permission from Buckenmaier and Bleckner [71]
Intralipid (KabiVitrum, Inc., Alameda, California) 20 % 1 mL/kg every 3–5 min, up to 3 mL/kg, administered during ACLS for local anesthetic toxicity can be lifesaving. Follow this bolus with an Intralipid 20 % infusion of 0.25 mL/kg/min for 2.5 h

vigilance is required for signs and symptoms of developing local anesthetic toxicity. Slow injections with frequent aspirations for blood are one of the best defenses against this complication. The preferred local anesthetic injection procedure used at Walter Reed Army Medical Center is provided in Fig. 46.1. Recommended techniques and conditions to minimize local anesthetic toxicity from intravascular injection for all blocks are provided in Table 46.1.

Anatomy of the Brachial Plexus

The brachial plexus is commonly formed from the five roots (anterior rami) of vertebrae C5 through T1 (Fig. 46.2). Considerable morphological variations in brachial plexus formation have been described, even on contralateral sides of the same individual, though sex, race, or side of the body does not appear to influence this variation [6]. The brachial plexus can be described as "prefixed" when C4 brachial plexus contributions occur or "postfixed" when T2 contributions are noted. Uysal et al. [7] surveyed 200 fetuses noting the common C5 through T1 contribution that occurred 71.5 %, prefixed plexuses were observed 25.5 %, and the postfixed plexus was noted in 2.5 %.

The brachial plexus is typically further categorized into four major components or sections as it passes into the upper extremity (Fig. 46.2). Each of these components is bounded by distinct anatomical structures [8]:

- Three trunks. The anterior rami of the plexus roots commonly coalesce into three major trunks with roots: C5 and C6 forming the superior trunk, C7 contributing to the middle trunk, and C8 and T1 making up the inferior trunk. The trunks are most easily identified as they pass between the anterior and middle scalene muscles. Anatomical variation exists in the relationship between the scalene muscles and the trunks with the most common variation being penetration of the anterior scalene muscle by the C5 and/or C6 roots [9]. These anatomical variants can have clinical significant when performing regional anesthetic blocks of the brachial plexus trunks.
- Six divisions. Each trunk divides into an anterior division (anterior flexor nerves of the arm) and a posterior division (posterior extensor nerves of the arm) for a total of six divisions (three anterior, three posterior). The separation of the trunks into divisions occurs at the level of the first rib. The divisions then pass posterior to the midpoint of the clavicle through the cervicoaxillary canal.
- Three cords. The six divisions emerge posterior to the clavicle to coalesce once again to form three cords. The cords are named based on their position in relation to

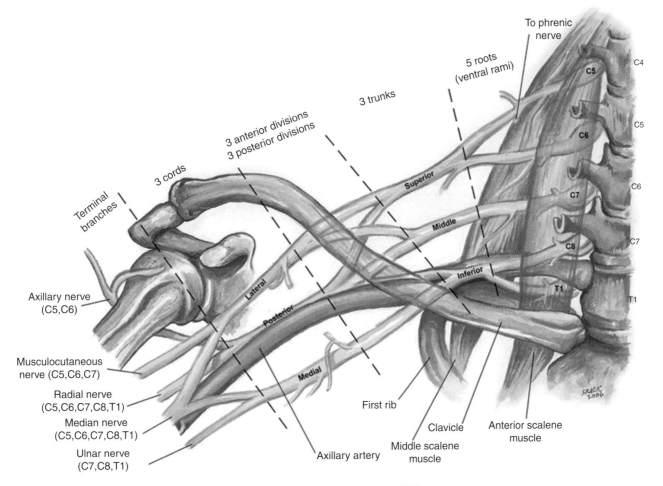

Fig. 46.2 Brachial plexus anatomy (With permission from Buckenmaier and Bleckner [71])

the axillary artery as this neurovascular bundle passes into the axilla. The *lateral cord* (lateral to the axillary artery) is composed of the anterior divisions of the superior and middle trunk. The *medial cord* consists of only a continuation of the anterior division of the inferior trunk. The lateral and medial cords therefore give rise to nerves that ultimately service the flexor surface of the arm. The *posterior cord* is formed from the posterior divisions of all three cords. The posterior cord contains all of the nerves that will supply the extensor surface of the arm.

- Five terminal branches. The five major nerves of the upper extremity are derived from the three cords. The *musculocutaneous nerve* (C5–C7) arises from the lateral cord and supplies the coracobrachialis, biceps brachii and brachialis muscles, and the skin to the lateral forearm. The lateral cord (C6–C7) and medial cord (C8–T1) both contribute to the formation of the *median nerve* which innervates anterior forearm muscles and the thenar half of the skin and muscles of the palm. The *ulnar nerve* is a branch of the medial cord (C7–T1) and supplies the forearm and hand medial to the midpoint of digit four. The shoulder joint and lateral skin over the deltoid muscle are innervated by

the *axillary nerve* that branches from the posterior cord. Finally, the largest branch of the posterior cord gives rise to the *radial nerve* (C5–T1) which supplies all of the posterior compartment muscles and most of the posterior skin of the arm. Numerous other named nerves branch off of the brachial plexus though knowledge of the five major nerves is adequate for most clinical blocks of the brachial plexus.

A discussion of brachial plexus anatomy would be incomplete without addressing the considerable controversy that surrounds the existence of a "sheath" surrounding the brachial plexus and includes the artery, vein, and investing connective tissue. Multiple authors have described the anatomical structure referred to as a sheath, perhaps most famously by Winnie [1] who noted the muscles surrounding the brachial plexus contribute fascia that we "conceive of as the 'sheath of the brachial plexus.'" Other authors have debated whether the sheath is a single tube or compartmented structure [10, 11]. Still others have rejected the existence of the sheath outright [12]. Recently, Franco et al. [13] performed systematic dissections on 11 embalmed cadavers and determined that a sheath-like structure surrounding the brachial plexus filled

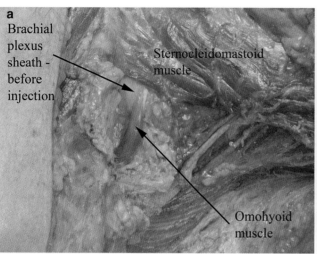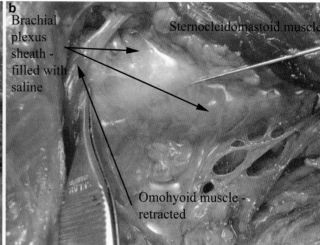

Fig. 46.3 (**a**) Brachial plexus sheath before and after injection with saline in a fresh cadaver specimen. Before: Prior to injection with saline. (**b**) Brachial plexus sheath before and after injection with saline in a fresh cadaver specimen. Before: prior to injection with saline (With permission from Buckenmaier and Bleckner [71])

with loose connective tissue could be demonstrated in every specimen (Fig. 46.3a, b). The clinical significance and existence of a structure enveloping the brachial plexus has been suggested by both radiopaque local anesthetic injections [14] and observations during injections under direct ultrasound guidance [15]. Regardless of the term used to describe the investment of fascia that surrounds neurovascular structures, the preponderance of evidence suggests the brachial plexus sheath is a reality. The clinical significance of this structure continues to be debated and is worthy of additional study.

Subsequent sections of this chapter will describe common regional anesthesia blocks for the brachial plexus to include interscalene, supraclavicular, infraclavicular, and axillary block. Each block will be presented with a discussion of pertinent anatomy, followed by approaches using both nerve stimulation and ultrasound guided. The approaches described in detail are preferred by the author and used in daily clinical practice. This should not deter the reader from exploring other methodologies that are referenced with no further explanation.

Interscalene Block of the Brachial Plexus

The interscalene block described by Winnie in 1970 [16] is performed at the level of the C6 vertebral body (Chassaignac's tubercle). At this level, the roots of the brachial plexus pass the transverse processes of the vertebral bodies where they are invested between the fascia of the anterior and middle scalene muscles as the plexus passes between these muscles (Fig. 46.4). This provides a convenient compartment that local anesthetic can be deposited, to bathe the C5–C7 roots, resulting in consistent block of the shoulder muscles to include the deltoid, supraspinatus infraspinatus, and teres major muscles. Therefore, interscalene block of the brachial plexus is most commonly selected for operations on the shoulder, clavicle, or upper arm. This block is typically not selected for operations of the hand or forearm due to unpredictable spread of local anesthetic to the C8–T1 nerve roots (ulnar nerve). Inconsistent spread of local anesthetic to C3–C4 can result in posterior shoulder (cape area) sparing that should be considered for large operations on the shoulder (Fig. 46.5). Supplemental blocks such as an intercostobrachial nerve block (subcutaneous injection of local anesthetic from the axilla to the midpoint of the clavicle) are used to supplement the interscalene block for major shoulder surgery. Paravertebral blocks at T1–T2 can be added for procedures that include significant posterior shoulder dissections.

The close proximity of the phrenic nerve lying anterior on the anterior scalene muscle usually results in paresis of the hemidiaphragm on the side blocked. Though most patients tolerate the loss of one hemidiaphragm with ease, the use of this block should be reconsidered in a patient that cannot tolerate a reduction in pulmonary function. Proximal spread of local anesthetic to the cervical plexus (C3, C4) and cervical sympathetic chain can result in a transient Horner's syndrome and vocal hoarseness in some patients [17]. While this condition is self-limited, patients can become unnecessarily concerned if the possible occurrence of this side effect is not part of pre-block counseling. Perhaps the most devastating complication associated with this block is the unintended injection of local anesthetic into the vertebral artery located posterior and medial to the brachial plexus at this level. This error can lead to rapid cardiovascular collapse with few, if any, clinical signs warning of systemic local anesthetic toxicity [18]. Proper slow injection technique, with frequent gentle aspiration for blood every 3–5 mL of local anesthetic injected, is critical to guard against intravascular needle placement.

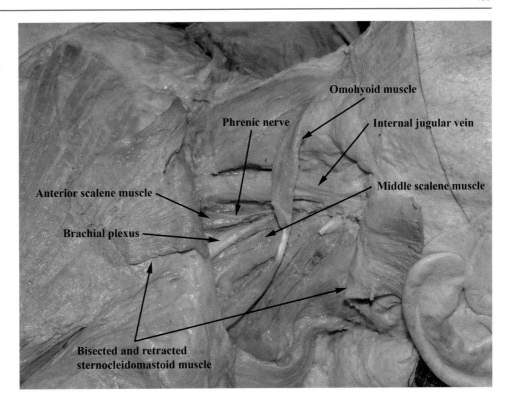

Fig. 46.4 Brachial plexus dissection above the clavicle (With permission from Buckenmaier and Bleckner [71])

Procedure

The patient is placed supine with the head turned to the nonoperative side. Major external landmarks include the lateral border of the sternocleidomastoid muscle (SCM – best defined by having the patient lift their head off the bed 1 in.), the external jugular vein, the cricoid cartilage which corresponds to the C6 level, and the clavicle (Fig. 46.6). Regardless of the technology used to perform any block of the brachial plexus, it is worthwhile to examine and mark the patient's pertinent anatomy prior to attempting needle placement. It is important not to confuse the more medial sternal head of the SCM with the clavicular head when palpating the lateral edge of this muscle, especially in obese patients. The jugular vein often crosses the lateral boarder of the SCM at the level of C6 (not the case in Fig. 46.6). At the level of C6, the lateral border of the SCM is gently palpated, and then fingers are moved just lateral to palpate the interscalene grove (between the anterior and middle scalene muscles). Initial needle placement is within the groove at the level of C6.

Stimulation blocks are typically performed with 22-gauge, 5-cm, insulated needles with the stimulator initially set at 1.0–1.2 mA (Fig. 46.7). References are available for the technique and clinical applications of peripheral nerve stimulation [19]. A muscle twitch of the deltoid, biceps, or triceps at 0.5 mA or less indicates adequate proximity of the needle tip to the plexus for local anesthetic injection [20]. In most adults, the brachial plexus is rarely deeper than 1–2 cm

below the skin. Trapezoid muscle stimulation suggests that the needle tip is posterior to the plexus while diaphragm stimulation indicates a needle tip that is too anterior. Local anesthetic volumes of 30–40 mL are sufficient to block the plexus in most adults. Modifications of the described interscalene method have been proposed to facilitate indwelling catheters [21], and posterior approaches have also been described [22]. Dagli et al. [23] compared the variations of the interscalene block and determined there was no reduction in complications and less satisfactory anesthesia compared to Winnie's classic approach.

Beginning with the last decade of the twentieth century, ultrasound technology has become a powerful tool to identify nerves and accurately place needles and local anesthetics. Preliminary data suggests that the addition of ultrasound to block procedures can improve success rates and decrease complications [15, 24, 25]. In some cases, ultrasound technology may be the only option available to place a regional anesthetic block when it is indicated [26]. A discussion on the physics and use of ultrasound is beyond the scope of this chapter though excellent references are available [27, 28]. The interscalene block is particularly well suited for ultrasound guidance due to the presence of good ultrasound landmarks and the superficial location of the brachial plexus at this level.

Preparation for an ultrasound-guided block is similar to a stimulation block. The use of external landmarks, when preparing for an ultrasound block, is no less important than when preparing for stimulation blocks. The external marks

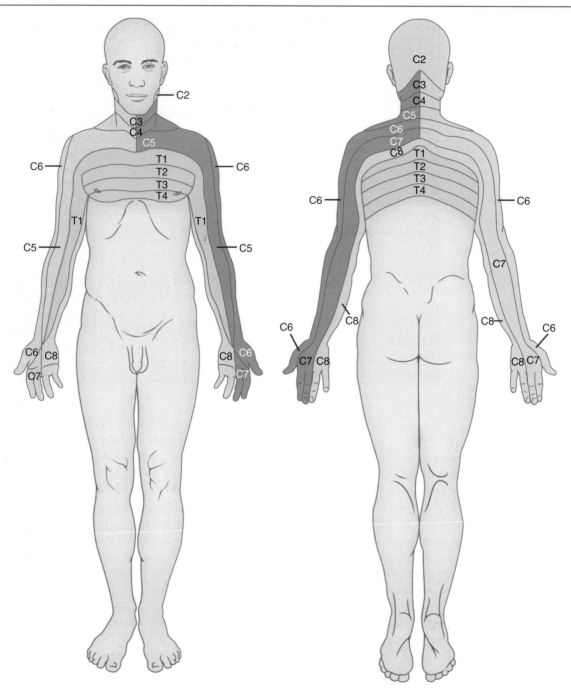

Fig. 46.5 Dermatomes anesthetized with the interscalene block (*dark blue*)

facilitate optimal ultrasound probe position and can reduce anatomy identification errors. The concurrent use of nerve stimulation with ultrasound can enhance block accuracy by providing objective evidence (motor nerve stimulation) that ultrasound-imaged targets are indeed nerves [29]. A high-frequency (5–12 MHz) linear probe is usually selected. Anatomical identification of the plexus at the C6 level is made easier if the probe is initially placed at the level of a supraclavicular block to identify the brachial plexus just lateral to the readily detectable subclavian artery. Once the plexus is located, it can be slowly traced cephalad to observe the three nerve trunks of the plexus as they pass between the middle and anterior scalene muscles (Fig. 46.8). The plexus is usually approached with the needle placed lateral within the plane of the ultrasound probe beam (Fig. 46.9). In-plane ultrasound-guided interscalene block allows real-time imaging of the needle in relation to target nerves and surrounding structures (Fig. 46.10). It also supports visualization of the local anesthetic injection allowing more accurate placement of medication around target nerves [30]. Many providers

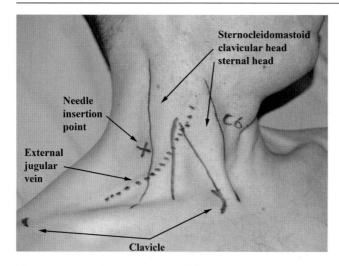

Fig. 46.6 External anatomy for interscalene block labeled (With permission from Buckenmaier and Bleckner [71])

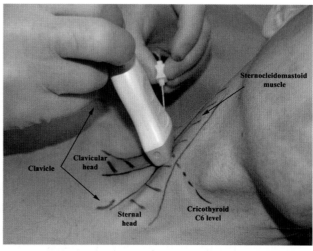

Fig. 46.9 Ultrasound-guided interscalene brachial plexus block (With permission from Buckenmaier and Bleckner [71])

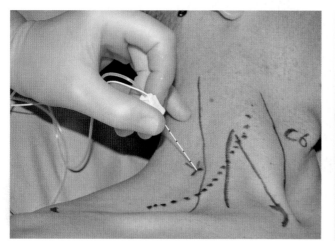

Fig. 46.7 Stimulating needle position for interscalene block (With permission from Buckenmaier and Bleckner [71])

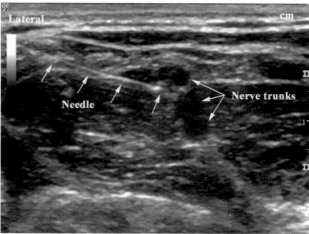

Fig. 46.10 In-plane needle placement during ultrasound-guided interscalene block (With permission from Buckenmaier and Bleckner [71])

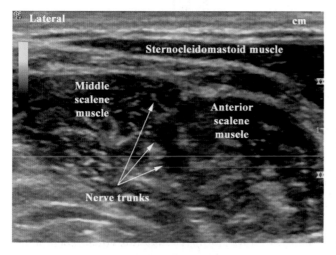

Fig. 46.8 Brachial plexus trunks at the level of C6 with ultrasound (With permission from Buckenmaier and Bleckner [71])

prefer out of plane needle placement when using ultrasound, though needle tip localization can be more difficult with this approach [31]. Practitioners often distribute local anesthetic to create the "donut sign" which is produced when hypoechoic local anesthetic surrounds the more echogenic nervous tissue. The most efficient block of the brachial plexus is produced when local anesthetic encircles the nerve structures. Authors have suggested that ultrasound guidance my also result in lower local anesthetic dosage requirements [32].

Supraclavicular Block of the Brachial Plexus

The supraclavicular approach, or subclavian perivascular technique [33], for blocking the brachial plexus is ideal for anesthesia and analgesia of the upper arm from the midhumeral level down to the hand (Fig. 46.11). If a tourniquet of the brachium

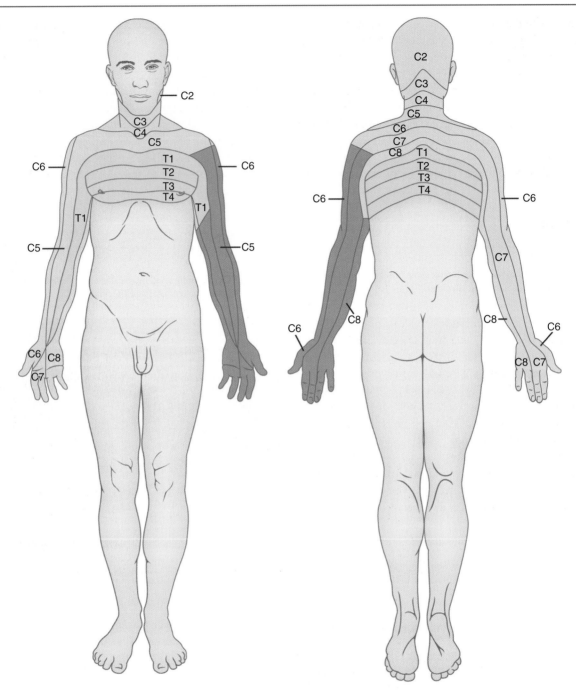

Fig. 46.11 Dermatomes anesthetized with the supraclavicular block (*dark blue*)

is planned for surgery, an intercostobrachial nerve block should be considered as a supplemental block. Anatomically, blockade of the brachial plexus just cephalad to the clavicle is facilitated by the compactness of the plexus trunks and divisions as these nerves pass under the midpoint of the clavicle. Packed together at this point, the brachial plexus is more easily surrounded by local anesthetic resulting in rapid block onset and high success rates. Franco et al. [34] determined that the unique supraclavicular anatomy of the brachial plexus allowed injection of local anesthetic during stimulation-assisted block at currents as high

as 0.9 mA rather than the typical 0.5 mA recommended for most stimulating blocks with no reduction in block success.

Unlike the interscalene approach which results in a 100 % incidence of hemidiaphragmatic paresis that can result in subjective symptoms of respiratory difficulty, the supraclavicular approach results in hemidiaphragmatic paresis only about 50 % of the time and is rarely associated with respiratory complaints [35]. At the level of the clavicle, the apex of the lung is just medial and posterior to the brachial plexus (deep to the first rib), so the complication most often associated with the supraclavicular block approach is pneumothorax. Using paresthesia techniques, authors in the 1960s described incidences of pneumothorax greater than 6 % [36]. For this reason, the technique fell out of favor until modern block technology and refinements in the approach reduced the incidence of this complication to less than 1 % [37–39]. Signs and symptoms of a large pneumothorax include sudden cough and shortness of breath. Should these symptoms manifest during the block procedure, the patient should undergo a chest X-ray prior to going to the operating room.

Procedure

The head of the supine patient is turned to the nonoperative side. External landmarks for the supraclavicular approach are similar to those used for the interscalene block (Fig. 46.12). The interscalene groove is palpated at the level of C6, and the fingers are then moved caudad within the groove to a point approximately 1 cm cephalad from the clavicle. This is the needle insertion point for stimulating blocks. The groove below C6 can sometimes be difficult to palpate due to the overlying omohyoid muscle. The subclavian arterial pulse is often palpable just medial to the needle insertion point by rolling the index finger over the top of the clavicle. This can be used as an additional confirmatory landmark.

Supraclavicular stimulation blocks are typically performed with 22-gauge, 5-cm, insulated needles with the stimulator initially set at 1.0–1.2 mA. The provider stands at the patients head and directs the needle toward the axilla

(Fig. 46.13). Proper needle placement in proximity to the brachial plexus is indicated by flexion or extension of the digits at 0.9–0.5 mA or less [34, 37]. Aspiration of blood or blood observed in the clear tubing suggests the needle tip is too medial and may have penetrated the subclavian artery. Persistent musculocutaneous nerve stimulation (biceps contractions) with needle advancement suggests too lateral a needle placement. Pectoralis muscle stimulation indicates anterior needle placement, and scapular stimulation suggests the needle is posterior to the brachial plexus. Local anesthetic volumes of 30–40 mL are usually injected to block the

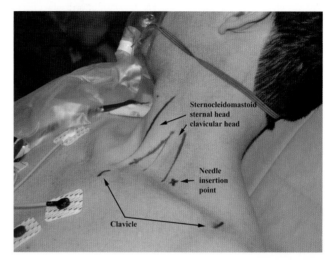

Fig. 46.12 External anatomy for the supraclavicular block labeled (With permission from Buckenmaier and Bleckner [71])

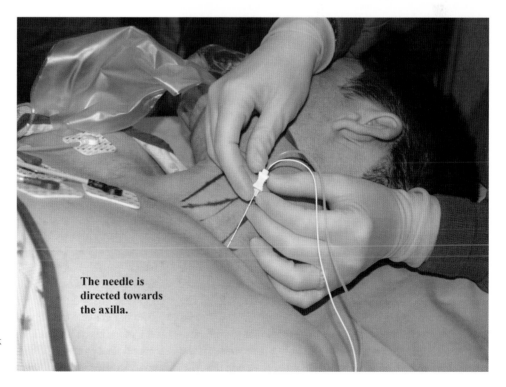

Fig. 46.13 Stimulating needle position for supraclavicular block (With permission from Buckenmaier and Bleckner [71])

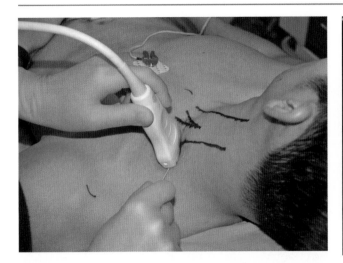

Fig. 46.14 Ultrasound-guided supraclavicular brachial plexus block (With permission from Buckenmaier and Bleckner [71])

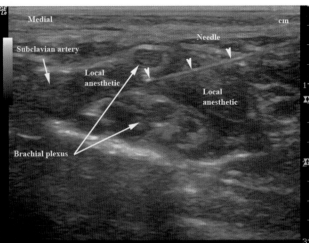

Fig. 46.16 In-plane needle placement for the supraclavicular block with ultrasound. Local anesthetic has been dynamically placed to surround the brachial plexus (With permission from Buckenmaier and Bleckner [71])

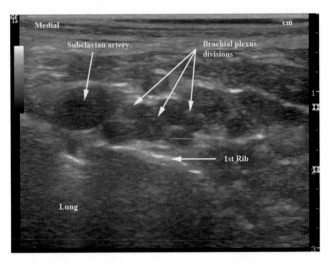

Fig. 46.15 Brachial plexus divisions in the supraclavicular fossa with ultrasound (With permission from Buckenmaier and Bleckner [71])

brachial plexus using this approach. Other stimulating supraclavicular block techniques have been described that purportedly reduce the risk of pneumothorax [40, 41].

Authors have suggested that the addition of ultrasound technology to the supraclavicular block has enhanced speed of block placement, improved block success, and provided superior anatomy identification compared to use of stimulation for the block [42, 43]. A high-frequency (5–12 MHz) linear probe is used for this block. The ultrasound probe is positioned directly above the clavicle in the supraclavicular fossa (Fig. 46.14). This plane gives the best transverse view of the brachial plexus, typically located lateral and slightly superior to the subclavian artery at a depth of 2–4 cm. The nerves appear as hypoechoic circles with hyperechoic rings that are sometimes described as a "bundle of grapes" (Fig. 46.15). The needle is inserted at the lateral end of the ultrasound probe and advanced under direct visualization of

the entire needle shaft down to the brachial plexus. It is very important to always keep the tip and shaft of the needle in clear view to ensure the needle is not being placed in areas that can result in pneumothorax or vascular puncture. The local anesthetic can be spread precisely by injecting small aliquots, observing spread, and adjusting the needle as necessary for complete envelopment of the brachial plexus (Fig. 46.16). Supraclavicular blocks can also be performed using out-of-plane approaches though there is no clinical data to support any particular out-of-plane technique [31].

Infraclavicular Block of the Brachial Plexus

The infraclavicular block of the brachial plexus is ideal for operations distal to the elbow (Fig. 46.17). In marked contrast to the quick onset of supraclavicular blocks placed with stimulation, infraclavicular blocks with stimulation take considerably longer to achieve the same level of block in most cases. This is explained by the less compact nature of the brachial plexus as it begins to spread around the axillary artery. The introduction of ultrasound-guided techniques that allow manipulation of anesthetic spread appears to have eliminated this difference between the two approaches [44, 45].

The infraclavicular block is performed at the level of the brachial plexus cords. The three cords – lateral, medial, and posterior – are named by their relation to the axillary artery at this level. When compared to the supraclavicular approach, local anesthetic injected for the infraclavicular block tends to remain below the clavicle, so clinical problems related to unintended block of the phrenic, recurrent laryngeal, or cervical sympathetic nerves do not tend to be issues [46]. The infraclavicular block is also associated with a lower incidence of pneumothorax [47].

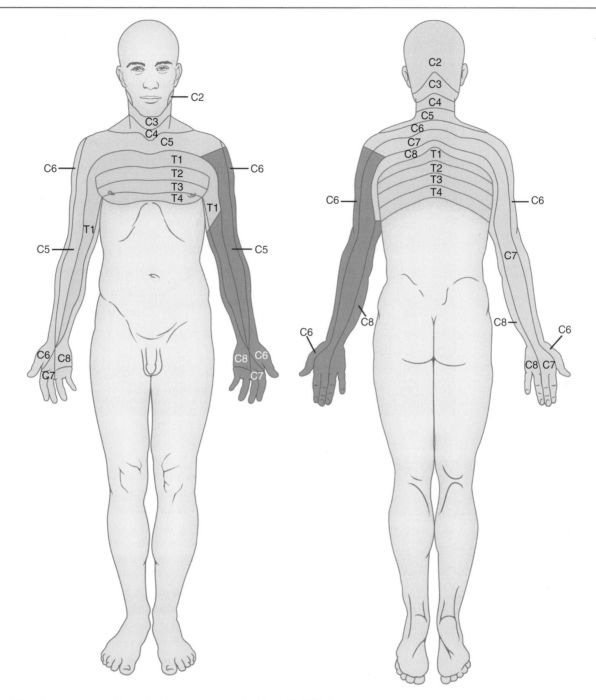

Fig. 46.17 Dermatomes anesthetized with the infraclavicular block (*dark blue*)

Excessive angulation of the block needle toward the axilla may result in inadequate blockade of the musculocutaneous and axillary nerves which can be a problem when stimulation is used.

Procedure

Multiple approaches to the brachial plexus from the infra-clavicular approach have been described [2, 47–49]. With the patient's arm externally rotated and abducted, the coracoid process can be palpated and a mark 2 cm medial and 2 cm caudal to the process is made for the initial needle position (Fig. 46.18). The axillary arterial pulse can be palpated in the axilla and is a useful landmark for aligning the needle with the brachial plexus as it passes into the brachium. A simple alternative to the coracoid landmark is the deltopectoral groove (Fig. 46.19). This approach does not necessitate manipulation of the patient's arm. The groove between the deltoid and pectoralis muscles is easily palpable in most patients. The needle is inserted

Fig. 46.18 External anatomy for
the infraclavicular nerve block
(With permission from
Buckenmaier and Bleckner [71])

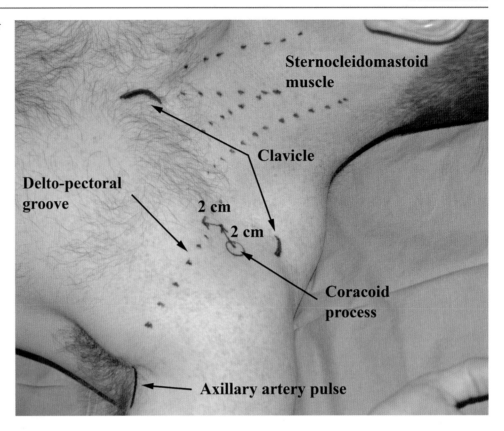

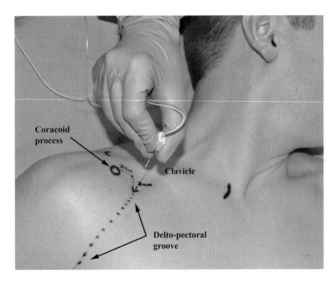

Fig. 46.19 Deltopectoral groove for the infraclavicular block (With
permission from Buckenmaier and Bleckner [71])

approximately 1 cm caudal to the clavicle within the
groove and directed deep toward the axilla.

Infraclavicular stimulation blocks are performed with
22-gauge, 10 cm, insulated needles with the stimulator initially
set at 1.0–1.2 mA. Stimulation of the posterior cord (extension
of the wrist/fingers) or stimulation of multiple cords simultaneously has been associated with high success rates for brachial
plexus block at this level using 30–40 mL of local anesthetic
[50]. Identification of which cord is being stimulated was elegantly described by Borene et al. [51] with their recognition
that the fifth digit (pinkie) moves "toward" the cord that is
being stimulated. With the arm positioned anatomically, lateral
cord stimulation will move the pinkie laterally (pronation of
the forearm), posterior cord posteriorly (extension), and medical cord medially (flexion). In most adults, 30–40 mL of local
anesthetic will block the plexus. As noted above, the latency of
this block can be long when stimulation alone is used.

As with other brachial plexus blocks, the introduction of
ultrasound technology has been suggested to improve the accuracy of local anesthetic injection, improve block success, and
decrease complication rates [52]. Though the preponderance
of evidence continues to support this hypothesis, large, controlled trials remain lacking, and the issue is controversial.

The linear, high-frequency (5–12 MHz) probe is again
selected for this approach. The needle is inserted in-plane at the
cephalad (lateral) aspect of the probe (Fig. 46.20). The primary
landmark for this block is the axillary artery. With the axillary
artery viewed in cross section, the cords of the plexus appear as
hyperechoic densities located lateral, medial, and posterior to
the artery (Fig. 46.21). The needle is inserted, under constant
visualization, to the posterior aspect of the axillary artery, and
local anesthetic is injected with the goal of surrounding the
artery with local. After the posterior portion of the artery is surrounded, it is often necessary to reposition the needle to the

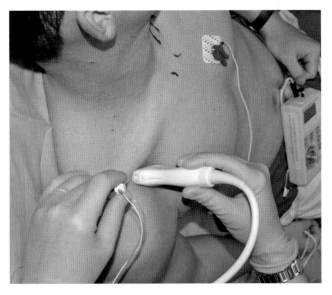

Fig. 46.20 Ultrasound-guided infraclavicular brachial plexus block (With permission from Buckenmaier and Bleckner [71])

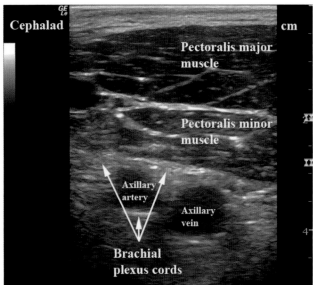

Fig. 46.21 Cords surrounding the axillary artery in the infraclavicular region (With permission from Buckenmaier and Bleckner [71])

anterior aspect of the artery to complete the injection. Care should be taken to ensure injected local anesthetic remains below the pectoralis muscle fascia, local injected above this plane will likely not contribute to the block. Furthermore, assiduous needle technique to maintain the needle under direct ultrasound view throughout the block to avoid vascular puncture is important to avert intravascular injection of local anesthetic or cause bleeding in this difficult to compress region of the body.

Axillary Block of the Brachial Plexus

The axillary block is the most distal block of the brachial plexus (Fig. 46.22). For a number of decades prior to widespread use of stimulation or ultrasound, the axillary block was considered the best block of the brachial plexus because it avoided the most feared complication of pneumothorax [53]. Considerable debate centered on the need to elicit needle paresthesias when performing the axillary block. Selander et al. [54] compared active paresthesia seeking blocks with blocks using only the arterial pulse as a landmark and noted a significant increase in postanesthetic nerve lesions in the paresthesia group prompting them to recommend avoidance of this paresthesia-seeking technique for nerve blocks. As nerve stimulation became more widely accepted, it was determined that paresthesia was related to motor responses using stimulation with currents less than 0.5 mA, which is the threshold current most often used today [55]. Paresthesia quickly fell out of general favor though providers continue to use the technique. Before the widespread availability of ultrasound, considerable debate surrounding the axillary brachial plexus block was common in the medical literature. Authors discussed virtues of single or multiple

injection techniques [56, 57] and transarterial [58, 59] and perivascular approaches [60]. Arguably, this debate was fueled by the negligible risks of respiratory compromise secondary to pneumothorax or phrenic nerve blockade that plagued other approaches. Notwithstanding this fact, the axillary brachial plexus block has the highest failure rate of the approaches discussed and was only appropriate for operations of the hand and forearm. As with other blocks of the brachial plexus, the advent of ultrasound technology has taken the "bite" out of much of this controversy with higher success levels and faster block onset being noted with ultrasound-guided axillary block [61, 62].

The anatomy of the brachial plexus at the level of the axilla explains why the block tends to enjoy less success compared to more proximal blocks. The plexus at this point has divided into the five individual nerves of the forearm that quickly diverge as they pass into the arm. The musculocutaneous nerve has already left the plexus at this level as it dives into the belly of the coracobrachialis muscle and must be blocked separately. Successful application of this block for surgery requires a clear understanding of surgical goals. Additionally, sufficient time must be incorporated into the analgesic plan to ensure all involved nerves are blocked or if some key nerves are spared, time is available for supplemental blocks.

Procedure

As noted, there are multiple approaches to the axillary block. The majority depend on the axillary arterial pulse as a landmark. The median, ulnar, and radial nerves can be anesthetized, as a group, with 30–40 mL of local anesthetic, with stimulation resulting in finger flexion and/or thumb opposition

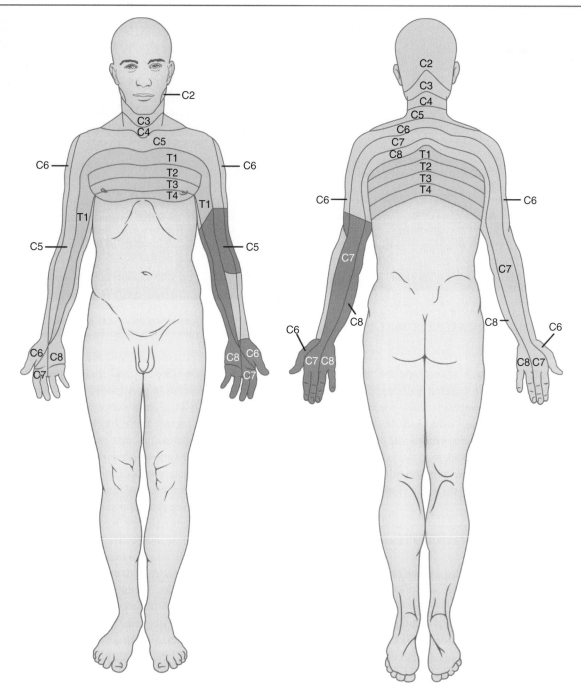

Fig. 46.22 The axillary block is the most distal block of the brachial plexus

at 0.5 mA or less. These nerves can also be individually stimulated and anesthetized, with both methods appearing equally successful. When using stimulation, it has been shown that actual stimulation of the musculocutaneous nerve, in addition to the nerves surrounding the axillary artery, is more successful than a simple injection into the coracobrachialis muscle [63]. It is important to note that local anesthetic spread within the axillary sheath may not consistently surround all the nerves within the compartment due to connective tissue barriers, positioning effects, or other factors [64]. Allowance for appropriate block

setup time and physical examination to determine block success is essential to avoid failed blocks in the operating room. Evidence suggests the application of ultrasound visualization can mitigate the majority of these anatomical issues that can complicate axillary stimulation blocks [65].

The patient is positioned supine with the operative arm abducted and externally rotated (Fig. 46.23). The axillary arterial pulse is palpated proximal in the axilla, and the needle is inserted superior to the axillary artery at a 45° angle (Fig. 46.24). The coracobrachialis muscle for the musculocutaneous block

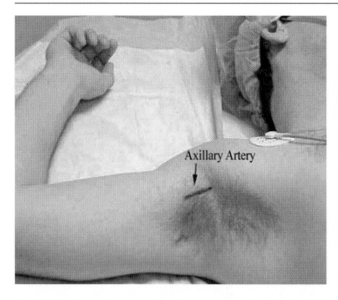

Fig. 46.23 External anatomy for axillary brachial plexus block (With permission from Buckenmaier and Bleckner [71])

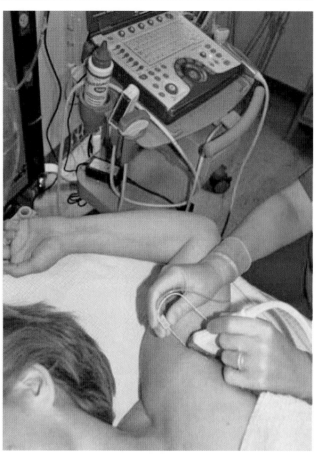

Fig. 46.25 Ultrasound-guided axillary brachial plexus block (With permission from Buckenmaier and Bleckner [71])

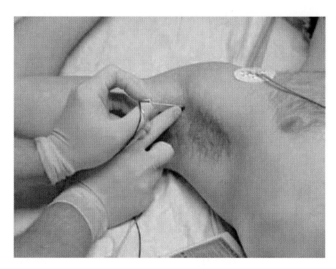

Fig. 46.24 Stimulating needle for axillary brachial plexus block (With permission from Buckenmaier and Bleckner [71])

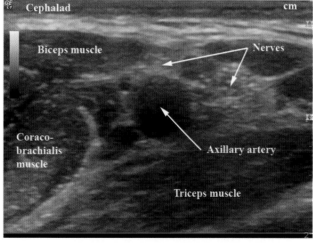

Fig. 46.26 Ultrasound view of the brachial plexus in the axilla (With permission from Buckenmaier and Bleckner [71])

is identified by displacing the biceps muscle laterally while the coracobrachialis muscle is palpable just medical to the biceps. A 22-gauge, 5 cm, insulated needle is used with the stimulator initially set at 1.0–1.2 mA.

For the ultrasound-guided axillary block, the patient is positioned the same as for stimulation. The high-frequency (5–12 MHz) linear probe and a 5-cm, 22-gauge needle are also used. The probe is placed high in the axilla, and the needle is directed from the cephalad end of the probe, in-plane (Fig. 46.25). Typical anatomical relations of the nerve to the axillary artery are as follows: the median nerve is located superficial and slightly cephalad to the artery, the radial nerve is located deep to the artery, and the ulnar nerve is located caudad to the artery (Fig. 46.26). Ultrasound allows dynamic injection of local anesthetic around the axillary artery to ensure adequate nerve exposure to the medication (Fig. 46.27). The musculocutaneous nerve can also be visualized within

Fig. 46.27 Ultrasound needle placement for axillary brachial plexus block (With permission from Buckenmaier and Bleckner [71])

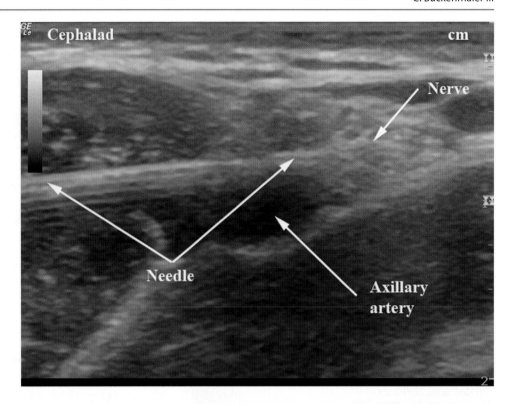

the substance of the coracobrachialis muscle and blocked separately under direct ultrasound visualization (Fig. 46.28). Once identified, 10 mL of local anesthetic is usually sufficient to block the musculocutaneous nerve.

Continuous Peripheral Nerve Block

All of the approaches to the brachial plexus are suitable for placement of continuous peripheral nerve block (CPNB) catheters. CPNB techniques provide superior analgesia compared to opioids [66, 67], have relatively few serious complications [68], maintain analgesia long after the trauma or surgical event [69], and can be used safely in the ambulatory patient population [70]. Approaches for placing needles for CPNB are the same as single injection blocks described above. A complete discussion on the placement of CPNB catheters is beyond the scope of this chapter, but technical aspects pertaining to CPNB catheters are available for download at Defense and Veterans Pain Management Initiative website (www.dvpmi.org/maraa-book-project.html) [71].

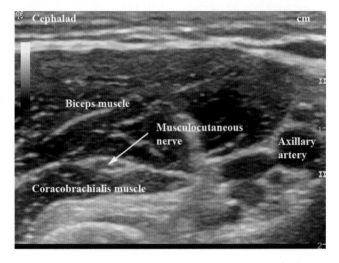

Fig. 46.28 Ultrasound anatomy of the musculocutaneous nerve (With permission from Buckenmaier and Bleckner [71])

Conclusion

Modern advances in needle, stimulator, and ultrasound technology have greatly enhanced the efficiency and safety of placing needles in proximity to the brachial plexus for anesthesia and analgesia. The ability to provide consistent and complete blockade of the brachial plexus has revolutionized

many operations of the upper extremity and enhanced recovery and rehabilitation from countless surgical procedures and traumatic events. Perhaps, one of the best examples of the advantages of regional anesthesia exists currently on the modern battlefield where the pain of traumatic extremity wounds is eased daily through the application of the techniques described here [72]. The clinical study of the anatomy and techniques for brachial plexus block is truly worth the clinician's effort and attention.

References

1. Winnie AP. Plexus anesthesia: perivascular techniques of brachial plexus block. Philadelphia: W.B. Saunders Co; 1993.
2. Raj PP. Infraclavicular approaches to brachial plexus anesthesia. Tech Reg Anesth Pain Manag. 1997;1:169–77.
3. Greengrass RA. Regional anesthesia for ambulatory surgery. Anesthesiol Clin North America. 2000;18:341–53, vii.
4. Exadaktylos AK, Buggy DJ, Moriarty DC, Mascha E, Sessler DI. Can anesthetic technique for primary breast cancer surgery affect recurrence or metastasis? Anesthesiology. 2006;105:660–4.
5. Gerancher JC. Upper extremity nerve blocks. Anesthesiol Clin North America. 2000;18:297–317.
6. Fazan VPS, Amadeu AS, Caleffi AL, Filho OAR. Brachial plexus variations in its formation and main branches. Acta Cir Bras. 2003;18:14–8.
7. Uysal II, Seker M, Karabulut AK, Buyukmumcu M, Ziylan T. Brachial plexus variations in human fetuses. Neurosurgery. 2003;53:676–84.
8. Moore KL, Dalley AF. Upper limb, clinically oriented anatomy. 5th ed. Philadelphia: Lippincott Williams & Wilkins; 2006. p. 725–884.
9. Harry WG, Bennett JD, Guha SC. Scalene muscles and the brachial plexus: anatomical variations and their clinical significance. Clin Anat. 1997;10:250–2.
10. Neal JM, Hebl JR, Gerancher JC, Hogan QH. Brachial plexus anesthesia: essentials of our current understanding. Reg Anesth Pain Med. 2002;27:402–28.
11. Thompson GE, Rorie DK. Functional anatomy of the brachial plexus sheaths. Anesthesiology. 1983;59:117–22.
12. Cornish PB, Leaper C. The sheath of the brachial plexus: fact or fiction? Anesthesiology. 2006;105:563–5.
13. Franco CD, Rahman A, Voronov G, Kerns JM, Beck RJ, Buckenmaier III CC. Gross anatomy of the brachial plexus sheath in human cadavers. Reg Anesth Pain Med. 2008;33:64–9.
14. Winnie AP, Radonjic R, Akkineni SR, Durrani Z. Factors influencing distribution of local anesthetic injected into the brachial plexus sheath. Anesth Analg. 1979;58:225–34.
15. Marhofer P, Chan VW. Ultrasound-guided regional anesthesia: current concepts and future trends. Anesth Analg. 2007;104:1265–9.
16. Winnie AP. Interscalene brachial plexus block. Anesth Analg. 1970;49:455–66.
17. Seltzer JL. Hoarseness and Horner's syndrome after interscalene brachial plexus block. Anesth Analg. 1977;56:585–6.
18. Tuominen MK, Pere P, Rosenberg PH. Unintentional arterial catheterization and bupivacaine toxicity associated with continuous interscalene brachial plexus block. Anesthesiology. 1991;75:356–8.
19. De AJ, Sala-Blanch X. Peripheral nerve stimulation in the practice of brachial plexus anesthesia: a review. Reg Anesth Pain Med. 2001;26:478–83.
20. Silverstein WB, Saiyed MU, Brown AR. Interscalene block with a nerve stimulator: a deltoid motor response is a satisfactory endpoint for successful block. Reg Anesth Pain Med. 2000;25:356–9.
21. Boezaart AP, de Beer JF, Du Toit C, van Rooyen K. A new technique of continuous interscalene nerve block. Can J Anaesth. 1999;46:275–81.
22. Rucci FS, Pippa P, Barbagli R, Doni L. How many interscalenic blocks are there? A comparison between the lateral and posterior approach. Eur J Anaesth. 1993;10:303–7.
23. Dagli G, Guzeldemir ME, Volkan AH. The effects and side effects of interscalene brachial plexus block by posterior approach. Reg Anesth Pain Med. 1998;23:87–91.
24. Denny NM, Harrop-Griffiths W. Location, location, location! Ultrasound imaging in regional anaesthesia. Br J Anaesth. 2005;94:1–3.
25. Marhofer P, Greher M, Kapral S. Ultrasound guidance in regional anaesthesia. Br J Anaesth. 2005;94:7–17.
26. Plunkett AR, Brown DS, Rogers JM, Buckenmaier III CC. Supraclavicular continuous peripheral nerve block in a wounded soldier: when ultrasound is the only option. Br J Anaesth. 2006;97:715–7.
27. Sites BD, Brull R, Chan VW, Spence BC, Gallagher J, Beach ML, Sites VR, Abbas S, Hartman GS. Artifacts and pitfall errors associated with ultrasound-guided regional anesthesia. Part II: a pictorial approach to understanding and avoidance. Reg Anesth Pain Med. 2007;32:419–33.
28. Sites BD, Brull R, Chan VW, Spence BC, Gallagher J, Beach ML, Sites VR, Hartman GS. Artifacts and pitfall errors associated with ultrasound-guided regional anesthesia. Part I: understanding the basic principles of ultrasound physics and machine operations. Reg Anesth Pain Med. 2007;32:412–8.
29. Peterson MK, Millar FA, Sheppard DG. Ultrasound-guided nerve blocks. Br J Anaesth. 2002;88:621–4.
30. Chan VW. Applying ultrasound imaging to interscalene brachial plexus block. Reg Anesth Pain Med. 2003;28:340–3.
31. Chin KJ, Perlas A, Chan VW, Brull R. Needle visualization in ultrasound-guided regional anesthesia: challenges and solutions. Reg Anesth Pain Med. 2008;33:532–44.
32. Eichenberger U, Stockli S, Marhofer P, Huber G, Willimann P, Kettner SC, Pleiner J, Curatolo M, Kapral S. Minimal local anesthetic volume for peripheral nerve block: a new ultrasound-guided, nerve dimension-based method. Reg Anesth Pain Med. 2009;34:242–6.
33. Winnie AP, Collins VJ. The subclavian perivascular technique of brachial plexus anesthesia. Anesthesiology. 1964;25:353–63.
34. Franco CD, Domashevich V, Voronov G, Rafizad AB, Jelev TJ. The supraclavicular block with a nerve stimulator: to decrease or not to decrease, that is the question. Anesth Analg. 2004;98:1167–71.
35. Neal JM, Moore JM, Kopacz DJ, Liu SS, Kramer DJ, Plorde JJ. Quantitative analysis of respiratory, motor, and sensory function after supraclavicular block. Anesth Analg. 1998;86:1239–44.
36. Brand L, Papper E. A comparison of supraclavicular and axillary techniques for brachial plexus blocks. Anesthesiology. 1961;22:226–9.
37. Franco CD, Vieira ZE. 1,001 subclavian perivascular brachial plexus blocks: success with a nerve stimulator. Reg Anesth Pain Med. 2000;25:41–6.
38. Franco CD, Gloss FJ, Voronov G, Tyler SG, Stojiljkovic LS. Supraclavicular block in the obese population: an analysis of 2020 blocks. Anesth Analg. 2006;102:1252–4.
39. Nielsen KC, Guller U, Steele SM, Klein SM, Greengrass RA, Pietrobon R. Influence of obesity on surgical regional anesthesia in the ambulatory setting: an analysis of 9,038 blocks. Anesthesiology. 2005;102:181–7.
40. Brown DL, Cahill DR, Bridenbaugh LD. Supraclavicular nerve block: anatomic analysis of a method to prevent pneumothorax. Anesth Analg. 1993;76:530–4.
41. Pham-Dang C, Gunst JP, Gouin F, Poirier P, Touchais S, Meunier JF, Kick O, Drouet JC, Bourreli B, Pinaud M. A novel supraclavicular approach to brachial plexus block. Anesth Analg. 1997;85:111–6.
42. Chan VW, Perlas A, Rawson R, Odukoya O. Ultrasound-guided supraclavicular brachial plexus block. Anesth Analg. 2003;97:1514–7.
43. Williams SR, Chouinard P, Arcand G, Harris P, Ruel M, Boudreault D, Girard F. Ultrasound guidance speeds execution and improves the quality of supraclavicular block. Anesth Analg. 2003;97:1518–23.
44. Arcand G, Williams SR, Chouinard P, Boudreault D, Harris P, Ruel M, Girard F. Ultrasound-guided infraclavicular versus supraclavicular block. Anesth Analg. 2005;101:886–90.

45. Koscielniak-Nielsen ZJ, Frederiksen BS, Rasmussen H, Hesselbjerg L. A comparison of ultrasound-guided supraclavicular and infraclavicular blocks for upper extremity surgery. Acta Anaesthesiol Scand. 2009;53:620–6.

46. Rodriguez J, Barcena M, Alvarez J. Restricted infraclavicular distribution of the local anesthetic solution after infraclavicular brachial plexus block. Reg Anesth Pain Med. 2003;28:33–6.

47. Borgeat A, Ekatodramis G, Dumont C. An evaluation of the infraclavicular block via a modified approach of the Raj technique. Anesth Analg. 2001;93:436–41, 4th.

48. Kapral S, Jandrasits O, Schabernig C, Likar R, Reddy B, Mayer N, Weinstabl C. Lateral infraclavicular plexus block vs. axillary block for hand and forearm surgery. Acta Anaesthesiol Scand. 1999;43: 1047–52.

49. Raj PP, Montgomery SJ, Nettles D, Jenkins MT. Infraclavicular brachial plexus block – a new approach. Anesth Analg. 1973;52:897–904.

50. Lecamwasam H, Mayfield J, Rosow L, Chang Y, Carter C, Rosow C. Stimulation of the posterior cord predicts successful infraclavicular block. Anesth Analg. 2006;102:1564–8.

51. Borene SC, Edwards JN, Boezaart AP. At the cords, the pinkie towards: interpreting infraclavicular motor responses to neurostimulation. Reg Anesth Pain Med. 2004;29:125–9.

52. Sandhu NS, Capan LM. Ultrasound-guided infraclavicular brachial plexus block. Br J Anaesth. 2002;89:254–9.

53. De Jong RH. Axillary block of the brachial plexus. Anesthesiology. 1961;22:215–25.

54. Selander D, Edshage S, Wolff T. Paresthesia or no paresthesia? Nerve lesions after axillary blocks. Acta Anaesthesiol Scand. 1979;23:27–33.

55. Choyce A, Chan VW, Middleton WJ, Knight PR, Peng P, McCartney CJ. What is the relationship between paresthesia and nerve stimulation for axillary brachial plexus block? Reg Anesth Pain Med. 2001;26:100–4.

56. Koscielniak-Nielsen ZJ, Stens-Pedersen HL, Lippert FK. Readiness for surgery after axillary block: single or multiple injection techniques. Eur J Anaesthesiol. 1997;14:164–71.

57. Lavoie J, Martin R, Tetrault JP, Cote DJ, Colas MJ. Axillary plexus block using a peripheral nerve stimulator: single or multiple injections. Can J Anaesth. 1992;39:583–6.

58. Koscielniak-Nielsen ZJ, Nielsen PR, Nielsen SL, Gardi T, Hermann C. Comparison of transarterial and multiple nerve stimulation techniques for axillary block using a high dose of mepivacaine with adrenaline. Acta Anaesthesiol Scand. 1999;43:398–404.

59. Winnie AP. Does the transarterial technique of axillary block provide a higher success rate and a lower complication rate than a paresthesia technique? New evidence and old. Reg Anesth. 1995;20:482–5.

60. Pere P, Pitkanen M, Tuominen M, Edgren J, Rosenberg PH. Clinical and radiological comparison of perivascular and transarterial techniques of axillary brachial plexus block. Br J Anaesth. 1993;70: 276–9.

61. Chan VW, Perlas A, McCartney CJ, Brull R, Xu D, Abbas S. Ultrasound guidance improves success rate of axillary brachial plexus block. Can J Anaesth. 2007;54:176–82.

62. Casati A, Danelli G, Baciarello M, Corradi M, Leone S, Di CS, Fanelli G. A prospective, randomized comparison between ultrasound and nerve stimulation guidance for multiple injection axillary brachial plexus block. Anesthesiology. 2007;106:992–6.

63. Coventry DM, Barker KF, Thomson M. Comparison of two neurostimulation techniques for axillary brachial plexus blockade. Br J Anaesth. 2001;86:80–3.

64. Vester-Andersen T, Broby-Johansen U, Bro-Rasmussen F. Perivascular axillary block VI: the distribution of gelatine solution injected into the axillary neurovascular sheath of cadavers. Acta Anaesthesiol Scand. 1986;30:18–22.

65. Perlas A, Chan VW, Simons M. Brachial plexus examination and localization using ultrasound and electrical stimulation: a volunteer study. Anesthesiology. 2003;99:429–35.

66. Richman JM, Liu SS, Courpas G, Wong R, Rowlingson AJ, McGready J, Cohen SR, Wu CL. Does continuous peripheral nerve block provide superior pain control to opioids? A meta-analysis. Anesth Analg. 2006;102:248–57.

67. Buckenmaier III CC, Rupprecht C, McKnight G, McMillan B, White RL, Gallagher RM, Polomano R. Pain following battlefield injury and evacuation: a survey of 110 casualties from the wars in Iraq and Afghanistan. Pain Med. 2009;10:1487–96.

68. Shinaman RC, Mackey S. Continuous peripheral nerve blocks. Curr Pain Headache Rep. 2005;9:24–9.

69. Stojadinovic A, Auton A, Peoples GE, McKnight GM, Shields C, Croll SM, Bleckner LL, Winkley J, Maniscalco-Theberge ME, Buckenmaier III CC. Responding to challenges in modern combat casualty care: innovative use of advanced regional anesthesia. Pain Med. 2006;7:330–8.

70. Grant SA, Nielsen KC, Greengrass RA, Steele SM, Klein SM. Continuous peripheral nerve block for ambulatory surgery. Reg Anesth Pain Med. 2001;26:209–14.

71. Buckenmaier III CC, Bleckner L. Continuous Peripheral Nerve Block. In: Buckenmaier III CC, Bleckner L, editors. Military advanced regional anesthesia and analgesia. Washington DC: Borden Institute; 2009. p. 83–90.

72. Buckenmaier III CC, Brandon-Edwards H, Borden Jr D, Wright J. Treating pain on the battlefield: a warrior's perspective. Curr Pain Headache Rep. 2010;14:1–7.

Suprascapular Nerve Block

47

Brian Belnap and Gagan Mahajan

Key Points

- The suprascapular nerve, due to its superficial location in the supraspinous fossa, is a readily accessible nerve that is easy and safe to block.
- The suprascapular nerve block (SSNB) can be a useful tool in the management of a variety of acute and chronic shoulder pain conditions.
- There is evidence that a SSNB may be effective in certain chronic shoulder conditions, e.g., glenohumeral degenerative joint disease, adhesive capsulitis, and rotator cuff degenerative tears.
- While the SSNB has been traditionally performed based on anatomic landmarks, imaging guidance utilizing fluoroscopy, CT, and ultrasound has been described.
- The suprascapular nerve block is a safe and effective procedure and should be considered in the management of postoperative pain following shoulder arthroscopy, scapular fractures, adhesive capsulitis, rotator cuff degenerative tears, and glenohumeral arthritis.

B. Belnap, DO (✉)
Department of Anesthesiology and Pain Medicine,
University of California Davis Medical Center,
Sacramento, CA, USA

3907 Waring Rd Suite #2, Oceanside, CA 92056, USA
e-mail: belnap2@gmail.com

G. Mahajan, M.D.
Department of Anesthesiology and Pain Medicine,
University of California, Davis School of Medicine,
4860 Y Street, Suite 3020, Sacramento, CA 95817, USA
e-mail: gmahajan@ucdavis.edu

Introduction and Historical Background

The suprascapular nerve, due to its superficial location in the supraspinous fossa, is a readily accessible nerve that is easy and safe to block [1–12]. The suprascapular nerve block (SSNB) has been utilized for well over 60 years to address various causes of shoulder pain. Early advocates of the SSNB reported its usefulness in treating shoulder pain secondary to rotator cuff degenerative tears [13]. Subsequent studies expanded its indications to include conditions such as glenohumeral degenerative joint disease, adhesive capsulitis, and postoperative shoulder pain following arthroscopic surgery [2, 4–11, 14–20]. The technique of the SSNB has evolved over the years. Early reports favored blocking the suprascapular nerve at the suprascapular notch; however, more recent advocates suggest blocking the nerve at the supraspinous fossa to minimize the risk of major complications.

Clinical Applications

The SSNB can be a useful tool in the management of a variety of acute and chronic shoulder pain conditions. For acute shoulder pain, reports have primarily described its use in postoperative pain management following arthroscopic shoulder surgery and shoulder dislocations [2, 6–8, 16, 18]. Ritchie and colleagues performed a prospective, double-blind, randomized controlled trial on 50 patients, half of whom received the SSNB and the other half a placebo injection of saline just prior to shoulder arthroscopy [2]. Both groups were given patient-controlled analgesic systems postoperatively. Compared to the placebo group, in the immediate postoperative period, the SSNB group demonstrated a 51 % reduction in demand and 31 % reduction in morphine use, a reduction in visual analog and verbal pain scores, and a more than fivefold reduction in the incidence of nausea. At 24-h follow-up, the SSNB group had a 40 % reduction in analgesic consumption and a reduction in verbal pain scores at rest and with abduction. Singelyn and colleagues performed a prospective, randomized placebo-controlled trial with 120 patients scheduled for elective arthroscopic shoulder acromioplasty and divided the patients into four groups: placebo, SSNB, interscalene brachial plexus block, and intra-articular shoulder injection with local anesthetic. Patients in the SSNB and interscalene brachial plexus block groups were found to have equally and significantly lower pain scores immediately after surgery when compared to placebo and intra-articular shoulder injection, but at 4-h follow-up, patients in the interscalene brachial plexus block group were found to have better pain relief and higher satisfaction scores when compared to all groups. The authors concluded that while the interscalene brachial plexus block was superior, the SSNB was an acceptable alternative in patients considered to be at higher risk for complications from the interscalene brachial plexus block, such as those with chronic obstructive pulmonary disease [18]. One retrospective review of 20 patients who received a SSNB combined with an axillary nerve block prior to arthroscopic shoulder surgery reported excellent results [8]. None of the patients required general anesthesia, opioids, or analgesics during the surgery. Fifteen of the 20 patients required NSAIDs for mild to moderate postoperative pain, but none required opioids. All were discharged the same day and were able to start physical therapy the following day. Randomized controlled trials are needed to confirm the effectiveness of the combined blocks.

One case report suggested that a SSNB may be helpful in addressing pain control for fractures of the scapula, but there were mixed results from case reports as to the effectiveness of the SSNB during reduction from an anterior shoulder joint dislocation [21–23]. A SSNB was not found to be helpful in treating shoulder tip pain following laparoscopic surgery or shoulder pain following thoracotomy, as both are considered to be referred pain to the shoulder [24, 25].

There is evidence that a SSNB may be effective in certain chronic shoulder conditions, e.g., glenohumeral degenerative joint disease, adhesive capsulitis, and rotator cuff degenerative tears [4, 5, 9–11, 14, 15, 17, 19, 23]. Shanahan et al. performed a randomized, double-blind, placebo-controlled trial evaluating 108 shoulders with chronic shoulder pain of at least 3-month duration due to osteoarthritis or rheumatoid arthritis. The SSNB group received 10 ml of 0.5 % bupivacaine and 40 mg of methylprednisolone, while the control group received 5 ml of saline infiltrated subcutaneously, well away from the suprascapular nerve [5]. Using the Shoulder Pain and Disability Index (SPADI), the authors evaluated the patients at 1, 4, and 12 weeks following the procedure. At week one, 67 % of the shoulders in the SSNB group showed at least a ten-point improvement on the overall SPADI score compared with 23 % in the control group. At week four, SPADI scores improved by 66 and 11 % in the SSNB and control groups, respectively. At week 12, SPADI scores improved by 55 and 18 % in the SSNB and control groups, respectively.

Gado and Emery conducted a double-blind study in 26 patients (52 shoulders) with bilateral rheumatoid arthritis, comparing the outcomes of a SSNB with 2 ml of bupivacaine 0.5 % on one side with 2 ml of bupivacaine 0.5 % plus 1 ml (40 mg) of methylprednisolone on the other side [19]. Significant improvements were made with both treatments in regards to pain, stiffness, and range of motion, but overall results favored the bupivacaine-only treatment. Thus, the inclusion of steroid offered no additional benefit.

The SSNB may have some usefulness in treating adhesive capsulitis [3, 4, 14]. Dahan et al. conducted a double-blind, placebo-controlled study on 34 patients with adhesive capsulitis for at least 4 weeks [4]. Patients received a series of three SSNBs at 7-day intervals with either 10 ml of 0.5 % bupivacaine or 10 ml of saline. Two weeks after the final injection, there was a 64 and 13 % reduction in pain (as measured by the McGill-Melzack Pain Questionnaire) for the treatment and control group, respectively. However, there was no statistically significant difference in shoulder range of motion. Jones et al. performed a randomized trial of 30 patients with chronic adhesive capsulitis and compared SSNB using 9.5 ml of 0.5 % bupivacaine and 20 mg triamcinolone with glenohumeral intra-articular joint injection using 20 mg triamcinolone and 4.5 ml of 2 % lidocaine [3]. Doing a SSNB one time was found to produce a faster and more complete resolution of pain and restoration of range of motion than a series of glenohumeral intra-articular injections.

Di Lorenzo et al. performed a prospective, randomized, crossover study on 40 patients who had chronic shoulder pain secondary to rotator cuff tear. Patients were randomized to receive physical therapy alone followed by physical therapy plus SSNB with 10 ml of 1 % lidocaine [17]. Patients who received a SSNB plus physical therapy had decreased severity and frequency of perceived pain, improved compliance with physical therapy, more normal sleep patterns, and increased compliance with their rehabilitation program in comparison to those who received physical therapy alone. Other studies that included chronic shoulder pain from multiple etiologies in their treatment groups also showed benefit from utilizing a SSNB [9, 11, 15, 26].

A few case series reported efficacy using pulsed mode radiofrequency of the suprascapular nerve in the treatment of chronic shoulder pain [27–29]. In their study of 13 shoulders with chronic pain of 3-month duration or longer, Liliang et al. showed that pulsed radiofrequency (38–42 °C and 45 V for 180 s) of the suprascapular nerve effectively treated chronic shoulder pain [28]. At 1- and 6-month follow-up, 76 and 69 % still had >50 % pain relief, respectively. Furthermore, mean SPADI scores at a 6-month follow-up showed a significant decrease along with 82 % of patients decreasing their pain medication requirements. Randomized controlled trials are needed to confirm these and other preliminary findings.

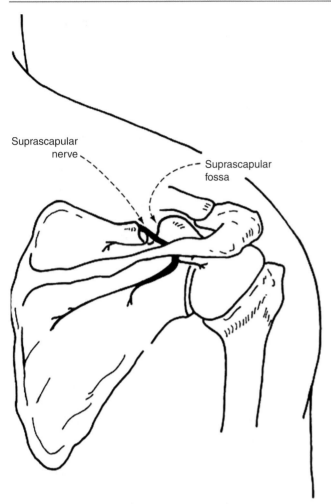

Fig. 47.1 Anatomy of the suprascapular nerve (From Waldman [31], with permission)

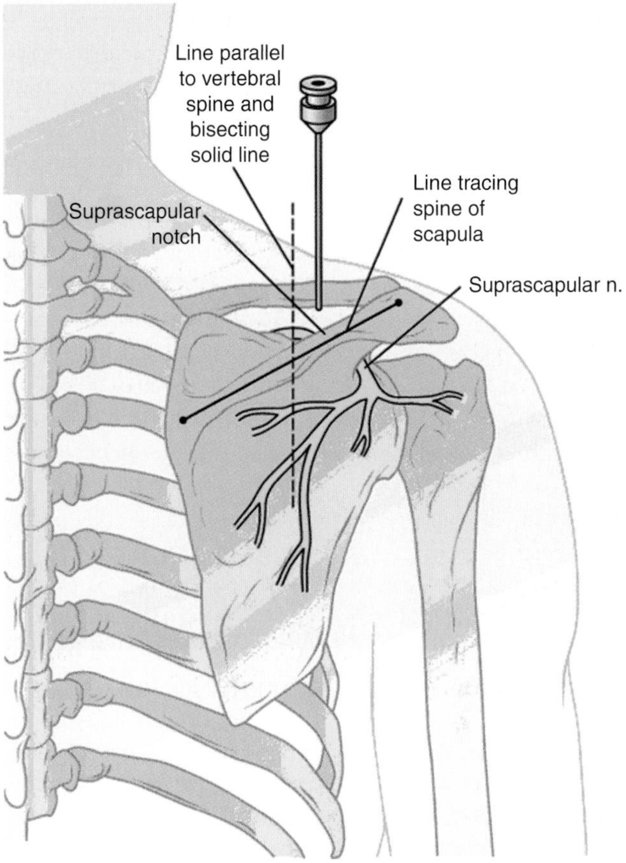

Fig. 47.2 Suprascapular nerve block. A *line* is drawn along the scapular spine and then bisected by a *second line* parallel to the vertebral spine. The entry point is 2–3 cm into the upper outer quadrant. The needle is directed from the top to avoid deep entry into the suprascapular notch, which could risk pneumothorax (From Rathmell et al. [35], with permission)

Suprascapular Nerve Anatomy

The suprascapular nerve originates from the upper trunk of the brachial plexus with major contributing fibers from the C5 and C6 nerve roots [11, 17, 30]. It travels posteriorly and laterally toward the supraspinous fossa and enters via the suprascapular notch (Fig. 47.1). Once it reaches the notch, it travels inferior to the superior transverse scapular ligament and laterally toward the base of the coracoid process where it splits into sensory and motor fibers. The motor fibers supply the supraspinatus muscle and then curve around the spinoglenoid notch to terminate in the infraspinatus muscle. The sensory fibers supply the acromioclavicular and glenohumeral joint capsules and the conoid, trapezoid, and coracoacromial ligaments. It is generally well accepted that the supraspinatus nerve provides approximately 70 % sensory innervation to the shoulder joint [11, 30].

Suprascapular Nerve Block Technique

The technique of the SSNB can be performed utilizing either a direct or indirect technique. The direct technique involves blocking the suprascapular nerve at the suprascapular notch, just as the nerve enters the supraspinous fossa [1, 21, 32–34]. The patient is placed in a seated position with the hands resting on the thighs. A line is drawn along the scapular spine from the tip of the acromion to the medial border of the scapula. After identifying the inferior angle of the scapula, a second line bisecting this angle is drawn and extended upward as far as the superior border of the scapula, intersecting the line drawn along the scapular spine and forming four quadrants (Fig. 47.2). The angle of the upper outer quadrant is bisected, and a point is marked on the line 1.5 cm from the apex of the angle. After the area is prepped and draped, the needle is advanced perpendicularly until the scapula is contacted and then redirected until it slides into the suprascapular

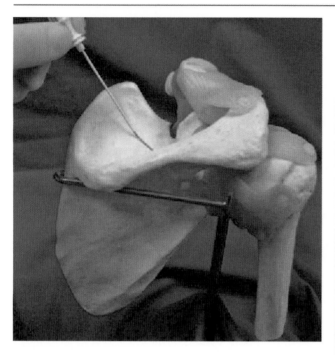

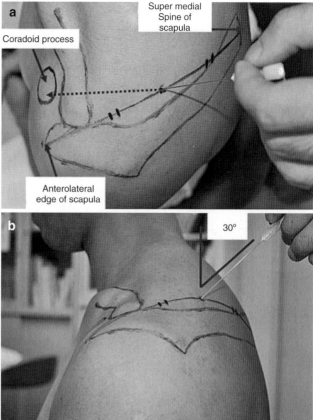

Fig. 47.3 The Meier technique (From Meier et al. [9], with permission)

notch. At this point, the needle is slightly withdrawn, aspiration is performed to rule out intravascular location, and local anesthetic is injected [1, 14]. Some authors describe utilizing a nerve stimulator to visually confirm contraction of the supraspinatus and infraspinatus muscles to verify proximity to the suprascapular nerve prior to placing the injectate. Keratas and Meray utilized EMG guidance with the direct technique to confirm proximity to the suprascapular nerve and reported superior results to traditional methods [14]. While the theoretical advantage of the direct technique includes placing the injectate immediately next to the suprascapular nerve as it emerges from the suprascapular notch, there is a slight increased risk of pneumothorax.

In more recent years, some investigators have advocated various versions of an indirect technique that involves placing the needle away from the suprascapular notch to avoid the risk of pneumothorax [36]. Dangiosse et al. described blocking the suprascapular nerve by injecting the local anesthetic into the floor of the suprascapular fossa [11]. The needle is introduced into the fossa 1 cm cephalad to the middle of the spine of the scapula, parallel to the blade, and until the bony floor of the supraspinous fossa is reached. Meier et al. described another variance to the indirect technique by drawing a line from the medial end of the spine of the scapula to the lateral posterior border of the acromion. After halving this line, the injection site is established 2 cm medial and 2 cm cranial from this point (Fig. 47.3). Using a 22-gauge, 6-cm needle, and nerve stimulator, the needle is advanced in a lateral direction on the floor of the fossa at an angle of 75° to the skin surface and toward the head of the humerus. Based on cadaveric studies showing the sensory branches of the suprascapular nerve course along the

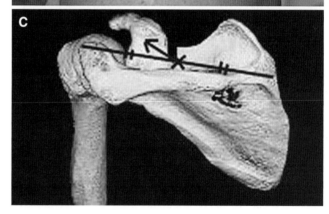

Fig. 47.4 (**a**) The needle is inserted to contact the bone toward the coracoid process from the midpoint of the anterolateral edge of the acromion and super medial angle of the scapular spine. (**b**) The needle is inclined at a 30° angle toward the dorsal direction from the axis of the body and inserted until it reaches the base of the coracoid process. (**c**) The needle can be inserted toward the sensory branch of the suprascapular nerve passing the base of the coracoid by the method shown in panels (**a**, **b**) (From Matsumoto et al. [6], with permission)

base of the coracoid process, Matsumoto et al. proposed blocking the nerve fibers at this location. The insertion point is the midpoint of the anterolateral angle of the acromion and the medial edge of the scapular spine. The needle is inclined at a 30° angle toward the dorsal direction from the axis of the body and inserted until it reaches the base of the coracoid process (Fig. 47.4). Preliminary results in eight patients experiencing severe pain after rotator cuff repair surgery resulted in effective

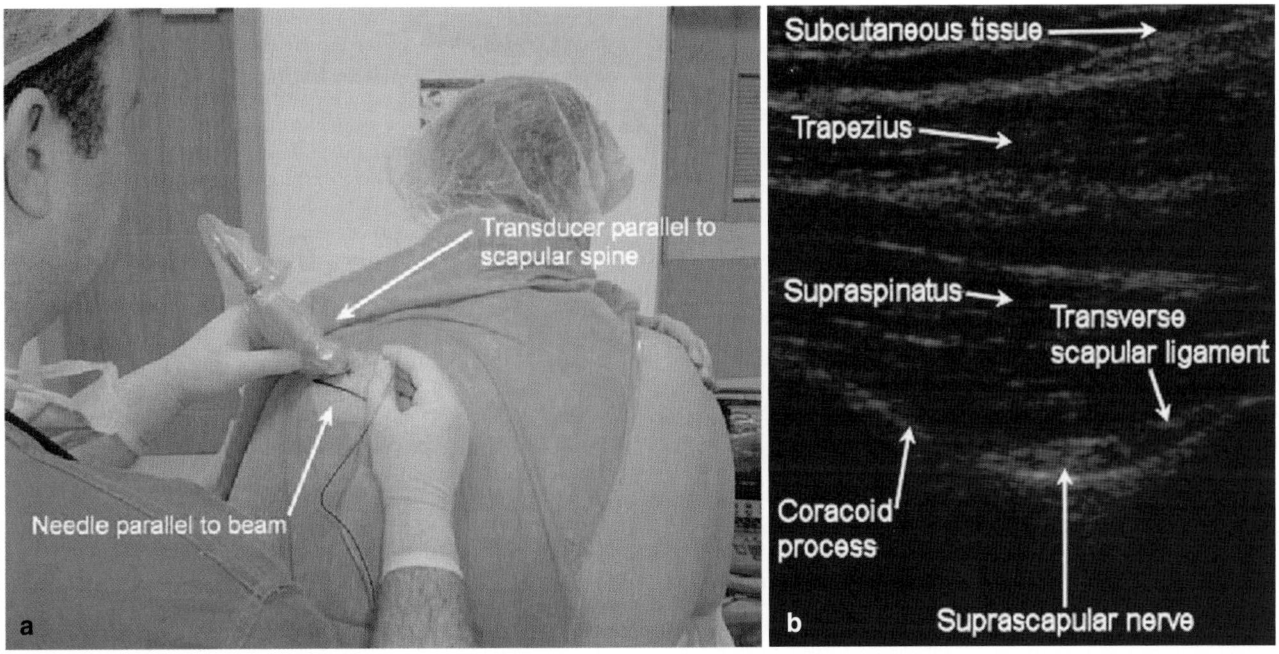

Fig. 47.5 (a) Ultrasound transducer and needle orientation for the ultrasound-guided suprascapular nerve block. (b) Transverse view of suprascapular fossa and scapular notch with a SonoSite ultrasound system and a 6–13-MHz linear transducer (From Harmon and Hearty [38], with permission)

pain relief. The average postoperative VAS scores of the eight patients were 5.4 ± 2.7. Notably, the volume of injectate varies in most reports from 5 to 15 ml while performing either the direct or indirect technique although most reported using a volume of 10 ml of local anesthetic.

While the SSNB has been traditionally performed based on anatomic landmarks, imaging guidance utilizing fluoroscopy, CT, and ultrasound has been described [26, 31, 37, 38]. One author recommended using fluoroscopy to identify the suprascapular notch when performing the direct technique, especially when it is difficult to locate the suprascapular notch via the anatomic approach. The patient should be placed in the prone position with the fluoroscope slightly lateral to midline at the T2–3 level with a slight cephalocaudad tilt [31]. In a non-randomized controlled trial of 40 patients with chronic shoulder pain, Schneider-Kolsky et al. performed a CT-guided SSNB with a direct approach and reported improvement in SPADI scores at 30 min, 3 days, weeks, and 6 weeks post injection [26]. While these results were encouraging, Shanahan et al.'s randomized controlled trial failed to show any difference in pain, disability, or patient satisfaction between CT-guided and traditional non-image-guided SSNBs [37]. Two case reports reported favorable results using ultrasound guidance. Harmon et al. described first placing the ultrasound transducer in a transverse orientation over the scapular spine (see Fig. 47.5) [38]. The transducer is then gradually moved in a cephalad and slightly lateral direction until the suprascapular notch and transverse scapular ligament are identified. The suprascapular nerve lies just inferior to the ligament. However, a subsequent cadaveric study revealed that the structure previously identified under ultrasound guidance as the transverse ligament was the fascia layer of the supraspinatus

muscle [39]. Therefore, an ultrasound-guided SSNB appears to be an indirect technique with the injectate placed near the nerve in the suprascapular fossa, rather than a direct technique in the suprascapular notch as previously believed.

The SSNB is considered a safe technique and is associated with few side effects and complications [1–12]. While pneumothorax is a possible serious complication, the incidence is less than 1 %. Furthermore, this complication has only been described with the direct technique in which the end of the needle is placed directly in the suprascapular notch and approximates the superior aspect of the lung [36]. In order to minimize this complication, Parris and colleagues suggest internally rotating the ipsilateral arm and placing the hand on the opposite shoulder in order to elevate the scapula away from the chest wall [12]. Most other complications described in the literature have been transient in nature and similar to minor complications associated with most other kinds of interventional procedures [1, 3–6, 9, 11, 12]. Goldner reported performing over 1,000 direct SSNBs, with the only occasional minor complication being temporary postinjection tenderness [34]. Dahan et al. reported performing over 2,000 indirect SSNBs and reported no significant complications other than a few vasovagal reactions and postinjection tenderness [4].

Conclusion

The suprascapular nerve block is a safe and effective procedure and should be considered in the management of postoperative pain following shoulder arthroscopy, scapular fractures, adhesive capsulitis, rotator cuff degenerative tears, and glenohumeral arthritis [1–12, 14–19]. Its low rate of complications and ease of use in the office setting make it a very useful procedure. It remains unclear whether the direct or indirect approach to blocking the suprascapular nerve is superior and whether the use of a nerve stimulator, EMG, or imaging guidance is essential to maximizing the effectiveness of the block. Clearly, recent trends have favored utilizing the indirect technique to minimize the risk of pneumothorax. Further randomized controlled trials are needed to compare the efficacy of the various SSNB techniques. The use of ultrasound guidance for SSNB is an area of particular interest for further studies. Ultrasound involves no radiation exposure to the patient or clinician and may facilitate an equally or more effective block as compared to other techniques. Furthermore, lower volumes of local anesthetic can be used due to the ability to visualize and inject immediately near the suprascapular nerve.

References

1. Vecchio PC, Adebajo AO, Hazleman BL. Suprascapular nerve block for persistent rotator cuff lesions. J Rheumatol. 1993;20(3):453–5.
2. Ritchie ED, et al. Suprascapular nerve block for postoperative pain relief in arthroscopic shoulder surgery: a new modality? Anesth Analg. 1997;84(6):1306–12.
3. Jones DS, Chattopadhyay C. Suprascapular nerve block for the treatment of frozen shoulder in primary care: a randomized trial. Br J Gen Pract. 1999;49(438):39–41.
4. Dahan TH, et al. Double blind randomized clinical trial examining the efficacy of bupivacaine suprascapular nerve blocks in frozen shoulder. J Rheumatol. 2000;27(6):1464–9.
5. Shanahan EM, et al. Suprascapular nerve block (using bupivacaine and methylprednisolone acetate) in chronic shoulder pain. Ann Rheum Dis. 2003;62(5):400–6.
6. Matsumoto D, et al. A new nerve block procedure for the suprascapular nerve based on a cadaveric study. J Shoulder Elbow Surg. 2009;18(4):607–11.
7. Jerosch J, et al. Suprascapular nerve block as a method of preemptive pain control in shoulder surgery. Knee Surg Sports Traumatol Arthrosc. 2008;16(6):602–7.
8. Checcucci G, et al. A new technique for regional anesthesia for arthroscopic shoulder surgery based on a suprascapular nerve block and an axillary nerve block: an evaluation of the first results. Arthroscopy. 2008;24(6):689–96.
9. Meier G, Bauereis C, Maurer H. The modified technique of continuous suprascapular nerve block. A safe technique in the treatment of shoulder pain. Anaesthesist. 2002;51(9):747–53.
10. Lewis RN. The use of combined suprascapular and circumflex (articular branches) nerve blocks in the management of chronic arthritis of the shoulder joint. Eur J Anaesthesiol. 1999;16(1):37–41.
11. Dangoisse MJ, Wilson DJ, Glynn CJ. MRI and clinical study of an easy and safe technique of suprascapular nerve blockade. Acta Anaesthesiol Belg. 1994;45(2):49–54.
12. Parris WC. Suprascapular nerve block: a safer technique. Anesthesiology. 1990;72(3):580–1.
13. Rose DL, Kelly CR. Shoulder pain. Suprascapular nerve block in shoulder pain. J Kans Med Soc. 1969;70(3):135–6.
14. Karatas GK, Meray J. Suprascapular nerve block for pain relief in adhesive capsulitis: comparison of 2 different techniques. Arch Phys Med Rehabil. 2002;83(5):593–7.
15. Taskaynatan MA, et al. Suprascapular nerve block versus steroid injection for non-specific shoulder pain. Tohoku J Exp Med. 2005;205(1):19–25.
16. Price DJ. The shoulder block: a new alternative to interscalene brachial plexus blockade for the control of postoperative shoulder pain. Anaesth Intensive Care. 2007;35(4):575–81.
17. Di Lorenzo L, et al. Pain relief in early rehabilitation of rotator cuff tendinitis: any role for indirect suprascapular nerve block? Eura Medicophys. 2006;42(3):195–204.
18. Singelyn FJ, Lhotel L, Fabre B. Pain relief after arthroscopic shoulder surgery: a comparison of intraarticular analgesia, suprascapular nerve block, and interscalene brachial plexus block. Anesth Analg. 2004;99(2):589–92, table of contents.
19. Gado K, Emery P. Modified suprascapular nerve block with bupivacaine alone effectively controls chronic shoulder pain in patients with rheumatoid arthritis. Ann Rheum Dis. 1993;52(3):215–8.
20. Emery P, et al. Suprascapular nerve block for chronic shoulder pain in rheumatoid arthritis. BMJ. 1989;299(6707):1079–80.
21. Edeland HG, Stefansson T. Block of the suprascapular nerve in reduction of acute anterior shoulder dislocation. Case reports. Acta Anaesthesiol Scand. 1973;17(1):46–9.
22. Gleeson AP, et al. Comparison of intra-articular lignocaine and a suprascapular nerve block for acute anterior shoulder dislocation. Injury. 1997;28(2):141–2.
23. Breen TW, Haigh JD. Continuous suprascapular nerve block for analgesia of scapular fracture. Can J Anaesth. 1990;37(7):786–8.
24. Hong JY, Lee IH. Suprascapular nerve block or a piroxicam patch for shoulder tip pain after day case laparoscopic surgery. Eur J Anaesthesiol. 2003;20(3):234–8.
25. Tan N, et al. Suprascapular nerve block for ipsilateral shoulder pain after thoracotomy with thoracic epidural analgesia: a double-blind comparison of 0.5 % bupivacaine and 0.9 % saline. Anesth Analg. 2002;94(1):199–202, table of contents.
26. Schneider-Kolsky ME, Pike J, Connell DA. CT-guided suprascapular nerve blocks: a pilot study. Skeletal Radiol. 2004;33(5):277–82.
27. Gurbet A, et al. Efficacy of pulsed mode radiofrequency lesioning of the suprascapular nerve in chronic shoulder pain secondary to rotator cuff rupture. Agri. 2005;17(3):48–52.
28. Liliang PC, et al. Pulsed radiofrequency lesioning of the suprascapular nerve for chronic shoulder pain: a preliminary report. Pain Med. 2009;10(1):70–5.
29. Keskinbora K, Aydinli I. Long-term results of suprascapular pulsed radiofrequency in chronic shoulder pain. Agri. 2009;21(1):16–21.
30. Price DJ. What local anesthetic volume should be used for suprascapular nerve block? Reg Anesth Pain Med. 2008;33(6):571; author reply 571–3.
31. Waldman S. Chapter 11: Somatic blocks of the thorax. In: Raj P, editor. Interventional pain management: image-guided procedures. 2nd ed. Philadelphia: Saunders/Elsevier; 2008. p. 252.
32. Carron H. Relieving pain with nerve blocks. Geriatrics. 1978;33(4):49–57.
33. Rabson M, Auday JH. Suprascapular nerve block for painful shoulder. J Albert Einstein Med Cent (Phila). 1960;8:39–42.
34. Goldner JL. Suprascapular nerve block for the painful shoulder. South Med J. 1952;45(12):1125–30.
35. Rathmell JP, et al. Requisites in anesthesiology: regional anesthesia. Philadelphia: Elsevier-Mosby; 2004. p. 69.
36. Moore DC, editor. Regional nerve block, Block of the suprascapular nerve, vol. 9. 4th ed. Springfield: Thomas CC; 1979. p. 300–3.
37. Shanahan EM, et al. Suprascapular nerve block in chronic shoulder pain: are the radiologists better? Ann Rheum Dis. 2004;63(9):1035–40. http://www.ncbi.nlm.nih.gov/pubmed/15308514.
38. Harmon D, Hearty C. Ultrasound-guided suprascapular nerve block technique. Pain Physician. 2007;10(6):743–6.
39. Peng PW, et al. Ultrasound-guided suprascapular nerve block: a correlation with fluoroscopic and cadaveric findings. Can J Anaesth. 2010;57(2):143–8.

Intradiscal Annuloplasty for the Treatment of Discogenic Pain

48

Leonardo Kapural

Key Points

- Establishing diagnosis of discogenic pain remains difficult secondary to lack of studies explaining clear mechanisms of pain generation and its nonspecific clinical features.
- Provocation discography remains the only available test linking the morphologic abnormalities seen on MRI with clinically observed pain, and its predictive value can be improved using a strict guideline.
- Several new minimally invasive intradiscal techniques for discogenic LBP control have been introduced, but sufficient clinical evidence is lacking.
- DiscTRODE annuloplasty and conventional nuclear RF seem to be ineffective in reducing pain and improving functional capacity in patients with discogenic LBP.
- IDET and intradiscal biacuplasty can provide positive therapeutic effect in well-selected patient groups.
- Strict clinical selection criteria significantly improve results of annuloplasty for lower back discogenic pain.
- Patients with presence of one or two levels of disc degeneration on magnetic resonance imaging (MRI) and one or two disc levels positive on provocation discography are appropriate candidates for annuloplasty.
- Serious complications following percutaneous interventional procedures for back or leg pain are infrequent.

L. Kapural, M.D., Ph.D.
Department of Carolinas Pain Institute
and Center for Clinical Research,
Wake Forest Baptist Medical Center,
145 Kimel Park Drive, Winston-Salem, NC 27103, USA
e-mail: lkapural@wfubmc.edu

Introduction

The term discogenic pain refers to pain arising from the disc itself. Discogenic pain is cited as the most common cause of chronic low back pain, accounting for approximately 26–39 % of patients with such pain etiology [1]. Internal disc disruption (IDD) is the most common diagnosis leading to chronic low back pain and one of the major causes of chronic neck pain [1, 2]. Discogenic pain is a significant medical challenge, in terms of its clinical, social, economic, and public health implications. An extensive body of literature suggests that discogenic pain is likely to be multifactorial. The most significant risk factors are genetic inheritance, environmental influences, and lifestyle choices. Although available literature supports hypothesis that the intervertebral disc is an independent chronic pain generator, research related to the epidemiology of discogenic pain is still in its formative stage [1–3].

Establishing Diagnosis of Discogenic Pain

Establishing diagnosis of discogenic pain remains difficult secondary to its nonspecific clinical features. Patient frequently describes more typical features of such pain as being persistent low back, groin, and/or leg pain that worsens with axial loading and improves with recumbency. These features alone, however, are frequently insufficient to establish an accurate diagnosis as many factors contribute to the complexity of this condition. These include other potential sources of pain in the spine causing symptoms of similar distribution area and character, present psychosocial factors and clear limitations of available diagnostic tools. In addition, different specialties dealing with the lower back pain employ various diagnostic approaches without clear consensus in diagnosing discogenic pain.

In the absence of signs or symptoms related to neurologic deficit, imaging should be utilized when the pain remains persistent despite continuous conservative management. MRI (magnetic resonance imaging) is frequently employed

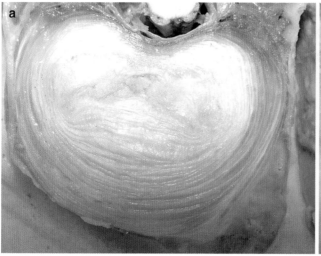
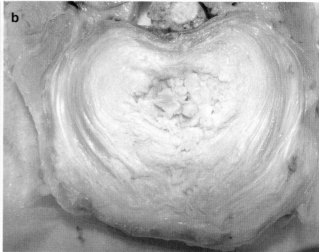

Fig. 48.1 Degenerative changes in the lumbar intervertebral discs. Human lumbar spine fixed in 10 % neutral buffered formalin for 1 week is shown. Individual lumbar segments were prepared, taking care to preserve the posterior elements. (**a**) Mostly intact annulus with minor lamellar disorganization in a minimally degenerated disc with the absence of fissuring. (**b**) Lamellar disorganization in a degenerated lumbar disc with presence of radiating tear extending to the outer 1/3 of the annulus. There may be some loss of the nucleus on this gross dissection of the human spine (With permission from Baylis Medical Company © Copyright)

imaging test to evaluate intervertebral discs. Three changes detected on MRI could be of interest: low signal intensity of the disc on T2 weighting, high-intensity zone (HIZ), and vertebral and/or end-plate changes. Disc degeneration with reduced water content within the disc produces a low signal intensity, or "black disc," on T2-weighted images. Such change is associated with disc degeneration and correlates poorly with the presence of discogenic pain versus any other pain in the lower back. The high-intensity zones (HIZ) are associated with presence of annular fissures within the disc, but it is not clear if they correlate with the presence of discogenic pain. Positive predictive value of HIZ to suggest that the pain origin is within the disc could be as high as 87–90 % [4–6]. HIZ are, however, present in a large number of asymptomatic discs as well (25–39 %) [7]. In addition, degenerative disc disease is often associated with nearby bone sclerosis, so-called modic type I–III changes [8, 9]. Those could be more prevalent in patients with low back pain and positive discography. Modic changes appear to have a high sensitivity, but low specificity for discogenic pain [10].

To date, provocation discography is the only available method linking the morphologic abnormalities seen on MRI with clinically observed pain, and its predictive value has been repeatedly questioned mainly as a result of reported higher false-positive rates [11–13]. Based on currently published data, it is difficult to draw any conclusion on predictive value of MRI findings and the presence of concordant pain on provocation discography. There are several reasons for that: defining disc degeneration on MRI may vary significantly, and the criteria used to establish presence of discogenic pain during provocative discography are still evolving [14].

Once the diagnosis of discogenic pain has been suggested, the next challenge involves instituting an effective therapy. Traditionally, surgical approaches of lumbar fusion with instrumentation and various disc arthroplasties were utilized. Common characteristic of those surgical approaches is an extensive surgery in the lower back with prolonged recovery interval and questioned efficacy in treating pain of discogenic origin. In an effort to provide percutaneous, minimally invasive treatment for discogenic pain in patients with relatively well-maintained disc height, several therapies were developed utilizing heat in the annulus fibrosus (annuloplasty procedures). Such therapeutic modalities have been used despite a somewhat poorly understood relationship between the therapeutic effects and, if any, histologic changes observed [15–18]. Most clinicians believe that the likely mechanism of pain relief by annuloplasty is denervation of the tissue or destruction of the nociceptors and less likely any alteration of the collagen fiber structure in the annulus, like collagen denaturation and coalescence [15–18]. Three annuloplasty technologies still available in clinical practice are intradiscal electrothermal therapy (IDET; Smith & Nephew, London, UK), discTRODE (Radionics Inc., Burlington, MA), and intradiscal biacuplasty (Baylis Medical, Montreal, Canada).

Mechanisms of the Pain Relief by Annuloplasty

Disc degeneration is associated with significant changes within the disc nucleus and annulus (Fig. 48.1a, b), like delamination or tearing of the lamellar layer of the annulus and dehydration and loss of nuclear material. Those physical changes are frequently associated with biochemical and cellular changes. Production of inflammatory cytokines, including tumor necrosis factor-α (TNF-α), nitric oxide, and matrix metalloprotineases (MMPs), is increased [19, 20]. Extensive vascularization in degenerated disc, mostly along annular fissures, may facilitate introduction of these inflammatory cytokines [19]. Nociceptors that are normally limited to the outer third of the annulus penetrate further into the degenerated disc along neovascularization of the areas around the newly formed fissures [21–24]. Immunohistochemical studies confirmed nociceptive origin (C- and Aδ-fibers) of newly formed neural tissue, thought to be responsible for the presence of discogenic pain [20, 23]. In addition, it is possible that inflammatory cytokines provide further sensitization of these ingrown nerves. Therefore, destroying these nociceptive fibers may eliminate, at least partially, possible source of the lower back pain.

Temperatures reached during biacuplasty or IDET may be sufficient to cause nerve destruction which occurs at 42–45 °C or higher [25–27]. However, evidence from the basic science studies to demonstrate neuroablation by delivered heat as the mechanisms of action for discogenic pain relief remains unavailable until this date.

The temperature profiles of the latest intradiscal heating procedure and one with most promising clinical data, intradiscal biacuplasty, were investigated in both porcine and human cadaveric lumbar discs. Histological examination could not detect signs of tissue degradation due to heating or changes in the collagen structure in both degenerated and nondegenerated intervertebral discs [28, 29].

Intradiscal Electrothermal Therapy (IDET)

The first effective minimally invasive therapeutic alternative to fusion surgery or arthroplasty came in the form of intradiscal electrothermal therapy (IDET) [30, 31]. IDET is performed using a thermal catheter, resistive coil (SpineCATH, Smith & Nephew Endoscopy, Andover, MA), that is percutaneously introduced to the interface between the posterior annulus and nucleus under multiplanar fluoroscopic control (Figs. 48.2a–d and 48.3a, b).

There are dozens of prospective case series and reports and a single, randomized, controlled trial that provided data on the IDET efficacy ([30–41]; Table 48.1). However, one, randomized, controlled trial and several published case series failed to demonstrate any clinical benefit of the IDET procedure [37, 41]. The first randomized, sham-controlled trial provided class I evidence that IDET is an efficacious annuloplasty procedure in properly selected patients [36]. It seems that IDET could provide rather long-term pain relief as evidenced at 1-year and 2-year follow-ups ([30–41]; Table 48.1). When used in general population of the patient with lower back pain,

it seems that those with overlapping inflammatory arthritides or nonspinal conditions that may mimic lumbar discogenic pain and those patients with multilevel degenerative disc disease do not benefit from the IDET annuloplasty [39, 42, 43]. It seems that the variation in patient selection and provided heating techniques are thought to account for most of the differences seen in clinical results [30, 31, 36, 37, 39, 41–50]. Pauza and colleagues' use of provocation discography, rather than MRI/discography combined criteria for the patients enrollment, may have contributed to high number of patients needed to treat – five to achieve >75 % improvement in one patient [36]. Overweight patients [42] and patients receiving workers' compensation benefits [43, 50] represent additional patient subsets that are unlikely to benefit from the IDET.

Technique

The IDET procedure is performed under local anesthesia and mild intravenous sedation in sterile conditions. IV antibiotics, most frequently 1 g of cefazolin or 1 g of vancomycin, should be given 30–60 min before the procedure. Patients are positioned prone using midabdomen support to correct for the lumbar lordosis. Using local anesthesia, a 17-gauge needle is inserted under fluoroscopic guidance into the targeted disc. Through that same needle, a catheter with thermal resistive coil is navigated until positioned appropriately within the disc. The key is to position such catheter across all of the semicircumference delineated by the interphase of the posterior annulus and nucleus (Fig. 48.3a, b). The thermal resistive coil generates gradual rising temperature inside the disc up to 90 °C in 0.5 °C increments. The temperature is then maintained at 90 °C for 4 min according to manufacturer protocol (Smith & Nephew, London, UK). Patient is then brought to the recovery area and discharged home with instructions regarding functional rehabilitation program. The goals of such rehabilitation after the annuloplasty are pain control and reduction of inflammation, providing early supervised stretching and mobilization of tissue. In order to achieve functional restoration, addressed are extensor muscles, which may be deconditioned, as well as abdominals, trunk rotator, and trunk/hip flexors. During that time interval of 4–6 weeks, manual manipulative therapy is avoided.

Intradiscal Biacuplasty

Intradiscal biacuplasty employs bipolar RF electrodes to heat posterior annulus of the intervertebral disc. Although recently described, it could be the most promising of all annuloplasty methods [33, 34, 51]. This method works specifically by concentrating RF current between the

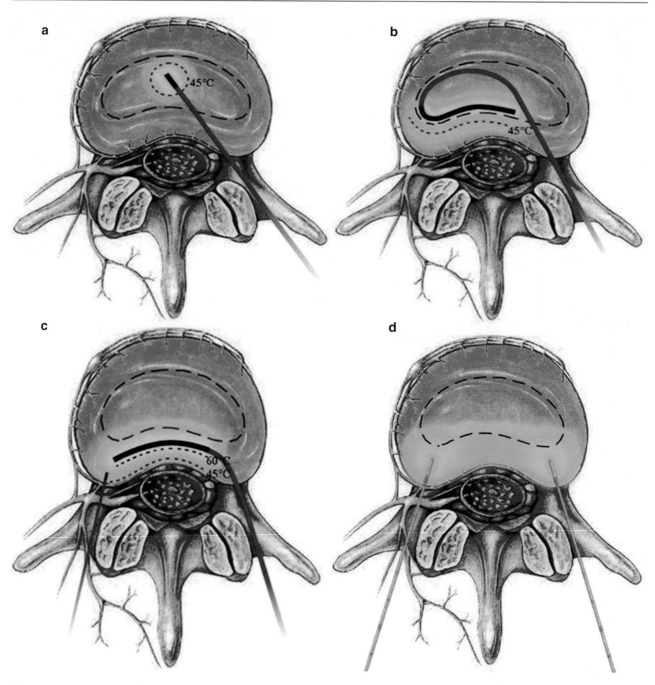

Fig. 48.2 Diagram of the heat-delivering electrodes within the intervertebral disc and approximate temperature that can be produced during four different minimally invasive procedures aimed to treat discogenic pain. (**a**) Intranuclear radio frequency. The RF electrode is positioned in the middle of the nucleus. Temperature achieved may not be sufficient to denervate posterior annulus when the heat source is inside the nucleus. (**b**) Intradiscal electrothermal therapy (IDET). Resistive coil is placed between the annulus and nucleus and along the posterior annulus. Optimal temperature dissipates several millimeters and may affect a very limited area of the annulus. (**c**) DiscTRODE™ (radio-frequency electrode) is positioned within the posterior annulus. (**d**) Intradiscal biacuplasty. Radio-frequency electrodes are positioned inside the posterior annulus to achieve optimal bipolar heating and possible nociceptor denervation (With permission from Baylis Medical Company © Copyright)

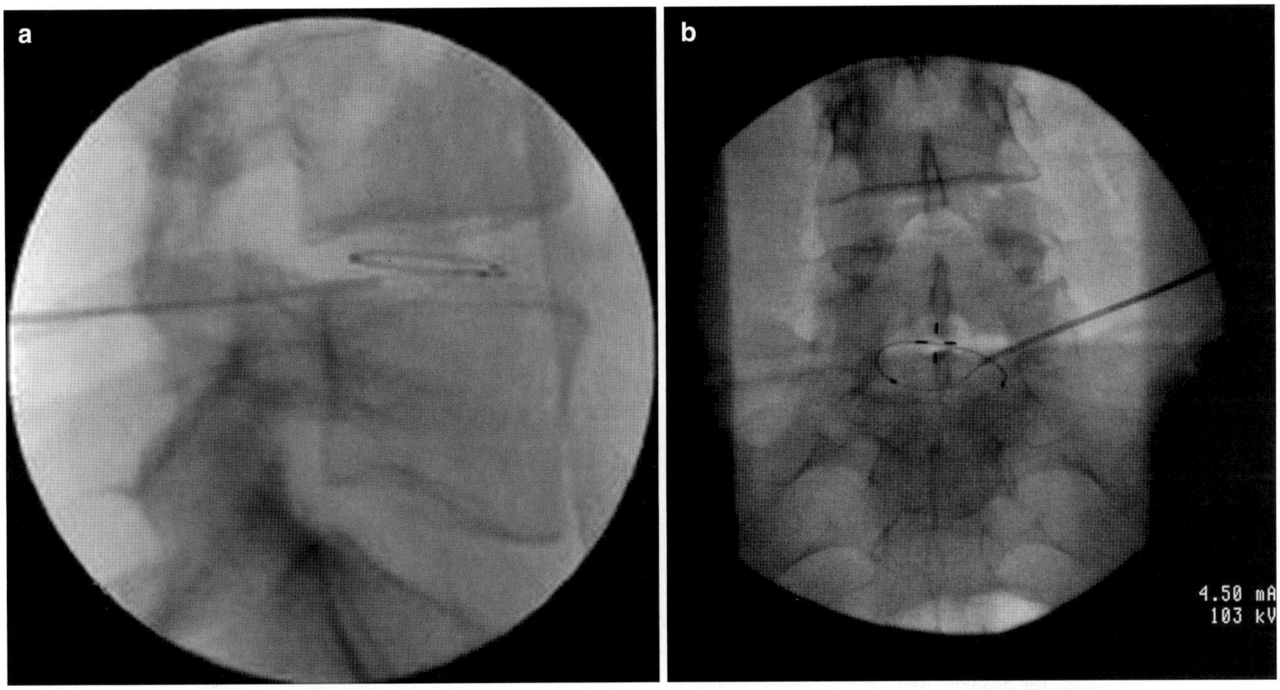

Fig. 48.3 The fluoroscopic views of the final electrode position during IDET procedure used for the treatment of discogenic pain. IDET resistive coil properly positioned just between annulus and nucleus of the lumbar intervertebral disc. (**a**) Lateral view of the final coil position within L4–5 lumbar disc. (**b**) Anterior view of the IDET coil when cranial tilt of the fluoroscope is used to clearly show a full circle of the coil placed inside the disc at the interphase between the annulus and nucleus (With permission from Baylis Medical Company © Copyright)

active electrodes placed on the tip of two straight probes (Fig. 48.4a, b). The larger area of the posterior annulus is ablated by internally cooling the electrodes [29, 52] (Figs. 48.2a, b and 48.4a, b). Two intradiscal electrodes are first placed bilaterally in the posterior annulus of the intervertebral disc, and then generator temperature is increased gradually over a period of 10 min to 50 °C with final heating for another 5 min. Additional two monopolar lesions over 2.5 min are then produced bilaterally at 60 °C in order to extend lesion laterally and to achieve appropriate temperature increase to extended area of posterior annulus. During this time, the patient should be awake and communicating to the physician.

The first case report on biacuplasty documented significant improvements in functional capacity and VAS pain score at 6 months following the procedure with no perioperative complications. Later, three prospective case series involving 8, 15, and 15 patients, respectively, were completed, during which significant pain relief and improvement in the function were achieved at 3, 6, and 12 months after biacuplasty [33, 34, 40, 53]. In the European case series [53] involving eight patients, there was an average of 50 % pain reduction at 3 months with an overall good patient satisfaction. No patients reported any post-procedural pain, often associated with other therapies,

and there were no reported complications. During the prospective pilot study involving 15 patients, reported were improvements in several functional capacity measures after the procedure with no complications [33, 34]. Improvements in Oswestry index were sustained from 23.3 at baseline to 16.5 points at 1 month and stayed same at 12 months. The prospective, randomized sham study is being currently completed in order to accept or refute results achieved during pilot study.

The latest prospective, observational study showed that 78.6 % of the patients had Oswestry score improvement of 10 points or more with 57 % of the patients having 50 % or more pain relief at 6 months after the procedure [40]. Authors concluded that their data are in agreement with other two studies data published earlier [33, 40, 53].

Intradiscal biacuplasty seems to provide several improvements over the IDET. There is minimal disruption to the native tissue architecture, and thus the biomechanics of the spine is less affected. The relative ease of electrode placement eliminates the need to thread a long resistive coil like in IDET procedure. Lower peak heating temperatures within the disc annulus compared to IDET do allow better patient tolerance. In addition, internal cooling of the probes limits excessively high temperatures in the disc that may cause tissue adherence [29, 52].

Table 48.1 Pertinent studies on various types of annuloplasties when used for the treatment of discogenic lower back pain

Author name	Year	Type of intervention	Indications of procedure	Patients (#)	Type of study	Outcomes	Complications	Conclusions
Assietti et al. [32]	2010	IDET	Single-level DDD and discogenic pain, >60 % disc height	50	Prospective	VAS 68 % decrease, ODI from 59.0 ± 7.6 % to 20.1 ± 11 % at 24 m	None	Safe and effective
Kapural et al. [33, 34]	2008	Biacuplasty	Single- or two-level DDD and discogenic pain, >50 % disc height	15	Prospective pilot	7 of 13 >50 % VAS, ODI to 17.5, and SF-36-PF from 51 to 67 at 12 m	None	Safe and effective
Kvarstein et al. [35]	2009	DiscTRODE™	Chronic LBP, discogenic pain	23	Prospective randomized, double-blind	No improvement study or sham at 12 m	None	Do not recommend use of discTRODE
Pauza et al. [36]	2004	IDET	DDD and discogenic pain, >80 % disc height	64	Randomized sham-controlled prospective	56 % >2 VAS change, 50 % patients >50 % relief at 6 m	None	Safe and effective
Freeman et al. [37]	2005	IDET	Multilevel DDD, workers' comp included		Randomized sham-control prospective	Oswestry unchanged	None	Ineffective
Jawahar et al. [38]	2008	IDET	DDD and discogenic pain, >80 % disc height, WC patients	53	Prospective	VAS reduction 63 %, ODI 70 %	None	Useful in carefully selecting WC patients
Kapural et al. [39]	2004	IDET	Single- or two-level DDD and discogenic pain, >50 % disc height vs. multilevel DDD	34	Prospective matched study	1.2-DDD >50 % improvement in VAS and PDI	None	IDET procedure effective only in one- or two-level DDD
Karaman et al. [40]	2011	Biacuplasty	Single- or two-level DDD and discogenic pain,, >50 % disc height	15	Prospective observational	78.6 % >10 points Oswestry; >2 points VAS	None	Safe and effective

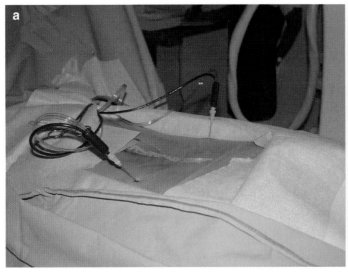
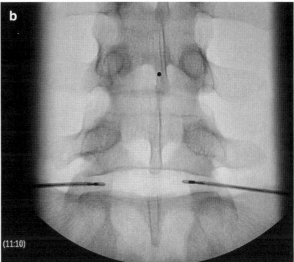

Fig. 48.4 Intradiscal biacuplasty electrodes properly positioned in bipolar fashion via introducers inside the patient's back (**a**) and shown in anterior-posterior view inside L5–S1 lumbar intervertebral disc (**b**). Note that the electrodes are positioned in the middle of the disc and away from the end plates and bony structures (With permission from Baylis Medical Company © Copyright)

Technique

The procedure is completed under fluoroscopy with the patient lying in the prone position. Light sedation and analgesia can be provided for relaxation and pain control before and during the procedure, but the patient should be able to communicate with physician throughout the procedure. Two 17-G TransDiscal introducers are introduced to annulus bilaterally (Fig. 48.4a, b). Oblique view similar to optimal lumbar discography view is achieved. The introducer should be directed along the SAP (superior articular process) and enters the disc in the lower half. This will ensure the electrodes are sufficiently far away from the end plates and exiting nerve root. The introducers are advanced into the disc until the tips appear to be aligned with the medial edge of the pedicles in an anterior-posterior (AP) image and in the lateral fluoroscopic view just piercing the disc. Two 18-G TransDiscal probes are then placed inside the disc through provided introducers. Probe placement should be checked in the AP and lateral views to ensure appropriate disc entry points and depth of the probe. The generator controls delivery of RF energy by monitoring the temperature at the tip of the probe. The temperature increases gradually over the period of 10 min to 50 °C with final heating at 50 °C for another 5 min. Following completion of the procedure, patient is required to wear a brace and follow physical therapy instructions over a rehabilitation period with same rehabilitation goals as listed above for the IDET procedure.

Other Annuloplasty and Nucleoplasty Procedures for Treatment of Discogenic Back Pain

Several other intradiscal radio-frequency methods to treat discogenic pain are approved for use in the United States. The original Sluijter radio-frequency (RF) technique in which the nucleus (and not the annulus) is heated to 70 °C for 90s was proven ineffective in a randomized trial [54]. The novel annular probe termed "discTRODE" has been also shown ineffective in improving pain or function in patients with lumbar discogenic pain and during comparison study shown inferior to the IDET procedure (Fig. 48.5) [35, 55].

Complications

Rare complications of the lumbar annuloplasty procedures can be divided into infectious, hemorrhagic, neurological, allergic, and other less specific complications [56, 57]. Most frequent are minor procedure-related side effects like temporary pain exacerbation and vasovagal reactions. More serious complications include discitis, spinal abscesses, and vertebral osteomyelitis. Other serious neurological complications such as cauda equina and nerve root damage are exclusively caused by misplacement of trocars, probes, or heating elements [58–61].

Fig. 48.5 The mean pain disability index (*PDI*) scores and 95 % confidence intervals by group at each time point following either intradiscal thermal annuloplasty (*IDET*) or radio-frequency posterior annuloplasty (*RFA*) using mixed-effects model analysis.
The IDTA and RFA treatment groups did not differ significantly in their baseline PDI scores. By 3 months and at all subsequent time points, the IDTA group had significantly lower mean PDI scores than the RFA group (With permission from Kapural et al. [55])

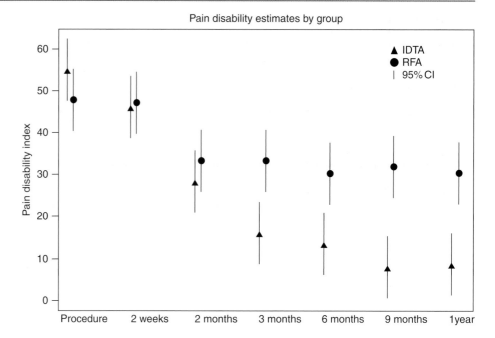

Conclusions

Several new minimally invasive intradiscal techniques for pain control have been introduced recently, but sufficient clinical evidence of their efficacy and extent of application is still lacking. While discTRODE™ annuloplasty and conventional nuclear radiofrequency are ineffective in reducing the pain and improving functional capacity in patients with discogenic back pain, IDET and intradiscal biacuplasty may produce positive therapeutic effect in appropriately selected patients.

References

1. Manchikanti L. Epidemiology of low back pain. Pain Physician. 2000;3(2):167–92.
2. Keshari KR, Lotz JC, Link TM, et al. Lactic acid and proteoglycans as metabolic markers for discogenic back pain. Spine. 2008;33(3): 312–7.
3. Coté P, Cassidy JD, Carroll L. The Saskatchewan Health and Back Pain Survey. The prevalence of neck pain and related disability in Saskatchewan adults. Spine. 1998;1(23):16789–98.
4. Braithwaite IJ, White A, et al. Vertebral end-plate (Modic) changes on lumbar spine MRI: correlation with pain reproduction at lumbar discography. Eur Spine J. 1998;7:363–8.
5. Kokkonen S, Kurunlahti M, Tervonen O, et al. Endplate degeneration observed on magnetic resonance imaging of the lumbar spine. Spine. 2002;27(20):2274–8.
6. Aprill C, Bogduk N. High-intensity zone: a diagnostic sign of painful lumbar disc on magnetic resonance imaging. Br J Radiol. 1992;65(773):361–9.
7. Ricketson R, Simmons J, Hauser W. The prolapsed intervertebral disc: the high intensity zone with discography correlation. Spine. 1996;21(23):2758–62.
8. Peng B, Hou S, Wu W. The pathogenesis and clinical significance of a high-intensity zone (HIZ) of lumbar intervertebral disc on MRI imaging in the patient with discogenic low back pain. Eur Spine J. 2006;15(5):583–7.
9. Korecki C, Costi J, Iatridis J. Needle puncture injury affects intervertebral disc mechanics and biology in an organ culture model. Spine. 2008;33(3):235–41.
10. Esposito P, Pinheiro-Franco JL, Froelich S, et al. Predictive value of MRI vertebral end-plate signal changes (Modic) on outcome of surgically treated degenerative disc disease: results of a cohort study including 60 patients. Neurochirurgie. 2006;52:315–22.
11. Carragee EJ, Tanner CM, Khurana S, Hayward C, Welsh J, Date E, et al. The rates of false-positive lumbar discography in select patients without low back symptoms. Spine. 2000;25:1373–80.
12. Walsh TR, Weinstein JN, Spratt KF, Lehmann TR, Aprill C, Sayre H. Lumbar discography in normal subjects. A controlled, prospective study. J Bone Joint Surg Am. 1990;72:1081–8.
13. Derby R, Howard MW, Grant JM, Lettice JJ, Van Peteghem PK, Ryan DP. The ability of pressure-controlled discography to predict surgical and nonsurgical outcomes. Spine. 1999;24:364–71.
14. Kapural L. Indications for minimally invasive disk and vertebral procedures. Pain Med. 2008;9(S1):S65–72.
15. Freeman BJ, Walters RM, Moore RJ, Fraser RD. Does intradiscal electrothermal therapy denervate and repair experimentally induced posterolateral annular tears in an animal model? Spine. 2003; 28:2602–8.
16. Kleinstueck FS, Diederich CJ, Nau WH, Puttlitz CM, Smith JA, Bradford DS, Lotz JC. Temperature and thermal dose distributions during intradiscal electrothermal therapy in the cadaveric lumbar spine. Spine. 2003;28:1700–8.
17. Shah RV, Lutz GE, Lee J, Doty SB, Rodeo S. Intradiskal electrothermal therapy: a preliminary histologic study. Arch Phys Med Rehabil. 2001;82:1230–7.
18. Smith HP, McWhorter JM, Challa VR. Radiofrequency neurolysis in a clinical model. J Neurosurg. 1981;55:248–53.
19. Podichetty VK. The aging spine: the role of inflammatory mediators in intervertebral disc degeneration. Cell Mol Biol (Noisy-le-Grand). 2007;53(5):4–18.

20. Ashton IK, et al. Neuropeptides in the human intervertebral disc. J Orthop Res. 1994;12(2):186–92.

21. Johnson WE, et al. Immunohistochemical detection of Schwann cells in innervated and vascularized human intervertebral discs. Spine. 2001;26(23):2550–7.

22. Melrose J, et al. Increased nerve and blood vessel ingrowth associated with proteoglycan depletion in an ovine anular lesion model of experimental disc degeneration. Spine. 2002;27(12):1278–85.

23. Palmgren T, et al. An immunohistochemical study of nerve structures in the anulus fibrosus of human normal lumbar intervertebral discs. Spine. 1999;24(20):2075–9.

24. Jackson 2nd HC, Winkelmann RK, Bickel WH. Nerve endings in the human lumbar spinal column and related structures. J Bone Joint Surg Am. 1966;48(7):1272–81.

25. Kleinstueck FS, et al. Acute biomechanical and histological effects of intradiscal electrothermal therapy on human lumbar discs. Spine. 2001;26(20):2198–207.

26. Troussier B, et al. Percutaneous intradiscal radio-frequency thermocoagulation. A cadaveric study. Spine. 1995;20(15):1713–8.

27. Smith HP, McWhorter JM, Challa VR. Radiofrequency neurolysis in a clinical model. Neuropathological correlation. J Neurosurg. 1981;55(2):246–53.

28. Pauza K. Cadaveric intervertebral disc temperature mapping during disc biacuplasty. Pain Physician. 2008;11(5):669–76.

29. Kapural L, Mekhail N, Sloan S, Moghal N, Kapural M, Hicks D, Petrinec D. Histological and temperature distribution studies in the lumbar degenerated and non-degenerated human cadaver discs using novel transdiscal radiofrequency electrodes. Pain Med. 2008;9(1):68–75.

30. Saal JA, Saal JS. Intradiscal electrothermal treatment for chronic discogenic low back pain: prospective outcome study with a minimum 2-year follow-up. Spine. 2002;27:966–73.

31. Saal JA, Saal JS. Intradiscal electrothermal treatment for chronic discogenic low back pain: a prospective outcome study with minimum 1-year follow-up. Spine. 2000;25:2622–7.

32. Assietti R, Morosi M, Block JE. Intradiscal electrothermal therapy for symptomatic internal disc disruption: 24-month results and predictors of clinical success. J Neurosurg Spine. 2010;12(3):320–6.

33. Kapural L, De la Garza M, Ng A, Kapural M, Mekhail N. Novel transdiscal biacuplasty for the treatment of lumbar discogenic pain: a 6 months follow-up. Pain Med. 2008;9(1):60–7.

34. Kapural L. Intervertebral disc cooled bipolar radiofrequency (intradiscal biacuplasty) for the treatment of lumbar discogenic pain: a 12 month follow-up of the pilot study. Pain Med. 2008;9(4):464.

35. Kvarstein G, Mawe L, Indahl A, Hol PK, Tennoe B, Digernes R, Stubhaug A, Tonnessen TI, Beivik H. A randomized double-blind controlled trial of intra-annular radiofrequency thermal disc therapy-a 12-month follow-up. Pain. 2009;145:279–86.

36. Pauza KJ, Howell S, Dreyfuss P, Peloza JH, Dawson K, Bogduk N. A randomized, placebo-controlled trial of intradiscal electrothermal therapy for the treatment of discogenic low back pain. Spine J. 2004;4:27–35.

37. Freeman BJ, Fraser RD, Cain CM, Hall DJ, Chapple DC. A randomized, double-blind, controlled trial: intradiscal electrothermal therapy versus placebo for the treatment of chronic discogenic low back pain. Spine (Phila Pa 1976). 2005;30:2369–77.

38. Jawahar A, Brandao SM, Howard C, Nunley PD. Intradiscal electrothermal therapy (IDET): a viable alternative to surgery for low back pain in workers' compensation patients? J La State Med Soc. 2008;160(5):280–5.

39. Kapural L, Korunda Z, Basali AH, et al. Intradiscal thermal annuloplasty for discogenic pain in patients with multilevel degenerative disc disease. Anesth Analg. 2004;99:472–6.

40. Karaman H, Tufek A, Kavak GO, Kaya S, Yildirim ZB, Uysal E, Çelik F. 6-Month results of transdiscal biacuplasty on patients with discogenic Low back pain: preliminary findings. Int J Med Sci. 2011;8(1):1–8.

41. Appleby D, Andersson G, Totta M. Meta-analysis of the efficacy and safety of intradiscal electrothermal therapy (IDET). Pain Med. 2006;7:308–16.

42. Cohen SP, Larkin T, Abdi S, Chang A, Stojanovic M. Risk factors for failure and complications of intradiscal electrothermal therapy: a pilot study. Spine. 2003;28:1142–7.

43. Webster BS, Verma S, Pransky GS. Outcomes of workers' compensation claimants with low back pain undergoing intradiscal electrothermal therapy. Spine. 2004;29:435–41.

44. Bogduk N, Karasek M. Two-year follow-up of a controlled trial of intradiscal electrothermal annuloplasty for chronic low back pain resulting from internal disc disruption. Spine J. 2002;2:343–50.

45. Endres SM, Fiedler GA, Larson KL. Effectiveness of intradiscal electrothermal therapy in increasing function and reducing chronic low back pain in selected patients. WMJ. 2002;101:31–4.

46. Wetzel FT, McNally TA, Phillips FM. Intradiscal electrothermal therapy used to manage chronic discogenic low back pain: new directions and interventions. Spine. 2002;27:2621–6.

47. Derby R, Eek B, Chen Y, O'Neill C, Ryan D. Intradiscal electrothermal annuloplasty (IDET): a novel approach for treating chronic discogenic back pain. Neuromodulation. 2000;3:82–8.

48. Lutz C, Lutz GE, Cooke PM. Treatment of chronic lumbar diskogenic pain with intradiskal electrothermal therapy: a prospective outcome study. Arch Phys Med Rehabil. 2003;84:23–8.

49. Lee MS, Cooper G, Lutz GE, Lutz C, Hong HM. Intradiscal electrothermal therapy (IDET) for treatment of chronic lumbar discogenic pain: a minimum 2-year clinical outcome study. Pain Physician. 2003;6:443–8.

50. Mekhail N, Kapural L. Intradiscal thermal annuloplasty of discogenic pain: an outcome study. Pain Pract. 2004;4:84–90.

51. Kapural L, Mekhail N. Novel transdiscal biacuplasty for the treatment of lumbar discogenic pain: a case report. Pain Pract. 2007;7(2):130–4.

52. Petersohn JD, Conquergood LR, Leung M. Acute histologic effects and thermal distribution profile of disc biacuplasty using a novel water-cooled bipolar electrode system in an in vivo porcine model. Pain Med. 2008;9(1):26–32.

53. Cooper AR. Disc biacuplasty for treatment of axial discogenic low back pain- initial case series, in British Pain Society Annual General Meeting. Glasgow; 2007.

54. Barendse GA, van Den Berg SG, Kessels AH, et al. Randomized controlled trial of percutaneous intradiscal radiofrequency thermocoagulation for chronic discogenic back pain: lack of effect from a 90-second 70 C lesion. Spine. 2001;26:287–92.

55. Kapural L, Hayek S, Malak O, Arrigain S, Mekhail N. Intradiscal thermal annuloplasty versus intradiscal radiofrequency ablation for the treatment of discogenic pain: a prospective matched control trial. Pain Med. 2005;6:425–31.

56. Kapural L, Cata J. Complications of minimally invasive procedures for discogenic pain. Tech Reg Anesth Pain Med. 2007;11(3): 157–63.

57. Cohen SP, Larkin T, Abdi S, et al. Risk factors for failure and complications of intradiscal electrothermal therapy: a pilot study. Spine. 2003;28:1142–7.

58. Djurasovic M, Glassman SD, Dimar JR, et al. Vertebral osteonecrosis associated with the use of intradiscal electrothermal therapy: a case report. Spine. 2002;27:E325–8.

59. Wetzel FT. Cauda equina syndrome from intradiscal electrothermal therapy. Neurology. 2001;56:1607.

60. Orr RD, Thomas SA. Intradural migration of broken IDET catheter causing a radiculopathy. J Spinal Disord Tech. 2005;18:185–7.

61. Hsia AW, Isaac K, Katz JS. Cauda equina syndrome from intradiscal electrothermal therapy. Neurology. 2000;55:320.

Percutaneous Disc Decompression

49

Stanley Golovac, Salim M. Hayek, and Fnu Kailash

Key Points

- At any time during the procedure, if a patient reports any lower extremity sensation (radicular pain or burning foot), the procedure should be stopped and the position of the trocar or probe assessed with anteroposterior and lateral fluoroscopic views and repositioned as necessary.
- Like all intradiscal procedures, multiplanar fluoroscopy should be used for confirmation of needle and probe placement. Sedation should be optimized to maintain meaningful communication between the operator and patient.
- If back pain occurs during PLDD, it may be due to the heating of adjacent vertebral end plates or increased pressure within the disc from trapped gas. In such cases, the position of the optical fiber should be checked to ensure it is away from the end plates,

and the interval between the pulses should be increased. Aspiration could also be applied through the sidearm fitting to avoid the trapping of gas.
- If no aspirated material is present in the Dekompressor probe after 3 min of activation, the procedure should be discontinued.

Introduction

Approximately two-thirds of individuals living in western countries suffer from an episode of low back pain during their lifetimes [1]. Low back pain is one of the leading reasons for multiple visits to physicians, and its rising prevalence is a significant factor in lost productivity, disability, and increased healthcare use [2–4]. Further, low back pain has had a substantial impact on the US economy, with healthcare expenditures swelling by 65 % from 1995 to 2005 [5].

"Nonspecific" low back pain with an unexplained etiology is currently the most prevalent low back pain group [6]. According to the best available evidence and proven diagnostic techniques, structural disorders of intervertebral discs, facet joints, and the sacroiliac joint are the three most important etiologies of the types of low back pain collectively known as "specific" low back pain [7]. Based on studies that employed controlled diagnostic injections, the relative prevalence of intervertebral discs, facet joints, and the sacroiliac joint as a source of low back pain has been estimated at 39 % [8], 15 % [9], and 19 % [10], respectively.

Lumbar disc prolapse accounts for less than 5 % of all low back problems, yet is the most common cause of radicular symptoms [11]. Given the incomplete understanding of the exact natural course of disc herniation and inconsistent findings in trials that compared surgery and conservative care, clinicians are often faced with the challenging choice of surgery versus nonsurgical care for the treatment of patients.

S. Golovac, M.D.
Department of Anesthesia, Pain Management, Surgery,
Cape Canaveral Hospital,
Cocoa Beach, FL, USA

Space Coast Pain Institute,
4770 Honeyridge Lane, Merritt Island, FL 32952, USA
e-mail: sgolovac@mac.com

S.M. Hayek, M.D., Ph.D. (✉)
Division of Pain Medicine, Department of Anesthesiology,
Case Western Reserve University,
University Hospitals Case Medical Center,
11100 Euclid Ave., Clevland, OH 44106, USA
e-mail: salim.hayek@uhhospitals.org

F. Kailash, M.D.
Department of Pain Management, Institute of Pain Diagnostics
and Care, Ohio Valley General Hospital,
1104 Ventana Drive, McKees Rocks, PA 15136, USA
e-mail: kachandwani@gmail.com

T.R. Deer et al. (eds.), *Comprehensive Treatment of Chronic Pain by Medical, Interventional, and Integrative Approaches*,
DOI 10.1007/978-1-4614-1560-2_49, © American Academy of Pain Medicine 2013

Historical Background

Historically, there have been paradigm shifts between operative and nonoperative treatment, and no single modality has been proven superior in long-term studies. In 1934, William Jason Mixter, a neurosurgeon, and Joseph Barr, an orthopedic surgeon, published a landmark article in the *New England Journal of Medicine* that established an association between the intervertebral disc and sciatica [12]. Their work led to a paradigm shift from conservative to surgical management for sciatica. This shift spurred innovations in diagnostic and surgical techniques designed to minimize the trauma of therapeutic interventions.

Conversely, the famous retrospective study of Saal and Saal supported conservative management and showed the resolution of pain in more than 90 % of the subjects treated nonoperatively [13]. This result is comparable to the 4-year outcomes in the nonoperative arm of a landmark study by Henrik Weber [14]. However, in a combined (randomized and observational cohort) as-treated 4-year analysis of large multicenter trial (Spine Patient Outcomes Research Trial: SPORT), patients who underwent surgery for lumbar disc herniation fared better than patients treated nonoperatively in all primary and secondary outcomes except work status [15]. Unfortunately, methodological weaknesses in both trials, including significant crossover between the operative and nonoperative arms and the use of as-treated analysis (vs. intention to treat analysis), undermine the validity of any conclusions drawn from this analysis.

Hence, in light of the generally favorable natural course of lumbar radiculopathy associated with lumbar disc herniation, conservative care and minimally invasive treatment modalities should be considered as the first-line treatment options, while an immediate referral to surgery should be made if the patient exhibits a progressive neurologic deficit or the signs and symptoms of cauda equina syndrome. The relative advantages for surgical decompression include rapid pain relief and functional improvement in those who have failed conservative management.

Evolution of Minimally Invasive Percutaneous Disc Decompression

Traditionally, conventional discectomy has been the gold standard treatment for sciatica refractory to conservative management. With the introduction of surgical microscopes in the 1970s, comparable results could be achieved with "microdiscectomy," which has the advantages of a smaller surgical incision and enhanced operative field view [11].

In the 1960s, three decades after Mixter and Barr's publication, there was once again a paradigm shift, as the field returned to a minimally invasive approach in the treatment of lumbar disc disease. Lyman Smith was the first to perform percutaneous injection of chymopapain (a proteolytic enzyme) for the treatment of unrelenting sciatica, a technique he called chemonucleolysis (CNL) [16]. In 1975, Japanese orthopedic surgeon Hijikata introduced "percutaneous manual nucleotomy," a technique that decompressed a herniated disc by the fenestration of the annulus and the partial resection of the nuclear material [17].

Over time, CNL and percutaneous manual nucleotomy fell out of favor due to fatal enzymatic complications and technical limitations, respectively. However, the desire of clinicians for minimally invasive therapies in the field of spine surgery has continued to lead to breakthroughs in percutaneous intradiscal therapies.

Minimally Invasive Percutaneous Disc Procedures

As one would expect, minimally invasive procedures are associated with smaller surgical scars, rapid convalescence, less postoperative analgesic consumption, lower costs, and less spinal instability. In an updated Cochrane review, Gibson and Waddell concluded that, in general, surgical discectomy procedures are superior to chemonucleolysis and other forms of percutaneous discectomy [11]. However, in several trials, most nonrandomized and uncontrolled, the success rate of percutaneous disc decompression ranged from 50 to 90 % [18–20].

Percutaneous Disc Decompression

The postulated mechanism of indirect decompression techniques entails that the excision or degradation of a portion of the central nucleus results in the reduction of intradiscal pressure and prolapsed disc retraction, thus allowing for indirect nerve decompression and the potential resolution of radicular pain [21].

Understandably, the selection of the appropriate patients with specific disc pathoanatomy would be crucial in a study to obtain successful outcomes with the chosen percutaneous disc decompression technique. Carragee and others have demonstrated that clinical (symptom duration, litigation status), demographic (age), morphometric (disc size and shape evident on MRI/CT scans), and intraoperative (type of disc herniation) variables have prognostic significance in terms of treatment outcomes [22, 23]. Small (<6 mm) and contained disc protrusions (intact outer annulus and posterior longitudinal ligament) are less likely to resorb spontaneously and are associated with fair or worse surgical outcomes after discectomy [22–24]. Individuals with contained disc protrusions may potentially benefit from percutaneous disc decompression. Percutaneous decompression can be accomplished through several techniques, including chemical (chemonucleolysis and ozone), thermal (Radiofrequency Coblation®, Acutherm®, and light amplification by stimulated emission of radiation (laser)), and mechanical (automated percutaneous lumbar discectomy and Dekompressor®) means. However, each technique has its limitations, and the full efficacy of each is unknown due to a paucity of high-quality evidence.

Procedural Anatomy

For any percutaneous disc procedure, access to the intervertebral disc is achieved with an extrapedicular posterolateral approach performed under fluoroscopic guidance (an oblique view) through a triangular working zone known as Kambin's triangle [25]. The exiting nerve root, superior articular process of the facet joint, and superior end plate of the distal vertebra make the three dimensions: more specifically, the hypotenuse, perpendicular, and base, respectively, of Kambin's triangle. Further fluoroscopic maneuvers are performed to access the disc as follows:

1. The target disc is identified via fluoroscopy with an anteroposterior view in which the vertebral end plates are aligned perfectly ("squared off view").
2. An oblique view of the target disc is obtained in which the superior articular process (SAP) of the facet joint of the target segment lies against the midpoint of the intervertebral disc.
3. A puncture point is identified over the target point at the mid-height of the target disc and ventral to the SAP projection. The introducer (trocar) entered in a coaxial fashion at this insertion point should avoid the spinal nerve as the nerve passes superolaterally.

Patient Selection

The radiologic identification of a disc herniation congruent with a patient's history and physical examination is mandatory before the contemplation of a percutaneous disc procedure. Magnetic resonance imaging (MRI) is both sensitive and specific and has been reasonably reliable in the diagnosis of lumbar disc herniation [26]. Additionally, as mentioned above, MRI findings (the size of disc herniation and the containment status of the herniation) have been found to have significant impact on surgical outcomes. In a prospective study by Weiner et al., MRI was found to be 70 % accurate in identifying the containment status of a lumbar disc herniation [27].

The other important prerequisite is the demonstration that a patient's symptoms emanate from the level of the disc proposed to be targeted for decompression. In the case where morphological changes are evident on MRI at multiple disc levels, the culprit level can be determined by the performing of selective nerve root blocks and the identification of the nerve root block that leads to the resolution of pain symptoms. In cases where there are equivocal findings on MRI or a lack of pain relief after selective nerve root block, provocative discography is warranted to find the symptomatic disc and assess its containment [28].

Indications [28]

1. Predominately radicular pain lasting more than 6 months.
2. The failure of conservative treatment.
3. A small contained disc herniation evident on MRI or computed tomography (CT)/discography.
4. The residual disc height of the involved disc is more than 50 % of the original disc height.

Contraindications [28]

In addition to the usual contraindications for any neuraxial intervention (such as systemic infection, local infection, coagulopathy, and patient refusal), contraindications particular to percutaneous disc decompression are as follows:

1. Severe disc degeneration, as evidenced by residual disc height <50 % of the original disc height on imaging
2. Large disc herniation that occupies more than one-third of the spinal canal
3. Extruded or sequestered nucleus pulposus at the proposed level of intervention
4. Previous lumbar back surgery (laminectomy, discectomy, or fusion) at the proposed level of intervention
5. Progressive neurologic deficit
6. Structural deformities such as spondylolisthesis, spinal canal stenosis, scoliosis, tumor, or fracture

Automated percutaneous lumbar discectomy, laser discectomy, Radiofrequency Coblation®, and Disc Dekompressor are the most common percutaneous disc decompression techniques used and are discussed below.

Automated Percutaneous Lumbar Discectomy (APLD)

After "percutaneous manual nucleotomy" fell out of favor and the use of CNL diminished due to adverse effects, refinements in surgical techniques led to the emergence of APLD in 1984. To overcome the inherent limitations of manual nucleotomy with a large cannula (5–8 mm diameter) and the cumbersome manual removal of nucleus pulposus, Onik et al. developed a smaller 2-mm probe with a single side port that potentially reduces the risk of nerve root injury and facilitates the easier removal of tissue with an all-in-one suction cutting device [29].

Procedure

After adequate preparation, the aspiration probe is placed through a 2.5-mm-sized cannula that had been positioned against the annulus over the affected side of the protrusion as outlined above (posterolateral approach under fluoroscopic guidance). The aspiration probe is a sharpened cannula that is pneumatically driven and fitted through an outer needle. Disc fragments are aspirated by the combination of irrigation and suction through an inner cannula connected to a collection bottle. The procedure is discontinued when aspiration ceases to be productive. The patient is then allowed to recover and discharged home on the day of the procedure.

Evidence of Efficacy

Clinical studies have yielded conflicting results about this procedure, and thus its effectiveness is yet to be determined. The initial prospective evaluations and case series reported promising outcomes and had success rates of 75–85 % [18, 30]. However, later randomized trials reported lower success rates of 29–37 % and the inferiority of APLD to techniques such as surgical discectomy and CNL [31, 32], although it should be noted that Revel's study [32] was subsequently criticized for inappropriate patient selection. In their systematic review, Hirsh and coworkers identified four randomized controlled trials and reported there was modest evidence that supported the use of APLD in properly selected patient populations with contained disc herniation [33].

Percutaneous Laser Disc Decompression (PLDD)

The declining popularity of chemonucleolysis and APLD led to the emergence of alternative techniques that employed thermal energy techniques such as laser and radiofrequency nucleotomy. Arguably, the advantage of thermal techniques is that they provide a combination of mechanical decompression and modification of intradiscal biochemical milieu, which can lead to the reduction of neuropathic (radiculopathic) and nociceptive pain, respectively [21, 34].

Procedure

The first clinical application of PLDD occurred in 1986 [35]. Various types of lasers have since been described in the literature, including those with wavelengths close to the infrared region (Nd:YAG, Ho:YAG, and diode lasers) and those with visible green radiation (potassium-titanyl-phosphate (KTP) laser) [36].

The working principle of PLDD is similar to other decompression techniques; access to intervertebral disc is achieved as outlined above except with a smaller diameter needle (18-gauge needle), followed by the introduction of 400-µm optical fiber for transmission of laser energy. The fiber optic channel is often used for visualization (LASE® endoscopic discectomy). If the endoscope is used for visualization, dilators are advanced over the guide needle for the introduction of the endoscope. Different protocols have been reported in the literature in terms of the type of laser, duration of the treatment, and impulsion energy

used to achieve decompression. Gangi and coworkers [37] reported that the application of a 1,064-nm Nd:YAG laser in short pulses of 0.5–1 s with pauses of 4–10 s was effective, while Choy and coworkers [38] reported the use of a 1,064-nm Nd:YAG laser in short pulses of 1 s and pauses of 1 s led to a favorable outcome. As with APLD, the patient is then allowed to recover and discharged home on the day of the procedure.

Evidence of Efficacy

To date, most observational studies on PLDD have reported favorable outcomes. Tassi, Choy, and coworkers reported a success rate of 70–89 % based on the results from multiple centers and approximately 20,000 procedures. The complication rate (complications were mainly discitis) ranged from 0.3 to 1.0 %, and there was a recurrence rate of 4–5 % over a 23-year follow-up period [19]. In a systematic review that encompassed 14 observational studies, Singh and coworkers reported that there was only modest evidence that the use of PLDD led to short- and long-term pain relief and that the procedure had a success rate of 56–87 % [39]. However, the lack of well-designed randomized clinical trials and the methodological weakness of the above studies question the validity of these conclusions.

Radiofrequency Coblation® [Plasma Disc Decompression (PDD)/Nucleoplasty]

PDD is a technique that uses bipolar radiofrequency energy and is based on the principle of the Coblation® (controlled ablation) technology patented by ArthroCare Corp. (Sunnyvale, CA, USA). This technology leads to the formation of a precisely focused plasma field of high-energy ionized particles close to the tip of an RF electrode (SpineWand™) that causes the dissolution and vaporization of nearby nucleus tissue [40]. Compared to laser discectomy (which has a high thermal output), plasma-based disc ablation works at a lower range of temperatures (40–70 °C), which could potentially result in minimal tissue charring and less collateral tissue damage [41].

Procedure

After adequate preparation, the appropriate intervertebral disc is accessed with a 17-gauge obturator stylet through the extrapedicular posterolateral approach mentioned above. A SpineWand™ device is advanced through the introducer needle, and a pathway is established between the anterior and posterior annular margins that establishes the proximal and distal limits of the excursion. Thereafter, Coblation® is commenced and typically consists of six alternative cycles of ablation and coagulation that cause the excavation of the cavity and a volumetric reduction of approximately 1 ml nuclear tissue. During ablation mode, the SpineWand® is advanced. This creates a plasma field and causes a molecular dissociation process that converts the tissue into a gas that exits through the introducer needle. During coagulation mode, the SpineWand® is retracted along the same pathway. This induces collagen shrinkage, which consolidates the ablation process. The patient is then allowed to recover and discharged home on the day of the procedure.

Evidence of Efficacy

Despite the favorable results from preclinical and observational studies in terms of the safety profile and clinical outcomes, the paucity of well-designed methodologically sound clinical trials makes the true efficacy of this modality questionable. Gerges and coworkers reported modest evidence of its efficacy in a pooled analysis of 14 publications (one randomized trial and 13 observational studies) in terms of various outcome measures of pain and function and showed a median percentage of improvement of 62.1 % (range: 6.25–84 %) [42]. It should be noted that the trial that reported the 6.25 % improvement was criticized for inappropriate patient selection, including the inclusion of patients with moderately degenerated discs and noncontained disc herniation [43]. Further, a prospective nonrandomized uncontrolled comparative study reported favorable outcomes in terms of analgesic consumption and degree of disability [44].

Mechanical Disc Decompression

Advancements in automated discectomy led to Dekompressor® (Stryker Corporation, Kalamazoo, MI, USA) being added to the armamentarium of mechanical decompression in 2002. This device is a disposable, battery-operated, handheld rotational motor that is attached to a helical probe. The outer cannula measures 1.5 mm and contains an inner rotating probe. The benefits of Dekompressor include its smaller profile than other devices, the ability to obtain a disc sample for biopsy, and the avoidance of thermal damage to neural structures.

Procedure

The system is deployed into the affected side of the disc of interest through a 17-gauge introducer needle previously positioned under fluoroscopic guidance as mentioned above. When fully advanced, the base of the probe locks onto the hub of the introducer needle in a manner in which at least one full thread length of the probe tip extends beyond the end of the cannula. The probe is activated and advanced slowly ($\approx$1 cm/10 s) under fluoroscopic guidance and draws out tissue based on Archimedes' screw pump principle. Approximately 0.5–2 cc nucleus pulposus is removed. The

patient is then allowed to recover and discharged home on the day of the procedure.

Evidence of Efficacy

Scientific evidence supporting the use of Dekompressor is very limited. Two observational studies and one prospective nonrandomized uncontrolled comparative study have reported favorable outcomes in regard to short- and long-term pain relief [44–46]. A systematic review of percutaneous lumbar mechanical disc decompression with the Dekompressor published in 2009 indicated level III (weak) evidence for Dekompressor having a positive effect on both short- and long-term pain relief due to a lack of high-quality studies [47].

Post-procedural Care [28]

Post-procedural rehabilitation protocols vary according to the type of procedure as follows:

1. Generally, sitting, bending, twisting, and lifting more than 10 lb is limited for the first week or so.
2. Patients may experience flare-ups of back pain, especially after thermal ablation, for several days after the procedure. Analgesics can be prescribed according to patient needs. Patients who experience discomfort at the site of insertion after the local anesthetic wears off may use an ice pack at the insertion site the day of the procedure and warm moist heat the following day.
3. Activity restriction is generally prophylactic in nature to prevent reherniation. The return to activity varies on a case-by-case basis. Many patients resume work and daily activities by 1 week after mechanical disc decompression. The average times to resume activities after a thermal ablation procedure such as laser are as follows:
   (a) Sedentary activity: 1–2 weeks after the procedure
   (b) Light duty: 2–4 weeks, depending upon activity
   (c) Resumption of full duty: 6–10 weeks

Complications

In general, complication rates of the percutaneous disc decompression procedures themselves appear low. The most common complications that follow are due to improper needle placement, a complication that could occur in any intradiscal therapy:

1. Transient paresthesias and the exacerbation of back pain during the first several days post-procedure are the most common complications that require supplemental analgesics.
2. Superficial skin infection.
3. Paraspinal abscess.

4. Discitis.

Potential complications due to intradiscal procedures are:
1. Reflex sympathetic dystrophy or causalgia
2. Vascular injury
3. Abdominal perforation [48]
4. Aseptic spondylodiscitis (presumably from heat damage to a disc or the adjacent vertebral end plate)
5. Cauda equina syndrome [48]
6. Epidural fibrosis after Coblation® [49]
7. Breakage of the probe needle

Conclusion

With innovative refinements in intradiscal techniques and a better understanding of the disease process, minimally invasive techniques for the treatment of lumbar disc herniation associated with lumbar radiculopathy will continue to evolve as a viable alternative to more invasive surgical options in the appropriate clinical setting. As in all of pain medicine, improved patient selection and robust blinded clinical trials are needed to properly evaluate the efficacy of these techniques and establish their place in the paradigm of lower back pain treatment.

In the era of technology-driven surgical techniques in which the field is driven by the notion of "less is more," I believe that endoscopic techniques will be the predominant technique used in future spine procedures. Refinements in endoscopic techniques, in conjunction with further developments in gene therapy and application of biomaterials, may further revolutionize spine procedures and lead to better outcomes.

References

1. Andersson GB. Epidemiological features of chronic low-back pain. Lancet. 1999;354:581–5.
2. Deyo RA, Mirza SK, Martin BI. Back pain prevalence and visit rates: estimates from U.S. National surveys, 2002. Spine (Phila Pa 1976). 2006;31:2724–7.
3. From the Centers for Disease Control and Prevention. Prevalence of disabilities and associated health conditions among adults – United States, 1999. JAMA. 2001;285:1571–2.
4. Manchikanti L, Singh V, Datta S, Cohen SP, Hirsch JA. Comprehensive review of epidemiology, scope, and impact of spinal pain. Pain Physician. 2009;12:E35–70.
5. Martin BI, Turner JA, Mirza SK, Lee MJ, Comstock BA, Deyo RA. Trends in health care expenditures, utilization, and health status among US adults with spine problems, 1997–2006. Spine (Phila Pa 1976). 2009;34:2077–84.
6. Deyo RA, Weinstein JN. Low back pain. N Engl J Med. 2001;344:363–70.
7. Manchikanti L, Boswell MV, Singh V, Benyamin RM, Fellows B, Abdi S, Buenaventura RM, Conn A, Datta S, Derby R, Falco FJ, Erhart S, Diwan S, Hayek SM, Helm S, Parr AT, Schultz DM, Smith HS, Wolfer LR, Hirsch JA. Comprehensive evidence-based guidelines for interventional techniques in the management of chronic spinal pain. Pain Physician. 2009;12:699–802.
8. Schwarzer AC, Aprill CN, Derby R, Fortin J, Kine G, Bogduk N. The prevalence and clinical features of internal disc disruption in patients with chronic low back pain. Spine (Phila Pa 1976). 1995;20:1878–83.
9. Schwarzer AC, Aprill CN, Derby R, Fortin J, Kine G, Bogduk N. Clinical features of patients with pain stemming from the lumbar zygapophysial joints. Is the lumbar facet syndrome a clinical entity? Spine (Phila Pa 1976). 1994;19:1132–7.
10. Maigne JY, Aivaliklis A, Pfefer F. Results of sacroiliac joint double block and value of sacroiliac pain provocation tests in 54 patients with low back pain. Spine (Phila Pa 1976). 1996;21:1889–92.
11. Gibson JN, Waddell G. Surgical interventions for lumbar disc prolapse: updated Cochrane Review. Spine (Phila Pa 1976). 2007;32:1735–47.
12. Parisien RC, Ball PA. William Jason Mixter (1880–1958). Ushering in the "dynasty of the disc". Spine (Phila Pa 1976). 1998;23:2363–6.
13. Saal JA, Saal JS. Nonoperative treatment of herniated lumbar intervertebral disc with radiculopathy. An outcome study. Spine (Phila Pa 1976). 1989;14:431–7.
14. Weber H. Lumbar disc herniation. A controlled, prospective study with ten years of observation. Spine (Phila Pa 1976). 1983;8:131–40.
15. Weinstein JN, Lurie JD, Tosteson TD, Tosteson AN, Blood EA, Abdu WA, Herkowitz H, Hilibrand A, Albert T, Fischgrund J. Surgical versus nonoperative treatment for lumbar disc herniation: four-year results for the Spine Patient Outcomes Research Trial (SPORT). Spine (Phila Pa 1976). 2008;33:2789–800.
16. Raj PP. Intervertebral disc: anatomy-physiology-pathophysiology-treatment. Pain Pract. 2008;8:18–44.
17. Hijikata S. Percutaneous nucleotomy. A new concept technique and 12 years' experience. Clin Orthop Relat Res. 1989;238:9–23.
18. Onik G, Mooney V, Maroon JC, Wiltse L, Helms C, Schweigel J, Watkins R, Kahanovitz N, Day A, Morris J. Automated percutaneous discectomy: a prospective multi-institutional study. Neurosurgery. 1990;26:228–32.
19. Tassi GP, Tassi GP, Choy Daniel SJ, Choy DSJ, Hellinger J, Hellinger J, Hellinger S, Hellinger S, Lee S, Lee SH. Percutaneous laser disc decompression (PLDD): experience and results from multiple centers and 19,880 procedures. AIP Conf Proc. 2010;1226:69–75.
20. Singh V, Piryani C, Liao K. Evaluation of percutaneous disc decompression using coblation in chronic back pain with or without leg pain. Pain Physician. 2003;6:273–80.
21. Hirsch C, Ingelmark BE, Miller M. The anatomical basis for low back pain: studies on the presence of sensory nerve endings in ligamentous, capsular and intervertebral disc structures in the human lumbar spine. Acta Orthop Scand. 1963;33:1–17.
22. Carragee EJ, Kim DH. A prospective analysis of magnetic resonance imaging findings in patients with sciatica and lumbar disc herniation. Correlation of outcomes with disc fragment and canal morphology. Spine (Phila Pa 1976). 1997;22:1650–60.
23. Carragee EJ, Han MY, Suen PW, Kim D. Clinical outcomes after lumbar discectomy for sciatica: the effects of fragment type and anular competence. J Bone Joint Surg Am. 2003;85-A:102–8.
24. Saal JA, Saal JS, Herzog RJ. The natural history of lumbar intervertebral disc extrusions treated nonoperatively. Spine (Phila Pa 1976). 1990;15:683–6.
25. Kambin P, Brager MD. Percutaneous posterolateral discectomy. Anatomy and mechanism. Clin Orthop Relat Res. 1987;223:145–54.
26. Jackson RP, Cain Jr JE, Jacobs RR, Cooper BR, McManus GE. The neuroradiographic diagnosis of lumbar herniated nucleus pulposus: II. A comparison of computed tomography (CT), myelography, CT-myelography, and magnetic resonance imaging. Spine (Phila Pa 1976). 1989;14:1362–7.
27. Weiner BK, Patel R. The accuracy of MRI in the detection of lumbar disc containment. J Orthop Surg Res. 2008;3:46.
28. Pomerantz SR, Hirsch JA. Intradiscal therapies for discogenic pain. Semin Musculoskelet Radiol. 2006;10:125–35.

29. Onik G, Helms CA, Ginsburg L, Hoaglund FT, Morris J. Percutaneous lumbar diskectomy using a new aspiration probe. AJR Am J Roentgenol. 1985;144:1137–40.
30. Davis GW, Onik G, Helms C. Automated percutaneous discectomy. Spine (Phila Pa 1976). 1991;16:359–63.
31. Chatterjee S, Foy PM, Findlay GF. Report of a controlled clinical trial comparing automated percutaneous lumbar discectomy and microdiscectomy in the treatment of contained lumbar disc herniation. Spine (Phila Pa 1976). 1995;20:734–8.
32. Revel M, Payan C, Vallee C, Laredo JD, Lassale B, Roux C, Carter H, Salomon C, Delmas E, Roucoules J. Automated percutaneous lumbar discectomy versus chemonucleolysis in the treatment of sciatica. A randomized multicenter trial. Spine (Phila Pa 1976). 1993;18:1–7.
33. Hirsch JA, Singh V, Falco FJ, Benyamin RM, Manchikanti L. Automated percutaneous lumbar discectomy for the contained herniated lumbar disc: a systematic assessment of evidence. Pain Physician. 2009;12:601–20.
34. O'Neill CW, Liu JJ, Leibenberg E, Hu SS, Deviren V, Tay BK, Chin CT, Lotz JC. Percutaneous plasma decompression alters cytokine expression in injured porcine intervertebral discs. Spine J. 2004;4:88–98.
35. Choy DS, Case RB, Fielding W, Hughes J, Liebler W, Ascher P. Percutaneous laser nucleolysis of lumbar disks. N Engl J Med. 1987;317:771–2.
36. Goupille P, Mulleman D, Mammou S, Griffoul I, Valat JP. Percutaneous laser disc decompression for the treatment of lumbar disc herniation: a review. Semin Arthritis Rheum. 2007;37:20–30.
37. Gangi A, Dietemann JL, Ide C, Brunner P, Klinkert A, Warter JM. Percutaneous laser disk decompression under CT and fluoroscopic guidance: indications, technique, and clinical experience. Radiographics. 1996;16:89–96.
38. Choy DS, Ascher PW, Ranu HS, Saddekni S, Alkaitis D, Liebler W, Hughes J, Diwan S, Altman P. Percutaneous laser disc decompression. A new therapeutic modality. Spine (Phila Pa 1976). 1992;17:949–56.
39. Singh V, Manchikanti L, Benyamin RM, Helm S, Hirsch JA. Percutaneous lumbar laser disc decompression: a systematic review of current evidence. Pain Physician. 2009;12:573–88.
40. Stalder KR, et al. Electrosurgical plasmas. J Phys D Appl Phys. 2005;38(11):1728. Ref type: abstract.
41. Chen YC, Lee SH, Saenz Y, Lehman NL. Histologic findings of disc, end plate and neural elements after coblation of nucleus pulposus: an experimental nucleoplasty study. Spine J. 2003;3:466–70.
42. Gerges FJ, Lipsitz SR, Nedeljkovic SS. A systematic review on the effectiveness of the nucleoplasty procedure for discogenic pain. Pain Physician. 2010;13:117–32.
43. Cohen SP, Williams S, Kurihara C, Griffith S, Larkin TM. Nucleoplasty with or without intradiscal electrothermal therapy (IDET) as a treatment for lumbar herniated disc. J Spinal Disord Tech. 2005;18(suppl):s119–24.
44. Lemcke J, Al-Zain F, Mutze S, Meier U. Minimally invasive spinal surgery using nucleoplasty and the Dekompressor tool: a comparison of two methods in a one year follow-up. Minim Invasive Neurosurg. 2010;53:236–42.
45. Alo KM, Wright RE, Sutcliffe J, Brandt SA. Percutaneous lumbar discectomy: one-year follow-up in an initial cohort of fifty consecutive patients with chronic radicular pain. Pain Pract. 2005;5:116–24.
46. Lierz P, Alo KM, Felleiter P. Percutaneous lumbar discectomy using the Dekompressor system under CT-control. Pain Pract. 2009;9:216–20.
47. Singh V, Benyamin RM, Datta S, Falco FJ, Helm S, Manchikanti L. Systematic review of percutaneous lumbar mechanical disc decompression utilizing Dekompressor. Pain Physician. 2009;12:589–99.
48. Quigley MR. Percutaneous laser discectomy. Neurosurg Clin N Am. 1996;7:37–42.
49. Smuck M, Benny B, Han A, Levin J. Epidural fibrosis following percutaneous disc decompression with coblation technology. Pain Physician. 2007;10:691–6.

The Racz Procedure: Lysis of Epidural Adhesions (Percutaneous Neuroplasty)

50

Gabor B. Racz, Miles R. Day, James E. Heavner, and Jeffrey P. Smith

Key Points

- Back pain and radiculopathy are identifiable by epidurogram and provocative tests (i.e., neural mapping and saline distention).
- Neural mapping is stimulating the nerve roots one by one to the point of paresthesia. Patients inevitably recognize the pain when the appropriate pain-generating nerve root is stimulated.
- Injection target sites for epidural lysis of adhesion procedures is the ventral-lateral epidural space, whereas the injection target site for back pain is the ventral midcanal that is achieved through percutaneous neuroplasty and can be provocated with saline distention.
- The "dural tug" is a provocative clinical test which is performed while the patient is sitting with straight legs on the examination table. The thoracolumbar spine is actively flexed by the patient with the neck in neutral position. At the end of thoracolumbar active range, the cervical spine is passively flexed by the examiner in a rapid manner. This maneuver pulls on the dura and reproduces pain at the site of pathology.
- Physicians who possess three-dimensional procedural skills typically have a shorter duration learning curve for lysis of adhesions and percutaneous neuroplasty which result in improved patient outcomes.

G.B. Racz, M.D., DABIPP, FIPP
4608-15TH Street, Lubbock, TX 79416, USA

Department of Anesthesiology,
Texas Tech University School of Medicine,
Lubbock, TX, USA

International Pain Center,
Texas Tech University Health Sciences Center,
Lubbock, TX, USA
e-mail: enidracz@yahoo.com, paula.brashear@ttuhsc.edu

M.R. Day, M.D., DABIPP, FIPP (✉)
Department of Anesthesiology,
Texas Tech University School of Medicine,
Lubbock, TX, USA

International Pain Center,
Texas Tech University Health Sciences Center,
Lubbock, TX, USA

3601 4th Street, MS: 8182, Lubbock, TX 79430, USA
e-mail: miles.day@ttuhsc.edu

J.E. Heavner, DVM, Ph.D.
Department of Anesthesiology,
Texas Tech University School of Medicine,
Lubbock, TX, USA

Department of Anesthesia, University Medical Center,
3601 4th Streest MS: 8182, Lubbock, TX 79430, USA
e-mail: james.heavner@ttuhsc.edu

J.P. Smith, M.D., MBA
Department of Anesthesiology and Pain Management,
Texas Tech University School of Medicine,
Lubbock, TX, USA

221 Genoa Avenue, Lubbock, TX 79415, USA
e-mail: jeffprestonsmith@gmail.com

Introduction

Back pain is an exceedingly common condition and is often treated with surgery when patients have failed traditional conservative treatment. Despite the best efforts of treating surgeons, these patients are often left with significant postoperative pain, and reoperation or chronic opiate therapy is frequently felt to be the only alternative. A large portion of pain in this patient population is directly attributable to epidural adhesions that prevent normal nerve root movement along with adhesions affecting the ventral epidural structures. Lysis of adhesions is a minimally invasive procedure that was initially developed to spare patients from an additional surgery. Since its inception, the procedure has proved effective for a variety of additional etiologies beyond postsurgical back pain. Through site-specific targeting, lysis of adhesions involves the placement of a catheter in the neuroforamen of the affected nerve root. A fluid foraminotomy is performed when hyaluronidase, local anesthetic, corticosteroid, and hypertonic sodium chloride are injected through the catheter. This releases the nerve root from epidural adhesions and increases neuroforaminal cross-sectional area. Additionally, adhesiolysis opens venous runoff and decompresses high-pressure epidural veins.

Percutaneous neuroplasty via a transforaminal approach evolved from the caudal approach. Lysis of adhesions via the caudal approach involves introducing a catheter through the sacral hiatus and advancing it to the affected nerve root in the ventral-lateral epidural space. On the other hand, transforaminal percutaneous neuroplasty achieves a midline catheter placement in the epidural space that is able to target the two most heavily innervated structures in the spine—the posterior annulus fibrosus and the posterior longitudinal ligament [1]. Apart from a surgical approach, the ventral epidural structures have been otherwise inaccessible.

The benefits of lysis of adhesions and percutaneous neuroplasty have been demonstrated in numerous studies including case series, observational studies, and randomized-controlled trials leading to an evidence rating of "strong" (SORT 1B or 1C) for post–lumbar surgery syndrome in the most recent American Society of Interventional Pain Physicians evidence-based guidelines. In addition to an evidence rating of strong, recommendation was also made that this procedure could be used without reservation in most circumstances.

Adhesiolysis will be used interchangeably with lysis of adhesions and percutaneous neuroplasty throughout the remainder of the chapter.

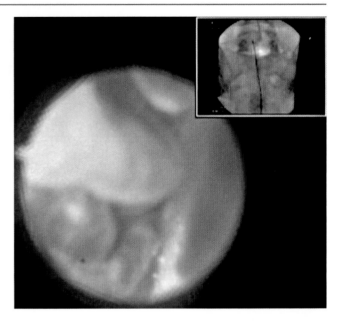

Fig. 50.1 Engorged blood vessels in the epidural cavity as observed during epiduroscopy. Inserted in upper right corner is fluoroscopy showing location for epiduroscopy tip (left anterior border of L5)

[4–7]. While epidural fibrosis itself is not a pain generator, it serves to entrap nerve roots making them more susceptible to compressive forces and tension [8]. For example, Ross et al. [9] correlated extensive peridural scarring with a 3.2-fold increase in recurrent radicular pain.

CPT Codes

There are two current procedural terminology (CPT) codes assigned to adhesiolysis depending on the number of infusions. CPT 62263 is used for a staged three-series infusion over 2–3 days; CPT 62264 denotes a one-time infusion in an outpatient surgery center model.

Low Back Pain and Radiculopathy Secondary to Epidural Adhesions

Kuslich et al. demonstrated that sciatica could only be produced by stimulation of a swollen, stretched, restricted (i.e., scarred), or compressed nerve root [1]. Contrary to all sciatica relating to the nerve root, back pain was found to be the result of multiple tissues—most commonly the posterior longitudinal ligament and the outer layer of the annulus fibrosus. Additionally, Kuslich demonstrated that the facet joint capsule and synovium were rarely indicated as an etiology of back pain [2].

Epidural fibrosis is caused by surgical trauma, annular tears, infection, hematoma, or intrathecal contrast [3]. Its indisputable presence has been demonstrated in many studies

Fluid Foraminotomy

Foraminal stenosis secondary to epidural fibrosis with corresponding nerve root entrapment is frequently evident after an epidurogram and signified by lack of epidural contrast flow at those levels. The lysis procedure effectively serves as a fluid foraminotomy reducing foraminal stenosis caused by epidural fibrosis. In addition to increasing foraminal cross-sectional area, adhesiolysis serves to decompress distended epidural venous structures that may exert compression at nearby spinal levels (Fig. 50.1) and inevitably cause needlestick-related epidural hematomas. Adhesiolysis has led to the development of flexible epiduroscopy that was primarily initiated, pursued, and to this day supported by Dr. James Heavner [10–12].

The Diagnosis of Epidural Fibrosis (Adhesions)

As with any patient, a thorough musculoskeletal and neurologic examination should be performed. In addition to standard dural tension provocative tests, we recommend a provocative test called "dural tug." To perform the test, the patient should be made to sit up with a straight leg, bend forward until their back pain starts to become evident, and rapidly flex the head and neck forward. During this maneuver, the dura is stretched cephalad and if adhered to structures such as the posterior longitudinal ligament, the most heavily innervated spinal canal structure, the movement of the dura will elicit back pain that is localized to the pain generator. The dural tug maneuver is no longer provocative after percutaneous neuroplasty (Fig. 50.2a–e).

Imaging modalities with utility in the diagnosis of epidural fibrosis include MRI, computed tomography (CT), and epiduroscopy; however, the best way to diagnosis epidural fibrosis is through an epidurogram [13–16]. In contrast to MRI or CT, an epidurogram is able to demonstrate filling defects which can be correlated with a patient's symptoms in real time. The sensitivity and specificity of MRI and CT for detecting epidural fibrosis are 50 and 70 %, respectively [17].

Patient Selection

There are many conditions for which the lysis of adhesions procedure may be appropriate for. The most common indication is for neck or back pain and radiculopathy secondary to postsurgical epidural fibrosis. Other indications include disk disruption, metastatic carcinoma of the spine leading to compression fracture, multilevel degenerative spondylosis, spinal stenosis, and pain unresponsive to spinal cord stimulation and spinal opioids [18].

Contraindications

Absolute contraindications to adhesiolysis include sepsis, chronic infection, coagulopathy, local infection at procedure site, syrinx formation, and patient refusal. Although not an absolute contraindication, arachnoiditis poses significant risk when performed by interventional pain physicians with limited experience with adhesiolysis. In arachnoiditis, the risk of loculation and subdural or subarachnoid spread is significantly increased; it is for this reason that we suggest the referral of these patients to a more experienced physician if doubt should arise.

Benefits and Risks

In order to obtain informed consent, risks and benefits should be discussed with the patient prior to performing adhesiolysis. Potential benefits of the procedure include pain relief, increased function, and the possible reversal of neurologic symptoms. Risks include, but are not limited to, bruising, bleeding, infection, reaction to medications used (i.e., hyaluronidase, contrast, local anesthetic, corticosteroids, hypertonic saline), damage to nerves or blood vessels, no or little pain relief, bowel/bladder

incontinence, worsening of pain, and paralysis. In our practice, we have never seen an allergic reaction to hyaluronidase and neither was any reported on a survey of large groups of ophthalmic anesthesiologists in its use with retrobulbar blocks [28]. Additionally, patients with a history of urinary incontinence should have urodynamic evaluation by a urologist before the procedure to document the preexisting urodynamic etiology and pathology.

Anticoagulant Medication

Any medication that prolongs bleeding and/or clotting should be held prior to performing adhesiolysis. We suggest contacting the physician prescribing the anticoagulant prior to holding it for adhesiolysis—typically the patient's primary care physician or cardiologist. We suggest the following times to withhold anticoagulant or antiplatelet medications prior to adhesiolysis: nonsteroidal anti-inflammatory 4 days, aspirin 7–10 days, clopidogrel (Plavix) 7 days, ticlopidine (Ticlid) 10–14 days [19], warfarin (Coumadin) 5 days [18], subcutaneous heparin a minimum of 12 h, and low-molecular-weight heparin 24 h [19]. Nonprescription homeopathic medications that prolong bleeding should also be withheld for approximately 2 weeks. These include fish oil, vitamin E, Gingko biloba, garlic, ginseng, and St. John's wort. We also routinely perform laboratory analysis as close to the day of the procedure as possible. Laboratory studies to ensure adequate coagulation status that we use include a complete blood count, prothrombin time, partial thromboplastin time, and a platelet function assay, or bleeding time.

Preoperative Laboratory Evaluation

In addition to the aforementioned coagulation parameters discussed, each patient should undergo a complete blood count and clean-catch urinalysis to rule out any underlying infection. As with all elective procedures, any abnormal laboratory value should warrant cancellation of adhesiolysis and further workup by the patient's primary care physician.

Technique

Adhesiolysis is most routinely performed in the lumbar and caudal regions of the spine, but can also be performed in the cervical and thoracic regions. This chapter will provide detailed explanation of the caudal and lumbar transforaminal placement of catheters.

Adhesiolysis is performed under strict sterile conditions in the operating room with prophylactic broad-spectrum

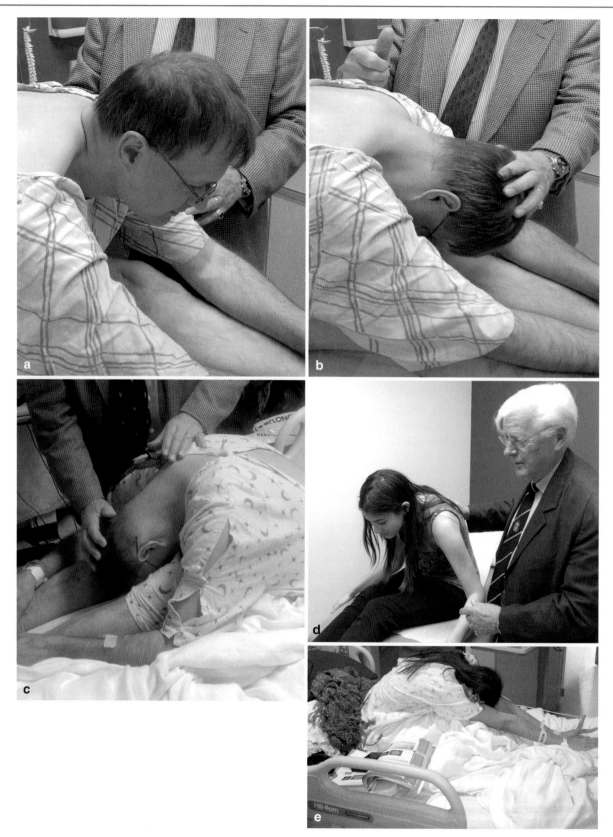

Fig. 50.2 (**a**) The "dural tug" maneuver being performed prior to percutaneous neuroplasty. (**b**) Note pain reproduction prior to full neck flexion secondary to dural adhesions. (**c**) Patient after percutaneous neuroplasty with pain-free neck and back flexion due to treatment of dural adhesions. (**d**) There is decreased spine flexion prior to treatment secondary to dural adhesions. (**e**) After treatment, the same patient demonstrates increased painless flexion of the spine

antibiotics given prior to the procedure and on postoperative day 1. We currently prefer cefazolin 1 g intravenously or clindamycin 600 mg intravenously for those allergic to penicillin. All procedures are performed with an anesthesiologist or nurse anesthetist providing monitored anesthesia care and/or appropriate sedation.

Lysis of Adhesions via a Caudal Catheter

The patient is placed in the prone position on the operating room table. Lumbar lordosis is minimized through the use of pillows placed under the abdomen. The patient's low back and buttocks are sterilely prepped and draped. To begin the procedure, the sacral hiatus is identified through palpation or with AP fluoroscopic guidance. If using palpation, the sacral hiatus can be identified slightly caudal to the sacral cornu and mimics the feel of the area between two knuckles on the dorsum of the hand. A skin wheal should be made approximately 5 cm caudal and 2.5 cm lateral to the sacral hiatus over the contralateral buttock to the targeted nerve root. The distal approach is advocated to reduce the frequency of meningitis by effectively tunneling the catheter. The skin wheal is then superficially punctured with an 18-gauge needle; through the same puncture site, a 15- or 16-gauge RX Coudé 2 needle is inserted and directed toward the sacral hiatus. The RX Coudé 2 is initially advanced at a 45° angle via fluoroscopic guidance or by palpation of sacral hiatus with the left index finger (Figs. 50.3 and 50.4). Once through the sacral hiatus, the needle angle is then dropped to 30° and advanced under lateral fluoroscopic guidance into the caudal epidural space. AP fluoroscopic views should also be obtained to assure midline needle placement which will assist in directing the catheter. The needle should be advanced no further cephalad than the S3 level to prevent inadvertent dural puncture in patients with low-lying dura.

The RX Coudé 2 needle is used as opposed to other needles for several reasons including an angled tip, slightly blunted distal tip, and a non-cutting back edge of the needle opening. The non-cutting back edge of the needle opening allows for catheter manipulation with minimal risk of shearing. Tuohy needles have a cutting back edge of the needle opening which increases the risk of catheter shear.

Once midline in the caudal epidural space, an epidurogram is performed using 10 mL of nonionic, water-soluble contrast. Omnipaque and Isovue are typically the contrast agents of choice and are suitable for myelography. Ionic water-insoluble contrast agents (Hypaque or Renografin) or ionic water-soluble contrast agents (Conray) must never be used. Injection of ionic contrast can result in seizures and death—inspect your contrast agent carefully prior to use. Additionally, aspiration prior to contrast injection should be performed to rule out intravascular or intrathecal injection.

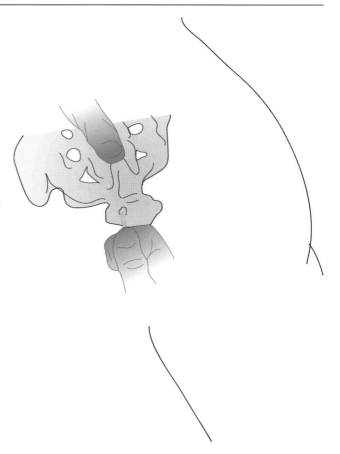

Fig. 50.3 Caudal lysis sequence—first find sacral hiatus and tip of coccyx

Slowly inject the contrast agent and observe for filling defects. A normal epidurogram will have a "Christmas tree" pattern with the central canal being the trunk and the outline of the nerve roots making up the branches. An abnormal epidurogram will have areas where the contrast does not fill (Fig. 50.5). These are the areas of presumed epidural fibrosis and typically correspond to the patient's radicular complaints. If vascular uptake is observed, the needle needs to be redirected.

After turning the distal opening of the needle ventral-lateral, insert a TunL Kath or TunL-XL-24 (stiffer) catheter with a bend on the distal tip through the needle (Fig. 50.6). The bend should be 1 in. from the tip of the catheter and at a 30° angle (Fig. 50.7). The bend will enable the catheter to be steered to the target level. Under continuous AP fluoroscopic guidance, advance the tip of the catheter toward the ventral-lateral epidural space of the desired level (Fig. 50.8). The catheter can be steered by gently twisting the catheter in a clockwise or counterclockwise direction. Avoid "propelling" the tip (i.e., twisting the tip in circles) because this makes it more difficult to direct the catheter. Do not advance the catheter up the middle of the sacrum because this makes guiding the catheter to the ventral-lateral epidural space more difficult. Ideal location of the tip of the catheter in the AP projection is

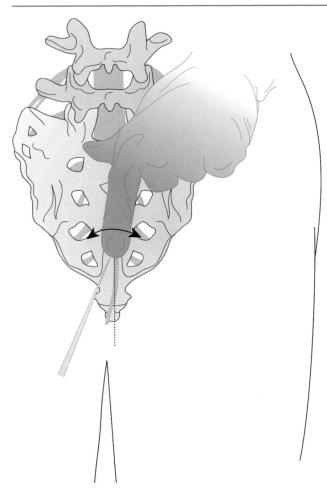

Fig. 50.4 Roll palpating index finger to identify the sacral cornua and thus the target sacral hiatus

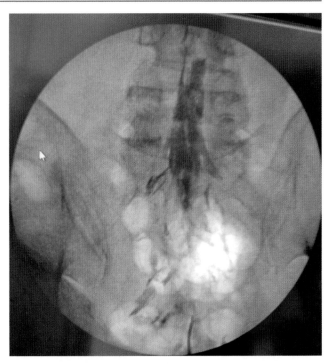

Fig. 50.5 Initial dye injection Omnipaque 240 (10 mL) in a patient with multilevel spinal stenosis showing filling defects bilaterally; pain worse on right side

in the foramen just below the midportion of the pedicle shadow (Figs. 50.9 and 50.10). Check a lateral projection to confirm that the catheter tip is in the ventral epidural space.

Once at the target, inject 2–3 mL of additional contrast through the catheter under real-time fluoroscopy in an attempt to outline the "scarred in" nerve root. If vascular uptake is noted, reposition the catheter and reinject contrast. Preferably, there should not be vascular runoff, but infrequently secondary to venous congestion, an epidural pattern is seen with a small amount of vascular spread. This is acceptable as long as the vascular uptake is venous in nature and not arterial. Extra caution should be taken when injecting the local anesthetic to prevent local anesthetic toxicity. Any arterial spread of contrast always warrants repositioning of the catheter. We have never observed intra-arterial placement in over 25 years of placing soft spring-tipped catheters.

Inject 1,500 U of hyaluronidase dissolved in 10 mL of preservative-free normal saline. A newer development is the use of Hylenex or human-recombinant hyaluronidase, which carries the advantage of a reportedly increased effectiveness at the body's normal pH compared to bovine-recombinant

hyaluronidase [20]. This injection may cause some discomfort, so slow injection is preferable. Observe for "opening up" (i.e., visualization) of the "scarred in" nerve root. A 3-mL test dose of a 10-mL local anesthetic/steroid (LA/S) solution is then given. Our institution used 4 mg of dexamethasone mixed with 9 mL of 0.2 % ropivacaine. Ropivacaine is used instead of bupivacaine for two reasons: the former produces a preferential sensory versus a motor block, and it is less cardiotoxic than a racemic bupivacaine. Doses for other corticosteroids commonly used are 40–80 mg of methylprednisolone (Depo-Medrol), 25–50 mg of triamcinolone diacetate (Aristocort), 40–80 mg of triamcinolone acetonide (Kenalog), and 6–12 mg of betamethasone (Celestone Soluspan). If, after 5 min, there is no evidence of intrathecal or intravascular injection of medication, inject the remaining 7 mL of the LA/S solution. Remove the needle under continuous fluoroscopic guidance to ensure the catheter remains at the target level (Fig. 50.11). Secure the catheter to the skin using nonabsorbable suture and coat the skin puncture site with antimicrobial ointment. Apply a sterile dressing and attach a 0.2-μm filter to the end of the catheter. Affix the exposed portion of the catheter to the patient with tape and transport the patient to the recovery area.

A 20- to 30-min period should elapse between the last injection of the LA/S solution and the start of the hypertonic saline (10 %) infusion. This is necessary to ensure that a subdural injection of the LA/S solution has not occurred. A subdural block mimics a subarachnoid block, but it takes longer to

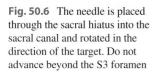

Fig. 50.6 The needle is placed through the sacral hiatus into the sacral canal and rotated in the direction of the target. Do not advance beyond the S3 foramen

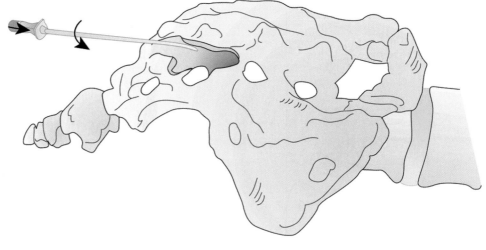

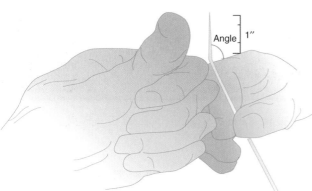

Fig. 50.7 The Epimed Racz catheter is marked for the location of the bend, or use the thumb as reference for the 15° angle bend

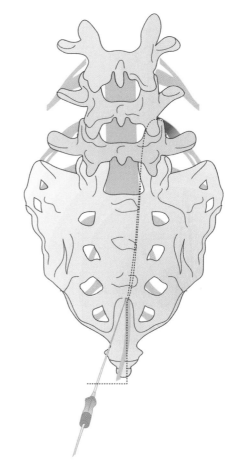

Fig. 50.8 The direction of the catheter is just near the midline, direct the curve under continuous fluoroscopic guidance to the ventral-lateral target site. The needle rotation, as well as the catheter navigation, may need to be used to reach the target

establish, usually 16–18 min. Evidence for subdural or subarachnoid spread is the development of motor block. If the patient develops a subarachnoid or subdural block at any point during the procedure, the catheter should be removed and the remainder of the adhesiolysis canceled. The patient needs to be observed to document the resolution of the motor and sensory block. If no difficulty with the catheter is noted, 10 mL of the hypertonic saline (assuming single catheter placement) is then infused through the catheter over 30 min. If the patient complains of increased pain at any point during the hypertonic saline infusion, the infusion is stopped and an additional 2–3 mL of 0.2 % ropivacaine is injected and the infusion is restarted. Alternatively, 50–75 μg of fentanyl can be injected epidurally in lieu of the local anesthetic. After completion of the hypertonic saline infusion, the catheter is slowly flushed with 2 mL of preservative-free normal saline and the catheter is capped.

Our policy is to admit the patient for 23-h observation status and do a second and a third hypertonic saline infusion the following day. On the day after the procedure, the catheter is twice infused (separated by 4- to 6-h increments) with 10 mL of 0.2 % ropivacaine without steroid and 10 mL of hypertonic saline (10 %). Using the same technique as the first infusion, a 3-mL test dose of ropivacaine 0.2 % is injected. If after 5 min, no signs or symptoms of catheter migration are evident (i.e., motor block), the remaining 7 mL of ropivacaine 0.2 % is injected. An additional 20 min is allowed prior to infusion

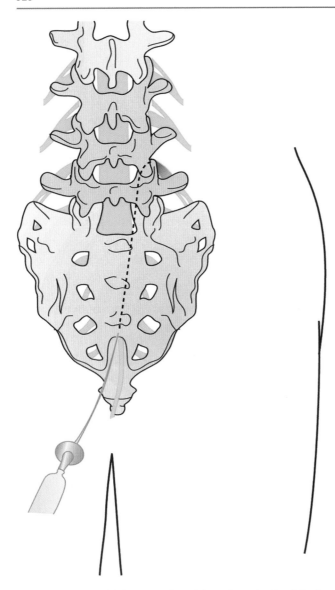

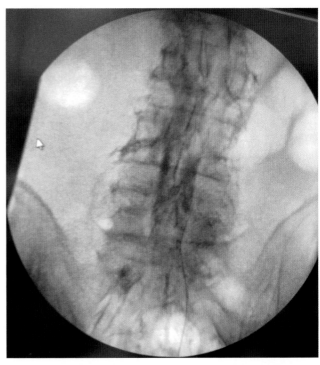

Fig. 50.10 Catheter (24×L) is threaded to right lateral L4 neural foramen

Fig. 50.9 The needle is removed, and the catheter is placed in the ventral-lateral epidural space ventral to the nerve root

of 10 mL of hypertonic saline (10 %) over 30 min. At the end of the third infusion, the catheter is removed, tip inspected for intactness, and a sterile dressing applied. The patient is discharged home with 5 days of oral cephalexin at 500 mg twice a day or oral levofloxacin (Levaquin) at 500 mg once a day for penicillin-allergic patients. Clinic follow-up is in 30 days.

Caudal Lysis of Adhesions Technique Tips

Occasionally, interventional pain physicians with limited experience performing caudal lysis of adhesions may experience difficulty with catheter advancement and placement. It is recognized that there is a learning curve encountered and the following tips are offered. First, the placement of the needle should be such that easy access is gained for the procedure. While this tip seems self-evident, the initial skin

wheal placed for caudal access is extremely important to ensure appropriate needle placement. As previously mentioned, the skin entry site should be approximately 5 cm caudal and 2.5 cm lateral to the sacral hiatus on the opposite buttock of the target. Failure to start at this location results in an angle that makes initial midline catheter advancement difficult. Second, the tip of the needle should be precisely in the midline of the caudal epidural space as viewed on AP fluoroscopic images. Again, off-center needle tip location predisposes the catheter to premature deviation and difficulty with proper advancement. Lastly, take your time when advancing the needle into the caudal epidural space and advancing the catheter. Remember, immediately ventral to the sacrum is the lower abdominal cavity and caution should be taken to prevent inadvertent bowel puncture. Advancing and steering the catheter should be performed slowly and with finesse to ensure an appropriate path to the target.

The initial catheter advancement is near the midline and the steering starts at the S3 level. The most difficulty comes from a catheter going to the lateral sacral wall and bouncing off.

Lysis of Adhesions and Percutaneous Neuroplasty via Transforaminal Catheters

Transforaminal catheters can be used to perform lysis of adhesions for levels difficult to access from the caudal approach or to perform percutaneous neuroplasty. Lysis of

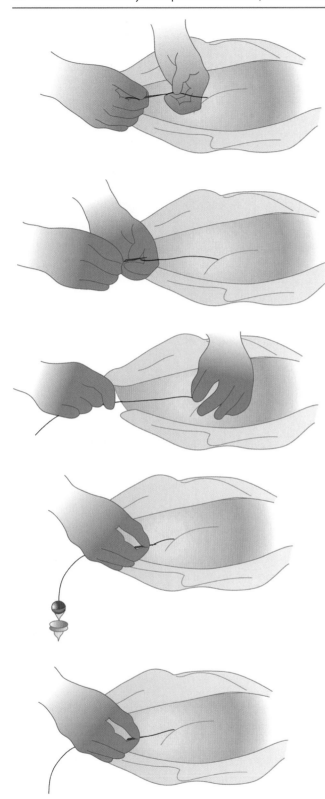

Fig. 50.11 Five picture sequence of removal of the needle to prevent dislodging the catheter from target site before suturing and application of dressing

adhesions is performed when the catheter is placed in the ventral-lateral epidural space and is used to target epidural

fibrosis associated with nerve roots. Percutaneous neuroplasty, on the other hand, is performed when the catheter is advanced from the foramen cephalad into the ventral epidural space. The percutaneous neuroplasty catheter position allows interventions to be directed at pain associated with the posterior annulus fibrosus and/or the posterior longitudinal ligament.

The following steps detail lumbar transforaminal catheter introduction for both lysis of adhesions and percutaneous neuroplasty. After the target level is identified with an AP fluoroscopic image, the superior vertebral end plates are superimposed ("squared off"), which is usually achieved with 15–20° of caudocephalad tilt of the fluoroscope. The fluoroscope is then obliqued approximately 15° to the side of the target and adjusted until the spinous process is rotated to the opposite side. This fluoroscope positioning allows the best visualization of the superior articular process (SAP) that forms the inferoposterior portion of the targeted foramen. The image of the SAP should be superimposed on the shadow of the disk space on the oblique view. The tip of the SAP is the target for the needle placement (Fig. 50.12). Raise a skin wheal slightly lateral to the shadow of the tip of the SAP. Pierce the skin with an 18-gauge needle and then insert a 15- or 16-gauge RX Coudé 2 needle and advance using gun-barrel technique toward the tip of the SAP. Continue to advance the needle medially toward the SAP until the tip contacts bone. Rotate the tip of the needle 180° laterally and advance about 5 mm (Fig. 50.13). Rotate the needle back medially 180° (Fig. 50.14) and place the second protruding stylet. This stylet is designed to prevent nerve root damage as the needle is advanced into the neuroforamen. As the needle is advanced slowly under lateral fluoroscopic guidance, a clear "pop" is felt as the needle penetrates the intertransverse ligament. The tip of the needle should be just past the SAP in the posterior foramen. In the AP plane, insert the catheter slowly into the foramen. Advance catheter to the midcanal position; the catheter tip is between the dura and the posterior longitudinal ligament. Injection of 2 mL of preservative-free saline produces pain on the same side as the catheter tip, indicating this to be the back pain generator (Figs. 50.15, 50.16, and 50.17). The injection of preservative-free normal saline during percutaneous neuroplasty allows reproduction and provocation of the patient's low back pain creating better understanding of its elusive mechanism and helps to point to appropriate therapy.

The target position of the transforaminal catheter for lysis of adhesions should be the ventral-lateral epidural space along the path of the exiting nerve root. The target position of the percutaneous neuroplasty catheter will be slightly cephalad to the level of the foramen of entry and in the midline of the spinal canal as demonstrated on AP fluoroscopic views. Confirm that the catheter is in the anterior epidural space with a lateral image. Anatomically, the catheter is in the foramen

Fig. 50.12 Transforaminal lateral-oblique view. Target the SAP with the advancing RX Coude needle

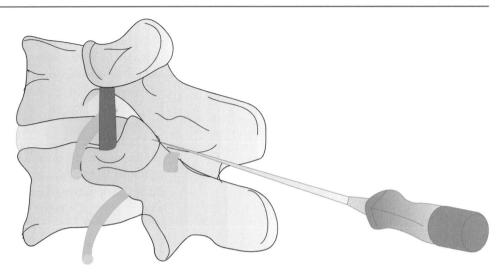

Fig. 50.13 Following bony contact with SAP. Lateral rotation of 180° to allow passage toward the target

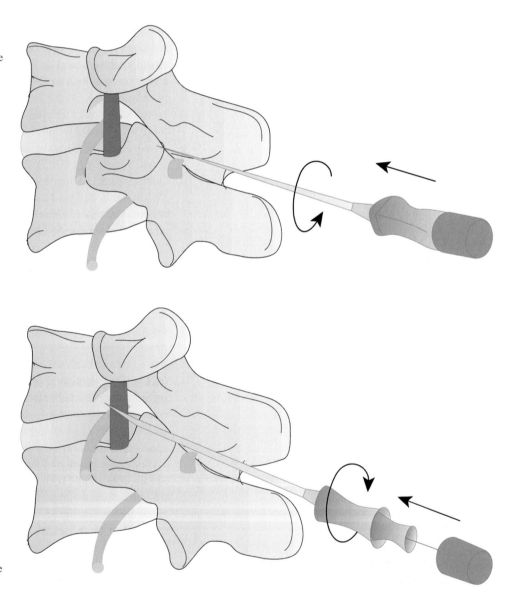

Fig. 50.14 Note the intertransverse ligament. The needle tip with the RX Coude 2 that has 1-mm protruding blunt stylet will pass through the ligament and will be less likely to damage the nerve

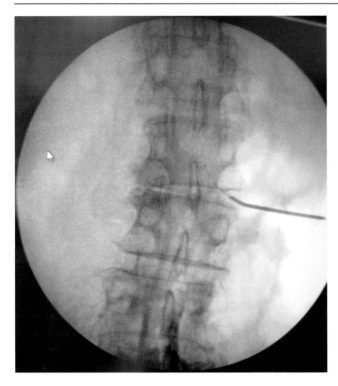

Fig. 50.15 RX Coude 2 needle is navigated around superior pars of L3 in the posterior neuroforamen, and a 24 × L catheter is threaded into the ventral midcanal epidural space

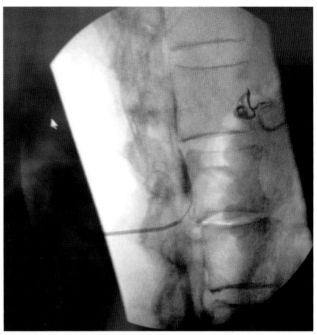

Fig. 50.17 Injection of 5 mL of Omnipaque 240 followed by 5 mL of 750 U of hyaluronidase (bovine compounded) and 5 mL 0.2 % ropivicaine with 20 mg of triamcinolone

too lateral to the foramen. It can also indicate that the foramen is too stenotic to allow passage of the catheter. The needle can be advanced a few millimeters anteriorly in relation to the foramen, and that will also move it slightly medial into the foramen. If the catheter still will not pass, the initial insertion of the needle will need to be more lateral. Therefore, the fluoroscope angle will be about 20° instead of 15°. The curve of the needle usually facilitates easy catheter placement.

Inject 1–2 mL of contrast to confirm epidural spread (Fig. 50.18). When a caudal and a transforaminal catheter are placed, the 1,500 U of hyaluronidase is divided evenly between the two catheters (5 mL of the hyaluronidase/saline solution into each). The LA/S solution is also divided evenly, but a volume of 15 mL (1 mL steroid and 14 mL 0.2 % ropivacaine; of the total volume, 5 mL is transforaminal and 10 mL is caudal) is used instead of 10 mL. Remove the needle under fluoroscopic guidance to make sure the catheter does not move from the original position in the epidural space. Secure and cover the catheter as described previously. The hypertonic saline solution is infused at a volume of 4–5 mL per transforaminal level and 8–10 mL per caudal catheter over 30 min. The hypertonic saline injection volume should always be less than or equal to the local anesthetic volume injected to avoid pain from injection. The second and third infusions should be performed as detailed above in the section "Lysis of Adhesions via a Caudal Catheter" with the adjusted volume of injectate for multiple catheters. It behooves the practitioner to check the position of the transforaminal catheter under fluoroscopy before performing the second and third infusions. The catheter may advance

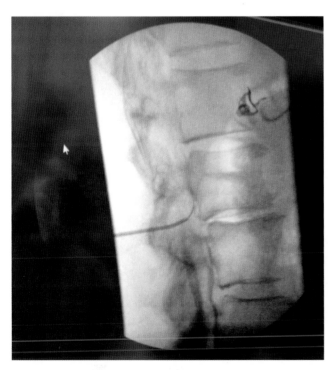

Fig. 50.16 Injection of 2 mL of preservative-free normal saline produces right-sided back pain

above or below the exiting nerve root. If the catheter cannot be advanced, it usually means the needle is either too posterior or

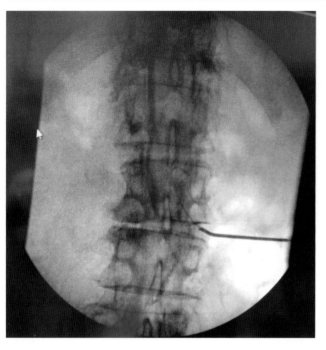

Fig. 50.18 AP view following contrast injection

across the epidural space into the contralateral foramen or paraspinous muscles or more commonly back out of the epidural space into the ipsilateral paraspinous muscles. This results in deposition of the medication in the paravertebral tissue rather than in the epidural space. As with the caudal approach, remove the transforaminal catheter after the third infusion.

Cervical and Thoracic Approaches: Epidural Mapping

Cervical and thoracic approaches to the aforementioned procedures, in addition to epidural mapping, are beyond the scope of this chapter due to chapter length limitations. Recommended reading Intech Article Open Access [21, 22].

Neural Flossing

The protocol for epidural adhesiolysis has been aided by neural flossing exercises that were designed to mobilize nerve roots by "sliding" them in and out of the foramen (Fig. 50.19).

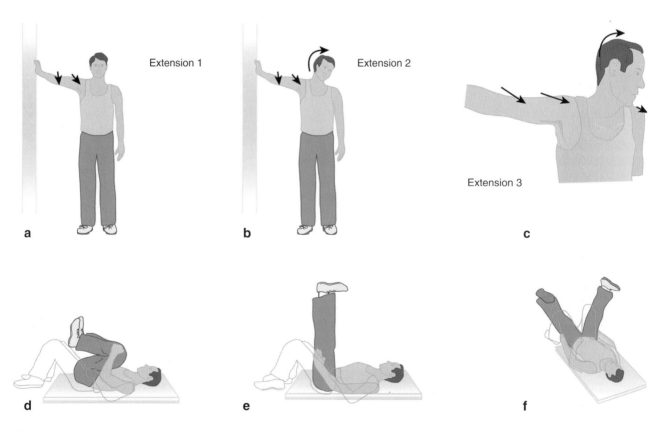

Fig. 50.19 Neural flossing exercises. (**a**) Standing erect, firmly grasp a stable surface (e.g., a door frame) with outstretched arm. Press elbow and shoulder forward. (**b**) Next, slowly tilt head in opposite direction from outstretched arm to achieve gentle tension. (**c**) Finally, rotate chin toward opposite shoulder as is comfortable. Hold this final position for approximately 20–30 s. (**d**) Lay down supine on an exercise mat without a pillow. Slowly bring both knees close to the chest with bent legs, and hold this position for 20 s. Release and assume a neutral position. (**e**) Again in supine position, raise both legs to 90°, with knees straight while lying flat on a firm surface. Hold for 20 s. Assume a neutral position and rest briefly. (**f**) Bring both legs to a 90° angle while lying supine. Slowly spread legs in a V shape, as much as is comfortable, and hold for 20 s

This breaks up weakened scar tissue from the procedure and prevents further scar tissue deposition. If these exercises are done effectively three to four times per day for a few months after the procedure, the formation of scar tissue will be severely restricted.

Complications

As with any invasive procedure, complications are possible. These include bleeding, infection, headache, damage to nerves or blood vessels, catheter shearing, bowel/bladder dysfunction, paralysis, spinal cord compression from loculation of the injected fluids or hematoma, subdural or subarachnoid injection of local anesthetic or hypertonic saline, and reactions to the medications used. We also include on the consent form that the patient may experience an increase in pain or no pain relief at all. Although the potential list of complications is long, the frequency of complications is very rare and the risk decreases significantly with experience performing the procedure.

Subdural spread is a complication that should always be watched for when injecting local anesthetic. During the caudal adhesiolysis, particularly if the catheter is advanced along the midline, subdural catheter placement is a risk (Figs. 50.20 and 50.21). Identification of the subdural motor block should occur within 16–18 min. Catheters used for adhesiolysis should never be directed midline in the epidural space.

Conclusion

Epidural adhesiolysis has evolved over the years as an important treatment option for patients with intractable cervical, thoracic, and low back and leg pain. Studies show that patients are able to enjoy significant pain relief and restoration of function. Manchikanti's studies show that the amount and duration of relief can be achieved by repeat procedures [23]. Recent prospective randomized double-blind studies on failed back surgery and spinal stenosis show 75 and 80 % improvement in visual analog scale scores and functional improvements at 12 months' follow-up [24, 25]. The evolution in the recognition of the site-specific importance of the catheter and medication delivery together with the fact that physicians need to acquire the skills to be able to carry out the procedure led to the improved outcomes seen in recent prospective randomized studies. Contradictory opinion usually originates from physicians who have never done the procedure or have never learned how to navigate the epidural space and quote earlier information that was published along the evolutionary trail.

This is evidenced by the fact that results seen at the Texas Tech International Pain Center surpass even the strongest randomized-controlled trials and may be related to both how the procedure is performed and patient

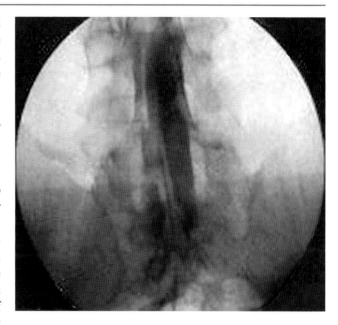

Fig. 50.20 Midline catheter placement enters subdural space. There is also some epidural dye spread. But the patient starts to complain of bilateral leg pain

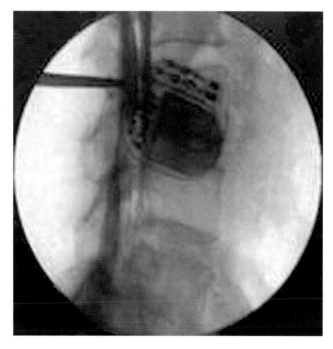

Fig. 50.21 A marker on the skin surface indicates subdural accumulation of contrast. A 22-gauge spinal needle and extension set with syringe was placed in the subdural space, and 12 mL fluid was aspirated (not seen on image). The patient reported immediate reversal of bilateral leg pain

involvement including doing "neural flossing" exercises. This is due to both familiarity with the procedure itself and combining the procedure with aggressive neural flossing exercises. Large numbers of patients have been spared unnecessary surgery or repeat surgery by the use of adhesiolysis and at tremendous cost savings, which is based on the cost-effectiveness studies [26, 27].

Facet pain is commonly encountered approximately 1 month post-adhesiolysis and can be confirmed with provocative testing and diagnostic facet blocks. Radiofrequency facet denervation gives us the best long-term outcome. Recognition of the above has led to the algorithmic thought process where disc- and facet-related therapeutic considerations always follow adhesiolysis. Patients who have undergone both lysis of adhesions and percutaneous neuroplasty experience reduction of pain-related radiculopathy and back pain. Lumbar disc-related procedures are extremely rare in the post-adhesiolysis period as some of the pathology causing back pain and radiculopathy is reversed. Spinal cord stimulation does not preclude the effectiveness of adhesiolysis. Spinal cord stimulation is either more effective following adhesiolysis or, if adhesiolysis is performed post-spinal cord stimulation, is equally effective in achieving enhanced pain relief.

References

1. Kuslich S, Ulstrom C, Michael C. The tissue origin of low back pain and sciatica. Orthop Clin North Am. 1991;22:181–7.
2. Racz G, Noe C, Heavner J. Selective spinal injections for lower back pain. Curr Rev Pain. 1999;3:333–41.
3. Manchikanti L, Staats P, Singh V. Evidence-based practice guidelines for interventional techniques in the management of chronic spinal pain. Pain Phys. 2003;6:3–81.
4. LaRocca H, Macnab I. The laminectomy membrane: studies in it evolution, characteristics, effects and prophylus in dogs. J Bone Joint Surg. 1974;5613:545–50.
5. Cooper R, Freemont A, Hoyland J, et al. Herniated intervertebral disc-associated periradicular fibrosis and vascular abnormalities occur without inflammatory cell infiltration. Spine. 1995;20:591–8.
6. McCarron R, Wimpee M, Hudkins P, et al. The inflammatory effects of nucleus pulposus; a possible element in the pathogenesis of low back pain. Spine. 1987;12:760–4.
7. Parke W, Watanabe R. Adhesions of the ventral lumbar dura: an adjunct source of discogenic pain? Spine. 1990;13:300–3.
8. Straus B. Chronic pain of spinal origin: the costs of intervention. Spine. 2002;27(22):2614–9.
9. Ross J, Robertson J, Frederickson R, et al. Association between peridural scar and recurrent radicular pain after lumbar discectomy; magnetic resonance evaluation. Neurosurgery. 1996;38:855–63.
10. Heavner JE, Chokhavatia S, Kizelshteyn G. Percutaneous evaluation of the epidural and subarachnoid space with a flexible fiberscope. Reg Anesth. 1991;15(1S):85.
11. Bosscher HA, Heavner JE. Incidence and severity of epidural fibrosis after back surgery: an endoscopic study. Pain Pract. 2010;10(1):18–24.
12. Manchikanti L, Pampati V, Bakhit CE, et al. Non-endoscopic and endoscopic adhesiolysis in post-lumbar laminectomy syndrome: a one-year outcome study and cost effectiveness analysis. Pain Phys. 1999;2(3):52–8.
13. Hatten Jr H. Lumbar epidurography with metrizamide. Radiology. 1980;137:129–36.
14. Stewart H, Quinnell R, Dann N. Epidurography in the management of sciatica. Br J Rheumatol. 1987;26(6):424–9.
15. Devulder J, Bogaert L, Castille F, et al. Relevance of epidurography and epidural adhesiolysis in chronic failed back surgery patients. Clin J Pain. 1995;11:147–50.
16. Manchikanti L, Bakhit C, Pampati V. Role of epidurography in caudal neuroplasty. Pain Dig. 1998;8:277–81.
17. Viesca C, Racz G, Day M. Special techniques in pain management: lysis of adhesions. Anesthesiol Clin North Am. 2003;21:745–66.
18. Day M, Racz G. Technique of caudal neuroplasty. Pain Dig. 1999;9(4):255–7.
19. Horlocker T, Wedel D, Benzon H, et al. Regional anesthesia in the anticoagulated patient: defining the risks (the second ASRA consensus conference on neuraxial anesthesia and anticoagulation). Reg Anesth Pain Med. 2003;28:172–97.
20. Racz G, Day M, Heavner J, et al. Hyaluronidase: a review of approved formulations, indications and off-label use in chronic pain management. Expert Opin Biol Ther. 2010;10(1):127–31.
21. Racz GB, Day MR, Heavner JE, et al. 2012. Epidural Lysis of Adhesions and Percutaneous Neuroplasty, Racz GB, Day MR, Heavner JE, Smith JP, Scott J, Noe CE, Nagy L, Ilner H (Ed.), http://www.intechopen.com/books/pain-management-current-issues-and-opinions/epidural-lysis-of-adhesions-and-percutane-ous-neuroplasty
22. Larkin T, Carragee E, Cohen S: A novel technique for delivery of epidural steroids and diagnosing the level of nerve root pathology, J Spinal Disord Tech. 2003;16(2):186–192.
23. Gerdesmeyer L, Lampe R, Veihelmann A, Burgkart R, Göbel M, Gollwitzer H, Wagner K. Chronic radiculopathy. Use of minimally invasive percutaneous epidural neurolysis according to Racz. Schmerz 2005;19:285–295.
24. Manchikanti L, Singh V, Cash KA, Pampati V, Datta S. A comparative effectiveness evaluation of percutaneous adhesiolysis and epidural steroid injections in managing lumbar post surgery syndrome: A randomized, equivalence controlled trial. Pain Physician 2009;12:E355–E368.
25. Manchikanti L, Cash KA, McManus CD, Pampati V, Singh V, Benyamin R. The preliminary results of a comparative effectiveness evaluation of adhesiolysis and caudal epidural injections in managing chronic low back pain secondary to spinal stenosis: A randomized, equivalence controlled trial. Pain Physician 2009;12:E341–E354.
26. Heavner JE, Racz GB, Raj P. Percutaneous epidural neuroplasty: Prospective evaluation of 0.9% NaCl versus 10% NaCl with or without hyaluronidase. Reg Anesth Pain Med. 1999;24:202–207.
27. Matsumoto, Tomikichi. Percutaneous Epidural Neuroplasty Using the Epimed Spring Guide Catheter (100 cases of Failed Back and Neck Surgery Syndrome). Presented at the American Japanese Society.
28. Lecture, Racz GB. Therapeutic and neurolytic blocks for the management of facial pain. Ophthalmic Anesthesia Society 8th Scientific Meeting, San Antonio, Texas. (unpublished).

Sacroiliac Joint Injection and Radiofrequency Denervation

Sunil J. Panchal

Key Points

- Sacroiliac joint pain is often a problem that is mimicking of other conditions which may delay the diagnosis.
- The SI joint as a pain generator is confirmed by appropriate response to fluoroscopically guided local anesthetic injection.
- Treatment of the joint is most commonly performed with injection of steroid by fluoroscopic guidance accompanied by physical medicine.
- Radiofrequency ablation should be considered in recurrent joint pain that is not resolved with steroid injection, physical medicine, and other conservative measures.
- New methods of radiofrequency ablation are evolving, and the physician should be well versed in options to treat this common malady.

Introduction

Sacroiliac (SI) joint pain is an often under-recognized condition affecting a significant number of patients with axial low back pain. Mapping studies have demonstrated that the SI joint can cause radiation of pain to the hip, groin, and posterior leg to the knee. This pattern of pain overlaps that of lumbar facet referral maps and also has been confused by clinicians with sciatica. Studies have demonstrated that historical and physical examination findings and radiological imaging are insufficient to diagnose SI joint pain. Most commonly, the method used to diagnose the SI joint as a pain generator is with fluoroscopic-guided local anesthetic blocks.

S.J. Panchal, M.D.
National Institute of Pain,
4911 Van Dyke Road, Tampa, FL 33558, USA
e-mail: sunilpanchal2000@yahoo.com

Treatment initially consisted of intra-articular steroid injections but has evolved to include radiofrequency denervation, with a variety of techniques that will be discussed in further detail in this chapter.

Anatomy

The sacroiliac (SI) joint is the largest axial joint in the body, with an average surface area of 17.5 cm^2 [1].

There is significant variability in the size, shape, and contour of the SI joint, even from one side versus the other within the same individual [2, 3]. The SI joint is commonly described as a large, auricular-shaped, diarthrodial synovial joint, but only the anterior third of the interface between the sacrum and ilium is a true synovial joint. The rest of the junction is created from a complex set of ligamentous connections. Due to an absent or rudimentary posterior capsule, the SI ligamentous structure is more extensive dorsally and functions as a connecting band between the sacrum and ilia [4]. The primary function of this ligamentous system is to limit motion in all planes of movement. During pregnancy, the ligaments are looser due to elevated levels of relaxin and thus allow the mobility necessary for vaginal delivery [5]. The SI joint is also supported by a network of muscles that create stabilizing forces to the pelvic bones. Some of these muscles, such as the gluteus maximus, piriformis, and biceps femoris, are functionally connected to SI joint ligaments, so their actions can affect joint mobility. The potential for vertical shearing is present in approximately 30 % of SI joints, owing to the more acute angulation of the short, horizontal articular component [6].

Age-related changes in the SI joint begin in puberty and continue throughout life. During adolescence, the iliac surface becomes rougher, duller, and coated in some areas with fibrous plaques. Surface irregularities, crevice formation, fibrillation, and the clumping of chondrocytes manifest in individuals in their 30s and 40s. By the time individuals reach their 60s, motion at the joint may become markedly restricted as the capsule becomes increasingly collagenous and fibrous ankylosis occurs [4].

SI Joint Innervation

The innervation of the SI joint is complex and variable in several reports in the literature. The lateral branches of the L4–S3 dorsal rami are described as composing the major innervation to the posterior SI joint [1]. Some investigators claim that L3 and S4 also contribute to the posterior nerve supply [7, 8]. The anterior joint is innervated by L4–S2 ventral rami [9–12], but some reports include ventral rami from as high as L2. It is important to note that there is significant variability of the posterior lateral branch nerves in regard to location and number in each patient, as well as side to side in the same individual. These nerves vary in regard to the tissue plane, with some directly on bone and others in the soft tissue. This variability will have strong implications in assessing results from denervation techniques. It is also important to understand that nociception in this area may originate from more than the synovial joint. Animal and human cadaver studies have identified nociceptors in the joint capsule and also in the surrounding ligaments [13].

Functional Role of the SI Joint

The SI joints provide stability and are involved in the transmission and dissipation of truncal loads to the lower extremities, limiting x-axis rotation and facilitating parturition. The SI joint rotates about all three axes, approximately 1–2° in each direction [14–16]. Sturesson et al. [17] measured multiple SI joint movements in 25 patients diagnosed with SI joint pain. No differences were found between symptomatic and asymptomatic joints, with the conclusion that three-dimensional motion analysis was not useful for identifying painful SI joints in most patients. However, hypermobility has been associated as a cause of SI joint pain in patients with traumatic instability, multiparity, muscular atrophy, and lower motor neuron disease [18].

Prevalence

The prevalence of LBP emanating from the SI joints has been reported to be as high as 30 %. The methodology of prevalence studies has included either physical examination findings and/or radiological imaging techniques to arrive at a diagnosis of SI joint pain. A retrospective study by Bernard and Kirkaldy-Willis [19] found a 22.5 % prevalence rate in 1,293 adult patients presenting with LBP based predominantly on physical examination. Schwarzer et al. [20] conducted a prevalence study involving 43 consecutive patients with

chronic LBP principally below L5–S1 using fluoroscopically guided SI joint injections. With significant pain relief after LA injection as the sole criterion for diagnosis, the prevalence of SI joint pain was determined to be 30 %. The presence of groin pain was the only referral pattern found to distinguish patients with SI joint pain from those with LBP of non-SI joint origin. Maigne et al. [21] conducted a prevalence study in 54 patients with unilateral LBP using a series of blocks done with different LA based on International Spinal Injection Society guidelines [22]. Nineteen patients had a positive response (≥75 % pain relief) to the lidocaine screening block. Among these patients, 10 (18.5 %) responded with ≥2-h pain relief after the confirmatory block with bupivacaine and were considered to have true SI joint pain (95 % CI, 9–29 %). SI joint injury has previously been described as a combination of axial loading and abrupt rotation. This may result in capsular or synovial disruption, capsular and ligamentous tension, hypomobility or hypermobility, extraneous compression or shearing forces, abnormal joint mechanics, microfractures or macrofractures, chondromalacia, soft tissue injury, and inflammation. The experience of pain in this region from a variety of associated structures is confirmed from studies that demonstrated significant pain relief after both intra-articular and periarticular SI joint injections [23–26]. Risk factors for SI joint pain include leg length discrepancy [27], gait abnormalities [28], prolonged vigorous exercise [29], scoliosis [30], and spinal fusion to the sacrum [31]. Lumbar spine surgery has been associated as well due to SI ligament weakening and/or surgical violation of the joint cavity during iliac graft bone harvest [32] and postsurgical hypermobility [33]. Pregnancy increases risk in women for SI joint pain due to increased weight gain, exaggerated lordotic posture, mechanical trauma of parturition, and hormone-induced ligamental laxity [5, 34]. Inflammation of the SI joints occurs early in all seronegative and HLA-B27-associated spondylarthropathies [35]. In a subset of patients with Reiter's syndrome/reactive arthritis, the disease is due to infection [36]. A retrospective study by Chou et al. [37] assessed the inciting events in 54 patients with injection-confirmed SI joint pain and found that trauma was the cause in 44 % of patients, 35 % were idiopathic, and 21 % were attributed to the cumulative effects of repeated stress. Of the 24 patients who reported trauma as the cause of their pain, the most common events were motor vehicle accidents ($n=13$), falls onto the buttock ($n=6$), and childbirth ($n=3$).

Diagnosis

Many physical examination tests have been promoted as diagnostic tools in patients with presumed SI joint pain [38]. Several involve distraction of the SI joints, such as Patrick's test and Gaenslen's test. However, clinical studies have demonstrated that medical history or physical examination findings are not consistently reliable in identifying dysfunctional SI joints as pain generators [20, 39, 40]. Also, Dreyfuss et al. [41] found 20 % of asymptomatic adults had positive findings on three commonly performed SI joint provocation tests. Provocative SI joint maneuvers and alignment/mobility tests are also unreliable [42–49], but reproducibility has been found to be greater for provocative tests than for mobility and alignment assessments. In the Dreyfuss et al. study [40] conducted in 85 patients with injection-confirmed SI joint pain, there was moderate agreement among clinicians with regard to provocative maneuvers of painful joints but were still found to lack diagnostic utility.

Radiologic studies of patients with SI joint pain have limited benefits as well. Maigne et al. [50] and Slipman et al. [51] found sensitivities of 46 and 13 %, respectively, for the use of radionuclide bone scanning in the identification of SI joint pain. Even though these studies had high specificites (89.5 % for Maigne et al. [50] and 100 % for Slipman et al. [51]), the low sensitivities lead to the conclusion that bone scans are a poor screening test for SI joint pain. Diagnostic injections and symptoms have correlated poorly with CT and radiographic stereophotogrammetry [17, 52]. A retrospective analysis by Elgafy et al. [52] found CT imaging to be 57.5 % sensitive and 69 % specific in diagnosing SI joint pain.

Mapping studies of pain referral patterns from SI joints provide some useful information. Fortin et al. [53] performed provocative SI joint injections using contrast and lidocaine in ten asymptomatic volunteers. Sensory changes were localized to the ipsilateral medial buttock inferior to the posterior superior iliac spine in six of the ten subjects. In two subjects, the area of hyperesthesia extended to the superior aspect of the greater trochanter. The last two subjects experienced sensory changes radiating into the upper thigh. Then in a follow-up study, independent examiners selected 16 individuals among 54 with chronic LBP whose pain diagrams most closely resembled the pain referral patterns obtained in the first study [54]. These 16 patients proceeded to undergo provocative SI joint injections with contrast and LA. All 16 experienced concordant pain during the injection, with 14 obtaining pain relief after deposition of LA. Ten patients reported ≥50 % pain reduction. Six of the 16 patients had ventral capsular tears revealed during arthrography. After the SI joint injections, provocative discography and lumbar facet joint injections were performed in nine patients each. No one had a positive response to either. Slipman et al. [55] conducted a retrospective study to determine the pain referral patterns in 50 patients with injection-confirmed SI joint pain. In contrast to the findings by Fortin et al. [53] and Schwarzer et al. [20], the authors found the most common referral patterns for SI joint pain to be radiation into the buttock (94 %), lower lumbar region (72 %), lower extremity (50 %), groin area (14 %), upper lumbar region (6 %), and abdomen (2 %). Twenty-eight percent of patients experienced pain radiating below their knee, with 12 % reporting foot pain. Based on the existing data, the most consistent factor for identifying patients with SI joint pain is unilateral pain (unless both joints are affected) localized predominantly below the L5 spinous process [20, 40, 53–55].

Diagnostic Blocks

An analgesic response to a properly performed diagnostic block is the most reliable method currently available to confirm SI joint pain. However, there are several factors to take into consideration when interpreting the results of a diagnostic intra-articular local anesthetic block. These factors include a possible placebo response, extravasation of local anesthetic to surrounding pain-generating structures such as muscles, ligaments, and lumbosacral nerve roots. Other factors that may lead to unimpressive responses include inadequate spread of local anesthetic to the anterior and cephalad portions of the SI joint as well as pain from coexisting lumbar facet arthropathy. A pilot study by Fortin et al. [53] attempted to map SI joint referral patterns in asymptomatic volunteers, in which extravasation of contrast (mean volume of 1.6 mL) occurred in 9 of 10 subjects during SI joint injection, with half having at least moderate spread outside the joint. Following injection of local anesthetic, lower extremity numbness occurred in 40 % of the subjects, indicating unintended neural blockade of the lumbosacral nerve roots. In the Maigne et al. [21] study, 3 of the initial 67 patients were excluded because of "sciatic palsy" after the screening block, and another 7 were excluded because penetration of the SI joint was unable to be performed. Others have reported less frequent (≤5 %) failure rates with fluoroscopically guided SI joint injections [20, 40, 56]. More pronounced degenerative changes in the elderly and those with spondylarthropathies may lead to greater technical challenges. CT imaging may be another option for difficult cases [24, 57]. Blind SI joint injections are unreliable as demonstrated by Rosenberg et al. [58] who performed a double-blind study in 37 patients (39 joints) to determine the accuracy of clinically guided SI joint injections using CT imaging for confirmation. The authors found that intra-articular injection was accomplished in only 22 % of patients, whereas sacral foraminal spread occurred 44 % of the time. In three patients, no contrast was seen on CT scanning, indicating likely vascular uptake. In 24 % of injections, contrast extended into the epidural space (Figs. 51.1 and 51.2).

In order to reduce the incidence of false-positives, it is appropriate to consider a series of SI joint blocks. In a prospective study of 67 patients with unilateral LBP, SI joint-compatible referral patterns, and joint tenderness, Maigne et al. [21] investigated the prevalence of SI joint pain using a series of blocks with two different local anesthetics. Of the 54 patients who completed the study, 19 obtained ≥75 % pain relief with the lidocaine screening block. After the confirmatory block with bupivacaine, only 10 of the 19 patients achieved ≥75 % pain relief lasting 2 or more hours, resulting in a prevalence rate of 18.5 %. The false-positive rate of 17 % in this study is less than

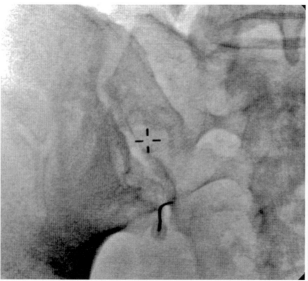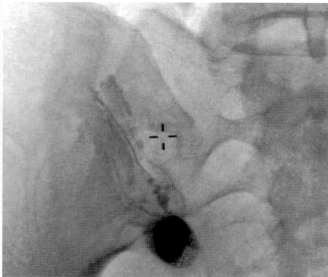

Figs. 51.1 and 51.2 SI Joint intra-articular injection before and after 1-ml nonionic contrast injection

that previously reported for lumbar facet blocks [59]. Since there is not another methodology to serve as a diagnostic "gold standard," we cannot determine the true sensitivity or specificity of intra-articular blocks. However, from a practical standpoint, with a low-risk profile of SI joint blocks, it is appropriate to proceed with this methodology and base treatment plans from the information gleaned. It is important to point out that while a series of blocks to demonstrate a consistent response may represent an ideal, it also incurs increased costs and an increased length of time until the patient is adequately treated.

Treatment

Non-interventional management of SI joint pain may include the use of shoe inserts to address leg length discrepancies as well as physical therapy and osteopathic or chiropractic manipulation to address altered gait mechanics and spine malalignment [60, 61]. However, there are no prospective, controlled studies supporting these modalities. Nonsurgical stabilization programs have been advocated including the application of pelvic belts that reduce the sagittal rotation of presumed incompetent SI joints in pregnant women [62, 63] to exercise-induced pelvic stabilization programs [64]. Ankylosing spondylitis (AS), an inflammatory rheumatic disease with spine and SI joint involvement that manifests as spondylitis and sacroiliitis, has been treated with pharmacologic approaches, but the results are muddled due to systemic involvement and cannot give specific conclusions as to the SI joints.

Intra-articular injections with steroid and LA can serve the dual function of being therapeutic and aiding in diagnosis. It is beneficial to blind the patient to the local anesthetic chosen, use a pain diary to assess the first phase response to local anesthetic, and then assess the second phase response to the anti-inflammatory effect of the steroid. Controlled studies demonstrate good relief for a majority of patients from a single dose of fluoro-guided intra-articular or periarticular steroid 1–2 months after injection, with a limited number of individuals still showing benefit at 3 or 6 months. Prospective observational studies of image-guided SI joint injections to demonstrate good to excellent pain relief lasting from 6 months to 1 year. As with any pharmacologic treatment, the length of duration of response to a single-dose steroid is less of a function of the effectiveness of the drug but rather an issue of how long other factors cause symptomatic inflammation to recur. Therefore, the decision to utilize steroid injections as a long-term treatment plan depends on the interval needed to maintain improvement, quality of relief, and potential adverse effects related to the cumulative dose of corticosteroids.

Radiofrequency Denervation Procedures

Radiofrequency (RF) denervation procedures are utilized to provide prolonged pain relief to patients with injection-confirmed SI joint pain. The techniques used have ranged from denervating the joint by performing intra-articular lesions, lesioning the lateral branches that provide a portion of the SI joint innervation [65–68], to the combination of ligamentous as well as neural RF ablation [69]. All of the techniques described cannot completely denervate the SI joint, and an analysis of the methodology of the techniques is important to place the published success rates in proper perspective as well as provide insight as how to possibly improve results. It is important to remember that percutaneous RF denervation procedures should not be expected to alleviate pain emanating from the ventral SI joint. In one study [20], ventral capsular pathology was shown to account for 69 % of all CT pathology in the 13 patients with a positive response to diagnostic SI joint blocks. Also, nociceptors have been confirmed to exist on the ligamentous tissue and likely need to be addressed as well (Table 51.1).

Table 51.1 Published clinical studies of radiofrequency treatment of sacroiliac joint pain

Author, year	Technique	Study design	N	Treatment	Outcomes	Key details
Ferrante et al. (2001) [68]	Intra-articular	Retrospective	33 (50 joints)	Multiple, 90 °C, 90-s lesions at approx. 1-cm intervals	At 6 months, 36.4 % had >50 % pain relief, average duration of responders was 12 months	Only the postero-inferior joint was lesioned
Cohen and Abdi (2003) [65]	Lateral branch	Retrospective	18 (9 underwent RF)	80 °C, 90-s lesions of L4 and L5 dorsal rami and S1–S3 lateral branches	13/18 had 50 % pain relief from prognostic blocks, 8/9 of RF-treated patients had >50 % pain relief at 9 months	Criteria for RF treatment were >50 % pain relief from prognostic blocks
Yin et al. (2003) [67]	Lateral branch	Retrospective	14	80 °C, 60-s lesions of L5 dorsal ramus and variably the S1–S3 lateral branches	At 6 months, 64 % had >50 % pain relief, 36 % had complete relief	Criteria for RF treatment were >70 % pain relief after 2 separate SI joint deep interosseous ligament injections
Cohen et al. (2009) [79]	Lateral branch	Retrospective	77	80 °C, 90-s lesions of L4 and L5 dorsal rami and S1–S3 lateral branches	At 6 months, 52 % had ≥50 % pain relief	Criteria for RF treatment were >50 % pain relief from intra-articular SI joint block. Limitations include variable technique (conventional and cooled RF treatments)
Burnham and Yasui (2007) [80]	Lateral branch	Prospective	9	3 conventional lesions at L5 and 3 bipolar strip lesions for S1–S3 dorsal rami	67 % success rate at both 6 months and at 12 months	Criteria for RF treatment were >50 % pain relief for both an SI joint block and a prognostic lateral branch block
Cohen et al. (2008) [81]	Lateral branch	Randomized, placebo controlled	28	Conventional lesions at L4 and L5 and cooled probable lesions at S1 and S2, and some at S3 or S4	At 6 months, 57 % had >50 % pain relief, 14 % success at 12 months	Criteria for RF treatment were >75 % pain relief from SI joint block. Only 14 % of control patients had relief at 1 month, none beyond that
Buijs et al. (2004)	Lateral branch	Prospective observational	38 (43 joints)	80 °C, 60-s lesions of S1–S3 lateral branches in all subjects, and L4–L5 dorsal rami in half of subjects	At 12 weeks, complete pain relief at 34.9 % sites and >50 % pain relief at 32.6 % sites	Criteria for RF treatment were >50 % pain relief from SI joint blocks. No difference in outcomes with or without L4 and L5 lesions
Vallejo et al. (2006) [82]	Pulsed RF of lateral branches	Prospective	22	39–42 °C, pulsed RF lesions of L4 and L5 medial branches and S1–S2 lateral branches	16 patients (73 %) had >50 % pain relief for a short time: 6–9 weeks (4 patients), 10–16 weeks (5 patients), 17–32 weeks (7 patients)	Criteria for RF treatment were >75 % pain relief after >2 SI joint injections
Kapural et al. (2008) [83]	Cooled RF	Retrospective case series	26	Lesion at L5 and 2–3 lesions at S1–S3	At 3–4 months, 50 % had >50 % pain relief	Criteria for RF treatment were 2 SI joint blocks with >50 % pain relief
Gevargez et al. (2002) [69]	CT-guided RF lesion of L5 dorsal ramus and posterior interosseous SI ligaments	Prospective observational	38	90 °C, 90-s lesions	At 3 months, 34.2 % were pain-free, 31.6 % reported substantial decrease in pain	Criteria for RF treatment were response to CT-guided SI joint injections

Intra-articular Approach

The first study of RF denervation of the SI joint utilized the intra-articular approach. In this study, 33 patients were treated, some on both sides, for a total of 50 joints. The patients underwent diagnostic SI joint injections to determine eligibility. RF lesions were performed with a bipolar technique with probes placed approximately 1 cm apart and leapfrogged for each lesion. Patients were assessed for VAS scores, pain diagrams, physical exam changes, and change in opioid consumption. A successful result was defined as a ≥50 % decrease in VAS for at least 6 months. With this definition, 36.4 % were considered responders, and in this group, the average duration of response was 12 months and also demonstrated a normalization of SI joint pain provocation tests as well as a reduction in opioid consumption. An in vitro study suggests that success rates could be improved upon by reducing the distance between the cannulae when performing bipolar RF lesions, as spacing the cannulae 4–6 mm apart maximized the surface area of the lesion [70]. Another factor to take into consideration is that when bipolar lesioning is performed, the power output is regulated to maintain the desired temperature at one of the cannulae, and there is often a difference in the temperature achieved at the other cannula, often being 5–10° lower, which also affects the size of the area lesioned. Therefore, monopolar lesions placed closely together may provide a more consistent result.

Lateral Branch Approach

This technique involves lesioning of the L4 and L5 dorsal rami as well as the lateral branches from S1 to S3 (or S4). Studies utilizing this approach have some variability as to the methods and results. Retrospective studies had a range of results including one with 8 of 9 patients with ≥50 % relief after 9 months and another with 64 % of 14 patients achieving >50 % relief at 6 months. A larger retrospective study had 52 % of 77 patients achieve at least 50 % relief at 6 months, but had variability in technique, as conventional as well as cooled RF treatments were included. The prospective studies performed are all very small in size (n=9, 28) and had success rates at 6 months at 67 and 57 %, respectively. Another prospective study reported success rates as high as 70 % in 38 patients, but only reported results at 3 months post-procedure (Fig. 51.3).

Emerging Concepts

Other techniques which have been reported on a limited basis in the literature include a prospective trial in 22 patients of pulsed RF lesions from 39 to 42 °C of the L4 and L5 medial branches and the S1 and S2 lateral branches. A >50 % reduction in pain was achieved in 73 % of patients for a short time. Only seven patients had relief that lasted from 17 to 32 weeks. A

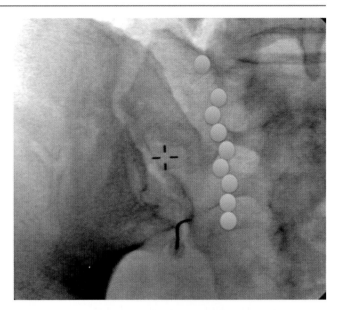

Fig. 51.3 Lesion sites on the sacrum for the lateral branch approach (sites for L5 dorsal rami and lateral branches from S1 to S3 are marked in *blue*)

retrospective case series of 26 patients was reported using cooled RF probes with the theoretical benefit of achieving larger sized lesions. In this study, lesions were performed at L5 and 2–3 lesions at the S1–S3 neuroforamina. This technique had 50 % of the patients achieve ≥50 % relief at 3–4 months posttreatment. There are no other reports to date that have investigated outcome at 6 months or greater. Gervagez et al. [69] utilized CT-guided RF treatment with denervation of the L5 dorsal ramus and the interosseous SI ligaments at three locations in 38 patients. After 3 months, 34.2 % of patients were pain-free, and 31.6 % had a substantial decrease in pain.

Conclusions

The SI joint is a common cause of axial low back pain which may also radiate to the hips, groin, and posteriorly to the knee in up to 30 % of patients. Historical and physical examination findings have limited reliability as tools in the diagnosis of SI joint pain, thus diagnostic blocks remain the most commonly used method for diagnosing this disorder. While there may be debate as to validity of utilizing injections as a diagnostic tool, they are useful as a prognostic tool prior to performing denervation treatments. Intraarticular and periarticular corticosteroid injections have been shown to provide benefit lasting from 1 month to 1 year in patients with and without spondylarthropathy [71–78]. Like any pharmacologic treatment, this is less a function of the duration of action of the corticosteroid but rather a reflection of the variability of recurrence of inflammation. Over the last decade, the emergence of RF denervation techniques has provided a useful option in providing longer lasting relief in patients with SI joint pain. All of the techniques described only partly denervate the SI joint and the surrounding tissue with nociceptors and can be improved upon. The concept of bipolar strip lesioning has been found to require close proximity of probe placement, which at that distance will provide equivalent lesions with monopolar lesioning at the same interval. Future research will need to be done to determine if success rates may be improved upon by utilizing this methodology to more completely denervate both the articular joint as well as the ligamentous nociceptors. This could be promising as responders to this approach have been documented to maintain benefits for at least 1 year. RF lesioning of the lateral branches results in a successful outcome in slightly greater than 50 % of patients, but follow-up has been limited, and longer term studies are needed. Pulsed radiofrequency lesioning has been unimpressive for this indication. The utilization of emerging tools to create larger lesions may simplify the denervation of a large target region but needs to be more fully investigated in regard to safety.

References

1. Bernard TN, Cassidy JD. The sacroiliac syndrome. Pathophysiology, diagnosis and management. In: Frymoyer JW, editor. The adult spine: principles and practice. New York: Raven; 1991. p. 2107–30.
2. Dijkstra PF, Vleeming A, Stoeckart R. Complex motion tomography of the sacroiliac joint: an anatomical and roentgenological study [in German]. Rofo. 1989;150:635–42.
3. Ruch WJ. Atlas of common subluxations of the human spine and pelvis. Boca Raton: CRC Press; 1997.
4. Bowen V, Cassidy JD. Macroscopic and microscopic anatomy of the sacroiliac joint from embryonic life until the eighth decade. Spine. 1981;6:620–8.
5. Berg G, Hammar M, Moller-Nielsen J, et al. Low back pain during pregnancy. Obstet Gynecol. 1988;71:71–5.
6. Mitchell Jr FL. The muscle energy manual, vol. 1. East Lansing: MET Press; 1995.
7. Murata Y, Takahashi K, Yamagata M, et al. Sensory innervation of the sacroiliac joint in rats. Spine. 2000;16:2015–9.
8. Grob KR, Neuhuber WL, Kissling RO. Innervation of the sacroiliac joint in humans [in German]. Z Rheumatol. 1995;54:117–22.
9. Solonen KA. The sacroiliac joint in the light of anatomical, roentgenological and clinical studies. Acta Orthop Scand. 1957;27(suppl):1–27.
10. Ikeda R. Innervation of the sacroiliac joint: macroscopic and histological studies. J Nippon Med Sch. 1991;58:587–96.
11. Fortin JD, Kissling RO, O'Connor BL, Vilensky JA. Sacroiliac joint innervation and pain. Am J Orthop. 1999;28:68–90.
12. Dreyfuss P, Park K, Bogduk N. Do L5 dorsal ramus and S1–4 lateral branch blocks protect the sacroiliac joint from an experimental pain stimulus? A randomized, double-blinded controlled trial. In: Presented at the international spinal injection society 8th annual scientific meeting. San Francisco, 8–10 Sept 2000.
13. Sakamoto N, Yamashita T, Takebayashi T, et al. An electrophysiologic study of mechanoreceptors in the sacroiliac joint and adjacent tissues. Spine. 2001;26:E468–71.
14. Brunner C, Kissling R, Jacob HA. The effects of morphology and histopathologic findings on the mobility of the sacroiliac joint. Spine. 1991;16:1111–7.
15. Egund N, Olsson TH, Schmid H, Selvik G. Movements in the sacroiliac joints demonstrated with roentgen stereophotogrammetric analysis. Acta Radiol Diagn. 1978;19:833–45.
16. Jacob H, Kissling R. The mobility of the sacroiliac joints in healthy volunteers between 20 and 50 years of age. Clin Biomech. 1995;10: 352–61.
17. Sturesson B, Selvik G, Uden A. Movements of the sacroiliac joints: a roentgen stereophotogrammetric analysis. Spine. 1989;14:162–5.
18. Harrison DE, Harrison DD, Troyanovich SJ. The sacroiliac joint: a review of anatomy and biomechanics with clinical implications. J Manipulative Physiol Ther. 1997;20:607–17.
19. Bernard TN, Kirkaldy-Willis WH. Recognizing specific characteristics of nonspecific low back pain. Clin Orthop. 1987;217:266–80.
20. Schwarzer AC, Aprill CN, Bogduk N. The sacroiliac joint in chronic low back pain. Spine. 1995;20:31–7.
21. Maigne JY, Aivaliklis A, Pfefer F. Results of sacroiliac joint double block and value of sacroiliac pain provocation tests in 54 patients with low back pain. Spine. 1996;21:1889–92.
22. Bogduk N. International Spinal Injection Society guidelines for the performance of spinal injection procedures. Part I: zygapophysial joint blocks. Clin J Pain. 1997;13:285–302.
23. Maugars Y, Mathis C, Berthelot JM, Charlier C, Prost A. Assessment of the efficacy of sacroiliac corticosteroid injections in spondyloarthropathies: a double-blind study. Br J Rheumatol. 1996;35:767–70.
24. Braun J, Bollow M, Seyrekbasan F, et al. Computed tomography guided corticosteroid injection of the sacroiliac joint in patients with spondyloarthropathy with sacroiliitis: clinical outcome and follow-up by dynamic magnetic resonance imaging. J Rheumatol. 1996;23:659–64.
25. Luukkainen R, Nissila M, Asikainen E, et al. Periarticular corticosteroid treatment of the sacroiliac joint in patients with seronegative spondyloarthropathy. Clin Exp Rheumatol. 1999;17:88–90.
26. Luukkainen R, Wennerstrand PV, Kautiainen HH, et al. Efficacy of periarticular corticosteroid treatment of the sacroiliac joint in non-spondyloarthropathic patients with chronic low back pain in the region of the sacroiliac joint. Clin Exp Rheumatol. 2002;20:52–4.
27. Schuit D, McPoil TG, Mulesa P. Incidence of sacroiliac joint malalignment in leg length discrepancies. J Am Podiatr Med Assoc. 1989;79:380–3.
28. Herzog W, Conway PJ. Gait analysis of sacroiliac joint patients. J Manipulative Physiol Ther. 1994;17:124–7.
29. Marymont JV, Lynch MA, Henning CE. Exercise-related stress reaction of the sacroiliac joint: an unusual cause of low back pain in athletes. Am J Sports Med. 1986;14:320–3.
30. Schoenberger M, Hellmich K. Sacroiliac dislocation and scoliosis. Hippokrates. 1964;35:476–9.
31. Katz V, Schofferman J, Reynolds J. The sacroiliac joint: a potential cause of pain after lumbar fusion to the sacrum. J Spinal Disord Tech. 2003;16:96–9.
32. Ebraheim NA, Elgafy H, Semaan HB. Computed tomographic findings in patients with persistent sacroiliac pain after posterior iliac graft harvesting. Spine. 2000;25:2047–51.
33. Frymoyer JW, Hanley E, Howe J, et al. Disc excision and spine fusion in the management of lumbar disc disease: a minimum ten-year follow-up. Spine. 1978;3:1–6.
34. Albert H, Godskesen M, Westergaard J. Prognosis in four syndromes of pregnancy-related pelvic pain. Acta Obstet Gynecol Scand. 2001;80:505–10.
35. Bollow M, Braun J, Hamm B. Sacroiliitis: the key symptom of spondylarthropathies. 1. The clinical aspects [in German]. Rofo. 1997;166:95–100.
36. Cush JJ, Lipsky PE. Reiter's syndrome and reactive arthritis. In: Koopman WJ, editor. Arthritis and allied conditions: a textbook of rheumatology, vol. 1. 14th ed. Philadelphia: Lippincott Williams & Wilkins; 2001. p. 1324–44.
37. Chou LH, Slipman CW, Bhagia SM, et al. Inciting events initiating injection-proven sacroiliac joint syndrome. Pain Med. 2004;5:26–32.
38. Cohen SP, Rowlingson J, Abdi S. Low back pain. In: Warfield CA, Bajwa ZA, editors. Principles and practice of pain medicine. 2nd ed. New York: McGraw-Hill; 2004. p. 273–84.

39. Slipman CW, Sterenfeld EB, Chou LH, et al. The predictive value of provocative sacroiliac joint stress maneuvers in the diagnosis of sacroiliac joint syndrome. Arch Phys Med Rehabil. 1998;79:288–92.

40. Dreyfuss P, Michaelsen M, Pauza K, et al. The value of medical history and physical examination in diagnosing sacroiliac joint pain. Spine. 1996;21:2594–602.

41. Dreyfuss P, Dreyer S, Griffin J, et al. Positive sacroiliac screening tests in asymptomatic adults. Spine. 1994;19:1138–43.

42. Laslett M, Williams M. The reliability of selected pain provocation tests for sacroiliac joint pathology. Spine. 1994;19:1243–9.

43. McCombe PF, Fairbank JC, Cockersole BC, Pynsent PB. Reproducibility of physical signs in low-back pain. Spine. 1989;14:908–18.

44. Kokmeyer DJ, Van der Wurff P, Aufdemkampe G, Fickenscher TC. The reliability of multitest regimens with sacroiliac pain provocation tests. J Manipulative Physiol Ther. 2002;25:42–8.

45. Riddle DL, Freburger JK. Evaluation of the presence of sacroiliac joint region dysfunction using a combination of tests: a multicenter intertester reliability study. Phys Ther. 2002;82:772–81.

46. Potter NA, Rothstein JM. Intertester reliability for selected clinical tests of the sacroiliac joint. Phys Ther. 1985;65:1671–5.

47. Freburger JK, Riddle DL. Measurement of sacroiliac joint dysfunction: a multicenter intertester reliability study. Phys Ther. 1999;79:1134–41.

48. Carmichael JP. Inter- and intra-tester reliability of palpation for sacroiliac joint dysfunction. J Manipulative Physiol Ther. 1987;10:164–71.

49. Meijne W, van Neerbos K, Aufdemkampe G, Van der Wurff P. Intraexaminer and interexaminer reliability of the Gillet test. J Manipulative Physiol Ther. 1999;22:4–9.

50. Maigne JY, Boulahdour H, Chatellier G. Value of quantitative radionuclide bone scanning in the diagnosis of sacroiliac joint syndrome in 32 patients with low back pain. Eur Spine J. 1998;7:328–31.

51. Slipman CW, Sterenfeld EB, Chou LH, et al. The value of radionuclide imaging in the diagnosis of sacroiliac joint syndrome. Spine. 1996;21:2251–4.

52. Elgafy H, Semaan HB, Ebraheim NA, Coombs RJ. Computed tomography findings in patients with sacroiliac pain. Clin Orthop. 2001;382:112–8.

53. Fortin JD, Dwyer AP, West S, Pier J. Sacroiliac joint: pain referral maps upon applying a new injection/arthrography technique. Part I: asymptomatic volunteers. Spine. 1994;19:1475–82.

54. Fortin JD, Aprill CN, Ponthieux B, Pier J. Sacroiliac joint: pain referral maps upon applying a new injection/arthrography technique. Part II: clinical evaluation. Spine. 1994;19:1483–9.

55. Slipman CW, Jackson HB, Lipetz JS, et al. Sacroiliac joint pain referral zones. Arch Phys Med Rehabil. 2000;81:334–8.

56. Dussault RG, Kaplan PA, Anderson MW. Fluoroscopy-guided sacroiliac joint injections. Radiology. 2000;214:273–7.

57. Bollow M, Braun J, Taupitz M, et al. CT-guided intraarticular corticosteroid injection into the sacroiliac joints in patients with spondyloarthropathy: indication and follow-up with contrast enhanced MRI. J Comput Assist Tomogr. 1996;20:512–21.

58. Rosenberg JM, Quint DJ, de Rosayro AM. Computerized tomographic localization of clinically-guided sacroiliac joint injections. Clin J Pain. 2000;16:18–21.

59. Schwarzer AC, Aprill CN, Derby R, et al. The false-positive rate of uncontrolled diagnostic blocks of the lumbar zygapophysial joints. Pain. 1994;58:195–200.

60. Cibulka MT, Delitto A. A comparison of two different methods to treat hip pain in runners. J Orthop Sports Phys Ther. 1993;17:172–6.

61. Osterbauer PJ, De Boer KF, Widmaier R, et al. Treatment and biomechanical assessment of patients with chronic sacroiliac joint syndrome. J Manipulative Physiol Ther. 1993;16:82–90.

62. Vleeming A, Buyruk HM, Stoeckart R, et al. An integrated therapy for peripartum pelvic instability: a study of the biomechanical effects of pelvic belts. Am J Obstet Gynecol. 1992;166:1243–7.

63. Damen L, Spoor CW, Snijders CJ, Stam HJ. Does a pelvic belt influence sacroiliac joint laxity? Clin Biomech. 2002;17:495–8.

64. Mooney V, Pozos R, Vleeming A, et al. Exercise treatment for sacroiliac pain. Orthopedics. 2001;24:29–32.

65. Cohen SP, Abdi S. Lateral branch blocks as a treatment for sacroiliac joint pain: a pilot study. Reg Anesth Pain Med. 2003;28:113–9.

66. Buijs EJ, Kamphuis ET, Groen GJ. Radiofrequency treatment of sacroiliac joint-related pain aimed at the first three sacral dorsal rami: a minimal approach. Pain Clin. 2004;16:139–46.

67. Yin W, Willard F, Carreiro J, Dreyfuss P. Sensory stimulation-guided sacroiliac joint radiofrequency neurotomy: technique based on neuroanatomy of the dorsal sacral plexus. Spine. 2003;28:2419–25.

68. Ferrante FM, King LF, Roche EA, et al. Radiofrequency sacroiliac joint denervation for sacroiliac syndrome. Reg Anesth Pain Med. 2001;26:137–42.

69. Gevargez A, Groenemeyer D, Schirp S, Braun M. CT-guided percutaneous radiofrequency denervation of the sacroiliac joint. Eur Radiol. 2002;12:1360–5.

70. Pino CA, Hoeft MA, Hofsess C, et al. Morphologic analysis of bipolar radiofrequency lesions: implications for treatment of the sacroiliac joint. Reg Anesth Pain Med. 2005;30:335–8.

71. Maugars Y, Mathis C, Vilon P, Prost A. Corticosteroid injection of the sacroiliac joint in patients with seronegative spondylarthropathy. Arthritis Rheum. 1992;35:564–8.

72. Gunaydin I, Pereira PL, Daikeler T, et al. Magnetic resonance imaging guided corticosteroid injection of the sacroiliac joints in patients with therapy resistant spondyloarthropathy: a pilot study. J Rheumatol. 2000;27:424–8.

73. Hanly JG, Mitchell M, MacMillan L, et al. Efficacy of sacroiliac corticosteroid injections in patients with inflammatory spondyloarthropathy: results of a 6 month controlled study. J Rheumatol. 2000;27:719–22.

74. Pereira PL, Gunaydin I, Duda SH, et al. Corticosteroid injections of the sacroiliac joint during magnetic resonance: preliminary results [in French]. J Radiol. 2000;81:223–6.

75. Pereira PL, Gunaydin I, Trubenbach J, et al. Interventional MR imaging for injection of sacroiliac joints in patients with sacroiliitis. AJR Am J Roentgenol. 2000;175:265–6.

76. Ojala R, Klemola R, Karppinen J, et al. Sacro-iliac joint arthrography in low back pain: feasibility of MRI guidance. Eur J Radiol. 2001;40:236–9.

77. Karabacakoglu A, Karakose S, Ozerbil OM, Odev K. Fluoroscopy-guided intraarticular corticosteroid injection into the sacroiliac joints in patients with ankylosing spondylitis. Acta Radiol. 2002;43:425–7.

78. Fischer T, Biedermann T, Hermann KG, et al. Sacroiliitis in children with spondyloarthropathy: therapeutic effect of CT guided intra-articular corticosteroid injection [in German]. Rofo. 2003;175:814–21.

79. Cohen SP, Strassels SA, Kurihara C, et al. Outcome predictors for sacroiliac joint (lateral branch) radiofrequency denervation. Reg Anesth Pain Med. 2009;34(3):206–14.

80. Burnham RS, Yasui Y. An alternate method of radiofrequency neurotomy of the sacroiliac joint: a pilot study of the effect on pain, function, and satisfaction. Reg Anesth Pain Med. 2007;32(1):12–9.

81. Cohen SP, Hurley RW, Buckenmaier CC 3rd, et al. Randomized placebo-controlled study evaluating lateral branch radiofrequency denervation for sacroiliac joint pain. Anesthesiology. 2008;109(2):279–88.

82. Vallejo R, Benyamin RM, Kramer J, et al. Pulsed radiofrequency denervation for the treatment of sacroiliac joint syndrome. Pain Med. 2006;7(5):429–34.

83. Kapural L, Nageeb F, Kapural M, et al. Cooled radiofrequency system for the treatment of chronic pain from sacroiliitis: the first case-series. Pain Pract. 2008;8(5):348–54.

Vertebral Augmentation: Vertebroplasty and Kyphoplasty

52

Philip S. Kim

Key Points

- Vertebral compression fractures are a common painful condition of osteoporosis.
- Metastatic disease can also lead to painful compression fractures.
- Although most fractures heal over time, some patients experience pain even with conservative therapy.
- The consequence of vertebral fractures can lead to increased mortality and morbidity.
- The psychosocial consequences of multiple fractures lead to poor self-esteem, depression, social isolation, and, ultimately, a poor quality of life.
- A detailed history and physical imaging evaluation are standard in confirming the diagnosis of acute compression fractures.
- Open surgical fixation is rarely utilized, given the poor quality of bone and anchoring for surgical hardware.
- Advanced age makes most patients poor surgical and anesthesia candidates.
- Percutaneous vertebral augmentation or vertebroplasty can be performed by the injection of cement into fractured trabecular bone to stabilize and relieve pain.
- Kyphoplasty is an alternative approach.

Summary

Vertebral compression fractures are a common painful condition of osteoporosis. Metastatic disease can also lead to painful compression fractures. Although most fractures heal over time, some patients experience pain even with conservative therapy. The consequence of vertebral fractures can lead to increased mortality and morbidity [1]. The psychosocial consequences of multiple fractures lead to poor self-esteem, depression, social isolation, and, ultimately, a poor quality of life [1–3]. A detailed history and physical imaging evaluation are standard in confirming the diagnosis of acute compression fractures. Open surgical fixation is rarely utilized, given the poor quality of bone and anchoring for surgical hardware. Advanced age makes most patients poor surgical and anesthesia candidates. Percutaneous vertebral augmentation or vertebroplasty can be performed by the injection of cement into fractured trabecular bone to stabilize and relieve pain. Kyphoplasty is an alternative approach. A balloon is placed in the compressed fracture to create a cavity where cement is placed to stabilize the fracture and restore vertebral height. Recent randomized studies have suggested limited effectiveness of vertebroplasty over controls [4, 5]. Thus, academic controversy has ensued over these negative results [6–9]. Modifications in the vertebral augmentation has been developed in sacroplasty and technical components of lumbo-thoracic augmentation.

Introduction

Osteoporosis is manifested by low mineral density or by the presence of fragility fractures. The occurrence of an atraumatic vertebral fracture is sufficient enough to establish a diagnosis of osteoporosis. In 1996, the incidence of osteoporotic vertebral compression fractures was 700,000 which surpasses the combined fractures of the ankle and the hip [10]. For several decades, vertebral compression fractures were thought to be benign and self-limited. This view evolved

P.S. Kim, M.D.
Center for Interventional Pain & Spine,
Newark, DE, and Bryn Mawr, PA, USA
e-mail: phshkim@yahoo.com

T.R. Deer et al. (eds.), *Comprehensive Treatment of Chronic Pain by Medical, Interventional, and Integrative Approaches*,
DOI 10.1007/978-1-4614-1560-2_52, © American Academy of Pain Medicine 2013

from at least two-thirds of fractures never being reported by patients to their physicians [11]. If diagnosed, most patients underwent conservative treatment.

Over 90% of patients with metastatic or advanced stage cancer will experience significant pain [12]. Approximately, half of these patients experience bone pain [46]. That is roughly 400,000 US citizens annually. Majority of the metastasis comes from breast, lung, and prostate cancers. Bone metastasis of the spine may lead to significant pain, poor quality of life, and morbidity. Treatments for painful osseous metastases include analgesics, glucocorticoids, radiation, ablative techniques, surgical approaches, and vertebral augmentation.

PMMA (polymethylmethacrylate) has been used in orthopedic treatment and dentistry to fill voids and grout. Specific uses include fixation in total joint arthroplasty. In spine surgery, PMMA has been used to reconstruct defects from open corpectomy and transpedicular application of PMMA to improved screw purchase in osteoporotic bone. The first reported use of percutaneous application of PMMA was performed in 1984 by Galibert and Deramond for C2 hemangioma [13]. The use of modified angioplasty balloon to reduce a vertebral fracture and create a cavity for placement of PMMA was described by Mark Reiley, MD [14]. Over decades, the technique of percutaneous vertebral augmentation has evolved with large-bore needles and modified PMMA.

Other fillers and cement have been proposed beyond PMMA. The concerns of PMMA are the high temperature that rises during the polymerization which can cause tissue damage and the lack of bioactivity [13, 15]. Bioactive composite materials such as calcium phosphate cement and Cortoss have been developed. These cements have varying elastic modulus and compressive strengths. It is thought stiffer cements can lead to increase stress on endplates of adjacent vertebrae, leading to higher fracture rate [16]. An interesting blood-mixed polymethylmethacrylate (PMMA) mechanical study was done to modify properties of PMMA (ahn). This mix was found to have a lower elastic modulus due to the higher porosity, less heating, and ease of placement through the trocar [17].

Pathophysiology and Patient Evaluation

Vertebral compression fractures occur due to weakened bone, causing severe pain and morbidity. These compression fractures are typically induced by osteoporosis, tumors, or traumatic injury. Typically, these fractures occur where load bearing is the greatest. Certain factors and habits which may frequently result in a loss of bone mass frequently may lead to osteoporosis. These factors include women of increased age, lack of calcium and vitamin D in the diet, and the high intake of cigarettes and coffee [18].

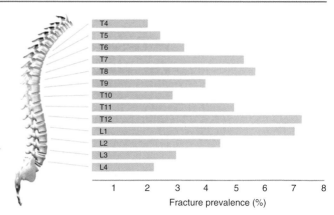

Fig. 52.1 Vertebral compression fractures typically occur spontaneously or as a consequence of minimal trauma, resulting from spinal loading during daily activities such as bending, lifting, and climbing stairs [19]. The most common locations are the midthoracic region (T7–T8) and the thoracolumbar junction

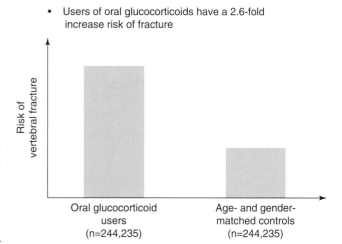

Fig. 52.2 When thoracic kyphosis develops, the midthoracic region receives tremendous load during flexion of the spine leading to potential compression fractures. Secondary contributors to osteoporosis include hypercalcemia, abnormal thyroid, and renal functions [18]. Users of oral glucocorticoids have a 2.6-fold increase risk of fracture

Vertebral compression fractures typically occur spontaneously or as a consequence of minimal trauma, resulting from spinal loading during daily activities such as bending, lifting, and climbing stairs [19]. The most common locations are the midthoracic region (T7–T8) and the thoracolumbar junction (see Fig. 52.1) [19]. These correspond to areas of the spine where there is the greatest burden during these common daily activities. When thoracic kyphosis develops, the midthoracic region receives tremendous load during flexion of the spine leading to potential compression fractures. Secondary contributors to osteoporosis include hypercalcemia, abnormal thyroid, and renal functions [18]. Users of oral glucocorticoids have a 2.6-fold increase risk of fracture (see Fig. 52.2) [20].

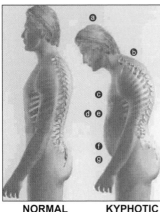

a. Height loss
b. Upright posture becomes impossible
c. Pulmonary volume loss due to anterior wedging of the spine
d. 12 rib rests on the iliac crest
e. Narrowed gab between ribs and ilium
f. Protruding abdomen
g. Distension, constipation, early satiety, eructation

NORMAL   KYPHOTIC

Fig. 52.3 As the spine changes with significant kyphosis, the downward angulation of the ribs leads to the 12th rib resting on the iliac crest. This results in the abdomen protruding and can lead to symptoms of distension, constipation, early satiety, and eructation

Osteolytic metastases and myeloma can cause the destruction of vertebral bodies and fractures, leading to pain and disability. Patients with advanced cancer can present with bone metastases to the vertebral bodies. The incidence of metastatic lesion to the spine depends on the primary cancer: 80% of patients with prostate cancer, 50% with breast cancer, 30% with lung, thyroid, or renal cell cancer [21]. Rarely, benign tumors such as spinal osteoid osteoma and aneurismal bone cysts can lead to instability and painful compression fractures. Vertebral augmentation can be used to reinforce and stabilize fractures related to tumors.

The multiple consequences of vertebral fractures can lead to increased morbidity and mortality. Pain and disability increases with kyphosis and vertebral compression fracture [1]. The physical consequences include pulmonary compromise. Studies suggest that there is decreased lung capacity and reduced pulmonary function with vertebral height loss and decreased lung volume [2]. As the spine changes with significant kyphosis, the downward angulation of the ribs leads to the 12th rib resting on the iliac crest. This results in the abdomen protruding and can lead to symptoms of distension, constipation, early satiety, and eructation (see Fig. 52.3). Above all, the forward position of the thoracic spine leads to strain of the posterior elements of the thoracic spine as the patient attempts to straighten his or her spine.

As seen by the author, the forward expansion of the abdomen leads to forward loading of the lumbar sacral spine, thereby exacerbating discogenic pain. The limited ability of the sacrum to flex and extend may load the sacroiliac joint and cause pain. Weakened physical function can lead to restricted daily activities, resulting in required assistance from family or hired help. The psychosocial consequences of the limitation of activities are seen with their reduced ability to fulfill their accustomed social roles and dependency upon others. This leads to poor self-esteem, depression, and social isolation [1, 3, 22]. There is also increased incidence of sleep disturbances. The number of depressive symptoms rises with the increased number of fractures. Studies reveal high mortality and reduced quality of life years (QALY) with vertebral compression fractures [1].

In addition to a detailed history and examination, imaging evaluations are standard in confirming the diagnosis of acute compression fractures. The radiologic findings on plain films may show subtle height loss changes. Comparison films are helpful to determine acute versus chronic fractures. Unfortunately, occult vertebral fractures are common with false-negative rates of 27–45% by radiologists [23].

MRI is the study of choice with T1 and STIR sagittal sequences. Acute vertebral compression fractures are revealed with marrow edema within the vertebral body. Assessment of spinal canal compromise and fractures of the pedicles is important. CT scan may be a useful alternative combined with a nuclear bone scan when the patient is not a good candidate for MRI. Bone scan may be helpful in fractures greater than 3–4 months in age where there is no marrow edema on MRI.

Treatment Goals

The treatment goals of vertebral compression fractures include pain management, rest, rehabilitation, and restoration of mechanical stability. Pain management usually involves use of opioids and nonsteroidal anti-inflammatories (NSAIDS). Medical management may also include treatments for osteoporosis: calcium, vitamin D, bisphosphonates, or nasal Miacalcin.

Prolong bedrest may allow the compression fracture to stabilize but can lead to fatigue and loss of muscle strength and bone density in elderly patients [24]. Other concerns of patients in prolonged bed rest are pressure sores and deep vein thrombosis in older patients. Back braces may offer support and stabilize the vertebral compression fractures. Limited contact orthoses such as the tri-pad Jewett extension brace are commonly used. Many patients do not tolerate the braces, citing discomfort and difficulty when putting on and removing them. Rehabilitation should be planned to strengthen bone density and increase core strength.

Mechanical instability of vertebral fractures with neurologic compromise is possible. Open surgery such as anterior decompression and stabilization may be needed. Stable, painful compression fractures may be treated by vertebral augmentation either vertebroplasty or kyphoplasty.

The mechanism of pain relief associated with vertebroplasty and kyphoplasty is unknown. Fractured vertebral bodies lose both strength and stiffness. Strength is related to the ability of the vertebral body to bear load, and

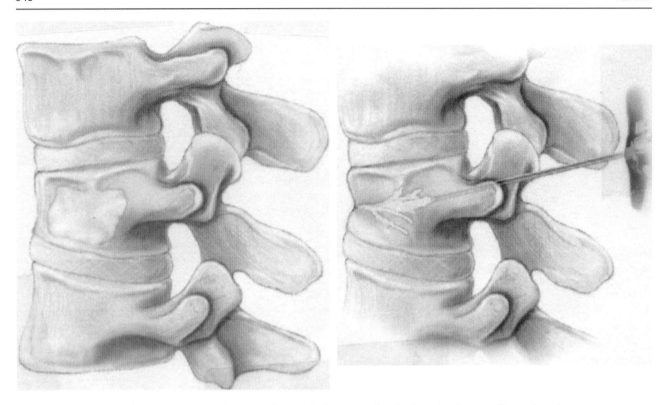

Fig. 52.4 Vertebroplasty is the percutaneous placement of cement in fractured trabecular bone, leading to an "internal cast"

stiffness limits micromotion within the compromised vertebral body. Restoration of stiffness and strength is augmented by placement of PMMA, reducing painful micromotion [25]. Large amounts of cement are needed to restore stiffness and less for strength [25]. Other mechanisms of pain relief may involve the thermal and cytotoxic reaction of PMMA. It has been hypothesized that the heat of polymerization causes thermal necrosis of neural tissue, explaining pain relief in patients. In vivo studies mapping temperatures from polymerization may rise greater than 50 °C leading to potential damage to interosseous nerves, periosteal nerves [26]. Temperature may also play a role in slowing tumor growth and apoptosis in osteoblasts exposed to 48 °C for 10 min or more. The cytotoxicity of PMMA may also have an antitumoral effect and could be potentially neurotoxic [27].

Vertebroplasty is the percutaneous placement of cement in fractured trabecular bone, leading to an "internal cast" [27] (see Fig. 52.4). The standard indication is for painful compression fractures refractory to medical therapy. The typical causes include osteoporosis, metastatic disease, multiple myeloma, and osteonecrosis. The contraindications are systemic and local infection, uncorrectable coagulopathy, retropulsion of vertebral body or tumor, posterior wall destruction, and radicular symptoms. Benefits for the patients are increased range of motion with pain relief. The procedure is typically done under monitored anesthesia care and as an outpatient procedure.

The alternatives are poor. These are conservative medical management, i.e., opioid therapy, physical therapy, bracing, and potential open surgery fixation. The cement is placed through fluoroscopically or CT-guided trocars.

The most common access is the transpedicular approach. Other approaches can be parapedicular, anterolateral (cervical), and posterior (sacral). The complications may include the following: infection, bleeding, pulmonary embolus, local trauma, paralysis, and even death. Fortunately, these complications are rare.

Kyphoplasty has been introduced as an alternative approach [28] (see Fig. 52.5). It is considered a "balloon-assisted vertebroplasty." This procedure involves percutaneous placement of a balloon in the vertebral body. Through the same large-bore needle, bone cement is placed into the cavity created by the balloon. The balloon is intended to restore vertebral body height in addition to creating the cavity.

Three new modifications on lumbo-thoracic augmentations have been reported. Vertebral body stenting is a new method for vertebral augmentation [29]. Once a compression fracture is reduced with a balloon, a vertebral body stent (VBS) is left in place to maintain the reduction and then stabilized with PMMA. This concept comes from peripheral artery stenting seen in interventional cardiac procedures. So far, it is only reported in human cadaveric specimens [29].

Another similar modification is vesselplasty [30]. The purpose is to obtain control of the volume of void created in the vertebral body, prevent the leakage of bone filler material,

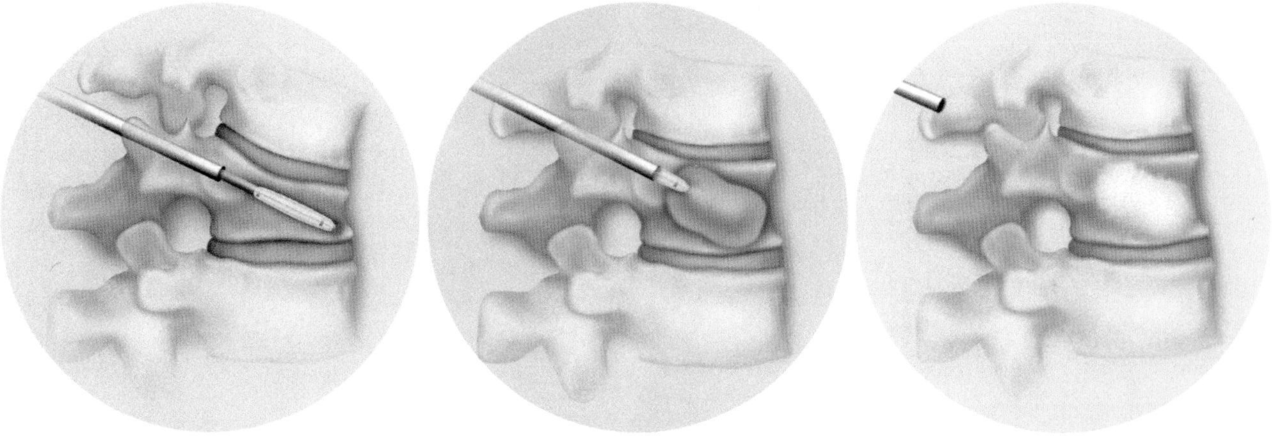

Balloon placement　　　　Cavity within vertebral body　　　　The internal cast

Fig. 52.5 Kyphoplasty has been introduced as an alternative approach [28]

and restore vertebral body height. Vesselplasty was designed by Jerry Lin, chairman of A-Spine Holding Group Corporation (Taipei, Taiwan), and was first performed in 2004 by Darwono [30]. A case series of 29 patients who underwent vesselplasty was performed with significant benefits of pain relief, improved mobility, and no complications [30].

Lordoplasty is a modification of vertebroplasty which has been developed as an alternative technique for the treatment of osteoporotic compression fractures [31]. It is known that percutaneous vertebroplasty is successful in producing pain relief but may not reduce the overloading of the anterior column of the spine and the height of the vertebral body. Kyphoplasty can restore the height and lordosis, but kyphotic angle is limited up to 6–9° due to collapse of height after deflating bone temps [31]. In lordoplasty, the vertebral body above and below the compression fracture is accessed with cannulae (see Fig. 52.6) [31]. Through the cannulae, cement is placed and allowed to harden. The compression fracture is also accessed. The fracture is reduced by ligamentotaxis with a lordosing force applied via the cannula in place and using the facet joints as a fulcrum (Fig. 52.7) [31]. The anterior height is reduced and maintained by a cross bolt. The vertebral fracture is augmented with PMMA. Once the cement hardens, the cannulae are removed (Fig. 52.8) [31]. To date, lordoplasty has been reported with successful case reports [31].

Sacral insufficiency fractures (SIFs) are being identified as a cause of back pain and disability in the elderly population [32]. The mainstay of treatment has been analgesics and physical therapy. Sacroplasty for SIFs evolved from the success of vertebroplasty and kyphoplasty in the treatment of compression fractures of lumbar and thoracic spine. Sacroplasty is the injection of PMMA cement into the fracture zone of the sacral ala with the purpose of pain relief with restoration of mechanical integrity. Using either fluoroscopic and CT guidance, various reported results have been published [32]. A review of

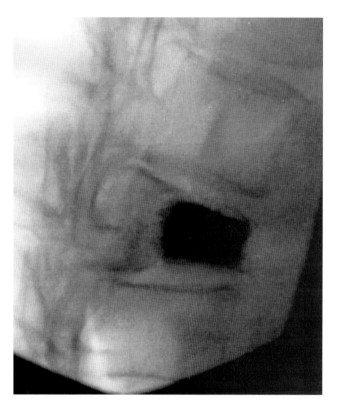

Fig. 52.6 In lordoplasty, the vertebral body above and below the compression fracture is accessed with cannulae

the literature reports a multitude of case reports and one prospective observational cohort study [32].

After reviewing published literature, a position statement on percutaneous vertebral augmentation by American Society of Interventional and Therapeutic Neuroradiology, American Association of Neurological Surgeons/Congress of Neurological Surgeons, and American Society of Spine Radiology has determined that the clinical response rate comparing kyphoplasty and vertebroplasty is similar [28].

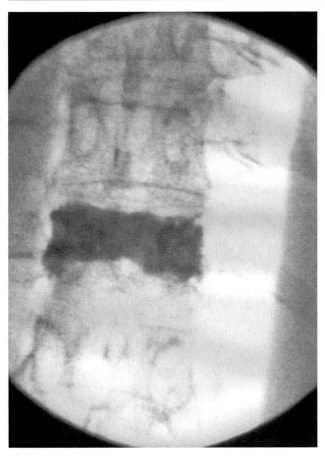

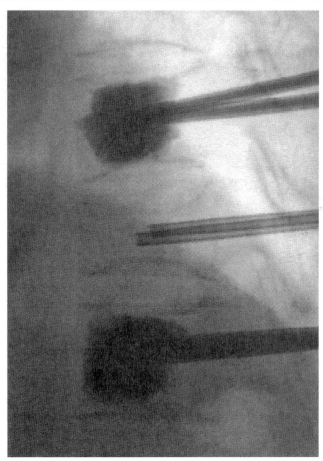

Fig. 52.7 Through the cannulae, cement is placed and allowed to harden. The compression fracture is also accessed. The fracture is reduced by ligamentotaxis with a lordosing force applied via the cannula in place and using the facet joints as a fulcrum

Fig. 52.8 The anterior height is reduced and maintained by a cross bolt. The vertebral fracture is augmented with PMMA. Once the cement hardens, the cannulae are removed

There is no proven advantage of kyphoplasty compared to vertebroplasty in regard to pain relief, height restoration, and complication rate [28].

Technique

Vertebroplasty and kyphoplasty rely on small incisions to place large-bore needles with radiographic guidance with fluoroscopy or CT guidance. These procedures are either done under general anesthesia or monitored anesthesia care. The procedure itself is not painful especially if local anesthesia is placed, but the duration of the procedure and position of the patient may necessitate at least intravenous sedation. Comorbidities such as poor cardiac dysfunction may need to be monitored. In patients with poor medical condition, medical clearance is advised. Anticoagulations are stopped prior to the procedure. Preoperative antibiotics are usually given as with many surgical implants. Sterile surgical preparation and draping are done.

The critical step is to have an understanding and visualization of the fractured vertebra. Poorly osteoporotic bone, especially in large patients, may offer a challenge. Spinal deformities such as scoliosis may hamper proper visualization of the bone landmarks to perform the procedure successfully. If the bone is not visualized with confidence under fluoroscopy, the case should be aborted. CT guidance is then suggested. The landmarks necessary to perform the procedure under fluoroscopy are the pedicles, vertebral bodies, and disc space in the anterior-posterior, lateral, and oblique views. Real-time three-dimensional fluoroscopic guidance using cone beam CT has been proposed to provide better accuracy and results [33]. A stereotactic guidance system using computer tomography is also proposed to improve accuracy and safety of procedure [34].

There are multiple approaches to access the thoracic and lumbar fractures' vertebral body [28]. The most common is posterior transpedicular approach. Bipedicular needles are usually placed at each level. Another approach is the parapedicular. For cervical, the anterolateral view is needed, a similar approach to cervical discography. For sacral fracture, a posterior approach is taken.

This author's approach to lumbar and thoracic fractures is to square the endplates of the fractured vertebral bone on an anterior-posterior view. On the oblique view, the pedicle is identified with clear definition of the medial border. The skin and tissue for the planned entry site are anesthetized with a local anesthetic. The needle will be placed at "eye of the scotty dog" and placed "straight down the barrel." The needle is gently tapped with a hammer staying lateral to the medial edge of the pedicle. Constant visualization of the needle is needed with fluoroscopy to stay away and lateral to the spinal canal. Needle position is usually anterior to the third of vertebral body on lateral view. PMMA is prepared to allow polymerization in a viscous consistency that still allows passage through the needle. This reduces risk of extravasation. Once confirmed in position on the anterior-posterior and lateral views, the prepared PMMA is injected slowly watching its spread within the vertebral body, under constant fluoroscopy. Once the spread is seen heading to the posterior third, the injection is completed (see Figs. 52.9 and 52.10).

Like vertebroplasty, the same approach is taken with kyphoplasty. Once access to the vertebral body is complete, a guide pin is placed where a large-bore (8 gauge) cannula is placed. Through this cannulae, an inflatable bone tamp or balloon is advanced. A bipedicular approach is recommended. Once both balloons are inflated and the fracture is realigned, a cavity is created. This is where PMMA is placed.

Standards and guidelines in the vertebroplasty can be found in the American College of Radiology's "Standards for the Performance of Percutaneous Vertebroplasty" and the Society of Interventional Radiology's "Quality Improvement Guidelines for Percutaneous Vertebroplasty" [35].

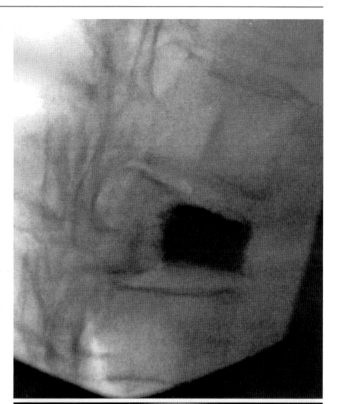

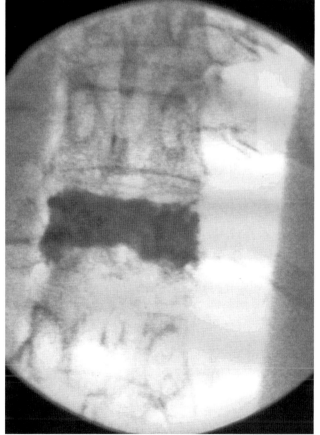

Figs. 52.9 and 52.10 PMMA is prepared to allow polymerization in a viscous consistency that still allows passage through the needle. This reduces risk of extravasation. Once confirmed in position on the ante rior-posterior and lateral views, the prepared PMMA is injected slowly watching its spread within the vertebral body, under constant fluoroscopy. Once the spread is seen heading to the posterior third, the injection is completed

Clinical Research

More than 100 studies have addressed the clinical outcomes of vertebroplasty [28]. The type of studies range from small, retrospective, uncontrolled case series to prospective randomized studies. Literary reviews about the efficacy of vertebroplasty conclude that when used for patients with osteoporotic compression fractures, substantial and immediate pain relief, improved functional status takes place. Minimal short-term complications have been noted. In 2007, there was a position statement on percutaneous vertebral augmentation. This consensus statement, developed by the American Society of Interventional and Therapeutic Neuroradiology, the Society of Interventional Radiology, the American Association of Neurologic Surgeons/Congress of Neurological Surgeons, and the American Society of Spine Radiology, concluded that the evidence supports vertebroplasty as being beneficial for the relief of pain and improved quality of life [28].

An example of a study supporting this statement was published in 2002 by Zoarski et al. In this study, a Musculoskeletal Outcomes Data Evaluation and Management Scale (MODEMS) spinal interventional questionnaire was done [36]. In the study, 30 patients with 54 symptomatic osteoporotic vertebral compression fractures had less than satisfactory response to conventional therapies. On the other hand, significant post-procedure benefits of vertebroplasty were demonstrated in four MODEMS modules: treatment score ($p < .0001$), pain and disability ($p < .0001$), physical function ($p = .0004$), and mental function ($p = .0009$). Long-term follow-up continued for 18 months. At the end of the study, 22 of 23 patients remained satisfied with their outcomes.

A recent prospective of randomized studies, published in the 2009 New England Journal of Medicine, showed that compared to control groups, vertebroplasty offered no proven advantage [4, 5]. The Buchbinder and Kallmes studies showed negative results which directly contradicts 100 of published studies showing positive outcomes. A common initial response to these findings was one of disbelief and surprise. A commentary by North American Spine Society serves to understand and explain the findings. In both studies, there are questions regarding patient selection, enrollment, control group, and outcomes.

Both studies accepted patients with fractures of less than 1 year, and it is known that pain from osteoporotic fractures diminishes over time. It is reasonable to conclude that in 3–6 months, fracture pain reduces naturally and would then be comparable to relief from vertebroplasty. The enrollment of patients was difficult in the Kallmes et al. study. Eighteen hundred and twelve were initially screened, and only 131 entered the study. The pain severity and functional compromise of those patients who refused participation were not reported. Thus, there exists an unquantifiable selection bias in the final patient group.

Both control groups in these studies were not really sham groups. Injection of anesthetic into the facet capsule and/or periosteum may have a beneficial effect in patients with facet mediated pain. Thus, another criticism takes us back to patient selection and outcomes. It is unclear if there was an effort to determine if the back pain originated from the osteoporotic fracture site. With experienced spine care providers, percussion and palpation of the spinous processes are critical to determine the level of maximum tenderness, i.e., painful compression fractures. History, physical examination, and imaging are critical to determine if pain is coming from a compression fracture, stenosis, facet, or degenerative disc.

The controversy of Kallmes and Buckbinder studies still remains. A meta-analysis of the combined individual patient-level data was performed on Kallmes and Buckbinder studies [9]. Powered by subgroup analysis, the two blinded trials of vertobroplasty failed to show advantage of vertebroplasty over placebo. Recent commentary is raised the concern that the reason why the sham-treatment group improved over time is that vertebral compression fractures heal naturally [6, 7]. Additionally, injections with local anesthetics can have long-lasting effect beyond the expected duration of local anesthetic as seen with selective nerve root blocks for lumbar radiculopathy [37]. Other practitioners have consternation and questions on the selection bias and statistical power of the studies [7].

The clinical outcome data for kyphoplasty are not as extensive as vertebroplasty [28]. Lieberman et al. reported in a phase I efficacy study of kyphoplasty in the treatment of painful compression fractures [38]. Thirty patients demonstrated significant improvements in Short Form (SF)-36 bodily pain scales from 11.6 to 58.7 ($p = .0001$). In 2009, a randomized controlled trial comparing nonsurgical treatment of vertebral compressions to balloon kyphoplasty showed the efficacy and safety of the procedure [39]. Three hundred patients were randomly selected to receive kyphoplasty versus nonsurgical treatment. Quality of life measures, SF-36, and safety measurements were taken over 12 months. Mean improvements in SF-36 physical components were seen. The frequency of adverse effects did not differ between groups. There were two serious complications noted (hematoma and urinary tract infection).

Currently, there is no published investigation which has compared vertebroplasty to kyphoplasty. Thus, the 2007 consensus statement on percutaneous vertebral augmentation developed by the American Society of Interventional and Therapeutic Neuroradiology, the Society of Interventional Radiology, the American Association of Neurologic Surgeons/Congress of Neurological Surgeons and the American Society of Spine Radiology concludes that the clinical response to kyphoplasty and vertebroplasty is equivalent [28]. There is no proven advantage in regard to pain relief, vertebral height restoration, or complication rate.

Complications

Vertebroplasty and kyphoplasty have identical complications [40]. With kyphoplasty, there is the reported spinal canal intrusion with the balloon tamp and cortical wall disruption from balloon misplacement. Complications can be divided into medical- and anesthesia-related complications, instrumentation, extravasation of PMMA, and adjacent segment spinal fractures.

Medical and anesthesia complications are uncommon as these minimal invasive procedures have minimal physiologic impact. In patients with severe cardiovascular compromise, laying in the prone position is difficult. Conversely, performing general anesthesia on these patients becomes a greater challenge. Cases of ileus, myocardial infarction, and congestive heart failure have been reported [13]. Careful attention to patient position is paramount as osteoporotic bones have fractured from sternum to ribs. Hemodynamic compromise has been associated with packing of the PMMA during hip replacement surgery. Transient systemic hypotension has been reported with packing cement in vertebroplasty [41].

Instrumentation complications exist from placing needles outside of the pedicles and into the spinal canal [40]. Operator inexperience, poor imaging equipment, and severe spinal deformity are the usual explanations. Uncontrolled bleeding and infection are extremely rare.

The most frequently reported complication is PMMA cement extravasation [40]. PMMA can exit out of any fracture line or cleft and vertebral venous plexus. Using viscous PMMA impregnated with barium, and under high-quality imaging, can reduce the incidence of these problems. The PMMA is injected slowly under live fluoroscopy. Extravasation of cement has flowed into the spinal canal with severe neurologic compromise. The rate of clinically significant leakage has been reported at up to 6% [42]. Higher rates of leakage have been identified when trying to treat fractures related to angiomas and metastatic disease, 2.5–10% [13]. It is likely that cortical destruction and occult fracture lines are to blame. PMMA leakage into the disc space may occur due to undetected fracture cleavage lines. Rates of 0–65% have been reported but most are considered clinically insignificant [13]. Epidural leakage is more of a concern leading to potential cytotoxic and exothermic damage to nerve roots. Liquid PMMA may leak out into the venous system, resulting in a rare case of pulmonary embolus. There is no published report of pulmonary embolus with kyphoplasty. The creation of a void in the vertebral body may compact the cancellous bone, causing it to act as a dam and prevent extravasation of the cement.

An issue of increased risk of fracture at an adjacent level has been raised. Grados et al. found a slight but statistically significant increase in adjacent segment fracture risk in a long-term vertebroplasty follow-up study [42]. It is not known if this is due to placing a hard material, PMMA, in close juxtaposition to the soft, osteoporotic bone of the adjacent vertebral levels. It is also possible that these adjacent fractures represent the natural progression of osteoporosis. Recent study has reviewed risk factors of compression fractures in adjacent vertebrae [43]. It appears lower bone mineral density, a preexisting fracture, a greater restoration rate of vertebral height after vertebroplasty, and intradiscal cement leakage during vertebroplasty are factors for future fracture of adjacent vertebral bodies [43]. On the other hand, another study suggests that percutaneous vertebroplasty is not a risk factor for new osteoporotic compression fractures [44]. VERTOS II is a prospective, multicenter randomized controlled trial comparing percutaneous vertebroplasty with conservative therapy. A total of 202 patients were studied looking at incidence, distribution, and timing of new vertebral compression fractures using spine radiographs [44].

Overall, the complication rates of vertebroplasty and kyphoplasty are reported similar [28]. Six major complications were reported in 531 patients (1.1%) treated with kyphoplasty in a multicenter study [45]. Four of these had neurologic complications. This is similar to the complication of vertebroplasty (1.3%) when used for osteoporotic fractures.

Recommendations and evaluations of complications can be found in the American College of Radiology's "Standards for the Performance of Percutaneous Vertebroplasty" and the Society of Interventional Radiology's "Quality Improvement Guidelines for Percutaneous Vertebroplasty" [35].

Conclusion

Vertebral augmentation with vertebroplasty or kyphoplasty is a medically appropriate treatment for painful vertebral compression fractures refractory to medical therapy [35]. Vertebral compression fractures are common and are often debilitating. Although most fractures heal within a few weeks to months, a minority of patients continue to suffer pain that does not respond to conservative therapy.

Vertebral compression fractures are often a leading cause of admission to nursing and intermediate care facilities. These patients are rarely provided with open surgical fixation due to the poor quality of bone for surgical fixation and the patient's tolerance of the surgery and anesthesia. Percutaneous vertebral augmentation is now an established therapy and should be reimbursed by payors as a safe and effective treatment of compression fractures.

Newer augmentation techniques are now available to treat sacral fractures and sacroplasty. Robotic assistance and alternative imaging may allow even safer placement of needles with reduced radiation exposure [40]. Currently, a number of alternative cements to PMMA are being tested. A number of companies have looked at alternatives to PMMA. A bioresorbable injectable cement called Cordis has been approved by the FDA. This bioactive material closely mimics the mechanical characteristic of bone.

Further clinical studies and econometric analysis are being done to determine the financial impact on society. Further prospective and randomized studies are needed to establish the benefits of vertebroplasty and kyphoplasty over standard conservative treatment.

References

1. Leidig-Bruckner G, et al. Clinical grading of spinal osteoporosis: quality of life components and spinal deformity in women with chronic low back pain and women with vertebral osteoporosis. J Bone Miner Res. 1997;12:663–75.
2. Leech JA, et al. Relationship of lung function to severity of osteoporosis in women. Am Rev Respir Dis. 1990;141:68–71.
3. Silverman SL. The clinical consequences of vertebral compression fracture. Bone. 1992;13 suppl 2:S27–31.
4. Buchbinder R, Osborne RH, Ebeling PR, Wark JD, Mitchell P, Wriedt C, Graves S, Staples MP, Murphy B. A randomized trial of vertebroplasty for painful osteoporotic vertebral fractures. N Engl J Med. 2009;361:557–68.
5. Kallmes DF, Comstock BA, Heagerty PJ, Turner JA, Wilson DJ, Diamond TH, Edwards R, Gray LA, Stout L, Owen S, Hollingworth W, Ghdoke B, Annesley-Williams DJ, Ralston SH, Jarvik JG. A randomized trial of vertebroplasty for osteoporotic spinal fractures. N Engl J Med. 2009;361:569–79.
6. Orr R. Vertebroplasty, cognitive dissonance, and evidence-based medicine: what do we do when the 'evidence' says we are wrong? Cleve Clin J Med. 2010;77:8–11.
7. Bolster M. Consternation and questions about two vertebroplasty trials. Cleve Clin J Med. 2010;77:12–6.
8. Kallmes D, Buchbinder R, Jarvik J, Heagerty P, Comstock B, Turner J, Osborne R. Response to "randomized vertebroplasty trials: bad news or sham news?". AJNR Am J Neuroradiol. 2009;30: 1809–10.
9. Staples MP, Kallmes DF, Comstock BA, Jarvik JG. Effectiveness of vertebroplasty using individual patient data from two randomised placebo controlled trials: meta-analysis. BMJ. 2011;343:d3952.
10. Wasnich U. Vertebral fracture epidemiology. Bone. 1996;18: 1791–6.
11. Nevitt M, et al. The association of radiologically detected vertebral fractures with back pain and function: a prospective study. Ann Intern Med. 1998;128:793–899.
12. Smith H. Painful osseous metastases. Pain Physician. 2011;14: E373–405.
13. Deramond H, et al. Percutaneous vertebroplasty with polymethylmethacrylate: technique, indication, and results. Radiol Clin North Am. 1998;36:533–6.
14. Belkoff S, et al. An ex vivo biomechanical evaluation of an inflatable bone tamp used in the treatment of compression fracture. Spine. 2001;26:151–6.
15. Huang K, Yan J, Lin R. Histopathologic findings of retrieved specimens of vertebroplasty with polymethylmethacrylate cement: case control study. Spine. 2005;30:E585–8.
16. Chevalier Y, Pahr D, Charlebois M, Heini P, Schneider E, Zysset P. Cement distribution, volume, and compliance in vertebroplasty: some answers from an anatomy-based nonlinear finite element study. Spine (Phila Pa 1976). 2008;33:1722–30.
17. Ahn SH, Lee S, Choi D, et al. Mechanical properties of blood-mixed polymethylmethacrylate in percutaneous vertebroplasty. Asian Spine J. 2009;3:45–52.
18. Tannenbaum C, et al. Yield of laboratory testing to identify secondary contributors to osteoporosis in otherwise healthy women. J Clin Endocrinol Metab. 2002;87:4431–7.
19. Cooper C, et al. Incidence of clinically diagnosed vertebral fractures: a population-based study in Rochester, Minnesota, 1985–1989. J Bone Miner Res. 1992;7:221–7.
20. Van-staa T, et al. Use of oral corticosteroids and risk of fractures. J Bone Miner Res. 2000;20:1487–94.
21. Malawer M, et al. Treatment of metastatic cancer to bone. In: DeVita V, Hellman S, Rosenberg S, editors. Principles and practice of oncology. 8th ed. Philadelphia: JB Lippincott; 1989. p. 2298–317.
22. Gold DT. The clinical impact of vertebral fractures: quality of life in women with osteoporosis. Bone. 1996;18:185S–9.
23. Group: T.E.P.O.S.E. J Bone Miner Res. 2002; 17:2214–21.
24. Babayev M, et al. The controversy surrounding sacral insufficiency fractures: to ambulate or not to ambulate? Am J Phys Med Rehabil. 2000;79:404–9.
25. Belkoff S, et al. Biomechanical evaluation of a new bone cement for use in vertebroplasty. Spine. 2000;25:1061–4.
26. Riggs B, et al. The worldwide problem of osteoporosis: insights afforded by epidemiology. Bone. 1995;17:505S–11.
27. Jensen ME, et al. Percutaneous polymethylmethacrylate vertebroplasty in the treatment of osteoporotic vertebral body compression fractures: technical aspects. AJNR Am J Neuroradiol. 1997;18: 1897–904.
28. Jensen ME, et al. Position statement on percutaneous vertebral augmentation: a consensus statement developed by the American Society of Interventional and Therapeutic Neuroradiology, Society of Interventional Radiology, American Association of Neurological Surgeons/Congress of Neurological Surgeons, and American Society of Spine Radiology. J Vasc Interv Radiol. 2007;18: 325–30.
29. Rotter R, Martin H, Fuerderer S, Gabl M. Vertebral body stenting: a new method for vertebral augmentation versus kyphoplasty. Eur Spine J. 2010;19:916–23.
30. Fiors L, Lonjedo E, Leiva-Salinas C, Martinez-Rodrigo JJ. Vesselplasty: a new technical approach to treat symptomatic vertebral compression fractures. AJR Am J Roentgenol. 2009;193: 218–26.
31. Jeon T, Kim S, Park WK. Lordoplasty: an alternative technique for the treatment of osteoporotic compression fracture. Clin Orthop Surg. 2011;3:161–8.
32. Bayley E, Srinivas S, Boszczyk BM. Clinical outcomes of sacroplasty in sacral insufficiency fractures: a review of the literature. Eur Spine J. 2009;18:1266–71.
33. Braal SJ, van Strijen MJL, van Leersum M, et al. Real-time 3D fluoroscopy guidance during needle interventions: technique, accuracy, and feasibility. Vasc Intervent Radiol. 2010;194: W445–51.
34. Patil A. Computed tomography-guided vertebroplasty using a stereotactic guidance system (stereo-guide). Surg Neurol Int. 2010; 1:17.
35. Mathias J, Deramond H, Belkoff S. Percutaneous vertebroplasty and kyphoplasty. 2nd ed. New York: Springer; 2006. p. 223–48.
36. Zoarski G, et al. Percutaneous vertebroplasty for osteoporotic compression fractures: quantitative prospective evaluation of long-term outcomes. J Vasc Interv Radiol. 2002;13:139–48.
37. Riew KD, Park J, Cho YS, et al. Nerve root blocks in the treatment of lumbar radicular pain: a minimum five-year follow-up. J Bone Joint Surg Am. 2006;88:1722–5.
38. Lieberman IH, et al. Initial outcomes and efficacy of "kyphoplasty" in the treatment of painful osteoporotic vertebral compression fractures. Spine. 2001;26:1631–8.

39. Wardlaw D, Cummings SR, Van Meirhaeghe J, Bastian L, Tillman JB, Ranstam J, Eastell R, Shabe P, Talmadge K, Boonen S. Efficacy and safety of balloon kyphoplasty compared with non-surgical care for vertebral compression fracture (FREE): a randomised controlled trial. Lancet. 2009;373:1016–24.

40. Truumees E, et al. Percutaneous vertebral augmentation. Contemporary concepts in spine care: NASS. 2004:1–16.

41. Vasconcelos S, et al. Transient arterial hypotension induced by polymethylmethacrylate injection during percutaneous vertebroplasty. J Vasc Interv Radiol. 2001;12:1001–2.

42. Grados F, et al. Long-term observation of vertebral osteoporotic fractures treated by percutaneous vertebroplasty. Rheumatology (Oxford). 2000;39:1410–4.

43. Kim M, Lee A, Min S, et al. Risk factors of new compression fractures in adjacent vertebrae after percutaneous vertebroplasty. Asian Spine J. 2011;5:180–7.

44. Klazen CA, Venmans A, de Vries J, et al. Percutaneous vertebroplasty is not a risk factor for new osteoporotic compression fractures: results from VERTOS II. AJNR Am J Neuroradiol. 2010;31: 1447–50.

45. Garfin S, et al. Minimally invasive treatment of osteoporotic vertebral body compression fractures. Spine. 2002;2:76–80.

46. Nevitt M, et al. Association of prevalent vertebral fractures, bone 720 density, and alendronate treatment with incident vertebral frac- 721 tures: effect of number and spinal location of fractures. Bone. 1999;25:613–619.

Piriformis Injection

53

Nathan J. Harrison and Gagan Mahajan

Key Points
- Piriformis syndrome is characterized by pain located in the buttock, with or without "sciatica," or radiation into the posterior thigh. It remains a controversial diagnosis of exclusion and debate continues due to a lack of consensus on its definition and pathophysiology.
- Before the diagnosis of piriformis syndrome is made, a broad differential should be considered in a patient presenting with "sciatica": lumbar disc herniation, facet arthropathy, sacroiliitis, myofascial pain and trochanteric bursitis.
- When the hip and knee are extended, as in standing, the piriformis muscle externally rotates the hip. When the hip is flexed to 90°, as in sitting, the piriformis muscle abducts the thigh.
- The sciatic nerve usually exits below the piriformis. However, variability exists in the exiting sciatic nerve in relation to the piriformis.
- There are no definitive laboratory tests and imaging tests that can unequivocally diagnose piriformis syndrome.
- Commonly used physical exam maneuvers include: Freiberg's sign, Pace's maneuver, Lasègue's sign, and Beatty's maneuver.

- Treatment of piriformis syndrome can include one or more of the following: activity modification and physical therapy, medicinal therapies, piriformis muscle injection, and surgery.

Introduction

In 1928, Yeoman described a condition of "sciatica" that he theorized occurred secondary to the close anatomic relationship of the piriformis muscle, anterior sacroiliac ligament, and adjacent branches of the sciatic nerve [1]. Frieberg and Vinke also believed that sacroiliac joint pathology could spread an inflammatory reaction to involve the piriformis muscle and sciatic nerve [2, 3]. In their 1934 study, they aimed to identify the physiologic mechanism of Lasègue's sign (buttock pain and tenderness with palpation in the greater sciatic notch while the hip is passively flexed to 90° and the knee is passively extended to 180°) and later introduced Freiberg's sign (buttock pain with passive, forced internal rotation of the hip), physical examination findings which they believed could identify the piriformis muscle as the source of sciatica [2, 3]. In 1934, Mixter and Barr described lumbar disc herniation as a cause of sciatica, calling into question the theories proposed by Yeoman and Frieberg [4]. In 1937 and 1938, Beaton and Anson described six possible variations of the exiting sciatic nerve in relation to the piriformis muscle and suggested that this relation could cause sciatic pain and coccydynia if the piriformis muscle was inflamed or in spasm [5, 6]. However, it was not until 1947 that Robinson first introduced the term "piriformis syndrome," which he found was associated with six signs and symptoms: (1) a history of trauma to the gluteal and sacroiliac regions; (2) pain in the region of the sacroiliac joint, greater sciatic notch, and piriformis muscle that may travel down the limb causing gait difficulties; (3) acute exacerbation of the pain with stooping or lifting with some relief of

N.J. Harrison, M.D. (✉)
Department of Anesthesiology, Ochsner Health System, New Orleans, LA, USA

1514 Jefferson Highway, New Orleans, LA 70121, USA
e-mail: nathanha504@gmail.com

G. Mahajan, M.D.
Department of Anesthesiology and Pain Medicine, University of California, Davis Medical Center, 4860 Y Street, Suite 3020, Sacramento, CA 95817, USA
e-mail: gmahajan@ucdavis.edu

T.R. Deer et al. (eds.), *Comprehensive Treatment of Chronic Pain by Medical, Interventional, and Integrative Approaches*,
DOI 10.1007/978-1-4614-1560-2_53, © American Academy of Pain Medicine 2013

Fig. 53.1 Relation of the sciatic nerve and its subdivisions to the piriformis muscle [6]. (**a**) The sciatic nerve exits below the piriformis muscle. (**b**) The sciatic nerve division passes both through and below the piriformis muscle. (**c**) The sciatic nerve division passes above and below the piriformis muscle. (**d**) The sciatic nerve passes through the piriformis muscle

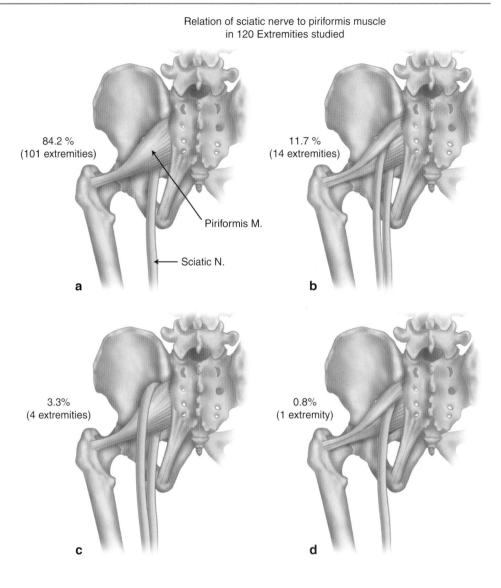

Relation of sciatic nerve to piriformis muscle
in 120 Extremities studied

84.2 %
(101 extremities)

Piriformis M.

Sciatic N.

a

11.7 %
(14 extremities)

b

3.3%
(4 extremities)

c

0.8%
(1 extremity)

d

pain by applying traction to the affected extremity; (4) a palpable, tender, sausage-shaped mass over the affected piriformis muscle; (5) a positive Lasègue's sign; and (6) depending on the duration of symptoms, gluteal atrophy [7].

Despite the advances in imaging and electrophysiological testing since piriformis syndrome was first described, it remains a diagnosis of exclusion with ill-defined clinical signs, diagnostic tests, and treatments.

Scientific Foundation

Anatomy

Branches of the ventral rami of the S1 and S2 nerve roots innervate the piriformis muscle. It is a pyramid or pear-shaped muscle that is superiorly co-localized with five short, external rotator muscles (superior and inferior gemmelli,

obturator internus and externus, and quadratus femoris) [8, 9]. The piriformis muscle originates medially from the ventrolateral surface of the second, third, and fourth sacral foramina and exits posterolaterally, filling most of the greater sciatic foramen as it passes to insert on the superior border of the greater trochanter [10]. When the hip and knee are extended, as in standing, the piriformis muscle functions synergistically with the five other external rotators to externally rotate the hip. When the hip is flexed to 90°, as in sitting, the piriformis muscle abducts the thigh. Along with several other external rotators, the piriformis muscle works to stabilize and steady the femoral head in the acetabulum. When the piriformis muscle contracts, its diameter may significantly increase and potentially lead to compression of the accompanying sciatic nerve, depending on its course through the greater sciatic foramen [11]. The sciatic nerve, which is a continuation of the sacral plexus and contains fibers from the L4–S3 nerve roots [10], usually exits below the piriformis and superior to the gemelli [6]. However, Beaton and Anson proposed that variability exists in the exiting sciatic nerve in relation to the piriformis muscle and described six possible arrangements [5, 6]. Of the six theoretical arrangements described, only four of these variations were actually found in their cadaveric studies: the sciatic nerve exited below the piriformis muscle in 84.2 %, the sciatic nerve divisions passed both through and below the piriformis muscle in 11.7 %, the sciatic nerve divisions passed above and below the piriformis muscle in 3.3 %, and the sciatic nerve passed through the piriformis muscle in 0.8 % (Fig. 53.1) [6].

Epidemiology and Pathophysiology

While an evolution of the definition of piriformis syndrome and its many etiologies has occurred, there has yet to be a clear, consensus definition. The lack of a consensus definition makes determining prevalence of piriformis syndrome difficult. Incidence rates range from 5 to 36 % of patients with buttock pain and sciatica symptoms [12]. Pace and Nagle described a 6:1 female to male ratio while others suggested a 1:1.4 female to male ratio [13, 14].

Attempts at classifying the various causes of piriformis syndrome include determining whether the symptoms are due to a primary or secondary piriformis syndrome. Primary piriformis syndrome refers to pathology intrinsic to the piriformis muscle, such as myofascial pain, pyomyositis, and myositis ossificans secondary to an inciting event such as direct trauma to the sciatic notch and gluteal region [7, 15]. This trauma may occur with prolonged sitting; prolonged and combined hip flexion, adduction and internal rotation; and certain sports activities [11, 16–18]. The latter include cyclists who ride for prolonged periods of time, tennis players who constantly internally rotate their hip with an overhead serve, and ballet dancers who constantly "turn out" or externally rotate their hip while dancing [11]. Pain may occur due to inflammatory and edematous changes in the muscle and surrounding fascia, which in turn cause a compressive neuropathy [18].

Secondary piriformis syndrome refers to all other cases in which the symptoms of posterior buttock pain and sciatica depend on the location of the pathology in relation to the structures adjacent to the sciatic notch, and includes the anatomic variations of the exiting sciatic nerve and piriformis muscle leading to sciatic nerve compression [5, 6, 15]. Such compression may occur with piriformis muscle hypertrophy, chronic inflammation, or muscle spasm which can then affect the sciatic nerve directly, especially with the nerve variations that pass through the muscle instead of beneath. Finally, secondary piriformis syndrome causes may include any lesions or structures causing a "pelvic outlet syndrome" such as pelvic tumors, endometriosis, and aneurysms or arterial malformations [15].

Clinical Examples

Diagnosis

Before the diagnosis of piriformis syndrome can be made, a broad differential should be considered in a patient presenting with sciatica. More common disorders, such as lumbar disc herniation, facet arthropathy, sacroiliitis, myofascial pain and trochanteric bursitis, can present with symptomatology similar to piriformis syndrome. There are no pathognomonic signs or symptoms, nor are there definitive laboratory tests and imaging tests that can unequivocally diagnose piriformis syndrome. However, numerous attempts have been made to describe the most common features and to provide diagnostic tools.

Symptoms and Physical Exam Findings

When he first introduced the term piriformis syndrome [7], Robinson assigned six signs and symptoms that are still widely regarded as useful today: (1) a history of trauma to the gluteal and sacroiliac regions; (2) tenderness in the region of the sacroiliac joint, greater sciatic notch, and piriformis muscle which often radiates to the hip; (3) acute exacerbations of pain with stooping or lifting and relief upon traction to the affected extremity; (4) a palpable, sausage-shaped mass over the piriformis muscle during an acute exacerbation; (5) a positive Lasègue's sign; and (6) depending on the duration of symptoms, gluteal atrophy.

Piriformis syndrome most commonly presents with a deep, aching buttock pain on the affected side. The pain may radiate to the hip, lower back and posterior thigh but rarely below the level of the knee. Squatting, prolonged sitting, and climbing stairs often exacerbate the pain. There may also be pain with bowel movements and dyspareunia in females. In physical exam, the ipsilateral foot may be noted to lie in an externally rotated position due to a contracted piriformis muscle [12, 19–22]. A contracted piriformis muscle may be elicited as a palpable mass on rectal exam [16].

The commonly used physical exam maneuvers are described here:

- *Freiberg's sign*: Buttock pain with passive, forced internal rotation of the hip [2].
- *Pace's maneuver*: Buttock pain with resisted abduction of the affected leg while in the seated position [13].
- *Lasègue's sign*: Buttock pain and tenderness to palpation in the greater sciatic notch with the hip passively flexed to 90° and the knee passively extended to 180° [3].
- *Beatty's maneuver*: While lying in a lateral decubitus position on the unaffected side, buttock pain is elicited in the affected extremity when the patient actively abducts the affected hip and holds the knee several inches off the table [23].

Table 53.1 Rehabilitation exercises for piriformis syndrome

1. *Piriformis stretch*: Supine position with knees flexed and feet flat on the floor. Rest the ankle of the injured leg over the knee of the uninjured leg. Grasp the thigh of the uninjured leg and pull that knee towards the chest. The patient will feel stretching along the buttocks and possibly along the outside of the hip on the injured side. Hold for 30 s. Repeat three times

2. *Standing hamstring stretch*: Place the heel of the patient's injured leg on a stool about 15 in. high. Lean forward, bending at the hips until a mild stretch in the back of the thigh is felt. Hold the stretch for 30–60 s. Repeat three times

3. *Pelvic tilt*: Supine position with the knees bent and feet flat on the floor. Tighten the abdominal muscles and flatten the spine on the floor. Hold for 5 s, then relax. Repeat ten times. Do three sets

4. *Partial curls*: Supine position with the knees bent and feet flat on the floor. Clasp hands behind the head to support it. Keep the elbows out to the side and do not pull with the hands. Slowly raise the shoulders and head off the floor by tightening the abdominal muscles. Hold for 3 s. Return to the starting position. Repeat ten times. Build up to three sets

5. *Prone hip extension*: Prone position. Tighten the buttock muscles and lift the right leg off the floor about 8 in. Keep the knee straight. Hold for 5 s and return to the starting position. Repeat ten times. Do three sets on each side

White [33]

- *FA(d)IR*: An acronym for flexion, adduction, and internal rotation of the affected hip. The maneuver prolongs the H (Hoffman)-reflex on nerve conduction studies [47].

Diagnostic Tests

In addition to clinical findings, numerous diagnostic tests have been proposed to identify piriformis syndrome. However, controversy remains regarding the true utility of these studies. Imaging studies of the lumbar and pelvic region are routinely obtained and best serve to exclude other well-defined causes of buttock and radicular leg pain such as lumbar disc herniations. MRI or CT of the pelvis may reveal inflammatory changes or edema of the affected muscle. While anatomic variations of the muscle and exiting sciatic nerve may be noted, the significance of these findings is unclear. Several case reports using MRI and CT have revealed unilateral hypertrophy of the piriformis muscle on the affected side in patients with piriformis syndrome [24, 25]. A study by Filler et al. examined MR neurography showing sciatic nerve hyperintensity at the sciatic notch in patients with hypertrophy (and occasionally atrophy) noted on MRI of the affected piriformis muscle [26]. The authors concluded that this additional imaging improved the sensitivity and specificity of identifying piriformis syndrome to 64 and 93 %, respectively [26]. However, others contend numerous theoretical and methodological flaws in this study. For instance, Beatty notes that the clinical diagnostic maneuver used by Filler et al. stretches the piriformis muscle, the sciatic nerve, and stresses the sacroiliac joint and thus constitutes a nonspecific sciatic nerve test [27]. Tiel et al. challenge that although pain relief may be obtained with injection of the piriformis muscle, this does not definitively diagnose piriformis syndrome [27, 28]. Furthermore, Tiel et al. state that the Filler study did not use a gold standard against which to compare the MR neurography and, therefore, true sensitivity and specificity measurements cannot be made [28].

Electrophysiologic testing in piriformis syndrome may represent a promising diagnostic tool. Fishman et al. have described prolongation (>3SD) of the posterior tibial or per-

oneal H-reflexes on FA(d)IR test and purport greater than 83 % sensitivity and specificity in diagnosing piriformis syndrome [29, 30]. While this would provide an effective objective diagnostic tool, critics disagree with the diagnostic criteria and methodology used in the study [31].

Treatment

After excluding other causes of low back, sciatica, and hip pain, piriformis syndrome can be diagnosed and therapy may begin. The mainstay treatment of piriformis syndrome consists of activity modification and physical therapy, with the goals of reducing pain and spasm of the piriformis muscle and correcting the pathology of compression of the sciatic nerve (Table 53.1) [32, 33]. The patient should be provided a home therapy program that may be combined with other modalities, such as heat, ultrasound, and manual techniques. Pharmacological treatments such as nonsteroidal anti-inflammatories (NSAIDs) and muscle relaxants may compliment physical therapy programs. Fishman et al. found 79 % of patients had symptom reduction with NSAIDs, muscle relaxants, ice, and rest [30].

If conservative therapy fails to provide adequate resolution of symptoms, intramuscular piriformis muscle injections may be warranted. Numerous injection techniques have been described utilizing CT guidance, fluoroscopic guidance, ultrasound, and combined fluoroscopic and EMG guidance (Table 53.2) [17, 34, 35]. Injected medications typically consist of local anesthetic and corticosteroid. Fishman et al. described injection of 2 % lidocaine 1.5 ml and triamcinolone 0.5 ml (20 mg) in patients with clinical criteria for piriformis syndrome and prolonged H-reflex on nerve conduction studies [30]. With an average follow-up of 10.2 months, 79 % of these patients reported at least 50 % improvement in symptoms [30].

Botulinum toxin represents an additional treatment alternative. Botulinum toxin is a potent neurotoxin with seven serotypes (A–G), all of which (except type G) are produced

Table 53.2 Piriformis injection techniques

Approach #1: Fluoroscopic guidance without EMG localization [17, 46]

1. The patient is placed in a prone position

2. The skin is prepared and draped in a sterile manner

3. The expected position of the piriformis muscle is identified under fluoroscopic guidance with the beam directed in an anteroposterior direction. The landmarks utilized include the greater trochanter relative to the lateral border of the sacrum and sacroiliac joint on the affected side

4. Visualize an imaginary line connecting the greater trochanter and the lower border of the sacrum

5. A superficial skin wheal is placed overlying the ischial, bone medial to the acetabulum and parallel to the target site of injection

6. A 22- or 25-gauge 3½-in. (6 in. if the patient is morbidly obese) spinal needle is advanced to a point along the imaginary line near the pelvic brim until the posterior ischium is contacted

7. Contrast media is injected to visually confirm a classic sausage-shaped piriformis myogram (Fig. 53.2)

Approach #2: Fluoroscopic and EMG guidance [17]

1. Repeat steps 1–3 as described in approach #1

2. A superficial skin wheal is placed overlying the 2 o'clock position (left side) or 10 o'clock position (right side) of the acetabulum of the affected leg

3. An EMG needle is advanced until the 2 or 10 o'clock position of the acetabulum is contacted (Fig. 53.3)

4. The patient is asked to contract the piriformis muscle by externally rotating and slightly abducting the affected hip

5. Placement of the EMG needle is adjusted until maximum motor unit action potentials (MUAPs) are demonstrated while the patient is externally rotating and abducting the hip. Once the MUAPs are localized, the patient is asked to stop contracting the piriformis muscle, and contrast media is injected to visually confirm a classic sausage-shaped piriformis myogram (Fig. 53.2)

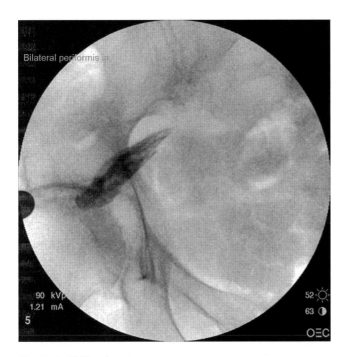

Fig. 53.2 Piriformis myogram

by the gram-negative anaerobic bacterium, *Clostridium botulinum* [36, 37]. The four clinically available forms of botulinumtoxin–onabotulinumtoxinA (Botox), abobotulinumtoxinA (Dysport), incobotulinumtoxinA (Xeomin), and rimabotulinumtoxinB (Myobloc), all inhibit presynaptic release of acetylcholine, thereby leading to muscle relaxation [36]. Studies in embryonic rat cells show that onabotulinumtoxinA may have a direct analgesic effect by inhibiting substance P from nerve terminals [38]. Food and Drug Administration (FDA) approval for onabotulinumtoxinA includes the treatment of strabismus, blepharospasm, upper limb spasticity, cervical dystonia, hyperhidrosis, chronic migraine headache, and frown lines [39]. FDA approval for abobotulinumtoxinA includes cervical dystonia and frown lines, while FDA approval for rimabotulinumtoxinB includes cervical dystonia only [40]. FDA approval for incobotulinumtoxinA includes cervical dystonia and blepharospasm [41]. Off-label uses include treatment of cervicogenic headaches, focal dystonias and spastic conditions due to cerebral palsy, stroke, and acquired brain injury [37]. Early investigations of intramuscular onabotulinumtoxinA for piriformis syndrome demonstrated improvement in symptoms. In their randomized, placebo-controlled crossover study involving nine patients, Childers et al. in 2002 demonstrated significant improvement in symptoms of pain intensity, distress, spasm, and interference of activities in all subjects of the onabotulinumtoxinA group [29]. Although the effects diminished, they persisted for all but one measure (spasm) at the end of 10 weeks [29]. In that same year, Fishman et al. reported a double-blind, placebo-controlled study comparing onabotulinumtoxinA (200 units mixed with preservative-free normal saline, 2 ml total volume) versus a combination of 2 % lidocaine 1.5 ml plus triamcinolone 0.5 ml (20 mg) versus preservative-free normal saline 2 ml [42]. Clinical improvement of at least 50 % on the VAS was reported in 65, 32, and 6 % of patients who received onabotulinumtoxinA, lidocaine plus triamcinolone, and placebo, respectively [42]. Most recently, Yoon et al. compared abobotulinumtoxinA (150 units in a 3 ml total volume) versus 1 % lidocaine and dexamethasone 5 mg in 20 patients [43]. Pain intensity scores were significantly lower in the onabotulinumtoxinA group at all follow-up time points. Because treatment in the experimental group was so much more effective, the control group was withdrawn at 4 weeks [43].

Fig. 53.3 Diagram of needle placement for piriformis injection (see Table 53.2) [17]

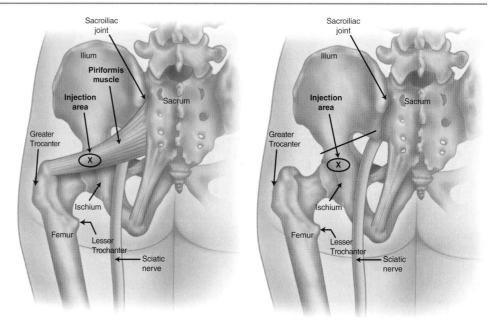

Finally, if all other conservative measures have proven inadequate, surgical management might be an option [7, 18, 44]. The procedure involves resecting the piriformis muscle itself or the muscle tendon near its insertion at the greater trochanter, and may include dissection of the sciatic nerve from the piriformis muscle if compression exists. While there is no definitive indication for proceeding to surgical management, outcome may be related to whether the etiology is secondary to trauma and/or the presence of electrodiagnostic abnormalities. Benson and Schutzer demonstrated excellent results in 11 of 14 patients with posttraumatic piriformis syndrome who underwent release of the piriformis tendon and sciatic neurolysis [18]. Of the 14 patients, preoperative electrodiagnostic studies were performed in only eight subjects who had obtained relief with surgical release [18]. Interestingly, however, six of these eight patients had definite findings of sciatic nerve compression at the level of the piriformis [18]. Conversely, Barton study showed relief in only one of four patients with non-traumatic piriformis syndrome who underwent piriformis tendon release [45].

Conclusion/Future Directions

Piriformis syndrome largely remains a diagnosis of exclusion. While its prevalence is not clear, there exist a certain number of patients whose "sciatica-type" symptoms are due anatomical variations causing compression or irritation of the sciatic nerve. Electrophysiologic tests and MR neurography may serve as accurate diagnostic tools in identifying piriformis syndrome, but more conclusive studies need to be performed. Conservative treatments including NSAIDs and physical therapy remain the first-line therapies for addressing piriformis syndrome. If these efforts are minimally successful or unsuccessful, patients may obtain relief with inclusion of piriformis muscle injections utilizing a combination of corticosteroid and local anesthetic. Recent studies with intramuscular botulinum toxin injections show promise for more long-term benefit, but larger studies with longer term follow-up need to be done. Surgical resection of the piriformis muscle has been performed successfully in cases of intractable pain, but comprehensive studies do not yet exist to support this intervention.

References

1. Yeoman W. The relation of arthritis of the sacroiliac joint to sciatica. Lancet. 1928;2:1119–22.
2. Freiberg AH, Vinke TH. Sciatica and the sacro-iliac joint. J Bone Joint Surg Am. 1938;16:126–36.
3. Freiburg AH. Sciatic pain and its relief by operations on muscle and fascia. Arch Surg. 1937;34:337–50.
4. Mixter WJ, Barr JS. Rupture of the intervertebral disc with involvement of the spinal canal. N Engl J Med. 1934;211:210–4.
5. Beaton LE, Anson BJ. The sciatic nerve and the piriformis muscle: their interrelation and possible cause of coccygodynia. J Bone Joint Surg. 1938;20:686–8.
6. Beaton LE, Anson BJ. The relation of the sciatic nerve and its subdivisions to the piriformis muscle. Anat Rec. 1937;70:1–5.
7. Robinson DR. Piriformis syndrome in relation to sciatic pain. Am J Surg. 1947;73:355–8.
8. Delagi EF, Perotto A, Iazzetti J, Morrison D. Anatomical guide for the electromyographer: the limbs and trunk. 3rd ed. Springfield: Charles C. Thomas, Publisher Ltd; 1994.

9. Jenkins DB. Hollingshead's functional anatomy of the limbs and back. 7th ed. Philadelphia: W.B. Saunders Company; 1998.

10. Moore KL, Dalley AF. Clinically oriented anatomy. 4th ed. Baltimore: Lippincott Williams & Wilkins; 1999.

11. Travell JG, Simons DG. Myofascial pain and dysfunction: the trigger point manual. Baltimore: Williams & Wilkins; 1992.

12. Boyajian-O'Neill LA, McClain RL, Coleman MK, Thomas PP. Diagnosis and management of piriformis syndrome: an osteopathic approach. J Am Osteopath Assoc. 2008;108(11):657–64.

13. Pace JB, Nagle D. Piriformis syndrome. West J Med. 1976;124:435–9.

14. Durrani Z, Winnie AP. Piriformis muscle syndrome: an undiagnosed cause of sciatica. J Pain Symptom Manage. 1991;6(6):374–9.

15. Papadopoulos EC, Khan SN. Piriformis syndrome and low back pain: a new classification and review of the literature. Orthop Clin North Am. 2004;35(1):65–71.

16. Thiele GH. Coccydgodynia and pain in the superior gluteal region. JAMA. 1937;109:1271–5.

17. Fishman SM, Caneris OA, Bandman TB, Audette JF, Borsook D. Injection of the piriformis muscle by fluoroscopic and electromyographic guidance. Reg Anesth Pain Med. 1998;23(6):554–9.

18. Benson ER, Schutzer SF. Posttraumatic piriformis syndrome: diagnosis and results of operative treatment. J Bone Joint Surg Am. 1999;81(7):941–9.

19. Chaitow L. Soft tissue manipulation: a practitioner's guide to the diagnosis and treatment of soft-tissue dysfunction and reflex activity. 3rd ed. Rochester: Healing Arts Press; 1988.

20. TePoorten BA. The piriformis muscle. J Am Osteopath Assoc. 1969;69:150–60.

21. Foster MR. Piriformis syndrome. Orthopedics. 2002;25:821–5.

22. Retzlaff EW, Berry AH, Haight AS, Parente PA, Lichty HA, Turner DM. The piriformis muscle syndrome. J Am Osteopath Assoc. 1974;73:799–807.

23. Beatty RA. The piriformis muscle syndrome: a simple diagnostic maneuver. Neurosurgery. 1994;34(3):512–4; discussion 514.

24. Jankiewicz JJ, Hennrikus WL, Houkom JA. The appearance of the piriformis muscle syndrome in computed tomography and magnetic resonance imaging. A case report and review of the literature. Clin Orthop. 1991;262:205–9.

25. Rossi P, Cardinali P, Serrao M, Parisi L, Bianco F, De Bac S. Magnetic resonance imaging findings in piriformis syndrome: a case report. Arch Phys Med Rehabil. 2001;82:519–21.

26. Filler AG, Haynes J, Jordan SE, et al. Sciatica of nondisc origin and piriformis syndrome: diagnosis by magnetic resonance neurography and interventional magnetic resonance imaging with outcome study of resulting treatment. J Neurosurg Spine. 2005;2(2):99–115.

27. Beatty RA. Piriformis syndrome. J Neurosurg Spine. 2006;5(1):101; author reply 101–2.

28. Tiel RL, Kline DG. Piriformis syndrome. J Neurosurg Spine. 2006;5(1):102–4; author reply 104–8.

29. Childers MK, Wilson DJ, Gnatz SM, Conway RR, Sherman AK. Botulinum toxin type A use in piriformis muscle syndrome: a pilot study. Am J Phys Med Rehabil. 2002;81(10):751–9.

30. Fishman LM, Dombi GW, Michaelsen C, et al. Piriformis syndrome: diagnosis, treatment, and outcome – a 10-year study. Arch Phys Med Rehabil. 2002;83(3):295–301.

31. Stewart JD. The piriformis syndrome is overdiagnosed. Muscle Nerve. 2003;28(5):644–6.

32. Kirschner JS, Foye PM, Cole JL. Piriformis syndrome, diagnosis and treatment. Muscle Nerve. 2009;40(1):10–8.

33. White T. Piriformis syndrome rehabilitation exercises. 2010. http://www.tzengs.com/health/Piriformis%20Syndrome/index.htm. Accessed 6 Jul 2010.

34. Fanucci E, Masala S, Sodani G, et al. CT-guided injection of botulinic toxin for percutaneous therapy of piriformis muscle syndrome with preliminary mri results about denervative process. Eur Radiol. 2001;11(12):2543–8.

35. Huerto APS, Yeo SN, Ho KY. Piriformis muscle injection using ultrasonography and motor stimulation – report of a technique. Pain Physician. 2007;10(5):687–90.

36. Davis LE. Botulism. Curr Treat Options Neurol. 2003;5(1):23–31.

37. Monnier G, Tatu L, Michel F. New indications for botulinum toxin in rheumatology. Joint Bone Spine. 2006;73(6):667–71.

38. Aoki KR, Guyer B. Botulinum toxin type A and other botulinum toxin serotypes: a comparative review of biochemical and pharmacological actions. Eur J Neurol. 2001;8 Suppl 5:21–9.

39. Medication guide: BOTOX® BOTOX® cosmetic (boe-tox) (onabotulinumtoxinA) for injection. 2010. http://www.fda.gov/downloads/Drugs/DrugSafety/UCM176360.pdf. Accessed 11 Nov 2010.

40. U.S. Food and Drug Administration. Information for healthcare professionals: Onabotulinumtoxina (marketed as botox/botox cosmetic), abobotulinumtoxina (marketed as dysport) and rimabotulinumtoxinb (marketed as myobloc). 2010. http://www.fda.gov/Drugs/DrugSafety/PostmarketDrugSafetyInformationforPatientsandProviders/DrugSafetyInformationforHeathcareProfessionals/ucm174949.htm. Accessed 19 Nov 2010.

41. Waknine Y. FDA approves incobotulinumtoxina for cervical dystonia and blepharospasm. 2010. http://www.medscape.com/viewarticle/726218. Accessed 19 Nov 2010.

42. Fishman LM, Anderson C, Rosner B. BOTOX and physical therapy in the treatment of piriformis syndrome. Am J Phys Med Rehabil. 2002;81(12):936–42.

43. Yoon SJ, Ho J, Kang HY, et al. Low-dose botulinum toxin type A for the treatment of refractory piriformis syndrome. Pharmacotherapy. 2007;27(5):657–65.

44. Freiberg AH. The fascial elements in associated low-back and sciatic pain. J Bone Joint Surg. 1941;23:478–80.

45. Barton PM. Piriformis syndrome: a rational approach to management. Pain. 1991;47:345–52.

46. Neural-scan helps identify piriformis syndrome. 2010. http://www.ndanerve.com/downloads/Axon_Piriformis_Syndrome.pdf. Accessed 14 Nov 2010.

47. Fishman LM, Zybert PA. Electrophysiologic evidence of piriformis syndrome. Arch Phys Med Rehabil. 1992;73(4):359–64.

Botulinum Toxin in the Management of Painful Conditions

54

Robert Gerwin

Key Points

- Botulinum toxin inhibits the release of neurotransmitters involved in the activation of sensory neurons.
- The release of substance P, glutamate, and calcitonin gene-related peptide is thought to be inhibited by botulinum toxin.
- Botulinum toxin is effective in reducing the frequency and intensity of migraine headaches. High-quality studies, class 1 data, A-level recommendation as effective.
- Botulinum toxin is effective in relieving nonspecific low back pain. High-quality, class 1 studies, A-level recommendation as effective.
- Botulinum toxin is possibly effective in treatment of neck and upper back pain, but results of studies are mixed. Class III studies, C-level recommendation as possibly effective.
- The studies of the use of botulinum toxin in myofascial trigger point pain are inconclusive due to the small number and poor quality of the studies. Class I studies but U-level recommendation of inadequate or conflicting studies.
- Studies of the treatment of pelvic pain are encouraging, but more and better studies need to be done (class III data and U-level recommendation of inadequate data).
- A variety of other painful conditions are now being investigated, including neuropathic pain. Results are mixed but this seems to be a promising area in need of more and better studies. Data is class III–IV and recommendation for use is level U (inadequate or conflicting data).

Introduction

Botulinum neurotoxin (BoNT) has been used clinically to impair muscle contraction and thereby has become useful in treating conditions characterized by persistent muscle spasticity, muscle spasm, or contraction. It has more recently been found to reduce pain in clinical pain syndromes. This chapter will present the current state of knowledge about the clinical use of BoNT in the treatment of painful conditions. It will also review the mechanism of action of BoNT with regard to inhibition of nociceptive activity.

Mechanism of Action of Botulinum Toxin

The activation of peripheral nociceptors and the subsequent activation of secondary neuronal pathways lead to pain perception. In a nutshell, nociceptive impulses from peripheral neurons are transmitted through the spinal cord to the brain where they activate a number of distinct centers including the somatosensory cortex where pain is perceived. The transmission of nociceptive impulses through the spinal cord are facilitated and inhibited by descending modulating impulses that pass through the spinal cord and have the potential to alter the quantity of ascending nociceptive impulses reaching the brain. BoNT can alter this process and dampen the cascade of events involved in pain perception, leading to a reduction in pain intensity. The mechanism of action of BoNT in this respect is partially understood and continues to be investigated. Botulinum toxin enzymatically cleaves the SNARE proteins that anchor synaptic vesicles to the cell membrane in the motor nerve terminal, allowing acetylcholine and other neurotransmitters to flow through the motor nerve terminal membrane fusion pore into the synaptic space. Botulinum toxin has an effect on sensory neurons and sensory perception as well, by inhibiting the release of neurotransmitters involved in activation of sensory neurons. This chapter will review what is known about the action of BoNT on pain perception. The work to be

R. Gerwin, M.D.
Department of Neurology, School of Medicine,
Johns Hopkins University School of Medicine,
7830 Old Georgetown Road, Suite C15, Bethesda, MD 20814, USA
e-mail: gerwin@painpoints.com

reviewed will focus on studies with botulinum neurotoxin type A (BoNT-A) unless otherwise specified, as most studies have been done with this subtype of BoNT.

Botulinum toxin is approved by the Food and Drug Administration (FDA) in the United States for the treatment of strabismus, blepharospasm associated with dystonia, cervical dystonia, upper limb spasticity, and axillary hyperhidrosis. All other uses of botulinum toxin in the United States are off-label uses. This chapter will report on the studies of BoNT in pain management and will discuss the results of studies of BoNT in certain pain states. The information in this article should not be construed to advocate the general off-label non-FDA-approved usage of BoNT.

Mechanism of Action of BoNT in Alleviation of Pain

The mechanism of action of BoNT on muscle contraction is the inhibition of the release of the neurotransmitter acetylcholine at the neuromuscular junction. The action of BoNT on nociception is mediated by a similar inhibition of neurotransmitter release from peripheral nociceptors [1]. The release of Substance P (sub P), glutamate, and calcitonin gene-related peptide (CGRP) are all thought to be inhibited by BoNT.

Patients suffering from dystonia and dystonia-related pain experienced pain relief when treated with BoNT [2, 3]. Moreover, pain relief generally occurred before onset of its effect on the dystonia itself [4, 5]. In addition, pain relief outlasts the effect of BoNT on muscle in a masticatory muscle model [6], indicating that botulinum toxin has an analgesic effect that is quite separate from its effect on acetylcholine at the neuromuscular junction.

In vitro studies have demonstrated that the release of sub P [7, 8] is inhibited by BoNT. The inhibition of sub P was directly related to the degree of SNAP-25 cleavage. These studies established the inhibition of neuropeptide release by BoNT in inflammatory pain models, an effect that is in addition to the inhibition of acetylcholine release in the motor nerve terminal.

BoNT was shown to inhibit phase 2 of formalin-induced nociceptive behavior in the rat model. There was no effect on acute thermal nociception, considered to be consistent with the lack of effect on phase 1 of the response. This is also true in humans. The effect was associated with a reduction in formalin-induced release of the excitatory amino acid glutamate [9].

Migraine headache involves activation of the trigeminovascular system. The interest in botulinum toxin as a treatment of migraine headache has led to its study in trigeminal sensitization. The action of BoNT has been studied in the skin, particularly with relation to the activation of peripheral nociceptors by capsaicin. Botulinum toxin administered subcutaneously inhibits the extent of capsaicin-induced perceived pain area, pain intensity, secondary hyperalgesia, flare area, blood flow, and skin temperature in male subjects [10, 11]. Neurogenic vasodilation is reduced as well as capsaicin-evoked pain in human skin [12]. An effect was observed on cutaneous heat thresholds but not on electrical or pressure pain thresholds. The effect of BoNT appears to be mediated through an action on C-fibers and on TRPV1-receptors. In contrast, in one study injection of BoNT-A subdermally in the forearm did not alter the pain response to capsaicin [13]. In summary, BoNT works in nociception much in the same way that it does at the neuromuscular junction, by preventing the release of neurotransmitters by sensory nerve endings.

Clinical Studies of Botulinum Toxin in Pain Syndromes

BoNT has been studied in a number of pain syndromes. There has been great interest in the possible benefit of BoNT in headache syndromes, and recent studies have supported that usage. Its role in musculoskeletal pain syndromes has been less thoroughly studied. The benefit of treatment with BoNT in low back pain and neck pain is better established than in myofascial pain syndromes, where the results of studies have been contradictory. There is clearly a role for BoNT in the treatment of pelvic pain syndromes. There are either too few studies or inadequate or negative studies in some other conditions. Randomized controlled studies (RCT) are presented where available. Open label and uncontrolled studies are generally not cited in this chapter.

BoNT in Musculoskeletal Pain Conditions

Low Back and Joint Pain (Table 54.1)

There have been several studies that have shown a beneficial effect of botulinum toxin on low back pain. The studies were done on individuals with chronic low back pain that was predominantly unilateral and who did not have an identifiable acute source of pain like a herniated disc. Back pain in this sense can be called nonspecific low back pain. Foster et al. [14] evaluated the effect of botulinum toxin A over 8 weeks on nonspecific low back pain in a randomized, double-blind study. Botulinum toxin type A 40 units or saline was injected unilaterally at five different lumbar levels. Relief was greater than 50 % (VAS score) in 73 % of the botulinum toxin type A-treated subjects compared to 25 % of the saline control group ($p=0.012$). A follow-up open-label study by the same group was conducted over 14 months. The outcomes in the open-label extension of the study included the change in the

Table 54.1 Low back treatment protocol

Muscles	Units of onabotulinumtoxinA (Botox)
Lumbar paraspinal muscles	5–50 units bilaterally at each vertebral level (includes the multifidi and the lumbar iliocostalis muscles)
Psoas muscle	50–100 units
Quadratus lumborum	25 units

Note: The dosages given here are specific for Botox® brand of onabotulinum toxin type A. The number of units to be used is specific for each type and brand of BoNT (onabotulinum toxin Botox®, Dysport® brand of botulinum toxin type A, and Myobloc® brand of botulinum toxin type B), and are not interchangeable. Clinicians should be familiar with reconstituting the freeze-dried onabotulinum toxin type A without denaturing it and should be familiar with the dosing schedules of any particular form of BoNT that is to be used in a given situation

Table 54.2 Injection dosing schedule recommended for chronic, intractable neck pain

Muscle	Units of BoNT-A
Upper trapezius	15–40 units distributed through the muscle
Splenius capitis	5–10 units
Splenius cervicis	5 units
Semispinalis	5–10 units as 5 units in each of 1–2 units sites
Oblique capitis inferior	5 units
Levator scapulae	25 units
Medial scalene	5 units

The doses recommended are for unilateral injection. The same doses are used on the contralateral side for bilateral treatment. The adverse side effect that is potentially of concern is neck weakness manifested by inability to maintain the neck in an erect, upright posture

VAS, the number of pain days, and the Oswestry functional status scale. Botulinum toxin type A was found to significantly reduce pain over a 14-month period of time during which repeated injections were given. Ninety-one percent of initial responders maintained responsiveness over the duration of the open-label trial [15].

Neck and Upper Back Pain (Table 54.2)

There are few randomized, controlled studies of the use of BoNT in neck and upper back pain. Göbel et al. [16] found that BoNT-A (Dysport®) significantly reduced or eliminated upper back myofascial pain compared to saline (51 vs. 26 %, $p = 0.002$) 5 weeks after injection. However, another study of BoNT-A treatment of pain emanating from cervicothoracic myofascial TrPs showed that low dose (50 units total), higher dose (100 units total), and saline all resulted in a decline in pain and disability scores, with no benefit of BoNT over placebo, but those in the subgroup of subjects who received a second injection of BoNT-A experienced such a high incidence of becoming asymptomatic that the authors concluded that further studies were warranted. In contrast, a RCT, double-blinded study of the effect of BoNT-A in the treatment of refractory neck pain, in which 33 of 47 subjects had neck injury (72 %), resulted in a significant number of subjects classified as excellent responders who had a ≥50 % decrease in VAS for pain, ≥30 % reduction in pain days, and 2 grades or more improvement in the Modified Oswestry Pain Questionnaire (6/23 in the BoNT-A group vs.1/21 in the control group). Pain intensity was greater in the BoNT-A group at baseline, but was significantly decreased at 2 months compared to the saline control group ($p < 0.0018$). Injections were made in the trapezius, splenius, and rhomboid muscles as clinically indicated, using 20 units per injection site and ranged in total from 150 to 300 units. No information was given about the criteria for selection of specific injection sites, but it appears that the injection sites were selected to give a general distribution of BoNT-A in the muscles treated, as opposed to injecting in myofascial trigger points. This well-designed and executed study clearly shows efficacy of BoNT-A treatment for chronic neck pain.

Myofascial Pain Syndromes

Pain in myofascial pain syndrome (MPS) is generated by a tender, taut band that is the fundamental feature of the myofascial trigger point (MTrP). It is thought that relaxation of the taut band through inhibition of acetylcholine release from the motor nerve terminal at the neuromuscular generation and inhibition of the release of neurotransmitters at the sensory nerve will result in decreased pain from MTrPs. However, the few studies that have looked at this have not supported this concept. Often-quoted studies include those of Ferrante et al. [17], Graboski et al. [18], Kamanli et al. [19], and Ojala et al. [20]. Ferrante et al. [17] stopped all pain medication prior to the trial injections, then gave all subjects amitriptyline, ibuprofen 800 mg qid, and prn propoxyphene/apap. In this RCT, subjects were given either BoNT-A (10, 25, or 50 units/trigger point) or saline in up to 5 trigger points. Patients were excluded if they had more than 5 trigger points or more than 2 trigger points in on trapezius muscle, or more than one trigger point in any other single surface muscle. There was no difference in rescue medication, or in pressure pain threshold between saline injected groups and those injected with BoNT-A. Both the lowest dose and highest dose BoNT-A outperformed saline, but not to a significant degree. Some of the possibilities include the fact that all subjects were treated with adjuvant pain medication and that saline is not an inactive control. Finally, the standard deviation of the sum of pain intensity differences, a reflection of the primary outcome measure, was so great that differences between the saline group and the BoNT-A were not significant. For these reasons, the results of this study cannot be seen as conclusive. Graboski et al. [18] compared BoNT-A to bupivicaine. A maximum of 8 trigger points were injected with either 25 units of BoNT-A or saline in this RCT. The end point was a return to 75 % of pre-injection pain. At that time, subjects were injected with the other substance (a crossover study). There was no statistically significant difference between the two treatments. Bupivicaine was considered cheaper. Outcome measures were changed in pain scores and duration of relief. Although there was no significant difference between groups, there was a definite trend toward greater decrease in pain and greater duration of effect with BoNT-A. Possible issues were the low number of subjects completing the trial (17 subjects in all) and the limited number of trigger points injected. Kamanli et al. [19] compared BoNT-A, lidocaine, and dry needling. Pain scores were lower in the subjects treated with BoNT-A and dry needling, and visual analogue scale significantly decreased in the lidocaine and BoNT-A groups at the single follow-up visit of 4 weeks. A single trigger point was treated. BoNT-A was not inferior to lidocaine or dry needling. However, in this study, as well as in the other two studies, no attempt was made to provide a comprehensive treatment to clear all relevant trigger points. In clinical practice, one would treat all of the trigger points deemed to be relevant in producing a pain syndrome. In this regard, inactive trigger points that are known to cause dysfunction [21] also need to be treated. In partial treatments, trigger points tend to recur more quickly. Studies that use pressure pain thresholds as a measure have not shown that this measurement reliably reflects inactivation of trigger points.

Ojala et al. [20] did a single-blind, RCT, crossover design, injecting either saline or BoNT-A in up to six neck and shoulder muscles bilaterally and then injecting the trigger points with the other substance 1 month later. There was no difference between groups 1 month after the second injection when subjects had received both saline and BoNT-A 1 month apart. However, after the first month, before the saline group received BoNT-A, subjects treated with BoNT-A had a significantly greater decrease in pain than those treated with saline. BoNT-A has a peak motor effect at about 6 weeks, and effectiveness is maintained from 10 to 14 weeks in most subjects. Hence, one would expect a difference 1 month after the first injection and no difference 1 month after the crossover injection.

There are a number of other studies that address this issue. Pain in patients with temporomandibular joint disorders was treated with BoNT-A injected into the masseter and temporalis muscles in a randomized, controlled study [22]. The result was a decrease in pain and an improvement in psychological status. Both the studies of Göbel et al. [16] and Wheeler et al. [23] were suggestive of a benefit for BoNT at a certain time and under certain circumstances.

It helps to be very clear in defining the desired outcome using BoNT. All studies show that BoNT treatment of myofascial trigger points can respond well to BoNT, but the placebo effect has also been striking. It is essentially like giving a lidocaine trigger point injection that lasts between 10 and 14 weeks in duration. The local twitch response that marks a successful trigger point injection with lidocaine is generally lost after BoNT injection. The number of lidocaine trigger point injections needed to treat an MPS is usually reduced and sometimes eliminated altogether for the duration of action of the toxin. The effectiveness of the toxin in MPS seems to depend on the care with which the trigger point zone is injected and the comprehensive clearing of TrPs in a functional muscle unit. Treatment of trigger points in only one muscle instead of a functional muscle unit may be a reason why spontaneous pain was not reduced 28 days after BoNT-A was injected in an infraspinatus muscle trigger point [24].

BoNT in Headache Management

Migraine Headache (Tables 54.3, 54.4, and 54.5)

The headache literature is very mixed on the issue of the effectiveness of BoNT in the treatment of headache in general, and migraine in particular. This literature was reviewed through 2007/2008 in Gerwin [25]. The literature prior to 2010 can be summarized by saying that the results of the many studies done in patients with migraine and other headaches varied in their outcome. One of the reasons for variability this is the lack of uniformity in subject selection, sites, and dosing schedules used. Silberstein et al. [26], in a RCT of chronic migraine showed that patients treated at predetermined fixed sites with low-dose onabotulinumtoxinA (25 units total) had a significantly reduced migraine frequency and a reduction in the use of medications compared to the carrier alone, but the higher dose of 75 units showed no benefit. A RCT using lower doses of BoNT in the temporalis muscles and omitting injection of glabellar muscles showed a 50 % reduction in headache days in 30 % of the active treatment group, but the 25 % of the placebo group showed the same response, so the results were not

Table 54.3 Treatment of migraine headache by Botox: migraine protocol

Muscle	Units of onabotulinumtoxinA (Botox)
Temporalis	25 in a linear or diamond grid
Procerus	5
Corrugator	5 each
Frontalis	10–20

Table 54.4 Follow-the-pain protocol for use in chronic tension-type headache and migraine

Muscle with trigger points referring pain to headache regions	Units of onabotulinum-toxinA (Botox)
Temporalis	25 in a linear or diamond grid
Masseter	2–4
Zygomaticus	2–3
Pterygoid	2–3
Sternocleidomastoid (inject only one side)	10–15
Splenius capitis	5
Splenius cervicis	5
Oblique capitis inferior	5
Semispinalis	5–10
Levator scapulae	10–25
Upper trapezius	25–40

Table 54.5 Combined migraine and follow the pain for most migraine headaches

Muscle	Units of onabotulinumtoxinA (Botox)
Upper trapezius	25–40
Sternocleidomastoid (inject only one side)	10–15
Temporalis	25 in a linear or diamond grid
Procerus	5
Corrugator	5
Splenius capitis and cervicis	5
Semispinalis	5
Oblique capitis inferior	5

significant [27]. A study using three different dosing schedules of BoNT-A and using a low dose (7.5 units) of BoNT as an active control showed equal reduction in headache frequency in all groups [28]. A small study failed to show benefit of BoNT-A in reduction of headache frequency or severity compared to placebo, but headache index worsened in the placebo group, but not in the active treatment group, suggesting that BoNT had a protective effect in headache severity. Studies of episodic migraine fared no better [29, 30]. However, there two studies that indicated that BoNT-A to be of benefit in the treatment of migraine [31, 32]. The largest and most comprehensive RCT, to date, of 1,384 subjects was done by the PREEMPT Chronic Migraine Study Group [33] and found that onabotulinumtoxinA (BoNT-A) was superior to placebo in the primary outcome measure of reduction in frequency of headache days at all time points in the 24-week double-blinded portion of the trial. In addition, onabotulinumtoxinA was superior to placebo in six secondary outcome measures: mean change from baseline in frequencies of headache days, moderate or severe headache days, cumulative hours of headache on headache days,

headache episodes, migraine episodes, and the proportion of patients with severe Headache Impact Test-6 score. Acute medication use in the treatment group was not statistically better than placebo. The size of the study and the thoroughness of evaluation make this a landmark study. The authors point out that the study was not made against a comparator. The authors themselves refer to a pilot study comparing onabotulinumtoxinA to topiramate [34], an FDA-approved drug for the prevention of migraine. In this study, subjects were randomly assigned to either onabotulinumtoxinA or to topiramate. The study was placebo controlled.

Technique

There are two approaches to treatment of migraine headache with BoNT. One is the so-called migraine protocol and the other has been called the "follow-the-pain" protocol. In practice, a third approach is often utilized, which is a combination of the two protocols. No uniform approach has been determined for either protocol, and the studies done to establish doses have been few and preliminary at best. Therefore, there is no established best practice based on acceptable medical evidence in terms of dosing or sites to be injected. What is recommended here is based on a combination what has been published and on the author's experience as to what has generally worked best. However, the recommendations in this chapter include the protocol in the largest trial to date that showed efficacy of onabotulinumtoxinA in the management of chronic migraine headache [33].

The "migraine protocol" involves injecting BoNT into the corrugator muscles, the procerus muscles, and the temporalis muscles (Fig. 54.1). Many physicians who treat migraine with BoNT include the frontalis muscle as well. I do not do that, but I combine the migraine protocol with the "follow-the-pain" protocol, instead.

The "follow-the-pain" protocol is best characterized as injecting sites in the neck and shoulders that refer to the places where headache pain is felt in the head. This is essentially treating regions in head, neck, and shoulder muscles that refer pain to various places in the head that are characteristic of that person's migraine headache. An early test of the concept of "follow the pain" is in the 1981 paper by Tfelt-Hansen et al. [35] in Denmark, in which the authors showed that headache could be decreased or eliminated in large percentage of subjects with migraine by injecting muscles outside of head, that is, muscles in the neck and shoulder, that cause pain. An elegant study that specifically looked at sites in muscle that cause pain to be referred specifically to places of headache complaint showed that injection of these referral sites in head, neck, and shoulder, done on a repeated basis, result in a significant reduction in migraine headache frequency and intensity [36].

The muscles and sites to be injected are those that harbor tight and tender taut bands. The taut bands are hardened regions

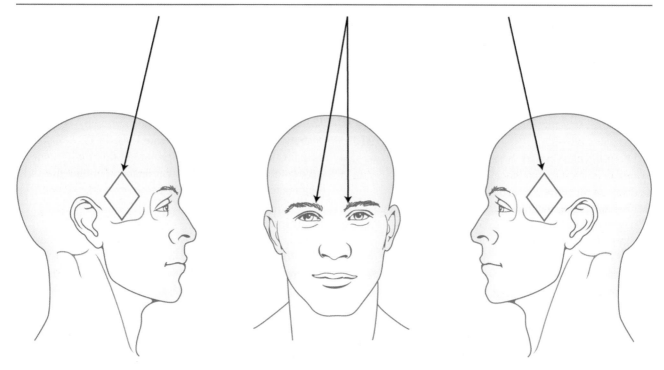

Fig. 54.1 Procerus: between and inferior to the corrugator muscle

of muscle that are tender to palpation. They are relevant to the patient's pain when they result in pain referred to the region of headache. This applies not only to migraine but also to tension-type headache and to cervicogenic headache. It also applies to involvement of masticatory muscles that not only directly cause headache pain but that indirectly affect headache by activating trigger points in the cervical musculature.

Chronic Tension-Type and Cervicogenic Headache (CTTH) (Table 54.4)

The headaches of interest in this headache subgroup are those of ≥15 headache days per month, the generally accepted headache frequency for chronic daily headache. There have been few studies of the effect of BoNT on headache that target this group specifically. Many of the studies of chronic daily headache did not distinguish between migraine headache and tension-type headache. Of the few studies that specifically targeted CTTH, three used fixed-dose and fixed-site injection of BoNT-A. They showed no significant reduction in headache frequency [37–39], although in one study, the BoNT-A-treated subjects showed a significantly greater percentage with ≥50 % reduction in headache days compared to the placebo group [39]. One pilot study [40] of great interest looked at the myofascial trigger points (MTrP) that referred pain to typical headache sites, a strategy that builds on many recent studies of the relationship of myofascial trigger points to headache symptomatology, a subject recently

summarized in the text by Fernandez-de-las-Peñas et al. [41]. Harden et al. [40] identified trigger points in the neck and upper shoulder, including the sternocleidomastoid and the upper trapezius muscles, and the splenius capitis muscle. They injected 25 units of BoNT-A into each of up to 4 MTrP per subject, using up to 100 units. This was a randomized, double-blinded, placebo-controlled study, but it was quite small, with only 12 subjects in the treated group and 11 subjects in the placebo group. There was a significant decrease in headache days in the BoNT-A-treated group through week 10, but the effect was gone by week 12. This is consistent with the expected duration of effect of BoNT-A on muscle. An open-label extension of the study included 12 subjects from both the BoNT-A and placebo groups. It again showed a significant reduction in headache frequency compared to the original placebo group, for the first 2 months. This study was limited by the small number of subjects and by the small selection of the muscles considered (there were no facial muscles like the masseter and temporalis muscles, and neither the splenius cervicis, oblique capitis inferior, nor semispinalis muscles were injected, although the authors implied that injection of the splenius capitis might have treated multiple underlying muscles). A randomized, single-blinded, placebo-controlled study utilizing a combination of a fixed injection site and "follow-the-pain" approaches also showed significant improvement in the subjects treated with BoNT-A at 1 month, in headache days per month, headache severity, and the in the Henry Ford Headache Disability Inventory [42]. In both the Harden et al. study [40] and the Hamdy et al.

study [42], side effects were minor and transient. Another small study of headache associated with myofascial trigger points randomized 45 subjects to treatment with dry needling, lidocaine injections, and botulinum toxin [43]. All three groups showed fewer headaches, shorter headache duration, and decreased pain intensity. Those treated by botulinum toxin also showed a decreased use of rescue medication and less post-injection soreness. The authors concluded that botulinum toxin is no better or worse than the other two treatment modalities, but that it is more expensive and should be reserved for refractory cases of headache.

The conclusion that one can draw from the studies is that treatment of chronic daily headache, particularly of the migraine headache type, with botulinum toxin type A is effective, but BoNT has not been shown to be necessarily more effective than treatment with lidocaine or intramuscular therapy (IMT) with solid, monofilament needles (dry needling). The role of botulinum toxin is uncertain if derived solely from these studies. It would seem sensible to use botulinum toxin only in those cases of chronic daily headache where conventional drug therapy is unsatisfactory either because of ineffectiveness of prophylactic drugs or because of unacceptable side effects, and when lidocaine injections or IMT are effective but too short lasting. Several unanswered questions remain. Is BoNT effective when lidocaine injections of trigger points fail to relieve headache? Should subjects first be treated with lidocaine injections or IMT before being treated with BoNT?

The protocol for treatment of headache generally follows a migraine protocol in those patients with migraine features (Tables 54.3 and 54.5). In both those patients with migraine and in those with tension-type and cervicogenic headache, BoNT is injected in the trigger points themselves. Injection of BoNT into trigger points is not as exacting as injection of lidocaine or IMT into trigger points, because BoNT spreads through tissues and will alter transmitter release over about a 2.5-cm diameter around the injection site. The area of spread is directly related to the concentration of BoNT, so that there is greater spread with greater dilution. A concentration of 5–2.5 units of BoNT-A is commonly used. This is achieved with 2–4 per 0.1 cc respectively of preservative-free saline/100 units in reconstituting the freeze-dried product. See Tables 54.3, 54.4, and 54.5 for recommendations of the number of units to be injected in trigger points in various muscles.

BoNT in Pelvic Pain Conditions (Table 54.6)

Botulinum toxin has been used to treat conditions of the pelvic/hip region, including piriformis syndrome, other gluteal muscle pain syndromes, and levator ani muscle pain syndromes. In addition, it has been used in viscerosomatic pain syndromes including the abdominal wall muscle pain

Table 54.6 Pelvic/hip pain protocol

Muscle	Units of onabotulinum toxinA (Botox)
Quadratus lumborum	25
Lumbar paraspinals	
Multifidi	5–10 per vertebral level
Lumbar iliocostalis	5–40 per vertebral level
Tensor fascia lata	15–25
Gluteus medius	25–50
Gluteus minimus	25–50
Piriformis	25 units proximally and 25 units distally
Obturator Internus	25 units medial to the ischial tuberosity
	25 units lateral posterior to the greater trochanter (the muscle is usually indistinguishable from the gemelli laterally)
Levator ani	25 units distributed in 5–10 unit aliquots, given with the needle inserted through the gluteus maximus with digital guidance (rectal or vaginal)
Gluteus maximus	25–50
Adductor magnus iliococcygeal head	25
Hamstrings (upper medial)	25
Pectineus	10–15
Adductor brevis/longus	25

component of endometriosis, interstitial cystitis, and irritable bowel syndrome. Botulinum toxin has been injected directly into the bladder in the treatment of interstitial cystitis and irritable bladder.

Treatment of the levator ani syndrome with botulinum toxin is reported to decrease coital pain (dyspareunia) and menstrual pain (dysmenorrheal), to increase sexual activity, and to produce relaxation of the pelvic floor muscles [44, 45]. In the Jarvis et al. [44] study, women were treated in the lithotomy position and given conscious sedation. The puborectalis and pubococcygeus muscles were identified by digital examination through the vagina. The needle is guided along the examining finger, the injection made through the vaginal mucosa. No woman experienced fecal incontinence from treatment with botulinum toxin. The amount of botulinum toxin type A that was injected was 10 units per side.

Botulinum toxin type A injected into the bladder wall in patients with painful bladder syndrome reduced mean VAS scores, and daytime and nighttime urinary frequency [46]. Daytime frequency and nocturia, and pain, decreased significantly after BoNT-A (Dysport and Botox) was injected into 20–30 sites in the trigone and floor of the bladder submucosally through a cystoscope in women with interstitial cystitis [47]. Studies done by a Urology Department failed to show such benefits to intravesical injection of BoNT-A [48], but when hydrodistension was added to intravesical BoNT-A treatment, there was a significant improvement in pain and urinary frequency [49].

Vestibulodynia is another distressing pain syndrome that is being approached by injection of BoNT. In one open-label study, the injection of BoNT-A 35 or 50 units into the pelvic floor muscles resulted in a significant decrease in pain [50]. An anecdotal report of two patients treated with BoNT-A injected into the levator ani muscle to reduce coital pain, reduce pelvic floor tension, and reduce vestibular hyperalgesia resulted in improvement in coital pain in one patient but no reduction in vestibular hyperalgesia [51].

Ureteral stent placement for the treatment of ureteral obstruction can result in postoperative pain, increased urinary frequency, and urgency. One postulated cause is detrusor muscle spasm at the site of the intramural ureter. A randomized, single-blind study of the periureteral injection of BoNT-A showed a significant decrease in postoperative pain with a corresponding decrease in the use of opiate medications in this condition [52]. Urinary function was no different among those treated with BoNT-A and those not so treated.

Pelvic/Hip Pain Injection Technique (Table 54.6)

Injection of the pelvis/hip muscles for mechanical and viscerosomatic pain syndromes requires the examination of the low back muscles, the gluteal region muscles, the adductor muscles, the pelvic floor muscles, and the adductor magnus muscle. The quadratus lumborum muscle can refer pain widely in the low back and the pelvic region. The lumbar multifidi and the lumbar iliocostalis muscles refer pain to the sacroiliac joint and widely in the gluteal region. The pelvic floor muscles can give rise to local pain as well as pain referred to the hip and to both the groin and to the gluteal fold. The piriformis muscle gives rise to local pain, pain at the sacroiliac joint, and pain at the trochanter region, and can compress the sciatic nerve giving rise to sacroiliac joint pain. Most of the muscles, including the piriformis, obturator internus, and levator ani, can be injected from the outside the pelvis, rather than intrapelvically. So that there is almost never a need to inject through the rectum, even if a flute is used to guide the needle. Digital guidance through the vagina or through the rectum can be used to direct the needle. A 1.5-in., 25-gauge needle can be used for the more superficial muscles, and a 3.5-in., 25-gauge needle is adequate for almost all of the deeper muscles, including the piriformis and gluteus minimus muscles. The obturator internus can be injected medial to the ischial tuberosity at a point where the ischial tuberosity is concave to the anus, about 5 cm rostral to the inferior tip of the tuberosity. To inject the portion of the obturator internus that covers the obturator foramen requires a transvaginal approach.

BoNT in Other Painful Conditions

There is one RCT, double-blinded study that shows BoNT-A to be effective in reducing pain in chronic neuropathic pain [53]. BoNT-A was injected intradermally (20–190 units) into the painful area. Pain and allodynia were significantly reduced from 2 to 14 weeks after injection, whereas thermal perception thresholds were not altered. The only notable adverse effect was pain during the injections.

Painful Knee Osteoarthritis

A pilot double-blinded, RCT of BoNT-A injected intra-articularly showed that BoNT-A was better than intra-articular corticosteroid at 8 weeks [54]. The author of this chapter has found that BoNT injected into myofascial TrPS of the vastus medialis and lateralis muscles reduces knee pain as well. Injection of BoNT-A into the vastus lateralis muscle significantly reduced refractory anterior knee pain [55], showing the benefit of treating referred pain from muscle to knee. Injection of BoNT-A 25 units is often enough to provide 10–14 weeks of knee pain relief, enough to allow adequate rehabilitation to take effect. In general, if a vastus medialis or lateralis muscle trigger point responds to lidocaine injection or IMT, but the relief is not maintained, the BoNT can be an effective alternative. However, part of the rehabilitation process is to strengthen the quadriceps muscle, and weakening the muscle with BoNT is theoretically counterproductive. There are no published studies that have examined this question.

Sacroiliac joint pain was relieved by injection of BoNT-A intra-articularly [56]. Other studies of the effectiveness of BoNT may be confounded by pain originating in structures that are not treated by intra-articular injections of BoNT-A but that neverthele cause knee pain, like tendons, ligaments, and referred pain from muscle.

Shoulder pain in spastic post-stroke hemiplegia (Table 54.7 and Fig. 54.2) was successfully treated with BoNT-A (Dysport) using 500 Speywood units injected into the subscapularis muscle [57]. Lateral rotation was also improved. However, another study using BoNT-A (Botox), 50 units injected into each of two sites in the subscapularis muscle, failed to show any greater improvement than placebo over 12 weeks [58]. Even though the placebo injection was not an inactive control (injection of saline and IMT are both active treatments), improvement with saline is not expected to last for 12 weeks. A third study showed a strong trend toward significant improvement in hemiplegic shoulder pain treated with intramuscular BoNT-A into three muscles and intra-articular saline compared to intra-articular injection of triamcinolone

Table 54.7 Injection of BoNT-A (Botox) in post-stroke spastic shoulder hemiparesis

Muscle	Units of onabotulinum toxin (Botox)
Subscapularis	25–50
Latissimus dorsi	25–50
Teres major	10–25
Infraspinatus	25–40
Supraspinatus	25–35
Levator scapulae	25
Pectoralis major	25–50
Pectoralis minor	25

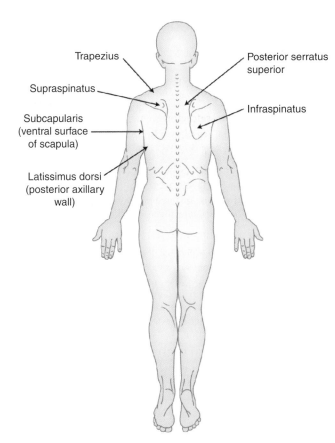

Fig. 54.2 Shoulder pain in spastic post-stroke hemiplegia

acetonide and saline injections into muscle ($p = 0.051$) [59]. Overall, it seems reasonable to treat pain associated with post-stroke spastic hemiplegia with BoNT if there is no response to conventional therapy. The key to successful treatment is the inclusion of all affected spastic muscles that includes the subscapularis, the pectoralis major and minor, the latissimus dorsi and teres major, and the supraspinatus muscle. None of the published studies included this wide a range of muscles.

Postwhiplash neck pain is a controversial area of treatment. Treatment of four sites in RCT trial, both acute and chronic, were treated with either BoNT-A or placebo and monitored to 24 weeks. Significantly greater reduction in pain was noted at 24 weeks in number of patients with greater than 50 % reduction of pain. This is not a clinically realistic treatment schedule. Treatment would be tailored to inject all muscles that have symptomatic trigger points, and to reinject trigger points that persist after the first injection. Physical therapy would be provided for subjects as well. Thus, this study does not give adequate guidance for clinical practice. Chronic facial pain associated with masticatory muscle overactivity responded well to BoNT-A injections into the masticatory muscles in a RCT [60].

Plantar fasciitis responded significantly to BoNT-A given as 40 units given close to the calcaneal tuberosity and 30 units given in the middle of the foot, in a RCT, double-blind, placebo-controlled trial [61].

Conclusion

Botulinum toxin has now been shown in many studies to be effective in reducing the intensity and frequency of pain in a variety of clinical pain syndromes. Much work still remains to define more specifically the conditions which are appropriately treated with BoNT and what treatment protocols are most effective.

References

1. Aoki KR. Evidence for antinociceptive activity of botulinum toxin type A in pain management. Headache. 2003;43 suppl 1:s9–15.
2. Tsui JK, Eisen A, Mak E, Carruthers J, Scott A, Calne DB. A pilot study on the use of botulinum toxin in spasmodic torticollis. Can J Neurol Sci. 1985;12:314–6.
3. Lew MF, Chinnapongse R, Zhang Y, Corliss M. RimabotulinumB effects on pain associated with cervical dystonia: results of placebo and comparator-controlled studies. Int J Neurosurg. 2010;120:2989–3000.
4. Brin MF, Fahn S, Moskowitz C, Friedman A, Shale HM, Greene PE, Lovelace RE, et al. Localized injections of botulinum toxin for the treatment of focal dystonia and hemifacial spasm. Mov Disord. 1987;2:237–54.
5. Jancovic J, Orman J. Botulinum toxin for cranial cervical dystonia: a double-blind, placebo controlled study. Neurology. 1987;37:616–23.
6. Freund B, Schwartz M. Temporal relationship of muscle weakness and pain reduction in subjects treated with botulinum toxin A. J Pain. 2003;4:159–66.
7. Purkiss J, Welch M, Doward S, Foster K. Capsaicin-stimulated release of substance P from cultured dorsal root ganglion neurons: involvement in two distinct mechanisms. Biochem Pharmacol. 2000;59:1403–6.
8. Durham PL, Cady R, Cady R. Regulation of calcitonin gene-related peptide secretion form trigeminal nerve cells by botulinum toxin type A. Implications for migraine therapy. Headache. 2004;44:35–43.

9. Cui M, Khanijou S, Rubino J, Aoki KR. Subcutaneous administration of botulinum toxin A reduces formalin-induced pain. Pain. 2004;107:125–33.

10. Gazerani P, Staahl C, Arendt-Nielsen L. The effects of botulinum toxin type A on capsaicin-evoked pain, flare, and secondary hyperalgesia in an experimental human model of trigeminal sensitization. Pain. 2006;122:15–25.

11. Gazerani P, Pedersen NS, Staahl C, Drewes AM, Arendt-Nielsen L. Subcutaneous botulinum toxin type A reduces capsaicin-induced trigeminal pain and vasomotor reactions in human skin. Pain. 2009; 141:60–9.

12. Tugnoli V, Capone JG, Eleopra R, Quatrale R, Sensi M, Gastaldo E, Tola MR, Geppetti P. Botulinum toxin type A reduces capsaicin-evoked pain and neurogenic vasodilation in human skin. Pain. 2007; 130:76–83.

13. Voller B, Sucha T, Gustorff B, Schmetterer L, Lehr S, Eichler HG, Auff E, Schider P. A randomized, double-blind, placebo controlled study on analgesic effects of botulinum toxin A. Neurology. 2003; 61:940–4.

14. Foster L, Clapp L, Erickson M, Jabbari B. Botulinum toxin A and chronic low back pain. Neurology. 2001;56:1290–3.

15. Jabbari B, Ney J, Sichani A, Monacci W, Foster L, Difazio M. Treatment of refractory, chronic low back pain with botulinum neurotoxin A: an open-label, pilot study. Pain Med. 2006;7:260–4.

16. Göbel H, Heinze A, Reichel G, Hefter H, Benecke R. Efficacy and safety of a single botulinum type A toxin complex treatment (Dysport) for the relief of upper back myofascial pain syndrome: results from a randomized double-blind placebo-controlled multicenter study. Pain. 2006;125:82–8.

17. Ferrante FM, Bean L, Rothrock R, King L. Evidence against trigger point injection techniques for the treatment of cervicothoracic myofascial pain with botulinum toxin type A. Anesthesiology. 2005; 103:377–83.

18. Graboski CL, Gray DS, Burnham RS. Botulinum toxin A versus bupivicaine trigger point injections for the treatment of myofascial pain syndrome: A randomized double blind crossover study. Pain. 2005;118:170–5.

19. Kamanli A, Kaya A, Ardicoglu O, Ozgocmen S, Zengin FO, Bayik Y. Comparison of lidocaine injection, botulinum toxin injection, and dry needling to trigger points in myofascial pain syndrome. Rheumatol Int. 2005;25:604–11.

20. Ojala T, Arokoski JPA, Partanen J. The effect of small doses of botulinum toxin A on neck-shoulder myofascial pain syndrome: a double-blind, randomized, and controlled crossover trial. Clin J Pain. 2006;22:90–6.

21. Lucas KR. The impact of latent trigger points on regional muscle function. Curr Pain Headache Rep. 2008;12:344–9.

22. Kurtoglu C, Gur OH, Kurkcu M, Sertdemir Y, Guler-Uysal F, Uysal H. Effect of botulinum toxin-A in myofascial pain patients with or without functional disc displacement. J Oral Maxillofac Surg. 2008;66: 1644–51.

23. Wheeler AH, Goolkasian P, Gretz SS. A randomized, double-blind, prospective pilot study of botulinum toxin injection for refractory, unilateral, cervicothoracic, paraspinal, myofascial pain syndrome. Spine. 1998;23:1662–6.

24. Qerama E, Fuglsang-Frederiksen A, Kasch H, Bach FW, Jensen TS. A double-blind, controlled study of botulinum toxin A in chronic myofascial pain. Neurology. 2006;67:241–5.

25. Gerwin R. Botulinum toxin A in the treatment of headaches. In: Fernádez-de-las-Peñas C, Arendt-Nielsen L, Gerwin RD, editors. Tension-type and cervicogenic headache. Boston: Jones and Bartlett; 2010. p. 431–46.

26. Silberstein SD, Mathew N, Saper J, Jenkins S, for the BOTOX Migraine Clinical Research Group. Botulinum toxin type A as a migraine preventative treatment. Headache. 2000;40:445–50.

27. Evers S, Vollmer-Haase J, Schwaag S, Rahman A, Husstedt I-W, Frese A. Botulinum toxin A in the prophylactic treatment of migraine: a randomized, double-blind, placebo-controlled study. Cephalagia. 2004;24:838–43.

28. Elkind AH, O'Carroll P, Blumendfeld A, DeGryse R, Dimitrova R, for the BoNTA-024—26—36 Study Group. A series of three sequential, randomized, controlled studies of repeated treatments with botulinum toxin type A for migraine prophylaxis. J Pain. 2006;7:688–96.

29. Saper J, Mathew NT, Loder EW, DeGryse R, VanDenburgh AM, for the BoNTA-009 study group. A double-blind, randomized, placebo-controlled comparison of botulinum toxin type a injection sites and doses in the prevention of episodic migraine. Pain Med. 2007;8:478–85.

30. Aurora SK, Gawel M, Brandes JL, Pokta S, VanDenburgh AM, for the BOTOX North American Episodic Migraine Study Group. Botulinum toxin type A treatment of episodic migraine: a randomized, double-blind, placebo-controlled exploratory study. Headache. 2007;47:486–99.

31. Anand KS, Prasad A, Singh MM, Sharma S, Bala K. Botulinum toxin type A in prophylactic treatment of migraine. Am J Ther. 2006;13:183–7.

32. Freitag FG, Diamond S, Diamond M, Urban G. Botulinum toxin type A in the treatment of chronic migraine without medication overuse. Headache. 2008;48:201–9.

33. Dodick DW, Turkel CC, DeGryse RE, Aurora SK, Silberstein SD, Lipton RB, Diener H-C, Brin MF. OnabotulinumtoxinA for treatment of chronic migraine: pooled results from the double-blind, randomized, placebo controlled phases of the PREEMPT clinical program. Headache. 2010;50:921–36.

34. Mathew NT, Jaffri SF. A double-blind comparison of onabotulinumtoxina (BOTOX) and topiramate (TOPAMAX) for the prophylactic treatment of chronic migraine: a pilot study. Headache. 2009;49(10):1466–78.

35. Tfelt-Hansen P, Lous I, Olesen J. Prevalence and significance of muscle tenderness during common migraine attacks. Headache. 1981;21(2):49–54.

36. Giamberardino MA, Tafuri E, Savini A, Fabrizio A, Affaitati G, Lerza R, Di Ianni L, Lapenna D, Mezzetti A. Contribution of myofascial trigger points to migraine symptoms. J Pain. 2007;8(11):869–78. Epub 2007 Aug 9.

37. Schmitt WJ, Slowey E, Fravi N, Weber S, Burgender JM. Effect of botulinum toxin A injections in the treatment of chronic tension type headache: a double-blind, placebo-controlled trial. Headache. 2001;41:658–64.

38. Schulte-Mattler WJ, Krack P, BoNTTH Study Group. Treatment of chronic tension type headache with botulinum toxin A: a randomized, double-blind, placebo-controlled multicenter study. Pain. 2004;109:110–4.

39. Silberstein SD, Göbel H, Jensen R, Elkind AH, Degryse R, Walcott JM, Turkel C. Botulinum toxin type A in the prophylactic treatment of chronic tension type headache: a multicenter, double-blind, randomized, placebo-controlled, parallel group study. Cephalagia. 2006;26:790–800.

40. Harden RN, Cottrill J, Gagnon CM, Smitherman TA, Weinland SR, Tann B, Joseph P, Lee TS, Houle TT. Botulinum toxin a in the treatment of chronic tension-type headache with cervical myofascial trigger points: a randomized, double-blind, placebo-controlled pilot study. Headache. 2009;49:732–43.

41. Fernandez-de-las-Peñas C, Arendt-Nielsen L, Gerwin RD. Tension-type and cervicogenic headache. Boston: Jones and Bartlett; 2010. p. 61–89.

42. Hamdy SM, Samir H, El-Sayed M, Adel N, Hasan R. Botulinum toxin: could it be an effective treatment for chronic tension-type headache? J Headache Pain. 2009;10:27–34.

43. Venancio RA, Alencar Jr FG, Zamperini C. Botulinum toxin, lidocaine, and dry needling injections in patients with myofascial pain and headaches. Cranio. 2009;27:46–53.
44. Jarvis SK, Abbott JA, Lenart MB, Steensma A, Vancaillie TG. Pilot study of botulinum toxin type A in the treatment of chronic pelvic pain associated with spasm of the levator ani muscles. Aust N Z J Obstet Gynaecol. 2004;44:46–50.
45. Romito S, Bottarnelli M, Pellegrini M, Vicentini S, Rizzulo N, Bertolasi L. Botulinum toxin for the treatment of genital pain syndromes. Gynecol Obstet Invest. 2004;58:164–7.
46. Giannantoni A, Mearini E, Del Zingaro M, Proietti S, Porena M. Two-year efficacy and safety of botulinum a toxin intravesical injections in patients affected by refractory painful bladder syndrome. Curr Drug Deliv. 2010;7:1–4.
47. Smith CP, Radziszewski P, Borkowski A, Somogyi GT, Boone TB, Chancellor MB. Botulinum toxin a has antinociceptive effects in treating interstitial cystitis. Urology. 2004;64:871–5.
48. Kuo HC. Preliminary results of suburothelial injection of botulinum a toxin in the treatment of chronic interstitial cystitis. Urol Int. 2005;75:170–4.
49. Liu HT, Kuo HC. Intravesical botulinum toxin A injections plus hydrodistension can reduce nerve growth factor production and control bladder pain in interstitial cystitis. Urology. 2007;70:463–8.
50. Dykstra DO, Presthus J. Botulinum toxin type A for the treatment of provoked vestibulodynia: an open-label, pilot study. J Reprod Med. 2006;51:467–70.
51. Brown CS, Glazer Hl, Vogt V, Menkes D, Bachman G. Subjective and objective outcomes of botulinum toxin type A treatment in vestibulodynia: pilot study. J Reprod Med. 2006;51:635–41.
52. Gupta M, Patel T, Xavier K, Maruffo F, Lehman D, Walsh R, Landman J. Prospective randomized evaluation of periureteral botulinum toxin type A injection for ureteral stent pain reduction. J Urol. 2010;183:598–602.
53. Wohlfarth K, Sycha T, Ranoux D, Naver H, Caird D. Dose equivalence of two commercial preparations of botulinum neurotoxin type A: time for a reassessment? Curr Med Res Opin. 2009;25(7):1573–84. Review.
54. Boon AJ, Smith J, Dahm DL, Sorenson EJ, Larson DR, Fitz-Gibbon PD, Dykstra DD, Singh JA. Efficacy of intra-articular botulinum toxin type A in painful knee osteoarthritis: a pilot study. PM R. 2010;2:268–76.
55. Singer BJ, Silbert PL, Song S, Dunne JW, Singer KP. Treatment of refractory anterior knee pain using botulinum toxin type A (Dysport) injection to the distal vastus lateralis muscle: a randomized placebo controlled crossover trial. Br J Sports Med. 2011;45(8):640–5. Epub 2010 Apr 23.
56. Lee JH, Lee SH, Song SH. Clinical effectiveness of botulinum toxin A compared to a mixture of steroid and local anesthetics as a treatment for sacroiliac joint pain. Pain Med. 2010;11(5):692–700.
57. Yelnik PP, Colle FM, Bonan IV, Vicaut E. Treatment of shoulder pain in spastic hemiplegia by reducing spasticity of the subscapular muscle: a randomized, double blind, placebo controlled study of botulinum toxin A. J Neurol Neurosurg Psychiatry. 2007;78:845–6.
58. de Boer KS, Arwert HJ, de Groot JH, Meskers CG, Mishre AD, Arendzen JH. Shoulder pain and external rotation in spastic hemiplegia do not improve by injection of botulinum toxin A into the subscapular muscle. J Neurol Neurosurg Psychiatry. 2008;79:581–3.
59. Lim JY, Koh JH, Paik NJ. Intramuscular botulinum toxin-A reduces hemiplegic shoulder pain. Stroke. 2008;39:126–31.
60. von Lindern JJ, Niederhagan B, Bergé S, Appel T. Type A botulinum toxin in the treatment of chronic facial pain associated with masticatory hyperactivity. J Oral Maxillofac Surg. 2003;61:774–8.
61. Babcock MS, Foster L, Pasquina P, Jabbari B. Treatment of pain attributed to plantar fasciitis with botulinum toxin A: a short-term, randomized, placebo-controlled, double-blind study. Am J Phys Med Rehabil. 2005;84:649–54.

Emerging Imaging Tools for Interventional Pain

55

Marc A. Huntoon

Key Points

- The earliest approaches to procedures in pain medicine were often hampered by the limitations of the sightless, surface landmark-driven "art of medicine." Imaging levels the playing field, as it were, by allowing all physicians to see exactly what was done.
- Image-guided options for the pain clinician included fluoroscopy, C-arm flat detector CT, ultrasound, and MRI.
- It is critical that image-guided procedures are used for proper medically indicated indications.
- New uses of imaging such as ultrasound may change the way we do current procedures. The placement of peripheral stimulation leads and the refill of difficult to access pumps are two examples of use of these emerging tools.

Introduction

The introduction of image guidance for precise targeting of anatomical structures, accurate reproduction of successful procedures, and storage of a procedural record was an important step forward for modern pain medicine. The earliest approaches to procedures in pain medicine were often hampered by the limitations of the sightless, surface landmark-driven "art of medicine." Imaging levels the playing field, as it were, by allowing all physicians to see exactly what was done. Obviously, the ability to review critical images as part of a quality management process might improve medical outcomes. However, as for many advances,

M.A. Huntoon, M.D.
Department of Anesthesiology,
Mayo Clinic, 200 1st Street SW, Rochester, MN 55905, USA
e-mail: huntoon.marc@mayo.edu

there are concerns that imaging could be used by government payers, insurers, or others to restrict one's ability to participate in procedural care or receive remuneration for the procedure if the stored image does not meet specific standards [1]. Additionally, at the start of the new decade, clinicians find that technologies of the future must prove to be cost-effective. It is possible that certain technologies might improve care outcomes, but not be widely adopted by the medical community due to the fact that they do not meet a certain value threshold. Simply put if a particular image-guidance technique produces only minimal improvements by some measure (clinical outcome, decreased complication rate, etc.) but at a greater cost, the best value alternative will survive [2]. Finally, many of the procedures in interventional pain have not yet been justified by medical evidence [3]. Thus, the question of which image-guidance technique is superior (fluoroscopy, computed tomography (CT), or ultrasound (US)) for a given procedure [4] may be mute if the guided procedure is medically futile.

There are currently many barriers to adoption of image-guidance technologies. These include not only up-front equipment acquisition costs but also a significant investment in time for the requisite imaging workshops and mentored skill acquisition ("on-the-job practice time") [2].

The risks of any image-guidance technique considered for routine use are also of significance. Recent scrutiny of the risk/benefit ratio of CT scanning relative to alternative techniques has been increasingly discussed in the literature. Several publications have suggested that the rate of increase in the number of annual CT scans (now over 72 million per year) has led to detrimental effects in human health, with hard to quantitate tangible benefits [5, 6]. Cancer risk relative to dose radiation from CT has been modeled after longitudinal population-based studies of cancer occurrences in atomic bomb survivors [6]. One study suggested that, based on year 2007 CT scans, one could anticipate about 14,000 or more future cancer deaths [5]. This chapter aims to describe some of the current work going on in image guidance and imaging in general as these topics relate to pain procedures. Specific areas where one technique may be superior to another or emerging techniques are also discussed.

C-Arm Flat Detector CT

A number of complex interventional pain procedures have emerged over the last decade, with new imaging modalities following suit. Simple target blocks such as interlaminar or transforaminal epidurals, facet procedures, and sacroiliac injections are quite easily accomplished with fluoroscopy. However, some procedures such as vertebral augmentation (vertebroplasty, kyphoplasty), celiac and hypogastric plexus neurolysis, diskography and other disk access procedures, and minimally invasive surgical procedures may be more easily accomplished with 3-dimensional fluoroscopy systems. In addition, some believe that neuromodulation procedures might be more readily accomplished with the capability to visualize in three dimensions. For example, peripheral neuromodulation procedures might be more facile with an imaging technique that showed soft tissue structures in three-dimensional or to similarly be able to detect if a spinal cord stimulation lead had migrated anteriorly. It would be an obvious advantage to avoid the hassle of bringing the conventional fluoroscopy unit back into the field and redraping it for sterility just to obtain a lateral image to verify a spinal stimulation leads location in the dorsal epidural space.

All of these modern three-dimensional systems have multifunctionality. C-arm flat detector CT (FDCT) or C-arm cone-beam CT (CBCT) may utilize different gantries but are essentially similar descriptions of these devices [7]. These systems offer what may be viewed as a "Star Wars" operating arena, where advanced optical tracking, integration of several imaging modalities (US, digital subtraction angiography, fluoroscopy, and CT) all occur in a single suite. Fluoroscopy works well to view bone structures, but in essence, there are very few procedures intended to target boney structures. Exceptions include vertebral and sacral augmentation, transpedicular fusion, etc. Yet, even in these cases where a bone target is sought, knowledge about the location and alignment of other structures such as the spinal canal, nerve roots, blood vessels, etc., is desirable to avoid complications. The limited CT scan capability of many of these systems is another plus. Instead of an image intensifier, most units have a flat detector computed tomography (FDCT) capability, which is not real time but delayed by only a few seconds. Flat panel detection enhances the accuracy and safety of the procedure as compared to plain fluoroscopy [7]. In general, interventional radiologists have been the main users of these systems, but at least two academic pain medicine practices in the United States are using equipment with these FDCT capabilities. FDCT utilizes a single rotation of

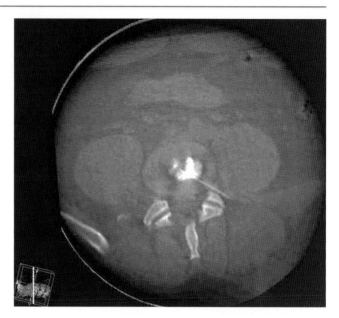

Fig. 55.1 Pictured is an axial CT acquisition with FDCT demonstrating a diskogram of a structurally normal disk. Provocative testing did not yield any pain at this level

the fluoroscope gantry, as opposed to conventional CT wherein there are multiple detectors and a requirement for several rotations of the gantry as the patient is moved in and out of the scanner [7]. The resulting volumetric data set from a FDCT is not as high quality as a modern 64 slice CT, but patient access is easier and more similar to conventional fluoroscopy. With FDCT, the patient stays in the same position through the imaging cycle. CT images are delayed by approximately 5–20 s. Although the images from FDCT scanning are of lower resolution, the images are most often quite adequate for the intended procedure. For example, at the author's institution, we are investigating the necessity for the traditional post-diskography CT, when compared to intraoperative FDCT images (Fig. 55.1).

FDCT systems produce increased scatter radiation, which can result in artifacts and inaccuracies in CT calculations. Anti-scatter grids that may increase patient radiation dose are commonly used to overcome this problem. However, radiation doses are less than that for a single helical CT [7].

Cone-beam CT/FDCT units are increasingly popular for intraoperative minimally invasive surgery [8]. Transpedicular fusions are one area where this technology is being used with success. Some of the touted advantages of modern imaging system use intraoperatively are (1) reduced time for image acquisition compared to repeatedly bringing a conventional fluoroscope into the field, (2) decreased incidence of transgression of the pedicle, (3) reduced overall operating time, and (4) reduced dose of radiation to both the surgeon and the patient. For example, a recent study compared intraoperative computer-assisted spinal navigation to serial radiography for posterior fusions at the L5/S1 level. The navigation system shortened the operative time by about 40 min compared to serial radiographs [9]. More recently, a Japanese group compared isocentric three-dimensional fluoroscopy with navigation to conventional fluoroscopy for percutaneous screw placements. This large study included 300 percutaneous screw placements of which half were inserted with the advanced imaging and half with conventional fluoroscopy. They then evaluated post-procedural accuracy with 2-mm axial slice CT imaging. The authors found that there were 7.3 % exposed screws and zero perforated pedicles in the three-dimensional image group compared to 12 % exposed screws and 3.3 % perforated pedicles in the conventional fluoroscopy group. This was a statistically significant difference for pedicle screw misplacement ($P < 0.05$) [10]. In a previous study of conventional two-dimensional fluoroscopy, Weinstein et al. noted a 21 % rate of misplaced pedicle screws, with the vast majority being on the medial side (towards the spinal canal) [11]. The performance of celiac or superior hypogastric plexus neurolytic blocks is potentially impeded by the size of the local tumor burden or lymphadenopathy which may limit spread of the alcohol or phenol neurolytic solution. Other soft tissue structures such as the renal cortex, thoracic duct, abdominal aorta, or inferior vena cava for celiac plexus blocks or the iliac veins, L5/S1 disk, and L5 nerve root for superior hypogastric plexus blocks may be injured by two-dimensional guidance alone. Thus, a three-dimensional imaging system may improve block accuracy and decrease potential complications. Goldschneider et al. [12] used a 3D-RA system to perform celiac plexus blocks in children with good outcomes.

When performing vertebral augmentation procedures, it is normally considered a contraindication to proceed if a retropulsed fragment is pushing posteriorly into the spinal canal, due to the risk of neurological injury as polymethyl methacrylate (PMMA) cement is injected into the vertebral body. Knight et al. demonstrated the utility of CBCT imaging for this exact scenario, however, with a successful vertebroplasty in a patient with a retropulsed bone fragment [13]. The utilization of three-dimensional technology to better treat patients seems likely to grow as the creativity of proceduralists catches up to the capability of the imaging.

Magnetic Resonance Guidance

The use of magnetic resonance imaging (MRI) has lagged behind some of the other imaging modalities but may have significant future uses. Most physicians who treat patients with complex spine disease appreciate the superiority of the imaging of soft tissue structures with MRI. However, the lack of real-time injection, the limited access to the patient, and the need for MRI-safe equipment were significant problems to overcome. Some of the advantages of MRI imaging are the lack of radiation risks (making it potentially superior for the care of pregnant women and children as well as decreasing risks to the operator), the familiarity of spinal injectionists with MRI images, and the ability to avoid contrast dyes for patients with allergies. Disadvantages of MRI-image guidance with optical tracking include distortion of imaging with needle bending, which may malposition the graphic overlay. This may increase the number of images necessary to accurately reach the target [14]. Sequeiros and colleagues evaluated the feasibility of MR guidance with an optical tracking system for diskography. The authors found that the results were similar to those with conventional fluoroscopy or CT. A 0.23 T open configuration MRI unit was utilized. Only one complication, a collapsed disk, occurred during their study of 35 patients, with 34 procedures completed [14]. In another study, Streitparth et al. studied the outcomes of spinal injection procedures such as nerve root injection, facet joint, and sacroiliac joint injections performed in an open-field MRI of 1.0 T with vertical field orientation [15]. The authors found that proton-density-weighted turbo spin-echo (PDw TSE) technique was optimal for the image guidance. They studied 183 total injections in 53 patients. Target delivery of injectate was achieved in 100 % of the nerve root blocks, but only 87 % of the facet and sacroiliac joint injections. Posterior osteophytes limited appropriate spread in some patients. There were no major complications. MRI-image guidance has not yet come of age but may continue to grow for particular procedures. Certainly, the advantages of soft tissue imaging and lack of radiation risks warrant ongoing research.

Ultrasound

Ultrasound is another technique that has become more popular with anesthesiologists for regional block procedures and with physiatrists for musculoskeletal diagnosis and joint injections over the last decade. Some chronic pain practitioners are advocating use of ultrasound for additional procedures [2]. The ability to visualize soft tissue targets (such as nerves, blood vessels, muscles, and ligaments), evaluate for anatomic variants, and the lack of risk from radiation are attractive reasons to use US. Multiple feasibility studies have been published examining the merits of various blocks of small sensory or mixed nerves, including the ilioinguinal/iliohypogastric, saphenous, lateral femoral cutaneous, suprascapular, pudendal, intercostal, and greater occipital nerves to name a few, have turned up in the last few years [16–21]. The advantage of many of these blocks is that they had previously been targeted mostly utilizing surface landmarks. Thus, the accuracy of blockade should be increased by any of the soft tissue image-guidance techniques. Some papers have examined the use of US for axial targets, but the deeper location of these blocks, the dropout (dark hypo-acoustic window causing poor visualization) caused by bone and lack of real-time contrast injection capability, renders procedures such as epidurals, selective spinal nerve blocks, facet joint blocks, lumbar, celiac and pelvic sympathetic blocks, and a few others extremely difficult and requiring of significant experience and skill.

Sympathetic Blocks

Stellate ganglion block is an example of one sympathetic block which may be advantageous for US blockade. Kapral et al. was the first to describe this technique and noted a decrease in the number of accidental vascular punctures in an ultrasound group compared to a surface landmark group [22]. Recently summarized risks of vertebral artery or deep/ascending cervical artery uptake or neck hematoma punctuate the seriousness of complications. A review from Japan reported 27 cases of retropharyngeal hematoma after stellate ganglion block (SGB) [23]. Narouze and colleagues have described the possibility of esophageal puncture as an additional risk [24]. Celiac plexus block has been studied using an anterior approach. Injury to bowel or organs is the main risks of anterior approaches. One study that is best characterized as US-assisted celiac plexus block had good success, but by today's standards, the imaging is poor [25]. As current CT and fluoroscopy techniques are good, it is unlikely that ultrasound will make great inroads in this area.

Trigger Point and Muscular Injections

There is little glamour in the performance of deep muscular and trigger point injections, which are usually office-based procedures. Only in the thoracic area or the abdomen is there any real risk of a major complication. Fluoroscopy is basically unnecessary for these soft targets. However, ultrasound may have real advantages, as the different muscle and fascial layers can be visualized well. A deep muscle like the piriformis muscle could be targeted more accurately using US. US offers the opportunity to perform a diagnostic exam (hip rotation) to aid needle localization in the correct muscle, whereby fluoroscopy could show a contrast-striated pattern, for example, but the needle could mistakenly be in a gluteal muscle. Studies suggest excellent accuracy [26]. Trigger points in other areas have been improved by US targeting [27]. Previous closed claim data shows the danger of pneumothorax from a misplaced trigger point in the thoracic area [28].

Zygapophyseal (Facet) Joint Injections and Medial Branch Blocks

Lumbar approaches to the facet joints and the medial branch nerves have been conducted. One trial compared ultrasound-guided facet joint injections to computed tomography (CT)-guided injections [29]. Ultrasound compared favorably to the outcomes from CT in this trial. The patients with larger body mass could not be performed with US, however. Ionizing radiation doses were reduced during the study, with the US group demonstrating a mean of 14.2 ± 11.7 versus 364.4 ± 213.7 mGy.cm for the group blocked utilizing CT. The US group was also blocked in a shorter time span, which may be advantageous in a busy practice [29]. Lumbar medial branch blocks have been investigated too. One study compared blocks of the medial branches performed with US or fluoroscopy. US consistently produced blocks at the correct level suggesting precise placement, with 95 % of the needles in correct anatomical position to effectively interrupt nerve conduction [30].

A study of US utilized for third occipital nerve block procedures in the cervical spine also demonstrated good results [3] as 23 of 28 needles were placed correctly [31]. Given the fact that fluoroscopically guided procedures targeting the third occipital nerve require a three-needle approach on or around the C2/3 zygapophyseal joint, the results are intriguing.

Epidural Blocks

Epidural injections are possible with US, but due to the high reliability of fluoroscopy, it is unlikely that significant change is imminent for the performance of these techniques. Likewise, CT is unlikely to induce a significant change in physician performance for these procedures with the possible exception of cervical transforaminal procedures. All the major approaches including interlaminar, caudal, transforaminal, and selective spinal root blocks have been studied using ultrasound guidance. The one area where change may occur in the short term is for caudal injections. The sacral hiatus is identified readily with US. Caudal needles placed with US in one study of 70 patients yielded 100 % accuracy as verified by caudal epidurogram [32]. Another study examined color flow Doppler as a surrogate for contrast injection with excellent reliability of the technique in most cases [33].

Neuromodulation

Ultrasound can also be utilized to target peripheral nerves at multiple sites including the upper and lower extremities, as well as epicranial sites such as the occipital and supraorbital nerves. Two anatomical feasibility studies of peripheral nerve stimulation electrode placement next to upper and lower extremity neural targets have been conducted [34, 35]. These were followed by an initial case series of nine patients showing that the majority of patients had good long-term stimulation [36]. In one study, simulated movement of the limbs after ultrasound-guided placements demonstrated resiliency of the placement despite continuous passive motion (CPM) [35]. Occipital nerve stimulation placement is also possible with US, either directly next to the artery and nerve or in a specific fascial layer [37]. Another target for peripheral nerve stimulation is the groin, for example, the ilioinguinal nerve [38].

Combination Imaging

Very limited study has been performed to date, but there may be some scenarios where two imaging modalities at once are used for additive or synergistic effects. For cancer therapy of bone tumors, percutaneous cryoablation is often utilized. Imaging with CT to visualize the external margins of the tumor and correlation with ice-ball formation are often used. CT-fluoroscopy technique is used to pass the cryoprobe, which may also be visualized with US [39]. Other combinations of imaging modalities may be used depending on the complexity of the procedure.

Conclusion

Pain medicine procedures are challenging, and most require some form of image guidance. Increasing attention to radiation risks, physician skill levels, and procedural outcomes and safety are important future considerations. As health-care costs rise, the relative value of imaging for individual procedural performance will be paramount. Ultrasound will have some utility, particularly for nerve, joint, and superficial targets. As the move to minimally invasive surgery takes hold, advanced FDCT systems may also be utilized with increasing frequency. But in the final analysis, best practice may continue to favor fluoroscopy for some procedures. It will likely fall to comparative outcomes researchers to answer the questions of which imaging is appropriate for a select procedure in the future.

References

1. American College of Occupational and Environmental Medicine. Chap. 12: Low back disorders. In: Occupational medicine practice guidelines. 2nd ed. Elk Grove Village: American College of Occupational and Environmental Medicine; 2008.
2. Huntoon MA. Ultrasound in pain medicine: advanced weaponry or just a fad? Reg Anesth. 2009;34:387–8.
3. Manchikanti L, Boswell MV, Singh V, et al. Comprehensive evidence-based guidelines for interventional techniques in the management of chronic spinal pain. Pain Physician. 2009;12:699–802.
4. el-Khoury GY, Ehara S, Weinstein JN, Montgomery WJ, Kathol MH. Epidural steroid injection: a procedure ideally performed with fluoroscopic control. Radiology. 1988;168:554–7.
5. Berrington de Gonzalez A, Mahesh M, Kim K-P, Bhargavan M, Lewis R, Mettler F, Land C. Projected cancer risks from computed tomographic scans performed in the United States in 2007. Arch Intern Med. 2009;169:2071–7.
6. Brenner DJ, Hall EJ. Computed tomography – an increasing source of radiation exposure. N Engl J Med. 2007;357:2277–84.
7. Orth RC, Wallace MJ, Kuo MD. C-arm cone-beam CT: general principles and technical considerations for use in interventional radiology. J Vasc Interv Radiol. 2008;19:814–21.
8. Siewerdsen JH, Moseley DJ, Burch S, et al. Volume CT with flat-panel detector on a mobile, isocentric C-arm: pre-clinical investigation in guidance of minimally invasive surgery. Med Phys. 2005;32:241–54.
9. Sasso RC, Garrido BJ. Computer-assisted spinal navigation versus serial radiography for posterior spinal fusion at L5/S1. J Spinal Disord Tech. 2007;20:118–22. http://www.ncbi.nlm.nih.gov/pubmed/17414979
10. Nakashima H, Sato K, Ando T, Inoh H, Nakamura H. Comparison of the percutaneous screw placement precision of isocentric C-arm 3-dimensional fluoroscopy-navigated pedicle screw implantation and conventional fluoroscopy method with minimally invasive surgery. J Spinal Disord Tech. 2009;22:468–72.
11. Weinstein JN, Spratt KF, Spengler D, et al. Spinal pedicle fixation: reliability and validity of roentgenogram-based assessment and surgical factors on successful screw placement. Spine. 1988;13:1012–8.
12. Goldschneider KR, Racadio JM, Weidner NJ. Celiac plexus blockade in children using a three-dimensional fluoroscopic reconstruction technique: case reports. Reg Anesth Pain Med. 2007;32:510–5.
13. Knight JR, Heran M, Munk PL, Raabe R, Liu DM. C-arm cone-beam CT: applications for spinal cement augmentation demonstrated by three cases. J Vasc Interv Radiol. 2008;19:1118–22.
14. Sequeiros RB, Klemola R, Ojala R, et al. Percutaneous MR-guided discography in a low-field system using optical instrument tracking: a feasibility study. J Magn Reson Imaging. 2003;17:214–9.
15. Streitparth F, Walter T, Wonneberger U, et al. Image-guided spinal injection procedures in open high-field MRI with vertical field orientation: feasibility and technical features. Eur Radiol. 2010;20:395–403.
16. Eichenberger U, Greher M, Kirchmair L, et al. Ultrasound – guided blocks of the ilioinguinal and iliohypogastric nerve: accuracy of a selective new technique confirmed by anatomical dissection. Br J Anaesth. 2006;97:238–43.
17. Gofeld M, Christakis M. Sonographically guided ilioinguinal nerve block. J Ultrasound Med. 2006;25:1571–5.
18. Rofaeel A, Peng P, Louis I, Chan V. Feasibility of real-time ultrasound for pudendal nerve block in patients with chronic perineal pain. Reg Anesth Pain Med. 2008;33:139–45.
19. Peng P, Narouze S. Ultrasound-guided interventional procedures in pain medicine. Part 1: non axial structures. Reg Anesth Pain Med. 2009;34:458–74.
20. Byas-Smith MG, Gulati A. Ultrasound-guided intercostal nerve cryoablation. Anesth Analg. 2006;103:1033–5.
21. Harmon D, Hearty C. Ultrasound guided suprascapular nerve block technique. Pain Physician. 2007;10:743–6.
22. Kapral S, Krafft P, Gosch M, Fleischmann M, Weinstabl C. Ultrasound imaging for stellate ganglion block: direct visualization of puncture site and local anesthetic spread. A pilot study. Reg Anesth. 1995;20:323–8.
23. Higa K, Hirata K, Hirota K, Nitahara K, Shono S. Retropharyngeal hematoma after stellate ganglion block. Anesthesiology. 2006;105:1238–45.
24. Narouze S, Vydyanathan A, Patel N. Ultrasound-guided stellate ganglion block successfully prevented esophageal puncture. Pain Physician. 2007;10:747–52.
25. Montero Matamala A, Vidal Lopez F, Aguilar Sanchez JL, Bach LD. Percutaneous anterior approach to the coeliac plexus using ultrasound. Br J Anaesth. 1989;62:637–40.

26. Smith J, Hurdle M-F, Locketz AJ, Wisnewski SJ. Ultrasound-guided piriformis injection: technique description and verification. Arch Phys Med Rehabil. 2006;87:1664–7.

27. Botwin KP, Sharma K, Saliba R, Patel BC. Ultrasound-guided trigger point injections in the cervicothoracic musculature: a new and unreported technique. Pain Physician. 2008;11:885–9.

28. Fitzgibbon DR, Posner KL, Domino KB, et al. Chronic pain management: ASA Closed Claims Project. Anesthesiology. 2004;100:98–105.

29. Galiano K, Obwegeser AA, Walch C, et al. Ultrasound – guided versus computed tomography- controlled facet joint injections in the lumbar spine: a prospective randomized clinical trial. Reg Anesth Pain Med. 2007;32:317–22.

30. Shim JK, Moon JC, Yoon KB, Kim WO, Yoon DM. Ultrasound-guided lumbar medial- branch block: a clinical study with fluoroscopy control. Reg Anesth Pain Med. 2006;31:451–4.

31. Eichenberger U, Greher M, Kapral S, et al. Sonographic visualization and ultrasound-guided block of the third occipital nerve: prospective for a new method to diagnose C2/3 zygapophysial joint pain. Anesthesiology. 2006;104:303–8.

32. Chen CP, Tang SF, Hsu TC, Tsai WC, Liu HP, Chen MJ, Date E, Lew HL. Ultrasound guidance in caudal epidural needle placement. Anesthesiology. 2004;101:181–4.

33. Yoon JS, Sim KH, Kim SJ, et al. The feasibility of color Doppler ultrasonography for caudal epidural steroid injection. Pain. 2005;118:210–4.

34. Huntoon MA, Huntoon EA, Obray JB, Lamer TJ. Feasibility of ultrasound guided percutaneous placement of peripheral nerve stimulation electrodes in a cadaver model: part one, lower extremity. Reg Anesth Pain Med. 2008;33(6):551–7.

35. Huntoon MA, Hoelzer BC, Burgher AH, Hurdle MF, Huntoon EA. Feasibility of ultrasound-guided percutaneous placement of peripheral nerve stimulation electrodes and anchoring during simulated movement: part two, upper extremity. Reg Anesth Pain Med. 2008;33(6):558–65.

36. Huntoon MA, Burgher AH. Ultrasound-guided permanent implantation of peripheral nerve stimulation (PNS) system for neuropathic pain of the extremities: original cases and outcomes. Pain Med. 2009;10:1369–77.

37. Hayek SM, Jasper JF, Deer TR, Narouze SN. Occipital neurostimulation-induced muscle spasms: implications for lead placement. Pain Physician. 2009;12:867–76.

38. Carayannopouos A, Beasley R, Sites B. Facilitation of percutaneous trial lead placement with ultrasound guidance for peripheral nerve stimulation trial of ilioinguinal neuralgia: a technical note. Neuromodulation. 2009;12:296–301.

39. Callstrom MR, Atwell TD, Charboneau JW, et al. Painful metastasis involving bone: percutaneous image-guided cryoablation-prospective trial interim analysis. Radiology. 2006;241:572–80.

Interventional Approaches: Neuromodulation

Asokumar Buvanendran, Sunil J. Panchal, and Philip S. Kim

Introduction

Interventional procedures are covered in three parts:
Part II reviews the anatomy and physiology of pain, as relevant to the practitioner
Part III details neural blockade and neurolysis blocks
Part IV provides guidance to the full range of neuromodulation techniques

As supported by this volume, comprehensive pain care is the optimal method to help patients progress to recovery. Interventional pain procedures are one part of the comprehensive approach. New procedures continue to be developed and established procedures continue to evolve as our understanding of the pathophysiology of pain grows. At the same time, the evidence base for interventional pain procedures is under intense scrutiny. The issue is a familiar one in the realm of interventional treatments. As with other surgical procedures, having a control group in a clinical study of interventions for patients with chronic pain presents significant ethical concerns.

The contributors to these parts and we share the belief that the decision to use a procedure solely on the basis of evidence misses the importance of the context of treatment. By the time a patient seeks out a pain medicine physician, he or she is looking for a practice that provides advanced and novel interventional treatments. The primary care physician has already started the patient on non-surgical approaches such as physical therapy and analgesics, and the interventional procedure acts as a therapeutic bridge between the patient's non-surgical management and psychological coping strategies, often significantly reducing the dose requirements of oral analgesics. From trigger point injections and epidural steroids, to radiofrequency ablation and implantable devices (for spinal cord stimulation, peripheral nerve stimulation, and intraspinal drug delivery), interventional procedures are among the most efficient ways of effecting change in pain reporting.

As the population of patients coping with pain grows older, maintenance on oral analgesics, particularly opioids for chronic non-cancer pain, becomes less of an option due to the development of comorbid medical conditions and the addition of other medications. Interventions for painful conditions, such as vertebral compression fractures, spondylosis, and spinal stenosis, can help older patients with acute pain and provide immediate and temporizing relief.

Given the fast evolutionary pace of technology, we expect that the chapter content in these parts will change significantly when the next edition of the book is published. In this inaugural edition, our aim is to provide you with up-to-the-minute expert guidance and practical tips for the current practice of simple and complex interventions for pain control. Furthermore, we hope to offer you a glimpse into the future, of therapies to come.

A History of Neurostimulation

56

Jeffrey T.B. Peterson and Timothy R. Deer

Key Points

- The earliest documented use of electricity to treat pain occurred around 63 AD.
- The Leyden jar made the storage of electrical current possible.
- Many early attempts at using electricity to treat pain were unsuccessful.
- Norman Shealy is credited with the development of modern neuromodulation.
- There are many new therapies on the horizon.

Discovery and Early Applications

The word "electricity" comes from the word "*ēlektron*," the Greek word for amber. Greek scientists found that when Amber, the fossilized resin of trees, was rubbed with another material, it created sparks of electricity. The capture or harnessing of these sparks led to the ability to utilize electricity in many applications, including the treatment of human disease conditions.

The earliest documented use of electricity to treat pain occurred around 63 AD. Scribonius Largus discovered that

J.T.B. Peterson (✉)
The Center for Pain Relief, Inc.,
400 Court Street, Suite 100, Charleston,
WV 25301, USA
e-mail: jpeterson@centerforpainrelief.com

T.R. Deer, M.D.
The Center for Pain Relief,
400 Court Street, Suite 302, Charleston,
WV 25301, USA

Department of Anesthesiology,
West Virginia University School of Medicine,
Charleston, WV, USA
e-mail: doctdeer@aol.com

pain from gout could be relieved by contact with a torpedo fish (Fig. 56.1) and suggested that this treatment would be effective for generalized pain relief and treatment:

> For any type of gout, a live black torpedo should, when the pain begins, be placed under the feet. The patient must stand on a moist shore, washed by the sea, and he should stay like this until the whole foot and leg up to the knee is numb. This takes away present pain, and prevents pain from coming on if it has not already arisen [1].

In the seventeenth century, Gilbert, a famous scientist of the time, described the use of lodestone, a piece of magnetic iron ore, to treat pain. He wrote that the electromagnetic qualities of the lodestone could be used to manage pain symptoms of headaches, mental disorders, and marital infidelities with varying degrees of success [2].

Dutch physicist Pieter van Musschenbroek, University of Leyden, is credited with a breakthrough in the storage of electrical charges. This device he developed, the Leyden jar (Fig. 56.2), stored an electrical charge that was constructed by placing water in a metal container suspended by insulating silk cords and placing a brass wire through a cork into the water. In 1746, Jean Jallabert employed a Leyden jar and discovered that electricity could be used to stimulate muscle fibers [3]. Jallabert treated a paralyzed limb in a locksmith causing involuntary contractions, regeneration of muscle, and increased blood flow. Jallabert's report inspired many scientists, and over the following two decades, there were several reports of successful treatment of neuromuscular disorders and disease. In 1756, Leopaldo Caldani noted that a Leyden jar could be discharged in the vicinity of a mounted and dissected frog's leg, which subsequently caused the leg to twitch. This discovery led many to proclaim electricity as a miracle cure for many diseases and that its use in stimulating areas of the body had far-reaching applications [4]. Benjamin Franklin, the first American credited with using neurostimulation, was intrigued by these experiments and conducted his own research on the treatment of painful conditions. After many failed experiments, Franklin concluded that successful claims of pain treatment were without merit

T.R. Deer et al. (eds.), *Comprehensive Treatment of Chronic Pain by Medical, Interventional, and Integrative Approaches*,
DOI 10.1007/978-1-4614-1560-2_56, © American Academy of Pain Medicine 2013

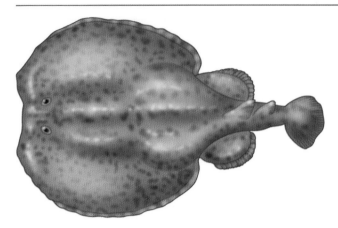

Fig. 56.1 The torpedo fish. An early treatment option

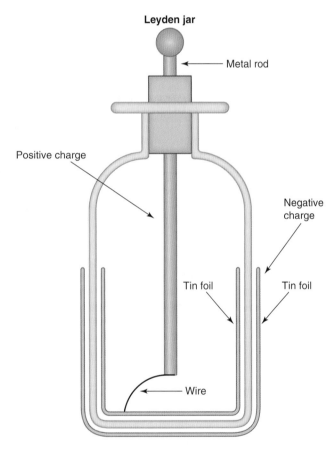

Fig. 56.2 The Leyden jar

and reported that his tests produced nothing more than discomfort for his subjects. It should be noted, however, that Franklin used high-voltage stimulation in his experiments, which caused true adverse effects of burning and injury to his test subjects.

In 1840, Guillaume Duchenne used a process of "electro puncture" to map muscle function, using electrically charge

needles that were inserted into the skin. Duchenne's book "De L'electrisation Localise" described direct muscle stimulation and indirect nerve stimulation and contributed to greater understanding of the effects of electrical current on these systems.

Between 1884 and 1886, Sir Victor Horsley introduced the first practical application of intraoperative neurostimulation when electrical stimulation was used to identify a specific cortical in a patient with epileptic foci [5].

Modern Treatment Protocols

By the beginning of 1900s, many devices were commercially available to treat painful conditions. Transcutaneous electrical nerve stimulation devices, comparable to today's TENS (Fig. 56.3) units, as well as devices like the Electreat (Fig. 56.4), which sold as many as 250,000 units over 25 years, were present in many physician's offices. These electrical devices were used to treat medical problems such as gout, baldness, arthritis, and marital "issues." Although these crude devices may have produced few positive results, they did foreshadow the development of today's common treatment options.

The breakthrough in the use of neurostimulation in modern medicine came about in the 1960s.

Norman Shealy and colleagues described the use of electrical current to modulate the nervous system and change the perception of pain and suffering [6]. Shealy codeveloped a stimulating "lead" that would work on the dorsal columns of the spinal cord. The device used a platinum electrode design with a positive and negative electrode to treat end of life cancer pain. Shealy referred to these devices as "dorsal column stimulators." The leads were attached to an external cardiac generator device. In 1968, Medtronic (Minneapolis, Minnesota) obtained FDA approval to market these devices for the treatment of pain (Fig. 56.5). This early development was not without difficulty, as many serious complications were associated with these early devices including spinal fluid leakage and compression of the spinal cord. These safety issues led many to believe that this type of treatment was not safe, and until the development of extradural placement, many were concerned about employing these treatment methods.

During the last three decades, there have been significant improvements in technology. Early systems employed two contact leads composed of platinum; newer leads use eight contact leads made from titanium, significantly reducing complications associated with lead migration or lead fracture (Fig. 56.6). Surgical laminotomy leads have been improved with the development of new configurations capable of giving more direct stimulation. Complex programming devices and

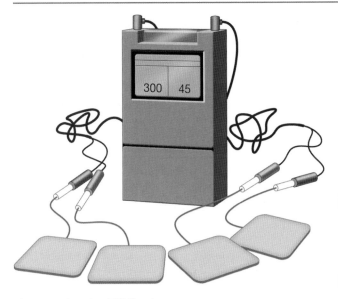

Fig. 56.3   A modern TENS unit

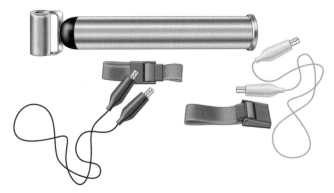

Fig. 56.4   The Electreat device

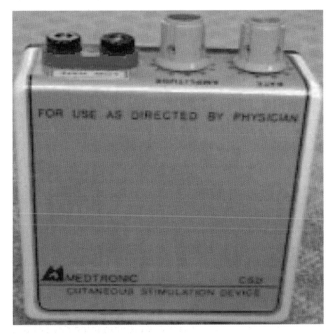

Fig. 56.5   Early Medtronic stimulation device

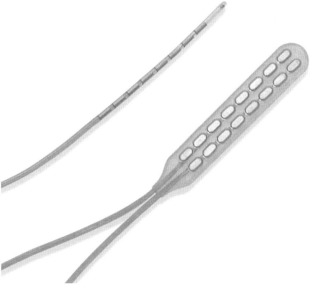

Fig. 56.6   Modern lead design

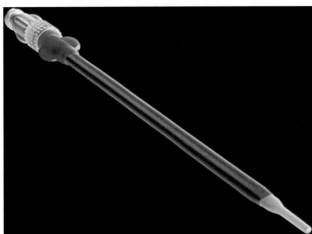

Fig. 56.7   The Epiducer lead delivery system

models, rechargeable batteries, and lower profile wire connectors and wiring are all now widely available. Other advanced technologies including the Epiducer (Fig. 56.7) (St. Jude Neurological, Minneapolis, MN), a percutaneous sheath that may simplify placement of paddle leads and complex percutaneous arrays, and Spinal Modulation's (Menlo Park, CA) DRG stimulation device (Fig. 56.8) are also rapidly expanding the neurostimulation options that are available to patients, while improving safety and patient outcomes.

In the future, physicians will be able to combine advanced imaging with these technologies and track the individual patients' response to neurostimulation. This pain response feedback may open a door to fully customizable treatment options and allow individualized medical therapies.

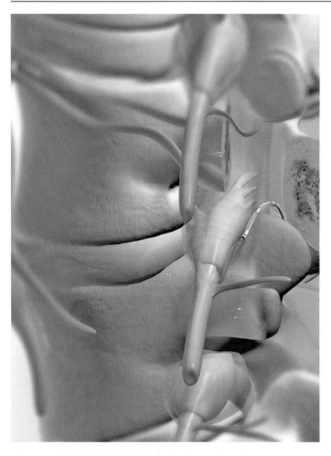

Fig. 56.8 Spinal modulation – DRG stimulation

References

1. Stillings D. The first use of electricity for pain treatment. Medtronic. Archive on Electro-Stimulation. 1971.
2. Pumfrey S, Tilley D. William Gilbert: forgotten genius. Phys World. 2003:15–6.
3. Experiments on electricity with some conjectures on the cause of its effects, vol. 8. 2nd ed. Geneva; 1749, Paris, 12 mo.
4. Cotti P. The discovery of the electric current. Physica B. 1995;204 (1–4):367–9; condensed matter.
5. Sakas D, Simpson A, Krames E. Operative neuromodulation, Functional neuroprosthetic surgery: an introduction, vol. 1. Vienna: Springer; 2007. 482 pages.
6. Shealy CN, Mortimer JT, Reswick JB. Electrical inhibition of pain by stimulation of the dorsal columns: preliminary clinical report. Anesth Analg. 1967;46:489–91.

Stimulation of the Peripheral Nerve and Peripheral Nerve Field

Jason E. Pope, Timothy R. Deer, Eric J. Grigsby, and Philip S. Kim

Key Points

- Stimulation of the peripheral nerve is a critical part of the pain treatment algorithm for neuropathic pain.
- Stimulation of the peripheral nerve field is helpful in conditions where the conventional SCS is not possible or contraindicated.
- These techniques may be used to supplement other implants such as spinal cord stimulation systems or intrathecal drug delivery.
- Complications of PNS and PNFS are limited and are generally much less of a risk than implants in the epidural space.
- The therapies continue to evolve, and further product development is needed to achieve optimal outcomes in a cost effective manner.

J.E. Pope, M.D. (✉)
Napa Pain Institute, Queen of the Valley,
St Helena Hospital, 3434 Villa Lane, Suite 150,
Napa, CA 94558, USA

Department of Anesthesiology,
Vanderbilt University School of Medicine,
Nashville, TN, USA
e-mail: popeje@me.com

T.R. Deer, M.D.
The Center for Pain Relief,
400 Court Street, Suite 302,
Charleston, WV 25301, USA

Department of Anesthesiology,
West Virginia University School of Medicine,
Charleston, WV, USA
e-mail: doctdeer@aol.com

E.J. Grigsby, M.D.
Napa Pain Institute, Queen of the Valley, St Helena Hospital,
3434 Villa Lane, Suite 150, Napa, CA 94558, USA
e-mail: sam@neurovations.com

P.S. Kim, M.D.
Center for Interventional Pain & Spine,
4701 Ogletown-Stanton Road, Suite 2131,
Newark, DE 19713, USA
e-mail: phshkim@yahoo.com

Introduction

Neuromodulation by stimulation is most likely active by changing the balance in excitatory and inhibitory fibers based on the theory of Melzak and Wall [1]. Since its introduction, neuromodulation strategies have progressively been advancing into the periphery. Peripheral nerve stimulation (PNS) is the direct electrical stimulation of named nerves outside of the neuroaxis. Peripheral nerve field stimulation (PNFS) is the stimulation of unnamed small nerves in the vicinity of pain by superficial, subcutaneous lead placement. Historically, PNS can be performed via an open surgical or percutaneous technique, well described by Stanton-Hicks [2, 3]. The percutaneous technique for both PNS and PNFS has now become more common and presents less risk and invasiveness to the patient. Because of this evolution to less invasive therapies, and the applicability to modern pain practice, this chapter will focus on these more practical approaches to targeting the nervous system.

Similar to spinal cord stimulation, patient selection is crucial to treatment success. PNS and PNFS are indicted for chronic neuropathic pain of peripheral nerve origin. Unlike the evidence supportive of spinal cord stimulation (SCS), peripheral nerve stimulation, and even less so for peripheral field stimulation, lacks strong leveled evidence from prospective, randomized, blinded studies. Further, many percutaneous neuromodulatory stimulation devices are not approved for PNS or PNFS by the FDA and are classified as "off label." Commonly accepted clinical indications for PNS include complex regional pain syndrome type II where there has been injury to the peripheral nervous system, neuropathic pain from mononeuropathy or plexopathy from a variety of causes, and headache (trigeminal neuralgia, occipital neuralgia, supraorbital neuralgia, cervicogenic headache, hemicrania continua, migraine) [4]. PNFS indications are less defined, as the mechanism is still being determined. Further, although spinal cord stimulation (SCS) for radicular pain secondary to failed back surgery syndrome (FBSS) is well accepted and validated, PNFS alone or in combination with epidural leads have anecdotal success for axial back pain for FBSS [5]. Sometimes conventional SCS may be contraindicated prior to PNFS. PNFS may be placed to supplement regions such as axial low back and neck that are not covered with SCS.

Comorbid psychiatric illness significantly reduces interventional treatment success rates [6], mindfully appreciating that approximately 20–45 % of chronic pain patients have accompanying psychopathology [7]. Subsequently, it is paramount to identify candidates suitable for concurrent treatment or exclude patients that require additional psychiatric treatment. Poor treatment outcome was identified in patients with presurgical somatization, depression, anxiety, and poor coping; however, some patients experience improvement in these factors once the pain is under better control, so these issues are not contraindicated [8].

Ideal candidacy for PNS and PNFS has yet to be determined. While some advocate a successful nerve block prior to the trial, others argue that a previous successful nerve block is unnecessary and is not predictive of outcome. Notwithstanding, a trial prior to implantation is mandatory. With the open technique (not described here), some advocate a direct to implant approach in an effort to reduce repetitive procedural morbidity [7]. This can be accomplished by a staged technique when indicated, with the initial implant of the lead prior to finalizing the system by generator placement at a later date. Failure of conservative and traditional management of neuropathic or mixed nociceptive/neuropathic pain is usually recommended.

Contraindications

Patients with local infection near the injection site, coagulopathy, allergy to injectate, or comorbidities/conditions that prevent fluoroscopic needle guidance or consent should be avoided. In regard to bleeding risk, the use of needles outside the neuroaxis makes the use of guides by the American Society of Regional Anesthesia less appropriate for guidance in these cases, despite their most recent argument [9]. Clinical judgment is required, as permanent neurologic sequela is less likely in the periphery.

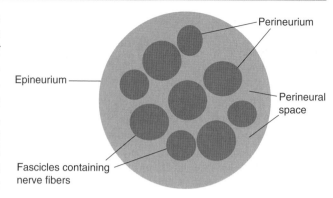

Fig. 57.1 Peripheral nerve architecture [12]

Scientific Foundation

Peripheral neuromodulatory success requires an anatomic appreciation for the architecture of the peripheral nerve. Peripheral nerves are composed of axons encased by Schwann cells, with or without a myelin sheath. The cell body of the sensory nerve is unipolar and is located in the dorsal root ganglion. Sensory afferent nerve cell bodies extend an axon and dendrites that permit synaptic communication with neighboring cells. In addition to creating a transmembrane potential essential for nerve conduction, they also provide a means for nutritional flow, an important rate-limiting step for nerve repair [10]. Axons enclosed in myelin have gaps, termed nodes of Ranvier, and are utilized to increase conduction velocity. The axons are encased within the endoneurium and bundled into fascicles and surrounded by perineurium. These fascicles divide and fuse to form multiple plexi along the nerve trunk, with discrete topographic architecture. The vasculature of the peripheral nerve resides in the perineurium [11]. The perineural bundles are then finally encased by epineurium (Fig. 57.1).

Peripheral nerves can be categorized based on their conduction velocity and diameter (Table 57.1).

The aforementioned nerve layers and inconsistent fascicular topographic arrangement provide an anatomic explanation not only for the impendence to overcome but also the cumulative effect of cathodal stimulation employed in peripheral neuromodulation [14]. PNS and PNFS directly inhibit primary nociceptive afferents and suggest central sensitization can be subverted by peripheral nociceptive suppression. Moreover, percutaneous PNS and PNFS approaches utilize devices that were designed for use in the epidural space, and therefore peripheral use is accompanied by frequent, although minor, complications.

Image guidance is recommended to perform percutaneous PNS. Unlike the spine, the use of imaging in the periphery is complex and is impacted by patient positioning, variation in bony landmarks, and obesity. Consequently, neuropathic pain peripheral nerve targets are only limited by the

Table 57.1 Nerve fiber classification, diameter, and conduction velocity [13]

Description of nerve fibers	Group		Diameter (μm)	Conduction velocity (m/s)
Myelinated somatic		Alpha α	20	120
		Beta β		
	A	Gamma γ		S-40 (pain fibers)
		Delta ∂	3–4	S-40 (pain fibers)
		Epsilone	2	5
Myelinated visceral (preganglionic autonomic)	B		<3	3–15
Unmyelinated somatic	C		<2	0.5–2 (pain fibers)

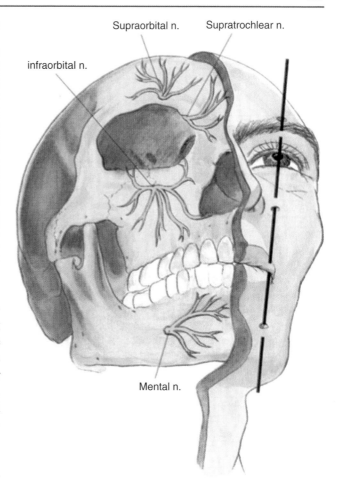

Fig. 57.2 Terminal branches of the trigeminal nerve [15]

ability to visualize them, either directly or indirectly (by anatomic correlation to well-defined osteal landmarks or using US guidance and/or fluoroscopy). Common sites include the supraorbital, the infraorbital, and the greater occipital nerves in the head and neck; the ulnar, median, and suprascapular nerves in the upper extremity; the intercostal, ilioinguinal, iliohypogastric, and genitofemoral nerves in the trunk; and the lateral femoral cutaneous, saphenous, sciatic, and posterior tibial nerves in the lower extremity.

Clinical Examples

PNS and PNFS trialing and permanent implantation require a meticulous sterile preparation and wide enough operative fields to visualize the necessary surgical targets. Further, peripheral nerve stimulation is only limited by the ability to visualize the target nerve and IPG implantation location. Peripheral nerve stimulation targets will be discussed separately.

Trigeminal Peripheral Nerve Stimulation

Terminal branch trigeminal targets include the supraorbital and infraorbital nerves, as illustrated in Fig. 57.2.

Infraorbital Nerve Stimulation Trial

The infraorbital nerve is one of the terminal branches of the maxillary division of the trigeminal nerve and exits via the infraorbital canal (please refer to Fig. 57.3).

The patient is positioned supine, prepped, and draped in sterile fashion (alcohol should be avoided in the face to avoid corneal irritation). Fluoroscopy is used in the anterior-posterior view to approximate the target. The target site is the infraorbital foramen on fluoroscopy. If it cannot be appreciated, the lead is placed approximately 1 cm below the orbit and just lateral to the ipsilateral nose, as described by Slavin et al. [16]. The entry point is lateral and inferior to the eye over the zygoma. Again, after judicious local anesthetic use at the entry point, a bent introducer needle to accommodate the contour of the face is inserted and directed to the target zone under fluoroscopy. Once the needle is in the correct position, the percutaneous cylindrical lead is introduced with care not to direct the distal tip of the needle too superficial to avoid lead tip erosion. The introducer needle is withdrawn slightly to allow intraoperative testing (Fig. 57.3).

Once therapeutic stimulation is achieved, the needle and stylet are removed, leaving the lead in place. After serial imaging to confirm placement, the lead is sutured in place, and a sterile dressing is applied and taken to the recovery area.

Supraorbital Nerve Stimulation Trial

Slavin et al. described the most commonly employed technique for terminal branch trigeminal nerve stimulation [16, 17]. The patient is positioned and prepared as discussed for

Fig. 57.3 Diagram of infraorbital lead placement (**a**) and fluoroscopic image (**b**) [12]

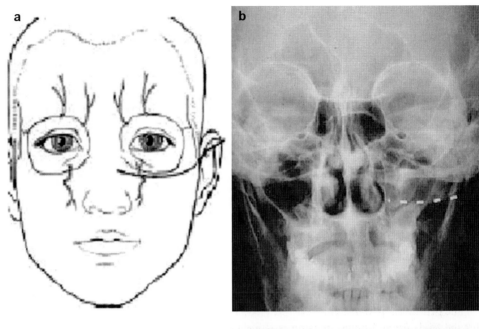

Fig. 57.4 Diagram of supraorbital lead placement [16] (**a**) and AP radiograph of electrode under fluoroscopy (**b**) [18]

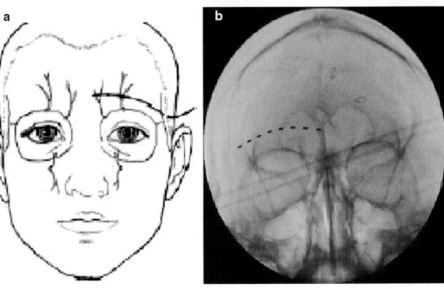

the infraorbital nerve stimulation. Fluoroscopy is used in the anterior-posterior view to approximate the target. A skin wheel is raised using 1 % lidocaine and is raised approximately 3–4 cm lateral to the lateral corner of the eye. An incision is then made, where a standard 14 G Tuohy needle (bent to allow and follow the contour of the face), is directed toward the midline approximately 1 cm above the supraorbital ridge until it is approximately 1 cm from the midline (Fig. 57.4). Avoiding too superficial trajectory will avoid lead tip erosion.

The stylet is removed, the percutaneous electrode is placed, and the needle is withdrawn to allow for intraoperative stimulation testing. Judicious use of local anesthetic at the puncture site will allow for intraoperative testing.

Once the desired therapeutic paresthesia overlying the patient's pain is achieved, the needle is withdrawn and removed while performing serial fluoroscopic guidance to ensure no inadvertent lead migration. The externalized lead is then secured with the supplied plastic anchor of the surgeon's choosing and nonabsorbable sutures. A sterile dressing is applied and the patient is taken to the recovery area.

Supra- and Infraorbital Nerve Permanent Implant

For the permanent implantation of both the infra- and supraorbital leads and IPG, general anesthesia is recommended (with laryngeal mask airway if feasible). The patient is again

Fig. 57.5 Greater occipital nerve diagram (**a**) and anatomic dissection (**b**) [15, 26]

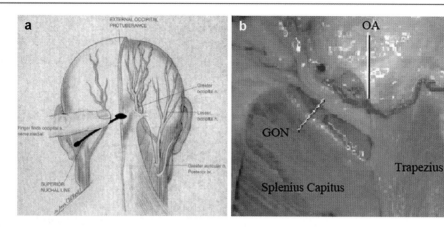

positioned supine with a slight contralateral head turn to provide access to the retroauricular location. A meticulous sterile prep and drape is required to accommodate tunneling and IPG site location. Commonly, the infraclavicular sight is chosen.

The permanent percutaneous lead is inserted as described for the trial. An additional incision is made in the ipsilateral retroauricular location after appropriate topicalization. Two techniques have been described for tunneling the lead's IPG connection portion. One is simply using the introducer needle with stylet in place (bent to accommodate the contour of the tunneling from the retroauricular incision to the anterior incision). The stylet is then removed, the lead introduced, and the needle withdrawn, leaving the tunneled lead.

From the retroauricular location, the lead is secured with the supplied plastic anchor using nonabsorbable suture. A stress loop is recommended (approximately 2–3 cm in diameter), and the lead is attached to the extension cable. It is recommended to place the extension cable connection in close approximation to the retroauricular incision to allow for easy access if reoperation is required.

IPG site location is largely the surgeon's preference [19]. In tunneling to infraclavicular and periscapular, one must remain in the posterior triangle of the neck and avoid the suprascapular nerve. Tremendous care is needed to avoid the external jugular which is adjacent to and superficial to the sternocleidomastoid muscle. Specifically, one must recognize the mobility of neck and shoulder especially if placing IPG in infraclavicular and periscapular. Measurement of length of extensions and electrodes is necessary to accommodate the flexion and extension of the neck. Avoidance of placement around osteal structures may reduce pain overlying the IPG device.

Regardless of IPG location, careful dissection (avoiding excessive blunt dissection), meticulous hemostasis, and anchoring to the perimuscular fascia are crucial to avoid IPG dislodgement. Anchoring to the perimuscular fascia is crucial and requires the use of tiny and soft or suture anchors given the limited subcutaneous tissue present.

Copious non-pressurized irrigation is performed at all incision sites, and layered closure is performed with absorbable suture. It is recommended to avoid placing sutures overlying the IPG, as this may impair wound healing and increase the chance of wound dehiscence. Sterile dressing is applied and the patient is recovered in the postoperative area.

Greater Occipital Nerve Stimulation Trial

The greater occipital nerve is also known as the second occipital nerve and is the medial branch of dorsal primary rami of C2. After discovery of the trigeminocervical complex, the greater occipital nerve has become a popular target for the treatment of headache [20–22]. Anatomic dissection characterizes the location from osteal landmarks, including the mastoid process and the occipital protuberance [23–25]. (It is generally found 1.4–1.6 cm lateral from the external occipital protuberance and 2.91–3.7 cm inferior). The nerve is consistently medial to the occipital artery (see Fig. 57.5).

There are multiple techniques described to stimulate the greater occipital nerve, with major differences centering on target location (C1–2 vs. nuchal ridge/retromastoid), lead trajectory orientation (medial to lateral or lateral to medial), and type (percutaneous cylindrical vs. paddle) (Fig. 57.6) [17, 26, 27].

Variation in location and lead type implantation for occipital nerve stimulation qualifies the initial high migration rates and aberrant muscular stimulation with percutaneous leads [17, 22, 26]. Proponents of paddle leads argue that less migration may occur because of the larger surface area of the lead and unidirectional current [27]. Muscle spasms of splenius capitis may be subverted by placement of the electrodes at or above the nuchal line, as opposed to the C1–2 level, where too superficial of a lead placement may increase the chance of erosion and burning sensations, while too deep a placement may cause aberrant muscular stimulation.

The trial is performed with the patient in the prone position. The surgical site is prepared by hair and meticulous

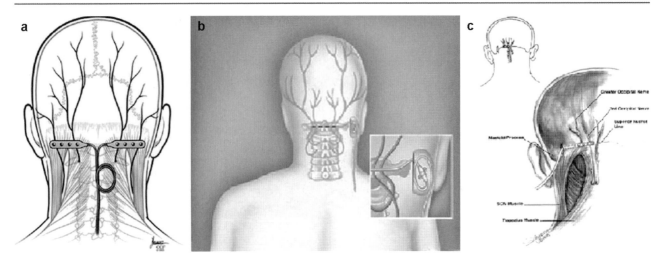

Fig. 57.6 Diagrams of percutaneous and paddle ONS lead placements (**a**) paddle placement (**b**) percutaneous placement (**c**) paddle placement [5, 17, 27]

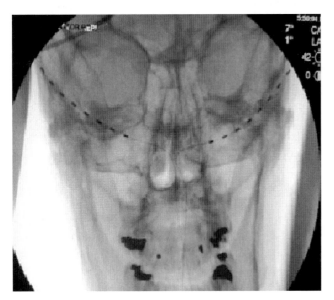

Fig. 57.7 Percutaneous cylindrical lead placement in AP fluoroscopic projection

sterile prep and drape in the normal fashion, leaving the entry site exposed. Image guidance is a prerequisite; fluoroscopy is commonly employed. After the target location is chosen, the incision site is identified. Care must be taken not to anesthetize the greater occipital nerve, and therefore judicious local anesthetic should be used at the incision site using 1 % lidocaine. The medial, nuchal line approach will be described here in further detail (Fig. 57.7).

An incision is made in the midline just caudal to the occipital protuberance. The needle is bent to accommodate the contour of the head. Under fluoroscopic guidance, lead is placed along the nuchal ridge ipsilateral to the target greater occipital nerve. Once appropriate lead position is achieved, the needle is withdrawn slightly to allow for intraoperative

stimulation testing. Once therapeutic stimulation is achieved, the needle is removed and the lead is secured using the plastic anchor provided and nonabsorbable suture. A sterile dressing is applied, and the patient is further recovered and programmed in the recovery room.

Greater Occipital Nerve Permanent Implant

Preparation and anesthesia and the lead placement procedure are largely the same for the occipital nerve trial and implant. The surgical prep site is extended to a larger area, however, to accommodate the IPG location. As discussed previously, IPG location and migration rates have been compared with superior outcomes suggested by infraclavicular and abdominal locations versus periscapular and gluteal sites, respectively. Like SCS, strain loops are created at the incision site by careful lateral dissection. Plastic anchors and nonabsorbable sutures are used to suture the lead to the dorsal fascia. A third incision is made and carefully dissected to accommodate the IPG. If extensions are needed and tunneling is required over a great distance, additional incisions with sequential tunneling may be required. Irrigation is performed at all incision sites, and layered closure is recommended, again, with care not to create a suture line overlying the implanted device. Sterile dressings are applied and further programming is performed in the recovery area.

Ulnar Nerve Stimulation Trial

The ulnar nerve is the most caudal portion of the brachial plexus, arising from the medial cord with nerve roots originating at C8–T1. The nerve descends medially to the brachial artery in the proximal arm, anterior to the medial triceps of the triceps, and at the elbow, it resides in the grove of the medial epicondyle.

Patient is positioned supine and patient preparation, including sterile prep and preoperative antibiotics, is performed in the usual manner. As described by Huntoon et al. [28] from the reliable and easily identified ulnar nerve location at the medial epicondyle, the nerve is traced in the axial sonographic view to approximately 9–13 cm proximal. Once the nerve is located, a skin wheel is raised with lidocaine 1 % and a skin nick is created. Under a live axial view of the ulnar nerve, the needle is then introduced via the long axis of the probe, placing the lead deep, adjacent, and perpendicular to the ulnar nerve. The needle is retracted and stimulation testing commenced. Anchoring of the lead to the skin was performed using the plastic anchors and nonabsorbable suture (Fig. 57.8).

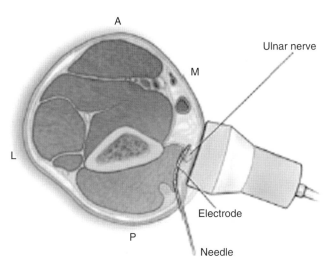

Fig. 57.8 The lead placement is aided by ultrasound guidance

Median Nerve Stimulation Trial

The median nerve arises from C5–8 and T1 roots and is more distal from the lateral and medial cords. It descends anterolateral to the axillary and brachial artery, where it lies medial to it and the biceps muscle tendon in the cubital fossa. Tracking distally in the forearm, the median nerve descends between the heads of the pronator teres muscle, and in the wrist, it resides between the tendons of the flexor carpi radialis and the flexor digitorum superficialis (Fig. 57.9).

The patient is positioned supine and preparation is performed in the usual manner. As described by Huntoon et al. [28] the ultrasound probe is placed in the transverse position and scanned distally until approximately 4–6 cm distal to the antecubital fossa between the pronator teres heads. After careful topicalization with 1 % lidocaine at the incision site only, a skin incision is made and under ultrasound guidance and 14-G needle is introduced in the longitudinal plane with the target nerve maintained in the axial plane with care to place it adjacent to the nerve. Once the needle is in the optimal position, the needle is retracted and stimulation testing is performed. Once therapeutic stimulation is achieved, anchoring of the lead to the skin is performed using the plastic anchors and nonabsorbable suture. A sterile dressing is applied. The patient is then transported to the recovery room for further programming.

Radial Nerve Stimulation Trial

The radial nerve has origins from the posterior cord from roots C5–8. Again, as described by Huntoon [28], the nerve travels obliquely to the humerus at the proximal arm, along with the deep brachii artery. The nerve is reliably located lateral to the humerus at approximately 10–14 cm proximal

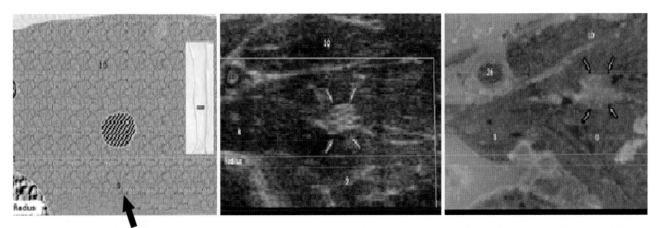

Middle third of the forearm (middle)

Fig. 57.9 Tracking distally in the forearm, the median nerve descends between the heads of the pronator teres muscle, and in the wrist, it resides between the tendons of the flexor carpi radialis and the flexor digitorum superficialis

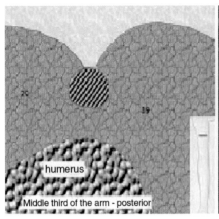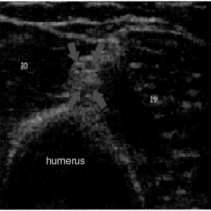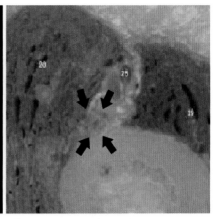

Fig. 57.10 The radial nerve is reliably located lateral to the humerus at approximately 10–14 cm proximal to the lateral epicondyle deep to the lateral head of the triceps. The radial nerve is outlined by the red *arrows* in the ultrasound image and the black arrows in the anatomic dissection. (Basic Human Anatomy. O'Rahilly, Muller, Carpenter and Swensen. Copyright © O'Rahilly 2009)

to the lateral epicondyle deep to the lateral head of the triceps (Fig. 57.10).

The patient is positioned supine and preparation is performed as described previously. As described by Huntoon et al. [28] the ultrasound probe is placed in the transverse position and scanned distally until approximately 10–14 cm proximal to the lateral epicondyle. After careful topicalization with 1 % lidocaine at the incision site only, a skin incision is made and under ultrasound guidance and 14-G needle is introduced in the longitudinal plane with the target nerve maintained in the axial plane with care to place it adjacent to the nerve. Once the needle is in the optimal position, the needle is retracted and stimulation testing is performed. Only after therapeutic stimulation is achieved, anchoring of the lead to the skin is performed using the plastic anchors and nonabsorbable suture to the skin. A sterile dressing is applied and the patient is transported to the recovery room for further programming.

Median, Ulnar, and Radial Permanent Implant

The patient preparation, anesthesia, and placement of the lead are the same as the trial procedure. The surgical prep site is extended to a larger area to accommodate the IPG location. Instead of anchoring to the skin for the permanent percutaneous placement, Huntoon recommends placement of the device in the upper chest (infraclavicular site) or abdomen for the upper extremity [28, 37].

Lead extensions and serial incisions are required to connect and tunnel the leads to the IPG. Sterile dressings are applied and programming is performed in the recovery room.

Peroneal Nerve Stimulation Trial

The sciatic nerve is formed from the L4 to S3 nerve roots and can be subdivided into medial and lateral compartments.

The medial portion of the sciatic nerve is functionally the tibial nerve, formed by the ventral branches of the L4–5 and S1–3, while the posterior branches of the ventral rami make up the peroneal nerve. The sciatic nerve descends and the rostral portion of the popliteal fossa, splitting formally into the tibial nerve medially and the common peroneal nerve laterally. The popliteal fossa's lateral boarders are the semimembranosus and semitendinosus medially, the biceps femoris laterally, and the gastrocnemius muscle caudally. The popliteal artery is medial to the neural targets (Fig. 57.11).

The patient is positioned to access the popliteal fossa of the afflicted leg after patient preparation, monitoring, and meticulous sterile prep and drape, as previously described. Axial ultrasound scanning is performed from the popliteal crease cephalad [37]. The tibial and peroneal nerves coalesce to from the sciatic nerve just cephalad to the aforementioned popliteal fossa. Identification of the popliteal artery is essential to avoid vascular entry. Once the desired nerve location is visualized, judicious topicalization of the skin entry site with 1 % lidocaine is performed. The introducer needle is then placed deep to the bifurcation of the sciatic nerve in a posterolateral to anteromedial direction [28]. Care to avoid muscular entry is essential. The electrode is introduced and the needle is retracted to allow for testing. Once therapeutic testing is achieved, the needle is withdrawn, the lead sutured to the fascia of the biceps femoris muscle using the plastic anchor and nonabsorbable suture, a sterile dressing applied, and the patient transported to the recovery room for further stimulation testing.

Saphenous Nerve Stimulation Trial

The saphenous nerve is a purely sensory nerve that is a distal cutaneous branch of the femoral nerve and therefore has contributions from the L2 to 4 nerve roots. It descends along the medial

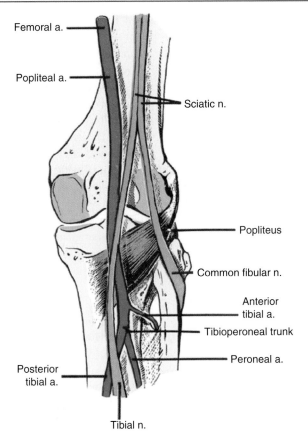

Fig. 57.11 The popliteal fossa's lateral boarders are the semimembranosus and semitendinosus medially, the biceps femoris laterally, and the gastrocnemius muscle caudally. The popliteal artery is medial to the neural targets

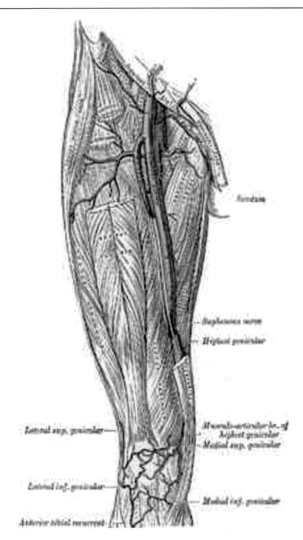

Fig. 57.12 Depiction of saphenous nerve [29]

aspect of the thigh and posterior to the sartorius muscle. In the caudal thigh, the nerve lies between the tendons of the sartorius and gracilis muscles (or vastus medialis muscle more distally), where it can be reliably located just proximal to the medial aspect of the knee and approximates the geniculate artery (Fig. 57.12).

The patient is positioned supine with slight ipsilateral extremity hip external rotation. After appropriate patient preparation, monitoring, and field prep and drape, axial scanning of the afflicted extremity is performed for an anatomic survey. The saphenous nerve is predominately hyperechoic, and Doppler survey to identify the geniculate artery may help identify the target. After needle entry topicalization with 1 % lidocaine, a small skin incision is made and the 14-G introducer needle is introduced and directed to the facial plane between the sartorius muscle and vastus medialis using an in-plane approach, avoiding muscle penetration. Once the needle approximates the nerve, the stimulation lead is placed and the needle retracted to allow for stimulation testing. Once therapeutic stimulation is achieved, the needle is removed and the lead is sutured to the vastus medialis fascia using a plastic anchor and nonabsorbable suture. A sterile dressing is applied and the patient is transported to the recovery area for further programming.

One author has placed electrodes to cover the saphenous and superficial peroneal nerves at the midpoint of the tibia. By placing medial and lateral to the tibia, stimulation is identified following the sensory coverage of the saphenous and superficial peroneal nerves (see Fig. 57.13). Successful trial with paresthesia coverage with pain relief have led to implantation of peripheral lead and generator placed in the medial calf.

Lateral Femoral Cutaneous Nerve (LFCN) Stimulation Trial

The lateral femoral cutaneous nerve is a branch of the posterior divisions of the L2–3 nerve roots and is also an exclusively sensory nerve. It travels lateral to the border of the psoas muscle and courses toward the anterior inferior iliac spine (ASIS), where it passes under the inguinal ligament, lying between the fascia lata (deep) and iliaca (superficial),

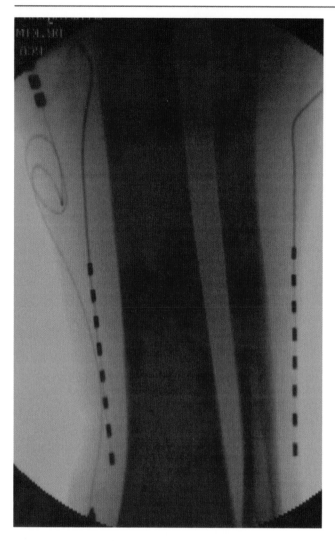

Fig. 57.13 Peripheral leads placed along the saphenous and superficial peroneal nerves

Intercostal Nerve Stimulation Trial

Intercostal nerves originate as the anterior rami of the paired exiting nerve roots and travel under the adjacent rib with close approximation to the intercostal vein and artery. Care must be taken not to violate the pleura. After aseptic preparation and monitoring as described previously, the patient is positioned either prone or in the lateral decubitus position. Under fluoroscopic guidance and after topicalization with 1 % lidocaine, a skin incision is made to accommodate the introducer needle. The needle should be bent to follow the curve of the rib. Once the needle is verified to be in the correct location, the lead is inserted and the needle retracted for stimulation testing. Once therapeutic stimulation is achieved, the needle is retracted and the lead is anchored with the supplied plastic anchor and nonabsorbable suture (Fig. 57.14).

Iliohypogastric, Ilioinguinal, Genitofemoral Nerves

The iliohypogastric and ilioinguinal nerves both arise from the L1 nerve root and emerge lateral to the psoas muscle. The nerves course in the anatomic plane of the internal oblique and transversus abdominal muscles. The genitofemoral nerve arises from the L1 and L2 nerve roots and emerges on the anterior surface of the psoas muscle. Its genital branch travels through the inguinal canal and, in males, supplies sensory information from the scrotal skin. In contrast, the ilioinguinal nerve supplies the groin. These nerves are amenable to peripheral stimulation, and care must be taken to ensure appropriate needle placement without violating the peritoneal cavity; image guidance via ultrasound is recommended. As these nerves are difficult to locate [31, 32], the line between PNS and PNFS begins to blur (Fig. 57.15).

providing sensory information from the lateral thigh. LFCN neuropathy is called meralgia paresthetica.

The patient is positioned supine with slight ipsilateral extremity in neutral position. After appropriate patient preparation, monitoring, and field prep and drape, axial scanning of the afflicted extremity is performed for an anatomic survey from the ASIS along the inguinal ligament. After appropriate needle entry site topicalization, a stab incision is made and the 14-G needle is introduced superficially along the longitudinal axis of the probe to lay in close proximity to the lateral femoral cutaneous nerve just caudal to the inguinal ligament. Once needle placement is optimized, the lead is introduced, placing the lead perpendicular to the course of the nerve. The needle is retracted and once therapeutic stimulation is achieved, the needle is retracted and the lead is anchored to the fascia lata with the supplied plastic anchor and nonabsorbable suture.

Peripheral Field Stimulation

As described previously, there is poor prospective data justifying PNFS. Nevertheless, the available evidence does suggest some efficacy in treating chronic neuropathic pain syndromes [33]. PNFS has also been used in conjunction with SCS to treat both back and leg pain, with inter- and intra-lead programming [34]. Common areas where PNFS has been employed include axial thoracic and lumbar back pain, failed back surgery syndrome (FBSS), greater trochanteric pain after total hip arthroplasty, post-herniorrhaphy pain, chronic abdominal pain, knee pain, and post-thoracotomy pain [5, 33, 35].

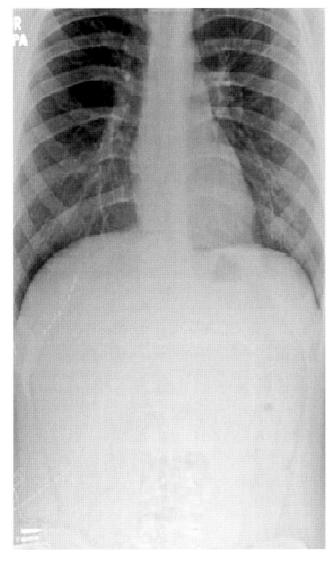

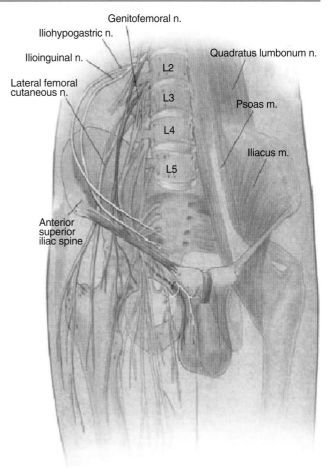

Fig. 57.15 Diagram of ilioinguinal, hypogastric and genitofemoral courses [15]

Fig. 57.14 Radiograph of T11 intercostal nerve percutaneous PNS [30]

Peripheral Field Stimulation Trial

The patient preparation and anesthesia are the same for the aforementioned named peripheral nerve neuromodulatory targets. Surgical site preparation is obviously dependent on the area of the painful area, and therefore the patient position needs to accommodate any easy operative field access. The leads are generally introduced to "bracket" the area of neuropathic pain, with the area of coverage approximately 180×90 mm, [36] while others advocate placing the lead centrally in the painful area [33].

Judicious anesthetizing is achieved at the desired entry site with 1 % lidocaine. A stab incision is created and the 14-G introducer needle is inserted near the target area subcutaneously under image guidance. After needle position finalized, the percutaneous lead is introduced, the needle is withdrawn, and stimulation testing commences. As described previously,

if unpleasant and burning sensations are reported, the lead is likely too deep and needs to be redirected more superficially. The lead is then secured to the skin using a plastic anchor and nonabsorbable suture and a sterile dressing is applied. The externalized lead is then connected to the externalized battery, and the patient is transported to the recovery room for more complex programming (Figs. 57.16, 57.17, and 57.18).

Peripheral Field Stimulation Permanent Implant

The peripheral nerve implant following a successful trial proceeds in the same manner as the trial with the additional prep and draping to include the battery site. The strategies and techniques that have been described previously can be translated to PNFS permanent placement.

Successful trial stimulation is defined as at least 50 % pain reduction and/or 50 % improvement in function. Trial periods commonly last for 5–7 days. Unlike spinal cord stimulator trials, PNS trials may be better tolerated for longer periods, as there is very low morbidity or mortality innate to

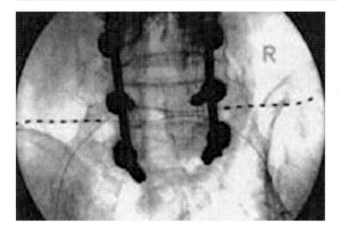

Fig. 57.16 PNFS for FBSS [33]

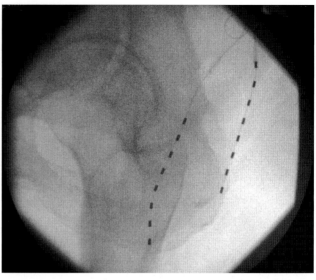

Fig. 57.17 PNFS for thigh pain following greater trochanteric bursectomy [5]

Fig. 57.18 Stimulator router

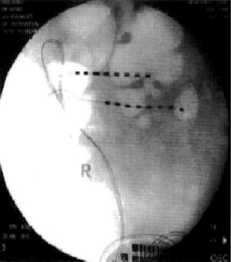
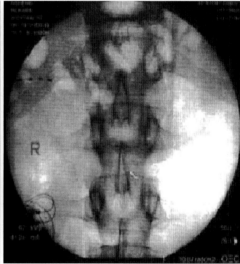

the superficial nature of the device placement. Once a trial is terminated and deemed successful, 3–4 weeks is usually allowed before permanent device placement.

Future Directions

Technical and surgical modifications of the leads and IPG originally designed for SCS are necessary. Further clinical and basic research is needed for the field to grow.

Stimulation in the periphery and centrally has been described working in parallel and concert. The StimRouter, designed to be a small self-contained lead with an external battery supply, is one example of the many advancements on the horizon (Fig. 57.18) [34].

References

1. Melzack R, Wall PD. Pain mechanisms: a new theory. Science. 1965;150:971–9.
2. Hassenusch SJ, Stanton-Hicks M, Schoppa D, Walsh JG, Covington EC. Long-term results of peripheral nerve stimulation for reflex sympathetic dystrophy. J Neurosurg. 1996;84(3):415–23.
3. Stanton-Hicks M, Salamon J. Stimulation of the central and peripheral nervous system for the control of pain. J Clin Neurophysiol. 1997;14(1):46–62.
4. Bittar RG, Teddy PJ. Peripheral neuromodulation for pain. J Clin Neurosci. 2009;16:1259–61.
5. Yakovlev AE, Resch BE, Karasev SA. Treatment of intractable hip pain after THA and GTB using peripheral nerve field stimulation: a case series. Wis Med J. 2010;109(3):149–52.
6. Fishbain D, Goldberg M, Meagher BR, et al. Male and female chronic pain patients characterized by DSMIII psychiatric diagnostic criteria. Pain. 1986;26:181–97.

7. Gallagher R. Primary care and pain medicine: a community solution to the public health problem of chronic pain. Med Clin North Am. 1999;83:555–83.

8. Celstin J, Edwards RR, Jamison RN. Pretreatment psychosocial variables as predictors of outcomes following lumbar surgery and spinal cord stimulation: a systematic review and literature synthesis. Pain Med. 2009;10(4):639–53.

9. Horlocker TT, Rowlingson JC, Enneking FK, Kopp SL, Benzon HT, Brown DL, Heit JA, Mulroy MF, Rosenquist RW, Tryba MT, Yuan CS. Regional anesthesia in the patient receiving antithrombotic or thrombolytic therapy: American society of regional anesthesia and pain medicine evidence – based guidelines (third edition). Reg Anesth Pain Med. 2010;35(1):64–101.

10. Thomas MA, Felsenthal G, Fast A, Yung M. Peripheral neuropathy, chap 39. In: Physical medicine and rehabilitation: principles and practice, vol. 1. 4th ed. Philadelphia: Lippincott Williams and Wilkins; 2005. p. 895.

11. Junqueira LC, Carneiro J, Kelley RO. Chap. 9: Nerve tissue and the nervous system. In: Basic histology. 9th ed. Norwalk: Appleton and Lange; 1995. p. 152–80.

12. Leng CL, Torrillo TM, Rosenblatt MA. Complications of peripheral nerve blocks. Br J Anaesth. 2010;105(S1):i97–107.

13. Johnson JO, Grecu L, Lawson NW: Autonomic nervous system. In: Barash PG, Cullen BF, Stoelting RK, Cahalan MK, Stock MC, Editors. Clinical Anesthesia. Philadelphia: Lippincott Williams & Wilkins, 2009, pp 326–368.

14. Grinberg Y, Schiefer MA, Tyler DJ, Gustafson KJ. Fascicular perineurium thickness, size, and position affect model predictions of neural excitation. IEEE Trans Neural Syst Rehabil Eng. 2008;16:572–81.

15. Brown DL. Atlas of regional anesthesia. 3rd ed. Philadelphia: Elsevier Inc; 2006. ISBN 13: 978-1-4160-2239-8.

16. Slavin KV, Wess C. Trigeminal branch stimulation for intractable neuropathic pain: technical note. Neuromodulation. 2005;8(1):7–13.

17. Jasper J, Hayek S. Implanted occipital nerve stimulator. Pain Physician. 2008;11:187–200.

18. Amin S, Buvanendran A, Park KS, Kroin JS, Moric M. Peripheral nerve stimulator for the treatment of supraorbital neuralgia: a retrospective case series. Cephalalgia. 2008;28:355–9.

19. Trentman TL, Mueller JT, Shah DM, Zimmerman RS, Noble BM. Occipital nerve stimulator lead pathway length changes with volunteer movement: an in vitro study. Pain Pract. 2010;10(1):42–8.

20. Goadsby PJ, Hoskin KL. The distribution of trigeminovascular afferents in the nonhuman primate brain Macaca nemestrina: a c-fos immunocytochemical study. J Anat. 1997;190:367–75.

21. Anthony M. Headache and the greater occipital nerve. Clin Neurol Neurosurg. 1992;94(4):297–301.

22. Schwedt TJ, Dodick D, Hentz J, Trentman TL, Zimmerman RS. Occipital nerve stimulation for chronic headache-long-term safety and efficacy. Cephalalgia. 2007;27:153–7.

23. Bovim G, Lucas B, Fredriksen TA, Lindboe CF, Stolt-Nielsen A, Sjaastad O. Topographic variations in the peripheral course of the greater occipital nerve: autopsy study with clinical correlations. Spine. 1991;16(4):475–8.

24. Mosser SW, Guyuron B, Janis J, Rohrich R. The anatomy of the greater occipital nerve: implications for the etiology of migraine headaches. Plast Reconstr Surg. 2004;114(2):693–7.

25. Loukas M. Identification of the greater occipital nerve landmarks for the treatment of occipital neuralgia. Folia Morphol. 2006;65(4):337–42.

26. Hayek SM, Jasper JF, Deer TR, Narouze SN. Occipital neurostimulation-induced muscle spasms: implications for lead placement. Pain Physician. 2009;12:867–76.

27. Oh MY, Ortega J, Bellotte JB, Whiting DM, Alo K. Peripheral nerve stimulation for the treatment of occipital neuralgia and transformed migraine using a C1–2–3 subcutaneous paddle style electrode: a technical report. Neuromodulation. 2004;7:103–12.

28. Huntoon MA, Burgher AH. Ultrasound-guided permanent implantation of peripheral nerve stimulation (PNS) system for neuropathic pain of the extremities: original cases and outcomes. Pain Med. 2009;10:1369–77.

29. Drake R, Vogl AW, Mitchell AWM. Slide 550 in Image Collection. Gray's Anatomy for Students, 2nd Edition 2009. Churchill Livingstone, Philadelphia.

30. Johnson RD, Green A, Aziz TZ. Implantation of an intercostal nerve stimulator for chronic abdominal pain. Ann R Coll Surg Engl. 2010;92:1–3.

31. Eichenberger U, Greher M, Kirchmair L, Curatolo M, Moriggl B. Ultrasound-guided blocks of the ilioinguinal and iliohypogastric nerve: accuracy of a selective new technique confirmed by anatomical dissection. Br J Anaesth. 2006;97:238–43.

32. Gofeld M, Christakis M. Sonographically guided ilioinguinal nerve block. J Ultrasound Med. 2006;25:1571–5.

33. Paicius RM, Bernstein CA, Lempert-Cohen C. Peripheral nerve field stimulation for the treatment of chronic low back pain: preliminary results of long-term follow-up: a case series. Neuromodulation. 2007;10(3):279–89.

34. Deer TR, Levy RM, Rosenfeld EL. Prospective clinical study of a new implantable peripheral nerve stimulation device to treat chronic pain. Clin J Pain. 2010;26:359–72.

35. Paicius RM, Bernstein CA, Lempert-Cohen C. Peripheral nerve field stimulation in chronic abdominal pain. Pain Physician. 2006;9:261–6.

36. Baralot G. Peripheral subcutaneous stimulation: a photographic surgical atlas. Denver: The Barolat Institute; 2009. p. 10.

37. Huntoon MA, Huntoon EA, Obray JB, Lamer TJ. Feasibility of ultrasound-guided percutaneous placement of peripheral nerve stimulation electrodes in a cadaver model: part one, lower extremity. Reg Anesth Pain Med. 2008;33(6):551–7.

Spinal Cord Stimulation

58

W. Porter McRoberts, Daniel M. Doleys,
and Kevin D. Cairns

Key Points

- While important, success in neuromodulation is dependent upon much more than technical aptitude. Of inestimable importance is awareness on the part of the implanter of the often surreptitious risks and elusive pitfalls in the process of patient selection, trialing, and implantation. This text seeks to expose, and then prepare the implanter for, those potential perils.
- Pain, being both multidimensional and multifactorial, has a significant psychological component. Therefore, a full understanding of the meaning of pain to the individual patient will provide the implanter with insights that may either doom or support the use of neuromodulation as a treatment.
- A multidisciplinary approach utilizing systematic behavioral and psychological treatment may sculpt patients with maladaptive coping skills or inappropriate expectations into better candidates with higher chances of treatment success.

- The mechanism of action of spinal cord stimulation (SCS) is not completely understood but likely involves several pathways including blocking nociceptive neurons at the level of the dorsal horn of the spinal cord, changes in neurotransmitters affecting supraspinal inhibitory pathways, and possible stimulation of spinothalamic tracts affecting blood flow, among other mechanisms.
- SCS has been shown to be a cost-effective and safe treatment, with several studies demonstrating superior efficacy as well as reduced cost compared to reoperation in patients who have already undergone spinal surgery.
- While the traditional approach of antegrade thoracic SCS may treat many patients, specific neural targets in the cervical cord, entering first-order sensory nerve roots or rootlets, or specific lumbar or sacral nerve root fibers require specialized techniques detailed here.

W.P. McRoberts, M.D. (✉)
Department of Interventional Spine and Pain Medicine,
Holy Cross Hospital, 4725 North Federal Highway,
Fort Lauderdale, FL 33308, USA
e-mail: portermcroberts@gmail.com

D.M. Doleys, Ph.D.
Pain and Rehabilitation Institute,
2270 Valley Road S-100, Birmingham, AL 35244, USA
e-mail: dmdpri@aol.com

K.D. Cairns, M.D., MPH
Department of Interventional Spine and Pain Medicine,
Florida Spine Specialists,6000 North Federal Highway,
Fort Lauderdale, FL, 33308USA

Division of PM&R, Nova Southeastern University,
3301 College Avenue, Fort Lauderdale, FL 33314, USA
e-mail: kcairnsmd@yahoo.com

Introduction

Since 1967, when Dr. Norman Shealy first demonstrated the temporary but complete abolition of pain implanting a dorsal column stimulator in a terminally ill cancer patient, great technological revolution and refinement has made spinal cord stimulation (SCS) widely available as a stable, long-term treatment option for chronic pain [1]. Compared to destructive techniques or other surgical approaches, SCS is unique in that it is both testable as a screening trial, using temporary percutaneous electrodes, and ultimately when implanted it is a reversible, augmentative treatment without damaging and thus permanent consequences.

SCS may represent the most stable and effective long-term treatment for pain yet devised, as increases in technology and miniaturization in the past 40 years led to implantable

T.R. Deer et al. (eds.), *Comprehensive Treatment of Chronic Pain by Medical, Interventional, and Integrative Approaches*,
DOI 10.1007/978-1-4614-1560-2_58, © American Academy of Pain Medicine 2013

methods and technology, yielding a treatment that is cost effective, ubiquitous, and effectual.

At least 116 million, or one in four, American adults suffer from chronic pain every year, costing as much as $635 billion annually [2]. The National Academy of Sciences in their recent publication, Relieving Pain in America: A Blueprint for Transforming, Prevention, Care, Education and Research, lists the first underlying principle as "effective pain management is a moral imperative, a professional responsibility, and the duty of people in the healing professions" [2]. In addition, as our population ages, so too does the prevalence of chronic pain and associated functional limitation and difficulty in performing activities of daily living. In a water-shed study investigating the incidence of chronic pain, von Korff et al. reported population data of 1,016 patient sample health maintenance organization enrollees, finding 45 % with persistent pain, 8 % with severe and persistent pain, and 2.7 % with severe, persistent pain-limiting activity for 7 days or greater [3]. Chronic neuropathic pain has a reported prevalence of 1.5–8 % in the general or primary care population [4]. The specialty of interventional pain medicine finds itself at a confluence of increasing societal awareness of chronic pain, rapidly evolving improvements in neuromodulation techniques and technology, and increasing demand for safe, effective, and cost-appropriate pain treatments.

The use of electrical measures to treat pain entered the treatment continuum early in medical history. Around 15 A.D., Scribonius Largus, a Roman physician, reported that a torpedo fish could be used to apply an electrical charge to patients to relieve pain [5]. The living fish was applied to the painful area to relieve pain treating such conditions as gout and headache [6]. Largus reported that Anteros, a freedman of Nero, was "cured" of the pains of gout using this technique, and Dioscorides, his contemporary, recommended "electroichthiotherapy" for headache [6]. Throughout the middle ages, the use of the torpedo fish persisted, treating chronic headache, unilateral headache as, well as vertigo [7]. Benjamin Franklin later experimented with electricity for pain relief and other afflictions [8]. Multiple other treatises were published on the use of electricity for pain relief as well as other medical and surgical applications, the most comprehensive authored by Beard and Rockwell [9].

In 1965, Ronald Melzack and Patrick Wall published their gate control theory, which adroitly departed from the popular theories of pain of Descartes, von Frey, and Goldscheider [10]. Their new paradigm not only set the stage for the development of SCS but also posited that pain was perceptual and modifiable through pathways of inhibition, both centrally and in the periphery. They surmised that the substantia gelatinosa acted as a form of central control summating the competing nociceptive and antinoceptive inputs and then sent the modified afferent signal rostrally (see Fig. 58.1).

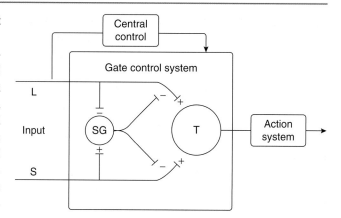

Fig. 58.1 Gate control theory

Building on the gate control theory, Shealy et al. [1] implanted a 70-year-old man dying of bronchogenic carcinoma via laminotomy, sewing the 3 × 4-mm electrodes to the dura. That evening in the postoperative setting, they began stimulation with 10–50-Hz and 400-ms pulse width at 0.8–1.2 V and 0.36–0.52 mA. Both his incisional pain and original chest pain were immediately abolished. Small changes were made throughout the remaining day and the next in response to discomforts. Eventually, the patient died on postoperative day 2 from a left hemispheric embolization from subacute bacterial endocarditis. Despite the abbreviated nature of this nascent trial, Shealy et al. [1] confirmed the suspicion that pain was not only modifiable at the spinal cord level, but that the clinical effect of electrical current in the spinal canal was of great importance to the human condition. Since that moment, SCS has undergone rapid evolution towards efficacy and safety.

This chapter will detail in short the scientific foundation of implantable SCS, the clinical use of SCS including patient selection and psychological screening, and trialing and implant techniques, with special attention to concepts that may diminish risk and complications and improve likelihood of success. Throughout the chapter, resources for further reader education will be included. Lastly, future directions for research surrounding spinal cord stimulation are summarized.

Patient Selection and Diagnostic Work-Up

Mechanism of Action

Chronic pain from injury to the central or peripheral nervous system can be managed by stimulating nerve fibers in the dorsal column via percutaneous or surgical electrode array placement, first described by Dr. Shealy in 1967 [1]. The exact mechanism of action of SCS is incompletely understood, however, likely involves both physiologic, orthodromic stimulation, and nonphysiologic, antidromic stimulation, respectively [11]. While several mechanisms of action have been described for SCS, the most accepted theory of pain relief can be explained by the gate theory first described by Melzack and Wall in 1965 [10]. This groundbreaking yet simplistic model describes the interaction of large sensory fibers and nociceptors and how they influence the transmission of neural impulses by second-order projection neurons in the dorsal horn. Placement of electrode arrays in the epidural space depolarizes A-beta nerves orthodromically in the posterior columns and antidromically via dorsal column collateral fibers, thereby inhibiting pain transmission to the brain [11]. Large, A-beta nerve activation causes depolarization of neurons in the dorsal horn and "closes the gate" for the transmission of A-delta and C-fibers to the projection neuron. In addition, large A-beta neuron activation inhibits GABAnergic pathways that influence wide dynamic range neurons that can become hyperexcitable in chronic pain states. Evoked paresthesia is targeted towards the specific region of pain, although the inhibition of pain is most likely related to activation of interneurons that suppress pain and not the antidromic depolarization resulting in the evoked paresthesia noted by the patient. Since the publication of the gate theory of pain transmission, it is clear that there are additional components to the transmission and processing of pain that include descending inhibitory pathways, alterations of neurotransmitters in the brain, as well as other tracts in the spinal cord that may be involved [12, 13]. The supraspinal descending inhibitory effects likely involve serotonin and norepinephrine and clinically may be related to patients noting pain relief several hours after the SCS system is turned off.

Inhibition of the sympathetic system by SCS is another potential mechanism to alleviate pain. Kemler et al. showed that in a group of patients with CRPS, pain relief did not depend on vasodilation, arguing against the inhibition of the sympathetic system by SCS to be vital for neuropathic pain relief [14]. It is possible, however, that stimulation-induced inhibition of the sympathetic system by SCS may be beneficial in patients with peripheral vascular disease where vasodilation may help with nociceptive pain related to ischemia, and it is likely that the underlying disease plays a large factor into the mechanism that ultimately results in pain relief [15].

The type of nerve population depolarized is determined by the placement of the electrode arrays and the stimulation parameters utilized. Different neural structures have different stimulation thresholds. The lowest threshold neural structures are located in the dorsal root entry zone, followed by the lateral fibers in the posterior columns, and the highest threshold fibers are the most medial. The somatotopic organization of the central nervous system persists in the dorsal columns and lead placement, and programming strategies are determined by the target neural element [16]. While importance has been historically placed on the cephalocaudal placement of SCS leads, more attention has been placed on the medial to lateral placement as well with multicolumn arrays, showing promise in more targeted stimulation given the medial to lateral somatotopic organization of nerves in the dorsal spinal cord and their ability to create guarded arrays. For that reason, placement of percutaneous SCS leads is generally preferred to be in the physiologic midline to maximize stimulation of the dorsal columns and minimize stimulation of the dorsal root entry zone. In addition, the frequency of SCS stimulation also effects which nerve population is depolarized [17]. Higher frequencies tend to stimulate a greater proportion of A-beta fibers, while lower frequencies stimulate more A delta and C fibers.

Functional MRI has demonstrated important changes in the way pain is processed in the brain in patients with chronic pain and how SCS may influence the central nervous system. The challenges with functional magnetic resonance imaging (fMRI) evaluating SCS and peripheral nerve field stimulation (PNfS) include minimizing heating of the contacts with pulsed radio frequency (RF) as well as fMRI, revealing widespread areas of activation and inhibition in the brain and the difficulty in interpretation [18]. In a healthy patient with an occipital nerve stimulator system, areas of activation were predominantly seen in the hypothalami, the thalami, the orbitofrontal and prefrontal cortex, the periaqueductal gray (PAG), the inferior parietal lobe, and the cerebellum. Deactivation was seen in primary areas (M1, V1, A1, and S1), the amygdala, the paracentral lobule, the hippocampus, S2, and SMA [19]. Kovaks et al. noted that the effects of stimulation were more pronounced with tonic stimulation rather than burst stimulation [19].

Patient Selection

Selecting the right patient is essential for a positive response to neuromodulation therapies. Among the diagnoses that have noted consistent benefit from SCS are lumbar post-laminectomy syndrome (PLS), radiculopathy, polyneuropathy, and complex regional pain syndrome (CRPS) [20, 21]. In general, patients with a history of spinal surgery with primarily leg pain have been shown to benefit significantly from SCS. North et al. [22, 23] in their seminal study randomized patients who had a history of lumbar surgery into repeat surgery and SCS groups and showed superiority of SCS to reoperation. In addition, in the same cohort of patients, North et al. demonstrated significant cost savings of SCS to repeat back surgery in intention to treat, treat as intended, and final treatment analysis [24]. The cause of post-laminectomy syndrome likely involves changes in peripheral sensitization as well as central windup phenomena in the spinal cord. Anatomically, these patients may present with epidural fibrosis, arachnoiditis, junctional

Table 58.1 SCS outcome data

References	Number of patients	Follow-up	Results
Kumar et al. [20]	410	8 years	74 % had >50 % relief
Cameron [32]	747	Up to 59 months	62 % had >50 % relief
Van Buyten et al. [31]	123	3 years	68 % had good to excellent relief
Aló et al. [93]	80	30 months	Mean pain scores declined from 8.2 at baseline to 4.8

stenosis above or below surgical site, or a completely normal MRI with normal postsurgical changes. In cases of instability with movement on flexion/extension x-rays, surgical referral is warranted. In addition, significant central canal stenosis in the thoracic or cervical spine impinging the spinal cord would be a contraindication for SCS implantation.

While in the USA the primary indications for SCS are radiculopathy, PLS, and polyneuropathy, emerging applications are being shown in Europe. The benefit of SCS in widespread small vessel coronary artery disease with chronic angina has been described [25]. In addition, there has been some evidence that the ability of SCS to cause vasodilation can potentially treat the underlying cause of peripheral vascular disease as well as mask its symptoms [26].

Case reports of more challenging diagnosis to treat with SCS have been reported including postherpetic neuralgia [27], post-thoracotomy syndrome [28], phantom limb pain, stroke central pain syndrome [29], spinal cord injury, and multiple sclerosis [30]. Case reports and small case series have been published describing benefit from SCS therapies in these patient populations, and it is unclear why these diagnoses have such variable response to treatment.

Outcomes/Cost-Effectiveness

Multiple studies have demonstrated clinical efficacy of SCS, with reduction in pain, improvement of function, and reduction in pain medicines well documented (see Table 58.1). In addition, SCS has been shown to be cost effective in several studies. North et al. [24] demonstrated significant cost savings in a cohort of patients who had spinal surgery when comparing SCS to repeat spine surgery. The cost for success for SCS was $48,357 compared to the cost for success with repeat spine surgery being $105,928 (treated as intended). Mekhail et al. compared patients with SCS systems to those without and noted a yearly cost savings of $30,221 per year attributed to less ER visits, less diagnostic tests, and lower utilization of health-care resources [31]. Of note, the timing of SCS implantation may be of great importance as Van Buyten et al. has shown a significant reduction in efficacy

when neuromodulation therapies are delayed with 85 % of patients realizing significant pain relief within 2 years of their pain beginning compared to 9 % of patients who have had pain for more than 15 years [32].

Psychological Evaluation for SCS

Background

Pain is well recognized as being multidimensional and multifactorial. Therefore, any therapy designed to affect pain, particularly in the chronic pain setting, should logically include a comprehensive or multidisciplinary evaluation. The psychological assessment should be considered as an integral and significant aspect of this evaluation process given the well-documented impact of psychosocial variables on the experience of pain.

Scores of studies involving thousands of chronic pain patients utilizing SCS therapy have been published. Although the results are touted as generally positive (the majority of patients report a 50 % or greater reduction is pain), reviews of the literature [33–35] have revealed a loss of pain relief in up to 50 % of patients at 1–2 years post-implant despite their having successfully "passed" a period of trial stimulation and the presence of a functional SCS unit. Indeed, one study [36] reported that 100 % of patients reported success at 16 months but only 59 % at 58 months. Psychological factors may play an important role in understanding this apparent loss of efficacy. An overemphasis on the SCS technology, while potentially economically rewarding (new power supplies, electrodes with more contacts, increased programming options, multiple electrode arrays), may come up short of a solution. In part, it may be equally advantageous to take the position of trying to discover "how to make what works, work better" rather than merely "tinkering with the technology." It is important to remember that the SCS trial is essentially an "acute" procedure being used to "predict" a "long-term" outcome with a "chronic disease." While computer modeling provides invaluable information about electrode disbursement patterns at the level of the spinal cord, it should not be mistaken to represent anything other than a guideline to achieving more specific patterns of stimulation, which may or may not be associated with greater and more prolonged pain relief.

Inclusion/Exclusion Criteria

Previous guidelines for "patient selection" have focused on exclusion criteria. For example, Daniel et al. [37] cited personality disorders [38], drug dependence, unstable family and personal relationships, poor vocational adjustment, and involvement in litigation/compensation as "red flags." Nelson et al. [39] suggested the presence of suicidality or homicidal, severe depression or other mood disorders, somatization/somatoform disorder, alcohol or drug dependency, unresolved compensation/litigation issues, lack of social support, and/or neurobehavioral cognitive deficits to be considered as contraindications of SCS therapy. In a conversation with Dr. Kumar (April 2004), he developed the "Kumar warning signs" which include K – "kannot" possibly live without this device; U – unlimited utilization, overuse of health-care resources; M – misunderstood, "nobody understands me, only you can help me doctor"; A – affective disorder, major psychopathology; and R – "REALLY…its only my pain I have no other problems," symptoms inconsistent with physical findings. The European Federation of IASP Chapters [51] declared major psychiatric disorders (active psychosis, severe depression or hypochondria, and somatization disorder), poor compliance and/or insufficient understanding of the therapy, lack of appropriate social support, and drug and alcohol abuse or drug-seeking behavior as contraindications.

Doleys [40] adopted a different approach when outlining 16 "hypothesized" positive indicators including a history of compliance with previous treatments, behavior and complaints consistent with pathology, behavioral/psychological evaluation consistent with patient complaints and reported psychosocial status, realistic concerns regarding "illness," mildly depressed, generally optimistic regarding outcome, and ability to cope with setbacks without responding in an emergent fashion. He went on described patient and physician beliefs "potentially" associated with positive and negative outcomes. In each of the cases above, the features outlined emerged from consensus, "common sense," clinical experience, and/or generalization of other literatures. None at this point has been experimentally validated and replicated.

The frequency with which a formal psychological assessment is carried out betrays what appears to be an almost universal acceptance of the role of psychological factors in chronic pain and pain therapies, including SCS. A Canadian survey [41] found that only 25 % of 13 participating centers reported routine psychological screening prior to SCS implantation, compared to 61 % of centers in a UK survey [42]. Although a "psychological screening" is required by Centers for Medicare & Medicaid Services (CMS) (Medicare health-care insurance) in the USA, the incidence of it in non-Medicare populations approximated 25 % [43]. The most common reasons given for the discrepancy between the support for psychological screening and its actual utilization were (a) lack of or inadequate insurance coverage, (b) lack of physician insistence, (c) patient refusal, and (d) lack of an appropriate evaluator. The cost of most psychological evaluations approximates 1–3 % or less of the total cost of the SCS trial and implantation in the USA. If screening/pretreatment prevented only 2–3/100 patients from failing treatment and the removal of the device, a cost savings would be realized [43].

Brief Literature Review

Celestin et al. [44] performed a systematic review of outcomes relating to lumbar surgery and SCS. They were able to identify only four SCS studies that met their criteria for the review. A successful outcome was defined as 6 months or more duration, decreased pain, increased function, and reduced health-care utilization. Depression, anxiety, somatization, poor coping, and hypochondriasis tended to be associated with poorer outcomes, but none was found to be statistically significant. Sparkes et al. [45] examined the literature on psychological variables affecting SCS outcomes spanning 1982–2008. In summarizing their review, they noted that the Minnesota Multiphasic Personality Profile (MMPI) [46] was the single most common test administered. The psychological variables studies included depression, hysteria, anxiety, mania, hypochondriasis, paranoia, defensiveness, joy, belief pain out control, catastrophizing, and psychopathic deviate. It was concluded that (a) depression probably correlates negatively, (b) mania possibly has a positive correlation, (c) hysteria was possibly negative, and (d) hypochondriasis was mixed [45].

One of the coauthors (DMD) recently participated as a member of group of clinicians and researchers organized by the American Pain Foundation to develop a consensus guideline for SCS therapy (in preparation). Nineteen studies from among several hundreds covering the period from 1990 to 2010 were selected on the basis of the information in their respective abstracts to be reviewed regarding their reported use of a psychological/psychiatric evaluation prior to SCS trialing or internalization. Twelve of the 19 studies noted using one or more psychometrically validated instruments or questionnaires. The content or makeup of the psychological screening was often based on theoretical bias. For example, Heckler et al. [47] and Molloy et al. [48] tended to favor behavioral/functionally oriented tests/questionnaires, Dumoulin et al. [49] a more psychoanalytic approach, and Lamé et al. [50] focused on the hypothesized impact of catastrophizing.

Only seven studies listed any psychological inclusion or acceptance criteria. Most often, the criteria was stated in the form of a very general statement, for example, "no contraindications," or "psychologically uncomplicated." Eight studies outlined psychological exclusion criteria. The often cited exclusion criteria were high levels of psychological distress, psychosis, somatization, alcohol/drug issues, and/or unresolved secondary gain issues, for example, pending litigation. Fourteen studies performed some type of pre post-internalization analysis on one or more of the tests results from the pre-implant screening. In nearly every case, this analysis was carried out for the purpose of determining the effect of SCS therapy. A few studies addressed psychological "predictors." In one, depression, especially when combined with age and the McGill score, predicted 88 % of 34 patients. Lamé et al. [50] found that catastrophizing did not predict outcomes in a group of CRPS patients. North et al. [51] reported that none of their psychological tests predicted the outcome, and Kupers et al. [52] and May et al. [36] noted that the patients with a "positive screen" did better than patients where caution or reservations were entered. In some cases, the emphasis was on predicting those who would proceed from trial to implant versus "outcome" predictors. A variety of tests/questionnaires were used. The MMPI, Beck Depression Inventory (BDI) [53], and the Oswestry Disability Questionnaire (ODQ) [54] were among the most common. It may be difficult to establish a commonly agreed upon interview format and battery of tests/questionnaires. Perhaps, the best approach at this point is to follow Deyo et al. [55] recommendation to obtain information regarding the qualitative/quantitative aspect of "pain," along with an assessment of mood, function, and personality features.

Elements of Psychological Evaluation

Unfortunately, the psychological evaluation is often construed as part of patient "selection." As such, the goal is seen as one of "clearing" the patient, a concept that has never been defined, clarified, or objectified [56]. This approach encourages a dichotomous decision of "go" or "no-go," with little regard to interventions that might improve the probability of a good long-term outcome [57]. It is herein suggested that the patient selection/evaluation aspect of SCS therapy should be considered as a *process* and not an event. The process begins with the review of records and the initial consultation and extends through the trial and up to the point that a decision is made to internalize or not. A systematic behavior/psychological assessment is part of the process. Patient selection is best conceptualized as longitudinal and focused on the identification of patient characteristics that implicates the patient as a good candidate for SCS or is potentially modifiable by psychological/behavioral interventions (CBT) designed to enhance the short- and long-term outcomes.

For the psychological evaluation to provide the most useful information and therefore to be of minimum benefit to the patient and clinician, the following components are recommended. First, the assessment should be conducted by an appropriately trained, knowledgeable, and experienced mental health clinician. Second, it should include a face-to-face interview with the patient and when possible the participation of a significant other. Data from the clinical interview should be supplemented by the use of well-known and validated test (s)/questionnaires. At least one of the clinical instruments employed should contain a mechanism for detecting dissimulation (i.e., a "fake-bad" or "fake-good"

scale). The use of generic (overall quality of life) and disease-specific (pain rating) measures should be considered. It would be important for the evaluator to have post-trial and/or post-internalization contact with the patients, or least the outcome data, to determine the accuracy of the recommendations generated by the evaluation.

Unfortunately, the psychological evaluation all too often is treated necessary nuisances. Patients are sent to "outside" consultants with little or no interest or experience in chronic pain or SCS therapy merely as a means of satisfying insurance or regulatory guidelines. Worse, computer-scored and interpreted tests are administered by the physician as a mechanism to satisfy the requirement. Even when such tests are administered by a psychologist, the American Psychological Association Ethical Guidelines [58] requires patient contact prior to rendering an interpretation of the test results. Finally, periodic updated brief assessments may well assist in adjustments of the therapeutic algorithm and improving long-term outcomes [59].

Despite the potential limited prognostic value, the evaluation process can and should serve several other functions [60]. First, it can be used to facilitate the development of an individualized treatment plan. Second, it provides an opportunity to properly prepare and educate the patient and significant other for the trial, possible internalization, and long-term treatment. Third, psychological interventions designed to mitigate the impact of maladaptive psychological issues (i.e., poor coping, limited acceptance, etc.) can be implemented and create a patient with a more favorable prognosis. And finally, the psychological evaluation process can be used as a means of addressing potentially modifiable problems and therefore may enhance the overall efficacy of therapy and prevent an overemphasis on the development of absolute exclusionary criteria. It can also help to fulfill the requirements of "informed consent"[61].

Our own approach to the evaluation process includes a clinical interview along with the administration of the BDI, McGill Pain Questionnaire, ODI, and MMPI. The assessment period is also used as an opportunity to educate the patients and significant other as to the various aspects of SCS therapy as well as allowing them to become familiar with the hardware by manipulating it. Addressing expectations that can be supported by the existing outcome literature and identifying functionally related goal which can be measured during the trial are fundamental. We also obtain a "functional level of pain" (FLOP). That is, the patient is asked at what level of pain do they feel they can be more accepting of their condition, existing residual pain, and more functional. Patients needing a pain level of less than 3/10 may be very unrealistic and require further education.

Table 58.2 Complications associated with spinal cord stimulation and their diagnosis and treatment

Complication	Diagnosis	Treatment
Complications involving the neuraxis		
Nerve injury	CT or MRI, EMG/NCS/physical exam	Steroid protocol, anticonvulsants, neurosurgery consult
Epidural fibrosis	Increased stimulation amplitude	Lead reprogramming, lead revision
Epidural hematoma	Physical exam, CT, or MRI	Surgical evacuation, steroid protocol
Epidural abscess	Physical exam, CT or MRI, CBC, blood work	Surgical evacuation, IV antibiotics, ID consult
Postdural puncture headache	Positional headache, blurred vision, nausea	IV fluids, rest, blood patch
Complications outside the neuraxis		
Seroma	Serosanguinous fluid in the pocket	Aspiration, if no response surgical drainage
Hematoma	Blood in pocket	Pressure and aspiration, surgical revision
Pain at generator	Pain on palpation	Lidoderm patches, injection, revision
Wound infection	Fever, rubor, drainage	Antibiotics, incision and drainage, removal
Device-related complications		
Unacceptable programming	Lack of stimulation in area of pain	Reprogramming of device, revision of leads
Lead migration	Inability to program, x-rays	Reprogramming, surgical revision
Current leak	High impedance, pain at leak site	Revision of connectors, generator or leads
Generator failure	Inability to read device	Replacement of generator

From Deer and Stewart [61]. With permission

CT computed tomography, *MRI* magnetic resonance imaging, *IV* intravenous, *CBC* complete blood count, *EMG* electromyography, *NCS* nerve conduction studies, *ID* infectious disease specialist

Summary

To the extent that "pain" remains a primary or significant outcome, and given the generally accepted multidimensional and biopsychosocial nature of pain, it seems logical and consistent to recommend a pre-SCS trial/implant psychological screening. In addition to pursuing the identification of "predictors," emphasis should also be given to the development of treatment algorithms based on the psychological evaluation. This algorithm may well call for pre- and/or post-implant psychological intervention(s).

Clinical Approaches to Spinal Cord Stimulation

Complications

Once the decision to trial SCS has been made, great attention to planning is required. Every effort, increasing awareness of risk, mitigates that risk and compounds the probability of success for the patient and surgeon. Despite a familiarity with the operating room, many implanting physicians' native medical training falls outside the surgical realm and thus attention to detail becomes paramount. Familiarity with the most common complications sharpens the implanter's level of surveillance for missteps and pitfalls. Deer and Stewart [61] familiarizes some of the more common complications of SCS in Table 58.2.

Reported complication rates are variable and difficult to interpret across populations and studies; however, Turner et al. [63] identified an overall complication rate of 34 %, a rate of surgical revision at 23 %, and deep infection at 0.1 %. Kumar et al. [64] found infection rate of 2.7 %, epidural fibrosis to affect 19 %, and a lead complication rate of 5.3 %. Cameron [33] summated that lead migration complicated 13.2 % of cases, infection affected 3.4 %, and lead fracture 9.1 %. Complication severity is highly variable varying from unwanted paresthesia to epidural abscess, hematoma, and paralysis. Nevertheless, careful preoperative risk assessment moderates risk and should begin not when entering the operating theater but with the patient and as soon as the treatment is considered.

Preoperative Risk Assessment

Risk reduction begins long before consideration of trial. Risk of neural injury is diminished by a thorough survey focusing on the anatomy of the spine and contents. The implanter needs awareness of anatomical or surgical changes, scarring or fibrosis, and canal stenosis or listhesis that could challenge the deployment of a percutaneous or possibly a paddle lead. Imaging, not only the spinal canal at the neural target, but also the approach will greatly aid in safety and avoidance of difficulty [65]. Anatomy may degrade or change and impair the safety of the implant in the years following implant and narrow cervical canals. For example, it may portend further degradation and stenosis with resultant cord compromise in time.

Concomitant disease states beg recognition and exploitation of treatment, and there should be a low threshold for involvement of primary care clinicians or specialists to assist in rejuvenation prior to surgery. Diseases of immunity such as diabetes as well as recent or ongoing infections such as human immunodeficiency virus increase the probability of infection. The bleeding profile should be assessed and any medications or interactions that influence bleeding appreciated and removed from the clinical setting in adequate time to allow normal hematologic function. New-generation anticoagulants without clear data regarding surgical bleeding risk, for example, should encourage partnership with cardiology or hematology. Education regarding preoperative prophylaxis against methicillin-resistant *Staphylococcus aureus* with antiseptic soaps and use of intranasal mupirocin may reduce operative infection [66, 67]. Hair clipping around the operative area may additionally be of benefit [68, 69]. Compliance issues need attention, and lastly, the patient needs adequate education regarding, and durable documentation reflecting, not only potential harms but also their role and responsibility in the endeavor in the short- and long-term.

The Percutaneous Trial of Spinal Cord Stimulation

The trial not only introduces the patient to the experience of paresthesia and tests the ability to meaningfully ameliorate pain but functions also as a provisional assessment of the technique as well: the appropriateness of neural targets and the approach to them. It is the primacy of pain location and thus neural targets that backwardly determine every part of the testing and implant process. Lastly, the trial serves as a team gathering, not only of the physician and patient, but also of the stimulator representative, nurses, and family members who will be assisting in the trial and in educating the patient about their new, potential treatment.

On the trial day, a concise but thorough pre-procedure review is prudent; the addition of a checklist will ensure thoroughness. Evaluate the patient's skin, not only at the planned operative site area, but also globally for infection. Begin preoperative IV antibiotics with efficacy against common skin pathogens in light of the local and hospital antibiogram. Within the cerebral spinal fluid (CSF) shunt literature, perioperative antibiotics administration is a significantly effective prophylactic measure [70]. Consultation with infectious disease colleagues is prudent regarding surgical standard of care especially in patients with suspect immunology or history of infection. Check coagulation status with a review of medicines taken and consider platelet count or bleeding profile if necessary. In addition, plan for positioning on the table in regards to the patient's habitus and the optimum amount of kyphosis at the level of entry [71]. Particularly, obese persons may require significant bolstering under the abdomen in thoracic lead placement. Whatever

time is lost in positioning is likely gained by facility of entry and lead positioning.

The skin is the major source of surgical pathogens, and optimization of preoperative skin antisepsis diminishes infection. Several choices of surgical preparatory agents with differing bacteriocidal specificity exist. Alcohols denature proteins and are highly effective against both gram-negative and gram-positive bacteria, even those multidrug resistant, as well as fungi, mycobacteria, and some viruses [72]. Iodine, most commonly Betadine, is effective against gram-positive, gram-negative, mycobacteria, and viruses and fungi [72]. Chlorhexadine gluconate is very effective against gram-positive bacteria, somewhat so against gram-negative bacteria, but minimally so against spores and tubercle bacilli. Chlorhexadine provides residual antiseptic activity and when combined with alcohol may be superior to iodine-based preparations [73]. Cleaning with multiple preparations may further diminish bacterial counts, due not only to the expanded action of the differing agents but also to the increased time of exposure to the agents. Prepping first with iodine-based preps followed by others may confer added benefit as blood, serum, and other protein-rich biomaterials diminish the antimicrobial effect of povidone-iodine [74]. The surgical skin preparation should extend at least 6 cm from the proposed surgical site [62], but there is no reason to limit the size of the prep. Draping with plastic adhesive border prior to the prep delineates the area to be prepped and prevents inadvertent contamination. After the skin preparation and then draping with sterile towels, taking great care not to contaminate the surgeon's gown, a laparotomy drape or other large surgical drape covers the remaining patient. Drying of the skin permits excellent adhesion for occlusive and impregnated plastic drapes like Ioban™ (3M Health Care, Inc). There is no consensus as to the degree of surgical operative preparation for the trial and permanent implant, but arguably, the greater the prophylaxis, the lower the risk for infection.

The aim of anesthesia, patient comfort and tranquility, must be balanced with the danger of oversedation, as the most sensitive neural monitoring equipment in the awake patient. The appropriate use of local anesthetic and limitation of sedation during periods of electrode placement renders the awake and conversant patient sensitive to minute changes in neurologic status, thus alerting the physician to avoid injury.

Regarding electrode placement, the aim should be to safely depolarize the nerves, which will present paresthesia to overlap the patient's pain. Holsheimer and Barolat have carried out significant work on neural mapping of the dorsal columns and likelihood ratios of paresthetic coverage in particular [75, 76, 77] (see Figs. 58.2 and 58.3). Alo and Holsheimer additionally summarize certain requirements for clinical efficacy:

1. The evoked paresthesia must consistently cover the entire painful area.

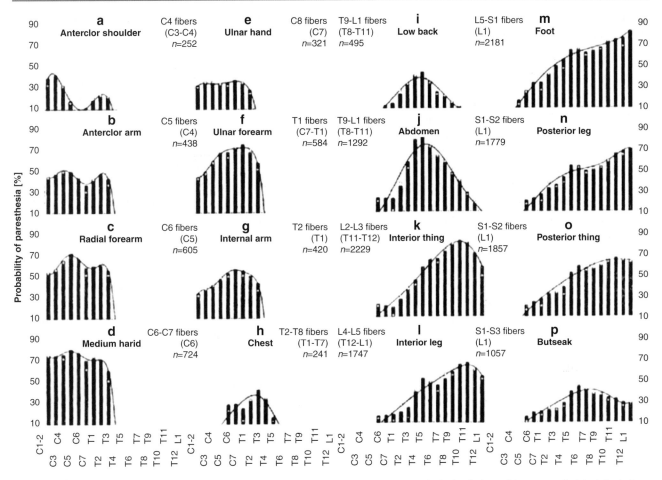

Fig. 58.2 Probability of paresthesia plots for 16 body areas as a function of the vertebral level of stimulation: *white squares* (original data), *bars* (averaged data), and curves fitting the averaged data (From Holsheimer and Barolat [75]. With permission)

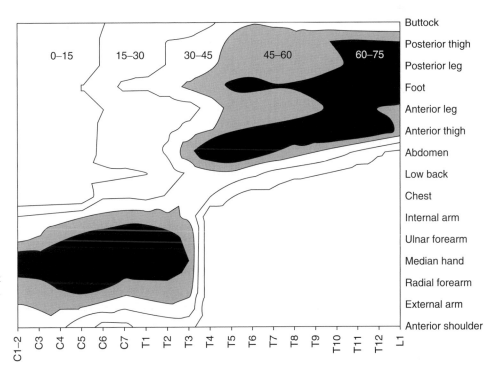

Fig. 58.3 Three-dimensional plot showing probability of paresthesia contours as a function of the vertebral level of stimulation (*x-axis*) and the body area (*y-axis*) (From Holsheimer [76]. With permission)

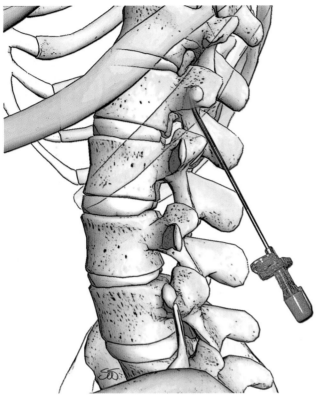

Fig. 58.4 Correct sagittal angle of incidence for thoracic spinal cord stimulator lead placement

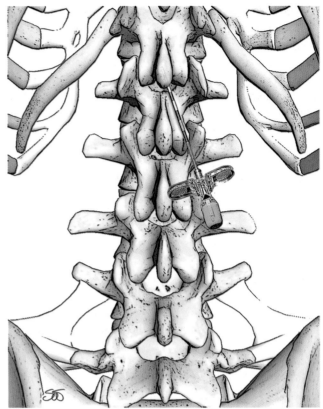

Fig. 58.5 Correct coronal angle of attack to allow midline lead deployment, and to allow for the anatomy of the spinous process

2. The cathode and resultant electrical field must focus on the corresponding dorsal column fibers to allow maximum paresthetic coverage of the painful area.
3. For coverage of bilateral pain, the cathode field should be focused on the "physiological" midline of the cord. In single-electrode SCS, by implication, this electrode should be centered on the spinal cord midline which may differ by up to 2 mm from the radiological midline.
4. If the pain is unilateral, the electrode may be displaced by up to 1 mm on the corresponding side of the physiological midline.
5. When the patient's pain is both unilateral and segmental, the electrode may be placed more laterally, thereby stimulating primarily the corresponding dorsal root fibers.
6. Even if requirements 1–5 are satisfied, anatomically precise paresthesia alone does not relieve pain as paresthesia is a necessary but often insufficient criterion for achieving relief.

Once the best location has been selected, then attention is turned to the site of ligamentum flavum entry. Enough lead length must lie in the epidural space proximal to the electrode array to provide stability of the lead in the space, and so entry through the flavum must occur at least one to two vertebral levels caudal to the anticipated array placement. Additionally, so as to allow for appropriate sagittal angle of incidence (less than 45°), appropriate skin entry

should occur about one to one-half vertebral bodies inferior to the interlaminar entry point (see Fig. 58.4) [76]. As the depth of the spine increases, as in obese persons, the skin entry site must move inferiorly to maintain the appropriately shallow angle of needle entry. The sagittal angle is important: the flatter angle greatly increases the ease of lead manipulation especially in the first few centimeters of travel from the needle. Additionally, as the angle of incidence, needle to dura, decreases, so too does the risk of neural injury. Too flat of a needle approach, however, blocks the needle's ability to pass under the inferior edge of the superior lamina and thus through the ligamentum flavum. Additionally, the coronal angle of the needle can be largely estimated by the angle of the chevron made by the spinous process of the inferior lamina usually 10–20° off of midline (see Fig. 58.5). If a lead persists in tracking to the contralateral side of entry, the implanter may halt attempts to pilot the lead and, if planned, introduce the second lead on the other side, providing a firm vector to recurve the lead back cephalad. If the interlaminar space permits, dual needle with unilateral approach may be also performed. While losing the benefit of "banking," the single-sided approach allows the implanter to easily visualize the depth of the first needle, thus allowing possibly more expeditious placement of the second needle.

After skin entry has been selected and cutaneous anesthesia provided, a small portal is suggested with a scalpel such as an 11 blade, so both the spinal needle used for deeper anesthesia and the introducer needle passes easily between the skin edges and avoid potential contamination with superficial and intradermal flora. Loss of resistance can be performed either with a medium such as saline or air, or conversely with the lead itself, carefully advancing the needle in either contralateral oblique or lateral view with constant exiting pressure placed on the lead tip with careful advancement of the needle [78]. Entry through the ligamentum flavum should be in the medial third of the interlaminar space, thus allowing the lead entry to be close to midline. This approach when combined with the rule that cephalad lead navigation remains within the confines of the lateral borders of the spinous process projection on anterior-posterior fluoro virtually guarantees posterior epidural lead placement. However, a low threshold for lateral and confirmative views is warranted.

Clearly, the entry through the ligamentum flavum and the initial lead entry into the spine is the most dangerous aspect of the entire procedure as injury to either the dura, nerve roots, or cord can result. To fail to recognize errant placement of either needle or lead and then to subsequently proceed greatly increases the consequences of the error. As noted above, safety and subsequently expediency are served by minimal use of sedation and excellent intra-trial communication between surgeon and patient regarding new paresthesias or pain in the extremities. Gentle loss of resistance, early use of transverse fluoro angles, negative aspiration of cerebral spinal fluid, as well as lead testing for perception amplitudes consistent with epidural placement further reduce risk.

Failure to recognize error compounds the consequences. If it becomes apparent that the dura has been compromised, the surgeon must stop, survey the degree of injury, and then make the decision to either proceed with a different approach or cease and allow the dura to heal before returning. There is no clear consensus on methodology of management. Eldrige et al. detail two cases of SCS lead placement complicated by CSF lead and postdural puncture headache [80]. Generally, in the setting of positive CSF return in the needle, the entry site is forfeited and another selected for entry. If the rent is large, this may also complicate the nearby attempt. Generally, if an epidural lead can be placed and an absence of CSF is seen at the skin despite different patient positions, and sufficient post-procedural time has elapsed, it is likely safe to send the patient home with education on surveillance and instruction on quick notification and return to the clinic for management if CSF is seen. Prophylactic blood patch is initially discouraged as may increase risk of infection.

Ease of lead manipulation increases with experience, but several tips aid the neophyte. Lead advancement generally occurs with the nondominant hand, and steering, either by manipulation of the steering stylette, or the lead body itself

with the other hand. As the degree of tip curvature increases, the lead turns more adroitly; however, once linear travel is desired, the curvaceous lead may become more fickle. Advancement in a less than satisfactory direction (even in settings where a return to midline is anticipated) should also be avoided as the wrong path in epidural fat can become established and new vectors more difficult to establish. Exiting the needle with the lead is the most difficult point at which to establish good lead control, and fortunately, when the lead tip is still close to the needle tip rotating, the bevel of the needle can provide additional control. If good lead control remains elusive early in the course, consider reestablishing the entrance in the epidural space more centrally.

Partial withdrawal of the stylette may allow a straighter tip for periods of linear advancement and may also allow easier entry from the needle into the epidural space in cases of steep needle angle, tender dura or nerve, or in cases where the lead prefers to steer laterally as opposed to midline. Occasionally, use of the straight stylette is suggested when axial lead integrity is required with a straight lead tip.

Once the desired location is reached, intraoperative testing ensues. Success is most likely when the target neural tissue is depolarized, generating paresthesia in the area of the patient's pain. The target should lie near the middle of the electrode array as if axial lead migration occurs reprogramming success is likely. Extensive work has been done not only with computer modeling but also with retrospective investigation regarding lead placement and neural recruitment [62, 80–91]. Ideally, the cathode should capture the target with low pulse width and amplitude, placing the paresthesia in the center of the pain. This will allow for wider paresthesia with increasing amplitude and pulse width. This concept is crucial, and testing is easily performed rapidly by the implanter and assistants using newer rapid programming algorithms, essentially trolling the lead for the best target and rapidly testing hundreds of permutations. If testing reveals paresthesia in the dermatome corresponding to the dorsal root entry zone fibers near the electrode, then the array may be too lateral, but this may be desirable as depolarization of first-order neurons may provide quite meaningful paresthesia. If very low amplitudes produce paresthesia, this signifies close and possibly undesirable proximity to either cord (in the intrathecal space) or nerve root itself.

Once the electrode array position is maximized, the needle and stylette are removed with attention to lead stability comparing pre- and post-removal fluoroscopic images. Prophylactic advancement of the lead by one to two electrodes prior to removal allows the implanter to pull down and reposition the lead back to the desired location with ease prior to anchoring. The methods for lead security or anchoring are multiple. Paramount in selection of technique is limitation of lead movement for the trial and especially limitation of cephalad movement as externalized; thus, contaminated lead can migrate into the patient. Because of this risk, often direct ligature of the lead to the skin is performed with direct tie to lead analogous to the technique used in securing a drain tube. Sacrifice of lead integrity for lead security may be warranted as trial leads are used for short duration. Significant work has been done on anchoring with several published approaches [92, 93]. Newer, titanium-sleeved, anchors from all companies may reduce likelihood of migration greatly.

After the completion of lead placement, there remain several important steps. Numerous and differing protocols for wound dressing exist; however, there are several universal maxims: patient comfort is paramount, strain relief coils protect inadvertent lead tension from influencing epidural movement, the location of lead taping should permit activities such as sleeping with minimal compromise, and most importantly, the dressing serves as a barrier to contamination of the operative site. Additionally, constant surveillance for infection, and education of the patient regarding such, is appropriate as epidural abscess demands early recognition and intervention [94]. The benefit of post-procedural oral antibiotics is unproven and debatable and, despite lack of evidence for use with most any surgery, remains a fairly common practice among American implanters. The main risk of indiscriminate use of postoperative antibiotics remains development of resistant strains of bacteria. The patient must additionally be educated regarding the sentinel signs of neural compromise as seen in evolving epidural hematoma as again early recognition and decompression radically improves outcomes [62, 95]. Lastly, the external pulse generator is programmed. Reprogramming soon after initial placement will be necessary, so prior to discharge tentative follow-up arrangement is made.

Dual and Triple Lead Techniques

While depolarization of target neural fibers is the aim, occasionally collateral and undesirable neural recruitment occurs. The clinical result is paresthesia outside the painful target, and while often tolerable, occasionally disagreeable stimulation limits the intensity and usefulness of the target paresthesia. Dual and triple lead approaches were developed not only to increase the redundancy and thus safety of the system but also to guard or hyperpolarize lateral fibers against the generated electrical field, or conversely to selectively activate those fibers [86, 96–101]. Percutaneous, three-lead arrays are thus a perfectly reasonable effort in spinal cord stimulation.

Single lead systems with expert placement satisfied many, but eventually gave way to transverse dual lead systems, allowing increased lateral control and with the introduction of lead splitters to transverse tripolar arrays and thus the ability to guard or hyperpolarize laterally entering dorsal roots and rootlets.

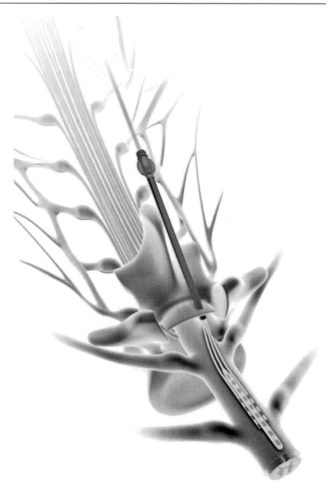

Fig. 58.6 Epiducer (St. Jude Neuromodulation) lead introducer

Technically, the introduction process into the epidural space of multiple leads is similar to a single lead. To pass all leads at the same interspace, however, requires either three separate needle placements or use of the Epiducer™ percutaneous lead delivery system (St. Jude Medical, Plano, TX) (see Fig. 58.6). Occasionally, the interlaminar space may be insufficiently accommodating for three leads, and multiple spaces must be used to complete access. Although using multiple spaces is acceptable practice, the efficacy of electrical field guarding is dependent upon the interelectrode proximity in separate leads acting in concert. Electrodes which are freely mobile *in relation to others in the same montage* present a dynamic and often ultimately confounding programming challenge. While trialing, the instability of the system may be overcome by frequent reprogramming; however, once permanently implanted, every effort should be made to ensure a rooted and immutable electrode array. Leads entering at the same interlaminar space permit anchoring to contiguous tissues and perhaps even to each other. As the superiority of tripolar arrays over dual column arrays has yet to be established, the Achilles heel of the percutaneous tripolar technique may lie in the inherent difficulty in producing montage stability. The Epiducer™ may greatly benefit this effort as it allows percutaneous, three-lead implantation all from the same site. Additionally, Epiducer™ allows placement of dual paddle lead or tripolar arrays, utilizing both paddle and percutaneous leads deployed through the same entry.

Electrode Placement in the Cervical Region

Electrical modulation of neuropathic pain in the upper extremities generally requires cervical lead placement. However, possibly, also treated by cervical neuromodulation may be intractable neck and upper extremity pain [102, 103], neuropathic facial pain [104], unstable angina [105], four-limb neuropathic pain [106], headache, craniocervical pain [107], as well as low-brain perfusion syndromes [108, 109]. In addition, some literature argues that cervical and lumbar devices for the treatment of chronic regional pain are similar in efficacy and safety [110]. With cervical stimulation, similarity exists in lead introduction and steering, but the architecture differs significantly from the more capacious canal of the thoracolumbar junction, where most implanters are comfortable. Entering the space at a level with posterior displacement of the cord, for example, places the patient at increased risk. Of additional concern is the increased mobility of the cervical canal, which may also increase the likelihood of lead migration, but also yield an unwanted higher variability in paresthesia intensity based on neck movement. Bracing in the postoperative weeks may limit movement and permit the leads to scar into place. Pre-procedural awareness and review of imaging of the canal and approach is required as well as attention to the dynamic nature of the anterior and posterior column, which may in time degrade further diminishing the available space for the cord. Entering the dorsal epidural space several levels caudal to the cervical spine allows the lead plenty of distance for stability. Many implanters enter the canal at the typical thoracolumbar junction and then tunnel cephalad all the way to the cervical cord. This approach minimizes the need for extensive extra-canal tunneling, but the increased distance from the lead array to the anchor may amplify the risk of lead migration. In addition, the implanter must have survey a completely patent canal from a low entry to high placement, and this may not always be present, especially in post-operative spines.

Similar to thoracic placement, cervical lead placement allows multiple locations for implantable pulse generator (IPG) implantation with the same aims: to minimize discomfort and likelihood for migration and complication. Many implanters continue to tunnel to the buttock, while others place the IPG in the precordial area, posterior axillary line, or even in the soft tissue of the high back. Success is largely dependent upon selecting a location which does not interfere with underwear, clothing, or sleep and allows the patient to manipulate programs and charge the IPG if appropriate. Lastly, it is advisable to confirm and document preoperative discussion with the patient with skin marking confirming the patient's choice of location.

Programming

It is beyond the scope of this chapter to attempt to fully present the depth of knowledge regarding stimulation of the dorsal columns. However, familiarization with several tenets of programming will serve the implanter well. Norman Shealy [1] nearly 45 years ago was restricted to the same parameters of stimulation as today: pulse amplitude (I) measured in either milliamperes (mA) or volts (V), pulse width (PW) measured in microseconds (ms), and frequency of pulse (F) measured in cycles per second or hertz (Hz). With conventional SCS systems available today, analgesia can only be provided when evoked paresthesia overlaps at least the majority of painful body areas and this should be the first aim [111–113]. Once the electrodes are placed, refinement of stimulation must occur via programming. Depolarization occurs secondary to electrical field generation near neural tissue.

Despite a long-held belief that the dorsal columnar fibers are activated in SCS enabling the gate control system and thus suppression of ascending afferent pain signals, most predictive models, however, suggest that secondary to their large size and the law of fiber recruitment, it is the dorsal root fibers that are first activated [10, 114, 115]. Stimulation of both cord and nerve root causes paresthesia and either may be useful, but generating useful paresthesia from depolarization of dorsal column fibers requires either medial electrode placement, guarding of lateral fibers, or lower energies.

Pulse energy and thus the threshold of neural depolarization is a product of the stimulus strength (amplitude) and stimulus duration (pulse width). A curvilinear strength-duration curve relationship exists between the two so that with increases in either amplitude or pulse width so too does the likelihood of neural recruitment [79, 116]. Holsheimer et al. show that increases in pulse energy translate into sequentially larger recruitment fields of neural fibers relative to the cathode resulting in increases in the perceived area of paresthesia [81]. Specific widening of pulse width translates into caudal extension of paresthesia area as the larger and smaller dorsal column fibers have a mediolateral distribution [79]. The limit to increasing energy and thus density of paresthesia is often painfully intense stimulation of lateral dorsal root fibers. To this end, bipolar, tripolar, and ultimately five-column arrays were developed in order to apply dense electrical fields to the cord with increasing specificity in medial to lateral arrangement while guarding the lateral entering dorsal root nerve fibers.

The majority of neuronal excitation occurs in the vicinity of the cathodal electrode, and with monopolar stimulation, the threshold stimulus of the anode is about five times that of the cathode [90]. Also determined by the same study was that the influence of the anode on recruitment area was negligible at any distance beyond 30 mm. The anode does, however, have significant impact on the shape of the cathodal field within that distance and can be used to "steer" or "block" the field. With bipolar stimulation, Holsheimer et al. [88] showed an ability to block the propagation of action potentials near the anode, thus guarding the lateral neural tissue from stimulation (see Fig. 58.7).

The Tunneled Trial

Performing a tunneled trial adds additional complexity and secondary to the use of an incision, possible infection risk, and therefore must be performed in a controlled operating environment. Prior to tunneled trialing, considerations usually saved for the permanent implant should be made preoperatively: IPG pocket placement and tunneling requirements should be anticipated; adequate lead lengths and extension lengths should be considered.

Lead placement is carried out in similar fashion to percutaneous trialing, but once the leads are placed, the incision is dissected down to thoracodorsal fascia and to the point of lead penetration. The leads are then anchored to the fascia using permanent anchoring techniques. Enough lead should remain to allow tunneling to the pocket with sufficient strain relief, or shorter leads are selected with anticipation of permanent extensions. Undermining, pocket creation and tunneling is then performed contralateral to the ultimate IPG pocket location. This pocket will house any redundant lead and lead extension. Often, the cutdown is performed with the needles in place if this is the case, either bipolar cautery is suggested or the epidural needles should be pulled sufficiently back to prevent electrical conduction to intraspinal contents. From this pocket, a tunnel is formed laterally away from the midline incision and ultimately out through the skin. Lead extensions, once connected, are passed out, and the midline incision is irrigated and closed.

If, upon completion of trialing, permanent implantation is desired, then the surgeon reopens the midline incision, disconnects the trialing extensions and removes them clean to dirty, irrigates clean to dirty, and then closes the proximal portal to the tunneling track. Pocket creation can be made from the midline incision using blunt dissection away from

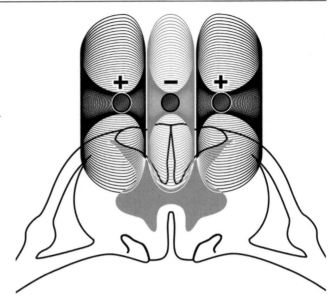

Fig. 58.7 A tripolar array demonstrating the effect of anodal blocking

the tunneled side, or an additional incision for pocket creation may be made opposite to the side of trial tunneling and then the leads either tunneled to the pocket or extensions used. Argument against use of extensions includes the possible increase in system complexity and points of failure as well as scar formation about the extension headers and thus increased lead strain [117]. If the trial fails the patient, then removal of the system is the aim. Reentry into the midline incision is required to dissect the anchors and remove the lead array.

Permanent stimulator implantation requires the same attention to detail, hemostasis, and sterility that any open spine procedure demands. If the trial is successful, it has not only shown the patient the possible impact neuromodulation can have in their life but it has also informed the surgeon regarding neural targets, ease of approach, and need for specific patient positioning.

Lead Selection

Neuromodulation's early history was forged with a bipolar array with often-excellent coverage and paresthesia. Simple elegance had limitations; however, lead migration led to surgical revision, and complex pain patterns were more difficult to treat. Today, there exists an ever-expanding compendium of options to help and possibly bewilder the implanter. Despite these options, the goal is unchanged: well-placed, stable, and useful paresthesia delivered safely. As the complexity of the pain pattern increases likely, too will the need for complex electrode arrays. Trialing will commonly take place with cylindrical leads as they confer the advantage of easy removal, lower cost, and the general ability to allow good testing of the eventual array. Lead selection for the ultimate array is commonly dependent on the training of the implanter. Percutaneous access has until recently only allowed cylindrical lead deployment; however, the Epiducer™ (St. Jude Neuromodulation™, Plano, TX) does allow slim, single-column paddle, and multiple-lead deployment through a single needle stick. The individual leads' properties influence the decision.

Cylindrical leads offer ease of deployment and steering, can be used in trialing and permanent implant settings, do not require laminotomy for placement of removal, are generally thinner than paddle leads, and take up less epidural space. They may be placed in single, dual-columnar, and "tripolar" arrays [118]. However, they require greater energies than paddles for similar paresthesia, are generally more likely to migrate (but the incidence may fall with new anchors), and in the setting of thick dorsal cerebral spinal fluid as seen in the lower thoracic levels may require energies which recruit lateral entering fibers at painful levels, and lastly, if placed proximal to sensitive ligamentum flavum, flaval stimulation may preclude tolerable dorsal column stimulation. Additionally, if "current steering" or anodal blocking is required, the stability of an array with three independent columnar leads placed in tripole is tenuous. Occasionally, however, multiple neural targets may beg stimulation, distant to each other, and demand the plasticity of an array spread over longer distances, for example, the high-thoracic cord, lumbar nerve root, and cervical cord. Lastly, percutaneous electrode arrays can be placed "cross midline" with excellent coverage of lower extremities as well as buttock pain [119].

Paddle leads when compared to cylindrical ones use less energy as a whole, resist migration, are stable across the midline, and easily placed by most surgeons, but require special surgical skill for laminotomy. They are thicker, with dorsal shielding protecting the possibly sensitive flavum. The electrodes lie more ventrally and closer to the cord, further increasing electrical economy and fidelity with less likelihood of undesired dorsal root or rootlet stimulation. Removal is dependent upon a surgeon, often at the expense of additional laminar bone.

Multicolumn paddle arrays allow for single lead placement and complex and accurate electrical fields that may allow coverage of more complex pain patterns with single lead deployment.

Percutaneous paddle leads, while single column in design, allow for significantly lower energies and thus the reconsideration of primary cell batteries as long-term power solutions.

The combination of percutaneous paddle leads with guarding cylindrical leads through a single needle stick may provide increased stability of a tripolar system.

Implantable Pulse Generator Selection (IPG)

As with leads design, innovation in IPGs has been rapid, with improvements in rechargeability, size, and contact number. Presently, each company makes a rechargeable IPG; however, only Medtronic™ and St. Jude Neuromodulation™ make primary cell IPGs, and St. Jude alone continues to make a radiofrequency-powered IPG.

Each has distinct advantages and disadvantages.

Smaller than conventional IPGs, radiofrequency-powered units such as the Renew™ radiofrequency system from St. Jude Medical™ offer high power in 8 and 16 contact designs and relatively high-frequency ceilings compared to conventional IPGs. They require for use, however, an external power source, which may be cumbersome. They usually cost less than battery-powered or rechargeable IPGs. Once implanted, they last decades as cell depletion or failure is of minimal concern.

Non-rechargeable battery-powered IPGs, produced by both Medtronic™ and St. Jude Medical™, generally confer most of the benefits of rechargeable IPGs, but lack the ability for charging. Useful in situations requiring low-power consumption as in efficient arrays, they may also be beneficial in persons who do not want to or may not have the cognitive discipline to tend the rechargeable battery. Additionally, they cost less than rechargeable IPGs.

Rechargeable programmable IPGs confer the benefit of high-power output with the ability to recharge and thus greatly lengthen the time between IPG failure and thus system revision. The majority of implanted systems utilize rechargeable IPGs, as with innovation, their size too has diminished making them quite comfortable housed in a variety of locations with minimal vexation.

Lumbosacral Nerve Root Stimulation and Retrograde Approaches and Technique

Stimulation of the sacral nerve roots can be performed with retrograde stimulation of the cauda equina and as well as in usual antegrade fashion overlying the conus at the terminal cord around T12–L1. The approach can be somewhat more challenging, however, secondary to the normal lumbar lordosis. Additionally, placing percutaneous leads sagittally over the conus at such a mobile segment makes stability difficult. Placing the lead across the midline, however, crossing over the conus and passing through the plica mediana dorsalis durae matris may stabilize the lead [120]. In order to selectively stimulate a nerve root, the lead and thus stimulating electrode must be close to either the exiting nerve at its corresponding foramen or along the descending course in the fan of cauda equina caudal to the conus medullaris. For lower

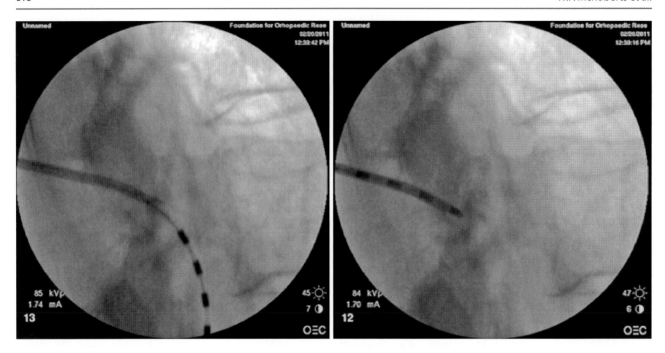

Figs. 58.8 and 58.9 A lateral fluoroscopic film demonstrating adequate angle for retrograde lead deployment

lumbar and for sacral nerve roots, this is best accomplished utilizing a retrograde needle approach and lead placement.

Sacral nerve root stimulation may be beneficial in the treatment of interstitial cystitis [121], painful bladder syndrome and chronic pelvic pain [122], fecal incontinence [123], and chronic anal fissures [124]. Similar to antegrade approaches, selection of interlaminar entry permits enough lead proximal to the electrode array for stability. As with every approach, planning begins with selection of neural target. The neural roots of L3 and roots caudad are most amenable to this technique. In the lumbar spine, the natural angle (in the cephalo-caudad dimension) of the laminar shingling steepens which each subsequent cephalad interlaminar space, limiting the easiest and functional entry points to just a few. This is clearly illustrated by the following technical description of technique.

Skin entry is determined by fluoroscopic angle. In terms of orbital travel angle, align the fluoroscope in sufficient caudo-cephalad angulation striving for maximum retrograde angulation, while allowing enough visual patency of the interlaminar space so as to permit passage of the usual 14-gauge introducer needle. Use of a coude-tipped introducer needle such as the 14-gauge epidural needle – RX Coudé® (Epimed, Irving, TX) allows a maximally diminished angle of incidence to the dura when entering into epidural space (see Figs. 58.8 and 58.9). Differing from antegrade needle introduction, the angle of fluoro greatly approximates the angle of needle introduction. Select for skin entry a site overlying the inferior edge of the superior lamina just paramedian to midline. From this point, guide the needle deeper to the superior laminar edge just selected. The needle will be very close, if not exactly in plane and on point with the x-ray

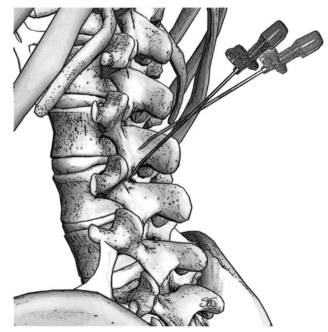

Fig. 58.10 Lateral view of "walking" the needle caudally off the inferior lamina before advancing through ligamentum flavum as used in retrograde lead deployment technique

beam. Once contact is made, increase the retrograde angle and walk inferiorly the needle tip off the inferior lamina into the interlaminar space (see Fig. 58.10). Advance as experience allows, confirming the depth on lateral projections if necessary. Once contact with ligamentum flavum is made, remove stylette and advance with loss of resistance technique. The steeper the angle, the less compliant the lead will be to direction towards the midline. It will want to fall off to either side, generating either advantage or frustration based on the selected target. Guidance to more caudal neural targets, such as sacral nerve fibers, will be best served by an initially midline approach with later ultimate vectoring to the targeted fibers.

As lead pliability is increased with temperature as well as de-styletting, when passing the lead through the rather acute angle encountered at the needle tip, wait a moment to warm the lead in the needle, and partially withdraw the stylette before advancing lead out the needle tip. Attentive advancement is warranted not only because of the aggressive angle to the dura mater but also as the initial course of the lead greatly predicts the ultimate course.

Lead stability and durability at this highly mobile segment is critical. Using an anchor with a nose, such as the Cinch™ and Swift-Lock™ anchor (St. Jude Neuromodulation, Plano, TX), when placing a permanent lead may protect the lead through the extreme angle encountered as the lead curves and dives deeply to the epidural space. Additionally, undermining the wound superiorly for a strain relief pocket allows for the lead to continue cephalad reducing the lead deviation and thus stress before recurving to the IPG pocket.

Long-term tenability of both the lead and electrode arrays in retrograde placement is more challenging, and every effort to diminish movement in the postoperative, healing phase will benefit stability. Lumbosacral bracing or use of a postoperative abdominal binder may limit movement to allow scarring to occur.

Percutaneous antegrade lumbar and sacral nerve root stimulation may be tempting via a caudal approach through the sacral hiatus; however, caution is advised as with any perirectal surgery or procedure, there is increased incidence of surgical infection, and with indwelling spinal hardware, the consequences can be disastrous. If lead migration plagues the retrograde approach, surgical consultation for sacral laminotomy or laminoplasty with paddle lead placement may be the most stable and sterile option.

The Permanent Implantation

The decision to permanently implant the electrode array is one made jointly with discussion between the patient and physician. Information obtained by the trial such as the appropriateness of neural targets, whether different lead locations would be more clinically useful, and the utility of the therapy for particular complaints influences planning for the permanent implantation. Additionally, configuration of the system and IPG placement must be discussed with the patient taking into account handedness, adiposity and body mass, and clothing preferences, especially important being constricting belt lines, dexterity, sleeping preferences, power

requirements, and IPG selection. The implanter may want to consider referral for surgical paddle lead implantation for a variety of reasons: while trialing, painful ligamentous stimulation was unavoidable, power requirements were very high, complex pain patterns demanded specifically focal paresthesia, or due to complex canal anatomy or cord rotation, consistent paresthesia was difficult to elicit. Variable intensity as a function of position is often secondary to thick dorsal cerebral spinal fluid at the thoracic levels; paddle leads may ventrally displace the dura diminishing the effect of position on paresthesia intensity. Lastly, if the physician is uncomfortable with, or inexperienced with permanent implantation, the surgery should be referred to a more seasoned implanter, or surgeon familiar with the process.

As previously mentioned, identification and then diminution of surgical risk is paramount especially in terms of infection, cardiac status, bleeding, and identification of postoperative compliance issues. Permanent implant begs a full preoperative clearance from the patient's primary physician. However, development and implementation of a preoperative information and risk-screening packet reviewed with the patient ensures consistency and lowers the likelihood of unforeseen circumstances affecting the implant.

In the preoperative holding area, the physician should mark the operative site, but more explicitly focusing on IPG location and lead pathways. Once preoperative antibiotics are infused, the patient is moved to the operative suite with attention to previously mentioned details.

Several variations in percutaneous implantation exist.

Leads placed first: With this approach, the introduction needles are deployed through the skin, much like a trial, and then after appropriate lead placement, the initial incisions are created. The midline incision either passes through both needle incisures, or is created along the sagittal midline between the needles down to the thoracodorsal fascia then undermining to access the needles as they pass through the fascia. Needles are then removed and leads anchored to fascia, ultimately tunneled to the pocket. Attractive with this approach is the ability to ensure lead placement prior to the committal that occurs with making an incision. However, the undermining process, which essentially must be made with the needles in place to protect the lead from the scalpel, is somewhat awkward and may increase risk of needle movement and possible dural injury. Also, the use of monopolar cautery is discouraged with needles passing to epidural space for risk of intraspinal conduction. This risk is minimized if nonconductive introduction devices are employed.

Incisions made first: Forming the pocket early in the surgery and then packing the pocket with gauze increases intrapocket pressure, limits bleeding, and may help prevent seroma formation later. Additionally, in making the incisions first, the use of cautery is limited only by the preoperative status of the patient, as no needles are yet intraspinal. The main drawback of the technique is the obvious: if spinal access is thwarted, then the patient has risked incision for nothing. However, experientially, if one level is particularly difficult, adjacent levels and patient perseverance often rewards with success.

Prior to incision, cutaneous and then deeper soft tissue anesthesia and hemostasis can be achieved with infiltration of local anesthetics with epinephrine. While there may be a dearth of literature supporting cutaneous anesthesia for control of postsurgical pain [125], preemptive analgesia has been shown to improve postoperative pain control [126]. More importantly, adequate local anesthesia promotes patient comfort thus diminishing patient movement and allows very light to no sedation during lead placement. Additionally, useful is infiltration with local anesthetic, appropriate for use in spinal blockade, all the way down to the lamina along the anticipated lead introducer track. With good local anesthesia, the patient can be surprisingly comfortable intraoperatively, allowing intimate and cogent feedback regarding the appropriateness of paresthesia coverage, as well as possible neural compromise.

Attention to hemostasis and development of a skill set with facility using electrocautery, intra-wound pressure, hemostatic agents, and vessel ligature is vital not only for patient safety during the operation, but also the elimination of dead space and loculated fluid or blood collection during wound closure diminishes infection and seroma risk postoperatively.

The parasagittal incision should be carried down all the way to the posterior thoracodorsal fascia and associated spinous processes. Some undermining may be needed to allow good angle for the lead and anchor, but it is important to expose fascia as anchoring must be to a stable substrate to minimize lead migration. Once the lead is deployed and testing confirms optimal placement, it is important to fluoroscopically confirm the lead has maintained location through the processes of de-styletting, needle removal, and anchoring. Saved fluoroscopic images document the placement.

Anchoring is a minimally studied component of the process, but it appears the inclusion of an internal, metal sleeve such as titanium improves stability compared to Silastic material alone [127]. All current companies now produce a metal-sleeved anchor. Nonabsorbable suture such as Nurolon™ or Ethibond Excel™ (Ethicon, New Jersey) provides excellent long-term strength with minimal tissue reaction, especially compared to silk [128].

Creation of the IPG pocket, despite being deceptively easy, merits attention. As noted previously, anatomic location and documented communication with the patient are essential. The pocket should be of sufficient depth to allow good protection from the skin and the external environment,

clothing, and bumps against hard objects, but still superficial enough to allow communication and charging. Too large a pocket encourages seroma formation and allows movement. Too small a pocket may predispose to wound dehiscence and poor wound edge approximation, so the pocket should be just large enough to house the IPG and associated redundant lead and connectors if used. Implanting particularly thin patients may present challenges regarding pocket pain in time. If during pocket creation there appears to be insufficient adipose to protect the IPG, incising and then undermining the thoracodorsal fascia, gluteal aponeurosis or local fascia, and placing the IPG sub-fascially may protect against painful trauma to the subdermis. Additionally, closing the fascia over the IPG improves wound and skin approximation and reduces tension upon the closure. While seromas are very rare with this technique, IPG migration may be a bit more common, so a stitch ligating the header to the fascia may be advantageous. Tunneling to the pocket can be quite painful requiring either deeper sedation or local anesthetic infiltration of the anticipated needle track.

While culminating the procedure, wound closure and wound dressing are critical last steps; done adeptly, they secure and protect the system from infection and migration. Seeing the approaching finish line, it may be tempting to rush the closure; but time and attention spent here will mature into dividends later. Wound irrigation diminishes bacterial counts [129] and reduces incidence of early and late postoperative infections [130]. Multilayer closure is used for gentle approximation without dead space until tissues restore their intrinsic strength and wound healing is complete. While the tissues undergo repair, the strength of the wound remains dependent upon the suture and thus the surgeon's attention to detail and discipline [131]. Running suture, while expedient, risks wound dehiscence as any compromise of part of the suture results in unraveling and large areas of wound compromise. Skin closure aims for excellent wound edge approximation and cosmesis.

Despite great variation in postsurgical wound dressing, the intention of the dressing is uniform: to protect the wound from soilage and bacterial contamination, to add integrity to the underlying wound closure if possible, to provide thermal regulation and an optimum environment for wound healing, and ultimately, to provide comfort to the patient.

Conclusion

The evolution of neuromodulation of the spinal cord has, if anything, been marked by rapid innovations, trials, failures, and often successes that astound even the most seasoned implanter. The majority of advancement arguably lies ahead. The expanding compendium of lead selection and power sources, refinement of new waveforms and high-frequency stimulation, percutaneous options for paddle lead placement, accelerometers for energy control,

MRI compatibility, systems that sense their environment, and innumerable other innovations all seek to expand the role and efficacy of SCS in the treatment of pain. What will challenge physicians and patients most in the coming years, however, will be the shifting financial substrate on which all of medicine rests. Payers will demand more rigorous evidence of fiscal rationality, and all will ask for more compelling scientific data supporting efficacy. While it may appear that our immediate responsibility of individual patient safety and outcomes is our sole concern, we have a deeper, collective accountability to judicious use, adherence to safe practices, and an empiric substantiation of our claims that SCS is safe, effective, and when appropriately paired, life changing.

References

1. Shealy CN, Mortimer JT, Resnick JB. Electrical inhibition of pain by stimulation of the dorsal columns: preliminary clinical reports. Anesth Analg. 1967;46(4):489–91.
2. Committee on Advancing Pain Research, Care, and Education; Institute of Medicine. Relieving pain in America: a blueprint for transforming prevention, care, education, and research. Washington, DC: The National Academies Press; 2011.
3. Von Korff M, Dworkin SF, Le Resche L. Graded chronic pain status: an epidemiologic evaluation. Pain. 1990;40(3):279–91.
4. Merskey H, Bogduk N. Classification of chronic pain. 2nd ed. Seattle: IASP Press; 1994.
5. Gildenberg PL. History of electrical neuromodulation for chronic pain. Pain Med. 2006;7(S1):S7–13.
6. Stillings D. A survey of the history of electrical stimulation for pain to 1900. Med Instrum. 1975;9(6):255–9.
7. Schechter DC. Origins of electrotherapy. Part 1. N Y State J Med. 1971;71(9):997–1008.
8. Miguel R. Interventional treatment of cancer pain: the fourth step in the World Health Organization analgesic ladder? Cancer Control. 2000;7:149–56.
9. Beard GM, Rockwell AD. A practical treatise on the medical and surgical uses of electricity. New York: William Wood & Co; 1871.
10. Melzack R, Wall PD. Pain mechanisms: a new theory. Science. 1965;150(699):971–9.
11. Buonocore M, Bonezzi C, Barolat G. Neurophysiological evidence of antidromic activation of large myelinated fibres in lower limbs during spinal cord stimulation. Spine. 2008;33(4):E90.
12. Song Z, Ultenius C, Meyerson BA, Linderoth B. Pain relief by spinal cord stimulation involves serotonergic mechanisms: an experimental study in a rat model of mononeuropathy. Pain. 2009; 147(1–3):241–8.
13. Song Z, Meyerson BA, Linderoth B. Spinal 5-HT receptors that contribute to the pain-relieving effects of spinal cord stimulation in a rat model of neuropathy. Pain. 2011;152(7):1666–73.
14. Kemler MA, Barendse GAM, van Kleef M, Egbrink MGA. Pain relief in complex regional pain syndrome due to spinal cord stimulation does not depend on vasodilation. Anesthesiology. 2000; 92(6):1653.
15. Meyerson BA, Linderoth B. Mode of action of spinal cord stimulation in neuropathic pain. J Pain Symptom Manage. 2006;31(4): S6–12.
16. Aló KM. Lead positioning and programming strategies in the treatment of complex pain. Neuromodulation. 1999;2(3):165–70.
17. De Ridder D, Vanneste S, Plazier M, van der Loo E, Menovsky T. Burst spinal cord stimulation: toward paresthesia-free pain suppression. Neurosurgery. 2010;66(5):986.
18. Kiriakopoulos ET, Tasker RR, Nicosia S, Wood ML, Mikulis DJ. Functional magnetic resonance imaging: a potential tool for the evaluation of spinal cord stimulation: technical case report. Neurosurgery. 1997;41(2):501.
19. Kovacs S, Peeters R, De Ridder D, Plazier M, Menovsky T, Sunaert S. Central effects of occipital nerve electrical stimulation studied by functional magnetic resonance imaging. Neuromodulation. 2011; 14(1):46–57.
20. Kumar K, Hunter G, Demeria D. Spinal cord stimulation in treatment of chronic benign pain: challenges in treatment planning and present status, a 22-year experience. Neurosurgery. 2006;58(3):481.
21. Kumar K, Toth C, Nath RK, Laing P. Epidural spinal cord stimulation for treatment of chronic pain–some predictors of success. A 15-year experience. Surg Neurol. 1998;50(2):110–21.
22. North RB, Kidd DH, Farrokhi F, Piantadosi SA. Spinal cord stimulation versus repeated lumbosacral spine surgery for chronic pain: a randomized, controlled trial. Neurosurgery. 2005;56(1):98–106.
23. Kumar K, Taylor RS, Jacques L, Eldabe S, Meglio M, Molet J, et al. The effects of spinal cord stimulation in neuropathic pain are sustained: a 24-month follow-up of the prospective randomized controlled multicenter trial of the effectiveness of spinal cord stimulation. Neurosurgery. 2008;63(4):762–70; discussion 770.
24. North RB, Kidd D, Shipley J, Taylor RS. Spinal cord stimulation versus reoperation for failed back surgery syndrome: a cost effectiveness and cost utility analysis based on a randomized, controlled trial. Neurosurgery. 2007;61(2):361–8; discussion 368–9.
25. Börjesson M, Andrell P, Lundberg D, Mannheimer C. Spinal cord stimulation in severe angina pectoris – a systematic review based on the Swedish Council on Technology assessment in health care report on long-standing pain. Pain. 2008;140(3):501–8.
26. Claeys LGY. Effects of spinal cord stimulation on nutritional skin blood flow in patients with ischemic pain. Neuromodulation. 2000; 3(3):123–30.
27. Yakovlev AE, Peterson AT. Peripheral nerve stimulation in treatment of intractable postherpetic neuralgia. Neuromodulation. 2007; 10(4):373–5.
28. Yakovlev AE, Resch BE, Karasev SA. Treatment of cancer-related chest wall pain using spinal cord stimulation. Am J Hosp Palliat Med. 2010;27(8):552–6.
29. Eisenberg E, Brecker C. Lumbar spinal cord stimulation for cervical-originated central pain: a case report. Pain. 2002;100(3):299–301.
30. Burkey AR, Abla-Yao S. Successful treatment of central pain in a multiple sclerosis patient with epidural stimulation of the dorsal root entry zone. Pain med. 2010 Jan;11(1):127–32.
31. Mekhail N, Wentzel DL, Freeman R, Quadri H. Counting the costs: case management implications of spinal cord stimulation treatment for failed back surgery syndrome. Prof Case Manag. 2011;16(1): 27–36.
32. Van Buyten JP, Van Zundert J, Vueghs P, Vanduffel L. Efficacy of spinal cord stimulation: 10 years of experience in a pain centre in Belgium. Eur J Pain. 2001;5(3):299–307.
33. Cameron T. Safety and efficacy of spinal cord stimulation for the treatment of chronic pain: a 20-year literature review. J Neurosurg. 2004;100(3 Suppl Spine):254–67.
34. Mailis-Gagnon A, Furlan A, Sandoval J, Taylor R. Spinal cord stimulation for chronic pain. Cochrane Database Syst Rev. 2004; (3):CD003783.
35. Taylor RS, Taylor RJ, Van Buyten JP, Buchser E, North R, Bayliss S. The cost effectiveness of spinal cord stimulation in the treatment of pain: a systematic review of the literature. J Pain Symptom Manage. 2004;27(4):370–8.

36. May MS, Banks C, Thomson SJ. A retrospective, long-term, third-party follow-up of patients considered for spinal cord stimulation. Neuromodulation. 2002;5(3):137–44.

37. Daniel MS, Long C, Hutcherson W, Hunter S. Psychological factors and outcome of electrode implantation for chronic pain. Neurosurgery. 1985;17(5):773–7.

38. American Psychiatric Association. Diagnostic and statistical manual of mental disorders. 4th ed (DSM–IV). Washington, DC: American Psychiatric Association; 1994.

39. Nelson DV, Kennington M, Novy DM, Squitieri P. Psychological selection criteria for implantable spinal cord stimulators. Pain Forum. 1996;5(2):93–103.

40. Doleys DM. Psychologic evaluation for patients undergoing neuroaugmentative procedures. Neurosurg Clin N Am. 2003;14(3):409–17.

41. Peng PWH, Fedoroff I, Jacques L, Kumar K. Survey of the practice of spinal cord stimulators and intrathecal analgesic delivery implants for management of pain in Canada. Pain Res Manag. 2007;12(4):281–5.

42. Ackroyd R, Bush DJ, Graves J, McVey J, Horton S. Survey of assessment criteria prior to implantation of spinal cord stimulators in United Kingdom pain management centres. Eur J Pain. 2005; 9(1):57–60.

43. Turner JA, Hollingworth W, Comstock BA, Deyo RA. Spinal cord stimulation for failed back surgery syndrome: outcomes in a workers' compensation setting. Pain. 2010;148(1):14–25.

44. Celestin J, Edwards RR, Jamison RN. Pretreatment psychosocial variables as predictors of outcomes following lumbar surgery and spinal cord stimulation: a systematic review and literature synthesis. Pain Med. 2009;10(4):639–53.

45. Sparkes E, Raphael JH, Duarte RV, LeMarchand K, Jackson C, Ashford RL. A systematic literature review of psychological characteristics as determinants of outcome for spinal cord stimulation therapy. Pain. 2010;150(2):284–9.

46. Butcher J, Dahlstrom W, Graham J, Tellegen A, Kaemmer B. Minnesota multiphasic personality inventory-2 (MMPI-2): manual for administration and scoring. Minneapolis: University of Minnesota Press; 1989.

47. Heckler DR, Gatchel RJ, Lou L, Whitworth T, Bernstein D, Stowell AW. Presurgical behavioral medicine evaluation (PBME) for implantable devices for pain management: a 1-year prospective study. Pain Pract. 2007;7(2):110–22.

48. Molloy AR, Nicholas MK, Asghari A, Beeston LR, Dehghani M, Cousins MJ, et al. Does a combination of intensive cognitive-behavioral pain management and a spinal implantable device confer any advantage? A preliminary examination. Pain Pract. 2006; 6(2):96–103.

49. Dumoulin K, Devulder J, Castille F, De Laat M, Van Bastelaere M, Rolly G. A psychoanalytic investigation to improve the success rate of spinal cord stimulation as a treatment for chronic failed back surgery syndrome. Clin J Pain. 1996;12(1):43–9.

50. Lamé IE, Peters ML, Patijn J, Kessels AG, Geurts J, van Kleef M. Can the outcome of spinal cord stimulation in chronic complex regional pain syndrome type I patients be predicted by catastrophizing thoughts? Anesth Analg. 2009;109(2):592–9.

51. North RB, Kidd DH, Wimberly RL, Edwin D. Prognostic value of psychological testing in patients undergoing spinal cord stimulation: a prospective study. Neurosurgery. 1996;39(2):301–10; discussion 310–1.

52. Kupers RC, Van den Oever R, Van Houdenhove B, Vanmechelcn W, Hepp B, Nuttin B, et al. Spinal cord stimulation in Belgium: a nation-wide survey on the incidence, indications and therapeutic efficacy by the health insurer. Pain. 1994;56(2):211–6.

53. Beck AT, Steer RA, Carbin MG. Psychometric properties of the Beck Depression Inventory: twenty-five years of evaluation. Clin Psychol Rev. 1988;8(1):77–100.

54. Fairbank JC, Couper J, Davies JB, O'Brien JP. The Oswestry low back pain disability questionnaire. Physiotherapy. 1980;66(8): 271–3.

55. Deyo RA, Battie M, Beurskens AJ, Bombardier C, Croft P, Koes B, et al. Outcome measures for low back pain research. A proposal for standardized use. Spine. 1998;23(18):2003–13.

56. Doleys DM. Psychological assessment for implantable therapies. Pain Dig. 2000;10:16–23.

57. Doleys DM. Preparing patients for implantable technology. In: Turk DC, Gatchel R, editors. Psychological aspect of pain management. New York: Guilford Press; 2002. p. 334–47.

58. American Psychological Association. Ethical Principles of Psychologists and Code of Conduct. www.apa.org/ethics/code2002. html. Accessed March 24, 2010.

59. Doleys DM. Psychological factors in spinal cord stimulation therapy: brief review and discussion. Neurosurg Focus. 2006;21(6):E1–6.

60. American Medical Association. Informed Consent. http://www.amaassn.org/ama/pub/physician-resources/legal-topics/patient-physician-relationshiptopics/informed-consent.page. Accessed March 24, 2010.

61. Doleys DM, Klapow J, Hammer M. Psychological evaluation in spinal cord stimulation. Pain Rev. 1997;4:186–207.

62. Deer TR, Stewart CD. Complications of spinal cord stimulation: identification, treatment, and prevention. Pain Med. 2008; 9(S1):S93–101.

63. Turner JA, Loeser JD, Deyo RA, Sanders SB. Spinal cord stimulation for patients with failed back surgery syndrome or complex regional pain syndrome: a systematic review of effectiveness and complications. Pain. 2004;108(1–2):137–47.

64. Kumar A, Felderhof C, Eljamel MS. Spinal cord stimulation for the treatment of refractory unilateral limb pain syndromes. Stereotact Funct Neurosurg. 2003;81(1–4):70–4.

65. Smith CC, Lin JL, Shokat M, Dosanjh SS, Casthely D. A report of paraparesis following spinal cord stimulator trial, implantation and revision. Pain Physician. 2010;13(4):357–63.

66. Edmiston Jr CE, Okoli O, Graham MB, Sinski S, Seabrook GR. Evidence for using chlorhexidine gluconate preoperative cleansing to reduce the risk of surgical site infection. AORN J. 2010; 92(5):509–18.

67. Epstein N. Preoperative, intraoperative, and postoperative measures to further reduce spinal infections. Surg Neurol Int. 2011;2:17.

68. Alexander JW, Fischer JE, Boyajian M, Palmquist J, Morris MJ. The influence of hair-removal methods on wound infections. Arch Surg. 1983;118(3):347–52.

69. Cruse PJ, Foord R. The epidemiology of wound infection. A 10-year prospective study of 62,939 wounds. Surg Clin North Am. 1980;60(1):27–40.

70. Follett KA, Boortz-Marx RL, Drake JM, DuPen S, Schneider SJ, Turner MS, et al. Prevention and management of intrathecal drug delivery and spinal cord stimulation system infections. Anesthesiology. 2004;100(6):1582–94.

71. Kumar K, Buchser E, Linderoth B, Meglio M, Van Buyten J. Avoiding complications from spinal cord stimulation: practical recommendations from an international panel of experts. Neuromodulation. 2007;10(1):24–33.

72. Centers for Disease Control and Prevention. Guideline for hand hygiene in health-care settings: recommendations of the Healthcare Infection Control Practices Advisory Committee and the HICPAC/SHEA/APIC/IDSA Hand Hygiene Task Force. MMWR. 2002; 51:1–45.

73. Darouiche RO, Wall Jr MJ, Itani KMF, Otterson MF, Webb AL, Carrick MM, et al. Chlorhexidine–alcohol versus povidone–iodine for surgical-site antisepsis. N Engl J Med. 2010;362(1):18–26.

74. Chaiyakunapruk N, Veenstra DL, Lipsky BA, Saint S. Chlorhexidine compared with povidone-iodine solution for vascular catheter-site care: a meta-analysis. Ann Intern Med. 2002;136(11):792–801.

75. Holsheimer J, Barolat G. Spinal geometry and paresthesia coverage in spinal cord stimulation. Neuromodulation. 1998;1(3):129–36.

76. Holsheimer J. Principles of neurostimulation. In: Simpson BA, editor. Electrical stimulation and the relief of pain, Pain research and clinical management, vol. 15. Amsterdam, Boston: Elsevier; 2003. p. 17–36.

77. Aló KM, Holsheimer J. New trends in neuromodulation for the management of neuropathic pain. Neurosurgery. 2002;50(4):690–703; discussion 703–4.

78. Zhu J, Falco F, Onyewu CO, Joesphson Y, Vesga R, Jari R. Alternative approach to needle placement in spinal cord stimulator trial/implantation. Pain Physician. 2011;14(1):45–53.

79. Eldrige JS, Weingarten TN, Rho RH. Management of cerebral spinal fluid leak complicating spinal cord stimulator implantation. Pain Pract. 2006;6(4):285–8.

80. Holsheimer J. Does dual lead stimulation favor stimulation of the axial lower back? Neuromodulation. 2000;3(2):55–7.

81. Holsheimer J, Buitenweg JR, Das J, de Sutter P, Manola L, Nuttin B. The effect of pulse width and contact configuration on paresthesia coverage in spinal cord stimulation. Neurosurgery. 2011;68(5):1452–61.

82. Holsheimer J, Struijk JJ, Wesselink WA. Analysis of spinal cord stimulation and design of epidural electrodes by computer modeling. Neuromodulation. 1998;1(1):14–8.

83. Feirabend HKP, Choufoer H, Ploeger S, Holsheimer J, van Gool JD. Morphometry of human superficial dorsal and dorsolateral column fibres: significance to spinal cord stimulation. Brain. 2002; 125(5):1137–49.

84. Holsheimer J. Concepts and methods in neuromodulation and functional electrical stimulation: an introduction. Neuromodulation. 1998;1(2):57–61.

85. Holsheimer J, Khan YN, Raza SS, Khan EA. Effects of electrode positioning on perception threshold and paresthesia coverage in spinal cord stimulation. Neuromodulation. 2007;10(1):34–41.

86. Holsheimer J. Which neuronal elements are activated directly by spinal cord stimulation. Neuromodulation. 2002;5(1):25–31.

87. Holsheimer J, Nuttin B, King GW, Wesselink WA, Gybels JM, de Sutter P. Clinical evaluation of paresthesia steering with a new system for spinal cord stimulation. Neurosurgery. 1998;42(3):541.

88. Holsheimer J, Struijk JJ, Rijkhoff NJM. Contact combinations in epidural spinal cord stimulation. Stereotact Funct Neurosurg. 1991; 56(4):220–33.

89. Holsheimer J, Wesselink WA. Effect of anode–cathode configuration on paresthesia coverage in spinal cord stimulation. Neurosurgery. 1997;41(3):654.

90. Holsheimer J. Effectiveness of spinal cord stimulation in the management of chronic pain: analysis of technical drawbacks and solutions. Neurosurgery. 1997;40(5):990.

91. Holsheimer J, Struijk JJ. How do geometric factors influence epidural spinal cord stimulation? Stereotact Funct Neurosurg. 1991; 56(4):234–49.

92. Renard VM, North RB. Prevention of percutaneous electrode migration in spinal cord stimulation by a modification of the standard implantation technique. J Neurosurg Spine. 2006;4(4):300–3.

93. Rosenow JM, Stanton-Hicks M, Rezai AR, Henderson JM. Failure modes of spinal cord stimulation hardware. J Neurosurg Spine. 2006;5(3):183–90.

94. Mackenzie A, Laing R, Smith C, Kaar G, Smith F. Spinal epidural abscess: the importance of early diagnosis and treatment. J Neurol Neurosurg Psychiatry. 1998;65(2):209–12.

95. Kloss BT, Sullivan AM, Rodriguez E. Epidural hematoma following spinal cord stimulator implant. Int J Emerg Med. 2010; 3(4):483–4.

96. Aló KM, Redko V, Charnov J. Four year follow up of dual electrode spinal cord stimulation for chronic pain. Neuromodulation. 2002; 5(2):79–88.

97. North RB, Kidd DH, Olin J, Sieracki JM, Farrokhi F, Petrucci L, et al. Spinal cord stimulation for axial low back pain: a prospective, controlled trial comparing dual with single percutaneous electrodes. Spine. 2005;30(12):1412–8.

98. Struijk JJ, Holsheimer J. Transverse tripolar spinal cord stimulation: theoretical performance of a dual channel system. Med Biol Eng Comput. 1996;34(4):273–9.

99. Struijk JJ, Holsheimer J, Spincemaille GHJ, Gielen FLH, Hoekema R. Theoretical performance and clinical evaluation of transverse tripolar spinal cord stimulation. IEEE Trans Rehabil Eng. 1998; 6:277–85.

100. Wesselink WA, Holsheimer J, King GW, Torgerson NA, Boom HBK. Quantitative aspects of the clinical performance of transverse tripolar spinal cord stimulation. Neuromodulation. 1999;2(1):5–14.

101. Oakley JC, Espinosa F, Bothe H, McKean J, Allen P, Burchiel K, et al. Transverse tripolar spinal cord stimulation: results of an international multicenter study. Neuromodulation. 2006;9(3): 192–203.

102. Simpson BA, Bassett G, Davies K, Herbert C, Pierri M. Cervical spinal cord stimulation for pain: a report on 41 patients. Neuromodulation. 2003;6(1):20–6.

103. Vallejo R, Kramer J, Benyamin R. Neuromodulation of the cervical spinal cord in the treatment of chronic intractable neck and upper extremity pain: a case series and review of the literature. Pain Physician. 2007;10(2):305–11.

104. Chang P, Levy MR. High lateral cervical spinal cord stimulation (SCS) for neuropathic facial pain: report of 10 cases. Neurosurgery. 2010;67(2):550.

105. González-Darder JM, Canela P, González-Martinez V. High cervical spinal cord stimulation f or unstable angina pectoris. Stereotact Funct Neurosurg. 1991;56:20–7.

106. Hayek SM, Veizi IE, Stanton-Hicks M. Four-limb neurostimulation with neuroelectrodes placed in the lower cervical epidural space. Anesthesiology. 2009;110(3):681–4.

107. Osenbach RK. High cervical spinal cord stimulation for refractory craniocervical pain. Neurosurgery. 1998;43(3):674.

108. Robaina F, Clavo B, Catalá L, Caramés MÁ, Morera J. Blood flow increase by cervical spinal cord stimulation in middle cerebral and common carotid arteries. Neuromodulation. 2004;7(1): 26–31.

109. Broseta J, García-March G, Sánchez-Ledesma MJ, Gonçalves J, Silva I, Barcia JA, et al. High-cervical spinal cord electrical stimulation in brain low perfusion syndromes: experimental basis and preliminary clinical report. Stereotact Funct Neurosurg. 1994;62(1–4):171–8.

110. Forouzanfar T, Kemler MA, Weber WEJ, Kessels AGH, van Kleef M. Spinal cord stimulation in complex regional pain syndrome: cervical and lumbar devices are comparably effective. Br J Anaesth. 2004;92(3):348–53.

111. Barolat G, Massaro F, He J, Zeme S, Ketcik B. Mapping of sensory responses to epidural stimulation of the intraspinal neural structures in man. J Neurosurg. 1993;78(2):233–9.

112. North RB, Fowler K, Nigrin DJ, Szymanski R. Patient-interactive, computer-controlled neurological stimulation system: clinical efficacy in spinal cord stimulator adjustment. J Neurosurg. 1992;76(6):967–72.

113. Nashold Jr BS, Friedman H. Dorsal column stimulation for control of pain. Preliminary report on 30 patients. J Neurosurg. 1972; 36(5):590–7.

114. Coburn B. A theoretical study of epidural electrical stimulation of the spinal cord – part II: effects on long myelinated fibers. IEEE Trans Biomed Eng. 1985;32(11):978–86.

115. Struijk JJ, Holsheimer J, Boom HBK. Excitation of dorsal root fibers in spinal cord stimulation: a theoretical study. IEEE Trans Biomed Eng. 1993;40:632–9.

116. Irnich W. The chronaxie time and its practical importance. Pacing Clin Electrophysiol. 1980;3(3):292–301.

117. Mironer YE. Response to Henderson et al. "Prevention of mechanical failures in implanted spinal cord stimulation systems". Neuromodulation. 2007;10(1):82–3.

118. Buvanendran A, Lubenow TJ. Efficacy of transverse tripolar spinal cord stimulator for the relief of chronic low back pain from failed back surgery. Pain Physician. 2008;11(3):333–8.

119. Mironer YE, Satterthwaite JR, Lewis EM, Haasis JC, LaTourette PC, Skoloff EM, et al. Efficacy of a single, percutaneous, across midline, Octrode® Lead using a "Midline Anchoring" technique in the treatment of chronic low back and/or lower extremity pain: a retrospective study. Neuromodulation. 2008;11(4):286–95.

120. Luyendijk W. The plica mediana dorsalis of the dura mater and its relation to lumbar peridurography (canalography). Neuroradiology. 1976;11(3):147–9.

121. Peláez E, Prieto Rodrigo MA, Muñoz Zurdo MM, Sánchez Montero FJ, Santos Lamas J, Muriel Villoria C. [Epidural spinal cord stimulation for interstitial cystitis]. Rev Esp Anestesiol Reanim. 2004;51(9):549–52.

122. Marcelissen T, Jacobs R, van Kerrebroeck P, de Wachter S. Sacral neuromodulation as a treatment for chronic pelvic pain. J Urol. 2011;186(2):387–93.

123. Pascual I, Gómez C de C, Ortega R, Toscano MJ, Marijuán JL, Espadas ML, et al. Sacral nerve stimulation for fecal incontinence. Rev Esp Enferm Dig. 2011; 103(7):355–9.

124. Yakovlev A, Karasev SA, Dolgich OY. Sacral nerve stimulation: a novel treatment of chronic anal fissure. Dis Colon Rectum. 2011; 54(3):324–7.

125. Møiniche S, Mikkelsen S, Wetterslev J, Dahl JB. A qualitative systematic review of incisional local anaesthesia for postoperative pain relief after abdominal operations. Br J Anaesth. 1998;81(3): 377–83.

126. Sekar C, Rajasekaran S, Kannan R, Reddy S, Shetty TAP, Pithwa YK. Preemptive analgesia for postoperative pain relief in lumbosacral spine surgeries: a randomized controlled trial. Spine J. 2004;4(3):261–4.

127. Raphael JH, Mutagi H, Hanu-Cernat D, Gandimani P, Kapur S. A cadaveric and in vitro controlled comparative investigation of percutaneous spinal cord lead anchoring. Neuromodulation. 2009; 12(1):49–53.

128. Postlethwait RW. Long-term comparative study of nonabsorbable sutures. Ann Surg. 1970;171(6):892–8.

129. Badia JM, Torres JM, Tur C, Sitges-Serra A. Saline wound irrigation reduces the postoperative infection rate in guinea pigs. J Surg Res. 1996;63(2):457–9.

130. Lord JW, Rossi G, Daliana M. Intraoperative antibiotic wound lavage: an attempt to eliminate postoperative infection in arterial and clean general surgical procedures. Ann Surg. 1977; 185(6):634–41.

131. Odland PB, Murakami CS. Simple suturing techniques and knot tying. In: Wheeland RG, editor. Cutaneous surgery. Philadelphia: WB Saunders; 1994. p. 178–88.

Brain Stimulation for Pain

59

Konstantin V. Slavin

Abbreviations

CCH	Chronic cluster headaches
CT	Computed tomography
DBS	Deep brain stimulation
DREZ	Dorsal root entry zone
ET	Essential tremor
FDA	US Food and Drug Administration
MCS	Motor cortex stimulation
MEG	Magnetoencephalography
MER	Microelectrode recording
MRI	Magnetic resonance imaging
OCD	Obsessive-compulsive disorder
PAG	Periaqueductal gray area
PD	Parkinson disease
PET	Positron-emission tomography
PNS	Peripheral nerve stimulation
PVG	Periventricular gray area
SCS	Spinal cord stimulation
STN	Subthalamic nucleus
TRD	Treatment-resistant major depression
VPL	Ventroposterolateral nucleus of thalamus
VPM	Ventroposteromedial nucleus of thalamus

Key Points
- Deep brain stimulation (DBS) in treatment of pain has a long and fascinating history that includes a decade and a half of its widespread use for variety of indications in the mid-1970s to the late 1980s.
- Use of DBS for pain greatly diminished after its approval for this indication was rescinded by FDA due to lack of conclusive evidence regarding its effectiveness.
- Most commonly used targets for DBS in treatment of pain include sensory nuclei of thalamus (primarily, ventroposteromedial and ventroposterolateral nuclei) and "central gray" matter (periaqueductal and periventricular gray areas).
- Currently, DBS is being explored as an option for otherwise refractory chronic cluster headaches, and the initial clinical results are quite encouraging.

Introduction

In the ever-advancing world of neuromodulation, use of electrical stimulation for pain relief has been a dominant theme – mainly due to wide acceptance of spinal cord stimulation (SCS) over the last four decades and, more recently, with rebirth of peripheral nerve stimulation (PNS) approach. The relative simplicity of these interventions resulted in a shift among practitioners who use it – and if in the beginning most neuromodulation procedures were done by neurosurgeons, vast majority of both SCS and PNS systems are now implanted by non-surgeons, primarily anesthesiologists and physiatrists who specialize in the field of pain medicine. Even those interventions that in the past required neurosurgical expertise – laminectomy for insertion of SCS paddles and nerve explorations for placement of PNS electrodes – are now frequently done by our orthopedic and plastic surgery colleagues.

K.V. Slavin, M.D., FAANS
Department of Neurosurgery, University of Illinois at Chicago, 912 South Wood Street, M/C 799, Chicago 60605, IL, USA
e-mail: kslavin@uic.edu

T.R. Deer et al. (eds.), *Comprehensive Treatment of Chronic Pain by Medical, Interventional, and Integrative Approaches,*
DOI 10.1007/978-1-4614-1560-2_59, © American Academy of Pain Medicine 2013

The only target of neuromodulation where neurosurgeons proudly keep their surgical monopoly is the brain. And when it comes to indications for cerebral neuromodulation procedures, one immediately thinks of movement disorders, Parkinson disease (PD), essential tremor (ET), and dystonia, all of which have been successfully treated with stimulation of thalamic nuclei or basal ganglia. More recently, this approach of electrical stimulation of deep cerebral structures – both in the white and gray matter, usually referred to as deep brain stimulation (DBS) – has been used in treatment of psychiatric conditions, primarily obsessive-compulsive disorder (OCD) and treatment-resistant major depression (TRD); mixed motor and behavioral disorders, such as Tourette syndrome; and refractory epilepsy. Gradually, DBS has become a standard in surgical treatment of some of these conditions – essentially replacing destructive interventions that were commonly used in the past.

In addition to stimulation of deep cerebral structures, surgical neuromodulation may also target surface of cerebral convexity. This approach, through either epidural or subdural electrodes, is referred to as cortical stimulation. While cortical stimulation has been tried for treatment of tinnitus, depression, poststroke weakness, tremor, and Parkinson disease, one of the best known indications is chronic neuropathic pain for which the contralateral motor cortex is stimulated with implanted electrode. Motor cortex stimulation (MCS) for treatment of pain is a subject of separate chapter in this book. Here, we focus on DBS procedures and their applications in treatment of chronic pain.

DBS for pain has long and fascinating history [27, 40, 69]. First mentions of electrical stimulation suppressing pain sensation came from laboratory animals in the 1950s [51, 61], and right around that time, first clinical experience in humans was reported by Heath [29, 30] and Pool et al. [57] when they investigated brain activity in variety of subjects. Soon thereafter, multiple publications described stimulation of deep cerebral structures in patients with different clinical conditions [22, 47, 75], primarily with cancer pain and other refractory pain syndromes.

Instead of discussing different mechanisms of action that have been proposed to explain DBS effects in chronic pain, we will briefly go over the targets for DBS interventions, some basic procedural details, and the reasons why DBS is rarely utilized in contemporary clinical practice. Interested readers may gather more in-depth information from multiple recently published reviews [12–14, 25–27, 36, 40, 53, 69] as with decline in number of DBS procedures worldwide and almost complete abandonment of this approach in the United States, detailed literature reviews seem to outnumber original case series.

Targets for Deep Brain Stimulation in Treatment of Pain

Over the several decades since DBS was introduced, multiple targets have been explored – frequently with very encouraging initial results. Published reports concentrated on various distinct cerebral regions that represent different components of the pain-processing system including sensory pathways of the midbrain and their relays in thalamus, parts of the limbic system, and connections between the sensory and limbic areas.

Among the most commonly used targets are lemniscal system and thalamic nuclei that were explored as early as the late 1960s due to their known involvement in the processing of somatic pain [31, 45, 46, 50, 65]. Around the same time, the septal area [22, 66] and the internal capsule [3, 18] were successfully tried for pain control. Somatotopic organization of the posterior thalamic nuclei allowed one to selectively stimulate those parts that correlated with location of pain [73]. Production of paresthesias in the region of pain distribution supported use of thalamic DBS in cases of neuropathic pain, with medial locations (ventroposteromedial (VPM) nucleus) used in treatment of facial pain [31] and lateral locations (ventroposterolateral (VPL) nucleus) used for treatment of pain in the extremities [45]. Similar to other neuromodulation approaches (SCS and PNS), VPM and VPL DBS elicit paresthesias in the contralateral face or body areas, and as long as the paresthesia location matches location of the neuropathic pain, the pain relief is expected. In addition to that, medial thalamic nuclei were stimulated due to known involvement of this part of the thalamus in pain and emotional processing [8, 65, 72].

Although this approach was effectively used for neuropathic pain and associated phenomena, it was less effective for truly nociceptive pain conditions. For this group of indications, stimulation of periaqueductal gray matter (PAG) and periventricular gray matter (PVG) was suggested and tried. Since PAG and PVG (so-called central gray) are involved in descending modulation of pain, it is indeed conceivable that stimulation of this region would suppress nociception and produce pain relief through either monoaminergic [4] or opioid-mediated pathways [63]. The opioid hypothesis was supported by finding both endorphin-like [6] and enkephalin-like [7] substances in ventricular cerebrospinal fluid during PAG/PVG stimulation and by reversal of analgesia that it produced with administration of naloxone [2, 5, 32]. However, since these findings were rather nonspecific and not consistent, it was concluded that the mode of DBS action in generation and suppression of chronic pain is so far unknown [33, 48, 76].

Finally, the last target from the traditional era of DBS for pain (before its approval was rescinded by US Food and Drug Administration (FDA)) was the medial parabrachial area of the rostral dorsolateral pons, particularly the Kölliker-Fuse nucleus [78]. Stimulation of this area was reserved for the patients who failed to improve or improved only temporarily with either thalamic or PVG/PAG DBS procedures.

The aforementioned decision of FDA to rescind approval of DBS for treatment of pain was based on less-than optimal results of two multicenter studies [13]. These studies were put together by Medtronic (Minneapolis, MN), the sole manufacturer of DBS equipment at that time, and failed to reach expected endpoints thereby negating positive findings reported in multiple large series published in the 1970s, 1980s, and 1990s [17, 26, 33, 35, 36, 41, 49, 50, 56, 60, 63, 64, 71, 77]. Nevertheless, the clinical experience continued to accumulate with several enthusiastic centers worldwide although most recent series came from outside of the United States [16, 28, 34, 53, 58, 59]. In addition to general series dealing with nonuniform cohorts of patients with neuropathic and nociceptive pain, there are now dedicated reports on use of DBS in treatment of poststroke pain [52], trigeminal postherpetic neuralgia [23], neuropathic pain in head and face [24], phantom limb pain [11], and pain due to spinal cord injury [58].

Low efficacy of DBS for pain and loss of its regulatory approval were not the only reasons for its gradual decline. The other treatment modalities such as improved nonsurgical means of pain control, more versatile spinal cord stimulation devices, and introduction of intrathecal opioids provided better choices for the patients and clinicians. In addition to that, not-so-low rate of complications made the entire modality less attractive, particularly when it is used exclusively on "off-label" status.

The concept of DBS for pain was reborn with discovery of discrete activation in hypothalamus during attacks of cluster headaches in 1998 [43]. Followed by discovery of similar pattern in patients with other painful conditions that involve face and head, such as short-lasting unilateral neuralgiform headaches with conjunctival injection and tearing, hemicrania continua, and paroxysmal hemicranias [42], a group of neurosurgeons implanted DBS into ipsilateral hypothalamus of a chronic cluster headache (CCH) patient [37]. This was followed by experience with bilateral implantation in a patient with bilateral symptoms [38] and then by several series of patients with intractable CCH [10, 19–21, 39, 67, 70] as well as other headache syndromes [9, 74]. Although the results were far from uniform with documented failure in some patients [55] – if anything, very similar to the past experience with DBS for other pain syndromes – and there was a mortality reported from DBS procedure in this otherwise nonfatal condition [67], hypothalamic DBS remains perhaps the most promising DBS application today, mainly due to severe disability and relative refractoriness of CCH and hemicranias to conventional, less invasive treatments.

Deep Brain Stimulation Procedure

Technically, DBS for pain uses very similar – or even identical – approach to DBS for movement disorders (PD and ET). The surgery usually consists of two parts with the first one done under local anesthesia and the second under general anesthesia. Stereotactic approach is used for implantation of DBS electrodes. The coordinates for stimulation target(s) are calculated based on MRI of the brain that is obtained prior to the surgery itself. Even though frameless DBS is gaining popularity, most centers continue using frame-based approaches for DBS when it comes to pain indications.

This means that the surgery starts with application of stereotactic frame. This is a metal contraption that is rigidly attached to the patient's head with several sharp pins. The frame serves as a reference for stereotactic coordinates and as a base for stereotactic surgical instruments. The pin insertion sites are anesthetized with local anesthetic, and then, once the frame is secured, the patient undergoes high-resolution stereotactic imaging, which may be either a brain MRI or a combination of CT scan with either MRI or ventriculography. In the past, ventriculography was the gold standard imaging modality, but it became replaced by CT and then by MRI as technology advanced. Currently, ventriculography is considered in surgical targeting for those patients who cannot have MRI and is used very rarely. The MRI may be done when the frame is already attached, or, alternatively, it may be obtained before the day of surgery and then "fused" with stereotactic CT of the brain. However, since the resolution of current MRI systems does not allow direct visualization of thalamic nuclei, the surgical planning is done based on the atlas coordinates that are referenced against classic landmarks. These landmarks include anterior and posterior commissures, height of the thalamus, and third ventricular width, all of which have been in use since the time of ventriculography. This atlas-based approach is expected to change once higher power MRI systems become available for clinical use as preliminary data from 7 T imaging indicate that direct visualization of thalamic nuclei is indeed feasible [1], similar to the change in DBS practice since the introduction of 3 T MRI allowed better direct visualization of subthalamic nucleus (STN) [68].

Once the imaging and subsequent surgical planning are completed, the electrodes are implanted using a standard approach, usually from pre-coronal burr hole, with trajectory planned in such a way that blood vessels and ventricles are avoided. Physiological confirmation of target correctness may include microelectrode recording (MER) depending on the target and the surgeon's preference, but must include macrostimulation in order to determine thresholds for desired effects and for side effects.

Once the physiological testing is completed, the DBS electrode gets inserted into desired location, and its position is routinely confirmed with intraoperative fluoroscopy and postoperative CT scan. The hardware for DBS is beyond the scope of this chapter – but it is worth mentioning that the originally used DBS electrode with four separate stimulating contacts (model 3380, Medtronic, Minneapolis, MN) was discontinued in the early 1990s. The next model of DBS electrode (3387) was eventually approved by FDA for ET and PD treatment. With this approval, DBS electrodes remain available for other indications such as treatment of pain but only on an "off-label" basis [13].

DBS electrodes that are implanted into desired location are secured to the skull with cement, metal plates, or special locking devices. For the purposes of stimulation trial, a temporary extension cable is then connected to each electrode and tunneled under skin to a distant exit site. During this trial, the patient and surgeon determine whether DBS results in expected improvement and if there are any side effects that would prevent long-term DBS use. In case of implantation of multiple electrodes, a decision is made whether all of them are needed for best clinical effects. Following this trial that usually lasts a week or so, the implanted electrodes are either removed if the trial fails or get internalized if the trial succeeds. Internalization is performed under general anesthesia, and the permanent extension cables are tunneled toward the generator site which usually gets implanted in the infraclavicular region.

Postoperative DBS Management

The programming of DBS devices implanted for treatment of pain is similar to other neuromodulation applications, such as SCS for pain and DBS for movement disorders. The parameters of stimulation greatly depend on location of the DBS electrode contacts. In the early days, these electrodes were placed either in the thalamic nuclei, in the internal capsule, or in the central gray areas (PAG/PVG). More recently, it has become a common practice to put electrodes into both thalamic nuclei and central gray and then decide which one of them will be internalized or whether both areas need to be stimulated for optimal pain relief. The choice of the best contacts and stimulation parameters is determined by degree of pain relief, but since it may not occur immediately, attention is paid to location of paresthesias, particularly in the case of thalamic sensory nuclei, and to presence and tolerability of side effects that may be quite pronounced. At the same time, there is certain "insertional effect" where almost a half of patients in one series had a substantial improvement in pain severity in the absence of stimulation [28]. This may necessitate certain delay in the beginning of active programming following device implantation.

Most common side effects of DBS for pain are relatively minor. The transient headache occurs in more than half of all patients [36]. In addition to this, there are multiple issues related to the location of the electrodes – the proximity of PAG/PVG to oculomotor centers explains complaints related to double vision, blurred vision, and oscillation of objects in the visual field (oscillopsia), as well as sensation of nausea. Objectively, these patients may present with nystagmus and gaze palsy. Most of these phenomena, however, are transient and short-lasting. The stimulation-related sense of impending doom and severe apprehension are sometimes observed in PAG stimulation therefore limiting the patient's willingness to use the device [77]. PVG stimulation, on the other hand, may produce sense of diffuse warmth and/or well-being – and in several cases, this difference in associated sensations necessitated electrode repositioning [77].

Technical complications related to the insertion procedure and to the presence of implanted hardware include hemorrhages, sometimes fatal, ranging in incidence between 2 and 4 %, and infections in 3–13 % of cases [40]. Permanent neurological deficits were reported in 2–3.4 % of cases with mortality between 0 and 1.6 % [40]. Interestingly enough, duration of externalized trial did not correlate with the incidence of infections [36].

Inevitable and unavoidable risks associated with DBS appear to be another deterrent to its wide acceptance (and to its regulatory approval for this indication). One, however, has to take into consideration that the alternative treatments of severe and chronic pain are not absolutely safe either – and the recently reported incidence of mortality from intrathecal morphine in non-cancer pain patients reaching 3.89 % in 1 year [15] is an example of dangers associated with "less invasive" treatment modalities.

Future of Deep Brain Stimulation for Pain

It appears that despite its long history, DBS for pain will remain a rarely used modality in foreseeable future. Things may change if a new study performed in accordance with modern standards and expectations [14] shows its effectiveness and safety. However, with a general lack of enthusiasm among device manufacturers and, more importantly, in the neurosurgical community, the chance of such study happening anytime soon is rather low. An "off-label" status plays a major role in this – but one has to keep in mind that this situation is not the main reason for low DBS for pain utilization. Rather, this "off-label" status is the reflection of low efficacy and even lower enthusiasm toward this modality.

Despite this, there may be several incentives for DBS development. First, there may be a better definition of surgical indications and associated targets – similar to what we saw when DBS was explored for treatment of cluster headaches after an imaging-derived abnormality became a target for surgical intervention.

Second, the better understanding of DBS mechanisms in treatment of pain may strengthen a rationale for its clinical application. In the past, this was done with magnetoencephalography (MEG) [34] and positron-emission tomography (PET) [16, 44, 54] whereas pursuit of MRI-based investigations [62] was hindered by MRI incompatibility of implanted hardware. With continuous strive toward development of MRI-compatible devices, it is conceivable that in the near future, we will be able to investigate DBS effects and perhaps define better responders during the stimulation trial or even preoperatively based on the imaging findings.

Lastly, new devices in the field of neuromodulation may be designed to specifically address needs of pain surgery – having multiple miniaturized contacts that may be stimulated simultaneously or independently from each other based on the patient's individualized and ever-changing requirements.

There is a definite need for more effective and safe pain interventions that may be used for a selected group of patients that are refractory to other modalities. As a part of busy pain surgery practice, I, like many others, frequently receive referrals for DBS or simply "brain stimulation," usually indicating that stimulation of everything "below the brain" has already been tried – and failed. Some of these patients, particularly those with intractable back pain, may qualify for intrathecal drug therapy. Others, like patients with brachial plexus avulsions and pain due to spinal cord injury, may require destructive interventions that include dorsal root entry zone (DREZ) and midline myelotomy. The patients with deafferentation pain including anesthesia dolorosa may be candidates for MCS. Similarly, some of the patients with intractable CCH and hemicranias may respond to PNS procedures that target their occipital and supraorbital nerves. Therefore, the resurrected DBS for pain will have to be compared with all these alternative approaches. And if DBS turns out to be safer and more effective, then it may replace some or all of them.

References

1. Abosch A, Yacoub E, Ugurbil K, Harel N. An assessment of current brain targets for deep brain stimulation surgery with susceptibility-weighted imaging at 7 Tesla. Neurosurgery. 2010;67:1745–56; discussion 1756.
2. Adams JE. Naloxone reversal of analgesia produced by brain stimulation in the human. Pain. 1976;2:161–6.
3. Adams JE, Hosobuchi Y, Fields HL. Stimulation of internal capsule for relief of chronic pain. J Neurosurg. 1974;41:740–4.
4. Akil H, Liebeskind JC. Monoaminergic mechanisms of stimulation-produced analgesia. Brain Res. 1975;94:279–96.
5. Akil H, Mayer DJ, Liebeskind JC. Antagonism of stimulation-produced analgesia by naloxone, a narcotic antagonist. Science. 1976;191:961–2.
6. Akil H, Richardson DE, Barchas JD, Li CH. Appearance of beta-endorphin-like immunoreactivity in human ventricular cerebrospinal fluid upon analgesic electrical stimulation. Proc Natl Acad Sci USA. 1978;75:5170–2.
7. Akil H, Richardson DE, Hughes J, Barchas JD. Enkephalin-like material elevated in ventricular cerebrospinal fluid of pain patients after analgetic focal stimulation. Science. 1978;201:463–5.
8. Andy OJ. Parafascicular-center median nuclei stimulation for intractable pain and dyskinesia (painful-dyskinesia). Appl Neurophysiol. 1980;43:133–44.
9. Bartsch T, Falk D, Knudsen K, Reese R, Raethjen J, Mehdorn H, Volkmann J, Deuschl G. Deep brain stimulation of the posterior hypothalamic area in intractable short-lasting unilateral neuralgiform headache with conjunctival injection and tearing (SUNCT). Cephalalgia. 2011;31:1405–8.
10. Bartsch T, Pinsker MO, Rasche D, Kinfe T, Hertel F, Diener HC, Tronnier V, Mehdorn HM, Volkmann J, Deuschl G, Krauss JK. Hypothalamic deep brain stimulation for cluster headache: experience from a new multicase series. Cephalalgia. 2008;28:285–95.
11. Bittar RG, Kar-Purkayastha I, Owen SL, Bear RE, Green A, Wang S, Aziz TZ. Deep brain stimulation for pain relief: a meta-analysis. J Clin Neurosci. 2005;12:515–9.
12. Bittar RG, Otero S, Carter H, Aziz TZ. Deep brain stimulation for phantom limb pain. J Clin Neurosci. 2005;12:399–404.
13. Coffey RJ. Deep brain stimulation for chronic pain: results of two multicenter trials and a structured review. Pain Med. 2001;2:183–92.
14. Coffey RJ, Lozano AM. Neurostimulation for chronic noncancer pain: an evaluation of the clinical evidence and recommendations for future trial designs. J Neurosurg. 2006;105:175–89.
15. Coffey RJ, Owens ML, Broste SK, Dubois MY, Ferrante FM, Schultz DM, Stearns LJ, Turner MS. Mortality associated with implantation and management of intrathecal opioid drug infusion systems to treat noncancer pain. Anesthesiology. 2009;111:881–91.
16. Davis KD, Taub E, Duffner F, Lozano AM, Tasker RR, Houle S, Dostrovsky JO. Activation of the anterior cingulate cortex by thalamic stimulation in patients with chronic pain: a positron emission tomography study. J Neurosurg. 2000;92:64–9.
17. Dieckmann G, Witzmann A. Initial and long-term results of deep brain stimulation for chronic intractable pain. Appl Neurophysiol. 1982;45:167–72.
18. Fields HL, Adams JE. Pain after cortical injury relieved by electrical stimulation of internal capsule. Brain. 1974;97:169–78.
19. Fontaine D, Lazorthes Y, Mertens P, Blond S, Géraud G, Fabre N, Navez M, Lucas C, Dubois F, Gonfrier S, Paquis P, Lantéri-Minet M. Safety and efficacy of deep brain stimulation in refractory cluster headache: a randomized placebo-controlled double-blind trial followed by a 1-year open extension. J Headache Pain. 2010;11:23–31.
20. Franzini A, Ferroli P, Leone M, Broggi G. Stimulation of the posterior hypothalamus for treatment of chronic intractable cluster headaches: first reported series. Neurosurgery. 2003;52:1095–9; discussion 1099–101.
21. Franzini A, Messina G, Cordella R, Marras C, Broggi G. Deep brain stimulation of the posteromedial hypothalamus: indications, long-term results, and neurophysiological considerations. Neurosurg Focus. 2010;29(2):E13.
22. Gol A. Relief of pain by electrical stimulation if the septal area. J Neurol Sci. 1967;5:115–20.
23. Green AL, Nandi D, Armstrong G, Carter H, Aziz T. Post-herpetic trigeminal neuralgia treated with deep brain stimulation. J Clin Neurosci. 2003;10:512–4.
24. Green AL, Owen SL, Davies P, Moir L, Aziz TZ. Deep brain stimulation for neuropathic cephalalgia. Cephalalgia. 2006;26:561–7.
25. Grover PJ, Pereira EA, Green AL, Brittain JS, Owen SL, Schweder P, Kringelbach ML, Davies PT, Aziz TZ. Deep brain stimulation for cluster headache. J Clin Neurosci. 2009;16:861–6.
26. Gybels J, Kupers R. Deep brain stimulation in the treatment of chronic pain in man: where and why? Neurophysiol Clin. 1990;20:389–98.

27. Hamani C, Fontaine D, Lozano A. DBS for persistent non-cancer pain. In: Lozano AM, Gildenberg PL, Tasker RR, editors. Textbook of stereotactic and functional neurosurgery. Berlin: Springer; 2009. p. 2227–38.

28. Hamani C, Schwalb JM, Rezai AR, Dostrovsky JO, Davis KD, Lozano AM. Deep brain stimulation for chronic neuropathic pain: long-term outcome and the incidence of insertional effect. Pain. 2006;125:188–96.

29. Heath RG. Studies in schizophrenia: a multidisciplinary approach to mind-brain relationships. Cambridge: Harvard University Press; 1954.

30. Heath RG, Mickle WA. Evaluation of seven years' experience with depth electrodes in human patients. In: Ramey ER, O'Doherty DS, editors. Electrical studies on the unanesthetized human brain. New York: Hoeber; 1960. p. 214–47.

31. Hosobuchi Y, Adams JE, Rutkin B. Chronic thalamic stimulation for the control of facial anesthesia dolorosa. Arch Neurol. 1973;29:158–61.

32. Hosobuchi Y, Adams JE, Linchitz R. Pain relief by electrical stimulation of the central gray matter in humans and its reversal by naloxone. Science. 1977;197:183–6.

33. Hosobuchi Y. Subcortical electrical stimulation for control of intractable pain in humans. Report of 122 cases (1970–1984). J Neurosurg. 1986;64:543–53.

34. Kringelbach ML, Jenkinson N, Green AL, Owen SL, Hansen PC, Cornelissen PL, Holliday IE, Stein J, Aziz TZ. Deep brain stimulation for chronic pain investigated with magnetoencephalography. Neuroreport. 2007;18:223–8.

35. Kumar K, Toth C, Nath RK. Deep brain stimulation for intractable pain: a 15-year experience. Neurosurgery. 1997;40:736–46; discussion 746–7.

36. Kumar K, Wyant GM, Nath R. Deep brain stimulation for control of intractable pain in humans, present and future: a ten-year follow-up. Neurosurgery. 1990;26:774–81; discussion 781–2.

37. Leone M, Franzini A, Bussone G. Stereotactic stimulation of posterior hypothalamic gray matter for intractable cluster headache. N Engl J Med. 2001;345:1428–9.

38. Leone M, Franzini A, Broggi G, May A, Bussone G. Long-term follow-up of bilateral hypothalamic stimulation for intractable cluster headache. Brain. 2004;127:2259–64.

39. Leone M, Proietti-Cecchini A, Franzini A, Broggi G, Cortelli P, Montagna P, May A, Juergens T, Cordella R, Carella F, Bussone G. Lessons from 8 years' experience of hypothalamic stimulation in cluster headache. Cephalalgia. 2008;28:787–97; discussion 798.

40. Levy R, Deer TR, Henderson J. Intracranial neurostimulation for pain control: a review. Pain Physician. 2010;13:157–65.

41. Levy RM, Lamb S, Adams JE. Treatment of chronic pain by deep brain stimulation: long term follow-up and review of the literature. Neurosurgery. 1987;21:885–93.

42. Matharu MS, Cohen AS, Frackowiak RS, Goadsby PJ. Posterior hypothalamic activation in paroxysmal hemicrania. Ann Neurol. 2006;59:535–45.

43. May A, Bahra A, Buchel C, Turner R, Goadsby PJ. Hypothalamic activation in cluster headache attacks. Lancet. 1998;352:275–8.

44. May A, Leone M, Boecker H, Sprenger T, Juergens T, Bussone G, Tolle TR. Hypothalamic deep brain stimulation in positron emission tomography. J Neurosci. 2006;26:3589–93.

45. Mazars GJ. Intermittent stimulation of nucleus ventralis posterolateralis for intractable pain. Surg Neurol. 1975;4:93–5.

46. Mazars G, Merienne L, Cioloca C. Treatment of certain types of pain with implantable thalamic stimulators. Neurochirurgie. 1974;20:117–24.

47. Mazars G, Rogé R, Mazars Y. Résultats de la stimulation du fasciceau spinothalamique et leur incidence sur la physiopathologie de la douleur [Results of the stimulation of the spinothalamic fasciculus and their bearing on the pathophysiology of pain]. Rev Prat. 1960;103:136–8.

48. Meyerson BA. Biochemistry of pain relief with intracerebral stimulation. Few facts and many hypotheses. Acta Neurochir Suppl (Wien). 1980;30:229–37.

49. Meyerson B, Boethius J, Carlsson A. Alleviation of malignant pain by electrical stimulation in the periventricular-periaqueductal region: pain relief as related to stimulation sites. In: Bonica J, editor. Advances in pain research and therapy. New York: Raven; 1979.

50. Mundinger F, Salomão JF. Deep brain stimulation in mesencephalic lemniscus medialis for chronic pain. Acta Neurochir Suppl (Wien). 1980;30:245–58.

51. Olds J, Milner P. Positive reinforcement produced by electrical stimulation of septal area and other regions of rat brain. J Comp Physiol Psychol. 1954;47:419–27.

52. Owen SL, Green AL, Stein JF, Aziz TZ. Deep brain stimulation for the alleviation of post-stroke neuropathic pain. Pain. 2006;120:202–6.

53. Owen SL, Green AL, Nandi DD, Bittar RG, Wang S, Aziz TZ. Deep brain stimulation for neuropathic pain. Acta Neurochir Suppl. 2007;97(Pt 2):111–6.

54. Pereira EA, Green AL, Bradley KM, Soper N, Moir L, Stein JF, Aziz TZ. Regional cerebral perfusion differences between periventricular grey, thalamic and dual target deep brain stimulation for chronic neuropathic pain. Stereotact Funct Neurosurg. 2007;85:175–83.

55. Pinsker MO, Bartsch T, Falk D, Volkmann J, Herzog J, Steigerwald F, Diener HC, Deuschl G, Mehdorn M. Failure of deep brain stimulation of the posterior inferior hypothalamus in chronic cluster headache – report of two cases and review of the literature. Zentralbl Neurochir. 2008;69:76–9.

56. Plotkin R. Results in 60 cases of deep brain stimulation for chronic intractable pain. Appl Neurophysiol. 1982;45:173–8.

57. Pool JL, Clark WK, Hudson P, Lombardo M. Steroid hormonal response to stimulation of electrodes implanted in the subfrontal parts of the brain. In: Fields WS, Guillermin R, Carton CA, editors. Hypothalamic-hypophyseal interrelationships, a symposium. Springfield: Charles C. Thomas; 1956. p. 114–24.

58. Prévinaire JG, Nguyen JP, Perrouin-Verbe B, Fattal C. Chronic neuropathic pain in spinal cord injury: efficiency of deep brain and motor cortex stimulation therapies for neuropathic pain in spinal cord injury patients. Ann Phys Rehabil Med. 2009;52:188–93.

59. Rasche D, Rinaldi PC, Young RF, Tronnier VM. Deep brain stimulation for the treatment of various chronic pain syndromes. Neurosurg Focus. 2006;21(6):E8.

60. Ray CD, Burton CV. Deep brain stimulation for severe, chronic pain. Acta Neurochir Suppl (Wien). 1980;30:289–93.

61. Reynolds DV. Surgery in the rat during electrical analgesia induced by focal brain stimulation. Science. 1969;164:444–5.

62. Rezai AR, Lozano AM, Crawley AP, Joy ML, Davis KD, Kwan CL, Dostrovsky JO, Tasker RR, Mikulis DJ. Thalamic stimulation and functional magnetic resonance imaging: localization of cortical and subcortical activation with implanted electrodes. Technical note. J Neurosurg. 1999;90:583–90.

63. Richardson DE, Akil H. Long term results of periventricular gray self-stimulation. Neurosurgery. 1977;1:199–202.

64. Richardson DE, Akil H. Pain reduction by electrical brain stimulation in man. Part 2: chronic self-administration in the periventricular gray matter. J Neurosurg. 1977;47:184–94.

65. Schvarcz JR. Chronic self-stimulation of the medial posterior inferior thalamus for alleviation of deafferentation pain. Acta Neurochir Suppl (Wien). 1980;30:295–301.

66. Schvarcz JR. Chronic stimulation of the septal area for the relief of neuropathic pain. Appl Neurophysiol. 1985;48:191–4.

67. Schoenen J, Di Clemente L, Vandenheede M, Fumal A, De Pasqua V, Mouchamps M, Remacle JM, de Noordhout AM. Hypothalamic stimulation in chronic cluster headache: a pilot study of efficacy and mode of action. Brain. 2005;128:940–7.

68. Slavin KV, Thulborn KR, Wess C, Nersesyan H. Direct visualization of the human subthalamic nucleus with 3 T MR imaging. AJNR Am J Neuroradiol. 2006;27:80–4.

69. Stadler 3rd JA, Ellens DJ, Rosenow JM. Deep brain stimulation and motor cortical stimulation for neuropathic pain. Curr Pain Headache Rep. 2011;15:8–13.

70. Starr PA, Barbaro NM, Raskin NH, Ostrem JL. Chronic stimulation of the posterior hypothalamic region for cluster headache: technique and 1-year results in four patients. J Neurosurg. 2007;106:999–1005.

71. Tasker RR, Vilela Filho O. Deep brain stimulation for neuropathic pain. Stereotact Funct Neurosurg. 1995;65:122–4.

72. Thoden U, Doerr M, Dieckmann G, Krainick JU. Medial thalamic permanent electrodes for pain control in man: an electrophysiological and clinical study. Electroencephalogr Clin Neurophysiol. 1979;47:582–91.

73. Turnbull IM, Shulman R, Woodhurst WB. Thalamic stimulation for neuropathic pain. J Neurosurg. 1980;52:486–93.

74. Walcott BP, Bamber NI, Anderson DE. Successful treatment of chronic paroxysmal hemicrania with posterior hypothalamic stimulation: technical case report. Neurosurgery. 2009;65:E997; discussion E997.

75. White JC, Sweet WH. Pain and the neurosurgeon. A forty-year experience. Springfield: Thomas; 1969.

76. Young RF, Chambi VI. Pain relief by electrical stimulation of the periaqueductal and periventricular gray matter. Evidence for non-opioid mechanism. J Neurosurg. 1987;66:364–71.

77. Young RF, Kroening R, Fulton W, Feldman RA, Chambi I. Electrical stimulation of the brain in treatment of chronic pain. Experience over 5 years. J Neurosurg. 1985;62:389–96.

78. Young RF, Tronnier V, Rinaldi PC. Chronic stimulation of the Kölliker-Fuse nucleus region for relief of intractable pain in humans. J Neurosurg. 1992;76:979–85.

Motor Cortex Stimulation

60

Chima O. Oluigbo, Mariel Szapiel, Alexander Taghva, and Ali R. Rezai

Key Points

- The management of central and peripheral neuropathic pain remains a daunting challenge for pain physicians in general and the functional neurosurgeon in particular.
- In spite of the increase in interest in motor cortex stimulation, its exact mechanism of action remains unknown.
- The main focus of preoperative planning is the localization of the motor cortex and its somatotopic arrangement and relationship to the relevant area of pain.
- Prediction of patient response to MCS is, at this time, based on response to a period of externalized trial stimulation. The development of techniques for predicting patient response to MCS noninvasively, such as the use of transcranial magnetic stimulation, will be an invaluable contribution to the management of these patients.
- Patients who have a successful trial are then returned to the operating room for internalization of the stimulator system. The scalp flap is only partially reopened during this second procedure to expose the MCS electrode lead that was coiled under the galea of the scalp at the first procedure.
- The outline of the precentral gyrus is projected onto the scalp using preoperative imaging fused with a frameless neuronavigation system. An appropriate incision centered over this region is made, and then, a 4-cm craniotomy, which is large enough to allow for epidural placement of a 4 × 4 electrode grid, is fashioned. The 16-electrode grid is then placed in the epidural space.

C.O. Oluigbo, M.D. (✉) • A. Taghva, M.D.
Department of Neurological Surgery,
The Ohio State University Medical Center,
410 West 10th Avenue, N-1014 Doan Hall,
Columbus, OH 43210, USA
e-mail: Chima.Oluigbo@osumc.edu; alextaghva@gmail.com

M. Szapiel, M.D.
Department of Neurological Surgery,
The Ohio State University Medical Center,
410 West 10th Avenue, N-1014 Doan Hall,
Columbus, OH 43210, USA

South Denver Neurosurgery,
Littleton, CO, USA
e-mail: mariel.szapiel@osumc.edu

A.R. Rezai, M.D.
Department of Neurological Surgery,
The Ohio State University Medical Center,
410 West 10th Avenue, N-1014 Doan Hall, Columbus,
OH 43210, USA

Center for Neuromodulation, The Ohio State University
School of Medicine, Columbus, OH, USA
e-mail: Ali.Rezai@osumc.edu

Background

The management of central and peripheral neuropathic pain remains a daunting challenge for pain physicians in general and the functional neurosurgeon in particular. The reasons are manifold. Pharmacological advances in the management of neuropathic pain have been glacial with the only relatively new developments being the use of antiepileptics and antidepressants. Furthermore, the subset of these patients who present to the neurosurgeon have had this distressing pain for a long period of time and, having usually tried and failed numerous pain medications over this period of time, have developed psychological overlays such as depression, hopelessness, anxiety, personality disorders, and substance abuse issues.

The management of patients with intractable neuropathic pain can be of great challenge. A number of neurosurgical

T.R. Deer et al. (eds.), *Comprehensive Treatment of Chronic Pain by Medical, Interventional, and Integrative Approaches*,
DOI 10.1007/978-1-4614-1560-2_60, © American Academy of Pain Medicine 2013

interventions involving various brain targets have been utilized to help these patients. These include deep brain stimulation (DBS), cranial nerve stimulation, lesioning, and motor cortex stimulation. DBS of the various regions of the somatosensory pathways has been performed, including the thalamic sensory relay nucleus – ventroposterolateral or ventroposteromedial (VPL/VPM) – periventricular and periaqueductal gray, internal capsule, and medial lemniscus. The outcomes have been mixed and in particular limited for central neuropathic pain. It was against this background that in 1991, Tsubokawa et al. first proposed the use of motor cortex stimulation for the treatment of central neuropathic pain [1]. Tsubokawa and colleagues were considering stimulation of the sensory and motor cortex as components of the somatosensory pathway and noted that stimulation of the motor cortex was more efficacious than the sensory cortex (REF). Tsubokawa's rationale for stimulation of the motor cortex was also based on observations in a cat model following deafferentation of the anterior spinothalamic tract. They initially noted burst hyperactivity of thalamic neurons recorded in these cats. However, complete, long-term inhibition of the burst hyperactivity was induced by stimulation of the motor cortex. Based on this experimental finding, they proposed that thalamic pain syndrome can be most effectively treated by chronic motor cortex stimulation. He then translated the procedure to seven human subjects with thalamic pain syndrome and reported "excellent" or "good" pain control in all cases without any complications or side effects.

Later, Tsubokawa et al. reported the use of motor cortex stimulation for the treatment of medically refractory central deafferentation pain in 12 patients with lasting pain improvement in 67 % of these patients [2].

In 1993, Meyerson confirmed the effectiveness of motor cortex stimulation in the treatment of neuropathic pain [3]. Importantly, he noted that all the patients with trigeminal neuropathic pain had significant improvement in their pain, while none of the patients with central neuropathic pain poststroke improved, in distinct contrast to Tsubokawa's results.

In any case, since these reports, the interest in motor cortex stimulation grew rapidly as a result of the need for another therapeutic option in the challenging management of these patients with neuropathic pain. This interest is illustrated by a recent critical review of the literature on the efficacy and safety of motor cortex stimulation for chronic neuropathic pain in which Fontaine et al. reported 244 articles in the literature over a 15-year period (1991–2006) [4].

Mechanism of Action

In spite of the increase in interest in motor cortex stimulation, its exact mechanism of action remains unknown. Functional imaging studies are, however, providing insights into the mechanisms by which motor cortex stimulation (MCS) works to inhibit pain signal transmission in patients with central neuropathic pain. Positron emission tomography (PET) studies have highlighted the thalamus as the key structure mediating functional MCS effects [5]. Using PET, Garcia-Larrea et al. studied regional changes in cerebral blood flow (rCBF) in ten patients undergoing motor cortex stimulation for pain control [6]. They noted that the most significant MCS-related increase in rCBF was in the ventrallateral thalamus, probably reflecting corticothalamic connections from motor areas. CBF increases were also observed in medial thalamus, anterior cingulate/orbitofrontal cortex, anterior insula, and upper brainstem; conversely, no significant CBF changes appeared in motor areas beneath the stimulating electrode. They therefore hypothesized that descending axons from the motor and premotor cortices are primarily activated by MCS, and these activate thalamic nuclei. The activation of these thalamic nuclei then initiate a downstream cascade of synaptic events in pain-related structures receiving afferents from these nuclei, including the medial thalamus, anterior cingulate, and upper brainstem. Through these connections, they reasoned that MCS could influence the affective-emotional component of chronic pain by way of cingulate/orbitofrontal activation and lead to descending inhibition of pain impulses by activation of the brainstem.

Recent evidence also points to a possible secretion of endogenous opioids triggered by chronic MCS. Using PET imaging and [(11)C]diprenorphine, an exogenous opioid receptor ligand, Maarrawi et al. studied the changes in opioid receptor availability induced by MCS in eight patients with refractory neuropathic pain. They noted significant decreases of [(11)C]diprenorphine binding in the anterior middle cingulate cortex (aMCC), periaqueductal gray (PAG), prefrontal cortex, and cerebellum which significantly correlated with pain relief. They concluded that the decrease in binding of the exogenous ligand was most likely explained by receptor occupancy due to enhanced secretion of endogenous opioids. This observation on the delayed release of endogenous opioids is consistent with the clinical effects of MCS, which may also last for hours or days after MCS discontinuation [7].

Indications

Motor cortex stimulation is finding increasing utility in the treatment of central and peripheral neuropathic pain. The main indications are central pain, especially pain related to a thalamic lesion, and trigeminal neuropathic pain since spinal cord stimulation is generally available for pain in the extremities or trunk. The central pain usually follows ischemic or hemorrhagic stroke in most cases but may be due to other rarer causes as multiple sclerosis and trauma. In a critical review of the literature on the efficacy and safety of motor cortex stimulation for chronic neuropathic pain, Fontaine et al. reported that of 210 cases identified who had undergone MCS, the most common indication was central pain (117 cases) followed by trigeminal neuropathic pain (44 cases) [4]. Other indications reported in the literature include phantom limb pain, brachial plexus avulsion, spinal cord injury, postherpetic neuralgia, and peripheral nerve lesions including nerve root or nerve trunk pain related to previously excised neurofibromas in patients with neurofibromatosis [8–13].

Outcome

Fontaine et al. reviewed the outcomes in 210 cases of MCS implanted for different conditions in 14 studies published in the literature between 1991 and 2006 and reported that overall, 57.6 % of the patients had a "good" postoperative pain relief (defined as pain relief ≥40 or ≥50 % depending on the studies) while about 30 % of the patients had ≥70 % improvement [4]. In the 152 patients in the studies who had a follow-up of ≥1 year, 45.4 % had a "good postoperative outcome." Outcomes are best in patients with trigeminal neuropathic pain. It is generally suggested that outcome is related to the relative position of the MCS electrodes over the somatotopically relevant part of the motor cortex, but this has not been proven. In any case, patients with lower extremity neuropathic pain are known to have poorer outcomes with MCS, and this is felt to be related to the difficulty encountered with placing the MCS electrode over the medial surface of the brain [4].

Unfortunately, the literature on MCS is heterogenous, and the number of clinical series is still relatively low. There are very few double-blinded evaluations of the efficacy of MCS. This is in spite of the fact that MCS offers a unique opportunity for blinded evaluations as it does usually induce perceptible sensations. A randomized double-blinded trial by Velasco et al. reported pain improvement of ≥40 % at 1 year in all of eight patients who were implanted with MCS [14]. Rasche et al. noted that under double-blinded "on-off" conditions, a placebo response could occur in up to 35 % of patients undergoing MCS [15]. In any case, a detailed review of the literature to date suggests that MCS is effective and safe in the treatment of medically refractory neuropathic pain in select patients.

The ability to predict the outcome of motor cortex stimulation even before embarking on an externalized MCS trial will be invaluable. It will prevent a surgical misadventure with potential risks to the patient and save time and resources which is expended in planning and executing the procedure. To this end, various investigators have looked into means of predicting the outcome of MCS. Predictive factors that have been investigated include a system of pharmacological classification of pain [16], degree of motor impairment (which is felt to correlate to extent of intact thalamocortical connections) [17], degree of alteration of non-nociceptive sensory modalities within the painful area [18], and response to transcranial magnetic stimulation [19]. Unfortunately, larger studies have failed to confirm these findings [8, 20].

Procedure

Preoperative Evaluation

A detailed clinical history and physical examination is the first step in the evaluation of these patients. A history of the nature of the pain to confirm a neuropathic character, an identification of the etiology, and an evaluation of pain medications and other interventions undertaken to treat the pain are warranted. Sometimes, in the course of this evaluation, it may become evident that motor cortex stimulation is not indicated in the particular clinical scenario and that other simpler and less invasive interventions may be all that is warranted.

A neuropsychological evaluation should also be performed. Some of these patients, in the course of the long duration of their pain, have developed associated psychological overlays such as depression, anxiety disorders, and substance abuse issues that need to be addressed. Patients with personality disorders and those who have adopted a sick role or are deriving secondary gain from their condition generally tend to have poor outcomes. Detailed neuropsychological assessment will identify this subpopulation of patients who may sometimes be excluded.

The patient and family should have a clear understanding of the details and steps of the procedure and should have realistic expectations of the outcome. The patient should understand that the first stage of the procedure consists of an externalized MCS trial period which lasts typically between 3 and 7 days. A positive response consists of a 40–50 % reduction in pain, and the patient should indicate that this degree of reduction in pain will significantly improve his or her quality of life to justify this invasive procedure. Patient should also be aware of the prolonged stimulation sessions involved during the externalized MCS trial period and following the implantation of the permanent device and should have the mental fortitude to undergo this. Generally, a strong social and emotional support network from the patient's family is important in this regard. The patient should understand and be willing to accept the fact that a failure of the externalized MCS trial implies that the electrodes will be removed and no further treatment with regard to MCS will be pursued.

Surgical Technique

The specific surgical technique varies significantly between different institutions, but constant themes are maintained in the sequence of events. The sequence of events are preoperative localization of the motor cortex, intraoperative electrophysiological mapping of the motor cortex, and implantation of the MCS electrodes followed by a variable period of externalized MCS trial and then internalization of the system following a successful trial.

Preoperative Localization of the Motor Cortex
The main focus of preoperative planning is the localization of the motor cortex and its somatotopic arrangement and relationship to the relevant area of pain (Fig. 60.1). Fusion of preoperative imaging with frameless neuronavigation system enables anatomical localization of the motor cortex. Reformatted volumetric T1 magnetic resonance images are superior in this regard, but stereotactically acquired CT scans may also be used. Functional MRI (fMRI) may also be used to map the motor cortex and has sufficient spatial resolution to define somatotopic maps. Transcranial magnetic stimulation and the use of skull landmarks are other methods of localizing the motor cortex.

Surgical Procedure and Intraoperative Electrophysiological Mapping
The placement of the MCS electrodes may be performed through a burr hole or a small craniotomy. Our preference is to perform it through a small craniotomy centered over the region identified as the precentral gyrus during preoperative planning. This larger access allows for placement of epidural electrodes and optimizes intraoperative electrophysiological evaluation.

The procedure is performed under general endotracheal anesthesia while avoiding paralytic agents as these can interfere with electrical cortical mapping using electromyographic (EMG) responses. Some centers elect to perform awake procedures with monitored anesthesia care (MAC). The head is fixed with a three-pin head holder. The outline of the precentral gyrus is projected onto the scalp using preoperative imaging fused with a frameless neuronavigation system. An appropriate incision centered over this region is made, and then, a 4-cm craniotomy, which is large enough to allow for epidural placement of a 4 × 4 electrode grid, is fashioned. The 16-electrode grid is then placed in the epidural space (Fig. 60.2).

There are two main objectives of intraoperative electrophysiological testing – (1) the confirmation of the position of central sulcus (following earlier localization using preoperative imaging) and (2) the confirmation of the position of the motor cortex by stimulation.

The position of the central sulcus may be confirmed using somatosensory evoked potentials (SSEPs). The site and ori-

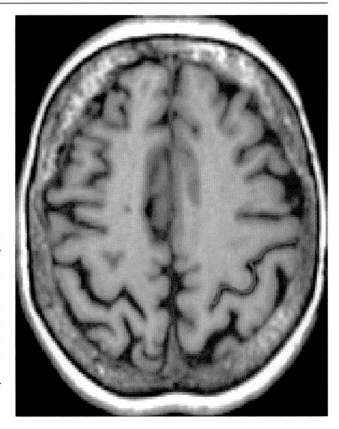

Fig. 60.1 MRI showing the central sulcus and the precentral gyrus

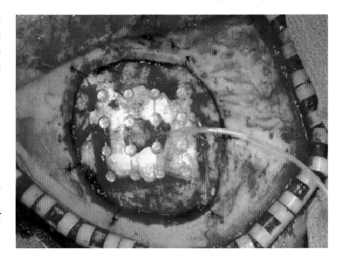

Fig. 60.2 16-Electrode grid placed in the epidural space

entation of the central sulcus is identified based on N20-P20 wave shift (phase reversal) obtained during SSEP recordings (Fig. 60.3). Following this determination, the position of the motor cortex is then confirmed by stimulation via the electrode grid. In performing this test, stimulation of increasing intensity is applied while watching for motor contractions at the lowest stimulation threshold in the zone corresponding to the region of pain in the non-paralyzed patient. It is important to note that motor seizures can be provoked by the cortical stimulation. Cold saline or lactated ringer's solution

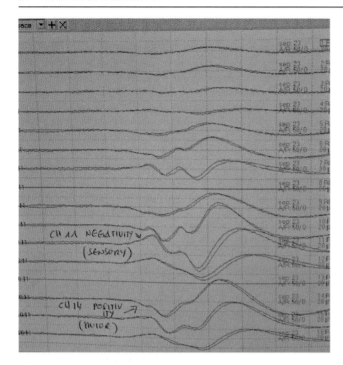

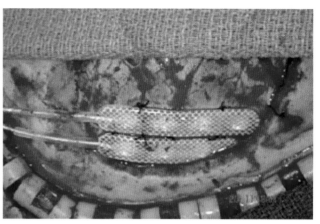

Fig. 60.4 Two two-plate Medtronic Resume paddle electrode arrays placed in the epidural space and oriented perpendicularly to the central sulcus and sutured to the dura

Fig. 60.3 The site and orientation of the central sulcus is identified based on N20-P20 wave shift (phase reversal) obtained during SSEP recordings

should be immediately available for irrigation of the motor cortex in case of a seizure. The position of the stimulating electrodes which produced motor contractions at the lowest threshold in the appropriate region of the body is noted and marked on the dura. This position defines the optimal site for motor cortex stimulation.

Implantation of MCS Electrodes

Two two-plate paddle electrode arrays are then placed in the epidural space in the previously determined optimal position and are oriented perpendicularly to the central sulcus and sutured to the dura (Fig. 60.4). Alternatively, a four-plate Resume electrode array may be used, and in this case, the electrodes may be placed perpendicularly or parallel to the central sulcus. Some investigators have placed these electrodes in the subdural space [21]. Following placement, the electrodes are connected to extension leads, which are tunneled externally and connected to an external pulse generator for testing of the efficacy of stimulation over several days.

Externalized MCS Trial, Stimulation Parameters, and Internalization of Stimulation System

The externalized MCS trial stimulation is generally performed over 3–5 days. Patient should be monitored during the trial in an epilepsy monitoring unit, an intensive care unit, or the neurosurgical floor. During the trial, the stimulation amplitude is set at a value of 80 % of the threshold for motor contraction. Typical stimulation parameters used are

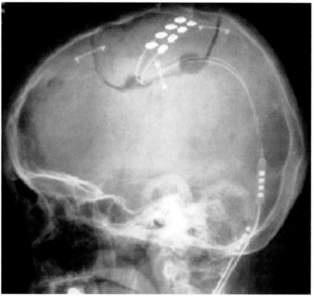

Fig. 60.5 The lead is connected to an extension wire which is tunneled under the skin and connected to an implantable pulse generator (*IPG*), which is typically placed in a subcutaneous or subfascial pocket created in the infraclavicular region

amplitudes of 1–3 V, frequency of 40 Hz, and pulse width of 90 ms. A trial is considered successful if patients report at least 50 % pain relief with stimulation.

Patients who have a successful trial are then returned to the operating room for internalization of the stimulator system. The scalp flap is only partially reopened during this second procedure to expose the MCS electrode lead that was coiled under the galea of the scalp at the first procedure. This lead is then connected to an extension wire which is tunneled under the skin and connected to an implantable pulse generator (IPG), which is typically placed in a subcutaneous or subfascial pocket created in the infraclavicular region (Fig. 60.5).

Conclusion

Motor cortex stimulation is safe and effective in the treatment of medically refractory neuropathic pain in select patients. Its main indications at this time are the treatment of medically refractory central and trigeminal neuropathic pain, but it is finding utility in other indications including treatment of phantom limb pain and complex regional pain syndromes. The mechanism of action is not yet fully elucidated, but may involve disruption of abnormal thalamic impulses by cortically mediated modulation.

Prediction of patient response to MCS is, at this time, based on response to a period of externalized trial stimulation. The development of techniques for predicting patient response to MCS noninvasively, such as the use of transcranial magnetic stimulation, will be an invaluable contribution to the management of these patients. Finally, more double-blinded randomized evaluations of this technique are indicated in view of its invasiveness and cost implications.

References

1. Tsubokawa T, Katayama Y, Yamamoto T, Hirayama T, Koyama S. Treatment of thalamic pain by chronic motor cortex stimulation. Pacing Clin Electrophysiol. 1991;14(1):131–4.
2. Tsubokawa T, Katayama Y, Yamamoto T, Hirayama T, Koyama S. Chronic motor cortex stimulation for the treatment of central pain. Acta Neurochir Suppl (Wien). 1991;52:137–9.
3. Meyerson BA, Lindblom U, Linderoth B, Lind G, Herregodts P. Motor cortex stimulation as treatment of trigeminal pain. Acta Neurochir Suppl (Wien). 1993;58:150–3.
4. Fontaine D, Hamani C, Lozano A. Efficacy and safety of motor cortex stimulation for chronic neuropathic pain: critical review of the literature. J Neurosurg. 2009;110(2):251–6.
5. Garcia-Larrea L, Peyron R, Mertens P, Laurent B, Mauguiere F, Sindou M. Functional imaging and neurophysiological assessment of spinal and brain therapeutic modulation in humans. Arch Med Res. 2000;31(3):248–57.
6. Garcia-Larrea L, Peyron R, Mertens P, et al. Electrical stimulation of motor cortex for pain control: a combined PET-scan and electrophysiological study. Pain. 1999;83(2):259–73.
7. Garcia-Larrea L, Peyron R. Motor cortex stimulation for neuropathic pain: from phenomenology to mechanisms. Neuroimage. 2007;37 Suppl 1:S71–9.
8. Nguyen JP, Lefaucheur JP, Decq P, et al. Chronic motor cortex stimulation in the treatment of central and neuropathic pain. Correlations between clinical, electrophysiological and anatomical data. Pain. 1999;82(3):245–51.
9. Smith H, Joint C, Schlugman D, Nandi D, Stein JF, Aziz TZ. Motor cortex stimulation for neuropathic pain. Neurosurg Focus. 2001;11(3):E2.
10. Saitoh Y, Shibata M, Sanada Y, Mashimo T. Motor cortex stimulation for phantom limb pain. Lancet. 1999;353(9148):212.
11. Sol JC, Casaux J, Roux FE, et al. Chronic motor cortex stimulation for phantom limb pain: correlations between pain relief and functional imaging studies. Stereotact Funct Neurosurg. 2001;77(1–4):172–6.
12. Son UC, Kim MC, Moon DE, Kang JK. Motor cortex stimulation in a patient with intractable complex regional pain syndrome type II with hemibody involvement. Case report. J Neurosurg. 2003;98(1):175–9.
13. Tani N, Saitoh Y, Hirata M, Kato A, Yoshimine T. Bilateral cortical stimulation for deafferentation pain after spinal cord injury. Case report. J Neurosurg. 2004;101(4):687–9.
14. Velasco F, Arguelles C, Carrillo-Ruiz JD, et al. Efficacy of motor cortex stimulation in the treatment of neuropathic pain: a randomized double-blind trial. J Neurosurg. 2008;108(4):698–706.
15. Rasche D, Ruppolt M, Stippich C, Unterberg A, Tronnier VM. Motor cortex stimulation for long-term relief of chronic neuropathic pain: a 10 year experience. Pain. 2006;121(1–2):43–52.
16. Yamamoto T, Katayama Y, Hirayama T, Tsubokawa T. Pharmacological classification of central post-stroke pain: comparison with the results of chronic motor cortex stimulation therapy. Pain. 1997;72(1–2):5–12.
17. Katayama Y, Fukaya C, Yamamoto T. Poststroke pain control by chronic motor cortex stimulation: neurological characteristics predicting a favorable response. J Neurosurg. 1998;89(4):585–91.
18. Drouot X, Nguyen JP, Peschanski M, Lefaucheur JP. The antalgic efficacy of chronic motor cortex stimulation is related to sensory changes in the painful zone. Brain. 2002;125(Pt 7):1660–4.
19. Migita K, Uozumi T, Arita K, Monden S. Transcranial magnetic coil stimulation of motor cortex in patients with central pain. Neurosurgery. 1995;36(5):1037–9; discussion 1039–40.
20. Nuti C, Peyron R, Garcia-Larrea L, et al. Motor cortex stimulation for refractory neuropathic pain: four year outcome and predictors of efficacy. Pain. 2005;118(1–2):43–52.
21. Saitoh Y, Hirano S, Kato A, et al. Motor cortex stimulation for deafferentation pain. Neurosurg Focus. 2001;11(3):E1.

Intrathecal Drug Delivery for Control of Pain

Brian M. Bruel, Mitchell P. Engle, Richard L. Rauck, Thomas J. Weber, and Leonardo Kapural

Key Points

- The utilization of intrathecal drug delivery has increased over the last two decades.
- Intrathecal delivery of analgesics provides another option for the treatment of both chronic and cancer-related pain.
- Appropriate selection of patients and competence in the implantation procedure are keys to successful therapeutic outcomes.
- There are numerous intrathecally delivered medications currently being utilized with different mechanisms of action for the treatment of pain.
- Guidelines for intrathecal drug delivery for pain are available, but further research is required in intrathecal pharmacology and physiology.

Introduction

Over the last two decades, the use of intraspinal drug delivery (ISDD) systems for the treatment of chronic pain and spasticity has increased [1]. The clinical practice varies from institution to institution as far as the utilization of different agents or routes of administration. The clinical approach for intraspinal drug delivery is influenced by the type of pain treated (e.g., chronic nociceptive vs. neuropathic). The choice depends on life expectancy as well as the planned time frame of treatment. Intraspinal catheter placement is frequently chosen for the treatment of cancer pain, spasticity (caused by cerebral palsy, multiple sclerosis, spinal cord injury, and other neurologic conditions), and intractable nonmalignant pain (severe post-laminectomy syndrome and arachnoiditis, vertebral compressive fractures resistant to other therapies, complex regional pain syndrome (CRPS), postherpetic neuralgia and other types of neuralgias), and the administration of intrathecal chemotherapy and CSF drainage [2]. Effective dosing through continuous intrathecal infusion is five to ten times less over 24 h when opioids are used.

Intrathecal (IT) drug delivery systems for the administration of opioids and non-opioids to treat intractable chronic pain have been used since late 1970s [3]. Technological improvements to intrathecal drug delivery systems throughout the 1980s and 1990s brought more sophisticated, totally implantable, and externally programmable devices [3]. The potential advantages of contemporary drug delivery systems include effective pain control by delivering opioids or non-opioids directly to the spinal cord, much lower doses of opioids and non-opioids required to control the pain, and fewer side effects in comparison with systemic drug delivery [3].

B.M. Bruel, M.D., MBA (✉) • M.P. Engle, M.D., Ph.D.
Department of Pain Medicine,
The University of Texas MD Anderson Cancer Center,
1515 Holcombe Boulevard, Unit 409, Houston, TX 77030, USA
e-mail: bbruel@mdanderson.org; mpengle@mdanderson.org

R.L. Rauck, M.D., FIPP • T.J. Weber, DO • L. Kapural, M.D., Ph.D.
Carolinas Pain Institute, Wake Forest University School of Medicine,
145 Kimel Park Drive Suite 330, Winston-Salem, NC 27103, USA
e-mail: rrauck@ccrpain.com; lkapural@wfubmc.edu

Brief History

In 1973, the opioid receptor was first identified [4]. This early research on the opioid receptor and its location in the dorsal horn of the spinal cord became the foundation for current intrathecal therapies. The first "permanent" catheter for intraspinal drug delivery was developed in the 1980s by Dupen and associates [5]. In the early 1980s, Coombs et al. pioneered the usage of continuous intraspinal morphine delivered by an implanted continuous system for chronic intractable pain. This small series of ten patients confirmed the efficacy of the sustained analgesic effects of the intrathecal route of opioids in treating cancer pain [6]. In 1991, Medtronic released the first FDA-approved externally programmable IDDS pump powered by batteries in the United States [3]. Since its FDA approval, more than 200,000 chronic pain patients have been treated with continuous intrathecal drug therapy.

Patient Selection and Workup

Proper patient selection is the cornerstone to successful intrathecal drug therapy. Appropriate patient selection is achieved by carefully choosing patients that may experience therapeutic success while experiencing minimal drug or procedural side effects. It is important to begin with a thorough history, physical exam, and psychological evaluation to develop an accurate diagnosis of the patient's pain condition. Another key step in successful implantable therapy is patient education. It is extremely important for the patient to have a thorough understanding of the procedure prior to implant and to have realistic expectations of pain relief post implantation.

Selection criteria for implantable therapies depend mainly upon the etiology of the patient's pain. It is important to differentiate between cancer pain and noncancer chronic pain. The strongest evidence in support of intrathecal therapy lies in the treatment of cancer pain patients [6–8]. Cancer pain is often associated with severe, debilitating pain. Oral opioid pain medications are often used in high dosages to treat cancer pain. Unfortunately, they are often associated with multiple side effects that negatively affect the patient's quality of life. Intrathecal opioids allow these patients to use lower overall amounts of opioids, allowing greater pain relief and the ability to minimize the side effects of excessive sedation, constipation, and respiratory depression, and to allow an improvement in overall function [7, 8].

In the United States, the most common indication for intrathecal therapy is chronic intractable noncancer pain that is not responsive to conservative therapy. Unfortunately, there are limited randomized controlled studies showing the long-term benefit of continuous intrathecal therapy in nonmalignant pain patients. Failed back surgery syndrome, spinal stenosis, intractable lower back pain, and other diseases of the spine are the most common indications for intrathecal therapy [2]. There is some general debate among pain physicians on who is an appropriate candidate for intrathecal therapy. Table 61.1 provides some general guidelines on selection criteria to intrathecal drug therapy [9].

Proper patient evaluation also requires knowledge of the contraindications of intrathecal therapy (see Table 61.2) [10, 11].

Prior to implant, it is important to perform thorough patient counseling on intrathecal therapy to ensure an appro-

Table 61.1 Selection criteria for intrathecal pump placement

Stable medical condition amenable to surgery	☐
Clear organic pain generator	☐
No psychological or sociological contraindication	☐
No familial contraindication such as severe codependent behavior	☐
Documented responsible behavior and stable social situation	☐
Good pain relief with oral or parenteral opioids	☐
Intolerable side effects from systemic opioid therapy	☐
Baseline neurological exam and psychological evaluation	☐
Failure of more conservative therapy including trials with non-opioid medications and nerve blocks	☐
Constant or almost constant pain requiring around-the-clock opioid therapy	☐
No tumor encroachment of thecal sac in cancer patients	☐
Life expectancy >3 months	☐
No practical issues that might interfere with device placement, maintenance, or assessment (e.g., morbid obesity, severe cognitive impairment)	☐
Positive response to an intrathecal trial	☐

Table 61.2 Contraindications for intrathecal (IT) therapy

Systemic infection
Coagulopathy
Allergy to medication being used
Inappropriate drug habituation (untreated)
Failure to obtain pain relief in a screening trial
Unusual observed behavior during screening trial
Poor personal hygiene

priate chance of success. The counseling process begins with detailed instruction on the entire procedural process, the risks and benefits of the procedure, and discussion on realistic expectations from the therapy. The patient must understand the signs and symptoms of potential under- and overdosages to minimize potential life-threatening problems (Table 61.3). The patient must also be instructed to avoid any strenuous and high-impact activities. Scuba diving at a depth of 2 ATA (atmospheres absolute) may damage the pump. These activities may potentially damage the intrathecal catheter or pump reservoir. Intrathecal catheter or battery malfunction may require revision secondary to catheter kinking or occlusion.

There is no standard interpretation of the efficacy and utility of an intrathecal trial. In general, minimal expected outcome is a >50 % reduction in patient's pain and absence of side effects. Trial techniques are based on individual physician preferences

Table 61.3 Drug concentrations and dosages

Drug	Maximum concentration	Maximum dose/day
Morphine	20 mg/mL	15 mg
Hydromorphone	10 mg/mL	4 mg
Fentanyl	2 mg/mL	No known upper limit
Sufentanil	50 µg/mL (not available for compounding)	No known upper limit
Bupivacaine	40 mg/mL	30 mg
Clonidine	2 mg/mL	1.0 mg
Ziconotide	100 µg/mL	19.2 µg (Elan recommendations)

and available resources. There is no convincing evidence that one technique is far superior to another; these include a single-shot injection of intrathecal opioids and non-opioids, multiple bolus injections, and continuous infusion of analgesics, either single or in combination, via an external catheter. There are pros and cons to each method.

A single intrathecal opioid injection involves the injection of intrathecal morphine or other opioids through a lumbar puncture. This is performed with a recommended 0.2–1 mg of intrathecal morphine or the daily equivalent intrathecal dose [12]. There are currently no standard conversion guidelines from systemic opioid doses to intrathecal dosing. Intrathecal boluses allow for a short trial period to evaluate the efficacy and safety of test medication. Long-term efficacy is not expected, and potential side effects of the therapy may occur but are usually short-lived. Multiple bolus injections can be performed through intrathecal or epidural injections, with or without the use of a catheter. This method allows the patient to experience a longer trial period to judge the efficacy of the therapy. The patient may also receive placebo injections to rule out any false positives or any underlying central mediated pain syndromes. The last method of trialing involves the use of continuous infusion of opioid therapy through an external intrathecal catheter. Continuous infusion occurs over several days at a low starting dose and increases every 6–12 h until pain relief is achieved [12, 13]. It is recommended that morphine be trialed in an inpatient or overnight setting to closely monitor for delayed onset adverse events, such as respiratory depression.

Non-opioids, such as ziconotide, may be trialed on an outpatient basis. Trialing of ziconotide is more complex and unpredictable mainly because of a narrow therapeutic window. Continuous infusion trials of ziconotide are traditionally utilized; however, some clinicians perform single bolus trials with varying dosages. Serious adverse side effects during a ziconotide trial, such as respiratory depression and death, are unlikely [13]. Although life-threatening adverse events are not expected with ziconotide, appropriate monitoring for cognitive and psychological effects, ataxia, nausea, and vomiting is recommended.

Psychological Evaluation for Implantable Devices

Currently, there is no large prospective study demonstrating positive predictive value of preoperative psychological testing prior to implantation of IT pump. However, most experts agree that psychological evaluations can improve the patient's chance of successful therapy by discovering untreated depression, anxiety, drug addiction, or/and underlying personality disorders. Patients with underlying personality disorders may have poor functional outcomes using implantable pain therapies [14]. Patients should understand possible outcomes and have realistic expectations for intrathecal therapy. A therapeutic partnership with the patient and physician should focus on adherence to the physician's recommendations and self-monitoring of efficacy and adverse events.

Intrathecal Delivery Systems Implantation Technique

The first step in the implant process is to appropriately prepare the patient for surgery. This begins by marking the potential pump reservoir site on the patient's abdomen. This should be performed with the help of the patient making sure that the site will not interfere with wheelchair use, patient's beltline, or any other activities of daily living. The most appropriate position in the abdomen would be below the lower costal margin and above the iliac crest and beltline and away from rectus abdominis muscle [15]. Chlorhexidine wash one night prior to implantation is recommended by some clinicians; however, there is no clear evidence that this reduces surgical site infection. After appropriate preoperative IV antibiotics are given, the patient is taken to the operating table and placed in the lateral decubitus position with the pump site in the nondependent position. Sterile prep and drape is then performed. A spinal needle is then placed at a shallow-angle (approximately 30° off the spine), paramedian oblique needle insertion trajectory (see Fig. 61.1). The entry point of the needle into the skin (or fascia if the needle insertion is performed through an open incision) should be approximately 1–1 1/2 vertebral levels below the interlaminar space selected for dural puncture and 1–2 cm lateral to the midline, on the side of the intended pump pocket.

The catheter guide wire is seated completely, with its hub against the proximal end of the catheter and remains in place during all maneuvers to insert or position the catheter. The needle bevel is oriented cephalad and the distal tip of the catheter is threaded through the needle to the desired location. One must be aware that if the catheter must be retracted during positioning, the needle tip can damage the catheter, requiring additional surgery to repair or replace the catheter. The needle is carefully removed, ensuring that the hub is orientated cephalad, with the guide wire removed simultaneously.

Fig. 61.1 Lateral and anterior-posterior model view of intrathecal needle placement using paramedian oblique approach. Note a significantly decreased angle to the lumbar spine. Such acute angle is needed to easily position catheter into posterior intrathecal space (Modified from the Medtronic IT implantation manual)

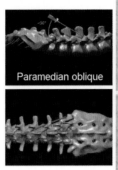
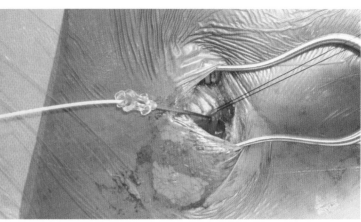

To prevent catheter damage or dislodgement during guide wire removal, the catheter is held straight and securely at the exit site. Minimal traction to avoid catheter twisting helps prevent damage to the catheter. A purse string suture is then tied around the fascia surrounding the catheter, and then, an anchor is attached to the fascia via nonabsorbable sutures.

A subcutaneous pocket is prepared that is large enough to accommodate the selected IT pump. The pocket size should be close-fitting to prevent flipping or migration of pump. Expert implanters recommend that the pocket size should be no more than 20 % larger than the size of the pump. Using the appropriate size catheter passer, a subcutaneous tunnel is formed from the spinal incision site directed toward the pump pocket. The residual catheter length should be noted for accurate programming if a programmable pump is implanted. Strain relief loops at the spinal incision site and behind the implanted pump will allow for patient movements.

Nonabsorbable sutures are placed in the pump pocket fascia closest to four different corners of the pump pocket. The pump is then positioned inside the pocket so that the catheter is not twisted or kinked and securely anchored (Fig. 61.2). Skin and underlying fascia are closed with sutures.

Basics Concepts of Intraspinal Drug Delivery Routes

Epidural versus intrathecal modes of delivery influences distribution of the delivered drugs. Drugs delivered epidurally must cross the dura and arachnoid and then diffuse to their site of action. Drugs delivered intrathecally diffuse directly into the spinal cord [18]. However, the location of the catheter is important even for intrathecal drug delivery. Adjustment of intrathecal medications may be required to achieve therapeutic concentrations at target sites in the spinal cord if the catheter is distal to the targeted spinal level [16, 17].

The hydrophilic medications circulate throughout the CSF. Their duration of action is longer, have relatively slow onset, rostral migration may be more predictable, and is dose dependent [18]. Drugs deposited intrathecally reach high CSF concentration rapidly before reaching any significant serum level and are dose dependent [19]. Morphine and other opioids diffuse to the substantia gelatinosa in the spinal cord – their primary site of action – and bind to opioid receptors there. The required dose to achieve pain relief epidurally is much higher than intrathecally, and systemic absorption is much higher for the same level of analgesia. There is approximately five to ten times reduction of required dose when the route of morphine delivery is changed from epidural to intrathecal [20].

Lipophilic medications remain closer to the catheter tip. For these medications, slow migration of the drug in the spinal space, combined with the rapid uptake by intrathecal tissues, produces large drug gradients within the intrathecal space. Lipophilic opioids (fentanyl and sufentanil) when used for epidural analgesia have significantly higher plasma levels and exhibit less rostral spread. Their spinal mechanism of action is uncertain [21]. The dose for epidural injection is higher than for intrathecal administration, and drug pharmacokinetics is more complex. Dural penetration, epidural fat deposition, and systemic absorption occur [21]. The extent of systemic absorption for epidural infusion is thus higher than with intrathecal administration.

Recent animal studies provided the evidence that the position of the infusion catheter orifice and its relationship to the targeted spinal cord segment are crucial. There is limited capacity of the CSF to distribute drugs away from the distal lumen of the catheter [22–24]. Inadequate pain relief following definitive pump implantation occurs frequently and often requires optimization, even after a successful trial.

The infusion velocity of the drug and the CSF motion are two elements that are critical in intrathecal pharmacokinetics. A bolus or a faster infusion rate shows wider CSF distribution compared with slower rates. The classic flow of CSF is caudad in the posterior surface of the spinal cord and cephalad along the anterior surface. However, this classic depiction is incorrect based on multiple MRI studies that have showed a to-and-fro

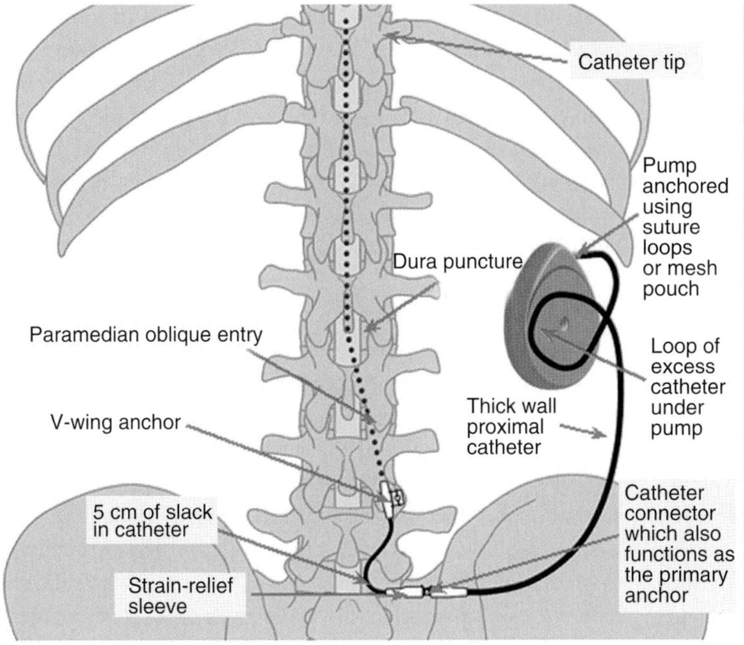

Key points of the low-complication implant technique include:

Paramedian oblique entry
- Reduced catheter fractures/breaks
- Eases catheter advancement

V-wing anchor at spinal entry point
- Reduces catheter dislodgements

Catheter connector/primary anchor
- Reduces catheter dislodgements

Strain-relief sleeve on catheter tubing
- Reduces catheter kinks and holes

Loop of catheter under pump
- Reduces catheter kinks

Slack in catheter by connector
- Reduces catheter kinks

Thick wall pump segment catheter
- Reduces catheter kinks and holes

Pump anchored using suture loops or mesh pouch
- Reduces catheter kinks and dislodgements

Fig. 61.2 Schematic and key points of what is called "low-complication implant technique" for intrathecal pump and catheter. Although such recommendations seem to represent common sense, there are no studies to support all of listed recommendations to prevent catheter kinks and migrations (Modified from the Medtronic IT implantation manual)

rostrocaudal movement, driven by the cerebrospinal vasculature during the cardiac cycle. This flow pattern is greatest in the upper cervical segments and decreases progressively, becoming negligible at the cauda equina. There are three channels of CSF flow. These are medial-ventral, medial-dorsal and lateral, and the most valuable is the undetected circumferential motion in between the anterior and posterior sides of the spinal cord. The dorsal horn is the target. A well-positioned posterior catheter tip is important for dorsal column flow; however, targeting the anterior horn via ventral placement of the catheter tip may provide a better drug response [24].

Intrathecal Versus Epidural Delivery Route

When compared to epidurally placed catheters, intrathecal catheters may last longer with lower rates of complications [25, 26]. In addition, side effects related to drug infusion are less frequent (lethargy, respiratory depression, dysphoria) when intrathecal route is used [27]. The development of tolerance in patients with chronic pain is less frequent when intrathecal route is used [28]. Moreover, the major reason to select the intrathecal route for delivery of opioids came from cancer pain research. Patients who converted from epidural to intrathecal morphine have somewhat better pain relief [25, 26]. This trend was most obvious when long-term externalized epidural catheters were followed by externalized and internalized intrathecal catheters [26]. In regard to medications used, epidural opioids either alone or combined with epidural bupivacaine provided significantly less pain relief than intrathecal opioids or intrathecal opioids and bupivacaine [26].

Intrathecally Delivered Medications

Morphine

Morphine is the prototypical opioid analgesic. It is the only opioid currently approved for intrathecal administration by the FDA. Morphine is a highly hydrophilic compound that is poorly metabolized in the CSF, leading to prolonged duration of effect when delivered intrathecally. Morphine works through activation of opioid receptors, most specifically the μ-opioid receptor. These receptors are located in both the superficial laminae of the spinal cord and supraspinal sites such as the periaqueductal gray matter and the raphe nuclei [29]. Mu opioid receptors are G protein-coupled receptors and are located at both pre- and postsynaptic sites in the spinal cord. On presynaptic terminals, activation of μ-opioid receptors leads to inhibition of voltage-gated calcium channels [30, 31]. In primary afferent neurons, this results in decreased substance P and excitatory amino acid release [32, 33]. Agonism of postsynaptic μ-opioid receptors activates G protein-coupled inwardly rectifying potassium (GIRK) channels leading to neuronal hyperpolarization [34, 35].

Hydromorphone

Hydromorphone is a semisynthetic derivative of morphine. Like morphine, it is a μ-opioid receptor agonist, but it also activates δ- and κ-opioid receptors. Hydromorphone is commonly used as a first-line drug for intrathecal delivery. In addition, due to its different chemical properties and receptor pharmacology, it is also used as a second-line agent when morphine fails to provide sufficient analgesia [36]. There is some evidence that hydromorphone is more lipophilic than morphine which may account for decreased distribution to supraspinal sites resulting in less side effects [37]. The potency of hydromorphone is five times that of morphine.

Fentanyl and Sufentanil

Fentanyl and sufentanil are synthetic anilinopiperidines that are μ-opioid receptor agonists. They are both highly lipophilic which results in segmental analgesia near the catheter tip due to rapid diffusion out of the CSF into the systemic circulation. Anilinopiperidines have higher intrinsic receptor activity than morphine, indicating that less receptors need to be occupied to generate the same physiological response [38, 39]. This property is likely related to the decreased tolerance seen with anilinopiperidine opioids compared to morphine. Relative to morphine, the potencies of fentanyl and sufentanil are 100 and 1,000 times greater, respectively.

Clinical Evidence for Intrathecal Opioids

Intrathecal opioids are currently used in the treatment of a broad spectrum of clinical conditions. Despite an extensive clinical literature detailing the usage of intrathecal opioids, only a relative handful of controlled prospective studies exist on the topic. The strongest evidence for the use of intrathecal opioid comes from the treatment of cancer pain. Rauck and colleagues published a multicenter prospective study of 119 cancer pain patients with data reported out to 16 months. Intrathecal morphine reduced the VAS from 6.1 to 4.2, and this effect continued through month 13. In addition, the patients had a reduction in both oral opioid consumption and the opioid complication severity index. The authors reported clinical successes of 83 % at 1 month and 91 % at 4 months with success defined as ≥50 % reduction in VAS, use of systemic opioids, or opioid complication severity [40]. Smith and colleagues published an important prospective multicenter randomized clinical trial comparing comprehensive medical management (CMM) versus CMM plus implantable drug delivery system (IDDS). With clinical success defined as ≥20 % reduction in VAS or equal VAS with ≥20 % reduction in toxicities, the CMM plus IDDS success rate was 84.5 versus 70.8 % for CMM alone. At 4 weeks, the CMM plus IDDS VAS was reduced by 52 versus 39 % for the CMM alone group. In addition, the CMM plus IDDS group had significant reductions in fatigue and depressed levels of consciousness. Finally, the CMM plus IDDS group had a trend toward increased survival at 6 months [7]. Collectively, these studies indicate a strong role for intrathecal opioids in managing cancer pain.

Evidence for the use of intrathecal opiates in noncancer pain is not quite as clear as with cancer pain in part because of a lack of randomized controlled trials. That said, several high-quality prospective studies have evaluated the effect of intrathecal opioids on neuropathic, nociceptive, and mixed noncancer pains [41–47]. Deer and colleagues reported a multicenter prospective registry of 136 patients with low back and leg pain who were implanted with intrathecal drug delivery systems. At 1 year, numeric pain ratings dropped by 47 % for back pain and 31 % for leg pain. In addition, there was a significant improvement in the Oswestry Low Back Pain Disability scores in implanted patients. Patients who had successful trials but were not implanted did not have similar improvements [48]. Thimineur and colleagues reported a prospective three-armed study of chronic nonmalignant pain. The first arm ($N=38$) were implanted with pumps, the second ($N=31$) either failed a trial or declined implantation, and the third ($N=41$) were newly referred patients. All participants filled out extensive questionnaires at baseline and every 6 months for 3 years. Intrathecal therapy had significant benefits on pain scores, functionality, and mood. The nonimplanted group declined in these functions despite escalation of oral opioids and injective therapies. Neither of the first two groups advanced as well as the new referral group indicating that although intrathecal therapy is associated with significant pain, functional, and mood improvements, the disease pain burden remains high [49]. Although ample evidence exists demonstrating the ability of intrathecal morphine to provide analgesia for chronic noncancer pain, randomized trials need to be conducted before it is considered standard care.

Non-opioids
Bupivacaine

Bupivacaine is the most commonly used local anesthetic for intrathecal administration. The drug is an amino amide that binds the intracellular portion of the α-subunit of voltage-gated Na^+ channels, inhibiting Na^+ influx into the neuron. This ultimately decreases the rate of neuronal depolarization, inhibiting action potential initiation and signal transduction [50]. For continuous intrathecal infusion therapy, bupivacaine is commonly combined with other agents and is rarely used alone. The drug is generally selected for neuropathic pain or when analgesic doses of opioids produce intolerable side effects. The data regarding the efficacy of intrathecal bupivacaine are mixed. In a retrospective analysis of 109 patients with failed back surgery syndrome or metastatic cancer, Deer and colleagues reported that patients with intrathecal opioids plus bupivacaine had better pain control, fewer physician visits, and higher overall satisfaction than patients with intrathecal opioids alone [51]. A single randomized, double-blind placebo-controlled crossover study has evaluated the effect of adding bupivacaine to intrathecal opioid therapy. Mironer and colleagues utilized 24 patients with chronic nonmalignant intractable pain and found no difference in mean pain scores with the addition of bupivacaine; however, there was a statistically significant improvement in quality of life scores [52]. Additionally, one prospective study in cancer patients by van Dongen and colleagues demonstrated that the addition of bupivacaine to morphine attenuated the dose progression of morphine over time, indicating a likely synergistic effect between the two drugs [53].

Ziconotide

Ziconotide is a selective N-type calcium channel blocker that was formerly known as SNX-111. It is a synthetic analog of the ω-conopeptide derived from the venom of the giant marine snail *Conus magus* [54, 55]. Ziconotide inhibits presynaptic N-type calcium channels, leading to decreased excitatory neurotransmitter release in the dorsal horn. Ziconotide is a permanently charged molecule with a molecular weight ten times that of morphine which provides relative confinement to the CSF. In addition, the molecule is relatively resistant to CSF peptidases. As such, clearance of the drug is mediated by CSF bulk flow and not by metabolism [56]. Common side effects include amblyopia, dizziness, nausea, nystagmus, urinary retention, and vomiting, which appear to be in part dose and titration schedule dependent. Ziconotide is approved for intrathecal administration by the FDA.

Three double-blind placebo-controlled studies examining the efficacy of ziconotide in the treatment chronic pain have been conducted. Staats and colleagues evaluated 111 patients with cancer or AIDS-related pain over an 11-day span. The study included a 5–6 day titration phase followed by a 5-day maintenance phase. The placebo group was crossed over into the ziconotide group after 5 days. Mean VAS reduction at the end of the titration phase was 53 % for ziconotide versus 18 % for the placebo group [57]. Wallace and colleagues evaluated 169 with nonmalignant mostly neuropathic pain over 11 days. Mean VAS reduction was 31 % for the ziconotide group versus 6 % for the placebo-treated group. Although both of these studies had significant reductions in pain scores with ziconotide therapy, they also had higher rates of serious adverse events and discontinuation [58]. Rauck and colleagues enrolled 248 patients with neuropathic, nociceptive, and mixed pain for randomization into either intrathecal ziconotide or placebo treatment. Unlike the previous two studies, the dose of ziconotide was gradually increased over 3 weeks to a low maximum dose. At week 3, the VAS decreased by 14.7 % in the ziconotide group compared to 7.2 % in the placebo group ($P=0.036$). Discontinuation rates for adverse events and serious adverse events were similar between the groups [59]. Collectively, these results demonstrate that intrathecal ziconotide is an effective analgesic for both cancer and noncancer pain and

that the adverse effects of the drug can be limited by careful titration and dosing.

Clonidine

Clonidine is a relatively selective α-2-adrenergic receptor agonist that produces dose-dependent analgesia when delivered intrathecally. It is FDA approved for epidural use in the treatment of cancer pain [60, 61] but is commonly used for intrathecal therapy [62]. Alpha-2-adrenergic receptors are located on both pre- and postsynaptic neurons in the dorsal horn [63–65]. The mechanism of action is mediated through inhibition of substance P and excitatory amino acid release from the primary afferent neurons and direct inhibition of second-order neurons [29, 66]. Clonidine synergistically augments the effect of morphine. It does not cause respiratory depression and does not potentiate opioid induced respiratory depression [67]. The major side effects of clonidine are bradycardia and hypotension. These effects tend to be dose related [68]. Abrupt cessation of intrathecal clonidine therapy may produce severe rebound hypertension [62]. Several studies have prospectively documented the efficacy of intrathecal clonidine in humans, particularly in the treatment of neuropathic pain. A small, prospective, randomized, double-blind, placebo-controlled trial in complex regional pain syndrome demonstrated significant benefit of epidural clonidine over placebo [69]. Eisenach and colleagues utilized a placebo-controlled trial to evaluate the efficacy of epidural clonidine for the treatment of severe cancer pain. Successful analgesia was more common in the clonidine (45 %) than saline group (21 %), with the effect being most pronounced in individuals with neuropathic pain [60]. Hassenbusch and colleagues evaluated intrathecal clonidine in the treatment of predominantly neuropathic pain at a large cancer center. Long-term success, defined as 50 % or greater reduction in pain intensity scores, was reported in 42 % of all patients enrolled in the study [62]. Taken together, these data indicate that intrathecal clonidine produces clinically significant analgesia, particularly with neuropathic pain.

Baclofen

Baclofen is a γ-amino butyric acid analog that is the prototypical $GABA_B$ receptor agonist. The receptor is expressed in the superficial laminae of the dorsal horn, appropriately situating it to modulate nociceptive information [70]. In rodent models, baclofen produces significant antinociception and analgesia [71, 72]. Unfortunately, the results in humans are less robust. A double-blind, randomized, placebo-controlled trial by Herman and colleagues reported the effect of intrathecal baclofen on pain associated with multiple sclerosis and spinal cord injury. Dysesthetic and spasm-related pain was significantly reduced, while pinch-induced pain was not [73]. In another study, intrathecal baclofen decreased painful muscle spasms in a population of women with complex regional pain syndrome [74]. Interestingly, intrathecal baclofen may augment the response to spinal cord stimulation [75]. The most common clinical utilization of intrathecal baclofen is for treatment of spasticity. However, in selected circumstances, intrathecal baclofen may be beneficial in managing centrally mediated pain. One concern of note with intrathecal baclofen is the life-threatening withdrawal that occurs with abrupt discontinuation of therapy. Physicians using intrathecal baclofen should be aware of this risk and understand appropriate treatment if accidental discontinuation should occur.

Adenosine

Adenosine is an endogenous purine nucleoside that is involved in multiple biological processes such as energy transfer and signal transduction. It activates four types of receptors in the spinal cord to modulate nociceptive transmission [76–78]. Several studies have examined the efficacy of intrathecal adenosine in humans. Following a dose-escalating phase I safety trial [79], Eisenach and colleagues reported a double-blind placebo-controlled study on the effects of intrathecal adenosine in 40 subjects. Adenosine did not modulate the response to acute thermal or chemical stimulation, but it did reduce mechanical hyperalgesia and allodynia following intradermal capsaicin injection. This effect lasted for at least 24 h even though adenosine levels in the CSF return to baseline by 4 h [80]. Belfrage and colleagues delivered intrathecal adenosine to 14 patients with chronic neuropathic pain, primarily of traumatic origin. The injection caused transient (<60 min) back pain in five patients. Spontaneous pain scores decreased by 63 %, while evoked pain scores dropped by 83 %. In addition, the area of allodynia and hyperalgesia decreased [81]. These studies indicate that intrathecal adenosine may be an effective treatment for neuropathic or centrally mediated pain syndromes, although further toxicity work is needed before adenosine can be recommended for widespread clinical use [37].

Gabapentin

Gabapentin is a γ-amino butyric acid analog that was originally approved for the treatment of epilepsy. Although initially thought to produce its pharmacological effect through GABA receptors, it has now been shown to bind the $\alpha_2\delta_1$ subunit of voltage-gated calcium channels, inhibiting channel function [82]. Gabapentin has both spinal and supraspinal effects. In the dorsal horn, it decreases the release of substance P [83] while supraspinal gabapentin activates descending inhibitory norepinephrine neurons [84]. Together, these effects are situated to dynamically modulate nociceptive transmission at the level of the spinal cord. Although gabapentinoids have increasingly diverse clinical indications, they have historically been a first-line treatment for neuropathic pain. Several recent rodent studies have demonstrated increased expression of the $\alpha_2\delta_1$ subunit in primary afferent neurons following nerve injury that is associated with allodynia [85, 86]. This upregulation may contribute to the initiation of neuropathic pain by altering voltage-gated calcium channel function and presents a putative mechanism for efficacious use of gabapentin in neuropathic pain. The intrathecal delivery of gabapentin has particular theoretical advantages. Following oral administration, the absorption of this drug is transporter dependent in the gastrointestinal tract and at the blood–brain barrier. As such, a "ceiling effect" is commonly seen clinically. Intrathecal delivery of gabapentin will bypass issues of absorption, possibly leading to less systemic side effects. Preliminary results of the phase II clinical trial of intrathecal gabapentin did not produce significant reduction in pain in humans.

Emerging Drugs

The field of emerging intrathecal drug therapies is continually expanding. Several drugs with particular promise include the ultrapotent capsaicin analog resiniferatoxin (RTX), the NMDA receptor antagonist ketamine, the synthetic analog of somatostatin octreotide, the COX inhibitor ketorolac, the benzodiazepine midazolam, the cholinesterase inhibitor neostigmine, the weak μ-opioid receptors agonist and serotonin/norepinephrine reuptake inhibitor tramadol, and the partial μ-opioid receptors agonist and κ-opioid receptors antagonist buprenorphine. For a more in-depth discussion of these compounds, we would refer the readers to the following reviews [37, 56].

The Polyanalgesic Consensus

In 2007, an expert multidisciplinary panel of clinicians convened to develop consensus guidelines for intraspinal therapy for pain. The panel convened on two separate occasions prior to 2007, and the latest published algorithm is shown in Fig. 61.3. Review of published preclinical and clinical data led to the development of these guidelines. This publication was not meant to be the "standard of care" for intrathecal therapy for pain. The document was composed to serve as a guide for safe and effective therapy based on available evidence at the time. In 2007, the panel upgraded ziconotide to a first-line therapy based on relevant literature and collective clinical experience. Catheter tip granulomas (intrathecal inflammatory mass) were identified as an ongoing clinical problem, and steps to mitigate and correct this issue were identified. Recommended concentrations of intrathecal medications were also published in the consensus paper (Table 61.3).

Complications

Most of the drug-related complications were already detailed in respective paragraphs; however, there are some general complications related to route of drug delivery, technique of

Fig. 61.3 Latest (2007) polyanalgesic consensus guidelines for management of pain by intraspinal drug delivery

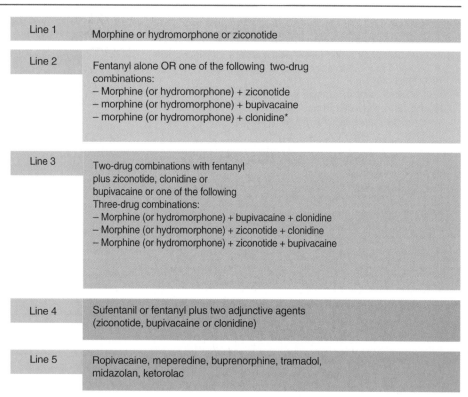

Line 1	Morphine or hydromorphone or ziconotide
Line 2	Fentanyl alone OR one of the following two-drug combinations: – Morphine (or hydromorphone) + ziconotide – morphine (or hydromorphone) + bupivacaine – morphine (or hydromorphone) + clonidine*
Line 3	Two-drug combinations with fentanyl plus ziconotide, clonidine or bupivacaine or one of the following Three-drug combinations: – Morphine (or hydromorphone) + bupivacaine + clonidine – Morphine (or hydromorphone) + ziconotide + clonidine – Morphine (or hydromorphone) + ziconotide + bupivacaine
Line 4	Sufentanil or fentanyl plus two adjunctive agents (ziconotide, bupivacaine or clonidine)
Line 5	Ropivacaine, meperedine, buprenorphine, tramadol, midazolan, ketorolac

*Consider clonidine as a line 2 single agent for neuropathic pain

implantation, maintenance of the IT pump, and characteristics of the spinal fluid.

Intrathecal continuous infusion is safer than epidural infusion if the treatment exceeds 20 days [25, 26]. A comparison of complications between these two routes of opioid delivery suggests more problems with the subarachnoid route in the first 20 days of infusion (25% versus 8%). However, long-term epidural delivery of analgesia is associated with catheter failure, possibly due to epidural fibrosis [26]. The incidence of this complication ranges from 19–41 % [87, 88]. After the 20th day to about 1 year, 55% of patients who received epidural morphine experienced complications compared to 5% in the subarachnoid group. On this basis, the subarachnoid route is preferred for patients expected to live longer than 1 month [25].

Leakage of cerebrospinal fluid (CSF) during the first weeks of intrathecal treatment and formation of a CSF hygroma are possible complications after implantation of an intrathecal drug delivery device. In most patients, symptoms abate within 2 weeks. Symptoms can range from mild postdural puncture headache to a severe postural headache and additional complications related to extensive external loss of cerebrospinal fluid.

Intrathecal infections are more frequent when an underlying disease process is present. Also, externalized catheters may result in more infections compared to internalized systems. Noninfectious fever spikes are possible within 72 hours of implantation, occasionally associated with mild neck stiffness.

Normal white blood cell count and some leukocytosis from CSF drawn from the pump side-port are common findings. Krames suggests that the management of these cases should be guided by the CSF analysis [11].

Conclusion

Intrathecal drug delivery for control of pain is an effective therapy for well-selected patients. Clinical experience, scientific investigations, and published reports have helped to elucidate practices that optimize intrathecal pain control while mitigating complications related to therapy. Current evidence supports intrathecal therapy for cancer-related pain, but there continues to be limited evidence for nonmalignant pain. Ziconotide has been added to the pharmacologic arsenal available for intrathecal infusion in the last decade. The introduction of ziconotide, a non-opioid analgesic, and the ongoing use of intrathecal opioids have led to a better understanding of pain modulation at the spinal level. Refinement of surgical techniques and early identification of potential complications of intrathecal therapy, such as the formation of inflammatory masses at the catheter tip, will improve overall safety of this important modality for pain control. Currently, there continue to be abundant unknowns in intrathecal therapy for pain, and the opportunity for further research will extend for many decades to come.

References

1. Paice JA, Penn RD, Shott S. Intraspinal morphine for chronic pain: a retrospective, multicenter study. J Pain Symptom Manage. 1996;11:71–80.

2. Manchikanti L, Staats PS, Singh V, Schultz DM, Vilims BD, Jasper JF, et al. Evidence-based practice guidelines for interventional techniques in the management of chronic spinal pain. Pain Physician. 2003;6:3–81.

3. Wallace M, Yaksh TL. Long-term spinal analgesic delivery: a review of the preclinical and clinical literature. Reg Anesth Pain Med. 2000;25:117–57.

4. Pert CB, Snyder SH. Opiate receptor: demonstration in nervous tissue. Science. 1973;179:1011–4.

5. Prager J, Jacobs M. Evaluation of patients for implantable pain modalities: medical and behavioral assessment. Clin J Pain. 2001;17:206–14.

6. Coombs DW, Saunders RL, Gaylor MS, Block AR, Colton T, Harbaugh R, et al. Relief of continuous chronic pain by intraspinal narcotics infusion via an implanted reservoir. JAMA. 1983;250: 2336–9.

7. Smith TJ, Staats PS, Deer T, Stearns LJ, Rauck RL, Boortz-Marx RL, et al. Randomized clinical trial of an implantable drug delivery system compared with comprehensive medical management for refractory cancer pain: impact on pain, drug-related toxicity, and survival. J Clin Oncol. 2002;20:4040–9.

8. Smith TJ, Coyne PJ. How to use implantable intrathecal drug delivery systems for refractory cancer pain. J Support Oncol. 2003;1:73–6.

9. Cohen SP, Dragovich A. Intrathecal analgesia. Anesthesiol Clin. 2007;25:863–82, viii.

10. Levy RM, Salzman D. Implanted drug delivery systems for control of chronic pain. In: North RB, Levy RM, editors. Neurosurgical management of pain. New York: Springer; 1997. p. 302–24.

11. Krames ES. Intraspinal opioid therapy for chronic nonmalignant pain: current practice and clinical guidelines. J Pain Symptom Manage. 1996;11:333–52.

12. Onofrio BM, Yaksh TL. Long-term pain relief produced by intrathecal morphine infusion in 53 patients. J Neurosurg. 1990;72:200–9.

13. Kapural L, Szabova A, Mekhail NA. Intraspinal drug delivery routes for treatment of chronic pain and spasticity. Semin Pain Med. 2003;1:254–9.

14. Brown J, Klapow J, Doleys D, Lowery D, Tutak U. Disease-specific and generic health outcomes: a model for the evaluation of long-term intrathecal opioid therapy in noncancer low back pain patients. Clin J Pain. 1999;15:122–31.

15. Narouze SN, Yonan S, Kapural L, Malak O. Erosion of the inferior epigastric artery: a rare complication of intrathecal drug delivery systems. Pain Med. 2007;8:468–70.

16. Ummenhofer WC, Arends RH, Shen DD, Bernards CM. Comparative spinal distribution and clearance kinetics of intrathecally administered morphine, fentanyl, alfentanil, and sufentanil. Anesthesiology. 2000;92:739–53.

17. Dobos I, Toth K, Kekesi G, Joo G, Csullog E, Klimscha W, et al. The significance of intrathecal catheter location in rats. Anesth Analg. 2003;96:487–92, table of contents.

18. Prager JP. Neuraxial medication delivery: the development and maturity of a concept for treating chronic pain of spinal origin. Spine (Phila Pa 1976). 2002;27:2593–605; discussion 606.

19. Samuelsson H, Nordberg G, Hedner T, Lindqvist J. CSF and plasma morphine concentrations in cancer patients during chronic epidural morphine therapy and its relation to pain relief. Pain. 1987;30: 303–10.

20. Gourlay GK, Plummer JL, Cherry DA, Onley MM, Parish KA, Wood MM, et al. Comparison of intermittent bolus with continuous infusion of epidural morphine in the treatment of severe cancer pain. Pain. 1991;47:135–40.

21. Rawal N. Epidural and spinal agents for postoperative analgesia. Surg Clin North Am. 1999;79:313–44.

22. Flack SH, Bernards CM. Cerebrospinal fluid and spinal cord distribution of hyperbaric bupivacaine and baclofen during slow intrathecal infusion in pigs. Anesthesiology. 2010;112:165–73.

23. Flack SH, Anderson CM, Bernards C. Morphine distribution in the spinal cord after chronic infusion in pigs. Anesth Analg. 2011;112:460–4.

24. Bernards CM. Cerebrospinal fluid and spinal cord distribution of baclofen and bupivacaine during slow intrathecal infusion in pigs. Anesthesiology. 2006;105:169–78.

25. Crul BJ, Delhaas EM. Technical complications during long-term subarachnoid or epidural administration of morphine in terminally ill cancer patients: a review of 140 cases. Reg Anesth. 1991;16:209–13.

26. Dahm P, Nitescu P, Appelgren L, Curelaru I. Efficacy and technical complications of long-term continuous intraspinal infusions of opioid and/or bupivacaine in refractory nonmalignant pain: a comparison between the epidural and the intrathecal approach with externalized or implanted catheters and infusion pumps. Clin J Pain. 1998;14:4–16.

27. Gestin Y, Vainio A, Pegurier AM. Long-term intrathecal infusion of morphine in the home care of patients with advanced cancer. Acta Anaesthesiol Scand. 1997;41:12–7.

28. Yaksh TL, Onofrio BM. Retrospective consideration of the doses of morphine given intrathecally by chronic infusion in 163 patients by 19 physicians. Pain. 1987;31:211–23.

29. Pan YZ, Li DP, Pan HL. Inhibition of glutamatergic synaptic input to spinal lamina II(o) neurons by presynaptic alpha(2)-adrenergic receptors. J Neurophysiol. 2002;87:1938–47.

30. Moises HC, Rusin KI, Macdonald RL. Mu- and kappa-opioid receptors selectively reduce the same transient components of high-threshold calcium current in rat dorsal root ganglion sensory neurons. J Neurosci. 1994;14:5903–16.

31. Wu ZZ, Chen SR, Pan HL. Differential sensitivity of N- and P/Q-type Ca^{2+} channel currents to a mu opioid in isolectin B4-positive and -negative dorsal root ganglion neurons. J Pharmacol Exp Ther. 2004;311:939–47.

32. Kohno T, Kumamoto E, Higashi H, Shimoji K, Yoshimura M. Actions of opioids on excitatory and inhibitory transmission in substantia gelatinosa of adult rat spinal cord. J Physiol. 1999;518(Pt 3):803–13.

33. Kondo I, Marvizon JC, Song B, Salgado F, Codeluppi S, Hua XY, et al. Inhibition by spinal mu- and delta-opioid agonists of afferent-evoked substance P release. J Neurosci. 2005;25:3651–60.

34. Marker CL, Lujan R, Loh HH, Wickman K. Spinal G-protein-gated potassium channels contribute in a dose-dependent manner to the analgesic effect of mu- and delta- but not kappa-opioids. J Neurosci. 2005;25:3551–9.

35. Marker CL, Stoffel M, Wickman K. Spinal G-protein-gated K+ channels formed by GIRK1 and GIRK2 subunits modulate thermal nociception and contribute to morphine analgesia. J Neurosci. 2004;24:2806–12.

36. Anderson VC, Cooke B, Burchiel KJ. Intrathecal hydromorphone for chronic nonmalignant pain: a retrospective study. Pain Med. 2001;2:287–97.

37. Deer T, Krames ES, Hassenbusch SJ, Burton A, Caraway D, Dupen S, et al. Polyanalgesic consensus conference 2007: recommendations for the management of pain by intrathecal (intraspinal) drug delivery: report of an interdisciplinary expert panel. Neuromodulation. 2007;10:28.

38. Sosnowski M, Yaksh TL. Differential cross-tolerance between intrathecal morphine and sufentanil in the rat. Anesthesiology. 1990;73:1141–7.

39. Krames ES, Harb M. Neuromodulation. London: Elsevier; 2009.

40. Rauck RL, Cherry D, Boyer MF, Kosek P, Dunn J, Alo K. Long-term intrathecal opioid therapy with a patient-activated, implanted delivery system for the treatment of refractory cancer pain. J Pain. 2003;4:441–7.

41. Hassenbusch SJ, Stanton-Hicks M, Covington EC, Walsh JG, Guthrey DS. Long-term intraspinal infusions of opioids in the treatment of neuropathic pain. J Pain Symptom Manage. 1995;10:527–43.

42. Tutak U, Doleys DM. Intrathecal infusion systems for treatment of chronic low back and leg pain of noncancer origin. South Med J. 1996;89:295–300.

43. Angel IF, Gould Jr HJ, Carey ME. Intrathecal morphine pump as a treatment option in chronic pain of nonmalignant origin. Surg Neurol. 1998;49:92–8; discussion 98–9.

44. Anderson VC, Burchiel KJ. A prospective study of long-term intrathecal morphine in the management of chronic nonmalignant pain. Neurosurgery. 1999;44:289–300; discussion 300–1.

45. Kumar K, Kelly M, Pirlot T. Continuous intrathecal morphine treatment for chronic pain of nonmalignant etiology: long-term benefits and efficacy. Surg Neurol. 2001;55:79–86; discussion 86–8.

46. Shaladi A, Saltari MR, Piva B, Crestani F, Tartari S, Pinato P, et al. Continuous intrathecal morphine infusion in patients with vertebral fractures due to osteoporosis. Clin J Pain. 2007;23:511–7.

47. Duse G, Davia G, White PF. Improvement in psychosocial outcomes in chronic pain patients receiving intrathecal morphine infusions. Anesth Analg. 2009;109:1981–6.

48. Deer T, Chapple I, Classen A, Javery K, Stoker V, Tonder L, et al. Intrathecal drug delivery for treatment of chronic low back pain: report from the National Outcomes Registry for Low Back Pain. Pain Med. 2004;5:6–13.

49. Thimineur MA, Kravitz E, Vodapally MS. Intrathecal opioid treatment for chronic non-malignant pain: a 3-year prospective study. Pain. 2004;109:242–9.

50. Reig E, Abejon D, Kranes ES. Neuromodulation. London: Elsevier; 2009.

51. Deer TR, Caraway DL, Kim CK, Dempsey CD, Stewart CD, McNeil KF. Clinical experience with intrathecal bupivacaine in combination with opioid for the treatment of chronic pain related to failed back surgery syndrome and metastatic cancer pain of the spine. Spine J. 2002;2:274–8.

52. Mironer YE, Haasis JC, Chapple I, Brown C, Satterthwaite JR. Efficacy and safety of intrathecal opioid/bupivacaine mixture in chronic nonmalignant pain: a double blind, randomized, crossover, multicenter study by the National Forum of Independent Pain Clinicians (NFIPC). Neuromodulation. 2002;5:6.

53. van Dongen RT, Crul BJ, van Egmond J. Intrathecal coadministration of bupivacaine diminishes morphine dose progression during long-term intrathecal infusion in cancer patients. Clin J Pain. 1999;15:166–72.

54. Olivera BM, Gray WR, Zeikus R, McIntosh JM, Varga J, Rivier J, et al. Peptide neurotoxins from fish-hunting cone snails. Science. 1985;230:1338–43.

55. Miljanich GP, Ramachandran J. Antagonists of neuronal calcium channels: structure, function, and therapeutic implications. Annu Rev Pharmacol Toxicol. 1995;35:707–34.

56. Lawson EF, Wallace MS. Current developments in intraspinal agents for cancer and noncancer pain. Curr Pain Headache Rep. 2010;14:8–16.

57. Staats PS, Yearwood T, Charapata SG, Presley RW, Wallace MS, Byas-Smith M, et al. Intrathecal ziconotide in the treatment of refractory pain in patients with cancer or AIDS: a randomized controlled trial. JAMA. 2004;291:63–70.

58. Wallace MS, Rauck R, Fisher R, Charapata SG, Ellis D, Dissanayake S. Intrathecal ziconotide for severe chronic pain: safety and tolerability results of an open-label, long-term trial. Anesth Analg. 2008;106:628–37, table of contents.

59. Rauck RL, Wallace MS, Leong MS, Minehart M, Webster LR, Charapata SG, et al. A randomized, double-blind, placebo-controlled study of intrathecal ziconotide in adults with severe chronic pain. J Pain Symptom Manage. 2006;31:393–406.

60. Eisenach JC, DuPen S, Dubois M, Miguel R, Allin D. Epidural clonidine analgesia for intractable cancer pain. The Epidural Clonidine Study Group. Pain. 1995;61:391–9.

61. Tamsen A, Gordh T. Epidural clonidine produces analgesia. Lancet. 1984;2:231–2.

62. Hassenbusch SJ, Gunes S, Wachsman S, Willis KD. Intrathecal clonidine in the treatment of intractable pain: a phase I/II study. Pain Med. 2002;3:85–91.

63. Stone LS, Broberger C, Vulchanova L, Wilcox GL, Hokfelt T, Riedl MS, et al. Differential distribution of alpha2A and alpha2C adrenergic receptor immunoreactivity in the rat spinal cord. J Neurosci. 1998;18:5928–37.

64. Stone LS, MacMillan LB, Kitto KF, Limbird LE, Wilcox GL. The alpha2a adrenergic receptor subtype mediates spinal analgesia evoked by alpha2 agonists and is necessary for spinal adrenergic-opioid synergy. J Neurosci. 1997;17:7157–65.

65. Sullivan AF, Dashwood MR, Dickenson AH. Alpha 2-adrenoceptor modulation of nociception in rat spinal cord: location, effects and interactions with morphine. Eur J Pharmacol. 1987;138:169–77.

66. Ono H, Mishima A, Ono S, Fukuda H, Vasko MR. Inhibitory effects of clonidine and tizanidine on release of substance P from slices of rat spinal cord and antagonism by alpha-adrenergic receptor antagonists. Neuropharmacology. 1991;30:585–9.

67. Bailey PL, Sperry RJ, Johnson GK, Eldredge SJ, East KA, East TD, et al. Respiratory effects of clonidine alone and combined with morphine, in humans. Anesthesiology. 1991;74:43–8.

68. Filos KS, Goudas LC, Patroni O, Polyzou V. Hemodynamic and analgesic profile after intrathecal clonidine in humans. A dose-response study. Anesthesiology. 1994;81:591–601; discussion 27A–8A.

69. Rauck RL, Eisenach JC, Jackson K, Young LD, Southern J. Epidural clonidine treatment for refractory reflex sympathetic dystrophy. Anesthesiology. 1993;79:1163–9; discussion 27A.

70. Engle MP, Gassman M, Sykes KT, Bettler B, Hammond DL. Spinal nerve ligation does not alter the expression or function of GABA(B) receptors in spinal cord and dorsal root ganglia of the rat. Neuroscience. 2006;138:1277–87.

71. Hammond DL, Drower EJ. Effects of intrathecally administered THIP, baclofen and muscimol on nociceptive threshold. Eur J Pharmacol. 1984;103:121–5.

72. Dirig DM, Yaksh TL. Intrathecal baclofen and muscimol, but not midazolam, are antinociceptive using the rat-formalin model. J Pharmacol Exp Ther. 1995;275:219–27.

73. Herman RM, D'Luzansky SC, Ippolito R. Intrathecal baclofen suppresses central pain in patients with spinal lesions. A pilot study. Clin J Pain. 1992;8:338–45.

74. van Hilten BJ, van de Beek WJ, Hoff JI, Voormolen JH, Delhaas EM. Intrathecal baclofen for the treatment of dystonia in patients with reflex sympathetic dystrophy. N Engl J Med. 2000;343:625–30.

75. Lind G, Meyerson BA, Winter J, Linderoth B. Intrathecal baclofen as adjuvant therapy to enhance the effect of spinal cord stimulation in neuropathic pain: a pilot study. Eur J Pain. 2004;8:377–83.

76. Yoon MH, Bae HB, Choi JI, Kim SJ, Chung ST, Kim CM. Roles of adenosine receptor subtypes in the antinociceptive effect of intrathecal adenosine in a rat formalin test. Pharmacology. 2006;78:21–6.

77. Lee YW, Yaksh TL. Pharmacology of the spinal adenosine receptor which mediates the antiallodynic action of intrathecal adenosine agonists. J Pharmacol Exp Ther. 1996;277:1642–8.

78. Sawynok J. Adenosine and ATP receptors. Handbook of Experimental Pharmacology. Berlin/Heidelberg: Springer; 2007.

79. Eisenach JC, Hood DD, Curry R. Phase I safety assessment of intrathecal injection of an American formulation of adenosine in humans. Anesthesiology. 2002;96:24–8.

80. Eisenach JC, Hood DD, Curry R. Preliminary efficacy assessment of intrathecal injection of an American formulation of adenosine in humans. Anesthesiology. 2002;96:29–34.

81. Belfrage M, Segerdahl M, Arner S, Sollevi A. The safety and efficacy of intrathecal adenosine in patients with chronic neuropathic pain. Anesth Analg. 1999;89:136–42.

82. Perret D, Luo ZD. Targeting voltage-gated calcium channels for neuropathic pain management. Neurotherapeutics. 2009;6:679–92.

83. Takasusuki T, Yaksh TL. The effects of intrathecal and systemic gabapentin on spinal substance P release. Anesth Analg. 2011;112:971–6.

84. Takeuchi Y, Takasu K, Honda M, Ono H, Tanabe M. Neurochemical evidence that supraspinally administered gabapentin activates the descending noradrenergic system after peripheral nerve injury. Eur J Pharmacol. 2007;556:69–74.

85. Luo ZD, Chaplan SR, Higuera ES, Sorkin LS, Stauderman KA, Williams ME, et al. Upregulation of dorsal root ganglion (alpha)2(delta) calcium channel subunit and its correlation with allodynia in spinal nerve-injured rats. J Neurosci. 2001;21: 1868–75.

86. Luo ZD, Calcutt NA, Higuera ES, Valder CR, Song YH, Svensson CI, et al. Injury type-specific calcium channel alpha 2 delta-1 subunit up-regulation in rat neuropathic pain models correlates with antiallodynic effects of gabapentin. J Pharmacol Exp Ther. 2002;303:1199–205.

87. Arner S, Rawal N, Gustafsson LL. Clinical experience of long-term treatment with epidural and intrathecal opioids – a nationwide survey. Acta Anaesthesiol Scand. 1988;32:253–9.

88. Nitescu P, Sjoberg M, Appelgren L, Curelaru I. Complications of intrathecal opioids and bupivacaine in the treatment of "refractory" cancer pain. Clin J Pain. 1995;11:45–62.

Clinical Applications of Neuromodulation: Radicular Pain and Low Back Pain

62

Thomas L. Yearwood

Key Points

- It is crucial to understand and appreciate the clinically relevant neuroanatomy of intraspinal and extraspinal components of the sensory nervous system in order to achieve therapeutic and durable neuromodulation in the treatment of neuropathic pain.
- Neurostimulation is a "surface" phenomenon, and in general, penetration of the neuronal tissues is limited to less than 0.5 mm of depth.
- The nervous system is characterized by a somatotopic arrangement of sensory fibers and tracts, each of which offers a statistically relevant population density of targets suitable for stimulation. The more "focal" the need for neurostimulation, the more important it becomes to find access to the CNS by way of these suitable targets, moving peripherally from the dorsal columns toward the dorsal root entry zone (DREZ), nerve roots, dorsal root ganglion (DRG), and named peripheral nerves. The more "regional" the need for neurostimulation, the more important it becomes to find access to the CNS centrally, beginning with the dorsal columns. The somatotopic arrangement of fibers and tracts greatly enhances appropriate targeting for neurostimulation.
- The important "tools of the trade" for neurostimulation therapy are contact placement, complex programming, blending of neurostimulation targets, and integration of neurostimulation therapy with all the other therapeutic modalities in a cohesive and complementary fashion.

- The ultimate goal of neurostimulation is not targeting a specific anatomical area of neuropathic pain with paresthesias, but targeting those locations within the CNS where the neuropathic pain is perceived and interpreted and results in a response. There are numerous "portals of access" to those locations in the CNS from the periphery, and these neuronal pathways provide our opportunities for therapeutic neurostimulation.

Introduction

Neuropathic pain in the upper or lower extremities, and axial spine, can result from numerous and diverse disease states and are some of the most difficult conditions to treat effectively. Neuropathic pain is particularly resistant to opioid therapy and at a minimum requires the balanced integration of polypharmaceutical techniques, functional rehabilitation (physical and occupational therapy), behavioral medicine, and other conservative techniques such as fluoroscopically guided spinal injections techniques. The addition of electrical neurostimulation to this overall treatment plan has proven to be of substantial benefit in reducing pain and restoring physical function for patients with debilitating neuropathic pain of one or more extremities.

As technology for the treatment modality has matured, the practical applications of physician-prescribed electrical fields to excitable neural targets within the spinal canal and in the periphery have expanded. For example, in the spinal canal, technological limitations of lead construction and implantable pulse generator (IPG) programmability and power capabilities limited the application of electrical fields to the largest targets, and the terms "spinal cord stimulation" (SCS) and "dorsal column stimulation" (DCS) were synonymous. However, recent technological advances in lead and IPG design, allowing the development of sophisticated programming of the areas' electrical field parameters (pulse

T.L. Yearwood, M.D., Ph.D.
Pain Consultants ASC, LLC,
4105 Hospital Road, Suite 112-A,
Pascagoula, MS 39581, USA
e-mail: tyearwood@nopaindr.com

T.R. Deer et al. (eds.), *Comprehensive Treatment of Chronic Pain by Medical, Interventional, and Integrative Approaches,*
DOI 10.1007/978-1-4614-1560-2_62, © American Academy of Pain Medicine 2013

width, frequency, intensity, and polarity: wide ranges of cathode and anode combinations), have enabled the clinician to effectively target a greater variety of sites within the intraspinal canal. This has resulted in extending the indications for this treatment modality. These targets now include the dorsal root entry zone (DREZ), the dorsal root ganglion (DRG), and the spinal nerve roots as well as the dorsal columns. Thus, the more appropriate term would be *intraspinal neurostimulation*. In the periphery, the largest targets were the "named" nerves and the early neurostimulator systems produced what is now called peripheral nerve stimulation (PNS). With more advanced technologies, smaller and more discrete targets can be activated; this has allowed the evolution of peripheral nerve field stimulation (PNFS), stimulation of small "unnamed" nerves. These small "unnamed" nerves may come from more than one "named" nerve, and thus, a "field" of neurostimulation can be achieved.

Etiology of Neuropathic Axial and Extremity Pain

Neuropathic pain represents the principal clinical manifestation of neuronal injury. It can involve peripheral mechanisms, which become centralized over a period to produce a clinical state of pain and impairment without regard to ongoing tissue damage or insult. Any disease process can result in a neuropathic pain phenomenon depending on the neurophysiologic status. Table 62.1 summarizes some of these disease processes relative to neuropathic axial and extremity pain with examples of typical clinical conditions.

In each of these scenarios, some pathological mechanism for peripheral or central nerve injury has created an ongoing, self-sustaining pain process. This involves processes imbedded within the central nervous system such as "central sensitization" and "windup," which can be substantially influenced by normal sensory signals resulting in painful sensations, dysesthesias, and paresthesias. The involvement of the sympathetic nervous system in response to these phenomena adds another layer of complexity and pain pathology, as alterations in global and local sympathetic tone can amplify the pain experience.

Typical manifestations of neuropathic extremity pain include burning, throbbing, aching, and boring pains accompanied by allodynia, dysesthesias, hyperalgesia, and temperature or blood flow alterations. These can result in abnormalities of perspiration and piloerection, and episodic muscle cramping and twitching [1, 2], ipsilateral blockade of the sympathetic ganglia of the affected extremity (for neuropathic extremity pain), or bilateral blockade of the sympathetic ganglion of the affected intervertebral disc level (for neuropathic axial pain) will often result in pain relief and a normalization of vascular abnormalities. This includes enhanced blood flow to distal sensory neurons (with an

Table 62.1 Disease processes relative to neuropathic axial and extremity pain with examples of typical clinical conditions

Congenital	1. Tethered cord syndromes
	2. Spina bifida
	3. Dural ectasia
	4. Spinal stenosis
Metabolic and inflammatory	1. Diabetic peripheral neuropathy
	2. Hyperthyroidism, hypothyroidism
	3. Ankylosing spondylitis
	4. Paget's disease
	5. Sarcoidosis
	6. Arachnoiditis
Traumatic	1. Traumatic disc disruption
	2. Complex regional pain syndrome (CRPS) types I and II
	3. Postsurgical nerve entrapment:
	(a) Post-laminotomy syndromes
	(b) Post-carpal tunnel/tarsal tunnel release-related CRPS-II
	(c) CRPS-II of the ulnar nerve postsurgical transposition
	(d) Chronic piriformis syndrome (sciatic neuralgia)
	(e) Brachial plexus avulsion
	(f) Electrical injury
	4. Traumatic amputation
Neoplastic	1. Chemotherapy-related peripheral neuropathy
	2. Peripheral nervous system malignancies
	3. Intraspinal malignancies
Infectious	1. Herpes zoster
	2. Epidural abscess
	3. HIV-related peripheral neuropathy
	(a) Primary
	(b) Secondary, related to antiretroviral chemotherapy
	4. Lyme's disease

increased sensitivity to light touch) and to muscle groups (with a relaxation of cramping and spasm). Those patients who respond well to sympathetic blockade tend to respond well to intraspinal neurostimulation, and many of these same features can be seen clinically.

Neuroanatomy and Neurostimulation

Nociceptive and neuropathic pain is carried to the central nervous system (CNS) from the periphery via sensory neurons, directly or indirectly. Beginning in small, microscopic ("unnamed") nerves, sensory information is transmitted to larger nerves and then to spinal nerves. These sensory neurons are incorporated into spinal nerves directly into the CNS by way of the dorsal root ganglia (DRG) and the dorsal root entry zone (DREZ) and, from there, into the dorsal horn to be incorporated into elements of the central nervous system. Sensory neurons can also enter the CNS indirectly by way of the autonomic nervous system (sympathetic or parasympathetic elements). At the level of the DRG, the spinal nerves are separated into ventral motor and dorsal sensory components before entering the spinal cord. The majority of sensory neuronal systems enter the spinal cord via the dorsal root entry zone (DREZ) and are distributed within the dorsal horn to ascending pathways in the dorsal columns (ipsilateral) and tracts of the ventrolateral quadrants (ventral spinothalamic tract and lateral spinothalamic tract) in both ipsilateral and contralateral manners via numerous interneuronal synapses [3, 4].

It is extremely important to understand that different ascending tracts within the spinal cord carry *qualitatively* different aspects of sensory information; this can have a bearing on the appropriate targeting for intraspinal neurostimulation. The dorsal columns carry the sensations of vibration, touch, proprioception, and pain to the thalamus; the lateral spinothalamic tract (part of the ventrolateral quadrants) carries sensations of pain and temperature, while the ventral spinothalamic tract carries sensations of visceral pain and temperature. Because of the profound neuroplasticity often associated with neuropathic pain, it is entirely possible that different qualitative pain sensations can be modulated with neurostimulation along tracts not traditionally associated with neuropathic pain. If this were not the case, it might very well be that neurostimulation of the dorsal columns alone would have minimal effect on neuropathic pain [4].

Since neuropathic pain frequently incorporates elements of both touch and temperature, it is often necessary to provide neurostimulation to both the dorsal columns and the ventral and lateral spinothalamic tracts in order to achieve optimal therapy. However, neurostimulator leads must be placed dorsally (e.g., dorsal columns and dorsal root entry zone), in order to avoid the motor stimulation that occurs with more ventral placements, and this substantially impedes access to the ventral and lateral spinothalamic tracts. The lateral spinothalamic tract is located too deeply within the spinal cord to be influenced directly by neurostimulation fields on the surface of the cord. The ventral spinothalamic tract is more superficial, and it can be influenced with neurostimulation. However, precise lead placement in this area can be quite difficult, dangerous, and complicated by motor recruitment. Thus, traditional dorsal column lead placement alone may miss some of the opportunities to adequately and more thoroughly affect the modulation of neuropathic sensory information traversing all three spinothalamic tracts.

Directly stimulating the DRG, or combining dorsal stimulation of the traversing and exiting spinal nerves (at the level of the neuroforamina), with/without DREZ stimulation, added to the more traditional approach of dorsal column stimulation (DCS), takes advantage of the neuroanatomy by incorporating additional spinal tracts in the total neuromodulation scheme of neuropathic pain. By appropriately targeting the DRG, individual spinal nerves, or the DREZ, electrical

neuromodulation of fibers can be achieved before they are anatomically distributed and reorganized within the dorsal horn to the various spinothalamic tracts. This can greatly augment the efficacy of neuromodulation achieved with DCS alone and can be referred to as *multi-target stimulation*.

It is thus extremely important for the implanter to have a thorough understanding of cranial, spinal, and peripheral neuroanatomy to appropriately take advantage of the wide variety of neuronal targets that are available for efficacious neurostimulation.

Lower amplitudes of stimulation than that needed for the dorsal columns are required for stimulation of the nerve roots and the DRG, because the CSF layer is quite thin at these locations. Thus, contact separation from the targeted tissues is quite small, and significantly less energy is required for activating the nerve fibers at these locations [5, 6]. The amplitudes involved to generate a "therapeutic window" for pleasant and efficacious neurostimulation in the general region of nerve roots and the DRG are extremely small. (This phenomenon is present in the periphery as well, where the distance of separation from the electrical contact to the targeted nerve, and local tissue electrical impedance, determines the amount of energy (amplitude of stimulation) required to obtain clinically relevant neuromodulation.) With the presence of a disease state creating neuropathic pain, these same neuronal pathways may actually be much more sensitive to stimulation as a result of "primary hypersensitivity". Thus, these exquisitely sensitive neuronal pathways may be recruited with even lower levels of amplitude than their adjacent, somatotopically arranged neighbors, and thereby provide more focal targeting of specific anatomical areas. This could have significant clinical ramifications for selective neurostimulation of peripheral nerves, spinal nerves, the DRG, traversing nerves, nerve rootlets and the DREZ.

The optimal contact locations that enable field exposure to a sufficiently wide range of sensory fibers suitable for stimulation tend to cluster in the dorsal aspects of the spinal canal and are the preferred region for therapeutic neurostimulation. To avoid motor stimulation when nerve root or ganglion stimulation is desired, the individual lead electrodes need to be placed quite dorsal to the targeted structure. At this location, the therapeutic effects of both sensory and subsensory stimulation can be obtained with greater precision and success.

Electrical neurostimulation is a surface phenomenon, and the depth of penetration into neural tissue is remarkably small (less than 0.25–0.5 mm) compared to the spread of the stimulating electrical field across the surface of the targeted structure [6]. The more superficial the individual neuron is to the surface of the neural structure being targeted, the greater will be its sensitivity to electrical stimulation. In view of this, it is important to take advantage of the neuroanatomical differentiation between motor and sensory fibers in the spinal nerve roots in the area of the dorsal root ganglion and between the DREZ and the dorsal columns in the cord itself. Precise anatomic placement of the electrical field is essential, and the tools to be used include amplitude, frequency, pulse width, and contact configuration of cathodes and anodes. Appropriate attention to the use of all of these tools is necessary to create a therapeutic electrical field.

Further features of the neuroanatomy of the dorsal columns also bear consideration in the clinical application of electrical fields. They include the concepts of somatotopic organization, surface area, fiber types, sizes, and speeds of conduction, and thickness of the dorsal CSF layer.

Somatotopic Organization

There is considerable somatotopic organization within the dorsal columns [7], and fibers consistent with a particular dermatome tend to ascend within an organized scheme. After entrance into the dorsal horn, fibers synapse with interneurons and are distributed to the various ascending tracts. Within the dorsal columns, fibers associated with individual dermatomes appear in the ventral areas, deep within the gray matter of the fasciculus gracilis (thoracic, lumbar, and sacral spine) or the more lateral fasciculus cuneatus (in the cervical spine). From there, these fibers ascend toward the thalamus and migrate dorsally within the lateral aspects of the fasciculus to gradually develop a "dorsal exposure at the lateral border with the DREZ (Fig. 62.1)" [7].

The dorsal exposure on the surface of the dorsal columns is extremely important, as the electrical field does not penetrate greater than 0.25–0.50 mm within the gray matter of the cord. Thus, until a particular dermatome has a "dorsal exposure," it cannot be affected by epidural neurostimulation. The electrical impedance of the CSF is so much greater than the conductivity of the gray matter of the cord that electrical current will more readily be shunted (following the "path of least resistance") into the CSF, away from penetration of gray matter. This causes the electrical field to extend into the area of the dorsal roots (producing "flank" stimulation), and motor activation can occur as stimulation amplitude is further increased.

As shown in Fig. 62.2, this somatotopic organization of dermatomes across the surface of the dorsal columns creates a "grain," much like what one would see within a plank of wood. Clearly, the geometry of the electrical field needs to be parallel to the "grain" to induce the greatest electrical influence over the parallel fibers ascending to the thalamus. Interestingly enough, the majority of neurostimulator leads have contacts with the long axis parallel to the "grain" of the dorsal columns.

This somatotopic organization in the dorsal columns also helps to explain the ability to recruit fibers to create therapeutic paresthesias in the lower extremities from distal sites of stimulation such as the cervical spine (fasciculus gracilis).

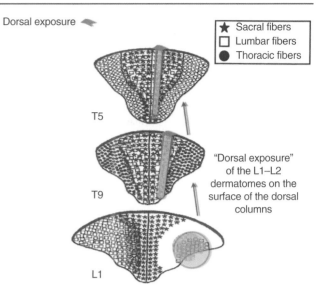

Dorsal exposure

★ Sacral fibers
☐ Lumbar fibers
● Thoracic fibers

T5

T9

L1

"Dorsal exposure" of the L1–L2 dermatomes on the surface of the dorsal columns

Fig. 62.1 Somatotopic representation of the dorsal columns. Note that after appearing in the deep tissues of the dorsal columns at lower spinal levels, the L1 and L2 dermatomes gradually develop a "dorsal exposure" at more cephalad spinal levels. This creates a superficial "rim" of somatotopic tissue for those specific dermatomes, which can respond to applied electrical fields. This rim of "dorsal exposure" migrates medially from the lateral edges of the dorsal columns along the borders of the dorsal root entry zone DREZ. They then "migrate" medially, as they ascend toward the foramen magnum, becoming thinner as the fibers decrease in size (Adapted from Smith and Deacon [7], with permission)

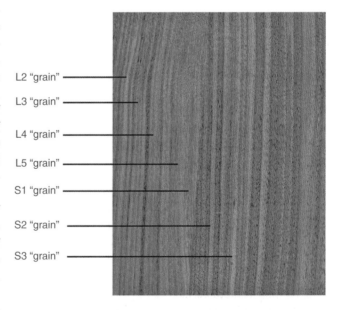

L2 "grain"

L3 "grain"

L4 "grain"

L5 "grain"

S1 "grain"

S2 "grain"

S3 "grain"

Fig. 62.2 Somatotopic representation of the dorsal columns. The striations of the dermatomes across the surface of the dorsal columns, moving lateral to medial, may well be a bit similar to the grain of wood as seen in this image of a walnut panel. Very little in nature is perfectly parallel, and individual variation between subjects appears to be the "norm." This concept helps to account for the high degree of variation between patients in programming neurostimulator leads over the Dorsal Columns, the DREZ, the DRG and even in the periphery

Fig. 62.3 Distribution of paresthesia from the dorsal columns. The ability to recruit stimulation of the lower extremities from cervical levels is well demonstrated in these figures. Barolat et al. noted that roughly 30 % of their subjects could obtain foot stimulation at C7 and nearly 60 % of their subjects could obtain stimulation of the low back at T5 under the right conditions (From Barolat et al. [8], with permission)

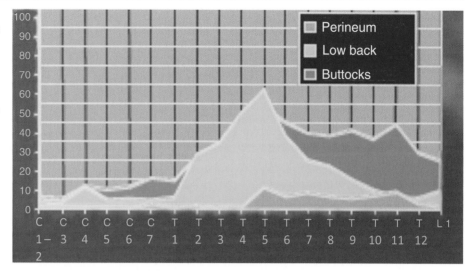

This is demonstrated by the ground-breaking work by Barolat et al. [8], shown in Fig. 62.3.

Somatotopic sensory organization is seen at all levels in the hierarchy of the nervous system, from the homunculus of the sensory cortex [9] to the ascending tracts in the cord [7], to the DRG [10–12], and within the peripheral nerves [13, 14]. Slipman et al. [15] carefully demonstrated with highly selective, fluoroscopically guided neural stimulation of cervical dorsal root ganglia the wide range of overlapping dermatomal stimulation associated with each DRG. This is a consequence of sensory input from multiple sensory nerve roots into adjacent and nearby dorsal root ganglia and enables a significantly robust interpretation of the sensory environment by the CNS. Thus, the whole concept of "two-point discrimination" is really a subtle and somewhat complex integration of sensory stimuli within the thalamus and higher centers. Obviously, this phenomenon is present throughout the peripheral nervous system, and while the classic dermatome maps are helpful, they are not to be interpreted in absolute terms. While there does appear to be a somatotopic distribution of dermatomal fibers within the DRG at any given level, for neurostimulation to be truly "focal" to a specific anatomic location, it is necessary to be "local" [16]. A conceptual schema of this is shown in Fig. 62.4.

Surface Area

The spinal cord varies in its cross-sectional area as it ascends from the conus medullaris to the foramen magnum. There are several remarkably important areas to be considered: the lumbosacral enlargement, the thoracic cord, the cervical enlargement, and the cervical cord. The lumbosacral and cervical enlargements are created by the immense number of additional neurons associated with motor, sensory, and autonomic functions within the lower and upper extremities, respectively, entering the spinal cord. This additional neuronal tissue

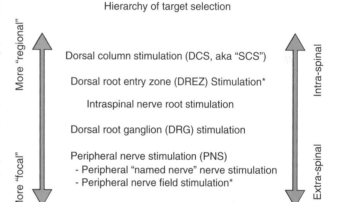

Fig. 62.4 Hierarchy of target selection in neurostimulation. As one moves from intraspinal to peripheral, the targets for neurostimulation change in complexity and specificity. There are always exceptions, especially with tremendous individual variation in patients. Two general exceptions are notable: (a) occasionally somewhat "focal" stimulation can be obtained with small electrical fields placed over rootlets at the DREZ and (b) peripheral nerve field stimulation (*PNFS*) is considerably broader than "named-nerve" peripheral nerve stimulation (*PNS*), as a result of the overlap of small branches from various separate "named-nerves"

enlarges the cross-sectional area of the cord over a portion of its distance, and thus, the total surface area of the dorsal columns is also increased. With this increase in the total surface area of the dorsal columns, a statistically greater opportunity exists for stimulating neurons within the dermatomal "grain."

Of particular interest is the fact that within the thoracic cord, above the lumbosacral enlargement, the cross-sectional area diminishes and the ability to stimulate sacral elements almost diminishes considerably. It is reasonable to conclude that the width of the "grain" for the sacral dermatomes becomes quite small for most patients and is thus potentially quite difficult to recruit from surface stimulation.

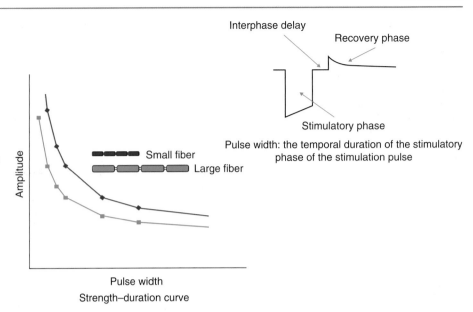

Fig. 62.5 Strength-duration curve. Larger diameter neuronal fibers are activated by applied electrical fields more easily than smaller fibers. Fiber sizes tend to be smaller nearer the midline of the dorsal columns. Increasing the pulse width of the stimulatory phase of the applied electrical field recruits more of these smaller diameter fibers and increases the area of perceived stimulation. *Inset*: A typical stimulation pulse for a neurostimulator contact

The opportunity to stimulate sacral and lower extremity dermatomes reappears at the cervical enlargement and continues some distance toward the foramen magnum [17]. It is almost as though fiber tracts "hidden" from an applied electrical field of stimulation within the fold of the dorsal median sulcus have blossomed back out onto the surface where they are again susceptible to stimulation. In many patients, there appears to be a slight contraction of the surface area of the dorsal columns within the cervical cord cephalad to the cervical enlargement, but in general, the surface area of the dorsal columns within the cervical cord is much greater than seen in the thoracic cord below the cervical enlargement. The cross-sectional geometry of the thoracic cord is virtually circular, whereas the cross-sectional geometry of the cervical cord resembles that of a lima bean, having a broader dorsal surface. With the cervical enlargement, the fasciculus cuneatus is formed lateral to the fasciculus gracilis, between which is the dorsal intermediate sulcus, and carries a "dorsal exposure" for dermatomes representing the upper extremities.

Fiber Types, Sizes, and Speeds of Conduction

There are different fiber types and sizes of fibers populating the dorsal columns. Both myelinated and unmyelinated fibers are found within the superficial layers of the dorsal columns, and they vary in size. Feirabend et al. [18] have shown by histological studies that Aβ-fibers having larger fiber diameters are found to recur more frequently along the lateral edges of the dorsal columns and near the center. Roughly 85 % of all fibers in the superficial dorsal columns are smaller than 7 μm, and only 1 % is larger than 10 μm, but these larger fibers occur with much greater frequency in the more lateral portions of the dorsal columns [18]. Aβ-fibers from a laterally placed dermatomal "grain" become smaller and migrate medially as they ascend toward the thalamus.

Of course, not all of the fibers are of a uniform size, nor are all the fibers myelinated. This has important consequence in neurostimulation because smaller fibers require greater amplitudes of stimulation intensity to trigger a response than larger fibers. This is demonstrated by a typical strength-duration curve shown in Fig. 62.5. Longer pulse width values promote the activation of smaller diameter fibers relative to larger diameter fibers, as found in other neurostimulation applications [19]. Thus, in dorsal column stimulation, longer pulse widths tend to increase the number of fibers activated, recruiting more of the smaller fibers toward the midline in the dorsal columns, where more sacral fibers are to be found, and producing a "sacral shift" in the perceived stimulatory pattern (Fig. 62.6) [20].

Also of note is the fact that the sensations created by neurostimulation of the dorsal columns traveling in myelinated fibers will reach the thalamus prior to those traveling in unmyelinated fibers. This is true whether the number of fibers recruited by any stimulatory pulse is sufficient to create a perceptible sensation within the thalamus, or remain as an imperceptible or "subliminal" influence upon the global sensory processing within the thalamus. Such a situation could perhaps block painful and erratic neuropathic signals from traversing the same individual neurons. With higher frequencies of stimulation, a greater number of fibers could potentially be slowly driven into a relative refractory phase, effectively rendering these fibers unavailable for pathologic signal transmission.

Finally, the absolute and relative refractory periods of the targeted neurons are in the time range of milliseconds, whereas stimulation duration and recovery phases of a typical neurostimulation system are in the time range of microseconds. This means that a typical neurostimulation system can deliver a number of stimulatory pulses of different contact configurations much more quickly than the CNS can process

Fig. 62.6 Clinical example of the "sacral shift." The clinical effect of increasing pulse width in the stimulation pulse is often to increase the incorporation of smaller, more medial fibers (typically in greater abundance in the midline of the dorsal columns: sacral dermatomes primarily) (From Yearwood et al. [20], with permission)

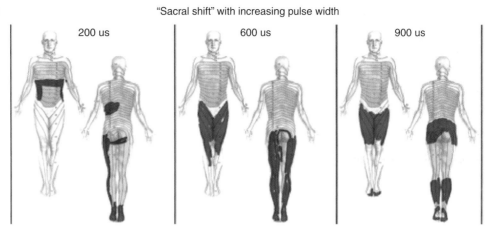

"Sacral shift" with increasing pulse width

200 us   600 us   900 us

the individual signals. The typical speed of cinema is roughly 24 frames/s. This enables the CNS to appreciate perceptions of smooth motions from rapidly displayed individual "still-shot" frames. Thus, it is not surprising that the neurostimulation systems presently available are able to provide considerable sophistication in perceived and subliminal signals to interrupt the interpretation and CNS response of painful stimuli resulting from neuropathic processes. A typical rate of 40 stimulatory pulses/s is certainly above the CNS processing speed, as noted by the sensation of constant stimulation by most patients and this frequency. As in cinema, however, it remains to be seen if even higher rates of stimulation (400–800 Hz) provide a sense of "high definition (HD)" to the CNS that could have therapeutic benefit.

Thickness of the Dorsal CSF Layer

The thickness of the CSF layer between the implanted epidural contacts and the surface of the dorsal columns or other neuronal structures varies considerably within each individual patient based on posture and location within the spinal canal [21]. With increasing thickness of the CSF (dCSF) between individual contacts and neuronal surfaces, there is increasing influence of the electrical impedance of the CSF, requiring increased intensity of stimulation to achieve paresthesias. However, with increased distance from the contact, coupled with increased amplitude, the size of the electrical field across the surface of the targeted neuronal structures becomes larger and optimal target stimulation is easily compromised. In transitioning from prone to supine, there is a dorsal movement of the spinal cord within the dural and the dCSF can decrease remarkably. Unless the amplitude of the stimulation is decreased concomitantly, the patient may feel too intense a stimulation, and be uncomfortable, or the patient may experience too wide a field of stimulation, with collateral paresthesias that are similarly uncomfortable. Alterations in the local dCSF are also seen with transitioning from laying to sitting, sitting to standing, extending and flexing the spine, and lateral bending or twisting. All these considerations are important during the

programming of the implanted device to assure optimal therapeutic benefit to the patient.

In summary, the efficacy of neurostimulation is dependent upon two fundamental concepts: appropriate placement of the electrode array (lead) in order to electrically modulate the bioelectric phenomena of the targeted neuronal tissue and the appropriate programming of the electrical neurostimulator system to control the style and character of the neuromodulation of the neuronal surfaces.

Lead Placement

Careful lead placement near the appropriate neuronal target(s) is essential in order to achieve the greatest likelihood of therapeutic stimulation within the superficial layers of the neuronal structure: peripheral nerve, DRG, dorsal roots, DREZ, dorsal columns, superficial motor cortex stimulation (MCS), or deep brain stimulation (DBS). It is crucial to remember the principle that the *ultimate target* of all of our neurostimulation efforts is the thalamus and that portion of the CNS involved in the perception of painful signals, and the response to pain.

Electrical Field Shaping (Programming)

Contact configuration and amplitude determine the size and shape of the stimulatory field. Pulse width can exert an influence on the total number of fibers stimulated by a specific stimulatory pulse by causing the stimulatory field to "linger" over the neuronal target, recruiting a greater number of fibers. Frequency can alter the repetition of activation and at higher rates (>1,000 Hz) can theoretically create a situation in which many fibers in the superficial layers of the dorsal columns can become relatively refractory.

Therapeutic Goals

The goal of therapy in electrical neurostimulation is to alter the pain state of the patient in such a way as to enhance the capability of achieving success with functional rehabilitation.

Neuropathic pain in the extremities is often accompanied by abnormal muscle tone, usually episodic in nature, as well as autonomic dysfunction: decreased blood flow to connective tissue, muscles, and neuronal tissues; temperature abnormalities; and perspiration dysfunction. To achieve improvement in physical function, these autonomic features must be addressed along with the underlying pain complaints, to improve the metabolic state of the affected extremity. For this reason, it is often not sufficient for the patient to "feel stimulation" in the affected area and yet still have the autonomic dysfunction.

It is quite important to realize that the role of electrical neurostimulation is not limited to "pain relief" per se but should serve as an important tool in the rehabilitation of the patient. As such, it becomes a part of the overall plan of therapy for the patient to be integrated with functional rehabilitation, oral medication management, behavioral therapy, and conservative spinal injection techniques.

Clinical Examples: Treatment of Radicular Pain Syndromes

The term "radiculitis" is from the Latin *radix* – root – and is defined as the inflammation or irritation of the nerve root between the spinal cord and the exit of the nerve root from the canal [22]. As such, any irritation of a lumbar nerve root would be expected to create sensations (often painful) that "radiate" from the axial spine to the periphery. But note that the emphases of the definition are on the nerve "*radix* – root"– and not on the concept of radiating (from Latin *radiare* – "to emit rays"). Thus, painful sensations perceived along the axial distribution of the spine can result from a radiculitis or a radiculopathy of the nerve roots. That can be a significant clinical challenge. It can also provide a significant advantage for the clinical application of neurostimulation.

As noted by Malik and Benzon [23], the clinical syndrome of radicular pain in a predictable dermatomal pattern, characterized by *subjective* reports of sensory disturbance (paresthesia, dysesthesias, numbness, hyperalgesia, allodynia, etc.), and typical *objective* signs of weakness, decreased reflexes, and positive dural tension signs is referred to by a variety of terms: radiculopathy, radiculitis, and radicular syndrome. However, as they point out, the term *radiculopathy* inappropriately implies the presence of objective signs of pathological nerve root damage, including loss of sensation, muscle weakness, and diminished reflexes. But all of these objective signs can occur without objective evidence of anatomical or pathological nerve damage. In a similar fashion, *radiculitis* inappropriately implies an inflammatory process as the sole etiology for the causation of the radicular signs and symptoms. The term *radicular pain syndrome* appears to be most appropriate and correctly suggests a con-

stellation of clinical signs and symptoms of variable etiology secondary to pathology or dysfunction of the sensory nerve roots or the dorsal root ganglia (DRG).

Thus, a radicular pain syndrome can be axial in distribution, or it can be manifested as radiating into an extremity, or a distribution of pain can occur in both the spinal axis and in the extremities concurrently.

Cervical Radicular Pain Syndrome

Post-laminotomy syndrome of the cervical spine s/p anterior cervical discectomy and fusion (ACDF), also known as failed neck surgery syndrome, often manifests itself with continued cervicogenic headache (CHA) [24–26], primary discogenic pain above and below the level of the fusion, axial neck pain, and upper extremity radiculitis/radiculopathy. Little is known about the neuropathic nature of primary discogenic pain in the cervical spine, but it has been well studied in the lumbar spine and has been found to have a nociceptive etiology with heavy autonomic nervous system transmission of sensory signals [27]. Thus, perceived pain within the axial spine, centrally and laterally, may have a neuropathic-like component susceptible to neurostimulation therapy; it is not necessarily always due to nociceptive facet arthropathy. Because it is neuropathic in nature, neurostimulation efforts can be of substantial benefit in treating this form of pain. Additionally, chemical radiculitis secondary to a disrupted cervical disc annulus can provoke tremendous neuropathic discomfort of the nerve roots, also suitably treated with neurostimulation. (This pattern of pain pathology is frequently seen with patients having a relatively normal MRI appearance of the cervical disc, but to exhibit significant leakage of radiocontrast material injected during provocative discography into the nucleus of the disc.)

In the example shown below (Fig. 62.7), neurostimulator leads have been placed in such a way as to garner the greatest degree of therapy for the various pain areas in this particular patient: cervicogenic headache (CHA), axial neck pain, and bilateral upper extremity radicular pain. Stimulation of the nerve roots at C2 and C3 by the most cephalad contacts places sensory stimulation into that part of the thalamus and CNS that processes pain interpreted as deriving from the occipital nerves bilaterally. Clinically, this pattern of stimulation over the C2 and C3 nerve roots has the ability to provide excellent control of suboccipital headache pain, remarkably similar to that seen with peripheral occipital nerve stimulation (ONS).

More proximal along the leads, the neurostimulator contacts diagonally traverse the bilateral dorsal root entry zones (DREZ). Contact configurations can be along each lead individually, or between the leads, to achieve lateral and posterior axial stimulation of the neck. This pattern of stimulation can often cover the lateral neck, posterior neck, and shoulder

Fig. 62.7 Antegrade leads for post-laminotomy syndrome – cervical. Leads have been advanced in such a way as to curve laterally from the area of the dorsal columns (proximally) to the area of the nerve roots at C2 and C3 (distally), traversing the dorsal root entry zone (*DREZ*) along the way. Thus, in this single-lead array, three different types of neuronal targets are available for therapeutic stimulation

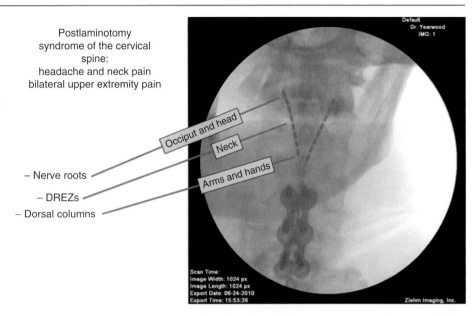

Postlaminotomy syndrome of the cervical spine: headache and neck pain bilateral upper extremity pain

Occiput and head

Neck

Arms and hands

– Nerve roots

– DREZs

– Dorsal columns

Fig. 62.8 Retrograde C1–C2 cylindrical leads ("perc" leads) for post-laminotomy syndrome – cervical (AP view)

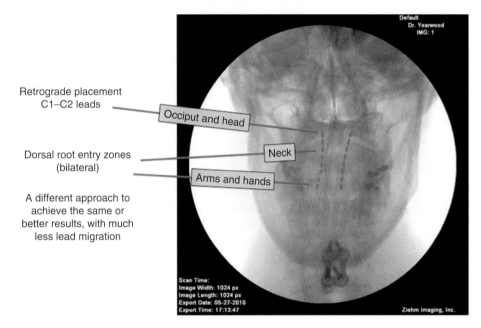

Retrograde placement C1–C2 leads

Occiput and head

Neck

Dorsal root entry zones (bilateral)

Arms and hands

A different approach to achieve the same or better results, with much less lead migration

girdle area: posteriorly (to the spine of the scapula) and anteriorly (to the infraclavicular area). Activation of the more caudal and medial contacts produces a dorsal column stimulation, affecting the upper extremities. Thus, all portions of the leads are used in a highly efficient manner.

An entirely different approach to the same clinical problem is shown in Figs. 62.8 and 62.9. In this case, retrograde C1–C2 cylindrical leads (euphemistically known as "percutaneous leads") have been placed over the area of the DREZ bilaterally, using an approach similar to that described by Whitworth and Feler [28]. In this case, the same results have been obtained. The advantages to this particular lead arrangement are the relative stability of the lead positions and their resistance to migration with active and dynamic

movement of the head and neck. Migration of antegrade-placed cylindrical leads in the cervical spine can be a frequent clinical complication, because anchoring to the supraspinous ligament to the level of T2 or T3 allows too large a range of motion for the cervical spine relative to the leads. While paddle lead placement is associated with less lead migration, the lack of lead flexibility encourages greater encapsulation than is seen in more flexible "percutaneous" leads and can create a greater degree of spatial "occupation" in an area of the spine at risk for spinal stenosis secondary to degenerative disc disease. Furthermore, with factory-specified contact configurations, the surgical-lead implant is less versatile for selection of neuronal targets within the cervical spine.

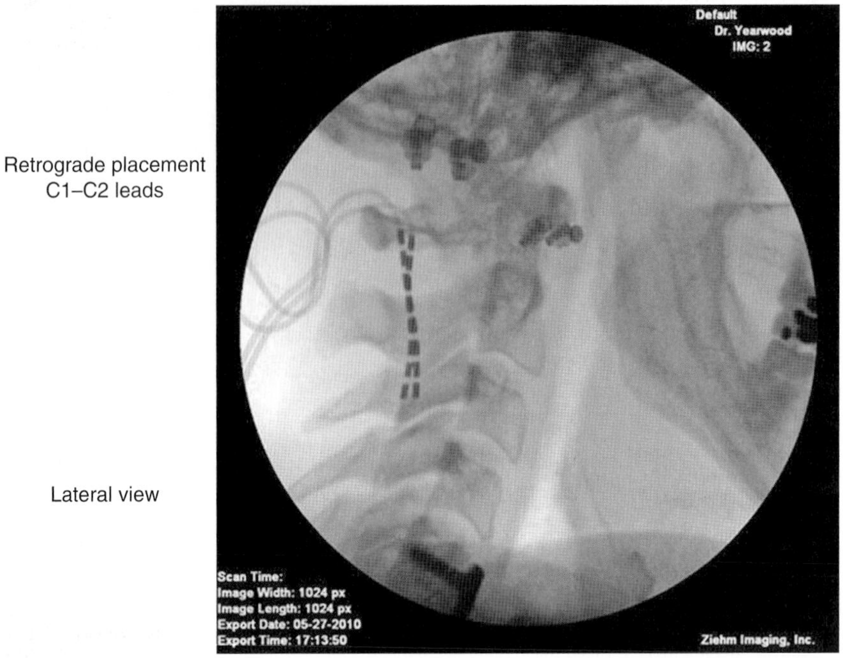

Fig. 62.9 Retrograde C1–C2 cylindrical leads ("perc" leads) for post-laminotomy syndrome – cervical (lateral view). Note that the leads have been surgically placed over the arch of C1, to which they have been anchored. The leads remain posterior and experience very little migration with this configuration

Retrograde placement C1–C2 leads

Lateral view

Thoracic Radicular Pain Syndrome

Thoracic radiculitis can arise from a number of pathological conditions, including trauma, surgical trauma, infection (most notably herpes zoster), chemical radiculitis from degenerating discs, mechanical nerve impingement related to discopathy, metabolic disease (i.e., diabetic mononeuritis), degenerative scoliosis, degenerative stenosis, and peripheral intercostal nerve trauma. Figure 62.10a, b show the lead configuration for a patient suffering from three-level intercostal neuralgia secondary to trauma. The patient has had open reduction and internal fixation (ORIF) of two ribs at T8 and T10 and a complete resection of the T9 rib, all on the right. The patient's neuropathic pain was widely distributed along the lateral chest wall and toward the upper abdomen. Repeated intercostal injections provide the patient with an excellent pattern of pain relief, but were not durable, and the patient went on for implantation of neurostimulation therapy. Because of the secondary hyperalgesia involved in this neuropathic pain problem, it was clear that dorsal column stimulation was needed to provide "regional" therapy, with nerve root/DREZ stimulation more "focal" intercostal nerve therapy.

"Multimodal" Targeting for Neurostimulation at Different Levels of the Sensory Processing Hierarchy

This particular case serves to illustrate the concept of combining the more direct *focal* therapy achieved by modulating nerve roots/DREZ (creating a pre-dorsal horn modulation of sensory signals) with more diffuse *regional* therapy achieved by modulating dorsal column fibers directly (post-dorsal horn modulation). This combination of nerve root/DREZ and dorsal column stimulation fields can be highly effective, especially in more difficult cases of radiculitis where a strong component of neuralgia is present in addition to the more diffuse aching and burning pain associated with secondary hyperalgesia. This technique can often succeed in other cases throughout the spinal canal where there is a strong component of peripheral neuralgia coupled with a more regional field of neuropathic pain (e.g., CRPS-II). In the thoracic spine specifically, this technique has proven to be highly effective for postherpetic neuropathy pain and intercostal neuralgia associated with post-thoracotomy syndrome [29–33], which can be quite refractory to dorsal column stimulation alone [34].

An excellent example of this situation is shown in Fig. 62.11. This patient sustained an electrocution injury of the right upper extremity and right chest wall while speaking on the telephone during a lightning storm. He developed severe neuropathic pain that was consistent with a CRPS-II ulnar nerve presentation, coupled with a large area of neuropathic pain in the right chest wall having a CRPS-I presentation. His ulnar nerve-related neuropathic pain spread over several dermatomes, but his trial with dorsal column stimulation alone failed to relieve him of the obvious and persistent neuralgia associated with the ulnar nerve. Thus, he required not only dorsal column stimulation (DCS) but also nerve root stimulation (NRS) for more durable and efficacious therapy in his right upper extremity. The ability to stimulate along neuronal traction specific to the ulnar nerve on the right with

Fig. 62.10 (**a**) Radiological view of rib pathologies leading to intercostal neuralgia in a young male patient after a motorcycle accident. (**b**) Staggered thoracic leads for intercostal neuralgia

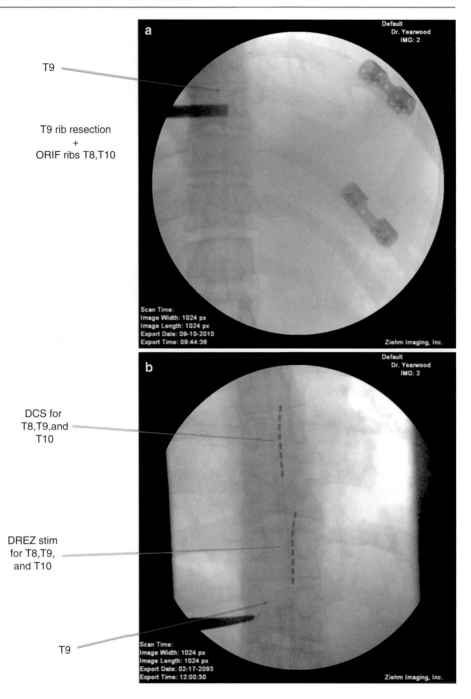

NRS enabled "focal" therapy to be added to "regional" therapy from the DCS. In addition, he required neurostimulation therapy over the dorsal root entry zone (DREZ) in the thoracic spine to achieve suitable therapeutic efficacy of a very "focal" region of secondary hyperalgesia over multiple dermatomes. This is demonstrated by the right DREZ lead over the T2 and T3 spinal levels in Fig. 62.11. Thus, three different levels of the sensory processing hierarchy are involved in providing the patient with suitable pain relief.

Axial thoracic spine pain from degenerative disc disease and chemical radiculitis, as would be expected from incompetent thoracic annuli fibrosis (as demonstrated by significant leakage of radiocontrast material during thoracic discography), is notoriously difficult to treat with neurostimulation. However, optimal lead placement and creative programming can be effective in this area as well. Figure 62.12a, b demonstrate lead placements over the lateral edges of the DREZ for a young male patient with debilitating thoracic axial pain and rather modest radicular pain secondary to chronic degenerative disc processes believed to be associated with sports injuries (football). Dorsal column stimulation alone proved to be very inadequate in covering this patient's

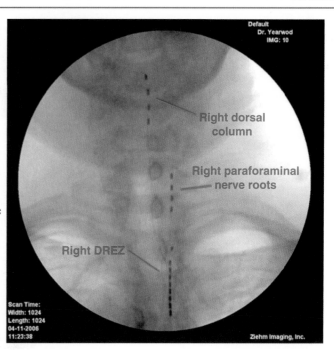

Electrocution injury, right upper extremity and right chest wall

1. Neuropathic pain in right upper extremity ≈ CRPS-II ulnar nerve presentation

2. Large area of neuropathic pain in right chest wall ≈ CRPS-I presentation

DCS plus NRS creates greater efficacy in CRPS-II, allowing a greater influence over multiple spinothalamic tracts: lateral, ventral and dorsal

DREZ stimulation across a wide swath of nerve rootlets influences larger areas of pain:
- Sympathetic fibers involved
- Total surface area is much greater than at the neuroforamen

Right dorsal column

Right paraforaminal nerve roots

Right DREZ

Fig. 62.11 Clinical application of "multimodal" neurostimulation at three different types of neuronal targets in the same patient

pain problems. A more lateral DREZ placement proved necessary, in order to obtain suitable therapeutic stimulation for his axial pain. Optimal programming for this lead involved the use of an "over-intensified anode" stimulation scheme.

"Over-intensified Anode" Stimulation Scheme

This case demonstrates the application of a single anode (+) coupled with seven cathodes (−) at three locations within a single stimulation program (Fig. 62.13). By carefully adjusting the amplitude and the pulse width of stimulation within these multiple, encompassing cathodes, "over-intensification" of the anode is achieved. This produces an area of hyperpolarization, surrounded by a very small area of the cathodic stimulation known as anodic "side lobes." This phenomenon is described in more detail by Rattay [35] and Struijk et al. [6]. As shown in Fig. 62.14, the highest current density is located at the anode. Fibers traversing "away" from the contacts with anodic side lobes are most responsive to this cathodic stimulation. The effects of the region of hyperpolarization may include denied access for neuropathic sensory signals along the neuronal structures in that "somatotopic grain." With this area surrounded by a very narrow field of cathodic activation, the net result arriving at the level of the thalamus is an interruption of neuropathic sensations with rather significant insertion of therapeutic, neuromodulating sensations. Clearly, stimulation from the caudal aspects of the cathodic field, which surrounds the area of hyperpolarization, will be partially blocked from the thalamus, but they

may play a dual role in retrograde (antidromic) interference with ascending neuropathic signals [36]. Considerably, more work is needed to tease these aspects out in detail, but multiple clinical applications of this programming scheme are currently under investigation. This programming scheme is also quite effective for other targets within the spinal canal:

(a) The C2–C3 nerve roots (for stimulation within the distribution of the occipital nerves), where recruitment of high cervical fibers beyond the "reach" of standard cathode field stimulation

(b) The S2 and S3 nerve roots and the dorsal root ganglia in the sacrum (for stimulation within the distribution of the pudendal nerve).

Lumbar Radicular Pain Syndrome

Lumbar radicular pain syndrome is a very common pain problem because of degenerative or traumatic structural changes in the lumbar spine. As a portion of the spine with the greatest biomechanical stresses imposed throughout a normal day of activity, the structures are generally larger, thicker, and more bulky and are held in alignment with some of the most structurally durable fascia anywhere to be found in the body. Because of the interrelatedness of these structures and the profuse neural supply that accompanies them, a physiologic or anatomic failure in any member of this articulated, weight-bearing complex of hard and soft tissues can have widespread consequences. Further, with the wide distribution of sensory neurons throughout this highly complex

Fig. 62.12 (**a**) Bilateral DREZ placement for axial mid-thoracic primary discogenic pain. (**b**) "Over-intensified" anode in thoracic DREZ lead for axial thoracic pain

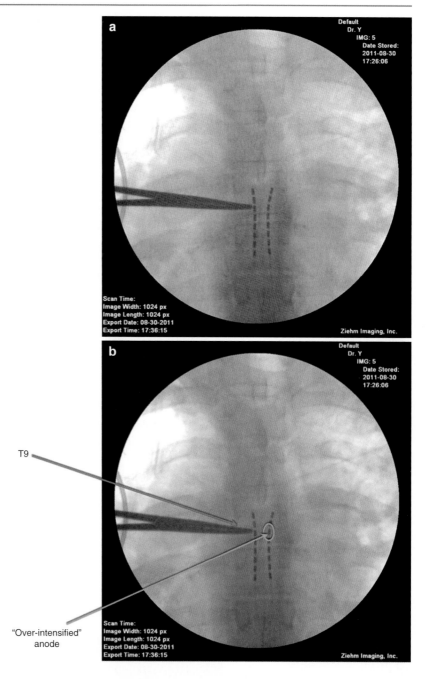

structure, the problems of referred pain can be tremendous. But, referred pain patterns can also offer an advantage to the clinical application of neurostimulation.

The appropriate intraspinal neuronal targets for the treatment of radicular pain syndrome with neurostimulation are as follows: the dorsal columns, the dorsal root entry zone, the nerve roots (traversing and exiting), and the dorsal root ganglion. These can be targeted individually, or more commonly, in combination. At nearly every target, the somatotopic distribution of sensory pathways offers opportunities and challenges.

Lower extremity radicular pain syndrome is easily addressed with dorsal column stimulation (DCS). The dermatomes of the lower extremities are L3, L4, L5, and S1, with portions of L2 and S2 that may be more pronounced or less pronounced within individual patients. The somatotopic distributions of these dermatomes are easily obtainable in most individuals between the superior endplate of T8 and the inferior endplate of T10. At these vertebral levels, midline placements of the contact arrays provide them with multiple available targets over the surface of the dorsal columns medial to the dorsal root entry zone (DREZ). If there is any correlation between the size of the homunculus and the density of the corresponding sensory neurons traversing the superficial layers of dorsal columns, it would be expected that there would be many more neurons available for stimulation of the lower extremities than for stimulation of the low back.

Multiple programming techniques can be highly useful in obtaining discrete areas of neurostimulation within this broadly distributed field of targets. As noted above, increasing pulse width can cause recruitment of smaller, more medial fibers associated with more sacral dermatomes (the sacral shift [14]). Discretely placed "over-intensified" anodes [30] can provide remarkable precision in obtaining relatively small areas of focal neurostimulation from the dorsal columns.

Figure 62.15 demonstrates lead placement for single lower extremity neuropathic pain secondary to post-laminotomy syndrome of the lumbar spine. In this clinical situation, the patient had severe neuropathic pain, responsive to lumbar sympathetic blockade, isolated to the entirety of the left

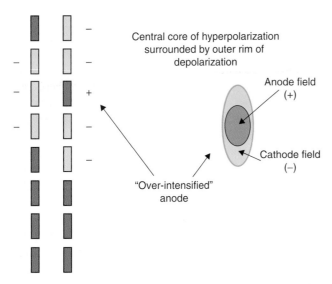

Fig. 62.13 Contact configuration for "over-intensified" anode programming scheme

lower extremity. The leads were place in such a manner to obtain the maximal stimulation over the available dermatomes based on the somatotopic organization of lower extremity fibers in the dorsal columns. The more caudal lead is slightly more laterally placed than the cephalad lead, and multiple vertebral levels are covered from the T9–T10 disc to the T11 vertebral body. This configuration provides neurostimulation across the full width of the left dorsal column, in the area of dorsal surface exposure of the dermatomes of the lower extremity. The patient experiences paresthesias throughout all areas of his leg, foot, and toes.

It is not always possible to obtain and maintain suitable stimulation of the foot from a dorsal column lead placement (Barolat personal communication, 2002; unpublished). From the discussion above, it should be apparent that this may be due more to the individual variations in the presence of sensory fibers that specifically represent the foot. A statistically sufficient number of targets within the area of "dorsal exposure" are required for those specific neuronal tracts on the surface of the dorsal columns specific for the foot to be available for DCS. Thus, it may be important to employ multi-target stimulation techniques, as described above, in order to achieve a more "focal" stimulation pattern.

Figure 62.16 shows lead placement for nerve root stimulation (NRS) to obtain suitable neurostimulation of the foot (plantar surface) for treatment of neuropathic pain. This patient had dorsal column neurostimulation leads for post-laminotomy syndrome but required supplemental stimulation of the L4 and L5 nerve roots in order to fully recruit efficacious paresthesias to areas of the foot. This lead was placed in a retrograde manner from the L1–L2 level, with entrance into the epidural space from the right, and dorsal placement maintained over the midline of the spinal canal, until the region of L4 was reached, at which point the lead

Fig. 62.14 "Side lobes" of depolarization associated with an "over-intensified" anode. Note that the rectangular geometry of the neurostimulator contacts, coupled with a decreased electrical impedance along the "grain" of the dorsal columns, causes the width of the electrical field on the surface of the spinal cord to be elongated in the cephalad-caudad dimension and narrowed laterally. This can be used to move the area of depolarization under the cathode away from the DREZ when attempting to avoid "flank" stimulation with the thoracic epidural lead placement (Adapted from Rattay [35], with permission)

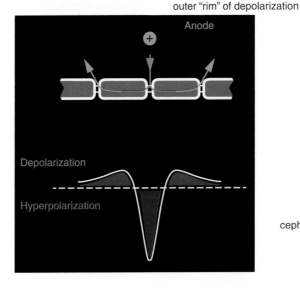

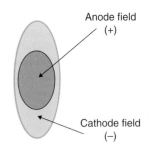

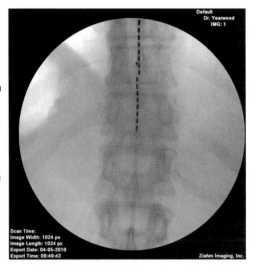

Dorsal column stimulator (DCS) lead placement for complex, unilateral left lower extremity pain

Fig. 62.15 Lead placement for multilevel dorsal column stimulation to an isolated lower extremity

Lead placement for plantar surface pain

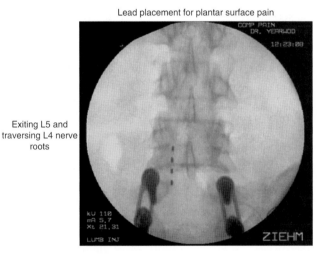

Exiting L5 and traversing L4 nerve roots

Fig. 62.16 Retrograde lead for plantar surface pain. This lead captures targets from the exiting L4 nerve and the traversing L5 and S1 nerves to provide stimulation to the plantar surface of the foot, achieving durable access to the CNS for neuromodulation of a specific anatomic location not well accessible in this particular patient from the dorsal columns

was gradually steered into the dorsal aspects of the lateral recess on the left.

Despite the excellent clinical results achieved by this method of neurostimulation in the short term, there has been at least one report in the literature to suggest that nerve root stimulation may ultimately prove to be nondurable solution [37]. Nevertheless, clinical experience indicates that nerve root stimulation can offer substantial benefit to the patient and has been maintained for over 5–6 years with sophisticated reprogramming (Yearwood, (2010) personal communication not published). When there has been progression of discopathy, creating further central and neuroforaminal

stenosis, the encapsulated lead itself can create a mechanical compression of the nerve root, evidenced by clinical signs of increased radicular pain. Judicious removal of the neurostimulation lead is then advised. This appears to be a rare phenomenon.

Low Back Pain: Lumbar Radicular Pain Syndrome Limited to the Axial Distribution

The treatment of axial pain that is predominantly centered about the lower lumbar and lumbosacral area has proven to be a considerable challenge. Many patients are able to experience therapeutic neurostimulation in this area from epidural lead arrays placed over the dorsal columns, yet often find that the pain is inadequately treated, and suffer from persistent "breakthrough" pain. Many patients cannot maintain an efficacious stimulation of this area, after having experienced substantial benefit initially, and only continue to receive paresthesias in the lower extremities. This all too often encountered clinical experience has led to increasingly sophisticated technologies to target the lower back from the epidural space. Some of these technologies are still "emerging" and have yet to prove themselves in the long run: subthreshold and high-frequency stimulation (Nevro Corporation, Menlo Park, CA), a new way to "program" epidural neurostimulation, and dorsal root ganglion stimulation (Spinal Modulation Inc., Menlo Park, CA), a new *location to target* from within the epidural space.

Deep spinal pain originating in the disc results from the transmission of nociceptive pain of inflammatory etiology by way of the sinuvertebral nerves. The sinuvertebral nerves also supply innervation to the longitudinal ligament and notably cross the midline of the posterior disc and ligament complex [38, 39]. Thus, right-sided annular disruption can at times be perceived as pain on the left lower back, as the depth and height of the annular tear progresses under the normal "wear and tear" of the activities of daily living. The primary nociceptive afferent fibers of the sinuvertebral nerve travel to the spinal cord by a dual pathway [40]: one route travels with fibers of the DRG and thus presents a segmental pattern of innervation from the disc to spinal cord. The other route travels in a non-segmental fashion with the sympathetic system by way of the gray ramus communicans to the sympathetic chain. From here, primary nociceptive afferent fibers ascend to the L2 level (and possibly to some other levels more cephalad), returning via the white ramus communicans nerve to the join the sensory fibers of the DRG and ascend into the cord in that manner (Fig. 62.17). Thus, the character and mechanisms of lumbar discogenic pain suggest it is a type of "visceral pain" (as suggested by others [27, 41, 42]) unique to the musculoskeletal system that is subject to "peripheral sensitization" and "central sensitization," leading to its chronic nature in an anatomically widespread presentation.

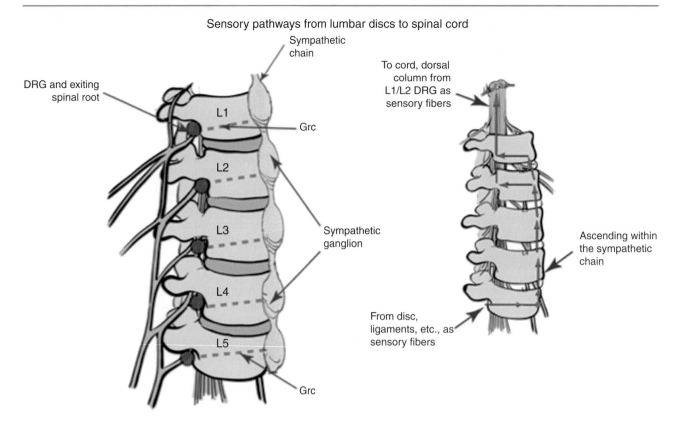

Fig. 62.17 GRC pathways for intradiscal nociceptive pain. The argument can be made that primary discogenic pain, secondary to inflammatory mechanisms within the disc annulus, is a type of "visceral" pain because of its close association and escort to the CNS by way of the sympathetic nervous system. This association gives discogenic pain an entry into a very wide distribution of influence within the dorsal horn, allowing a spread of sensory information over a relatively wide number of levels and producing a flood of neuronal signals to the CNS consistent with a very broad, diffuse anatomic location of the perceived discomfort. This is quite characteristic of "visceral" pain in general [27]

Clinical Applications of Central (Dorsal Column) Neurostimulation for Axial Low Back Pain

Two features of the neuroanatomy of lumbar discogenic pain lend itself to epidural neurostimulation as a reasonable therapeutic modality: the somatotopic distribution of dermatomes across the dorsal columns and the apparent concentration of afferent sensory fibers in association with L2 sensory input. This suggests that placement of electrical contacts over the region of the L2 "grain" should enable suitable neuromodulation along the sensory tract most associated with primary discogenic pain. Clinically, the dorsal exposure of the L2 "grain" can be found between T7 and T9, and this correlates very well with the work of Smith and Deacon [7].

Figure 62.18 demonstrates placement of dual neurostimulator leads over this area of the dorsal columns. Placed more cephalad, the targets for low back pain are lost in the midline and become too narrow; placed too caudal and the targets are too close to the DREZ to obtain efficacious paresthesia without stimulating flank. The somatotopic dermatomes of S1, L5, L4, and L3 already have a "dorsal exposure" by the time L2 develops one (in the region of T9). The width of this L2 "dorsal exposure" decreases in size as it ascends, as a result of fiber diameter contraction, and it migrates toward the midline. Thus, at all levels of the L2 "dorsal exposure," "leg" fibers greatly outnumber "back" fibers along the narrow L2 strip. For many patients, the physical dimensions of their L2 "grain" appear to be quite narrow, and the perceived paresthesia patterns appear to "jump" from flank stimulation to hip and thigh stimulation, without traversing the low back. This is due to individual variation, and many patients can achieve excellent stimulation of the lower back. The proximity of the L3, L4, and L5 fibers create an environment in which therapeutic stimulation of the low back is quite difficult to achieve without collateral stimulation of the lower extremities to some extent, and patient satisfaction will depend on the degree of that collateral stimulation.

Clinical Applications of Peripheral Neurostimulation for Axial Low Back Pain

Neurostimulation in the periphery appears to be most appropriate for peripheral nerve pathology which presents clinically as a neuralgia, and very "focal" neurostimulation is

Fig. 62.18 Dorsal column stimulation at T7–T8 for primary discogenic pain. The L2 dermatomal "grain" runs along the surface of the dorsal columns in most patients and can be accessed with this lead arrangement. When sensations of electrical paresthesias cannot be achieved in the lower back, it is occasionally possible to obtain relief of low back pain using subsensory stimulation of the L2 dermatomal "grain." Targeting the L2 dermatomal "grain" is accomplished by obtaining sensory paresthesias in the groins (See Yearwood and Foster [45])

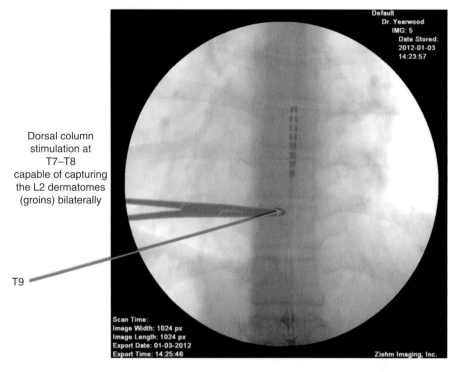

Dorsal column stimulation at T7–T8 capable of capturing the L2 dermatomes (groins) bilaterally

T9

Fig. 62.19 Typical subcutaneous lead placement schemes for peripheral nerve field stimulation (*PNFS*) to a "field" of neuropathic pain

Peripheral nerve field stimulation

Typical lead placement configurations through a field of neuropathic pain

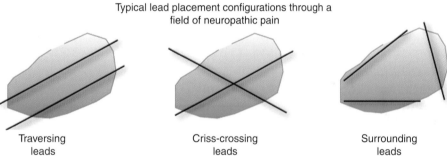

Traversing leads

Criss-crossing leads

Surrounding leads

needed. When secondary hyperalgesia accompanies the neuralgia, the patient experiences a field of neuropathic pain that extends beyond the distribution of the identifiable nerve [43]. For example, in the case of CRPS type II, dorsal column stimulation (DCS) in conjunction with peripheral neurostimulation (PNS) appears to be indicated, as discussed above (multi-target stimulation). Recognition of this fact has given rise to the increased interest in the clinical applications of peripheral nerve stimulation (PNS) of "named," macroscopic nerves, and peripheral nerve field stimulation (PNFS) of "unnamed" and microscopic nerves (assumed to be branches of one or more anatomically identifiable peripheral nerves).

The "unnamed" nerves most frequently targeted using this technique are in the subcutaneous tissues. But a major question has been exactly "where" and in what arrangement to place the leads to achieve optimal results. Typical lead arrangements relative to the geometry of a "field" of neuropathic pain are

shown in Fig. 62.19. Clearly, each of these lead arrangements takes advantage of garnering stimulation from many branches of one or more peripheral nerves as these branches ascend into the subcutaneous tissues from deeper levels. Optimal lead depth has also been studied [44], and it has been reported to be the best location for stimulating Aβ "fast adapt" and appears to be roughly 10–12 mm below the surface. The neuroanatomy of the dermis and subcutaneous tissue is such that Aδ fibers tend to concentrate closer to the dermis and within the dermis and produces a sensation of "sharp pain" and "stinging" by electrical fields. The Aβ "fast adapt" fibers are modestly deeper within the subcutaneous tissue and produce sensations of "tingling" and "tickling" (see Table 62.2). For programming algorithms utilizing subsensory stimulation, this is less important [45]. But for programming algorithms utilizing sensory stimulation, this can be quite important. It is essential to understand that the main goal is pain relief per se and not simply the production of sensory paresthesias. As with any other neuronal target suitable for neurostimulation, even the "unnamed nerves" provide a portal of entry for neuromodulation of the central nervous system. It is just a matter of finding most suitable "on-ramps" to the "interstate" to arrive at the optimal location within the CNS.

Of particular interest to peripheral neurostimulation for low back pain are the superior and middle cluneal nerves. These nerves are each derived from two spinal nerves: superior cluneal nerves (principally arising from L1, L2, and L3) in three separate branches over the posterolateral iliac crest and middle cluneal nerves (principally arising from S1, S2, and S3) in three separate branches about the posterior superior iliac spine (PSIS). Their locations relative to the bony ilium have been studied in detail by Tubbs et al. [46]. Figure 62.20 shows their distribution relative to the iliac crest. This is an area that is subject to surgical trauma during harvesting of bone for spinal fusions at L4 and L5 [47–49]. Further, the postsurgical biomechanics of the investing fas-

cial layers become altered with spinal surgery, deconditioning, loss of range of motion about the lumbosacral junction, and fascial degeneration [50]. As shown in Fig. 62.20, these nerves must penetrate the lumbosacral and sacroiliac fascial layers in order to pass over the iliac crest. Because of this, they are subject to any biomechanical alterations in these layers, and this can lead to biomechanically induced neuralgia and even neural entrapment. Cluneal nerve entrapment has been reported in the literature [51–53], as a clinical symptom characterized by persistent low back pain, aggravated by activity [50]. Thus, as noted by Vora et al., the discs, facet joints, and posterior spinal elements are interwoven in a dynamic biotensegrity network of ligaments, muscles, and fascia [50]. When this condition is chronic, there is potential for "central sensitization" within the dorsal horn of the spinal cord. Stretching exercises, which may keep these fascial layers and tissues flexible, are well noted to provide a reduction in low back pain [55] in patients who have not been treated by spinal fusion at the lumbosacral junction.

There are numerous reports in the literature of neuroablative efforts at relieving chronic low back pain within the distribution of the superior and middle cluneal nerves and their medially and laterally displaced branches. Neurostimulation along the anatomic pathways of the cluneal nerves is thus a highly rational approach to treating a peripheral neuralgia involving these nerves.

As of this writing, a retrospective study of ten patients with previously implanted epidural neurostimulator leads for failed

Table 62.2 Fiber types and associated sensation

Fiber types	Associated sensation
Aβ "fast" adapt	Tingling, tickling
Aβ "slow" adapt	Vibrating
Aδ	Sharp pain, stinging
C fibers	Burning, aching

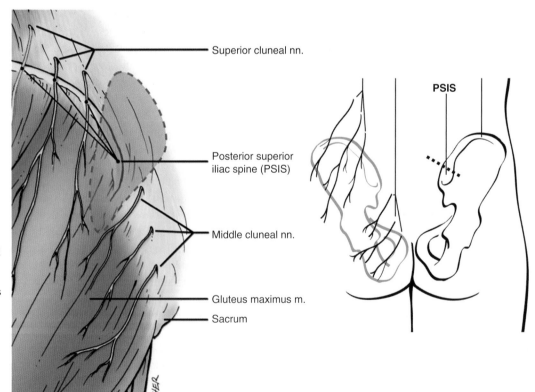

Fig. 62.20 Anatomical drawing (**a**) and Schematic drawing (**b**) of the cluneal nerves in the left gluteal region. The relative "safe zone" for bone harvesting is shown in *light red*. *M* muscle, *nn* nerves (Adapted from Tubbs et al. [46], with permission)

PNS of the right middle cluneal nerves
s/p Iliac crest bone harvesting

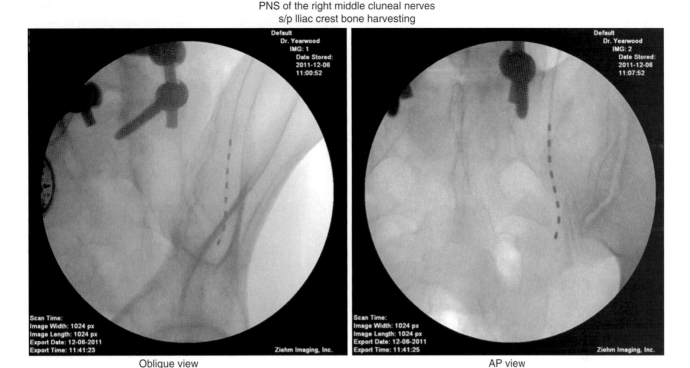

Oblique view   AP view

Fig. 62.21 PNS stimulation of the middle cluneal nerves on the right. Neurostimulation along the anatomic pathways of the cluneal nerves is thus a highly rational approach to treating a peripheral neuralgia involving these nerves

back surgery syndrome (FBSS) is currently underway in our clinic, in which a combined technique of fluoroscopy and ultrasound guidance was employed for PNS of the cluneal nerve lead placement. This configuration appears to demonstrate excellent pain relief in patients with and without previous iliac bone harvesting. Figure 62.21 demonstrates a typical lead placement along the iliac crest to a level slightly caudal to the PSIS. The fact that not all patients had previously undergone iliac crest bone harvesting for fusion underscores the potential for disuse atrophy and disruption of the dynamic biotensegrity network of ligaments, muscles, and fascia in the lumbosacral junction to create a peripheral neuralgia in this area that is resistant to epidural neurostimulation alone.

Sacroiliac joint dysfunction syndrome [57, 58] has a remarkably similar clinical presentation and is not well treated with epidural-based neurostimulation techniques. PNS stimulation of the primary dorsal rami of L5, S1, S2, and S3 gives an entirely similar pattern of stimulation, providing one with a suitable axial low back pain relief at the lumbosacral junction, hips, and buttocks. This is identical to the peripheral neurostimulation seen with PNS over the middle cluneal nerves described above and has been a target for recently developed "cooled-RF" neuroablative techniques in the treatment of sacroiliac joint dysfunction syndrome [59]. Figure 62.22 shows a typical arrangement of the leads in this case. Once again, this stimulation is much more "focal" in nature than can be achieved with epidural neurostimulation,

even in cases where a previously implanted epidural system provides some degree of paresthesia coverage to this difficult and hard-to-reach anatomical area.

Peripheral nerve field stimulation (PNFS) in the more superficial layers of the low back would appear to derive its success from utilizing anatomic pathways to the dorsal horn which are similar or identical to those used in PNS and intraspinal neurostimulation (DCS, DRG stimulation, and nerve root stimulation) for neuromodulation of painful neuropathic signals. The primary difference between PNS and PNFS appears to be the "focality" of the stimulation. PNFS offers access to the CNS for neuromodulation that is conceptually larger than PNS, as it may involve multiple "named" nerves, as noted above. This is an exploding area of interest, and excellent results have been reported for its use in many conditions, including chronic low back pain [60]. Figure 62.23 [61] shows typical lead placements for PNFS leads in treating axial low back pain. It should be noted that in each of these cases, the patient has undergone fusion of the L5 disc. Specific mention of bone harvesting was not made in this report, but direct surgical trauma to the iliac crest is not needed to produce chronic low back pain in this area, for biomechanical reasons noted above. Indirect effects can certainly result in cluneal neuralgia, and this is precisely the area where superior and middle cluneal involvement would be expected and where PNS stimulation of the primary dorsal rami of L5, S1, S2, and S3 is also effective.

Fig. 62.22 PNS stimulation of the primary dorsal rami of L5, S1, S2, and S3

PNS stimulation of the primary dorsal rami of L5, S1, S2, and S3

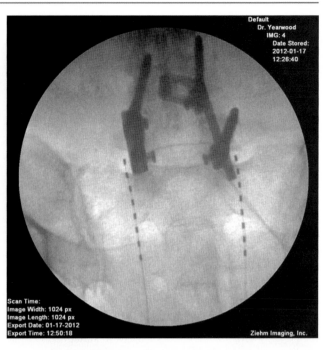

Peripheral field nerve stimulation (PNFS) for axial low back pain s/p spinal fusion

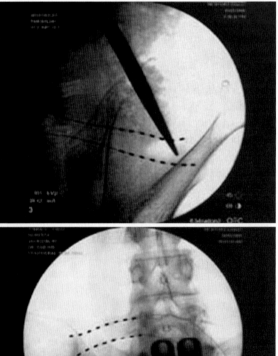

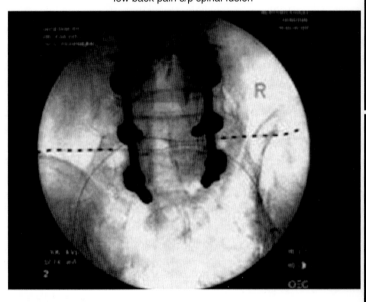

Fig. 62.23 Peripheral nerve field stimulation for low back pain in post-laminotomy syndrome ("FBSS") (From Paicius et al. [61], with permission)

PNFS has also been combined with intraspinal neurostimulation for the treatment of low back and leg pain [62]. This technique derives its clinical benefit from the advantages of multi-target stimulation, providing a modestly "focal" stimulation pattern when epidural-based "regional" DCS proves inadequate. It could be that similar neuroanatomical "conduits" of neurosensory input by these two different approaches result in modulating areas of the dorsal horn where wide dynamic range neurons play a role in central sensitization and "wind up" in chronic low back pain from both nociceptive and neuropathic sources.

In summary, neurostimulation can have significant benefit in treating radicular pain syndromes of the cervical, thoracic, and lumbar spine, including particularly difficult pain problems such as low back pain. Recognition of the capabilities of and limitations of each style of neurostimulation is necessary, as determined by the pathology of the targets involved, in achieving optimal clinical results. If secondary hyperalgesia and other "centrally mediated" neuropathic pain processes predominate in a given clinical situation, dorsal column stimulation may suffice. Where a peripheral neuralgia is superimposed on this clinical picture, combined techniques of intraspinal neurostimulation and peripheral neurostimulation (PNS, PNFS) may be required. The ultimate goal is to modulate those sensory signals that reach the thalamus which are disruptive to CNS as a whole and, in so doing, enable the patient to have a substantially greater clinical capacity for physical function and social engagement.

References

1. Merskey H, Bogduk N, editors. Classification of chronic pain: descriptions of chronic pain syndromes and definitions of pain terms. 2nd ed. Seattle: IASP Press; 1994.
2. Lindblum U. Analysis of abnormal touch, pain and temperature sensation in patients. In: Boivie J, Hansson P, Lindblum U, editors. Touch, temperature and pain in health and disease: mechanisms and assessments. Seattle: IASP Press; 1994. p. 63–84.
3. Willis WD, Coggeshall RE. Sensory mechanisms of the spinal cord. New York: Plenum; 1991. p. 79–132.
4. Sadde NE, Baliki M, El-Khoury C, Hawwa N, Atweh SF, Apkarian AV, Jabbur SJ. The role of dorsal columns and neuropathic behavior: evidence for plasticity and specificity. Neuroscience. 2002;115(2):403–13.
5. Struijk JJ, Holsheimer J, van der Heidi GG, Boom HBK. Recruitment of dorsal column fibers in spinal cord stimulation: influence of collateral branching. IEEE Trans Biomed Eng. 1992;39:903–12.
6. Struijk JJ, Holsheimer J, Boom HBK. Excitation of dorsal root fibers in spinal cord stimulation: a theoretical study. IEEE Trans Biomed Eng. 1993;40:632–9.
7. Smith MC, Deacon P. Topographical anatomy of the posterior columns of the spinal cord in man; the long ascending fibres. Brain. 1984;107:671–98.
8. Barolat G, Massaro F, He J, Zeme S, Ketcik B. Mapping of sensory responses to epidural stimulation of the intraspinal neural structures in man. J Neurosurg. 1993;78(2):233–9.
9. Nakamura A, Yamada T, Goto A, Kato T, Ito K, Abe Y, Kachi T, Kakigi R. Somatosensory homunculus as drawn by MEG. Neuroimage. 1998;7(4):377–86.
10. Puigdellívol-Sánchez A, Prats-Galino A, Ruano-Gil D, Molander C. Sciatic and femoral nerve sensory neurones occupy different regions of the L4 dorsal root ganglion in the adult rat. Neurosci Lett. 1998;251(3):169–72.
11. Wessels WJT, Feirabend HKP, Marani E. Evidence for a rostrocaudal organization in the dorsal root ganglia during development as demonstrated by intrauterine WGA-HRP injections into the hindlimb of rat fetuses. Dev Brain Res. 1990;54(2):273–81.
12. Feirabend HKP, Marani E. Dorsal root ganglion. In: Aminoff MJ, Daroff RB, editors. Encyclopedia of the neurological sciences. San Diego: Academic. 2003. p. 28–33 and 90 complaints of ISBN: 978-0-12-226870-0.
13. Kaas JH, Merzenich MM, Killackey HP. The reorganization of somatosensory cortex following peripheral nerve damage in adult and developing mammals. Annu Rev Neurosci. 1983;6:325–56.
14. Swett JE, Woolf CJ. The somatotopic organization of primary afferent terminals in the superficial laminae of the dorsal horn of the rat spinal cord. J Comp Neurol. 1985;231:66–77.
15. Slipman CW, Plastaras CT, Palmitier RA, Huston CW, Sterenfeld EB. Symptom provocation of fluoroscopically guided cervical nerve root stimulation: are dynatomal maps identical to dermatomal maps? Spine. 1998;23(20):2235–42.
16. Haque R, Winfree CJ. Spinal nerve root stimulation. Neurosurg Focus. 2006;216(E4):1–7.
17. Hayek SM, Veizi IEM, Stanton-Hicks M. Four-limb neurostimulation with neuroelectrodes placed in the lower cervical epidural space. Anesthesiology. 2009;110(3):681–4.
18. Feirabend HKP, Choufoer H, Ploeger S, Holsheimer J, van Gool JD. Morphology of human superficial dorsal and dorsolateral column fibres: significance to spinal cord stimulation. Brain. 2002;125:1137–49.
19. Gorman PH, Mortimer JT. The effect of stimulus parameters on the recruitment characteristics of direct nerve stimulation. IEEE Trans Biomed Eng. 1983;30:407–14.
20. Yearwood TL, Hershey B, Bradley K, Lee D. Pulse width programming in spinal cord stimulation: a clinical study. Pain Physician. 2010;13:321–35.
21. Holsheimer J, den Boer JA, Struijk JJ, Rozeboom AR. MR assessment of the normal position of the spinal cord in the spinal canal. AJNR Am J Neuroradiol. 1994;15:951–9.
22. Dorland's Medical Dictionary for Health Consumers. MSDict Viewer, v.4.0.2008-2011. Mobile Systems, Inc. www.multisystems.com. Accessed on Sep. 8 2011
23. Malik K, Benzon HT. Low back pain, chapter 17. In: Benzon: Raj's practical management of pain. 4th ed. Philadelphia: Mosby/Elsevier; 2008. 367.
24. Bogduk N. Cervicogenic headache: anatomic basis and pathophysiologic mechanisms. Curr Pain Headache Rep. 2001;5:382–6.
25. Bartsch T, Goadsby PJ. Anatomy and physiology of pain referral patterns in primary and cervicogenic headache disorders. Headache Curr. 2005;2:42–8.
26. Mørch CD, Hu JW, Arendt-Nielsen L, Sessle BJ. Convergence of cutaneous, musculoskeletal, dural, and visceral afferents onto nociceptive neurons in the first cervical dorsal horn. Eur J Neurosci. 2007;26(1):142–54.
27. Nakamura SI, Takahashi K, Takahashi Y, Yamagata M, Moriya H. The afferent pathways of discogenic low-back pain: evaluation of L2 spinal nerve infiltration. J Bone Joint Surg Br. 1996;78:606–12.
28. Whitworth LA, Feler CA. C1-C2 Sublaminar insertion of paddle leads for the management of chronic painful conditions of the upper extremity. Neuromodulation. 2003;6:153–7.

29. Hazelrigg SR, Cetindag IB, Fullerton J. Acute and chronic pain syndromes after thoracic surgery. Surg Clin North Am. 2002; 82:849–65.

30. Erdek M, Staats PS. Chronic pain after thoracic surgery. Thorac Surg Clin. 2005;15:123–30.

31. Merskey H. Classification of chronic pain: description of chronic pain syndromes and definitions of pain terms. Pain. 1986;3: S138–9.

32. Karmakar M, Ho A. Postthoracotomy pain syndrome. Thorac Surg Clin. 2004;14:345–52.

33. Gotoda Y, Kambara N, Sakai T, Kishi Y, Kodama K, Koyama T. The morbidity, time course and predictive factors for persistent post-thoracotomy pain. Eur J Pain. 2001;5:89–96.

34. McJunkin TL, Berardoni N, Lynch PJ, Amrani J. An innovative case report detailing the successful treatment of post-thoracotomy syndrome with peripheral nerve field stimulation. Neuromodulation. 2010;13:311–4.

35. Rattay AM. Modeling axon membranes for functional electrical stimulation. IEEE Trans Biomed Eng. 1993;40(12):1201–9.

36. Buonocore M, Bonezzi C, Barolat G. Neurophysiological evidence of antidromic activation of large myelinated fibers in lower limbs during spinal cord stimulation. Spine. 2008;33(4):E90–3.

37. Weigel R, Capelle HH, Krauss JK. Failure of long-term nerve root stimulation to improve neuropathic pain. J Neurosurg. 2008; 108(5):921–5.

38. Bogduk N, Tynan W, Wilson AS. The nerve supply to the human lumbar intervertebral discs. J Anat. 1981;132:39–56.

39. Groen GJ, Baljet B, Drukker J. Nerves and nerve plexuses of the human vertebral column. Am J Anat. 1990;188:282–96.

40. Edgar MA. The nerve supply of the lumbar intervertebral disc. J Bone Joint Surg Br. 2007;89(9):1135–9.

41. Suseki K, Takahashi Y, Takahashi K, Chiba T, Yamagata M, Moriya H. Sensory nerve fibers from lumbar intervertebral discs pass through rami communicantes. A possible pathway for discogenic low back pain. J Bone Joint Surg Br. 1998;80:737–42.

42. Aoki Y, Takahashi Y, Ohtori S, Moriya H, Takahashi K. Distribution and immunocytochemical characterization of dorsal root ganglion neurons innervating the lumbar intervertebral disc in rats: a review. Life Sci. 2004;74:2627–42.

43. Woolf CJ, Salter MW. Plasticity and pain: the role of the dorsal horn, chapter 5. In: McMahon SB, Koltzenburg M, editors. McMahon: Wall and Melzack's textbook of pain. 5th ed. Edinburgh: Churchill Livingstone, an imprint of Elsevier; 2006.

44. Verrills P, Bernard A. The effect of electrode lead depth distribution on paresthesia in peripheral nerve field stimulation and occipital nerve stimulation. In: From a paper delivered at the international neuromodulation society 10th world congress, London, 21–26 May 2011.

45. Yearwood T, Foster A. A prospective comparison of spinal cord stimulation (SCS) using dorsal column stimulation (DCS), intraspinal nerve root stimulation (INRS) and varying pulse width in the treatment of chronic low back pain. In: Digital abstract presented at CNS 56th annual meeting, Chicago, 2006.

46. Tubbs RS, Levin MR, Loukas M, Potts EA, Cohen-Gadol AA. Anatomy and landmarks for the superior and middle cluneal

nerves: application to posterior iliac crest harvest and entrapment syndromes; laboratory investigation. J Neurosurg Spine. 2010;133:356–9.

47. Figure of cluneal nerve distribution from Canale and Beaty: Campbell's operative orthopedics. 11th ed. Chapter 38: Scoliosis and kyphosis. Philadelphia: Mosby; 2007.

48. Goulet JA, Senunas LE, DeSilva GL, Greenfield ML. Autogenous iliac crest bone graft. Complications and functional assessment. Clin Orthop. 1997;83:76–81.

49. Summers BN, Eisenstein SM. Donor site pain from the ilium. A complication of lumbar spine fusion. J Bone Joint Surg. 1989; 71B:677–80.

50. Vora AJ, Doerr KD, Wolfer LR. Functional anatomy and pathophysiology of axial low back pain: disc, posterior elements, sacroiliac joint and associated pain generators. Phys Med Rehabil Clin N Am. 2010;21(4):679–709.

51. Talu GK, Ozyalçin S, Talu U. Superior cluneal nerve entrapment. Reg Anesth Pain Med. 2000;25(6):648–50.

52. Akbas M, Yegin A, Karsli B. Superior cluneal nerve entrapment eight years after decubitus surgery. Pain Pract. 2005;5(4):364–6.

53. Maigne JY, Doursounian L. Entrapment neuropathy of the medial superior cluneal nerve. Nineteen cases surgically treated, with a minimum of 2 years' follow-up. Spine. 1997;22(10):1156–9.

54. Kose KC, Altinel L, Isikb C, Komurcuc E, Mutlud S, Ozdemire M. Bilateral post-injection fibrosis of the gluteal region mimicking lumbar disc herniation: a case report. Orthop Rev. 2009;1:e25, 67–9.

55. Carragee EJ. Persistent low back pain. N Engl J Med. 2005;352: 1891–8.

56. Yearwood TL. Dorsal sacral rami and cluneal nerve peripheral neurostimulation for residual low back pain after epidural neurostimulation for FBSS: a report of 10 cases using combined fluoroscopy and ultrasound-guided lead placement (in preparation).

57. DonTigny RL. Anterior dysfunction of the sacroiliac joint as a major factor in the etiology of idiopathic low back pain syndrome. Phys Ther. 1990;70(4):250–62.

58. Slipman CW, Lipetz JS, Plastaras CT, Jackson HB, Vresilovic EJ, Lenrow DA, Braverman DL. Fluoroscopically guided therapeutic sacroiliac joint injections for sacroiliac joint syndrome. Am J Phys Med Rehabil. 2001;80(6):425–32.

59. Kapural L, Nageeb F, Kapural M, Cata JP, Narouze S, Mekhail N. Clinical study: cooled radiofrequency system for the treatment of chronic pain from sacroiliitis: the 1st case series. Pain Pract. 2008;8(5):348–54.

60. Verrills P, Vivian D, Mitchell B, Barnard A. Peripheral nerve field stimulation for chronic pain: 100 cases and review of the literature. Pain Med. 2011;12:1396–405.

61. Paicius RM, Bernstein CA, Lempert-Cohen C. Peripheral nerve field stimulation for the treatment of chronic low back pain: preliminary results of long-term follow-up: a case series. Neuromodulation. 2007;10:279–90.

62. Bernstein CA, Paicius RM, Barkow SH, Lempert-Cohen C. Spinal cord stimulation in conjunction with peripheral nerve field stimulation for the treatment of low back and leg pain: a case series. Neuromodulation. 2008;11:116–23.

Clinical Applications of Neuromodulation: Neurostimulation for Complex Regional Pain Syndrome

63

Michael Stanton-Hicks

Key Points

- Complex regional pain syndrome (CRPS) is defined, and criteria necessary to be satisfied for this diagnosis are addressed.
- A review of recent literature describing the use of spinal cord stimulation (SCS) in the management of CRPS is provided.
- The risk–benefit analysis, patient criteria, and conditions should be met before consideration of SCS is addressed including the need for psychometric testing and instruments that are used for this purpose.
- The multidisciplinary management of patients with CRPS is emphasized including how SCS may be introduced as either a temporary adjunct to functional restoration or its permanent implantation in cases that require the ongoing attributes of SCS as it serves to ameliorate pain and improve the microcirculation and functional improvement of motor function is emphasized.

Introduction

Complex regional pain syndrome (CRPS), formerly termed reflex sympathetic dystrophy (RSD), was introduced in 1994 by the International Association for the Study of Pain (IASP) [1, 2]. CRPS comprises two syndromes: type I, representing reflex sympathetic dystrophy, and type II referring to causalgia

M. Stanton-Hicks, M.D., MBBS, FRCA, ABPM, FIPP
Department of Pain Management, Cleveland Clinic,
9500 Euclid Ave, C-25, Clevland, OH 44195, USA

Department of Anesthesiology,
Cleveland Clinic Lerner College of Medicine,
Cleveland, OH, USA
e-mail: stanton@ccf.org

[3]. The hypothesis of sympathetically maintained pain (SMP), introduced by Roberts in 1986, represents a phenomenon that may be present in both syndromes and can be confirmed, when present, by sympathetic blockade [4].

As set forth by the IASP, the diagnostic criteria that must be satisfied comprise pain, impaired function in the region, trophic changes involving the nails, hair growth, and sudomotor dysfunction [2]. Sensory abnormalities such as hyperesthesia, hyperalgesia, and mechanical or thermal allodynia (or both) are also present (Table 63.1).

The fundamental signs and symptoms of CRPS entail sensory, motor, autonomic, and trophic changes. The IASP requires that these clinical features be identified under these four categories. No supportive clinical tests are included in the IASP classification. However, tests of sudomotor dysfunction, e.g., the quantitative sudomotor axon reflex test (QSART), quantitative sensory testing (QST), skin biopsy, and the use of sympathetic blocks to determine whether any significant autonomic dysfunction is evident, can be undertaken.

The differential diagnosis of CRPS requires the elimination of other clinical syndromes which share clinical features with CRPS but which are clearly distinct by virtue of their own unique constellation of signs and symptoms. Clinical features similar to those of CRPS include the pain, edema, and temperature asymmetry characteristic of trauma patients, but who nevertheless do not develop CRPS. Table 63.2 describes the clinical diagnostic criteria of CRPS, termed the "Budapest Criteria" and published in 2010.

Movement disorders, not previously associated with CRPS, are now well recognized (see Table 63.3) [8]. They include weakness, tremor, muscle spasms, dystonia, and inability to initiate movement. Occasionally sympathetic blockade, when undertaken soon after the onset of CRPS, may eliminate the movement disorder.

Contemporary thinking accepts that the initial clinical features of CRPS resemble a significant inflammatory disorder. However, this thinking has been shaped by studies revealing that free O_2 radical expression can sensitize activity in C and A-δ fibers. Continuous excitation of these

Table 63.1 Diagnostic criteria for complex regional pain syndrome (CRPS)

Factor 1	Factor 2	Factor 3	Factor 4
Hyperalgesia signs (0.75)	Temperature asymmetry symptoms (0.68)	Edema signs (0.69)	Decreased range of motion signs (0.81)
Hyperesthesia symptoms (0.78)	Color change signs (0.67)	Sweating asymmetry signs (0.62)	Decreased range of motion symptoms (0.77)
Allodynic signs (0.44)	Color change symptoms (0.52)	Edema symptoms (0.61)	Motor dysfunction signs (0.77) Motor dysfunction symptoms (0.61) Tropic symptoms (0.52) Trophic signs (0.51)

From Harden and Bruehl [5]. With permission

Table 63.2 Budapest clinical diagnostic criteria for complex regional pain syndrome (CRPS)

1. Continuing pain, which is disproportionate to any inciting event
2. Must report at least one symptom in *three of the four* following categories:
   Sensory: reports of hyperesthesia and/or allodynia
   Vasomotor: reports of temperature asymmetry and/or skin color changes and/or skin color asymmetry
   Sudomotor/edema: reports of edema and/or sweating changes and/or sweating asymmetry
   Motor/trophic: reports of decreased range of motion and/or motor dysfunction (weakness, tremor, dystonia) and/or trophic changes (hair, nail, skin)
3. Must display at least one sign at time of evaluation in *two or more* of the following categories:
   Sensory: evidence of hyperalgesia (to pinprick) and/or allodynia (to light touch and/or deep somatic pressure and/or joint movement)
   Vasomotor: evidence of temperature asymmetry and/or skin color changes and/or asymmetry
   Sudomotor/edema: evidence of edema and/or sweating changes and/or sweating asymmetry
   Motor/trophic: evidence of decreased range of motion and/or motor dysfunction (weakness, tremor, dystonia) and/or trophic changes (hair, nail, skin)
4. There is no other diagnosis that better explains the signs and symptoms

From Harden et al. [6]. Used with permission

nociceptors will in turn sensitize first-order and higher neurons in the central nervous system (CNS). Central sensitization can be demonstrated not only in the spinal cord but also at the supratentorial centers in the brain [9].

Rationale for the Use of Neurostimulation

Most pharmacologic treatments of CRPS target neurologic dysfunction. The treatments include membrane stabilizers, antidepressants, norepinephrine reuptake inhibitors, and NMDA antagonists—all of which are used to support a return of function by means of physiotherapeutic measures [10]. Two other measures used to support rehabilitation are (1) epidural infusions of local anesthetics with or without opioids and (2) the addition of alpha-2 agonists like clonidine. These techniques have proved very effective but are associated with a low incidence of infection as well as technical failure of the infusion system. They are also expensive because they require home health-care support and associated pharmaceuticals.

When sympathetically maintained pain (SMP) has been demonstrated by a sympathetic block, with almost complete symptomatic relief, a comparatively long duration of effect can be achieved by segmental radio frequency ablation (RFA) of the sympathetic trunk.

Increasing evidence now supports the use of neuroaugmentative procedures such as spinal cord stimulation (SCS) or peripheral nerve stimulation (PNS) [11–13]. This evidence includes randomized controlled trials (RCTs), several long-term studies, and several case studies. The first RCT, conducted by Kemler et al., was published in 2000 [14]. The patients in this study met the IASP diagnostic criteria for CRPS and were unresponsive to conventional medical management (CMM). Two randomly assigned groups comprised patients who undertook spinal cord stimulation (SCS) plus physical therapy and patients who received only physical therapy. All patients who successfully completed their trial underwent implantation of the neurostimulator. The subsequent intention-to-treat analysis demonstrated a significant reduction in pain in the SCS/physical therapy group [15]. Other measures showed that the SCS/physical therapy group experienced improvement both in the global perceived effect (GPE) and in quality of life (QOL). All patients underwent implantation of their SCS. The same authors demonstrated long-term improvement in pain relief and GPE among the SCS/physical therapy group, in comparison to the patients who received only physical therapy at 2 years. At 5 years, the GPE remained better than in patients who had received only physical therapy, although the "expressed" pain relief did not differ between the two groups. However, all the patients who had received an SCS stated they would repeat the treatment should the need arise.

In one study, carbamazepine and morphine were compared in patients previously implanted with an SCS [16]. This study,

Table 63.3 Prevalence of movement disorders in complex regional pain syndrome (CRPS)

N	Weakness (%)	Akinesia (%)	Dystonia (%)	Spasms (%)	Tremor (%)	Reference
200			22			Schwartzman and Kerrigan (1990)
829	95		36[a]	25	49	Veldman et al. (1993)
181	89	80			45	Blumberg and Jänig (1994)
123	75/76[b]				24/94[b]	Harden et al. (1999)
145	79	45	30[c]		48	Birklein et al. (2000)

From van Hilten et al. [7]. Used with permission
[a]Reflects involuntary movements
[b]Symptoms/signs
[c]Including myoclonia

divided into two phases, investigated the effect of administering carbamazepine or placebo in phase I and morphine and placebo in phase II after the patient's SCS system had been deactivated. Carbamazepine was superior to morphine in reducing the level of pain. However, only 2 of the 38 patients preferred to continue their treatment with carbamazepine; the remaining 36 preferred to continue their treatment with SCS. These results clearly demonstrated the successful symptomatic management of either neuropathic pain or CRPS.

Although most of the papers during the past 35 years have been case studies or retrospective reviews, a common thread of success runs through these works. The latest publication that supports the use of SCS is probably the 2009 Health Technology Assessment report, issued by the National Institute for Health and Clinical Excellence (NICE). This report reviewed 6,000 citations, including 11 RCTs of neuropathic pain and eight of ischemic pain [17], and concluded that SCS effectively decreases chronic neuropathic pain, and the results are more effective than those of conventional medical management (CMM). With regard to cost containment, the incremental cost-effectiveness ratio (ICER) described a range of $25,000–$30,000 per quality-adjusted life year (QALY), and if based on device longevity of 4 years, these figures were reduced to $20,000 per QALY.

It should be emphasized that most of the data reported so far have been obtained with comparatively unsophisticated systems. However, the efficacy of SCS, and in particular its effect on CRPS, has been improved by means of more modern neurostimulation systems with computerized programming capabilities, multiple arrays, and dual or multiple electrode systems. When the results of these latest systems are carefully studied, it becomes clear that early intervention is responsible for a much greater success rate in reversing or suppressing the symptoms.

The temporary use of SCS to provide analgesia in support of a physiotherapeutic program or a more comprehensive interdisciplinary treatment program was advocated by Prager and Chang in 2000 [18]. In this study, the authors described a triple-lead (tripolar) system that was temporarily implanted, and an "extended trial" was used to facilitate exercise therapy. The system was retained for 4 weeks, and if the patient required further analgesia after that time, it was implanted.

A second set of 16 patients, who had failed 4 weeks of comprehensive therapy, underwent permanent implant of SCS with continuing interdisciplinary treatment. Patients who no longer felt that SCS was necessary underwent explantation. Five of the original eight patients showed improvement in their symptoms sufficient to warrant removal of the system. The authors noted that SCS is a fairly inexpensive treatment compared to CMM or multiple sympathetic blocks. Finally, it should be noted that an implanted SCS lead with an externalized pulse generator could always be converted to a totally implanted system, circumstances prevailing.

Patient Selection

Appropriate selection of patients for SCS is essential to a successful outcome [11]. Most published treatment algorithms describe the use of SCS after simpler and more conservative therapies have been tried in a stepwise fashion although usually in support of an exercise therapy treatment program [19]. Conventional wisdom would suggest that any patient who is likely to need an implantable device such as an SCS must undergo a satisfactory behavioral assessment [20]. Such an assessment is essential for precluding those patients who might believe that a simple or rapid intervention such as SCS is most likely to cure their clinical problem, or who may have unrealistic expectations regarding the management of their syndrome. Although SCS is a minimally invasive procedure, it should always follow an adequate screening trial. The trial should demonstrate to the patient and to the treating physician that the activities of daily living (ADLs) can be improved and that notwithstanding improved symptoms, the patient should maintain their exercise therapy (Table 63.4).

In this respect, convention requires a 50% reduction of pain. If other comorbidities, or the possible anatomic anomalies, are suggested, preradiologic screening with MRI or CT scan is imperative. Additional selection criteria have been developed by several authors (see Table 63.3). In an effort to standardize criteria for the selection of patients for SCS, several scientific bodies, including the International Association for the Study of Pain (IASP), the International Neuromodulation

Table 63.4 Selection criteria for spinal cord stimulation in complex regional pain syndrome (CRPS)

Oakley [11]	
Inclusion	Exclusion
Diagnosis of CRPS	Absence of initial CMM
6-month pain duration	Previous failed SCS trial
Psychological clearance	Untreated axis I psychiatric disorder
Informed consent	Certain psychoses
Contraindications	
North et al. [21]	
Relative	Absolute
Medication dependence	Coagulopathy
Unresolved psychiatric disorder	Immunosuppressive therapy
Nonorganic signs (Waddell's)	Unacceptable surgical risk
Inconsistent history	Conflicting therapy diathermy
Anticoagulation therapy	Serial MRI requirements
Alternative therapy with lower risk/benefit ratio	Occupational risk

Minimally adapted from Prager [22]. Original used with permission

Society (INS), the North American Neuromodulation Society (NANS), and the American Academy of Pain Medicine (AAPM), are involved in the education and dissemination of guidelines to be met before patients are selected for neurostimulation. The requirement for psychological pretesting is addressed by the Centers for Medicare Services (CMS), the industrial commissions and state bureaus of workers compensation (BWC), and most health insurance agencies. Most contemporary psychological evaluation is based on an inventory of risk factors which, together with behavioral management, play a significant role in patient care that supports the use of SCS in selected patients [23, 24].

Risk–Benefit Analysis

The potential benefit of SCS as a treatment modality for CRPS has been described in the supporting literature. Table 63.5 identifies several observations that underscore the value of SCS; however, pain relief remains the most significant reason to consider SCS. For more than 30 years, success has been defined as a reduction of 50 % in pain [30]. However, pain reduction is subjective, and the level of pain is assessed by means of arithmetic scales such as the visual analog scale (VAS), verbal rating scale (VRS), and numerical rating scale (NRS). Unfortunately, because pain is subjective and is an exponential function, the values, expressed arithmetically, bear little resemblance to the constellation of symptoms about which the patient complains. Furthermore, chronicity and environmental factors materially impact the number chosen on any one of the above scales. Function

should become the standard by which the impact of pain can influence a variety of functional markers (Table 63.5).

The Neuromodulation Therapy Access Coalition identified studies that demonstrate the ability of patients to undertake their activities of daily living (ADL) and to improve quality of life (QOL). Although there are quite extensive data from patients in whom failed back surgical syndrome (FBSS) has been treated by SCS, other functional markers used are the Oswestry Disability Index and the Hospital Anxiety and Depression (HADS) Scale [27]. All measures showed significant reduction. In the single RCT on CRPS by Kemler et al., the QOL improved by 11 % [14]. Although patient satisfaction has never been standardized, several authors have indirectly described patient satisfaction as those patients who choose to cross over from CMM to SCS, or who choose to repeat implantation to achieve the same result, indicating the success of SCS [25, 31]. An interesting aspect of SCS that often escapes comment is its effect on depression. Several authors have noted that SCS patients manifest fewer symptoms of depression such as those measured by the Beck Depression Inventory (BDI) [29, 32, 33].

The greatest impediment to successful treatment stems from complications due to technical failure, or from infection, which occurs in as many as 30 % of all cases [34].

Under the best of circumstances, the incidence of perioperative infection is between 4 and 5 % of all cases [11, 34]. North, describing 20 years of experience with spinal cord stimulation, found 0 incidence of spinal cord injury, meningitis, or other life-threatening infection. An incidence of spinal fluid leak, neurologic injury, or hemorrhage has been reported in 0–42 % of cases [11].

Electrode displacement occurs in approximately 24 % of cases [34]. The subsequent loss of therapeutic stimulation requiring surgical revision occurs in approximately 50 % of cases. However, many of the foregoing data have been derived from older and simpler systems. Modern multichannel systems with computerized implanted pulse generators (IPGs) are significantly more reliable. Accordingly, the future of SCS should markedly improve as a result of technological advances in contemporary equipment.

In a review of 126 cases, Oakley found that 26 patients (20 %) requested that their system be explanted or discontinued [11]. The main reasons for failure were progression of disease, loss of therapeutic paresthesia, and discomfort at the implant site (primarily IPG). On the other hand, four patients (3 %) experienced such successful analgesia that they no longer used their system. When patients are being prepared to consider SCS, the relative merits of its use should be placed in the context of their treatment to date. It is critical that the patient be informed of the shortcomings associated with SCS (as described above), of the nature of the screening trial, and the reasons for it. The specific endpoints a patient should assess during a trial are (1) the degree of pain relief, (2) what functional improvements are experienced on the affected side, (3) whether activity

Table 63.5 Potential benefits of spinal cord stimulation in treating complex regional pain syndrome (CRPS)[a]

Benefit	Comments
Pain relief [25, 26]	The primary outcome measure of SCS success is patient-reported pain relief, generally using a standard pain scale such as the visual analog scale (VAS), functional rating index, McGill Pain Questionnaire [21]
	A majority of patients may experience at least 50 % reduction in pain
Increased activity levels or function [12, 26, 27]	As demonstrated by activities of daily living, such as walking, climbing stairs, sleeping, engaging in sex, driving a car and sitting at a table [28]
	Measured by the Oswestry Disability Index (specific for low back pain), the Sickness Impact Profile (for general health), Functional Rating Index, Pain Disability Index
Reduced use of pain medication (Harke et al. 2005)	Patients in whom SCS is successful should be able to reduce or eliminate their intake of pain medication [21]
Improvement in quality of life [21, 27] Patient satisfaction with treatment (Alo et al. 1999; Bennett et al. 1999; [12, 21, 27])	Would repeat treatment to achieve the same result [21]
Fewer symptoms of depression [12, 21, 27, 29]	Measured by the Beck Depression Inventory

From Prager [22]. Used with permission

[a]Original author's note: Consult "practice parameters for the use of spinal cord stimulation in the treatment of chronic neuropathic pain" [21] for a comprehensive bibliography of studies that support the benefits of spinal cord stimulation in treating complex regional pain syndrome (CRPS) Selected long-term or seminal studies are cited here; short-term studies and case reports are not

is facilitated, and (4) whether circulation, as determined by temperature change and skin color in the region, is improved. It is also important to allow the patient to continue their routine medical management—in particular, medication—so that any reduction in use may definitively reflect successful SCS. Finally, patients should be encouraged to increase daily activities and, if appropriate, maintain their exercise program.

Obviously, a detailed description of the risk–benefit aspects of SCS that can be experienced should be discussed with each patient. Moreover, long-term efficacy should be placed within the context of our cumulative experience of SCS.

Multidisciplinary Care: The Role of SCS

Experience gained during the past 20 years has clearly highlighted the need for multidisciplinary or interdisciplinary management of patients with CRPS. It has been determined that neurostimulation, in its various forms, is the single most successful modality to use in most patients. In 2002, a physiotherapeutic continuum involving multidisciplinary management for CRPS was published (see Fig. 63.1) [35]. This algorithm underscored that psychological, rehabilitative, and interventional pain management should be implemented in a time-contingent manner—sequentially, or at times simultaneously. The various behavioral and/or interventional approaches are introduced only if or when progress slows or stalls during the course of

psychotherapeutic measures. "Time contingency" as proposed by the international group that participated in the development of this algorithm was considered to be the sine qua non for promoting physical therapy and, when adopted, underscored the need to incorporate neurostimulation as a major component of therapy. In fact, during rehabilitation, desirable functional effects (e.g., vasodilatation and motor improvement) are most often conferred when interventions such as SCS are incorporated [36]. These effects obviously require validation.

Although SCS is usually introduced as an intervention during the course of treating neuropathic pain, contemporary experience would suggest that in some cases, because of its significant attributes, SCS should be introduced much earlier [37–42]. This point is already addressed in the treatment algorithm.

One thing is certain that previously used ablative measures such as sympathectomy—whether pharmacologic or surgical—have little part to play in the modern management of CRPS.

The SCS Trial

A trial of SCS offers patient and physician the opportunity to determine whether the patient's therapy can be continued without the restrictions of their disability and at the same time allows the physician to assess whether the patient might be able to successfully discontinue their medications if any. The trial should assess goals that the treating physician has proposed, and it

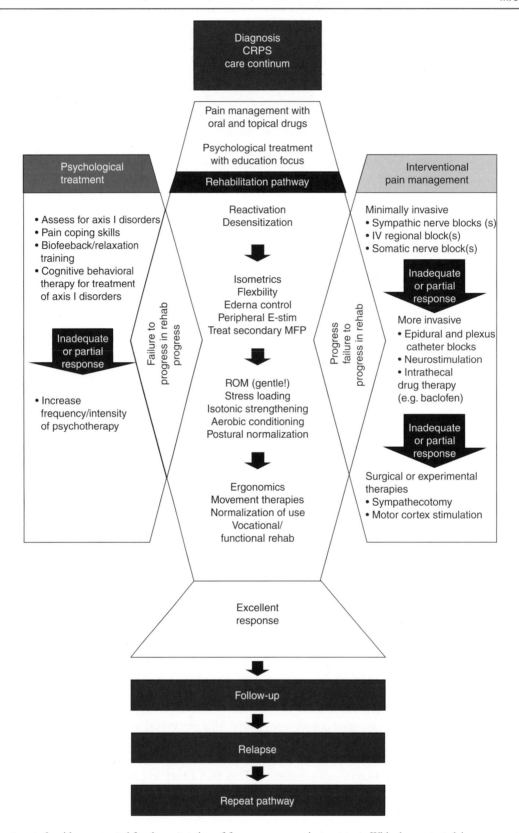

Fig. 63.1 Treatment algorithm suggested for the restoration of function using a stepwise approach and the introduction of behavioral or interventional measures that should be introduced in order to facilitate progress in treatment. With demonstrated improvement, the physiotherapeutic measures may be increased in intensity and frequency in order to achieve a final remission of this syndrome

should also aim to reduce pain symptoms by at least 50 %, while functional rehabilitation is still being undertaken [26, 29].

In addition to psychological assessment, a physical examination should be performed; this is also including a complete neurologic assessment to detect and evaluate other possible comorbidities [28]. Although many screening protocols are followed, a trial of SCS will be influenced by the site (upper vs. lower extremity), the patient's overall medical condition, the practice resources, geographic proximity to the patient's home, and economic issues related to the patient's reimbursement for their trial, e.g., private insurance, Medicare, BWC.

If the patient has certain anatomic abnormalities and/or prior adverse experience with neurostimulation, these aspects may require consultation with a neurosurgeon so that a percutaneous trial [28, 43, 44]. The customary duration of an SCS trial is 1 week, which is usually long enough for the patient and physician to evaluate the merits of SCS as a therapeutic modality. Longer periods are customary if a patient doubts the efficacy of their trial.

In certain cases, a so-called "extended" SCS trial is used to facilitate either rehabilitation or a comprehensive outpatient or inpatient multidisciplinary pain program [45, 46]. In such cases, the trial electrode is left in situ for periods of 6–8 weeks. In many of these cases, it is not intended that an SCS system be subsequently implanted; the trial merely serves as a means for facilitating their exercise program.

Surgical Implantation

Because SCS represents a radical departure from CMM, the patient should regularly be made aware that SCS will reduce, but in most cases will not completely eliminate, their pain. Patients must also understand that SCS will be a component of other therapies. Whenever practicable, patients should be followed at intervals of 3, 6, and 12 months so that any adjustments can be made prospectively or in response to the loss of therapeutic stimulation. Patients who are to undergo laminotomy placement of their SCS must be informed that greater discomfort and some morbidity are associated with the procedure but that within a reasonably short time, these symptoms should resolve [47]. Patients should also be counseled that lifelong exercise therapy will be needed to maintain optimal therapeutic support from the SCS. Moreover, they should be cautioned that over a 2-year period there will be about a 10 % loss in efficacy; after which, there will be no further loss for the life of the neurostimulator [48]. Finally, at no time should the relationship between the patient and the implanting physician be disrupted; for maintenance of the relationship allows subsequent technical issues or a breakdown in SCS efficacy to be addressed in a timely manner.

Cost-Effectiveness

Several studies in the USA, the Netherlands, the UK, Germany, and Canada have evaluated the cost of SCS treatment. Evidence from RCTs confirms the cost-effectiveness of SCS for treating CPRS. In the Netherlands, the 12-month cost of CRPS treatment by SCS was $4,000 greater than that for CMM but in an analysis over a lifetime; SCS was found to be $60,000 less than CMM per patient. In the UK, the lifetime cost savings was $60,800 for SCS compared to physical therapy alone. In Canada, Kumar et al. found that in a group of 104 patients, the cumulative cost of SCS was $29,123 compared to $38,029 for CMM [21, 48–53].

Summary

SCS is successful as an adjunct in the treatment continuum for CRPS. A trial of SCS is always necessary before implantation is considered or implemented. Not only analgesia but also improvement in function and in the ability to tolerate physical therapy should be determinants of a successful trial. Over the past 30 years, during which SCS has been used in the treatment of CRPS, no adverse effects have been reported on the central nervous system or neuroendocrine systems. SCS is cost-effective. Continuing improvements in the understanding of its mechanism of action, as well as improvements in technological developments, should anchor this modality as one of the most successful treatments for neuropathic pain. Thus, it plays a unique role in the management of and supportive of rehabilitation for CRPS.

References

1. Evans J. Reflex sympathetic dystrophy. Surg Clin North Am. 1946;26:780.
2. Merskey H, Bogduk N, editors. Classification of chronic pain: descriptions of chronic pain syndromes and definitions of pain terms. 2nd ed. Seattle: IASP Press; 1994.
3. Stanton-Hicks M, Janig W, Hassenbusch SJ, et al. Reflex sympathetic dystrophy: changing concepts and taxonomy. Pain. 1995;3: 127–33.
4. Roberts WJ. A hypothesis on the physiological basis for causalgia and related pains. Pain. 1986;24(3):297–311.
5. Harden RN, Bruehl SP. Chapter 4: Diagnostic criteria: the statistical derivation of the four criterion factors, page 49: Table II. Factors (and factor loadings) resulting from principal components factor analysis of diagnostic and associated signs and symptoms of CRPS. In: Wilson PR, Stanton-Hicks M, Harden RN, editors. CRPS: current diagnosis and therapy, Progress in pain research and management, vol. 32. Seattle: IASP Press; 2005. p. 45–58.
6. Harden RN, Bruehl S, Perez RS, et al. Validation of proposed diagnostic criteria (the "Budapest Criteria") for Complex Regional Pain Syndrome [page 274]. Pain. 2010;150:268–74.
7. Hilten JJ, Blumberg H, Schwartzman R. Chapter 8: Factor IV: movement disorders and dystrophy—pathophysiology and measurement,

page 120: Table 1. Prevalence of movement disorders in CRPS. In: Wilson P, Stanton-Hicks M, Harden RN, editors. CRPS: current diagnosis and therapy, Progress in pain research and management, vol. 32. Seattle: IASP Press; 1999. p. 120–37.

8. van Hilten J, Blumberg H, Schwartzman RJ. Factor IV: movement disorders and dystrophy – pathophysiology and measurement. In: Wilson PR, Stanton-Hicks M, Harden RN, editors. CRPS: current diagnosis and therapy, Progress in pain research and management, vol. 32. Seattle: IASP Press; 2005. 8:119–138.

9. Wolf CJ, Salter MW. Neuronal plasticity: increasing the gain in pain. Science. 2000;288(5472):1765–9.

10. Oaklander AL. Evidence-based pharmacotherapy for CRPS and related conditions. In: Wilson PR, Stanton-Hicks M, Harden RN, editors. CRPS: current diagnosis and therapy, Progress in pain research and management, vol. 32. Seattle: IASP Press; 2005. 12:181–200.

11. Oakley JC. Spinal cord stimulation for the treatment of chronic pain. In: Follett KA, editor. Neurosurgical pain management. Philadelphia: Saunders; 2004. p. 131–44.

12. Kumar K, Hunter G, Demeria D. Spinal cord stimulation in treatment of chronic benign pain: challenges in treatment planning and present status, a 22 year experience. Neurosurgery. 2006;58(3): 481–96.

13. Hassenbusch SJ, Stanton-Hicks M, Schoppa AD, et al. Long-term peripheral nerve stimulation for reflex sympathetic dystrophy. J Neurosurg. 1996;84:415–23.

14. Kemler MA, Barendse GAM, van Kleef M, et al. Spinal cord stimulation in patients with chronic reflex sympathetic dystrophy. N Engl J Med. 2000;343:618–24.

15. Kemler MA, De Vet HC, Barendse GA, et al. Effect of spinal cord stimulation for chronic complex regional pain syndrome type I: five-year final followup of patients in a randomized controlled trial. J Neurosurg. 2008;108:292–8.

16. Harke H, Gretenkort P, Ladleif HU, et al. The response of neuropathic pain and pain in complex regional pain syndrome I to carbamazepine and sustained-release morphine in patients pretreated with spinal cord stimulation: a double-blind randomized study. Anesth Analg. 2001;92(2):488–95.

17. Simpson EL, Duenas A, Holmes MW, Papaioannou D, Chilcott J. Spinal cord stimulation for chronic pain of neuropathic or ischemic origin: systematic review and economic evaluation. Health Technol Assess. 2009;13(17):iii, ix–x, 1–154.

18. Prager JP, Chang JH. Transverse tripolar spinal cord stimulation produced by a percutaneously placed triple lead system. Presented at the international neuromodulation society world pain congress, San Francisco, 2000 (Abstract)

19. North RB, Shipley J. The neuromodulation therapy access coalition. Practice parameters for the use of spinal cord stimulation in the treatment of chronic neuropathic pain. Pain Med. 2007;8: S200–75.

20. Doleys DM, Olson K. Psychological assessment and intervention in implantable pain therapies. Minneapolis: Medronic Neurologic; 1997.

21. North RB, Kidd DH, Shipley J, Taylor RS. Spinal cord stimulation versus reoperation for failed back surgery syndrome: a cost effectiveness and cost utility analysis based on a randomized, controlled trial. Neurosurgery. 2007;61(2):361–8.

22. Prager JP. Neurostimulation in the treatment of complex regional pain syndrome [Box 28.2, page 391]. In: Krames ES, Peckham PH, Rezai AR, editors. Neuromodulation, vol. 2. Oxford: Elsevier; 2009. p. 385–95.

23. Prager JP, Jacobs M. Evaluation of patients for implantable pain modalities: medical and behavioral assessment. Clin J Pain. 2001;3:206–14.

24. Turk DC, Gatchel R, editors. Psychological approaches to pain management, a practitioners' handbook. 2nd ed. New York: Guilford Publication; 2002.

25. Kumar K, Taylor RS, Jacques L, et al. Spinal cord stimulation versus conventional medical management for neuropathic pain: a multicentre randomized controlled trial in patients with failed back surgery syndrome. Pain. 2007;132(1–2):179–88.

26. North RB, Kidd DH, Zahurak M, et al. Spinal cord stimulation for chronic, intractable pain: two decades' experience. J Neurosurg. 1993;32:384–95.

27. May MS, Banks C, Thomson SJ. A retrospective, long-term, third-party follow-up of patients considered for spinal cord stimulation. Neuromodulation. 2002;5(3):137–44.

28. North RB, Kidd DH, Olin J, et al. Spinal cord stimulation for axial back pain: a prospective controlled trial comparing 16-contact electrode arrays with 4-contact percutaneous electrodes. Neuromodulation. 2006;9(1):56–67.

29. Oakley JC, Weiner RL. Spinal cord stimulation of complex regional pain syndrome: a prospective study of 19 patients at two centers. Neuromodulation. 1999;2:47–50.

30. Long DM, Erickson DE. Stimulation of the posterior columns of the spinal cord for relief of intractable pain. Surg Neurol. 1975;4:134–41.

31. North RB, Kidd DH, Farrokhi F, Piantadosi S. Spinal cord stimulation versus repeated lumbosacral spine surgery for chronic pain: a randomized, controlled trial. Neurosurgery. 2005;56(1):98–106.

32. Kumar K, Wilson JR. Factors affecting spinal cord stimulation outcome in chronic benign pain with suggestions to improve success rate. Acta Neurochir Suppl. 2007;97(PT1):91–9.

33. Burchiel K, Anderson VC, Brown FD, et al. Prospective, multicenter study of spinal cord stimulation for relief of chronic back and extremity pain. Spine. 1996;21(23):2786–94.

34. Turner JA, Loeser JD, Bell KG. Spinal cord stimulation for chronic low back pain: a systematic literature synthesis. Neurosurgery. 1995;37:1088–98; discussion 1095–6.

35. Stanton-Hicks M, Burton AW, Bruehl SP, et al. An updated interdisciplinary clinical pathway for CRPS: report of an expert panel. Pain Pract. 2002;2:1–16.

36. Croom JE, Foreman RD, Chandler MJ, et al. Cutaneous vasodilation during dorsal column stimulation is mediated by dorsal roots and CGRP. Am J Physiol. 1997;272:H950–7.

37. Linderoth B, Fedoresak I, Meyerson BA. Peripheral vasodilation after spinal cord stimulation: animal studies of putative effector mechanisms. Neurosurgery. 1991;28:187–95.

38. Barolat G, Massaro F, He J, et al. Mapping of sensory responses to epidural stimulation of the intraspinal neural structures in man. J Neurosurg. 1993;78:233–9.

39. Dubuisson D. Effect of dorsal-column stimulation on gelatinosa and marginal neurons of cat spinal cord. J Neurosurg. 1989;70: 257–65.

40. Roberts MHT, Rees H. Physiological basis of spinal cord stimulation. Pain Rev. 1994;1:184–98.

41. Foreman RD, Linderoth B, Ardell JL, et al. Modulation of intrinsic cardiac neurons by spinal cord stimulation: implications for its therapeutic use in angina pectoris. Cardiovasc Res. 2000;47: 367–75.

42. North RB, Kidd DH, Olin J, et al. Spinal cord stimulation for axial low back pain: a prospective, controlled trial comparing dual with single percutaneous electrodes. Spine. 2005;30(12): 1412–8.

43. North RB, Kidd DH, Olin J, Sieracki JN. Spinal cord stimulation electrode design: prospective randomized controlled trial comparing percutaneous and laminectomy electrodes: part I: technical outcomes. Neurosurgery. 2002;51(2):381–90.

44. North RB, Ewend MG, Lawton MT, Piantadosi S. Spinal cord stimulation for chronic, intractable pain: superiority of "multichannel" devices. Pain. 1991;44:119–30.

45. Stanton-Hicks M. Plasticity of complex regional pain syndrome (CRPS) in children. Pain Med. 2010;11:1216–23.

46. Prager JP, Stanton-Hicks M. Chapter 41: Neurostimulation. In: Cousins M, editor. Cousins and Bridenbaugh's neural blockade in clinical anesthesia and pain medicine. Philadelphia: Lippincott Williams & Wilkins; 2009. p. 948–90.

47. Ohnmeiss DD, Rashbaum RF, Bogdanffy GM. Prospective outcome evaluation of spinal cord stimulation in patients with intractable leg pain. Spine. 1996;21(11):1344–50.

48. Barolat G, Singh-Sahni K, Staas WE, et al. Epidural spinal cord stimulation in the management of spasms in spinal cord injury: a prospective study. Stereotact Funct Neurosurg. 1995;64(3): 153–64.

49. Budd K. Spinal cord stimulation: cost-benefit study. Neuromodulation. 2002;5(2):75–8.

50. Kumar K, Malik S, Demeria D. Treatment of chronic pain with spinal cord stimulation versus alternative therapies: cost-effectiveness analysis. Neurosurgery. 2002;51(1):106–15.

51. Taylor RS, Van Buyten JP, Buchser E. Spinal cord stimulation for complex regional pain syndrome: a systematic review of the clinical and cost-effectiveness literature and assessment of prognostic factors. Eur J Pain. 2006;10(2):91–101.

52. Kemler MA, Furnee CA. Economic evaluation of spinal cord stimulation for chronic reflex sympathetic dystrophy. Neurology. 2002;59:1203–9.

53. Bell GKK, Kidd DH, North RB. Cost-effectiveness analysis of spinal cord stimulation in treatment of failed back surgery syndrome. J Pain Symptom Manage. 1997;13(5):286–95.

Clinical Applications of Neuromodulation: Section on Angina and Peripheral Vascular Disease

64

Marte A. Martinez and Robert D. Foreman

Key Points

- The gate control theory of Melzack and Wall provided the backdrop for developing various forms of neuromodulation including spinal cord stimulation, but the exact mechanisms remain controversial.
- Spinal cord stimulation for treatment of ischemic conditions activates mechanisms that are fundamentally different from those activated for neuropathic pain.
- Every year, patients are treated worldwide with spinal cord stimulation to alleviate peripheral arterial occlusive disease and chronic refractory angina pectoris.
- The principal indication for using spinal cord stimulation to treat peripheral arterial occlusive disease is severe ischemic pain at rest (Fontaine classification stage 3).
- Spinal cord stimulation for ischemic pain is primarily mediated by suppressing efferent sympathetic activity and antidromic activation of the dorsal roots innervating blood vessels that release calcitonin gene-related peptide.
- Spinal cord stimulation is indicated for patients suffering from angina pectoris (NYHA classes III–IV or Canadian Cardiovascular Society classifications I–IV) and refractory to conventional treatment.
- Basic science research has suggested that angina pain is reduced because pain transmission is reduced in nociceptive pain pathways and cardiac function is improved as a result of stabilizing neurons of the intrinsic cardiac nervous system, activating adrenoreceptors that reduce infarct size, and reducing atrial arrhythmias.

M.A. Martinez, M.D. (✉)
Department of Anesthesiology,
University of Oklahoma Health Sciences Center,
940 SL Young Blvd, Oklahoma City, OK 73104, USA
e-mail: marte-martinez@ouhsc.edu

R.D. Foreman, Ph.D.
Department of Anesthesiology,
University of Oklahoma Health Sciences Center,
940 SL Young Blvd, Oklahoma City, OK 73104, USA

Department of Physiology,
University of Oklahoma College of Medicine,
Oklahoma City, OK, USA
e-mail: robert-foreman@ouhsc.edu

Background

Clinical neuromodulation refers to the use of electrical stimulation of a peripheral nerve, the spinal cord, or the brain for relief of pain. For centuries, physicians have been interested in deriving therapeutic benefit from the use of electrical impulses to treat a variety of diseases. In fact, the first medical use of electricity is credited to a Roman physician named Scribonius Largus who described the use of the electric torpedo fish in the treatment of headaches and gouty arthritis. In his work titled *Compositiones Medicae* [1], Scribonius described the placement of a fish across the forehead or affected area to deliver a shock that alleviated pain much like a modern transcutaneous electrical nerve stimulators (TENS). As human understanding and utilization of electricity evolved so did its use in the treatment of various disease states.

In the early twentieth century, Head and Thompson proposed the theory that certain discriminative sensations including touch could exert an inhibitory effect on pain impulses; furthermore, that this facilitation or inhibition of sensory impulses was mediated in the posterior horn before the signal was relayed to secondary interneurons [2]. The idea that chronic pain involved an imbalance between the epicritic and the protopathic components of pain in which the epicritic sensory system exerted an inhibitory influence over the protopathic sensations led, in part, to the modern era of neuromodulation [3]. This era moved forward with the first trials of sensory electrical thalamic stimulation via implanted electrodes for treating severe neuropathic pain conditions that were performed in Paris [4]. Mazars and colleagues hypothesized that sensory thalamic stimulation could compensate for a deficit of epicritic information by artificially enhancing the epicritic level [4].

In a 1965 *Science* article entitled "Pain Mechanisms: A New Theory," Melzack and Wall [5] proposed the gate control theory which allowed for significant advancement of our understanding about pain control over the next decades. This theory proposed that the balance of activity between large and small nerve fibers in the peripheral nervous system determines whether signals are transmitted centrally. According to the theory, small-diameter fibers, which carry nociceptive (pain) signals, impede inhibitory cells located in the dorsal horn (DH) and when small fiber input is dominant leads to central transmission of nociceptive stimuli ("open gate") to areas of the brain that interpret this information as painful. However, when large-diameter fiber input dominates, inhibitory cells are stimulated and hence "close the gate." Since electric stimulation depolarizes large-diameter fibers before small fibers are affected, Melzack and Wall stated that selective stimulation of larger-diameter fibers could have therapeutic implications in the treatment of pain. Based on this study, Shealy [6] delivered current directly to the spinal cord of a terminal cancer patient via an implanted electrode and an external pulse generator that he called a "dorsal column stimulator" successfully relieving the patient's otherwise intractable pain. Today, we refer to "dorsal column stimulation" as spinal cord stimulation (SCS).

The gate control theory was heavily criticized throughout the 1970s and remains controversial because of apparent inconsistencies noted during clinical experience. For example, according to the gate control theory, all pain should be inhibited by electrical stimulation; however, clinical studies have demonstrated that although SCS clearly demonstrates benefit in the treatment of neuropathic pain, acute and nociceptive pain signals are only minimally affected [7, 8]. Moreover, *large fiber activity* can itself signal pain during sunburns, for example, which is opposite with the view that all large/diameter fibers stimulate inhibitory cells and prevent central transmission of painful stimuli [9]. Although the gate control theory was not completely novel and has remained controversial, it is impossible to overstate its importance and impact on modern pain research [10]. In fact, today, neuromodulation involves the placement of a SCS for the treatment of neuropathic pain for which there may be only a few alternative therapies.

It is estimated that each year over 18,000 new SCS implantations are performed worldwide for a variety of conditions including peripheral arterial occlusive disease (POAD) and chronic refractory angina pectoris [11–13]. SCS implantation is a minimally invasive, reversible procedure that offers its candidates the advantage of undergoing a screening trial with a temporary SCS system to ensure efficacy of treatment before permanent implantation is performed. Unlike other surgical procedures that aim to ablate pain pathways, SCS implantation results in minimal anatomic changes. As such, SCS is expected to ameliorate but not eliminate neuropathic pain and can provide sustained pain relief for decades in some patients. The application of SCS at various levels along the dorsal aspect of the spinal cord has been found to have different effects and to affect function in different organ systems. For example, evidence suggests that mechanisms involved when SCS is utilized for treatment of ischemic conditions are fundamentally different than those for neuropathic pain [14, 15].

Spinal cord stimulation is a safe and effective therapy for a variety of patients; however, the lack of knowledge of its clinical usefulness and underlying mechanisms especially for treating cardiac diseases and peripheral vascular disease has deterred its dissemination into mainstream practice. The initial high cost of SCS implantation has been considered an initial deterrent, but recent studies have demonstrated the cost-effectiveness of SCS versus coronary artery bypass grafting in conditions such as cardiac ischemia [16]. One additional hurdle to mainstream acceptance of the use of SCS in conditions such as PAOD and refractory cardiac ischemia is a consistent referral of these patients from primary care and internal medicine physicians to a cardiologist. While cardiologists have used electrical stimulation for more than 50 years for cardiac rhythm management, the idea that SCS can alter and improve coronary blood flow and functional status is a novel idea [17]. To date, hesitance in referring patients to physicians who specialize in neuromodulation reflects a lack of knowledge and understanding of the therapy. Strides must be made to implement education programs that promote a shift in awareness that would allow primary care physicians, cardiologists, cardiovascular surgeons, and pain physicians to work hand in hand for the benefit of the patient [17].

Spinal Cord Stimulation for Peripheral Arterial Occlusive Disease (PAOD)

PAOD is responsible for the majority of ischemic conditions in the limbs [18]. In addition to its impairment of activity of daily living (ADL) and quality of life (QOL), PAOD is a major cause of disability, loss of work, and lifestyle changes in the United States [18, 19]. It is estimated that PAOD affects two million Americans with an incidence of 2 % in men under 50 years old and 5 % in men over 70 years old; although the incidence in women is similar, on average onset of disease is delayed by 10 years [20]. SCS has been used for the treatment of PAOD and vasospastic conditions, such as Raynaud's syndrome, for over 30 years and was originally described by Cook et al. in 1976 [21].

Table 64.1 The Fontaine classification of symptoms in peripheral vascular disease

Stage	Clinical features
I	Arteriosclerosis with no symptoms
II	Intermittent claudication with no symptoms at rest
IIa	Intermittent medium claudication (after 200 m of walking)
IIb	Intermittent severe claudication (before 200 m of walking)
III	Claudication, symptoms at rest and night pain without tissue involvement
IV	Grade III + tissue loss (ischemic ulceration; gangrene)
IVa	With local inflammation
IVb	With widespread inflammation

PAOD is usually caused by atherosclerosis leading to an imbalance between oxygen supply and demand. PAOD begins as intermittent claudication with only 1–2 % of cases progressing to critical ischemia classified as Fontaine stage III or IV (Table 64.1). With major advancements made in vascular surgery techniques allowing longer bypass grafting procedures, SCS implantation is considered only after vascular surgery and medications have failed to prevent the progress of PAOD. The principal indication for the use of SCS is severe ischemic pain at rest (stage III). SCS is not likely to relieve neuropathic pain associated with injury to peripheral nerves cause by ischemia and diabetes. Likewise, SCS is also not expected to alleviate peripheral nociceptive pain associated with ulcerations or edema from venous insufficiency. The patient should be made aware that only deep aching ischemic pain may respond to treatment [22]. Transcutaneous oxygen pressure (TcpO$_2$) measured on the diseased extremity should range between 10 and 30 mmHg; additionally, a TcpO$_2$ gradient of supine to sitting position measurements exceeding 15 mmHg predicts a greater benefit [22–24]. Patient ulcerations should not exceed 3 cm in diameter although benefit of SCS for arresting tissue loss may be the primary goal with the aim of permitting a more distal amputation site [25].

Exclusion Criteria (Adapted from [26])

1. Life expectancy <3 months.
2. Lack of patient compliance.
3. Ischemic ulcerations >3 cm.
4. Wet gangrene.
5. Presence of infection.
6. Imminent acute obliteration requiring emergency amputation.
7. The use of SCS in the presence of an on-demand pacemaker is relatively contraindicated.

8. MRI with body coil is absolutely contraindicated after SCS implantation.

Mechanism of Action

Ischemic pain is the only nociceptive pain that is proven to respond to SCS. As opposed to mechanisms involved in neuropathic pain attenuation, beneficial effect of SCS on ischemic pain involves attenuation of tissue ischemia as a result of increasing and/or redistributing blood flow to ischemic area or by decreasing tissue oxygen demand to the ischemic area. SCS has been shown to improve microcirculation in an animal model [27]. These effects appear to be mediated by two mechanisms: (1) suppression of efferent sympathetic activity (via nicotinic ganglionic receptors and mainly alpha-1 adrenoreceptors in the periphery) and (2) antidromic mechanisms involving the dorsal roots that stimulate the release of calcitonin gene-related peptide (CGRP) [15]. The balance of these mechanisms depends on a variety of factors including the tone of the sympathetic nervous system, patient factors (diet, genetic differences, etc.), and intensity of SCS [29]. Figure 64.1 illustrates the mechanisms and neurotransmitters known or hypothesized to be involved in the effects of SCS in PAOD. A thorough review of the putative mechanisms behind the effects of SCS on peripheral vascular disease is found in Wu et al. [29].

Spinal Cord Stimulation for Angina Pectoris

Angina usually occurs during episodes of vasospasm or occlusion of the coronary vessels that results in an imbalance between the supply and the demand of oxygen in the heart due to decreased blood flow to the heart. Patients with angina pectoris are often managed effectively through pharmacological treatment with beta-receptor blocking agents, long-acting nitrates, and calcium antagonists, by revascularization procedures such as coronary bypass surgery (CABG) or by percutaneous transluminal coronary angioplasty (PTCA); however, a segment of patients suffering from chronic angina pectoris does not respond to conventional treatments [30]. Many patients suffering from severe disabling angina (New York Heart Association (NYHA) classes III–IV) suffer from concurrent comorbidities, making them unsuitable for major invasive procedure. Other patients suffer from widespread obliteration or distal lesions that do not permit successful surgical interventions. Regardless of the etiology, these patients suffer from what is termed treatment refractory angina and have a low quality of life, limited physical capacity, and frequent hospital admissions representing a large costs for society [31]. Patients suffering from treatment refractory angina led clinicians to develop alternative strategies such as neuromodulation to provide pain relief. In

Fig. 64.1 (**a**, **b**) Illustrates the mechanisms and neurotransmitters known or hypothesized to be involved in the effects of SCS in PAOD

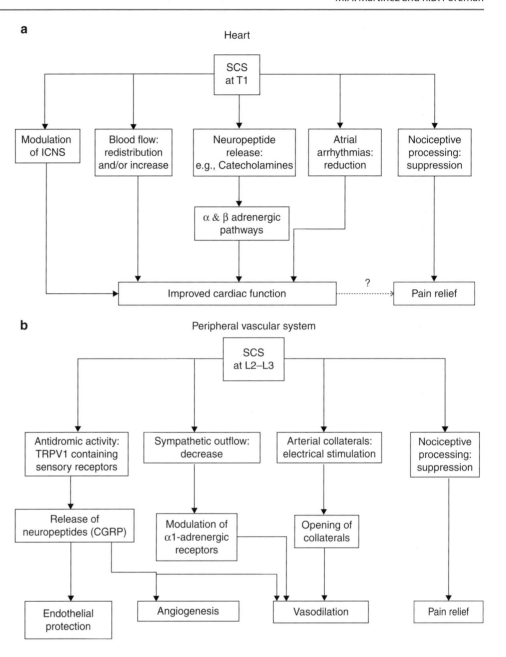

European estimates, refractory angina is a common condition with a prevalence of 100,000 patients [32]. SCS has been used to treat such therapy-resistant angina pectoris since the mid-1980s [33, 34]. The first ten cases of SCS directed specifically at the treatment of angina were reported in 1987 by Murphy and Giles [34].

Patient selection involves specific criteria that maximize the likelihood of clinical success and eliminates patients that are not likely to benefit in an effort to prevent these patients from undergoing an unnecessary procedure in lieu of their multiple comorbidities. The following inclusion and exclusion criteria are adapted from [26].

Inclusion Criteria

1. Severe angina pectoris (NYHA classes III–IV or Canadian Cardiovascular Society classifications I–IV) refractory to conventional treatment. Patients who have been subjected to thoracotomy may present with post-thoracotomy syndrome or intercostal neuralgia, so a careful pain assessment is mandatory. Efficacy of treatment is related to angina that is due to a reversible cardiac insult.
2. Significant coronary artery disease.
3. Demonstrated reversible myocardial ischemia as a cause of patient's symptoms.

4. Patients diagnosed as suffering from syndrome X.
5. Success of TENS in pain alleviation indicates a high likeliness for a positive response to SCS.

Exclusion Criteria

1. Acute myocardial infarction.
2. Presence of other ongoing heart diseases such as pericarditis or myocarditis.
3. Presence of on-demand pacemaker (relative contraindication).
4. MRI investigation with body coil is an absolute contraindication after implantation.

Mechanism of Action

Ischemic heart disease often presents as shortness of breath and angina pectoris, described clinically as an extremely intense substernal crushing pain and that usually radiates to the chest, shoulder and left arm, and occasionally to the neck and jaw [33, 35]. This nociceptive information is transmitted by sensory afferent fibers that enter the C7–T5 spinal segments and synapse on spinothalamic tract cells, and cells of other ascending pathways, that also receive converging cutaneous and muscle input from the overlying somatic structures such as the chest and upper arm [35]. This nociceptive information is also transmitted in nociceptive vagal afferent fibers that converge on spinothalamic tract cells in the upper cervical segments that also receive somatic convergent input from the neck and jaw [35].

Although investigators disagree about the mechanisms responsible for the alleviation of angina pain by SCS, human studies have shown that SCS reduces ischemia by redistributing coronary blood flow [36, 37] and also by decreasing cardiac myocyte oxygen demand [38]. Patients also benefit from increased time to angina in exercise tests [37], increased resistance to critical ischemia [38], and modulation of cardiac neurons leading to decreased dysrhythmias [14, 39]. Of particular importance is that SCS does not mask myocardial infarction [40, 41]. Animal studies have shown that SCS suppresses pain transmission in nociceptive pathways and improves cardiac function by stabilizing neurons of the intrinsic cardiac nervous system, reducing infarct size via adrenoreceptors, and reducing ST segment changes during ischemic episodes, and reducing atrial arrhythmias [42] (for review see Foreman et al. [43]; Wu et al. [29]). Figure 64.1 illustrates the mechanisms and neurotransmitters known or hypothesized to be involved in the effects of SCS in angina.

Preoperative Considerations

Careful preoperative evaluation of patients with PAOD and angina pectoris is mandatory since these patients often have an assortment of coexisting comorbidities that makes even a minimally invasive procedure a challenge. SCS requires active patient participation to ensure proper placement of electrodes with the goal of covering the patient's pain with a comfortable level of paresthesia that completely covers the affected area. During preoperative evaluation, a psychological evaluation performed by a psychologist or a pain-oriented psychiatrist may reveal certain psychological conditions that may exclude patient's from SCS treatment including major personality disorders, deficient capacity to collaborate and to communicate their pain, and drug-seeking behavior or abuse. A thorough analysis of the patient's pain is mandatory since many mixed pain conditions (i.e., coexisting neuropathic and nociceptive pains) may not respond to treatment and may result in clinical failure. Risks and benefits including spinal cord or nerve injury, dural puncture, epidural hematoma, headache, and infection should be discussed with the patient, and all questions and concerns should be answered or addressed appropriately.

Patients with chronic pain conditions are usually being treated with multiple pain medications, and in general, all pain medications should be continued until 2 h before the procedure is performed. Transdermal patches may be continued throughout the procedure. A majority of chronic pain patients do not respond well to increased or additional pain and are seemingly immune to normal doses of systemic analgesics. Caution should be used with liberal dosing of opioids as these patients remain vulnerable to overdose and oversedation may lead to difficulty in communicating with patient to ensure proper electrode placement. Copious use of local anesthetic may be utilized; however, the maximum dose of local anesthetic should be calculated preemptively to avoid toxic dosages. Patients on antipsychotic medications are at risk for developing neuroleptic malignant syndrome.

Chronic pain conditions are associated with numerous physiologic abnormalities of which the practitioner should remain vigilant. Patients will often be deconditioned and have a decreased respiratory reserve due to decreased physical activity caused by pain. As with all procedures involving prolonged immobility, a careful neurologic evaluation should be performed to detect preexisting deficits. Chronic opioid users have decreased gastric emptying and GI motility with superimposed chronic constipation. These patients are at an increased risk of aspiration, and care should be taken if emergency tracheal intubation becomes necessary. It is prudent to administer aspiration prophylaxis including 10–20 mg of intravenous metoclopramide 30 min before transport to the operating room and 30 mL oral Na citrate on transport to operating room.

Intraoperative Considerations and Technique

Following the placement of standard monitors and an intravenous catheter, sedation with midazolam is initiated as the patient is placed in the prone or lateral position. Antibiotic coverage with 1–2 g of cefazolin is administered. The majority of percutaneous SCS electrodes are placed in the prone position with the aid of frontal fluoroscopy. Sterile technique is mandatory as infection in the epidural space can lead to catastrophic consequences if an epidural abscess should develop. As previously discussed, the procedure is performed under copious local anesthesia.

Epidural puncture is usually performed 20 cm below the target level (C7–T2 for angina [usually slightly to the left] and T10–11 for PAOD); however, desired position of the active electrodes and the length of the leads must be taken into account. Thoracic SCS placement mandates a lateral-oblique approach that is also used for lumbar SCS placement. A loss-of-resistance technique with air or saline using a Tuohy needle is used to locate the epidural space. Fluoroscopic guidance may aid in determining correct location of the epidural space if location proves difficult. The lead is manipulated using fluoroscopy until desired position is obtained. Intraoperative test stimulation is used to finalize placement of the lead over the target area. The goal of stimulation should be to completely cover the painful area (or at least 75–80 %) with a tolerable level of paresthesia, which requires patient cooperation and interaction. Some clinicians recommend testing the electrode position in the sitting position because it may provide a more stable electrode position. Frequency of stimulation ranges between 50 and 120 Hz, with a pulse width between 100 and 500 μs. The effective amplitude can vary but usually falls in the range of 2–6 V. The effective amplitude should ultimately be set to produce comfortable effective stimulation. There are a variety of electrode designs and configurations to choose from, and ultimately, clinicians should use equipment which with they feel comfortable. To date, there is little evidence supporting that superiority of technically more advanced types of SCS over simple quadripolar, transcutaneously implantable electrodes [44].

Electrodes can migrate leading to loss of appropriate paresthesia coverage. Plate electrodes are less likely to dislocate; however, many physicians reserve plate electrodes for clinical situations in which a cable lead has been dislodged, dislocated, or when scar tissue creates technical difficulty in threading cable electrode to target area [25]. Occasionally, pain can change location leading to clinical failure; however, SCS systems allow postimplantation adjustment of stimulation parameters to recapture coverage or "steer" paresthesia to a new location [25]. Surgical intervention for readjustment of SCS is only occasionally encountered. Some patients do not tolerate or dislike paresthesia and do not continue SCS therapy.

Trial stimulation should be performed via temporary electrodes or via temporary, percutaneous connections with potentially permanent electrodes for PAOD [45]. Moreover, many health-care systems mandate a trial stimulation period as a requirement for reimbursement. Data on the predictive value of trial stimulation for long-term outcome of PAOD are conflicting, and there are no systematic, well-designed studies demonstrating the improvement of long-term outcome after success of trial stimulation. Trial stimulation period is performed for 1–2 weeks, and pain scores using visual analogue scale (VAS), opioid consumption, value for their daily life activities, as well as objective measures of peripheral blood flow should be assessed to indicate success of SCS. Because of the high success rate when SCS is applied for angina pectoris, systems can be applied in one session when being used for this purpose.

Postoperative Considerations

Postoperative complications include spinal cord injury, epidural hematoma, or abscess/other infection and require prompt postoperative neurologic assessment if suspected. Postoperative pain scores range from 3 to 8 on a VAS, and patients may require increased pain medication dosages as they are frequently intolerant of postoperative pain. Opioids should be used with caution as patients remain susceptible to narcotic overdose including respiratory distress in response to the patient's usual opiate dose if relief is achieved. If SCS has produced significant pain relief, patients may experience drug withdrawal symptoms from a rapid decrease in their opioid usage and may need to be tapered. A 50 % reduction in pain is generally considered as an accepted clinical goal of SCS treatment; however, most single measures of clinical success have limitations [46]. Hence, pain reduction needs to be coupled with functional capacity increase as well as improved quality of life to demonstrate success.

References

1. Largus S. Compositiones. In: Helmreick G, editor. Leipzig: Teubner; 1887.
2. Head H, Thompson T. The grouping of afferent impulses within the spinal cord. Brain. 1906;29:537–741.
3. Head H, Holmes G. Sensory disturbances from cerebral lesions. Brain. 1911;34:103–254.
4. Mazars G, Roge R, et al. Results of the stimulation of the spinothalamic fasciculus and their bearing on the physiopathology of pain. Rev Prat. 1960;103:136–8.
5. Melzack R, Wall PD. Pain mechanisms: a new theory. Science. 1965;150(699):971–9.
6. Shealy CN, Mortimer JT, Reswick JB. Electrical inhibition of pain by stimulation of the dorsal columns: preliminary clinical report. Anesth Analg. 1967;46(4):489–91.
7. Lindblom U, Meyerson BA. Influence on touch, vibration and cutaneous pain of dorsal column stimulation in man. Pain. 1975;1:257–70.
8. Linderoth B, Meyerson BA. Dorsal column stimulation: modulation of somatosensory and autonomic function. In: Mcmahon SB,

Wall PD, editors. The neurobiology of pain, Seminars in the neurosciences. London: Academic; 1995. p. 263–77.

9. Campbell JN, Davis KD, Meyer RA, et al. The mechanism by which spinal cord stimulation affects pain: evidence for a new hypothesis. Pain. 1990;5:S223.

10. Dickenson AH. Gate control theory of pain stands the test of time. Br J Anaesth. 2002;88(6):755–7.

11. Simpson B. Electrical stimulation and the relief of pain. Pain Res Clin Manag. 2003;15:131–42.

12. Eddicks S, Maier-Hauff K, Schenk M, Müller A, Baumann G, Theres H. Thoracic spinal cord stimulation improves functional status and relieves symptoms in patients with refractory angina pectoris: the first placebo-controlled randomised study. Heart. 2007; 93:585–90.

13. Hautvast RW, DeJongste MJ, Staal MJ, van Gilst WH, Lie KL. Spinal cord stimulation in chronic intractable angina pectoris: a randomized, controlled efficacy study. Am Heart J. 1988;136: 1114–20.

14. Myerson B, Linderoth B. Spinal cord stimulation: mechanisms of action in neuropathic and ischemic pain. In: Simpson B, editor. Electrical stimulation and relief of pain. New York: Elsevier; 2003. p. 161–82.

15. Linderoth B, Foreman R. Mechanisms of spinal cord stimulation in painful syndromes. Role of animal models. Pain Med. 2006;7 Suppl 1:14–26.

16. Andréll P, Ekre O, Eliasson T, et al. Cost-effectiveness of spinal cord stimulation versus coronary artery bypass grafting in patients with severe angina pectoris – long-term results from the ESBY study. Cardiology. 2003;99:20–4.

17. Levy RM. Spinal cord stimulation for medically refractory angina pectoris: can the therapy be resuscitated? Neuromodulation. 2011;14:1–5.

18. Garcia LA. Epidemiology and pathophysiology of lower extremity peripheral arterial disease. J Endovasc Ther. 2006;13:II3–9.

19. Golomb BA, Dang TT, Criqui MH. Peripheral arterial disease: morbidity and mortality implications. Circulation. 2006;114: 688–99.

20. Chochola M, Linhart A. Epidemiology of ischemic diseases of the lower extremities. Cas Lek Cesk. 2006;145:368–70.

21. Cook AW, Oygar A, Baggenstos P, et al. Vascular disease of extremities: electrical stimulation of spinal cord and posterior roots. N Y State J Med. 1976;76:366–8.

22. Klomp HM, Spincemaille GH, et al. Spinal-cord stimulation in critical limb ischaemia: a randomized trial ESES study group. Lancet. 1999;353(9158):1040–4.

23. Ubbink DT, Spincemaille GH, et al. Microcirculatory investigations to determine the effect of spinal cord stimulation for critical leg ischemia: the Dutch multicenter randomized controlled trial. J Vasc Surg. 1999;30(2):236–44.

24. Ubbink DT, Gersbach PA, et al. The best TcpO(2) parameters to predict the efficacy of spinal cord stimulation to improve limb salvage in patients with inoperable critical leg ischemia. Int Angiol. 2003;22(4):356–63.

25. Linderoth B, Meyerson BA. Spinal cord stimulation; techniques, indications and outcome. In: Lozano AM, Gildenberg PL, Tasker RR, editors. Textbook of stereotactic and functional neurosurgery. 2nd ed. Berlin/Heidelberg: McGraw Hill/Springer; 2009. p. 3288.

26. Linderoth B, Simpson BA, Myerson BA. Spinal cord and brain stimulation, Chap. 37. In: McMahon S, Kolzenburg M, editors. Wall and Melzack's textbook of pain. 5th ed. Amsterdam: Elsevier; 2005. p. 1–20.

27. Linderoth B. Spinal cord stimulation in ischemia and ischemic pain. In: Horsch S, Clayes L, editors. Spinal cord stimulation III: an innovative method in the treatment of PVD and angina. Darmstadt: Steinkopff Verlag; 1995. p. 19–35.

28. Foreman RD. The neurological basis for cardiac pain. In: Zucker IH, Gilmore JP, editors. Reflex control of the circulation. Boca Raton: CRC Press; 1991. p. 907.

29. Wu M, Linderoth B, Foreman RD. Putative mechanisms behind effects of spinal cord stimulation on vascular diseases: a review of experimental studies. Auton Neurosci. 2008;1381(1–20):9–23.

30. Mannheimer C, Camici P, Chester MR, et al. The problem of chronic refractory angina report from the ESC Joint Study Group on the treatment of refractory angina. Eur Heart J. 2002;23: 355–70.

31. DeJongste MJL, Haaksma J, Hautvast RW, et al. Effects of spinal cord stimulation on daily life myocardial ischemia in patients with severe coronary artery disease. A prospective ambulatory ECG study. Eur Heart J. 1994;71:413–8.

32. Mukherjee D, Bhatt DL, Roe MT, Patel V, Ellis SG. Direct myocardial revascularization and angiogenesis – how many patients might be eligible? Am J Cardiol. 1999;84(5):598–600.

33. Mannheimer C, Augustinsson LE, Carlsson CA, et al. Epidural spinal electrical stimulation in severe angina pectoris. Br Heart J. 1988;59:56–61.

34. Murphy DF, Giles KE. Dorsal column stimulation for pain relief from intractable angina. Pain. 1987;28:365–8.

35. Foreman RD. Mechanisms of cardiac pain. Annu Rev Physiol. 1999;61:143–67.

36. de Vries J, Anthonio RL, Dejongste MJ, Jessurun GA, Tan ES, de Smet BJ, van den Heuvel AF, Staal MJ, Zijlstra F. The effect of electrical neurostimulation on collateral perfusion during acute coronary occlusion. BMC Cardiovasc Disord. 2007;7:18.

37. Mannheimer C, Eliasson T, Andersson B, et al. Effects of spinal cord stimulation in angina pectoris induced by pacing and possible mechanisms of action. BMJ. 1993;307:477–80.

38. Hautwast RW, Blanksma PK, DeJongste MJ, et al. Effect of spinal cord stimulation on myocardial blood flow assessed by positron emission tomography in patients with refractory angina pectoris. Am J Cardiol. 1996;77:462–7.

39. Foreman RD, Linderoth B, Ardell JL, et al. Modulation of intrinsic cardiac neuronal activity by spinal cord stimulation: Implications for its therapeutic in angina pectoris. Cardiovasc Res. 2000;47(2): 367–75.

40. Eliasson T, Augustinsson LE, Mannheimer C. Spinal cord stimulation in severe angina pectoris: presentation of current studies, indications and practical experience. Pain. 1996;65:169–79.

41. Hautvast RW, Ter Horst GJ, DeJong BM, et al. Relative changes in regional blood flow during spinal cord stimulation in patients with refractory angina pectoris. Eur J Neurosci. 1997;9: 1178–83.

42. Cardinal R, Page P, Vermeulen M, Bouchard C, Ardell JL, Foreman RD, Armour JA. Spinal cord stimulation suppresses bradycardias and atrial tachyarrhythmias induced by mediastinal nerve stimulation in dogs. Am J Physiol Regul Integr Comp Physiol. 2006;291: R1369–75.

43. Foreman RD, DeJongste MJL, Linderoth B. Integrative control of cardiac function by cervical and thoracic spinal neurons. In: Armour JA, Ardell JL, editors. Basic and clinical neurocardiology. London: Oxford University Press; 2004. p. 153–86.

44. North RB, Kidd DH, et al. Spinal cord stimulation electrode design: a prospective, randomized, controlled trial comparing percutaneous with laminectomy electrodes: part II-clinical outcomes. Neurosurgery. 2005;57(5):990–6; discussion 990–6.

45. Richard BN, Linderoth B. Spinal cord stimulation: chapter 96. In: Rathmell J, Ballantyne J, Fishman S, editors. Bonica's management of pain. 4th ed. Philadelphia: Lippincott Williams & Wilkins; 2009. p. 16–48: chapter 95.

46. North RB. The glass is half full (commentary on the fallacy of 50% pain relief). Pain Forum. 1999;8:195–7.

Clinical Applications of Neuromodulation: Spinal Cord Stimulation for Abdominal Pain

65

Leonardo Kapural and Marc D. Yelle

Key Points

- Proper patient selection may result in better outcome when SCS is used to treat visceral abdominal pain.
- Team work with referring gastroenterologist and continued collaboration helps to elucidate main cause of the patient's pain and prevents us to conceal any serious symptomatology.
- Diagnostic retrograde differential epidural block can identify those patients who have predominantly visceral abdominal chronic pain.
- Careful placement of the epidural needle and lead is of greatest importance in thoracic area as of presence of the spinal cord.
- Most frequent tip of the lead positioning is around T5 area to achieve paresthesias within the area of abdomen.
- Further studies are needed to explain possible mechanisms of pain relief when spinal cord stimulation is used to treat painful gastrointestinal disorders and to provide more evidence that such treatment would produce long-term improvements in patients' chronic pain.

L. Kapural, M.D., Ph.D. (✉)
Department of Carolinas Pain Institute, Center for Clinical Research,
Wake Forest Baptist Medical Center,
145 Kimel Park Drive, Winston Salem, NC 27103, USA
e-mail: lkapural@wfubmc.edu

M.D. Yelle, M.D., Ph.D.
Department of Carolinas Pain Institute, Center for Clinical Research,
Wake Forest Baptist Medical Center,
145 Kimel Park Drive, Winston Salem, NC 27103, USA

Department of Anesthesiology, Wake Forest Baptist Medical Center,
Winston-Salem, NC, USA
e-mail: marc@yelle.net

Introduction

Chronic abdominal pain poses significant challenges to patients and physicians alike. For patients, pain can limit both professional and personal quality of life [1]. It results in increased doctor visits, imaging and surgery interventions that frequently fail to find a cause or provide relief [2, 3]. For physicians, identification of etiology is fraught with difficulty, largely due to the fact that visceral pain is frequently diffuse and is poorly localized and referred to somatic structures [4, 5]. Abdominal pain is one of the most common complaints for primary care visits [6] and is the leading reason for gastroenterological consultation. These challenges taken together with the high prevalence, frequent office visits and extensive work-up, as well as decreases in productivity, work hours [1, 3], and socioeconomic status, make chronic abdominal pain a significant burden on the patient, physician, healthcare system [1, 3], and society as a whole. In the United States alone, between 20 and 45 % of Americans will suffer from chronic visceral pain [7], of these only 50–70 % will have a definitive etiology of their pain identified [8]. Recent research has provided data helping to better elucidate visceral pain pathways and the dorsal column's role in not only transmission but also amplification of visceral pain. Exciting data in both animal models and human subjects has demonstrated that spinal cord stimulation of the dorsal horn can provide analgesia for chronic visceral pain and improve both quality of life and functional status.

Mechanisms of Abdominal Pain

Data from multiple disciplines have shown that the integration of peripheral (sensory, motor, and autonomic) and central nervous system (spinal cord as well as midbrain and cortex) input to end organs (GI mucosa, glands, muscles, etc.) is essential to normal gastrointestinal physiology. This bidirectional neural circuit has been referred to as the "brain-gut axis" [9, 10]. Imbalance within this system that links visceral sensation with intestinal function is fundamentally

T.R. Deer et al. (eds.), *Comprehensive Treatment of Chronic Pain by Medical, Interventional, and Integrative Approaches*,
DOI 10.1007/978-1-4614-1560-2_65, © American Academy of Pain Medicine 2013

linked to both functional GI disorders as well as chronic visceral pain [11–14]. Chronic visceral pain has been classically thought of as simply a nociceptive sensory disorder, but new evidence suggests that it may not only be entirely organic to the viscera but also neuropathic pain disorder [15, 16].

Peripheral Pathways

Visceral pain is not only difficult for patients to specifically localize to structures within the abdomen; the pain is frequently referred to various somatic structures. This is largely due to complex neurobiology of the visceral pain pathways. Visceral nociceptors are frequently polymodal and can respond to mechanical, thermal, and chemical stimulation [15], but are not uniformly distributed around the abdomen.

Autonomic and spinal nociceptors project on unmyelinated C- or lightly myelinated Aδ-fibers. Like somatic sensory afferents, the cell bodies of visceral afferent fibers are located in the spinal (or dorsal root) ganglia, with the exception of vagal afferents that have cell bodies located in the inferior ganglion of the vagus nerve (nodose ganglia). On their path to the dorsal horn, visceral spinal afferents project collaterals to both prevertebral and paravertebral ganglia allowing for modulation of autonomic response to sensory stimuli. Visceral spinal fibers then enter Lissauer's fasciculus followed by the dorsal gray matter, synapsing on second-order neurons in mostly the substantia gelatinosa (lamina II) and nucleus proprius (laminae IV–VI). These same second-order neurons also receive somatic sensory input. This convergent input explains, in part, why visceral pain is frequently referred to somatic structures [17–19].

Dorsal Horn: Neuromodulation and Hypersensitivity

Data from animal models as well as humans have long demonstrated alterations in activity of dorsal horn neurons in response to peripheral tissue injury [1, 3]; nerve damage [20, 21]; frequent, repeated sensory input [22]; and descending modulation (facilitatory and inhibitory) from midbrain and cortex [23]. Functional plasticity within dorsal horn neurons following sensitization results in enlargement of receptive fields, increased recruitment of peripheral fibers, increases in suprathreshold responses (both in intensity and duration) to sensory input, and even vigorous activation of neurons that are usually silent with normal nociceptive input. In somatic pain, central sensitization in the dorsal horn leads to leftward shift in the stimulus/response curve where normally innocuous stimuli cause painful responses (allodynia) and previously painful stimuli result in an exaggerated response (hyperalgesia). It seems that similar patterns of stimulus/response occur in visceral sensitivity and in functional bowel disorders [24] where exaggerated responses are not only intrinsic to the viscera but also get referred to somatic regions. In animal studies, repeated colonic distension results in the enlargement and convergence of visceral afferent receptive fields, demonstrating the central nervous system involvement in visceral hypersensitivity [25, 26]. In normal human subjects, repeated distension of the viscus results in increased reported pain intensity and referred somatic pain as well as changes in the reported quality of the sensation [27]. These data demonstrate how peripheral visceral input to the CNS can result in hypersensitivity and pain. This hypersensitivity has been shown to be involved in the pathophysiology of chronic visceral pain [28, 29].

Spinal Pathways of Visceral Pain: Spinothalamic Tract and Dorsal Column Pathway

Second-order neurons in the dorsal horn relay afferent (nociceptive) sensory information to thalamus mainly through two ascending pathways, the spinothalamic tract and the spinoreticular tract. Projection neurons, mostly in the substantia gelatinosa and nucleus proprius, project fibers across midline and ascend to thalamus and brainstem in the contralateral, anterolateral spinal cord. The spinothalamic tract is regarded to be the relay primary pathway for visceral nociceptive information [30]. However, dorsal column has been shown to not only transmit some visceral nociceptive information [31] but also modulate (amplify) visceral pain transmission [31]. Lesions in dorsal cervical spinal cord in primates altered responses to colorectal distension, demonstrating that nociceptive information ascends in not only the anterolateral spinal cord (STT) but also the dorsal column pathways [32], which usually thought to transmit purely innocuous sensory information. Anatomical studies identified fibers in both the STT and DC were activated by visceral peripheral nerve stimulation [30]. Other studies have carefully described the dorsal column pathway involvement in modulation of visceral sensory information. With chronic stimulation and/or inflammation of peripheral visceral nerves, plastic changes in receptors and signal transduction occur in postsynaptic dorsal column neurons [33–37].

In several animal studies, visceral pain caused by direct stimulation of organs including the ureter, pancreas, stomach, and colon diminished after DC lesion [30, 38, 39]. This hypothesis is supported by substantial clinical data. In a study conducted in patients with visceral pain related to colon cancer, small midline lesions (either mechanical or radio-frequency myelotomy) relieved pain in 71.5 % (10 or 14) patients [40]. This data has been replicated by multiple surgeons for chronic visceral pain from multiple locations within the abdomen (stomach, liver, pancreas, bowels) and pelvis with considerable success and few complications [4, 41–46]. Patient not only had reductions in reported pain but also decreases in opioid use [46]. Investigations into the exact role of the DC in the processing of visceral information have shown that while the STT tract is central to the relay of sensory information, the DC pathway appears more important than the STT in the modulation of this information [42, 46–48]. These studies suggest that such pathway is an excitatory and central to the visceral pain processing; it may play a critical role in mediating the changes in sensory processing associated with peripheral inflammation and central sensitization. Moreover, it seems likely that the neurons in this DC pathway comprise the ascending arm of the amplification loop by activating descending facilitatory influences from the rostroventral medulla [48]. While surgical lesions have provided significant improvements in patients with cancer-related abdominal and pelvic pain, less invasive treatment options would benefit a larger patient population with more varied and benign pain etiologies.

Spinal Cord Stimulation for Visceral Pain

The use of electrical stimulation of the dorsal horns has been for years to treat numerous chronic pain syndromes [49], originally indicated for back and extremity pain including radicular low back pain, post-laminectomy syndrome [50], complex regional pain syndrome [51, 52], and peripheral vascular disease [53, 54]. Spinal cord stimulation involves delivery of the low current from implantable generator to the epidural leads and contacts, protecting a small electrical field into and around the spinal cord at that level. The mechanism of SCS neuromodulation resulting in pain relief is not completely understood; however, a number of hypotheses have been proposed [49, 55]. Activation of supraspinal pain modulatory pathways by SCS could account for its analgesic effects [56]. It is possible that the SCS modulates the afferent signal in the dorsal horn by "closing the spinal gate" by activating large, myelinated that inhibit small nociceptive fibers [57] or by the release of inhibitory neuromodulators, such as GABA [58, 59]. Alternatively, SCS could provide blockade of nerve conduction [60, 61], possible by antidromic activation. Neurosurgical data (discussed above) suggests that lesioning the postsynaptic DC pathway via midline myelotomy interferes with the generation and maintenance of chronic visceral pain by removing the ascending limb of a facilitatory pain loop. It is possible that the electrical field from SCS also interrupts this ascending limb without physical lesioning of the pathway. Another possible mechanism for SCS is downregulation of intersegmental or supraspinal sympathetic outflow [59, 62–64]. Regardless of the exact mechanism of SCS, the resultant neuromodulation in the dorsal horn provides great potential for the treatment of chronic abdominal pain.

Basic Science

SCS has been studied in rats with and without post-inflammatory visceral hypersensitivity during colonic distention. The visceromotor response (VMR) elicited by colonic distention was suppressed by SCS in both normal and sensitized rats [65]. In addition, the authors reported that the effect of SCS on VMR continued to be observed for a prolonged duration, even after SCS was discontinued. These data are consistent with previous SCS data for treatment of refractory angina pectoris [66] and suggest that SCS may result in persistent, complex alterations of the neural activity and neurotransmitter release. SCS electrodes placed in either cervical or lumbar regions have been shown to inhibit lumbosacral neural responses to colonic distention in rats [67]. These data lead the authors to hypothesize that SCS may cause antidromic activation of peripheral sensory fibers negating the afferent input [67].

Clinical Evidence in Humans

At this time, there is very compelling yet limited data demonstrating the significant improvements, both in reported decreased pain intensity and increased functional capacity in patients with a wide variety of chronic visceral pain syndromes. Level A clinical evidence and recommendations remain years away; still numerous case reports and case series have demonstrated significant clinical improvements and positive treatment outcomes for chronic visceral syndromes including mesenteric ischemic pain [68], esophageal dysmotility [69], gastroparesis [70], IBS [71], chronic pancreatitis [72–75], familial mediterranean fever [76], posttraumatic splenectomy [74], generalized chronic abdominal pain [74], and chronic pelvic pain [62]. While these studies provide encouraging results, the full significance of their findings needs to be validated.

The first reported use of SCS in the treatment of chronic abdominal pain was in an elderly patient with refractory pain secondary to chronic mesenteric ischemia. Transient relief of severe postprandial pain was reported after celiac plexus block; however, the pain quickly returned. In order to provide a long-term relief, SCS system was trialed. Leads were placed in the epidural space at T6 spinal level. Following the procedure, the patient reported paresthesia across her abdomen and complete relief of the pain [68]. Thoracic SCS was also used to treat visceral pain related to inflammatory bowel syndrome (IBS). The patient reported a robust initial reduction in pain. However, this effect was not sustained. The patient experienced paresthesias in distal extremities, but not in the region of her abdominal pain [71]. While the pain relief was transient, immediate and sustained relief of frequent diarrheal episodes was achieved. These data taken together with case studies in esophageal dysmotility [69] and gastroparesis [70] suggest that, in addition to providing visceral pain relief, SCS may improve dysmotility of the functional gastrointestinal disorders. Khan and colleagues [74] reported significant pain relief (mean VAS decrease of 4.9) in long-standing chronic pancreatitis patients using less than half the narcotics required prior to the procedure. These findings were corroborated a later case study of a 38-year-old female with a 13-year history of recalcitrant, chronic pancreatitis [73] who had undergone multiple surgeries and frequent [22] endoscopic retrograde cholangiopancreatography without relief.

Recently, a several much larger case series provided evidence that chronic pancreatitis, but also multiple other chronic abdominal pain and dysmotility syndromes, could be controlled using SCS. Those treatable causes of chronic abdominal pain studied included gastroparesis, mesenteric ischemia, post-gastric bypass chronic epigastric pain, and chronic visceral pain after various intra-abdominal surgeries with present evidence of abdominal adhesions [72, 77, 78].

A first larger study examined 35 patients with chronic visceral pain who underwent SCS trial [72]. The etiology of these patients' pain was confirmed to be visceral ($n=32$) or mixed visceral and central ($n=3$) in origin by retrograde differential epidural block. Five of these patients failed SCS trial. The 30 remaining patients reported at least a 50 % reduction in their pain with significant reductions in pain scores (average pretrial VAS rating of 8.1 ± 1.6 to 3.1 ± 1.6 cm) and an average opioid use (110 ± 119 to 70 ± 68 mg morphine sulfate equivalents). Nineteen patients were followed for 1 year; the remainder were either followed for less than a year ($n=3$); had the SCS removed due to infection or lead migration ($n=4$), were lost to follow-up ($n=1$), or passed SCS trial, but did not have improvement at 6 months and requested explant ($n=1$). The 19 patients that were followed for 1 year following SCS implant maintained low pain rating (VAS of 3.8 ± 1.9 cm and opioid use (38 ± 48 mg morphine equivalents)) [72].

To elucidate further specifics of the technical aspects of SCS when used for chronic abdominal pain, survey was conducted across the United States. Twenty-two physicians reported 70 cases of SCS for various chronic abdominal pain syndromes [77]. The technical characteristics of SCS when used to achieve the optimal spinal cord stimulation in this study were consistent with the data that we collected in above-described retrospective study on 35 consecutive patients [72]. The most frequent placement of the lead (mainly two octrode leads) was posterior epidural midline, and the most frequent vertebral level where the lead tip was positioned was T5 (see Figs. 65.1 and 65.2) [77].

Most recently reported was a clinical experience using SCS in 30 patients with chronic pancreatitis [78]. Patient

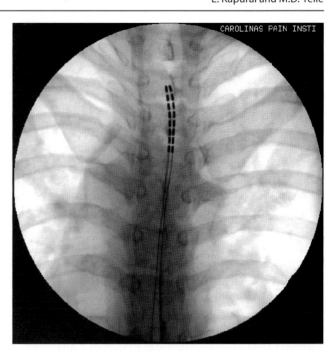

Fig. 65.1 Fluoroscopic anterior-posterior (*AP*) radiograph of thoracic spine with appropriately positioned two octrode leads midline and with the tips positioned at T5. This is the most frequent lead positioning when used for the SCS in painful gastrointestinal disorders

population was somewhat different, as there were 9 out of 30 patients with previous alcohol or opioid abuse. Similar SCS lead placement was required to achieve appropriate paresthesias (T5 ($N=10$) or T6 ($N=10$)). Twenty-four patients (80 %) had >50 % pain relief during the trial. Improvements in VAS pain scores were substantial: from 8 ± 1.6 to 3.6 ± 2 cm at 1 year (same as decrease in opioid use from 165 ± 120 to 48.6 ± 58 mg of morphine equivalents). SCS was very useful therapeutic option for >70 % of trialed patients with severe visceral pain from chronic pancreatitis [78].

Conclusion

When SCS is used in the animal models of colorectal distension and irritant-induced colonic sensitization, data suggest that the SCS may suppress visceromotor reflex in rats [65]. Recent study results suggest that SCS may be a very useful therapeutic option when trialed in patients with various chronic visceral pain conditions [72, 77]. In order to elucidate mechanisms behind such modulatory effect, additional basic science research is required. In addition, prospective, randomized studies are needed to determine the long-term clinical efficacy of SCS (Fig. 65.3).

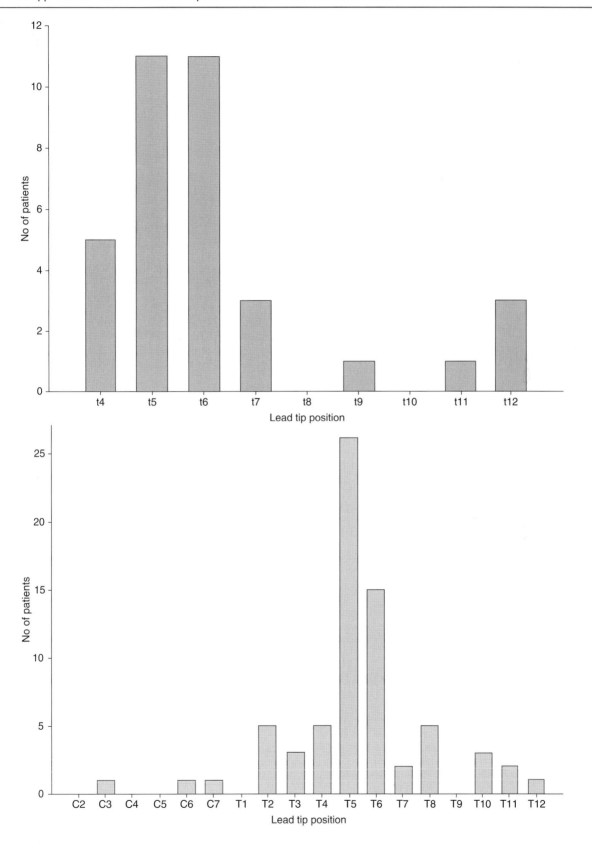

Fig. 65.2 Two graphs below illustrate distribution of the lead tip positions when SCS used for treatment of chronic visceral hyperalgesia. Graphs shown are from two published studies: (**a**) a retrospective larger case series on 35 patients with various causes of abdominal pain and (**b**) a survey that collected data on 70 SCS cases. More than two-thirds of the patients were able to achieve optimal paresthesias to cover the area of abdominal pain when leads were positioned midline and up to T5 or T6 vertebral level (With permission from *Pain Medicine* [72, 77])

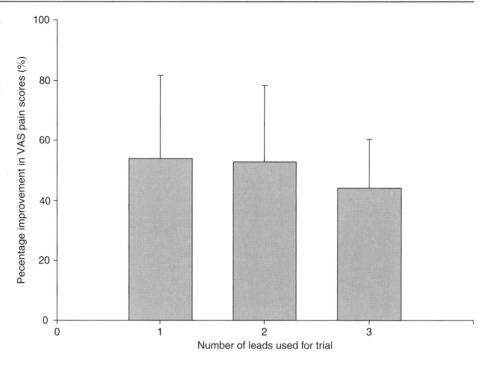

Fig. 65.3 Additional published data on spinal cord stimulation for chronic abdominal pain. It appears that the number of leads used does not influence improvements in pain relief, at least not in below-presented small study. If one, two, or three leads are used in order to provide an optimal trialing, pain relief was comparable at the end of the trial (With permission from Kapural et al. [72])

References

1. Pare P, et al. Health-related quality of life, work productivity, and health care resource utilization of subjects with irritable bowel syndrome: baseline results from LOGIC (Longitudinal Outcomes Study of Gastrointestinal Symptoms in Canada), a naturalistic study. Clin Ther. 2006;28(10):1726–35; discussion 1710–1.

2. Derbyshire SW. Imaging visceral pain. Curr Pain Headache Rep. 2007;11(3):178–82.

3. Russo MW, et al. Digestive and liver diseases statistics, 2004. Gastroenterology. 2004;126(5):1448–53.

4. Giamberardino MA, Vecchiet L. Pathophysiology of visceral pain. Curr Pain Headache Rep. 1997;1(1):23–33.

5. Grundy D. Neuroanatomy of visceral nociception: vagal and splanchnic afferent. Gut. 2002;51 Suppl 1:i2–5.

6. Everhart J. Digestive diseases in the United States: epidemiology and impact, P.H.S. US Department of Health and Human Services, National Institute of Diabetes and Digestive and Kidney Diseases, NIH publication No. 94–1447. p. 3–53.

7. Graney DO. General considerations of abdominal pain. In: Loesser JD, editor. Bonica's management of pain. Philadelphia: Lippincott, Williams & Williams; 2001. p. 1235–68.

8. Klinkman MS. Episodes of care for abdominal pain in a primary care practice. Arch Fam Med. 1996;5(5):279–85.

9. Camilleri M, Ford MJ. Functional gastrointestinal disease and the autonomic nervous system: a way ahead? Gastroenterology. 1994;106(4):1114–8.

10. Mayer EA, Raybould HE. Role of visceral afferent mechanisms in functional bowel disorders. Gastroenterology. 1990;99(6):1688–704.

11. Elsenbruch S. Abdominal pain in Irritable Bowel Syndrome: a review of putative psychological, neural and neuro-immune mechanisms. Brain Behav Immun. 2011;25(3):386–94.

12. Mertz H. Review article: visceral hypersensitivity. Aliment Pharmacol Ther. 2003;17(5):623–33.

13. Wood JD. Neuropathophysiology of irritable bowel syndrome. J Clin Gastroenterol. 2002;35(1 Suppl):S11–22.

14. Wood JD. Neuropathophysiology of functional gastrointestinal disorders. World J Gastroenterol. 2007;13(9):1313–32.

15. Gebhart GF. Visceral pain-peripheral sensitisation. Gut. 2000;47 Suppl 4:iv54–5; discussion iv58.

16. Gebhart GF. Pathobiology of visceral pain: molecular mechanisms and therapeutic implications IV. Visceral afferent contributions to the pathobiology of visceral pain. Am J Physiol Gastrointest Liver Physiol. 2000;278(6):G834–8.

17. Cervero F, Janig W. Visceral nociceptors: a new world order? Trends Neurosci. 1992;15(10):374–8.

18. Kasparov SA. Viscerosomatic convergence on the lumbar interneurons of the dorsal horn of the spinal cord in cats and rats. Neirofiziologiia. 1992;24(1):3–11.

19. Milne RJ, et al. Convergence of cutaneous and pelvic visceral nociceptive inputs onto primate spinothalamic neurons. Pain. 1981;11(2):163–83.

20. D'Mello R, Dickenson AH. Spinal cord mechanisms of pain. Br J Anaesth. 2008;101(1):8–16.

21. Wall PD, Woolf CJ. The brief and the prolonged facilitatory effects of unmyelinated afferent input on the rat spinal cord are independently influenced by peripheral nerve section. Neuroscience. 1986;17(4):1199–205.

22. Woolf CJ, Fitzgerald M. The properties of neurons recorded in the superficial dorsal horn of the rat spinal cord. J Comp Neurol. 1983;221(3):313–28.

23. Millan MJ. Descending control of pain. Prog Neurobiol. 2002;66(6):355–474.

24. Price DD, et al. Peripheral and central contributions to hyperalgesia in irritable bowel syndrome. J Pain. 2006;7(8):529–35.

25. Cervero F, Laird JM, Pozo MA. Selective changes of receptive field properties of spinal nociceptive neurons induced by noxious visceral stimulation in the cat. Pain. 1992;51(3):335–42.

26. Hylden JL, et al. Expansion of receptive fields of spinal lamina I projection neurons in rats with unilateral adjuvant-induced inflammation: the contribution of dorsal horn mechanisms. Pain. 1989;37(2):229–43.

27. Ness TJ, Metcalf AM, Gebhart GF. A psychophysiological study in humans using phasic colonic distension as a noxious visceral stimulus. Pain. 1990;43(3):377–86.

28. Verne GN, et al. Central representation of visceral and cutaneous hypersensitivity in the irritable bowel syndrome. Pain. 2003;103(1–2):99–110.

29. Verne GN, Robinson ME, Price DD. Hypersensitivity to visceral and cutaneous pain in the irritable bowel syndrome. Pain. 2001;93(1):7–14.

30. Palecek J, Paleckova V, Willis WD. Fos expression in spinothalamic and postsynaptic dorsal column neurons following noxious visceral and cutaneous stimuli. Pain. 2003;104(1–2):249–57.

31. Palecek J, Willis WD. The dorsal column pathway facilitates visceromotor responses to colorectal distention after colon inflammation in rats. Pain. 2003;104(3):501–7.

32. Al-Chaer ED, Feng Y, Willis WD. A role for the dorsal column in nociceptive visceral input into the thalamus of primates. J Neurophysiol. 1998;79(6):3143–50.

33. Ishigooka M, et al. Spinal NK1 receptor is upregulated after chronic bladder irritation. Pain. 2001;93(1):43–50.

34. Okano S, Ikeura Y, Inatomi N. Effects of tachykinin NK1 receptor antagonists on the viscerosensory response caused by colorectal distention in rabbits. J Pharmacol Exp Ther. 2002;300(3):925–31.

35. Palecek J, Paleckova V, Willis WD. Postsynaptic dorsal column neurons express NK1 receptors following colon inflammation. Neuroscience. 2003;116(2):565–72.

36. Wu J, et al. The role of c-AMP-dependent protein kinase in spinal cord and post synaptic dorsal column neurons in a rat model of visceral pain. Neurochem Int. 2007;50(5):710–8.

37. Polgar E, et al. GABAergic neurons that contain neuropeptide Y selectively target cells with the neurokinin 1 receptor in laminae III and IV of the rat spinal cord. J Neurosci. 1999;19(7): 2637–46.

38. Feng Y, et al. Epigastric antinociception by cervical dorsal column lesions in rats. Anesthesiology. 1998;89(2):411–20.

39. Houghton AK, Kadura S, Westlund KN. Dorsal column lesions reverse the reduction of homecage activity in rats with pancreatitis. Neuroreport. 1997;8(17):3795–800.

40. Gildenberg PL, Hirshberg RM. Limited myelotomy for the treatment of intractable cancer pain. J Neurol Neurosurg Psychiatry. 1984;47(1):94–6.

41. Becker R, Sure U, Bertalanffy H. Punctate midline myelotomy. A new approach in the management of visceral pain. Acta Neurochir (Wien). 1999;141(8):881–3.

42. Hirshberg RM, et al. Is there a pathway in the posterior funiculus that signals visceral pain? Pain. 1996;67(2–3):291–305.

43. Hwang SL, et al. Punctate midline myelotomy for intractable visceral pain caused by hepatobiliary or pancreatic cancer. J Pain Symptom Manage. 2004;27(1):79–84.

44. Kim YS, Kwon SJ. High thoracic midline dorsal column myelotomy for severe visceral pain due to advanced stomach cancer. Neurosurgery. 2000;46(1):85–90; discussion 90–2.

45. Nauta HJ, et al. Surgical interruption of a midline dorsal column visceral pain pathway. Case report and review of the literature. J Neurosurg. 1997;86(3):538–42.

46. Nauta HJ, et al. Punctate midline myelotomy for the relief of visceral cancer pain. J Neurosurg. 2000;92(2 Suppl):125–30.

47. Ness TJ. Evidence for ascending visceral nociceptive information in the dorsal midline and lateral spinal cord. Pain. 2000;87(1): 83–8.

48. Palecek J. The role of dorsal columns pathway in visceral pain. Physiol Res. 2004;53 Suppl 1:S125–30.

49. Krames ES, Foreman R. Spinal cord stimulation modulates visceral nociception and hyperalgesia via the spinothalamic tracts and the postsynaptic dorsal column pathways: a literature review and hypothesis. Neuromodulation. 2007;10(3):224–37.

50. North RB, Kidd DH, Piantadosi S. Spinal cord stimulation versus reoperation for failed back surgery syndrome: a prospective, randomized study design. Acta Neurochir Suppl. 1995;64:106–8.

51. Kumar K, Nath RK, Toth C. Spinal cord stimulation is effective in the management of reflex sympathetic dystrophy. Neurosurgery. 1997;40(3):503–8; discussion 508–9.

52. Stanton-Hicks M. Complex regional pain syndrome: manifestations and the role of neurostimulation in its management. J Pain Symptom Manage. 2006;31(4 Suppl):S20–4.

53. Jivegard LE, et al. Effects of spinal cord stimulation (SCS) in patients with inoperable severe lower limb ischaemia: a prospective randomised controlled study. Eur J Vasc Endovasc Surg. 1995;9(4):421–5.

54. Reig E, et al. Spinal cord stimulation in peripheral vascular disease: a retrospective analysis of 95 cases. Pain Pract. 2001;1(4):324–31.

55. Linderoth B, Foreman R. Mechanisms of spinal cord stimulation in painful syndromes: role of animal models. Pain Med. 2006;7 Suppl 1:S14–26.

56. Saade NE, et al. Inhibition of nociceptive evoked activity in spinal neurons through a dorsal column-brainstem-spinal loop. Brain Res. 1985;339(1):115–8.

57. Linderoth B, Meyerson BA. Physiology of spinal cord stimulation: mechanism of action. In: Burchiel K, editor. Surgical management of pain. Stuttgart: Thieme Medical Publisher Inc; 2002. p. 505–26.

58. Cui JG, et al. Spinal cord stimulation attenuates augmented dorsal horn release of excitatory amino acids in mononeuropathy via a GABAergic mechanism. Pain. 1997;73(1):87–95.

59. Linderoth B, et al. Gamma-aminobutyric acid is released in the dorsal horn by electrical spinal cord stimulation: an in vivo microdialysis study in the rat. Neurosurgery. 1994;34(3):484–8; discussion 488–9.

60. Campbell JN. Examination of possible mechanisms by which stimulation of the spinal cord in man relieves pain. Appl Neurophysiol. 1981;44(4):181–6.

61. Larson SJ, et al. Neurophysiological effects of dorsal column stimulation in man and monkey. J Neurosurg. 1974;41(2):217–23.

62. Kapural L, et al. Spinal cord stimulation is an effective treatment for the chronic intractable visceral pelvic pain. Pain Med. 2006;7(5):440–3.

63. Linderoth B, Fedorcsak I, Meyerson BA. Peripheral vasodilatation after spinal cord stimulation: animal studies of putative effector mechanisms. Neurosurgery. 1991;28(2):187–95.

64. Steege JF. Superior hypogastric block during microlaparoscopic pain mapping. J Am Assoc Gynecol Laparosc. 1998;5(3): 265–7.

65. Greenwood-Van Meerveld B, et al. Attenuation by spinal cord stimulation of a nociceptive reflex generated by colorectal distention in a rat model. Auton Neurosci. 2003;104(1):17–24.

66. Linderoth B, Foreman R. Physiology of spinal cord stimulation: review and update. Neuromodulation. 1999;2:150–64.

67. Qin C, et al. Spinal cord stimulation modulates intraspinal colorectal visceroreceptive transmission in rats. Neurosci Res. 2007;58(1):58–66.

68. Ceballos A, et al. Spinal cord stimulation: a possible therapeutic alternative for chronic mesenteric ischaemia. Pain. 2000;87(1):99–101.

69. Jackson M, Simpson KH. Spinal cord stimulation in a patient with persistent oesophageal pain. Pain. 2004;112(3):406–8.

70. Tiede JM, et al. The use of spinal cord stimulation in refractory abdominal visceral pain: case reports and literature review. Pain Pract. 2006;6(3):197–202.

71. Krames ES, Mousad DG. Spinal cord stimulation reverses pain and diarrheal episodes of irritable bowel syndrome: a case report. Neuromodulation. 2005;8:82–8.

72. Kapural L, Sessler D, Tluczek H, Nagem H. Spinal cord stimulation for visceral abdominal pain. Pain Med. 2010;11(3):347–55.

73. Kapural L, Rakic M. Spinal cord stimulation for chronic visceral pain secondary to chronic non-alcoholic pancreatitis: a case report. Clin Gastroenterol Hepatol. 2008;42(6):750–1.

74. Khan Y, Raza S, Khan E. Application of spinal cord stimulation for the treatment of abdominal visceral pain syndromes: case reports. Neuromodulation. 2005;8:14–27.

75. Kim JK, et al. Spinal cord stimulation for intractable visceral pain due to chronic pancreatitis. J Korean Neurosurg Soc. 2009;46(2):165–7.

76. Kapur S, Mutagi H, Raphael J. Spinal cord stimulation for relief of abdominal pain in two patients with familial Mediterranean fever. Br J Anaesth. 2006;97(6):866–8.

77. Kapural L, Deer T, Yakovlev A, Bensitel T, Hayek S, Pyles S, Narouze S, Khan Y, Kapural A, Cooper D, Stearns L, Zovkic P. Spinal cord stimulation for visceral abdominal pain: results of the national survey. Pain Med. 2010;11(5):685–91.

78. Kapural L, Cywinski J, Sparks D. Spinal cord stimulation for visceral pain from chronic pancreatitis. Neuromodulation. 2011;14(5):423–7.

Cost-Effectiveness of Interventional Techniques

66

Krishna Kumar, Syed Rizvi, Sharon Bishop, and Mariam Abbas

Key Points

- Intrathecal drug therapy (IT) and spinal cord stimulation (SCS) therapy are robust, cost-effective therapies for management of chronic pain and are superior to conventional medical management (CMM).
- From a cost-effectiveness standpoint, it is better to have failed SCS and IT than to be maintained on CMM alone.
- An integrated approach to the treatment of chronic pain will result in improved utilization of limited health-care resources.
- Technological advances that increase hardware lifespan and improve catheter and electrode design will reduce complication rates, further bolstering the already favorable cost profile of these interventions.

K. Kumar, M.B.B.S., M.S., FRCSC (✉)
Department of Neurosurgery, Regina General Hospital,
University of Saskatchewan, Medical Office Wing, 1440-14th Ave,
Regina, SK, S4P 0W5, Canada
e-mail: krishna.kumar902@gmail.com

S. Rizvi, M.D.
Department of Neurosurgery, Regina General Hospital,
c/o Dr. Kumar, 1440-14th Ave, Regina, SK, S4P 0W5, Canada
e-mail: rizvi20s@gmail.com

S. Bishop, BScN, MHlthSci
Department of Neurosurgery, Unit 5A, Regina General Hospital,
1440-14th Ave, Regina, SK, S4P 0W5, Canada
e-mail: sharon.bishop@rqhealth.ca

M. Abbas
Department of Neurosurgery, Regina General Hospital,
1440-14th Ave, Regina, SK, S4P 0W5, Canada
e-mail: maryam14@gmail.com

Introduction

The field of neurostimulation has matured over the past decade to emerge as an important modality for the treatment of intractable chronic pain. Despite relatively high initial costs, a breadth of evidence exists, and extensive clinical experience suggests that spinal cord stimulation and intrathecal drug delivery systems are safe, effective, and economical. The benefits of neuromodulation are manifested in improved functional capability, health-related quality of life (HRQoL), and reduced demand for health-care resources. This results in long-term economic benefit and cost saving. Neuromodulation is a viable option for the early treatment of patients with intractable pain syndromes.

This chapter profiles the development, clinical utility, and cost-effectiveness of two popular neuromodulatory modalities: intrathecal drug therapy (IT) for the management of intractable chronic nonmalignant pain (CNMP) and the role of spinal cord stimulation (SCS) in the treatment of failed back surgery syndrome (FBSS).

Spinal Cord Stimulation

Background

SCS is a safe, reversible, cost-effective, and minimally invasive intervention capable of generating superior outcomes for the treatment of neuropathic pain [1–17]. A large body of evidence supports the application of SCS in a diverse array of clinical scenarios [18–21]. The role of SCS is well established in the treatment for pain resulting from FBSS, complex regional pain syndrome, diabetic neuropathy, and peripheral vascular disease. The beneficial effects of SCS on pain, function, and depression are widely acknowledged [3–5, 22, 23]. It is now recommended that SCS be considered earlier in the treatment continuum in order to maximize patient outcomes and improve the opportunity for successful rehabilitation [2, 13].

T.R. Deer et al. (eds.), *Comprehensive Treatment of Chronic Pain by Medical, Interventional, and Integrative Approaches*,
DOI 10.1007/978-1-4614-1560-2_66, © American Academy of Pain Medicine 2013

Low back pain is extremely common, trailing only hypertension and diabetes as the reason behind most physician office visits [24]. It accounts for a large proportion of healthcare expenditure without clear evidence of improvement in health status. Ten to forty percent of patients undergoing lumbosacral spinal surgery for low back pain (with or without radicular symptoms) fail to achieve satisfactory outcomes and develop persistent or recurrent pain – referred to as FBSS [25]. In this scenario, SCS has proven superior to reoperation, both in terms of pain relief and cost [8, 9].

At present, only three published, randomized, controlled trials have evaluated the impact of SCS in management of FBSS and CRPS [4, 5, 8, 26]. These investigations demonstrate that SCS offers superior pain relief, HRQoL, and functional capacity and is cost-effective compared to conventional medical management (CMM).

Technological innovation, in terms of leads (type and variety), pulse generators (rechargeable and non-rechargeable), and programming capability, facilitates enhanced pain control and outcomes. This has improved the management of axial pain, which has historically defied harnessing.

Scientific Rationale

Through epidural electrode placement, SCS electrically stimulates dorsal columns of the spinal cord. The exact mechanism(s) by which SCS achieves pain control remains unclear. Several experimentally supported theories have been propagated. Initially, the effects of SCS were explained on the basis of Melzack–Wall's gate control theory [27]. However, this explanation proved inadequate and does not fully account for the differential success of SCS in neuropathic pain management.

Mechanisms at play during stimulation may include (1) suppression of the hyperexcitability of wide dynamic range neurons and high-threshold nociceptive-specific spinothalamic neurons in the dorsal column, (2) activation of interneurons at or in close proximity to the substantia gelatinosa which consequently inhibits the deeper laminae III–V in the dorsal horn, and (3) excitation of supraspinal sites such as the pretectal nucleus which in turn produces analgesia by inhibiting nociceptive dorsal horn neurons. The long-lasting effects are thought to be mediated via the dorsolateral funiculus because sectioning of this tract abolishes this beneficial effect. Moreover, SCS is known to produce electrical and chemical alterations as it induces the release of neurotransmitters such as adenosine, glycine, and 5-hydroxytryptamine, while also activating gamma-aminobutyric acid beta-receptors, which in turn decrease excitatory amino acids at the level of the dorsal horn cells [28–32].

Early SCS employed the use of unipolar electrodes. Technological advances have led to the introduction of multichannel quadripolar and octapolar leads which enable bipolar stimulation and are superior to single-channel devices. Single-electrode arrays have been used successfully to produce pain relief, in both unilateral and bilateral pain of the upper or lower extremities [33–40]. At present, dual-electrode arrays (either percutaneously implanted (placed parallel to each other on either side of the midline) or surgically implanted) are more often used in this role. Clinical reports indicate that patients with FBSS, experiencing predominant radicular symptoms, respond well to dual quadripolar or octapolar lead arrays [4, 5, 34, 35, 41]. Computer modeling suggests that patients with predominant axial pain may benefit from the enhanced current steering capabilities offered by tripolar lead configurations [33]. Lead choice primarily depends on surgeon preference taking into consideration underlying pathology. The octapolar lead has an advantage over the quadripolar lead in cases where migration occurs resulting in loss of stimulation-induced paresthesia and recurrence of pain. In these circumstances, pain relief can be restored by reprogramming rather than resorting to surgical intervention. Advances in lead and pulse generator technology have improved clinical outcomes by enabling programming of each individual contact which allows for more accurate and consistent stimulation of the desired body region [36, 37].

In the mid-1970s, the first fully implantable pulse generator (IPG) was introduced and was powered by a non-rechargeable primary cell battery [38]. The disadvantage of this system is that battery life is limited to 2–5 years. When battery exhaustion occurs, a surgical procedure is required for replacement. The first rechargeable IPG was approved by the Federal Drug Administration (FDA) in 2004 (Advanced Bionics, Valencia, California, USA). Bench testing reveals that rechargeable IPGs could last 10–25 years, necessitating fewer replacements and consequently improving morbidity and resulting in cost saving [38].

Intrathecal Drug Therapy

Background

In 1979, Wang, Nauss, and Thomas reported the first human study demonstrating safe, effective intrathecal administration of morphine [42]. Soon thereafter, Behar and associates [43] and Lund [44] demonstrated the efficacy of epidural morphine in pain management. Since the 1980s, IT has been successfully used for the management of CNMP and spasticity [45–64]. IT becomes a valuable tool for patients who have failed multidisciplinary, multimodal treatment algorithms. Over the lifetime of IT, some patients develop tolerance or experience disease progression and have to contend with drug dosage escalation and associated side effects in an attempt to maintain adequate pain control. In these situations, polyanalgesic regimens become necessary [65–68].

As several delivery systems exist, the choice of system is dictated by patients' clinical need. A percutaneous catheter (tunneled or not tunneled) or a catheter with a subcutaneous injection port, connected to an external pump, is suitable for patients with limited life expectancy. However, percutaneous catheters require frequent monitoring for infection and migration. This mode of delivery also restricts patient mobility. For long-term use, a fully implantable system is required. This has the advantage of retaining mobility and functional activity. Fixed-rate delivery systems are less expensive than variable-rate systems but lack flexibility of drug delivery. In fixed-rate systems, dosage adjustments require that drug concentration be changed, which necessitates an additional pump refill. In contrast, programmable systems allow for easy dose alteration without invasive intervention and enable bolus programs (practitioner and/or patient-activated) [62, 63].

The first fully implantable and programmable infusion pump (Medtronic Inc., Minneapolis, MN, USA) became available in 1988 [64]. Technological advances have been paralleled by the availability of pharmaceutical agents for IT use, resulting in the expansion of this field. Presently, opioids are used as single agents or in combination with adjuvant pain medications such as anesthetic or antispasticity drugs [62].

Presently, there are no standard guidelines for patient selection [46, 47]. Common indications for IT include CNMP due to FBSS, mixed neuropathic–nociceptive pain, complex regional pain syndrome, and certain neuropathies including diabetic and small-fiber neuropathy. IT is also utilized to control severe spinal and supraspinal spasms and rigidity which may occur with multiple sclerosis, cerebral palsy, stroke, brain injury, or spinal cord injury [49–61]. It is safe, effective, and cost-efficient [46, 54–58, 69–73].

In 2000, the first expert panel convened to develop basic guidelines for administration and use of IT pharmacotherapy [65]. The consensus statements for intrathecal drug delivery were revised in 2003 and again in 2007 to incorporate new evidence, recently approved medications, and safety warnings [67, 68]. To date, only morphine, ziconotide, and baclofen acquired FDA approval for intrathecal use [68]. However, other agents are used frequently and are done so "off-label."

Scientific Rationale

IT primarily relies on an implantable (programmable) pump which is connected to an intrathecal catheter. This system allows the administration of analgesics directly into the intrathecal space at a specified concentration and rate. The advantage of IT being that analgesia may be obtained at dose levels significantly below those needed if oral therapy is used. This is accompanied by a reduction in dose-related side effects. For instance, subarachnoid delivery has a two orders of magnitude (100-fold) dose advantage over oral delivery [74].

Opioid receptors were originally identified in the spinal cord in 1973 [75]. Cousins in 1979 used the phrase "selective spinal analgesia" to describe the phenomenon that spinally administered opioids could produce a specific analgesic effect with few motor, sensory, or autonomic side effects [76, 77]. Intrathecal opioids exert their analgesic effect pre- and post-synaptically by reducing neurotransmitter release and by hyperpolarizing the membranes of neurons in the dorsal horn, thus inhibiting pain transmission [78].

Intrathecally, local anesthetics exert their effect by sodium channel blockade, which inhibits the action potential in neural tissue in the dorsal horn, producing a reversible analgesic effect. Intrathecal clonidine, an $\alpha2$ agonist, modulates pain transmission by depression of the release of (1) C-fiber neurotransmitters, (2) substance P, and (3) calcitonin gene-related peptide. It has been hypothesized that clonidine also suppresses preganglionic sympathetic outflow [79].

Ziconotide is a calcium channel antagonist specific to the presynaptic terminals in the dorsal horn of the spinal cord. Intrathecal ziconotide is thought to produce its analgesic effects by blocking neurotransmitter release in primary nociceptive afferent fibers [80].

Polyanalgesia is therapeutically beneficial and modulates the various components of pain, with each agent serving to attenuate a specific mechanism involved in producing the pain state. Combinations of different drug classes such as opioids plus local anesthetics (±clonidine) are currently being used in clinical practice. The basis for polyanalgesic therapy includes the following: (1) Multiple agents with different mechanisms of action can more effectively combat clinical pain states which are themselves an amalgam of several mechanisms implicating both central and peripheral neuronal circuits. (2) There is strong evidence that several agents may attenuate the tolerance otherwise associated with an equipotent dose of a monodrug regime. (3) Even if various pain states are produced by a single underlying mechanism, agents acting on different elements of the system may exhibit a synergistic interplay that improves the therapeutic effect [79–81].

Methods

At our multidisciplinary pain clinic, we maintain a database of more than 500 patients. Our present analysis is based on the results of earlier studies in which we compared intervention (SCS or IT) to CMM [4, 5, 16, 72, 73]. A decision analytic model was constructed to examine the cost-effectiveness of intervention versus CMM. We have updated financial data to reflect current economic realities. Additionally, we reexamined patients' charts to verify accuracy of outcomes and utilization of health-care resources.

Tabulation of Costs

The cost basis for each group was calculated by tabulating costs of the initial evaluation, physician visits, diagnostic procedures, adjunctive therapies, medications, and hospital stays for the treatment of breakthrough pain. In addition to this common base cost, the intervention groups incurred additional expenses including the costs of hardware, hospital, and surgical fees for implantation, complications related to the implant procedure and its maintenance, and pharmacotherapy.

All actual costs are based on the year 2011 Canadian dollar which is presently trading at par with the US dollar (March 29, 2011: $1 CDN = $1.02 US). As this study was conducted in Regina, Saskatchewan, Canada, all cost references are taken from that province's fee schedule. The costs of the implantable devices were obtained from the manufacturer's price list for the year 2011 (Medtronic of Canada, Ltd., Brampton, ON). Markup of these products is not permissible under Canadian law. The costs for each category were calculated on an annual basis, extrapolated for the 10-year study period, applied to each group, and then compared. Cost data were organized into the following categories:

1. Pre-implant costs: including professional fees and diagnostic procedures such as magnetic resonance imaging (MRI), computed tomography (CT) scanning, myelography, and lumbar spine x-ray films.
2. Implant procedure costs: including professional surgical fees, operating room fees, hospital stay, and equipment costs.
3. Maintenance costs: consisting of nursing contact, physician consults, medication, associated complications (for intervention groups), and hospitalizations for acute exacerbation of pain.
4. Adjunctive therapy costs: such as acupuncture, physiotherapy, massage, and chiropractic therapy.
5. Pharmacotherapy costs include drug and dispensing costs.

Personnel Cost Analysis

Health-care professional fees are determined through negotiations between various professional groups and the provincial health department. Professional fees calculated in this study are based on the actual year 2011 payments. The costs associated with nursing contacts were calculated according to the hourly wage earned by the neuromodulation nurse. Similarly, costs calculated for contact with physiotherapists, chiropractors, massage therapists, and acupuncturists reflect actual therapy costs.

Diagnostic Costs

The frequency of the imaging procedures performed was extracted from all patients' charts. The cost of each imaging procedure was derived from the actual costs incurred to the hospital as determined by the finance department of the Regina Qu'Appelle Health Region.

Hospitalization Costs

Hospitalization costs at the Regina General Hospital, where the study was based, are $1,500/patient/day.

Oral Pharmacotherapy Costs

The commonly used drugs prior to and following implantation were opioid, antidepressant, nonsteroidal anti-inflammatory, analgesic, or muscle relaxant agents. Costs of pharmacotherapy for each patient were calculated according to the Saskatchewan Health Formulary, allowing a predetermined government-approved pharmacist markup schedule and a flat rate for dispensing according to pharmaceutical standards. From this, we calculated a monthly and subsequently yearly cost, which was then extrapolated to a 10-year period.

Decision Analysis Model

We constructed a Markov-based decision model to simulate the course of events for patients undergoing intervention. We applied the cost–utility guidelines developed by the United Kingdom's National Institute of Clinical Excellence to compare the cost-effectiveness of intervention versus CMM [82]. In each case, the model assumes that CMM remains available as an adjunct treatment. Cost-effectiveness analysis (CEA) was performed to optimize (maximize) effectiveness and minimize cost.

We conducted probabilistic sensitivity analysis (PSA) to account for underlying parameter uncertainty. In a PSA, each parameter is given a probability distribution, and uncertainty in all model parameters was then explored simultaneously using 100,000 Monte Carlo simulations. Medical treatment decisions are subject to uncertainty. Thus, Markov models are preferred over conventional decision trees to avoid unrealistic simplifying assumptions.

The variables we subjected to PSA include clinical success, resource use, complication rate, and hardware failure rate over time. We calculated the cost-effectiveness of each strategy and ranked them accordingly. We also plotted the results as acceptability curves, sensitivity analyses, and net monetary benefit (NMB) graphs and judged them to be cost-effective on the basis of maximum willingness to pay (WTP) thresholds of $20,000/quality-adjusted life year (QALY). We discounted costs and QALYs at an annual rate of 3.5 %.

Spinal Cord Stimulation

All patients were initially managed in a multidisciplinary pain clinic where CMM failed to provide adequate relief. In the previous study, data of 122 consecutive patients with FBSS was utilized. The data were derived from chart reviews and follow-up appointments, supplemented with telephone interviews. The patients were then subdivided into two groups. The groups were matched with respect to age, sex, mean number of operations performed before enrollment into the study (3.3 operations), and time away from work since injury (minimum of 1 year). All patients were evaluated by the same multidisciplinary pain specialist group.

All patients underwent a SCS trial and received permanent implants if they reported ≥50 % pain relief on the visual analogue scale (VAS). While these patients were awaiting trial stimulation, 18 patients either moved or refused to participate in the study and thus were lost to follow-up. These exclusions left a working group of 104 patients who were monitored for a minimum of 5 years. The SCS group consisted of 60 patients (57.7 %; 28 female patients [47 %] and 32 male patients [53 %]), with a mean age of 52.3 years. The CMM group included 44 patients (42.3 %; 21 female patients [48 %] and 23 male patients [52 %]), with a mean age of 51.4 years [16].

At our center, the neuromodulation nurse is responsible for device programming. The cost of SCS is predicated, in part, on the longevity of the IPG which is approximately 4 years in the case of non-rechargeable systems and 9 (Medtronic Inc.), 10 (St. Jude Medical), and 5 (Boston Scientific) years for the various rechargeable IPGs as conservatively provisioned by the FDA. It should be noted that bench testing of the Boston Scientific IPG reflects a lifespan of 10–25 years [38]. In our present analysis, we subsume the cost of IPG replacement at 4 years postimplantation for non-rechargeable systems, and at 9 years for rechargeable ones, these costs are amortized accordingly.

To reflect the current trends in lead choice for implantation, we reviewed our current implant practices over the past 3 years. Accordingly, we apply the present breakdown: 50 % receive a percutaneous octapolar or a 16-contact paddle lead. The remaining 50 % receive dual octapolar leads. Similarly, half of patients are now receiving rechargeable IPGs while the other half have new generation non-rechargeable IPGs such as the Prime-Advanced™ (Medtronic Inc., Minneapolis, MN, USA). These trends are influenced by patient need and choice as well as by budgetary constraints as the hardware is financed through the publically funded Canadian health-care system.

Decision Analytic Model

The model was developed by using software (Excel, Microsoft, Seattle, WA). A decision tree reflects possible initial responses to SCS and a Markov model which simulates costs and QALYs over a 10-year time span (Fig. 66.1).

In this model, patients were divided into three cohorts, each undergoing a different strategy:
1. Successful treatment with SCS (success-SCS).

2. Failed SCS after 3 years of intervention had hardware explanted and were subsequently maintained on CMM (failed-SCS).
3. CMM.

During the simulation, there were four mutually exclusive health states in which patients could exist: optimal HRQoL (with or without complications), suboptimal HRQoL, or death. Each health state was associated with a utility value and probability taken from the literature [7–10]. In health economics, a utility value is a number that represents a given quality of life or state of health. An individual with a medical condition can be assigned a utility value between 0 (death) and 1 (perfect health) depending on how substantially the disease affects quality of life. Patients first undergo a screening trial. Those who achieve optimal pain relief proceed to a permanent implant, and the rest receive CMM.

During each 1-year Markov cycle, patients allocated to SCS are assumed to remain in their health state unless they (1) experience a complication or (2) move from optimal to suboptimal HRQoL [7–10]. Table 66.1 indicates the values assigned to model probabilities, utilities, and costs. EuroQoL-5Dimension (EQ-5D) scores were 0.598 for optimal pain relief without a complication, 0.258 for suboptimal pain relief (with or without complications), and 0.168 for no pain relief. In calculating the results of the failed-SCS group, we utilize the success-SCS group data for the first three cycles and CMM results for the remaining cycles. The model assumes that long-term SCS complications will occur at a rate of 18 % per annum [14]. It is assumed that any complications incurred in the CMM strategy do not impact cost or quality of life. We also modeled the impact of non-rechargeable versus rechargeable IPGs (Table 66.1).

Intrathecal Drug Therapy

To investigate IT cost-effectiveness, we utilized the data of 88 patients with FBSS who underwent SCS and subsequently failed to achieve satisfactory pain relief. These patients had their SCS electrodes explanted. The 88 patients were randomly divided into two groups of 44 patients each and were matched, in the same manner described earlier. Patients in the IT group received an IT morphine trial. Twenty-three patients (11 female [48 %] and 12 male [52 %]) were selected to undergo implantation of a permanent SynchroMed™ pump (Medtronic of Canada Ltd., Brampton, ON, Canada) as they met the outcome criteria of ≥50 % pain relief. The remaining 21 patients were excluded from study. In the original investigation as in the current study, anticipated costs of these patients were not factored, as they received no further treatment of any kind and thus incurred no further expenses [72].

Pump refills are performed by a neuromodulation nurse, the frequency of which is dictated by the medication dose

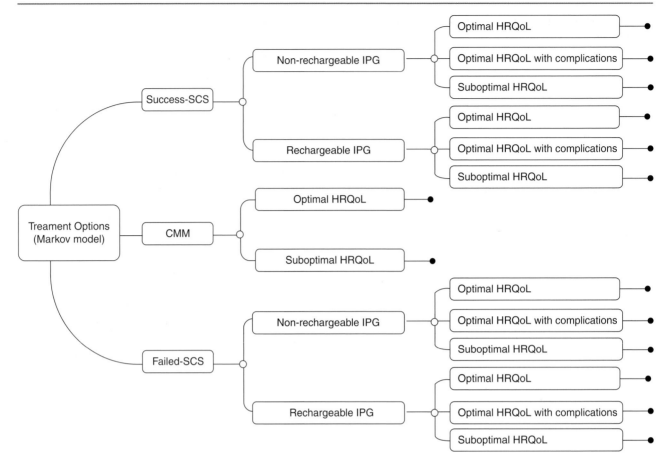

Fig. 66.1 Markov model, SCS analysis

and concentration. The dose escalation required with time for each patient was averaged. In this study, we found that the pumps had to be replaced in the sixth year of life due to battery depletion and amortized the cost accordingly. In the context of IT, costs include those associated with intrathecal agents, pharmacy costs for compounding and dispensing, refill costs, and physician contacts for dose adjustment.

Decision Analytic Model

This model was developed to compare costs and outcomes over a 10-year span for three strategies and is structured similarly to the abovementioned Markov process for SCS (Fig. 66.2). It is assumed that a patient always exists in one discrete health state during each 1-year Markov cycle. In this model, patients were divided into three cohorts, each undergoing a different strategy:

1. Successful treatment with IT which is initiated by monotherapy. If monotherapy results in suboptimal pain relief, the patients are sequentially advanced to dual- and triple-drug admixtures (success-IT).

2. Failed IT after 3 years and subsequent maintenance on CMM (failed-IT).
3. CMM.

During the simulation, patients could exist in three mutually exclusive health states, optimal HRQoL, suboptimal HRQoL, or death. Each health state was associated with a utility value and probability taken from the literature and patient chart reviews [72, 73]. Patients first undergo a screening trial. Those who achieve optimal pain relief proceed to a permanent implant, and the rest receive CMM.

Utility values were 0.521, 0.617, 0.603, and 0.405 for optimal improvement in HRQoL with IT mono-, dual-drug, triple-drug therapy, and CMM, respectively. EQ-5D scores for suboptimal improvement were 0.250. In calculating the outcomes of the failed-IT group, we utilized the success-IT group data for the first three cycles and CMM results for the remaining cycles. Our model assumes that the pump will remain functional for an average of 6 years, after which a replacement will be necessary. Furthermore the model assumes that CMM complications will not impact cost or quality of life. The model subsumes an overall rate of 24 % per annum for IT-related complications (Table 66.2) [84].

Table 66.1 Costs, utility, and probability distribution pertaining to SCS analysis

Procedure	Cost	Sensitivity analysis range	
SCS			
Implantation			
Rechargeable system	$23,160	$18,528	$27,792
Non-rechargeable system	$29,162	$23,330	$34,994
Annual maintenance			
Rechargeable system	$2,786	$2,229	$3,343
Non-rechargeable system	$3,732	$2,985	$4,478
Trial	$1,930	$1,544	$2,316
Explantation	$529	$423	$635
Adjunct drug therapy with SCS	$1,692	$1,354	$2,030
CMM	$7,988	$6,390	$9,586
Utility score (EQ-5D)			
Optimal HRQoL			
Success-SCS			
Without complications	0.598	0.478	0.718
With complications	0.528	0.422	0.634
CMM	0.396	0.317	0.475
Suboptimal HRQoL			
Success-SCS			
Without complications	0.258	0.206	0.310
With complications	0.258	0.206	0.310
CMM	0.205	0.164	0.246
Probability			
Complication rate (SCS)	0.180	0.144	0.216
Complication rate (CMM)	0.000	0.000	0.000
Death rate	0.009	0.007	0.011
Optimal HRQoL			
Success-SCS	0.585	0.468	0.702
CMM	0.100	0.080	0.120
Suboptimal HRQoL			
CMM	0.900	0.720	1.000
Strategy			
Success-SCS			
Cost	$104,197	$83,357	$125,036
Effectiveness (QALY)	5.63	4.50	6.76
Cost/effectiveness	$18,504	$14,803	$22,205
CMM			
Incremental cost	−$7,197	−$5,757	−$8,636
Incremental effectiveness	−3.51	−2.81	−4.21
Cost/effectiveness	$46,180	$36,944	$55,416
Failed-SCS			
Incremental cost	$67,628	$54,103	$81,154
Incremental effectiveness	−1.34	−1.07	−1.60
Cost/effectiveness	$39,998	$31,998	$47,997

Modified from Kumar et al. [83]

Interpretation

Spinal Cord Stimulation

Cost-Effectiveness

The analysis confirms that success-SCS is the most cost-effective strategy with a cost-effectiveness ratio (CER) of $18,504 followed by failed-SCS (CER: $39,998). Clinically, even if the effectiveness of SCS dissipates over 3 years requiring hardware removal and reversion to CMM, it is a more acceptable alternative to CMM which is least cost-effective (CER: $46,180) (Table 66.1). The CER for successful SCS therapy is well below the societal WTP thresholds of $20,000–$50,000.

In addition to the Markov model, we re-tabulated cumulative costs for a 10-year period by updating our previously published 2002 analysis [16] to reflect 2010 values. Costs are calculated as described above in methods: tabulation of costs (Fig. 66.3). The graph reflects that the higher initial cost of SCS, due largely to hardware costs, is recovered by 2.25 years after which CMM becomes more costly than SCS.

The one-way sensitivity analyses (using CMM, failed-SCS, or success-SCS as baseline) revealed that the cost-effectiveness of success-SCS was exceptionally resistant to parameter uncertainty, as it remained cost-effective compared with the other two strategies (i.e., CER < $20,000/QALY) throughout all of the sensitivity analyses.

Net Monetary Benefit

A positive NMB implies that the cost of a new therapy is less than the value of the additional benefit achieved. Conversely, a negative NMB implies that an intervention should be rejected, as its costs are higher than the value of the benefit achieved. The NMB analysis showed substantial savings over a relevant range of WTP for a QALY in the case of success-SCS where the NMB becomes positive at a WTP of $18,501. For failed-SCS and CMM, the NMB thresholds were much higher at WTP of $40,000 and $48,000, respectively. For all commonly accepted values of WTP, SCS represents the optimal strategy (Fig. 66.4).

Impact Analysis

The tornado diagram shows the impact of the most influential individual parameters on the incremental CER for base-case analysis. Impact analysis determined that the most significant factor affecting the model was IPG costs.

Acceptability of Treatment

The acceptability curve represents the probability that the intervention is cost-effective, given a varying threshold for the willingness to pay for each QALY gained. The success-SCS strategy had a 50 % probability of being cost-effective

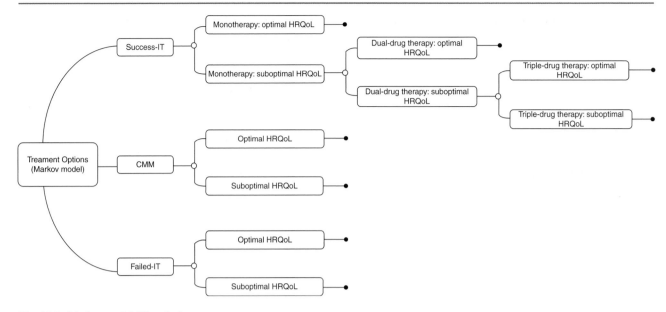

Fig. 66.2 Markov model, IT analysis

even under the conservative assumption that there exists no WTP ($0) for a gain of one QALY which subsequently increases to 99 % at a WTP of $5,500.

Rechargeable Versus Non-rechargeable IPG

One-way sensitivity analysis shows that the rechargeable IPG is relatively less costly than a rechargeable one. However, both strategies are cost-effective with a CER of $15,672/QALY for the rechargeable system and $16,439/QALY for the non-rechargeable IPG.

Future Directions

Advances in hardware technology and surgical technique will ensure that both clinicians and patients continue to benefit. Computer-interactive programming is gaining popularity, especially due to the increasing sophistication of implanted devices. Spinal cord stimulators now offer the ability to independently stimulate individual contacts as well as multiple arrays of electrodes [33]. This allows for accurate direction of current flow and more consistent overlapping paresthesia, resulting in better pain control and improved clinical outcomes [38]. SCS will undoubtedly move up several steps in the treatment ladder of chronic pain conditions as new applications are realized [40].

The limitations of current literature present an opportunity for researchers to generate robust, hypothesis-driven studies. This is a challenging and potentially rewarding undertaking. To date, most studies with SCS are not controlled. It is difficult to find a control group, let alone perform adequate randomization, because by definition the patients have often failed all other available treatments and

are reluctant to enroll. A sham procedure presents its own set of ethical predicaments. Similarly, investigations are virtually impossible to blind because the patient can detect the stimulation-induced paresthesia created by the system.

Intrathecal Drug Therapy

Cost-Effectiveness

The analysis confirms that success-IT is the most cost-effective strategy with a CER of $18,532 followed by failed-IT of $34,363 and CMM of $41,772 (Table 66.2). Clinically, even if the effectiveness of IT dissipates over 3 years requiring hardware removal and reversion to CMM, it is a more acceptable alternative to CMM which is least cost-effective. The CER for success-IT is well below societal WTP thresholds of $20,000–$50,000/per QALY.

In addition to the Markov model, we re-tabulated cumulative costs for a 10-year period by updating our previously published 2002 analysis [72] to reflect 2010 values. Costs are calculated as described above in methods: tabulation of costs (Fig. 66.5). The graph reflects that the higher initial cost of IT, due largely to hardware costs, is recovered by 2.5 years, after which CMM becomes more costly than SCS. The one-way sensitivity analyses (using CMM, failed-IT, or success-IT as baseline) demonstrated that the cost-effectiveness of success-IT was exceptionally resistant to parameter uncertainty, as it remained cost-effective compared with the other two strategies (i.e., CER < $20,000/QALY) throughout all of the sensitivity analyzes except in the single case when the probability of obtaining optimal HRQoL in the success-IT

Table 66.2 Cost, utility, and probability distribution pertaining to IT analysis

Procedure	Cost	Sensitivity analysis range	
IT			
Implantation	$16,140	$12,912	$19,368
Annual maintenance			
Polyanalgesia and supplemental oral drug costs	$6,157	$4,926	$7,389
Monotherapy and supplemental oral drug costs	$3,700	$2,960	$4,440
Trial	$4,535	$3,628	$5,442
Explantation	$636	$509	$763
CMM	$7,988	$6,390	$9,586
Utility score (EQ-5D)			
Optimal HRQoL			
Success-IT	0.527	0.422	0.632
CMM	0.400	0.320	0.480
Suboptimal HRQoL			
Failed-IT	0.310	0.248	0.372
CMM	0.205	0.164	0.246
Probability			
Complication rate – IT	0.240	0.192	0.288
Complication rate – CMM	0.000	0.000	0.000
Death rate	0.009	0.007	0.011
Optimal HRQoL			
Success-IT			
Monotherapy	0.571	0.457	0.685
Dual-drug therapy	0.797	0.638	0.956
Triple-drug therapy	0.789	0.631	0.947
CMM	0.150	0.120	0.180
Suboptimal HRQoL			
Failed-IT			
Monotherapy	0.429	0.343	0.515
Dual-drug therapy	0.203	0.162	0.244
Triple-drug therapy	0.211	0.169	0.253
CMM	0.850	0.680	1.000
Strategy			
Success-IT			
Cost	$92,798	$74,239	$111,358
Effectiveness (QALY)	5.01	4.01	6.01
Cost/effectiveness	$18,532	$14,825	$22,238
CMM			
Incremental cost	$1,414	$1,131	$1,696
Incremental effectiveness	−2.75	−2.20	−3.30
Cost/effectiveness	$41,772	$33,418	$50,127
Failed-IT			
Incremental cost	$14,958	$11,967	$17,950
Incremental effectiveness	−1.87	−1.50	−2.25
Cost/effectiveness	$34,363	$27,490	$41,236

arm is less than 10 %. Failed-IT was more cost-effective than CMM when the probability of an optimal outcome with CMM is less than 30 %.

Net Monetary Benefit

Single-drug IT generates the greatest NMB. The success-IT NMB is positive for WTP > $18,500. For failed-IT and CMM, the NMB threshold is much higher at WTP > $39,000 and > $42,000, respectively (Fig. 66.6). The difference between the averages of NMB between two strategies is equivalent to the incremental NMB. The incremental NMB for IT is approximately 2.9 times WTP.

Impact Analysis

Impact analysis determined that the most significant factors affecting the model were costs for success-IT and the probability of optimum pain relief with intrathecal monotherapy.

Acceptability of Treatment

The acceptability curve shows that the success-IT strategy had a 100 % probability of being more acceptable than the comparator condition (CMM) from a cost-effectiveness point of view, even under the conservative scenario that there is no ($0) WTP for a gain of one QALY.

Future Directions

Considerable progress has been made in the field of IT since the 2000 Polyanalgesic Consensus Conference (PACC) survey [65]. Ziconotide was approved by the FDA in 2004, making it the first new IT analgesic in more than a decade to gain approval. Today, it is considered first-line therapy. IT drug selection algorithms developed by the 2000, 2003 PACCs, and again updated in 2007 have aided physicians in choosing the safest and most effective drugs and their dosages for their patients [65–68]. Strides have also been made in the prevention and treatment of granulomas [67]. In 2011, the American Pain Foundation will publish new consensus guidelines.

The past 20 years have provided significant advances in the systemic and spinal approaches to analgesic drug delivery. Since the initial description of the spinal action of opioids and alpha-2 agonists 25 years ago (and demonstration of human efficacy), many spinal targets have been elucidated; some have been validated in human pain states [85]. Intrathecal delivery enables clinicians to target specific sites where nociceptive signals are encoded. However, the full potential of therapy is limited by the lack of clinical investigation of available agents. Researchers should prioritize the identification of new central targets and the development of new formulations and concentrations of known agents for intrathecal administration. The investigation of the stability

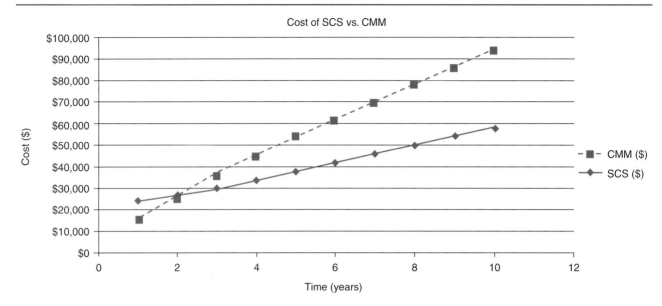

Fig. 66.3 Cumulative cost comparison SCS and CMM over a 10-year period. The 2.25-year payoff period should be noted

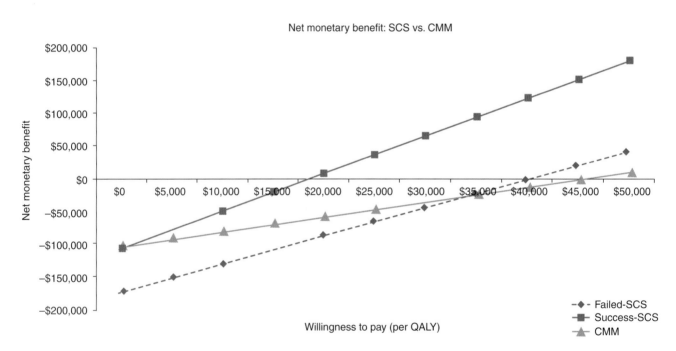

Fig. 66.4 Net monetary benefit (*NMB*), SCS versus comparator treatment. In the case of success-SCS, the NMB becomes positive at a WTP of $18,501. For failed-SCS and CMM, the NMB thresholds were much higher at WTP of $40,000 and $48,000, respectively. Thus, success-SCS represents the optimal strategy

and compatibility of single and combinations of multiple agents must be attuned to the physiologic conditions that exist in pump environment. Clinical inquiry should focus on well-designed randomized controlled clinical trials. In this context, multicenter collaboration and standardized clinical trials merit strategic priority.

In spite of significant advances on the therapeutic side, results of a recent survey suggest that economic and reimbursement difficulties continue to constrain IT use [86]. Clinicians, researchers, and advocacy groups must further evaluate the effects of economic trends on patient access to treatment [86].

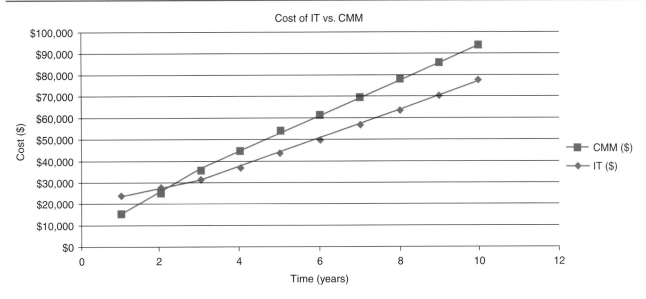

Fig. 66.5 Cumulative cost comparison IT and CMM over a 10-year period. The 2.5-year payoff period should be noted

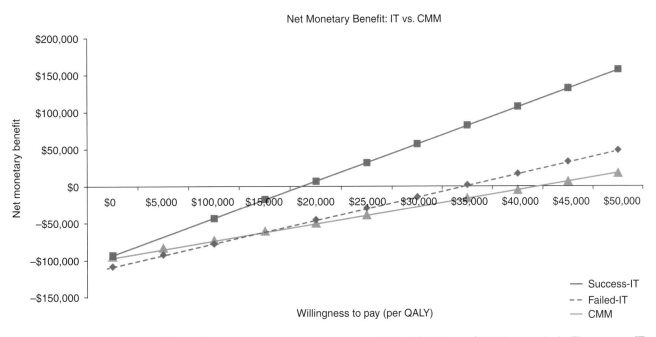

Fig. 66.6 Net monetary benefit (*NMB*), IT versus comparator treatment. In the case of success-IT, the NMB becomes positive at a WTP of $18,500. For failed-IT and CMM, the NMB thresholds were much higher at WTP of $39,000 and $42,000, respectively. Thus, success-IT represents the optimal strategy

Conclusion

IT and SCS are robust, cost-effective therapies. Significant cost savings can be attained with the use of these therapies in patients with CNMP secondary to FBSS when compared to CMM. Additional benefits may include an increased rate of return to work, better pain control, and quality of life. An integrated approach to the treatment of FBSS will result in improved utilization of scarce healthcare resources. Technological advances that increase hardware lifespan and improve catheter and electrode design will reduce complication rates, further bolstering the already favorable cost profile.

References

1. De Andres JM, Van Buyten JP. Neural modulation by stimulation. Pain Pract. 2006;6(1):39–45.
2. Grabow TS, Tella PK, Raja SN. Spinal cord stimulation for complex regional pain syndrome: an evidence-based medicine review of the literature. Clin J Pain. 2003;19(6):371–83.
3. Harke H, Gretenkort P, Ladleif HU, et al. Spinal cord stimulation in sympathetically maintained complex regional pain syndrome type I with severe disability. A prospective clinical study. Eur J Pain. 2005;9(4):363–73.
4. Kumar K, Taylor RS, Jacques L, et al. Spinal cord stimulation versus conventional medical management for neuropathic pain: a multicentre randomised controlled trial in patients with failed back surgery syndrome. Pain. 2007;132(1–2):179–88.
5. Kumar K, Taylor RS, Jacques L, et al. The effects of spinal cord stimulation in neuropathic pain are sustained: a 24-month follow-up of the PROCESS trial. Neurosurgery. 2008;63:762–70.
6. Manca A, Kumar K, Taylor RS, et al. Quality of life, resource consumption and costs of spinal cord simulation versus conventional medical management in neuropathic pain patients with failed back surgery syndrome (PROCESS trial). Eur J Pain. 2008;12:1047–58.
7. North RB, Kidd DH, Zahurak M, James CS, et al. Spinal cord stimulation for chronic, intractable pain: experience over two decades. Neurosurgery. 1993;32(3):384–94; discussion 394–95.
8. North RB, Kidd DH, Farrokhi F. Spinal cord stimulation versus repeated lumbosacral spine surgery for chronic pain: a randomized, controlled trial. Neurosurgery. 2005;56:98–107.
9. North RB, Kidd DH, Shipley J, et al. Spinal cord stimulation versus reoperation for failed back surgery syndrome: a cost effectiveness and cost utility analysis based on a randomized, controlled trial. Neurosurgery. 2007;61:361–9.
10. Kemler MA, Furnee CA. Economic evaluation of spinal cord stimulation for chronic reflex sympathetic dystrophy. Neurology. 2002;59(8):1203–9.
11. Kemler MA. The cost-effectiveness of spinal cord stimulation for complex regional pain syndrome. Value Health. 2010;13(6):735–42.
12. Mailis-Gagnon A, Furlan AD, Sandoval JA, Taylor R. Spinal cord stimulation for chronic pain. Cochrane Database Syst Rev. 2004;(3):CD003783.
13. Stanton-Hicks M. Complex regional pain syndrome: manifestations and the role of neurostimulation in its management. J Pain Symptom Manage. 2006;31(4S):20–4.
14. Taylor RJ, Taylor RS. Spinal cord stimulation for failed back surgery syndrome: a decision-analytic model and cost-effectiveness analysis. Int J Technol Assess Health Care. 2005;21:351–8.
15. Taylor RS, Buyten JPV, Buchser E. Spinal cord stimulation for complex regional pain syndrome: a systematic review of the clinical and cost-effectiveness literature and assessment of prognostic factors. Eur J Pain. 2006;10(2):91–101.
16. Kumar K, Malik S, Demeria D. Treatment of chronic pain with spinal cord stimulation versus alternative therapies: cost-effectiveness analysis. Neurosurgery. 2002;51(1):106–16.
17. Kumar K, Bishop S. Financial impact of spinal cord stimulation on the healthcare budget: a comparative analysis of costs in Canada and the United States. J Neurosurg. 2009;10:564–73.
18. Tesfaye S, Watt J, Benbow SJ, Pang KA, Miles J, MacFarlane IA. Electrical spinal-cord stimulation for painful diabetic peripheral neuropathy. Lancet. 1996;348(9043):1698–701.
19. Jivegard LEH, Augustinsson LE, Holm J, Risberg B, Örtenwall P. Effects of spinal cord stimulation (SCS) in patients with inoperable severe lower limb ischaemia: a prospective randomised controlled study. Eur J Vasc Endovasc Surg. 1995;9(4):421–5.
20. Hautvast RWM, DeJongste MJL, Staal MJ, van Gilst WH, Lie KI. Spinal cord stimulation in chronic intractable angina pectoris: a randomized, controlled efficacy study. Am Heart J. 1998;136(6):1114–20.
21. Kumar K, Toth C, Nath RK, Laing P. Epidural spinal cord stimulation for treatment of chronic pain – some predictors of success. A 15-year experience. Surg Neurol. 1998;50(2):110–20.
22. May MS, Banks C, Thomson SJ. A retrospective, long-term, third-party follow-up of patients considered for spinal cord stimulation. Neuromodulation. 2002;5(3):137–44.
23. National Institute for Clinical Excellence. Pain (chronic neuropathic or ischaemic) - spinal cord stimulation: guidance (TA159). London: National Institute for Clinical Excellence; 2008.
24. Martin BI, Deyo RA, Mirza SK, et al. Expenditures and health status among adults with back and neck problems. JAMA. 2008;299:656–64.
25. Hazard RG. Failed back surgery syndrome: surgical and nonsurgical approaches. Clin Orthop Relat Res. 2006;443:228–32.
26. Kemler MA, Barendse GA, Van Kleef M, et al. Spinal cord stimulation in patients with chronic reflex sympathetic dystrophy. N Engl J Med. 2000;343:618–24.
27. Melzack R. Pain mechanisms: a new theory. Science. 1965;150(699):971–9.
28. Roberts MH, Rees H. Physiological basis of spinal cord stimulation. Pain Rev. 1994;1:184–98.
29. Raslan AM, McCartney S, Burchiel KJ. Management of chronic severe pain: spinal neuromodulatory and neuroablative approaches. Acta Neurochir Suppl. 2007;97(1):33–41.
30. Dubuisson D. Effect of dorsal-column stimulation on gelatinosa and marginal neurons of cat spinal cord. J Neurosurg. 1989;70(2):257–65.
31. Cui J, O'Connor W, Ungerstedt U, Linderoth B, Meyerson B. Spinal cord stimulation attenuates augmented dorsal horn release of excitatory amino acids in mononeuropathy via a GABAergic mechanism. Pain. 1997;73(1):87–95.
32. Wallin J, Cui JG, Yakhnitsa V, Schechtmann G, Meyerson BA, Linderoth B. Gabapentin and pregabalin suppress tactile allodynia and potentiate spinal cord stimulation in a model of neuropathy. Eur J Pain. 2002;6(4):261–72.
33. Krames E. Overview of spinal cord stimulation: with special emphasis on a role for dual spinal cord stimulators. Pain Digest. 2000;10:6–12.
34. Holsheimer J, Wesselink WA. Effect of anode-cathode configuration on paresthesia coverage in spinal cord stimulation. Neurosurgery. 1997;41:654–60.
35. North RB, Ewend ME, Lawton MA, et al. Spinal cord stimulation for chronic, intractable pain: superiority of `multi-channel' devices. Pain. 1991;44(2):119–30.
36. Barolat G, Massaro F, He J, et al. Mapping of sensory responses to epidural stimulation of the intraspinal neural structures in man. J Neurosurg. 1993;78(2):233–9.
37. Shatin D, Mullett K, Hults G. Totally implantable spinal cord stimulation for chronic pain: design and efficacy. Pacing Clin Electrophysiol. 1986;9:577–83.
38. Hornberger J, Kumar K, Verhulst E, et al. Rechargeable spinal cord stimulation versus non-rechargeable system for patients with failed back surgery syndrome: a cost-consequence analysis. Clin J Pain. 2009;24:244–52.
39. North RB, Shipley J, Prager J. Practice parameters for the use of spinal cord stimulation in the treatment of chronic neuropathic pain. Pain Med. 2007;8(4):S200–75.
40. Barolat G, Sharan AD. Future trends in spinal cord stimulation. Neurol Res. 2000;22:279–84.
41. Kumar K, Hunter G, Demeria D. Spinal cord stimulation in treatment of chronic benign pain: challenges in treatment planning and present status, a 22-year experience. Neurosurgery. 2006;58:481–96.
42. Wang J, Nauss LA, Thomas JE. Pain relief by intrathecally applied morphine in man. Anesthesiology. 1979;50:149–51.
43. Behar M, Magora F, Olshwang D, et al. Epidural morphine in treatment of pain. Lancet. 1979;1:527.

44. Lund PC. Reflections upon the historical aspects of spinal anesthesia. Reg Anesth. 1983;8:89–98.

45. Ghafoor VL, Epshteyn M, Carlson GH, Terhaar DM, Charry O, Phelps PK. Intrathecal drug therapy for long-term pain management. Am J Health Syst Pharm. 2007;64(23):2447.

46. Prager J, Jacobs M. Evaluation of patients for implantable pain modalities: medical and behavioral assessment. Clin J Pain. 2001;17:206–14.

47. Krames ES, Olson K. Clinical realities and economic considerations: patient selection in intrathecal drug therapy. J Pain Symptom Manage. 1997;14:S3–13.

48. Krames ES. Spinal administration of opioids and other analgesic compounds. In: Waldman SD, editor. Interventional pain management. 2nd ed. Philadelphia: W. B. Saunders; 2001. p. 593–603.

49. Lance JW. Synopsis. In: Feldman RG, Young RR, Koella WP, editors. Spasticity: disordered motor control. Chicago: Year Book Medical Publishers; 1980. p. 480–5.

50. Sanger TD, Delgado MR, Gaebler-Spira D, Hallet M, Mink JW, Task Force on Childhood Motor Disorders. Classification and definition of disorders causing hypertonia in childhood. Pediatrics. 2003;111(1):e89–97.

51. Francisco GC, Boake C. Improvement in walking speed in poststroke spastic hemiplegia after intrathecal baclofen therapy: a preliminary study. Arch Phys Med Rehabil. 2003;84(8):1194–9.

52. Meythaler JM, Guin-Refroe S, Brunner RC, Hadley MN. Intrathecal baclofen for spastic hypertonia from stroke. Stroke. 2001;32(9):2099–109.

53. Ivanhoe CB, Francisco GE, McGuire JR, Subramanian T, Grissom SP. Intrathecal baclofen management of poststroke spastic hypertonia: implications for function and quality of life. Arch Phys Med Rehabil. 2006;87(11):1509–15.

54. Gilmartin R. Intrathecal baclofen for management of spastic cerebral palsy: multicenter trial. J Child Neurol. 2000;15(2):71–7.

55. Penn RD. Intrathecal baclofen for spasticity of spinal origin: seven years of experience. J Neurosurg. 1992;77(2):236–40.

56. Albright AL, Gilmartin R, Swift D, Krach LE, Ivanhoe CB, McLaughlin JF. Long-term intrathecal baclofen therapy for severe spasticity of cerebral origin. J Neurosurg. 2003;98(2):291–5.

57. Coffey RJ, Cahill D, Steers W. Intrathecal baclofen for intractable spasticity of spinal origin: results of a long-term multicenter study. J Neurosurg. 1993;78(6):226–32.

58. Ordia JI, Fischer E, Adamski E, Chagnon KG, Spatz EL. Continuous intrathecal baclofen infusion by a programmable pump in 131 consecutive patients with severe spasticity of spinal origin. Neuromodulation. 2002;5(1):16–24.

59. Becker R, Alberti O, Bauer BL. Continuous intrathecal baclofen infusion in severe spasticity after traumatic or hypoxic brain injury. J Neurol. 1997;224(3):160–6.

60. Clinical reference guide. Intrathecal baclofen for the management of severe spasticity. Minneapolis: Medtronic; 2004.

61. Dario A, Tomei G. A benefit-risk assessment of baclofen in severe spinal spasticity. Drug Saf. 2004;27:799–818.

62. Intrathecal drug delivery for the management of pain and spasticity in adults; Recommendations for best clinical practice. British Pain Society. Grady K, Raphael J editors. British Pain Society. 2008. http://www.britishpainsociety.org/book_ittd_main.pdf. Web 8 Aug 2010.

63. Mercadante S. Problems of long-term spinal opioid treatment in advanced cancer patients. Pain. 1999;79:1–13.

64. Heruth K. Medtronic synchromed drug administration system. Annals of the New York Academy of Sciences 1988;531:72–75.

65. Bennett G, Burchiel K, Buchser E, et al. Clinical guidelines for intraspinal infusion: report of an expert panel. J Pain Symptom Manage. 2000;20:S37–43.

66. Hassenbusch SJ, Portenoy RK. Current practices in intraspinal therapy – a survey of clinical trends in decision making. J Pain Symptom Manage. 2000;20:S4–11.

67. Hassenbusch S, Portenoy RK, Cousins M, et al. Polyanalgesic consensus conference 2003: an update on the management of pain by intraspinal drug delivery – report of an expert panel. J Pain Symptom Manage. 2004;27:540–63.

68. Deer T, Krames ES, Hassenbusch SJ, et al. Polyanalgesic consensus conference 2007: recommendations for the management of pain by intrathecal (intraspinal) drug delivery: report of an interdisciplinary expert panel. Neuromodulation. 2007;10: 300–28.

69. Postma TJ, Oenema D, Terpstra S, Bouma J, Keipers-Upmeier H, Staal MJ, Middel B. Cost analysis of the treatment of severe spinal spasticity with continuous intrathecal baclofen infusion system. Pharmacoeconomics. 1999;15:395–404.

70. Sampson FC, Hayward A, Evans G, Morton R, Collett B. Functional benefits and cost/benefit analysis of continuous intrathecal baclofen infusion for the management of severe spasticity. J Neurosurg. 2002;96:1052–7.

71. Hassenbusch SJ, Paice JA, Patt RB, et al. Clinical realities and economic considerations: economics of intrathecal drug therapy. J Pain Symptom Manage. 1997;14:S36–48.

72. Kumar K, Hunter G, Demeria DD. Treatment of chronic pain by using intrathecal drug therapy compared with conventional pain therapies: a cost effectiveness analysis. J Neurosurg. 2002;97: 803–10.

73. Kumar K, Bodani V, Bishop S, Tracey S. Use of intrathecal bupivacaine in refractory chronic nonmalignant pain. Pain Med. 2009;10: 819–28.

74. Royal MA, Wiesemeyer DL, Gordin V. Intrathecal opioid conversions: the importance of lipophilicity. Neuromodulation. 1998;1:195–7.

75. Yaksh TL, Rudy TA. Narcotic analgesia produced by a direct action on the spinal cord. Science. 1976;192:1357–8.

76. Cousins MJ, Mather LE, Glynn CJ, Wilson PR, Graham JR. Selective spinal analgesia. Lancet. 1979;1:1141–2.

77. Gourlay GK, Cherry DA, Cousins MJ. Cephalad migration of morphine in CSF following lumbar epidural administration in patients with cancer pain. Pain. 1985;23:317–26.

78. Dickenson AH. Recent advances in the physiology and pharmacology of pain: plasticity and its implications for clinical analgesia. J Psychopharmacol. 1991;5:342–51.

79. Eisenach JC. Three novel spinal analgesics: clonidine, neostigmine, amitriptyline. Reg Anesth. 1996;21:81–3.

80. Staats P. Intrathecal ziconotide in the treatment of refractory pain in patients with cancer or AIDS. JAMA. 2004;291:63–70.

81. Yaksh TL. Pharmacology of spinal adrenergic systems which modulate spinal nociceptive processing. Pharmacol Biochem Behav. 1985;22:845–58.

82. National Institute for Health and Clinical Excellence. Guide to the methods of technology appraisal. London: National Institute for Health and Clinical Excellence; 2004.

83. Kumar K, Abbas M, Rizvi S. The use of spinal cord stimulation in pain management. Pain Management. 2012;2:2, 125–134.

84. Turner JA, Sears JM, Loeser JD. Programmable intrathecal opioid delivery systems for chronic non-malignant pain: a systematic review of effectiveness and complications. Clin J Pain. 2007;23: 180–95.

85. Bennett G, Deer T, Du Pen S, et al. Future directions in the management of pain by intraspinal drug delivery. J Pain Symptom Manage. 2000;20:S44–50.

86. Deer TR, Krames E, Levy RM, Hassenbusch SJ, Prager JP. Practice choices and challenges in the current intrathecal drug therapy environment: an online survey. Pain Med. 2009;10:304–9.

Neurosurgical Techniques for Pain Management

67

Hendrik Klopper and Kenneth A. Follett

Key Points

- Augmentative neuromodulation techniques have supplanted ablative procedures as treatments of choice for intractable pain.
- Augmentative techniques are effective in well-selected patients and are associated with a low risk of complications.
- Augmentative techniques are superior to ablative techniques in the treatment of neuropathic pain that has a continuous, dysesthetic component.
- Ablative techniques may be appropriate for individuals such as those with cancer-related pain who have short life expectancies, patients with a predominant nociceptive component of pain, and those with neuropathic pain with paroxysmal or evoked components.
- Ablative techniques are very useful for certain pain syndromes: rhizotomy for trigeminal neuralgia, DREZ lesioning for "end-zone" or "boundary" pain associated with spinal cord injury or phantom-limb pain associated with avulsion of cervical or lumbosacral spinal nerve roots, and cordotomy or myelotomy for treatment of intractable cancer pain in individuals with short life expectancies or who have failed treatment with neuraxial analgesics.

- Pain management physicians should be familiar with the variety of neurosurgical techniques available for the treatment of pain, the general indications, and the general outcomes, and incorporate these treatments in the care of their patients when appropriate.

H. Klopper, M.D. (✉)
Department of Neurosurgery,
University of Nebraska Medical Center,
982035 Nebraska Medical Center, Omaha, NE 68198, USA
e-mail: hklopper@unmc.edu

K.A. Follett, M.D., Ph.D.
Department of Neurosurgery,
University of Nebraska College of Medicine,
982035 Nebraska Medical Center, Omaha,
NE 68198, USA

Introduction

Surgical procedures have been important tools for the treatment of pain for many years. Until the 1980s, most surgical therapies for pain treatment were anatomic (e.g., decompressive or reconstructive) or ablative in nature. Ablative procedures, based on knowledge of the anatomy and physiology of nociception and aimed at interrupting pain pathways, were the mainstay of surgical treatment of intractable pain for decades. The past few decades have witnessed the introduction of the gate control theory and an awareness of intrinsic pain-modulating systems, leading to the advent of neuroaugmentative therapies. In most instances, neuroaugmentative therapies, including neurostimulation and neuraxial analgesic infusion, have supplanted ablative techniques as the procedures of choice for the treatment of chronic pain. These therapies are discussed in detail in Chaps. 39, 40, 41, 42, 43, 44, 45, 46, and 47 of this book. Although ablative therapies have largely fallen by the wayside, pain providers should retain a general familiarity with them because they may be procedures of choice for certain pain syndromes and certain patients. Unfortunately, as augmentative therapies increasingly supplant ablative neurosurgical techniques, fewer neurosurgeons have the expertise or equipment to perform traditional neuroablative surgeries. This requires that in some instances, patients may need to be referred to a neurosurgical center with special expertise in pain therapy. In this chapter, the authors discuss pain procedures provided primarily or exclusively in the neurosurgical domain of pain treatment, including anatomic, ablative, and augmentative therapies.

T.R. Deer et al. (eds.), *Comprehensive Treatment of Chronic Pain by Medical, Interventional, and Integrative Approaches*,
DOI 10.1007/978-1-4614-1560-2_67, © American Academy of Pain Medicine 2013

Table 67.1 Anatomic procedures and their primary indications

Procedure	Indication
Spinal decompression and reconstruction	Progressive myelopathy or radiculopathy resulting from compression of neural structures (e.g., from intervertebral disk herniation, osteophyte, spondylolisthesis, ligamentous hypertrophy)
Microvascular decompression	Classical trigeminal, glossopharyngeal, or nervus intermedius neuralgia (i.e., paroxysmal, lancinating pain)

As with all other pain treatments, the basic tenets of pain care must be observed during the delivery of neurosurgical pain therapies. The treatment offered should be selected according to the needs of each individual patient and the skills of the treating physician. Patient-related factors must be taken into consideration including the pain etiology, location, and characteristics (nociceptive or neuropathic); life expectancy; and psychological, social, and economic factors that could impact the pain complaint. The relative advantages and disadvantages of anatomic, augmentative, and ablative therapies should be weighed in view of these factors, and a choice between these three general approaches should be made before choosing a specific intervention.

Anatomic Therapies

The anatomic therapies are aimed at correcting underlying structural abnormalities that cause specific pain syndromes. These procedures include spinal decompressive or reconstructive techniques for spinal pain syndromes and microvascular decompression for cranial neuralgias (e.g., trigeminal neuralgia). The anatomic therapies and their primary indications are summarized in Table 67.1.

Spinal Decompressive and Reconstructive Procedures

This group of procedures encompasses a range of operations aimed at decompression of the spinal cord and spinal nerve roots for the treatment of structural abnormalities that result in neurological deficit or intractable pain. Procedures in this category include cervical, thoracic, and lumbar diskectomy, laminectomy, and spinal fusion. They are performed routinely in the practice of general neurosurgery with minimal morbidity and mortality and – provided treatment is directed at a structural abnormality that is concordant with the pain

syndrome – are for the most part quite successful in relieving axial and/or radicular pain resulting from the structural abnormality. The discussion of these procedures is beyond the scope of this chapter, and the interested reader is referred to any of a number of general neurosurgical textbooks for a more detailed treatment of these operations and outcomes.

Microvascular Decompression

Microvascular decompression is one of the most important techniques for the treatment of intractable trigeminal neuralgia, glossopharyngeal neuralgia, and nervus intermedius neuralgia [1, 2]. It is indicated for the treatment of classical neuralgia (paroxysmal, lancinating pain, often described as "electrical shocks") that is refractory to pharmacological treatment. It is most appropriate for healthy patients, generally under the age of 65 or 70, with no medical contraindications to craniotomy.

The rationale of microvascular decompression is to eliminate compression of the affected cranial nerve by a blood vessel (usually an artery), which generally occurs near the entry of the nerve into the brainstem. Microvascular decompression has the advantage of the absence of a postoperative sensory deficit, which is an obligate outcome of percutaneous or open ablative procedures (e.g., radiofrequency rhizotomy or ganglionectomy for trigeminal neuralgia). Early pain relief is achieved in more than 90 % of patients. Pain may recur over the course of months or years, but microvascular decompression is regarded generally as providing the most durable pain relief of the various procedures, and most patients obtain lasting pain relief [1, 2]. Microvascular decompression is much less successful in treating atypical facial pain (i.e., constant, burning pain, typically not involving a clear trigeminal sensory distribution). In general, the less the degree of paroxysmal pain and the greater the degree of constant, burning, dysesthetic pain in a given individual, the less likely a good long-term outcome will be achieved with surgical intervention [3].

Ablative Therapies

Ablative therapies are often viewed as treatments of last resort for intractable pain, but in some instances, they remain the procedures of choice and should not be forgotten or overlooked by pain care providers. Important examples include dorsal root entry zone (DREZ) lesioning for treatment of phantom-limb pain following spinal nerve root avulsion or "end-zone" pain arising from spinal cord injury and cordotomy, which may be preferable to intrathecal analgesic administration for the treatment of cancer-related pain in a patient with a short life expectancy.

Table 67.2 Ablative procedures and their primary indications

Procedure	Indication
Sympathectomy	Visceral, cancer-related pain
Neurectomy	Identifiable neuroma following peripheral nerve injury (e.g., following limb amputation); meralgia paresthetica; inguinal pain syndromes (e.g., post-herniorrhaphy pain)
Dorsal rhizotomy/ganglionectomy	Cancer-related trunk/abdominal pain
Cranial nerve rhizotomy	Classical trigeminal and glossopharyngeal neuralgia when microvascular decompression is contraindicated
C2 ganglionectomy	Occipital neuralgia
DREZ lesioning	Localized neuropathic pain following spinal nerve root avulsion; "end-zone" pain following spinal cord injury
Cordotomy	Cancer-related pain below mid- to low cervical dermatomes
Myelotomy	Cancer-related abdominal, pelvic, perineal, or lower extremity pain

Ablative therapies have been developed which target almost every level of the peripheral and central nervous system: eripheral techniques that interrupt or alter nociceptive input into the spinal cord (e.g., neurectomy, ganglionectomy, rhizotomy), spinal interventions that alter afferent input or rostral transmission of nociceptive information (e.g., DREZ lesioning, cordotomy, myelotomy), and supraspinal intracranial procedures that may interrupt transmission of nociceptive information (e.g., mesencephalotomy, thalamotomy) or influence perception of painful stimuli (e.g., cingulotomy).

Ablative therapies tend to be most appropriate for the treatment of nociceptive pain rather than neuropathic pain. Neuropathic pain that is intermittent, paroxysmal, or evoked (e.g., allodynia and hyperpathia) may improve after an ablative procedure, but continuous, dysesthetic neuropathic pain tends to respond much less favorably in long-term follow-up [4]. The ablative therapies are summarized along with their primary indications in Table 67.2.

Sympathectomy

Sympathectomy is indicated for the treatment of visceral pain associated with certain cancers [5, 6]. It can alleviate non-cancer pain such as that associated with vasospastic disorders or sympathetically maintained pain (when sympathetic blocks reliably relieve the pain), but it has generally fallen into disfavor as a treatment for intractable pain of nonmalignant origin because of inconsistent results [5–8]. Some data indicate that SCS provides better long-term outcomes with lower morbidity and SCS may replace sympathectomy in the treatment of sympathetically maintained pain of non-

cancer origin [9]. Sympathectomy is commonly and successfully used in the treatment of intractable hyperhidrosis.

Neurectomy

Neurectomy may be useful in individuals who develop pain following peripheral nerve injury, including that associated with limb amputation. If an identifiable neuroma is the cause of pain, its resection can provide significant relief [10]. In the absence of an identifiable neuroma, neurectomy is unlikely to provide pain relief. In this regard, neurectomy is not useful for treatment of nonspecific stump pain after amputation, and it is not generally useful for the treatment of other nonmalignant peripheral pain syndromes. The utility of neurectomy is limited because pain arising from a pure sensory nerve is uncommon, and sectioning of mixed sensory-motor nerves is associated with significant risk of neurologic deficit and resultant functional impairment. There may be several exceptions to this rule. For example, section of the lateral femoral cutaneous nerve has been reported to provide long-lasting relief of meralgia paresthetica [11], and section of the ilioinguinal and/or genitofemoral nerves has been reported to provide relief of certain inguinal pain syndromes (e.g., post-herniorrhaphy pain) in properly selected individuals [12].

Dorsal Rhizotomy/Ganglionectomy

Dorsal rhizotomy and ganglionectomy serve similar purposes in denervating somatic and/or visceral tissues, but ganglionectomy may produce more complete denervation than can be accomplished by dorsal rhizotomy. Some afferent fibers enter the spinal cord through the ventral root [13] and are not affected by dorsal rhizotomy. In contrast, ganglionectomy effectively eliminates input from dorsal and ventral root afferent fibers by removing their cell bodies, which are located within the dorsal root ganglion.

Rhizotomy and ganglionectomy can be used to treat pain in the trunk or abdomen. Neither procedure is useful for treatment of pain in the extremities unless function of the extremity is already lost because denervation removes proprioceptive as well as nociceptive input and produces a functionless limb. Limited denervation (e.g., a single level) does not generally provide adequate pain relief because segmental innervation of dermatomes overlaps with adjacent levels. Therefore, these procedures typically must be performed at several adjacent spinal levels. Multilevel denervation increases the sensory loss and risk of functional impairment of an extremity.

These procedures are most useful for the treatment of cancer-related pain, as non-cancer pain does not improve consistently [14, 15]. When used for treatment of neuropathic pain (e.g., postherpetic neuralgia of the trunk), lancinating, paroxysmal, or evoked pain may improve but continuous dysesthetic pain does not typically improve. In the setting of cancer, these procedures can be useful for thoracic or abdominal wall pain; for perineal pain in patients with impaired bladder, bowel, and sexual function; or for the treatment of pain in a functionless extremity. Multiple sacral rhizotomies can be performed (e.g., to treat pelvic pain from cancer) by passing a ligature around the thecal sac below S1 [16].

Cranial Nerve Rhizotomy

Rhizotomy is especially useful as a treatment of cranial neuralgias, especially trigeminal and glossopharyngeal neuralgia [17, 18]. Classical trigeminal and glossopharyngeal neuralgia are unique among neuropathic pain syndromes in their uniformly good response to ablative procedures. This reflects the general utility of ablative techniques in relieving lancinating, paroxysmal pain. In contrast, atypical facial pain syndromes (constant, burning, dysesthetic pain) do not improve with ablative techniques and may be worse following denervation by rhizotomy or other ablative techniques, either from worsening of the pain, per se, or superimposition of potentially unpleasant sensory loss on the original pain.

Percutaneous trigeminal rhizotomy can be accomplished with thermal radiofrequency (RF), glycerol injection, or balloon compression. These techniques are performed on an outpatient basis, are well tolerated, and have high success rates in relieving paroxysmal pain of cranial neuralgias. Early pain relief is almost universal, but pain can recur over months or years (in which case the same procedure or another surgical treatment can be offered) [18]. These techniques are especially useful in treating elderly, medically infirm patients who are not good candidates for craniotomy for microvascular decompression of a cranial nerve. Postoperative sensory deficit is an obligate outcome of successful rhizotomy, so candidates should be counseled accordingly. Postoperative sensory loss may render this procedure undesirable for treatment of pain around the eye because corneal sensory loss may lead to keratitis and impaired vision. Open rhizotomy (i.e., via craniotomy or craniectomy) is usually performed for treatment of glossopharyngeal and nervus intermedius neuralgia and may be useful for treatment of some trigeminal neuralgias.

Stereotactic radiosurgery rhizotomy for the treatment of trigeminal neuralgia is an alternative to percutaneous or open rhizotomy or microvascular decompression for some individuals [19]. Radiosurgery is performed on an outpatient basis as a single procedure. In contrast to percutaneous rhizotomy and other surgical treatments for cranial neuralgias, which have a high likelihood of providing immediate postoperative pain relief, pain relief may not occur for several weeks

following radiosurgical treatment. Radiosurgery is, therefore, not appropriate for individuals with severe acute pain that cannot be controlled adequately with medications. Pain may recur over months or years in some patients, but relief is maintained in many patients [17, 18]. Unlike percutaneous or open rhizotomy, sensory loss after radiosurgery is uncommon. Radiosurgery is most useful for individuals who desire a relatively noninvasive treatment and whose pain is sufficiently well controlled that they can tolerate the postprocedure delay in pain relief.

C2 Ganglionectomy

C2 ganglionectomy is indicated for the treatment of occipital neuralgia. It is especially effective for individuals with posttraumatic occipital neuralgia who have no migraine component to their headache [20]. Pain relief may be comparable to that achieved with occipital nerve stimulation (see Chaps. 40 and 47) but without the need for implanted devices and long-term follow-up.

Dorsal Root Entry Zone (DREZ) Lesioning

DREZ lesioning of the spinal cord (for trunk or extremity pain) [21–23] or nucleus caudalis (for facial pain) [22, 24] can provide significant relief of neuropathic pain in properly selected individuals. The rationale of DREZ lesioning is to disrupt input into and outflow from the superficial layers of the spinal cord dorsal horn, which are the sites of termination of afferent nociceptive fibers and sites of origin of some of the nociceptive fibers that ascend within the spinal cord. DREZ lesioning may also disrupt spontaneous abnormal activity and hyperactivity that develops in spinal cord dorsal horn neurons in the setting of neuropathic pain.

DREZ lesioning is best reserved for localized pain with a neuropathic component. Certain types of cancer pain can be treated effectively with DREZ lesioning (e.g., neuropathic arm pain associated with Pancoast tumor). The most successful applications are related to treatment of neuropathic pain arising from spinal nerve root avulsion (cervical or lumbosacral) and "end-zone" or "boundary" pain following spinal cord injury. These pain syndromes sometimes respond to spinal cord stimulation or intrathecal drug infusion, but DREZ lesioning can provide a similar result without the need for long-term maintenance required by an augmentative device.

DREZ lesioning has been used for the treatment of other neuropathic pain syndromes (e.g., postherpetic neuralgia), but good pain relief is not achieved consistently. DREZ lesioning of nucleus caudalis can provide relief of deafferentation pain affecting the face (including postherpetic neuralgia), but outcomes are inconsistent. It is less helpful for facial pain of peripheral origin (e.g., traumatic trigeminal neuropathy). As with other ablative procedures, DREZ lesioning is most effective for relieving paroxysmal or evoked neuropathic pain rather than continuous neuropathic pain [23].

Cordotomy

Cordotomy can be an effective method of pain control, especially when pain is related to malignancy, and especially for individuals with short life expectancies for whom it is difficult to justify the costs of implantation of drug infusion systems. The rationale of cordotomy is to disrupt nociceptive afferent fibers ascending in the spinothalamic tract in the anterolateral quadrant of the spinal cord. Cordotomy offers the advantage, compared to neuraxial analgesic administration, of being a onetime procedure with no required long-term follow-up or maintenance. This is important for individuals who may find it difficult to return to a medical facility for refilling of an infusion system or for whom costs of ongoing medical care can become burdensome. Cordotomy is used most commonly for the treatment of cancer-related pain below mid- to low cervical dermatomes. It is not generally used for treatment of patients with pain of non-cancer origin because pain typically recurs over months to years in patients with long life expectancies, and there is significant risk of post-cordotomy dysesthesias or neurological complication [25]. Cordotomy can be performed as an open [25] or closed (percutaneous) [26, 27] procedure. Percutaneous techniques are less invasive, but open techniques remain viable options because most surgeons lack the expertise and equipment required for percutaneous procedures.

Pain relief varies with pain characteristics and location. Laterally located pain responds better than midline or axial pain (e.g., visceral pain). Midline and axial pain may require bilateral procedures to achieve pain relief. Lancinating, paroxysmal neuropathic pain and evoked (allodynic or hyperpathic) pain that sometimes occurs following spinal cord injury or as part of peripheral neuropathic pain syndromes can improve following cordotomy, but continuous neuropathic pain does not improve [26].

There is a significantly greater risk of complication with bilateral procedures, including weakness, bladder, bowel, and sexual dysfunction, and respiratory depression (if the procedure is performed bilaterally at cervical levels) [25, 26]. Bilateral percutaneous cervical cordotomies are usually staged at least 1 week apart to reduce the likelihood of a serious complication. The risk of respiratory depression subsequent to a unilateral high cervical procedure mandates that pulmonary function be acceptable on the contralateral side. For example, a patient who has undergone a previous pneu-

monectomy for lung cancer should not be subject to cordotomy that would compromise pulmonary function on the side of the remaining lung [26].

Cordotomy provides good pain relief in approximately 60–80 % of patients [26, 28], but loss of pain relief tends to occur over time. Approximately, one-third of patients have recurrent pain in 3 months, half at 1 year, and two-thirds at longer follow-up intervals [28, 29].

Myelotomy

As with many other traditional ablative neurosurgical therapies, myelotomy has become an uncommon procedure since the advent of neuroaugmentative therapies, but it can provide significant pain relief in properly selected individuals, including some who fail treatment with intrathecal analgesia [30]. Commissural myelotomy was developed to provide the benefits of bilateral cordotomy without the inherent risks of lesioning both anterior quadrants of the spinal cord [30–32]. This is accomplished by sectioning spinothalamic tract fibers from both sides of the body simultaneously with one lesion where they decussate in the anterior commissure. The advantage compared to cordotomy is that bilateral and midline pain can be treated with a single operative procedure, with lower morbidity and mortality.

Clinical observations revealed that a limited midline cordotomy (a lesion of a few millimeters in length vs. the several centimeter length lesion of commissural myelotomy) [33] or high cervical myelotomy [28, 34] can be as effective as classical commissural myelotomy in relieving abdominal, pelvic, and lower extremity pain. Identification of a dorsal column visceral pain pathway has lead to the development of punctuate midline myelotomy [32].

These procedures are indicated primarily for the treatment of cancer-related pain, generally in the abdomen, pelvis, perineum, and legs. They are most effective for nociceptive rather than neuropathic pain. Early complete pain relief is achieved in most patients (greater than 90 %), but pain tends to recur over time such that approximately 50–60 % of patients have good long-term pain relief [28]. The risk of bladder, bowel, and/or sexual dysfunction is less than that associated with bilateral cordotomy, but still remains sufficiently high that use of these procedures is restricted in most instances to patients with cancer-related pain who have preexisting dysfunction.

Brainstem Ablative Procedures

Ablative neurosurgical procedures directed at the brainstem are not in widespread use, in part because relatively few patients require such interventions and because relatively

Table 67.3 Brainstem ablative procedures and their primary indications

Procedure	Indication
Mesencephalotomy	Cancer-related pain involving the head, neck, or upper extremities
Thalamotomy	Widespread cancer-related pain (e.g., diffuse metastatic cancer); midline, bilateral, or head/neck pain with contraindications to other procedures (e.g., cordotomy, neuraxial analgesic infusion)

few neurosurgeons have the expertise to perform these interventions. These procedures are mostly of historical interest, but rarely may be considered for patients who fail more conservative therapies or who are not candidates for less invasive procedures. These procedures and their indications are summarized in Table 67.3.

Mesencephalotomy

Mesencephalotomy is indicated for the treatment of intractable pain involving the head, neck, shoulder, and arm [4, 35]. Most commonly, the procedure is used for the treatment of pain related to cancer. The rationale for mesencephalotomy is disruption of nociceptive fibers ascending in the brainstem, in which sense it can be viewed as a supraspinal version of cordotomy [4]. Early pain relief is achieved in 85 % of patients [28]. It does not provide consistent long-term relief of central neuropathic pain [35]. Side effects and complications are common, especially oculomotor dysfunction [4, 28, 35].

The utility of mesencephalotomy has diminished subsequent to the advent of neuraxial analgesic administration. Intraventricular morphine infusion can provide good relief of head, neck, shoulder, and arm pain with a lower incidence of complications. Mesencephalotomy may be preferable for some individuals, for example, those with short life expectancies or for whom the costs or long-term follow-up required with neuraxial analgesic administration become a burden.

Thalamotomy

Thalamotomy has been used for the treatment of cancer-related and non-cancer-related pain [36, 37]. In the setting of cancer, thalamotomy is most appropriate for individuals who have widespread pain (e.g., from diffuse metastatic disease) or who have midline, bilateral, or head/neck pain, for which other procedures may not be likely to provide relief [36].

The success rate of thalamotomy in relieving pain is slightly lower than that achieved with mesencephalotomy, but the incidence of complications is lower with thalamotomy [38], so thalamotomy may be preferable for the treatment of head, neck, shoulder, and arm pain in individuals who are not candidates for neuraxial analgesic administration. It can also be useful for individuals who are not candidates for cordotomy, for example, those with pain above the C5 dermatome or with pulmonary dysfunction [38]. The procedure can be accomplished via stereotactic radiofrequency [4, 28, 38, 39] or radiosurgical techniques [37]. Medial thalamotomy appears most effective for treating nociceptive pain (e.g., cancer pain), with acceptable long-term pain relief obtained in approximately 30–50 % of patients [4, 36, 39]. Overall, neuropathic pain syndromes respond less consistently to thalamotomy, with only about one-third of patients improving long term [4, 39]. As with other ablative procedures, paroxysmal, lancinating neuropathic pain or neuropathic pain with elements of evoked pain (i.e., allodynia and hyperpathia) may improve following thalamotomy, whereas continuous neuropathic pain tends not to improve [4].

Cingulotomy

Cingulotomy is used less commonly for treatment of intractable pain than for management of psychiatric disorders. It is applied most commonly to the treatment of cancer pain but has been used for non-cancer pain as well [28, 40, 41]. Approximately, 50–75 % of patients benefit from the procedure, at least short-term. In the cancer population, pain relief is maintained generally at least 3 months. The utility of cingulotomy for chronic non-cancer pain is less certain, with some studies indicating relatively good long-lasting pain relief [28, 41] and others indicating only 20 % long-term success [36]. Because cingulotomy is performed for treatment of psychiatric disease and carries the stigma of "psychosurgery," formal review by institutional ethics committees may be warranted if this procedure is being considered as a treatment for intractable pain.

Hypophysectomy

Hypophysectomy (surgical, chemical, or radiosurgical) can provide good relief of cancer-related pain. It is traditionally felt to be most effective for hormonally responsive cancers (e.g., prostate, breast cancer) but may relieve pain associated with other tumors as well. It is indicated primarily for the treatment of diffuse pain associated with widespread disease. Pain is alleviated in 45–95 % of patients. Pain relief is independent of tumor regression, and the specific mechanism of pain relief is unknown [28, 42–44].

Stimulation Therapies

Stimulation therapies provided by neurosurgeons include spinal cord stimulation, peripheral nerve stimulation, deep brain stimulation (DBS), and motor cortex stimulation (MCS). These therapies are presented in detail elsewhere in this chapter. A brief overview of intracranial stimulation therapies, which lie exclusively in the neurosurgical pain management domain, is presented here.

Intracranial stimulation therapies include DBS of the somatosensory thalamus, hypothalamus, and periventricular-periaqueductal gray [45–51] and MCS [52–55]. Deep brain stimulation and motor cortex stimulation are not approved for use by the United States Food and Drug Administration, but have been incorporated into pain management strategies in some centers. DBS and MCS are used primarily for treating pain of nonmalignant origin, such as pain associated with failed back surgery syndrome, neuropathic pain following central or peripheral nervous system injury, or trigeminal pain or cluster headache.

Stimulation sites for DBS are chosen generally on the basis of the pain characteristics. Nociceptive pain and paroxysmal, lancinating, or evoked neuropathic pain (e.g., allodynia, hyperpathia) tend to respond to PVG-PAG stimulation. Continuous neuropathic pain responds most consistently to paresthesia-producing stimulation of the sensory thalamus (nucleus ventrocaudalis) [48]. Because many pain syndromes (e.g., failed back surgery syndrome) have mixed components of nociceptive and neuropathic pain, some physicians offer the patient a screening trial using electrodes in both regions to determine which provides the best pain relief. A morphine-naloxone test has been used by some providers to clarify the extent of nociceptive and neuropathic pain components and facilitate selection of the best stimulation target [46].

Success rates of DBS for the treatment of intractable pain are difficult to determine because patient selection, techniques, and outcomes assessments vary substantially among studies. Approximately 60–80 % of patients undergoing a screening trial with DBS will have pain relief sufficient to warrant implantation of a permanent stimulation system. Of those who receive a permanent stimulation system, approximately 25–80 % (generally 50–60 %) [45] will gain acceptable long-term pain relief [45–49]. Patients with cancer pain [48], FBSS, peripheral neuropathy, and trigeminal neuropathy (not anesthesia dolorosa) [45, 46, 48] tend to respond to DBS more favorably than patients with central pain syndromes (e.g., thalamic pain, spinal cord injury pain, anesthesia dolorosa, postherpetic neuralgia, or phantom-limb pain) [45, 46, 48]. The incidence of serious complications of DBS is low, but the combined incidence of morbidity, mortality, and technical complications can approach 25–30 % [45, 48].

In contrast to reports that describe utility of DBS for treatment of chronic pain, others indicate little if any long-term benefit [51], and the procedure remains uncommon even in neurosurgical circles.

MCS has been proposed as an alternative to deep brain stimulation [52–55]. MCS is used primarily for treatment of neuropathic pain syndromes and seems most effective for certain types of facial pain (e.g., trigeminal neuropathic pain), in part because the cortical region of interest for treatment of facial pain is relatively easy to target [53]. Approximately 50 % of patients undergoing MCS have good long-term pain relief. As with DBS, MCS appears most effective in the absence of anesthesia in the distribution of pain being treated. Compared with DBS, the overall clinical efficacy of MCS is similar, but the complications associated with MCS might be less serious because the electrode is placed epidurally rather than within the brain parenchyma. MCS shows some promise, but long-term efficacy remains to be determined.

Summary

In general, augmentative neuromodulation techniques have supplanted ablative procedures as treatments of choice for intractable pain. The augmentative techniques are quite effective in well-selected patients, and the risk of complication is low, making them the first choice for many patients. They are also superior to ablative techniques in the treatment of neuropathic pain that has a continuous, dysesthetic component. Ablative therapies may be appropriate for some individuals, for example, individuals with cancer-related pain who have short life expectancies, patients with a predominant nociceptive component of pain, and those with neuropathic pain with paroxysmal or evoked components. Furthermore, ablative techniques are very useful for certain pain syndromes: rhizotomy for trigeminal neuralgia, DREZ lesioning for "end-zone" or "boundary" pain associated with spinal cord injury or phantom-limb pain associated with avulsion of cervical or lumbosacral spinal nerve roots, and cordotomy or myelotomy for treatment of intractable cancer pain in individuals with short life expectancies or who have failed treatment with neuraxial analgesics.

As attention is focused increasingly on augmentative therapies for the treatment of intractable pain, ablative therapies that might be appropriate for some individuals may be overlooked as treatment options. Pain management physicians should be familiar with the variety of neurosurgical techniques available for the treatment of pain, the general indications, and the general outcomes, and incorporate these treatments in the care of their patients when appropriate.

References

1. Barker II FG, Janetta PJ, Bissonette DJ, et al. The long-term outcomes of microvascular decompression for trigeminal neuralgia. N Engl J Med. 1996;334:1077–83.

2. Kasam PA, Horowitz M, Chang YF. Microvascular decompression in the management of glossopharyngeal neuralgia: analysis of 217 cases. Neurosurgery. 2002;50:705–10.

3. Miller JP, Burchiel K. Classification of trigeminal neuralgia: clinical, therapeutic, and prognostic implications in a series of 144 patients undergoing microvascular decompression. J Neurosurg. 2009;111:1231–4.

4. Tasker RR. Stereotactic surgery. In: Wall PD, Melzack R, editors. Textbook of pain. 3rd ed. Edinburgh: Churchill Livingstone; 1994. p. 1137–58.

5. Hardy Jr RW, Bay JW. Surgery of the sympathetic nervous system. In: Schmidek HH, Sweet WH, editors. Operative neurosurgical techniques: indications, methods, and results. 3rd ed. Philadelphia: WB Saunders; 1995. p. 1637–46.

6. Wilkinson HA. Sympathectomy for pain. In: Youmans JR, editor. Neurological surgery. Philadelphia: WB Saunders; 1996. p. 3489–99.

7. Johnson JP, Obasi C, Hahn MS, et al. Endoscopic thoracic sympathectomy. J Neurosurg Spine. 1999;91:90–7.

8. Schwartzman RJ, Liu JE, Smullens SN, et al. Long-term outcome following sympathectomy for complex regional pain syndrome type I (RSD). J Neurol Sci. 1997;150(2):149–52.

9. Kumar K, Nath RK, Toth C. Spinal cord stimulation is effective in the management of reflex sympathetic dystrophy. Neurosurgery. 1997;40(3):503–9.

10. Burchiel KJ, Johans TJ, Ochoa J. The surgical treatment of painful traumatic neuromas. J Neurosurg. 1993;78:714–9.

11. Van Eerten PV, Polder TW, Broere CAJ. Operative treatment of meralgia paresthetica: transection versus neurolysis. Neurosurgery. 1995;37(1):63–5.

12. Starling JR, Harms BA. Diagnosis and treatment of genitofemoral and ilioinguinal neuralgia. World J Surg. 1989;13(5):586–91.

13. Hosobuchi Y. The majority of unmyelinated afferent axons in human ventral roots probably conduct pain. Pain. 1980;8:167–80.

14. Onofrio BM, Campa HK. Evaluation of rhizotomy: review of 12 years' experience. J Neurosurg. 1972;36:751–5.

15. North RB, Kidd DH, Campbell JN, et al. Dorsal root ganglionectomy for failed back surgery syndrome: a 5-year follow-up study. J Neurosurg. 1991;74:236–42.

16. Saris SC, Silver JM, Vieira JFS, et al. Sacrococcygeal rhizotomy for perineal pain. Neurosurgery. 1986;19(5):789–93.

17. Tew Jr JM, Taha JM. Percutaneous rhizotomy in the treatment of intractable facial pain (trigeminal, glossopharyngeal, and vagal nerves). In: Schmidek HH, Sweet WH, editors. Operative neurosurgical techniques: indications, methods, and results. 3rd ed. Philadelphia: WB Saunders; 1995. p. 1469–84.

18. Taha JM, Tew Jr JM. Comparison of surgical treatments for trigeminal neuralgia: reevaluation of radiofrequency rhizotomy. Neurosurgery. 1997;38:865–71.

19. Maesawa S, Salame C, Flickinger JC, et al. Clinical outcomes after stereotactic radiosurgery for idiopathic trigeminal neuralgia. J Neurosurg. 2001;94:14–20.

20. Lozano AM, Vanderlinden G, Bachoo R, et al. Microsurgical C-2 ganglionectomy for chronic intractable occipital pain. J Neurosurg. 1998;89:359–65.

21. Rath SA, Seitz K, Soliman N, et al. DREZ coagulations for deafferentation pain related to spinal and peripheral nerve lesions: indication and results of 79 consecutive procedures. Stereotact Funct Neurosurg. 1997;68(1–4 Pt 1):161–7.

22. Nashold JRB, Nashold Jr BS. Microsurgical DREZotomy in treatment of deafferentation pain. In: Schmidek HH, Sweet WH, editors. Operative neurosurgical techniques: indications, methods, and results. 3rd ed. Philadelphia: WB Saunders; 1995. p. 1623–36.

23. Sindou MP. Microsurgical DREZotomy. In: Schmidek HH, Sweet WH, editors. Operative neurosurgical techniques: indications, methods, and results. 3rd ed. Philadelphia: WB Saunders; 1995. p. 1613–21.

24. Bullard DE, Nashold Jr BS. The caudalis DREZ for facial pain. Stereotact Funct Neurosurg. 1997;68(1–4 Pt 1):168–74.

25. Poletti CE. Open cordotomy and medullary tractotomy. In: Schmidek HH, Sweet WH, editors. Operative neurosurgical techniques: indications, methods, and results. 3rd ed. Philadelphia: WB Saunders; 1995. p. 1557–71.

26. Tasker RR. Percutaneous cordotomy. In: Schmidek HH, Sweet WH, editors. Operative neurosurgical techniques: indications, methods, and results. 3rd ed. Philadelphia: WB Saunders; 1995. p. 1595–611.

27. Kanpolat Y, Akyar S, Caglar S, et al. CT-guided percutaneous selective cordotomy. Acta Neurochir. 1993;123(1–2):92–6.

28. Gybels JM, Sweet WH. Neurosurgical treatment of persistent pain: physiological and pathological mechanisms of human pain. Basel: Karger; 1989.

29. Rosomoff HL, Papo I, Loeser JD, et al. Neurosurgical operations on the spinal cord. In: Bonica JJ, editor. The management of pain. 2nd ed. Philadelphia: Lea & Febiger; 1990. p. 2067–81.

30. Watling CJ, Payne R, Allen RR, et al. Commissural myelotomy for intractable cancer pain: report of two cases. Clin J Pain. 1996;12(2):151–6.

31. King RB. Anterior commissurotomy for intractable pain. J Neurosurg. 1977;47:7–11.

32. Nauta HJW, Hewitt E, Westlund KN, et al. Surgical interruption of a midline dorsal column visceral pain pathway. Case report and review of the literature. J Neurosurg. 1997;86:538–42.

33. Hirshberg RM, Al-Chaer ED, Lawand NB, et al. Is there a pathway in the posterior funiculus that signals visceral pain? Pain. 1996;67:291–305.

34. Hitchcock ER. Stereotactic cervical myelotomy. J Neurol Neurosurg Psychiatry. 1970;33:224–30.

35. Bullard DE, Nashold Jr BS. Mesencephalatomy and other brain stem procedures for pain. In: Youmans JR, editor. Neurological surgery. Philadelphia: WB Saunders; 1996. p. 3477–88.

36. Jannetta PJ, Gildenberg PL, Loeser JD, et al. Operations on the brain and brain stem for chronic pain. In: Bonica JJ, editor. The management of pain. 2nd ed. Philadelphia: Lea & Febiger; 1990. p. 2082–103.

37. Young R. Technique of stereotactic medial thalamotomy with the Leksell Gamma Knife for treatment of chronic pain. Neurol Res. 1995;17:59–65.

38. Tasker RR. Thalamotomy. Neurosurg Clin N Am. 1990;1(4):841–64.

39. Tasker RR. Thalamic stereotaxic procedures. In: Schaltenbrand G, Walker AE, editors. Stereotaxy of the human brain: anatomical physiological and clinical applications. Stuttgart: Georg Thieme Verlag; 1982. p. 484–97.

40. Hassenbusch SJ, Pillay PK, Barnett GH. Radiofrequency cingulotomy for intractable cancer pain using stereotaxis guided by magnetic resonance imaging. Neurosurgery. 1990;27(2):220–3.

41. Bouckoms AJ. Limbic surgery for pain. In: Wall PD, Melzack R, editors. Textbook of pain. 3rd ed. Edinburgh: Churchill Livingstone; 1994. p. 1171–87.

42. Levin AB, Katz J, Benson RC, et al. Treatment of pain of diffuse metastatic cancer by stereotactic chemical hypophysectomy: long term results and observations on mechanism of action. Neurosurgery. 1980;6(3):258–62.

43. Ramirez LF, Levin AB. Pain relief after hypophysectomy. Neurosurgery. 1984;14(4):499–504.

44. Hayashi M, Taira T, Chernov M, et al. Gamma Knife surgery for cancer pain – pituitary gland-stalk ablation: a multicenter prospective protocol since 2002. J Neurosurg. 2002;97 Suppl 5:433–7.

45. Levy RM, Lamb S, Adams JE. Treatment of chronic pain by deep brain stimulation: long term follow-up and review of the literature. Neurosurgery. 1987;21(6):885–93.

46. Kumar K, Toth C, Nath RK. Deep brain stimulation for intractable pain: a 15-year experience. Neurosurgery. 1997;40:736–47.

47. Richardson DE. Intracranial stimulation therapies: deep brain stimulation. In: Follett KA, editor. Neurosurgical pain management. Philadelphia: Elsevier; 2004. p. 156–9.

48. Kaplitt M, Rezai AR, Lozano AM, et al. Deep brain stimulation for chronic pain. In: Winn HR, editor. Youmans neurological surgery. Philadelphia: Elsevier; 2004. p. 3119–31.

49. Bittar RG, Kar-Purkayastha I, Owen SL, et al. Deep brain stimulation for pain relief: a meta-analysis. J Clin Neurosci. 2005;12(5):515–9.

50. Leone M, Proietti Cecchini A, et al. Lessons from 8 years' experience of hypothalamic stimulation in cluster headache. Cephalalgia. 2008;28(7):787–97.

51. Coffey RJ. Deep brain stimulation for chronic pain: results of two multicenter trials and a structured review. Pain Med. 2001;2: 183–92.

52. Nguyen J-P, Lefaucheur J-P, Decq P, et al. Chronic motor cortex stimulation in the treatment of central and neuropathic pain. Correlations between clinical, electrophysiological and anatomical data. Pain. 1999;82:245–51.

53. Henderson JM, Lad SP. Motor cortex stimulation and neuropathic facial pain. Neurosurg Focus. 2006;21(6):E6.

54. Lima MC, Fregni F. Motor cortex stimulation for chronic pain: systematic review and meta-analysis of the literature. Neurology. 2008;70(24):2329–37.

55. Velasco F, Argüelles C, Carrillo-Ruiz JD, et al. Efficacy of motor cortex stimulation in the treatment of neuropathic pain: a randomized double-blind trial. J Neurosurg. 2008;108(4): 698–706.

Spinal Cord Stimulation in the Treatment of Postherpetic Neuralgia

68

Stanley Golovac and Louis Raso

- Postherpetic neuralgia is a painful condition affecting your nerve fibers and skin.
- The burning pain associated with postherpetic neuralgia can be severe enough to interfere with sleep and appetite.
- Postherpetic neuralgia is a complication of shingles, which is caused by the chickenpox virus.
- Most cases of shingles clear up within a few weeks. But if the pain lasts long after the shingles rash and blisters have disappeared, it is called postherpetic neuralgia.
- The risk of postherpetic neuralgia increases with age, primarily affecting people over the age of 60. Effective treatment of postherpetic neuralgia is difficult, and the pain can last for months or even years.
- Cases in which pain persists can be treated with spinal cord stimulation.

Introduction

In the pain clinic setting, one of the most difficult pain syndromes to treat is postherpetic neuralgia (PHN). Recent advances in the treatment of an acute infection with the

herpes zoster virus have lowered the incidence of PHN. The pain specialist needs to treat the acute episode aggressively and early, if he is to be successful in reducing the onset of PHN. It is well known that PHN continues to be a common reason for suicide in the elderly population [1]. In most patients with an acute herpes zoster infection, the disease is self-limiting, and the rash and pain disappear completely. In some patients, however, the pain can persist for many years. This chapter will review the cause, clinical course, and current treatments including the use of spinal cord stimulation in the treatment of PHN.

Epidemiology

Acute herpes zoster infection is a reemergence of the varicella zoster virus, or chickenpox virus, which has been lying dormant in the dorsal root ganglion of the nervous system since it became infected during childhood. The reactivation of the virus occurs with the loss of immune surveillance and cell-mediated immunity due to aging [1]. Therefore, the disease is one of the elderly. It starts as a ganglionitis and progresses to an inflammation of the sensory root with eventual skin involvement with the classic vesicular rash [2]. This classic vesicular rash that follows one or two dermatomes is so unique that once seen, it is easily recognizable in future clinical situations. The immune system is usually able to limit the disease process to one or two dermatomes. The most common area for the outbreak is the thoracic area followed by the ophthalmic division of the trigeminal nerve [3].

In patients of any age with a significant immune deficiency, the disease is more common. Examples of such include patients with AIDS, lymphoma, leukemias, corticosteroid dependency, and chemotherapeutic immune suppression. In patients with PHN, there is irreversible skin and sensory damage when the dorsal root ganglion and its processes are attacked by varicella zoster virus and may be severely damaged from the spinal cord to the epidermis [1–3].

S. Golovac, M.D. (✉)
Department of Anesthesia, Pain Management, Surgery,
Cape Canaveral Hospital,
Cocoa Beach, FL 32952, USA

Space Coast Pain Institute,
4770 Honeyridge Lane, Merritt Island, FL, USA
e-mail: sgolovac@mac.com

L. Raso, M.D.
CEO Jupiter Interventional Pain Management Corp,
2141 South Alternate A1A, Suite 110, Jupiter, FL 33477, USA
e-mail: lraso@aol.com

T.R. Deer et al. (eds.), *Comprehensive Treatment of Chronic Pain by Medical, Interventional, and Integrative Approaches,*
DOI 10.1007/978-1-4614-1560-2_68, © American Academy of Pain Medicine 2013

721

Patients with PHN collectively describe three distinct components to their disorder:

A constant, usually deep pain

A brief, recurrent shooting or shocking tic-like pain

A sharp, radiating dysesthetic sensation evoked by very light touching of the skin (allodynia)

The probability that an acute herpes zoster episode will result in PHN increases with increasing age. PHN occurs in less than 8 % of zoster cases in patients under age 30, 50 % in patients aged 50, 60 % in patients aged 60, 70 % in patients aged 70, etc. [3].

PHN is defined as pain lasting more than 6 weeks after the acute onset of zoster. In the past, with standard treatment, patients were generally not satisfied and they were unable to achieve any significant reduction in their pain levels and any improvement in their quality of life [3]. Generally, after an acute episode of zoster, only 5–8 % of patients will have a recurrence, implying that immune system is able to keep the virus in check for the remainder of the patient's life. Ten to 15 % of patients may present with the classic pain without the classic rash (sine herpete).

Generally, the pain precedes the rash, and it is not unusual for a patient to get a complete work-up prior to the emergence of a rash. There are many patients that have been treated for a herniated disk, acute cholecystitis, myocardial infarction, or other pain syndrome prior to confirming the diagnosis. If the patient is given any corticosteroid therapy, it can even further confuse the clinical picture [1–3].

Treatment of PHN

In a survey conducted in 2002 in 385 patients ≥65 years of age with persistent pain after shingles (PHN) and receiving prescription medication, only 14 % were highly satisfied with their treatment. A majority of patients had moderate to severe pain. Treatment of the acute phase with medical therapy has the ability to decrease viral shedding and the development of new lesions, while also it has the ability to potentially decrease the duration of the outbreak [4].

There have been numerous treatments for PHN cited in the literature. They have included corticosteroids, opioids, antiviral agents, and topical agents. They are tried after aggressive treatment of the acute phase has failed. Some of the common medications used in the past include the following:

• Anticonvulsants
• Antidepressants – tricyclics, serotonin-norepinephrine reuptake inhibitors (SNRIs)
• Opioid analgesics
• Dermal and topical treatments [5]

Recently, a chickenpox vaccine has been instituted into society to reduce both the acute and chronic episodes of varicella infection. As the population ages, we will see the impact of this vaccine [6]. The acute phase is mediated via the sympathetic nervous system and the chronic phase being a sympathetically independent phase. The chronic or PHN phase is very difficult to treat. Numerous treatments have been tried with a very low success rate and a low percentage of patient satisfaction. This ineffective therapy has led to the high incidence of suicide in the elderly population.

Interventional Therapy

It has been thought for a long time that if the sympathetic outflow could be disrupted to the nerves involved, the occurrence of PHN could be reduced. The interventional pain community has embraced this concept and is aggressive with neural blockade early in the treatment of the acute phase. There are numerous references as far back as 1938 continuing to the present day [7]. It has been proven in these studies that if you are able to intervene early during the acute phase, you can prevent the onset of PHN in up to 95 % of the patients. Dr. Alon Winnie published one of the largest studies that revealed the drop-off time in order to reduce the incidence of PHN at approximately 8 weeks. By instituting sympathetic blockade, you are able to reduce the duration of the acute phase and the progression to PHN [8]. PHN is thought to be due to neural ischemia and intraneural capillary blood flow, and by 8 weeks, the ischemic changes become irreversible, especially in the larger nerve fibers [9]. The large nerve fibers are more prone to the ischemic changes due to their higher metabolic rate. These changes result in the allodynia, resulting from activation of the nonmyelinated C-nociceptive fibers along with a loss of large myelinated fibers [9]. The large myelinated fibers normally suppress the activation of the small nonmyelinated and therefore the pain transmission. It is this loss of suppression that leads to the sharp lancinating pain and allodynia that is closely associated with acute herpes zoster and postherpetic neuralgia [9].

Evidence is scant for the value of surgical and procedural interventions in general, although there are numerous small studies supporting the use of specific interventions such as nerve blocks, neurosurgical procedures, and neuro-augmentation.

Conventional methods are used daily in order to blunt and force the viral entity that most patients desire to avoid. Many patients elect to apply creams with antiviral components, tricyclic antidepressants (TCAs), neuroleptic medications, and some unfortunately with opioid medications such as hydrocodone, oxycodone, and morphine sulfate [10]. Each of these forms of treatments may help to a degree, but without interventional treatments, procrastination is enviable.

Epidural steroids is a treatment form that helps reduce swelling, inflammation, and pain sensation from the nerve endings located at the dorsal root ganglion (DRG), where the varicella zoster virus is located.

Neurostimulation is the application of precise targeted electrical stimulation on nociceptive pathways. Electric stimulation has a long history in medicine for treating various ailments [11]. The nociceptive pathways are made up of tracts in the central and peripheral nervous systems. The central nervous system includes nociceptive pathways in the spinal cord and brain, specifically the dorsal roots, dorsal ganglion, spinothalamic tracts, and all ascending neural tracts to the cerebrum. The peripheral nervous system includes pathways outside the spinal cord, specifically various plexuses and peripheral nerves.

Components of the System

Spinal cord stimulation involves the placement of an electrical system to block nociception. The system comprises the surgical placement of epidural electrodes, cables, and radiofrequency transmitter or battery. Much of this method has evolved from cardiac pacemaker technology. The minimal invasiveness and trialing has led to the success of this approach. Neurostimulation can be placed during an outpatient procedure, with local anesthesia and sedation. The patient experiences minimal discomfort when the system is placed and during the postoperative period [12–16].

Before the system is placed, a simple trial of percutaneous lead placement can be performed. In this case, the patient goes home with the lead connected to a screener box. No incision is necessary, and the procedure is performed using only local anesthesia. The purpose of the trial is to determine the effectiveness of the stimulation for relieving pain and improving the patient's quality of life. If this temporary method allows the patient to sleep better, use less pain medication, and sit and stand longer, then it becomes more convincing to place an internalized spinal cord stimulation system.

Leads of various types are commonly used by all three companies: Boston Scientific, St. Jude Medical, and Medtronic. There is an array of various leads from percutaneous to paddles (Fig. 68.1). Figure 68.2 demonstrates two leads placed slightly off the midline toward the left dorsal root entry zone. This allows segmental stimulation over the roots affected by the viral injury.

Mechanism of Action

The mechanism of action of spinal cord stimulation is based on the placement of epidural electrodes along the dorsal columns. Originally, spinal cord stimulation was called dorsal column stimulation. It is thought that spinal cord stimulation works through the gate-control theory of Melzack and Wall [13] which theorizes that stimulating large nerve fibers (A beta fibers) can inhibit or modulate smaller nerve fibers (A delta or C fibers), transmitting nociceptive input possibly at the dorsal root or horn of the spinal cord. Strategically placed epidural electrodes stimulate the dorsal columns (A beta fibers) to inhibit or modulate incoming nociceptive input through the A delta or C fibers. Ongoing research suggests

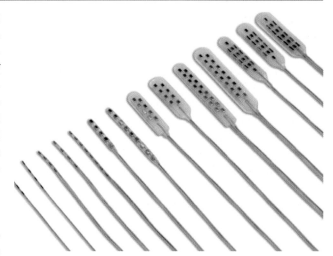

Fig. 68.1 Array of various leads from percutaneous to paddles

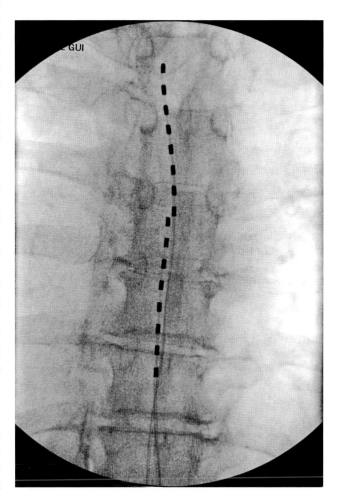

Fig. 68.2 Two leads placed slightly off the midline toward the left dorsal root entry zone. This allows segmental stimulation over the roots affected by the viral injury

that spinal cord stimulation may inhibit transmission in the spinothalamic tract, activation of central inhibitory mechanisms influencing sympathetic efferent neurons, and release of various inhibitory neurotransmitters.

Pain Conditions

Spinal cord stimulation can be applied to treat neuropathic pain conditions, including arachnoiditis, complex regional pain syndrome (formerly called reflex sympathetic dystrophy), neuropathies, brachial and lumbosacral plexopathies, radiculopathies, deafferentation syndromes, phantom limb pain, and postherpetic neuralgia. Clinical studies and 30 years of clinical experience have continued to show efficacy in these conditions. Visceral syndromes such as interstitial cystitis, chronic abdominal pain, and chronic pancreatitis have been treated with limited success.

Most randomized controlled trials of chronic neuropathic pain have examined only two pain syndromes: PHN and diabetic neuropathy [17]. In the Practice Parameter: Treatment of Postherpetic Neuralgia, an evidence-based report of the quality standards subcommittee of the American Academy of Neurology, published in Neurology in September 2004, excellent overview of treatment options is provided. Overall, the group with the best efficacy with low side effects included gabapentin, lidocaine patch, pregabalin, and tricyclic antidepressants. Opiates remain a controversial option for treatment of PHN or any chronic pain syndrome. In severe cases of either shingles or PHN, epidural steroid injection can be helpful.

Limited success of spinal cord stimulation may depend on the extent of peripheral vascular disease. Based on one study, spinal cord stimulation does not reduce the incidence of amputation in the lower extremities. The same rationale for using spinal cord stimulation for treating peripheral vascular disease is now being applied in clinical trials of patients with intractable angina, including those with patent coronary vessels who continue to have intractable angina and patients who are not candidates for coronary bypass and stent procedures. It is theorized that these patients have a neuropathic condition and microvascular blood flow deficiency.

Some painful conditions cannot be stimulated along the spinal cord and therefore are not responsive to spinal cord stimulation. Thus, peripheral nerve and plexus stimulation has evolved as a complementary neurostimulation approach. The mechanism of peripheral nerve and plexus stimulation is unclear since the electrodes are not stimulating the dorsal columns. Some postulate that a variation of the gate-control theory is involved at the peripheral nervous system level. Moreover, peripheral nerve stimulation may activate central structures, leading to inhibition of various nociceptive pathways, similar to the way acupuncture results in somatosensory cortex activation.

Postherpetic Neuralgia

The effectiveness of SCS in postherpetic neuralgia remains controversial. Meglio et al. reported good success in six of ten implanted patients [17]. Other authors have been unable to reproduce this success rate. None of the published series contain more than a handful of patients with this condition. In the senior author's experience, postherpetic neuralgia has not been very responsive to stimulation. The stimulation-induced paresthesias are often felt as sharp and annoying and not tolerated by these patients.

Conclusion

Neurostimulation of the central and peripheral nervous systems is playing a vital role in the treatment of various intractable pain conditions, including conditions for which we have limited pathophysiologic understanding, such as complex regional pain syndrome. Until we develop treatments that truly eliminate pain, neurostimulation can play a major role in improving the quality of life for pain patients. These systems do not damage neural pathways and could be removed when curative therapy becomes available.

References

1. Burgoon Jr CF, Burgoon JS. The natural history of herpes zoster. JAMA. 1957;164:265–9.
2. Juel-Jensen BE, MacCalum FO. Herpes simplex varicella and zoster. Clinical manifestations and treatment. Philadelphia: JB Lippincott Company; 1972. p. 44, 79–116.
3. Bonica JJ. Chapter 26: thoracic segmental and intercostal neuralgia. In: The management of pain. Philadelphia: Lea & Febiger; 1953. p. 865.
4. Bonezzi C, Demartini L. Treatment options in postherpetic neuralgia. Acta Neurol Scand. 1999;100:25–35.
5. Ashburn MA, Staats PS. Management of chronic pain. Lancet. 1999;353(9167):1865–9.
6. Brisson M, Edmunds W, Gay N. Varicella vaccination: impact of vaccine efficacy on the epidemiology of VZV. J Med Virol. 2003;70:S31–7.
7. Colding A. The effect of regional sympathetic blocks in the treatment of herpes zoster. Acta Anaesthesiol Scand. 1969;13:133–41.
8. Winnie AP, Hartwell PW. Relationship between time of treatment of acute herpes zoster with sympathetic blockade and prevention of post-herpetic neuralgia: clinical support for a new theory of the mechanism by which sympathetic blockade provides therapeutic benefit. Reg Anesth Pain Med. 1993;18(5):271–329.
9. Selander D, Mansson LG, Karisson L, Svanvic J. Adrenergic vasoconstriction in peripheral nerves of the rabbit. Anesthesiology. 1985;62:6–10.
10. Bokai J. Das auftreten der schafblattern unter be sonderen umstanden. Ungar Arch Med. 1892;1:159–61.
11. Stankus SJ, Dlugopolski M, Packer D. Management of herpes zoster (shingles) and postherpetic neuralgia. Am Fam Physician. 2000;61(8):2437–44, 2447–8.
12. Cruccu G, Aziz TZ, Garcia-Larrea L, Hansson P, Jensen TS, Lefaucheur JP, Simpson BA, Taylor RS. EFNS guidelines on neurostimulation therapy for neuropathic pain. Eur J Neurol. 2007;14(9):952–70.
13. Melzack R, Wall PD. Pain mechanisms: a new theory. Science. 1965;150:971–9.
14. Tesfaye S, Stevens LK, Stephenson JM, Fuller JH, Plater M, Ionescu-Tirgoviste C, Nuber A, Pozza G, Ward JD. Prevalence of

diabetic peripheral neuropathy and its relation to glycaemic control and potential risk factors: the EURODIAB IDDM Complications Study. Diabetologia. 1996;39(11):1377–84.

15. Tölle T, Xu X, Sadosky AB. Painful diabetic neuropathy: a cross-sectional survey of health state impairment and treatment patterns. J Diabetes Complications. 2006;20(1):26–33.

16. van Seventer R, Sadosky A, Lucero M, Dukes E. A cross-sectional survey of health state impairment and treatment patterns in patients with postherpetic neuralgia. Age Ageing. 2006;35(2):132–7.

17. Meglio M, Cioni B, Prezioso A, Talamonti G. Spinal cord stimulation (SCS) in deafferentation pain. Pacing Clin Electrophysiol. 1989;12(4 Pt 2):709–12.

Complications of Interventional Pain Management Techniques

69

Marco Araujo and Dermot More O'Ferrall

Key Points

- The most common reported complications are medication-related misuse, pneumothorax, spinal cord injury, and nerve damage.
- Intrathecal injection of 10 ml of preservative-free normal saline can reduce the potential for post-dural-puncture headache after a dural puncture.
- Other causes of headache following epidural steroid injection include intracranial or subdural hematoma, epidural abscess, meningitis, and pneumocephalus.
- Frequently, the ligamentum flavum is adherent to the dura above C5 spinal level.
- Injection of particulate steroids can lead to anterior spinal cord syndrome. Use of nonparticulate steroids and inferoposterior foraminal needle placement reduces the risk of paraplegia after transforaminal epidurals.
- The use of lateral fluoroscopic guidance for trigger point injections of the thoracic wall musculature reduces the risk of pneumothorax.
- Radiofrequency needle placement close to the nerve root can cause severe postoperative dysesthesia and nerve root and spinal cord injury.
- Right-sided SGB may cause sinus arrhythmias, while left-sided SGB can cause left ventricular dysfunction in patients with preexisting left ventricular disease.
- Contrast volume should be maximum of half (0.5) ml/disc in cervical discography.
- Warfarin should be stopped five (5) days prior to neuraxial procedure, and the INR should be less than 1.4 before proceeding.

M. Araujo, M.D., FACIP (✉)
Pain Clinic Advanced Pain Management,
4131 W. Loomis Rd Ste 300, Greenfield, WI 54301, USA
e-mail: sirmarcoarauvo@hotmail.com

D.M. O'Ferrall, M.D.
Pain Clinic Advanced Pain Management,
4131 W. Loomis Rd Ste 300, Greenfield, WI 53221, USA
e-mail: doferrall@wi.rr.com

Introduction

Several textbooks cover the techniques, indications, contraindications, and the mechanism of action of the interventional pain management techniques, but only few textbooks have focused on the complications and on their consequences. Interventional pain management has evolved tremendously since the first described therapeutic nerve block, performed by Tuffer in 1899 [1, 2]. The combination of Interventional Pain Physicians with small amount of experience in the field and the recent significant increase in the utilization of interventional diagnostic and therapeutic techniques raises the potential for increased complications.

Unfortunately, there are major limitations in the analysis of complications. Historically, physicians have a tendency to report no poor outcomes; therefore, only few complications are reported. Health privacy issues and fear of litigation prevent several physicians from reporting the complications of interventional techniques. Furthermore, the complications may be reported to different databases, making the analysis even more difficult.

The American Society of Anesthesiologists (ASA) Closed Claims Project Database can provide valuable information on the adverse outcomes in chronic pain management from 1970 through December 2000 [3]. During this time period, 284 chronic pain management claims were reported. 276 (96 %) claims were related to interventional pain management techniques including nerve blocks, epidural steroid injections, trigger point injections, tendon or joint injections, neuroablation procedures, and neuromodulation implant techniques. 78 % claims were related to nerve blocks and injections. The most common complications were pneumothorax and spinal cord-nerve injury [3]. There were 18 (6 %) claims for paraplegia or quadriplegia with four caused by epidural abscess, eight caused by chemical injury from injection into the spinal cord, and six caused by epidural hematoma. Even more alarming, 5 % of claims were related to brain damage, while 4 % were related to death.

While the overall incidence of significant complications in interventional pain medicine is low, some catastrophic complications do occur as ASA Close Claims Project Database shows. Physicians need to be familiar with current literature and to be aware of potential complications. With the advent of interventional pain medicine as a recognized subspecialty of medicine, more formal and standardized interventional training must occur in the academic setting, which will hopefully reduce the likelihood of complications [2–6]. This chapter will focus on procedure-specific complications and on ways to improve safety and minimize complications, by addressing issues pertinent to the patient, the physician, the nursing staff, the equipment, and the medications utilized.

Procedure-Related Complications

As the practice of pain medicine grows, there is a need for greater awareness of potential injuries to patients. Interventional pain management physicians and staff must explain clearly these complications in layman's terms to the patient in order to reduce the occurrence of claims. Written preoperative instructions explaining the procedure and potential complications should be given and signed by the patient prior to the procedure, allowing time for its review. The *informed* consent prior to all procedures should include a discussion about the indication, complications, risks, and available alternative therapies. Ideally, additional consent should also be obtained prior to utilizing medication for off-label, non-FDA (Food and Drug Administration)-approved use.

Epidural Injection

Absolute contraindications to epidural steroid injections include local or systemic infection and bleeding diathesis. Severe central spinal stenosis may be a relative contraindication, and caution must be taken if the injection is being performed interlaminarly at the severe spinal stenosis level. Pregnancy may be a contraindication if fluoroscopy is used.

The documented incidence of dural puncture is anywhere from 0.5 to 5 % in the literature, although this is unacceptably high, especially with the use of fluoroscopy [7–9]. Potential complications of dural puncture include spinal headache, subdural hematoma, and potential for spinal anesthesia or spinal-neural injury. When the rate of cerebral spinal fluid (CSF) loss exceeds CSF production, a downward shift of the brain in the skull may occur, placing traction on the meningeal nerves and subdural veins resulting in spinal headache or subdural hematoma, respectively. Post-dural-puncture headache may follow dural puncture in up to 75 % of cases [10].

If, while performing an interlaminar epidural injection, an inadvertent dural puncture is obtained and confirmed with injection of contrast, producing a myelogram, then without needle movement, an intrathecal injection of 10 cc of preservative-free normal saline can reduce the potential for post-dural-puncture headache significantly [11]. The injection should be performed at another level, or via a different route, such as transforaminal, but without local anesthetic because of the potential for spinal anesthesia.

One epidural blood patch can result in complete, almost instantaneous relief of spinal headache in up to 75 % of patients. If the first epidural blood patch was not successful, the second epidural blood patch can relieve the spinal headache in up to 95 % of patients [12]. Dural puncture brings the risk of subdural hematoma, which can be seen intracranially or spinally [13–15].

It is important to understand that there are many, potentially serious causes of headache following epidural steroid injection, including intracranial or subdural hematoma, epidural abscess, meningitis, pneumocephalus, and spinal headache from dural puncture. A thorough history and physical examination will usually yield a diagnosis, although occasionally imaging studies will be warranted. An epidural abscess, subdural or epidural hematoma resulting in spinal cord compression, needs to be recognized early, and surgical intervention within 8 h is mandatory in order to prevent a permanent neurological injury (Fig. 69.1a, b) [16–25]. Epidural abscess, bacterial meningitis, and aseptic meningitis have all been described [17, 23, 26, 27]. Pneumocephalus produces an immediate and severe headache when patient is allowed to sit. Pneumocephalus is diagnosed with CT scan, and the headache usually resolves as the air is absorbed, over a period of 5–7 days.

Other documented complications of interlaminar epidural injections include arachnoiditis, intrinsic spinal cord injury, spinal anesthesia, transient paralysis, arterial gas embolism, and transient blindness [28, 29]. Controversy exists over whether arachnoiditis can complicate epidural steroid injection [19, 20].

Anatomy

Understanding the anatomy of the epidural space is important. It is triangular in shape, and 1–2 mm in depth in the upper cervical spine, with 3 mm in depth in the lower cervical

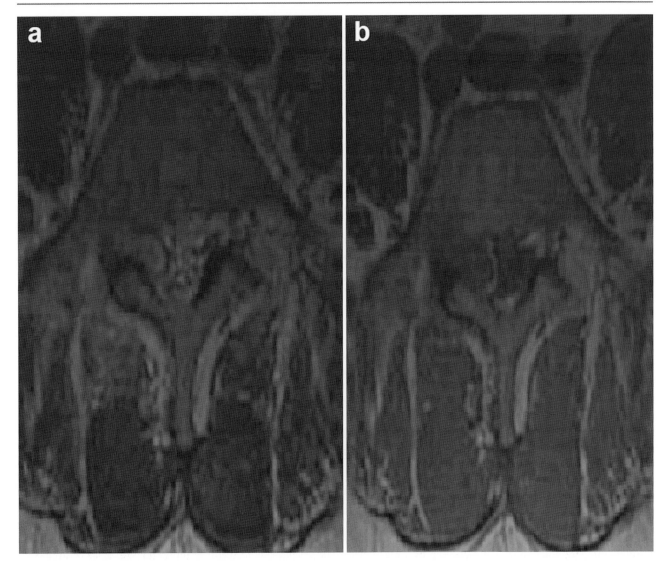

Fig. 69.1 (**a**, **b**) Epidural abscess seen on the above T2 and T1 axial images of the lumbar spine resulting in compression of the exiting right L5 spinal nerve. It occurred following a right L5/S1 intra-articular zygapophysial joint injection

spine, this increases to up to 5 mm in the upper thoracic spine and is 5–6 mm in depth in the midlumbar spine. Thirty-four percent of the time, the ligamentum flavum is adherent to the dura above C5 [30].

Recommendation

The needle entry point for cervical interlaminar epidural steroid injections should be at the C7/T1 level or below, and the epidural space should be entered in the midline where depth is greatest. The needle should be anchored at the skin with the nondominant hand and advanced with the dominant hand.

When the epidural space is identified with the loss of resistance technique, a catheter should be thread to the appropriate level and contrast injected to confirm the correct level, no vascular uptake and an epidurogram (Figs. 69.2 and 69.3)

[31–34]. One should minimize the volume injected to 2–3 cc, and the solution should be injected slowly. AP, oblique, and lateral fluoroscopic views should be taken to document unequivocal epidural spread of contrast prior to injection of medication. Contrast should be injected under live fluoroscopy to confirm no concomitant vascular uptake (Fig. 69.4). Sedation should also be minimized because oversedation may cause loss of communication and the ability to monitor the patient. Oversedation also increases the potential for unintentional patient movement or startle and increases the potential for cardiopulmonary complications. It is generally accepted in the pain medicine community that oversedation or deep monitored anesthesia care (MAC) should not be utilized because it increases the potential for catastrophic complications as spinal cord trauma.

The advantage of this technique is to reduce the chance of dural puncture, spinal anesthesia, and spinal cord injury.

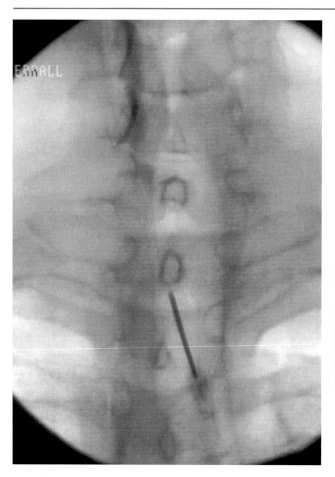

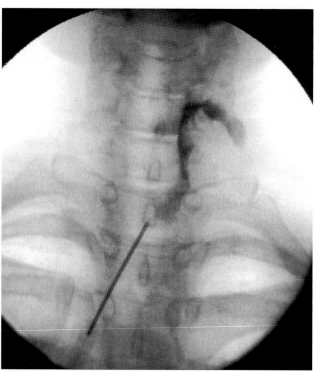

Fig. 69.3 AP fluoroscopic image of a cervical interlaminar epidural steroid injection with a catheter thread to C5/6 in a patient with a right C6 radiculopathy. Note needle entry at T1/2

Fig. 69.2 AP fluoroscopic image of a cervical interlaminar epidural steroid injection with a catheter thread to C6/7 in a patient with a left C7 radiculopathy. Note needle entry at T2/3

Entering the epidural space at the midline position, where there are fewer epidural veins, will also reduce the potential risk of epidural hematoma.

Transforaminal epidural steroid injections are felt in general to be safe, although the prevalence of complications remains underreported [35]. Complications from the transforaminal approach are similar to interlaminar epidural steroid injections but also include the catastrophic complication of anterior spinal cord syndrome. This can follow inadvertent injection into the radiculomedullary artery (Adamkiewicz) in the lumbar or thoracic spine or cervical radicular artery in the cervical spine. Locked-in syndrome or brain stem infarct may follow unrecognized vertebral artery injection during cervical transforaminal injection (Fig. 69.4).

In the thoracic and lumbar spines, two unfortunate circumstances need to be present. Firstly, the artery of Adamkiewicz (radicular medullary artery) needs to be present at the symptomatic level and, secondly, undetected arterial penetration with subsequent injection. The artery of Adamkiewicz usually arises on the left between T7 and L4

but may be as low lying as S1 on the left or right. It runs with the spinal nerve in the anterosuperior aspect of the foramen and therefore may be penetrated inadvertently at this site [36, 37].

Proposed theories for this include intravascular injection of particulate steroid, resulting in spasm or thrombosis, which results in anterior spinal cord infarction because of the absence of collateral circulation. In the cervical spine, the sole vascular supply to the anterior spinal cord again comes from the anterior spinal artery, and the feeding radicular arteries are highly variable in number, location, and side. Similarly, the presence of a radicular artery at the symptomatic level, and undetected interarterial injection, can result in anterior spinal cord infarction and quadriplegia [38–47].

Strategies to reduce the chance of this catastrophic complication include the following: (1) understanding the fluoroscopic anatomy; (2) understanding contrast flow patterns; (3) optimizing interventional skills; (4) use of extension tubing and injection of contrast under live fluoroscopy to avoid the need to recannulate the needle after contrast is injected; (5) use of digital subtraction imaging; (6) use of nonparticulation solution such as dexamethasone and betamethasone; (7) in addition, some experts have recommended using blunt tip needles, as these are less likely to

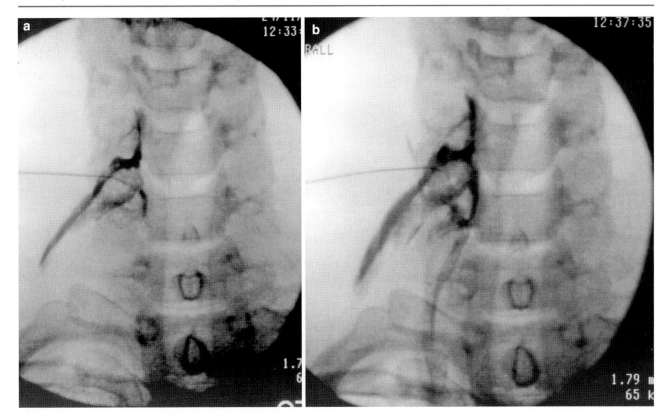

Fig. 69.4 (**a**) AP fluoroscopic image of a right C5/6 transforaminal epidural steroid injection. (**b**) AP fluoroscopic image of a right C5/6 transforaminal epidural steroid injection. Please note the vascular uptake not seen on the previous image is apparent with contrast injection under live fluoroscopy

penetrate an artery [48, 49]; and (8) needle placement in the posteroinferior aspect of the foramen (lumbar, thoracic) to avoid the artery of Adamkiewicz which runs with the spinal nerve in the anterosuperior aspect of the foramen.

Trigger Point Injection

Trigger point injections are generally considered to be fairly straightforward; however, some catastrophic complications have been described in cases without fluoroscopy. In a closed claims study, the second most common cause of pneumothorax behind intercostal nerve block was trigger point injection, being responsible for 21 % of cases [5].

Other documented complications include local infection, cellulitis, hematoma, epidural abscess, pneumothorax, spinal anesthesia, spinal cord injury, anaphylaxis, and death.

Use of fluoroscopy for trigger point injections in the cervical or thoracic area will help reduce needle misplacement, either into the epidural, subdural, subarachnoid space, or into the spinal cord, which has occurred with trigger point injections of paraspinal muscles. The use of lateral fluoroscopic guidance for trigger point injections of any

posterior thoracic wall musculature will document needle depth and prevent pneumothorax by remaining superficial to the ribs [50–52].

Zygapophysial Joint Injection/ Medial Branch Block

In general, lumbar zygapophysial (facet) joint injection is a safe procedure, although complications similar to epidural steroid injections have been described. These include infection with resulting cellulitis or epidural abscess, epidural hematoma, intravascular injection, dural puncture, spinal anesthesia, spinal cord trauma, neural trauma, chemical meningitis, and pneumothorax. Vertebral artery damage or injection is a potential risk with cervical facet joint injections [53–59]. With the use of fluoroscopy and contrast injection in experienced hands, serious complications should not occur. In the cervical spine, a posterior parasagittal approach to the medial branch nerves or posterior approach to the interarticular z-joint injection is safer than a lateral approach (Fig. 69.5). A lateral approach brings the contents of the spinal canal potentially into the path of the needle, especially if

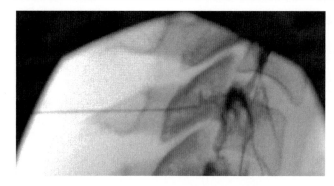

Fig. 69.5 Lateral cervical spine fluoroscopic image of C4 medial branch block showing vascular uptake

the clinician is unable to eliminate parallax and get a true lateral fluoroscopic image. Potential for going through and through a facet joint is real if needle depth is not checked frequently as the needle is advanced. Ideally, under tunnel vision, the periosteum of the adjacent articular process should be intentionally contacted prior to entering the joint to confirm depth and then the needle rotated into the joint. This will help prevent the needle going through the joint to the adjacent tissue [60].

Stellate Ganglion Block

Many techniques have been described for stellate ganglion block, some of which are without fluoroscopic guidance [61–63]. Multiple complications have been described, most of which have occurred from nonfluoroscopically guided injections that have resulted in inadvertent needle placement into the vertebral artery, adjacent disc, neurotissue, esophagus, intrathecal space, or pleura. These complications have included seizures from intravascular injection, spinal anesthesia, cervical epidural abscess, brachial plexus block, intercostal neuralgia, locked-in syndrome, pneumochylothorax, pneumothorax, reversible blindness, hoarseness, dysphagia, and death [64–74]. These complications can be reduced or hopefully eliminated with a technique described by Abdi et al. [75].

Under ipsilateral oblique fluoroscopic guidance, the respective endplates are squared off, and the C-arm is obliqued until a crisp C7 uncinate process is visualized. Then a 25-gauge spinal needle is advanced down, under tunnel vision, to the base of the uncinate process at the junction of the vertebral body. Under live fluoroscopic guidance with extension tubing, injection of contrast is performed to confirm appropriate nonvascular contrast flow. The needle will lie anterior to the vertebral artery, posterior to the common carotid artery, and lateral to the esophagus. A total of 5 cc should be adequate to obtain stellate ganglion blockade.

Discography

In experienced hands, discography is safe, whether that be in the cervical, lumbar, or thoracic spine. Understanding indications and contraindications to discography is important. Coagulopathy and active infection are general contraindications, but central spinal stenosis, myelopathy, and large disc protrusion are contraindications to cervical or thoracic discography [76].

Potential and described complications pertinent to all three areas include superficial infection, epidural abscess, discitis, or nerve root injury. In the cervical or thoracic spine, the potential for spinal cord injury exists. Quadriplegia has been described following epidural hematoma, epidural abscess, and from subdural empyema [77–84]. It has also occurred secondary to cervical disc herniation from disc pressurization at discography. Keeping the contrast volume in cervical or thoracic discography to a minimum is also important, with less than 0.5 cc/disc usually sufficient for cervical discography.

While infection is a real concern, the administration of preoperative intravenous antibiotics, intradiscal antibiotics, and/or a coaxial needle technique has been described in the literature to be able to reduce the incidence of infection (Fig. 69.6).

A coaxial needle technique has been shown to reduce the chance of discitis from 2.7 to 0.7 % in 220 patients [85]. Preoperative intravenous cefazolin has been shown to reduce the chance of disc infection from 1 to 4 % down to 0 %. Utilizing cefazolin in a concentration of 1 mg/cc intradiscally resulted in no intradiscal infections of 127 patients [86, 87].

The prophylactic antibiotics commonly utilized do not prevent anaerobic discitis, which may occur with the anterior approach to cervical discography, where esophageal penetration is possible. Utilizing a right anterolateral (oblique) approach reduces the chance for esophageal perforation and consequent potential anaerobic discitis. Auscultation of the carotid artery should be performed and ultrasound ordered if carotid bruits are heard prior to discography if an oblique approach is utilized, because of the potential of the needle traversing the carotid and dislodging an unstable plaque.

Patients with discitis usually present with pain and fever, 3 days to 2 weeks post-discography. Erythrocyte sedimentation rate, white cell count, and C-reactive protein are usually positive within the first week. It may take anywhere from 2 to 5 weeks for a bone scan to become positive. MRI with or without gadolinium is now considered the gold standard imaging study. If discitis is suspected, infectious disease consultation, disc biopsy, and culture should be taken. IV antibiotics should be started, and consideration should be given for surgical exploration and/or bracing.

Many of the complications reported with lumbar discography were reported prior to 1970, with many of them

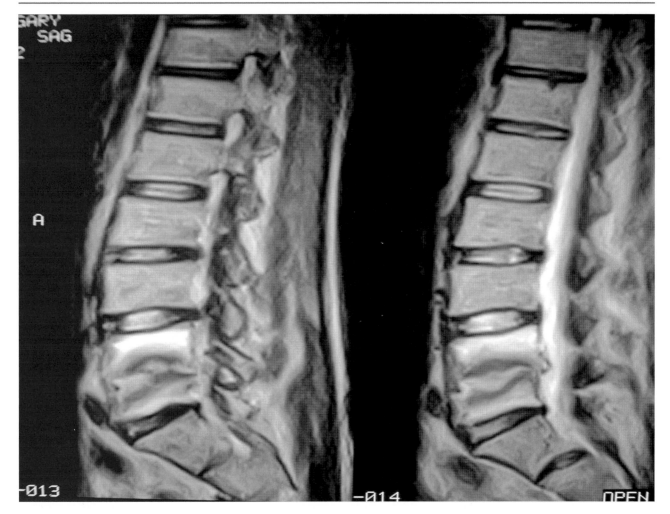

Fig. 69.6 T2-weighted MRI scan of lumbar spine demonstrating L4/5 discitis

in the 1950s. Today with preoperative intravenous antibiotics, intradiscal antibiotics, and a coaxial needle technique, with extrapedicular, extradural fluoroscopically guided approach, these complications should be minimal [88, 89].

If a posterior transdural approach to a disc is planned, then it is important not to utilize intradiscal cefazolin because of the potential for intractable seizures with inadvertent intrathecal cefazolin injection. Therefore, in a patient with previous posterolateral intratransverse bony fusion mass, when posterior transdural approach is considered, or if inadvertent dural puncture occurs with extrapedicular, extradural approach to the disc, then contrast should be mixed with another antibiotic besides cefazolin, such as ceftriaxone, gentamicin, or clindamycin [90].

Pneumothorax has been described as a complication of thoracic discography but could also occur with cervical discography at the C7/T1 level.

In general, cervical or thoracic discography, because of the more challenging technical aspects, and potential for

more catastrophic complications, should only be performed by highly skilled and experienced interventionalists.

Summary

It is important to know the literature on current technical standards, modify practice accordingly, and understand that many complications are never published. History and physical examination should be performed on all patients prior to spinal injections. Physicians should review pertinent imaging studies, understand indications and contraindications of procedures, and obtain informed consent. Knowledge of regional and fluoroscopic anatomy is important before attaining technical expertise in a supervised training environment. Familiarization with all contrast flow patterns under live fluoroscopy is imperative. Above all, understand that complications are inevitable, and it is imperative to identify and treat these problems promptly to minimize their impact when they occur and communicate these issues with the patient.

Patient Pertinent Issues

A thorough history and physical examination is vital on all patients prior to neuraxial blockade, regardless of practice set-up or referral pattern. Important points of the history of a patient undergoing an interventional procedure will be addressed.

Past Medical History

This should include any bleeding diathesis, any immune suppressive disorder, history of allergy, anaphylaxis or asthma, and whether they have valvular heart disease.

Medications

It is important to note whether the patient is taking any oral steroid, antibiotics, anticoagulants, or Glucophage, as these will impact patient outcome. Glucophage is generally considered safe in patients with normal renal function when a small amount of nonionic contrast is utilized. It should be temporarily discontinued in patients with impaired renal function undergoing procedures requiring larger amounts of contrast, as it may result in the patient developing lactic acidosis.

Patients taking oral steroids will not only be immunosuppressed but also at increased risk of potential side effects from steroids [91].

Anticoagulants will clearly put patients at risk for hemorrhagic complications. Knowledge of prescription and over-the-counter medications and herbal remedies is important in risk-stratifying patients.

Neuraxial blocks on patients with an active infection requiring antibiotics should be postponed because of the potential for bacteremia and introduction of bacteria to the epidural space.

Allergies

Knowledge of patient allergic to medications that may be utilized in a procedure such as steroid, local anesthetic, or antibiotics is important in reducing the chance of anaphylactic reaction. It is also important to document any known allergy to shellfish or iodine if contrast is to be utilized and any latex allergy, as these procedures need to be done, first case of the day, in a latex-free environment. (Gadolinium may be used in iodine-allergic patients, although there is a documented cross allergy to gadolinium.)

Review of Systems

Thorough review of systems should help rule out any occult coagulopathy, infection, cord compression, malignancy, or pregnant state.

Social History

This should include any prior litigation as even more thorough documentation and informed consent may be required.

Physical Examination

A general but also procedure-specific physical examination should be performed. Attention should be paid to whether the patient is hemodynamically unstable or febrile, as elective procedures should be rescheduled in that event.

A thorough neurological examination is important to establish as a baseline, especially in the event of an adverse neurological outcome. Knowledge of a carotid bruit and subsequent Doppler study result is vital in patients undergoing procedures, in which the carotid artery may be penetrated, such as cervical discography, as the potential for dislodging a mobile thrombus is real. A thorough cardiopulmonary assessment is important in patients undergoing conscious sedation.

Imaging Study

Interventional pain physicians should be to the spine, what the cardiologist is to the heart. They should be comfortable with not only the medical and interventional management of these patients but as good, if not better, than the radiologist in interpreting pertinent spinal imaging studies. Reviewing the imaging prior to procedure in all patients is important [30, 76].

The Nurse

Time should be taken to train nursing staff and allied health professionals in interventional pain medicine, as they play a vital role in reducing significant complications.

Probably the most important *checklist* that medical assistants, nurses, and surgical technicians should review with all patients includes:

1. *Allergies* – Knowledge of nonmedication (shellfish, latex, iodine) and medication allergies is imperative as outlined above.

2. *Pregnancy* – Documentation of the last menstrual period and a pregnancy test if there is any concern should be required if fluoroscopy is utilized.
3. *Anticoagulants* – Prescription anticoagulation or over-the-counter medication or herbal remedies taken by the patient, which have potential for impairing normal coagulation, need to be known. This will be discussed in more detail later.
4. *Diabetes* – If the patient is a diabetic, knowledge of their finger-stick blood glucose is important, as they may be hypoglycemic if fasting or at risk of hyperglycemic complication if steroid injection is planned.
5. *Fever* – Elective spinal injections should be postponed in a febrile patient, as the risk of infectious complication increases.
6. *Fasting* – Knowledge of the last time a patient ate or drank is important if conscious sedation is anticipated.
7. *Side* – The side of the patient's symptoms should be marked with an X to help reduce one of the more common preventable surgical errors.

This *checklist* should be issued to all staff members who interact with the patient and should be communicated to the physician in the operating room prior to each procedure.

Nurse/Surgical Technician Preparation

If the physician is not drawing up the medications for injection, then appropriate education and training of the surgical staff is vital in reducing medication errors. Medication should be drawn up by a surgical technician with nursing supervision. All syringes should be labeled, and clearly, sterile precautions must be followed.

If you practice in a setting that is used by different specialists, such as a radiology suite at a hospital, it is important that the physician reviews all the medications prior to each procedure, to ensure no medication error. Specifically, that preservative-free local anesthetics are utilized (for epidural injections), and nonionic contrast that is safe for intrathecal use, such as Omnipaque or Isovue, and not an ionic contrast medium that may be used for urologic or gastrointestinal imaging.

Appropriate sterile preparation is mandatory and should include povidone-iodine preparation, allowing it to dry. In patients with iodine allergy, chlorhexidine gluconate and/or isopropyl alcohol may be used. For more invasive procedures such as implant or discography, some practices utilize a triple scrub, including isopropyl alcohol, chlorhexidine gluconate, and povidone-iodine. While sterile towels are adequate for draping an area for most procedures, in the case of more invasive spinal procedures, full-body draping with iodine-impregnated fenestrated adhesive biodrapes, sterile towels, and half sheets should be used [92, 93].

Patient Monitoring

Appropriate perioperative monitoring is important for all procedures and should include IV access, pulse oximetry, cardiac monitoring with ECG tracing, and blood pressure and heart rate monitoring. A fully stocked, regularly updated crash cart should be easily accessible. ACLS-trained personnel should be available. Mock codes should be run at least quarterly. This will help minimize the impact of an adverse reaction or complication.

In the postoperative patient recovery room, trained staff knowledgeable in recognizing post-procedural complications should be available. Such complications include hypotension, vasovagal reactions, sensory motor blockade, excessive somnolence, respiratory suppression, and cardiovascular complications.

Depending upon the procedure and the amount of sedation utilized, patients will be in a monitored postoperative setting, anywhere from 20 min to 8 h, until discharge criteria are met. These include an alert, oriented patient who is hemodynamically stable, with stable cardiovascular and neurologic examination and ambulating as well as expected, with someone else to drive them home if they have had sedation.

Physician

Physicians from numerous subspecialties have converged on the field of interventional pain medicine, all with varying levels of training and competence. Until recently, the standard interventional pain training occurred in the fellowship setting. Interventional pain medicine, now a recognized subspecialty of medicine, will soon have formal residency training programs.

There are still physicians performing interventional pain techniques that were learned at weekend courses. While these courses are helpful, they are by no means sufficient. A thorough understanding of spinal anatomy and how that relates to fluoroscopic anatomy is vital. Unfortunately, at these conferences, the optimum fluoroscopic image is already set, and physicians may struggle with reproducing this in their clinical practice. Contrast flow patterns are not generally taught, and therefore, the ability to recognize vascular uptake or to differentiate between a myelogram, epidurogram, or subdural contrast flow is not learned.

Physicians should be cognizant of all potential complications pertinent to a given procedure being performed. The mindset of anticipating complications will hopefully lead to earlier recognition, a more prompt and appropriate response, and minimize the effect of that complication. It is inevitable that a complication will occur to every interventionalist. How it is dealt with will frequently determine the outcome.

The physician should not be afraid to reschedule the procedure if difficulties are encountered with a particular procedure on a given day. If, for example, while performing a cervical transforaminal epidural steroid injection, vascular uptake is noted despite repositioning the needle multiple times in the foramen, the appropriate course of action may be to reschedule the patient or consider an interlaminar approach.

The minimum experience level required for certain procedures is somewhat controversial. Clearly the level of expertise required to perform an uncomplicated interlaminar lumbar epidural steroid injection on a healthy patient is far less than that required for a cervical transforaminal epidural steroid injection. Cadaver courses may help develop some of those skills, but supervised training in the clinical setting is strongly advised.

Equipment

The physician should be familiar with all equipment that may be required for a given procedure. They should be able to operate all the equipment independently and problem solve in the event of equipment malfunction. Reliance on company representatives or surgical technicians may result in operator error and avoidable complication. The physician should know how to run the fluoroscope and obtain optimal fluoroscopic images and minimize radiation exposure to all personnel.

Needle

Three basic types of needles are utilized in interventional pain practice, including a ramped needle such as a Tuohy needle which is utilized for interlaminar epidural steroid injections, a Quincke or standard spinal needle, which is used for most common spinal injections, and the third type, a pencil-point needle, which is used far less frequently (Fig. 69.7). The pencil-point needle was developed to reduce the incidence of post-dural-puncture headaches for patient undergoing spinal anesthesia and is not used frequently in interventional pain procedures.

Understanding the needle dynamics and bevel control is vital to facilitate precise needle placement. The direction of needle deviation is governed by the design of the needle tip (Fig. 69.7). Ramped needles (Tuohy) deviate away from the ramp. Pencil-point needles (Sprotte or Whitacre) only deviate a minimal amount, although not in a specific direction. Beveled needles (Quincke) consistently deviate away from the bevel. Experienced interventionalists usually accentuate this natural tendency of the beveled needle by placing a 15-degree curve, just proximal to the distal end of the needle.

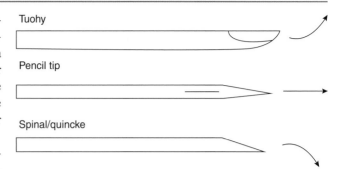

Fig. 69.7 Examples of needle types and deviation direction: Tuohy/ramped utilized for interlaminar epidurals. Pencil tip utilized for spinal anesthesia and lumbar punctures. Spinal/Quincke utilized for most interventional procedures

The degree to which a needle deflects depends on the density and distance of tissue traversed, the needle type and gauge, with 25-gauge needles deflecting more than 22 gauge [94–98].

Regardless of what needle is utilized, a two-handed needle technique should be used on all interventional procedures, with the nondominant hand anchoring the needle at the skin, and the dominant hand advancing the needle. Anchoring the needle at the skin will prevent inadvertent excessive needle advancement in the case of a patient making a sudden move which, in the case of a thoracic or cervical interlaminar epidural steroid injection, may result in spinal cord injury.

Complications resulting from interventional pain procedures have raised the issue of safety of blunt versus sharp needles for doing these procedures [45]. Some experts have recommended using blunt tip needles, rather than traditional sharp needles when performing transforaminal ESIs, with the hope of reducing the catastrophic complications of vascular penetration and anterior spinal cord infarction. This may occur with inadvertent and unrecognized injection of medication into an artery, such as radiculomedullary artery (Adamkiewicz), which may be encountered with thoracic or lumbar transforaminal injections. It may also occur with penetration of a cervical radicular artery with cervical transforaminal epidural steroid injections. Blunt needles have been unable to directly puncture the renal artery or penetrate the spinal nerve in animal models and are therefore felt by some to be safer [40, 99, 100].

Needle Placement

It is very important for the interventionalist to understand the concept of a three-dimensional object, such as the spine, being projected in two dimensions on the fluoroscope. The principle of direction, depth, direction is vital. Once the fluoroscopic working view is obtained and needle entry point determined, then the needle is directed in the sagittal or coronal plain with the needle advancing in the caudad/cephalad or medial/lateral direction. Needle depth is then checked by switching the fluoroscope to a different view, for example, by switching from an AP view to a lateral view. After assessing depth, the fluoroscope is then changed back to the original working view and redirected. Frequent checks of needle depth are vital to avoid potential needle misplacement with resultant potential complication.

Medications

The interventionalist should be very familiar with all medications utilized, including various steroid formulations, and which ones are deemed safe and appropriate for epidural use. Understanding the appropriate dosage, duration of action, potency, and side effect profile is important [19, 20, 101, 102]. This is beyond the scope of this chapter. Utilizing the smallest particle size steroid may help reduce the potential for vascular thrombotic complications. Betamethasone is of smaller particle size than triamcinolone and dexamethasone, respectively. Ideally steroid in solution and not suspension should be used.

If compounded medications are being utilized, be aware of the practices of your pharmacy, as US Pharmacopeia guidelines should be followed. There have been numerous deaths throughout the United States linked to contaminated compounded betamethasone, resulting from meningitis, encephalitis, and septic shock. If compounding medications are being utilized, it behooves the interventionalist to check the pharmacy's practice and track record.

Contrast agents are used for accurate localization of needle placement, to confirm no vascular uptake and to delineate pertinent anatomy and appropriate contrast flow pattern. Nonionic and ionic contrast agents are available. Nonionic contrast agents are more hydrophilic, and this reduces subarachnoid and intravenous toxicity. They also have a lower osmolality and produce fewer adverse effects. All epidural and intrathecal procedures should be performed with nonionic contrast agents. Commonly used nonionic contrast agents in interventional pain include iohexol (Omnipaque) and iopamidol (Isovue).

For patients who are iodine allergic and who require contrast, either gadolinium or premedication and nonionic iodinated contrast can be utilized. Premedication should include corticosteroid and an antihistamine combination, such as prednisone, 50 mg by mouth, 13, 7, and 1 h before injection with diphenhydramine (Benadryl) 50 mg IV or by mouth, 1 h prior to the injection. Other experts also include H2 blockers such as Zantac taken 1 h before and following the injection. If premedication with steroid alone is utilized, methylprednisolone, 32 mg orally, 12 and 2 h prior to the contrast agent is sufficient [103, 104].

It is generally accepted in the radiology community that it is safe to administer gadopentetate dimeglumine in patients with a known allergy to an iodinated contrast agent. In one study, however, 6.3 % of iodine-allergic patients experienced an adverse reaction to gadopentetate dimeglumine, and therefore, some degree of caution is still warranted [105].

Knowledge of anesthetic type, whether it be an amino amide, such as lidocaine or bupivacaine or an amino ester such as 2-chloroprocaine, as well as the usual concentration, onset, duration of action, and maximal single dosage is required. Caution should be exercised not to exceed the maximum dose which could occur, especially with larger procedures such as spinal cord stimulation or perhaps multilevel bilateral radiofrequency medial branch neurolysis.

Toxic CNS effects include confusion, convulsions, respiratory arrest, seizures, and even death. Other potential adverse reactions include cardiodepression, anaphylaxis, and malignant hypothermia. The patient should be monitored for signs of toxicity including restlessness, anxiety, incoherent speech, light-headedness, numbness and tingling of the mouth and lips, blurred vision, tremors, twitching, depression, or drowsiness. Injections in the cervical spine require the utmost care, as even a small dose of local anesthetic injected intravascularly may result in significant systemic toxicity and deaths have been reported [106, 107].

All local anesthetics injected into the epidural space should be preservative-free.

Resuscitative equipment and medication should be immediately available when local anesthetics are being utilized. Central nervous system toxicity by 1 % lidocaine has an onset at plasma concentrations of 5–10 mcg/ml which equates to slightly more than 400 mg (40 cc) of total bolus. Bupivacaine is about four times more toxic than lidocaine, with a toxic bolus of 100 mg (10 cc) [108].

Volume and Rate of Injection

There is some controversy as to the optimum volume for epidural injection. As a general rule in a young patient with no central or foraminal stenosis, large volumes of contrast can be injected safely without any neurocompressive complications. However, in the cervical spine in someone with multilevel moderate to severe central and foraminal stenosis, where limited run off is available, then compressive complications may occur with as small volume as 3 ml, especially if injected quickly.

As a general rule, target-specific epidural injections delivered transforaminally at the symptomatic level or interlaminarly with a catheter advanced to the appropriate level can be achieved with volumes of 2 or 3 ml. High volume, rapid epidural steroid injection can result in large increases of intraspinal pressure, with the risk of cerebral hemorrhage, retinal hemorrhage, visual disturbance, headache, and compromise of spinal cord blood flow. A retinal hemorrhage has been described and felt to be secondary to a sudden increase in intracranial pressure from a rapid epidural steroid injection, resulting in increase in retinal venous pressure [109–114].

Fluoroscopy

Fluoroscopy should be used for all spinal injections, including discography, diagnostic intra-articular facet joint injections, diagnostic medial branch blocks, diagnostic sacroiliac joint injections, radiofrequency medial branch neurolysis, and all transforaminal epidural steroid injections. For these, no controversy should exist. Surprisingly, however, controversy still abounds regarding the need for fluoroscopy with interlaminar or caudal epidural steroid injections. This, despite the fact that needle misplacement occurs 25–40 % of the time with caudal injections and about 30 % of the time with interlaminar lumbar epidural injections, and up to 53 % of the time with cervical epidural steroid injections without fluoroscopy [115–117]. Fredman reported more than 50 % of blind lumbar epidural steroid injections were performed at the wrong level [118–120].

Surprisingly, the results of a national survey of private and academic practices demonstrated that for cervical interlaminar epidural steroid injections, only 39 % of academic practice versus 73 % of private practitioners utilize fluoroscopy [121].

There are multiple studies showing that negative aspiration is unreliable for vascular uptake and the high incidence of vascular penetration with transforaminal lumbar and cervical epidural steroid injections which if unrecognized could result in catastrophic spinal cord infarction [122–124].

The use of fluoroscopy and contrast injection can demonstrate precise needle placement at the correct level and appropriate contrast flow. Injection of contrast under live fluoroscopy with extension tubing can help confirm there is no vascular uptake prior to injection of medication.

Many of the published complications of interventional pain procedures including sympathetic blocks and trigger point injections are because of needle misplacement with *blind* techniques and are eminently avoidable with fluoroscopy. These will be discussed in more detail later in this and other chapters.

Unrecognized inadvertent subdural injection may occur in close to 1 % of injections without fluoroscopy [125]. A hard copy confirming accurate needle placement can also be kept in the file. Fluoroscopy should be used for all interventional spine procedures except during pregnancy.

Anticoagulation

Significant bleeding following interventional pain procedures is extremely rare but may have catastrophic outcome. These procedures carry an inherent risk of bleeding, but the real extent of this risk is unknown. Bleeding complications will increase with poor technique, the presence of high procedure or patient-associated bleeding risk factors, and anticoagulation. Many prescription or over-the-counter medications and even herbal remedies such as garlic, ginkgo, ginseng, and ginger may impair coagulation [126].

Published guidelines from European and American Anesthesiology societies exist but only define the risk of significant bleeding complications for neuraxial procedures in the presence of anticoagulation [127–129]. The incidence of spinal hematoma is rare. In fact, the published incidence is 1/150,000–1/190,000 for epidurals, and 1/220,000 for spinals [130–132].

The authors as well as the German and the Spanish Society of Anesthesiology recommend that aspirin and nonsteroidal anti-inflammatory drug (NSAID) should be held prior to elective spinal injections. In the presence of increased procedure and patient-related bleeding risk factors, aspirin should be held 7 days and NSAIDs for 72 h prior to these procedures. The American Society of Regional Anesthesia and Pain Medicine (ASRA) states this practice as controversial.

In general, little controversy surrounds ticlopidine which should be held for 14 days and clopidogrel which should be held for 7 days prior to neuraxial block [130–132]. Warfarin should be stopped 4–5 days prior to neuraxial procedure, and the INR should be less than 1.4 prior to proceeding according to ASRA guidelines.

Prophylactic or therapeutic dose low molecular weight heparins should be held at least 12 or 24 h, respectively, before an epidural. Understand, however, that there are newer, longer-acting LMWHs that may need to be held longer [133].

COX-2 inhibitors such as celecoxib and valdecoxib do not need to be stopped perioperatively.

The ASA recommends discontinuing herbal medicines for 2–3 weeks prior to elective surgery. The authors suggest that vitamin E and herbal medications like garlic, ginseng, ginger, and ginkgo may increase the patient risk for bleeding, and consideration should be given to stop them, especially if there is other associated patient or procedure-related risk factors present.

Acknowledgment I would like to thank Advanced Pain Management staff and physicians for all support.

References

1. Machikanti L, Bowell M, Raj P, Racz GB. The evolution of interventional pain management. Pain Physician. 2003;6:485–94.
2. Schweitzer A. On the edge of primeval forest. New York: MacMillan; 1931. p. 62.
3. Machikanti L. The growth of interventional pain management in the new millennium; a critical analysis of utilization in the Medicare population. Pain Physician. 2004;7:465–82.
4. Brown DL, Fink BR. The history of neuroblockade and pain management. In: Cousins MJ, Bridenbaugh PO, editors. Neuroblockage

and clinical anesthesia and management of pain. 3rd ed. Philadelphia: Lippencott, Raven; 1998. p. 3–34.

5. Kalawokalani D. Malpractice claims for non-operative pain Management: a growing pain for Anesthesiologists. ASA Professional Information, 1999.

6. Fitzgibbon DR. Chronic pain management: ASA closed claims project. Anesthesiology. 2004;100:98–105.

7. Purkis IE. Cervical epidural steroids. Pain Clin. 1986;1:3–7.

8. Okell RW, Sprigge JS. Unintentional dural puncture. A survey of recognition and management. Anaesthesia. 1987;42:1110–3.

9. Bogduk N, Cherry D. Epidural cortico steroid agents for sciatica. Med J Aust. 1985;143:402–6.

10. Deisenhammer E. Clinical and experimental studies on headache after myelography. Neuroradiology. 1985;9:99–102.

11. Charlsley MM, Abram SE. The injection of intrathecal normal saline reduces the severity of post dural puncture headache. Reg Anesth Pain Med. 2001;26(4):301–5.

12. Soffa TV. Effectiveness of epidural blood patch in the management of post Dural puncture headache. Anesthesiology. 2001;95(2):334–49.

13. Reitman CA. Subdural hematoma after cervical epidural steroid injection. Spine. 2002;27(6):174–6.

14. Vos PE. Subdural hematoma after lumbar puncture; Two case reports and review of the literature. Clin Neurol Neurosurg. 1991;93(2):127–32.

15. Tekkok IH. Spinal subdural hematoma as a complication of immediate epidural blood patch. Can J Anaesth. 1996;43(3):306–9.

16. Williams KN. Epidural hematoma requiring surgical decompression following repeated cervical epidural steroid injection for chronic pain. Pain. 1990;42(2):197–9.

17. Chan ST, Leung S. Spinal epidural abscess following steroid injection for sciatica. Case report. Spine. 1989;14(1):106–8.

18. Goris H, Wilms G, Hermans B, Schillebeeckx J. Spinal epidural abscess complicating epidural infiltration: CT and MR findings. Eur Radiol. 1998;8(6):1058.

19. Abram S, O'Connor T. Complications associated with epidural steroid injections. Reg Anesth. 1996;21(2):149–62.

20. Manchikanti L. Role of neuraxial steroids in interventional pain management. Pain Physician. 2002;5(2):182–99.

21. Hodges SD. Cervical epidural steroid injection with intrinsic spinal cord damage; two case reports. Spine. 1998;23(19):2137–42.

22. Katz JA, Lukin R, Bridenbaugh PO, Gunzenhauser L. Subdural intracranial air; unusual cause of headache after spinal epidural steroid injection. Anesthesiology. 1991;75:615–8.

23. Dougherty JH, Fraser RAR. Complications following intraspinal injections to steroid. J Neurosurg. 1978;48:1023–5.

24. Mateo E, López-Alarcón MD, Moliner S, Calabuig E, Vivó M, De Andrés J, Grau F. Epidural and subarachnoid pneumocephalus after epidural technique. Eur J Anaesthesiol. 1999;16(6):413–7.

25. Krisanda TJ, Laucks SO. Pneumocephalus following epidural blood patch procedure; unusual cause of severe headache. Ann Emerg Med. 1994;23:129–31.

26. Gutknecht DR. Chemical meningitis following epidural injections with corticosteroids. Am J Med. 1987;82:570.

27. Plumb VJ, Dismukes WE. Chemical meningitis related to intrathecal corticosteroid therapy. South Med J. 1977;70:1241.

28. Adriani J, Naragi M. Paraplegia associated with epidural anesthesia. South Med J. 1986;79:1350–5.

29. Bomage PR, Benumof JL. Paraplegia following intracord injection during attempted epidural anesthesia under general anesthesia. Reg Anesth Pain Med. 1998;23:104–7.

30. Derby R. Procedural safety training guidelines for performance of interlaminar cervical epidural steroid injections. ISIS Newsl. 1998;3(1):17–21.

31. Darvy R. Procedural safety training guidelines for the performance of interlaminar cervical epidural steroid injections. Isis Newsl. 1998;3(1):17–21.

32. Bogduk N. Spine update; epidural steroids. Spine. 1998;20:845–8.

33. Cicala RS, Westbrook A, Angel JJ. Side effects and complications of cervical epidural steroid injections. J Pain Symptom Manage. 1998;4:64–6.

34. Derby R. Point of view. Spine. 1998;2:2141–2.

35. Botwan KP, Gruber RD, Bouchlas CG, Tores-Ramos FN. Complications of fluoroscopically-guided transforaminal lumbar epidural steroid injections. Arch Phys Med Rehabil. 2000;81(8):1045–50.

36. Houten JK, Errico TJ. Paraplegia after lumbosacral nerve root block; report of three cases. Spine J. 2002;2:70–5.

37. Windsor RE, Falco FJE. Paraplegia following selective nerve root blocks. ISIS Newsl. 2001;4(1):53–4.

38. Kloth DS. Risk of cervical transforaminal epidural injections by anterior approach. Pain Physician. 2003;6(2):392–3.

39. Helm S, Jasper JF, Racz GB. Complications of transforaminal epidural injections. Pain Physician. 2003;6:389–94.

40. Schultz DM. Risk of transforaminal epidural injections. Pain Physician. 2003;6(2):390–1.

41. Derby R, Lee SH, Kim BJ, Chen Y, Seo KS. Complications following cervical epidural steroid injections by expert interventionalists in 2003. Pain Physician. 2004;7:445–9.

42. Windsor RE, Storm S, Sugar R. Prevention and management of complications resulting from common spinal injections. Pain Physician. 2003;6:473–83.

43. Windsor RE, Storm S, Sugar R, Negula D. Cervical transforaminal injection; review of the literature, complications and a suggested technique. Pain Physician. 2003;6:457–65.

44. Brouwers P, Kottink E, Simon M, Prevo R. A cervical anterior spinal artery syndrome after diagnostic blockade of the right C6 nerve root. Pain. 2001;91:397–9.

45. Nelson J. Letter to the editor. Spine. 2002;3:1–2.

46. Nelson JW. Letter to the editor. In response to Hauten JK, Erico TJ. Paraplegia of the Lumbosacral Nerve Block. Spine J. 2003;2:88–9.

47. Baker R, Dreyfus P, Mercer S. Cervical transforaminal injection with corticosteroids into a radicular artery; a possible mechanism for spinal cord injury. Pain. 2003;103:211–5.

48. Heavner James E, Racz GB, Jenigiri B, Lehman T, Day MR. Sharp vs. Blunt needle; a comparative study of penetration of internal structures on bleeding in dogs. Pain Pract. 2003;3(3):226–31.

49. Burger JJ, Hawkins IF. Celiac plexus injection. Use of a blunt Tip needle. Reg Anesth. 1995;20(2S):25.

50. Nelson LS, Hoffman RS. Intrathecal injection; unusual complication of trigger point injection therapy. Ann Emerg Med. 1998;32(4):506–8.

51. Elias M. Trigger point injections; are they a simple procedure. Isis Newsl. 1999;3(3):13–8.

52. Fischer AA. Trigger point needling with infiltration and somatic blocks. Phys Med Rehabil Clin North Am. 1995;6(4):851–70.

53. Stolker RJ. Percutaneous facet denervation and chronic thoracic spinal pain. Acta Neurochir (Wien). 1993;122:82–90, 107.

54. Dreyfus P, Kaplan M, Dreyer S. Zygapophysial joint injection techniques in the spinal axis. Pain procedures and clinical practice, vol. 27. 2nd ed. Philadelphia: Hanley and Belfus Inc; 2000. p. 276–308.

55. Goldstone JC, Pennant JH. Spinal anesthesia after facet joint injection. Anaesthesia. 1987;42:754–6.

56. Marks R, Semple AJ. Spinal anesthesia after facet joint injection. Anaesthesia. 1988;43:65–8.

57. Thompson SJ, Lomax DM, Collett BJ. Chemical meningism after lumbar facet joint block with local anesthetic and steroids. Anaesthesia. 1991;46:563–4.

58. Cook NJ, Hanrahan P, Song S. Paraspinal abscess following facet joint injection. Clin Rheumatol. 1999;18(1):52–3.

59. Magee M, Kannangara S, Dennien B, Lonergan R, Emmett L, Van der Wall H. Paraspinal abscess complicating facet joint injection. Clin Nucl Med. 2000;25(1):71–3.

60. Machikanti L, Statz PS, Singh V, et al. Evidence-based practice guidelines for interventional techniques in the management of chronic spinal pain. Pain Physician. 2003;6:3–81.

61. Moore DC, Bridenbaugh LD. The anterior approach to the stellate ganglion. JAMA. 1956;160:158–62.

62. Moore DC. Anterior (paratracheal) approach for block of the stellate ganglion. In: Moore DC, editor. Regional block. Springfield: Charles C. Thomas; 1981. p. 123–37.

63. Ellis H, Feldman S. Anatomy for anesthetists. 3rd ed. Oxford: Blackwell Scientific Publication; 1979. p. 256–62.

64. Mahli A, Coskun D, Akcali DT. Aetiology of convulsions due to stellate ganglion block: a review and report of two cases. Eur J Anaesthesiol. 2002;19(5):376–80.

65. Forrest JB. Total spinal block at C4. Can J Anaesth. 1976;23(4):435–9.

66. Bruins T, Devulder J. Inadvertent subdural block, following attempted stellate ganglion block. Anaesthesia. 1991;46(9):747–9.

67. Whitehurst L. Brainstem anesthesia; an unusual complication of stellate ganglion block. J Bone Joint Surg Am. 1977;59(4):541–2.

68. Makiuchi T. Stellate ganglion blocks at the suspected source of infection in a case of cervical epidural abscess. No Shinkei Geka. 1993;21(9):805–8.

69. Caron H, Litwiller R. Stellate ganglion block. Anaesth Analg. 1975;54(5):567–70.

70. McCallum MI, Glyn CJ. Intercostal neuralgia following stellate ganglion block. Anaesthesia. 1986;41(8):850–2.

71. Dukes RR, Alexander LA. Transient locked-in syndrome after vascular injection during stellate ganglion block. Reg Anesth. 1993;18(6):378–80.

72. Thompson KJ. Pneumochylothorax; a rare complication of stellate ganglion block. Anaesthesiology. 1981;55(5):589–91.

73. Seinfeld M. Total reversible blindness following attempted stellate ganglion block. Anesth Anal. 1981;60(9):689–90.

74. Hardy PA, Wells JC. Extent of sympathetic blockade after stellate ganglion block with bupivacaine. Pain. 1989;36:190–6.

75. Abdi S, Zhou Y, Patel N, Saini B, Nelson J. A new and easy technique to block the stellate ganglion. Pain Physician. 2004;7: 327–31.

76. Fortin JD. Cervical discography with CT and MRI correlations. In: Pain procedures in clinical practice. Philadelphia: Hanley and Belfus; 2000. p. 230–41.

77. Zeidman SM, Thompson K, Ducker TB. Complications of cervical discography; analysis of 400 diagnostic disc injections. Neurosurgery. 1995;37:414–7.

78. Grubb SA, Kelly CK. Cervical discography; clinical implications from 12 years of experience. Spine. 2000;25:1382–9.

79. Guyer RD, Ohnmeiss DD, Mason SL, et al. Complications of cervical discography; findings in a large series. J Spinal Disord. 1997;10:95–101.

80. Guyer RD, Collier R, Stith WJ, et al. Discitis after discography. Spine. 1998;13:1352–4.

81. Lownie SP, Furgeson GG. Spinal subdural empyema complicating cervical discography. Spine. 1989;14:1415–7.

82. Connor PM, Darden BV. Cervical discography; complications of clinical efficacy. Spine. 1993;18(14):2053–8.

83. Laun A. Complications of cervical discography. J Neurosurg Sci. 1981;25(1):17–20.

84. Smith MD, Kim SS. Herniated cervical disc resulting from discography; an unusual complication. J Spinal Disord. 1990;3(4):392–4.

85. Fraser RD. Discitis after discography. J Bone Joint Surg Br. 1997;69(1):26–35.

86. Osti OL, Fraser RD, Vernon-Roberts B. Discitis after discography. The role of prophylactic antibiotics. J Bone Joint Surg Br. 1990;72(2):271–4.

87. Fraser RD, Osti OS, Vernon-Roberts B. Iatrogenic discitis; the role of intravenous antibiotics in prevention and treatment. Spine. 1989;14(9):1025–32.

88. Goldie I. Intervertebral disc changes after discography. Acta Chir Scand. 1957;113:438–9.

89. DeSeze S, Levernieux J. Lesaccidents De La Discographie. Rev Rheum Mal Osteoartic. 1952;19:1027–33.

90. Klessig HT, Showsh SA, Sekorski A. The use of intradiscal antibiotics for discography: an invivo study of gentamicin, cephazolin, and clindamycin. Spine. 2003;28:1735–8.

91. Machikanti L. Role of neuraxial steroids in interventional pain management. Pain Physician. 2002;5(2):182–99.

92. Windsor RE, Storm SR. Prevention and management from complications resulting from common spinal injections. Pain Physician. 2003;6:473–83.

93. Windsor RE, Pinzon EG, Gore HC. Complications of common selective spinal injections; prevention and management. In: Pain procedures and clinical practice. 2nd ed. Philadelphia: Hanley and Belfus, Inc; 2000. p. 10–24.

94. Kopacz DJ, Allen HW. Comparison of needle deviation during regional anesthetic techniques in a laboratory model. Anesth Analg. 1995;81:630–3.

95. Baumgarten RK. Importance of needle bevel during spinal and epidural anesthesia. Reg Anesth. 1995;20(3):234–8.

96. Drummond GB, Scott DHT. Deflection of spinal needles by the bevel. Anesth Analg. 1980;35:854–7.

97. Hart JR, Whitacre RJ. Pencil point needle and prevention of post spinal headaches. J Am Med Assoc. 1951;147:657–8.

98. Dreyfus P. The power of beveled control. Isis Newsl. 1998;3(1): 16–7.

99. Heavner JE, Racz GB, Jenigiri B, Lehman T, Day MR, Sharp Vs. Blunt needle; a comparative study of penetration of internal structures and bleeding in dogs. Pain Pract. 2003;3(3):226–31.

100. Helm S, Josper JF, Racz GB. Complications of transforaminal epidural steroid injections. Letters to the editor. Pain Physician. 2003;6:389–90.

101. Andre SA. Steroid side effects of epidurally administered celestone. Int Spinal Inject Soc. 1993;1:5.

102. Kay J, Findling JW, Raff H. Epidural triamcinolone suppresses the pituitary-adrenal axis in human subjects. Anesth Analg. 1994;79(3):501–5.

103. Chopra P, Smith H. Use of radiopaque contrast agents for the interventional pain physician. Pain Physician. 2004;7:459–63.

104. Woodward JL, Herring SA, Windsor RE. Epidural procedures in spine pain management. In: Pain procedures in clinical practice, vol. 2. Philadelphia: Hanley and Belfus; 2000. p. 341–77.

105. Nelson KL, Gifford LM, Lauber-Huber C, Gross CA, Lasser TA. Clinical safety of gadopentetate dimeglumine. Radiology. 1995;196:439–43.

106. Olin BR. Miscellaneous products; local anesthetics, injectable. In: Olin BR, editor. Facts and comparisons. St. Louis: Wolters Kluwer; 1993. p. 2654–65.

107. Kovino BG. Clinical pharmacology of local anesthetic agents. In: Cousins MJ, Bridenbaugh PO, editors. Neuroblockade and clinical evidence in pain management. Philadelphia: JB Lippincott; 1996. p. 111–44.

108. Kovino BG. Clinical pharmacology of local anesthetic agents. In: Cousins MJ, Bridenbaugh MJ, Philip O, editors. Neuroblockade in clinical anesthesia and management of pain. Philadelphia: Lippincott; 1998. p. 111–44.

109. Cyriax JH. Epidural anesthesia and bed rest in sciatica. Br Med J. 1961;1:20–4.

110. Kushner FH, Olson JC. Retinol hemorrhage as a consequence of epidural steroid injection. Arch Ophthalmol. 1995;113:309–13.

111. Ling C, Atkinson PL, Muntol CG. Bilateral retinol hemorrhages following epidural injection. Br J Ophthalmol. 1993;77:316–7.

112. Purdy EP, Haimal GS. Vision loss after lumbar epidural steroid injection. Anesth Analg. 1998;86:119–22.

113. Victory RA, Hassett P, Morrison G. Transient blindness following epidural analgesia. Anesthesia. 1991;46:940–1.

114. Flock CJ, Whitwell J. Intraocular hemorrhage after epidural injection. Br Med J. 1961;2:1612–3.
115. Renfrew DL, Moore TE, Cathol MH. Correct placement of epidural steroid injections: fluoroscopic guidance and contrast administration. AJNR Am J Neuroradiol. 1991;12:1003–7.
116. White AH, Derby R, Winne G. Epidural injections for the diagnosis and treatment of low-back pain. Spine. 1980;5:78–86.
117. Stojanovic MP, Vu TN, Caneras O. The role of fluoroscopy in cervical epidural steroid injections: an analysis of contrast dispersal patterns. Spine. 2002;27:509–14.
118. Fredman B, Nun MB, Zohar E, et al. Epidural steroids for "failed back surgery syndrome". is fluoroscopy really necessary. Anesth Analg. 1999;88:367–72.
119. Mehta M, Salmon N. Extradural block. Confirmation of the injection site by X-ray monitoring. Anaesthesia. 1985;40:1009–12.
120. Burn JM, Guyer PB, Langdon L. The spread of solutions injected into the epidural space: a study using epidurograms in patients with lumbosciatic syndrome. Br J Anaesth. 1973;43:338–45.
121. Cluff R. The technical aspects of epidural steroid injections: a national survey. Anesth Analg. 2002;95(2):403–8.
122. Furman MB, Giovanniello MT, O'Brien EM. Incidence of intravascular penetration in transforaminal cervical epidural steroid injections. Spine. 2003;28:21–5.
123. Furman MB, Giovanniello MT, O'Brien EM. Incidence of vascular penetration in transforaminal lumbar epidural steroid injections. Spine. 2000;25:2628–32.
124. Sullivan WJ. Incidence of intravascular uptake in lumbar spinal injection procedures. Spine. 2000;25:481–6.
125. Lubenow T, Keh-Wong E, Kristof K, Ivankovich O. Inadvertent subdural injection: a complication of epidural injection. Anesth Analg. 1988;67:175–9.
126. Raj PP, Shah RV, Kaye AD, Denaro S, Hoover JM. Bleeding risk in interventional pain practice: assessment, management, and review of the literature. Pain Physician. 2004;7(1):3–51.
127. Horlocker TT, Wedel DJ, Benzon HFL. Regional anesthesia in the anticoagulated patients: defining the risks (2nd ASRA CCNAA). Reg Anesth Pain Med. 2003;28:172–97.
128. Llau JV, de Andres J, Gomar C, et al. Drugs that alter hemostasis and regional anesthetic techniques: safety guidelines. Consensus conference. Rev Esp Anestesiol Reanim. 2001;48:270–0278.
129. Gogarten W, VanAken H, Wulf H, et al. Paraspinal regional anesthesia and prevention of thromboembolism/anticoagulation: recommendations of the German Society of anesthesiology and intensive care medicine. Anesthesiol Intensive Med Notfallmed Schmerzther. 1997;38:623–8.
130. Horlocker TT, Tyagi A, Bhattacharya A. Central neuraxial blocks in anticoagulation. A review of current trends. Eur J Anaesthesiol. 2002;19:317–29.
131. Wulf H. Epidural anesthesia and spinal hematoma. Can J Anaesth. 1996;43:1260–71.
132. Vandermeulen EP, Van Aken H, Vermylen J. Anticoagulants and spinal epidural anesthesia. Anesth Analg. 1994;79:1165–77.
133. Fox J. Spinal and epidural anesthesia and anticoagulation. Int Anesthesiol Clin. 2001;39(1):51–61.

Part V

Integrative Approaches

Albert L. Ray

Introduction

It has been my privilege and honor to serve as the editor for the part on Integrative Approaches, and to have been able to work with a superb Editor-in-Chief, Tim Deer, and the publisher's staff. We have assembled a significant number of chapters that will give our readers an opportunity to understand the importance of treating a person in pain, not merely a body part.

Pain is a complex perceptual experience involving multiple brain areas simultaneously being influenced and directed to contribute to what each individual person's pain experience is like, and further hinting as to what can be done about it. The goals of all pain treatment are to restore a person's ability to function, to take charge of their lives, and to gain the maximum fulfillment from life, with as little influence from pain as possible.

The other two parts of this book offer significant information on pharmacological approaches and interventional approaches to managing pain. The Integrative Approaches part is intended to round out how the specialty of Pain Medicine can offer comprehensive help to those living and/or suffering with persistent pain.

From the perspective that pain perception can be likened to a hologram with "laser" inputs from: the physical body, including nervous system, muscle, and fascial systems; the cognitive and emotional brain systems; the body and brain memory systems; the mind, which includes all of one's values (both cultural and personal); the meaning of the pain; and one's spiritual beliefs and strengths, we offer a part in this book that will address this complex subject. Although chapter subjects may initially seem disparate, all chapters are linked by the concept of treating "whole" people, and I have asked all authors to discuss the concept of how neuroplasticity may be part of their subject. We have tried to look at what components are important to understanding pain perception, how persistent pain becomes a disease process, and what can be addressed for help, both within the person and from the world around them.

To that goal, we begin our part with a chapter on Neuroplasticity and Sensitization to give a foundation for what we consider the basic characteristics of normal and abnormal nervous system anatomy and physiology. This is followed by a chapter on Pain Perception, which details the complex involvement of how a person feels (perceives) pain.

From the foundation of these two chapters, we will then have chapters on Muscle Pain and its treatments, Manual Therapies, and Regenerative Injection Therapies. Additionally, to further address the complexities of pain, we offer chapters on Psychological Testing; Psychological Treatments; The "Five-minute" Mental Status Examination of Persons with Pain, which serves as a quick and simple mental status exam for non-psychiatric practitioners; and a chapter on Coding for Psychiatric/Psychological Treatments, including medical codings for psychological services that can help those without direct mental health insurance benefits. Further treatments that help address pain include chapters on Acupuncture, Hypnosis, Interdisciplinary Functional Restoration/Pain Programs, and Primary Care Pain Perspectives.

Because abuse and diversion can become so entwined with other, more legitimate, forms of aberrant pain behaviors, we have included a chapter on Addictive Disorders and Pain. In order to help cover some potential legal issues, there are chapters on Failure to Treat, The Double Effect, and Assessing Disability in the Pain Patient.

Some issues relate to special populations and/or special aspects of pain perception that we felt deserve individual attention. These include chapters on Spirituality and Pain, a very important topic which is frequently overlooked, Sleep and Pain, Pain in the Elderly, Disparate Populations and Pain, and Neonatal Pain.

Finally, we have tried to incorporate a new perspective for clinical pain textbooks: what is living with pain like for the person experiencing it and for their caretakers, and what public support systems are available for persons in pain and those in their worlds? To this end, we offer chapters on Personal Pain Perspectives, Pain Caretaker Perspectives, and Public Support Systems for everyone. These chapters are intended to enlighten pain practitioners, and offer them helpful organizational referrals for their patients in need.

We offer to our readers through this Integrative Approaches part a three-dimensional description of the pain experience, and multiple treatment alternatives to address this three-dimensional perspective. The chapters have all been written by authors with exceptional expertise in their respective subjects, and we have all tried to discuss the state of the art within these topics. I respectfully thank all of the dedicated authors who have contributed their knowledge and created a very high level of information in order to help those who live with pain, and those who are in their worlds, to find joy and peace in their lives.

Pain as a Perceptual Experience

Albert L. Ray, Rhonwyn Ullmann, and Michael C. Francis

Key Points
- Human perception
- Pain perception
- Physical contribution, including nervous system and fascial network
- Cognitive contribution
- Memory contribution
- Emotional contribution
- Mind contribution

Definitions

Hologram: A three-dimensional image created by intersecting two or more laser beams of light. The more laser beams intersecting, the richer the image.

Pain hologram: A perceptual experience likened to a hologram comprised of "laser beam" inputs from physical nervous system and fascia, cognitions, emotions, memory, and mindful contributions, differing in intensity from person

A.L. Ray, M.D. (✉)
The LITE Center,
5901 SW 74 St, Suite 201, South Miami, FL 33143, USA

University of Miami Miller School of Medicine,
Miami, FL, USA
e-mail: aray@thelitecenter.org

R. Ullmann, BS, M.S.
The LITE Center,
5901 SW 74 St, Suite 201, South Miami, FL 33143, USA
e-mail: bearrab@aol.com

M.C. Francis, M.D.
St. Jude Medical, New Orleans, LA, USA

Integrative Pain Medicine Center, New Orleans, LA, USA
e-mail: integrativepmc@gmail.com

to person, thereby creating the uniqueness to each person's pain experience.

Neuroplasticity: The ability of the nervous system to change itself throughout the entire life cycle. The operating system by which the nervous system develops its patterns of functioning in both states of health and illness and by which it maintains the balance between sensory and motor function.

Sensitization: A process by which the neuroplastic nature of the nervous system alters normal transmission into an abnormal state. This can occur in pain states and result in pain as a disease state (maldynia), rather than as a normal occurrence (eudynia). It can also happen in other sensory states, as well, such as auditory, visual, olfactory, and tactile sensations.

Eudynia: Normal nociceptive pain; warning pain; pain as a symptom; has value to the person.

Maldynia: Abnormal pain; pain as a disease state and not a symptom; has no value to the person.

Persistent pain: A state of unremitting maldynia, with or without the additional input of eudynia.

TANS: Tonically active neurons; an area in the caudate that modulates cognitive input with emotional input, interacting with memory and having output to the thalamus and basal ganglia and eventually to the motor cortex. TANS are also responsive to auditory or visual stimuli that are linked to reward.

Tensegrity: A term derived from a contraction of "tensional integrity"; a term to describe a structural relationship that allows for a system to yield without breaking; a term used to describe how the fascial system maintains its integrity while allowing movement of its encapsulated structures, such as muscle; a term that allows for an understanding of why the fascial system could stand on its own, if the bones and muscles were removed from the body.

Price's Two Dimensions of All Pains

Sensory-discriminative: Highly localized; discrete; signal transmitted from dorsal horn via spinothalamic tract to thalamus and contralateral sensory cortex; we call it the "ouch" portion of pain.

Affective-motivational: Vague; not localized; signal transmitted from dorsal horn via parabrachial tract to limbic system, ACC, insula and prefrontal cortex and distributed bilaterally throughout brain; we call it the "yuck" portion of pain.

Introduction

"The mind creates the brain." J. Schwartz, MD, PhD: The Mind and the Brain

Human perception has been likened to a hologram [1]. A hologram exists by converging two or more laser beams together, producing a three-dimensional vision that is very real, but does not really exist. You can put your hand right through a hologram, yet it is quite visible and not disturbed by your hand. The more laser beams we add to the hologram, the richer the vision. This analogy is often used to address human perception [1–3].What our brain creates as a perception and how we project these perceptions onto the outside world are called qualia [4]. The qualia we call our conscious experience of pain cannot be fully explained by neurophysiological events only [5, 6]. Some qualia, or perceptions, can be up to 90 % memory [7]. Thus, our qualia are produced by a dynamic interaction between mind and brain and most likely through the mechanics of quantum physics [6, 8].

In this chapter, we will look at what component "laser beams" comprise our "holographic" perception of pain, and we will understand why each person's pain perception is unique to them. Even with the addition of *f*MRIs, which can demonstrate confluence of multiple brain areas utilized during pain perception [9], the experience on the part of the person in pain remains unique to them [10]. The goal of our treatment of pain, then, is to deconstruct as much of the pain hologram as possible, by reducing or eliminating as many laser beams as possible. The weakening of the hologram can come about by reducing laser beams from any number of perspectives, as we will see below, and this accounts for why interdisciplinary/multidisciplinary treatment is so often the best choice.

Doidge said, "When we wish to prefect our senses, neuroplasticity is a blessing; when it works in the service of pain, plasticity can be a curse" [11]. We now understand how sensitization, through neuroplastic reorganization, can also influence and change perceptions [12, 13]. In abnormal pain states, these neuroplastic changes cause a sensitization which enhances pain perceptions in a negative way, by increasing either the sensory-discriminative dimension or the affective-motivational dimension of pain, or both. In the previous chapter, we have reviewed the issue of neuroplasticity, "for better or for worse," and its role in the production of abnormal pain perception. However, to understand the ultimate perceptual experience of abnormal pain, we must look beyond just the physical neuroplastic sensitization of the nervous system and incorporate the role of the mind and its effect on the physical system. What we will see is that mindful will and attentional focus also can actually change the neuroplastic structure of the brain [6].

Pain Perception

Price has identified two dimensions to all pain [14, 15]: the sensory-discriminative and the affective-motivational dimensions, and these have been further discussed by others [12, 16, 17]. The sensory-discriminative dimension is perceived as a highly localized sensation and is processed via the spinothalamic tract through the thalamus and up to the contralateral somatosensory cortex. This part of the pain experience we refer to as the "ouch" portion of pain. The affective-motivational dimension contributes the vague coloration to pain and is processed via the spinoparabrachial tract to the amygdala, hippocampus, prefrontal cortex, insula anterior cingulate gyrus (ACC), etc., and is distributed bilaterally throughout the brain. This part of the pain experience we refer to as the "yuck" portion of pain. Obviously, these two separate dimensions of pain are perceived as one final integrated perception [18–21]. In our experience, the affective-motivational dimension of pain is the most difficult for people to tolerate. In other words, the "suffering" component of pain is harder to live with than the "ouch" portion [22, 23].

Price's concepts are applicable to all pain, whether it be eudynia (acute nociceptive warning pain) or maldynia (pain as a disease process unto itself which is not useful to the person) [13, 24–27]; Rome and Rome [28] have previously described LAPS (limbically augmented pain syndrome) in terms of sensitization of the nervous system through neuroplastic reorganization resulting in a condition in which the pain perception is "out of proportion" to physical findings. Previously, these pain sufferers have been labeled as hysterics, "crocks," and even malingerers. However, we now understand that the intensity of their pain perception is quite genuine and real.

In addition, we do know that the brain is similarly activated by actual events or by imagined events within one person [29–31], and this brain activation function has also been demonstrated between two different persons who are highly sympathetic with each other [32]. "Performing" an activity in our mind's eye causes brain function to occur as if we were actually doing that same activity [6, 29]. The development of new neuroplastic patterns in the brain or the arousal of previously established patterns can be excited by imagination. This is a well-documented happening with musicians and athletes, who "practice" at times even when they are away from their actual activity. Brain activity on *f*MRIs is identical whether visualizing or actually playing. In terms of pain perception, this concept was very nicely demonstrated by Krämer et al. in a rather enlightening experiment with imagined allodynia in subjects who had a history of allodynia, but no current allodynia. fMRIs done while touching the subjects' hands demonstrated excitation of S_1 and S_2 somatosensory cortices bilaterally. However, when the subjects imagined their allodynia while having their hand touched, their simultaneous fMRIs indicated activity of brain areas congruent with those of someone experiencing "real" allodynia [29].

Turning to the pain hologram produced by the neuromatrix network and the mind, besides the "physical" laser beam input from the peripheral and/or central nervous system to the brain or via the fascial network [2], there are multiple other major laser beam inputs which have a

significant influence on the ultimate perception of "I hurt." These inputs can include, but are not limited to, emotional, cognitive, memory, and mindful contributions, and these other inputs can frequently be of greater significance to our pain hologram [4, 12, 20]. We will now discuss the components of a hypothetical painful hologram (Table 70.1).

Physical Laser Beams

We live with and through a dynamically fluctuating nervous system, one which has a marvelously complex functioning in terms of pain transmission [13, 18, 19]. To briefly review, eudynia starts with stimulation of chemical, mechanical, or temperature nociceptors in the periphery [33, 34]. Via transduction, an action potential is created, and this electrical signal is conducted to the spinal dorsal horn (Fig. 70.1). Here, a complex series of interactions occur, with Aδ and C fibers working to enhance the signal strength, while Aβ fibers and descending inhibitory fibers work to inhibit the signal, and all of this interaction receives an additional excitatory influence from the glial cells [35, 36] within the dorsal horn. Once the dorsal horn interactions reach a final summation of factors, the remaining signal is then transmitted via the spinothalamic and spinoparabrachial tracts to the brain

Table 70.1 Contributions to a pain hologram

Physical neuromatrix, including peripheral and central nervous systems plus fascial network:
• Emotional
• Cognitive
• Memory
• Mind

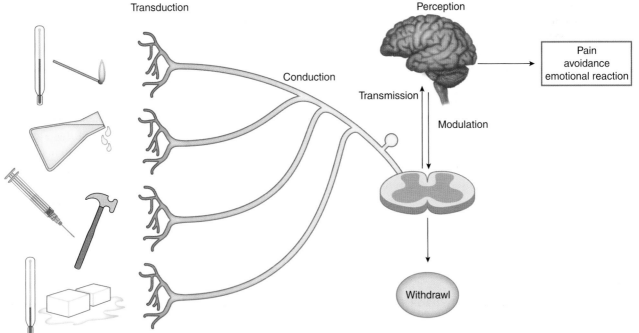

Nociceptive pain processing*: Transduction to perception

*The stimulus is well localized; its duration, intensity, and quality are clear

Fig. 70.1   Nociceptive pain processing. Transduction to perception

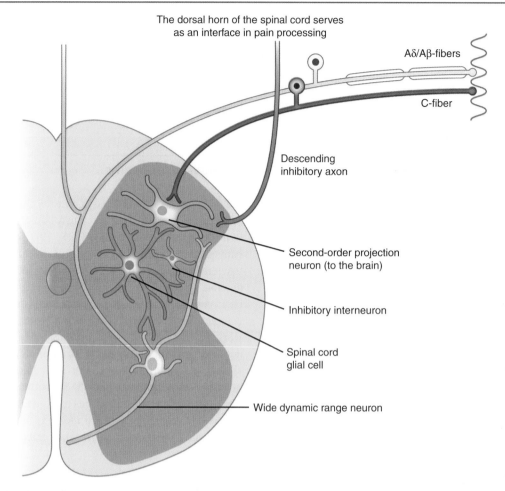

The dorsal horn of the spinal cord serves
as an interface in pain processing

Aδ/Aβ-fibers

C-fiber

Descending
inhibitory axon

Second-order projection
neuron (to the brain)

Inhibitory interneuron

Spinal cord
glial cell

Wide dynamic range neuron

Fig. 70.2 The dorsal horn of the spinal cord serves as an interface in pain processing

(Fig. 70.2). The spinothalamic transmission is delivered to the thalamus and is processed on to the contralateral somatosensory cortex. The spinoparabrachial transmission is processed through the hippocampus, amygdala, and onward to the prefrontal cortex, ACC, and other areas of the brain bilaterally (Fig. 70.3) [13, 26, 27, 37–40].

Intensification of the laser beam being generated by the periphery or spinal cord can occur via sensitization of the peripheral nociceptors, which increases the intensity of the signal reaching the spinal cord [12]. At the spinal level, we can experience recruitment of new nociceptive inputs or even non-nociceptive fibers (as with Aβ fibers) when the signals are strong enough. When enough stimulation has occurred via root input or dorsal horn sensitization, the spinal cord can go into "automatic" mode, where it no longer needs peripheral input to fire. Thus, we can wind up with very strong and enduring laser beams from the physical generators below the brain [13, 38, 39, 41].

Within the brain, adding further to this complex process which happened in the dorsal horn, an area of the caudate contains TANS (tonically active neurons). It is in this area of the brain where a confluence of signals from the hippocam-

pus (memory), our emotions (amygdala), and our cognitions are processed, with the resultant signals being sent to the globus pallidus and up to the motor cortex. Thus, messages that come from areas of our brain that are overlapping and interacting with pain signals can incorporate cognitive, emotional, and memory inputs that have a direct effect on our motor system as well as our sensory system [6]. This provides an understanding to the concept that our brain processing is geared to result in "action" and is responsive to our sensory perceptions such as pain. We do not experience sensory perceptions for the sake of experiencing alone [6, 14, 22, 42, 43].

In addition to the neural network, physical input to our pain hologram can be strongly influenced by the fascial system, described as the organ system of stability and mechano-regulation [44], and wherein lies ten times more sensory nerve endings than in muscle [45, 46]. Fascia lines all body parts, as John Barnes puts it: "fascia is a tough connective tissue that spreads throughout the body in a three-dimensional web from head to foot functionally, without interruption" [2]. The purpose of fascia is to maintain body shape and keep organs in their proper positions,

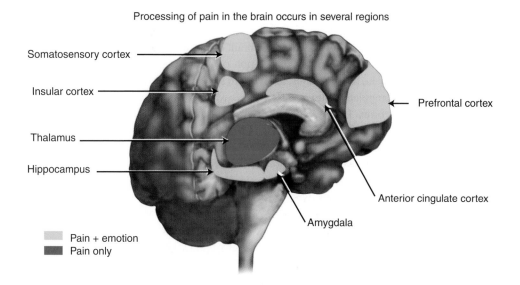

Processing of pain in the brain occurs in several regions

Somatosensory cortex

Insular cortex

Thalamus

Hippocampus

Prefrontal cortex

Anterior cingulate cortex

Amygdala

Pain + emotion
Pain only

Fig. 70.3 Processing of pain in the brain occurs in several regions

as well as resist mechanical stresses from any source such as trauma and inflammation [47]. This function of fascia is best understood through the construct of tensegrity, a concept that explains the relationship between skeleton, tensional forces of the fascia, contractility of muscle, and hydrostatic pressure of fascial compartments [48]. Restrictions of the fascia have been found to cause limitations in movement and pain which can have non-dermatomal referral patterns [49, 50], thus demonstrating that the physical input to our pain hologram from fascia is not by activation of peripheral nociceptors. While often ignored in evaluating a person's pain perception, fascial contribution to pain has been demonstrated in such diverse problems as Achilles tendinopathy [51], plantar fasciitis [52], systemic lupus erythematosus [53], and acute compartment syndrome of the upper extremity [54].

Researchers have demonstrated an energy transmission system throughout fascial planes. This energy wave is faster than neural transmission and is very nicely visually demonstrated by Guimberteau [55]. Body memory of past events or trauma (physical, emotional, or sexual) [3] can be stored in the fascia, similarly to neural storage, and this stored memory can interrupt the smooth flow of energy via the fascial system [2, 55–57]. We do know that traumatic events are processed by the person immediately after they happen. However, what is not totally processed at that time is stored in cellular body memory traces that become like a three-dimensional photo (although the storage is in energy units and not pictures) and incorporates all contingencies of that event, placing them in "storage" at an unconscious level. Barnes has found that a part of these stored memory traces in the fascial network are positionally dependent [2]. Through Barnes' unwinding technique, bodily positions that can rep-

licate the same body part position at the time of the trauma can release and make conscious the stored unconscious memories and allow the person to finish working through that event [2].

Other therapeutic applications that take advantage of this fascial network input to pain are being used for surgical anesthesia and post-op pain control. Fascial iliaca compartment block has been used in fractured neck of femur [58], hip arthroplasty [59], and this same block has been shown to reduce emergence agitation in children having thigh surgery [60]. One study cited has replaced epidural anesthesia with fascial anesthesia in prostatectomies [61]. Although the fascial network is not processed via the peripheral nociceptors, there is some recent animal research to indicate some dorsal horn activity via the fascial network in addition to fascial activation itself, and this article concludes that fascial input is a significant contributing force to painful syndromes [62].

Emotional Laser Beams

We are all familiar with the fact that people with persistent pain frequently have complaints of anger, anxiety, depression, and sometimes fear attached to their pain experience. These reactions have been categorized into phasic, acute, and chronic by Craig, with phasic and acute representing anticipatory fear and relief, while chronic represents depression, fear, anger, disgust, social distress, guilt, subservience, resignation, and abandonment [63]. The question then arises as to whether these emotional complaints are representative of primary psychological illnesses or are they part and parcel of normal and/or dysfunctional brain activity relative to pain perception? Do people living with maldynia have multiple illnesses or was Osler correct to have us think of "one person, one disease"?

Perhaps we can make more sense of this question by looking at brain function. Brain areas significantly involved in emotion in the brain include the amygdala, hippocampus, lateral hypothalamus, caudate, anterior cingulate cortex (ACC), supraorbital cortex, and prefrontal cortex [13, 37]. These same areas have been well documented in depression, anxiety, obsessive-compulsive disorder, and fear among others [4, 6, 11]. Interestingly, if we look at the affective dimension of pain, according to Price and the Rome article, these same brain areas are the ones involved [14, 15, 28]. Thus, what we are beginning to identify is that pain perception and emotional problems share some of the same "brain railroad tracks." The brain doesn't "know" what it is doing, it just does. Therefore, if the brain is utilizing the same tracks for two different types of perception, it cannot tell which train is riding that track at any given time, nor does it care. In fact, two trains can use the same tracks at the same time, and by so doing, they can signal a "go" to each other. This mixed signaling helps us understand why people in pain, especially those with maldynia, will report that stressful or depressing events can exacerbate their pain. In our holographic analogy, this would be equivalent to adding strength to some of the laser beams making up our pain hologram, by non-painful inputs. This could be likened to "recruitment" in the spinal cord, where we intensify a pain signal through recruitment of non-nociceptive fibers. (Spinal recruitment is a lower level route to add strength to the "physical" pain laser beam being fed into our hologram.)

The medical literature supports the reverse concepts to also be a frequent occurrence; that is, psychiatric patients with affective disorders often have pain as a symptom of their affective disorder. Phillips and Hunter identified an increased prevalence and intensity in tension-type headaches in a psychiatric population compared to the general population [64]. Melzack and Katz have discussed that stressful events have been associated with angina pectoris, ulcers, rheumatoid arthritis, painful menses, ulcerative colitis, and regional enteritis [20].

In addition, some psychiatrists have taken the position that pain is no more than a symptom of psychiatric disease and is not a disease unto itself. We believe the distinction is better conceived by understanding perception rather than disease states. For example, Romano and Turner have written that approximately 50 % of all patients with pain and depression develop the two "disorders" simultaneously [65]. In view of brain imaging studies and our current understanding of overlapping brain areas in pain and depression, it makes sense that some patients may experience pain and depression simultaneously, while others may feel one or the other first. If both perceptions are utilizing the same brain areas and reinforcing each other, then it becomes easier to understand why depression could stimulate a pain perception, pain could stimulate depression, or both could start together. Remember, the brain is the only part of the body that can "perceive," and since the brain only "does," without understanding, then any combination of perceptions can take place if the same areas of the brain are being utilized for them.

Cognitive Laser Beams

Marcus Aurelius [66] once said:

> If you are distressed by anything external, the pain is not due to the thing itself, but to your estimate of it. THIS you have the power to revoke at any time.

Our brain is structured such that the most primitive areas, in terms of development, are lower in location. Our cortex has been described as having evolved to be sitting on top of the older brain. Thus, the areas that are so highly integrated into the affective dimension of pain, as well as much of the pain areas associated with maldynia, are for the most part sub/lower cortical. As mentioned above, the TANS is the location where the cognitive areas meet the emotional areas, which have had input already from memory. Like so many of our sensory perceptions, the lower brain takes charge rather than the logical inputs we are capable of. It is often said that in most any issue between emotions and logic, the emotions will win out, that is, we will default to the "heart." This is another way of saying that decisions and responses, unless consciously influenced, will include "unconscious" influences that are more emotionally driven. Perlmutter and Villodo discuss the role of prefrontal cortex in reasoning and creative thinking and how changes in prefrontal functioning can lead to a "dysregulation" of the balance necessary for optimum brain function [67].

This "default" system can often lead us into difficulty. For example, when a person takes a medication for pain relief, the feeling of relief ("feels good") can easily lead us into the behavior of "if one feels good, then two or three must be even better." And hence, we can wind up with a patient developing significant adverse medication reactions by their instinctual (unconscious) desire to be pain free. Too much NSAID, acetaminophen, antidepressant, antiepileptic, etc., can produce physical harm to the body. Too much controlled substance can produce adverse bodily reactions and/or behaviors that result in legal trouble as well. The ultimate expression of this "action without thinking" response can be the development of pseudoaddiction, where the perception of pain relief is the desired goal, and our behaviors can mimic those of someone with a true addictive disorder. One person's actions are driven by the desire to relieve pain, while the person with an addictive disorder demonstrates behavior driven by the need to get high and, further into the disease, by the need to avoid crashing and experiencing withdrawal. The behaviors may be very similar on the part of those two different people, with lack of demonstrable control in following prescription directions, drug seeking behaviors, actually placing themselves in harm's way at times, lying to those around them in order to obtain more medications, etc. (see Chap. 75 on Addictive Disorders and Pain). What we experience in situations where the lower brain centers are controlling our responses are cognitive rationalizations, that is, "if one pill works, two is better" as a way to justify our desire to have less pain. This kind of cognitive laser beam is one in which the cognition follows the affective dimension rather than lead it.

Various issues regarding the cognitive input to pain perception have been described [4]. These contributions have looked at such issues as the roles of language descriptors [68], emotion and attitudes [69], culture and attention [70], ethnicity [71], gender differences [72], and age differences (see Chap. 88, Pain in the Elderly Population) [73]. The literature also supports the significance of the affective dimension through the cognitive inputs [23]. These contributions from mind and cognition support Schwartz's description of processing the affective, memory, and cognitive processes through the TANs, described earlier.

Conversely, when cognitive-behavioral therapies are utilized in treating pain or other problems such as depression or OCD, the success of the patient depends on their ability, through much practice, to have the cognitive abilities of the higher cortex take charge and present alternative "thinking" to the patient. This change allows for a reframing of thoughts and a refocusing of attention as well as the consequent behaviors away from the "painful" thoughts, that is, "I hurt," "I am suffering," "I will never be able to enjoy family picnics again," etc [4, 74]. These examples are of our cognitive system in a passive mode (default system). The alternatives, through cognitive-behavioral approaches, would be to assertively place into consciousness such concepts as "this pain has no beneficial meaning to me, therefore, I will focus on the love I have for antique cars and review some pictures of old convertibles now," or "since this pain is meaningless to me, I choose to breathe deep ten times and allow my body to feel the flow of positive energy course through me," etc. Utilizing our higher cortical powers assertively, then, allows us to change the "default" system by building in new neuroplastic patterns. We literally can control our lives by creating the new set of railroad tracks we want our train to utilize and set up the switching mechanisms by practicing, until the new track becomes our "default." This becomes active mode for our cognitive inputs [6].

Thus, the cognitive contribution to pain lasers can be positive or negative and can be minimal when in passive mode (old default), or when in active mode, the cognitive input has the potential, in many instances, to become the most powerful influence to overcome adverse emotional reactions [23]. As we will see below, the cognitive force from our mind through our cortical thinking brain can become a valuable source of positive neuroplastic retraining of our brain. Cognitive-behavioral processes have been shown to be the most effective in helping people with maldynia to restore their functional status and maximize their abilities to take charge of their lives again [4, 74]. Our developmentally highest level of brain function is often needed to help us deal with our most significant life problems, when our lower brain levels that normally run on automatic default fail us. The paradox is that it so often requires professional help to teach us how to utilize these higher level approaches to alter our life experiences, which are our perceptions (see Chap. 76).

Another example of how we can utilize our higher cognitive power to defeat pain is through hypnosis. Rainville et al. have demonstrated that if we use hypnosis to alter the affective-motivational dimension of pain first, there is often a reduction in the sensory-discriminative pain dimension that follows it [75]. However, this approach makes changes in brain function through the lower centers which mediate the affective dimension of pain and does not involve the somatosensory cortex. On the other hand, the reverse is not true. If we utilize hypnosis to alter the sensory-discriminative dimension of pain first, the process does involve the somatosensory cortex, but even if we alter the pain intensity, the affective dimension (the "yuck") doesn't change [75]. Thus, how we build our new railroad tracks and which "switchers" we utilize can have a rather dramatic effect on the "retraining" process of the brain (see Chap. 78).

Memory Laser Beams

Memory in humans is a complex process, which involves multiple inputs to go from immediate memory to long-term memory. Memory is made in the body cells [7, 56] as well as in the brain, but it is not made in pictures. It is made in mnemonics, with different memory storage for each part of the memory. For example, the memory for a traumatic event (painful or not) will have memory traces for the event itself, the place it happened, the smells involved, the sounds heard, the sights seen, the emotions perceived, the thoughts associated with the event, our judgment of what has happened, etc. The memory is made and stored according to events and patterns. The memory may or may not remain in our conscious awareness, but long-term memory is permanent [76, 77].

Brain areas involved in memory involve left prefrontal, temporal, and parahippocampal cortices. The level of activation of these areas predicts which memory becomes long term or not [78, 79]. The hippocampus and amygdala relate to emotional memory (remember the TANS) via NMDA and dopamine, and long-term potentiation in the hippocampus may underlie learning and memory [76, 77, 80]. Prefrontal cortex is involved with object identity, spatial locations, memory and coding, and analysis of the meaning of items

[81–83]. Prefrontal cortical involvement increases as the semantic complexity rises [78, 79]. Thus, we can begin to see how memory becomes entwined with the confluence of brain patterning involved in pain perception. Through the TANS, the feed-in of memory, emotions, and meaning all meld together. When the input is of sufficient intensity, memory will be made [83].

When we want to actively recall a memory, such as "what did I eat for lunch today," our brain must activate these brain areas, pull up the mnemonic for each part of that hologram for "lunch," and converge them all to produce the three-dimensional holographic picture in my mind's eye of lunch today. This will include all my senses, including taste, color, food presentation, sounds in the room where lunch was eaten, the conversation that took place, who was there, the temperature of the food and room, how much comfort or discomfort was involved both physically and emotionally, etc.

Thus, memory is made in parallel for the events and for the emotional and other components [15, 28]. Hence, when we have to converge multiple mnemonics to produce our pain perception hologram, the mnemonic for any portion of the pain (sensory-discriminative, affective, memory, or both) can be overloaded by previous memory mnemonics for that particular quality of the pain [4, 84]. If the affective component is overloaded, we can see the limbically augmented pain syndrome (LAPS) described by Rome and Rome. Thus, memory, and sensitization of the memory system, can result in augmentation of the pain perception. This accounts for why sufferers of persistent pain often have a more frequent history of trauma compared to the general population.

Returning to our great Roman emperor, Marcus Aurelius [66], we can again quote him:

> As for pain, a pain that is unbearable carries us off; but that which lasts a long time is bearable; the mind retires into itself, and the ruling faculty is not injured. As for the parts which are hurt by the pain, let them, if they can, give their opinion of it.

If we view this memory system through the lenses of the brain areas involved, and realize those same brain areas are involved with the physical, emotional, cognitive, and meaningfulness of any perception, including pain, we can see the genius behind Marcus Aurelius' two observations about pain perception. He demonstrated a far-reaching wisdom about pain perception, without any scientific knowledge of how accurate his statements have turned out to be in terms of modern investigations into brain functioning.

Mind Control and Mind Laser Beams

Building on the foundation that our mind is something different from our brain, even though it operates through the brain, we can add some very powerful laser beams and control over the entire system through mindfulness.

As Schwartz has described, "quantum theory creates a causal opening for the mind, a point of entry by which mind can affect matter, a mechanism by which mind can shape brain. That opening arises because quantum theory allows intention, and attention, to exert real, physical effects on the brain…" [6].

This same author has brought together the work of many neuroscientists, such as William James, Henry Stapp, and Benjamin Libet in order to demonstrate how the mind can physically affect the brain. It has been demonstrated that a wave of "readiness" energy appears in the brain about 350–550 ms before a motor movement occurs. In addition, the sense of will occurs 150–200 ms prior to a movement. This free will offers an opportunity to make the movement a "go" or "not go" [6]. Stowell has previously described a similar time delay in pain perception [85], and the impact of psychosocial feedback has been investigated in the timing of events by Lee and colleagues [42].

Hence, the understanding of free will becomes a process by which the brain "bubbles up" unconscious thoughts that could lead to action; but free will, as a conscious system, provides an opportunity to screen these bubbling ideas and exert control over which ones are a go or not. It has been proposed that the initiatives that bubble up in the brain are based on the person's past memories, experiences, values inculcated from society, and present circumstances. Interestingly, studies of brain function in relationship to free will demonstrate that the prefrontal cortex is activated as a primary area. Disorders such as schizophrenia, which is marked by autistic behavior and inactivity, and clinical depression, one symptom of which is lack of initiative, demonstrate a consistently low level of activity in the prefrontal cortex [6].

Additionally, studies cited by Schwartz have demonstrated activation of brain regions which affect perception, such as auditory-language association cortices in the temporal lobe without any associated activity of the auditory cortex in schizophrenic patients who are having active auditory hallucinations. In fact, the hippocampus (retrieving contextual information), ventral striatum (integrating emotional experience with perception), and thalamus (maintaining conscious awareness) were also involved in these patients, but the frontal cortex remained quiet. Another example of a patient with amyotrophic lateral sclerosis (ALS) showed that by implanting electrodes into his motor cortex, he was able to will his brain to activate his motor cortex by imagining his finger moving. This enabled him to be able to move a cursor on his computer through brain activation via his imagination [6]. We have previously discussed in this chapter how imagination also activates brain function consistent with allodynia, in people without any current allodynia, but only a history of same.

It has been shown that long-standing pain can interrupt time perception, causing a disorganization of the patient's being in the world [86]. Spatial additivity and attention also had impact on the mind-pain relationship [87]. One of the most powerful demonstrations of mindfulness "power" is presented by Fitzgibbon and colleagues, in which "synesthesia" is used to explain how, if we experience another person's pain, similar brain areas that are activated in the pain person are activated in the sympathetic person as well [32]. Rainville et al. [75]. have shown the brain activation associated with hypnosis, and Krämer's group has shown brain activation through imagination, another mindful activity [29].

Our spiritual perspectives also contribute to our mindful contributions to our pain lasers. Perlmutter and Villoldo describe nicely the relationship between our spiritual beliefs and brain function (see also Chap. 83, for a more comprehensive discussion of this important input to our pain hologram) [67].

Another area that deserves discussion in terms of mind laser beam input to our pain hologram is that of post-traumatic stress disorder (PTSD). We have long known of an association between PTSD, either military or civilian, and pain perception. The trauma, which can be due to physical calamity, emotional abuse, sexual abuse, or combinations of these, results in neuroplastic changes causing a sensitization in brain regions overlapping with some of those involved in pain perception [88–92]. The limbic system, especially amygdala, demonstrates hypersensitivity, while the medial frontal cortex fails to exert governance [93]. For example, loud noise results in a more severe and exaggerated effect in people with PTSD [94]. Other clinical symptoms, such as intrusive rethinking of the traumatic event, intrusive dreaming of same, diminished interests, constriction of affective responses, as well as heightened responses to events that arouse recollections of the trauma, are all congruent with the dysfunction of the limbic and prefrontal cortex areas seen in chronic pain sufferers. As we discuss in this chapter, the more attention we pay to things that activate similar areas of the brain, the more intensely those brain areas react to less intense stimuli or even imagined stimuli. Thus, we can see why trauma and maldynia so frequently coexist and how two seemingly different happenings can serve to reinforce each other. Treatments directed at one, can conversely, reduce the intensity of the perceptual experience of the other. Perception within PTSD victims has been described as "you can never feel just a little bit: it is all or nothing" [95]. This is very similar to the heightened pain perceptions in such painful conditions as limbically augmented pain syndrome (LAPS) [28], phantom pain [11, 96, 97], irritable bowel syndrome (IBS) [98, 99], chronic daily headache [100, 101], chronic depression [102, 103], and fibromyalgia [104–106]. Dohrenbusch et al. have also demonstrated the heightened sensory system in general in patients with fibromyalgia [106]. Hence, in all of these conditions, our mindful perception is increased secondary to the neuroplastic sensitization of the brain.

Finally, Schwartz has discussed how volitional attention is the key to inducing neuroplastic changes through mindfulness. Attention determines brain activity, through the selection process discussed earlier. "Attention can do more than enhance the responses of selected neurons. It can also turn down the volume in competing regions" [6]. "When it comes to determining what the brain will process, the mind (through the mechanism of selective attention) is at least as strong as the novelty or relevance of the stimulus itself" [6]. This attention seems to originate in the frontal and parietal lobes, but like other functions, imaging studies show that there is no attention center in the brain. Rather, we see similar patterns as those associated with pain perception, that is, prefrontal cortex and anterior cingulate. In addition, parietal cortex, basal ganglia, and cerebellum are involved. Furthermore, studies have shown that when you pay attention to something, the brain parts involved in processing that something become more active. "Attention, then, is not some fuzzy, ethereal concept. It acts back on the physical structure and activity of the brain" [6]. Indeed, hypnosis, one of our potentially powerful treatment tools, is best understood as focused awareness (highly selective attention) with a resulting reduction in peripheral awareness (see Chap. 80, Hypnosis and Pain Control) [107]. Tai Chi, another mindfulness system, also incorporates attentional focus to utilize slow movements that promote balance, agility, flexibility, and strength to develop synergy of mind and body [108].

In creating neuroplastic changes to aid control over pain holograms, repeatedly utilizing patterns of attention will actually result in changes in patterns of sensory processing, and this remapping of sensory cortex has been demonstrated. Animal studies that have documented these neuroplastic changes in primary auditory cortex, somatosensory cortex, and motor cortex support the position that it is the attentional state of the animal which is crucial to make the change, not the sensory input itself. "Every stimulus from the world outside impinges on a consciousness that is predisposed to accept it, or to ignore it. We can therefore go further: not only do mental states matter to the physical activity of the brain, but they can contribute to the final perception even more powerfully than the stimulus itself" [6]. In fact, it has been shown that when stimuli identical to those inducing neuroplastic changes in an attending brain are delivered to a nonattending brain, there is no induction of neuroplastic cortical change [6]. Hence, "the willful focusing of attention is not only a psychological intervention. It is also a biological one" [6].

Schwartz nicely summarizes the contribution of mind via quantum brain functioning in the following quote [6]:

> Our will, our volition, our karma, constitutes the essential core of the active part of mental experience. It is the most important, if not the only important, active part of consciousness. We generally think of will as being expressed in the behaviors we exhibit: whether we choose this path or that one, whether we

make this decision or that. Even when will is viewed introspectively, we often conceptualize it in terms of an externally pursued goal. But I think the truly important manifestation of will, the one from which our decisions and behaviors flow, is the choice we make about the quality and direction of attentional focus. Mindful, or unmindful, wise or unwise--- no choice we make is more basic, or important, than this one.

Pain Holograms

We have looked at how perception is analogous to holograms. When we want to evaluate a person's pain, we need to just look at what laser beam is part of the pain hologram. Is there a contribution to their pain perception from physical inputs, emotional inputs, cognitive inputs, mindful inputs, memory inputs, or multiple sources linked together by brain function? Only by understanding their entire hologram can we then begin to devise the appropriate treatments to deconstruct as much of their hologram as possible.

The importance of evaluating and treating a person's pain by identifying what laser beams may be contributing to their pain hologram is critically important to our success in finding them relief. For example, a 34-year-old female migraine sufferer had been averaging 2–3 headaches/month, relieved by an injection at local emergency rooms, for years. One evening, she suffered a severe headache, went to an emergency room for treatment, and was told "you're having a migraine; go home and go to bed." The patient, who sought treatment at a different hospital, was found to have a ruptured brain aneurysm, which was successfully surgically repaired. However, she began to experience a daily headache from that time forward. She had been to several headache clinics and neurologists, all of whom treated her for "transformed migraine" for over 2 years with multiple classes of migraine pharmacological treatments, biofeedback, acupuncture, and meditation without success. She was referred to our clinic for treatment of the PTSD from the night of the ruptured aneurysm, as she clearly thought she was going to die that night. Processing the PTSD with eye movement desensitization and reprocessing (EMDR), a psychological treatment that seems to "delink" linked memories and possibly reverse the long-term potentiation associated with this memory storage, was successful in alleviating her PTSD symptoms completely. However, her headache continued. EMDR was then used to target the daily headache itself, and after six sessions, her daily headache was resolved and has not returned in over 8+ years. She does continue with her 2–3 migraines/month. Her daily headache hologram appears to have been a "phantom headache." EMDR is a useful treatment for phantom pain and can resolve it permanently, as it did in this case, unless the person is re-traumatized [109]. Thus, only by continuing to search for what laser beams may have been underlying her pain hologram were we able to identify and treat her with a treatment that allowed deconstruction of that hologram and resolution of her daily headache.

John Barnes has said that, "prior to seeing any patient that day, if we believe we know what we are going to do based on their diagnosis, then we don't know what we are doing." This is not only an observation, but we consider it to be a medical principle [2, 3]. Our patients' pain holograms are dynamic, not static, just like our physical nervous system. Thus, we owe it to ourselves and our patients to find out what that pain hologram is comprised of and the importance of each contributing factor on any given day in order to properly plan treatment. This approach allows us to treat people, not body parts. Pain holograms are three-dimensional, just like any other hologram, and we can be more successful with pain sufferers if we approach pain perception through those lenses.

Summary

In this chapter, we have explored human perception and pain as a perceptual experience. We have looked at how individual parts of pain perception are processed in the brain, with overlapping of multiple different inputs within brain regions resulting in the enabling, enhancement, sensitization, and altered perceptions which can result from this. This perspective allows a better understanding of why pain has so many comorbid psychological consequences, as well as altered motor behaviors.

By utilizing an analogy to holograms, we have discussed how various sources of input into a pain hologram can come from physical inputs, including the nervous system and fascial tissue energy, and/or from emotional, cognitive, memory, as well as mindful sources. These different inputs, which operate via the brain, are best explained through both traditional and quantum physics. Traditional physics can help us understand some of the hard-wiring nervous system (peripheral, spinal, and brain) functions. However, it is only through a "quantum brain" perspective that we can make sense out of the perspectives of mind, thoughts, fascial energies, memory, and our cognitions which include our social, cultural, familial, spiritual, and personal values. Through these traditional and quantum brain approaches, we can understand why each person's pain hologram is unique to them, regardless of the type of pain. If five people all suffered a tibial fracture in an auto accident, there would be five different holograms created, and those five individuals' experiences with "tibial fracture pain" would all be different from each other.

Our ultimate formula for successful treatment is to restore a sense of balance to the system [110]. An example of this is seen in intracranial electrical stimulation for chronic depression and pain control. Here, the stimulation, which reduces brain activity, is applied to the motor cortex and not the sensory cortex, thus reestablishing a better balance within the brain [111]. The results are immediate.

Through comprehensive exploration of our patients' pain holograms, we are better able to identify appropriate treatments [21]. Patients who don't respond "as expected" may well have laser beams that we have not yet found or perhaps undervalued. If we keep in mind our old adage that the patient is always "right," it can lead us to unexplored paths to seeing their pain hologram differently and allow us newer approaches to those "difficult" cases. It can help us to keep in our consciousness, as pain treaters, the opening thought to this chapter: *the mind creates the brain.*

References

1. Talbot M. The holographic universe. New York: HarperCollins; 1991.
2. Barnes J. Myofascial release: the missing link in traditional treatment. In: Davis C, editor. Complementary therapies in rehabilitation, evidence for efficacy in treatment, prevention, and wellness. 3rd ed. Thorofare: Slack In; 2009. p. 89–112.
3. Barnes JF. Myofascial release: the search for excellence-A comprehensive evaluatory and treatment approach. Paoli: Rehabilitation Services Inc; 1990.
4. Ray A, Zbik A. Cognitive behavioral therapies and beyond. In: Tollison CD, editor. Practical pain management. 3rd ed. Philadelphia: Lippincott Williams and Wilkins; 2002. p. 189–208.
5. Benini A. Pain as a biological phenomenon of consciousness. Praxis. 1998;87(7):224–8.
6. Schwartz J, Begley S. The mind and the brain neuroplasticity and the power of mental force. New York: Harper Perennial; 2002. p. 372–7.
7. Gregory R. Brainy mind. BMJ. 1999;317:1693–5.
8. Satinover J. The quantum brain. New York: Wiley; 2001.
9. Schweinhardt P, Lee M, Tracey I. Imaging pain in patients: is it meaningful? Curr Opin Neurol. 2006;19:392–400.
10. Songer D. Psychotherapeutic approaches in the treatment of pain. Psychiatry. 2005;2(5):19–24.
11. Doidge N. The brain that changes itself. New York: Penguin Books; 2007.
12. Stohler C, Kowalski C. Spatial and temporal summation of sensory and affective dimensions of deep somatic pain. Pain. 1999;79(2–3):165–73.
13. Apkarian A, Bushnell M, Treede R-D, Zubieta J. Human brain mechanisms of pain perception and regulation in health and disease. Eur J Pain. 2005;9:463–84.
14. Price D. Psychological mechanisms of pain and analgesia. Seattle: IASP Press; 1999.
15. Price D, Harkins S. The affective-motivational dimension of pain: a two-stage model. APS J. 1992;1:229–39.
16. Auvray M, Myin E, Spence C. The sensory-discriminative and affective-motivational aspects of pain. Neurosci Biobehav Rev. 2010;34(2):214–23.
17. Gracely R. Affective dimensions of pain: how many and how measured? APS J. 1992;1:243–7.
18. Melzack R. Evolution of the neuromatrix theory of pain: the Prithvi Raj Lecture. Presented at the third world congress of World Institute of pain, Barcelona, Spain, 2004. Pain Pract. 2005;5(2):85–94.
19. Melzack R. Pain – an overview. Acta Anaesthesiol Scand. 1999;43(9):880–4.
20. Melzack R, Katz J. Pain assessment in adult patients. In: McMahon S, Koltzenburg M, editors. Wall and Melzack's textbook of pain. 5th ed. Oxford: Elsevier Churchill Livingstone; 2006. p. 291–304.
21. Pesut B, McDonald H. Connecting philosophy and practice: implications of two philosophic approaches to pain for nurses' expert clinical decision making. Nurs Philos. 2007;8(4):256–63.
22. Sitges C, Garcia-Herrera M, Pericas M, et al. Abnormal brain processing of affective and sensory pain descriptors in chronic pain patients. J Affect Disord. 2007;104(1–3):73–82.
23. Mialet J. From back pain to life-discontent: a holistic view of psychopathological contributions to pain. Ann Med Interne (Paris). 2003;154(4):219–26.
24. Bonica J. Neurophysiologic and pathologic aspects of acute and chronic pain. Arch Surg. 1977;112(6):750–61.
25. Lippe P. An apologia in defense of pain medicine. Clin J Pain. 1998;14:189–90.
26. Casey K, Tran T. Cortical mechanisms mediating acute and chronic pain in humans. In: Cervero F, Jensen T, editors. Handbook of clinical neurology. Boston: Elsevier; 2006. p. 159–77.
27. Voscopoulos C, Lema M. When does acute pain become chronic? Br J Anaesth. 2010;105 Suppl 1:i69–85.
28. Rome H, Rome J. Limbically augmented pain syndrome (LAPS): kindling, corticolimbic sensitization, and convergence of affective and sensory systems in chronic pain disorders. Pain Med. 2000;1:7–23.
29. Krämer H, Stenner C, Seddigh S, et al. Illusion of pain: pre-existing knowledge determines brain activation of 'imagined allodynia. J Pain. 2008;9(6):543–51.
30. Fontani G, Migliorini S, Benocci R, et al. Effect of mental imagery on the development of skilled motor actions. Percept Mot Skills. 2007;105(3 Pt 1):803–26.
31. Sanders CW, Sadoski M, Bramson R, et al. Comparing the effects of physical practice and mental imagery rehearsal on learning basic surgical skills by medical students. Am J Obstet Gynecol. 2004;191(5):1811–4.
32. Fitzgibbon B, Giumarra M, Georgiou-Karistianis N, et al. Shared pain: from empathy to synaesthesia. Neurosci Biobehav Rev. 2010;34(4):500–12.
33. Meyer R, Ringkamp M, Campbell J, Raja S. Peripheral mechanisms of cutaneous nociception. In: McMahon S, Koltzenburg M, editors. Wall and Melzack's textbook of pain. 5th ed. London: Elsevier; 2006. p. 3–34.
34. Julius D, McCloskey E. Cellular and molecular properties of primary afferent neurons. In: McMahon S, Koltzenburg M, editors. Wall and Melzack's textbook of pain. 5th ed. London: Elsevier; 2006. p. 35–48.
35. Ji R, Kawasaki Y, Wen Y, Decostrel I. Possible role of spinal astrocytes in maintaining chronic pain sensitization: review of current evidence with focus on bFGF/JNK pathway. Neuron Glia Biol. 2006;2:259–69.
36. Hertz L, Hansson E. Roles of astrocytes an microglia in pain memory. In: DeLeo J, Sorkin L, Watkins L, editors. Immune and glial regulation of pain. Seattle: IASP Press; 2007. p. 21–41.
37. Woolf C. Pain: moving from symptom control toward mechanism specific pharmacological management. Ann Intern Med. 2004;140:441–51.
38. Baron R. Mechanisms of disease: neuropathic pain – a clinical perspective. Nat Clin Pract Neurol. 2006;2(2):95–106.
39. Basbaum A, Jessell T. The perception of pain. In: Kandel E et al., editors. Principles of neural science. 4th ed. New York: Oxford University Press; 2000. p. 472–91.
40. Fields H, Heinricher M, Mason P. Neurotransmitters in nociceptive modulating circuits. Annu Rev Neurosci. 1991;14:219–45.
41. Kuner R. Central mechanisms of pathological pain. Nat Med. 2010;16(11):1258–66.

42. Lee M, Mouraux A, Iannetti G. Characterizing the cortical activity through which pain emerges from nociception. J Neurosci. 2009;29(24):7909–16.

43. Nicolelis M, Katz D, Krupa D. Potential circuit mechanisms underlying concurrent thalamic and cortical plasticity. Rev Neurosci. 1998;9(3):213–24.

44. Varela F, Frenk S. The organ of form. J Soc Biol Struct. 1987;10(1):1073–83.

45. Myers T. Fascial fitness: training in the neuromyofascial web. Fitness J. 2011:36–43.

46. Myers T. Anatomy trains: myofascial meridians for manual and movement therapists. New York: Churchill Livingstone; 2009.

47. Scott J. Molecules that keep you in shape. New Sci. 1986;111:49–53.

48. Juhan D. Job's body. Barrytown: Station Hill Press; 1987.

49. Travell J. Myofascia pain and dysfunction. Baltimore: Williams and Wilkins; 1983.

50. Hackett G, Hemwall G, Montgomery G. Ligament and tendon relaxation treated by prolotherapy. 5th ed. Oak Park: Beulah Land Press; 2002.

51. van Sterkenburg M, et al. The plantaris tendon and a potential role in mid-portion Achilles tendinopathy: an observational anatomical study. J Anat. 2011;218(3):336–41.

52. Sahin N, Oztürk A, Atici T. Foot mobility and plantar fascia elasticity with plantar fasciitis. Acta Orthop Traumatol Turc. 2010;44(5):385–91.

53. Ball T. Structural integration-based fascial release efficacy in systemic lupus erythematosus (SLE): two case studies. J Bodyw Mov Ther. 2011;15(2):217–25.

54. Prasarn ML, Oullette EA. Acute compartment syndrome of the upper extremity. J Am Acad Orthop Surg. 2011;19(1):49–58.

55. Guimberteau J. Strolling under the skin. New York: Elsevier SAS; 2004.

56. Pert C. The molecules of emotion. New York: Touchstone; 1999.

57. Oschman J. Energy medicine: the scientific basis. New York: Churchill Livingstone; 2000.

58. Elkhodair S, et al. Single fascia iliaca compartment block for pain relief in patients with fractured neck of femur in the emergency department: a pilot study. Eur J Emerg Med. 2011;18:340–3.

59. Kearns R, et al. Intrathecal opioid versus ultrasound guided fascia iliaca plane block for analgesia after primary hip arthroplasty: study protocol for a randomized, blinded, noninferiority controlled trial. Trials. 2011;21:12–51.

60. Kim HS, et al. Fascia iliaca compartment block reduces emergence agitation by providing effective analgesic properties in children. J Clin Anesth. 2011;23(2):119–23.

61. Boström P, Karjalainen V. Epidural or fascial anesthesia for postoperative pain? Duodecim. 2011;127(3):281–3.

62. Hoheisel U, Taguchi T, Treede RD, Mense S. Nociceptive input from the rat thoracolumbar fascia to lumbar dorsal horn neurones. Eur J Pain. 2011;15(8):810–5. Epub 2011 Feb 16.

63. Craig K. Emotions and psychobiology. In: McMahon S, Koltzenburg M, editors. Wall and Melzack's textbook of pain. 5th ed. Philadelphia: Elsevier Churchill Livingstone; 2006. p. 231–9.

64. Phillips HC, Hunter M. Headache in a psychophysical population. J Nerv Ment Dis. 1982;170:1–12.

65. Romano J, Turner J. Chronic pain and depression: does the evidence support a relationship? Psychol Bull. 1985;97:18–34.

66. Aurelius M. The meditations of Marcus Aurelius. In: Eliot C, editor. Plato, Epictetus, Marcus Aurelius the Harvard Classics. New York: Collier & Son; 1937. p. 245–61.

67. Perlmutter D, Villoldo A. Power up your brain the neuroscience of enlightenment. Carlsbad: Hay House; 2011. p. 26–31.

68. Kusumi T, Nakamoto K, Koyasu M. Perceptual and cognitive characteristics of metaphorical pain language. Shinrigaku Kenkyu. 2010;80(6):467–75.

69. Moroni C, Laurent B. Pain and cognition. Psychol Neuropsychiatr Vieil. 2006;4(1):21–30.

70. Kirmayer L. Culture and the metaphoric mediation of pain. Transcult Psychiatry. 2008;45(2):318–38.

71. Campbell C, France C, Robinson M, et al. Ethnic differences in the nociceptive flexion reflex (NFR). Pain. 2008;134(1–2):91–6.

72. Fillingham R. Sex differences in analgesic responses: evidence from experimental pain models. Eur J Anaesthesiol. 2002;26(suppl):16–24.

73. Gibson S, Farrell M. A review of age difference in the neurophysiology of nociception and the perceptual experience of pain. Clin J Pain. 2004;20(4):227–39.

74. Turk D, Flor H. The cognitive-behavioral approach to pain management. In: McMahon S, Koltzenburg M, editors. Wall and Melzack's textbook of pain. 5th ed. New York: Elsevier Churchill Livingstone; 2006. p. 339–48.

75. Rainville P, Hofbauer RK, Paus T, et al. Cerebral mechanisms of hypnotic induction and suggestion. J Cogn Neurosci. 1999;11(1):110–25.

76. Malenka R, Nicoll R. Long-term potentiation – a decade of progress. Science. 1999;285:1870–4.

77. Engert F, Bonhoeffer T. Dendritic spine changes associated with hippocampal long-term synaptic plasticity. Nature. 1999;399:66–70.

78. Wagner A, Schacter D, Rotte M, et al. Building memories: remembering and forgetting of verbal experiences as predicted by brain activity. Science. 1998;281:1188–91.

79. Brewer J. Making memories: brain activity that predicts how well visual experience will be remembered. Science. 1998;281:1185–7.

80. Shi S, Hayashi Y, Petralia R, et al. Rapid spine delivery and redistribution of AMPA receptors after synaptic NMDA receptor activation. Science. 1999;284:1811–6.

81. Damasio A. On some functions of the human prefrontal cortex. Ann N Y Acad Sci. 1995;769:241–51.

82. Owen A, Herrod N, Menon D, et al. Redefining the functional organization of working memory processes with human lateral prefrontal cortex. Eur J Neurosci. 1999;11:567–74.

83. D'Esposito M, Detre J, Alsop D, et al. The neural basis of the central executive system of working memory. Nature. 1995;378:279–81.

84. Shapiro F. Eye movement desensitization and reprocessing. New York: Guilford Press; 1995.

85. Stowell H. Event related brain potentials and human pain: a first objective overview. Int J Psychophysiol. 1884;1(2):137–51.

86. Hellström C, Carlsson S. The long-lasting now: disorganization in subjective time in long-standing pain. Scand J Psychol. 1996;37(4):416–23.

87. Lautenbacher S, Prager M, Rollman G. Pain additivity, diffuse noxious inhibitory controls, and attention: a functional measurement analysis. Somatosens Mot Res. 2007;24(4):189–201.

88. van der Kolk B. The psychobiology of posttraumatic stress disorder. J Clin Psychiatry. 1997;58 Suppl 9:16–24.

89. van der Kolk B, Fisler R. Childhood abuse and neglect and loss of self-regulation. Bull Menninger Clin. 1994;58(2):145–68.

90. van der Kolk B, Greenberg M, Boyd H, et al. Inescapable shock, neurotransmitters, and addiction to trauma: toward a psychobiology of post-traumatic stress. Biol Psychiatry. 1985;20(3):314–25.

91. van der Kolk B, Greenberg M, Orr S, et al. Endogenous opioids, stress induced analgesia, and posttraumatic stress disorder. Psychopharmacol Bull. 1989;25(3):417–21.

92. van der Kolk B, Pelcovitz D, Roth S, et al. Dissociation, somatization, and affect dysregulation: the complexity of adaptation of trauma. Am J Psychiatry. 1996;153(7 Suppl):83–93.

93. Rauch S. Neuroimaging and the neuroanatomy of PTSD. CNS Spectr. 1998;3 Suppl 2:31–3.

94. Shalev A, Peri T, Brandes D, Freedman S, Orr SP, Pitman RK. Auditory startle response in trauma survivors with PTSD: a prospective study. Am J Psychiatry. 2000;157:255–61.

95. van der Kolk B. Psychological trauma. Washington: American Psychiatric Press; 1987.

96. Ramachandran V, Rogers-Ramachandran D. Phantom limbs and neural plasticity. Arch Neurol. 2000;57(3):317–20.

97. Wade N. Beyond body experiences: phantom limbs, pain and the locus of sensation. Cortex. 2009;45(2):243–55.

98. Kwan C, Diamant N, Mikula K, Davis K. Characteristics of rectal perception are altered in irritable bowel syndrome. Pain. 2005;113(1–2):160–71.

99. Pain Giamberardino M, et al. Referred muscle pain and hyperalgesia from viscera. J Musculoskeletal Pain. 1999;7(1–2):61–9.

100. Silberstein S, et al. Neuropsychiatric aspects of primary headache disorders. In: Yudofsky S, Hales R, editors. Textbook of neuropsychiatry. 3rd ed. Washington: American Psychiatric Press; 1997. p. 381–412.

101. Burstein R, Strassman A. Peripheral and central sensitization during migraine. In: Devor M et al., editors. Proceedings of the 9th world congress on pain. Seattle: IASP Press; 2000. p. 589–602.

102. Post R, Weiss S, Smith M. Sensitization and kindling: implications for the evolving neural substrates of post-traumatic stress disorder. In: Friedman M, Charney D, Deutch A, editors. Neurobiological and clinical consequences of stress: from normal adaptation to post-traumatic stress disorder. Philadelphia: Lippincott-Raven; 1995. p. 203–24.

103. Weiss S, Post R. Caveats in the use of the kindling model of affective disorders. Toxicol Ind Health. 1994;10:421–7.

104. Vecchiet L, Giamberardino M. Muscle pain, myofascial pain, and fibromyalgia: recent advances. J Musculoskeletal Pain. 1999;7(1–2).

105. Graven-Nielson T. Central hyperexcitability in fibromyalgia. J Musculoskeletal Pain. 1999;7(1–2):261–72.

106. Dohrenbusch R, Sodhi H, Lamprecht J, Genth E. Fibromyalgia as a disorder of perceptual organization? An analysis of acoustic stimulus processing in patients with widespread pain. Z Rheumatol. 1997;56(6):334–41.

107. Spiegel H, Spiegel D. Trance and treatment: clinical uses of hypnosis. 2nd ed. Washington: American Psychiatric Publishing Inc; 2004.

108. Francis M. Mindfulness exercises may help chronic pain patients. In: Pain medicine network. Spring; 2011: p. 6–7.

109. Schneider J, Hofmann A, Rost C, Shapiro F. EMDR in the treatment of chronic phantom limb pain. Pain Med. 2008;9(1):76–82.

110. Sumatani M, Miyachi S, Uematsu H, et al. Phantom limb pain originates from dysfunction of the primary motor cortex. Masui. 2010;59(11):1364–9.

111. Levy R, Deer T, Henderson J. Intracranial neurostimulation for pain control: a review. Pain Physician. 2010;13(2):157–65.

Neuroplasticity, Sensitization, and Pain

71

Albert L. Ray

Key Points

- Neuroplasticity is the "operating system" for the nervous system.
- Eudynia: "the good"; acute nociceptive pain; a symptom; useful; warning pain
- Maldynia: "the bad"; sensitized system at peripheral nerves, cord, and/or brain; no benefits to the person; pain becomes the disease process itself
- Persistent pain: "the ugly"; continual maldynia; LAPS, CRPS, phantom pain, myofascial pain, IBS, fibromyalgia, chronic headaches, chronic mood changes

Introduction

Neuroplasticity is a term that is used quite frequently these days in pain-related literature, and in many ways, it has come to be a term especially associated with maldynia [1, 2]. However, neuroplasticity is a term that more accurately delineates the way our nervous system operates, peripherally and centrally, and it should have no intrinsic judgment placed upon it. It simply is what it is.

Neuroplasticity implies a mechanism whereby the physical anatomy and physiological workings of our nervous systems happen, both in normal and pathological conditions. It is the operating system for our nervous system "computer." It is like a combined hardware and software program. It is programmable, and when neuroplastic changes occur, they cause both physical changes, that is, anatomical changes to neurons, and physiological changes in the neurological patterns of operation. In many ways, these changes are analogous to laying down a set of railroad tracks. Once the tracks are in place, a train has no options but to follow the tracks, unless a switcher makes a change in the track and sends the train onto another set of tracks. In a similar way, once neuroplastic changes occur, our nervous system has no option but to follow these tracks, unless something causes a switch onto new tracks. However, the old tracks remain available indefinitely, and certain circumstances can switch our neurological train back onto the old track again.

In normal conditions, we foster the utilization of neuroplastic development to not only develop "railroad tracks" but also to polish them. For example, we develop the ability to walk from about 1 year of age, and hence, we lay down some early tracks for mobilization. As we age, and as we utilize walking in our everyday life, we polish those tracks till we become adept at walking. Eventually, we finely polish the system to allow for balance, mobility at low speed (walking) or high speed (running), and we develop variations on the mobility theme, such as skipping and hopping. With practice, we become better and better at it, adding more and more polished tracks as we develop. Later, we utilize neuroplasticity to accomplish more sophisticated tasks, such as developing the ability to play musical instruments, develop craft skills, or become athletes. In these situations, we merrily go our way without paying much attention to the fact that we are building new neurons devoted to the task at hand, and then, we are polishing and fine-tuning how the neurons work together in patterns that allow us to become proficient and efficient at what our task is. These neuroplastic changes are what allows us to become very accomplished at "within-self" activities, such as practicing at a musical instrument until the finger movements become "automatic," thus allowing the musician to concentrate on how they want the music to sound rather than on how to move fingers to produce the desired sound. But practicing also allows for neuroplastic changes to affect social activities with others, for example, when linemen

A.L. Ray, M.D.
Medical Director, The LITE Center,
5901 SW 74 St, Suite 201, South Miami, FL 33143, USA

University of Miami Miller School of Medicine,
Miami, FL, USA
e-mail: aray@thelitecenter.org

members of a football team describe the state of being where they "know" what their teammates will do without having to verbally communicate during plays. This happens from concentrated practice until the neuroplastic tracks for working together are highly polished.

Certain principles have been attributed to neuroplastic development and functioning [3–5]:

1. Our brain is constantly changing, based on our current experiences.
2. Cells that fire together, wire together, and, through practice, stay together.
3. "Use it or lose it" works for brain activity and numbers of neurons.
4. Our brain works best when the system is "balanced."
5. The left and right hemispheres work together within this balance, under normal conditions, as a whole and not separately.
6. The corpus callosum is the bridge between hemispheres, and it is denser in females than in males, making the female brain more symmetrical and women more intuitive.
7. Male brains have an asymmetrical torque, with a right frontal lobe larger than the left and the left occiput larger than the right.
8. Right hemispheres process visual and spatial information related to the big picture and is more active while we are learning something new, while left hemispheres are more adept at details, categories, and linearly arranged information such as language, and the left hemisphere becomes more involved once something is "overlearned" and is now routine.
9. Right brain makes more connections with centers below the cortex and hence has more to do with emotional things.
10. Women have a greater density of neurons in the temporal lobe, which specializes in language, and in developing language skills; they activate the left hippocampus (related to memory) more than men do, while men generally have greater visual and spatial skills, because they show greater activity in the right hippocampus.
11. Prefrontal cortex provides our most complex cognitive, behavioral, and emotional capacities. The dorsolateral prefrontal cortex is involved in higher-order thinking, attention, and short-term memory, while the orbital frontal cortex processes emotions via connections through the amygdala and is involved in social issues. Right prefrontal cortex develops foresight and "gets the gist of it," allowing us to stay on course to our goals and understand metaphor, whereas left prefrontal cortex focuses on details of individual events.
12. The major neurotransmitters function in coordination with each other according to the following general understandings:

    (a) Gamma-aminobutyric acid (GABA) is inhibitory and quiets the brain, while glutamate is excitatory and stirs it up. These neurotransmitters account for about 80 % of brain signaling.
    (b) Serotonin, norepinephrine, and dopamine act more as neuromodulators, alter sensitivity of receptors, make transmission more efficient, and instruct neurons to make more glutamate. They also have other modulating duties: serotonin helps the system stay in control, norepinephrine activates attention and amplifies signals for perception, arousal, and motivation, and both serotonin and norepinephrine are associated with mood. Dopamine sharpens and focuses attention and is involved with reward, movement, learning, and pleasure.
13. Neuroplastic development and changes occur via long-term potentiation (LTP). This happens through electrochemical changes. Glutamate in presynaptic cells builds up, while the postsynaptic cell increases receptivity of receptor sites, increasing the voltage to attract more glutamate. If the increased firing continues, the genes within neurons turn on and build more infrastructures to enhance the system. This occurs via brain-derived neurotrophic factor (BDNF). BDNF increases gene activation, voltage, serotonin, and even more of itself. It also regulates apoptosis.

Under normal conditions, the system described above works in harmony within the brain to regulate our learning, emotions, thinking, and controls through a marvelous balance of a feedback system of neurophysiology. Through the development of neuroplastic brain anatomy and physiology, we function in a state of health.

However, when we are dealing with neuroplastic changes that have negative consequences for our lives, we tend to place a "black cloud" value onto them. For example, the neuroplastic changes that account for fibromyalgia, complex regional pain syndrome, and neuropathic pain are all understood through negative lenses. In these painful conditions, we focus our understandings on how neuroplastic changes produce such ravaging conditions that account for so much human suffering.

Neuroplasticity, then, can account for "the good, the bad, and the ugly" of pain perception. In the remainder of this chapter, we will focus on how neuroplasticity can result in the normal transmission of pain and how sensitization of the nervous system, peripherally and centrally, can alter a rather magnificent "pain system" and place the pain train on different tracks. Through the remainder of this chapter, we will describe what happens in terms of normal pain transmission and the neuroplastic changes of the nervous system in the disease of pain and principles of treatment applications designed to retrain the brain for health, by taking advantage of the principles listed above.

Neuroplasticity in Pain

Eudynia: The "Good"

In our normal development, our nervous system becomes wired and develops the ability to transmit pain as a warning symptom. For example, if we fall down and break a bone, the warning pain says "something is wrong; fix it and I will go away." This transmission of a warning signal comes about through what we consider the "normal" development of our nervous system, but this is accomplished via our neuroplastic system of development. That system is a most complex and wonderful system that helps protect us.

It begins with transduction from nociceptors in the skin. These nociceptors respond to mechanical, chemical, and temperature extremes of hot or cold. They turn their response into an electrical/chemical signal that conducts information to the dorsal horn of the spinal cord (see Fig. 70.1).

At the dorsal horn, multiple inputs can have an effect on that information signal, some acting to enhance and some acting to diminish it. Once these influences occur, a final summated signal is then sent up to the brain, where it is further processed (see Fig. 70.2). Some of the signal passes up the spinothalamic tract, through the thalamus, and on to the contralateral somatosensory cortex, while some of it passes via the parabrachial tract to be distributed to multiple brain regions including the limbic system, the anterior cerebral cortex (ACC), the prefrontal cortex, the amygdala, and the striatum and on to the somatosensory cortex and also the motor cortex via the basal ganglia. The first part accounts for Price's sensory-discriminative dimension (the ouch) of pain, while the latter accounts for Price's affective-motivational dimension (the yuck) of pain (see Fig. 70.3) [6–9].

Overall, this system of eudynia offers us the security and protection against many threats, including injury, infection, and tumors, by alerting us to the pain associated with these threats. (The details of normal pain transmission are covered elsewhere in this book.) Hence, our system, through helpful neuroplastic development, will continue to serve us well indefinitely, unless something goes awry.

Sensitization of the System

Maldynia: The "Bad"

Negative changes in the transmission of pain tend to occur through a process of sensitization. The nervous system can become sensitized at peripheral sites as well as centrally at dorsal horn and/or brain. Hence, a system that once worked to protect us can transform into one that produces ongoing pain [10]. Long-term potentiation (LTP) is the cellular model for sensitization [2, 11], whereas long-term depression (LTD) inhibits pain [12].

For example, peripheral sensitization is known to happen at trigger point sites in muscle. Trigger points have been described as consisting of sensory (sensitive locus) and motor (active locus) combinations with sensitized nociceptors [13]. Allodynic and hyperalgesic areas have been found in trigger points secondary to peripheral sensitization in chronic muscle pain [14, 15], tension-type headaches [16], and postmastectomy pain [17]. Both nociceptor and non-nociceptor sensitization secondary to ischemia due to sustained contraction have been identified in trigger points [18]. The peripheral sensitization of trigger points feeds into the dorsal horn and contributes to the beginning of central sensitization. However, this peripheral sensitization resolves with treatment of the trigger points, whereas the central sensitization appears to continue if LTP has occurred.

Likewise, plastic changes have been noted in peripheral nerve injuries, and these injuries also contribute to spinal and brain sensitizations [19]. The plasticity of the peripheral system is not quite as well identified as that of the central system.

Central sensitization is more studied, especially at the spinal dorsal horn level and, more recently, brain level, which has been undervalued in the past. "Central sensitization represents an enhancement in the function of neurons and circuits on nociceptive pathways caused by the increases in membrane excitability and synaptic efficacy as well as to reduced inhibition and is a manifestation of the remarkable plasticity of the somatosensory nervous system in response to activity, inflammation, and neural injury" (Fig. 71.1) [20].

At the cord level, many interactions can lead to sensitization, both in terms of functional and structural changes [21]. Voltage-gated calcium channels (VGCC) [22, 23], transient receptor potential vanilloid type 1 (TRPV1) receptors [24, 25], glutamate [7, 26–29], protein kinases [30, 31], serotonin, and N-methyl-D-aspartate (NMDA) [32] have all been described in functional roles within both the spinal cord and brain for sensitization (Figs. 71.1 and 71.2).

Structural and functional changes also occur in the spinal cord level regarding astrogliosis, and this effect seems to be mediated through secretion of diffusible transmitters, such as interleukins, ATP, and nitric oxide. The glial cells, via glutamate release, are thought to sensitize second-order neurons. However, they may also have a direct effect via the astrocytic networks that can transduce signals intrinsically [33, 34]. Additionally, animal studies have demonstrated an increase in the number of synapses within the dorsal horn in neuropathic pain [35].

Within the brain, reduced opioid neurotransmission has been noted in animal studies of spinal LTP, especially in brain areas associated with pain modulation and affective-emotional response [36]. LTP in the hippocampus is also involved with memory [37] and fear changes [38].

Fig. 71.1 Mechanisms contributing to peripheral sensitization

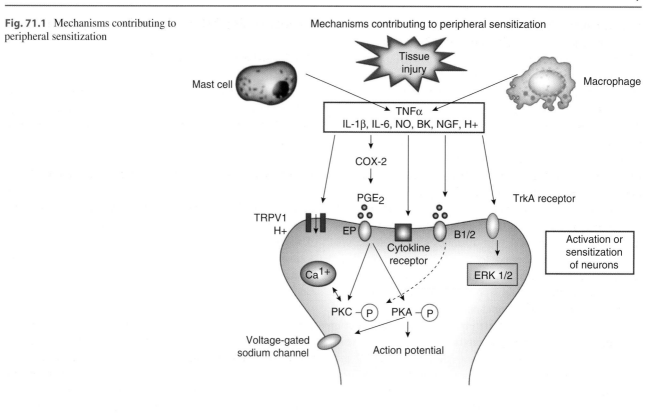

Fig. 71.2 Initiation of transmission at the level of the second-order neuron in the dorsal horn

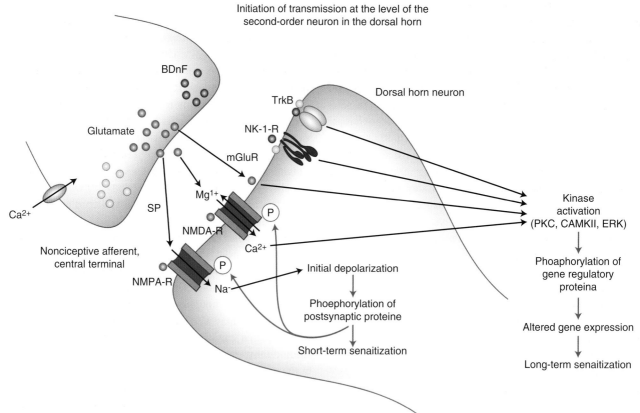

Spatiotemporal hippocampal changes have been observed in response to persistent nociception [39]. Tetanic stimulation of the ACC increased neurons in the central lateral nucleus of the medial thalamus [40]. fMRI, magnetoencephalography (MEG), positron emission tomography (PET), and voxel-based morphometry (VBM) studies in neuropathic pain have also shown reorganization of cortical somatotropic maps in sensory and motor areas, increased activity in nociceptive areas, recruitment of new cortical areas usually not activated by nociceptive stimuli, aberrant brain behavior normally involved with descending inhibitory pathways, changes in excitatory and inhibitory transmitter systems, and significant structural changes of neurodegeneration (use it or lose it) [41, 42]. These changes have been noted in phantom pain, chronic back pain, irritable bowel syndrome (IBS), fibromyalgia (FM), and two types of headaches. The alterations were different for each pain syndrome but overlapped in the cingulated cortex, the orbitofrontal cortex, the insula, and the dorsal pons [43]. These recent studies support an earlier proposition that the syndromes of chronic daily headache, chronic depression, IBS, and FM may all be different "phenotypes" of one "genotype" secondary to central sensitization [44]. Also, in post-spinal cord injury-related neuropathic pain, VBM studies have shown anatomical changes in pain-related and classic reward circuitry, including the nucleus accumbens, orbitofrontal, dorsolateral prefrontal, and posterior parietal cortices, and the right posterior parietal cortex projected to most of these affected areas [45]. Emotional-affective and cognitive dimensions of pain seem to also demonstrate structural and functional changes in maldynia, especially amygdala and prefrontal cortical areas [46, 47]. In fact, animal models for the amygdala-medial prefrontal cortex-driven pain-related cognitive deficits, including decision making, demonstrated that the cortical deactivation resulted from a shift of balance between excitatory and inhibitory transmission [47]. Hormones may have a role in neuroplasticity as well. Changes in neuroactive steroids during the estrous cycle have been shown to affect GABA-A receptor expression in female rats, resulting in an upregulation of GABA-A receptors late diestrus causing an increased excitability of output neurons in the periaqueductal gray (PAG) and clinically resulting in hyperalgesia [48].

Hence, we now have seen a neuroplastic transformation within the nervous system from a marvelous eudynic pain transmission model to one which demonstrates anatomic cellular changes, chemical transmitter and neuromodulator changes, and physiological functional changes via the process of sensitization. Indeed, our pain train now has different numbers of cars, different speeds at which to travel, changes in the stations along the way, and different tracks upon which it must now travel. It is what it has become!

Neuroplastically Remodeled Pain System

Persistent Pain: The "Ugly"

We will now turn more toward the clinical side of neuroplasticity and look at some specific pain problems. Ultimately, we will look at what can be done about them to ease our patient's suffering.

Limbically Augmented Pain Syndrome (LAPS) [49]

LAPS was described in a seminal pain paper to account for people who demonstrate more pain and pain behaviors than would be expected based solely on physical findings. These patients had previously been labeled as "hysterics," "crocks," and malingerers. Their presentation was usually affectively colorful, intense, and consisted of dramatic levels of dysfunction based on what previously looked like very little wrong physically. Through a very extensive comparison of clinical symptoms to sensitization research work, this paper clarified the role of central sensitization in both the traditional pain pathways and non-pain pathways regarding the affective-motivational and cognitive dimensions to pain perception. LAPS provides a foundational understanding of how sensitization presents clinically and why the primary pain and secondary non-pain complaints make sense. This includes many maldynia-accompanying complaints such as memory problems, slower thinking, non-restful sleep, decreased energy, lack of drive, decreased mental concentration and focus, anxiety, depression, anger, irritability, social isolation, a marked change in self-perception, and other frequent complaints we hear from our patients. The neuroplastic changes secondary to sensitization which account for decreased pain threshold, increased pain perception, recruitment, amplification of pain signaling within the central nervous system, and the intertwined role of pain- and non-pain-related inputs to pain have all been borne out and clarified through the research that has progressed since LAPS was identified, primarily due to improved technologies, but based on the core principles presented in the LAPS paper.

Through the LAPS foundation, we can make more sense out of the two dimensions of pain: the sensory-discriminative and affective-motivational dimensions described by Price [8]. Understanding these two dimensions and the overlapping brain functions involved with both helps unify our understanding of a person's pain perception, again reminding us of Osler's decree: one person, one disease. Rather than separate the two dimensions of pain and their respectively related symptoms, we can now focus on one person with all those complaints related to alterations in neuroplastic changes of the brain.

Fibromyalgia

Clinical aspects of neuroplastic changes in fibromyalgia are easily delineated, including many of those identified by the LAPS paper. However, peripheral evidence of change is basically lacking, in spite of much research on the peripheral tissues and peripheral pain transmissions. Within the central nervous system, however, much has been demonstrated. Fibromyalgia sufferers demonstrate hyperalgesia and allodynia, and this seems to result from an abnormal temporal summation of pain [50]. Changes in both sensory and motor brain have been found. One MRI and VBM study showed decreases in gray matter in the right superior temporal gyrus and left posterior thalamus, with increased gray matter in the left orbitofrontal cortex, left cerebellum, and striatum [51]. Another study found increased levels of serum BDNF in 30 female fibromyalgia patients, with no correlation to age, disease duration, pain score, number of pain tender points, or depression rating scores (HAM-D) [52].

Some of the treatments for fibromyalgia include pharmacological approaches designed to lower the level of pain transmission secondary to the neuroplastic sensitization by "calming down" the system at spinal and brain levels (see Part I. Medical Approaches). Other treatments include mind-body paradigms, as well as physical modalities. One study demonstrated benefit with a mind-body treatment utilizing psychosocial genomic postulates coupled with ideodynamic hand movements [53]. One study is being planned to utilize virtual exercise for those fibromyalgia patients who tend to avoid exercise as part of a catastrophizing style [54]. Moderate exercise for 24 weeks has been shown to have benefit for those able to tolerate it, resulting in improved health status and quality of life [55]. A separate 10-week exercise study demonstrated reduction in anxiety, improved sleep, and improved quality of life [56]. However, a group who had demonstrated improved daily step count by 54 %, improved functioning by 18 %, and reduced pain by 54 % in a 12-week trial found poor sustainability at 12-month follow-up, at which time the patients did not differ from controls on pain, physical activity, tenderness, fatigue, depression, the 6-min walk test, or self-reported functioning [57]. These findings would raise question as to what could be done to maintain the home treatment strategies long enough, or what could be added to them, in order to establish positive neuroplastic changes (i.e., what fires together wires together and what fires apart, wires apart).

Phantom Pain

Phantom limb sensations and pain have become more prominent in the literature since the incidence of amputation has increased as a result of the recent wars throughout the world [58]. The most recent successful treatments for phantom pain have also been based on what can change the brain LTP, hence, utilizing neuroplasticity to understand the pathophysiology of phantom pain and also to reverse it.

Studies have shown changes in the cortical representation of the affected limb and a correlation between these changes and the phantom pain. Mechanisms for the phantom pain are thought to relate to a loss of gamma-amino-butyric acid (GABA)-ergic inhibition, glutamate-mediated LTP changes, and structural changes such as axonal sprouting, and furthermore, these changes and consequent pain seem to be more extensive if chronic pain precedes the amputation [59].

One proposal suggests the imbalance of the system to be part of the problem. Specifically, the motor cortical body-representation cells involute, while the sensory cortical body-representation cells remain, the resulting imbalance producing the phantom pain. Reconciliation of this imbalance produces relief [60]. In fact, one treatment protocol utilizing imagined amputated limb movement coupled with existing counterpart limb movement resulted in fMRI evidence of elimination of the cortical reorganization and a reduction in constant pain and exacerbation pain [61]. Eye movement desensitization and reprocessing (EMDR) has also been shown to virtually eliminate phantom pain, without return barring further trauma to the body, through a similar process of alternating sensory input coupled with mental processing of the phantom pain [62, 63].

Complex Regional Pain Syndrome (CRPS)

CRPS is currently understood to be a complex of altered somatosensory, motor, autonomic, and inflammatory systems. But the central feature is both peripheral and central sensitization. Especially important to this sensitization is the neuroplastic alterations in the dorsal horn of postsynaptic NMDA receptors via chronic C-fiber input, among other changes. Motor changes are effected by calcitonin gene-related peptide (CGRP), substance P, and pro-inflammatory cytokines involved in the inflammatory process. Recent evidence implicates sensitization of adrenergic receptors in the sympathetic system having an influence on the C-fibers [64]. In animal studies, chronic peripheral inflammation has been shown to increase AMPA receptor-mediated glutamergic transmission in the ACC, which then increases the central excitatory transmission [65].

Visceral Pain

Visceral pain drives many doctor visits by patients, and it is one of the most common complaints in primary care offices. Visceral afferents have been found to play a role in tissue homeostasis by monitoring the viscera and contributing efferent functions via the release of small molecules such as CGRP that can drive inflammation. These afferents are highly plastic and are responsive to their cellular environment. They are quite susceptible to long-term changes associated with irritable bowel syndrome (IBS), pancreatitis, and visceral cancers [66]. In fact, recent work on chronic pancreatitis links sensitization to this syndrome, with descriptions of temporal and spatial alterations of intrapancreatic nerves and central neuroplastic consequences [67]. This process in chronic pancreatitis, then, seems to involve peripheral nociception, peripheral pancreatic neuropathy and neuroplasticity, and central neuroplastic changes as follows: sustained sensitization of pancreatic peripheral nociceptors by neurotransmitters and neurotrophic factors following neural damage, resulting in intrapancreatic autonomic "neural remodeling," which in turn causes our familiar hyperexcitability of second-order dorsal horn neurons, followed by viscerosensory cortical spatial reorganization [68].

Headache

Much work has been done regarding sensitization involving headache [69]. Recent understanding of sensitization in migraine considers peripheral sensitization leading to intracranial hypersensitivity (worsening the headache with cough and activity) and sensitized neurons becoming hyperresponsive to normally innocuous and unperceived fluctuations in intracranial pressure changes from arterial pulsation, resulting in the throbbing sensation. Central sensitization results in hyperexcitability of second-order neurons in the trigeminocervical complex, again a result of increased glutamate sensitivity of NMDA receptors and neuronal nitric oxide synthase activity. Clinically, this is manifested by facial and scalp allodynia along with neck stiffness [70].

Additionally, in chronic posttraumatic headache, a VBM study found spatial cortical reorganization to include decreased gray matter in the ACC and dorsolateral prefrontal cortex after 3 months. After resolution of the headache, at 1-year follow-up, patients who had developed the chronic headaches also showed an increase in gray matter in antinociceptive brainstem centers, thalamus, and cerebellum [71].

Postsurgical Pain

Chronic postoperative pain is becoming more prominently recognized. It is again thought to follow sensitization of the peripheral and central system by persistent acute postoperative pain. In most patients, it resembles neuropathic pain and occasionally follows continuous post-op inflammation [72]. This problem is estimated at between 10 and 80 %, and increased risk is associated with the existence of preoperative pain, the intensity and duration of post-op pain, and the type of surgery (high-risk surgeries) such as thoracotomy, breast, inguinal herniorrhaphy, and amputations [73]. The use of perioperative regional anesthesia has been shown to reduce the incidence, compared with intravenous morphine [74].

What to Do About It: Retraining the Brain

Multiple treatment approaches have been investigated for persistent pain, some designed to reduce the pain, others to improve functional status, and still others to reestablish a sense of contentment with life. The main theme behind all treatments is to try to establish a reversal of the neuroplastic sensitization or find ways to diminish its significance [75, 76].

Low back pain has been improved utilizing a training program model of delayed postural activation of the deep abdominal muscle, the transverse abdominis (TrA). Motor skill training induced an anterior and medial shift in motor cortical representation of the TrA, more closely resembling that of healthy persons. This training reversed the neuroplastic reorganization associated with chronic low back pain [77]. Other paradigms for chronic musculoskeletal pain also identify the need for motor learning as an important component for success, secondary to their ability at cortical reorganization [78]. One example is the use of peripheral electrical stimulation, which has been shown to develop rapid plastic change in the motor cortex, with parameters of variation in intensity of stimulation and longer periods of stimulation having the most sustained effects [79]. A fMRI study involving low-frequency electrical stimulation of cutaneous afferents in healthy volunteers resulted in pain relief and increased activity in the ACC, anterior insula, striatum, and frontal and temporal cortices, demonstrating long-term depression (LTD) of pain-related cerebral activation involving sensory, affective, cognitive, and attentional processes [80].

Acupuncture (see Chap. 79 for a detailed analysis of the approach) and massage have also been found to be peripheral stimulations which can cause central reorganizations. This has been described in terms of changing the neuroplastic adaptations associated with pain and addictive disorders [81].

Other therapeutic approaches include training of perceptual abilities, motor function, direct cortical stimulation, and behavioral approaches. Treatments that combine several modalities, such as imagery, mirror treatment, and prostheses, have been shown to have benefit [82]. For example, mirror therapy has been utilized for phantom pain, hemiparesis from stroke, and CPRS [83]. A somatosensory evoked potential (SEP) study involving chiropractic manipulation of the neck in subjects without current pain, but a history of chronic cervical pain, suggested alteration of the cortical integration of dual somatosensory input [84]. Paired associative stimulation in which peripheral nerve stimulation is followed by transcranial magnetic stimulation resulted in increased volleys of the descending inhibitory pathways [85], resulting in apparent LTD [86]. Even such techniques such as caloric restriction, via reduced intake of calories or intermittent fasting, have been shown to stimulate neurogenesis, enhance plasticity affecting pain sensation, cognitive function, and possibly resist brain aging. This is felt to occur through neurotrophic factors, neurotransmitter receptors, protein chaperones, and mitochondrial biosynthesis regulators which contribute to stimulation of the neuronal plasticity and resistance to oxidative metabolic insults [87]. Interestingly, one of the three worldwide characteristics of people who live the longest is eating 25 % less than the rest of their community members (caloric restriction) [4]. Cognitive-behavioral approaches have included somatosensory amplification associated with training in affect differentiation and the interaction of somatoform pain and interpersonal relationships [88].

It has been the clinical experience of the current author that the most effective treatment for maldynia or maldynia-eudynia combinations is a comprehensive approach designed to *retrain the brain*. This includes the utilization of some/all of the below modalities, individualized for each patient, such as myofascial release, unwinding, movement, electrical stimulations, muscle and ligament injections, exercising, postural training, guided imagery, body manipulations, visualization, meditation, spiritual healing, energy work, hypnosis, use of appropriate medications, inappropriate medication reductions, low-glycemic load nutritional approaches, nutritional supplements, bioidentical hormones, aroma therapy, graduated functional increases, massage and therapeutic touch, acupuncture, cognitive-behavioral treatment, Eye Movement Desensitization and Reprogramming (EMDR), NeuroEmotional Technique (NET), music therapy, family therapy and education, and patient education including neuroplasticity and brain function and how they are affecting their lives. The author of this chapter also utilizes written materials, some self-created and some published. Patients are referred to such items such as the American Pain Foundation (APF) website, the American Chronic Pain Association (ACPA) website, The Brain That Changes Itself [5], Rewire Your Brain [3], The Mind and the Brain [4], You Can Heal Your Life [89], The Quantum Brain [90], Power versus Force [91], and Healing and Recovery [92], among others.

These various therapies, educational materials, and philosophical approaches are often delivered individually, but sometimes simultaneously in a dual stimulatory approach through co-treatment (i.e., two therapists utilizing different treatments simultaneously, often incorporating two different senses/physical modalities at the same time). Treatments such as EMDR and NET incorporate two types of brain activity within one treatment approach. Some of these modalities take time and ritualistic practice in order to make neuroplastic changes (LTD, depotentiation of the LTP that occurred, or new LTD which is positive), while others, such as EMDR and NET, can have a rapid and lasting response, implying a neuroplastic reorganization that is immediate. Most of the therapeutic approaches mentioned above, however, must be done extensively and relatively frequently to make cortical changes permanently. We view ALL of these possible treatment modalities to have the same ultimate goal: RETRAINING THE BRAIN!

Summary

In this chapter, we have discussed the concept of neuroplasticity as the operating system of our nervous system computer. Without judgment, neuroplasticity can be of extreme usefulness, or it can produce, via sensitization, an "altered computer program" with devastating life effects of pain and suffering.

We have looked at the normal neuroplastic pain system for eudynia and what can go awry to result in maldynia, a disease. We have seen how neuroplasticity and sensitization can account for the good, the bad, and the ugly for pain transmission.

Although the mechanisms involved with neuroplastic sensitization of peripheral and central nervous components have been studied and continue to be researched, we still do not know which is the chicken or the egg. Exactly why this sensitization occurs, and who are the vulnerable people, is still a mystery. We do know that the brain can undergo neuroplastic reorganization from lower level (peripheral and spinal) changes or from higher level (mind) inputs. The system remains plastic throughout time and is responsive to inputs from any level.

However, successful treatment approaches all seem to be explained in terms of their effect on the neuroplastic changes (i.e., LTP that have happened). Successful treatments either seem to cause LTD, dampen the sensitized transmission of the disordered system, or cause new LTP that results in positive change rather than negative change.

Ultimately, however, the most significant changes appear to be related to those that occur in the brain. The brain has the ability to respond to the mind inputs and/or peripheral and spinal inputs. This input from above and below the brain can result in devastating negative changes in pain and suffering perception. However, effective treatment modalities seem to be those that can take advantage of the plastic nature of the brain to utilize those same higher and lower inputs to the brain to resolve and lessen pain and increase joy in life (see Chap. 70 on Pain as a Perceptual Experience for an extension of this topic).

References

1. Lippe P. An apologia in defense of pain medicine. Clin J Pain. 1998;14:189–90.
2. AMA Council on Science and Public Health Report 5. Maldynia: pathophysiology and non-pharmacologic treatment. 2010.
3. Arden J. Rewire your brain. New York: Wiley; 2010.
4. Schwartz J, Begley S. The mind and the brain: neuroplasticity and the power of mental force. New York: Harper Collins; 2002.
5. Doidge N. The brain that changes itself. New York: Penguin Group; 2007.
6. Voscopoulos C, Lema M. When does acute pain become chronic? Br J Anaesth. 2010;105 Suppl 1:169–85.
7. Apkarian A, Bushnell M, Treede R-D, Zubieta J. Human brain mechanisms of pain perception and regulation in health and disease. Eur J Pain. 2005;9:463–84.
8. Price D, Harkins S. The affective-motivational dimension of pain: a two-stage model. APS J. 1992;1:229–39.
9. Reichling DB, Levine JD. Critical role of nociceptor plasticity in chronic pain. Trends Neurosci. 2009;32(12):611–8.
10. Basbaum AI, Bautista DM, Scherrer G, Julius D. Cellular and molecular mechanisms of pain. Cell. 2009;139(2):267–84.

11. Descalzi G, Kim S, Zhuo M. Presynaptic and postsynaptic cortical mechanisms of chronic pain. Mol Neurobiol. 2009;40(3):253–9.

12. Treede RD. Highly localized inhibition of pain via long-term depression (LTD). Clin Neurophysiol. 2008;119(8):1703–4.

13. Hong CZ. New trends in myofascial pain syndrome. Zhonghua Yi Xue Za Zhi (Taipei). 2002;65(11):501–12.

14. Nielsen LA, Henriksson KG. Pathophysiological mechanisms in chronic musculoskeletal pain (fibromyalgia): the role of central and peripheral sensitization and pain disinhibition. Best Pract Res Clin Rheumatol. 2007;21(3):465–80.

15. Henrikssen KG. Hypersensitivity in muscle pain syndromes. Curr Pain Headache Rep. 2003;7(6):426–32.

16. Bendtsen L, Fernández-de-la-Peñas C. The role of muscles in tension-type headache. Curr Pain Headache Rep. 2011;15(6):451–8.

17. Fernández-Lao C, Cantarero-Villanueva I, Fernández-de-la-Peñas C, et al. Myofascial trigger points in neck and shoulder muscles and widespread pressure pain hypersensitivity in patients with postmastectomy pain: evidence of peripheral and central sensitization. Clin J Pain. 2010;26(9):798–806.

18. Ge HY, Fernández-de-la-Peñas C, Yue SW. Myofascial trigger points: spontaneous electrical activity and its consequences for pain induction and propagation. Chin Med. 2011;6:3.

19. Navarro X. Neural plasticity after nerve injury and regeneration. Int Rev Neurobiol. 2009;87:483–505.

20. Latremoliere A, Woolf CJ. Central sensitization: a generator of pain hypersensitivity by central neural plasticity. J Pain. 2009;10(9):895–926.

21. Kuner R. Central mechanisms of pathological pain. Nat Med. 2010;16(11):1258–66.

22. Park J, Luo ZD. Calcium channel functions in pain processing. Channels (Austin). 2010;4(6):510–7.

23. Tuchman M, Barrett JA, Donevan S, et al. Central sensitization and Ca(V)α₂δ ligands in chronic pain syndromes: pathologic processes and pharmacologic effect. J Pain. 2010;11(12):1241–9.

24. Palazzo E, Luongo L, de Novellis V, et al. Moving towards supraspinal TRPV1 receptors for chronic pain relief. Mol Pain. 2010;6:66.

25. Alter BJ, Gereau RW. Hotheaded: TRPV1 as mediator of hippocampal synaptic plasticity. Neuron. 2008;57(5):629–31.

26. Adedoyin MO, Vicini S, Neale JH. Endogenous N-acetylaspartylglutamate (NAAG) inhibits synaptic plasticity/transmission in the amygdala in a mouse inflammatory pain model. Mol Pain. 2010;6:60.

27. Larsson M, Broman J. Synaptic plasticity and pain: role of ionotropic glutamate receptors. Neuroscientist. 2011;17(3):256–73. Epub 2010 Apr 1. Review.

28. Zhou HY, Chen SR, Chen H, Pan HL. Functional plasticity of group II metabotropic glutamate receptors in regulation spinal excitatory and inhibitory synaptic input in neuropathic pain. J Pharmacol Exp Ther. 2011;336(1):254–64.

29. Liu XJ, Salter MW. Glutamate receptor phosphorylation and trafficking in pain plasticity in spinal cord dorsal horn. Eur J Neurosci. 2010;32(2):278–89.

30. Sanderson JL, Dell'Acqua ML. AKAP signaling complexes in regulation of excitatory synaptic plasticity. Neuroscientist. 2011;17(3):321–36. Epub 2011 Apr 15.

31. Li XY, Ko HG, Chen T, et al. Alleviating neuropathic pain hypersensitivity by inhibiting PKMzeta in the anterior cingulated cortex. Science. 2010;330(6009):1400–4.

32. Maneepak M, le Grand S, Srikiatkhachorn A. Serotonin depletion increases nociception-evoked trigeminal NMDA receptor phosphorylation. Headache. 2009;49(3):375–82.

33. Hald A. Spinal astrogliosis in pain models: cause and effects. Cell Mol Neurobiol. 2009;29(5):609–19.

34. Gwak YS, Hulsebosch CE. GABA and central neuropathic pain following spinal cord injury. Neuropharmacology. 2011;60(5):799–808.

35. Peng B, Lin JY, Shang Y, et al. Plasticity in the synaptic number associated with neuropathic pain in the rat spinal dorsal horn: a stereological study. Neurosci Lett. 2010;486(1):24–8.

36. Hjornevik T, Schoultz BW, Marton J, et al. Spinal long-term potentiation is associated with reduced opioid neurotransmission in the rat brain. Clin Physiol Funct Imaging. 2010;30(4):285–93.

37. Blanchard J, Chohan MO, Li B, et al. Beneficial effect of a CNTF tetrapeptide on adult hippocampal neurogenesis, neuronal plasticity, and spatial memory in mice. J Alzheimers Dis. 2010;21(4):1185–95.

38. Zhuo M. A synaptic model for pain: long-term potentiation in the anterior cingulate cortex. Mol Cells. 2007;23(3):259–71. Review.

39. Zhao XY, Liu MG, Yuan DL, et al. Nociception-induced spatial and temporal plasticity of synaptic connection and function in the hippocampal formation of rats: a multi-electrode array recording. Mol Pain. 2009;5:55.

40. Zhang L, Zhao ZQ. Plasticity changes of neuronal activities on central lateral nucleus by stimulation of the anterior cingulate cortex in rat. Brain Res Bull. 2010;81(6):574–8.

41. Maihöfner C. Neuropathic pain and neuroplasticity in functional imaging studies. Schmerz. 2010;24(2):137–45.

42. Teutsch S, Herken W, Bingel U, et al. Changes in brain gray matter due to repetitive painful stimulation. Neuroimage. 2008;42(2):845–9.

43. May A. Chronic pain may change the structure of the brain. Pain. 2008;137(1):7–15.

44. Ray A, Zbik A. Cognitive therapies and beyond. In: Tollison CD, editor. Practical pain management. 3rd ed. Philadelphia: Lippincott Williams and Wilkins; 2002. p. 189–208.

45. Gustin SM, Wrigley PJ, Siddall PJ, Henderson LA. Brain anatomy changes associated with persistent neuropathic pain following spinal cord injury. Cereb Cortex. 2010;20(6):1409–19.

46. Neugebauer V, Galhardo V, Maione S, Mackey SC. Forebrain pain mechanisms. Brain Res Rev. 2009;60(1):226–42.

47. Ji G, Sun H, Fu Y, et al. Cognitive impairment in pain through amygdala-driven prefrontal cortical deactivation. J Neurosci. 2010;30(15):5451–64.

48. Lovick TA, Devall AJ. Progesterone withdrawal-evoked plasticity of neural function in the female periaqueductal grey matter. Neural Plast. 2009;2009. doi:10.1155/2009/730902;730902. Epub 2008 Dec 2. Review.

49. Rome H, Rome J. Limbically augmented pain syndrome (LAPS): kindling, corticolimbic sensitization, and convergence of affective and sensory symptoms in chronic pain disorders. Pain Med. 2000;1(1):7–23.

50. Staud R, Spaeth M. Psychophysical and neurochemical abnormalities of pain processing in fibromyalgia. CNS Spectr. 2008;13(3 Suppl):12–7.

51. Schmidt-Wilcke T, Luerding R, Weigand T, et al. Striatal grey matter increase in patients suffering from fibromyalgia— a voxel-based morphometry study. Pain. 2007;132 Suppl 1:s109–16.

52. Haas L, Portela LV, Böhmer AE, et al. Increased plasma levels of brain derived neurotrophic factor (BDNF) in patients with fibromyalgia. Neurochem Res. 2010;35(5):830–4.

53. Cuadros J, Vargas M. A new mind-body approach for a total healing of fibromyalgia: a case report. Am J Clin Hypn. 2009;52(1):3–12.

54. Morris LD, Grimmer-Somers KA, Spottiswoode B, Louw QA. Virtual reality exposure therapy as a treatment for pain catastrophizing in fibromyalgia patients: proof-of-concept study (study protocol). BMC Musculoskelet Disord. 2011;12(1):85.

55. Sañudo B, Galliano D, Carrasco L, et al. Effects of prolonged exercise program on key health outcomes in women with fibromyalgia: a randomized controlled trial. J Rehabil Med. 2011;43(6):521–6.

56. Arcos-Carmona IM, Castro-Sánchez AM, Matarán-Peñarrocha GA, Gutiérrez-Rubio AB, Ramos-González E, Moreno-Lorenzo C. Effects of aerobic exercise program and relaxation techniques on anxiety, quality of sleep, depression, and quality of life in patients with fibromyalgia: a randomized controlled trial. Med Clin (Barc). 2011;137(9):398–401. doi:10.1016/j.medcli.2010.09.045. Epub 2011 Feb 22 [Article in Spanish].

57. Fontaine KR, Conn L, Clauw DJ. Effects of lifestyle physical activity in adults with fibromyalgia: results at follow-up. J Clin Rheumatol. 2011;17(2):64–8.

58. Weeks SR, Anderson-Barnes VC, Tsao JW. Phantom limb pain: theories and therapies. Neurologist. 2010;16(5):277–86.

59. Flor H. Maladaptive plasticity, memory for pain and phantom limb pain: review and suggestions for new therapies. Expert Rev Neurother. 2008;8(5):809–18.

60. Sumitani M, Miyauchi S, Uematsu H, et al. Phantom limb pain originates from dysfunction of the primary motor cortex. Masui. 2010;59(11):1364–9.

61. MacIver K, Lloyd DM, Kelly S, et al. Phantom limb pain, cortical reorganization and the therapeutic effect of mental imagery. Brain. 2008;131(Pt 8):2181–91.

62. Shapiro F. Eye movement desensitization and reprocessing. New York: Guilford; 1995.

63. Schneider J, Hofmann A, Rost C, Shapiro F. EMDR in the treatment of chronic phantom limb pain. Pain Med. 2008;9(1):76–82.

64. Nickel FT, Maihöfner C. Current concepts in pathophysiology of CRPS I. Handchir Mikrochir Plast Chir. 2010;42(1):8–14.

65. Bie B, Brown DL, Naguib M. Increased synaptic Glur1 subunits in the anterior cingulated cortex of rats with peripheral inflammation. Eur J Pharmacol. 2011;653(1–3):26–31.

66. Christianson JA, Bielefeldt K, Altier C, et al. Development, plasticity and modulations of visceral afferents. Brain Res Rev. 2009;60(1):171–86.

67. Ceyhan GO, Demir IE, Maak M, Friess H. Fate of nerves in chronic pancreatitis: neural remodeling and pancreatic neuropathy. Best Pract Res Clin Gastroenterol. 2010;24(3):311–22.

68. Demir IE, Tieftrunk E, Maak M, et al. Pain mechanisms in chronic pancreatitis: of a master and his fire. Langenbecks Arch Surg. 2011;396(2):151–60.

69. Silberstein S, et al. Neuropsychiatric aspects of primary headache disorders. In: Yudofsky S, Hales R, editors. Textbook of neuropsychiatry. 3rd ed. Washington DC: Amer Psychiatric Press; 1997. p. 381–412.

70. Tajti J, Vécsei L. The mechanism of peripheral and central sensitization in migraine. A literature revie. Neuropsychopharmacol Hung. 2009;11(1):15–21.

71. Obermann M, Nebel K, Schumann C, et al. Gray matter changes related to chronic posttraumatic headache. Neurology. 2009;73(12):978–83.

72. Nau C. Pathophysiology of chronic postoperative pain. Anasthesiol Intensivmed Notfallmed Schmerzther. 2010;45(7–8):480–6.

73. Schnabel A, Pogatzki-Zahn E. Predictors of chronic pain following surgery. What do we know? Schmerz. 2010;24(5):517–31.

74. Chauvin M. Chronic pain after surgery. Presse Med. 2009;38(11):1613–20.

75. Berger JV, Knaepen L, Janssen SP, et al. Cellular and molecular insights into neuropathy-induced pain hypersensitivity for mechanism-based treatment approaches. Brain Res Rev. 2011;67(1-2):282–310.

76. Engineer ND, Riley JR, Seale JD, et al. Reversing pathological neural activity using targeted plasticity. Nature. 2011;470(7332):101–4.

77. Tsao H, Galea MO, Hodges PW. Driving plasticity on the motor cortex in recurrent low back pain. Eur J Pain. 2010;14(8):832–9.

78. Boudreu SA, Farina D, Falla D. The role of motor learning and neuroplasticity in designing rehabilitation approaches for musculoskeletal pain disorders. Man Ther. 2010;15(5):410–4.

79. Chipchase LS, Schabrun SM, Hodges PW. Peripheral electrical stimulation to induce cortical plasticity: as systematic review of stimulus parameters. Clin Neurophysiol. 2011;122(3):456–63.

80. Rottmann S, Jung K, Vohn R, Ellrich J. Long-term depression of pain-related cerebral activation in healthy man: an fMRI study. Eur J Pain. 2010;14(6):615–24.

81. Zhao HY, Mu P, Dong Y. The pathological neural plasticity and its applications in acupuncture. Zhen Ci Yan Jiu. 2008;33(1):41–6.

82. Flor H, Diers M. Sensorimotor training and cortical reorganization. NeuroRehabilitation. 2009;25(1):19–27.

83. Ramachandran VS, Altschuler EL. The use of visual feedback, in particular mirror visual feedback, in restoring brain function. Brain. 2009;132(Pt 7):1693–710.

84. Taylor HH, Murphy B. Altered central integration of dual somatosensory input after cervical spine manipulation. J Manipulative Physiol Ther. 2010;33(3):178–88.

85. Di Lazzaro V, Dileone M, Profice P, et al. Associative motor cortex plasticity: direct evidence in humans. Cereb Cortex. 2009;19(10):2326–30.

86. Di Lazzaro V, Dileone M, Profice P, et al. LTD-like plasticity induced by paired associative stimulation: direct evidence in humans. Exp Brain Res. 2009;194(4):661–4.

87. Fontán-Lozano A, López-Lluch G, Delgado-Garcia JM, et al. Molecular bases of caloric restriction regulation of neuronal synaptic plasticity. Mol Neurobiol. 2008;38(2):167–77.

88. Lahmann C, Henningsen P, Noll-Hussong M. Somatoform pain disorder-overview. Psychiatr Danub. 2010;22(3):453–8.

89. Hay L. You can heal your life. Carlsbad: Hay House; 1999.

90. Satinover J. The quantum brain. New York: Wiley; 2001.

91. Hawkins D. Power vs Force. New York: Hay House; 2002.

92. Hawkins D. Healing and recovery. Sedona: Veritas Publishing; 2009.

Muscle Pain Treatment

Norman Marcus and Jason Ough

Key Points

- Muscle pain: history and nomenclature
- Assessment of the community standard of care for muscle pain
- Epidemiology
- Pathophysiology: muscle nociceptors, clinical mediators
- Peripheral and central sensitization and conditioned pain modulation—the mechanisms of chronicity and referred pain patterns
- Trigger points
- History, physical examination, and treatments
- Atypical muscle pain presentations
- Future directions

The greatest enemy of knowledge is not ignorance…it is the illusion of knowledge

—Stephen Hawking

Introduction

Muscles represent approximately 40 to 50 % of the body by weight yet are generally absent from our evaluation and treatment protocols for common pain syndromes. This chapter will provide a brief background on the history of the understanding of muscle pain, its epidemiology and pathophysiology,

N. Marcus, M.D. (✉)
Division of Muscle Pain Research, Departments of Anesthesiology and Psychiatry, New York University Langone School of Medicine, 30 East 40th Street, New York 10016, NY, USA
e-mail: njm@nmpi.com

J. Ough, M.D.
Department of Pain Management/Anesthesiology, New York University Langone Medical Center,
317 E. 34th Street, Suite 902, New York 10016, NY, USA
e-mail: jkough@gmail.com

problems in implementing a universally accepted approach to its diagnosis and treatment, and a suggested protocol for the inclusion of muscle evaluation and treatment in all instances of subacute and chronic pain presentations.

Background and Historical Perspectives

Muscle pain and tenderness interfering with physical function has been observed for centuries. However, its etiology has been elusive. The understanding of pain mechanisms in general has been helped from experiments on cutaneous pain fibers and our understanding of obvious neuronal pathways. For example, we know that damage to skin will start a cascade of neurochemical events that results in stimulation of cells in the dorsal horn of the spinal cord and possibly goes on to be consciously experienced as a generally unpleasant sensation. Likewise, we recognize that compression of a spinal nerve can produce pain in the distribution of that nerve. However, medical training has generally not shown us how mechanisms in muscles can generate local pain, which in turn may refer pain to adjacent and distant regions. Muscle nociceptors actually excite spinal cord neurons more than cutaneous nociceptors [1].

A review of comprehensive pain treatment textbooks [2–5] finds no chapters dealing with muscle pain aside from sections on "myofascial pain syndrome" discussing "trigger points" as the defining characteristic of syndromes with painful muscles.

A fundamental problem in discussing and understanding clinical muscle pain is the lack of agreed terminology to describe clinical findings. To better appreciate this obstacle, the history of muscle pain should be reviewed.

The same confusion encountered today is found as early as the sixteenth century when Guillaume de Baillou first referred to a clinical entity, *muscular rheumatism*, while describing diffuse soft tissue pain [6]. Other clinicians subsequently offered their explanations, inventing new terms along the way. In the nineteenth century, many believed that muscle pains were a disease of the muscle itself (a "serous exudative process") [7]. Tender nodules were thought to be a clinical manifestation of this disease and were first reported during this period. In 1919, Schade also observed muscle nodules and coined the term *myogelosen* (muscle gelling), and in 1921, Max Lange used the term *muskelhärten*, meaning hardened muscle [8]. Various other authors referred to some type of muscular or fibrous inflammation and used terms such as *fibrositis* and *myofibrositis*, but with the absence of clear signs of inflammation, these terms eventually lost favor. The debate on the importance of tender nodules in muscles, which began at the turn of the last century [7], continues [9], with some authors denying their importance and observing their presence in patients who are otherwise without pain complaints [10].

Muscle Pain Referral Patterns

A distinct aspect of painful muscles is the referring of pain to adjacent and distant muscles. Pioneering work regarding muscle pain and referral patterns was conducted in the 1930s when Jonas Kellgren, a student in the laboratory of Sir Thomas Lewis, performed experiments on approximately 1,000 patients over a 3-year period [11–13]. Kellgren's initial groundbreaking observations showed that muscle can refer pain to another region, and preclinical studies since the 1970s have demonstrated that the mechanisms of referred pain and windup are related to peripheral sensitization of muscle nociceptors and central sensitization of spinal cord neurons [14, 15].

The term "trigger points" was introduced in the literature as early as 1921 [16], elaborated on by Lange in 1931 [17], and in 1940, first used by Steindler [18] to describe tender areas in muscles that referred pain to other muscles. It was Janet Travell (and later, with David Simons), however, who popularized its use when she published papers describing the treatment of trigger points with injection of local anesthetic [19] and in the 1950s also popularized the term myofascial pain syndrome [20]. Travell and Simons played an important role in teaching colleagues about the presence of trigger points and typical patterns of referred pain from specific muscles [21]. Although myofascial pain syndrome (MPS) refers generically to pain from muscle and connective tissue, it is frequently used to infer that the muscle pain is the result of trigger points (TrPs) and tender points, contributing to the conceptual distortion that all muscle pain is from TrPs or tender points. A noteworthy episode in the muscle pain saga is the contrasting treatment approaches of Janet Travell and Hans Kraus who both treated President John F. Kennedy [22] for his low back pain. When Kennedy had been unable to walk without pain for months, trigger point injections were ineffective. Providing exercises addressing his weakness, stiffness, and tension resulted in pain reduction and restoration of function. Dr. Kraus shared with the senior author (NM) (1995) that JFK was planning to establish a national back pain institute so that his own experience of success and failure with various interventions could be studied. Following the death of Kennedy, two phenomena would interfere with the acceptance of muscles as a legitimate area of interest for pain-treating clinicians: (1) muscle pain treatment overemphasizing TrPs became the world community standard rather than a comprehensive muscle evaluation and treatment approach, thus laying the foundation for the overemphasis of trigger points as the sole area of interest in clinical muscle pain, and (2) the introduction of sophisticated imaging (e.g., CT scans, MRI) allowed clinicians to believe that the source of pain could be visualized, minimizing the importance of the physical examination [22] and relegating it frequently to a perfunctory ritual.

Chronic Widespread Pain (CWP) and Fibromyalgia Syndrome (FMS)

A subset of patients with muscle pain has diffuse pain and tenderness. The cause of widespread pains has been debated. Is the origin in the soft tissues in the periphery or in the central nervous system? Smythe and Moldofsky reintroduced the term fibrositis to describe patients with widespread pain and later renamed it fibromyalgia syndrome (FMS), when they described a collection of symptoms that included persistent widespread pain, fatigue, nonrestorative sleep, and multiple tender points at specific locations in the body [23, 24]. FMS was originally thought to be related to peripheral muscle pain generators [25], but research suggesting central dysregulation [26] as the cause has moved the entire field toward the concept that FMS is a CNS phenomenon typified by lowered thresholds to painful stimuli, accounting for the muscle pain. Peripheral pain generators have been recently reintroduced as important causes of FMS [27–30].

Psychogenic Muscle Pain

The debate over central versus peripheral origins of muscle pain includes the concept that in patients with widespread regional pain, the underlying problem may be psychiatric (*psychogenic rheumatism*) [31]. The concept of psychiatric/psychological etiologies of muscle-related pain may not properly distinguish neurophysiological effects of emotion on brain function from psychodynamic aspects of pain initiation and perpetuation. Chronic pain patients will frequently report that their pain is increased when they experience stressful events or feelings. Psychological factors producing specific physiological changes, including muscle tension patterns, have been described [32–34]. Denial or repression of uncomfortable feelings appears to be an important aspect in perpetuating pain in some patients with chronic pain syndromes [35]. Kasamatsu showed how CNS adaptation to interrupting stimuli could easily block out (deny) the presence of the stimulus in novices but not in seasoned meditaters, and Asendorpf demonstrated the deleterious physiological effects of denial of affect [36, 37]. The effectiveness of various psychological interventions associated with enhancing the patient's capacity to tolerate uncomfortable thoughts and feelings may operate in part by reducing or eliminating sustained muscle tension patterns, relieving discomfort in chronic muscular-related pain syndromes [38–43]. The reduction in pain will produce decreased emotional discomfort; decreased emotional discomfort will decrease the perception of pain [44, 45].

Present Terminology

The term myofascial pain syndrome is used in lieu of muscle pain in most articles and textbooks on chronic pain, and multiple theories have been offered to explain myofascial pain syndromes [46–56]. The resultant confusion in the literature prevents the creation of universally accepted approaches to study painful muscles.

Review of Muscle Pain in the Literature

According to the core curriculum of the International Association for the Study of Pain, myofascial pain is defined as pain emanating from muscle and connective tissue that causes pain in common clinical regional pain syndromes and "lacks reliable means [for physicians] to identify, categorize, and treat such pain" [57, 58]. Studies of clinicians attempting to identify painful muscles demonstrate poor inter-rater reliability in the identification of myofascial trigger points [59–64]. Clinicians will frequently and mistakenly use the terms "myofascial trigger point" and "myofascial pain" interchangeably. Myofascial trigger points are only one possible source of myofascial pain. Muscle and other soft tissue pain are thought to be responsible for most acute back pain [91] and yet muscle pain evaluation and treatment are absent in low back treatment guidelines [66]. Failure to agree on nomenclature and methods of evaluation and treatment and the absence of valid RCTs to provide evidence of effective-

ness of specific treatment approaches, has contributed to the rejection of trigger point injections (TPIs) and sclerosant injections as recommended treatment options for low back pain [67]. Ignoring muscle facilitates an overemphasis on structural abnormalities demonstrated on imaging and not necessarily identifying the true source of the patient's pain. Subsequent inappropriate treatments contribute to the $86 billion spent in 2005 on neck and back pain in the United States [68].

Possible Etiologies of Myofascial Pain Are Not Fully Recognized by Clinicians

Myofascial pain can be caused by various etiologies. However, the current community standard of establishing the diagnosis is limited to palpating the putative muscle causing regional pain and identifying any TrPs. The standard treatment is to give TPIs to the putative muscle, injecting into a discrete area that includes only the TrPs and associated taut bands. The evaluation of TrPs without a complete assessment of muscle conditioning contributes to unexplainable variability in treatment outcomes because diagnoses are confounded when clinicians fail to consider weakness, stiffness, spasm, or tension as a primary source of pain [69]. Therefore, even if the putative muscle is correctly identified and injection is effective, failure to acknowledge and/or appropriately treat pain from these other causes of myofascial pain may leave the patient with persistent discomfort, and clinically unchanged.

Limits of Palpation as a Diagnostic Tool

Palpation alone used to detect areas of muscle pain introduces two confounding variables. First, varying amounts of pressure may be applied, diminishing the reliability of the examination. Pressure-recording devices have been introduced to determine more accurately the amount of applied pressure necessary to elicit discomfort in the patient [70, 71]. However, the accuracy of these devices is compromised because examiner preconceptions have been reported to influence the assessment [72]. Second, palpation to elicit a subjective experience of pain is often performed in a sedentary muscle. Most functional muscle pain is experienced with muscle activity versus rest. Therefore, an examination of a resting muscle is likely to be less accurate in determining the source of the muscle pain, frequently identifying a referred pain pattern, compared with an examination utilizing movement of discrete muscles [73, 74].

Two technologies to image muscles thought to harbor taut bands and TrPs have been suggested as possible means to more objectively identify the presence of pain-generating structures. Magnetic resonance elastography (MRE) allows visualization and identification of tissues with varied elasticity and has been shown to be reliable than palpation in identifying taut bands [75]. Visualization of TrPs is more elusive, but recent studies have demonstrated the use of ultrasound in identifying TrPs [76, 77]. Both of these techniques may help to objectify the identification of taut bands and TrPs but have not yet been clinically tested to determine if they will improve the effectiveness of treatment for muscle pain.

Injection Techniques

The description of TPIs and the assessment of their effectiveness in the literature has great variability. At least one published study used the return of 75 % of the pre-injection pain as a measure of success in studying TPIs using different injectates [78], and other studies have commented on the need to reinject TrPs [79, 80].

Other studies address the specific number of trigger points in a muscle [81], the importance of eliciting a "twitch response" [79] or of thoroughly injecting the "taut band" [82]. We suggest an approach modeled on that of Kraus who had originally thought that injecting TrPs when present could successfully diminish or eliminate muscle pain. Kraus observed that many of his patients treated with TPIs would frequently return with the need for reinjection in the same muscle. He speculated that as the muscle-tendon and bone-tendon attachments had the least blood supply versus the muscle tissue, these areas might also be the source of the recurrent pain pattern, and therefore modified his injection technique so that it always included the origin and the insertion of the identified painful muscle. Gibson et al. [83] has reported that the tendon-bone junction is more sensitive and susceptible to sensitization by hypertonic saline than muscle tissue. This observation would support our clinical impression of the importance of the tendon-bone junction in the course of muscle needling [84].

Exercise

Exercise is defined as a "series of movements to promote good physical health." Therefore almost any activity can be defined as an exercise protocol, thus accounting for the wide variety of outcomes achieved through "exercise" [85]. The existing protocols for MPS (and for diagnoses of regional pain that are relied upon to support the use of prolotherapy) usually include some general prescription for "exercise." The utility of exercise

in the treatment paradigm makes sense, and a systematic review has concluded that a variety of nonspecific exercises has produced long-term results in NSLBP patients [86, 87]. A problem in the exercise literature is the general absence of subgroups of patients [88] based on psychosocial variables and specific assessments for level of conditioning (strength and flexibility). Trigger point injection therapy and prolotherapy protocols suggest the generic use of exercise following injections [89]. Idiosyncratic provision of exercise protocols without patient subclassification may confound outcome data and eliminate the possibility of valid systematic review or meta-analysis.

Statistically significant effects of exercise in pain populations may not reflect clinical significance. Van Tulder et al. [85] found that of 43 Cochrane-reviewed trials on exercise for the treatment of low back pain, 18 of the trials reported a positive response, but only four showed any statistically significant reduction of pain. We believe that the absence of specific goals based in part on the results of specific muscle testing which could provide subclassification of patients, along with the nonspecific nature of the exercise protocols administered in conjunction with muscle injections, contributes to the inconsistent outcomes, even when apparently similar injection techniques are used.

Epidemiology

Difficulty in Obtaining Accurate Survey Data

The search for the incidence of muscular pain leads to a confusing array of concepts. Musculoskeletal pain is an umbrella term that describes pain originating in bones, joints, and muscles. Low back, neck, and shoulder pains are frequently thought to be caused by soft tissue [90]. Chronic widespread pain and fibromyalgia may have peripheral muscle pain generators contributing to the pain presentation.

Therefore, the interpretation of incidence and prevalence data for muscle-related pain is confounded. In addition, patients diagnosed with other comorbidities may indeed have muscles as the source of their pain but may be excluded from survey data. Indeed, it is the premise of this chapter that muscles are an overlooked contributing etiology of many common pain syndromes which are incorrectly attributed to only nonmuscular causes.

Low back pain is an example of the difficulty encountered. The most frequent diagnosis for low back pain in an ambulatory setting is nonspecific or idiopathic low back pain, generally referred to as sprains or strains of soft tissue, and represents 70–80 % of patients seen in large-scale studies [91], yet soft tissue-/muscle-generated pain is a small percentage (which has been diminishing over time) of all causes in a large national study [68].

Prevalence and Incidence of Musculoskeletal Low Back and Shoulder Pain

Adolescent Data

Musculoskeletal pain is frequently experienced in adolescence. Multinational surveys report lifetime prevalence rates of approximately 50 % when patients are queried on their past experience of low back pain, chronic widespread pain (CWP), fibromyalgia, shoulder or musculoskeletal pain with similar rates for prospective studies lasting 1–5 years [92]. When pain occurs at more than one site and at least once a week, there is a significant reduction in health-related quality of life scores [93]. A 2009 European study reported a 1-month period prevalence of LBP of nearly 40 % in adolescents [94].

Adult Data

According to the 2008 National Health Interview Survey report, 27 % of adults reported low back pain in the preceding 3 months and 14 % reported neck pain [95]. A 2009 study demonstrated a rising prevalence of chronic LBP across all age groups over a 14-year period [96]. The lifetime prevalence of chronic LBP in the UK general population is estimated to be 6.3–11.1 % [97].

In 2008, The Bone and Joint Decade 2000–2010 Task Force on Neck Pain and Its Associated Disorders reported the 12-month prevalence of neck pain was 30–50 % [98]. The 1-month period prevalence of shoulder pain is between 20 and 33 % [99].

Data for CWP (US and UK) shows 10–11 % point prevalence with females affected 1.5 times more often than males [100–102]. The same data shows 0.5–4 % point prevalence for FMS, with females affected 10 times more often than males. Lawrence et al. in 2008 estimated that approximately five million American adults over 18 years of age have primary fibromyalgia (this data was extrapolated from Wolfe's Wichita survey in 1993 and another from London, Ontario) [103]. Another study in 2009 reported that chronic widespread pain had a lifetime prevalence of 5–10 % of the general population [104].

Data also show that patients with FMS may have a history of work-related neck and shoulder pain, whiplash, low back pain, and muscle tension [105, 106], and therefore, the authors believe that many of these patients have undetected and potentially treatable muscles as a source of pain.

No matter how the data is analyzed, muscles appear to be a significant source of pain in a wide range of diagnoses and age groups.

Pain in Cancer Patients

Ten percent of patients diagnosed with cancer have pain unrelated to their disease, and it is generally related to muscles and connective tissue [107] and often overlooked in practice [108].

Pathophysiology and Scientific Foundations

Much of the preclinical data in the literature on the pathophysiology of muscle pain is based on animal studies, and therefore much of our knowledge in humans is extrapolative. This section can only provide a limited introduction to the existence of known mechanisms that account for the presence of pain originating in muscles. Therefore, the reader is encouraged to refer directly to source material on muscle pain and at least review the 2009 IASP textbook, *Fundamentals of Musculoskeletal Pain*, edited by Arendt-Nielsen, Graven-Nielsen, and Mense, and *Muscle Pain: Understanding the Mechanisms,* edited by Mense and Gerwin.

Neurologic Mechanisms of Pain Originating in Muscle

Morphology of Muscle Nociceptors

The structure typically mediating muscle pain is free nerve endings that have a high mechanical threshold in the noxious range/and or respond to pain producing chemicals [109]. Whereas cutaneous pain is localized to an injury site, muscle pain tends to be diffuse, based on the fact that muscle nociceptors have a larger receptor field and lower innervation densities [14].

Neuropeptide Content of Nociceptors

Dorsal root ganglion cells projecting into muscle contain substance P, calcitonin gene-related peptide, and somatostatin, which may be released when nociceptors are sensitized, causing further stimulation of the nociceptor.

Functional Types of Muscle Nociceptors

There are three types of muscle nociceptors:
1. High-threshold mechanoreceptors, activated by tissue-threatening mechanical stimuli, which allow the organism to respond to threats of damage as well as actual damage.
2. Chemonociceptors which respond to algesic substances but not to mechanical stimuli. For example, a receptor would respond to ischemic contraction of the muscle but not normal contraction.
3. Polymodal nociceptors which respond to both mechanical and chemical stimuli.

Nociceptors Are Equipped with Specific Molecular Receptors for Various Ligands

Inflammatory Chemical Mediators

These particular nociceptors may respond to a variety of chemical mediators, including inflammatory mediators released by damaged muscle tissue (bradykinin, serotonin, and prostaglandin E2).

Proton Receptors

These receptors respond to lowered pH (e.g., due to exhausting muscle work), which excites acid-sensing ion channels. With aggressive work or exercise, the pH may be less than 5.0 and in extreme conditions as low as 4.0 with resultant severe pain [110].

Vanilloid receptors are specific for capsaicin and are also sensitive to protons and heat.

Purinergic receptors bind ATP and its metabolites.

Excitatory amino acid receptors bind glutamate.

Nerve growth factor (NGF) exclusively excites high-threshold mechanoreceptors. Mense cautions that since multiple mediators are present at the same time, it is not possible to determine which are key mediators since there are important synergies among them [111].

Pathophysiological Mechanisms That Produce Spread of Muscle Pain

Nerve Growth Factor (NGF)

Experimental evidence suggests that NGF may be important in the production of certain chronic muscle pain syndromes, such as work-related musculoskeletal pain. NGF, released by a repetitively used inflamed muscle, may painlessly sensitize spinal neurons and ultimately lead to chronic muscle pain [110, 112, 113].

Peripheral Sensitization

Nociceptors in muscles become sensitized following a variety of events such as repetitive strain (overuse), direct trauma, and ischemia. These events all produce sensitization of type III and IV nerve fibers through stimulation of the aforementioned receptors, which lowers the stimulation threshold for pain, with resultant tenderness (hyperalgesia) and pain with movement (muscle allodynia) [114]. Axonal reflexes will then excite previously uninvolved branches of the same nerve (that were not directly stimulated by the tissue damage), with a spread of sensitization so that adjacent areas will also be experienced as tender.

Central Sensitization

Central sensitization may also result in muscle allodynia and hyperalgesia. Mense and his colleagues have shown that experimental inflammation in the leg muscles of rats produced three observable changes in the excitability of dorsal horn neurons [115]:

1. An increase in the spontaneous activity of the dorsal horn neurons.
2. An increase in the response of neurons in spinal segments L4 and L5 (the segments to which gastrocnemius/soleus (GS) muscle afferents travel for the rat; in human L5–S1) to mechanical stimulation of the GS. If there is persistent stimulation of the GS, neuroplastic changes will occur in the dorsal horn.
3. Excitation of adjacent spinal segments that are not usually stimulated by the GS.

Previously ineffective connections that become effective in pathological conditions may become opened, leading to a larger number of neurons being excited in response to an input which was previously nonexciting. The clinical significance of these changes is seen in the development of pain with movement of a sensitized muscle (muscle allodynia) and exaggerated pain (hyperalgesia) with painful stimuli. In addition, the opening of previously unaffected channels connected to adjacent spinal segments may be another mechanism of referred pain often seen in muscle pain syndromes. Central sensitization should not be confused with windup—although they have similarities in transmitters and neuronal pathways responsible for the heightened responsiveness to stimuli, they are not identical. Windup does not persist for a long time after stimulation unlike central sensitization, which can be long lasting [15].

Clinical Significance of Conditioned Pain Modulation (CPM) - formerly known as Diffuse Noxious Inhibitory Control, in the Treatment of Muscle Pain Syndromes and in the Relationship of FMS to Regional Muscle Pain

Central sensitization is known to be a normal event in acute pain [116], but it becomes pathologic when it is long standing or permanent. There is now ample evidence for central sensitization in fibromyalgia [117]. However, there have been differing schools of thought on the role peripheral generators play in the maintenance and development of central sensitization in a chronic pain syndrome such as fibromyalgia. While some scholars focus on the lack of direct evidence of peripheral input as proof that there is no true muscular pathology in FMS, others believe that peripheral generators should be considered the primary cause of pain in FMS unless proven otherwise [25, 116]. In a 2006 review article,

Vierck offers several examples of possible muscle pathology supporting a peripheral generator theory, including red, ragged fibers on muscle biopsy, constricting band-like structures, mitochondrial abnormalities, metabolic changes, and vascular effects [25]. In further support of the idea that FMS can develop from a local or peripheral source, Arendt Nielsen points out that most patients diagnosed with fibromyalgia initially present with localized or regional pain, which subsequently leads to chronic, widespread pain [116].

It is already understood that in certain diseases, continuous peripheral input maintains central sensitization, resulting in painful conditions such as hyperalgesia and allodynia [118]. Studies have been done which continue to support the idea of peripheral generators playing a significant role in central sensitization in fibromyalgia. A randomized, double-blind, placebo-controlled study by Staud and others in 2009 showed that lidocaine injections into the trapezius muscle increased local pain thresholds and, in cases of FM, decreased remote secondary heat hyperalgesia [118]. Ignoring potential primary afferent mechanisms may lead to the mistaken impression that all FMS patients have a chronic intractable condition and deprive those with treatable peripheral pain generators the chance to eliminate an actual pain source and avoid the prolonged administration of serotonin/norepinephrine reuptake inhibitors or anticonvulsants.

Loss of centrally mediated inhibitory pain modulation is a proposed mechanism of pain in fibromyalgia. Two mechanisms have been discussed: (1) Fields and Basbaum described a tonic descending inhibitory mechanism that when impaired decreases pain thresholds and may be associated with the pain seen in FMS [119]. (2) In experiments performed on healthy controls, normally functioning central pain inhibitory mechanisms were demonstrated when a secondary tonic stimulation reduced brief episodes of experimentally induced pain. This pain modulation, referred to as diffuse noxious inhibitory control (DNIC) and recently renamed conditioned pain modulation (CPM) [120], was not observed in patients with FMS, and there is evidence suggesting that this mechanism is impaired or deficient in a chronic pain state such as FMS [121, 122]. The functional role of CPM is still unclear, but it is possible that lack of CPM may play a role in central sensitization itself and may further be involved in the transformation of acute pain to chronic pain [122].

Observations by the senior author (NM) suggest that both central sensitization and CPM may be evident in the course of treatment of patients with multiple painful muscles requiring needling. Approximately 20 % of muscles identified in the initial consultation of patients with pain duration of more than 1 year and with more than five muscles identified as sources of regional pain were found not to be present in the course of ongoing muscle injections [57]. Conversely, muscles that did not test positive on the initial consultation sometimes would become painful over the course of injections, reflecting the belief of NM that this may be a function of CPM, i.e., when the most painful area is eliminated, a less painful area can be identified. Based on these observations, after the first muscle is injected, a reevaluation should be performed prior to each additional muscle injection.

Prolonged inactivity results in weakness and stiffness and diminished endurance, all contributing to the overall pain experience in FMS. A recent Cochrane review of exercise in FMS concluded that exercise was effective as related in part to improved muscle conditioning rather than decreased pain or tender points [123]. Another small study by E. Ortega et al. [124] suggests that exercise reduces inflammation as measured by inflammatory markers in FMS.

Trigger Points (TrPs) or Myofascial Trigger Points

Trigger points are tender nodular spots in muscles that are frequently associated with a taut band of muscle fibers and when palpated will frequently radiate pain to a distant site. Laboratory studies have found evidence of dysfunctional neuromuscular end plates [55], and recent studies have reported alteration in the biochemical milieu of the TrPs [125]. Although numerous articles have been written on the evaluation and treatment of trigger points, there is diminishing interest in their importance and even disbelief in the construct [9] based in part on the inconsistency of evaluation and treatment methodology and relative transient relief of pain following injection of TrPs. It does appear that TrPs are important sources of localized and diffuse [126, 127] muscle pain [10], but the lack of agreed nomenclature and treatment approaches has rendered the available clinical literature unusable for meta-analyses, systematic reviews, and inclusion as a validated approach [128] in published guidelines for common pain syndromes such as low back pain [129]. Altered muscle tissue is not only present in TrPs in the belly of the muscle but has been noted by Simons et al. [130] as occurring in the muscle attachments as well. The typical examination using palpation will frequently miss these areas of tenderness especially in deep muscles. NM has used electrical stimulation to contract discreet muscles. When a muscle is painful to stimulation, in contrast to surrounding muscles that are nonpainful to stimulation, it is considered a putative source of pain in that region of the body. An important aspect of the examination is the production of pain along the entire course of a suspected muscle, from origin to insertion, in order to unambiguously identify that muscle as a source of pain.

Peripheral Nerve Entrapments

Muscle spasm, either in the entirety of the muscle or in a small region, may result in compression of an adjacent nerve (e.g., the piriformis muscle compressing the sciatic nerve). Kopell and Thompson [131] report on the "fall from grace" of the diagnosis of the "piriformis syndrome," which had been an important explanation for sciatic pain in the mid-twentieth century, because surgical sectioning of the muscle to release the sciatic nerve was often unsuccessful, but the practice of sectioning the piriformis muscle persists [132, 133]. The piriformis syndrome is an important consideration in the differential diagnosis of apparent lumbosacral radicular pains, and proper identification and nonsurgical treatment of a painful piriformis muscle may result in sciatic pain relief. Other referral patterns of pain associated with peripheral entrapment neuropathies are reported [131] and in the author's opinion are important sources of apparent "radicular" patterns of pain.

Impediments to Creating a Reliable, Valid Muscle Pain Protocol

General absence of education in medical school and postgraduate training of the published basic science mechanisms of muscle pain has lead to the perpetuation of the belief that muscle pain is only a response to problems in the spine or the CNS [9]. Functional muscle pain from tension, weakness, stiffness, and spasm should be part of the standard assessment leading to specific diagnosis-driven treatments of patients presenting with regional pain syndromes. Absence of these functional pain categories leads to overdiagnosis and treatment of trigger points and the ensuing suboptimal results.

The Need for a Protocol That Recognizes and Incorporates Muscle Pain and Physical Function into the Evaluation and Treatment of Common Pain Syndromes

We have an obligation to come together as a discipline and attempt to formulate testable protocols that could facilitate reasonably equivalent data collection. This could lead to valid meta-analyses and systematic reviews of the evaluation and treatment of muscles as a source of pain in a variety of chronic pain syndromes. In this spirit, the authors present the following protocol for consideration as a comprehensive model of evaluation and treatment for all persistent pain presentations to facilitate the study of muscle as a putative source of pain.

History

When taking a patient's history, clinicians should always inquire about the presence and duration of any muscle tenderness. Pre- and posttreatment use of a self-administered test instrument for assessment of pain and its effect on daily function, such as the Brief Pain Inventory [134], is encouraged. The history should gather appropriate data to establish possible habits, postures, and activities that could contribute to and perpetuate muscle dysfunction and pain. For example, patients can be asked if pain is worsened with prolonged positioning (such as sitting or standing in one place for too long), or if movements such as walking diminish pain, which suggests that a muscle pain component is present. For headaches or pain in the upper body, neck or shoulder, some common habits may contribute to the perpetuation and exacerbation of pain: (A) reading or watching TV in bed (causing a stiffening isometric contraction of the muscles of the shoulder and neck), (B) typing with a keyboard placed too high (causing a nonergonomic elbow bend of less than 90°), (C) not positioning a computer monitor straight ahead and at eye level or slightly below and not using a telephone head set to avoid isometric contraction of the neck and shoulder muscles.

Physical Exam

The physical examination should contain a method to establish whether or not the patient has an acceptable minimal level of strength and flexibility in the upper and/or lower body. The Kraus-Weber (KW) (see Fig. 72.1) test is proposed for key trunk muscle strength and flexibility. An examination for neck and shoulder range of movement, a neurological examination, and palpation for muscle tenderness and resilience are all suggested evaluation tools. If available, an evaluation with an electrical instrument to stimulate specific muscles (NM uses the MPDD [SPOC, Inc. Stamford, CT]) to locate those producing pain is also recommended. The MPDD is thought to work by contracting a specific muscle, which stimulates nociceptors in (1) the muscle attachments and (2) in the muscle belly in trigger points when deformed by the muscle contraction. In the practice of NM, palpation for tenderness and resilience is performed to identify presumptive sources of muscle pain, but the diagnosis of muscle pain amenable to injection (MPAI) is only made with the MPDD. For MPAI to be diagnosed in a muscle, the entire course of the muscle from origin to insertion must be experienced as painful (tender, aching, or sore) during the stimulation. Sustained pain produced by MPDD in only a portion of the muscle suggests that another muscle is the true source of the pain.

In the absence of an electrical device to identify the muscular source of pain, manual palpation can sometimes correctly identify the muscle where the tenderness originates

Fig. 72.1 KW test for strength and flexibility of key postural muscles; failure—inability to perform any of the tasks (Courtesy of the Norman Marcus Pain Institute)

Six Basic Muscle Tests

These six standardized tests of musular function may help to "pinpoint" deficiencies of strength or flexibility (Test 6). They are done as slowly and smoothly as possible. Avoid jerky movements. Do not strain. Stop and rest briefly after each test.

Test 1. Lie on your back, hands behind your neck, legs straight. Keeping your legs straight, raise both feet 10 inches off the floor and hold for 10 seconds. This is a test of your hip-flexing muscles.

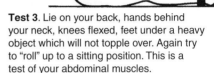

Test 2. Lie on your back, hands behind your neck, feet under a heavy object which will not topple over. Try to "roll" up to a sitting position. This tests your hip-flexing and abdominal muscles.

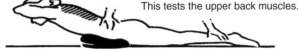

Test 3. Lie on your back, hands behind your neck, knees flexed, feet under a heavy object which will not topple over. Again try to "roll" up to a sitting position. This is a test of your abdominal muscles.

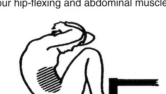

Test 4. Lie on your stomach with a pillow under your abdomen, hands behind your neck. With someone holding your feet and hips down, raise your trunk and hold for 10 s. This tests the upper back muscles.

Test 5. Taking the same position as that used for Test 4, but this time having someone holding your shoulders and hips down, try to raise your legs and hold for 10 s. This test the muscles of the lower back.

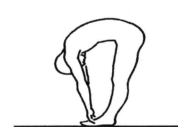

Test 6. Stand erect with shoes off, feet together, knees stiff, hands at sides. Try to touch the floor withe your fingertips. If you can not, try it again. Relax, drop your head forward, and try to let your torso "hang" from your hips. Keep your knees stiff. Chances are you'll do better the second time. This is a test of muscle tension or flexibility.

versus a referred muscle pain. To maximize the accuracy of the manual examination, an instrument that facilitates the application of a standard amount of pressure is suggested [135–137].

Treatment Protocols

Patients who are diagnosed with muscle pain that does not lend itself to injection should receive treatment appropriate to the diagnosis. Therefore, patients who have stiffness, but not weakness, should not be given strengthening exercises since this will only further stiffen their muscles. The current nostrum (following the fads of low-impact aerobics [138–140] and then closed-chain exercises [141, 142]) using

core strengthening for back pain without any test of strength and flexibility is ill-founded [143].

Injection Technique

When muscle involvement is suggested and the evaluation protocol finds that injections are indicated, the authors suggest the use of the term Muscle Pain Amenable to Injection (MPAI), as opposed to "trigger point pain." Suggested treatment consists of muscle-tendon injections (MTIs) instead of only TrP injections (TPIs), in order to include the regions (the entheses) with possibly the greatest density of sensitized nociceptors, followed by a structured physical therapy protocol which includes a validated set of exercises [144].

Patients should not be injected if they have a concurrent physical diagnosis (including morbid obesity, profound weakness and/or stiffness, Parkinson's disease, severe peripheral neuropathy, or significant psychological comorbidities) that discourages aggressive treatment of the diagnosed muscle pain until the underlying problem is adequately addressed.

We suggest that only one muscle is injected during a given injection treatment. A needle that is long enough to reach the bony attachment of the muscle (between 25 gauge × 5/8 in. and 20 gauge × 3½ in.) is used, depending on the size and depth of the identified muscle. The treatment is the needle disrupting the muscle tissue with particular attention to the origin and insertion. NM refers to the injection as a muscle-tendon injection (MTI) because of the significant difference in location of the injections versus TPIs. An entire muscle, and not just a "point or taut band," is injected.

The patient will typically first receive an intravenous analgesic. After seeing ketamine used for minor procedures at Walter Reed Army Medical Center, NM routinely uses it at a dose of <1 mg/kg, with total doses between 15 and 50 mg maximum, along with Midazolam 1–2 mg IV, with patients experiencing no pain from the procedure. Patients are counseled prior to the use of ketamine that they will have an unusual experience but that they will be able and are encouraged to keep discussing with me what they are feeling and thinking. Most patients elect to have ketamine on subsequent injections. The few that do not because of discomfort from the psychological effects of the ketamine, or lack of available recovery time, will be given a low-dose opioid, determined by the patient's past response to opioids.

The area to be injected is swabbed with iodine. Next, up to 10 ml of 0.5 % lidocaine is injected into the subcutis overlying the indexed muscle (5 ml for muscles in the neck and above). After 5–8 min, the muscle is needled from its origin to its insertion point (including the muscle belly) with an additional 10 ml of 0.5 % lidocaine (5 ml for muscles in the neck and above) for comfort, down to the bony attachment. With such doses of lidocaine, NM has never produced a systemic lidocaine reaction.

To illustrate the treatment technique, consider the example of giving an MTI to the infraspinatus (see Figs. 72.1 and 72.2). After instilling subcutaneous lidocaine, the muscle is injected at the vertex of the scapula with a 22-gauge × 1½-in. needle, and with the needle still inserted, it is moved along the medial and lateral borders of the scapula, withdrawing and reinserting the needle as one proceeds up toward the spine of the scapula and the rotator cuff. Ice is applied for 4 min after the injection. The area is cleansed, and when all bleeding stops, the stable patient is released.

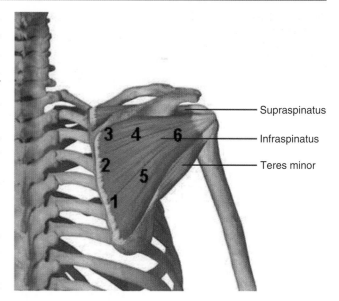

Fig. 72.2 The numbers represent the suggested sequence of muscle-tendon injections into the infraspinatus muscle down to the periosteum (With permission from the University of Washington)

Postinjection Physical Therapy

The MTI procedure causes some degree of pain both during and after the procedure. In order to facilitate additional injections and subsequent mobilization, the patient receives physical therapy on the day following the MTI. The physical therapy lasts for three consecutive days postinjection and consists of the patient receiving neuromuscular sine-wave stimulation (with ice) to a visible contraction, 2 seconds on and 2 seconds off, for a total of 15–20 min. This is followed by the first seven Kraus exercises for the lower body or the eight exercises for the upper body (see Figs. 72.3 and 72.4). Treatment always commences on a Monday to allow more than one muscle to be injected per week and to allow time for the three required post-MTI physical therapy sessions to be completed for each MTI. Therefore, treatment is considered complete on the final day of the post-MTI physical therapy session, of the last week that injections are given. Patients are given further instructions on the final day of physical therapy for the remaining 14 additional lower body exercises.

Summary of Suggestions for the Inclusion of Muscle Assessment in All Patients with Persistent Pain

1. Any patients with persistent pain should undergo a thorough examination of all muscles that could possibly contribute to the pain complaint.
2. Distinguish injectable muscle pain from pain related to tension, deficiency (weakness and/or stiffness), and spasm. We suggest the Kraus-Weber test for strength and flexibility

Fig. 72.3 Kraus-Marcus level 1 exercises for the relaxation and limbering of the lower body musculature (Courtesy of the Norman Marcus Pain Institute)

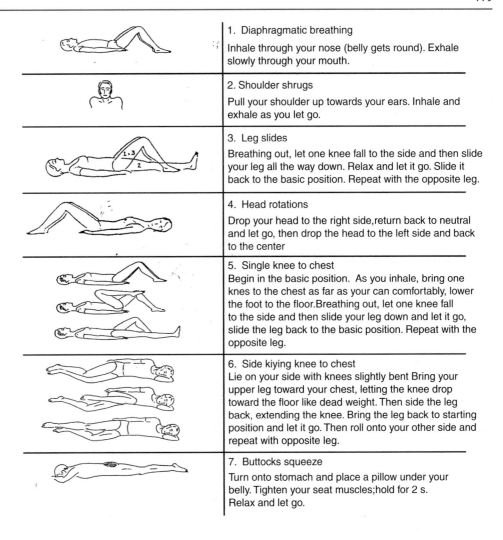

	1. Diaphragmatic breathing Inhale through your nose (belly gets round). Exhale slowly through your mouth.
	2. Shoulder shrugs Pull your shoulder up towards your ears. Inhale and exhale as you let go.
	3. Leg slides Breathing out, let one knee fall to the side and then slide your leg all the way down. Relax and let it go. Slide it back to the basic position. Repeat with the opposite leg.
	4. Head rotations Drop your head to the right side, return back to neutral and let go, then drop the head to the left side and back to the center
	5. Single knee to chest Begin in the basic position. As you inhale, bring one knes to the chest as far as your can comfortably, lower the foot to the floor. Breathing out, let one knee fall to the side and then slide your leg down and let it go, slide the leg back to the basic position. Repeat with the opposite leg.
	6. Side kiying knee to chest Lie on your side with knees slightly bent Bring your upper leg toward your chest, letting the knee drop toward the floor like dead weight. Then side the leg back, extending the knee. Bring the leg back to starting position and let it go. Then roll onto your other side and repeat with opposite leg.
	7. Buttocks squeeze Turn onto stomach and place a pillow under your belly. Tighten your seat muscles; hold for 2 s. Relax and let go.

of key postural muscles for low back and lower extremity pain. We suggest standard tests of upper body strength along with assessment of forward elevation and abduction of the arm and functional internal and external rotation of the shoulder (scapulohumeral and scapulothoracic motion) to find asymmetries of motion in the shoulder girdles which may suggest which muscle(s) may be involved.

3. Attempt to identify primary versus referred muscle pain. (Identification through muscle stimulation appears to be more accurate than palpation.)

4. Utilize a standardized exercise program to correct muscle deficiencies. We recommend the Kraus exercises: 8 for the upper body and 21 for the lower body.

5. When injecting a specific muscle, pay particular attention to the entheses of the identified muscle rather than just TrPs and taut bands. Consider injecting only one muscle at a given injection session.

6. If you use an injection procedure that targets the entire muscle, we recommend following up with 3 days of a postinjection physical therapy protocol to minimize postinjection soreness and stiffness.

7. If more than one MPAI is identified and multiple treatments are planned, reassess the patient for continued presence of MPAI prior to injecting the next planned muscle. It is possible that changes may have taken place as a result of successful injection. These changes may be related to central sensitization (the next muscle is no longer painful to manual or electrical stimulation) or CPM (a new muscle is painful after the previous; most severely painful muscle was successfully treated).

In future editions of this textbook, we hope to be able to publish head-to-head comparisons of other proposed and published comprehensive protocols.

Unusual Clinical Presentations in Which Muscles Played a Role

The following extraordinary case examples are presented not as a suggestion that all patients with the initial putative diagnoses below have muscle pain, but rather that we do not know whether any of our patients with persistent pain

Fig. 72.4 Kraus upper quadrant exercises for flexibility of the neck and shoulder girdle (Courtesy of the Norman Marcus Pain Institute)

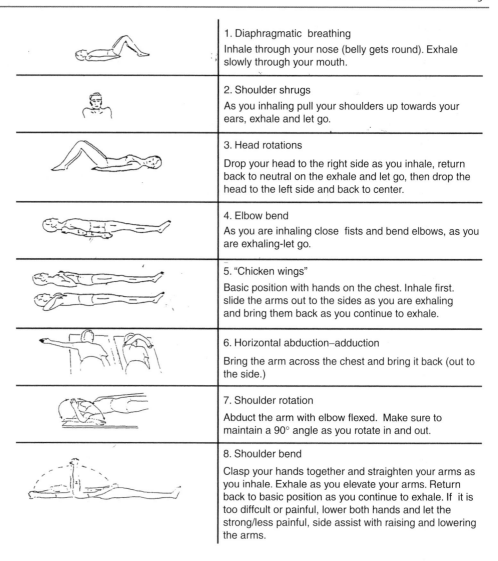

1. Diaphragmatic breathing
Inhale through your nose (belly gets round). Exhale slowly through your mouth.

2. Shoulder shrugs
As you inhaling pull your shoulders up towards your ears, exhale and let go.

3. Head rotations
Drop your head to the right side as you inhale, return back to neutral on the exhale and let go, then drop the head to the left side and back to center.

4. Elbow bend
As you are inhaling close fists and bend elbows, as you are exhaling-let go.

5. "Chicken wings"
Basic position with hands on the chest. Inhale first. slide the arms out to the sides as you are exhaling and bring them back as you continue to exhale.

6. Horizontal abduction–adduction
Bring the arm across the chest and bring it back (out to the side.)

7. Shoulder rotation
Abduct the arm with elbow flexed. Make sure to maintain a 90° angle as you rotate in and out.

8. Shoulder bend
Clasp your hands together and straighten your arms as you inhale. Exhale as you elevate your arms. Return back to basic position as you continue to exhale. If it is too diffcult or painful, lower both hands and let the strong/less painful, side assist with raising and lowering the arms.

complaints have an overlooked, treatable muscle pain because we are not routinely and systematically looking at their muscles as a possible source of pain. Ignoring muscles in patients with chronic pain may lead to unnecessary treatment failures and, in some cases, exacerbation rather than elimination of the pain complaint.

Complex Regional Pain Syndrome (CRPS)

A 50-year-old woman suffered a right-sided tibia/fibula fracture requiring open reduction and internal fixation and postoperatively developed complex regional pain syndrome in her foot and lower leg with discoloration, swelling, restricted range of motion, allodynia, and decreased temperature. Her initial diagnosis was made at a prominent New York City hospital. She received ketamine infusions, spinal cord stimulation, and a variety of traditional medications utilized for CRPS. She was unable to wear a sock or a closed-toe shoe.

She was severely depressed. She was seen for assessment five and a half years after the onset of her symptoms. Examination revealed pain emanating from the bilateral quadratus lumborum, left piriformis, left peroneus, left tibialis posterior, left soleus, left extensor hallucis longus, and left extensor digitorum longus muscles. The muscles were treated in the fashion previously described. She was pain free for approximately 4 months after her last treatment, with no restrictions and no medication, wearing a normal shoe and playing golf.

Her pain then returned, coincident with failed rotator cuff surgery and cessation of her prescribed lower body exercises, as well as the onset of wintry weather. Interestingly, only the dysesthetic pain and allodynia at the surgical scar site returned and not the skin color, temperature, and sweat changes. She was found to have MPAI in the following muscles: right quadratus lumborum (pain reduced 50 % after injection), piriformis (pain reduced 30 % after injection), extensor digitorum longus (pain reduced 10 % after injection), and extensor hallucis longus (complete relief of pain after injection). At the time of this writing, the patient has been essentially pain free for more than two years.

Failed Back Surgery Syndrome (FBSS)/ Spinal Stenosis

A 65-year-old entrepreneur with a 15-year history of back and leg pain was diagnosed with spinal stenosis and underwent two failed lumbar spine fusions at a prominent surgically oriented hospital. He was told that his only option for his persistent pain, which prevented him from leaving his home and socializing with friends and family, was a spinal cord stimulator or an epidural morphine pump. He was on round-the-clock opioid analgesia. In November 2005, he was evaluated for the presence of muscles as a source of his now persistent bilateral anterior thigh pain. Three muscles were identified—the right gluteus maximus and the left tensor fascia lata and vastus lateralis—and injected. One month after, he was essentially pain free and ambulating normally and remains pain free 5 years after his last injection. He has been able to travel to Vietnam and China and reports no impairments secondary to back or proximal leg pain.

FBSS is generally considered to be only amenable to palliative interventions such as spinal cord stimulation and/or lifelong delivery of potent analgesics, orally or parenterally. We have previously reported on a series of patients with FBSS successfully treated for muscle pain in the same fashion [145].

Fibromyalgia/Disk Protrusion

A 42-year-old woman with a 2-year history of neck, head, back, and lower extremity pain following an auto accident (causing her to spend days and weeks in bed with severe pain) was evaluated by multiple physicians and diagnosed with fibromyalgia. It was suggested that she undergoes cervical/lumbar spinal fusion as well. She was evaluated for the presence of muscle pain, and 13 muscles were identified—in the upper body, bilateral frontalis, infraspinatus, pectoralis minor, and left anterior/medial scalenes; and in the lower body, bilateral quadratus lumborum, gluteus medius, and right gluteus maximus, and piriformis. Since the most intense and disabling pain was in her head and neck, this region was treated first. After five muscles had been injected in her upper body (bilateral infraspinatus, frontalis, and left pectoralis minor), she reported that nearly all of the upper and lower body pain was eliminated. No other muscle injections needed to be done. She

is now without any pain-related impairment, 1 year after her last treatment.

Patients with imaging studies suggesting clinically meaningful spinal pathology may also present with diffuse pain diagnosed as FMS. Spinal fusion may be suggested. Some of these patients may have treatable muscle pain.

Rotator Cuff Tear

A 60-year-old medical assistant with a 2-year history of severe right shoulder pain and markedly restricted of range of motion was found to have a full-thickness buttonhole tear of the supraspinatus tendon on MRI. He was scheduled for rotator cuff surgery repair but was evaluated prior to surgery for muscle-based pain and found to have tenderness in six muscles of his shoulder girdle—coracobrachialis, trapezius, levator scapula, posterior para-cervicals, biceps brachii, and pectoralis major—which were successfully injected with elimination of all pain and total restoration of his range of motion (and subsequent cancellation of his surgery). He remained without pain or restriction for the 1 year he was followed.

Shoulder pain is inconsistently evaluated and treated [146–148]. Including the routine examination for specific shoulder muscle pain and dysfunction could decrease unnecessary surgeries and long-term use of analgesics.

Future Directions

The addition of a muscle protocol into the standard pain treatment paradigm should be supported by adequate RCTs to establish the validity of any intervention. In the realm of injection techniques to treat NSCLB, such a formidable task has uniquely been done by Francisco Kovacs.

Neuroreflexotherapy (NRT)

Neuroreflexotherapy (NRT) consists of the temporary implantation of a number of epidermal devices (surgical staples and small "burins" implanted subcutaneously) in trigger points in the back at the site of dermatomes and at the referred tender points located in the ear. The purpose is to "deactivate" neurons assumed to be involved in the persistence of pain, neurogenic inflammation, muscle dysfunction, and contracture.

As recognized by the Cochrane Back Review Group, NRT is one of the few technologies which has shown to be effective through high-quality, randomized, controlled trials and to provide "unusually positive" results [149]. This technology is currently implemented in Spain through the Spanish National Health System [150], and its evaluation in other countries is warranted.

Fascial Pain

Muscles do not function in a vacuum, and the relationship of muscle to its adjacent fascia and ligaments has not been systematically explored. As obscure as the data on muscle pain may be, fascial pain is even more so. The dynamic structure and function of fascia has not been appreciated. Fascia appears to have contractile properties that make it integral to efficient muscle contraction [151], as well as mechanosensitive properties which provide important information to surrounding muscles. Fascia has been shown to refer pain to different structures [152]. Therefore, damaged fascia may play an important role in chronic and recurrent low back pain [153, 154].

Stretching of injured muscle and tendon appears to inhibit scarring, which may be related to the production of transforming growth factor (TGF) beta 1 by damaged fascia [155]. In surgical procedures where fascia is resected, one should at least consider preservation of functional integrity whenever possible.

Regional Nonspecific Neck Pain

Regional pain such as neck pain is loosely defined [156], and although muscles are acknowledged as one of the pain-producing structures, little data exist on their importance. Andersen et al. [157] demonstrated that when pain was predominantly from the trapezius muscle (i.e., trapezius myalgia), strength training of the trapezius and surrounding muscles resulted in large decreases in pain that were sustained months after cessation of the study. Vuillerme and Pinsault [158] demonstrated the importance of intact nonpainful neck muscles in maintaining normal balance. In using manual palpation to identify muscle-related neck pain, facet arthropathy may be confused with pain associated with muscle attachments on the cervical spine [159]. Multifaceted treatment remains the norm for generic neck pain. In a systematic review, Chow found low-level laser therapy (LLLT) to be effective for acute- and moderate-duration neck pain [160], although a recent Cochrane review found that LLLT appeared to be ineffective [161].

Summary

Muscle and other soft tissue may be a primary source of common pain complaints and, if consistently acknowledged in our evaluation and treatment protocols, could result in improved treatment outcomes.

References

1. Wall PD, Woolf CJ. Muscle but not cutaneous C-afferent input produces prolonged increases in the excitability of the flexion reflex in the rat. J Physiol. 1984;356:443–58.
2. Fishman SM, Ballantyne JC, Rathmell JP, editors. Bonica's management of pain. 4th ed. Philadelphia: Lippincott Williams & Wilkins; 2009.
3. McMahon SB, Koltzenburg M, editors. Wall and Melzack's textbook of pain. 5th ed. Philadelphia: Elsevier/Churchill Livingstone; 2005.
4. Aronoff GM. Evaluation and treatment of chronic pain. 3rd ed. Baltimore: Lippincott Williams & Wilkins; 1999.
5. Benzon H, Rathmell J, Wu C, Turk D, Argoff C, editors. Raj's practical management of pain. 4th ed. St. Louis: Mosby; 2008.
6. Wallace DJ. The history of fibromyalgia. In: Wallace DJ, Clauw DJ, editors. Fibromyalgia and other central pain syndromes. 1st ed. Philadelphia: Lippincott Williams & Wilkins; 2005. p. 1–5.
7. Reynolds MD. The development of the concept of fibrositis. J Hist Med Allied Sci. 1983;38(1):5–35.
8. Inanici F, Yunus MB. History of fibromyalgia: past to present. Curr Pain Headache Rep. 2004;8:369–78.
9. Cohen M, Quintner J. The horse is dead: let myofascial pain syndrome rest in peace [letter]. Pain Med. 2008;9(4):464–5.
10. Marcus N. Response to letter to the editor by Dr. Cohen and Dr. Quintner [letter]. Pain Med. 2008;9(4):466–8.
11. Kellgren JH. Observations on referred pain arising from muscle. Clin Sci. 1938;3:174–90.
12. Kellgren JH. On distribution of pain arising from deep somatic structures with charts of segmental pain areas. Clin Sci. 1939; 4:35–6.
13. Lewis T, Kellgren JH. Observations relating to referred pain, visceromotor reflexes and other associated phenomena. Clin Sci. 1939;4:47–71.
14. Mense S, Hoheisel U. Central hyperexcitability and muscle nociception. In: Graven-Nielsen T, Arendt-Nielsen L, Mense S, editors. Fundamentals of musculoskeletal pain. 1st ed. Seattle: IASP; 2008. p. 61–73.
15. Arendt-Nielsen L, Graven-Nielsen T. Translational aspects of musculoskeletal pain. In: Graven-Nielsen T, Arendt-Nielsen L, Mense S, editors. Fundamentals of musculoskeletal pain. 1st ed. Seattle: IASP; 2008. p. 347–66.
16. Schade H. Untersuchungen in der Erkaltungsfrage. III: Ueber den rheumatismus, insbesondere den muskelrheumatismus (myogelose). Munch Med Wschr. 1921;68:418–20.
17. Lange M. Die Muskelhärten (Myogelosen): Ihre Entstehung und Heilung. Munich: Lehmann; 1931.
18. Steindler A. The interpretation of sciatic radiation and the syndrome of low-back pain. J Bone Joint Surg Am. 1940;22: 28–34.
19. Travell JG, Rinzler SH, Herman M. Pain and disability of the shoulder and arm: treatment by intramuscular infiltration with procaine hydrochloride. JAMA. 1942;120:417–22.
20. Travell JG, Rinzler SH. The myofascial genesis of pain. Postgrad Med. 1952;11:425–34.
21. Simons DG, Travell JG. Myofascial origins of low back pain. 1. Principles of diagnosis and treatment. Postgrad Med. 1983;73(2): 66–73.
22. Reeves R. President Kennedy: profile of power. New York: Simon and Schuster; 1993. p. 15, 82–85, 120, 242–3.
23. Smythe H. Tender points: the evolution of concepts of the fibrositis/fibromyalgia syndrome. Am J Med. 1986;81(3A):2–6.
24. Moldofsky H, Scarisbrick P, England R, Smythe H. Musculoskeletal symptoms and non-REM sleep disturbance in patients with "fibrositis syndrome" and healthy subjects. Psychosom Med. 1975; 37:341–51.

25. Vierck CJ. Mechanisms underlying development of spatially distributed chronic pain (fibromyalgia). Pain. 2006;124(3):242–63.

26. Mease PJ. Fibromyalgia syndrome: review of clinical presentation, pathogenesis, outcome measures, and treatment. J Rheumatol Suppl. 2005;75:6–21.

27. Borg-Stein J. Management of peripheral pain generators in fibromyalgia. Rheum Dis Clin North Am. 2002;28(2):305–17.

28. Ge HY, Nie H, Madeline P, Danneskiold-Samsøe B, Graven-Nielsen T, Arendt-Nielsen L. Contribution of the local and referred pain from active myofascial trigger points in fibromyalgia syndrome. Pain. 2009;147(1–3):233–40.

29. Stein C, Clark JD, Oh U, et al. Peripheral mechanisms of pain and analgesia. Brain Res Rev. 2009;60(1):90–113.

30. Staud R. The role of peripheral input for chronic pain syndromes like fibromyalgia syndrome. J Musculoskelet Pain. 2008;16(1–2):67–74.

31. Ellman P, Shaw D. The "chronic rheumatic" and his pains; psychosomatic aspects of chronic non-articular rheumatism. Ann Rheum Dis. 1950;9(4):341–57.

32. Sarno JE. Etiology of neck and back pain. An automatic myoneuralgia? J Nerv Ment Dis. 1981;169(1):55–9.

33. Burns JW. Arousal of negative emotions and symptom-specific reactivity in chronic low back pain patients. Emotion. 2006;6(2):309–19.

34. Cathcart S, Petkov J, Winefield AH, Lushington K, Rolan P. Central mechanisms of stress-induced headache. Cephalalgia. 2010;30(3):285–95.

35. Asendorpf JB, Scherer KR. The discrepant repressor: differentiation between low anxiety, high anxiety, and repression of anxiety by autonomic-facial-verbal patterns of behavior. J Pers Soc Psychol. 1983;45(6):1334–46.

36. Kasamatsu A, Hirai T. An electroencephalographic study on the zen meditation (Zazen). Folia Psychiatr Neurol Jpn. 1966;20(4):315–36.

37. Weinberger DA, Schwartz GE, Davidson RJ. Low-anxious, high-anxious, and repressive coping styles: psychometric patterns and behavioral and physiological responses to stress. J Abnorm Psychol. 1979;88(4):369–80.

38. Budzynski TH, Stoyva JM, Adler CS. EMG biofeedback and tension headache: a controlled outcome study. Psychosom Med. 1973;35(6):484–96.

39. Jacobson E. The technique of progressive relaxation. J Nerv Ment Dis. 1924;60(6):568–78.

40. Luthe W. Autogenic training: method, research and application in medicine. Am J Psychother. 1963;17:174–95.

41. Holroyd KA, Andrasik F, Westbrook T. Cognitive control of tension headache. Cogn Ther Res. 1977;1(2):121–33.

42. Stenn PG, Mothersill KJ, Brooke RI. Biofeedback and a cognitive behavioral approach to treatment of myofascial pain dysfunction syndrome. Behav Ther. 1979;10(1):29–36.

43. Kabat-Zinn J, Lipworth L, Burney R. The clinical use of mindfulness meditation for the self-regulation of chronic pain. J Behav Med. 1985;8(2):163–90.

44. Campbell C, Edwards R. Mind-body interactions in pain: the neurophysiology of anxious and catastrophic pain-related thoughts. Transl Res. 2009;153(3):97–101.

45. Martenson M, Cetas J, Heinricher M. A possible neural basis for stress-induced hyperalgesia. Pain. 2009;142(3):236–44.

46. Gunn CC. Radiculopathic pain: diagnosis and treatment of segmental irritation or sensitization. J Musculoskelet Pain. 1997;5(4):119–43.

47. Gunn CC. Reply to Chang-Zern Hong [letter]. J Musculoskelet Pain. 2000;8(3):137–42.

48. Gunn CC, Milbrandt WE, Little AS, Mason KE. Dry needling of muscle motor points for chronic low-back pain: a randomized clinical trial with long-term follow-up. Spine. 1980;5(3):279–91.

49. Hong CZ. Comment on Gunn's radiculopathy model of myofascial trigger points [letter]. J Musculoskelet Pain. 2000;8(3):133–5.

50. Hong CZ. Treatment of myofascial pain syndrome. Curr Pain Headache Rep. 2006;10(5):345–9.

51. Hopwood MB, Abram SE. Factors associated with failure of trigger point injections. Clin J Pain. 1994;10(3):227–34.

52. Kraus H, Fischer AA. Diagnosis and treatment of myofascial pain. Mt Sinai J Med. 1991;58(3):235–9.

53. Marcus N, Kraus H. Letter to the editor in response to article by Hopwood and Abram [letter]. Clin J Pain. 1995;11(1):84.

54. Rachlin E, Rachlin I. Myofascial pain and fibromyalgia. St. Louis: Mosby; 2002. p. 234–44.

55. Simons DG, Travell J. Myofascial pain and dysfunction (the trigger point manual). 2nd ed. Baltimore: Lippincott Williams & Wilkins; 1999.

56. Tough EA, White AR, Richards S, Campbell J. Variability of criteria used to diagnose myofascial trigger point pain syndrome – evidence from a review of the literature. Clin J Pain. 2007;23(3):278–86.

57. Marcus NJ, Gracely EJ, Keefe KO. A comprehensive protocol to diagnose and treat pain of muscular origin may successfully and reliably decrease or eliminate pain in a chronic pain population. Pain Med. 2010;11(1):25–34.

58. International Association for the Study of Pain (IASP). Core curriculum. 3rd ed. Seattle: IASP; 2005.

59. Christensen HW, Vach W, Manniche C, et al. Palpation for muscular tenderness in the anterior chest wall: an observer reliability study. J Manipulative Physiol Ther. 2003;26(8):469–75.

60. Levoska S. Manual palpation and pain threshold in female office employees with and without neck-shoulder symptoms. Clin J Pain. 1993;9(4):236–41.

61. Maher C, Adams R. Reliability of pain and stiffness assessments in clinical manual lumbar spine examination. Phys Ther. 1994;74(9):801–9; discussion 9–11.

62. Marcus N, Kraus H, Rachlin E. Comments on K.H. Njoo and E. Van der Does, pain 58 (1994) 317–323 [letter]. Pain. 1995;61(1):159.

63. Njoo KH, Van der Does E. The occurrence and inter-rater reliability of myofascial trigger points in the quadratus lumborum and gluteus medius: a prospective study in non-specific low back pain patients and controls in general practice. Pain. 1994;58(3):317–23.

64. Wolfe F. Stop using the American College of Rheumatology criteria in the clinic. J Rheumatol. 2003;30(8):1671–2.

65. Kraus H. Diagnosis and treatment of muscle pain. Chicago: Quintessence Books; 1988. p. 11–37.

66. Chou R, Qaseem A, Snow V, et al. Diagnosis and treatment of low back pain: a joint clinical practice guideline from the American College of Physicians and the American Pain Society. Ann Intern Med. 2007;147(7):478–91.

67. Van Tulder MW, Koes B, Seitsalo S, Malmivaara A. Outcome of invasive treatment modalities on back pain and sciatica: an evidence-based review. Eur Spine J. 2006;15 suppl 1:S82–92.

68. Martin BI, Deyo RA, Mirza SK, et al. Expenditures and health status among adults with back and neck problems. JAMA. 2008;299(6):656–64.

69. Rachlin E, Rachlin I. Myofascial pain and fibromyalgia. 2nd ed. St. Louis: Mosby; 2002. p. 438.

70. Fischer AA. Documentation of myofascial trigger points. Arch Phys Med Rehabil. 1988;69(4):286–91.

71. Jensen K, Andersen HO, Olesen J, Lindblom U. Pressure-pain threshold in human temporal region. Evaluation of a new pressure algometer. Pain. 1986;25(3):313–23.

72. Orbach R, Crow H. Examiner expectancy effects in the measurement of pressure pain thresholds. Pain. 1988;74:163–70.

73. Hunter C, Dubois M, Zou S, Oswald W, Coakley K, Shehebar M, Conlon AM. A new muscle pain detection device to diagnose muscles as

a source of back and/or neck pain. Pain Med. 2010;11(1): 35–43.

74. Simons D, Travell J. Myofascial pain and dysfunction (the trigger point manual). 2nd ed. Baltimore: Lippincott Williams & Wilkins; 1999. p. 166.

75. Chen Q, Basford J, An K-N. Ability of magnetic resonance elastography to assess taut bands. Clin Biomech. 2008;23(5):623–9.

76. Sikdar S, Shah JP, Gebreab T, et al. Novel applications of ultrasound technology to visualize and characterize myofascial trigger points and surrounding soft tissue. Arch Phys Med Rehabil. 2009;90(11):1829–38.

77. Park G-YMDP, Kwon DRMDP. Application of real-time sonoelastography in musculoskeletal diseases related to physical medicine and rehabilitation. Am J Phys Med Rehabil. 2011;90(11): 875–86.

78. Graboski CL, Gray DS, Burnham RS. Botulinum toxin a versus bupivacaine trigger point injections for the treatment of myofascial pain syndrome: a randomized double blind crossover study. Pain. 2005;118(1–2):170–5.

79. Hong CZ. Lidocaine injection versus dry needling to myofascial trigger point. The importance of the local twitch response. Am J Phys Med Rehabil. 1994;73(4):256–63.

80. Hong CZ. Consideration and recommendation of myofascial trigger point injections. J Musculoskelet Pain. 1994;2:29–59.

81. Kamanli A, Kaya A, Ardicoglu O, et al. Comparison of lidocaine injection, botulinum toxin injection, and dry needling to trigger points in myofascial pain syndrome. Rheumatol Int. 2005;25(8): 604–11.

82. Fischer AA. New injection techniques for treatment of musculoskeletal pain. Philadelphia: Mosby; 2002.

83. Gibson W, Arendt-Nielsen L, Graven-Nielsen T. Referred pain and hyperalgesia in human tendon and muscle belly tissue. Pain. 2006;120(1–2):113–23.

84. Starr M. Theory and practice of myofascial pain as both practicing clinician and patient. J Back Musculoskelet Rehabil. 1997;8(2): 173–6.

85. Van Tulder M, Malmivaara A, Hayden J, Koes B. Statistical significance versus clinical importance: trials on exercise therapy for chronic low back pain as example. Spine. 2007;32(16): 1785–90.

86. Hayden JA, van Tulder MW, Malmivaara A, Koes BW. Exercise therapy for treatment of non-specific low back pain. Cochrane Database Syst Rev. 2005;(3):CD000335.

87. Abenhaim L, Rossignol M, Valat JP, et al. The role of activity in the therapeutic management of back pain. Report of the International Paris Task Force on Back Pain. Spine. 2000;25 suppl 4:1S–33.

88. Fersum KV, Dankaerts W, O'Sullivan PB, Maes J, Slcouen JS, Bjordal JM, Kvale A. Integration of sub-classification strategies in RCTs evaluating manual therapy treatment and exercise therapy for non-specific chronic low back pain (NSLBP): a systematic review Br J Sports Med. 2010;44(14):1054–62.

89. Van Tulder M, Malmivaara A, Esmail R, Koes B. Exercise therapy for low back pain. Spine. 2000;25(21):2784–96.

90. Natvig B, Picavet HS. The epidemiology of soft tissue rheumatism. Best Pract Res Clin Rheumatol. 2002;16(5):777–93.

91. Deyo RA, Weinstein JN. Low back pain. N Engl J Med. 2001;344(5):363–70.

92. McBeth J, Jones K. Epidemiology of chronic musculoskeletal pain. Best Pract Res Clin Rheumatol. 2007;21(3):403–25.

93. Petersen S, Hägglöf BL, Bergström EI. Impaired health-related quality of life in children with recurrent pain. Pediatrics. 2009; 124(4):e759–67.

94. Pellisé F, Balagué F, Rajmil L, et al. Prevalence of low back pain and its effect on health-related quality of life in adolescents. Arch Pediatr Adolesc Med. 2009;163(1):65–71.

95. Pleis JR, Lucas JW, Ward BW. Summary health statistics for U.S. adults: National Health Interview Survey, 2008. National Center for Health Statistics. Vital Health Stat. 2009;10(242):6–7.

96. Freburger JK, Holmes GM, Agans RP, et al. The rising prevalence of chronic low back pain. Arch Intern Med. 2009;169(3): 251–8.

97. Juniper M, Le TK, Mladsi D. The epidemiology, economic burden, and pharmacological treatment of chronic low back pain in France, Germany, Italy, Spain and the UK: a literature-based review. Expert Opin Pharmacother. 2009;10(16):2581–92.

98. Hogg-Johnson S, van der Velde G, Carroll LJ, et al. The burden and determinants of neck pain in the general population: results of the bone and joint decade 2000–2010 task force on neck pain and its associated disorders. Spine. 2008;33(4 Suppl):S39–51.

99. Pope DP, Croft PR, Pritchard CM, Silman AJ. Prevalence of shoulder pain in the community: the influence of case definition. Ann Rheum Dis. 1997;56(5):308–12.

100. Croft P, Rigby AS, Boswell R, Schollum J, Silman A. The prevalence of chronic widespread pain in the general population. J Rheumatol. 1993;20(4):710–3.

101. Wolfe F, Ross K, Anderson J, Russell IJ, Hebert L. The prevalence and characteristics of fibromyalgia in the general population. Arthritis Rheum. 1995;38(1):19–28.

102. Weir PT, Harlan GA, Nkoy FL, et al. The incidence of fibromyalgia and its associated comorbidities: a population-based retrospective cohort study based on international classification of diseases, 9th revision codes. J Clin Rheumatol. 2006;12(3):124–8.

103. Lawrence RC, Felson DT, Helmick CG, et al. Estimates of the prevalence of arthritis and other rheumatic conditions in the United States. Part II. Arthritis Rheum. 2008;58(1):26–35.

104. Staud R. Chronic widespread pain and fibromyalgia: two sides of the same coin? Curr Rheumatol Rep. 2009;11(6):433–6.

105. Buskila D, Neumann L. The development of widespread pain after injuries. J Musculoskelet Pain. 2002;10:261–7.

106. Littlejohn G. Regional pain syndrome: clinical characteristics, mechanisms and management. Nat Clin Pract Rheumatol. 2007;3(9):504–11.

107. Marcus N. Pain in cancer patients unrelated to the cancer or treatment. Cancer Invest. 2005;23(1):84–93.

108. Marcus N. Treating nonacute pain in the cancer population [letter]. Pain Med. 2007;8(6):539.

109. Stacey M. Free nerve endings in skeletal muscle of the cat. J Anat. 1969;105:231–254.

110. Mense S. Algesic agents exciting muscle nociceptors. Exp Brain Res. 2009;196(1):89–100.

111. Mense S, Hoheisel U. Morphology and functional types of nociceptors. In: Graven-Nielsen T, Arendt-Nielsen L, Mense S, editors. Fundamentals of musculoskeletal pain. 1st ed. Seattle: IASP; 2008. p. 14–5.

112. Svensson P, Wang K, Arendt-Nielsen L, Cairns BE. Effects of NGF-induced muscle sensitization on proprioception and nociception. Exp Brain Res. 2008;189(1):1–10.

113. Nie H, Madeleine P, Arendt-Nielsen L, Graven-Nielsen T. Temporal summation of pressure pain during muscle hyperalgesia evoked by nerve growth factor and eccentric contractions. Eur J Pain. 2009;13(7):704–10.

114. Mense S. Muscle pain: mechanisms and clinical significance. Dtsch Arztebl Int. 2008;105(12):214–9.

115. Mense S, Simons DG, Hoheisel U, Quenzer B. Lesions of rat skeletal muscle after local block of acetylcholinesterase and neuromuscular stimulation. J Appl Physiol. 2003;94(6): 2494–501.

116. Nielsen LA, Henriksson KG. Pathophysiological mechanisms in chronic musculoskeletal pain (fibromyalgia): the role of central and peripheral sensitization and pain disinhibition. Best Pract Res Clin Rheumatol. 2007;21(3):465–80.

117. Yunus MB. Role of central sensitization in symptoms beyond muscle pain, and the evaluation of a patient with widespread pain. Best Pract Res Clin Rheumatol. 2007;21(3):481–97.

118. Staud R, Nagel S, Robinson ME, Price DD. Enhanced central pain processing of fibromyalgia patients is maintained by muscle afferent input: a randomized, double-blind, placebo-controlled study. Pain. 2009;145(1–2):96–104.

119. Fields HL, Basbaum Al. Central nervous system mechanisms of pain modulation. In: Wall PD, Melzack R, editors. Textbook of pain. Edinburgh: Churchill Livingstone; 1999. p. 309–29.

120. Moont R, Pud D, Sprecher E, Sharvit G, Yarnitsky D. 'Pain inhibits pain' mechanisms: is pain modulation simply due to distraction? Pain. 2010;150(1):113–20.

121. Lautenbacher S, Rollman GB. Possible deficiencies of pain modulation in fibromyalgia. Clin J Pain. 1997;13(3):189–96.

122. Staud R, Robinson ME, Vierck CJ, Price DD. Diffuse noxious inhibitory controls (DNIC) attenuate temporal summation of second pain in normal males but not in normal females or fibromyalgia patients. Pain. 2003;101(1–2):167–74.

123. Busch AJ, Barber KA, Overend TJ, Peloso PM, Schachter CL. Exercise for treating fibromyalgia syndrome. Cochrane Database Syst. Rev. 2007;(4):CD003786.

124. Ortega E, García JJ, Bote ME, Martín-Cordero L, Escalante Y, Saavedra JM, Northoff H, Giraldo E. Exercise in fibromyalgia and related inflammatory disorders: known effects and unknown chances. Exerc Immunol Rev. 2009;15:42–65.

125. Shah JP, Gilliams EA. Uncovering the biochemical milieu of myofascial trigger points using in vivo microdialysis: an application of muscle pain concepts to myofascial pain syndrome. J Bodyw Mov Ther. 2008;12(4):371–84.

126. Ge H, Nie H, Madeleine P, Danneskiold-Samsøe B, Graven-Nielsen T, Arendt-Nielsen L. Contribution of the local and referred pain from active myofascial trigger points in fibromyalgia syndrome. Pain. 2009;147(1–3):233–40.

127. Staud R. Are tender point injections beneficial: the role of tonic nociception in fibromyalgia. Curr Pharm Des. 2006;12(1):23–7.

128. Scott NA, Guo B, Barton PM, Gerwin RD. Trigger point injections for chronic non-malignant musculoskeletal pain: a systematic review. Pain Med. 2009;10(1):54–69.

129. Chou R, Qaseem A, Snow V, et al. Diagnosis and treatment of low back pain: a joint clinical practice guideline from the American College of Physicians and the American Pain Society. Ann Int Med. 2007;147(7):478–91.

130. Simons D, Travell J, Simons L. Myofascial pain and dysfunction: the trigger point manual. 2nd ed. Baltimore: Williams & Wilkins; 1999. p. 122.

131. Kopell HP, Thompson WA. Peripheral entrapment neuropathies of the lower extremity. N Engl J Med. 1960;262:56–60.

132. Byrd JW. Piriformis syndrome. Oper Tech Sports Med. 2005;13(1):71–9.

133. Fishman LM, Dombi GW, Michaelsen C, et al. Piriformis syndrome: diagnosis, treatment, and outcome – a 10-year study. Arch Phys Med Rehabil. 2002;83(3):295–301.

134. Tan G, Jensen MP, Thornby JI, Shanti BF. Validation of the brief pain inventory for chronic nonmalignant pain. J Pain. 2004;5(2):133–7.

135. Fischer AA. Pressure algometry over normal muscles. Standard values, validity and reproducibility of pressure threshold. Pain. 1987;30(1):115–26.

136. Kinser AM, Sands WA, Stone MH. Reliability and validity of a pressure algometer. J Strength Cond Res. 2009;23(1):312–4.

137. Bendtsen L, Jensen R, Jensen NK, Olesen J. Pressure-controlled palpation: a new technique which increases the reliability of manual palpation. Cephalalgia. 1995;15(3):205–10.

138. Neuberger GB, Press AN, Lindsley HB, et al. Effects of exercise on fatigue, aerobic fitness, and disease activity measures in persons with rheumatoid arthritis. Res Nurs Health. 1997;20(3):195–204.

139. Liemohn W. Exercise and arthritis. Exercise and the back. Rheum Dis Clin North Am. 1990;16(4):945–70.

140. Mannion AF, Müntener M, Taimela S, Dvorak J. A randomized clinical trial of three active therapies for chronic low back pain. Spine. 1999;24(23):2435–48.

141. Graham VL, Gehlsen GM, Edwards JA. Electromyographic evaluation of closed and open kinetic chain knee rehabilitation exercises. J Athl Train. 1993;28(1):23–30.

142. Kibler WB. Closed kinetic chain rehabilitation for sports injuries. Phys Med Rehabil Clin North Am. 2000;11(2):369–84.

143. Lederman E. The myth of core stability. J Bodyw Mov Ther. 2010;14(1):84–98.

144. Kraus H, Nagler W, Melleby A. Evaluation of an exercise program for back pain. Am Fam Physician. 1983;28(3):153–8.

145. Hunter C, Marcus N, Shehebar M. Muscles as a treatable pain source in patients with failed back surgery syndrome. Poster session presented at: American Academy of Pain Medicine (AAPM) 25th Annual Meeting; 2009 Jan 28 – 31; Honolulu, HI.

146. Bamji A. Interventions to treat shoulder pain. Lack of concordance between rheumatologists may render multicentre studies invalid. BMJ. 1998;316(7145):1676–7.

147. Szebenyi B, Dieppe P. Interventions to treat shoulder pain. Review was overly negative. BMJ. 1998;316(7145):1676; author reply 1677.

148. Green S, Buchbinder R, Glazier R, Forbes A. Systematic review of randomized controlled trials of interventions for painful shoulder: selection criteria, outcome assessment, and efficacy. BMJ. 1998;316(7128):354–60.

149. Urrútia G, Burton AK, Morral Fernández A, Bonfill Cosp X, Zanoli G. Neuroreflexotherapy for non-specific low-back pain. Cochrane Database of Syst Rev. 2009;(2):CD003009.

150. Corcoll J, Orfila J, Tobajas P, Alegre L. Implementation of neuroreflexotherapy for subacute and chronic neck and back pain within the Spanish public health system: audit results after one year. Health Policy. 2006;79:345–57.

151. Schleip R, Klingler W, Lehmann-Horn F. Active fascial contractility: fascia may be able to contract in a smooth muscle-like manner and thereby influence musculoskeletal dynamics. Med Hypotheses. 2005;65(2):273–7.

152. Hackett GS, Hemwall GA, Montgomery GA. Ligament and tendon relaxation treated by prolotherapy. Oak Park: Beulah Land Press; 2002.

153. Langevin HM, Sherman KJ. Pathophysiological model for chronic low back pain integrating connective tissue and nervous system mechanisms. Med Hypotheses. 2007;68(1):74–80.

154. Langevin HM. Potential role of fascia in chronic musculoskeletal pain. In: Audette JF, Bailey A, editors. Integrative pain medicine: the science and practice of complementary and alternative medicine in pain management. Totowa: Humana; 2008. p. 123–32.

155. Bouffard NA, Cutroneo KR, Badger GJ, et al. Tissue stretch decreases soluble TGF-beta1 and type-1 procollagen in mouse subcutaneous connective tissue: evidence from ex vivo and in vivo models. J Cell Physiol. 2008;214(2):389–95.

156. Ariëns GAM, Borghouts JAJ, Koes BW. Neck pain. In: Crombie IK, Croft PR, Linton SJ, LeReseche L, Von Korff M, editors. Epidemiology of pain. London: IASP; 1999.

157. Andersen LL, Kjaer M, Søgaard K, Hansen L, Kryger AI, Sjøgaard G. Effect of two contrasting types of physical exercise on chronic neck muscle pain. Arthritis Rheum. 2008;59(1):84–91.

158. Vuillerme N, Pinsault N. Experimental neck muscle pain impairs standing balance in humans. Exp Brain Res. 2009;192(4):723–9.

159. Bogduk N, Simons DG. Neck pain: joint pain or trigger points? Pain Res Clin Manag. 1993;6:267–73.

160. Chow RT, Johnson MI, Lopes-Martins RA, Bjordal JM. Efficacy of low-level laser therapy in the management of neck pain: a systematic review and meta-analysis of randomised placebo or active-treatment controlled trials. Lancet. 2009;374(9705):1897–908.

161. Gross AR, Aker PD, Goldsmith CH, Peloso P. Physical medicine modalities for mechanical neck disorders. Cochrane Database Syst Rev. 2000;(2):CD000961.

Addictive Disorders and Pain

Lynn Webster and Stuart Gitlow

Key Points

- Patients with chronic pain occupy a subset of the general population as do patients with addictive disorders. The two subsets sometimes overlap, an occurrence that cannot be judged solely by the quantity of opioid consumption.
- Addiction requires genetic vulnerability, conducive environmental conditions, and exposure to a chemical that triggers expression of the disorder, which itself results in a compromised reward system.
- Problematic drug-related behaviors and medication-induced side effects do not necessarily indicate addiction. Substance-induced disorders and substance-related symptoms may, therefore, arise in the absence of addictive disease and require a different treatment approach.
- Components of effective opioid therapy include screening patients for drug-related risks and psychiatric comorbidities and monitoring patients for regimen adherence, pain control, and stressors that could compromise treatment.
- Patients with histories of substance-use disorders may benefit from strong support systems, including 12-step groups.
- Patients who exhibit continued nonadherence to medical direction and inadequate analgesia may be humanely tapered from opioids.

L. Webster, M.D. (✉)
Clinical Research,
3838 South 700 East, Suite 200,
Salt Lake City, UT 84106, USA
e-mail: lynnw@lifetreepain.com

S. Gitlow, M.D., MPH, M.B.A.
Clinical Professor of Medicine, Mount Sinai School of Medicine,
153 Gaskill Street, Woonsocket, RI 02895, USA

Mount Sinai School of Medicine,
New York, NY, USA
e-mail: drgitlow@aol.com

Introduction

People consume opioids for many reasons, some medically beneficial and others harmful to themselves and to society. It is difficult to conclude that opioid use is harmful by evaluating consumption alone. Consider Fig. 73.1, in which we first have a population of individuals none of whom have been exposed to opioid use. Within that population are those who do not have addictive disease involving opioids; these individuals will not demonstrate signs and symptoms of addiction whether exposed to opioids or not. A smaller group within the population, shown in red and blue, has addictive disease. Those shown in blue do not know they have addictive disease simply because they have never been exposed to opioids. Phenotypically, then, they do not have addiction despite the underlying physiology. The group of individuals depicted in red, however, will show signs of addiction, resulting from medical or nonmedical use of opioids.

The two populations can be subdivided differently. Users of any substance, for medical or nonmedical reasons, do so with a range of frequency and quantity (addicted people have a further non-correlated range of disease severity). People with addictive disease might actually use less of the substance less frequently than those without addictive disease, particularly when those without addiction use the substance because they have been prescribed it. It is equally critical to realize that patients with addictive disease and with pain might use opioids precisely as prescribed with close monitoring and that in such cases the signs and symptoms of addiction may be absent despite the development of physiologic dependence.

Clinical evaluation and treatment are complicated when pain and addiction coexist. When addiction is present without the added component of pain, the focus is not on dissecting what a patient means by terms such as "occasional" or "experimental" use but on why the patient has used at all. When pain is added to the equation, that signal is valueless, because the patient has been prescribed the substance and is expected to use it. Furthermore, because denial is inherent to

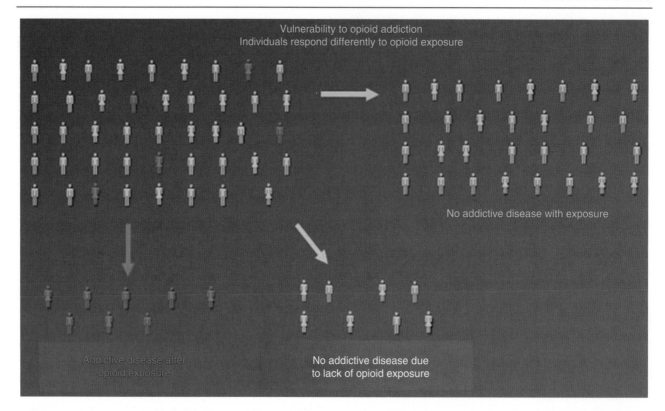

Fig. 73.1 First, we have a population of individuals none of whom have been exposed to opioid use. Within that population are those who do not have addictive disease involving opioids; these individuals will not demonstrate signs and symptoms of addiction whether exposed to opioids or not. A smaller group within the population, shown in *red* and *blue*, has addictive disease. Those shown in *blue* do not know they have addictive disease simply because they have never been exposed to opioids. Phenotypically, then, they do not have addiction despite the underlying physiology. The group of individuals depicted in *red*, however, will show signs of addiction, resulting from medical or nonmedical use of opioids

addictive illness, one always questions subjectively provided information when a patient is being treated for addiction but not pain. When pain is added, detective work is needed to determine whether the patient has taken the amount prescribed; whether he has doctor shopped to gain access to additional medication; whether he is taking the opioid only to avoid withdrawal; whether objective data exist to support the subjective report of pain; and many other factors.

Background

A subset of patients who are prescribed opioids for pain will eventually use their medication in ways not intended by their prescribing clinicians. Addiction is one reason why. Addiction prevalence among opioid-treated pain patients has been reported between 2 and 5 % [1, 2]; however, the prevalence of problematic opioid use is far higher. A prospective cohort study showed that 62 of 196 (32 %) patients enrolled in a chronic pain disease management program had at least one episode of opioid misuse after 1 year [3].

Patients who engage in multiple, repeated, or egregious aberrant drug-related behaviors are in danger of self-harm and are nearly certain to realize poor outcomes from pain

therapy. Many problematic drug-related behaviors can be handled by screening opioid candidates, stratifying patients by risk category, monitoring them closely, and treating them for comorbid depression, anxiety, and other mental conditions. Patients with strong risk factors for problematic opioid use, such as a family history of addiction or a personal history of addictive disease, present a special challenge because the potential for triggering or reactivating a substance-use disorder is real. Another reality is the frequent overlap of pain and addiction. In a study of patients receiving methadone for chemical dependency, 37 % experienced chronic, severe pain [4]. In a separate study, an association between chronic pain and self-reported prescription drug abuse was confirmed in veterans referred for a behavioral health evaluation [5]. Given the subjective nature of pain, these studies suggest the possibility that those with addictive disease are either more aware of painful stimuli or more susceptible to a subjective experience of pain than those without addictive illness when exposed to identical stimuli. This is consistent with Hennecke's findings with respect to stimulus augmentation in children of alcoholic fathers [6].

Failure to treat pain is poor medical practice as is failure to treat addiction, including opioid use disorders. Physicians, however, often receive little medical training on addiction or

Table 73.1 Definitions associated with opioid use and misuse [8, 9]

Misuse	Use of a medication for a medical purpose other than as directed or as indicated, whether willful or unintentional and whether harm results or not
Abuse	Any use of an illegal drug; the intentional self-administration of a medication for a nonmedical purpose such as altering one's state of consciousness (e.g., getting high)
Addiction	A primary, chronic neurobiologic disease influenced by genetic, psychosocial, and environmental factors. It is characterized by impaired control over drug use, compulsive use, continued use despite harm, and craving
Tolerance	A physiologic state resulting from the regular use of an opioid where increased doses are needed to maintain the same effects. In *analgesic tolerance*, increased opioid doses are needed to maintain pain relief
Physical dependence	A physiologic state characterized by abstinence syndrome (withdrawal) if an opioid is stopped or decreased abruptly or if an opioid antagonist is administered. It is an expected result of opioid therapy and does not, by itself, equal addiction

clinical pain treatment [7]. The treatment plan for chronic nonmalignant pain may include opioids, even for patients with substance-abuse histories or strong risk factors, if accompanied by careful screening, medication selection, and monitoring. However, some patients cannot be managed with opioid therapy, because their nonadherence or lack of analgesic response renders opioid therapy more harmful than helpful. In such cases, compassionate discontinuation of opioids can improve outcomes. The key is to personalize the treatment plan and to adjust when needed.

Scientific Foundation of Addiction

Definitions

The field of addictive disease suffers from a plethora of terminology, much of which has been defined and redefined over the years by different groups of specialists. Use, abuse, misuse, heavy use, dependence, and addiction: these terms are all in general use. Dependence carries a specific meaning to the pain physician as it refers to a physiologic neuroadaptation of the central nervous system to the effects of a given substance, in which an individual will experience objective physiologic symptoms of withdrawal should the substance use be terminated without tapering. Dependence has a different meaning to the reader of *DSM-IV-TR* where it refers to the medical disorder in which an individual repetitively uses an addictive substance despite that person's best interest. This latter definition is more widely applied to the class of disease known as addiction, with the acknowledgment that consensus among experts regarding terminology is not complete. Table 73.1 contains suggested definitions to clarify opioid use and misuse [8, 9].

The critical point is that, whatever terminology you choose, addictive disease is an illness or class of illnesses of the brain in which one marker is that of repetitive substance use; this approach simplifies the concept of pre-addiction, in which an individual is predisposed to the development of observable symptoms but has not yet developed them as a result of not having been exposed to the drug.

Neurobiology of Addiction

As addiction develops, changes occur within neuroanatomic structures, communication pathways, and neurochemical processes of the nervous system. Drugs of abuse impact the mesolimbic dopaminergic system, the region of the brain linked to basic emotions, by activating the ventral tegmental area and releasing dopamine into the nucleus accumbens, amygdala, prefrontal cortex, and ventral palladium [10]. Dopamine has been called the master molecule of addiction, but glutamate and gamma-amino butyric acid (GABA) also play key roles [10]. Opioids and other drugs decrease GABA activity in the ventral tegmental area, causing an increase in glutamate release in the nucleus accumbens which increases dopamine release. The release of dopamine in the nucleus accumbens appears to reinforce memories of pleasant drug experiences, boosting craving.

The amygdala mediates anxiety and other strong emotions. Not only does it help to regulate craving and relapse in addicted people, but amygdala stimulation may partially explain why certain chronic pain patients overuse opioids or anxiolytics, looking for relief from the stress and fear associated with chronic pain.

The activation of the reward pathway from the ventral tegmental area to the nucleus accumbens is crucial to the formation of addiction but is not in itself sufficient to cause addiction. Changes, which are both structural and functional, create in the vulnerable individual a behavioral compulsion to use drugs. With repeated use, the brain experiences neuroadaptive changes that can include tolerance, necessitating larger quantities of the substance to achieve the desired effects, and sensitization or heightened reward. Chronic drug abuse results in neuroplastic learning and altered brain systems with results that are observable in behavior. The brain becomes unable to distinguish between stimuli to engage in behaviors related to survival, such as eating, and the reward incentive delivered by addictive drugs. The result is a compromised reward system, and the changes are long term.

Observing the addicted brain is easier than understanding how it got that way, and the reason why some people become addicted while others do not must remain the subject of ongoing inquiry. Genetic and environmental vulnerabilities exist for the individual, who, in order to trigger the underlying neurobiologic mechanisms that lead to addiction, must be exposed to a drug of abuse. According to the National Institute on Drug Abuse, changes in frontal activity that accompany loss of control and compulsive drug intake are observable in addicted people during brain imaging studies [11]. What is still unclear is whether the changes preceded or followed drug use. Young people, whose central nervous systems are still developing, appear to be at particular risk for sustaining changes to the prefrontal cortex that could lead to compulsive drug behaviors when drug use is initiated early [12]. A study conducted by researchers at Rockefeller University in New York City found that adolescent mice allowed to self-administer oxycodone took less of the drug than adult mice did; however, when reexposed as adults, they exhibited increased striatal dopamine levels at the lowest dose [13]. Neither effect was found in the adult mice studied, and investigators concluded that both effects suggest greater sensitivity to oxycodone's effects in younger mice [13].

Disorders such as posttraumatic stress disorder, depression, and anxiety disorders also frequently coincide with substance abuse [12]. Whether psychiatric disorders confer vulnerability to addiction or vice versa – or whether both proceed from a common genetic vulnerability – is a question still to be answered.

Clinical Practice

Screening Opioid-Treated Patients for Risk of Abuse or Addiction

The universal precautions of opioid prescribing include initial screening and ongoing assessment for the presence of substance-use disorders [14]. High-risk patients, those likely to fit in the right-hand circle of Fig. 73.1, generally display risk factors such as personal or family history of substance abuse [2, 5], younger age [2, 5], history of preadolescent sexual abuse [2], mental disease [2, 5], social patterns of drug use [15], psychological stress [15], lack of a 12-step program [16], polysubstance abuse [16], poor social support [16], cigarette dependency [5, 17], and repeated drug or alcohol rehabilitations [17]. Conversely, low-risk patients, those likely to fit in the left-hand circle of Fig. 73.1, are those with fewer risk factors. Perhaps, they have completed a regimen of opioids in the past without difficulty or evidence of addiction.

Several tools are available to screen for the risk of opioid abuse. Opioid guidelines jointly released by the American Pain Society (APS) and the American Academy of Pain Medicine (AAPM) [18] endorse the Opioid Risk Tool (ORT) [2], the Screener and Opioid Assessment for Patients with Pain (SOAPP) [19], and the Diagnosis, Intractability, Risk, Efficacy (DIRE) [20]. Unlike the ORT and the SOAPP, which guide risk stratification, the DIRE purports to identify who would not be a suitable candidate. Other opioid-specific tools include the Screening Instrument for Substance Abuse Potential (SISAP) [21] and the Pain Medication Questionnaire (PMQ) [22].

A comparison study of the SOAPP, the ORT, and the DIRE found the SOAPP to be the most sensitive, followed by the ORT and then the DIRE [23]. Little data exist to differentiate the validity of self-administered vs. clinician-administered tools, although face-to-face interviews may give the clinician opportunity to gauge the patient's reactions and facial cues. However, self-administered tools are more practical for most clinical environments, and the choice is likely to be influenced by the time available.

The possibility of deception always exists when a patient is asked to share sensitive information. It is important to build trust and rapport during the assessment process to encourage honesty. The validity of the information provided is enhanced when [10]:

- Confidentiality is observed.
- Patients fear no negative consequences from disclosing information.
- The information disclosed has a likelihood of subsequent verification.
- The clinician is nonjudgmental and matter of fact.
- The clinician treats substance-use questions as an important, routine component of the medical history, no different than data on diet, exercise, and smoking.

Management of High-Risk, Opioid-Treated Patients

Screening can help clinicians to stratify and monitor patients by risk level – usually high, moderate, or low risk. There is a triage associated with chronic pain treatment [14]. The highest-risk patients who also experience moderate-to-severe chronic pain should be treated only by physicians trained to care for this complex population. In moderate-to-high-risk patients, care may be coordinated with appropriate specialists in addiction, pain, and mental health. Low-risk patients typically may be treated by primary care physicians.

All patients should receive at least the routine level of monitoring with monitoring measures intensifying as the level of risk rises (Table 73.2) [10]. Patients with histories of substance-use disorders require the strictest monitoring measures. In addition to cooperation with the high-risk measures listed in Table 73.2, patients with addiction histories should provide proof of continuing involvement with substance-related treatment, including 12-step programs or some equivalent. Deviations from the treatment program should result in a tightening of monitoring measures such as increased clinic visit frequency, reduced prescription quantities, and

Table 73.2 Monitoring methods according to patient risk for drug abuse [10]

Low-risk (routine)	Pain assessment
	Substance-abuse assessment
	Informed consent
	Signed treatment agreement
	Regular follow-up visits, prescriptions
	Initial prescription database check
	Medical reports
	Initial UDT
	No specialist consult required
	Med type, unrestricted
	Document 4A's
	Document patient/physician interactions
Moderate risk	Biweekly visits
	Biweekly prescriptions
	Regular prescription database check
	Verification via family members/ friends
	Random UDT
	Question comorbid disease
	Consider psychiatry/pain specialist evaluation
	Consider medication counts
	Consider limiting RO analgesics
High risk	Weekly visits
	Weekly prescriptions (on attendance)
	Quarterly prescription database check
	Friend/family member controls medication
	UDT: scheduled and random
	Consider blood screens
	Psychiatry/addiction specialist evaluation
	Consider pain specialist evaluation
	Limit RO analgesics
	Consider limiting SAO

RO rapid onset, *SAO* short-acting opioids, *UDT* urine drug testing, *4A's* analgesia, activities, adverse events, and aberrant drug taking

the involvement of a third party to control the dispensing. Patients with psychiatric comorbidities should receive treatment in tandem with addiction and pain treatment as these can worsen addiction-related behaviors involving opioids.

Choice of pain therapy is influenced by substance-related risk and pain condition. In high-risk patients with chronic pain, rapid-onset and short-acting opioids possess the potential to produce more rapid effects, including the potential for a reward that could prove reinforcing. If the pain severity allows, non-opioid therapies should be tried first. Medications with properties similar to drugs abused in the past should be avoided. Clinical decisions must be reached based on the individual patient; however, slow-release opioids that are

difficult to alter or manipulate are preferred for high-risk patients with pain.

Ongoing monitoring of the patient and clear documentation of the treatment process must take place at every clinic visit. Useful clinical monitoring tools include the Pain Assessment and Documentation Tool (PADT) [24] and the Current Opioid Misuse Measure (COMM) [25]. Urine drug screens (administered according to risk as shown in Table 73.2) and opioid treatment agreements that spell out the terms of treatment and the consequences for failure to comply are particularly valuable for patients at high risk for nonadherence. Agreements clarify expectations and also provide for early intervention if a high-risk patient exhibits problems managing opioid use. Prescription monitoring programs (PMPs), in the states where they are available, enable clinicians to ascertain whether patients are obtaining unauthorized prescriptions from more than one provider.

Any patient being considered for chronic opioid treatment should be screened for the history and presence of psychiatric comorbidities, and care should be coordinated with experts in mental-health fields when indicated. Recently, investigators have concluded that mental disorders among pain patients place them at special risk for abusing their medications [26]. A history of substance-use disorders is a red flag for potential abuse of prescription medications [10]. Patients with a trio diagnosis of chronic pain, addictive disorder, and psychiatric comorbidity should be treated for all three problems simultaneously. Agreement should be reached on the medications to be prescribed by each provider. It is vital to know what is being prescribed and by whom in order to manage medication use as safely and effectively as possible. Whenever possible, one physician should prescribe all medications with additional specialists to contribute consultations and recommendations as needed. Bipartite or tripartite management requires clear, timely, and complete communication for maximum success.

Support Systems

Addictive disease, as with many disease states, has two components that must be addressed: the genetic and the environmental. We can look at the genetic component as being phenotypically expressed in terms of a patient's heightened level of discomfort with life. We can look at the environmental expression as the patient's failure to learn a coping mechanism that does not involve self-medication for dealing with the discomfort.

Twelve-step programs and equivalent self-help groups are methods of providing patients with new coping mechanisms. This fresh approach to dealing with discomfort, which should not be confused with treatment, provides a helpful adjunct at every stage of addiction therapy. Indeed, patients who attend

12-step meetings achieve rates of abstinence that are nearly double that of patients who do not attend such meetings [27]. Furthermore, higher levels of attendance are related to higher rates of abstinence [27]. Given the significant improvement in addiction treatment efficacy provided by attendance at 12-step meetings, an important area of focus for treating clinicians is to facilitate meeting attendance. It has been demonstrated that it is possible to increase such involvement and that this increase directly leads to reduced use [28].

Narcotics Anonymous (NA), started in 1947, has since become international just as Alcoholics Anonymous (AA) has. NA is open to users of any drug regardless of whether the drug is a narcotic. NA promotes a spiritual awakening; some think of this as a religious experience, while others disregard any religious overtones. While NA started in part due to concern about drugs other than sedatives within AA, nearly all of the NA traditions, steps, and policies are based upon those of AA. The groups have a history of cooperating with one another.

Patients should be encouraged to build support systems in all areas of their lives. Factors that can contribute to first-time abuse or relapse include unrelieved pain, family difficulties, unemployment, and financial strain. Patients should be counseled to avoid social and family contacts that could influence them to misuse opioids or any other substance. Encourage the patient to seek help if stressors tempt him or her to overuse medication or lead to drug cravings. Facilitation of involvement with 12-step programs can be helpful here as well.

Discontinuation

A patient with an addictive disorder may be successfully treated with opioids given strict monitoring by the treating clinician and the patient's commitment to adherence. A poor candidate for opioid therapy is one whose physical functioning and quality of life continues to deteriorate and whose adherence to the treatment regimen cannot be established despite stringent measures. Clinical indications that it may be time to consider cessation of opioid therapy include the following [29]:

- Lack of benefit despite dose adjustment, side effect management, and/or opioid rotation
- Poor tolerance at analgesic dose
- Persistent adherence problems
- Presence of a comorbid condition that makes opioid therapy more likely to harm than help (e.g., sleep apnea, addiction)

Tapering from opioids is performed to prevent a physically dependent patient from going through withdrawal and to allow the clinician to observe the effect of tapering on pain level. Table 73.3 contains a suggested exit strategy [10].

Table 73.3 Exit strategy to discontinue opioid therapy [10]

Meet with the patient and review exit criteria agreed on in treatment agreement
Clarify that exit is for the patient's benefit
Clarify that exiting opioid therapy is not synonymous with abandoning pain management
Consider tapering opioids gradually over 1 month
Implement non-opioid pain strategies, including:
Psychiatric/behavioral therapies
Physical therapy
Non-opioid analgesics
Treatment for insomnia, anxiety, or depression
Consideration of interventional procedures
If patient does not cooperate with outpatient taper:
Do not provide additional opioids.
Refer to inpatient program or comprehensive outpatient program for opioid discontinuation as available.
Provide non-opioid medical maintenance until admission.
If addiction is the problem, refer for addiction management or comanagement.

Future Directions

No one argues that opioids are a panacea, certainly not doctors who frequently treat chronic pain. Medical research is currently focused on finding less abusable opioid formulations and testing alternatives to opioids. Much exciting research is being done in the field of genetics as it impacts pain perception and response to analgesic medication. Individuals demonstrate wide variations in responses to morphine and other opioids, and research implicates slight variations in DNA sequencing as a reason [30]. Opioids produce very effective pain control for some people and not for others. Science is moving in the direction of creating drugs that are tailored for individual genetic makeup.

Buprenorphine, a partial mu-receptor agonist, is being considered as an alternative to full mu agonists for certain types of pain [31]. Although buprenorphine has long been available, increased interest in its use has resulted from the possibility it could control pain while posing a reduced risk for addiction. Its value in addressing perioperative pain has also been broadly recognized [32]. Buprenorphine is available as a sublingual agent combined with naloxone. In this formulation, when used as directed, the naloxone has little-to-no direct effect. As a result, this combination drug works as one would expect buprenorphine to work while further reducing the potential misuse of the agent. Specific studies looking at the combination drug as a method of treating chronic pain have found it to be efficacious [33]. However, as a partial mu agonist, buprenorphine has limited analgesic potency. Used alone, it may not provide adequate analgesia for many patients with moderate-to-severe pain.

Summary

The overlap of pain and addiction presents special challenges to the clinical treatment of both disorders. Some patients with histories of substance-use disorders or other risk factors for addiction who also suffer moderate-to-severe pain may be successfully managed using opioids when alternative treatments would be ineffective. For other patients, opioids may be ineffective, retrigger abuse, and clearly be the wrong treatment for the individual patient. Every clinician who provides opioids should be familiar with risk factors for opioid addiction and screen patients for possible addictive disorders, remembering that the spectrum of aberrant behaviors ranges from misuse to the disease of addiction. Effective ongoing management requires an understanding of the motivations underlying drug-related behaviors and a recognition that not all substance use is addiction. Ongoing management is then tailored by setting the level of clinical monitoring appropriate to the degree of risk, reassessing the patient frequently, and being prepared to humanely taper the patient from opioids if necessary.

Acknowledgment   Technical writing and manuscript review are provided by Beth Dove of Medical Communications, Salt Lake City, Utah.

References

1. Fleming MF, Balousek SL, Klessig CL, Mundt MP, Brown DD. Substance use disorders in a primary care sample receiving daily opioid therapy. J Pain. 2007;8(7):573–82.
2. Webster LR, Webster RM. Predicting aberrant behaviors in opioid-treated patients: preliminary validation of the opioid risk tool. Pain Med. 2005;6(6):432–42.
3. Ives TJ, Chelminski PR, Hammett-Stabler CA, et al. Predictors of opioid misuse in patients with chronic pain: a prospective cohort study. BMC Health Serv Res. 2006;6:46.
4. Rosenblum A, Joseph H, Fong C, Kipnis S, Cleland C, Portenoy RK. Prevalence and characteristics of chronic pain among chemically dependent patients in methadone maintenance and residential treatment facilities. JAMA. 2003;289(18):2370–8.
5. Becker WC, Fiellin DA, Gallagher RM, Barth KS, Ross JT, Oslin DW. The association between chronic pain and prescription drug abuse in veterans. Pain Med. 2009;10(3):531–6.
6. Hennecke L. Stimulus augmenting and field dependence in children of alcoholic fathers. J Stud Alcohol Drugs. 1984;45(6):486–92.
7. Public policy statement on the rights and responsibilities of healthcare professionals in the use of opioids for the treatment of pain: a consensus document from the American Academy of Pain Medicine, the American Pain Society, and the American Society of Addiction Medicine. Adopted 2004. Available at http://www.ampainsoc.org/advocacy/pdf/rights.pdf. Accessed 7 Jan 2010.
8. Katz NP, Adams EH, Chilcoat H, et al. Challenges in the development of prescription opioid abuse-deterrent formulations. Clin J Pain. 2007;23(8):648–60.
9. Federation of State Medical Boards of the United States, Inc. Model policy for the use of controlled substances for the treatment of pain. 2004. Available at: http://www.fsmb.org/pdf/2004_grpol_Controlled_Substances.pdf. Accessed 7 Jan 2010.
10. Webster LR, Dove B. Avoiding opioid abuse while managing pain: a guide for practitioners. 1st ed. North Branch: Sunrise River Press; 2007. p. 145.
11. National Institutes of Health, U.S. Department of Health and Human Services. Drugs, brains, and behavior: the science of addiction. NIH Pub No. 07–5605. Printed Apr 2007.
12. National Institutes of Health, U.S. Department of Health and Human Services. Research report series. Comorbidity: addiction and other mental illnesses. NIH Pub No. 08–5771. Printed Dec 2008.
13. Zhang Y, Picetti R, Butelman ER, Schlussman SD, Ho A, Kreek MJ. Behavioral and neurochemical changes induced by oxycodone differ between adolescent and adult mice. Neuropsychopharmacology. 2009;34(4):912–22.
14. Gourlay DL, Heit HA, Almahrezi A. Universal precautions in pain medicine: a rational approach to the treatment of chronic pain. Pain Med. 2005;6(2):107–12.
15. Savage SR. Assessment for addiction in pain-treatment settings. Clin J Pain. 2002;18(4 Suppl):S28–38.
16. Dunbar SA, Katz NP. Chronic opioid therapy for nonmalignant pain in patients with a history of substance abuse: report of 20 cases. J Pain Symptom Manage. 1996;11(3):163–71.
17. Friedman R, Li V, Mehrotra D. Treating pain patients at risk: evaluation of a screening tool in opioid-treated pain patients with and without addiction. Pain Med. 2003;4(2):182–5.
18. Chou R, Fanciullo GJ, Fine PG, et al. Clinical guidelines for the use of chronic opioid therapy in chronic noncancer pain. J Pain. 2009;10(2):113–230.
19. Butler SF, Budman SH, Fernandez K, Jamison RN. Validation of a screener and opioid assessment measure for patients with chronic pain. Pain. 2004;112(1–2):65–75.
20. Belgrade MJ, Schamber CD, Lindgren BR. The DIRE score: predicting outcomes of opioid prescribing for chronic pain. J Pain. 2006;7(9):671–81.
21. Coambs RB, Jarry JL. The SISAP; a new screening instrument for identifying potential opioid abusers in the management of chronic nonmalignant pain in general medical practice. Pain Res Manag. 1996;1(3):155–62.
22. Adams LL, Gatchel RJ, Robinson RC, et al. Development of a self-report screening instrument for assessing potential opioid medication misuse in chronic pain patients. J Pain Symptom Manage. 2004;27:440–59.
23. Moore TM, Jones T, Browder JH, Daffron S, Passik SD. A comparison of common screening methods for predicting aberrant drug-related behavior among patients receiving opioids for chronic pain management. Pain Med. 2009;10(8):1426–33.
24. Passik SD, Kirsh KL, Whitcomb L, et al. A new tool to assess and document pain outcomes in chronic pain patients receiving opioid therapy. Clin Ther. 2004;26(4):552–61.
25. Butler SF, Budman SH, Fernandez KC, et al. Development and validation of the current opioid misuse measure. Pain. 2007;130(1–2):144–56.
26. Wasan AD, Butler SF, Budman SH, Benoit C, Fernandez K, Jamison RN. Psychiatric history and psychologic adjustment as risk factors for aberrant drug-related behavior among patients with chronic pain. Clin J Pain. 2007;23(4):307–15.
27. Kaskutas LA. Alcoholics anonymous effectiveness: faith meets science. J Addict Dis. 2009;28(2):145–57.
28. Donovan DM, Floyd AS. Facilitating involvement in twelve-step programs. Recent Dev Alcohol. 2008;18:303–20.
29. Katz N. Patient level opioid risk management: a supplement to the PainEDU.org manual. Newton: Inflexxion, Inc; 2007.
30. Webster LR. Pharmacogenetics in pain management: the clinical need. Clin Lab Med. 2008;28(4):569–79.
31. Induru RR, Davis MP. Buprenorphine for neuropathic pain: targeting hyperalgesia. Am J Hosp Palliat Care. 2009;26(6):470–3.
32. Vadivelu N, Hines RL. Buprenorphine: a unique opioid with broad clinical applications. J Opioid Manag. 2007;3(1):49–58.
33. Malinoff HL, Barkin RL, Wilson G. Sublingual buprenorphine is effective in the treatment of chronic pain syndrome. Am J Ther. 2005;12(5):379–84.

The "Five-Minute" Mental Status Examination of Persons with Pain

74

J. David Haddox and Barry Kerner

Key Points
- Mental status findings are common in patients with pain.
- Many medicines employed in pain care can induce or worsen underlying psychiatric problems.
- Examining the mental status in routine pain care requires little additional work.
- Pain physicians should understand the well-defined terms to describe mental status findings.

Introduction

The mental status examination (MSE) is just that – a set of processes that systematically examine various aspects of a person's mental functioning – in essence, a physical examination of the mind. A complete MSE constitutes a distinct portion of a complete psychiatric assessment. In practice, whether in psychiatry or other specialties, the MSE can be less comprehensive than a complete MSE, according to the clinical setting. MSEs can be partial – focusing only a particular aspect, such as mood or intelligence, or can be exhaustive. Abbreviated MSEs can range anywhere from keen observations of people, to structured interviews (e.g., Structured Clinical Interview for DSM-IV (SCID)), to the use of validated instruments for the assessment of a specific aspect of the mental status (e.g., Profile of Mood States,

J.D. Haddox, DDS, M.D., DAPBM, MRO (✉)
Tufts University School of Medicine,
Boston, MA, USA

Department of Health Policy, Purdue Pharma L.P.,
One Stanford Forum, Stanford, CA 06901, USA
e-mail: dr.j.david.haddox@pharma.com

B. Kerner, M.D., DABPM
Silver Hill Hospital,
208 Valley Road, New Canaan, CT 06840, USA
e-mail: bkerner@silverhillhospital.org

Wechsler Adult Intelligence Test, Minnesota Multiphasic Personality Inventory, State-Trait Anxiety Inventory), and to multi-hour assessments of specific functions (e.g., Halstead-Reitan Neuropsychological Test Battery) [1]. MSEs can involve standardized clinical assessment techniques (e.g., "serial sevens" or copying a figure) or can be less formal. Incorporating certain aspects of the MSE into clinical pain assessment and care is important because persons in pain may present with mental status findings that (a) predate the onset of pain (e.g., the presence of generalized anxiety disorder long before a cancer diagnosis), (b) date to the onset of pain (e.g., posttraumatic stress disorder initiated by the same motor vehicle accident that caused the spinal fracture that gave rise to the pain for which they are being evaluated or treated), (c) follow the onset of, but are related to, the pain syndrome (e.g., depression or anxiety due in part or in whole to chronic, unremitting pain), or (d) are related to treatment (e.g., cognitive impairment due to medications prescribed). Because virtually all medications used to treat pain have the potential for significant effects on various aspects of a patient's mental status, it is important to assess the mental status at baseline and note any changes over time. The thorough way to do this is to learn how to observe patients in clinical interactions while keeping the potential MSE findings in mind, to record the findings using precise, unambiguous, and proper terms, and to interpret these findings in the assessment and plan.

An abbreviated MSE in pain practice does not necessarily have to take a lot of time, or even be a separate part of the initial or ongoing evaluation of patients undergoing treatment for pain. Certain aspects of mental function can have significant influences on the course of treatment and potential treatment outcomes. Documenting important aspects of the patient's mental status can be very helpful in the overall assessment by affording a chronology of the presence, absence, improvement, or worsening of specific symptoms and signs from visit to visit. The inclusion or absence of documentation of important MSE findings can have significant medical/legal consequences as well.

Fortunately, once the physician has learned the principles of an abbreviated MSE, most information needed to document MSE findings can be readily obtained as part of the normal conversation and observation that occurs during a typical clinical encounter. Just as a pain physician begins their observation of pain behaviors immediately upon seeing the patient and ends it as the patient leaves their sight (e.g., walking down the hall to schedule an appointment), the abbreviated MSE becomes part of the entire interaction, to be separately described and interpreted in the health record.

The "Five-Minute Mental Status Examination for Persons in Pain" (5-MSEPP) is a distillation of some salient aspects of the MSE that the authors have found useful from decades of direct clinical care of persons in pain and is specifically aimed at assisting the nonpsychiatrist in routine care of their patients (see Table 74.1). There will, of course, be cases in which a more structured, formal MSE is indicated, but these should be done by a psychiatrist or psychologist, rather than the pain physician without such qualification.

In this chapter, the authors will review the various aspects of the mental status that can be assessed during the provision of clinical pain care, provide precise terminology and definitions for the phenomena commonly encountered, suggest some methods for mental status assessment that can easily

be incorporated into clinical routines, and provide a framework for how to document such findings in the health care record.

The MSE includes assessment and interpretation of both subjective and objective aspects of the person's mental function. The subjective aspects are called *symptoms* and represent experiences, beliefs, thoughts, feelings, etc., which are *reported* by the patient. The objective findings are referred to as *signs* and are those phenomena and behaviors that are directly *observed* by the practitioner. Just as during the physical examination a physician would note and record the speed and amplitude of the biceps tendon reflex objectively (e.g., "3+, normal recovery, no clonus"), so, too, should the findings of the MSE be recorded objectively, leaving the interpretation of the constellation of history, MSE, physical examination, and laboratory findings to the assessment section of consultation, initial visit, or progress note.

As will be clear from the information that follows, the traditional separation of "mental status" from "neurological" findings is somewhat arbitrary and may be of questionable clinical relevance, since both are ways of assessing the function and abnormalities of the same nervous system. For example, if a person with dementia (a "neurological" diagnosis) presents with psychosis (a "psychiatric" diagnosis), both need addressing, whether by a psychiatrist, a neurologist, a geriatrician, or a family physician.

Table 74.1 5-MMSEPP – key points to observe and describe

Appearance
Development
Nutritional status – including change over time
Dress/grooming
Level of consciousness – alert, somnolent, lethargic, obtunded, stuporous, comatose
Orientation – person, place, time, situation
Motor activity
Quantity – hypoactive, normoactive, hyperactivity, agitation
Quality – altered gait (antalgic, ataxic, festinating, etc.)
Fluidity – tremors
Spontaneity
Speed
Abnormal signs – cogwheel rigidity, tics, stereotypies, chorea, athetosis
Affect and mood – range, amplitude, stability, appropriateness, relation to examiner
Suicidality – ideation, plans, intent, threats, gestures, attempts
Homicidality – ideation, plans, intent, threats, attempts, duty to protect intended victim
Thought process
Speech – spontaneity, rate, amount, rhythm, articulation, idiosyncrasies
Associations – fragmentation, derailment, non sequiturs, flight of ideas, circumlocution, tangential
Thought content – delusions, hallucinations (sensory modality), illusions
Memory – registration, short-term, long-term, confabulation
Judgment and insight

Background Concepts and Terms

There are well-defined aspects of an abbreviated MSE that can be readily assessed in the provision of pain care. The following are the various domains assessed as part of a typical MSE: appearance, level of consciousness, orientation, motor activity, affect and mood, thought content and processes, intellect, memory, and judgment.

Appearance

The first thing typically noticed is the patient's *appearance*. Aspects of appearance that warrant observation and characterization include the apparent degree of development (i.e., the patient is well developed or, if not, describes what aspects of development deviate from normal), the nutritional status (i.e., well nourished, overweight, cachectic, emaciated, etc.), and the degree of grooming/dress/hygiene (i.e., well groomed, appropriately dressed, disheveled, poor hygiene, etc.). Because various drugs encountered in pain care can directly or indirectly cause either weight gain (increased body mass from antidepressants or fluid retention from corticosteroid injections) or weight loss (stimulant use/abuse, cocaine abuse, opioid abuse), note should be made of changes in appearance over time.

Eye contact can be revealing, but like many signs, whether a patient makes good eye contact with the examiner can have different meanings. For example, it is common, in Western cultures, to infer that someone not making good eye contact is being evasive. However, this behavior must be interpreted carefully because in certain cultures, looking at an authority figure, such as a physician, directly in the eye is considered disrespectful or sexually provocative [2, 3].

Overall comments about the nature of the interaction deserve documentation, such as the patient's demeanor, courtesy, and cooperativeness. The term *guarded* is used to describe a person who appears to be *inappropriately* cautious or reserved about the interaction or reluctant to provide information.

Level of Consciousness

This aspect of a patient's presentation is virtually always perceived by the clinician, but is often not reported. The normal level of consciousness in a clinical situation is, of course, is *alert* (which implies that the person being evaluated is also awake). Other descriptors commonly employed included *somnolent* (i.e., drowsy, or sleepy), *lethargic* (i.e., very sleepy, in which the person can be verbally or physically aroused to a level of communication, but when unprovoked, will drift back to sleep), *obtunded* (i.e., more sleepy than lethargic), *stuporous* (i.e., repeated, vigorous stimuli can arouse the person, but ceasing the stimuli results in immediate return to sleep), and *comatose* (i.e., unresponsive to any stimulus mode – auditory, tactile, etc.) [4]. Degree of attention or engagement is important to observe and report. For example, an alert patient can be disengaged from the interaction (e.g., a person with drug-induced hallucinations may be alert, but completely or intermittently disengaged with the clinician because they are attending to the hallucinations).

Orientation

Orientation is typically assessed and described in four domains: orientation to *person*, *place*, *time*, and *situation*. A patient who is oriented to person knows who they are and who others they should know are. Orientation to place is the ability to indicate where they are. With organic brain syndromes, whether degenerative, metabolic, traumatic, infectious, or drug-induced, orientation to time can be an especially sensitive indicator. In a rapidly changing organic brain syndrome (e.g., a person who is admitted to hospital for an overdose of a tricyclic antidepressant), incremental improvement in orientation to time can be a useful adjunct to monitoring progress, as the toxicity resolves, in that the person may initially be disoriented with respect to time, then may know what year it is, but still be disoriented to season or month and will gradually regain orientation to month and date. Orientation to situation is sometimes referred to as situational insight and is used to describe the person who demonstrates an understanding of the context of what is happening at that time.

Motor Activity

The *quantity*, *quality*, *fluidity*, *spontaneity*, and *speed* of motor activity should be described, as should the presence of any *abnormal motor signs*. The terms used to quantify activity include normoactive, hypoactive (less spontaneous or responsive activity than normally observed, as might be seen in a patient with drug-induced Parkinsonian syndrome or a person with chronic benzodiazepine toxicity), and hyperactive. *Hyperactivity* specifically describes an excess amount of *goal-directed* activity, such as might be seen in a child with attention deficit hyperactivity disorder, in which the clinical presentation may include the child hopping out of their chair, opening and closing the examining room door or drawers in the cabinetry, taking off their shoes, etc.

Excess, purposeless, voluntary motor activity is referred to as *agitation*. Agitation is often associated with alteration in affect or mood. Pacing, frequently switching positions, hand wringing, finger drumming, or pulling on one's hair are all examples of agitation. Purposeless, involuntary motor activity, such as *tremors*, should be described. Tremors can be characterized with regard to their *location* (e.g., finger, arm), *amplitude* (small or large), *frequency* (low or high), whether they are *resting* or *intention* (intention tremors appear when an action is attempted, such as reaching for a pencil), and whether they *diminish* or *disappear* with distraction. A well-described tremor of note is the *pill-rolling tremor*, which describes a low-amplitude, high-frequency resting tremor involving the thumb and index finger (with possible involvement of other digits, as well), that is named because it is reminiscent of the rolling of medicinal compounds into round pills by early apothecaries (the dominant technique of creating oral formulations before tableting presses were invented). Another tremor equivalent is that of constant or nearly constant head bobbing or low-amplitude shaking (as if one was repeatedly signaling "no") that is referred to as *titubation*. This is seen in a variety of neurodegenerative diseases and drug-induced neurological syndromes.

Drugs may induce several disorders of motor activity, including agitation (e.g., cocaine, stimulants), cogwheel rigidity, tics, and stereotypies. *Cogwheel rigidity* is the term used to describe a ratchet-like quality of the muscles when flexing and extending a joint. This can be visually observed in some cases, with the hand moving through the flexion-extension arc in a jerky or "start-and-stop" fashion, but often is detectable only by placing the examiner's thumb over, for example, the biceps tendon and asking the patient to allow the examiner to smoothly, but relatively quickly, flex and extend the elbow (passive flexion and extension). It results in a subtle "bumping" or "ratcheting" feeling of the tendon under the thumb, likened by some to feeling as though a string of pearls is being pulled subcutaneously under the examiner's thumb. Cogwheel rigidity is an *extrapyramidal* phenomenon (i.e., it is mediated via neural pathways that are *outside* of the corticospinal tracts – most of which cross the midline in the medulla oblongata at the pyramidal decussation). *Drug-induced* extrapyramidal side effects (EPSE) result from dopamine antagonism. Extrapyramidal findings can also occur with disease processes that cause the loss of dopaminergic neurons in the basal ganglia, such as Parkinson's disease. In general, the corticospinal tracts mediate coarse motor activity and the extrapyramidal paths mediate fluidity and "fine-tuning" of movement. A person with basal ganglia dysfunction may be able to reach for a glass of water, but the movement will be so coarse that they will overshoot the target or knock the glass over. Other features of the Parkinsonian syndrome, whether drug-induced or naturally occurring, include gait abnormalities (see below), masklike facies (i.e., far less activity in the muscles of facial expression than is normal – which can also be seen in chronic depression resulting in so-called *pseudodementia* and myotonic dystrophy), general hypoactivity, and difficulty initiating an activity or initiating a change in activity. For example, a person with Parkinsonian syndrome may appear to sit comfortably in an examination room chair, but at the conclusion of the visit demonstrate significant difficulty rising from the chair. This difficulty initiating or changing movement is often reported to the physician as difficulty rising from the toilet, or going up stairs (which requires initiation of change of activity with every step). Another characteristic presentation that can be induced by administration of dopamine antagonists is *tardive dyskinesia* (Fr, *tardif*, late, as in *tardy*, + Gk, *dys*+*kinesia*, movement). Tardive dyskinesia usually affects the muscles of the head, causing involuntary lip pursing or tongue protrusion, but can affect other muscle groups, as well, even creating restrictive pulmonary compromise.

Drug-induced EPSE can also occur acutely, following the administration of dopamine antagonists used as antiemetics (e.g., droperidol, promethazine), and can manifest as an overwhelming urge to move, or restlessness, called *akathisia* (Gk, *a*+*kathízein*, to sit). This phenomenon can typically be treated with the administration of a drug with antimuscarinic properties, such as diphenhydramine or benztropine. It is important to remember that akathisia refers to the *urge* to move, not to the movement itself, which may take the form of agitation or hyperactivity. Administration of dopamine antagonists (e.g., some antiemetics or antipsychotics) rarely results in *acute dystonias*, or sudden increased tone of certain muscles, but not their antagonist muscles, such that the person presents, for example, with their head painfully rotated to one side, and is unable to voluntarily rotate it to a neutral, forward-looking position. The most dramatic of the drug-induced acute dystonias is opisthotonos (Gk, *opistho*, behind+*tonos*, tension) in which the extensor muscles of the axial spine and extremities are acutely contracted such that the only contact with the floor is the occiput and the heels – a bridging or arching posture.

Tic (Fr, from It, *ticchio*) is the term used to describe a rapid, involuntary, repetitive movement of small muscles, such as it can involve the muscles of facial expression. Common tics are throat clearing, blinking, and nose twitching. Tics often disappear during sleep, and can be exacerbated in frequency with anxiety. It is common for persons with tics to describe increasing emotional discomfort the longer they consciously suppress a tic, which discomfort is relieved when they allow the tic to reemerge.

Complex, repetitive, voluntary movements of larger muscle groups are referred to as *stereotypies* (pronounced "stereo-TIP-eez") (Gk, *stereos*, hard or fixed+type). Stereotypies can involve many muscle groups, including muscles involved in speech. They can appear almost mechanical in their repetition and can be difficult for a patient to consciously suppress. A stereotypy can take the form of assuming a particular posture, movements that appear almost purposeful (crossing and uncrossing legs, periodic rubbing a body part not due to pain, rocking, arm flapping), or utterances as one might observe in Tourette's syndrome. Abusers of methamphetamine or amphetamines may engage in sterotypies that involve picking at their skin, excessive grooming, and disassembling and reassembling or plucking at things. These stereotypies are sometimes referred to in the addiction community as *tweaking* or *punding*. Tweaking may also occur in patients treated for Parkinson's disease with ₗ-DOPA.

Chorea, or choreia, (Gk, *choreia*, a circle dance) is used to describe brief, irregular contractions that are not repetitive or rhythmic, but appear to flow from one muscle to the next [5]. Chorea is common in Huntington's disease, but can also occur following infection with group A beta-hemolytic streptococci (GABHS) which cause rheumatic fever; some cases of which can present with *Sydenham chorea*, which is characterized by rapid, irregular, and aimless involuntary movements of the arms and legs, trunk, and facial muscles, affecting females more often and typically occurring between the ages of 5 and 15 years. The etiology is likely via an autoimmune reaction from infection-induced antibodies that attack neurons [6]. Chorea can also present in Wilson's disease, can be drug-induced (dopamine agonists and antagonists, and anticonvulsants), or can be due to cerebrovascular accidents.

Not infrequently, chorea is accompanied by *athetosis* (Gk, *a*+*thetos*, not placed), which is the term used to describe writhing, twisting movements involving multiple muscle groups. When chorea is accompanied by athetosis, the term *choreoathetosis* is used.

One aspect of a patient's motor behavior typically observed by pain physicians is gait. A normal gait includes a reasonable stride length, a fluid shift from leg to leg, a moderate arm swing, and an upright or nearly upright posture. A common gait abnormality encountered in care of persons with pain is referred to as *antalgic* (literally, "against pain," in clinical use, "pain avoiding") gait which is characterized by limping, guarding, one lower extremity consistently moving more rapidly than the contralateral extremity to reduce the amount of time weight is borne on the painful side, or significant flexion of the lumbar spine or hips, any of which is done to avoid or minimize pain on ambulation. Ankylosing spondylitis resulting in a fused vertebral column presents with the so-called *simian* ("apelike") gait in which there is prominent, fixed flexion of the spine, which pitches the upper body well forward of the feet. A simian gait, because of the forward position of the torso, is also characterized by arms dangling in front of the feet. A person with a simian gait who is wearing a coat or jacket may not be able to see their feet because the forward position of the torso causes the jacket to drape in front of the person and obscures their view of their feet. This can, of course, make the person prone to trips and falls, especially when descending stairs.

An *ataxic* gait is an unsteady or uncoordinated manner of walking that often includes a *broad-based* gait (i.e., the lateral distance between the feet is greater than normal and often exceeds the shoulder-to-shoulder width). Ataxic gaits can result from inherited or acquired neurodegenerative conditions (e.g., Friedreich's ataxia, cerebellar ataxia from inhalant toxicity), acute or chronic drug exposure (e.g., ethanol, benzodiazepines), may be due to conditions affecting the vestibular system (e.g., Meniere's disease, drug-induced vertigo from calcium antagonists, orthostatic hypotension), or may be due to cerebrovascular disease.

A *festinating* gait is characterized by short, staccato, accelerating steps in an effort to move forward, almost as if the person is falling forward in order to move and they are having trouble making their feet keep pace with their body. It is often seen in Parkinsonian conditions, as well as other neurological syndromes.

Fortunately, neurologic complications from *syphilis* infection are currently rare in the USA, but its prevalence is rising. Persons who have *tabes dorsalis* (peripheral neuropathy, ataxia, autonomic dysfunction) have a characteristic gait due to dorsal column disease causing them to lose proprioception. The tabetic gait is characterized by several distinct components – an inordinate degree of hip flexion, resulting in a high lift of the knee (to ensure that the foot clears the floor, since the lack of proprioception prevents the person from sensing if their ankle is flexed or extended), followed by a forceful "slapping" of the foot on the floor wherein the entire plantar surface contacts the floor at or nearly at once

(instead of a normal gait, wherein the heel strikes the floor and the rest of the sole "rolls" down to the floor as weight is shifted). The forceful slapping, in addition to accommodating for a partial or complete foot drop, also provides a supranormal amount of proprioception, so that the person perceives some feedback with regard to position in space, even though dorsal columnar function is impaired. Dorsal spinal space tumors, hematomas, and infection can cause a tabetic-like presentation. Persons with unilateral foot drop, due to tibial nerve injury or early amyotrophic lateral sclerosis, may exhibit features of a tabetic-like gait only in the affected extremity.

A *hemiplegic* gait, as might be seen following a cerebrovascular accident, is typified by lower extremity circumduction (swinging it laterally as it is brought forward) and exaggerated hip flexion, both of which combine to ensure the foot clears the floor. A *spastic* gait is that in which the lower extremities are stiff and do not flex normally, causing a "stiff-legged" walking pattern.

Affect and Mood

Surprisingly, there is some disagreement over the precise constructs referred to as *affect* and *mood*. Some authors consider mood to be a parameter of affect (e.g., "affect is the emotional tone underlying all behaviors" and "mood is only one facet of affect") [7]. Other authors prefer the convention of affect being the immediately observable expression of emotion which typically changes during a conversation, while mood is the prevailing or underlying emotional state. In other words, affect is to weather as mood is to climate. For example, a person could be in a bad mood, yet still respond with an affective change to something they found very humorous [8]. Others would describe them by analogy, as mood being the channel a person is watching on television, while affect is the color saturation of the image (Ray A, 2011, personal communication).

The parameters of affect that are typically described include the range, amplitude, stability, appropriateness, and ability to relate to the examiner (which is inferred from the affect observed).

Range of affect refers to the person's emotional repertoire. A person who does not react much to various emotionally laden comments during a clinical encounter would be described as having a *constricted* range, whereas a *full* range of affect is the societal norm. With a full range of affect, the person exhibits transient changes in the immediate emotional state the course of an interaction (e.g., frowning when describing the intensity and impact of their pain, furrowing their brow while listening intently to counseling instructions, and smiling at the conclusion of the visit as they are leaving the office and saying their goodbyes).

Amplitude, or intensity, is the degree to which a particular affective vector is expressed. The difference between a chuckle and guffaw is a difference in range along the same vector, as is the difference between indicating annoyance with a scowling expression and screaming at someone, which is an affective vector of a very different nature than laughing. Affect may be of normal amplitude, exaggerated (e.g., in mania or intoxication with certain substances), diminished, blunted, or *flat* (e.g., schizophrenics, when their psychotic symptoms are not prominent, exhibit a marked and characteristic reduction in affective amplitude).

Stability refers to the rapidity with which the affect changes during a clinical encounter. If the person is doing well, with their pain under good control, it is likely that their affect will be relatively stable. If, on the other hand, a person is laughing or smiling one moment, crying the next, and appears irritable the next, their affect is described as *labile*. Labile affect can be observed in drug-induced conditions (e.g., steroid use, intoxication) or in idiopathic or reactive mental diagnoses, such as depression, mania, or dementia.

Appropriateness refers to the degree of correlation of affect to the content of conversation or situation. Usually, what is appropriate for the examiner is appropriate for the patient. Therefore, if the patient describes getting into a serious automobile accident in which they and others were injured and is smiling during the description, the patient's affect would be described as *inappropriate*.

The *ability to relate* to the examiner refers to the patient's ability to express emotional warmth, establish rapport, and interact with the examiner. When a patient does this, they are described *relating well*. When a patient remains cold or unfeeling and no rapport is apparent, they are described as exhibiting *relating poorly*. Due to the flat affect that characterizes schizophrenia, examiners typically describe a poor ability to relate. Historically, this was referred to as the *praecox feeling*, a reference to an obsolete term once used to describe schizophrenia, *dementia praecox* (premature dementia, i.e., "dementia" occurring in a young person, when schizophrenia typically manifests) [9].

Mood is the prevailing or underlying emotional state being experienced by the patient. Mood generally falls into one of these classifications: sad, happy, angry, anxious, or apathetic. A person who has what is considered a normal mood is described as *euthymic* (Gk, *eu*, true or normal + *thymia*, mood; ancient practitioners believed the function of the thymus gland was to control mood). Mood on the depressed side of normal is designated as *dysthymic*. Excessive mood on the happy side of euthymia is referred to as *hypomania* (Gk, *hypo*, beneath or under + via L, *mania*, loss of reason, from Gk, *mainesthai*, to rage).

Anger is a common concomitant of chronic, unrelenting pain [10]. It is strongly related to self-reported assessments of pain intensity, pain behaviors, and perceived pain interference in activities of daily living. In the person with chronic pain, anger is often diffuse and nondirected, such that they lash out at the examiner for asking a simple question. This is often followed by guilt, which can then contribute to sadness.

Anxiety often occurs in patients with acute or chronic pain [11]. As noted at the beginning of the chapter, it may antedate, co-occur, or follow the onset of a chronic pain condition.

Depression and depressive spectrum disorders (pervasive sad mood, loss of interest in social interactions, etc., but not to the degree as is seen in clinically diagnosable depression) frequently accompany persistent pain [11].

Suicidality should be regularly assessed as part of the mental status examination of persons with persistent pain [12–18]. Depression is prevalent among this population, and it, coupled with the loss of hope that so commonly occurs as a result of repeated treatment failures, can cause patients with chronic pain to have thoughts of killing themselves. Treatments used for certain chronic or recurrent conditions (e.g., β-adrenergic antagonists for migraine prophylaxis) can also cause depression through alteration of the brain neurochemistry, as can antidepressants, themselves, as noted in the boxed warning most antidepressants now carry. The motivation for suicidal thoughts can range from ideas of stopping suffering once and for all, to simply giving up ("I just don't have the energy to go on."), to getting even with someone who the person feels has wronged them ("I'll show them!"). The assessment of suicidality is often overlooked or avoided by practitioners not trained in the behavioral sciences. Inquiring about suicide does not increase the risk of suicidal thoughts [19]. Since the best predictor of future risk of successful suicide is a history of suicide attempts, it is important to assess this in providing clinical pain care. When assessing and characterizing suicidal thoughts and behaviors, one should document *suicidal ideation* (i.e., *thoughts* of suicide), *suicidal plans* (the more detailed and thought-out the plan, the greater the risk of completion), *suicidal intent* (a person could have thought about suicide and formulated a plan, but have no intent to carry it out), *suicidal threats* (i.e., communication to others of the intent to commit suicide – sometimes used to manipulate, sometimes a serious plea for help), *suicidal gestures* (i.e., actions without lethal intent that are intended to appear lethal – which may also be manipulation or a genuine call for help), or *suicidal attempts* (i.e., actions with sincere intent to end one's life). The process of suicidal thoughts represents a psychiatric emergency and should be referred immediately to a psychiatrist/hospital emergency department for further assessment.

Similarly, *homicidal* ideation or plans should be assessed [20]. Unfortunately, a not uncommon occurrence is the plan of a desperate person to "take out" someone they hold responsible for harm or wrong, followed by taking their own life or, in some cases, "suicide by police" (constructing a situation in which there is a high probability that the police will use lethal force to protect the public or themselves). Case law has established an affirmative duty to protect the intended victim when the examiner believes the homicidal threat is credible [21].

Thought Processes and Content

The content of a patient's thoughts and their thought processes are inferred largely from their speech, although some other behaviors may provide clues to thought content or process (e.g., a person suffering from paranoid delusions may present as electively mute, anxious, and hypervigilant with an exaggerated startle response). Thought processes refer to how the patient is thinking; what the patient is thinking (talking) about is called content.

Speech qualities that can be characterized include *spontaneity*, *rate*, *amount*, *rhythm*, *articulation*, *idiosyncratic* word usage, and the tightness and form of *associations*.

Spontaneous speech is typical in a normal clinical interaction; however, the lack of spontaneity, as with all mental status signs, must be interpreted in the totality of the presentation. As with eye contact, in some cultures, a sign of deference to an authority figure is to "speak only when spoken to." Thus, the lack of spontaneous speech in a person from such a culture, in the absence of other findings, may be of no clinical significance from the standpoint of assessing their mental state.

The *rate* of speech can be described as normal, slow, or rapid. *Pressured speech* refers to the behavior which results from an apparent drive to keep talking. A person with pressured speech is difficult to interrupt. Persons with pressured speech often "do all the talking" (i.e., in addition to the rate and uninterruptability of speech, the *amount* of speech is also abnormal) or appear that their thoughts are coming faster than their mouth can get them out. In the latter presentation, the presence of *racing thoughts* can be inferred. Racing thoughts are common in mania, whether endogenous (e.g., bipolar disorder) or drug-induced (e.g., methamphetamine abuse). Abnormally slow or labored speech can be a feature of benzodiazepine or opioid toxicity [22].

Most patients speak with a *normal rhythm*; however, certain clinical conditions exhibit unusual rhythm of speech. *Scanning speech*, where certain words or syllables are stressed, producing a slow, sliding cadence is observed in multiple sclerosis. *Hesitant speech* can accompany Huntington's disease. Persons with early Huntington's disease or other incipient dementias can appear normal until exposed to drugs with antimuscarinic properties, after which the disease will become manifest. *Staccato speech*, which is abrupt and clipped, can be present in temporal lobe epilepsy. *Stuttering or stammering speech* can be a persistent problem for some persons. The acute onset of stammering during a

procedure, however, may be an indication of systemic toxicity of a local anesthetic.

Articulation, or the accuracy with which syllables and words are pronounced, can be affected by numerous diseases and drugs. Acute intoxication with ethanol, sedative-hypnotics, or marijuana can induce *slurring of speech* (a form of *dysarthria*). Cerebrovascular accidents in different parts of the brain can affect most speech in various ways, including the ability to articulate words.

Some patients may use words or word-like sounds in idiosyncratic ways. A person who repeatedly uses approximations of or substitution of correct words is described as having *paraphasia* (Gk, *para*, to one side of + *phrasein*, to utter). In *verbal* or *semantic paraphasia*, there is a complete word substitution (e.g., the person says "dog" when referring to a photograph of a cat). *Literal* or *phonemic paraphasia* is characterized by substitution or addition of syllables ("phonemes") or letters (e.g., the use of "rice" instead of "nice" or "shoots" to mean "shoes"). The term *neologism* is used to describe a new word created by the patient. Neologisms often sound-like words or are composed of parts of existing words. The apparent meaning of a neologism may vary during a conversation. Anomia (Gk, *a* + L, *nom*, name), or nominal aphasia, refers to the inability to find the right word for an object. A person with expressive anomia when asked, "Can you tell me what this is?" (with the examiner pointing to their watch), may answer, "Oh, it's … you know … it's …, it's a time-telling thing." Paraphasic speech often indicates an organic brain lesion, such as a cerebrovascular accident, but can also be observed in some primary mental disorders. When caused by the former, the type of dysfluency of speech can facilitate anatomic localization of the lesion. *Complete aphasia* is the apparent inability to speak despite an effort to do so (as contrasted with *elective mutism*, where the examiner has reason to believe the person can speak, but is choosing not to). Complete aphasia is most commonly due to cerebrovascular accidents.

The *tightness and form of associations* refer to the way in which ideas or concepts are linked together. Normal speech manifests tight associational linkages, that is, each element of speech is logically linked to the previous ones and the thought behind the speech is goal-directed. In some conditions, there is a disruption of the tightness of association, which is referred to as *loose association*. The form of thought disorder can be partially determined by where the loosening of the association occurs. In the most severe form, called *word salad*, sometimes called *gibberish*, or *jargon* (old Fr, *jargoun*, gibberish) speech, the loosening of associations occurs between words, such that consecutive words seem to have no relationship (e.g., "red up tolerable cloud fine want"). *Fragmentation* is defined as a loosening of associations that occurs between clauses or sentences. In fragmentation, a person begins to relate a thought in a sequential, coherent manner, but winds up changing the content within a sentence or a paragraph. *Derailment* refers to a sudden switch from one line of thinking to a new parallel line of thought. A *non sequitur* (L, "it does not follow") refers to a totally unrelated response. *Flight of ideas* is characterized by rapid switching of the line of thought which may be somewhat understandable but is often interpreted as reflecting the patient's distraction by external or internal stimuli. *Circumstantial speech*, also called *circumlocution* (L, *circum*, around + *locutio*, speech), has tightly linked associations, but contains extraneous, nonessential material that is interspersed throughout before ultimately reaching its goal. *Tangential speech* refers a series of tightly linked associations which never reach a goal.

Thought content can be inferred by listening to and probing the drive behind speech content. A patient's thought content may indicate preoccupation with a particular issue, paranoia, guilt, shame, etc. A *delusion* is a fixed, false belief, which is held by the person despite evidence to the contrary. The presence of delusions is considered to represent a *psychotic* state (i.e., an inability to relate to reality). Delusions are described by their content, for example, *delusions of guilt*, *persecutory delusions*, *religious delusions*, etc. *Perceptual disorders* are those in which there is an abnormality manifesting as a report of alteration of or interference with one of the senses. A hallucination is a perception in any sensory modality in the absence of a stimulus. When a patient reports having a hallucination while fully awake with a clear *sensorium* (consciousness and connectedness to the environment), he or she is said to have reported a psychotic symptom. Hallucinations can be *visual* (most commonly encountered with intoxication (e.g., antimuscarinic toxicity), withdrawal (e.g., ethanol), or diffuse Lewy body disease, which typically presents with the triad of dementia, Parkinson's syndrome, and psychosis, involving delusions and hallucinations, especially visual ones), *auditory* (the most prevalent type of hallucination in idiopathic psychotic disorders, such as schizophrenia), *olfactory*, *gustatory* (reports of which can also be due to *candidiasis*, vitamin or mineral deficiency (e.g., zinc), medications, or pyorrhea), or *tactile*, or *haptic*, a particular form of which *formication* (L, *formica*, ant), is association with abuse of certain substances ("*coke* (or *crack*) *bugs*," or ethanol withdrawal) and is so named because the person reports the sensation of ants or other insects crawling on or underneath their skin [23]. With the so-called phenomenon of coke bugs, rarely does the individual report actually seeing the insects (which would be a visual hallucination) or report believing that there are bugs crawling beneath the skin (which would be a delusion). When a hallucination is present, it is important to explore it further to determine its form; for example, an olfactory hallucination of the smell of sulfur or burning rubber may indicate the presence of a temporal lobe lesion. Also, hearing voices telling the patient to kill himself or somebody else clearly has important implications in terms of intervention. Auditory hallucinations that are ordering a person to do something are referred to as *command hallucinations*. Most people have experienced at some time a specific kind of hallucination usually during the transition period between sleep and wakefulness. A hallucination while falling asleep is called a *hypnagogic* (Gk, *hypno*, sleep + *agogos*, leading) hallucination, and a hallucination that occurs while awakening is called *hypnopompic* (Gk, *hypno*, sleep + *pompe*, sending forth) hallucination. These can emerge or become more prevalent when a person is taking medicines that alter sleep architecture, especially those that cause REM sleep rebound, such as tricyclic antidepressants.

Because so many drugs have significant antimuscarinic properties, especially in situations of multiple medications or overdoses, the pain clinician should be aware of the presentations of persons so affected [24, 25]. Drugs with antimuscarinic properties include some antidepressants (e.g., tricyclic antidepressants), skeletal muscle relaxants (e.g., cyclobenzaprine), medicines used for urinary incontinence (e.g., oxybutynin), antidiarrheals (e.g., diphenoxylate + atropine), antiemetics (e.g., promethazine, transdermal scopolamine), antipsychotics (e.g., chlorpromazine), drugs used to treat dopamine antagonist-induced movement disorders or Parkinson's disease (e.g., benztropine), cardiovascular drugs (e.g., nifedipine), antispasmodics (e.g., dicyclomine), antiulcer drugs (e.g., cimetidine), and antihistamines (both prescription and over-the-counter). The features of the antimuscarinic syndrome can include tachycardia; blurred vision (especially difficulty with accommodation); worsening of narrow-angle glaucoma; larger than normal pupils; visual hallucinations or other psychotic symptoms and signs; delirium; impaired memory; ataxia; hyperthermia; urinary retention; constipation; xerostomia; fever; and warm, red, and dry skin. All these effects are mediated by blockade of the actions of acetylcholine upon muscarinic receptors.

If a person misperceives a real sensory stimulus, the reported perception is called an *illusion*. For this same reason, magicians who do coin tricks, etc., are referred to as illusionists because adults know the coin has not, in fact, disappeared, but our eyes tell us it did. An illusion is often associated with an intense affective state (e.g., when walking past a cemetery at midnight, one may perceive shadows to be objects).

Assessment of *intellect* can be initially done during the general conversation with the patient. Noted are whether the patient's vocabulary is consistent with their educational background. The ability to think abstractly and form concepts by the use of words, numbers, and other symbols is also assessed. Subtraction of serial sevens from 100 to 75 is a way to assess the patient's ability to concentrate. If the person has difficulty with the arithmetic, one can assess concentration by asking them to add 3 to 20, and then keep adding 3 to the resultant sum. A useful clinical tool is the mini-mental state exam, which is a brief, structured, valid procedure to assess cognitive function, when impairment is suspected from the clinical encounter [26]. The MMSE is sensitive to changes in cognitive function, such as might occur when a person is recovering from a concussion or drug-induced cognitive decrements.

Memory is typically assessed conversationally by paying attention to the person's ability to recall for recent and remote events. If impairment of memory is suspected during the interview, a more formal assessment of memory can easily be performed in the clinical setting. Memory functions are generally divided into *registration, immediate recall*, and *long-term recall*. The ability to register information can be tested by naming three unrelated objects and asking the patient to repeat them as soon as you finish. Once that has occurred, ask the patient to remember those three objects while you continue the interview. The continuation of the interview serves as a distraction, preventing them from simply repeating the names of the objects to themselves repeatedly. About three minutes later, ask the patient to repeat those objects named earlier, which assesses *immediate recall*. Long-term memory can be assessed by asking them to recall the last three US presidents or some similar well-known but sequential information that spans several years. People with organic causes for memory gaps will sometimes fill in those gaps with so-called false memories, which they believe to be real. This is referred to as *confabulation* [27–29].

Fibromyalgia syndrome and chronic fatigue syndrome are both associated with a particular, but vaguely defined, cluster of cognitive deficits known among patients as "brain fog" [30]. Interestingly, neuropsychological testing does not always confirm the degree of memory dysfunction reported by patients. Recent research suggests that short-term memory is worsened by distraction in persons with fibromyalgia syndrome, which may explain common complaints in this population, such as, "I walk from the kitchen to the living room to get something and then can't remember what I went to get" [31].

Judgment refers to the ability to evaluate various situations and information and reach an effective conclusion. Decisions about the patient's real-life situations are the best way to evaluate judgment. Asking the patient, "What are you going to tell your boss about this?" or "What are your plans for dealing with this problem?" assists in evaluating the patient's judgment. Judgment is described as good, fair, or poor. Some choose to describe judgment as intact or impaired and modify how impaired it is, for example, mildly impaired, moderately impaired, or severely impaired.

Performing the 5-MSEPP

As can be inferred from the information presented in this chapter, much of the 5-MSEPP is accomplished merely by being attuned to the patient's presentation during the clinical encounter and using precise terminology to document it. In actual practice, observing and describing various aspects of mental functioning do not add much time to a typical interac-

tion. Yet, doing so can have important ramifications for clinical care, as well as in the medicolegal realm.

Documentation of findings is relatively simple and can constitute one additional paragraph in the progress note. For example, during asking how a person is doing since the last visit, one can make many observations. It is human nature to only recall or document those observations which catch one's attention. However, it is just as important in a clinical practice dealing with persons in pain to document normal findings, instead of believing that someone else reading a progress note in which normal findings were not documents will assume they were observed and interpreted as within normal limits. Thus, for an uncomplicated visit in a patient with low back pain and unilateral, chronic lumbar radiculopathy who is stable on a medication regimen, a typical 5-MMSEPP comment would be:

> The patient is alert and oriented in all spheres (or: oriented × 4, which refers to person, place, time, and situation). They are well-nourished, well-developed, dressed appropriately, and well-groomed. The patient relates well, and affect is slightly constricted, stable, and appropriate. Mood is slightly depressed. Speech is fluid, articulate, and reveals no indication of disorder of thought process or content. Memory appears intact × 3 (referring to registration, immediate recall, and long-term recall). Judgment appears unimpaired. Other than an antalgic gait, favoring the affected side, there is no evidence of abnormal motor activity. The patient denies suicidal and homicidal ideation at this time.

Conclusion

The astute pain practitioner unwittingly performs aspects of a mental status examination as part of everyday clinical encounters. Learning the material presented in this chapter and incorporating a conscious assessment of these parameters into routine pain care will translate to better diagnoses, improved documentation, more precise and thorough documentation, and enhanced care for patients presenting with pain.

References

1. Pull CB, Cloos J-M, Pull-Erpelding M-C. Clinical assessment instruments in psychiatry. In: Maj M, Gaebel W, López-Ibor JJ, Sartorius N, editors. Psychiatric diagnosis and classification. Chichester: Wiley; 2002.
2. Galanti G-A. Caring for patients from different cultures. Philadelphia: University of Pennsylvania Press; 2004. p. 33–4. http://books.google.com/books?id=nVgeOxUL3cYC&pg=PA34#v=onepage&q&f=false. Accessed 2 Oct 2011.
3. Teal CR, Street RL. Critical elements of culturally competent communication in the medical encounter: a review and model. Soc Sci Med. 2009;68:533–43.
4. Tindall SC. Level of consciousness. In: Walker HK, Hall WD, Hurst JW, editors. Clinical methods: the history, physical, and laboratory examinations. 3rd ed. Boston: Butterworths; 1990. p. 296–9. http://www.ncbi.nlm.nih.gov/books/NBK380/#A1732. Accessed 2 Oct 2011.

5. NINDS. Chorea information page. http://www.ninds.nih.gov/disorders/chorea/chorea.htm. Accessed 2 Oct 2011.
6. NINDS. Sydenham chorea information page. http://www.ninds.nih.gov/disorders/sydenham/sydenham.htm. Accessed 2 Oct 2011.
7. Taylor MA. The neuropsychiatric mental status examination. New York: SP Medical & Scientific Books; 1981. p. 36–8.
8. Sadock BJ, Sadock VA, Ruiz P. Kaplan & Sadock's comprehensive textbook of psychiatry. 9th ed. Philadelphia: Lippincott Williams & Wilkins; 2009. 1083p.
9. Ungvaria GS, Xianga Y-T, Hong Y, et al. Diagnosis of schizophrenia: reliability of an operationalized approach to 'praecox-feeling'. Psychopathology. 2010;43:292–9.
10. Bruehl S, Burns JW, Chung OY, Chont M. Pain-related effects of trait anger expression: neural substrates and the role of endogenous opioid mechanisms. Neurosci Biobehav Rev. 2009;33:475–91.
11. Tsang A, von Korff M, Lee S, et al. Common chronic pain conditions in developed and developing countries: gender and age differences and comorbidity with depression-anxiety disorders. J Pain. 2008;9(10):883–91.
12. Fishbain DA. The association of chronic pain and suicide. Semin Clin Neuropsychiatry. 1999;4(3):221–7.
13. Cheatle MD. Depression, chronic pain, and suicide by overdose: on the edge. Pain Med. 2011;12:S43–8.
14. Edwards RR, Smith MT, Kudel I, Haythornthwaite J. Pain-related catastrophizing as a risk factor for suicidal ideation in chronic pain. Pain. 2006;126:272–9.
15. Ilgen MA, Zivin K, McCammon RJ, Valenstein M. Pain and suicidal thoughts, plans and attempts in the United States. Gen Hosp Psychiatry. 2008;30:521–7.
16. Braden JB, Sullivan MD. Suicidal thoughts and behavior among adults with self-reported pain conditions in the National Comorbidity Survey Replication. J Pain. 2008;9(12):1106–15.
17. Smith MT, Edwards RR, Robinson RC, Dworkin RH. Suicidal ideation, plans, and attempts in chronic pain patients: factors associated with increased risk. Pain. 2004;111:201–8.
18. Tang NKY, Crane C. Suicidality in chronic pain: a review of the prevalence, risk factors and psychological links. Psychol Med. 2006;36:575–86.
19. Gould MS, Frank A, Marrocco FA, Kleinman M, et al. Evaluating iatrogenic risk of youth suicide screening programs: a randomized controlled trial. JAMA. 2005;293(13):1635–43.
20. Fishbain DA, Bruns D, Lewis JE, et al. Predictors of homicide – suicide affirmation in acute and chronic pain patients. Pain Med. 2011;12:127–37.
21. Tarasoff v. Regents of the University of California, 17 Cal. 3d 425, 551 P.2d 334, 131 Cal. Rptr. 14 (Cal. 1976).
22. Mokhlesi B, Leiken JB, Murray P, Corbridge TC. General approach to the intoxicated patient. Part I. Chest. 2003;123:577–92.
23. Crack Cocaine. http://www.cesar.umd.edu/cesar/drugs/crack.asp. Accessed 2 Oct 2011.
24. Mokhlesi B, Leiken JB, Murray P, Corbridge TC. General approach to the intoxicated patient. Part II. Chest. 2003;123:897–922.
25. Examples of medications with anticholinergic properties. In: Center for Medicare and Medicaid Services. State operations manual, appendix PP – Guidance to surveyors for long term care facilities. p. 410–412. https://cms.gov/manuals/Downloads/som107ap_pp_guidelines_ltcf.pdf. Accessed 2 Oct 2011.
26. Folstein MF, Folstein SE, McHugh PR. Mini-mental state. A practical method for grading the cognitive state of patients for the clinician. J Psychiatr Res. 1975;12(3):189–98.
27. DeLuca J, Cicerone KD. Confabulation following aneurysm of the anterior communicating artery. Cortex. 1991;27(3):417–23.
28. Gundogar D, Demirci S. Multiple sclerosis presenting with fantastic confabulation. Gen Hosp Psychiatry. 2006;28(5):448–51.
29. Schnider A. Spontaneous confabulation, reality monitoring, and the limbic system – a review. Brain Res Rev. 2001;36:150–60.
30. Jason LA, Boulton A, Porter NS, et al. Classification of myalgic encephalomyelitis/chronic fatigue syndrome by types of fatigue. Behav Med. 2010;36(1):24–31.
31. Leavitt F, Katz RS. Distraction as a key determinant of impaired memory in patients with fibromyalgia. J Rheumatol. 2006;33(1):127–32.

The Psychological Assessment of Patients with Chronic Pain

Daniel Bruns and John Mark Disorbio

Key Points

- There is strong evidence that the biopsychosocial model does not apply only to dysfunctional patients with chronic pain, but rather represents the inherent nature of pain.
- There is strong evidence that psychological tests are scientifically as valid and reliable as medical tests with regard to diagnostics and predicting a patient's response to treatments for pain.
- As many payors and guidelines require psychological evaluations prior to authorizing certain treatments for pain, pain clinics increasingly use some form of psychological assessment.
- While there are a large number of psychometric questionnaires used to assess patients with chronic pain, only a few have undergone the rigorous process required to become standardized tests, and these are reviewed.
- Both evidence and opinion are converging on a set of psychosocial variables that should be assessed when treating patients with chronic pain, and these can all be organized within a biopsychosocial "vortex" paradigm.
- A standardized method of psychological assessment can identify patients who are at low, moderate, and high risk, and this is illustrated with three case vignettes.

Introduction

There is strong evidence that the biopsychosocial model does not apply only to dysfunctional patients with chronic pain, but rather represents the inherent nature of pain. Research has determined that psychological tests are scientifically as valid and reliable as medical tests with regard to diagnostics and predicting a patient's response to treatments for pain. As many payers and guidelines now require psychological evaluations prior to authorizing certain treatments for pain, pain clinics increasingly use some form of psychological assessment. While there are a large number of psychometric questionnaires used to assess patients with chronic pain, only a few have undergone the rigorous process required to become standardized tests, and these are reviewed. Both evidence and opinion are converging on a set of psychosocial variables that should be assessed when treating patients with chronic pain, and these can all be organized within a biopsychosocial "vortex" paradigm. A standardized method of psychological assessment can identify patients who are at low, moderate, and high risk, and this is illustrated with three case vignettes.

A review of the research reveals strong evidence that pain is a biopsychosocial phenomena, having biological, psychological, and social components [2, 3]. In addition to biological components of pain being the product of pathophysiology, the experience and report of pain are also strongly influenced by psychosocial factors. As the IASP notes, while pain often has a physical cause, pain can also occur in the absence of any likely pathophysiological explanation. Further, since pain is a subjective, psychological

D. Bruns, PsyD (✉)
Health Psychology Associates,
1610 29th Avenue Place, Suite 200, Greeley, CO 80634, USA
e-mail: daniel.bruns@healthpsych.com

J.M. Disorbio, EdD
Independent Practice,
225 Union Blvd. Suite 150, Lakewood, CO 80228, USA
e-mail: jmdisorbio@earthlink.net

T.R. Deer et al. (eds.), *Comprehensive Treatment of Chronic Pain by Medical, Interventional, and Integrative Approaches*,
DOI 10.1007/978-1-4614-1560-2_75, © American Academy of Pain Medicine 2013

state, we are dependent on the patient's report of pain to guide our treatments [1]. However, there are a variety of psychological and social variables that affect what patients say about their pain.

The Natural History of Biopsychosocial Pain Disorders

The biopsychosocial model does not apply only to dysfunctional patients with chronic pain, but rather represents the inherent nature of pain [2, 3]. Over the natural history of chronic pain disorders, the biological, psychological, and social aspects of these conditions interact in complex ways. Some psychosocial factors may lead to the onset of a pain condition, while others may arise as a reaction to a pain condition. The subsequent medical treatment of chronic pain may also be complicated by interactions with preexisting psychological vulnerabilities or conflicts in the social environment. Thus, complex biopsychosocial pain disorders do not simply appear, but rather tend to evolve over the course of their natural history.

Psychosocial Factors That Lead to the Onset of Pain Conditions

A variety of psychosocial factors have been associated with the onset of a variety of medical painful conditions (Fig. 75.1). Life stress has been associated with the onset of musculoskeletal pain [4, 5] and functional gastrointestinal pain [6], and one prospective study of workers found that the variable most predictive of the future report of back pain was job dissatisfaction [7].

Psychological dysfunction can also lead to the onset of painful conditions. A systematic review of the literature determined that risk-taking is influenced by mood and personality disorder, and associated with an increased chance of injury [8], while another study determined that risk-taking is influenced by personality type [9]. One study found that half of all traumatic brain injury hospitalizations were associated with alcohol intoxication [10], while another study found that patients reporting drug or alcohol abuse were more likely to sustain violent injuries [11]. Consequently, it is not surprising that some research has found that the prevalence of substance abuse disorders in patients with chronic pain is twice as high as that observed in the normal population [12]. Another study of patients being treated in an interventional pain medicine setting explored the prevalence of substance abuse problems. Of those patients with a prior history of drug abuse, 34 % of those who were being treated with controlled substances for pain were simultaneously abusing illicit drugs [13].

Overall, a multitude of psychosocial variables may influence lifestyle, risk-taking behaviors, and health habits that can act to increase or decrease the risk of onset of a medical condition.

Psychological Reactions to a Pain Condition

Serious illness and injury are often life-altering conditions, with a profound psychosocial impact (Fig. 75.1). Not surprisingly, in a study of patients with pain-related disability, 64 % reported one or more diagnosable psychiatric disorders, compared to a prevalence of 15 % in the general population. In this sample, the prevalence of major depression was 25 times higher than that seen in the general population. This finding is especially significant as even minimal levels of depression have been associated with increased rates of service utilization [14] and poorer adherence to treatment [15]. In many cases, though, the direction of the arrow of causality is not clear. For example, while in some cases, depression could be a reaction to a severe injury, in other cases, depression that preexisted an injury may increase the risk that the pain will become chronic [16].

Pain can alternately be associated with anxiety, depression, or anger, depending upon how pain is perceived [17]. Laboratory experiments in pain perception suggest that the presence of depression tends to magnify the perception of pain [18]. Additionally, affective distress combines with pain to produce suffering, and ultimately, this suffering may be more closely associated with the patient's level of functioning than is the pain itself [19]. Research also suggests that a number of other psychological variables are associated with poor treatment outcome. These include anger [20, 21], neuroticism [22], psychological distress [23–27], relationship with spouse [28, 29], positive or negative perceptions prior to treatment [30–32], maladaptive beliefs [33, 34], and fears of reinjury [31].

Psychological Vulnerability Risk Factors

A review of the literature on psychopathology and chronic pain concluded that psychological vulnerabilities of various types could both increase the risk of onset of chronic pain, plus shape how the pain disorder was manifested. This review also concluded that the dominant emerging perspective is that preexisting but dormant vulnerabilities of the individual may be activated by the stress of an illness or injury [35]. If this proves to be true, this would mean that some patients are inherently at increased risk for disability, but this vulnerability may not appear until an environmental event precipitates it. Consequently, understanding preexisting vulnerabilities is an important part of chronic pain assessment (Fig. 75.1).

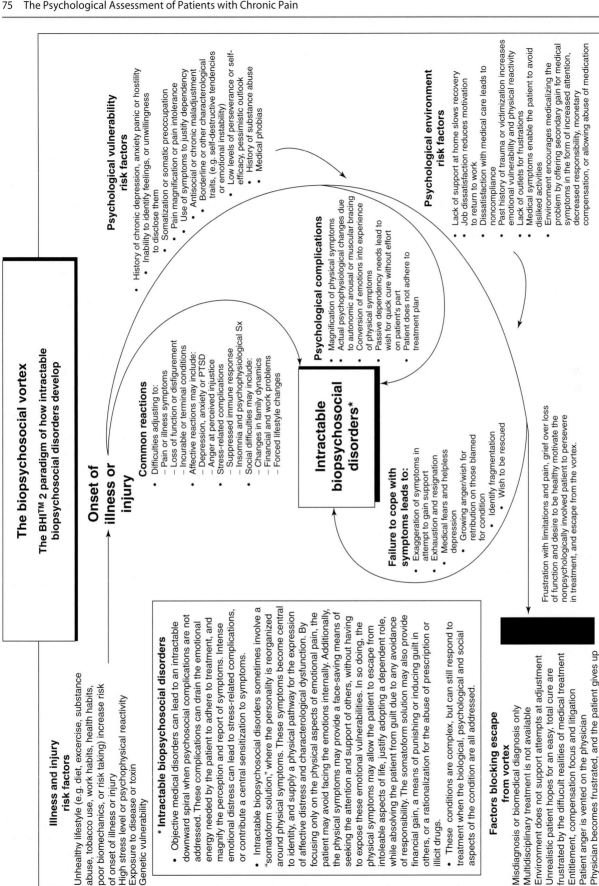

Fig. 75.1 A variety of psychosocial factors have been associated with the onset of intractable chronic pain (Biopsychosocial Vortex © 2008 by Daniel Bruns, PsyD and John Mark Disorbio, EdD. All Rights Reserved. Reprinted with permission. BHI 2 © 2003 by Pearson Assessments)

If a person who is prone to chemical dependency becomes injured, any subsequent pain could become a rationalization for excessive opioid use [36, 37]. Under such circumstances, the possibility of opioid abuse must be addressed [38]. Similarly, patients may be at increased risk for excessive opioid abuse if they are pain intolerant or feel entitled to be pain-free [39]. Although concerns about regulatory scrutiny can sometimes complicate the clinical decision-making process when prescribing opioids, carefully designed interdisciplinary programs can successfully treat patients at risk for addiction [38, 40]. One study found that patients with histories of substance abuse report higher levels of pain [41], and so distinguishing true pain from drug-seeking behavior becomes a matter of great importance [42]. Related to this, a review of the research determined that positive scores on substance abuse screening measures could identify patients who were at significantly higher risk for aberrant drug-related behaviors in treatment [43].

Patients with personality disorders may have an aberrant reaction to pain and may be at increased risk for chronicity. This hypothesis is supported by five studies of patients with chronic pain. These studies found the prevalence rate of personality disorders to range from 40 to 77 % [12, 16, 44–46], far higher than the estimated 5.9–13.5 % prevalence rate found in the general population [47]. However, a recent study reviewed psychological characteristics of patients with chronic pain and determined that a decrease in pain tends to produce a decrease in signs of personality disorder as well [48]. Thus, dysfunctional traits observed in patients with chronic pain may be partially attributable to the destabilizing effect of pain rather than to an enduring personality disorder. This suggests that estimates of personality disorders in patients with chronic pain could be spuriously inflated.

Non-characterological personality traits or cognitive styles can also constitute risk factors for recovery. For example, patients who are prone to catastrophizing [49, 50] have a low sense of self-efficacy [51], and who are prone to pessimism [52] are at risk for failing to make needed behavioral changes and for generally poor functioning. Conversely, positive personality traits such as perseverance have been found to be associated with favorable outcomes from pain conditions [53]. In general, a history of maladjustment [28], low educational level [54], or the presence of a personality disorder can undermine a patient's ability to cope satisfactorily with an illness or injury, increase the risk of noncompliance, and thus increase the risk of delayed recovery [47, 55]. Severe psychopathology may sometimes affect pain reports in mysterious ways. For example, patients with dissociative disorders often present with psychogenic pain symptoms [56, 57], and in patients with dissociative identity disturbance (multiple personality), each personality may manifest different pain and disability symptoms [58, 59].

Social Environment Risk Factors

Environmental stressors are known to be associated with numerous psychophysiological reactions (Fig. 75.1). A patient's social environment includes relationships with family, friends, professionals in the medical setting, and supervisors and coworkers in the workplace. The onset of a disabling condition can stress the family system [60, 61] and leads to family conflicts if the disability prevents the patient from performing expected family responsibilities [62, 63]. The problems arising from these changes can be overcome if the patient is a member of a healthy, supportive family. However, in response to disability, an overly solicitous family may reinforce patient passivity and encourage the patient to adopt a disabled role [64, 65], while a dysfunctional family may exacerbate a patient's condition.

For example, patients who have experienced adverse childhood experiences, such as childhood abuse, have been found to exhibit increased pituitary-adrenal and autonomic responses to stress compared with controls [66–71] and suppressed immunological resistance to cancer and infection [72–74]. These findings may help to explain the association between stress and poor surgical outcome [75], increased mortality [76–78], and slowed speed of wound recovery [79, 80] observed in numerous studies. Consistent with this, studies have found that psychological traumas in childhood are associated with a poor treatment outcome [75, 81].

Within the medical setting, research has found that the therapeutic alliance between the physician and the patient strongly influences the course of treatment [82, 83]. If the physician is perceived as competent and empathic, a positive relationship can develop. This can facilitate the flow of information between physician and patient and promote patient compliance. In contrast, these studies have found that a poor physician/patient relationship can complicate the recovery process and increase the risk of noncompliance. A history of physical or sexual abuse has also been found to increase the risk of delayed recovery [84, 85], as patients reporting a history of assault may feel more physically vulnerable, exhibit more stress-related symptomatology, and resist examinations that they find threatening [86].

Disability is most often considered in the context of the patient's ability to be gainfully employed. Consequently, the psychological assessment of disability needs to be especially sensitive to social aspects of the workplace that could influence disability behaviors. For example, escape from a disliked workplace environment may offer considerable secondary gain for the report of medical symptoms, and this may influence the course of recovery. In a longitudinal, prospective study of back pain, job dissatisfaction was determined to be the strongest predictor of future back pain reports [87]. This suggests that the avoidance of a disliked workplace may be a powerful negative reinforcer for both pain and disability behaviors [29].

In addition to avoidance of an aversive workplace, other types of reinforcers are also present in the social environment. Studies have shown that both litigation [88–93] and compensation play a role in treatment outcome [25, 88, 90, 92, 94–98]. In some contexts, an injury can socially empower a patient or increase the attention and support from others. Pain can cause the patient to be assigned to lighter job tasks in the workplace or avoid undesirable chores at home. However, once disability appears, the inability of the patient to function in the workplace often leads to financial distress [99] and a continuation of a downward spiral. Overall, it is not surprising that psychosocial variables have been found to be important predictors of the cost of medical treatment [100].

The lack of English proficiency can impact treatment outcome and disability [101] in a number of ways. The inability to speak English in the USA can make it much more difficult to communicate with caregivers, understand how to fill out paperwork, or in other ways access care. In the immigrant community, though, the effects of a lack of English proficiency may be confounded by a low level of education, and low education has been found to be a separate risk factor for poor medical treatment outcome [54].

Etiologically, while some biopsychosocial disorders have their origin in biology or pathophysiology, others have psychosocial origins. Thus, the assessment of biopsychosocial conditions requires not only assessing biomedical variables but also assessing the psychosocial aspects as well. These assessments are facilitated by the use of psychometric tools.

The Psychological Assessment of Patients with Pain

In a survey performed in 1996, some type of psychological screening was performed in about 70 % of surveyed pain clinics using implantable devices [102]. Since that time, multiple evidence-based medical guidelines have recommended psychological evaluation prior to SCS [103–105], and many insurers now require psychological assessment prior to implantation. More generally, multiple evidence-based medicine guidelines now recommend psychological evaluation for all patients with chronic pain [103–105]. As a result, a similar survey in 2005 found that 100 % of surveyed clinics used some type of psychological assessment for patients being considered for implantable devices for pain [106].

The reason for the increased use of psychological tests for patients with pain is the growing evidence of their utility. A recent extensive review of the literature compared the scientific merits of psychological tests to traditional medical tests [107]. After reviewing 125 meta-analyses and 800 samples, this seminal study concluded that psychological tests are scientifically as good as medical tests and can sometimes predict the outcome of medical treatment as well as medical tests. Specifically, this study of psychological tests concluded that (a) there is strong evidence for psychological test validity, (b) the evidence for psychological test validity is comparable to that of medical tests, (c) psychological test provides a unique source of information, and (d) psychological tests supply information beyond what can be obtained by an interview.

In the assessment of patients with back pain, psychological tests are sometimes stronger predictors of treatment outcome than medical tests. For example, a recent study found that psychometric assessment was better than either MRIs or discography in predicting future back pain disability [108] while another study found that psychosocial variables predicted delayed recovery from back pain correctly 91 % of the time, without using any medical diagnostic information [109]. Multiple research studies have shown that psychosocial factors can predict the results of lumbar surgery [28, 54, 75, 90, 110, 111] or spinal cord stimulation [112] correctly over 80 % of the time, and there is evidence that protocols which integrate psychological and medical assessments can provide improved care at reduced cost [196]. Beyond back pain, research sponsored by the World Health Organization found that psychopathology was a stronger contributor to disability than was disease severity [113].

Psychological Testing Concepts

Psychological tests are developed using the science of psychometrics, which is a mathematical approach to measuring intangible human abilities (such as intelligence or memory), traits (such as personality), and subjective experiences (such as sadness or pain). Bruns and Warren have noted that the science of psychometrics is less esoteric than it would first appear:

> Although psychometrics sounds mysterious, it is a science that Western society has come to rely on heavily. Perhaps the most common example of this is that on almost every edition of the news on television, the results of a poll are reported. Scientific surveys, which employ psychometric principals, have an established ability to accurately predict the sentiments of a population, with a known degree of error. In manner analogous to the way that scientific questioning of voters can assess their subjective opinions and predict voting behavior, standardized psychometric instruments can assess subjective states in patients that predict disability [114].

To use an analogy, before a medication is ready for clinical use, rigorous scientific testing is needed to show that it is safe and effective. Similarly, before a psychological test is ready for clinical use, it should be psychometrically *standardized*. While informal questionnaires may be developed without any scientific method at all, a standardized psychological test is developed using the psychometric principles outlined in a work called the *Standards for Educational and Psychological Testing* [115]. When a questionnaire has been developed to meet the criteria listed in the *Standards*, it is said to be a *standardized test*. Standardized tests offer an efficient and scientific means of gathering information about psychological, social, and medical variables.

To illustrate the impact of a lack of standardization, consider the numerical pain rating scale. Although it may have been used in over 1,000 research studies, it is not standardized, and the following clinical vignette illustrates the effect of this: Suppose a clinician asks a patient, "On a 1–10 scale, how would you rate your pain?" How should the clinician respond if the patient responds with the following questions:

1. What is a pain level of 10? My other doctor defines a pain level of 10 as pain like having a baby, but you say it is pain so bad I want to die. Which one is correct?
2. Rate my pain from 1 to 10? Does 1 mean no pain, or is that 0? Should I rate my pain from 0 to 10?
3. Do you mean my back pain, my leg pain, or my headaches? Or do you want the average of all three? Or maybe the highest?
4. Do you mean right this second while I am sitting? As soon as I stand up, it is worse.
5. My pain is a 5 – Is that high? What does the average patient say?

Since the numerical pain rating scale is not standardized, there is no test manual to supply the correct answer to the above questions. Consequently, the clinician could respond to the questions in any number of ways, and this would significantly influence which number the patient chooses to describe the pain. As a result, it has been noted that without a more rigorous method, scores returned by measures such as informal pain rating scales are essentially meaningless [116]. In contrast, with a standardized measure of pain like the BBHI 2, all of the above questions would have a definitive answer [117]. This illustrates the advantage of standardized tests. By imposing a carefully standardized method of asking questions, scoring the responses in a standardized way, and having a norm group to which the scores can be compared, a much more meaningful result is obtained.

Characteristics of a Standardized Test

The characteristics of standardized tests are defined in the *Standards for Educational and Psychological Testing*, which states that standardized psychological tests are characterized by having a number of features:

1. Standardized tests are developed to be used for a defined purpose and may have less applicability outside of that purpose.
2. A standardized test reduces error by having standardized testing materials, standardized administration procedures, standardized instructions, and standardized scoring and interpretation methods, and may even require a standardized type of writing instrument, such as a #2 pencil.
3. A standardized test must have evidence of validity, demonstrating that the test measures what it intends to measure (e.g., the report of medication side effects such as fatigue and weight gain can cause false-positive findings for depression on some psychological tests).
4. A standardized test must have evidence of reliability, demonstrating that if the test is administered twice in a short time frame, the results will be very similar.
5. Standardized tests use one or more reference groups called norm groups, which make it possible to have standardized scores with percentile ranks.
6. A standardized test takes steps to eliminate gender, race, age, and other biases.
7. A standardized test has an official manual that has recorded the psychometric details of the standardization process and provides the information needed to use the test appropriately.
8. The content of standardized tests is controlled by copyright and other methods and cannot be modified by end users, as this would destroy the standardization.
9. Standardized tests are subject to test security or trade secret restrictions, keeping the details of the test confidential (e.g., if the answers on an I.Q. test were made public, a test subject could appear to be a genius by studying the answers beforehand, and this would invalidate the test).

In addition to meeting the criteria specified by the *standards*, others have suggested that a standardized psychological test should also be peer reviewed, either by the Mental Measurements Yearbook [105, 118] or in a scientific journal [118].

What Psychosocial Variables Need to Be Assessed in Patients with Chronic Pain?

A recent review proposed what it termed the "convergent model" of biopsychosocial assessment. The term "convergent model" was intended to reflect that while at this time the field has yet to achieve any final determinations about how to perform biopsychosocial assessments, evidence and opinion are beginning to converge [119]. This review identified both cautionary risk factors or "yellow flags" (Table 75.1) and

Table 75.1 "Yellow flag" cautionary risk factors suggested by literature review

Type of risk	Potential cautionary factors	
Affective	Depression	
	Anger	
	Anxiety (fears, phobias, PTSD, etc.)	
Psychological vulnerability	History of substance abuse	
	Personality disorder	
	Cognitive disorder or low education	
	Poor coping	
	Diffuse somatic complaints	
Social	Conflict with physicians	
	Job dissatisfaction	
	Family dysfunction	
	History of being abused	
	Worker compensation	
	Compensation focus	
	Represented by attorney	
Biological	Pain and disability	Extreme pain
	Pain sensitivity	Dysfunctional pain cognitions
	Pain invariance	Diffuse pain
		Pain > 2 years
		Unexplained disability
	Exam	Degree to which patient does not meet medical criteria for procedure
		No medical necessity of procedure to preserve life or function
		Destructive/high-risk elective medical procedure
		Procedure specific risks: smoking, diet, attitude toward implant, etc.
	History	Similar procedure failed previously
		No response to any treatment
		History of nonadherence to conservative care
		No objective medical findings
	Science	Insufficient evidence that the proposed medical treatment would be effective

Adapted from Bruns and Disorbio [121]

exclusionary risk factors or "red flags" (Table 75.2), and these risk factors were organized within the framework of a biopsychosocial paradigm (Fig. 75.1). Exclusionary risk factors were defined as extreme concerns (e.g., imminent risk of suicide or homicide, active psychosis, or intoxicated at medical appointments), any one of which could be sufficient to delay or exclude a patient from elective medical treatment. In contrast, cautionary risk factors were less extreme concerns (e.g., depression, poor pain tolerance), which, in combination, could negatively impact prognosis.

The convergent model was tested using 2264 US subjects obtained from 106 sites, and the demographics of the norm groups approximated US census data for gender, race, education, and age. The risk factors identified by the convergent model were assessed in a standardized manner, using the Battery for Health Improvement 2 [120] and the shorter Brief Battery for Health Improvement 2 [117]. US national norms for the prevalence of these risk scores were generated for two groups: community members and patients with a variety of diagnoses being treated in a variety of treatment settings. The norms obtained from these samples allowed the calculation of a risk score percentile rank, which was used to establish empirical benchmarks. This made it possible to answer the question, at what point can the risk factors present be regarded as clinically elevated [119]? Using this method, standardized cautionary risk and exclusionary risk scores were shown to predict both work status and satisfaction with care for patients in multiple treatment groups (spinal surgery, upper extremity surgery, brain injury, work hardening, chronic pain, acute injury, and injured litigants). Repeat testing showed these risk scores demonstrated test-retest reliabilities ranging from 0.85 to 0.91, with no indications of race or gender bias.

Table 75.2 "Red flag" exclusionary risk factors suggested by literature review

Type of risk	Potential exclusionary factors	
Affective	Active suicidal urges	
	Active homicidal urges	
	Severe depression	
	Severe anxiety (generalized, panic, PTSD, medical phobia/death fears, etc.)	
	Severe anger	
	Mood elevation/mania	
Other psychological risks	Psychosis/delusions/hallucinations	
	Active substance abuse	
	Severe somatization	
	Pain-focused somatoform disorder	
	Severe personality disorder	
	Extremely poor coping	
	Severe social isolation, family dysfunction, or current severe abuse	
Social	Litigation for pain and suffering and pain-related treatment	
	Intense doctor/patient conflict	
Biological	Pain	Bizarre pain reports
		Dysfunctional pain cognitions
		Extreme, invariant pain
		Extreme pain sensitivity
	Exam	Medically impossible symptoms
		Gross inconsistencies between objective findings, symptom reports, and patient behavior
		Falsifying information, malingering, or factitious symptoms
		Inability to cooperate with treatment due to cognitive or other problems
	History	Same treatment failed multiple times in past
		Abuse of prescription medications, violation of opioid contracts
		History of gross noncompliance
	Science	Evidence that the proposed medical treatment would be injurious or ineffective given the circumstances

Adapted from Bruns and Disorbio [121]

Commonly Used Tests for Assessing Patients with Chronic Pain

There are a large number of psychometric tests and questionnaires commonly used to assess patients with chronic pain [121]. When determining what psychological tests to review here, a number of factors were taken into consideration. One evidence-based panel concluded that a psychological test battery for the evaluation of patients with chronic pain would include one or more tests designed for the assessment of medical patients with pain and one or more tests of personality and psychopathology [105]. With regard to selecting each of these types of tests, we would suggest the following criteria, which are that the tests (a) are standardized measures, (b) have been peer reviewed by the Burrows Institute of Mental Measures, (c) have been the subject of multiple empirical research articles in peer-reviewed journals, (d) have been vetted by multiple evidence-based medicine panels reviewing the psychological assessment of chronic pain, (e) [if a pain-related measure] should have been designed and developed for pain assessment, and (f) [if a pain-related

measure] should have standardized scores based on a norm group consisting of medical patients, and especially medical patients suffering from chronic pain. Reviews of other psychological tests for pain assessment are available elsewhere [105, 121, 122].

When you apply these criteria to measures of personality and psychopathology, four tests are identified. These are the MMPI-2, MMPI-2-RF, MCMI-III, and the PAI. If you apply these criteria to measures used for the assessment of medical patients and chronic pain, the tests identified are the BBHI 2, the BHI 2, the BSI-18, the MBMD, and the P-3.

The Three MMPIs

The three MMPI (Minnesota Multiphasic Personality Inventory) tests are arguably the most used and most researched psychological tests in existence. The original MMPI™ was published in 1943 and remained in use until the MMPI-2™ was published 1986, after which the original MMPI was phased out [123, 124]. Over the last several decades, the MMPI (and to a lesser degree, the MMPI-2) has been used in numerous studies related to patients with chronic pain and surgical outcome. Overall, the MMPI-2 is currently the most widely used measure of psychopathology and is also a well-researched measure of malingering. With regard to the evaluation of patients with pain and injury, the MMPI/MMPI-2 have historically been the most commonly recommended tests [28, 33, 125–129].

However, the MMPI-2 (Minnesota Multiphasic Personality Inventory-2) also has a number of significant weaknesses. First of all, the MMPI-2 scales are aging and are based on archaic psychiatric constructs dating back to the 1930s, such as hysteria, psychopathic deviate, and psychasthenia. Secondly, the MMPI was developed in a time when much less was known about psychometrics and test construction. As a result, all of the clinical scales contained items that later research concluded should not have been on the scale [130]. Third, it has been noted that the MMPI-2 is a lengthy test [126], sometimes prohibitively so [125], as it commonly takes up to 90 min to administer [131], and it takes considerable skill to interpret [126]. Fourth, as the MMPI-2 is not normed or designed for patients with pain, it is prone to over-pathologize them [126], especially on its primary scales for assessing depression and somatization [127]. Fifth, despite the length of the MMPI-2, it does not assess many of the variables relevant to medical patients and must be combined with other measures for chronic pain assessment. To this end, Block et al. recommends that the MMPI-2 be used with three other tests [125], Burchiel et al. employed the MMPI-2 and five other tests [33], Doleys and Olson discussed the use of the MMPI-2 and seven other tests [126], Beltrutti et al. discussed the MMPI-2 and eight other tests [129], and Olson et al. employed the MMPI-2 and 10 other tests [128]. Given that the MMPI-2 is already a long test, this makes for a very lengthy test battery.

After much debate, the MMPI-2-RF™ (Minnesota Multiphasic Personality Inventory-2-Revised Form) was published in 2008 [130, 132]. This test has been called a radical departure from the MMPI-2 [133]. While most of the MMPI-2-RF scales were derived from MMPI-2 scales, none are identical, many are markedly different, while others are totally new [130, 132]. In addition to about 80 measures of psychopathology, the MMPI-2 has 15 "validity scales" used to detect exaggerating or concealing information. In contrast, the MMPI-2-RF has 50 scales including eight validity scales. The term "validity scale" is used to convey that these scales attempt to determine if the patient's test responses are valid representations of his or her true feelings or if the patient is attempting to "fake" or appear better or worse than he or she actually is by biasing the information that is presented [114]. The goal of the MMPI-2-RF development was to address the MMPI-2 shortcomings mentioned above and produce a shorter and more psychometrically sound test. Unfortunately, while there were 60 years of research on the original MMPI/MMPI-2 scales, the changed scales in the MMPI-2-RF mean that these decades of research have at best only moderate applicability to the MMPI-2-RF test.

The difference between the MMPI-2 and the MMPI-2-RF is illustrated in one study of 7,330 patients, which found that the "code type" (traditionally used to determine how the test was interpreted) agreed only 14.6 % of the time [134]. Additionally, research suggests that the MMPI-2 is substantially more likely to return a profile suggestive of psychopathology [134] or somatoform disorder [135] than the MMPI-2-RF. Overall, even though these two tests share the same name, it is probably better to think of the MMPI-2-RF as a distinctly different test. At the date of this writing, no published studies were found that utilized the MMPI-2-RF to assess patients with chronic pain. Further, it has been noted that the MMPI-2-RF Revised Clinical Scales were optimized for psychiatric assessment, and without consideration for use with medical patients or assessing somatic symptoms, possibly making them less useful for that purpose than the MMPI-2 [135]. Overall, while the relative merits of the MMPI-2 and the MMPI-2-RF tests remain the subject of ongoing debate [136, 137], both tests will likely remain popular measures of psychopathology.

The MCMI-III

The MCMI-III™ (Millon Clinical Multiaxial Inventory III) is another widely used measure of general psychopathology [138]. One of the MCMI-III's most distinctive features is that among its 25 scales are scales for the assessment of a variety of types of personality disorders, which is helpful for differential diagnosis. While the MCMI-III has the distinct advantage that its scales are keyed to DSM-IV diagnostic criteria, this will be less of an advantage once DSM-5 is released.

A feature of the MCMI-III that could be seen as either a strength or a weakness is its utilization of what are called "base rate" scores. These scales employ a psychometric method where a base rate score of above 75 suggests that some aspects of a syndrome are present, while base rates scores above 85 suggest that the full syndrome is present. While this represents an advantage in some respects, on the negative side, this psychometric method is not based on the normal curve and cannot be used to generate a percentile rank. This makes it somewhat more difficult to identify statistical outliers, but easier to identify the degree to which a particular syndrome might be present. Another feature is three validity scales and one measure random responding.

With regard to its applicability to patients with chronic pain, there is some research on the MCMI-III with regard to its use with chronic pain patients [139–141]. However, it was developed with and normed on psychiatric patients. Consequently, while the MCMI-III is a valuable measure of psychopathology, it must be remembered that like the

MMPI-2 and MMPI-2-RF, its use with patients with objective physical disease or injury may lead to spuriously elevated scales scores, as patient reports of physical symptoms may inflate some of its measures of psychopathology.

The PAI

The PAI™ (Personality Assessment Inventory) is also a popular measure of general psychopathology. Psychometrically, the PAI is a carefully constructed measure, whose 22 scales assess a broad cross section of affective, characterlogical, and psychotic conditions. Like the MMPI-2, the PAI uses standardized T-scores based on community norms, which allows it to identify statistical outliers. The PAI, however, is substantially shorter than the MMPI-2, about the length of the MMPI-2-RF, but considerably longer than the MCMI-III. The PAI has four validity scales.

Some research has studied the applicability of the PAI to assess chronic pain patients [142, 143]. Like other psychological inventories designed for assessing psychiatric patients, it utilizes items about physical symptoms to diagnose depression, anxiety, and other conditions. Consequently, as with the MMPIs and the MCMI-III, it will tend to overestimate some forms of psychopathology in patients with chronic pain.

Psychological Measures for Medical Patients

As noted above, while the MMPIs, the MCMI-III, and the PAI are well-established measures of psychopathology, they are at risk for overestimating psychopathology when used with medical patients. One reason that this happens has been called the "psychological fallacy" [117], which is a problem that occurs when psychological measures intended for psychiatric patients are given to medical patients.

Most psychological tests of psychiatric conditions utilize items about physical symptoms. For example, a measure of depression might contain items about psychological symptoms (e.g., negative thoughts and sad feelings) and physical symptoms as well (e.g., fatigue, loss of libido, changes in weight). However, it has been noted that physical symptoms of this type can also be the product of injury, disease, or medication side effects. Thus, when patients report their medical symptoms on such measures, it can spuriously increase their scores on measures of psychiatric conditions. This is true not only of the MMPIs, MCMI-III, and PAI but also other common measures such as the Beck Depression Inventory [144]. In contrast, a few tests, such as the State Trait Anxiety Inventory [145] or the Battery for Health Improvement 2 [120], control this problem by avoiding the use of items containing physical symptoms to assess emotions. Another important difference in psychological measures designed for medical patients is that they are normed on medical patients,

rather than psychiatric patients or community members. By comparing a patient to a group of other patients, it is much easier to identify the unusual, at risk patient [105].

The BHI 2

The BHI 2™ (Battery for Health Improvement 2) is a test designed for the biopsychosocial assessment of medical patients [120]. This test had its origins in a biopsychosocial paradigm (Fig. 75.1) and as such attempts to assess the medical, psychological, and social aspects of a patient's condition. A strength of the BHI 2 is its norms, which include both patient and community samples. Beyond this, however, the patient norms are broken down into a number of subcategories. About half of the BHI 2 patient norm group consisted of patients with acute injury or other conditions, while the other half consisted of patients with chronic conditions including patients with orthopedic injury, brain injury, headache, fibromyalgia, CRPS, and other conditions. Further, diagnosis-specific pain norms were developed for six groups, which were chronic pain, lower extremity injury, low back injury, upper extremity injury, neck injury, headache, and head injury. This allowed for many patients' pain reports to be compared to other patients in their own diagnostic category. While the BHI 2 uses pain norms for a variety of injury types, other aspects of the BHI 2 were designed to assess conditions unrelated to injury, such as somatic preoccupation and somatization, death fears, the perception of addiction to prescription medication, the tendency to become physically tense when under stress, the perception of disability, and negative attitudes toward physicians that have been found to be associated with thoughts of litigation [146, 147] and violence [148, 149]. Additionally, in order to avoid the psychological fallacy, the BHI 2's 18 scales and 40 subscales assess the thoughts and feelings associated with depression and anxiety separately from the physical symptoms associated with depression and anxiety. Overall, since the BHI 2 was designed to assess medical patients in general and patients with chronic pain in particular, it assesses most of the risk factors identified in the literature [119]. The BHI 2 has a measure of random responding and two bidirectional validity scales, giving it two measures of exaggerating complaints and two measures of concealing information.

Weaknesses of the BHI 2 include that while it assesses some aspects of psychopathology, especially relevant to medical patients, it was not intended to assess the breadth of psychiatric conditions assessed by inventories designed for psychiatric patients. For example, it uses only critical items to assess psychosis and makes no attempt to assess mania, obsessive-compulsive disorder, and some other types of severe psychopathology. Additionally, while there is a growing body of BHI 2 research related to chronic pain [39, 119, 146–161], its research base is not as extensive as that of the MMPI/MMPI-2.

The MBMD

The MBMD™ (Millon Behavioral Medicine Diagnostic) is a psychological test designed for use with medical patients [162]. Like the BHI 2, the MBMD is theory driven, being based in part on Millon's "Evolution-based Personality Theory" [163], with the resulting coping styles being applied to the medical setting. The MBMD could be said to be the psychometric cousin of the MCMI-III, as it adapts many of the MCMI-III scales for use in a medical setting. Like the MCMI-III, the MBMD uses base rate scores. As with the MCMI-III, the strength of this approach is that it attempts to identify patients above a certain level of symptomatology, at the expense of being unable to identify statistical outliers or generate a percentile rank. The MBMD differs from the MCMI-III, however, in that while the MCMI-III attempts to assess psychopathology, the MBMD is designed to assess less extreme aspects of the same constructs that are likely to be observed in a nonpsychiatric population. For example, while the MCMI-III has a scale measuring schizoid tendencies, a similar scale on the MBMD assesses introversive tendencies.

The MBMD is a test designed for medical patients and was constructed using patients with heart disease, diabetes, HIV, and neurological problems. However, only 9 % of patients in the original patient normative group were reported to be suffering from chronic pain. More recently, bariatric and chronic pain norms for this test were also developed. The MBMD pain patient computerized interpretive report displays both the original general medical norm profile using *base rate* scores and a pain patient norm profile using *normative* scores. This produces a pain patient profile that is far less elevated than that produced by the original norm groups and adds a measure of complexity to the interpretation. Perhaps because of this, the pain patient interpretive report continues to be based on the original general medical norms. At the time of this writing, no research studies were found that applied the MBMD to patients with chronic pain.

The MBMD's 38 scales excel at describing the patient's coping style, health habits, potential for certain types of negative reactions to treatment, and factors which may potentiate the patient's distress. It also excels at the psychological assessment of medical patients who are more or less psychologically normal and is also unique in that it offers a brief assessment of spiritual resources for coping. The MBMD also has three validity measures for assessing a patient's test-taking attitude.

The BBHI 2

The BBHI 2™ (Brief Battery for Health Improvement 2) is a short (10-min) version of the BHI 2. The BBHI 2's six scales measure a number of concerns commonly seen in medical patients and especially those with chronic pain: depression, anxiety, somatization, pain, functioning, and utilization of the same norms as the BHI 2 [117]. With regard to pain, the BBHI 2 assesses pain preoccupation, pain tolerance, pain location, pain variability, and dysfunctional pain cognitions. Additionally, it uses critical items to screen for 15 other concerns such as satisfaction with care, home life problems, addiction, psychosis, sleep disorders, panic, compensation focus, and suicidality.

A strength of the BBHI 2 is that it assesses a wide variety of risk factors in a short amount of time [119] and it is the shortest psychological inventory to have validity measures for exaggerating, concealing information, and random responding, and a critical item for psychosis as well. In addition to being used diagnostically, the BBHI 2 can also be used in a serial fashion to track changes in pain, function, depression, anxiety, and somatic distress over the course of time in treatment. A weakness of the BBHI 2 is that outside of its core scales, it screens for a number of concerns using critical items, which is a less reliable method than that which can be obtained with a longer instrument.

The P-3

The P-3™ (Pain Patient Profile) is a short measure useful within pain practices [164]. The strength of the P-3 is its parsimony. The P-3 assesses three critically important variables: depression, anxiety, and somatization. Although the P-3 is tightly focused on these three scales, one strength is that these scales have unusually high reliability. Another strength is that the P-3 utilizes both chronic pain and community norms in interpreting these scales. The appeal of the P-3 is its elegant simplicity, the strength of its norms, and its intended use with patients with chronic pain. The P-3 also has a growing base of empirical research studies pertaining to chronic pain [141, 165–173]. The primary weakness of the P-3 is that there are many risk factors it does not assess, such as coping, pain, functioning, and substance abuse.

The BSI-18

The BSI-18® (Brief Symptom Inventory 18) [174] is an 18-item version of the much longer Brief Symptom Inventory [175], which in turn was derived from the SCL-90 test [176]. Like the P-3, the BSI-18 has three scales: depression, anxiety, and somatization. Thus, it shares the P-3's parsimonious, straightforward approach, and on the surface, the BSI-18 appears identical to the P-3. However, these tests differ in three important respects. First of all, BSI-18 is much shorter than P-3, taking only about one-third of the time to complete. Secondly, while the BSI-18 scales are shorter, they also have lower reliability than the P-3 scales.

A third difference is that while the P-3 was normed on both community members and patients with chronic pain generally, the BSI-18 was normed on patients suffering from cancer-related pain. Thus, while both tests have pain norms, the two normative groups were quite different. Overall, the meaningfulness of a patient's scores on a standardized test is influenced by the degree of similarity between the patient and the norm group to which the patient is compared. Overall, the strength of the BSI-18 is assessing the psychological distress of patients with cancer [177–180].

Other Noteworthy Pain-Related Questionnaires

There are a multitude of other questionnaires pertaining to pain [121] which did not meet all of the criteria for review here, but which are nevertheless noteworthy. Three of these are the West Haven-Yale Multidimensional Pain Inventory (WHYMPI or MPI) [181], the Chronic Pain Coping Inventory (CPCI) [182], and the Survey of Pain Attitudes (SOPA) [183]. The MPI is a well-researched questionnaire that offers scales to assess attitudes about pain, the perceived attitudes of others toward the patient's pain, and the impact of pain on functioning. Weaknesses of the test include that it is not a standardized test: It does not have a formal test manual and has multiple versions [184] with alternate instructions, which have been found to significantly alter the results [185].

Conversely, the CPCI and the SOPA are both questionnaires used in research that evolved into different, standardized versions that kept the same name. Both tests are also similar in that they assess a number of variables directly related to pain. As aptly suggested by its name, the CPCI assesses a variety of strategies patients may use to cope with pain, which include three illness-focused coping strategies and six wellness-focused strategies. A weakness of this test is that it lacks a pain catastrophizing measure. The SOPA is also well researched and assesses a patient's beliefs about pain, which include two scales assessing adaptive beliefs and five scales assessing maladaptive beliefs. Both of the CPCI and the SOPA perform the important task of assessing attitudes, beliefs, and behaviors about pain. A weakness of both the CPCI and the SOPA is that their norms lack diversity in several respects, such as including less than 2 % African-American and Hispanic patients. Overall, the CPCI, SOPA, and MPI are all alike in that they all measure variables directly related to pain. However, none of these scales assess psychopathology or faking, and so they would probably best be paired with another measure.

Validity Assessment

Patients are sometimes motivated to falsely report pain or disability. Incentives range from primary gain (i.e., the individual finds some intrinsic satisfaction in being a patient, such as in being a suffering, tragic hero), secondary gain (i.e., the patient receives monetary, opiate, or other rewards for reporting pain), or tertiary gain (i.e., someone the patient cares about, often a family member, receives monetary or other rewards when the patient reports pain). Since pain is a subjective experience, reports of pain are easily faked [186], and false reports

of pain are sometimes associated with malingering. An extensive review of pain-related malingering examined 68 studies and concluded that malingering was present in 1.25–10.4 % of patients with chronic pain [187]. Other more recent studies have suggested that there may be a 30–40 % incidence of malingering of pain or other symptoms in patients who were litigating or seeking benefits [188, 189] and that reports of symptoms increase when monetary compensation for them is present [190–192]. To detect these tendencies, psychometric measures called validity scales are used.

Validity measures are common features on major psychological inventories, and the MMPI-2, MMPI-2-RF, MCMI-III, PAI, BHI 2, and MBMD all have multiple validity scales. Of these, the MMPI-2 and MMPI-2-RF easily have the greatest number of and the most researched validity measures. With regard to brief psychological measures for pain, only the BBHI 2, P-3, and SOPA have validity measures. The BBHI 2 includes assessments of exaggerating, denial, random responding, and psychosis, while the P-3 has a measure of bizarre responding and the SOPA has a measure of inconsistent responding. Validity measures in general look for patterns of complaints that are so strange, improbable, or extreme as to be extraordinarily unlikely. This could involve claiming on a questionnaire to have never had a bad feeling or reporting a pattern of symptoms that is extraordinarily unlikely.

Relative Merits of the Tests Reviewed

In consideration of the relative merits of the tests above, the following observations are offered. While the MMPI-2-RF is shorter than the MMPI-2-RF and has improved psychometrics, the MMPI-2 has a far larger research base. In contrast, the MCMI-III has the advantage of being keyed to DSM-IV diagnoses and is only about 1/3 the length of the MMPI-2. When time is a factor, this is a considerable advantage. Lastly, the PAI is about the same length as the MMPI-2-RF, but about twice the length of the MCMI-III. The PAI is a well-designed measure of psychopathology and is a reasonable alternative to the other tests mentioned.

With regard to measures of chronic pain, the BHI 2 has the advantage of being intended for the assessments of patients with chronic pain. It includes standardized measures of pain, function, and most of the risk factors identified by the convergent model. The other major health psychology inventory reviewed here, the MBMD, has surprisingly little overlap with the BHI 2. While the MBMD was developed using a disease model and does not measure pain per se, it does measure some attitudes toward pain. If an assessment of how relatively normal patients cope with pain is desired, the MBMD is particularly strong. In contrast, the BHI 2 assesses a greater number of aberrant traits that may be problematic in treatment.

With regard to brief measures for medical patients, the P-3 offers a straightforward assessment of three factors

Table 75.3 Subacute low back pain: good candidate

BBHI 2 results					
Global pain complaint		*Pain complaints areas*		*Scale ratings and percentile ranks*	
Overall pain at testing:	4	Head (headache pain):	0	Defensiveness:	Average 48 %
High pain last month:	8	Jaw or face:	0	Somatic complaints:	Average 63 %
Low pain last month:	2	Neck or shoulders:	0	Pain complaints:	Average 66 %
Peak pain:	8	Arms or hands:	0	Functional complaints:	Mod high 78 %
Pain range	6	Chest:	0	Depression:	High 88 %
Max tolerable pain	5	Abdomen or stomach:	0	Anxiety:	Average 71 %
Pain tolerance index	3	Genital area:	0	*Summary*	
Number of body areas with pain	10	Middle back:	6	Exclusionary risks=0	
Critical concerns		Lower back:	8	Cautionary risks=1	
Sleep disorder		Legs or feet:	3	Cautionary risk rank: 17th percentile	

known to play an important role in chronic pain in a manner that is easily understood. While the BBHI 2 is a test of similar length to the P-3, these two tests approach the assessment of pain patients differently. While the P-3 prefers the elegance of parsimony, the BBHI 2 assesses a much broader range of variables and paints a more detailed picture of the patient. Both of these tests can be used to track changes in treatment over time. The BSI-18 offers the same three scales as the P-3. However, the BSI-18 was developed and normed on patients with cancer, and so this measure has particular strengths if pain is associated with that condition.

It should be noted, however, that the final decision about tests should rest with the examiner, as unique features of a particular case or future research might indicate that a different set of tests would be warranted. At this point, however, given the current state of knowledge, the tests above meet the criteria specified.

Referral for Psychological Assessment

A multidisciplinary panel, following rules of evidence-based medicine, explored the question of when psychological assessments should be conducted in patients suffering from chronic pain [105]. The conclusion was that, given the biopsychosocial nature of pain, psychological assessment is generally indicated. Beyond this, specific indications for evaluation were also identified. These were as follows:
1. When psychological dysfunction is observed or suspected
2. When there has been inadequate recovery, as indicated by the duration of symptoms beyond the usual time, failure to benefit from all treatment, or pain complaints that cannot be explained by the patient's physical findings
3. Substance abuse and/or aberrant use of prescription medication
4. Premorbid history of major psychiatric symptoms
5. Lack of adherence to medical treatment
6. When cognitive impairment is suspected, especially if related to the medical condition or adverse effect of medications

7. When a patient has been judged to have a catastrophic medical condition
8. Prior to major surgical or invasive procedures, such as spinal cord stimulation, and prior to initiation of chronic opioid treatment

Chronic Pain Case Vignettes

For heuristic purposes, in the case vignettes below, the convergent model described above is used to assess three patients, whose biopsychosocial risk levels range from mild to extreme. It should be noted that there are other psychometric assessment protocols, and these are reviewed elsewhere [119]. However, analyzing these cases with multiple protocols would add a level of complexity that goes well beyond the vision of this chapter. In each case vignette to follow, there is both a standardized assessment of the risk factors described in Tables 75.1 and 75.2 and a clinical narrative. The first two cases assess biopsychosocial risk factors using the BBHI 2 test, while the third uses the longer BHI 2.

Case History One: Neuropathic Pain with Low Biopsychosocial Risk Level

Ms. A was a 26-year-old female college graduate and sports enthusiast, who injured her back while skiing. Initially, she had been diagnosed with a lumber strain. Later, she was determined by MRI to have bulging discs at L3-L4 and L4-L5. Ms. A wished to avoid lumbar surgery and was being evaluated for alternate treatment options. As part of a comprehensive assessment, Ms. A was administered a BBHI 2 test.

Table 75.3 summarizes the results of Ms. A's standardized testing with the BBHI 2. These results show a distribution of pain that is confined to the area near the injury, with only three body areas being involved. The pain level at testing was a four, with a high of eight and a low of two in the last month. These pain complaints were judged to be consistent with her

Table 75.4 Subacute whiplash condition: moderate risk patient

BBHI 2 results					
Global pain complaint		*Pain complaints area*		*Scale ratings and percentile ranks*	
Overall pain at testing:	9	Head (headache pain):	8	Defensiveness:	Average 42 %
High pain last month:	10	Jaw or face:	6	Somatic complaints:	Very high 96 %
Lowest pain last month:	6	Neck or shoulders:	9	Pain complaints:	High 88 %
Peak pain:	10	Arms or hands:	4	Functional complaints:	Mod high 76 %
Pain range	8	Chest:	9	Depression:	High 90 %
Max tolerable pain	6	Abdomen or stomach:	5	Anxiety:	Very high 96 %
Pain tolerance index	−4	Genital area:	0	*Summary*	
Number of body areas with pain	6	Middle back:	0	Exclusionary risks = 0	
Clinical concerns		Lower back:	0	Cautionary risks = 5	
Panic		Legs or feet:	0	*Cautionary risk rank* = 80th percentile	
PTSD/dissociation					
Perceived disability					

objective medical findings. Using the convergent model to summarize Ms. A's level of risk, she had none of the extreme exclusionary risk factors and only one cautionary risk factor. This produced a cautionary risk score at the 17th percentile rank or well below average. It should be noted that these risk scores are generated solely from the testing, without any interview or chart review. Following the testing, an interview identified additional information. The overall results of the evaluation are below.

On the BBHI 2 test, Ms. A's sole cautionary risk factor was that her level of depression was higher than that seen in 88 % of a national sample of patients with pain and injury, which is significantly elevated (Table 75.3). During the interview, she reported a low mood and was very concerned that she may have to give up her active lifestyle. Additionally, her score on the functional complaints scale was in the "moderately high" range. With regard to functioning, Ms A was reporting more difficulties with functioning than was 78 % of a national sample of patients and above 98 % of a national sample of persons in the community. While this is at the upper end of the average range for patients who are in rehabilitation, it is far higher than that of the average healthy person. This indicates that while a significant problem exists, it is still in the average range for patients with serious injuries. Thus, with regard to perceptions of disability and functioning, Ms. A was not an unusual patient. Additionally, Ms. A's BBHI 2 results determined that her pain, somatization, and anxiety were all in the average range. The only other significant problem reported was that the patient was having difficulty sleeping.

Importantly, the BBHI 2 Pain Tolerance Index was only −3, meaning that the patient felt that her worst pain must only be reduced by three points in order to function normally. Overall, this patient was judged to have localized back pain and a relatively low level of psychosocial complications. She was started on a trial of medications for depression and insomnia and was judged to be an excellent candidate for conservative treatment.

Case History Two: Whiplash with Moderate Biopsychosocial Risk Level

Ms. B was a 52-year-old patient who had sustained a whiplash injury in a motor vehicle accident and who had been exhibiting poor attendance in treatment. This patient complained of pain in her neck, head, and mid- to upper back, and this was judged to be consistent with the whiplash injury. In contrast, other aspects of Ms. B's pain complaints, such as the facial and jaw pain, were of uncertain etiology. It was possible that the latter pain complaints were indicative of other injuries that may have been overlooked during the acute phase or may have been attributable to dental or other conditions. Given the uncertain nature of some of her pain complaints and her lack of improvement with treatment, Ms. B was referred for psychological assessment.

Table 75.4 lists the BBHI 2 tests results of Ms. B. She had no exclusionary risk factors and five cautionary risk factors, producing a cautionary risk score at the 80th percentile rank, which is somewhat elevated. The "high" rating on the BBHI 2 pain complaints scale indicates that Ms. B's overall pain reports were substantially higher (elevated more than one standard deviation) than that seen in 88 % of patients with pain and injury. These test results also showed that Ms. B was extremely anxious, somatically preoccupied, and was reporting symptoms of panic and PTSD. This gave rise to an alternate interpretation of some of these symptoms. The interview determined that the patient was having PTSD flashbacks when driving in traffic and had also developed agoraphobia secondary to panic attacks. It was discovered that her poor attendance in treatment was not attributable to low motivation, but rather to her fear of leaving the house. Additionally, her jaw and facial pain were later determined to be associated with bruxing secondary to severe anxiety.

Ms. B's Pain Tolerance Index of −4 indicates that she felt she needed to reduce her worst pain by four points to make normal functioning possible. On the positive side, given that the patient reported that pain sometimes dropped as low as a

Table 75.5 Chronic low back pain: high-risk candidate

BHI 2 results							
Global pain complaints		*Pain complaints area*		*Scale ratings and percentile ranks*	
Overall pain at testing:	10	Headache:	10	Defensiveness:	Ext low 28 %
High pain last month:	10	Jaw/face:	6	Self-disclosure:	Mod high 80 %
Lowest pain last month:	10	Neck/shoulders:	5	Somatic complaints:	High 91 %
Peak pain:	10	Arms/hands:	2	Pain complaints:	Ext high 99 %
Pain range	0	Chest:	9	Functional complaints:	Very high 95 %
Max tolerable pain	0	Abdomen/stomach:	5	Muscular bracing	Average 58 %
Pain tolerance index	−10	Genital area:	2	Depression:	High 88 %
Number of body areas with pain	10	Middle back:	8	Anxiety:	Average 56 %
Clinical concerns		Lower back:	10	Hostility	Very high 96 %
Pain fixation		Legs or feet:	10	Borderline	Mod high 82 %
Rx addiction				Symptom dependency	Average 44 %
Violent ideation				Chronic maladjustment	Very high 95 %
Medical dissatisfaction				Substance abuse	Very high 96 %
Compensation focus				Perseverance	Average 62 %
Entitlement				Family dysfunction	Low 5 %
Cynical beliefs				Survivor of violence	Low 16 %
Aggressiveness				Doctor dissatisfaction	Ext high 99 %
Impulsiveness				Job dissatisfaction	High 84 %
Vegetative depression				*Summary*	
Autonomic anxiety				Exclusionary risks = 6	
Death anxiety				Cautionary risks = 18	
Sleep disorder				Exclusionary risk rank: 99th percentile	
Work disability				Cautionary risk rank: 99th percentile	

two and a pain of six could be tolerated, it would appear that at times, the pain was quite tolerable.

In cases like this, it is important to determine the physical and psychological causes of the reported symptoms and provide appropriate treatment. If the symptoms are determined to be heavily influenced by psychosocial factors, early intervention can prevent these psychosocial complications from delaying recovery. In this case, Ms. B was referred for treatment for PTSD and agoraphobia. Later, after the PTSD and anxiety symptoms were brought under control, Ms. B no longer exhibited attendance problems. Following a two-level cervical rhizotomy, her pain symptoms decreased markedly, and she began progressing in physical therapy.

Case History Three: Chronic Low Back Pain with Extreme Biopsychosocial Risk Level

Mr. C was a 44-year-old male with failed back surgery syndrome, who was being considered for spinal cord stimulation and other treatments. Mr. C presented as a patient who had injured himself 3 years earlier while working on an oil-drilling rig. The patient reported that following the injury, there was an immediate onset of severe lumbar pain, which radiated into his left leg. A subsequent MRI revealed an L5–S1 lumbar disc herniation. Mr. C was a two to three pack a day smoker and was instructed to stop smoking prior to

undergoing a lumbar fusion. He reported that he had quit, but later, after the surgery, it was discovered that he had not been honest about this. Mr. C complained that his pain after the surgery was far worse, and he increased his dose of opioid pain medications without consulting his surgeon.

Mr. C was referred for physical therapy, where he attended poorly and failed to progress. He was very pain affected, exhibited a hostile attitude, and complained that none of the treatments that had been offered to him had helped. Mr. C was offered light duty at his employer's office, which he refused. By this time, his use of opioid medication was excessive, and Mr. C became belligerent when an early refill of this medication was not allowed.

Three years postinjury, and after all other treatments had failed, Mr. C was referred to an interventional pain specialist to be evaluated for spinal cord stimulation, with hopes that this would help him decrease his opioid use. Prior to trial, Mr. C was referred for a psychological evaluation, but he regarded a referral to a psychologist as an insult, saying, "My pain is real. It is not in my head!" The physician explained that behavioral health services are a standard part of interdisciplinary care and persuaded Mr. C to attend the appointment. During the psychological evaluation, the patient was administered the BHI 2, and Table 75.5 lists Mr. C's BHI 2 results. Using the convergent model, he had 18 cautionary risk factors, producing a cautionary risk score at the 99th percentile rank, which is extremely high. Further, he also had six of the extreme exclusionary risk factors, producing an exclusionary risk score at the 99th percentile rank as well.

At the time of the psychological evaluation, Mr. C was reporting a pain of 10 in the low back, mid-back, and lower extremities, and the intensity of the pain reports was judged by his physicians to exceed what was expected. More significant perhaps was the report of pain in all seven other body areas, his report that his overall pain was a constant "10," with his pain range score of 0 indicating that he was reporting totally invariant pain over the last month. More importantly, his Pain Tolerance Index score was −10, indicating that the patient believed he needed to reduce the level of all his pains to 0 before he could function. Relative to this, he claimed that he had no pain at all before he was injured and he deserved to have no pain now. He stated that if spinal cord stimulation would reduce all of his pain to 0, he would have no need for medication. Overall, this patient reported more pain than did 99 % of a national sample of patients with pain and injury, including chest pain as high as 9. Given the fact that he was a heavy smoker, he was referred for coronary assessment, with negative findings. Overall, as there was no pathophysiological explanation for many of Mr. C's pain reports, therefore, psychophysiological reasons were explored.

The BHI 2 test results determined that Mr. C was at the 96th percentile rank for hostility and the 95th percentile for panic symptoms. This combination of anger and anxiety suggests extreme elevation of the fight-or-flight response, with the "fight" component being associated with anger and the "flight" component being associated with anxiety. Further, Mr. C's depression scale score was above that seen in 88 % of patients, and his depression appeared to manifest itself primarily in terms of anger and irritability. It was determined that Mr. C's reports of chest pain were associated with high levels of autonomic arousal and panic-like symptoms. Mr. C also reported a level of somatic preoccupation that was at the 91st percentile, and he was convinced that he had a severe heart condition, which his doctors were ignoring. Mr. C's BHI 2 profile also indicated that he was reporting more functional impairment than 95 % of patients, indicating that he saw himself as having a severe disability.

On the BHI 2, Mr. C also reported some violent thoughts, supported by a cynical view of others. He felt entitled to both special treatment and to financial compensation. With a level of job dissatisfaction at the 84th percentile, this patient was at odds with his employer, whom he blamed for his injury. He reported fantasies of harming his boss, "to make him feel pain the way I do." With a level of doctor dissatisfaction at the 99th percentile, he had even more negative attitudes toward physicians, who he accused of "working for the system." On the BHI 2, Mr. C reported an extensive history of substance abuse and chronic maladjustment. Overall, his BHI 2 test profile was one that has been found to be associated with thoughts of litigation [146, 147] and of assaultive behavior [148, 149, 155]. During the interview, he revealed

that he had been in jail previously for domestic violence and in prison for drug-related charges.

Mr. C stated that because of his extreme pain, he needed more opioids and blamed his physicians for not increasing his dosage saying, "There is no reason why doctors couldn't cure my pain if they wanted to." Mr. C also demanded "natural" treatments, rationalizing that he should be prescribed morphine as it was a "natural treatment made from flowers." Paradoxically, though, Mr. C refused treatment with antidepressant medications out of a fear that they were "addictive" and because they were "unnatural." Similarly, he refused behavioral pain management training with a psychologist. Despite being off of work, he was often "too busy" to attend physical therapy, yet he never missed an appointment for an opioid prescription refill. Although multiple treatment referrals were offered to this patient, he did not accept them. Overall, Mr. C had unrealistic expectations of being totally cured through surgery and opioids, without effort on his own part and without changing his dysfunctional behaviors. Despite the warnings of his physicians, though, he continued to smoke heavily. It was later determined that he was combining his pain medications with methamphetamines and large amounts of alcohol. Mr. C claimed he was using both "medicinally." Mr. C did not take responsibility for his behavior, though. Instead, he blamed his orthopedic surgeon for his pain and was discussing a malpractice lawsuit.

The psychologist concluded the following:

1. Even if Mr. C did undergo spinal cord stimulation, he would almost certainly be dissatisfied with his outcome. The possibility that this patient's back pain would be reduced to 0 by spinal cord stimulation was judged to be extremely unlikely. Even if spinal cord stimulation did totally eliminate all low back and lower extremity pain, it was unlikely that it would alleviate his multitude of other pain complaints, and so the overall reported pain level would be unlikely to change.

2. Even if treatment with spinal cord stimulation was successful, it is unlikely that it would change Mr. C's demands for opioids. Spinal cord stimulation is not a treatment for addiction, which was what Mr. C was suffering from.

3. Mr. C hated his job and had no desire to return there. It was judged unlikely that spinal cord stimulation would alter Mr. C's motivation to return to work.

4. Given the fact that Mr. C was pursuing litigation, he may be reluctant to admit to any gains in treatment, as it might weaken his lawsuit against his surgeon. Additionally, since his expectation of a totally pain-free outcome was so unrealistic, Mr. C would be probably extremely unhappy with his spinal cord stimulation as well.

5. The psychologist suggested the following treatment plan for Mr. C. First of all, Mr. C should be referred to an inpatient drug rehabilitation program for polysubstance abuse. Once he had completed that, he could then benefit from an interdisciplinary treatment program for pain, which

studies have shown can be effective, even for patients with personality disorders [193]. After consulting with the physician, it was decided that the interdisciplinary treatment should avoid opioids and include medical treatment as indicated, physical therapy with a focus on exercise and improving function, cognitive behavioral therapy for managing pain and emotional dysfunction, and other psychological treatments including relaxation, sleep hygiene, and mindfulness training.

After consulting with the psychologist, the pain physician felt she had a much deeper understanding of the scope of the problem and later met with Mr. C. She told Mr. C that spinal cord stimulation did not appear to be a viable treatment for him and that it was very likely that Mr. C would be unhappy with the results. The physician also said that she was committed to doing nothing to harm him and that given Mr. C's pattern of polysubstance abuse, treatment with opioids was dangerous and no longer an option. The physician said that instead, she was recommending the drug rehabilitation and interdisciplinary pain treatment program described above. The physician told Mr. C that this treatment program would not work unless he was fully invested in it and that if he faithfully adhered to it, they could continue working together. However, she also explained that if Mr. C refused this treatment, or did not adhere to it, he would be advised to seek treatment elsewhere, as this was the only treatment plan she thought was viable.

High-risk patients like Mr. C are challenging to treat. His initial injury was a serious one, but one which should have responded better to treatment. Unfortunately, Mr. C's entitled expectations, hostile attitude, noncompliance, and addictive behavior undermined the work of his treating professionals, and he suffered the consequences of his own dysfunctional tendencies.

If Mr. C followed through with the treatment plan above, one part of a 12-step treatment program for addiction would probably be a spiritual meditation commonly known as the Serenity Prayer: *God grant me the strength to change the things I am able to change, the ability to accept the things I cannot change, and the wisdom to know the difference.* Applying this approach to the treatment of pain generally, while the goal of changing physical pain is the domain of pain medicine, the emotional acceptance of having pain and coping with it is the domain of pain psychology. Knowing how to integrate these two approaches in the clinical setting requires a holistic understanding of how the patient's medical and psychological conditions interact. While events in life sometimes lead to pain, suffering comes from what you do to yourself. Thus, as the Buddha concluded, "Pain is inevitable. Suffering is optional."

Conclusions

Based on the studies reviewed here, it is evident that there is a growing consensus in the literature regarding the importance of assessing pain from a biopsychosocial perspective, which integrates both medical and psychological testing. At first glance, the specialties of pain medicine and pain psychology could seem worlds apart. Beneath the surface, though, they share a deep commonality, as both specialties focus on the assessment of subjective experiences and the attempt to alleviate painful feelings. While pain often has its origins in physical states, psychological forces can act either to alleviate or to compound the individual's suffering. Chronic pain may thus evolve into a complex biopsychosocial state, and depending upon the case, biological, psychological, or social factors may play the predominant causal role.

Given the complex nature of pain, success in treatment depends upon a full understanding of why the patient reports pain or requests opioids or other treatments. The dictum that "diagnosis precedes treatment" is nowhere more true than with the practice of pain medicine. While reports of pain are often the product of pathophysiology, they are sometimes the product of psychopathology. Consequently, when extreme pain is reported in the absence of any obvious pathophysiological explanation, tension can arise between patient and doctor. It has been said: "To have great pain is to have certainty. To hear that another has pain is to have doubt" [194]. Ultimately, successful assessment of chronic pain requires not only medical diagnostics but also a systematic investigation of the subjective world of the patient, which seeks to understand the origins of the pain reports.

From the perspective of patients, chronic pain often involves not just a loss of function but also a loss of one's future dreams and aspirations. The onset of a disabling condition may bring an abrupt end to a patient's assumptions about what the future holds, and the loss of this assumptive world can elicit profound grief [195]. Because of this, success in treatment cannot occur without addressing both medical and psychological concerns. Overall, the value of knowing one's patient, both medically and psychologically, cannot be overstated. To this end, and when integrated with medical diagnostics, psychological assessment can make an invaluable contribution to the understanding of the patient with chronic pain. In this manner, and through a determined blend of both science and humanity, more effective treatments may be identified.

References

1. International Association for the Study of Pain. Task Force on Taxonomy, Merskey H, Bogduk N. Classification of chronic pain. 2nd ed. Seattle: IASP Press; 1994.
2. Gatchel RJ, Peng YB, Peters ML, Fuchs PN, Turk DC. The biopsychosocial approach to chronic pain: scientific advances and future directions. Psychol Bull. 2007;133(4):581–624.
3. Melzack R. From the gate to the neuromatrix. Pain. 1999;Suppl 6:S121–6.

4. Joksimovic L, Starke D, v d Knesebeck O, Siegrist J. Perceived work stress, overcommitment, and self-reported musculoskeletal pain: a cross-sectional investigation. Int J Behav Med. 2002;9(2):122–38.

5. Chen WQ, Yu IT, Wong TW. Impact of occupational stress and other psychosocial factors on musculoskeletal pain among Chinese offshore oil installation workers. Occup Environ Med. 2005;62(4):251–6.

6. Bhatia V, Tandon RK. Stress and the gastrointestinal tract. J Gastroenterol Hepatol. 2005;20(3):332–9.

7. Bigos SJ, Battie MC, Spengler DM, et al. A longitudinal, prospective study of industrial back injury reporting. Clin Orthop. 1992; 279:21–34.

8. Turner C, McClure R, Pirozzo S. Injury and risk-taking behavior-a systematic review. Accid Anal Prev. 2004;36(1):93–101.

9. Levenson MR. Risk taking and personality. J Pers Soc Psychol. 1990;58(6):1073–80.

10. Corrigan JD. Substance abuse as a mediating factor in outcome from traumatic brain injury. Arch Phys Med Rehabil. 1995; 76(4):302–9.

11. Drubach DA, Kelly MP, Winslow MM, Flynn JP. Substance abuse as a factor in the causality, severity, and recurrence rate of traumatic brain injury. Md Med J. 1993;42(10):989–93.

12. Dersh J, Gatchel RJ, Mayer T, Polatin P, Temple OR. Prevalence of psychiatric disorders in patients with chronic disabling occupational spinal disorders. Spine (Phila Pa 1976). 2006;31(10):1156–62.

13. Manchikanti L, Damron KS, Beyer CD, Pampati V. A comparative evaluation of illicit drug use in patients with or without controlled substance abuse in interventional pain management. Pain Physician. 2003;6(3):281–5.

14. Broadhead WE, Blazer DG, George LK, Tse CK. Depression, disability days, and days lost from work in a prospective epidemiologic survey. JAMA. 1990;264(19):2524–8.

15. Gehi A, Haas D, Pipkin S, Whooley MA. Depression and medication adherence in outpatients with coronary heart disease: findings from the Heart and Soul Study. Arch Intern Med. 2005;165(21): 2508–13.

16. Polatin PB, Kinney RK, Gatchel RJ, Lillo E, Mayer TG. Psychiatric illness and chronic low-back pain. The mind and the spine – which goes first? Spine. 1993;18(1):66–71.

17. Turk DC, Monarch ES. Biopsychosocial perspective on chronic pain. In: Turk DC, Gatchel RJ, editors. Psychological approaches to pain management: a practitioner's handbook. 2nd ed. New York: The Guilford Press; 2002. xviii, 590p.

18. Carter LE, McNeil DW, Vowles KE, et al. Effects of emotion on pain reports, tolerance and physiology. Pain Res Manag. 2002;7(1): 21–30.

19. Fordyce WE. Pain and suffering. A reappraisal. Am Psychol. 1988; 43(4):276–83.

20. Dvorak J, Valach L, Fuhrimann P, Heim E. The outcome of surgery for lumbar disc herniation. II. A 4–17 years' follow-up with emphasis on psychosocial aspects. Spine. 1988;13(12):1423–7.

21. Herron L, Turner J, Weiner P. Does the MMPI predict chemonucleolysis outcome? Spine. 1988;13(1):84–8.

22. Hagg O, Fritzell P, Ekselius L, Nordwall A. Predictors of outcome in fusion surgery for chronic low back pain. A report from the Swedish Lumbar Spine Study. Eur Spine J. 2003;12(1):22–33.

23. Andersen T, Christensen FB, Bunger C. Evaluation of a Dallas Pain Questionnaire classification in relation to outcome in lumbar spinal fusion. Eur Spine J. 2006;10:1–15.

24. Derby R, Lettice JJ, Kula TA, Lee SH, Seo KS, Kim BJ. Single-level lumbar fusion in chronic discogenic low-back pain: psychological and emotional status as a predictor of outcome measured using the 36-item Short Form. J Neurosurg Spine. 2005;3(4):255–61.

25. Deyo RA, Mirza SK, Heagerty PJ, Turner JA, Martin BI. A prospective cohort study of surgical treatment for back pain with degenerated discs; study protocol. BMC Musculoskelet Disord. 2005;6(1):24.

26. Graver V, Haaland AK, Magnaes B, Loeb M. Seven-year clinical follow-up after lumbar disc surgery: results and predictors of outcome. Br J Neurosurg. 1999;13(2):178–84.

27. Van Susante J, Van de Schaaf D, Pavlov P. Psychological distress deteriorates the subjective outcome of lumbosacral fusion. A prospective study. Acta Orthop Belg. 1998;64(4):371–7.

28. Block AR, Ohnmeiss DD, Guyer RD, Rashbaum RF, Hochschuler SH. The use of presurgical psychological screening to predict the outcome of spine surgery. Spine J. 2001;1(4):274–82.

29. Schade V, Semmer N, Main CJ, Hora J, Boos N. The impact of clinical, morphological, psychosocial and work-related factors on the outcome of lumbar discectomy. Pain. 1999;80(1–2):239–49.

30. Cashion EL, Lynch WJ. Personality factors and results of lumbar disc surgery. Neurosurgery. 1979;4(2):141–5.

31. den Boer JJ, Oostendorp RA, Beems T, Munneke M, Evers AW. Continued disability and pain after lumbar disc surgery: the role of cognitive-behavioral factors. Pain. 2006;123(1–2):45–52.

32. Katz JN, Stucki G, Lipson SJ, Fossel AH, Grobler LJ, Weinstein JN. Predictors of surgical outcome in degenerative lumbar spinal stenosis. Spine. 1999;24(21):2229–33.

33. Burchiel KJ, Anderson VC, Wilson BJ, Denison DB, Olson KA, Shatin D. Prognostic factors of spinal cord stimulation for chronic back and leg pain. Neurosurgery. 1995;36(6):1101–10; discussion 1110–1.

34. Samwel H, Slappendel R, Crul BJ, Voerman VF. Psychological predictors of the effectiveness of radiofrequency lesioning of the cervical spinal dorsal ganglion (RF-DRG). Eur J Pain. 2000;4(2): 149–55.

35. Dersh J, Polatin PB, Gatchel RJ. Chronic pain and psychopathology: research findings and theoretical considerations. Psychosom Med. 2002;64(5):773–86.

36. Spengler DM, Freeman C, Westbrook R, Miller JW. Low-back pain following multiple lumbar spine procedures. Failure of initial selection? Spine. 1980;5(4):356–60.

37. Uomoto JM, Turner JA, Herron LD. Use of the MMPI and MCMI in predicting outcome of lumbar laminectomy. J Clin Psychol. 1988;44(2):191–7.

38. Passik SD, Kirsh KL. Opioid therapy in patients with a history of substance abuse. CNS Drugs. 2004;18(1):13–25.

39. Bruns D, Disorbio JM, Bennett DB, Simon S, Shoemaker S, Portenoy RK. Degree of pain intolerance and adverse outcomes in chronic noncancer pain patients. J Pain. 2005;6(3S):s74.

40. Compton P, Athanasos P. Chronic pain, substance abuse and addiction. Nurs Clin North Am. 2003;38(3):525–37.

41. Brennan PL, Schutte KK, Moos RH. Pain and use of alcohol to manage pain: prevalence and 3-year outcomes among older problem and non-problem drinkers. Addiction. 2005;100(6):777–86.

42. Mitchell AM, Dewey CM. Chronic pain in patients with substance abuse disorder: general guidelines and an approach to treatment. Postgrad Med. 2008;120(1):75–9.

43. Chou R, Fanciullo GJ, Fine PG, Miaskowski C, Passik SD, Portenoy RK. Opioids for chronic noncancer pain: prediction and identification of aberrant drug-related behaviors: a review of the evidence for an American Pain Society and American Academy of Pain Medicine clinical practice guideline. J Pain. 2009;10(2):131–46.

44. Large RG. DSM-III diagnoses in chronic pain. Confusion or clarity? J Nerv Ment Dis. 1986;174(5):295–303.

45. Okasha A, Ismail MK, Khalil AH, el Fiki R, Soliman A, Okasha T. A psychiatric study of nonorganic chronic headache patients. Psychosomatics. 1999;40(3):233–8.

46. Fishbain DA, Goldberg M, Meagher BR, Steele R, Rosomoff H. Male and female chronic pain patients categorized by DSM-III psychiatric diagnostic criteria. Pain. 1986;26(2):181–97.

47. Dersh J, Gatchel RJ, Polatin P, Mayer T. Prevalence of psychiatric disorders in patients with chronic work-related musculoskeletal pain disability. J Occup Environ Med. 2002;44(5):459–68.

48. Fishbain DA, Cole B, Cutler RB, Lewis J, Rosomoff HL, Rosomoff RS. Chronic pain and the measurement of personality: do states influence traits? Pain Med. 2006;7(6):509–29.

49. Swinkels-Meewisse IE, Roelofs J, Oostendorp RA, Verbeek AL, Vlaeyen JW. Acute low back pain: pain-related fear and pain catastrophizing influence physical performance and perceived disability. Pain. 2006;120(1–2):36–43.

50. Smeets RJ, Vlaeyen JW, Kester AD, Knottnerus JA. Reduction of pain catastrophizing mediates the outcome of both physical and cognitive-behavioral treatment in chronic low back pain. J Pain. 2006;7(4):261–71.

51. Rapley P, Fruin DJ. Self-efficacy in chronic illness: the juxtaposition of general and regimen-specific efficacy. Int J Nurs Pract. 1999; 5(4):209–15.

52. Brenes GA, Rapp SR, Rejeski WJ, Miller ME. Do optimism and pessimism predict physical functioning? J Behav Med. 2002;25(3): 219–31.

53. Lin CC, Ward SE. Perceived self-efficacy and outcome expectancies in coping with chronic low back pain. Res Nurs Health. 1996;19(4):299–310.

54. den Boer JJ, Oostendorp RA, Beems T, Munneke M, Oerlemans M, Evers AW. A systematic review of bio-psychosocial risk factors for an unfavourable outcome after lumbar disc surgery. Eur Spine J. 2006;15(5):527–36.

55. Weisberg JN. Personality and personality disorders in chronic pain. Curr Rev Pain. 2000;4(1):60–70.

56. Naring GW, van Lankveld W, Geenen R. Somatoform dissociation and traumatic experiences in patients with rheumatoid arthritis and fibromyalgia. Clin Exp Rheumatol. 2007;25(6):872–7.

57. Fishbain DA, Cutler RB, Rosomoff HL, Rosomoff RS. Pain-determined dissociation episodes. Pain Med. 2001;2(3):216–24.

58. McFadden IJ, Woitalla VF. Differing reports of pain perception by different personalities in a patient with chronic pain and multiple personality disorder. Pain. 1993;55(3):379–82.

59. Packard RC, Brown F. Multiple headaches in a case of multiple personality disorder. Headache. 1986;26(2):99–102.

60. Hamberg K, Johansson E, Lindgren G, Westman G. The impact of marital relationship on the rehabilitation process in a group of women with long-term musculoskeletal disorders. Scand J Soc Med. 1997;25(1):17–25.

61. MacGregor EA, Brandes J, Eikermann A, Giammarco R. Impact of migraine on patients and their families: the Migraine And Zolmitriptan Evaluation (MAZE) survey – Phase III. Curr Med Res Opin. 2004;20(7):1143–50.

62. Kemler MA, Furnee CA. The impact of chronic pain on life in the household. J Pain Symptom Manage. 2002;23(5):433–41.

63. Harris S, Morley S, Barton SB. Role loss and emotional adjustment in chronic pain. Pain. 2003;105(1–2):363–70.

64. Kerns RD, Haythornthwaite J, Southwick S, Giller Jr EL. The role of marital interaction in chronic pain and depressive symptom severity. J Psychosom Res. 1990;34(4):401–8.

65. Block AR, Kremer EF, Gaylor M. Behavioral treatment of chronic pain: the spouse as a discriminative cue for pain behavior. Pain. 1980;9(2):243–52.

66. Heim C, Ehlert U, Hanker JP, Hellhammer DH. Abuse-related post-traumatic stress disorder and alterations of the hypothalamic-pituitary-adrenal axis in women with chronic pelvic pain. Psychosom Med. 1998;60(3):309–18.

67. Rubin RT, Phillips JJ, McCracken JT, Sadow TF. Adrenal gland volume in major depression: relationship to basal and stimulated pituitary-adrenal cortical axis function. Biol Psychiatry. 1996;40(2):89–97.

68. Heim C, Newport DJ, Bonsall R, Miller AH, Nemeroff CB. Altered pituitary-adrenal axis responses to provocative challenge tests in adult survivors of childhood abuse. Am J Psychiatry. 2001;158(4): 575–81.

69. Heim C, Newport DJ, Heit S, et al. Pituitary-adrenal and autonomic responses to stress in women after sexual and physical abuse in childhood. JAMA. 2000;284(5):592–7.

70. Bremner JD, Vythilingam M, Anderson G, et al. Assessment of the hypothalamic-pituitary-adrenal axis over a 24-hour diurnal period and in response to neuroendocrine challenges in women with and without childhood sexual abuse and posttraumatic stress disorder. Biol Psychiatry. 2003;54(7):710–8.

71. De Bellis MD, Chrousos GP, Dorn LD, et al. Hypothalamic-pituitary-adrenal axis dysregulation in sexually abused girls. J Clin Endocrinol Metab. 1994;78(2):249–55.

72. Kiecolt-Glaser JK, Glaser R. Psychoneuroimmunology and cancer: fact or fiction? Eur J Cancer. 1999;35(11):1603–7.

73. Miller GE, Dopp JM, Myers HF, Stevens SY, Fahey JL. Psychosocial predictors of natural killer cell mobilization during marital conflict. Health Psychol. 1999;18(3):262–71.

74. Takahashi K, Iwase M, Yamashita K, et al. The elevation of natural killer cell activity induced by laughter in a crossover designed study. Int J Mol Med. 2001;8(6):645–50.

75. Schofferman J, Anderson D, Hines R, Smith G, White A. Childhood psychological trauma correlates with unsuccessful lumbar spine surgery. Spine. 1992;17(6 Suppl):S138–44.

76. Cossette S, Frasure-Smith N, Lesperance F. Clinical implications of a reduction in psychological distress on cardiac prognosis in patients participating in a psychosocial intervention program. Psychosom Med. 2001;63(2):257–66.

77. Donker FJ. Cardiac rehabilitation: a review of current developments. Clin Psychol Rev. 2000;20(7):923–43.

78. Frasure-Smith N, Lesperance F, Gravel G, et al. Social support, depression, and mortality during the first year after myocardial infarction. Circulation. 2000;101(16):1919–24.

79. Kiecolt-Glaser JK, McGuire L, Robles TF, Glaser R. Psychoneuroimmunology and psychosomatic medicine: back to the future. Psychosom Med. 2002;64(1):15–28.

80. Marucha PT, Kiecolt-Glaser JK, Favagehi M. Mucosal wound healing is impaired by examination stress. Psychosom Med. 1998;60(3):362–5.

81. Schofferman J, Anderson D, Hines R, Smith G, Keane G. Childhood psychological trauma and chronic refractory low-back pain. Clin J Pain. 1993;9(4):260–5.

82. Vermeire E, Hearnshaw H, Van Royen P, Denekens J. Patient adherence to treatment: three decades of research. A comprehensive review. J Clin Pharm Ther. 2001;26(5):331–42.

83. Lieberman 3rd JA. Compliance issues in primary care. J Clin Psychiatry. 1996;57 Suppl 7:76–82; discussion 83–75.

84. Green CR, Flowe-Valencia H, Rosenblum L, Tait AR. The role of childhood and adulthood abuse among women presenting for chronic pain management. Clin J Pain. 2001;17(4):359–64.

85. Winfield JB. Psychological determinants of fibromyalgia and related syndromes. Curr Rev Pain. 2000;4(4):276–86.

86. Roberts SJ. The sequelae of childhood sexual abuse: a primary care focus for adult female survivors. Nurse Pract. 1996;21(12 Pt 1):42, 45, 49–52.

87. Bigos SJ, Battie MC, Spengler DM, et al. A longitudinal, prospective study of industrial back injury reporting. Clin Orthop Relat Res. 1992;279:21–34.

88. Bernard Jr TN. Repeat lumbar spine surgery. Factors influencing outcome. Spine. 1993;18(15):2196–200.

89. DeBerard MS, Masters KS, Colledge AL, Schleusener RL, Schlegel JD. Outcomes of posterolateral lumbar fusion in Utah patients receiving workers' compensation: a retrospective cohort study. Spine. 2001;26(7):738–46; discussion 747.

90. Epker J, Block AR. Presurgical psychological screening in back pain patients: a review. Clin J Pain. 2001;17(3):200–5.

91. LaCaille RA, DeBerard MS, Masters KS, Colledge AL, Bacon W. Presurgical biopsychosocial factors predict multidimensional

patient: outcomes of interbody cage lumbar fusion. Spine J. 2005;5(1):71–8.

92. Taylor VM, Deyo RA, Ciol M, et al. Patient-oriented outcomes from low back surgery: a community-based study. Spine. 2000;25(19):2445–52.

93. Junge A, Dvorak J, Ahrens S. Predictors of bad and good outcomes of lumbar disc surgery. A prospective clinical study with recommendations for screening to avoid bad outcomes. Spine. 1995;20(4):460–8.

94. Greenough CG, Taylor LJ, Fraser RD. Anterior lumbar fusion. A comparison of noncompensation patients with compensation patients. Clin Orthop Relat Res. 1994;300:30–7.

95. Groth-Marnat G, Fletcher A. Influence of neuroticism, catastrophizing, pain duration, and receipt of compensation on short-term response to nerve block treatment for chronic back pain. J Behav Med. 2000;23(4):339–50.

96. Mannion AF, Elfering A. Predictors of surgical outcome and their assessment. Eur Spine J. 2006;15 Suppl 1:S93–108.

97. Glassman SD, Minkow RE, Dimar JR, Puno RM, Raque GH, Johnson JR. Effect of prior lumbar discectomy on outcome of lumbar fusion: a prospective analysis using the SF-36 measure. J Spinal Disord. 1998;11(5):383–8.

98. Klekamp J, McCarty E, Spengler DM. Results of elective lumbar discectomy for patients involved in the workers' compensation system. J Spinal Disord. 1998;11(4):277–82.

99. Feuerstein M, Callan-Harris S, Hickey P, Dyer D, Armbruster W, Carosella AM. Multidisciplinary rehabilitation of chronic work-related upper extremity disorders. Long-term effects. J Occup Med. 1993;35(4):396–403.

100. DeBerard MS, Masters KS, Colledge AL, Holmes EB. Presurgical biopsychosocial variables predict medical and compensation costs of lumbar fusion in Utah workers' compensation patients. Spine J. 2003;3(6):420–9.

101. Marquez de la Plata C, Hewlitt M, de Oliveira A, et al. Ethnic differences in rehabilitation placement and outcome after TBI. J Head Trauma Rehabil. 2007;22(2):113–21.

102. Nelson DV, Kennington M, Novy DM, et al. Providers' Attitudes and practices regarding psychological selection criteria for spinal cord stimulation. Seattle: International Association for the Study of Pain (IASP) Press; 1996.

103. Work Loss Data Institute. Official Disability Guidelines. Encinitas: Work Loss Data Institute; 2008.

104. Colorado Division of Worker Compensation. Chronic Pain Task Force. Rule 17, Exhibit 9: Chronic Pain Disorder Medical Treatment Guidelines: Colorado Department of Labor and Employment: Division of Worker Compensation 2007.

105. American College of Occupational and Environmental Medicine. Chronic pain treatment guidelines. In: Hegmann K, editor. Occupational medicine practice guidelines. 2nd ed. Beverly Farms: OEM Press; 2008.

106. Giordano N, Lofland K, Guay J, et al. Utilization of and beliefs about presurgical psychological screening: a national survey of anesthesiologists. J Pain. 2005;6(3 Suppl):S67.

107. Meyer GJ, Finn SE, Eyde LD, et al. Psychological testing and psychological assessment. A review of evidence and issues. Am Psychol. 2001;56(2):128–65.

108. Carragee EJ, Alamin TF, Miller JL, Carragee JM. Discographic, MRI and psychosocial determinants of low back pain disability and remission: a prospective study in subjects with benign persistent back pain. Spine J. 2005;5(1):24–35.

109. Gatchel RJ, Polatin PB, Mayer TG. The dominant role of psychosocial risk factors in the development of chronic low back pain disability. Spine. 1995;20(24):2702–9.

110. Block AR, Gatchel RJ, Deardorff WW, Guyer RD. The psychology of spine surgery. Washington, D.C.: American Psychological Association; 2003.

111. Gatchel RJ. A biopsychosocial overview of pretreatment screening of patients with pain. Clin J Pain. 2001;17(3):192–9.

112. Giordano N, Lofland K. A literature review of psychological predictors of spinal cord stimulator outcomes. American Pain Society 24th annual scientific meeting, Boston, 2005.

113. Ormel J, VonKorff M, Ustun TB, Pini S, Korten A, Oldehinkel T. Common mental disorders and disability across cultures. Results from the WHO Collaborative Study on Psychological Problems in General Health Care. JAMA. 1994;272(22): 1741–8.

114. Bruns D, Warren PA. The assessment of psychosocial contributions to disability. In: Warren PA, editor. Handbook of behavioral health disability. New York: Springer; 2010.

115. American Educational Research Association, American Psychological Association, National Council on Measurement in Education, Joint Committee on Standards for Educational and Psychological Testing (U.S.). Standards for educational and psychological testing. Washington, D.C.: American Educational Research Association; 1999.

116. Turk DC, Melzack R. Trends and future directions in human pain assessment. In: Turk DC, Melzack R, editors. Handbook of pain assessment. New York: Guilford Press; 1992. p. 473–9.

117. Disorbio JM, Bruns D. Brief battery for health improvement 2 manual. Minneapolis: Pearson; 2002.

118. Mitrushina M, Boone D, Razani J, D'Elia L. Handbook of normative data for neuropsychological assessment. 2nd ed. New York: Oxford University Press; 2005.

119. Bruns D, Disorbio JM. Assessment of biopsychosocial risk factors for medical treatment: a collaborative approach. J Clin Psychol Med Settings. 2009;16(2):127–47.

120. Bruns D, Disorbio JM. Battery for health improvement 2 manual. Minneapolis: Pearson; 2003.

121. Turk DC, Melzack R. Handbook of pain assessment. 2nd ed. New York: Guilford Press; 2001.

122. Bruns D. Psychological tests commonly used in the assessment of chronic pain patients. 2002. http://www.healthpsych.com/testing/psychtests.pdf. Accessed 7 July 2012.

123. Butcher JN, American Psychological Association. MMPI-2: a practitioner's guide. 1st ed. Washington, D.C.: American Psychological Association; 2006.

124. Butcher JN, Graham JR, Ben-Porath YS, Tellegen A, Dahlstrom WG, Kaemmer B. Minnesota Multiphasic Personality Inventory–2 (MMPI–2): manual for administration, scoring and interpretation. Rev. ed. Minneapolis: University of Minnesota Press; 2001.

125. Block A. The psychology of spine surgery. 1st ed. Washington, D.C.: American Psychological Association; 2003.

126. Doleys DM, Klapow JC, Hammer M. Psychological evaluation in spinal cord stimulation therapy. Pain Rev. 1997;4:189–207.

127. Nelson DV, Kennington M, Novy DM, Squitieri P. Psychological selection criteria for implantable spinal cord stimulators. Pain Forum. 1996;5(2):93–103.

128. Olson K, Bedder MD, Anderson VC, Burchiel KJ, Villaneuva MR. Psychological variables associated with outcome of spinal cord stimulation trials. Neuromodulation. 1998;1:6–13.

129. Beltrutti D, Lamberto A, Barolat G, et al. The psychological assessment of candidates for spinal cord stimulation for chronic pain management. Pain Pract. 2004;4(3):204–21.

130. Tellegen A, Ben-Porath YS, McNulty JL, Arbisi PA, Graham JE, Kaemmer B. The MMPI-2 restructured clinical (RC) scales. Minneapolis: Pearson Assessments; 2003.

131. Butcher JN. MMPI-2: Minnesota Multiphasic Personality Inventory-2: manual for administration, scoring, and interpretation. Rev.th ed. Minneapolis: University of Minnesota Press; 2001.

132. Ben-Porath YS, Tellegen A. MMPI-2-RF™ manual. Minneapolis: University of Minnesota; 2008.

133. Rogers R, Sewell KW. MMPI-2 at the crossroads: aging technology or radical retrofitting? J Pers Assess. 2006;87(2):175–8.

134. Rogers R, Sewell KW, Harrison KS, Jordan MJ. The MMPI-2 restructured clinical scales: a paradigmatic shift in scale development. J Pers Assess. 2006;87(2):139–47.

135. Butcher JN, Hamilton CK, Rouse SV, Cumella EJ. The deconstruction of the Hy Scale of MMPI-2: failure of RC3 in measuring somatic symptom expression. J Pers Assess. 2006;87(2):186–92.

136. Tellegen A, Ben-Porath YS, Sellbom M. Construct validity of the MMPI-2 restructured clinical (RC) scales: reply to Rouse, Greene, Butcher, Nichols, and Williams. J Pers Assess. 2009;91(3):211–21; discussion 222–6.

137. Rouse SV, Greene RL, Butcher JN, Nichols DS, Williams CL. What do the MMPI-2 restructured clinical scales reliably measure? Answers from multiple research settings. J Pers Assess. 2008;90(5):435–42.

138. Millon T, Davis R, Millon C. Millon clinical multiaxial inventory-III manual. 2nd ed. Minneapolis: Pearson Assessments; 1997.

139. Manchikanti L, Pampati V, Beyer C, Damron K. Do number of pain conditions influence emotional status? Pain Physician. 2002;5(2):200–5.

140. Manchikanti L, Fellows B, Pampati V, Beyer C, Damron K, Barnhill RC. Comparison of psychological status of chronic pain patients and the general population. Pain Physician. 2002;5(1):40–8.

141. Rivera JJ, Singh V, Fellows B, Pampati V, Damron KS, McManus CD. Reliability of psychological evaluation in chronic pain in an interventional pain management setting. Pain Physician. 2005;8(4):375–83.

142. Hopwood CJ, Creech SK, Clark TS, Meagher MW, Morey LC. Predicting the completion of an integrative and intensive outpatient chronic pain treatment with the personality assessment inventory. J Pers Assess. 2008;90(1):76–80.

143. Karlin BE, Creech SK, Grimes JS, Clark TS, Meagher MW, Morey LC. The personality assessment inventory with chronic pain patients: psychometric properties and clinical utility. J Clin Psychol. 2005;61(12):1571–85.

144. Williams AC, Richardson PH. What does the BDI measure in chronic pain? Pain. 1993;55(2):259–66.

145. Spielberger CD, Gorsuch RL, Lushene RE. Manual for the state-trait anxiety inventory. Palo Alto: Consulting Psychologists Press; 1970.

146. Fishbain DA, Bruns D, Disorbio JM, Lewis JE. What patient attributes are associated with thoughts of suing a physician? Arch Phys Med Rehabil. 2007;88(5):589–96.

147. Fishbain DA, Bruns D, Disorbio JM, Lewis JE. What are the variables that are associated with the patient's wish to sue his physician in patients with acute and chronic pain? Pain Med. 2008;9(8):1130–42.

148. Bruns D, Fishbain DA, Disorbio JM, Lewis JE. What variables are associated with an expressed wish to kill a doctor in community and injured patient samples? J Clin Psychol Med Settings. 2010;17(2):87–97.

149. Bruns D, Disorbio JM. Hostility and violent ideation: physical rehabilitation patient and community samples. Pain Med. 2000;1(2):131–9.

150. Freedenfeld RN, Bailey BE, Bruns D, Fuchs PN, Kiser RS. Prediction of interdisciplinary pain treatment outcome using the Battery for Health Improvement. Paper presented at proceedings of the 10th world congress on pain, San Francisco, 2002.

151. Bruns D, Disorbio JM, Hanks R. Chronic nonmalignant pain and violent behavior. Curr Pain Headache Rep. 2003;7(2):127–32.

152. Bruns D, Disorbio JM. Chronic pain and biopsychosocial disorders. Pract Pain Manag. 2005;5(7):52–61.

153. Disorbio JM, Bruns D, Barolat G. Assessment and treatment of chronic pain: a physician's guide to a biopsychosocial approach. Pract Pain Manag. 2006;6(2):11–27.

154. Bruns D, Disorbio JM, Hanks R. Chronic pain and violent ideation: testing a model of patient violence. Pain Med. 2007;8(3):207–15.

155. Fishbain DA, Bruns D, Disorbio JM, Lewis JE. Correlates of self-reported violent ideation against physicians in acute – and chronic-pain patients. Pain Med. 2009;10(3):573–85.

156. Fishbain DA, Bruns D, Disorbio JM, Lewis JE. Risk for five forms of suicidality in acute pain patients and chronic pain patients vs pain-free community controls. Pain Med. 2009;10(6):1095–105.

157. Fishbain DA, Bruns D, Disorbio JM, Lewis JE, Gao J. Variables associated with self-prediction of psychopharmacological treatment adherence in acute and chronic pain patients. Pain Pract. 2010;10(6):508–19.

158. Portenoy RK, Bruns D, Shoemaker B, Shoemaker SA. Breakthrough pain in community-dwelling patients with cancer pain and noncancer pain, part 2: impact on function, mood, and quality of life. J Opioid Manag. 2010;6(2):109–16.

159. Tragesser SL, Bruns D, Disorbio JM. Borderline personality disorder features and pain: the mediating role of negative affect in a pain patient sample. Clin J Pain. 2010;26(4):348–53.

160. Fishbain DA, Bruns D, Disorbio JM, Lewis JE, Gao J. Exploration of the illness uncertainty concept in acute and chronic pain patients vs community patients. Pain Med. 2010;11(5):658–69.

161. Fishbain DA, Lewis JE, Bruns D, Disorbio JM, Gao J, Meyer LJ. Exploration of anger constructs in acute and chronic pain patients vs community patients. Pain Pract. 2011;11(3):240–51.

162. Millon T, Antoni M, Millon C, Meagher S, Grossman S. Millon behavioral medicine diagnostic manual. Minnealpolis: Pearson Assessments; 2001.

163. Millon T. Toward a new personology: an evolutionary model. New York: Wiley; 1990.

164. Tollison D, Langley JC. Pain patient profile manual. Minneapolis: Pearson Assessments; 1995.

165. Willoughby SG, Hailey BJ, Wheeler LC. Pain patient profile: a scale to measure psychological distress. Arch Phys Med Rehabil. 1999;80(10):1300–2.

166. McGuire BE, Harvey AG, Shores EA. Simulated malingering in pain patients: a study with the pain patient profile. Br J Clin Psychol. 2001;40(Pt 1):71–9.

167. McGuire BE, Shores EA. Pain patient profile and the assessment of malingered pain. J Clin Psychol. 2001;57(3):401–9.

168. Manchikanti L, Pampati V, Beyer C, Damron K, Barnhill RC. Evaluation of psychological status in chronic low back pain: comparison with general population. Pain Physician. 2002;5(2):149–55.

169. Manchikanti L, Fellows B, Singh V, Pampati V. Correlates of non-physiological behavior in patients with chronic low back pain. Pain Physician. 2003;6(2):159–66.

170. Hankin HA, Killian CB. Prediction of functional outcomes in patients with chronic pain. Work. 2004;22(2):125–30.

171. Manchikanti L, Manchikanti KN, Damron KS, Pampati V. Effectiveness of cervical medial branch blocks in chronic neck pain: a prospective outcome study. Pain Physician. 2004;7(2):195–201.

172. Manchikanti L, Manchikanti KN, Manchukonda R, Pampati V, Cash KA. Evaluation of therapeutic thoracic medial branch block effectiveness in chronic thoracic pain: a prospective outcome study with minimum 1-year follow up. Pain Physician. 2006;9(2):97–105.

173. Noble J, Gomez M, Fish JS. Quality of life and return to work following electrical burns. Burns. 2006;32(2):159–64.

174. Derogatis LR. Brief symptom inventory 18 manual (BSI® 18). Minneapolis: Pearson Assessments; 2001.

175. Derogatis LR. Brief symptom inventory manual (BSI®). Minneapolis: Pearson Assessments; 2001.

176. Derogatis LR. SCL–90: Administration, scoring, and procedures manual for the revised version. Baltimore: Clinical Psychometric Research; 1983.

177. Clark KL, Loscalzo M, Trask PC, Zabora J, Philip EJ. Psychological distress in patients with pancreatic cancer-an understudied group. Psychooncology. 2010;19(12):1313–20.

178. Zeltzer LK, Recklitis C, Buchbinder D, et al. Psychological status in childhood cancer survivors: a report from the Childhood Cancer Survivor Study. J Clin Oncol. 2009;27(14):2396–404.

179. Gessler S, Low J, Daniells E, et al. Screening for distress in cancer patients: is the distress thermometer a valid measure in the UK and does it measure change over time? A prospective validation study. Psychooncology. 2008;17(6):538–47.

180. Mertens AC, Sencer S, Myers CD, et al. Complementary and alternative therapy use in adult survivors of childhood cancer: a report from the Childhood Cancer Survivor Study. Pediatr Blood Cancer. 2008;50(1):90–7.

181. Kerns RD, Turk DC, Rudy TE. The West Haven-Yale Multidimensional Pain Inventory (WHYMPI). Pain. 1985;23(4):345–56.

182. Jensen M, Turner J, Romano JM, Nielson WR. Chronic pain coping inventory manual. Lutz: Psychological Assessment Resources; 2010.

183. Jensen M, Karoly P. Survey of pain attitudes manual. Lutz: Psychological Assessment Resources; 2010.

184. Rudy TE. Multidimensional pain inventory (MPI) computer program, version 3.0. 2009. http://www.pain.pitt.edu/mpi/. Accessed 18 Sept 2010.

185. Okifuji A, Turk DC, Eveleigh DJ. Improving the rate of classification of patients with the multidimensional pain inventory (MPI): clarifying the meaning of "significant other". Clin J Pain. 1999;15(4):290–6.

186. Hall RC. Detection of malingered PTSD: an overview of clinical, psychometric, and physiological assessment: where do we stand? J Forensic Sci. 2007;52(3):717–25.

187. Fishbain DA, Cutler R, Rosomoff HL, Rosomoff RS. Chronic pain disability exaggeration/malingering and submaximal effort research. Clin J Pain. 1999;15(4):244–74.

188. Aronoff GM, Mandel S, Genovese E, et al. Evaluating malingering in contested injury or illness. Pain Pract. 2007;7(2):178–204.

189. Mittenberg W, Patton C, Canyock EM, Condit DC. Base rates of malingering and symptom exaggeration. J Clin Exp Neuropsychol. 2002;24(8):1094–102.

190. Binder LM, Rohling ML. Money matters: a meta-analytic review of the effects of financial incentives on recovery after closed-head injury. Am J Psychiatry. 1996;153(1):7–10.

191. Rohling ML, Binder LM, Langhinrichsen-Rohling J. Money matters: a meta-analytic review of the association between financial compensation and the experience and treatment of chronic pain. Health Psychol. 1995;14(6):537–47.

192. Bianchini KJ, Curtis KL, Greve KW. Compensation and malingering in traumatic brain injury: a dose–response relationship? Clin Neuropsychol. 2006;20(4):831–47.

193. Gatchel RJ, Polatin PB, Mayer TG, Garcy PD. Psychopathology and the rehabilitation of patients with chronic low back pain disability. Arch Phys Med Rehabil. 1994;75(6):666–70.

194. Scarry E. The body in pain: the making and unmaking of the world. New York: Oxford University Press; 1985.

195. Kauffman J. Loss of the assumptive world: a theory of traumatic loss. New York: Brunner-Routledge; 2002.

196. Bruns D, Mueller K, Warren PA. Biopsychosocial law, health care reform, and the control of medical inflation in Colorado. Rehabilitation psychology. 2012;57(2):81–97.

Psychological Therapies

Leanne R. Cianfrini, Cady Block, and Daniel M. Doleys

Key Points

- When we critically analyze reciprocal and plastic connections between limbic, thalamic, and sensorimotor areas of the brain, it becomes obvious that what we experience as *pain* is larger than the sum of its sensory, affective, and cognitive components.
- Acknowledging that psychological factors are involved with the pain experience does not mean that the pain is "in the patient's head."
- Cognitive behavioral therapy (CBT) is a cost-effective adjunct to medical interventions and is backed by strong empirical evidence for positive changes in health-related quality of life, coping and depression, social support, subjective pain intensity, and pain-related activity interference.
- While the cognitive techniques involve modifying pain-related maladaptive thoughts and aim to create realistic appraisals, the behavioral "conditioning" and physiological relaxation techniques can affect activity engagement, treatment adherence, overt pain behaviors, and muscle tension.
- Physicians can implement many of these basic cognitive techniques and offer potent behavioral suggestions during even the briefest of consultations;

practical tips for setting appropriate expectations and encouraging self-management are suggested.
- The incremental benefit of combined treatments can address the limitations that we have seen with pain monotherapies.
- The more advanced cognitive and behavioral techniques can be secured through collaboration with mental health providers in the community or by employing a qualified therapist in the office for a seamless interdisciplinary and biopsychosocial therapeutic approach.

Introduction

Pain is a more terrible lord of mankind than even death itself.
– Albert Schweitzer, *On the Edge of the Primeval Forest*, 1914

Although the tenor of that oft-quoted sentence is dramatic, the rest of the sentiment from the humanitarian and physician reads: "We must all die. But that I can save him from days of torture, that is what I feel is my great, ever-new privilege." In the early twentieth century, Dr. Schweitzer elegantly described in three sentences the destructive nature of pain and the obligation and privilege of the physician to relieve it. He continues, "So, when the poor, moaning creature comes, I lay my hand on his head and say to him: 'Don't be afraid! In an hour's time, you shall be put to sleep, and when you wake you won't feel any more pain.'" So begins the promise of the interventionalist.

One undercurrent of this chapter is to demonstrate the *power* of such words—contained within self-reported pain descriptors and our own well-intentioned assurances—to influence pain processing and modulation. We will reveal the impact of cognitive processes (e.g., expectations, interpretations) on pain, pain-related mood issues, and behavioral responses. We will also explore the evidence-based psychological methods designed to

L.R. Cianfrini, Ph.D. (✉) • D.M. Doleys, Ph.D.
The Doleys Clinic / Pain & Rehabilitation Center, Inc.,
2270 Valleydale Road, Suite 100,
Birmingham, AL 35244, USA
e-mail: lcianfrini@gmail.com; dmdpri@aol.com

C. Block, M.S.
Department of Psychology,
University of Alabama at Birmingham,
1300 University Boulevard, Campbell Hall Ste 415,
Birmingham, AL 35294, USA
e-mail: cblock@uab.edu

T.R. Deer et al. (eds.), *Comprehensive Treatment of Chronic Pain by Medical, Interventional, and Integrative Approaches*,
DOI 10.1007/978-1-4614-1560-2_76, © American Academy of Pain Medicine 2013

treat unrealistic patient outcomes expectations, maladaptive pain behaviors, and the general physical and emotional consequences of chronic pain. We will examine not just the specialized techniques used within the purview of trained pain/health psychologists but will also introduce brief therapeutic strategies that can be implemented within any medical practice.

Background and History

> The mind is its own place and in itself, can make a Heav'n of Hell, a Hell of Heav'n.
> – John Milton, *Paradise Lost*

Like in the old Hallmark card commercial, we now accept readily that, "It's the thought that counts." A person can make what they will of any given situation. We have all seen friends, loved ones, coworkers, and patients exacerbate stress through worry, rumination, passivity, or aggression. Conversely, we have witnessed inspiring resilience in the face of personal traumas, environmental disasters, and debilitating chronic illnesses. Although laypersons, the medical pain management community, and third-party payors have increasingly recognized the impact of psychosocial factors and behavioral medicine interventions on the pain experience over the past 30 years, this was actually a battle long fought.

Historically, the biomedical, dualistic disease model of pain, dating back to the ancient Greeks and promulgated by Descartes in the seventeenth century, was the dominant conceptualization. Depending on philosophical and career orientation, pain was typically viewed in one of two ways: (a) as an organic phenomenon solely within the sensory domain of the body, to be treated by physicians and surgeons, or (b) as uniquely "of the mind" and thus beyond the scope of physical treatment. Philosophers, religious leaders, and physicians of each era provoked a pendulum swing from one extreme perspective to the other. Integrative models of pain have followed several key paradigm shifts throughout the last several decades, away from the unidimensional physiological model to the gate control theory conceived of by Melzack and Wall [1] to the more broadly encompassing biopsychosocial perspective of illness [2], to the current zeitgeist regarding the dynamic and elegant concept of neuroplasticity.

Scientific Foundation

> When we wish to perfect our senses, neuroplasticity is a blessing; when it works in the service of pain, plasticity can be a curse.
> – Norman Doidge

To understand the role of psychology in the treatment of pain, we must rewind and first clarify the difference between nociception and pain. Nociception begins with the activation of peripheral nociceptors via the process of transduction. Impulses are transmitted to the dorsal horn of the spinal cord where they can and often do undergo modulation. Depending upon the particular set of circumstances, these impulses may be up- or downregulated. The gate control theory introduced by Melzack and Wall [1], and later refined by Melzack and Casey [3], provided a heuristic foundation for understanding some of the sources of nociceptive modulation, including "top-down" cognitive processes such as anxiety, attention, or distraction that may influence the gate. The resulting nociceptive activity is propagated to higher centers via ascending tracts. Somatotopic organization is carried out in thalamic structures with subsequent activation of multiple higher cortical centers including the somatosensory, cingulate, and prefrontal cortices. The dynamic interplay among the various cortical structures involved as well as stimulation of the descending modulatory system influences an individual's overall experience of pain, which is subject to change *despite* stable peripheral stimulation. Put simply, the scientific evidence suggests that pain isn't pain until the brain *says* it's pain. Indeed, one can experience "pain" without the activation of peripheral nociceptors. While we understand nociception to be the electrochemical journey of impulses working toward the brain, the noted neurologist V.S. Ramachandran clarified that "Pain…is created by the brain and projected onto the body" ([4], p. 190).

As early as 1959, Beecher advanced the realization that pain is influenced by more than pure nociceptive input. In the context of his study with wounded World War II soldiers, secondary gain and cognitive appraisals (e.g., the wound pain is tolerable because it represents a reprieve from the battlefield) emerged as strong correlates of self-reported pain intensity and requests for opioid analgesia [5]. Almost 40 years later, Rainville and colleagues [6] demonstrated through a unique hypnosis study design that an emotional or affective component of pain could be independently manipulated from the sensory or intensity component.

These early studies, taken together with our increased understanding of anatomical brain structure and function assisted by advances in technology [e.g., functional magnetic resonance imaging (fMRI)], the mapping of interconnecting neural pain pathways, and our ever-expanding awareness of the plasticity of neuronal connections, help to account for some of the vast intra- and interindividual differences in the perception of and reaction to pain. When we pause to critically analyze the reciprocal connections between limbic, thalamic, and sensorimotor areas of the brain (see Fig. 76.1), it becomes obvious that what we experience as *pain* is larger than the sum of its sensory-discriminative, affective-motivational, and cognitive-evaluative components. The pain "maps" in the brain are in constant flux secondary to both afferent and efferent processes, including peripheral injury, continued nociceptive input, central and peripheral sensitization, and input fed from the limbic system and higher cortical connections.

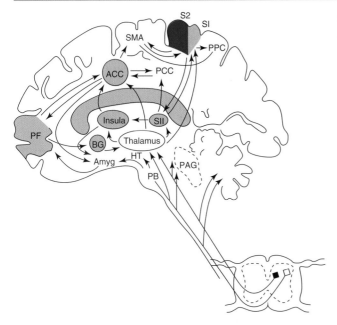

Fig. 76.1 The pain matrix (Reprinted with permission from Bushnell and Apkarian [7]). *ACC* anterior cingulate cortex, *Amyg* amygdala, *BG* basal ganglia, *HT* hypothalamus, *PAG* periaqueductal gray matter, *PB* parabrachial nucleus, *PCC* posterior cingulate cortex, *PF* prefrontal cortex, *PPC* posterior parietal cortex, *S1* primary somatosensory cortex, *S2* secondary somatosensory cortex, *SMA* supplementary motor area

Given the significant degree of reciprocal overlap between the limbic/emotional and pain-processing areas of the cortex evident in Fig. 76.1, intuitively, any treatment which influences one is likely to affect the other. Pharmacological therapies are well known to influence neurotransmitter activity. But, what about the psychological/behavioral therapies? Over a decade ago, psychiatrist and Nobel Laureate Eric Kandel ([8], p. 460) proposed the following:

> Insofar as psychotherapy or counseling is effective and produces long-term changes in behavior, it presumably does so through learning, by producing changes in gene expression that alters the strength of synaptic connections and structural changes that alter the anatomical pattern of interconnections between nerve cells of the brain. As the resolution of brain imaging increases, it should eventually permit quantitative evaluation of the outcome of psychotherapy.

This assertion was certainly prescient, given what we now know about the influence of psychological techniques on brain neuroplasticity. For example, using PET scan technology, Goldapple and colleagues [9] compared the effects of antidepressant treatment with paroxetine to that of cognitive behavioral therapy (CBT). CBT was found to have a modality-specific effect, producing unique blood flow changes in the frontal cortex, anterior cingulate cortex, and hippocampus. Thus, the effect of CBT was largely to normalize the metabolic activity of the prefrontal lobes. Other studies have also documented similar cortical changes

facilitated by psychotherapeutic intervention for disorders including posttraumatic stress disorder, specific phobia, depression, and anxiety [10–14]. Such studies led to Dr. Kandel's revised view, several years later, that "There is no longer any doubt that psychotherapy can result in detectable changes in the brain" [15].

Despite the appeal of the biopsychosocial model, medical pain specialists often unwittingly promote the "pain-as-functional-or-structural-abnormality" concept. The hope of surgeons and patients alike is that once the physical cause of the pain is identified and treated appropriately, the pain will be eliminated. The focused quest for a "pain generator" as well as the predominance of purely medical/physical modalities suggested as first-line options in published treatment guidelines from medical societies can lead some patients down an unsatisfying and incomplete path. This occurs especially if the somatic treatment recommended and attempted is ineffective, partially effective, or when a direct physiological cause cannot be immediately localized. Patients are often left to "just deal with" the residual, incurable symptoms on their own.

Psychological processes of learning and memory, mood and affect, social withdrawal and isolation, past traumatic events, pain beliefs, anticipation of pain exacerbation, and coping style can all play a role in an individual's adjustment to chronic pain. All of these factors have the potential to influence the pain experience at several phases: at the onset of pain, during the seeking and receiving of healthcare and support, and in the development of chronic pain-related disability and work loss [16]. Recognizing the contribution of psychosocial factors to an individuals' pain opens the door for the implementation of psychologically oriented cognitive and behavioral self-management strategies to address the remaining pain complaints and provide a more comprehensive, holistic approach to improving quality of life despite persistent pain.

Of note, acknowledging that psychological factors are involved with the pain experience does not mean that the pain is "in the patient's head," that is to imply, psychogenic or factitious in origin. As expressed by Andrew Miller in his novel *Ingenious Pain*, "All pain is real enough to those who have it; all stand equally in need of compassion" [17]. International studies show that nearly half of people with chronic pain still experience negative cognitive, emotional, and physical effects despite conventional medical therapies, as well as poor social and occupational functioning and overall lower quality of life [18, 19]. For example, the most potent drugs only decrease pain levels by 30–40 % in fewer than half of patients [20]. Surgical techniques such as artificial disk implantation or implantable drug delivery systems also provide modest pain reduction [20]. In addition to pain relief of limited clinical significance in inadequately screened patients, implantable devices also run the risk of adverse side effects [20, 21]. However, patients who participate in various forms of psychological interventions as a complement or adjunct to medical treatment have been found to significantly improve. Improvements in pain intensity, mood, coping, daily activity, and social functioning have all been reported [22, 23] without the risk of adverse physical consequences.

The inefficiency of even our best medical interventions may be due, in part, to the fact that many of the reasons for the inadequate responses to medical treatments are indeed psychological. Relevant psychological factors may include underreporting or exaggeration of pain intensity, inadequate communication skills between physician and patient, unrealistic or inappropriate expectations for outcomes, fears of addiction, fear of stigma, noncompliance to physical therapy exercise regimens, or other health behaviors. Addressing these psychological barriers can improve medical treatment outcomes and assist the patient in coping with any residual pain in the long term. Put simply, the goal of the psychological therapies is to help patients develop a satisfactory quality of life, whatever they define that to be within their own values and abilities, *despite* the persistent pain.

Clinical Examples and Usefulness in Clinical Practice

There are several evidence-based psychological therapies effectively implemented in clinical pain populations. These include but are not limited to (a) behavioral therapies modeled on operant and classical conditioning paradigms, such as exposure and desensitization to avoided activities; (b) cognitive behavioral therapy and acceptance-based therapies; (c) biofeedback and relaxation training; (d) group therapies; and (e) motivational enhancement therapy. Another technique that falls under the "psychological therapy" umbrella is hypnosis, which is covered elsewhere in this book. Insight-oriented and psychodynamic approaches, which are predicated on the belief that pain may be a manifestation of emotional distress and which emphasize the influence of early childhood experiences on the experience of pain in adulthood, will not be reviewed here in the interest of space and paucity of well-designed outcomes studies in pain populations. Some newer therapies such as narrative

therapy [24] show promise in the management of chronic mental and medical illnesses, but as of yet there is very little literature on the efficacy of this modality among individuals with chronic physical pain. We will begin with some of the classic behavioral psychology conceptualizations and associated therapies.

Classical and Operant Conditioning Techniques

The most useful piece of learning for the uses of life is to unlearn what is untrue.

– Antisthenes

Most everyone with an undergraduate Psych 101 class under their belt is familiar with the concept of Pavlovian conditioning, also known as "classical" conditioning. In the landmark experiment, dogs were trained to salivate (conditioned response) at the sound of a ringing bell (conditioned stimulus) after numerous repeated pairings of the bell with meat powder (unconditioned stimulus). Thus, the dogs were eventually conditioned to anticipate food and salivate at the mere sound of the bell. Pavlov's studies supported Aristotle's observations of the "law of association by contiguity," essentially paraphrased as "If a person experiences two environmental events (stimuli) at the same time or one right after the other (contiguously), those events will become associated in the person's mind, such that the thought of one will, in the future, tend to elicit the thought of the other."

This type of associative learning occurs in patients with chronic pain as well. Take, for example, a patient who has an unpleasant reaction like a spinal headache following a lumbar epidural block. This patient may develop a conditioned fear response to further epidurals, and the fear may even generalize to other contextual cues (e.g., needles) or other stimuli (e.g., other suggested interventional procedures). See Table 76.1 for an overview of classical conditioning terminology.

Therapeutic interventions based upon the premise of classical conditioning aim to replace the conditioned response through techniques that involve gradual exposure to the feared stimulus paired instead with a neutral or calming

Table 76.1 Classical conditioning basic terminology and examples

Term	Definition	Example
Unconditioned stimulus (US)	A stimulus that naturally triggers a response	A dental procedure that involves drilling
Unconditioned response (UR)	A response that occurs naturally in response to the unconditioned stimulus	The increased heart rate and muscle tension that arises during the painful dental procedure
Conditioned stimulus (CS)	A neutral stimulus, that when paired with an unconditioned stimulus, begins/triggers a conditioned response	The smell and sounds of the dentist's office experienced during the procedure
Conditioned response (CR)	A learned response to a previously neutral (conditioned) stimulus	Increased heart rate and muscle tension while sitting in the dentist's waiting room at the next visit, exposed only to the smell and sounds of the office

Table 76.2 Operant conditioning basic terminology and examples

Term	Definition	Example	Potential result
Positive reinforcement	An increase in the probability of a behavior being repeated due to the addition of a positive consequence	After Mr. Smith *displayed several verbal and nonverbal pain behaviors* (B), his wife pays him *increased attention* (C)	Increased likelihood that Mr. Smith will display pain behaviors in order to solicit support and attention
Negative reinforcement	Increase in the probability of a behavior being repeated due of the stopping or avoiding of a negative consequence	Mr. Smith *takes a few extra oxycodone* (B) which *reduces his pain* (C)	Increased likelihood that Mr. Smith will continue to self-adjust his medications in order to avoid anticipated pain
Extinction	Decreases the probability of a behavior being repeated due to absence of expected consequence	Rather than responding to Mr. Smith's pain behaviors, his wife instead *ignores them* (B)	Decreased likelihood that Mr. Smith will display pain behaviors around his wife
Punishment	Decreases the probability of the behavior being repeated due to application of negative consequence	Mr. Smith's physician, upon seeing another *failed urine drug screen* (B), *declines to prescribe* (C) Mr. Smith opioid medications any longer	Decreased likelihood that Mr. Smith will violate his pain treatment contract in the future

B behavior, *C* consequence

stimulus. In other words, individuals are taught to "unlearn" the anxiety symptoms. Techniques such as systematic desensitization are often and effectively used to treat panic disorder, specific phobias, and posttraumatic stress disorder [25]. Together with the provider, the patient who fears a needle would develop a hierarchy of increasingly anxiety-provoking scenarios (e.g., seeing a needle in the room, watching others receive a needle stick, feeling the prick on their own skin, and so on) and would be guided through the steps combined with deep breathing, other relaxation techniques, or pleasant thoughts. These steps are initially performed covertly using imagined scenarios until the patient's subjective ratings of distress are tolerable; the patient then progresses to in vivo exposure to real-life situations.

Another promising desensitization therapy, called eye movement desensitization and reprocessing (EMDR), is also described by its developer [26] as both an information processing and an "integrative" form of psychotherapy. It was developed initially for work with specific traumas, involves multiple phases of therapy, and can lead to rapid resolution of negative emotions. The goal is to associate/ pair calmer emotions with the traumatic memories and images; the individual recalls the event, but it is less upsetting. Techniques such as bilateral stimulation (alternating taps or auditory tones) or rapid lateral eye movements and substitution of neutral beliefs regarding the trauma are used. Most of the applied research and randomized controlled trials have been conducted with trauma samples like adult survivors of sexual abuse or assault, as well as natural disaster- and combat-related posttraumatic stress disorder [27–29]. However, there is some compelling early evidence that EMDR may be successful in the reduction and elimination of phantom limb pain and associated psychological consequences of amputation [30–33]. While intriguing, most of the studies using EMDR to treat pain have been case series with small sample sizes, and large-scale randomized controlled studies are, to date, lacking.

> The consequences of an act affect the probability of it's occurring again.
>
> – B.F. Skinner

If you have ever disciplined a child, either through time-outs, spanking, taking away TV or video game time, or raising your voice, or if you've given in to a demand for a toy in a store checkout line to avoid a tantrum and stares of passersby, you have felt the influence of another type of conditioning known as operant conditioning. Operant conditioning involves the use of reinforcement-based techniques—giving praise, taking away aversive conditions—to either increase the likelihood of a future positive behavior (e.g., doing homework) through reward or to decrease the potential for a negative behavior (e.g., checkout line tantrums) through aversive consequences. There is evidence indicating that, compared to healthy controls, patients with chronic pain have increased sensitivity to operant conditioning factors such as reinforcement and punishment [34]. Indeed, the word "pain" has etymological roots with the words *punishment* and *penalty* [35]. Table 76.2 provides an overview of operant conditioning principles.

One of the most common applications of operant conditioning in chronic pain patients is in the behavioral modification of overt pain behaviors. William Fordyce [36] was the first to recognize the effects of environmental factors in shaping the pain experience and to apply these principles to the treatment of chronic pain. Without standardized diagnostic procedures to quantify an individual's unique experience of pain, clinicians are compelled to ask for self-reports, monitor overt signals (e.g., in-office postures, facial expressions, and affect), and make inferences about the patient's pain from their verbal comments and observable behaviors.

Pain behaviors include (a) *verbal responses* such as moaning or gasping; (b) *nonverbal responses* including limping, grimacing, guarding painful limbs, and wincing; (c) *generally reduced activity level* including sitting and lying down; and (d) *increased or prolonged use of therapies* such as medications or a TENS unit to control pain [37]. These behaviors, either with conscious intent or more often unwittingly, elicit responses from observers. Family members may then acknowledge the patient's pain through overly solicitous attentive responses, for example, taking over chores or rubbing the patient's back. Physicians may respond with ordering unnecessary procedures or increasing medication doses. As a result of receiving these desirable consequences (i.e., positive reinforcement), the patient learns that their message has been received and the likelihood is increased that the patient will continue to exhibit the behaviors to obtain desired responses in the future. In addition, more adaptive well behaviors (e.g., working, doing laundry) may be overlooked and may extinguish with time.

Therapy based on operant conditioning principles has multiple goals: (a) making patients aware of their overt behaviors, (b) helping them realize more assertive ways of communicating about their pain, (c) educating spouses and families on how to respond with positive attention to desirable well behaviors or ignore/withdraw attention from unhealthy behaviors, and (d) reducing maladaptive or ineffective overt pain behaviors. Efficacy has been observed for this therapy across several chronic pain disorders, including low back pain [38] and fibromyalgia [39], although a more recent review indicates that it is not superior to cognitive or cognitive behavioral treatments for low back pain [40].

Interestingly, solicitous responses from spouses to nonverbal pain behaviors have been shown to be significant predictors of greater pain and physical disability in patients [41]. For example, women with chronic pain who have highly solicitous husbands show lower pain tolerance, greater pain-related interference, poorer performance on functional activity tasks, and greater use of opioid medications [42]. These results underscore the need to include the spouse/partner in clinical interviews and observe the interpersonal interactions. Intervention using couples therapy is warranted for patients with aggressive or overly solicitous spouses; couples can be educated on the operant conditioning model, and spouses can be trained to respond in more appropriate ways to improve the function of the patient.

Over time, you may notice that some patients start to restrict an expanding number of situations and activities (e.g., leave work, stop engaging in hobbies). Not only is an activity like work or exercise *associated* with an exacerbation of pain, the active person is, in effect, *punished* by the increase in pain intensity and discomfort. The individual learns to anticipate and fear the consequence and may choose to avoid the pain-provoking activity. Obviously, this process

may reduce compliance to exercise and physical therapy and prevent engagement in adaptive household chores and social activities. The restricted movement may then become reinforcing because the aversive stimulus is avoided, increasing the likelihood of further activity avoidance.

A team of neuroscientists recently presented evidence that fear memories in adult rats are protected from erasure by compounds in the extracellular matrix of the amygdala [43]. In adult animals, fear conditioning induces a permanent memory that is resilient to erasure. In contrast, during early postnatal development, extinction of conditioned fear leads to memory erasure. This suggests that fear memories are actively protected in adults. Compounds called chondroitin sulfate proteoglycans (CSPGs) organize into perineuronal nets in the amygdala, and this coincides with the developmental switch in fear memory resilience. So, not only can avoidance of pain lead to worse functional outcomes, but the avoidance behavior can also strengthen the fear of pain, and our adult brains may take over to actively protect and preserve these fear memories.

Intuitively, avoidance may subsequently lead to muscle deconditioning, increased muscle tension, and amplification of pain. This concept has been promoted in the literature under a variety of constructs: anticipatory avoidance, fear-avoidance, and kinesiophobia, among others. The fear-avoidance model has been used to explain why a minority of acute low back pain sufferers develop a chronic pain problem [44]. It is also the force behind the use of quota-based exercise programs that proliferated in the early multidisciplinary behavioral pain programs [45], in which there is a gradual buildup of exposure to exercises and repetitions. However, more recent studies have called into question the hypothesized consequences of fear-avoidance for daily functioning [46], and sophisticated longitudinal design and statistical analysis suggest that fear-avoidance beliefs do not limit activity and cause pain/disability in a global manner [47].

Traditionally, operant conditioning therapies took place within inpatient pain rehabilitation environments to promote consistency, but there are no limitations to the settings where operant and classical conditioning can be effectively applied. Mental health providers may work with patients individually or with couples in outpatient or residential therapy settings. Physical therapists can apply reinforcement techniques and graded exposure during exercise sessions. Nurses and medical assistants often talk a patient through blood draws in a calming manner to reduce fear associations.

There are several ways for physicians to implement these behavioral techniques during office visits, on rounds, or even during quick consultations:

- Avoid basing treatment plans solely on patient pain behaviors (e.g., "She's not writhing on the floor, so she must not be a 9/10") and conversely attempt to attend to and praise well behaviors. It has been shown that pain severity and other physical symptoms were significantly underestimated in patients with major depressive episode or panic disorder symptoms [48], who may appear excessive in their behavioral presentations. We do not want to reward or punish the patient with dramatic presentation nor undertreat the stoic patient.

- Suggest time-contingent medication dosing rather than pain-contingent dosing and clearly explain the rationale and recommended time schedule (e.g., write q8h rather than t.i.d.).
- Encourage activity pacing (remember the motto "Take a break *before* you need a break and then get back to it") to break up the overactivity-pain-rest cycle and reassociate activity with positive outcomes.
- Consider playing comforting music in post-procedure recovery rooms to associate a calming stimulus with a possibly uncomfortable and disorienting experience.

Classical and operant conditioning and their associated therapies are primarily subsumed under the umbrella of behavioral theories. You may be using them already more than you realize. While these therapies can be quite useful in addressing specific activity avoidance, overt pain behaviors, and overly solicitous spousal reactions, they fail to address an important factor in the development of maladaptive adjustment to chronic pain: cognition. This "second wave" of psychological therapies incorporates mental processes and responses and is known as cognitive behavioral therapy.

Cognitive Behavioral Therapy for Pain

If you don't like something, change it; if you can't change it, change the way you think about it.
— Mary Engelbreit

Imagine that you're sitting in a chair in the corner of a dimly lit room, ruminating on life's burdens, financial and social stressors, and uncomfortable physical symptoms. It's not difficult to imagine that your mood would change, posture might slump, facial expression draw into a frown, and muscles become tense. Why, then, is it such a surprise that the opposite is true—that one's mood could lift while in a sunny space, surrounded by supportive friends, distracted by enjoyed activities, or with kind words of self-encouragement? However, individuals with chronic pain often get stuck in a habitual cycle of negative thoughts about themselves, the world around them, and the future.

The cognitive part of cognitive behavioral therapy (CBT) for chronic pain management involves modifying such negative and maladaptive thoughts related to pain. Familiar negative statements include "This pain is killing me," "I'm worthless because of the pain," "No one understands my pain," and "I can't do *anything* because of this pain."

CBT also focuses on increasing a person's productive functioning in rewarding activities—the behavioral part, if you will. Cognitive behavioral treatment emphasizes active patient participation. Both didactic methods and Socratic dialogue are employed between therapist and patient. The four essential components of all CBT interventions are reviewed in further detail below and include (a) education, (b) skills acquisition, (c) cognitive and behavioral rehearsal, and (d) generalization and maintenance.

The best prescription is knowledge.
— C. Everett Koop

The *education* phase presents a credible rationale for the CBT intervention for chronic pain, encourages patients to believe they can actively manage their pain and mood, and integrates the CBT model with general health issues. Educational topics might cover pain mechanisms, activity pacing, sleep hygiene, proper use of pain medications, the pain-mood-behavior interaction, barriers to compliance, stress management, weight management, assertiveness and other communication skills, smoking cessation, and other health-related topics. In addition, before CBT techniques are implemented, the patient must learn and accept the cognitive behavioral model and be trained to identify thoughts, moods/emotions, environmental triggers, behavioral response patterns, and habitual belief systems.

During the next therapeutic phase called *skills acquisition*, maladaptive thoughts, feelings, and behaviors are slowly replaced with healthier and more effective alternatives. Behavioral skills include active relaxation training and controlled diaphragmatic breathing exercises to target reductions in autonomic arousal (discussed later in this chapter), attentional diversion from pain, training in assertiveness and problem-solving skills, pleasant activity scheduling, pacing activities to break the overactivity-pain-rest cycle, and other active health behavior strategies (e.g., implementing an exercise program, smoking cessation).

The negative thoughts of pain patients commonly fall into one or more of several categories. Some of the most common forms of distorted thinking or erroneous beliefs are seen in Table 76.3. One type of distorted negative thinking warrants special mention. You have seen a patient who is engaging in pain *catastrophizing* if you've heard the phrases, "My pain is killing me," "I can't cope with this," and/or "My pain is always a 10 out of 10 and will never get better." Defined both as a maladaptive appraisal or coping style and a stable dispositional trait, pain catastrophizing is most readily defined by its three components [49]: (a) magnification (exaggerated symptom perception), (b) rumination (inability to direct attention away from painful sensations), and (c) helplessness (feeling unable to cope with the pain given one's present resources).

Pain catastrophizing is a particularly influential construct that has been shown to be a potent predictor of pain-related

Table 76.3 Common types of pain-related cognitive distortions

Cognitive distortion	Examples
Dichotomous/all-or-none thinking	"Unless my pain is cured, my life will never be good"
	"If I can't dig in my garden, I won't get outside at all"
Fortune telling/prediction	"I can't go to church because I will end up experiencing more pain and be miserable the entire time"
Mind reading	"Everyone at the store thought I was lazy because I was using the scooter"
Imperative thinking/shoulds and musts	"I shouldn't have to ask for help"
	"I should be able to mow my lawn in an hour like I used to"

disability [50], quality of life [51], suicidal ideation [52], observable pain behavior and spousal response [53, 54], as well as postsurgical pain ratings and narcotic usage [55], often exceeding the contribution of depression itself to these outcomes. Pain catastrophizing has also been implicated as a predictor for poor response to minimally invasive procedures such as radiofrequency lesioning and injection treatments [56], as well as a predictor or persistent pain at two years following total knee arthroscopy [57]. With regard to mechanism of action, there is recent evidence that catastrophizing affects supraspinal endogenous pain-inhibitory and pain-facilitatory processes [58], is associated with dysfunctional cortisol responses [59], and may be linked to altered neuroimmunologic responses to pain [for an excellent critical review of the pain catastrophizing literature [60]].

Thus, during the cognitive skills acquisition phase, the patient is taught to monitor their thoughts, identify any irrational beliefs or thought distortions, and restructure the thought pattern toward more adaptive and realistic appraisals of the situation. For example, to "decatastrophize," a patient would be guided to evaluate the realistic probability of her worst case imagined scenario and identify resources to cope with it. A therapist might ask, "What's the worst thing that could happen with your pain?" "How sure are you that this will occur?" and "If so, then what? Could you cope with that?" With a teamwork approach and techniques such as modeling, role-playing exercises, and a careful questioning dialogue, a therapist will assist the patient with challenging their negative thoughts and encourage them to create alternatives. It is important to note that CBT is not about "putting on rose-colored glasses" and adopting a "Pollyanna personality," which is just as distorted as one who habitually thinks through a negative filter. Rather, it is about adopting a realistic and neutral view of the pain and other situations.

> Act the way you'd like to be and soon you'll be the way you act.
> – George W. Crane

The *cognitive and behavioral rehearsal* phase is a practice component to help the patient consolidate and master the newly learned skills in their natural environment. Homework assignments are often used with graded tasks to enhance the patient's sense of self-efficacy or confidence in one's abilities to use the new skills effectively and to reinforce their efforts.

The ultimate goal is *generalization and maintenance*, in which skills used for specific situations, such as coping with pain, generalize to everyday stressors across multiple environmental and social settings.

For example, we recall one particular patient who insisted that she felt angry and depressed following any type of exercise session. When asked what she was thinking about during her time on the treadmill, she responded that she aimed a rhythmic mantra toward the machine, "I hate this thing. I hate this thing. I hate this thing." One may then see how this became a self-fulfilling prophecy in which the patient essentially talked herself into "hating" the exercise session and her mood shortly followed suit. Once she identified the negative thought, she was guided to create an alternative to use during her exercise sessions, for example, "This is good for me, I'm proud of myself for exercising." She was asked to experiment with the alternative mental tapes during her session and track her thoughts, physical sensations, and mood before and after the exercise sessions in a diary format. When presented with the evidence that she felt better both physically and emotionally when she substituted the positive mantra, her efforts were reinforced and she began to look forward to the exercise sessions.

Evidence for Cognitive Behavioral Efficacy

The application of CBT for patients with chronic pain began nearly simultaneously with its advent in the early 1970s, although CBT and its close theoretical companion, rational emotive behavior therapy (REBT), were originally created with the intent to address more traditional psychological problems [61–63]. According to a review by Turk and colleagues [20], CBT—as a stand-alone treatment or when embedded within the framework of an interdisciplinary pain rehabilitation program—has shown strong empirical evidence of success in the treatment of chronic pain.

Several meta-analyses have indicated medium to large effect sizes for CBT-based interventions in both adult and child chronic pain populations [23, 64]. In addition to statistical significance by means of effect sizes, these studies also demonstrate clinical significance for pain reduction. For example, in one study a reduction of up to 68 % in headache frequency was observed from pre- to post-CBT treatment, as compared to 56 % for biofeedback and 20 % for a wait-list control condition [65].

CBT has been noted to produce significant changes in cognitive coping and appraisals, health-related quality of life, depression, social support, reported pain intensity, pain-related interference, return to work, and reductions in the behavioral expression of pain [22, 23, 65]. Improvements in physiological measures like heart rate, both at rest and in response to stress, have also been observed [65]. In general, CBT has strong empirical support as an effective treatment for chronic pain patients across a variety of conditions, including cancer pain [66], sickle-cell pain [67], low back pain [68–70], knee pain [71], rheumatoid arthritis [72, 73], vulvodynia [74], and temporomandibular joint pain [75], among others. Studies have compared treatment groups to waiting list controls, placebo medication conditions, and other treatment conditions such as physical therapy alone, education alone, and medical interventions alone. Improved outcomes have been shown to last at least 1 year or more, even among patients reporting long-term, preintervention disability [22, 23, 65, 76, 77]. There is also evidence from cross-lagged panel design studies that positive changes in cognitive process variables—including pain catastrophizing, helplessness, and pain anxiety—*precede* changes in pain-related outcomes in the context of multidisciplinary pain management programs [78].

CBT is also a cost-effective adjunct to medical interventions, associated with shorter hospital stays [79], and particularly when offered in group format. Brach and colleagues [80] performed an economic evaluation of 174 patients with rheumatoid arthritis randomly and blindly assigned to either a CBT group or client-centered supportive-experiential group (SET). Each group was performed as an adjunct module to a standard 2-week inpatient rehabilitation program. At 12-month follow-up, patients in the CBT group had fewer internist visits, fewer inpatient days, fewer day-care treatments, utilized fewer assistive devices, had lower medication costs, had fewer sick days, and required less caregiving from friends/relatives as compared to the SET group. All in all, the cost of adding either the CBT or SET group to the rehabilitation program was €47 per patient or about €282 per group [80].

Evidence for the efficacy of CBT has also come in the form of neuroimaging. Techniques such as magnetic resonance imaging (MRI), functional magnetic resonance imaging (fMRI), and positron-emission tomography (PET) have documented neuroplastic changes produced by components of CBT. deLange and colleagues [81] examined volumetric changes after CBT in 22 patients with chronic fatigue syndrome (CFS) and 22 healthy controls. At baseline, CFS patients had significantly lower gray matter volume than controls. After CBT, these patients experienced an increase in gray matter volume, specifically in the lateral prefrontal cortex. Neuroplasticity secondary to cognitive behavioral treatment has been observed for a variety of disorders including specific phobia [13, 14] as well as depression, anxiety, post-traumatic stress disorder, and obsessive-compulsive disorder

[10, 12, 82]. More specific to chronic pain, observed neuroplastic changes have been shown to especially involve neural regions implicated in the descending pain-inhibitory system: the anterior cingulate cortex (ACC), medial and lateral prefrontal cortex (particularly the dorsal lateral PFC), insula, periaqueductal gray, and ventromedial hypothalamus.

For example, enhanced perceived self-control over pain has been associated with increased activation of the prefrontal cortex in addition to attenuated activation in the ACC, insula, and secondary somatosensory centers, associated with reduced subjective pain perception [83]. Similarly, Salomons and colleagues [84] observed that individuals with greater perceived controllability of pain showed activation of the ventral lateral prefrontal cortex and reported less pain. Research indicates that endogenous opioid systems may be involved in cognitive pain coping—the opioid antagonist naloxone has been shown to block the beneficial analgesic effects of cognitive pain coping [85].

> Pain is inevitable; suffering is optional
>
> – Unknown

> …You have already borne the pain. What you have not done is feel all you are beyond the pain.
>
> – Saint Bartholomew [c. 1st century]

Acceptance-Based Therapy

As noted above, the traditional focus in CBT has been on teaching coping methods that emphasize control or change in the content of psychological experiences. The connotation of cognitive and behavioral coping skills training is that pain is an entity against which we must fight, control, or win. The constant struggle against pain is understandably exhausting and often frustrating. Acceptance and Commitment Therapy (ACT) is a recently evolved treatment model, one of the "third wave" or "third generation" behavioral and cognitive therapies that encompasses and extends CBT processes to instead engender a goal of "psychological flexibility" rather than control [86]. There are six important processes utilized in ACT, three of which have been studied in the context of chronic pain, including (1) *acceptance* [87, 88], (2) *mindfulness-based methods* that support awareness without judgment and "contact with the present moment" [89], and (3) *values-related processes* in relation to patient functioning [90] (for a full description of the six specific processes used in ACT, see [91]). In each of these studies, the ACT processes are significantly associated with improved emotional, physical, and social functioning [92].

In summary, CBT can target maladaptive thoughts and dysfunctional behaviors in a time-limited manner, either individually in outpatient therapy sessions or in a group setting. However, there are several brief interventions available to physicians in clinical practice:

- Listen to the content *and* context of patient's words. Suggest that they replace "shoulds and musts" with phrases that begin with "I'd like to." Model for them to replace "I can't…" with "I could if…."
- If they are being particularly harsh on themselves or indecisive, ask them to identify how they might talk to a friend with a similar problem.
- Ask them to rank their most cherished values (e.g., family, church, creative pursuits) and encourage them to focus their efforts on those goals despite pain.
- Consider giving a brief screening instrument for depression, anxiety, or catastrophizing in your office.
- Most importantly, be aware of the power of *your own* descriptors and prognostic statements.

During a recent intake interview, one of our patients commented, "My doctor told me he didn't think the SI joint injection would work, but he'd do it anyway. He was right… it didn't work." That patient was unwittingly set up ahead of time for a treatment failure simply from the force of the physician's comment. Similarly, phrases such as "You have the back of an 85-year-old," or "Your back is crumbling to dust" can create powerful and persistent imagery, and said to a patient already prone to catastrophizing, might influence patient mood, behaviors, and future treatment outcomes.

Biofeedback and Relaxation Therapies

We have writing and teaching, science and power;
we have tamed the beasts and schooled the lightning… but we have still to tame ourselves.
                                                                                        – Wells, H.G.

Head and feet keep warm, the rest will take no harm.
                                                                                        – Thomas Fuller

Stare into a mirror and smile. Adjust your facial muscles until you create the most comfortable looking smile. Congratulations, you've just performed biofeedback. Biofeedback and the various forms of self-management relaxation therapies are generally classified as psychophysiological interventions. These therapies involve a systematic approach to increasing awareness of one's cognitive and physiological responses to achieve a state of full body and mental relaxation and peace. Biofeedback is a procedure in which the therapist monitors an individual's physiological responses through a feedback device (e.g., a computer, temperature gauge, heart rate monitor). Processes such as heart rate variability, electrodermal responses, skin temperature, brain waves through electroencephalography (EEG), and respiratory rate can all be tracked. The feedback is provided in real time as the patient uses various cognitive and behavioral techniques to learn how to control the bodily response. Forms of relaxation therapy include autogenic training, diaphragmatic breathing, guided imagery, and progressive muscle relaxation.

Biofeedback has been shown to be especially effective in the treatment of migraine, tension-type, and vascular headaches [93, 94]. A recent meta-analysis [95] revealed medium to large effect sizes, as well as reductions in frequency of headache attacks. Biofeedback promotes higher perceived self-efficacy and reductions in anxiety, depression, muscle tension, and analgesic use [64, 96]. Intention-to-treat and publication-bias analyses have also shown that these treatment effects remain stable for at least 14 months posttreatment, even when patients who withdrew were treated as nonresponders [64, 96]. Research in this area has demonstrated that biofeedback is more effective than headache monitoring, placebo, and other relaxation therapies, and its effects are enhanced when home training is combined with clinic-based therapies [97]. Biofeedback is effective for a variety of other conditions, including temporomandibular disorders, arthritis, fibromyalgia, and traumatic brain injury [98, 99].

Biofeedback involving electromyographical (EMG) responses has been used as an adjunct therapy to standard exercise in patients experiencing low back pain [100, 101], with resulting improvement in the strength and tone of lumbar paraspinal muscles. However, some evidence is suggestive that EMG biofeedback is not superior to other relaxation treatments or even treatment as usual [102, 103]. Neurofeedback, which involves control over neuroelectrophysiological processes, has primarily been used to treat attention deficit/hyperactivity disorder (ADHD), learning disabilities, seizures, depression, head injury, substance abuse, and anxiety; however, it has also been recently applied to chronic pain. For example, Siniatchkin and colleagues [104] utilized neurofeedback in ten children suffering from migraine without aura. During these sessions, participants attempted to self-regulate slow cortical potentials. Results indicated reductions in cortical excitation and in number of days with migraines. Two recent studies using neurofeedback with fibromyalgia patients were equivocal. In one study [105], neurofeedback was shown to produce improvements in pain intensity, fatigue, depression, and anxiety ratings and scores on the Fibromyalgia Impact Questionnaire compared with patients taking escitalopram (Lexapro). However, in a study using a sham control group versus treatment with an EEG biofeedback system [106], no significant differences were observed at 3- and 6-month follow-up. For additional information on neurofeedback, see Evans and Abarbanel [107] and Demos [108].

In a novel application of real-time fMRI, deCharms and colleagues [109] first utilized thermal heat stimulus to show eight healthy participants activation in the rostral anterior cingulate cortex. During intermittent pain stimuli, participants were asked to change their brain activity while watching a visual representation of their rACC activation, using suggestions such as changing focus of attention or altering the pain's emotional value. Eight participants with chronic pain were also run through the training, using their own spontaneous pain rather than externally induced pain. By the end of the experiment, pain participants (vs. control) experienced a 64 % decrease in pain ratings on the McGill pain questionnaire as well as 44 % decrease in pain ratings on a visual analogue scale. Healthy participants (vs. control) experienced a 23 % enhancement in control over pain intensity as well as a 38 % enhancement in control over pain unpleasantness. Although the research is compelling that individuals can gain such control over brain activation and pain control [109–112], widespread clinical use of this method is not realistic or cost-effective at this time.

Additional reviews have evidenced efficacy for other relaxation therapies that do not use the equipment of biofeedback. One study of postoperative outcomes for 44 adults undergoing head and neck procedures found that listening to a 28-min guided imagery CD prior to the procedure resulted in reduced postoperative anxiety, pain intensity, and shorter length of stay in the postoperative anesthesia care unit [113]. Another study examined 15 women with interstitial cystitis (IC) who listened to a 25-min guided imagery CD twice a day for 8 weeks versus a group of women with IC instructed to rest; results indicated reductions in mean pain scores as well as reductions in reported IC-related symptoms [114]. Other studies have shown guided imagery to be effective for increasing self-efficacy for managing pain and fibromyalgia symptoms although no effect was noted for reduction in pain intensity [115].

Another form of relaxation therapy is *progressive muscle relaxation* (PMR), or the systematic tensing and relaxing of sets of muscle groups to decrease overall muscular tension. While some research has not shown any beneficial effects for PMR [116], other studies have demonstrated efficacy, for example, in reducing pain intensity for hip/knee osteoarthritis after 2 months of weekly 30-min PMR sessions [117]. Emery and colleagues [118] examined the effects of PMR on descending modulation of nociception, as measured by the nociceptive flexion reflex, in 55 healthy young adults. Compared with controls, participants in the PMR group experienced a significant increase in their reflex threshold and reported reduced stress, although pain ratings themselves did not change. Patients with certain types of chronic musculoskeletal pain should be cautioned against vigorously engaging in this form of relaxation since overtensing muscles in terms of both duration and intensity may exacerbate their pain.

Autogenic training (AT) combines elements of deep breathing, progressive relaxation, and guided imagery, whereby the patient attends to various muscle groups and visualizes sensations of warmth, tension reduction, or calm to induce feelings of relaxation—for example, noting internally "my legs feel heavy and warm" and/or "my heartbeat is gradually slowing down." This type of relaxation therapy may be more amenable to patients with chronic pain who cannot engage in PMR. However, research is equivocal to date. One study found no difference between AT groups and usual care groups for the treatment of reflex sympathetic dystrophy [119], while another study revealed significantly decreased mean headache frequency and intensity in women who suffered from migraine without aura [120].

Neuroimaging research utilizing MRI indicated that expert mindfulness meditation practitioners showed enhanced thickness in regions of the prefrontal cortex [121]. Similar research has also associated meditation with increased gray matter density in the brainstem [122], as well as increased gray matter concentration in the right anterior insula, left inferior temporal gyrus, and right hippocampus [123]. Using fMRI, transcendental meditation practitioners showed 50 % less activation of pain-processing brain regions during painful heat stimulation than controls, even when not in a meditative state. Even more interesting was the finding that controls could achieve the same results with just 5 months of training [124]. Xiong and Doraiswamy [125] suggest several potential mechanisms for these beneficial effects, including reduced stress-induced cortisol secretion, neuroprotection via increased levels of brain-derived neurotrophic factor, reduced oxidative stress, improved lipid profiles, and/or strengthened neuronal connections with increased cognitive reserve capacity.

Johnston and Vogele [126] examined 38 preparation-for-surgery outcomes studies grouped by type of intervention (e.g., procedural, sensory, behavioral, cognitive, relaxation) and found that an array of therapies such as relaxation, guided imagery, hypnosis, and education had an average effect size of 0.85 for pain reduction and 0.61 for improvements in recovery time. However, as helpful as these therapies may be for general stress reduction and pain coping, we still need to further our understanding in terms of their mechanisms of action and potential role in pain modulation.

There are a number of ways physicians can provide relaxation resources to complement existing medical therapies:

- Monitor blood pressure in-office while having the patient perform deep breathing.
- Purchase inexpensive finger temperature monitors and have patients attempt to raise their own hand temperature by a few degrees in the waiting area.
- Recommend portable biofeedback devices such as the *RESPeRATE* breathing trainer or the *emWave* personal stress reliever for use at home. These are moderately expensive options but may help with practice in between in-office biofeedback sessions.

- Research and locate a certified biofeedback therapist in your area through organizations such as the Biofeedback Certification International Alliance (BCIA, www.bcia.org).
- Educate patients on the physical and psychological benefits of relaxation. This can be done easily by providing educational literature in the form of flyers and handouts in your clinic waiting room that include brief "how to" guidelines for practice at home and contact information for local resources (e.g., yoga or Tai Chi classes, massage).

Pain Groups

'Tis not enough to help the feeble up, but to support them after.
– William Shakespeare

Individual commitment to a group effort -- that is what makes a team work, a company work, a society work, a civilization work.

– Vince Lombardi

As mentioned above, CBT and education can also be conducted in a cost-effective manner within group settings. This may be particularly important for chronic pain populations, as individuals with pain often gravitate to patient-led support groups. There are some advantages to using group therapy or support forums compared to individual counseling. Pain is often an isolating and alienating experience, and groups provide a sense that patients are not alone in this endeavor. The realization that one shares common problems (e.g., recurrent depression, physiological dependency on pain medications, unsupportive family members) can reduce the experience of helplessness and provide a sense of belonging. Patients may accept suggestions from others they perceive as sharing and appreciating their daily suffering, although they may resist similar feedback from therapists who they perceive as healthy.

Additionally, groups can serve as a place for sharing information about helpful procedures, treatments, specific skills for management of pain, tangible support, and to disconfirm chronic pain biases and myths. Research shows that social support has a beneficial impact on reducing morbidity and mortality from chronic health conditions [127–130]. For example, Holt-Lundstad and colleagues [127] performed a meta-analysis involving 148 studies and 308,849 total participants, followed for an average of 7.5 years. Results indicated a 50 % greater likelihood of survival (OR = 1.5; 95 % CI = 1.42–1.59) in individuals with increased social relationships as compared to those with poor/insufficient relationships. The authors noted that the magnitude of the observed effect was not only comparable to quitting smoking but exceeded many other renowned risk factors for mortality such as obesity and sedentary lifestyle.

Although reimbursement for group therapy and educational sessions varies widely, pain groups provide the opportunity for enhanced cost-effectiveness by allowing the therapist to treat a greater number of patients than would be feasible with more individualized treatment approaches [131]. Studies have shown pain groups to be effective across a variety of pain populations, including mixed chronic pain conditions [132], low back pain [133], rheumatoid arthritis [72], sickle-cell disease [134], fibromyalgia [135], and for subgroups of individuals with migraine headaches [136]. The group modality was found to be efficacious for adolescents [134], for the elderly [132, 137], and even for couples [138]. Pain groups have been shown to reduce reported pain intensity and disability scores [139]. Although formal group therapy is often conducted within the context of residential pain program or grant-funded projects, physicians can do the following to promote the benefits of supportive group settings:

- Let patients know they are not alone in coping with this chronic condition. Assist in normalizing some of the associated emotions and thoughts.
- Use your local resources, such as newspapers, city guides, recreational centers, or local chapters of national organizations to find the patient-led chronic pain support groups in your area.
- Contact the American Chronic Pain Association (ACPA; www.acpa.org) to find local group leaders—this organization will provide training and excellent materials for interested patient group leaders. Post flyers or brochures advertising the local groups in your waiting room.

Motivational Interviewing

Motivation is like food for the brain. You cannot get enough in one sitting.
It needs continual and regular top ups.

– Peter Davies

Motivation is the art of getting people to do what you want them to do because they want to do it.

– Dwight D. Eisenhower

For many chronic pain patients, making the required substantial lifestyle changes such as starting an exercise program, learning to pace daily activities, taking medications on a time-contingent regimen, and practicing relaxation techniques constitutes an overwhelming hurdle. As health providers, we hope and expect that patients who sought our expertise and advice will automatically be compliant with the agreed-upon treatment plan. However, in clinical practice, we also realize that absolute adherence is the ideal and not reality. Medication compliance, even for short-term antibiotic regimens, is notoriously low [140]. Simple strategies (e.g., varying type of exercise, providing incentives) for improving adherence to physical therapy have been largely unsuccessful, especially for home-based exercise programs [141]. We also understand the limitations in being able to predict and identify aberrant opioid-related behaviors, despite the availability of reasonable risk screening measures [142]. Treatment dropout is also a common problem in psychotherapy, due to low motivation, external social difficulties, dissatisfaction with the therapist, or feelings of improvement [143]. Some individuals just need an extra "push" to engage in necessary self-management approaches.

Motivational interviewing (MI) is an evidence-based clinical treatment approach initially developed for the treatment of alcoholic patients [144, 145] that has been adapted to help pain patients explore and resolve ambivalence about behavior change and boost their intrinsic motivation to adopt a self-management approach to their pain concerns [146]. Motivation is loosely defined by Miller and Rolnick [144] as "the probability that a person will enter into, continue, and adhere to a specific strategy" and is emphasized by the patient's actions rather than verbal assurances. One of the key assumptions of MI is that people already know *how* to engage in adaptive behaviors—they simply vary in the degree to which they are *prepared* to engage in those behaviors [147]. In the case of chronic pain, for example, one may assume that nearly all patients know how to walk for exercise, and thus, a lack of knowledge does not sufficiently explain the lack of exercise behavior. Motivational interviewing, then, can work synergistically with CBT to address lack of motivation or behavioral readiness by providing an environment conducive to increased readiness for change [148].

Prochaska and DiClemente [149] developed a *Stages of Change* model for identifying the specific stages people go through as they change from maladaptive to adaptive behaviors. According to this transtheoretical model, each stage poses a set of different challenges that must be addressed before progressing to the next stage (Fig. 76.2) [150]. Although there is a conflicting evidence regarding the exact number, nature, and clinical relevance of subscales using the primary measure called the Pain Stages of Change Questionnaire (PSOCQ) [151], five subscales generally emerge that are consistent with the original stages of change model as applied to chronic pain populations [152, 153]. The beginning stage, *precontemplation*, describes patients who do not see the need for change and may even be resistant to change. For example, a pain patient who smokes 2 packs of cigarettes per day may irritably resist the surgeon's recommendation to quit smoking prior to a lumbar fusion. *Contemplators*, on the other hand, see the need for change but have not yet committed to action. In our current example, perhaps the patient understands and accepts that their tobacco use is why the surgery has been delayed. In the *preparation* phase, there exists both the intent to change and initial steps

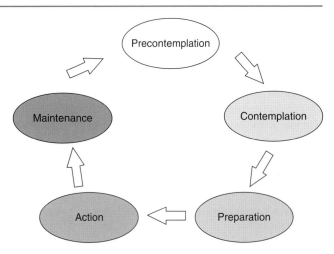

Fig. 76.2 Stages of change model (Adapted from Jensen [147], Miller and Rollnick [144], and Prochaska and DiClemente [149])

to do so, although the full range of self-care behaviors is absent. Here, the smoker may verbalize their intent to quit and set a target quit date. In the final stage, *action*, patients take on modification of their behavior and/or environment with the intent of creating change. The smoker throws away the final pack of cigarettes, buys some chewing gum, and stops smoking. This stage may either be maintained (*maintenance* stage) or individuals are susceptible to *relapse*, where they may exit the cycle and reenter at any point. Although the clinical utility of the stage classification has been questioned in use with chronic pain patients [154], identification with the various stages, as measured by scores on the PSOCQ, has been associated with pain intensity reports, disability, and depression [151, 155].

Treatment is longitudinal in nature given that a patient's stage of change is dynamic across time. MI is problem-focused, clinician-directed but patient-centered, interpersonal in nature, and can be tailored to the individual's stage of readiness with increasingly specific recommendations as the stages progress. At early stages, a supportive environment is key; the therapist must exhibit empathy and reflect patients' emotions. MI techniques help patients clearly recognize their problems, perform personal cost-benefit analyses of their behaviors (i.e., "decisional balance analysis"), develop consistency between their therapeutic goals and motivation, and increase patient's sense of self-efficacy and personal responsibility.

Meta-analytic review has indicated that MI is effective in improving both physiological (72 %) and psychological symptoms (73 %) [156], as well as health behaviors such as diet and exercise [157]. Changes in readiness to self-manage pain have been seen post-multidisciplinary pain treatment programs, with increases in action and maintenance behaviors over the course of the program, concurrent with changes in pain coping strategies and function [154].

Table 76.4 Using the neuropsychological model of pain in treatment planning

Behavioral/psychological symptom	Associated brain area	Appropriate psychological intervention
Maladaptive pain-related cognitions or treatment goals	Prefrontal cortex	Cognitive restructuring Operant conditioning Motivational interviewing Acceptance-based therapy
Elevated affective pain component ("suffering")	Anterior cingulate cortex (ACC)	Operant conditioning Motivational interviewing Acceptance-based therapy
Perceptions of physical pathology that needs to be fixed; feelings that the sensory experience is inconsistent with physical safety	Insula	Self-hypnosis Relaxation training
Reports of very high pain intensity	Sensory cortex	Self-hypnosis Relaxation training

Summarized from Jensen [158]

In summary, MI is a useful complementary set of techniques to enhance patient motivation, promote adherence to treatment recommendations, and increase readiness to adopt self-driven health and pain management behaviors. Mental health professionals often weave in MI techniques during a course of cognitive behavioral therapy, teach the skills during educational sessions, or focus on them during a multidisciplinary pain program. However, physicians can be a powerful source of encouragement and motivation in their office visits or pre-procedure consultations:

- By simply asking the patient what their goals are (in person or even on a medical visit paper-and-pencil form), you are heightening their awareness of what is important to them.
- Ask them about both their healthy and not-so-healthy coping behaviors (*we must admit that even smoking, overeating, and social withdrawal are still attempts to cope, albeit maladaptive*) and listen without judgment.
- Patients expect their physician to educate them about the negative consequences of their unhealthy behaviors (e.g., nicotine has a damaging effect on discs, bone, and wound healing) but consider turning the advice on its head. That is, focus on the "pros" of adopting the healthier behavior (e.g., "If you quit smoking, you are more likely to have faster postsurgical healing and bone fusion"). This subtle twist on the necessary health advice can help frame the desired behavior in a more positive light.
- Allow room within the traditionally paternalistic physician-patient relationship for the patient to take more personal responsibility for their behaviors and hold them accountable for their actions.

Conclusions

It is our duty to remember at all times and anew that medicine is not only a science, but also the art of letting our own individuality interact with the individuality of the patient.

– Albert Schweitzer

It would be a great thing to understand pain in all its meanings.
– Peter Mere Latham

This chapter has highlighted the need to consider pain as a personal experience influenced not only by physical pathology but also synergistically by prior learning history, cognitive belief systems, social influences, and behavioral motivators. These factors help to explain the wide variability of patient's responses to pain that we see in clinical practice. Given the strength of the emotional and psychosocial components involved in pain perception and modulation, it is critical to give the evidence-based psychological therapies a place in the whole-person management of pain.

One interesting recent suggestion is to match our knowledge of the primary cortical areas involved in the processing and modulation of pain with the goals of psychological pain therapies to provide a thoughtful scientific-based treatment plan for each individual patient. Jensen [158] called this a "neuropsychological model of pain," and some examples are summarized in Table 76.4.

We all have that "Oh no, so-and-so's on the schedule today" gut-drop feeling from time to time. Of course, psychological referrals for patients with suicidal ideation and disruptive personality disorders are certainly warranted, but the scope of psychological therapy for pain is much broader. Collaborate not only with the mental health providers in your area but also with the patient. Several studies have demonstrated that patients who are involved in making medical decisions fare better and are more satisfied than patients who do not [159–161]. Explain to your patient that your recommendation for a psychological referral does not mean you think the pain is "all in their head." Help them set realistic expectations for their treatment and frame the psychological therapies as additional neuroplastic modifiers.

Whether you collaborate with psychologists in the community through a referral process, or if you have one on staff, the integration of therapeutic modalities within the biopsychosocial perceptive is the goal. The incremental benefit of combined treatments can address the limitations that we have seen with pain monotherapies. Instead of the traditional step approach of progressing to more invasive treatments in a sequential manner after each successive treatment failure, consider using psychological treatments as an adjunct all the way through the process, from initial assessment to opioid monitoring to improving compliance with physical therapy recommendations to preinterventional screening, and so on. As you have also noticed in this chapter, you are likely already using some of these techniques in a modified way on a daily basis in your practice. As Dennis Turk stated simply in reference to the integration of medical and psychological therapies for pain, "Perhaps 1+1 does = 3" [162].

References

1. Melzack R, Wall PD. Pain mechanisms: a new theory. Science. 1965;150:971–9.
2. Engel GL. The clinical application of the biopsychosocial model. Am J Psychiatry. 1980;137:535–44.
3. Melzack R, Casey KL. Sensory, motivational, and central control determinants of pain. In: Kensalo DR, editor. The skin sense. Springfield: Thomas; 1968. p. 423–39.
4. Doidge N. The brain that changes itself: stories of personal triumph from the frontiers of brain science. New York: Penguin; 2007.
5. Beecher HK. Measurement of subjects responses. New York: Oxford University Press; 1959.
6. Rainville P, Duncan GH, Price DD, Carrier B, Bushnell MC. Pain affect encoded in human anterior cingulate but not somatosensory cortex. Science. 1997;277:968–71.
7. Bushnell MC, Apkarian AV. Representation of pain in the brain. In: McMahon SB, Koltzenburg M, editors. Wall and Melzack's textbook of pain. 5th ed. Philadelphia: Churchill Livingstone (Elsevier); 2005. p. 107–24.
8. Kandel E. A new intellectual framework for psychiatry? Am J Psychiatry. 1998;155:457–69.
9. Goldapple K, Segal Z, Garson C, et al. Modulation of cortical-limbic pathways in major depression. Arch Gen Psychiatry. 2004;61:34–41.
10. Frewen PA, Dozois DJ, Lamius RA. Neuroimaging studies of psychological interventions for mood and anxiety disorders: empirical and methodological review. Clin Psychol Rev. 2008;28:228–46.
11. Letizia B. Neuroanatomical changes after Eye Movement Desensitization and Reprocessing (EMDR) treatment in posttraumatic stress disorder. J Neuropsychiatry Clin Neurosci. 2007;19:475–6.
12. Linden DEJ. How psychotherapy changes the brain – the contribution of functional neuroimaging. Mol Psychiatry. 2006;11:528–38.
13. Paquette V, Levesque J, Mensour B, et al. Change the mind and you change the brain: effects of cognitive-behavioral therapy on the neural correlates of spider phobia. Neuroimage. 2003;18:401–9.
14. Straube T, Glauer M, Dilger S, Hans-Joachim M, Miltnera WHR. Effects of cognitive-behavioral therapy on brain activation in specific phobia. Neuroimage. 2006;29:125–35.
15. Etkin A, Pittenger C, Polan HJ, Kandel ER. Toward a neurobiology of psychotherapy: basic science and clinical applications. J Neuropsychiatry Clin Neurosci. 2005;17(2):145–58.
16. Barker S. Pain and psychosocial factors. In: Van Griensven HV, editor. Pain in practice: theory and treatment strategies for manual therapists. New York: Elsevier; 2005. p. 107–30.
17. Miller A. Ingenious pain. London: Sceptre; 1997.
18. Breivik H, Collett B, Ventafridda V, Cohen R, Gallacher D. Survey of chronic pain in Europe: prevalence, impact on daily life, and treatment. Eur J Pain. 2006;10:287–333.
19. Moulin DE, Clark AJ, Speechley M, Morley-Forster PK. Chronic pain in Canada – prevalence, treatment, impact, and the role of opioid analgesia. Pain Res Manag. 2002;4:179–84.
20. Turk DC, Swanson KS, Tunks ER. Psychological approaches in the treatment of chronic pain patients – when pills, scalpels, and needles are not enough. Can J Psychiatry. 2008;53:213–23.
21. Ives TJ, Chelminsky PR, Hammett-Stabler CA, et al. Predictors of opioid misuse in patients with chronic pain: a prospective cohort study. BMC Health Serv Res. 2006;4:46.
22. Hoffman BM, Papas RK, Chatkoff DK, Kerns RD. Meta-analysis of psychological interventions for chronic low back pain. Health Psychol. 2007;26:1–9.
23. Morley S, Eccleston C, Williams A. Systematic review and meta-analysis of randomized controlled trials of cognitive behaviour therapy and behaviour therapy for chronic pain in adults, excluding headache. Pain. 1999;80:1–13.
24. Roe D, Hasson-Ohayon I, Kravetz S, Yanos PT, Lysaker PH. Call it a monster for lack of anything else: narrative insight in psychosis. J Nerv Ment Dis. 2008;196:859–65.
25. Olatunji BO, Cisler JM, Deacon BJ. Efficacy of cognitive behavioral therapy for anxiety disorders: a review of meta-analytic findings. Psychiatr Clin North Am. 2010;33(3):557–77.
26. Shapiro F. Eye movement desensitization and reprocessing: basic principles, protocols, and procedures. 2nd ed. New York: Guilford Press; 2001.
27. Taylor S, Thordarson DS, Maxfield L, Fedoroff IC, Lovell K, Ogrodniczuk J. Comparative efficacy, speed, and adverse effects of three PTSD treatments: exposure therapy, EMDR, and relaxation training. J Consult Clin Psychol. 2003;71:330–8.
28. Bradley R, Greene J, Russ E, Dutra L, Westen D. A multidimensional meta-analysis of psychotherapy for PTSD. Am J Psychiatry. 2007;162(2):214–27.
29. Bisson J, Andrew M. Psychological treatment of post-traumatic stress disorder (PTSD). Cochrane Database Syst Rev. 2007;(3):CD003388. doi:10.1002/14651858.CD003388.pub3.
30. Ray AL, Zbik A. Cognitive behavioral therapies and beyond. In: Tollison CD, Satterthwaite JR, Tollison JW, editors. Practical pain management. 3rd ed. Philadelphia: Lippincott; 2001. p. 189–208.
31. Russell M. Treating traumatic amputation-related phantom limb pain: a case study utilizing eye movement desensitization and reprocessing (EMDR) within the armed services. Clin Case Stud. 2008;7:136–53.
32. Schneider J, Hofmann A, Rost C, Shapiro F. EMDR in the treatment of chronic phantom limb pain. Pain Med. 2008;9:76–82.
33. Wilensky M. Eye movement desensitization and reprocessing (EMDR) as a treatment for phantom limb pain. J Brief Ther. 2006; 5:31–44.
34. Flor H, Knost B, Birbaumer N. The role of operant conditioning in chronic pain: an experimental investigation. Pain. 2002;95:111–8.
35. Bingham B, Ajit SK, Blake DR, Samad TA. The molecular basis of pain and its clinical implications in rheumatology. Nat Clin Pract Rheumatol. 2009;5:28–37.
36. Fordyce WE. Behavioral methods for chronic pain and illness. Saint Louis: The C.V. Mosby Company; 1976.
37. Stiles TC, Wright D. Cognitive-behavioural treatment of chronic pain conditions. Nord J Psychiatry. 2008;62:30–6.
38. Vlaeyen JW, Haazen IW, Schuerman JA, Kole-Snijders AM, van Eeek H. Behavioural rehabilitation of chronic low back pain: comparison of an operant treatment, an operant-cognitive treatment and an operant-respondent treatment. Br J Clin Psychol. 1995;34:95–118.
39. Thieme K, Gromnica-Ihle E, Flor H. Operant behavioral treatment of fibromyalgia: a controlled study. Arthritis Rheum. 2003;49:(3)314–20.

40. Henschke N, Ostelo RW, van Tulder, MW, et al. Behavioural treatment for chronic low-back pain. Cochrane Database Syst Rev. 2010;(7):CD002014.

41. Romano JM, Turner JA, Jensen MP, et al. Chronic pain patient-spouse behavioral interactions predict patient disability. Pain. 1995;63:353–60.

42. Fillingim RB, Doleys DM, Edwards RR, Lowery DD. Spousal responses are differentially associated with clinical variables in women and men with chronic pain. Clin J Pain. 2003;19:217–24.

43. Gogolla N, Caroni P, Lüthi A, Herry C. Perineuronal nets protect fear memories from erasure. Science. 2009;325:1258–61.

44. Vlaeyen JW, Linton SJ. Fear-avoidance and its consequences in chronic musculoskeletal pain: a state of the art. Pain. 2000;85:317–32.

45. Doleys DM, Crocker MF, Patton D. Responses of patients with chronic pain to exercises quotas. Phys Ther. 1982;62:1111–4.

46. Hasenbring MI, Verbunt JA. Fear-avoidance and endurance-related responses to pain: new models of behavior and their consequences for clinical practice. Clin J Pain. 2010;26(9):747–53.

47. Leonhardt C, Lehr D, Chenot JF. Are fear-avoidance beliefs in low back pain patients a risk factor for low physical activity or vice versa? A cross-lagged panel analysis. Psychosoc Med. 2009;29:1–12.

48. Zastrow A, Faude V, Seyboth F, Niehoff D, Herzog W, Lowe B. Risk factors of symptom underestimation by physicians. J Psychosom Res. 2008;64(5):543–51.

49. Sullivan MJ, Bishop SR, Pivik J. The Pain Catastrophizing Scale: development and validation. Psychol Assess. 1995;7:524–32.

50. Severeijns R, Vlaeyen JW, van den Hout MA, Weber WE. Pain catastrophizing predict pain intensity, disability, and psychological distress independent of the level of physical impairment. Clin J Pain. 2001;17(2):165–72.

51. Lame IE, Peters ML, Vlaeyen JW, Kleef M, Patijn J. Quality of life in chronic pain is more associated with beliefs about pain, than with pain intensity. Eur J Pain. 2005;9:15–24.

52. Edwards RR, Smith MT, Kudel I, Haythornthwaite J. Pain-related catastrophizing as a risk factor for suicidal ideation in chronic pain. Pain. 2006;126:272–9.

53. Sullivan MJ, Adams H, Sullivan ME. Communicative dimensions of pain catastrophizing: social cueing effects on pain behavior and coping. Pain. 2004;107(3):220–6.

54. Keefe FJ, Lefebvre JC, Egert JR, Affleck G, Sullivan MJ, Caldwell DS. The relationship of gender to pain, pain behavior, and disability in osteoarthritis patients: the role of catastrophizing. Pain. 2000;87(3):325–34.

55. Roth ML, Tripp DA, Harrison MH, et al. Demographic and psychosocial predictors of acute perioperative pain for total knee arthroplasty. Pain Res Manag. 2007;12(3):184–94.

56. Van Wijk RM, Geurts JW, Lousberg R, et al. Psychological predictors of substantial pain reduction after minimally invasive radiofrequency and injection treatments for chronic low back pain. Pain Med. 2008;9(2):212–21.

57. Forsythe ME, Dunbar MJ, Hennigar AW, Sullivan MJ, Gross M. Prospective relation between catastrophizing and residual pain following knee arthroplasty: Two-year follow-up. Pain Res Manag. 2008;13(4):335–41.

58. Weissman-Fogel I, Sprecher E, Pud D. Effects of catastrophizing on pain perception and pain modulation. Exp Brain Res. 2008;186(1):79–85.

59. Johansson AC, Gunnarsson LG, Linton SJ, et al. Pain, disability and coping reflected in the diurnal cortisol variability in patients scheduled for lumbar disc surgery. Eur J Pain. 2008;12(5):633–64.

60. Quartana PJ, Campbell CM, Edwards RR. Pain catastrophizing: a critical review. Expert Rev Neurother. 2009;9(5):745–58.

61. Beck AT. Cognitive therapy and the emotional disorders. New York: Penguin; 1979.

62. Beck AT, Rush AJ, Shaw BF, et al. Cognitive therapy of depression. New York: Guilford; 1979.

63. Ellis A, Grieger RM. Handbook of rational-emotive therapy. New York: Springer; 1977.

64. Trautmann E, Lackschewitz H, Kröner-Herwig B. Psychological treatment of recurrent headache in children and adolescents – a meta-analysis. Cephalalgia. 2006;26:1411–26.

65. Martin PR, Forsyth MR, Reece J. Cognitive-behavioral therapy versus temporal pulse amplitude biofeedback training for recurrent headache. Behav Ther. 2007;38:350–63.

66. Syrjala KL, Donaldson GW, Davis MW, Kippes ME, Carr JE. Relaxation and imagery and cognitive-behavioral training reduce pain during cancer treatment: a controlled clinical trial. Pain. 1995;63:189–98.

67. Chen E, Cole SW, Kato PM. A review of empirically supported psychosocial interventions for pain and adherence outcomes in sickle cell disease. J Pediatr Psychol. 2004;29:197–209.

68. Bland P. Group CBT is a cost-effective option for persistent back pain. Practitioner. 2010;254:7.

69. Lamb SE, Hansen Z, Lall R, et al. Group cognitive-behavioral treatment improves chronic low back pain in a cost-effective manner. Lancet. 2010;375:916–23.

70. Turner JA, Clancy S. Comparison of operant behavioral and cognitive-behavioral group treatment for chronic low back pain. J Consult Clin Psychol. 1988;56:261–6.

71. Keefe FJ, Caldwell DS, Williams DA, et al. Pain coping skills training in the management of osteoarthritis knee pain: a comparative study. Behav Ther. 1990;21:49–62.

72. Bradley LA, Young LD, Anderson KO, et al. Effects of psychological therapy on pain behavior of rheumatoid arthritis patients: treatment outcome and six-month follow-up. Arthritis Rheum. 1987;30:1105–14.

73. Sharpe L, Sensky T, Timberlake N, Ryan B, Brewin CR, Allard S. A blind, randomized, controlled trial of cognitive-behavioural intervention for patients with recent onset rheumatoid arthritis: preventing psychological and physical morbidity. Pain. 2001;89:275–83.

74. Masheb RM, Kerns RD, Lozano C, Minkin MJ, Richman S. A randomized clinical trial for women with vulvodynia: cognitive-behavioral therapy vs. Supportive psychotherapy. Pain. 2009;141:31–40.

75. Turner JA, Mancl L, Aaron LA. Short-and long-term efficacy of brief cognitive-behavioral therapy for patients with chronic temporomandibular disorder pain: a randomized, controlled trial. Pain. 2006;12:181–94.

76. Nicholas MK. On adherence to self-management strategies. Eur J Pain. 2009;13:113–4.

77. Williams AC, Nicholas MK, Richardson PH, Pither CE, Fernandes J. Generalizing from a controlled trial: the effects of patient preference versus randomization on the outcome of inpatient versus outpatient chronic pain management. Pain. 1999;83:57–65.

78. Burns JW, Glenn B, Bruehl S, et al. Cognitive factors influence outcome following multidisciplinary chronic pain treatment: a replication and extension of a cross-lagged panel analysis. Behav Res Ther. 2003;41(10):1163–82.

79. Thomas VJ, Wilson-Barnett J, Goodhart F. The role of cognitive-behavioural therapy in the management of pain in patients with sickle cell disease. J Adv Nurs. 1998;27:1002–9.

80. Brach M, Sabariego C, Herschbach P, Berg P, Engst-Hastreiter U, Stucki G. Cost-effectiveness of cognitive-behavioral group therapy for dysfunctional fear of progression in chronic arthritis patients. J Public Health. 2010;32(4):547–54. Epub 2010 Apr 8.

81. deLange FP, Koers A, Kalkman JS. Increase in prefrontal cortical volume following cognitive behavioural therapy in patients with chronic fatigue syndrome. Brain. 2008;131:2172–80.

82. Roffman JL, Marci CD, Glick DM, Dougherty DD, Rauch SL. Neuroimaging and the functional neuroanatomy of psychotherapy. Psychol Med. 2005;35:1385–98.

83. Wiech K, Kalisch R, Weiskopf N, Pleger B, Stephan KE, Dolan RJ. Anterolateral prefrontal cortex mediates the analgesic effects of expected and perceived control over pain. J Neurosci. 2006; 26:11501–9.

84. Salomons TV, Johnstone T, Backonia MM, Shackman AJ, Davidson RJ. Individual differences in the effects of perceived controllability on pain perception: critical role of the prefrontal cortex. J Cogn Neurosci. 2007;19:993–1003.

85. Bandura A, O'Leary A, Taylor CB, Gauthier J, Gossard D. Perceived self-efficacy and pain control: opioid and nonopioid mechanisms. J Pers Soc Psychol. 1987;53:563–71.

86. Hayes SC. Acceptance and commitment therapy, relational frame theory, and the third wave of behavior therapy. Behav Ther. 2004; 35:639–65.

87. McCracken LM, Eccelston C. A prospective study of acceptance of pain and patient functioning with chronic pain. Pain. 2005;118:164–9.

88. McCracken LM, Vowles KE. Acceptance of chronic pain. Curr Pain Headache Rep. 2006;10:90–4.

89. McCracken LM, Gauntlett-Gilbert J, Vowles KE. The role of mindfulness in a contextual cognitive-behavioral analysis of chronic pain-related suffering and disability. Pain. 2007;131: 63–9.

90. McCracken LM, Yan SY. The role of values in a contextual cognitive-behavioral approach to chronic pain. Pain. 2006;123: 137–45.

91. Hayes SC, Luoma J, Bond F, Masuda A, Lillis J. Acceptance and commitment therapy: model, processes, and outcomes. Behav Res Ther. 2006;44:1–25.

92. Vowles KE, Wetherell JL, Sorrell JT. Targeting acceptance, mindfulness, and values-based action in chronic pain: findings of two preliminary trials of an outpatient group-based intervention. Cogn Behav Pract. 2009;16:49–58.

93. Andrasik F. Biofeedback in headache: an overview of approaches and evidence. Cleve Clin J Med. 2010;77:S72–6.

94. Cott A, Parkinson W, Fabich M, Bédard M, Marlin R. Long-term efficacy of combined relaxation: biofeedback treatments for chronic headache. Pain. 1992;51:49–56.

95. Nestoriuc Y, Martin A, Rief W, Andrasik F. Biofeedback treatment for headache disorders: a comprehensive efficacy review. Appl Psychophysiol Biofeedback. 2008;33:125–40.

96. Nestoriuc Y, Rief W, Martin A. Meta-analysis of biofeedback for tension-type headache: efficacy, specificity, and treatment moderators. J Consult Clin Psychol. 2008;76:379–96.

97. Nestoriuc Y, Martin A. Efficacy of biofeedback for migraine: a meta-analysis. Pain. 2007;128:111–27.

98. Yucha C, Montgomery D. Evidence-based practice in biofeedback and neurofeedback. Wheat Ridge: Association for Applied Psychophysiology and Biofeedback; 2008.

99. Pulliam CB, Gatchel RJ. Biofeedback 2003: its role in pain management. Crit Rev Phys Rehab Med. 2003;15:65–82.

100. Asfour SS, Khalil TM, Waly SM, Goldberg ML, Rosomoff RS, Rosomoff HL. Biofeedback in back muscle strengthening. Spine. 1976;15:510–3.

101. Nouwen A, Bush C. The relationship between paraspinal EMG and chronic low back pain. Pain. 1984;20:109–23.

102. Bush C, Ditto B, Feuerstein M. A controlled evaluation of paraspinal EMG biofeedback in the treatment of chronic low back pain. Health Psychol. 1985;4:307–21.

103. Stuckey SJ, Jacobs A, Goldfarb J. EMG biofeedback training, relaxation training, and placebo for the relief of chronic back pain. Percept Mot Skills. 1986;63:1023–36.

104. Siniatchkin M, Hierundar A, Kropp P, Kuhnert R, Gerber WD. Self-regulation of slow cortical potentials in children with migraine: an exploratory study. Appl Psychophysiol Biofeedback. 2000;25:13–32.

105. Kayiran S, Dursun E, Dursun N, Ermutlu N, Karamürsel S. Neurofeedback intervention in fibromyalgia syndrome: a randomized, controlled, rater blind clinical trial. Appl Psychophysiol Biofeedback. 2010;35(4):293–302.

106. Nelson DV, Bennett RM, Barkhuizen A, et al. Neurotherapy of fibromyalgia? Pain Med. 2010;11:912–9.

107. Evans JR, Abarbanel A. Introduction to quantitative EEG and neurofeedback. San Diego: Academic; 1999.

108. Demos JN. Getting started with neurofeedback. New York: WW Norton; 2005.

109. deCharms RC, Maeda F, Flover GH. Control over brain activation and pain learned by using real-time functional MRI. Proc Natl Acad Sci USA. 2005;102:18626–31.

110. Caria A, Veit R, Sitram R, et al. Regulation of anterior insular cortex activity using real-time fMRI. Neuroimage. 2007;35:1238–46.

111. deCharms RC, Christoff K, Glover GH, Pauly JM, Whitfueld S, Gabrieli JD. Learned regulation of spatially localized brain activation using real-time fMRI. Neuroimage. 2004;21:436–43.

112. Weiskopf N, Sitaram R, Josephs O, et al. Real-time functional magnetic resonance imaging: methods and applications. Magn Reson Imaging. 2007;25:989–1003.

113. Gonzalez EA, Ledesma RJ, McAllister DJ, Perry SM, Dyer CA, Maye JP. Effects of guided imagery on postoperative outcomes in patients undergoing same-day surgical procedures: a randomized, single-blind study. AANA J. 2010;78:181–8.

114. Carrico DJ, Peters KM, Diokno AC. Guided imagery for women with interstitial cystitis: results of a prospective, randomized controlled pilot study. J Altern Complement Med. 2008;14:53–60.

115. Menzies V, Taylor AG, Bourguignon C. Effects of guided imagery on outcomes of pain, functional status, and self-efficacy in persons diagnosed with fibromyalgia. J Altern Complement Med. 2006; 12:23–30.

116. Hasson D, Arnetz B, Jelveus L, Edelstam B. A randomized clinical trial of the treatment effects of massage compared to relaxation tape recordings on diffuse long-term pain. Psychother Psychosom. 2004;73:17–24.

117. Gay MC, Philippot P, Luminet O. Differential effectiveness of psychobiological interventions for reducing osteoarthritis pain: a comparison of Erickson hypnosis and Jacobsen relaxation. Eur J Pain. 2002;6:1–16.

118. Emery CF, France CR, Harris J, Norma G, Vanarsdalen C. Effects of progressive muscle relaxation on nociceptive flexion reflex threshold in healthy young adults: a randomized trial. Pain. 2008;138:375–9.

119. Fialka V, Korpan M, Saradeth T, et al. Autogenic training for reflex sympathetic dystrophy: a pilot study. Complement Ther Med. 1996;4:103–5.

120. Juhasz G, Zsombok T, Gonda X, Nagyne N, Modosne E, Bagdy G. Effects of autogenic training on nitroglycerin-induced headaches. Headache. 2007;47:371–83.

121. Lazar SW, Kerr CE, Wasserman RH, et al. Meditation experience is associated with increased cortical thickness. Neuroreport. 2005;16:1893–7.

122. Vestergaard-Poulsen P, van Beek M, Skewes J, et al. Long-term meditation is associated with increased gray matter density in the brainstem. Neuroreport. 2009;20:170–4.

123. Hölzel BK, Ott U, Gard T, et al. Investigation of mindfulness meditation practitioners with voxel-based morphometry. Soc Cogn Affect Neurosci. 2008;3:55–61.

124. Orme-Johnson DW, Schneider RH, Son YD. Neuroimaging of meditation's effect of brain reactivity to pain. Neuroreport. 2006;17:1359–63.

125. Xiong GL, Doraiswamy PM. Does meditation enhance cognition and brain plasticity? Ann N Y Acad Sci. 2009;1172:63–9.

126. Johnston M, Vogele C. Benefits of psychological preparation for surgery: a meta-analysis. Ann Behav Med. 1993;15:245–56.

127. Holt-Lundstad J, Smith TB, Layton B. Social relationships and mortality risk: a meta-analytic review. PLoS Med. 2010;7:1–20.

128. House JS, Landis KR, Umberson D. Social relationships and health. Science. 1988;241:540–5.

129. Mookadam F, Arthur HM. Social support and its relationship to morbidity and mortality after acute myocardial infarction. Arch Intern Med. 2004;164:1514–8.

130. Pinquart M, Duberstein PR. Associations of social networks with cancer mortality: a meta-analysis. Crit Rev Oncol Hematol. 2010; 75:122–37.

131. Thorn BE, Kuhajda MC. Group cognitive therapy for chronic pain. J Clin Psychol. 2006;62:1355–66.

132. Ersek M, Turner JA, McCurry SM, Gibbons L, Kraybill BM. Efficacy of a self-management group intervention for elderly persons with chronic pain. Clin J Pain. 2003;19:156–67.

133. Cole JD. Psychotherapy with the chronic pain patient using coping skills development: outcome study. J Occup Health Psychol. 1998;3:217–26.

134. Thomas VJ, Dixon AL, Milligan P. Cognitive-behaviour therapy for the management of sickle cell disease pain: an evaluation of a community-based intervention. Br J Health Psychol. 1999;4:209–29.

135. Keel PJ, Bodoky C, Gerhard U, Müller W. Comparison of integrated group therapy and group relaxation training for fibromyalgia. Clin J Pain. 1998;14:232–8.

136. Thorn BE, Pence LB, Ward LC, et al. A randomized clinical trial of targeted cognitive behavioral treatment to reduce catastrophizing in chronic headache sufferers. J Pain. 2007;8:938–49.

137. Ersek M, Turner JA, Cain KC, Kemp CA. Results of a randomized controlled trial to examine the efficacy of a chronic pain self-management group for older adults. Pain. 2008;138:29–40.

138. Langelier RP, Gallagher RM. Outpatient treatment of chronic pain groups for couples. Clin J Pain. 1989;5:227–31.

139. Bezalel T, Carmeli E, Katz-Leurer M. The effect of a group education programme on pain and function through knowledge acquisition and home-based exercise among patients with knee osteoarthritis: a parallel randomised single-blind clinical trial. Physiotherapy. 2010;96:137–43.

140. Greenberg RN. Overview of patient compliance with medication dosing: a literature review. Clin Ther. 1984;6(5):592–9.

141. McLean SM, Burton M, Bradley L, Littlewood C. Interventions for enhancing adherence with physiotherapy: a systematic review. Man Ther. 2010;15(6):514–21. Epub 2010 Jul 14.

142. Chou R, Fanciullo GJ, Fine PG, Miaskowski C, Passik SD, Portenoy RK. Opioids for chronic noncancer pain: prediction and identification of aberrant drug-related behaviors: a review of the evidence for an American Pain Society and American Academy of Pain Medicine clinical practice guidelines. J Pain. 2009;10(2):131–46.

143. Bados A, Balaguer G, Saldana C. The efficacy of cognitive-behavioral therapy and the problem of drop-out. J Clin Psychol. 2007;63(6):585–92.

144. Miller WR, Rollnick S. Motivational interviewing: preparing people to change addictive behavior. 2nd ed. New York: Guilford Press; 2002. p. 33–42.

145. Miller WR, Zweben A, DiClemente CC, Rychartik RG. Motivational enhancement therapy manual: a clinical research guide for therapists treating individuals with alcohol abuse and dependence (DHHS publication no. ADM 92–1894). Washington, D.C.: U.S. Government Printing Office; 1992.

146. Kerns RD, Rosenberg R. Predicting responses to self-management treatments for chronic pain: application of the pain stages of change model. Pain. 2000;84:49–55.

147. Jensen MP. Enhancing motivation to change in pain treatment. In: Gatchel RJ, Turk DC, editors. Psychological approaches to pain management: a practitioner's handbook. New York: Guilford Press; 1996. p. 78–111.

148. Hettema J, Steele J, Miller WR. Motivational interviewing. Annu Rev Clin Psychol. 2005;1:91–111.

149. Prochaska JO, DiClemente CC. Stages of change in the modification of problem behaviors. In: Hersen M, Eisler RN, Miller PN, editors. Progress in behavior modification. Sycamore: Sycamore Press; 1982. p. 184–214.

150. Prochaska JO, DiClemente CC, Norcross JC. In search of how people change: applications to addictive behaviors. Am Psychol. 1992;47:1102–14.

151. Kerns RD, Rosenberg R, Jamison RN, Caudill MA, Haythornthwaite J. Readiness to adopt a self-management approach to chronic pain: the Pain Stages of Change Questionnaire (PSOCQ). Pain. 1997;72(1–2): 227–34.

152. Keefe FJ, Lefebvre JC, Kerns RD, Rosenberg R, Beaupre P, Prochaska J, et al. Understanding the adoption of arthritis self-management: stages of changes profiles among arthritis patients. Pain. 2000;87:303–13.

153. Dijkstra A, Vlaeyen JWS, Rijnen H, Nielson W. Readiness to adopt the self-management approach to cope with chronic pain in fibromyalgic patients. Pain. 2001;90:37–45.

154. Jensen MP, Nielson WR, Turner JA, Romano JM, Hill ML. Changes in readiness to self-manage pain are associated with improvement in multidisciplinary pain treatment and pain coping. Pain. 2004;111:84–95.

155. Strand EB, Kerns RD, Haavik-Nilsen K, et al. Higher levels of pain readiness to change and more positive affect reduce pain reports – a weekly assessment study on arthritis patients. Pain. 2007;127(3):204–13.

156. Rubak S, Sandbæk A, Lauritzen T, Christensen B. Motivational interviewing: a systematic review and meta-analysis. Br J Gen Pract. 2005;55:305–12.

157. Burke B, Arkowitz H, Mechola M. The efficacy of motivational interviewing: a meta-analysis of controlled clinical trials. J Consult Clin Psychol. 2003;71:843–61.

158. Jensen MP. A neuropsychological model of pain: research and clinical implications. J Pain. 2010;11(1):2–12.

159. Singh JA, Sloan JA, Atherton PJ, Smith T, Hack TF, Huschka MM, et al. Preferred roles in treatment decision making among patients with cancer: a pooled analysis of studies using the Control Preferences Scale. Am J Manag Care. 2010;16(9): 688–96.

160. Petrella RJ, Petrella M. A prospective, randomized, double-blind, placebo controlled study to evaluate the efficacy of intraarticular hyaluronic acid for osteoarthritis of the knee. J Rheumatol. 2006;33(5):951–6.

161. Greenfield S, Kaplan S, Ware Jr JE. Expanding patient involvement in care: effects on patient outcomes. Ann Intern Med. 1985;102(4):520–8.

162. Turk DC. Combining somatic and psychosocial treatment for chronic pain patients: perhaps 1+1 does=3. Clin J Pain. 2001;17:281–3.

Billing Psychological Services for Patients with Chronic Pain*

77

Geralyn Datz and Daniel Bruns

Key Points

- It is important for mental health professionals to be knowledgeable about current regulations and rationale for psychological billing in the context of pain management.
- Understanding of correct billing procedures allows psychologists to accurately code their services, as well as receive reimbursement.
- Health and behavior codes provide an opportunity for psychologists delivering primarily medically related services, including psychological pain treatment, to accurately code and receive reimbursement.
- Psychological testing is an essential component in assessing surgical readiness, psychiatric comorbidity, and/or risk evaluation for chronic opioid use. It is vital for psychologists to be informed of appropriate coding and recording procedures of this service.
- Correct documentation is a valuable tool for obtaining timely reimbursement, as well as successfully capturing the patient encounter. Incorrect docmentation can result in denial of services.

Money is better than poverty,
if only for financial reasons.

– Woody Allen

G. Datz, Ph.D. (✉)
Southern Behavioral Medicine Associates,
1 Commerce Drive, Suite 106,
Hattiesburg, MS 39402, USA
e-mail: southernbmed@gmail.com

D. Bruns, PsyD
Health Psychology Associates,
1610 29th Avenue Place, Suite 200,
Greeley, CO 80634, USA
e-mail: daniel.bruns@healthpsych.com

Introduction

Billing and coding is the means through which a clinical service gains economic value. Within the practice of pain medicine, knowledge of psychological billing methods is a matter of particular importance to anyone wishing to employ a psychologist or provide psychological services within a pain medicine practice, medical center, outpatient health services, or surgery center. Unfortunately, billing for psychological services is poorly understood Understanding of correct billing procedures allows psychologists to accurately code their services, as well as receive reimbursement. Health and behavior codes provide an opportunity for psychologists delivering primarily medically related services, including psychological pain treatment, to accurately code and receive reimbursement. Psychological testing is also an essential component for developing treatment plans, and appropriate coding and recording procedures of this service are also reviewed. Psychologists, medical providers, billing agencies, and the insurance companies that reimburse psychological services all may be confused or differ with regard to billing for psychological procedures. At minimum, this leads to delays in patient care, inconvenience to patients and providers, and lost revenue. At worst, a lack of billing knowledge leads to psychological services not being reimbursed and as a result not being provided. Without the availability of psychological evaluation services to address psychological screening requirements for various medical treatments, these treatments might not be funded either. Beyond that, without these psychological services, there is an increased risk of improper selection of patients for procedures or therapies, patient nonadherence to medical instructions, decline of patient health or recovery due to undetected or untreated psychiatric comorbidity, or worsening of chronic pain due to influences of biopsychosocial factors.

---

*Billing codes and requirements are subject to change and modification. The authors would recommend conversations with your local carrier for billing updates and clarification.

T.R. Deer et al. (eds.), *Comprehensive Treatment of Chronic Pain by Medical, Interventional, and Integrative Approaches,*
DOI 10.1007/978-1-4614-1560-2_77, © American Academy of Pain Medicine 2013

Psychological Assessment of Patients with Chronic Pain

Surprisingly, despite the essential nature of billing knowledge, most psychologists and medical professionals graduate with no training at all about billing for psychology services in a medical setting. Psychological services are products whose nature is defined by the Current Procedural Terminology (CPT) [1]. The CPT, somewhat ironically, is a work in which psychologists have extremely limited input. As a result, the rules and procedures of billing for psychological services are sometimes counterintuitive. As such, understanding the methods of billing and the perspective of business is essential to enable psychologists and their colleagues to define a suite of services that not only meet the needs of patients but also conform to established requirements of billing procedures. Only then can psychological services become the foundation of an economically viable practice.

The rationale for this chapter is to educate providers about the role and practice of psychological billing in the pain medicine environment. A caveat here is that the information below may change over time and may vary by region, payor, and policy. While the information below is believed to be accurate at the time of this writing, a cornerstone of business practice is that a clinician should verify the terms of a particular policy before service delivery and, as is often necessary, preauthorize the services requested.

Business Considerations

It has been noted that at the present time, most of health care remains divided between general medicine and mental health. This distinction permeates our culture to a remarkable degree, manifesting itself in the form of professional organizations (American Medical Association vs. American Psychological Association), treatment guidelines (medical treatment guidelines vs. mental health treatment guidelines), and law (medical laws vs. mental health laws). Unfortunately, the science is clear that this premise is not true for chronic medical conditions generally [2, 3] and for chronic pain in particular [4]: Medical health and mental health are not separate and distinct, but are inseparably intertwined.

Traditionally, psychologists have provided psychotherapy as a separate service from medical care. When physicians referred medical patients to psychologists, or psychiatrists, it was after no organic cause had been found. In those cases, it was assumed that lacking an obvious medical cause, the report of symptoms must be due to psychopathology, drug seeking, attention-seeking, or malingering. This belief arose from seeing the body and mind as separate, a direct result of the biomedical model of training that many physicians receive [5]. The biomedical model also influences reimbursement, as most private insurance policies employ a two-payor system, which separates or "carves out" mental health services from medical services and creates separate funding sources for each of these types of services. This can create challenges for the psychologist who is treating patients with pain, as the psychologist is using psychological methods to treat a medical condition. These techniques, which are often referred to as "behavioral medicine," include psychological methods that identify, diagnose, treat, and rehabilitate illness and disease. Several of the psychological specializations that use behavioral medicine techniques are health psychologists, pain psychologists, medical psychologists, behavioral health consultants, and behavioral medicine specialists.

Beyond psychologists, physicians, nurse practitioners, and other professionals may also use some or all of psychological procedure codes to supplement the practice of pain medicine. The purpose of this chapter is to educate healthcare professionals working in the pain medicine environment about two of the most useful but often misunderstood areas of psychological services to pain medicine: health and behavior (H&B) code services and psychological testing services. H&B services are reimbursed for several non-physician specialists. In contrast, psychological testing codes may be used by psychologists, physicians, and sometimes other professions as well. In pain medicine specifically, physicians will benefit from becoming familiar with psychological evaluation and treatment practices and billing methods. Together, these will make it possible to develop an economically sustainable means of detecting significant adjustment issues [6] or comorbid psychopathology [7–9] and to develop strategies for risk mitigation in patients with chronic pain [10]. In the text that follows, the background and logistics of code usage will be explained, and clinical vignettes will illustrate their proper use.

Health and Behavior Codes

The belief that psychological and physical health is entirely separate leads to the mistaken assumption that psychological services would have no impact on "real" medical conditions. Nothing could be further from the truth. A recent study determined that the leading causes of death in this country are modifiable behaviors, such as smoking, improper diet, lack of physical activity, and substance abuse, which in turn cause heart disease, stroke, pulmonary disease, diabetes, and many forms of cancer [11]. Because of this, for 7 of the top 10 leading causes of death, the primary means of prevention and/or treatment involves behavior change [12]. Since psychologists specialize in assessing and modifying behaviors, they can play a valuable role in the treatment of medical disorders. The application of psychological services to the treatment of medical disorders is called "behavioral medicine."

In January 2002, the Centers for Medicaid and Medicare services adopted six new codes reflecting health and behavior intervention services, and these were added to the Current

Table 77.1 Health and behavior code descriptions and reimbursement estimates

Service	CPT code	Description	Approximate Medicare 2012 payment
Assessment – initial	96150	An assessment service that includes a clinical interview, behavioral and psychophysiological assessment, and the administration of health-oriented questionnaires	15 min (1 unit): $20.42 1 h (4 units): $81.68
Reassessment	96151	A reassessment to evaluate the patient's condition and determine the need for further treatment	15 min (1 unit): $19.74 1 h (4 units): $78.96[a]
Intervention – individual	96152	Intervention services provided to an individual to modify the psychological, behavioral, cognitive, and social factors affecting the patient's physical health and well-being	15 min (1 unit): $18.72 1 h (4 units): $74.88
Intervention – group (per person)	96153	An intervention service provided to a group Group must be two or more people	15 min (1 unit): $4.42 60 min (4 units): $17.68 10 members (4 units): $176.80
Intervention – family with patient present	96154	An intervention service provided to family to improve patients health and well-being, with education and skills training of family members	15 min (1 unit): $18.38 1 h (4 units): $73.52
Intervention – family without patient present	96155	An intervention service provided to family members of a patient, designed to improve patient health, adaptation to illness, and enhance familial coping	15 min (1 unit): $0[a] 1 h (4 units): $0

[a]Note: Medicare and some private payors do not currently reimburse this service

Procedural Terminology (CPT®) code book (Table 77.1) [1, 13]. These "health and behavior" (H&B) codes are designed to address the behavioral, social, and psychophysiological procedures to prevent, treat, or manage physical health problems and are intended for use by non-physician healthcare clinicians operating within their scope of practice. This includes psychologists (PhDs), nurses (RN, NPs), and other non-physician specialists.

The H&B assessment procedures are offered to patients with an established illness or medical symptoms. The codes make it possible for psychologists and others to provide services to patients with chronic pain without having to diagnose the patient with some type of psychological disorder. In contrast to traditional psychological services, which must be paired with psychiatric diagnosis for billing, the H&B codes are psychological services that are paired with a medical diagnosis for billing. Consequently, it has been noted that, "Clinically, for the first time, practitioners working inside of medicine now have a tool to conceptualize psychology as medical service and have a mechanism to pay for it" [14].

It is noteworthy that, prior to CPT 2002, there was no way for psychologists to adequately capture these types of services. This sometimes led to ethical and professional quandaries for psychologists who worked in medical settings [15]. Medicare and other insurance companies have disallowed psychologists from using evaluation and management (E/M) codes, CPT 99201–99205; 99211–99215; all CPT codes ©2012 American Medical Association. All rights reserved) on the basis of their training and the fact that these codes require medical management. Neuropsychological test codes (CPT 96100–96117) are not appropriate because they reflect testing of cognitive function and response of the central nervous system, which does not necessarily pertain to physical illness. Psychotherapy codes (CPT 90801–90809) are

designed for use by psychologists and psychiatrists, but require a mental health diagnosis, which may not be present in medical patients. "The difficulties associated with acute or chronic medical illness, prevention of physical illness and disability, and maintenance of health, in many instances, do not meet criteria for a psychiatric diagnosis" [15]. Nonetheless, traditional psychotherapy codes were often used in this context, which could create a clinical dilemma. In the past, some providers used psychotherapy codes to bill for behavioral medicine services, as it was "administratively mandated," while observing that it was also "not an accurate reflection of the patient encounter" [14]. Counseling and risk factor reduction codes (CPT 99401–99429) are not useful in this context as they require the *absence* of a physical health diagnosis, illness, or symptoms, which is clearly contraindicated for health and behavior interventions. In any case, these procedure codes are generally not reimbursable for psychologists. Similarly, psychological assessment codes (CPT 90801 for the interview and 96101–96103 for testing and report) were also developed in the context of a mental illness/psychiatric diagnosis. While appropriate for some clinical assessments of medical patients, they may be problematic if the primary assessment is related only to the medical condition and its impact on functioning (e.g., herniated lumbar disc, cancer-related pain), as opposed to identifying psychiatric disorders (e.g., depression, anxiety, addiction, or PTSD) or psychiatric complications (e.g., malingering or symptom magnification). It should be noted here though that the ICD-9-CM, the ICD-10-CM, and the DSM-IV-TR all include a diagnosis for "pain disorder," which includes those patients whose pain reports are judged to be affected by psychosocial factors. Thus, for those patients exhibiting chronic pain with symptoms that exceed what would be expected given the objective medical findings, a diagnosis of pain disorder coupled with

Table 77.2 Commonly used diagnoses for patients with pain

ICD-9-CM/ICD-10-CM diagnosis[a]	DSM-IV-TR diagnosis[b]	ICD-9-CM/ICD-10-CM diagnostic code
Pain disorder related to psych. factors/pain disorder with related psych. factors	Pain disorder with associated [psychological factors] and [medical condition] (code physical diagnosis on Axis III)	307.89/F45.42
Psychogenic pain/pain disorder exclusively related to psychological factors	Pain disorder associated with psychological factors	307.80/F45.41
Somatization disorder [Briquet's disorder]	Somatization disorder	300.81/F45.0
Undifferentiated somatoform disorder	Undifferentiated somatoform disorder	300.82/F45.1
Other specified psychophysiological malfunction/somatoform autonomic dysfunction		306.8/F45.8
Unspecified adjustment reaction	Adjustment disorder unspecified	309.9/F43.20
Psychic factors associated with diseases classified elsewhere/psychosomatic disorder, NOS	[specified psychological factor] Affecting [indicate medical condition]	316.00F45.9
Other unknown and unspecified causes of morbidity and mortality	Diagnosis deferred	799.90
Noncompliance with medical treatment	Personal history of noncompliance with treatment, presenting hazards to health	V15.81
	DSM 5[c]: Proposed Complex Somatic Symptom Disorder will incorporate previous diagnoses of somatization disorder, undifferentiated somatoform disorder, hypochondriasis, pain disorder associated with both psychological factors and a general medical condition, pain disorder associated with psychological factors, and factitious disorder, and has no equivalent in the ICD-9 or ICD-10	

DSM-IV-TR © 2000 American Psychiatric Association. All rights reserved
DSM 5 © 2010 American Psychiatric Association. All rights reserved
[a]Note: ICD-10-CM scheduled to become effective October 1, 2013 [44]
[b]Note: All DSM-IV-TR Dx use the equivalent ICD-9-CM Dx codes
[c]Note: DSM-IV-TR is current APA manual for psychiatric disorders. DSM 5 is currently in revision and expected to become effective in 2013

psychological assessment CPT codes may be applicable. These are discussed in greater detail below.

The principle advantage of health and behavior coding is that they allow psychologists to provide behavioral medicine services without utilizing psychiatric diagnoses. These codes were intended to be funded through medical, not mental, health carve outs, and this offers several advantages over traditional psychological service codes (CPT 90801–90806 and 96101–96103). Most importantly, health and behavior codes are not subject to Medicare's "Outpatient Mental Health Treatment Limitation," whereby Medicare reduces its copayment for mental health services from 80 to 50 %. This reduction only applies to services provided to outpatients with a "mental, psychoneurotic, or personality disorder identified by an ICD-9-CM diagnosis code between 290 and 319" [16]. As such, reimbursement for H&B codes occurs at a rate of 80 %, as it is considered a covered service under the medical portion of insurance. By 2014, though, it is expected that mental health services will be paid at the same 80 % level as physical health services [17]. Secondly, outside of Medicare, the use of psychological codes by psychologists will generally involve billing the mental health insurer, not the medical insurer, and the involvement of a second insurance company can add an additional complication administratively. Third, as above, the use of psychological codes requires a psychiatric diagnosis, and while psychiatric disorders are common in patients with chronic pain, they are not always present.

Logistics of Code Use

There are six H&B codes: two for assessment (initial and reassessment) and four for intervention (individual, group, family with and without patient present). All health and behavior codes only account for face-to-face time spent between a provider and patient. H&B codes are billed in 15-min increments, with no "rounding up." Therefore, if less than 15 min of services is provided the lesser increment must be used (e.g., 28 min of intervention = 1 unit = 15 min). Under Medicare rules, psychiatric treatment codes (CPT 90801–90809 and 96101–96103) and H&B treatment codes cannot be billed on the same day. If both services are needed on the same day, only the predominant service should be billed. With respect to identifying physical health diagnosis, only existing medical diagnoses as reported by the patient's physician should be reported. These codes rely on coding a physical health diagnosis from the International Classification of Diseases, 9th Edition [18]. Obtaining the physical diagnosis requires a review of medical records or communication with the patients' referring physician. While multiple ICD-9-CM diagnoses may also be present (e.g., 722.81 post laminectomy syndrome, lumbar, 723.1 cervicalgia), the physical diagnosis that is primary focus of treatment that day should be reported. While a direct referral from a physician is not necessary to utilize these codes, non-physician practitioners should not attempt to diagnose a patient's medical condition without medical collaboration as that is outside the scope of practice. Table 77.2 provides a description of Axis I diagnoses codes that are typically used with these codes.

With respect to goals of these codes, "The elements of a health and behavior assessment and intervention are designed to improve a patient's health, ameliorate specific disease processes, and improve overall well-being" [15]. Performance of an H&B *assessment* may include a health-focused clinical interview, behavioral observations, psychophysiological monitoring, use of health-oriented questionnaires, and assessment data interpretation. Elements of a H&B *intervention* may include cognitive, behavioral, social, and psychophysiological procedures that are designed to improve the patient's health, ameliorate specific disease-related problems, and improve overall well-being. A detailed description of these services is provided below in clinical vignettes. The patients with chronic pain who may benefit from use of these codes include those with needs for monitoring adherence to medical treatment and medication regimens, overall adjustment issues secondary to pain diagnosis, and those suffering from the physical and emotional discomfort of chronic pain. In addition, patients suffering from chronic pain with a need for training in adaptive coping behaviors (i.e., relaxation, biofeedback, pacing, problem solving), and/or reduction in potentially harmful or risk taking behaviors (including overmedicating, excessive sedentary behavior, and social isolation), would also be excellent candidates for treatment with these codes. Established illnesses that may benefit from use of these codes include cancer, low back pain, neck pain, shoulder pain, postsurgical pain, post laminectomy syndrome, fibromyalgia, phantom limb pain, and myofascial pain, to name a few.

Since 2006 almost all medicare-assisted contractors reimburse H&B codes. In addition, although many private carriers also reimburse these codes, there are exceptions, so it is always recommended to check with the specific carriers in the state of practice. It is notable that Medicare, and most private carriers, does not reimburse for services provided without the patient present (CPT 96155), despite the fact that a fee has been established for this code. As a guideline, nationwide Medicare reimbursement rates, without geographic adjustments, are listed in Table 77.1.

Troubleshooting Issues

Psychiatric Comorbidity. Use of the H&B codes is not precluded in a patient with an existing mental health diagnosis. However, H&B treatment in a patient with comorbid psychopathology must focus on the physical illness/disease that is present and the patients' biopsychosocial adjustment to their disease/illness, *not* their needed mental health treatment. A general rule of thumb is that if you spend greater than 50 % of time discussing concerns and offering treatment for physical illness, bill the H&B code. Conversely, if greater

Table 77.3 Commonly used non- and partly standardized assessment tools

Assessment tool	Abbreviation
Beck Anxiety Inventory	BAI
Beck Depression Inventory – II	BDI-II
Brief Pain Inventory	BPI
Coping Strategies Questionnaire	CSQ
Current Opioid Misuse Measure	COMM
Chronic Pain Acceptance Questionnaire	CPAQ
McGill Pain Questionnaire	MPQ
Multidimensional Pain Inventory	MPI
Numerical Rating Scales	NRS
Opioid Risk Tool	ORT
Oswestry (Low Back Pain) Disability Questionnaire	ODQ
Pain Anxiety Symptoms Scale	PASS
Pain Catastrophizing Scale	PCS
Patient Health Questionnaires	PHQ
Screener and Opioid Assessment for Patients in Pain – Revised	SOAPP-R
Visual Analog Scales, Verbal Rating Scales	VAS, VRS

Table 77.4 Resources for psychologists

APA Practice Directorate: Phone number: 202-336-5889. For advocacy and support with claims denials of H&B codes by managed care companies
APA Practice Central: www.apapractice.org includes section on H&B coding, psychological testing, and practice tips. Look under the "Reimbursement" and "Billing and Coding" subsections
Health Psychology and Rehabilitation: www.healthpsych.com go to the "Practitioner's Toolbox" for valuable strategies about "Resolving Issues with Medical Payors"
2006 Psychological Testing Codes Toolkit from the APA Practice Organization, available at http://www.apapractice.org/apo/toolkit.html#

than 50 % of time is spent in counseling and providing support and techniques for treatment of mental illness, then the psychotherapy codes should be used, and the documentation should reflect this.

Assessment. When using the H&B assessment or reassessment codes (96150, 96151), a variety of health-oriented questionnaires can be included along with a clinical interview. These can include traditional standardized psychological measures, along with a variety of nonstandardized checklists and physical and coping strategy measures. A few examples of nonstandardized measures specific to pain assessment are included in Table 77.3, and standardized measures are listed in Table 77.4. Note that this code does not include indirect, or non-face-to-face time, and as a result, measures used in this assessment are generally brief and focused and may include nonstandardized clinical checklists. When more extensive testing (personality, psychopathology) is warranted, the psychological testing codes (96101–96103) should be employed.

Group Therapy. H&B groups provide psychoeducation and social support as relating to physical health, health behaviors, and medical illness (e.g., distinguishing acute from chronic pain, explaining the pathophysiology of pain signal, teaching how to increase activity level despite pain), not mental health (e.g., management of depression, anxiety, trauma). H&B group therapy is reasonable in medical or psychological settings that already use group-based treatments, including intensive outpatient pain management settings, multidisciplinary pain programs, medical or mental health-based office-based settings, and hospital settings. H&B groups often have a cognitive behavioral component, instructing patients how to practice psychological coping skills for modulating chronic pain, improving quality of life despite pain, or for coping with functional limitations. This treatment is different than mental health groups (CPT 90853) that focus on mental illness and may use non-evidence-based methods (e.g., process, support, or psychodynamic approaches).

Payor Issues. While H&B services are sorely needed in the field of pain medicine, in practice, reimbursement problems can occur. In most insurance policies, mental health reimbursement has been "carved out" of the medical insurance contract and provided for under a separate contract. This sometimes creates a problem when attempting to get H&B services authorized, as H&B services can violate contractual boundaries. The mental health insurer will say "We can't reimburse you for this because [contractually] we can't pay for medical diagnoses or medical CPT codes. You should call the medical insurer." Similarly, the medical insurer will say "We can't reimburse you for this because [contractually] we can't reimburse psychologists. Call the mental health insurer." If these problems occur, several resources are available to support and advocate for practitioners and are listed in Table 77.4 and are also available online [19]. In practice, handling this issue sometimes entails educating the payors about these codes and their purpose and pointing out any discrepancy in their policy. In particular, it is ironic that while many payors now require psychological evaluations prior to spinal surgery, spinal cord stimulator implants, or inrathecal pump implants, these same payors may not have made arrangements to reimburse these evaluations. When this type of difficulty is encountered, it is often useful to begin by speaking with the payor's provider relations representative and to inquire about gaining in-network status for providing health and behavior services or making other arrangements for reimbursement. In the case of some private payors, reimbursement of H&B services for psychologists must go through the mental health payor. Paradoxically, this will require the assignment of a DSM-IV-TR psychiatric diagnosis for a medical patient who may have no known psychiatric condition. A method of addressing this matter suggested by some payors is to assign a DSM-IV-TR diagnosis as follows: On Axis III, list the medical diagnosis and ICD-9-CM code. On Axis I and II, list "DSM-IV 799.90 Diagnosis Deferred," as the purpose

of H&B services are neither to assess nor treat psychiatric disorders. Having this DSM-IV code on the forms, however, may facilitate the mental health payor's ability to process the claim.

Clinical Vignettes

96150 Initial Evaluation

A 42-year-old male, military veteran, undergoing treatment for irritable bowel syndrome and fibromyalgia pain is referred for biopsychosocial assessment of pain and psychological distress that developed after fibromyalgia diagnosis. Reduced quality of life due to pain and inability to return to work are also noted.

A 56-year-old male who fell 200 ft off of an oil rig, sustained injuries to both cervical and lumbar spine regions, and is status post two cervical spine surgeries and a lumbar discectomy. He is referred for persisting distress and refractory pain that has not optimally responded surgical and pharmacological interventions. The patient feels worthless and useless as he has never been unemployed before and strongly identifies with his work.

A 16-year-old female is referred for chronic pelvic pain secondary to endometriosis and has dropped out of school due to constant pain and embarrassment over her condition. She has trouble tolerating short-acting opioid analgesics, and her family also has cultural discomfort with the use of pain medicines.

Procedure Description

Patients are assessed with either standardized tests or less formal clinical questionnaires, and a structured clinical interview, which includes both the patient and family members. The clinician assesses the impact of pain condition on activities of daily living, sleep, mood, and quality of life in the following ways. During the interview, medical, psychiatric, and substance abuse histories are assessed, and behavioral observations are made. Medical records are also reviewed, and the overall impressions are formulated into a case conceptualization and treatment plan that is made explicit in the documentation. When appropriate, patients are recommended for individual and/or group cognitive behavioral therapy services emphasizing non-pharmacological coping skills, psychological adjustment to chronic pain and disability, and relaxation training or biofeedback for chronic pain.

96152 Individual Intervention

A 35-year-old female, diagnosed with ankle pain after a fall at work, is referred for assessment and follow-up treatment including coping strategies for chronic pain and assistance in return to work. Initial assessment included clinical interview, psychosocial assessment, and review of medical records. It was determined that the patient had significant concerns about returning to work due to the possibility of re-injury, as well as conflicts with her employer over requested accommodations, and a concern about lax safety policies that led to her injury in the first place.

A 68-year-old male who is status post 5 lumbar surgeries, most recently a fusion of L5 to S1, is seen for 8 months of cognitive behavioral therapy focusing on his distress at his inability to perform daily activity including yard work and manual tasks related to the maintenance of his 75-acre farm. Initial assessment via clinical interview, test results, and corroboration from medical providers revealed him as resistant to taking any form of pain medication and to have continual problems in pacing and accepting his pain diagnosis.

Procedure Description

Patients are provided weekly or bimonthly cognitive behavioral therapy, relaxation response training, and cognitive restructuring focused on teaching abilities to self-manage pain. Patients are taught how to adjust activity level, take medications correctly, and address psychological maladjustment (anger, denial) regarding injuries. Patients are given knowledge about their disease process and educated about which factors assist and limit their recovery. Weekly assessments demonstrate progress in treatment and individualized therapy goals.

96153 Group Intervention

A psychologist runs an 8-week outpatient H&B pain management group that meets twice a week for 90 min. The psychologist uses a treatment manual [20] to design a cognitive behavioral intervention for 8–10 chronic patients with chronic pain who are referred by their physicians for learning problem solving and self-management strategies for adapting to their chronic pain conditions. The psychologist treats a variety of pain syndromes in the group including low back, neck, and leg pain.

A psychologist runs a 12-week outpatient H&B treatment group for 60 min once weekly for patients with chronic pain secondary to fibromyalgia. The group consists of four to eight female patients referred by a rheumatologist who observed that many of her female patients were suffering with a variety of behavioral and psychological issues including sleep disturbance, depression secondary to pain and disability, poor pacing, and chronic tension which appeared to worsen the patients underlying pathology. Topics include activity scheduling, cognitive restructuring, relaxation training, and cognitive behavioral therapy for insomnia.

A psychologist runs a six-session medication compliance group for patients with chronic pain being maintained on

chronic opioid therapy. A board-certified pain physician who offers long-term medication management for patients with chronic pain and requires the group as part of his opioid treatment agreement. The group meets once weekly for 6 weeks for 60 min. Topics include explaining risks and side effects of medications, medical adherence principles, motivational enhancement strategies, and discussing the concepts of addiction, tolerance, withdrawal, and physical dependence. Strategies for safeguarding medications and how to report and manage side effects are also discussed.

A psychologist runs a biweekly 12-session smoking cessation group for patients with chronic pain who are being considered for chronic opioid therapy. Internal medicine and pain medicine specialists in a hospital-based setting provide referrals. Based on evidence that nicotine use in this population is correlated with greater presence of aberrant opioid behaviors, the physician group requires abstinence from nicotine prior to initiating pharmacotherapy. The group occurs once weekly for 8 weeks, 60 min per session, and topic includes identifying smoking triggers, how to develop a quitting plan, and preventing relapse. Referring physicians also collaborate in prescribing nicotine replacement therapies and/or pharmacotherapies for smoking cessation.

Procedure Description

For each group, the rationale for the group is fully explained in the documentation. Each group includes psychoeducation, cognitive behavioral components, and social support elements. Patients are given outcome assessments prior to, during, and at the termination of the group, and these are recorded in the patients' therapy notes. Behavioral observations are made of the patients, their responses to the treatments, and their completion of assignments and behavioral tasks. Topics covered at each session and the progress of each patient are recorded and individualized.

96151 Reassessment

A 52-year-old male, a former commercial builder who fell off a roof, received 8 months of cognitive behavioral (96152) therapy and made significant gains in treatment. He recently reinjured his low back while vacationing with his son. His pain increased, and he began to regress, exhibiting unsanctioned dose escalations of his Lortab. He admits he became very anxious when realizing his physical limitations outside of work and states, "I wasn't going to just give into the pain." He is referred for reevaluation of psychosocial adjustment and coping skills training.

A 25-year-old female nurse who sustained a crush injury to her right upper extremity as a result of a mounted television falling on her while at work is being treated as an individual in an outpatient mental health setting. She is reassessed after

6 months of treatment, as she is not progressing as expected. Additionally, FCE results indicate she has significant upper extremity impairment and may not be able to return work in her former capacity. She has significant catastrophizing and is developing psychosocial distress at the prospect of not returning to work, as she is a single mother.

Procedure Description

Initial assessment measures are reviewed on both patients. Additional tests are administered based on the patients' reactions to new stressors. Patient's psychological status, medical compliance, use of cognitive behavioral strategies, relaxation and meditation practices are assessed. Current functioning is compared to initial evaluation and last outcome measurement. The need for further treatment is evaluated and supported.

96154 Family with Patient Present

A 21-year-old male who was run over by a commercial forklift. He sustained significant and debilitating injuries to right lower extremity and is status post nine leg surgeries. Although his limb was preserved, the patient was having significant difficulty adjusting to his injury. His mother encourages his passivity, bringing him everything he needs, and even bathing and clothing him, activities his physical therapist states he can do on his own with adaptations which were ordered for the home (rails and supports). The mother reported feeling extreme sympathy for son. The father and older sister have become resentful of patient and mother, stating that they feel "ignored" and "unimportant." At the same time, the mother feels unsupported by family members and appears to increase her focus on son in response to reactions from husband and daughter. The sister and the patient frequently fight, with the sister calling him a "baby," and the patient feeling shamed by his sisters' judgments and experiencing self-pity stating, "No one will ever marry me."

Procedure Description

A family systems approach is sometimes utilized to treat the multiple interactions of the patient's pain problem with the family of origin. For example, a mother could be taught which activities require the most assistance and how to emotionally support her son without catering to his every whim. At the same time, her son could be encouraged to develop physical as well as emotional independence from his mother, which is something that he wants, but does not know how to implement. The son's recreational activity is also increased including church attendance and community involvement. During treatment, the sister and father's feelings of resentment and frustration are openly aired and cognitive restructuring and behavioral assignments are used to assist

family members in developing new relationships with each other. Communication skills and assertiveness techniques are also emphasized which reduce conflicts at home.

96155 Family Without Patient Present

A 49-year-old female diagnosed with metastatic breast cancer is being aggressively treated with both pharmacotherapy and radiation therapy status post right-sided mastectomy. The patient is referred for treatment by her oncologist for pain management via behavioral methods including biofeedback and imagery, as well as impact of disease on her quality of life, physical image, and family of two teenage sons and husband.

Procedure Description

The patient's husband and sons are enrolled in treatment as the patient has trouble attending psychologist appointments due to the distance that she lives from the treatment facility and the severity of her pain. The husband works approximately 1 mile from treatment facility and is able to come for therapy in the mornings prior to his workday, while the sons attend as they are able. In treatment, the family members are taught relaxation, communication strategies, emotional support, and cognitive restructuring techniques to assist the patient in managing her pain at home. This allows family members to become active agents in the treatment of their mother's problem, as previously they felt marginalized and helpless as they watched their mother suffer.

Psychological Assessment

In pain medicine, the purposes of psychological assessment include (1) assessing the patient for presence of psychopathology, (2) as a supplement to determining surgical readiness (which may also be required by the insurance carrier), and (3) for assessing potential substance abuse, including any aberrant behaviors or personality variables associated with increased risk of medication misuse.

The prevalence of psychopathology in patients with chronic pain is well recognized [7, 8, 21]. In one study, 77 % of patients with chronic pain met lifetime diagnostic criteria for at least one Axis I diagnosis, and 59 % demonstrated current symptoms [22]. The most common diagnoses preceding chronic low back pain were major depression (54 %), substance abuse (94 %), and anxiety disorders (95 %). Beyond affective disturbances, at least one personality disorder was present in 51 % of the patients [22]. Other studies show that anxiety decreases pain thresholds and tolerances [23], depression is linked to poor treatment outcome with traditional medical approaches [24], and anxiety and depression are associated with magnification of medical symptoms [25]. In general, psychopathology increases pain intensity and disability, contributing to a negative cycle, where functional limitations are perpetuated [26]. As a result, it is not surprising that unrecognized and untreated psychopathology can interfere with successful rehabilitation [27].

The concept of psychological testing for use in assisting medical decision-making is not new. Psychological selection has been used in several arenas for assessing surgical appropriateness and readiness, including for spinal cord stimulation [9], bariatric surgery [28, 29], spine surgery [9, 30], heart surgery [31, 32], and intrathecal pump placement [33]. Overall, results suggest that attitudinal (e.g., expectations) and mood factors (e.g., depression, anxiety) are strongly predictive of surgical outcome, including need for anesthesia, length of hospital stay, functional recovery, and patient ratings of recovery [34]. Recently, Wasan and colleagues utilized psychological assessment to identify outcome for medial branch nerve blocks [35]. They found that the presence of psychiatric comorbidity, in particular high levels of depression and anxiety, predicted diminished pain relief from steroid injection at 1-month follow-up.

In addition, the use of psychological assessment is part of an emerging application of patient selection methodology that is helpful in identifying patients most appropriate for opioid use. Several guidelines have recognized that a comprehensive opioid screening requires assessment of substance abuse, addiction potential, psychopathology, and medical compliance [35–38]. In practice, this is achieved via a multifaceted approach that includes psychological testing, as part of a "universal precautions" approach to risk assessment [39, 40]. In summary, there is a strong rationale for the use of psychological testing to pain medicine, and physicians are encouraged to use experienced assessment practitioners to supplement their chronic pain treatments in this way.

Although either a clinical psychologist or a physician can bill psychological testing codes and perform supervision for these types of tests, psychologists generally have the greatest expertise in the area. Clinical psychologists must indicate who ordered the testing on the bill for services, however. Some other non-physician practitioners are also allowed to conduct these tests, including nurse practitioners, clinical nurse specialists, and physician assistants, but doing so must be consistent with their training and experiences and within their scope of practice as defined in their state. For example, nurse practitioners and specialists offering this service typically must do so in collaboration with a physician.

The CPT codes for psychological assessment include 90801 (diagnostic interview) and three codes for psychological testing (see Table 77.5). CPT 96101 was revised in 2008 to distinguish the actual services of the psychologist or the

Table 77.5 Psychological testing codes and use

96101	Psychological testing, per hour, and interpretation and reporting, per hour, by a qualified professional (clinical or independent psychologist, physician, nurse, clinical nurse specialist, or physician assistant)
96102	Psychological testing per hour by a technician, with per hour interpretation and reporting by a qualified professional (psychologist of physician)
96103	Psychological testing per unit by a computer, with interpretation and reporting by a psychologist or physician. Can only be billed once no matter how many instruments are administered

Table 77.6 Commonly used standardized psychological tests used for pain assessment

Assessment tool	Abbreviation
Battery Health Improvement-2	BHI2™
Brief Battery for Health Improvement	BBHI2™
Millon Behavioral Medicine Diagnostic	MBMD™
Minnesota Multiphasic Personality Inventory-2	MMPI-2™
Minnesota Multiphasic Personality Inventory-2 Revised Form	MMPI-2-RF™
Millon Multiaxial Clinical Inventory-III	MCMI-III™
Pain Patient Profile	P3®

physician (interview, report writing, integration) from those performed by technicians (96102) or computers (96103 for unassisted computer administration and scoring). In theory, all of these codes can be used in various combinations for an evaluation. In practice, however, some private payors and policies have idiosyncratic rules, including ones that may redefine CPT codes and how they are used. For example, the policy of some payors dictates that while they will preauthorize multiple hours of testing during an evaluation, their system does not allow reimbursement of more than one psychological service on any given day. This policy requires the clinician to bill all hours under a single CPT code, such as 96101. Another area of variance is that the definition of "technician" varies under differing states and coverage policies and should be investigated prior to billing these codes. Types of psychological tests that pertain to psychological evaluations for pain medicine that commonly meet the standards of utilization review are listed in Table 77.6. When submitting psychological testing claims for payment, physicians, psychologists, and non-physician practitioners must use both the CPT codes utilized reporting the healthcare practitioner service(s) and the DSM-IV-TR/ICD-9-CM diagnosis codes for documenting the suspected or diagnosed mental illness condition. In addition, the medical necessity of these tests must be established (see Documentation section for meeting these criteria). The ICD-9-CM diagnosis code ranges that can be used to support psychological testing codes and medical necessity include 290.0–299.80 (dementias through pervasive developmental disorders), 300.00–319 (anxiety, dissociative, and somatoform disorders through unspecified mental retardation), and 347.00–347.01 (narcolepsy and aphasia through aphonia).

The CPT codes of 96101 and 96102 are based on 1-h units of service. In practice, though, the actual amount of time spent providing the service will vary and will need to be rounded off. The accepted means of rounding the time for these codes for some payors is as follows: If the actual time spent providing the service is 31–90 min, 1 h is charged. Similarly, if the actual time spent providing the service is 91–150 min, 2 h are charged. Since under these rules, the reimbursement for 31 min of time is the same as for 90 min, clinicians need to be mindful of the financial impact of rounding rules. Sometimes, though, a brief psychological assessment may take less than 31 min. Is this case, the modifier "-52" can be appended to the code (e.g., 96101–52). This modifier indicates a reduced service and thus allows for billing for the use of brief measures when less than 31 min is spent. This practice can make it possible to get reimbursed for the use of brief psychological tests, and this is especially useful in medical offices where patients are seen at a fast pace.

Case Vignettes

A patient is referred to a psychologist for a presurgical spinal cord stimulator evaluation. The patient cannot tolerate oral medication and severe neuropathic pain in left lower extremity. The psychologist spends 60 min in face-to-face contact with the patient, taking a psychological and medical history, a substance use history, and assessing motivation and understanding of procedure. In addition, 135 min is spent reviewing medical records, report writing, and integration. The MMPI-2-RF and the BHI 2 tests are administered via computer and scored on the computer. Billing: 90801 is billed for the interview, 1 unit of 96103–59 computer administration is billed for the testing [note that Medicare and others may require the modifier "-59" to be appended to this procedure code when it is used on the same day as 96101 to indicate that it is a separate service], and 2 units of 96101 are billed of psychologist time to write the report that integrates the test results with the interview and the medical records.

A physician is considering a patient for an intrathecal pump placement. The patient has exhausted all conservative treatments. The patient is administered a MMPI-2-RF via paper and pencil, unattended, for 2 h. The results are scored via computer, entered by a nurse. The report is given to the physician, who interprets profile, discusses the results with the patient, and determines that the patient is appropriate for the procedure, given test results and the patients history, which is well known to the provider. Under this scenario, no units could be billed. As no report is generated and no integration of results occurs, 96101 cannot be billed. As the computer is only used for scoring and not for administration, 96103 cannot be billed either. Consideration of additional data, however, and additional time spent with the patient may allow the MD to bill for a more extensive E/M service.

A patient is being considered for chronic opioid therapy. She evidences aberrant behavior in the form of recent unsanctioned dose escalations. The patient is referred to a psychologist for assessment of risk for medication misuse. The MBMD, PAI, and SOAPP-R are administered via paper, for 3 h, while a technician observes patient and is available to assist the patient as needed. The technician scores the measures and presents to psychologist. The psychologist interviews patient for 90 min and spends 2 h in report writing, integration, and consultation with the referring provider about patient behavior. Billing: 90801 is billed for a 75 min interview, 96101 is billed for 2 h of testing of psychologist time (2 units), and 96102 is billed for 3 h of technician time (3 units).

A patient being treated for fibromyalgia has not responded as expected to treatment and cries frequently during the interview. The physician suspects depression and uses a computer-administered BBHI 2 to assess the patient. Since the patient is a delayed recoverer (which could suggest a DSM-IV pain disorder) and also exhibits signs of depression, there are two separate justifications for ordering a psychological test. The physician bills for 96103 computerized test administration in addition to the E&M code.

Documentation

The importance of proper documentation cannot be overemphasized. Documentation substantiates the services being billed, quantifies the payment being billed, and may be requested by the carrier in many cases. In the case of H&B codes, documentation should include stating the medical necessity of services, outlining a plan of care and its specific elements, monitoring progress in treatment, and documenting the outcome of services provided. For psychological testing, the need for testing should be provided (e.g., suspicion of depression, anxiety, addictive behavior), test results should be summarized, and recommendation for treatment should be made. For all codes used, it is important that the general structure of each clinical contact should include a discussion of the rationale for service, the primary diagnosis being treated, the intervention provided, the overall plan of care, and either the start and end times or duration of visit (Tables 77.7 and 77.8).

Table 77.7 Health and behavior documentation guidelines

Session start and end time	Behavioral factors affecting physiological function
Estimated # of sessions	Emotional factors affecting physiological function
Presence of physical illness	Cognitive factors affecting physiological function
Psychological factor/status	Social factors affecting physiological function
Measurement of goals	Treatment, prevention, and management of physical health problem or disability

Table 77.8 Psychological testing guidelines

Where testing and interview (if applicable) occurred	Patient has symptoms consistent with mental illness
Test administrator	Interpretation of test(s): if by computer, add summary of test administrator
Face-to-face time spent administering, interpreting, and reporting test results	Summarize results including:
Time spent incorporating test results, clinical interpretation, and writing report	1. Treatment, including how test results affect the prescribed treatment
Appropriate test(s) selected and how tests scored	2. Follow-up/administration of test to measure efficacy of procedure
Medical necessity of test(s) described (supported through documented diagnosis)	3. Outcomes/measurement
	4. Any recommendation for further testing
Documentation of physical condition(s)	

Medical Necessity

In many cases, establishing medical necessity is required. CMS defines medical necessity as "always based on the patient's condition. When documenting medical necessity, identify the skilled service and the reason this skilled service is necessary for the beneficiary in objective terms." Services are medically necessary if they are (a) proper and needed for diagnosis and treatment of a medical condition; (b) furnished for the purpose of diagnosis, direct care, and treatment of a medical condition; (c) meet good clinical practice standards; and (d) are not primarily for the convenience of the patient [41].

If medical necessity is not established, claims for services will be denied. Further, if Medicare or another payor determines that services were medically unnecessary after payment has already been made, it will be treated as an overpayment and the payer will insist that the money be refunded, typically with interest. Additionally, if a provider routinely demonstrates a pattern of delivering services that

are not medically necessary, the provider may face monetary penalties, exclusion from insurance programs, and even criminal prosecution.

Notes Versus Records

When documenting health and behavior interventions, practitioners must decide whether they wish to keep additional psychotherapy notes. Under the Privacy Rule of the Health Insurance Portability and Accountability Act (HIPAA), behavioral therapy and psychotherapy notes have special status, while psychotherapy records do not. *Psychotherapy notes* means "notes recorded (in any medium) by a health care provider who is a mental health professional documenting or analyzing the contents of conversation during a private counseling session or a group, joint, or family counseling session" and that are separated from the rest of the individual's medical record. "Such notes are to be used only by the therapist who wrote them, maintained separately from the medical record, and not involved in the documentation necessary for health care treatment, payment, or operations" [42].

Psychotherapy notes "exclude medication prescription and monitoring, counseling session start and stop times, the modalities and frequencies of treatment furnished, results of clinical tests, and any summary of the following items: diagnosis, functional status, the treatment plan, symptoms, prognosis, and progress" to date. These elements are referred to as psychotherapy records (see Table 77.7) [43]. HIPAA singles out behavioral therapy notes for special handling and leaves all other types of psychotherapy records to be handled the same as all other protected health information (PHI). If a provider chooses to also keep psychotherapy notes, these must be kept separate from the rest of patients' medical records, which can make patients feel more secure about their privacy. Note that even though H&B treatment may not be psychotherapy from the clinical perspective, notes generated from H&B services can still be classified as psychotherapy notes as defined by HIPAA.

Conclusion

This chapter reviews the use of two groups of psychological treatment codes, H&B and psychological testing, as they pertain to pain medicine. Assessments and interventions that these codes support are reviewed, and case discussions are provided. Psychologists can offer a valuable service to medical providers. Although it is doubtful that anyone goes into the field of medicine with hopes of mastering the CPT, doing so is a practical necessity, without which services cannot be reimbursed. When the complexities of billing and coding for psychological services are mastered, the rendering of mental health care is able to become an economically sustainable and integral aspect of pain treatment.

References

1. Beebe M, Dalton JA, Espronceda M. CPT 2009 professional edition (current procedural terminology, professional ed.). Washington, D.C: American Medical Association; 2008.

2. Havelka M, Lucanin JD, Lucanin D. Biopsychosocial model – the integrated approach to health and disease. Coll Antropol. 2009; 33(1):303–10.

3. Adler RH. Engel's biopsychosocial model is still relevant today. J Psychosom Res. 2009;67(6):607–11.

4. Gatchel RJ, Peng YB, Peters ML, Fuchs PN, Turk DC. The biopsychosocial approach to chronic pain: scientific advances and future directions. Psychol Bull. 2007;133(4):581–624.

5. American College of Occupational and Environmental Medicine. Occupational medicine practice guidelines. 2nd ed. Beverly Farms: OEM Press; 2004.

6. Turner JA, Jensen MP, Romano JM. Do beliefs, coping, and catastrophizing independently predict functioning in patients with chronic pain? Pain. 2000;85(1–2):115–25.

7. Dersh J, Polatin PB, Gatchel RJ. Chronic pain and psychopathology: research findings and theoretical considerations. Psychosom Med. 2002;64(5):773–86.

8. McWilliams LA, Cox BJ, Enns MW. Mood and anxiety disorders associated with chronic pain: an examination in a nationally representative sample. Pain. 2003;106(1–2):127–33.

9. Bruns D, Disorbio JM. Assessment of biopsychosocial risk factors for medical treatment: a collaborative approach. J Clin Psychol Med Settings. 2009;16(2):127–47.

10. Ives TJ, Chelminski PR, Hammett-Stabler CA, et al. Predictors of opioid misuse in patients with chronic pain: a prospective cohort study. BMC Health Serv Res. 2006;6:46.

11. Mokdad AH, Marks JS, Stroup DF, Gerberding JL. Actual causes of death in the United States, 2000. JAMA. 2004;291(10):1238–45.

12. Wiggins JG. Would you want your child to be a psychologist? Am Psychol. 1994;49(6):485–92.

13. APA Government Relations Staff. Health and behavior assessment and intervention CPT codes. 2010. http://www.apapracticecentral.org/reimbursement/billing/health-behavior.aspx. Accessed 21 Oct 2010.

14. Kessler R. Integration of care is about money Too: the health and behavior codes as an element of a new financial paradigm. Fam Syst Health. 2008;26(2):207–16.

15. American Medical Association. Health and behavior assessment/intervention. CPT assistant, vol. 15. Washington, DC: AMA Press; 2005. p. 1–15.

16. Department of Health and Human Services: Centers for Medicare and Medicaid Services. CMS manual system. Transmittal 1843. Outpatient mental health treatment limitation. Washington, D.C.: Department of Health and Human Services; 2009.

17. Department of Health and Human Services: Centers for Medicare & Medicaid Services (CMS). CMS manual system: Transmittal #1843. Outpatient mental health treatment limitation. 2009. https://www.cms.gov/transmittals/downloads/R1843CP.pdf. Accessed 1 Nov 2010.

18. American Medical Association. ICD-9-CM, 1996: international classification of diseases, 9th revision, clinical modification : volumes 1 and 2, color-coded, illustrated ICD-9 CM codes. Dover: American Medical Association; 1995.

19. Bruns D. A step-by-step guide to obtaining reimbursement for services provided under the health and behavior codes. 2009; http://www.healthpsych.com/tools/resolving_h_and_b_problems.pdf. Accessed 5 Nov 2010.

20. Thorn BE. Cognitive therapy for chronic pain: a step-by-step guide. New York: Guilford Press; 2004.

21. Dersh J, Gatchel RJ, Polatin P, Mayer T. Prevalence of psychiatric disorders in patients with chronic work-related musculoskeletal pain disability. J Occup Environ Med. 2002;44(5):459–68.

22. Polatin PB, Kinney RK, Gatche RJ, Lillo E, Mayer TG. Psychiatric illness and chronic low-back pain. The mind and the spine – which goes first? Spine. 1993;18(1):66–71.

23. Cornwall A, Donderi DC. The effect of experimentally induced anxiety on the experience of pressure pain. Pain. 1988;35(1): 105–13.

24. Burns JW, Johnson BJ, Mahoney N, Devine J, Pawl R. Cognitive and physical capacity process variables predict long-term outcome after treatment of chronic pain. J Consult Clin Psychol. 1998; 66(2):434–9.

25. Katon W, Ciechanowski P. Impact of major depression on chronic medical illness. J Psychosom Res. 2002;53(4):859–63.

26. Holzberg AD, Robinson ME, Geisser ME, Gremillion HA. The effects of depression and chronic pain on psychosocial and physical functioning. Clin J Pain. 1996;12(2):118–25.

27. Gatchel R. Psychological disorders and chronic pain: cause and effect relationships. In: Gatchel RJ, Turk DC, editors. Psychological approaches to pain management: a practitioner's handbook. New York: Guilford; 1996. p. 33–54.

28. Sarwer DB, Thompson JK, Mitchell JE, Rubin JP. Psychological considerations of the bariatric surgery patient undergoing body contouring surgery. Plast Reconstr Surg. 2008;121(6):423e–34.

29. Mechanick JI, Kushner RF, Sugerman HJ, et al. Executive summary of the recommendations of the American Association of Clinical Endocrinologists, the Obesity Society, and American Society for Metabolic & Bariatric Surgery medical guidelines for clinical practice for the perioperative nutritional, metabolic, and nonsurgical support of the bariatric surgery patient. Endocr Pract. 2008;14(3):318–36.

30. den Boer JJ, Oostendorp RA, Beems T, Munneke M, Oerlemans M, Evers AW. A systematic review of bio-psychosocial risk factors for an unfavourable outcome after lumbar disc surgery. Eur Spine J. 2006;15(5):527–36.

31. Burg MM, Benedetto MC, Soufer R. Depressive symptoms and mortality two years after coronary artery bypass graft surgery (CABG) in men. Psychosom Med. 2003;65(4):508–10.

32. Burg MM, Benedetto MC, Rosenberg R, Soufer R. Presurgical depression predicts medical morbidity 6 months after coronary artery bypass graft surgery. Psychosom Med. 2003;65(1): 111–8.

33. Van Dorsten B. Psychological considerations in preparing patients for implantation procedures. Pain Med. 2006;7(s1):S47–57.

34. Rosenberger PH, Jokl P, Ickovics J. Psychosocial factors and surgical outcomes: an evidence-based literature review. J Am Acad Orthop Surg. 2006;14(7):397–405.

35. Wasan AD, Jamison RN, Pham L, Tipirneni N, Nedeljkovic SS, Katz JN. Psychopathology predicts the outcome of medial branch blocks with corticosteroid for chronic axial low back or cervical pain: a prospective cohort study. BMC Musculoskelet Disord. 2009;10:22.

36. Trescot AM, Helm S, Hansen H. Opioids in the management of chronic non-cancer pain: an update of American Society of the Interventional Pain Physicians' (ASIPP) guidelines. Pain Physician. 2008;11(2S):S5–62.

37. Federation of State Medical Boards. Model policy for the use of controlled substances for the treatment of pain. J Pain Palliat Care Pharmacother. 2004;19:73–8.

38. Chou R, Fanciullo GJ, Fine PG, et al. Clinical guidelines for the use of chronic opioid therapy in chronic noncancer pain. J Pain. 2009;10(2):113–30.

39. Gourlay DL, Heit HA, Almahrezi A. Universal precautions in pain medicine: a rational approach to the treatment of chronic pain. Pain Med. 2005;6(2):107–12.

40. Passik SD, Kirsh KL. The interface between pain and drug abuse and the evolution of strategies to optimize pain management while minimizing drug abuse. Exp Clin Psychopharmacol. 2008;16(5): 400–4.

41. Department of Health and Human Services: Centers for Medicare & Medicaid Services (CMS). Medicare glossary: definition of medically necessary. 2010. http://www.medicare.gov/Glossary/ShowTerm.asp?Language=English&term=medically+necessary. Accessed 1 Nov 2010.

42. Department of Health and Human Services. Federal Register. 1999;64(212):59938. http://frwebgate2.access.gpo.gov/cgi-bin/PDFgate.cgi?WAISdocID=zT6q9W/1/2/0&WAISaction=retrieve. Accessed 1 Nov 2010.

43. Department of Health and Human Services. Federal Register. 2000;65(250):82497. http://frwebgate2.access.gpo.gov/cgi-bin/PDFgate.cgi?WAISdocID=zT6q9W/1/2/0&WAISaction=retrieve. Accessed 1 Nov 2010.

44. World Health Organisation. ICD-10 Classifications of Mental and Behavioural Disorder: Clinical Descriptions and Diagnostic Guidelines. 1992. Geneva. World Health Organisation.

Hypnosis and Pain Control

78

David Spiegel

Key Points

- Hypnosis is a state of highly focused attention, coupled with dissociation of peripheral awareness and heightened response to suggestion.
- Hypnotizability is a stable trait – most children and about two-thirds of the adult population are hypnotizable. Hypnosis can help people establish control over both acute and chronic pain.
- Hypnosis reduces pain perception in parts of the brain that affect both sensation and suffering.
- Hypnotic analgesia involves sensory transformation via change in perception of the nature of the pain (temperature, etc.) sensory accommodation, inducing physical relaxation rather than fighting the pain.
- Patients can be taught self-hypnosis and learn to manage pain on their own.

Introduction

Hypnosis, begun as a therapeutic discipline in the eighteenth century, was the first Western conception of psychotherapy [1]. It is a powerful analgesic, and there is compelling clinical documentation of its effectiveness as far back as the mid-nineteenth century. The British surgeon James Esdaile reported that 80 % of subjects obtained anesthesia with hypnosis during major surgical procedures such as amputations [2]. Hypnosis has been proven effective in treating pain and anxiety in the medical setting using randomized prospective trial methodology among both adults [3] and children [4]. Hypnosis is a state of highly focused attention coupled with a suspension of

peripheral awareness [5, 6]. This ability to attend intensely while reducing awareness of context allows one to alter the associational network linking perception and cognition. The hypnotic narrowing of the focus of attention [7] is analogous to looking through a telephoto lens rather than a wide-angle lens – one is aware of content more than context. This can also facilitate reduced awareness of unwanted stimuli, such as pain, or of problematic cognitions, such as depressive hopelessness, that can amplify pain [5, 8]. Such a mental state enhances openness to input from others – often called suggestibility – and can increase receptivity to therapeutic instruction. Yet despite much clinical and neurobiological evidence, hypnosis is rarely used as an analgesic for adults or children.

Background or History That Makes This Chapter Significant

Pain can be either exacerbated or diminished by the emotional, cognitive, and social environment that surrounds it. As Fig. 78.1 illustrates, pain signals can be modulated from the top down as well as the bottom up. When Melzack and Wall [9, 10] promulgated their "gate control" theory of pain, antedating the discovery of endogenous opiate receptors in the spinal cord and periaqueductal gray, they emphasized bottom-up modulation of pain signals. Yet they had noticed that in Pavlov's original experiments, dogs seemed to habituate to constant pain, implying a top-down pain modulation system as well. Cortical signals can amplify or inhibit pain input. Indeed, pain usually occurs within the context of subjective distress that is associated with a major medical illness or physical trauma. Thus, the "pain experience" represents a combination of both tissue damage and the emotional reaction to it. In fact, the intensity of pain is directly associated with its meaning, as Beecher showed when comparing opiate levels required to control post-injury pain on the Anzio Beachhead (very low levels) and among less seriously injured civilian trauma casualties (high levels) [11]. Those cancer patients who believe the pain represents a worsening of their

D. Spiegel, M.D.
Department of Psychiatry and Behavioral Sciences,
Stanford School of Medicine,
40th Quarry Road, Stanford, CA 94305, USA
e-mail: aspiegel@stanford.edu

T.R. Deer et al. (eds.), *Comprehensive Treatment of Chronic Pain by Medical, Interventional, and Integrative Approaches*,
DOI 10.1007/978-1-4614-1560-2_78, © American Academy of Pain Medicine 2013

Fig. 78.1 Pain processing

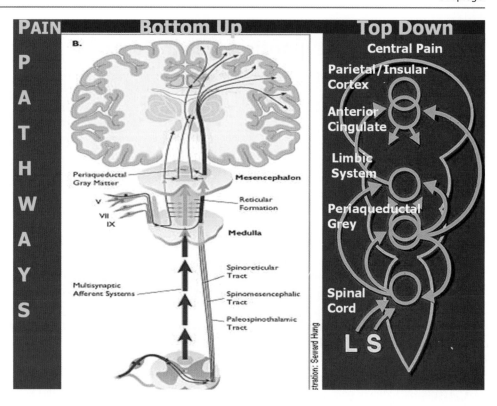

disease experience more pain [12]. Indeed, the meaning of the pain and associated anxiety and depression accounts for more variance in pain than site of metastasis. Pain is often intensified by the helplessness that accompanies it. Many chronic pain patients acknowledge that they could live with their discomfort if they could just keep it within certain boundaries. The combination of pain and its perceived uncontrollability serves to amplify it. The desire for control is a critical component of pain management. Hypnosis provides an excellent opportunity for many to modulate or even eliminate pain.

While there is a common misperception that hypnosis primarily involves relinquishing control and constitutes mindless submission to suggestion, hypnosis is actually a normally occurring state of highly focused attention, with a relative diminution in peripheral awareness [4–6]. Being hypnotized is akin to being so caught up in a good movie, play, or novel that one loses awareness of surroundings and enters the imagined world, a state termed "absorption" [7]. Indeed, people who have such states spontaneously are more likely to be highly hypnotizable on formal testing, indicating that native hypnotic ability is mobilized spontaneously in the service of intense engagement in a variety of activities [8]. Although the suspension of disbelief involved in such absorption may make hypnotized people appear more suggestible, that is, responsive to the instructions of the person inducing hypnosis, in fact all hypnosis is self-hypnosis, a means of focusing attention, whether self-induced or suggested by someone else. Thus, the very state that would appear to

engender loss of control can be utilized quite effectively to enhance control, especially over unwanted sensations such as pain, which can be placed at the periphery of awareness, altered, or even eliminated.

Pain is the ultimate psychosomatic phenomenon. It is composed of both a somatic signal that something is wrong with the body and interpretation of the meaning of that signal involving attentional, cognitive, affective, and social factors. Many athletes and soldiers sustain serious injuries in the heat of sport or combat and are unaware of the injury until someone points out bleeding or swelling. On the other hand, others with comparatively minor physical damage report being totally overcome with pain. A single parent with a sarcoma complained of severe unremitting pain as well as concern about her failure to discuss her terminal prognosis with her adolescent son. When an appropriate meeting was arranged to plan for his future and discuss her prognosis with him, the pain resolved [11].

Indeed, anxiety and depression are often associated with pain [13–15]. Depression is the most frequently reported psychiatric diagnosis among chronic pain patients. Reports of depression among chronic pain populations range from 10 to 87 % [16]. Patients with two or more pain conditions have been found to be at elevated risk for major depression, whereas those patients with only one pain condition did not show such an elevated rate of mood disorder in a large sample of health maintenance organization (HMO) patients. The relative severity of the depression observed in chronic pain patients was illustrated by Katon and Sullivan [17] who showed that 32 % of a sample of 37 pain patients met criteria for major depression and 43 % had a past episode of major depression.

Anxiety is especially common among those with acute pain. Like depression, it may be an appropriate response to serious trauma through injury or illness. Pain may serve a signal function or be part of an anxious preoccupation, as in the case of the woman with the sarcoma cited above. Similarly, anxiety and pain may reinforce one another, producing a snowball effect of escalating and mutually reinforcing central and peripheral symptoms.

Scientific Foundation of This Topic to Pain Care

There is considerable evidence that hypnosis affects clinically important aspects of somatic functioning. The oldest and best established effect is on pain, dating back to the pioneering work of Esdaile [2]. This finding has been replicated in numerous studies [3, 12–15, 18–23]. We conducted a randomized controlled clinical trial among 241 patients undergoing invasive radiological procedures and demonstrated that, compared to either routine care or structured attention, hypnosis produced significant reductions in pain, anxiety, complications, and procedure time while requiring only half of the total analgesic medication (Fig. 78.2a, b) [3].

Hypnosis in combination with group therapeutic support has been proven highly effective in reducing chronic pain as well. In two randomized clinical trials involving women with metastatic breast cancer, this treatment resulted in a significant reduction in pain over a 1-year period while patients were on the same and low amounts of analgesic medication (Fig. 78.3) [16, 24].

Neuroimaging and Hypnosis

Hypnotic analgesia results in reduced amplitude of the somatosensory event-related potential, including early (p100) as well as later (p200 and p300) components [17]. There is evidence from other laboratories that hypnotic analgesia involves both sensory and affective aspects of pain and that changes in the wording of hypnotic instructions alter parts of the brain involved in hypnotic analgesia, from reduced perception (somatosensory cortex) to reduced concern with the pain (anterior cingulate cortex) [25–27]. Many studies have demonstrated that hypnotic alteration of perception changes perceptual processing in the brain. Changing the wording of a pain-directed hypnotic instruction from "you will feel cool, tingling numbness more than pain" to "the pain will not bother you" shifts activation from the somatosensory cortex to the dACC [25, 27]. Similarly, in a PET study, hypnotic suggestion to add or subtract color was shown to alter blood flow in color processing regions of the brain in comparable

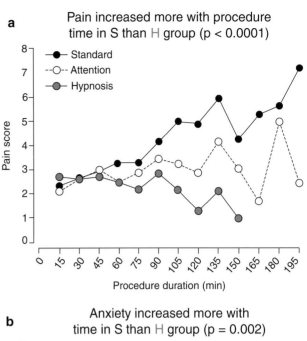

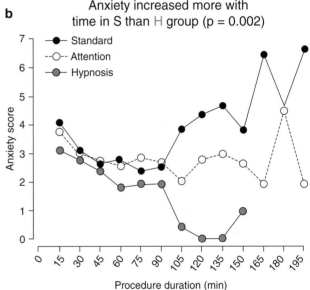

Fig. 78.2 (**a**) Pain increased more with procedure time in S than H group, and (**b**) anxiety increased more with time in S than H group (Adapted from Lang et al. [3])

directions [28]. Hypnotized subjects were asked to see a grayscale pattern in color; under hypnosis, color areas in the ventral visual processing stream were activated, whether they were shown colors or the grayscale stimulus. Believing was seeing. Raij et al. found that DLPFC, dACC, and fronto-insular activation correlated with the degree of pain experienced under hypnotic suggestion [29]. Using PET, Faymonville implicated many regions including the dACC and DLPFC in hypnosis and hypnotic reduction in pain perception [30].

Several studies have tested the idea that endogenous opiates account for hypnotic analgesia. But, with one partial exception [31], studies with both volunteers [32] and patients

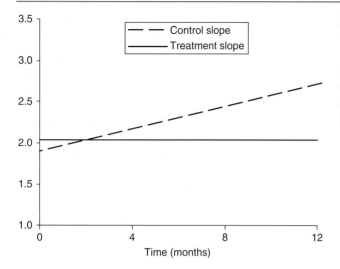

Fig. 78.3 Slopes and mean scores for pain and suffering over the first 12 months and analyzed separately for education only (control) and group therapy plus education (treatment) conditions

in chronic pain [33] have shown that hypnotic analgesia is not blocked and reversed by a substantial dose of naloxone, an opiate receptor blocker, given in double-blind, crossover fashion. Therefore, the cortical attention deployment mechanism is at the moment the most plausible explanation for hypnotic reduction of pain.

Clinical Examples and Usefulness in Clinical Practice

Utilizing Hypnosis

It is wise to commence pain treatment utilizing hypnosis with two types of measurement: of pain and of hypnotizability. Patients can reliably report their pain experience on a 0–10 analog scale, and this provides a benchmark for assessing the subsequent effectiveness of various hypnotic techniques.

The term "hypnotizability" refers to the individual's degree of responsiveness to suggestion during hypnosis [34]. Hypnotizability is a highly stable and measurable trait [5]. In one study, hypnotizability was found to have a 0.7 test-retest correlation over a 25-year interval, making it a more stable trait than IQ over such a long period of time [34]. The trait of hypnotizability is a crucial moderating variable in pain treatment response, both that involving hypnosis directly [35] and in augmenting placebo response [36]. Although not all patients are sufficiently hypnotizable to benefit from these techniques, two out of three adults are at least somewhat hypnotizable [4], and it has been estimated that hypnotic capacity is correlated at a 0.5 level with effectiveness in medical pain reduction [37]. Furthermore, clinically effective

hypnotic analgesia is not confined to those with high hypnotizability [25].

One especially useful way of introducing hypnosis into the therapy is through the use of a clinical hypnotizability scale, such as the Hypnotic Induction Profile [5] or the Stanford Hypnotic Clinical Scale [38]. This form of initial hypnotic induction has several advantages:

1. It provides useful information about the patient's degree of hypnotizability. About one in four adults are not hypnotizable, and one in ten is extremely responsive [5]. Patients' performance on a hypnotizability test provides either a tangible demonstration of their hypnotic ability, which is a good starting point for therapy and is often surprising to patients, or it demonstrates that hypnosis is unlikely to be useful, in which case other techniques can be employed. Thus, the hypnotic induction can be turned into a rational deduction about the patient's resources for change [37].

2. The atmosphere of testing enhances the treatment alliance and defuses anxieties about loss of control. The therapist's responsibility is to provide a clinically appropriate setting and give instructions for the systematic exploration of the patient's hypnotic capacity. This is not a power struggle in which the therapist tries to "get the patient into a trance" and the patient succumbs or resists. The therapist is interested in finding out the results of the test, not in proving how successful he or she is at hypnotizing a patient. Thus, the atmosphere becomes something of a Socratic dialogue, in which both discover what the patient already "knows" (hypnotic capacity) but about which there may be little conscious awareness or prior experience. The hypnotic test can be used as a means of providing a sense of physical comfort and safety that is dissociated from the pain experience itself, demonstrating to the patient in a neutral way their ability to alter perception and motor function. It is also useful to teach patients from the beginning to enter the state of hypnosis as a state of self-hypnosis so that they feel in control of the transition to this altered mental state. The instructions can be simple: "All hypnosis is really self-hypnosis." Now that we have demonstrated that you have a good capacity to use hypnosis, let me show you how to use it to work on a problem. While there are many ways to enter a state of self-hypnosis, one simple means is to count from one to three. On "one," do one thing: look up. On "two," do two things: slowly close your eyes, and take a deep breath. On "three," do three things: let the breath out, let your eyes relax but keep them closed, and let your body float. Then, let one hand or the other float up in the air like a balloon, and that will be your signal to yourself and to me that you are ready to concentrate [5]. Once in a state of self-hypnosis, patients can be taught to produce a physical sensation of floating, lightness, or buoyancy. Their sense of physical

comfort can be reinforced by having them initially imagine that they are somewhere safe and comfortable, such as floating in a bath, a lake, a hot tub, or space. This enhances their sense of control over their body.

Hypnotic Analgesia

Hypnosis and similar techniques work through three primary mechanisms: muscle relaxation, perceptual alteration, and cognitive distraction. Pain is often accompanied by reactive muscle tension. Patients frequently splint the part of their body that hurts. Yet, because muscle tension can by itself cause pain in normal tissue and because traction on a painful part of the body can exacerbate pain, techniques that induce greater physical relaxation reduce pain. Therefore, having patients enter a state of hypnosis and concentrate on an image that connotes physical relaxation such as floating or lightness often produces physical relaxation and reduces pain.

The second major component of hypnotic analgesia is perceptual alteration. Patients can be taught to imagine that the affected body part is tingling or numb. Temperature metaphors are often especially useful, which is not surprising since pain and temperature sensations are part of the same neurosensory system, conducted through small poorly myelinated C fibers to the lateral spinothalamic tract in the spinal cord. Thus, imagining that an affected body part is cooler or warmer using an image of dipping it in ice water or warming it in the sun can often help patients transform pain signals. This is especially useful for extremely hypnotizable individuals who can, for example, relive an experience of dental anesthesia and reproduce the drug-induced sensations of numbness in their cheek, which they can then transfer to the painful part of their body. Rather than "fighting" the pain, they can transform it, concentrating on competing sensations. The third approach involves cognitive alteration, changing the context in which pain is experienced or understood. They can also simply "switch off" perception of the pain with surprising effectiveness [27, 28]. Some patients prefer to imagine that the pain is a substance with dimensions that can be moved or can flow out of the body as if it were a viscous liquid. Others like to dissociate, imagining that they can step outside their body to, for example, visit another room in the house. Less hypnotizable individuals often do better with distraction techniques that help them focus on competing sensations in another part of the body.

The effectiveness of the specific technique employed depends upon the degree of hypnotic ability of the subject. For example, while most patients can be taught to develop a comfortable floating sensation on the affected body part, highly hypnotizable individuals may simply imagine a shot of Novocain (procaine hydrochloride) in the affected area, producing a sense of tingling numbness similar to that experienced in dental work. Other patients may prefer to move the pain to another part of their body or to dissociate the affected part from the rest of the body. As an extreme form of hypnotically induced, controlled dissociation, some highly hypnotizable patients may imagine themselves floating above their own body, creating distance between themselves and the painful sensation or experience. To some more moderately hypnotizable patients, it may be easier to focus on a change in temperature, either warmth or coolness. Low hypnotizable subjects often do better with simple distraction, focusing on sensations in another part of their body, such as the delicate sensations in their fingertips.

It is useful to take stock both during and after the hypnotic session regarding pain ratings: "Now with your eyes closed, and remaining in this state of concentration, please describe how your body is feeling." Then ask, "On a scale of 0–10, please rate your level of discomfort right now."

The images or metaphors used for pain control employ certain general principles [1]. Sensory transformation. The first is that the hypnotically controlled image may serve to "filter the hurt out of the pain." They learn to transform the pain experience. They acknowledge that the pain exists, but there is a distinction between the signal itself and the discomfort the signal causes. The hypnotic experience, which they create and control, helps them transform the signal into one that is less uncomfortable. So patients expand their perceptual options by having them change from an experience in which either the pain is there or it is not to an experience in which they see a third option, in which the pain is there but transformed by the presence of such competing sensations as tingling, numbness, warmth, or coolness [2]. Sensory accommodation. Patients are taught not to fight the pain. Fighting pain only enhances it by focusing attention on the pain, enhancing related anxiety and depression, and increasing physical tension that can literally put traction on painful parts of the body and increase the pain signals generated peripherally.

For patients undergoing painful procedures, such as bone marrow aspirations, the main focus is on the hypnotic imagery per se rather than relaxation. This works especially well with children since they are so highly hypnotizable and easily absorbed in images [29, 30]. Patients may be guided through the experience while the procedure is performed, or a given scenario can be suggested, and later the patient can undergo the experience hypnotically while the procedure is under way. This enables them to restructure their experience of what is going on and dissociate themselves psychologically from pain and fear intrinsic to their immediate situation. A large-scale randomized trial compared hypnosis with nonspecific emotional support and routine care during invasive radiological procedures. All patients had access to patient-controlled intravenous analgesic medication consisting of midazolam and fentanyl. The hypnosis condition provided significantly greater analgesia and relief of anxiety, despite patient use of one-half the medication. Furthermore, with hypnosis, there were fewer procedural complications such as hemodynamic instability; the procedures took on average 18 min less time, and the overall cost was reduced by $348 per procedure [38].

Self-Hypnosis

Hypnotic techniques can easily be taught to patients for self-administration [5, 6]. Pain patients can be taught to enter a state of self-hypnosis in a matter of seconds with some simple induction strategies, such as looking up while slowly closing their eyes, taking a deep breath and then letting the breath out, their eyes relax, and imagining that there is body floating and that one hand is so light it can float up in the air like a balloon. They are then instructed in the pain control exercise, such as coolness or warmth, tingling, or numbness, and taught to bring themselves out by reversing the induction procedure, again looking up, letting the eyes open, and letting the raised hand float back down. Patients can use this exercise every 1–2 h initially and any time they experience an attack of pain [5, 13]. It is useful to provide them with a written summary of the hypnotic induction, analgesic technique employed, and means of exiting the hypnotic state. As with any pain treatment technique, hypnosis is more effective when employed early in the pain cycle, before the pain has become so overwhelming that it impairs concentration. Patients should be encouraged to use this technique early and often because it is simple and effective [34] and has no side effects [35].

Hypnotic Analgesia in Children

Hypnotic techniques are likely to be even more effective among children with pain than adults, since children are more hypnotizable than adults and are thus easily absorbed in images [39, 40]. In using hypnosis with children, some find it helpful to play in an imaginary baseball game and to picture themselves going to another room in the house or watching a favorite TV show. This enables children to restructure their experience of what is occurring and dissociate themselves psychologically from pain and fear of the procedure. This approach utilizes the intense focus in hypnosis to help children dissociate their attention and imagination from their immediate physical surroundings and experiences. It is also helpful to have parents assist and rehearse the procedure so that the children do not encounter anything unfamiliar.

There is evidence that hypnosis can provide anxiety and pain relief to children with medical conditions [41–43], including with cancer [31, 32, 44, 45], cystic fibrosis [33], pain problems [46, 47], pulmonary symptoms [48], abdominal pain [49–56], and postoperative course [57]. Additionally, hypnosis is a noninvasive intervention with minimal risk, which returns control of the experience to the child [58, 59].

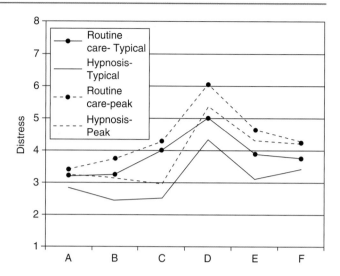

Fig. 78.4 Observer ratings of typical and peak distress levels over phases of the procedure by condition. *A* getting to the table, *B* initial x-ray, *C* catheterization, *D* cleaning and catheterization, *E* bladder infusion and x-rays, *F* voiding and catheter removal

We have considerable experience utilizing hypnosis as an analgesic with children experiencing acute pain. In one randomized clinical trial of the use of hypnosis for children undergoing voiding cystourethrograms, those randomized to the hypnosis condition were given a 1-h training session in self-hypnotic visual imagery by a trained therapist. Parents and children were instructed to practice using the imaginative self-hypnosis procedure several times a day in preparation for the upcoming procedure (Fig. 78.4). The therapist was also present during the procedure to conduct similar exercises with the child. Results indicate significant benefits for the hypnosis group, compared to the routine care group in the following four areas: (1) Parents of children in the hypnosis group, compared to those in the routine care group, reported that the procedure was significantly less traumatic for their children compared to their previous VCUG procedure. (2) Observational ratings of typical distress levels during the procedure were significantly lower for children in the hypnosis condition compared to those in the routine care condition. (3) Medical staff reported a significant difference between groups in the overall difficulty of conducting the procedure, with less difficulty reported for the hypnosis group. (4) Total procedural time was significantly shorter – by almost 14 min – for the hypnosis group compared to the routine care group (Fig. 78.5a, b). Moderate to large effect sizes were obtained on each of these four outcomes [4].

Future Directions for This Topic

Hypnosis is one of the oldest, safest, and most effective analgesic techniques, and there is growing evidence supporting its use [60, 61]. One interesting new direction is coupling

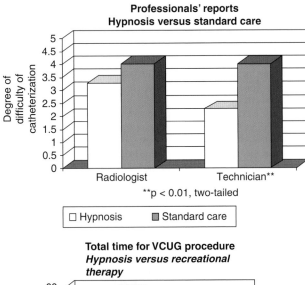

Professionals' reports
Hypnosis versus standard care

**p < 0.01, two-tailed

□ Hypnosis   ■ Standard care

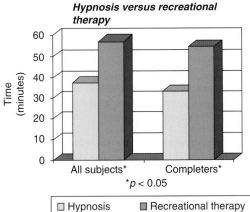

Total time for VCUG procedure
Hypnosis versus recreational therapy

*p < 0.05

□ Hypnosis   ■ Recreational therapy

Fig. 78.5 (**a**) Professional's reports: hypnosis versus standard care. (**b**) Total time for VCUG procedure: hypnosis versus recreational therapy

some benefit from it, and some will experience substantial relief. It is a means of teaching control over discomfort and can be coupled with other analgesic treatment approaches. Those clinicians utilizing hypnosis for analgesia should have training in this technique along with primary training and licensure in their clinical discipline, be it medicine, dentistry, psychology, or other health-care profession. Referral to a good clinician can be obtained from such professional organizations as the Society for Clinical and Experimental Hypnosis (www.SCEH.US) or the American Society of Clinical Hypnosis (www.ASCH. net). While many types of pain intervention are being developed, it is worth remembering that the strain in pain lies mainly in the brain.

References

1. Ellenberger HF. Discovery of the unconscious: the history and evolution of dynamic psychiatry. New York: Basic Books; 1970.
2. Esdaile J. Hypnosis in medicine and surgery (ed Reprinted 1957). New York: Julian Press; 1846.
3. Lang E, Benotsch E, Fink L, et al. Adjunctive non-pharmacological analgesia for invasive medical procedures: a randomised trial. Lancet. 2000;355:1486–90.
4. Butler LD, Symons BK, Henderson SL, et al. Hypnosis reduces distress and duration of an invasive medical procedure for children. Pediatrics. 2005;115:e77–85.
5. Spiegel H, Spiegel D. Trance and treatment: clinical uses of hypnosis. Washington, D.C.: American Psychiatric Press; 2004.
6. Spiegel D. The mind prepared: hypnosis in surgery. J Natl Cancer Inst. 2007;99:1280–1.
7. Spiegel D. Hypnosis and implicit memory: automatic processing of explicit content. Am J Clin Hypn. 1998;40:231–40.
8. Yapko M. Hypnotic intervention for ambiguity as a depressive risk factor. Am J Clin Hypn. 2001;44:109–17.
9. Melzack R. From the gate to the neuromatrix. Pain Suppl. 1999;6:S121–6.
10. Melzack R, Wall PD. Pain mechanisms: a new theory. Science. 1965;150:971–9.
11. Beecher HK. Relationship of significance of wound to pain experienced. J Am Med Assoc. 1956;161:1609–13.
12. Jensen M, Patterson DR. Hypnotic treatment of chronic pain. J Behav Med. 2006;29:95–124.
13. Patterson DR, Jensen MP. Hypnosis and clinical pain. Psychol Bull. 2003;129:495–521.
14. Frenay MC, Faymonville ME, Devlieger S, et al. Psychological approaches during dressing changes of burned patients: a prospective randomised study comparing hypnosis against stress reducing strategy. Burns. 2001;27:793–9.
15. NIH Technology AP. Integration of behavioral and relaxation approaches into the treatment of chronic pain and insomnia. NIH technology assessment panel on integration of behavioral and relaxation approaches into the treatment of chronic pain and insomnia. JAMA. 1996;276:313–8.
16. Butler LD, Koopman C, Neri E, et al. Effects of supportive-expressive group therapy on pain in women with metastatic breast cancer. Health Psychol. 2009;28:579–87.
17. Spiegel D, Bierre P, Rootenberg J. Hypnotic alteration of somatosensory perception. Am J Psychiatry. 1989;146:749–54.
18. Cardenas DD, Jensen MP. Treatments for chronic pain in persons with spinal cord injury: a survey study. J Spinal Cord Med. 2006;29:109–17.

hypnosis with technology that enhances sensory immersion, such as computer-based virtual reality systems [35, 62]. These can enhance analgesic effects and make the most of a given individual's hypnotizability.

Secondly, more can be learned about the neural basis of hypnotic trance and hypnotic analgesia. Knowing specific regions of the brain that are coactivated in hypnosis may help us to better design hypnotic techniques.

Third, application of hypnosis to novel settings can expand and improve its use. Recently, hypnosis has been effectively utilized during breast biopsy [61, 63], and even during lumpectomy for breast cancer [63, 64]. Such techniques have great promise in making medical treatment more effective and humane [6, 65].

Summary

Hypnosis is a safe, effective, and comforting adjunct to the management of both acute and chronic pain. Most individuals are sufficiently hypnotizable to obtain at least

19. Jensen MP, Barber J, Hanley MA, et al. Long-term outcome of hypnotic-analgesia treatment for chronic pain in persons with disabilities. Int J Clin Exp Hypn. 2008;56:156–69.

20. Jensen MP. The neurophysiology of pain perception and hypnotic analgesia: implications for clinical practice. Am J Clin Hypn. 2008; 51:123–48.

21. Molton IR, Graham C, Stoelb BL, et al. Current psychological approaches to the management of chronic pain. Curr Opin Anaesthesiol. 2007;20:485–9.

22. Oneal BJ, Patterson DR, Soltani M, et al. Virtual reality hypnosis in the treatment of chronic neuropathic pain: a case report. Int J Clin Exp Hypn. 2008;56:451–62.

23. Spiegel D. Hypnosis with medical and surgical patients. Gen Hosp Psychiatry. 1983;5:265–77.

24. Spiegel D, Bloom JR. Group therapy and hypnosis reduce metastatic breast carcinoma pain. Psychosom Med. 1983;45:333–9.

25. Rainville P, Duncan GH, Price DD, et al. Pain affect encoded in human anterior cingulate but not somatosensory cortex. Science. 1997;277:968–71.

26. Rainville P, Hofbauer RK, Paus T, et al. Cerebral mechanisms of hypnotic induction and suggestion. J Cogn Neurosci. 1999;11:110–25.

27. Rainville P, Carrier B, Hofbauer RK, et al. Dissociation of sensory and affective dimensions of pain using hypnotic modulation. Pain. 1999;82:159–71.

28. Kosslyn SM, Thompson WL, Costantini-Ferrando MF, et al. Hypnotic visual illusion alters color processing in the brain. Am J Psychiatry. 2000;157:1279–84.

29. Raij TT, Numminen J, Narvanen S, et al. Strength of prefrontal activation predicts intensity of suggestion-induced pain. Hum Brain Mapp. 2009;30:2890–7.

30. Faymonville ME, Laureys S, et al. Neural mechanisms of antinociceptive effects of hypnosis. Anesthesiology. 2000;92:1257–67.

31. Zeltzer L, LeBaron S. Hypnosis and nonhypnotic techniques for reduction of pain and anxiety during painful procedures in children and adolescents with cancer. J Pediatr. 1982;101:1032–5.

32. Zeltzer LK, Dolgin MJ, LeBaron S, et al. A randomized, controlled study of behavioral intervention for chemotherapy distress in children with cancer. Pediatrics. 1991;88:34–42.

33. Belsky J, Khanna P. The effects of self-hypnosis for children with cystic fibrosis: a pilot study. Am J Clin Hypn. 1994;36:282–92.

34. Green JP, Barabasz AF, Barrett D, et al. Forging ahead: the 2003 APA Division 30 definition of hypnosis. Int J Clin Exp Hypn. 2005; 53:259–64.

35. Patterson DR, Wiechman SA, Jensen M, et al. Hypnosis delivered through immersive virtual reality for burn pain: a clinical case series. Int J Clin Exp Hypn. 2006;54:130–42.

36. McGlashan TH, Evans FJ, Orne MT. The nature of hypnotic analgesia and placebo response to experimental pain. Psychosom Med. 1969;31:227–46.

37. Spiegel H, Spiegel D. Induction techniques. In: Burrows GD, Dennerstein L, editors. Handbook of hypnosis and psychosomatic medicine. Amsterdam: North-Holland/Biomedical Press; 1980.

38. Hilgard ER, Hilgard JR. Hypnosis in the relief of pain. Los Altos: William Kauffman; 1975.

39. Morgan AH, Hilgard ER. Age differences in susceptibility to hypnosis. Int J Clin Exp Hypn. 1972;21:78–85.

40. Hilgard JR. Personality and hypnosis: a study of imaginative involvement. Chicago: University of Chicago Press; 1970.

41. Kuttner L. Management of young children's acute pain and anxiety during invasive medical procedures. Pediatrician. 1989;16:39–44.

42. Kuttner L, Bowman M, Teasdale M. Psychological treatment of distress, pain, and anxiety for young children with cancer. J Dev Behav Pediatr. 1988;9:374–81.

43. Kuttner L. Managing pain in children. Changing treatment of headaches. Can Fam Physician. 1993;39:563–8.

44. Hilgard ER. Hypnotic susceptibility and implications for measurement. Int J Clin Exp Hypn. 1982;30:394–403.

45. Liossi C, Hatira P. Clinical hypnosis versus cognitive behavioral training for pain management with pediatric cancer patients undergoing bone marrow aspirations. Int J Clin Exp Hypn. 1999; 47:104–16.

46. Zeltzer L, Tsao JC, Stelling C, et al. A phase I study on the feasibility and acceptability of an acupuncture/hypnosis intervention for chronic pediatric pain. J Pain Symptom Manage. 2002;24:437–46.

47. Dinges DF, Whitehouse WG, Orne EC, et al. Self-hypnosis training as an adjunctive treatment in the management of pain associated with sickle cell disease. Int J Clin Exp Hypn. 1997;45:417–32.

48. Anbar RD. Hypnosis in pediatrics: applications at a pediatric pulmonary center. BMC Pediatr. 2002;2:11.

49. Vlieger AM, Menko-Frankenhuis C, Wolfkamp SC, et al. Hypnotherapy for children with functional abdominal pain or irritable bowel syndrome: a randomized controlled trial. Gastroenterology. 2007;133:1430–6.

50. Tsao JC, Zeltzer LK. Complementary and alternative medicine approaches for pediatric pain: a review of the state-of-the-science. Evid Based Complement Alternat Med. 2005;2:149–59.

51. Simons LE, Logan DE, Chastain L, et al. Engagement in multidisciplinary interventions for pediatric chronic pain: parental expectations, barriers, and child outcomes. Clin J Pain. 2010;26:291–9.

52. Kroner-Herwig B. Chronic pain syndromes and their treatment by psychological interventions. Curr Opin Psychiatry. 2009;22:200–4.

53. Kohen DP, Olness KN, Colwell SO, et al. The use of relaxation-mental imagery (self-hypnosis) in the management of 505 pediatric behavioral encounters. J Dev Behav Pediatr. 1984;5:21–5.

54. Jay SM, Elliott C, Varni JW. Acute and chronic pain in adults and children with cancer. J Consult Clin Psychol. 1986;54:601–7.

55. Galili O, Shaoul R, Mogilner J. Treatment of chronic recurrent abdominal pain: laparoscopy or hypnosis? J Laparoendosc Adv Surg Tech A. 2009;19:93–6.

56. Banez GA. Chronic abdominal pain in children: what to do following the medical evaluation. Curr Opin Pediatr. 2008;20:571–5.

57. Lambert SA. The effects of hypnosis/guided imagery on the postoperative course of children. J Dev Behav Pediatr. 1996;17:307–10.

58. Hockenberry MJ, Cotanch PH. Hypnosis as adjuvant antiemetic therapy in childhood cancer. Nurs Clin North Am. 1985;20:105–7.

59. Olness K, Kohen D. Hypnosis and hypnotherapy with children. 3rd ed. New York: Guilford; 1996.

60. Stoelb BL, Molton IR, Jensen MP, et al. The efficacy of hypnotic analgesia in adults: a review of the literature. Contemp Hypn. 2009; 26:24–39.

61. Lang EV, Berbaum KS, Faintuch S, et al. Adjunctive self-hypnotic relaxation for outpatient medical procedures: a prospective randomized trial with women undergoing large core breast biopsy. Pain. 2006;126:155–64.

62. Askay SW, Patterson DR, Sharar SR. Virtual reality hypnosis. Contemp Hypn. 2009;26:40–7.

63. Montgomery GH, Bovbjerg DH, Schnur JB, et al. A randomized clinical trial of a brief hypnosis intervention to control side effects in breast surgery patients. J Natl Cancer Inst. 2007;99:1304–12.

64. Schnur JB, Bovbjerg DH, David D, et al. Hypnosis decreases presurgical distress in excisional breast biopsy. Anesth Analg. 2008;106(2):440–4, table of contents.

65. Spiegel D. Wedding hypnosis to the radiology suite. Pain. 2006; 126:3–4.

Acupuncture

Ji-Sheng Han

Key Points

- The essence of acupuncture analgesia is to make use of endogenous neurotransmitters and neuropeptides, such as endorphins, to suppress pain and interrupt the vicious cycle of pain mechanisms with little aversive side effects.
- Aside from its placebo effect, acupuncture does have a strong physiological effect in the treatment of acute and chronic pain.
- Acupuncture significantly reduces, but not abolishes, surgically induced pain. Acupuncture can also significantly reduce postoperative pain and vomiting.
- The selection of an optimal frequency is a major issue for the effectiveness of electroacupuncture in the treatment of various kinds of chronic pain.
- Acupuncture-induced endogenously mobilized pain-killing mechanisms combined with exogenously induced pharmacological mechanisms can result in synergistic therapeutic effect for the best of pain patients.
- A design of a proper control group is important in the clinical study of acupuncture analgesia.

Introduction

Acupuncture is an ancient Chinese medical technique with a history of over 2,000 years. The term "acupuncture" is derived from the word *acus*, meaning a sharp point, and *punctura*, meaning to pierce. It can be defined as a technique of inserting and manipulating fine filiform needle into

J.-S. Han, M.D.
Department of Neurobiology, Neuroscience Research Institute, Peking University, 38 Xue Yuan Road, Beijing 100083, China
e-mail: hanjisheng@bjmu.edu.cn

specific points on the body to relieve pain and for various therapeutic purposes. According to the original acupuncture technique, after the insertion of the needle into the skin, it should be manipulated in an up-and-down and rotating movement, termed as "manual needling," in an attempt to reopen the hypothetical channel or meridian so that the obstructed Qi can resume its path. Since the hypothetical "meridian" has not been materialized so far, people tried to find other media for its execution, such as nerves, blood vessels, lymphatic, and connective tissues. In modern times, new methods of stimulating the acupuncture points (acupoints) have been introduced, including (a) applications of electric current to the needles inserted into the acupoints (electroacupuncture, EA), or via skin electrodes placed over the acupoints (transcutaneous electrical acupoint stimulation, TEAS); (b) injection of chemicals into the acupoints; or (c) finger-pressure massage on selected acupoints(acupressure). Concerning the site of stimulation, in addition to the original 362 acupoints, many new acupoints have been described on specific body parts, leading to, for instance, scalp acupuncture, hand acupuncture, and ear acupuncture.

Revival of acupuncture started in the late 1950s when a group of surgeons in China thought, if acupuncture can ameliorate the existing pain, why not use acupuncture preemptively to prevent the inevitable pain as a result of surgical procedures? The clinical trial of using acupuncture to replace anesthetics during surgical operations was termed "acupuncture anesthesia," now widely accepted as "acupuncture analgesia." Research in this field was encouraged by the Chinese medical authorities in the 1960s and being conducted in major hospitals and in most medical schools. A journalist, Mr. James Reston, reported in the *New York Times* on his own experience of having acupuncture to reduce the postoperative pain in Beijing in 1971. This was followed by the visit of the US President, Richard Nixon, to China in 1972, which then surged the popularity of acupuncture in the USA and around the world. The National Institute of Health (NIH)-sponsored Consensus Conference on Acupuncture held in Bethesda, Maryland, in 1997 marked

T.R. Deer et al. (eds.), *Comprehensive Treatment of Chronic Pain by Medical, Interventional, and Integrative Approaches*,
DOI 10.1007/978-1-4614-1560-2_79, © American Academy of Pain Medicine 2013

another milestone of acupuncture: treatment of pain, nausea, and vomiting was endorsed to acupuncture as clinically effective and scientifically valid [1].

Half a century has passed since the first practice of acupuncture anesthesia in a surgical theater in 1958. In this chapter, the established findings – both scientifically and in practice – will be summarized, starting from introduction of the scientific foundation of acupuncture effects, followed by some clinical applications. The key of this chapter is to capture the basic phenomena and the principal mechanisms of acupuncture analgesia and to help clinicians to decide whether they would like to try acupuncture and related techniques in their own practice. Several review articles are listed for the better understanding of the background and the general picture of acupuncture analgesia [2–6].

Scientific Foundation

Basic Phenomenon

To ascertain whether acupuncture stimulation would indeed lower pain sensitivity, acupuncture was administered to human volunteers [7]. To measure the nociceptive threshold of the skin, the potassium iontophoresis method was used, whereby the minimal intensity of an anode (5 mm diameter) current needed to produce a clear pain sensation was recorded, usually by 1 mA. A total of eight body sites, distributed over the head, neck, chest, abdomen, legs, and back, was selected to test pain sensitivity. An acupuncture needle was inserted into the Hegu (large intestine 4, LI4) point, located at the thenar muscle of the hand, considered to be the most powerful for its analgesic effect. Following the continuous manipulation of the needle, a gradual increase of the pain threshold was observed. It took 30 min for the pain threshold to increase from 1 to around 2 mA, and leveled off thereafter. When the needle was poured off, the pain threshold started to decrease exponentially, with a half-life of around 16 min. The time course of slow onset and slow decay, as well as an entire body elevation of the pain threshold, suggested a mechanism of chemical mediation (Fig. 79.1).

In above mentioned study, it was also noted that acupuncture did not work for every subject. While the majority (approximately 85 %) were responders, a small percentage were low or nonresponders, with no significant increase of the pain threshold during the period of stimulation. Interestingly, this type of distribution is reproducible, at least in a period of 1 week. Similar phenomena were observed in the rodent when they were administered with acupuncture at the Zusanli point (ST36) near the knee joint, and the nociceptive threshold was assessed by the tail-flick latency. The experiment was repeated within 1 week, and the results were highly reproducible. The closer the two tests, the higher the reproducibility. This suggests that the magnitude of the analgesic response toward acupuncture stimulation depends on constitutional factors on one hand, and some temporary acting factors on the other.

Preliminary Analysis of the Possible Mechanisms

While the nature of the "meridian" or the "channel" was still in question, one may ask whether the nervous system or chemical mediators were involved. The results obtained in the human study were so straightforward that the analgesic effect could be totally prevented when the local anesthetic procaine was infiltrated into the deeper structures under the point, but not by its subcutaneous injection. The results suggest that it is the nervous tissue in the muscle and tendon that senses the stimulation. It was later made clear that the small-myelinated nerve fibers (A_β fibers and a small part of the A_δ fibers) are responsible for the transmission of afferent impulses to the spinal cord [8].

Another important step made in the study of the mechanisms of acupuncture analgesia was the cerebrospinal fluid (CSF) cross-perfusion study [9]. In order to test the hypothesis of whether there are chemical mediators produced in the brain that may be responsible for the analgesic effect, stainless steel cannulae were implanted into the lateral ventricle of the rabbit so that the brain ventricle can be perfused with artificial CSF, and the perfusate was then infused immediately to the cerebroventricle of the recipient rabbit. When acupuncture was administered to the donor rabbit, the pain threshold increased dramatically. During this period, the CSF was drawn from the donor rabbit and injected into the brain of the recipient. A significant increase of the pain threshold was observed in the recipient rabbit (Fig. 79.2), although no acupuncture was given to this animal. These results suggested that during the acupuncture, some chemical substance(s) with analgesic potency might have been produced, which can be removed from the donor rabbit to the recipient. This finding triggered the interest to explore the neurochemical mechanisms of acupuncture effects.

Classical Neurotransmitters

A literature search revealed serotonin, or 5-hydroxytryptamine (5-HT), to be a candidate for the mediators of the analgesic effect. Studies performed in rats and rabbits showed that increase of the availability of 5-HT in brain or spinal cord potentiated acupuncture analgesia, whereas blockade of 5-HT synthesis or receptor activation resulted in a significant decrease of the analgesic effect. All of the results pointed to the conclusion that 5-HT in the central nervous system plays an important role in the mediation of acupuncture analgesia [10].

In contrast to the unique effect of 5-HT in the entire central nervous system, the role played by norepinephrine (NE)

Fig. 79.1 Pain threshold changes in response to acupuncture at LI4 point located at the thenar eminence. Eight representative skin points were identified for the measurement of pain threshold by potassium iontophoresis method. The needle was manipulated continuously for 50 min. The slow rising during the stimulation period and the slow decay after the removal of the needle suggest the involvement of neurochemical mechanisms (Modified from Research Group of Acupuncture Analgesia, Beijing Medical College [7])

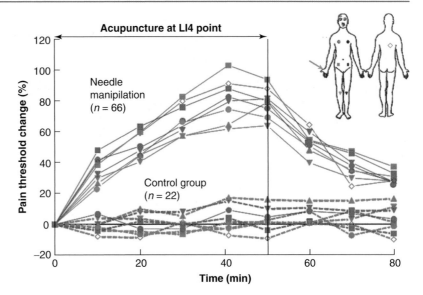

Fig. 79.2 Cross infusion of cerebroventricular fluid between two rabbits. The donor rabbit was subject to acupressure stimulation at the kunlun point near the Achilles tendon. The perfusate of the donor was injected into the lateral ventricle of the recipient rabbit. Latency of the radiant heat-induced head jerk was taken as the nociceptive threshold (Modified from Research Group of Acupuncture Anesthesia, Beijing Medical College [9])

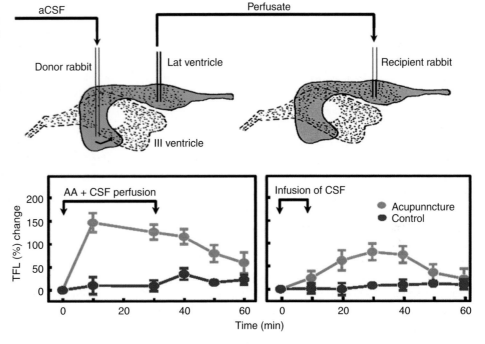

was much more complicated. Most of the information suggested that NE in the spinal cord played a facilitatory role for acupuncture analgesia, in contrast to the antagonistic role in the brain [11].

Opioid Peptides and the Frequency Specific Release (Fig. 79.3)

The discovery of enkephalins in the pig brain in 1975 triggered a huge storm in the biomedical field. Every researcher in this field tried to find some relation with endogenous opioid peptides, and there was no exception for researchers of acupuncture analgesia. David Mayor [12] was the first to

step into this field. He used the opioid receptor antagonist naloxone as the research tool and found that the analgesic effect of acupuncture for dental pain can be prevented by the subcutaneous injection of naloxone, suggesting the involvement of endogenous opioid substances. Since opioid receptors can be divided into three types, μ, δ, and κ, and naloxone is a nonspecific antagonist for all three kinds of opioid receptors, this pharmacological tool can hardly be used to make a further receptor-type differentiation. Using a specific antagonist for the three types of opioid receptor, Han and colleagues were able to find that the analgesic effect of 2-Hz stimulation is mediated by μ and δ receptor, whereas at 100 Hz, the effect is mediated by κ receptors [13]. Further studies using radioimmunoassay revealed that 2 Hz increased the release of

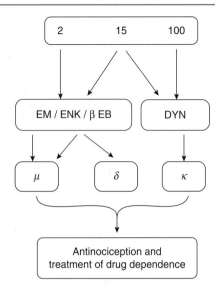

Fig. 79.3 Frequency-dependent release of opioid peptides in the central nervous system. Shown are four kinds of opioid peptides (*EM* endorphins, *ENK* enkephalins, *βEP* β-endorphin, *DYN* dynorphins), three kinds of opioid receptors (*μ*, *δ*, *κ*), and three representative frequency of electroacupuncture (2, 15, and 100 Hz)

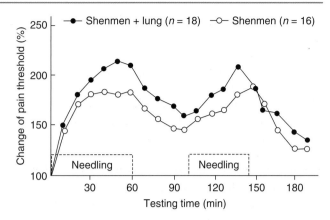

Fig. 79.4 Influence of manual needling at ear acupoint Shenmen ($n = 16$) or Shenmen plus lung ($n = 18$) on pain threshold of the skin over the chest and abdomen in humans. The pain threshold increased during the period of needle manipulation and started to decrease when the needle is staying in situ (Modified from Research Group of Ear Acupuncture, Jiangsu College of New Medicine [77])

enkephalins and endorphins in the CNS to interact with μ and δ receptors, whereas 100 Hz increased the release of dynorphin in the spinal cord to interact with κ receptors (Fig. 79.3) [13].

An interesting question was that if low- or high-frequency stimulation can only accelerate the release of a fraction of the opioid peptide family, can we design a pattern of frequency which can accelerate the release of all four kinds of opioid peptides. This may have a practical impact since there are reports showing that simultaneous activation of two types of opioid receptors may cause a synergistic effect [14, 15]. After a series of exhausting experiments performed in the rat, it was revealed that a frequency automatically alternating between 2 and 100 Hz, each lasting for 3 s, produced a significantly more potent analgesic effect than pure low or pure high frequency alone [13]. This is reasonable since a fraction of the enkephalins released during the low-frequency period may survive to the next period of high-frequency stimulation when dynorphin is released. The coexisting enkephalin and dynorphin may interact at the receptor sites to produce a synergistic effect.

Anti-opioid Peptides and Acupuncture Tolerance

In performing animal experiments of acupuncture analgesia, two basic phenomena called our attention. One is the marked individual variation or the unpredictability of the acupuncture effect, and the other is the gradual fading of the analgesic effect with time if acupuncture is administered too often in a

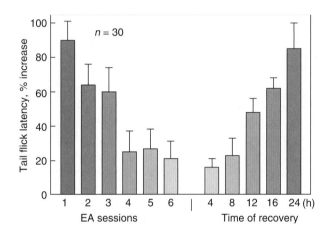

Fig. 79.5 Repeated electroacupuncture to the rat produced a decrease of the analgesic effect, referred to as acupuncture tolerance. It took 24 h for a full recovery of the acupuncture analgesia (Modified from Han et al. [16])

short period of time. As a general rule, acupuncture analgesia needs time (about 30 min) to build up to its full potential, and the effect would decay when the acupuncture needle is poured off (Fig. 79.1) or left unattended (Fig. 79.4). If EA is given 30 min/h, for 4–5 h, the analgesic effect would decrease gradually (Fig. 79.5) [16]. This is not due to the local tissue damage caused by repeated needle insertion and manipulation, since the situation would remain even if the needle is inserted into a new point of the body without any tissue damage.

In searching for the possible mechanisms, a hypothesis was raised that, according to the concept of Yin and Yang balance in the Chinese philosophy, the existence of a natural pain-killing substance (endorphin) might be accompanied by the existence of another substance with an antagonistic effect (anti-opioid substance). After a careful survey, this putative anti-opioid substance was identified as cholecystokinin octapeptide (CCK-8) [17]. In fact, repeated EA produced an increase of the production and release of opioid peptides, and in the same time, there is a gradual increase of the CCK-8 in the central nervous system which plays an antagonistic role against opioids, thereby reduces the effect of EA. This phenomenon is termed "acupuncture tolerance," to mimic the situation of "morphine tolerance" produced by repeated injection of morphine. It was interesting to find that for rats with CCK predominates over opioid peptides in the central nervous system, they can be a nonresponder toward acupuncture, or a weak responder but quickly developing into acupuncture tolerance. The situation can be reversed if (a) CCK antagonist is injected intracerebroventricularly or intrathecally to the rat, or (b) the gene expression of CCK is blocked by the antisense probe against preproCCK administered centrally. In that case, the nonresponder of acupuncture analgesia can be changed into responder and the diminished analgesic effect can be revived [17, 18]. The lesson learned from this mechanism is that acupuncture should not be given too often, or last too long in one session.

Neural Pathways

From neurophysiological point of view, acupuncture analgesia can be taken as a reflex action. The afferent comes from the nerve fibers (mostly Aβ fibers) innervating the acupoint, and the efferent is the descending pathway modulating the sensitivity of the dorsal horn neurons not only in the same segment but also in heterogenous segments. Studies in the rat revealed that 100-Hz stimulation of the acupoint would trigger the release of dynorphin in the spinal cord. After the destruction of the parabrachial nucleus of the brain stem, high-frequency EA would no longer produce an analgesic effect [19]. Conversely, 2-Hz EA induces the release of β-endorphin in the brain and enkephalin in the whole central nervous system. After the destruction of the arcuate nucleus of the hypothalamus (where β-endorphin neurons aggregated), 2-Hz EA would no longer elicit analgesic effect. Taken together, a diagram could be constructed to show the hypothetical neural pathway for acupuncture analgesia (Fig. 79.6). Neither low- nor high-frequency EA would work if a lesion is placed at the periaqueductal gray (PAG) of the midbrain [19].

Other neural pathways have also been proposed. For example, 100-Hz stimulation can evoke supraspinal long-term depression not only in normal rats [20] but also in sham operated rats subject to neuropathic pain [21], contributing to the mechanisms of high-frequency EA-induced analgesic effect.

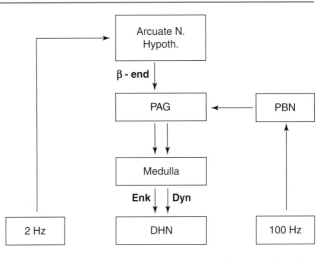

Fig. 79.6 The neural pathway for the analgesic effect induced by electroacupuncture of different frequencies. *Arcuate N. Hypoth.* arcuate nucleus of hypothalamus, *PAG* periaqueductal gray of the midbrain, *DHN* dorsal horn neuron of the spinal cord, *PBN* parabrachial nucleus, *β-end* β-endorphin, *ENK* Enkephalin, *DYN* dynorphin

A hypothetical diagram was proposed by Han, which gives a general picture of the neural network underlying acupuncture analgesia, at least for the control of the acute pain [6].

Functional magnetic resonance imaging (fMRI) was used to characterize the possible brain areas being involved in mediating the acupuncture effect. Since stimulation of any of the body sites would cause extensive changes in the brain MRI picture, it is hard to characterize the brain sites responsible for acupuncture-induced analgesic effect. Zhang et al. [22] tried to correlate the magnitude of acupuncture-induced BOLD signal change observed in identified brain area with the magnitude of the analgesic effect induced by 2- or 100-Hz EA stimulation, respectively. The results showed that the analgesic effect induced by low and high frequencies seems to be mediated by different, though partially overlapping brain networks. In either frequency, the averaged fMRI activation levels of bilateral secondary somatosensory area and insula, contralateral anterior cingulate cortex, and thalamus were positively correlated with the EA-induced analgesic effect. In the 2-Hz EA group, positive correlation was observed only in contralateral primary and supplementary motor areas, while negative correlation was observed in bilateral hippocampi. In 100-Hz EA group, positive correlations were observed in contralateral inferior parietal lobule and ipsilateral anterior cingulate cortex, while negative correlation was found in contralateral amygdale. These results suggest that functional activation of certain brain areas might be correlated with the effect of EA analgesia in a frequency-dependent manner. More work is needed in order to figure out the complicated neural network controlling acupuncture-induced analgesic effect.

Mode of Stimulation (MA, EA, TEAS)

In clinical practice, various kinds of methods have been used to secure the optimal stimulation of the acupoint. Manual needling (MA) is the classical technique, with the characteristics of preciseness, capable of directing the needle in various angles to find the maximal deqi sensation and freely adjusting the needle movement to obtain a specific effect termed "warm," "cold," etc.

Studies show that various kinds of manual needling produce different pattern of afferent impulses in the sensory nerves and activation of the dorsal horn neurons. Out of 12 different kinds of needle manipulation, Wang et al. [23] studied three most popularly used modes, that is, twist, drag-plug, and gradual mode, respectively. Single-unit recordings of the dorsal horn neuron of the rat showed clearly different patterns in the inter-spike intervals (ISI). Based on the reconstructed phase space, they analyzed the spatiotemporal behavior of the time series. The largest Lyapunov exponent, which is an important parameter for describing the nonlinear system behavior, varies significantly in different modes of acupuncture. However, various types of manual needling technique (e.g., "burning mountain" for hot, "frozen sky" for cold) need years to learn and to master.

Compared to manual needling, electroacupuncture (EA) is a modern approach based on the basic finding that the effect of acupuncture is relied on the integrity of the nervous system [7] and that delivering specific forms of electric impulses is the easiest way to activate the afferent nerves in a predictable manner, with the added advantage of time saving and very high reproducibility. Aside from the great time saving and the reproducibility of the treatment, a significant advantage of using EA is that you can try, in certain degree, to change the internal environment of the central nervous system according to the ever changing need of the body system, for example, the use of low frequency (2–4 Hz) for the production and release of enkephalins in the central nervous system and high frequency (80–120 Hz) for dynorphins in the spinal cord [13]. The clinical effects produced by EA of different frequencies can be very different. Study shows that for treatment of rat model of neuropathic pain produced by lumbar nerve ligation, 2 Hz is much effective than 100 Hz, with the involvement of mu opioid receptors [24]. In contrast, for the treatment of patients with spinal cord injury-induced muscle spasm, it is only 100 Hz, but not 2 Hz, which works [25], with the involvement of kappa opioid receptors [26]. In these extreme cases, one frequency may serve as the control of the other. Here, the credibility of the design for "control" is nearly perfect, since no one knows which frequency is better, even for the care provider. This frequency-specific design can be served as an example to show the specificity of the EA treatment, rather than a design of using a nonspecific skin touch for psychological "believing." However, the frequency specificity does not apply for every

disease. For example, for the treatment of rat model of complete adjuvant-induced arthritis, both high- and low-frequency EA work at a similar efficacy [27].

Unlike electroacupuncture (EA) which uses percutaneous (invasive) approach, the transcutaneous electric acupoint stimulation (TEAS) is a noninvasive way of stimulating the acupoint by the use of skin pads placed on the skin surface overlying the acupoint in lieu of the needle. This is also called "acupuncture without a needle." Since the skin electrode is usually 4×4 cm in size, it would never miss the "acupoint." Since all the parameters are shown on the LED screen precisely, it can also be used by the patient or family under the instruction of the acupuncturist or the physician, thereby reduces the number of visit to the doctor.

The efficacy of EA in pain control has repeatedly been shown to be no less than manual needling. Wang et al. [28] had done a careful study in the rat experiment, comparing the analgesic effect produced by EA or TEAS, with the conclusion that TEAS is at least as effective, if not more effective, than EA. The analgesic effect produced by either method can be blocked by naloxone at the same degree, suggesting a similar underlying mechanism of action. Given that these forms of acupoint stimulation may have similar therapeutic effect and underlying mechanisms, we will make clear statement separately for MA, EA, and TEAS in the following text when clinical applications are to be mentioned.

In the recent literature, there is another term called "percutaneous electrical nerve stimulation (PENS)" in contrast to "transcutaneous electrical nerve stimulation (TENS)" [29]. In a commentary put forwarded by Cummings [30], the author mentioned that "PENS is neither different in principle nor in practice from EA. While the term accurately reflects the nature of the treatment, there is no substantial justification for referring to PENS as a novel therapy."

Clinical Examples and the Usefulness in Clinical Practice

Acupuncture Anesthesia During the Surgical Procedure

In the late 1950s up to 1970s, there was a large-scale clinical practice in China of using acupuncture in lieu of anesthetics for surgical procedures, named "acupuncture anesthesia." In fact, in most hospitals, acupuncture was used in combination with anesthetics to form a "complex acupuncture anesthesia," or "acupuncture-assisted anesthesia (AAA)." To take a few examples, in the Tiantan hospital of Beijing specialized for brain surgery, Wang et al. [31] reported that in a series of cranial operations, they can reduce the dosage of enflurane by 45–48 % while fulfilling all the requirements of a successful anesthesia. This may be especially interested by the new trend of "anesthesia for awake neurosurgery" [32].

Qu et al. [33] performed kidney transplantation under combined acupuncture/epidural anesthesia in the Shanghai First People's Hospital. They reported a reduction of procaine usage for 48 % with robust satisfaction. Almost all the reports concerning the complex acupuncture anesthesia stressed the benefits of earlier recovery, less postoperative pain and other complications, and shortened hospitalization. Sim et al. [34] reported 90 patients randomly assigned to one of three groups: group I – placebo EA, group II – preoperative EA for 45 min, and group III – 45 min of postoperative EA. The results showed that preoperative EA leads to a reduced intraoperative alfentanil consumption and has a morphine-sparing effect during the early postoperative period. However, this was not universally confirmed by report from other group [35].

Postoperative Pain

In contrast to some controversy whether acupuncture can reduce the anesthetic use during the surgical procedure, there is a unanimous agreement that acupuncture could significantly reduce the postoperative pain. Paul White's group published the first paper of a series of studies in 1997 [36], using the electronic device (HANS) for transcutaneous electrical acupoint stimulation (TEAS) to assess if it can reduce the postoperative PCA requirement for hydromorphone (HM). In a single-blind controlled study, they found that compared to the blank control of "PCA only" group, the HM used in the sham TEAS group showed a 22 % reduction. For the real TEAS group, they used two levels of intensity, the threshold level (4–5 mA) and the double threshold level (9–12 mA), resulting in a 34 % ($P < 0.05$) and 65 % ($P < 0.001$) reduction, respectively. The postoperative side effects (nausea, dizziness, pruritis, and sedation) were also significantly reduced. Similar results were reported for reduction of postoperative pain [37–40], nausea, and vomiting [40–42].

Since acupuncture or its several variants are shown by evidence-based medicine to be so cost effective for controlling postoperative pain, nausea, vomiting, and lack of clinical toxicity, Dr. White called on more clinicians to incorporate these acustimulation techniques into their perioperative therapeutic armamentarium [43]. In an accompanying editorial, the editor in chief suggested that, "once the mechanism of action is understood, claims of clinical efficacy for acustimulation will no longer be extraordinary" [44].

Low Back Pain

Low back pain (LBP) is one of the most common causes for primary care clinic visits, only second to common cold, and it is the second most common cause of absence from work in adults who are over 55 years of age. According to the National Center of Complementary and Alternative Medicine (NCCAM), NIH, people use acupuncture for various types of pain, and back pain is the most commonly reported, followed by joint pain, neck pain, and headache [2].

In a study reported by Ghoname et al. [45], 60 patients of LBP were divided into four groups to compare the effectiveness of PENS (equivalent to EA) with sham-PENS, TENS, and exercise. PENS is significantly more effective in decreasing the VAS pain scores after each treatment than the other three groups. The average daily oral intake of nonopioid analgesics (2.6 ± 1.4 pills/day) was decreased to 1.3 ± 1.0 pills/day with PENS ($P < 0.008$) compared with 2.5 ± 1.1, 2.2 ± 1.0, and 2.6 ± 1.2 pills/day with sham-PENS, TENS, and exercise, respectively. Compared with the other three modalities, 91 % of the patients reported that PENS was the most effective in decreasing their LBP. The PENS therapy was also significantly more effective in improving physical activity, quality of sleep, and sense of well-being ($P < 0.05$ for each).

The SF-36 survey confirmed that PENS improved posttreatment function more than sham-PENS, TENS, and exercise [45]. In another study, 68 LBP patients secondary to degenerative lumbar disc diseases were treated with EA of different frequencies: 4 Hz, alternating 15 and 30 Hz, 100 Hz, and 0 Hz serving as control. Each treatment was administered for a period of 30 min, three times per week for 2 weeks. In contrast to the control group which produced little improvement, all other groups produced significant decreases in the severity of pain and improvement in the quality of life. Of the three frequencies, 15/30 Hz was the most effective in decreasing pain. Therefore, the alternative low and high frequency was more effective than with low or high frequency alone [46]. This replicates what we found in the rat experiment where 2/100 Hz was significantly better than only 2 or 100 Hz alone in the antinociceptive effect [47].

Further studies revealed that as far as analgesic effect is concerned, needle insertion plus electrical stimulation (EA) is much better than needle staying without stimulation [46, 48], acupuncture-like TENS is better than ordinary TENS [49], and dermatomal stimulation (lumbar region for back pain, neck region for neck pain) is better than stimulation at the distal sites [50].

In summary, while most of the studies showed that acupuncture or EA are effective for low back pain, there are negative reposts [51]. Concerning the life span of the therapeutic effect, it may be short lasting [52] or longer lasting for at least 3 months [48], depending on the design of the protocol, especially the number of treatment being used.

Osteoarthritis of the Knee

Acupuncture seems to be effective for osteoarthritis, especially in the area of the knee. However, controversy exists on

Table 79.1 Comparison of the conditions applied and results obtained by Berman et al. [53] and Scharf et al. [54], using acupuncture for the treatment of osteoarthritis of the knee joint

	Berman et al. [53]	Scharf et al. [54]
Treatment centers (number of physicians)	Three clinics in one University (7 acupuncturists)	Multicenters (320 physicians)
Trial size	570	1,039
% drops	31.4 % drop by 26 weeks	57.5 % drop by 26 weeks
Concealment of allocation	Letter from central statistical core	Centralized telephone randomization
Pain scale	WOMAC (0–10)	WOMAC (0–10)
Treatment duration (sessions)	26 weeks (23)	6 weeks (10)
Manual acupuncture group (depth of needle insertion)	4 distal points (1 in); 5 local points (1.5 in). Two points in abdominal area for non-insertion intervention	6 local obligatory points 2 of 16 defined acupoints could be chosen A maximum of 4 Ah shi points were allowed
EA	One point for EA (8 Hz, 20 min)	No EA
"No acupuncture" group	Six 2-h sessions of education	10 physician visits
Placebo acupuncture group	Mock needles on each of the 9 leg points, mock EA unit with light and sound 2 needle insertion in abdominal nonpoints	10 non-acupoints at lower and upper limb, superficial needling up to 5 mm without Qi, no manual needle movement
Standard care	Continue to receive analgesics from their primary care physicians	Oral NSAID, up to 6 physiotherapy
Summary for "true" group	Inserted needles with 2 manual stimulations, plus EA at one local point	Inserted needles with 2 manual stimulations, without EA
Summary for "placebo" group	9 placebo needles (no insertion) Only 2 true needles inserted in abdomen	10 needles inserted in upper and lower limbs
Evaluation	8th and 26th week	13th and 26th week
Primary outcomes	WOMAC and functional scores	WOMAC and functional scores
Secondary outcomes	Functional improvement: patient global assessment, 6 min walk, SF-36	Functional improvement: global patient assessment, SF-12 physical subscale, SF-12 mental subscale
Results	True acup > Placebo acup > No acup Pain improved in 14 week versus placebo. Improvement of functional score since 8th week, but not PGA score	Taking 36 % improvement in WOMAC as success: True acup (53.1) = Placebo acup (51.0) >No acup (29.1)

the clinical effectiveness. Moreover, difference in the design, sample size, and protocol of the studies made it hard to draw any definitive conclusions. Here, we make comparison of two articles using acupuncture for the treatment of osteoarthritis of the knee joint, both published in the Annals of Internal Medicine, one got negative result [52] and another positive result [53]. We hope to find out some meaningful differences in experimental design, data collection, and interpretation.

From the comparisons made above, we can see that in order to depict a difference between the true and placebo acupuncture groups, one should consider the following: (a) to strengthen the effect of true acupuncture by more treatment sessions. Compared to Berman et al. who used 23 sessions, Scharf et al. used only 10. (b) Berman et al. [53], but not Scharf et al. [54], used EA to supplement manual needling (1 vs. 0) and (c) to weaken the effect of placebo or sham acupuncture by reducing the number of needle insertion (2 vs. 10). Aside from that, there are

several related issues need to be considered in the future studies (Table 79.1).

Concerning the possible mechanisms of action, a recent publication [55] seemed to give some clue. Patients with chronic osteoarthritis were given EA of 20–25 min per session, once a day for 10 days, and the control group was given sham needle insertion at nonpoints without electrical stimulation. The EA group showed a significant improvement in pain, stiffness, and disability as shown by the WOMAX index and VAS value. In the meantime, there was a significant increase in plasma β-endorphin ($P=0.001$) and a significant fall in plasma stress hormone cortisol ($P=0.016$).

In February 2008, the OARSI recommendation for the management of hip and knee osteoarthritis, Part II: OARSI evidence-based, expert consensus guidelines, was released [56]. The purpose was to develop concise, patient-focused, up-to-date, evidence-based, expert consensus recommendations for the management of hip and knee osteoarthritis (OA). As a result, 20 out of 51 treatment modalities were universally recommended. The non-pharmacological modalities (totaling 12, including TENS and acupuncture) and the pharmacological (totaling eight) modalities were considered equally effective. Therefore, a combination of non-pharmacological and pharmacological treatments was recommended. Out of that, they also identified five surgical modalities. However, the National Institute of Health and Clinical Excellence (NICE) published a new guideline on the care and management of osteoarthritis, which stated that there is insufficient evidence to recommend acupuncture for the treatment of OA [57]. This raised controversy [58, 59] which needs time to reconcile with.

Diabetic Neuropathic Pain

Diabetic patient can develop neuropathic changes that affect peripheral nerve function, leading to symmetrical lower extremity pain. The pain could be very severe to affect a normal life, and no satisfactory treatment is currently available. Abuaisha et al. [60] conducted a relatively long-term study to explore the effectiveness of acupuncture for its treatment. Forty-six diabetic patients with chronic painful peripheral neuropathy were treated with classical acupuncture, 20 min per session, six sessions in 10 weeks. Seventy-seven percent showed significant improvement in their primary and/or secondary symptoms ($P < 0.01$). After 18–52 weeks of follow-up, 67 % were able to stop or significantly reduce their medication and only 24 % required further acupuncture treatment. These data suggest that acupuncture is a safe and effective therapy for painful diabetic neuropathy, although the mechanism of action remains speculative. Hamza et al. [61] used EA (PENS) at 15–30-Hz frequency for the treatment of 50 type 2 diabetic patients with peripheral neuropathic pain over 6-month duration, with sham EA (needle insertion without movement or electrical stimulation) as control. EA was given at 10 acupoints at the lower extremities, 30 min per session, three times a week, for 3 weeks. After a 1-week washout period, all patients were switched to the other modality. VAS was used to assess pain, physical activity, and quality of sleep before each session. A significant reduction of the pain score ($P < 0.001$) and improvement of physical activity, sense of well-being, and quality of sleep while reducing the need for oral non-opioid analgesic medication were observed in the EA group, whereas the control group was of no significant change. While the design of this study is more convincing than the previous one and the results are encouraging, more study is needed to uncover its long-term therapeutic effect.

Neuropathic pain is usually resulted from a nerve injury leading to the hypersensitivity or sensitization of the central nociceptive mechanisms. Acupuncture or electroacupuncture of low frequency (2 Hz) may produce a long-term depression at the spinal cord dorsal horn level [21], thereby reduces the sensitization, an effect mediated by opioid receptors and NMDA receptors.

Migraine

Migraine is a frequent and disabling episodic headache with autonomic disturbance. Pharmacological interventions are used to treat the acute attack and to prevent its relapse with limited success. Acupuncture has been reported to be effective in prophylactic and therapeutic purposes. Endres et al. [62] reviewed the existing data and came to the conclusion that a 6-week course (10 sessions) of acupuncture is not inferior to a 6-month prophylactic drug treatment, although the Chinese point selection and the depth of needle insertion is not as important as had been thought to be. They therefore suggested that acupuncture should be integrated into the existing migraine treatment protocol. For the treatment of acute attack of migraine, Li et al. [63] took 175 migraine patients and divided them into three groups. The verum group received acupuncture in 10 points with continuous manipulation for 30 min to induce deqi sensation, whereas the two control groups receive needle insertion in various nonpoints and staying there without movement, hence no deqi sensation. The degree of pain was assessed by the VAS (0–10) 0.5, 1, 2, and 4 h after the removal of the needles. A decrease of VAS by 1.0, 0.5, and 0.1 cm was observed after 4 h in the verum acupuncture group and the sham 1 and sham 2 acupuncture groups, respectively. Most patients in the acupuncture group experienced complete pain relief (40.7 %) and did not experience recurrence or intensification of pain (79.6 %). The results indicated that the true acupuncture group with deqi sensation is significantly better than the nonpoint groups. It is obvious that while the result of one treatment is moderate, the therapeutic effect may show a cumulative trend in the consecutive treatments.

Facco et al. [64] checked the effectiveness of a true acupuncture treatment in migraine without aura, comparing it to a standard mock acupuncture protocol, an accurate mock acupuncture-healing ritual and untreated controls. All groups were provided with standard rizatriptan treatment. The results showed that the true acupuncture group was significantly better than the control groups 6 months after the starting of the trial ($P < .0001$). Jena et al. [65] investigated the effectiveness of acupuncture in addition to routine care in patients with primary headache with more than 12-months history of two or more episodes per month. They found that acupuncture plus routine care was associated with marked clinical improvements compared with routine care alone ($P < .001$).

After reviewing all the reports, Diener [66] stated that application of the procedure in daily life would be impractical. The idea of patients leaving the workplace with a mild headache to see a person performing acupuncture is difficult to conceive. In fact, Diener's concern has been solved by technical improvement. It is time to try if transcutaneous electrical acupoint stimulation (TEAS) would induce similar therapeutic and prophylactic effect. If so, then it can be performed by the patient under the direction of the physician, saving a considerable amount of time, especially for the prophylactic purpose.

Muscle Spastic Pain

Spinal trauma is a condition often occurred in car accidents and falls. In the United States, the annual incidence of spinal cord injury (SCI) is around 12,000, with a prevalence of over 259,000 persons [67]. Severe spinal cord injury often induces flaccid muscle paralysis, which may turn into muscle spasm accompanied by cramping pain, and is hard to treat. Wang et al. [68] used transcutaneous electrical acupoint stimulation (TEAS) for the treatment of the spastic pain. The electrical stimulation was delivered to the skin over the two acupoints at the hand (LI4 on the dorsum of the hand and the other at the center of the palm) to form a circuit and two acupoints at the opposite leg (ST36 near the knee joint and BL57 at the calf muscle) to form a circuit. Wang et al. tried the low and high frequencies and found that only 100 Hz, but not 2-Hz stimulation, suppressed the muscle spasticity. The effect recorded at the end of one session (30 min) lasted for only 20–25 min. However, after a prolonged stimulation protocol (once a day, five times a week for 4 weeks), a cumulative therapeutic effect appeared in the second week, shown as a gradual decrease of the ankle clonus score and the Ashworth score accompanied by a reduction of pain score and an improvement of well-being. The therapeutic effect reached a plateau at the third and fourth week. The effect was sensitive to naloxone, suggesting that opioid peptides were involved. Animal studies revealed that implantation of a wax ball into the cervical spinal cord of the rat produced an increase of the muscle tonicity assessed by H reflex, accompanied by a decrease of the dynorphin content of the spinal cord [26]. Electroacupuncture at 100 Hz applied on the acupoint ST36 near the knee joint and SP6 near the ankle joint produced an increase of the dynorphin content and a decrease of the muscle tonicity. Intrathecal injection of the kappa opioid agonist U-50488 produced a similar spasmolytic effect [26]. Summarizing from the clinical observation and the rat experiment, we reached a hypothesis that spinal trauma produced a decrease of dynorphin in the spinal cord and an increase of muscle tonicity and the development of muscle spasm. This pathological status can be partially reversed by 100-Hz peripheral stimulation as a result of increased production and release of dynorphin which can be mimicked by the intrathecal injection of the kappa agonist U-50488. This preliminary study is certainly worth further clinical exploration.

Fibromyalgia

Fibromyalgia affect 2 % of population, with a man to women ratio of 1:7, and no cure is known. Acupuncture has been tried with uncertain effect. Four systemic reviews published in 2007–2009 showed pessimistic results, ranging from "no" to "mixed" or "moderate" effect. However, there are several papers showing optimistic results. One is from the Mayo Clinic [69]. They recruited 50 patients with fibromyalgia and evenly divided to two groups. One group used real acupuncture at 18–20 points, with 2- or 10-Hz stimulation for 20 min. The control group received mock needle without skin penetration. The patients received six sessions of treatment in a period of 2–3 weeks. The symptoms were measured by the Fibromyalgia Impact Questionnaire (FIQ) immediately, 1 and 7 months after the treatment. Acupuncture group showed a significant pain relief and a reduction of fatigue and anxiety. The effect was most marked in 1 month ($P=0.007$) and gradually faded in seventh month. Harris et al. [70] at the University of Michigan observed the severity of the symptom of FM and the availability of mu opioid receptors in the brain, assessed by the positron emission tomography (PET) using ^{11}C-labeled carfentanyl as the tracer. A negative correlation was revealed in the severity of the syndrome and the availability of mu receptors, especially in the brain region known to play a role in pain modulation, such as nucleus accumbens, the amygdale, and the dorsal cingulate gyrus. This result may explain why morphine is not very effective in reducing the pain of FM patients. In the second study [71], they observed the effect of acupuncture for the treatment of FM. In the meantime, they used PET scan to assess the ^{11}C carfentanyl-binding potential of the brain regions relevant to pain control (nucleus accumbens, cingulate, caudate, amygdale). Single session of manual acupuncture applied at nine acupoints located at the head and all four extremities produced a mild increase of the receptor-binding potential (short-term effect). After 1 month of acupuncture treatment (eight sessions), the brain binding potential of ^{11}C carfentanyl increased dramatically (long-term effect), which was associated with a decrease of the FM symptoms. These effects were not found in patients receiving sham acupuncture (skin pricking without needle penetration). The results indicate that the therapeutic effect of acupuncture for FM is related with the increase of the binding potential of the morphine receptors in the brain. The work of Harris and associates not only confirmed the therapeutic effect of acupuncture on FM but also demonstrated that the effect of acupuncture is related with its ability of increasing the binding potential of the brain to mu agonists.

Future Directions

Design of Appropriate Control Group

To make an overview on research in acupuncture analgesia, one can see that the main issues of controversy focused on the question whether the effect of acupuncture is superior over the control group. Unlike the pharmacological experiment where a pill or an injection which looks identical yet contains inert substance can be used to replace the real one, acupuncture is a sophisticated procedure which is extremely difficult to imitate. In designing a clinical trial, at least two factors should be considered. One is the selection of the site of stimulation (the right acupoint), and the other is the technique of needle manipulation. For the selection of the site of stimulation, one can use (a) the real acupoint, as documented in the ancient book marked with points along the hypothetical line on the skin, named "meridian"; (b) irrelevant point, which has been used for other purpose not related with the disease under study; and (c) non-acupoint, which can be located several millimeters away from the real acupoint, or midway between two meridians, or where no meridians are known, for example, in the area along the armpits where no meridians passing by. Acupuncture at (b) and (c) can be regarded as sham acupuncture. For the control of the stimulation, one can use (a) minimal stimulation, such as inserting the needle to a small depth, using a weak twisting, or even leaving the needle unattended so that no "deqi" sensation is produced; (b) a blunt needle or a tooth stick to prick the skin without penetration (placebo); and (c) a pseudo-intervention such as a beam of laser light which is switched off immediately. The procedure of placebo acupuncture can be done covert to the patient, or being done in an overt manner. In the later case, a special device is needed so that the patient sees the needle being taped into the skin but actually is withdrawn into a hollow space [72]. All these designs are considered inert to the subject, only to produce a psychological effect to imitate the acupuncture procedure. However, none of these are technically perfect. Lund et al. [73] pointed out that even light touch of the skin can stimulate the mechanoreceptors coupled to slow-conducting unmyelinated (C) afferent fibers, resulting in the activation of the insular region of the brain, but not in the somatosensory cortex. Activity in these C tactile fibers has been suggested to induce emotional and hormonal reactions commonly seen after caressing and a sense of well-being. In one word, they are not "inert." The authors listed results from published papers that for the treatment of migraine which has an important affective component, minimal acupuncture stimulation can produce the same therapeutic effect as real acupuncture. However, for the treatment of osteoarthritis of the knee with a more pronounced sensory component, minimal acupuncture is usually ineffective.

With the advance of technology, acupuncture has been developed into more sophisticated forms, such as EA and transcutaneous electric acupoint stimulation (TEAS). In these cases, the design of the control group has more flexibility. For example, in order to provide minimal electrical stimulation, one can use the threshold stimulation, that is, the intensity is adjusted to a level barely sensible to the patient. To further weaken the stimulation, one can adjust the current output to 1 min on and 2 min off, thereby to cut the time of stimulation to one third of the original level, yet the subject still feels the sensation come-and-go. In a study to test the feasibility of TEAS for reducing the urge to smoking, Han's group revealed that when they reduce the intensity from 10 to 5 mA, the effect remained. However, when the intermittent 5 mA is used, it could no longer reduce the urge to smoking [74].

Comparison of the neural correlates of acupuncture and placebo effect would show that while acupuncture pathway is from bottom up (afferent comes from spinal cord to brain), placebo effect is from up down (from brain to the cord). But they use similar descending pathways including opioid and monoaminergic mechanisms. Brain imaging study showed that amygdale, insula, and hypothalamus may demonstrate some acupuncture specificity, whereas dorsolateral prefrontal cortex (DLPFC) and rostral anterior cingulate cortex (rACC) may support nonspecific brain expectancy related with placebo effect [75].

To summarize, placebo effect is common in biomedical practice and acupuncture is of no exception. Therefore, great care should be taken for the interpretation of the experimental results. When one finds the effect of placebo acupuncture to be similar with verum acupuncture, it should not be simply interpreted to mean that acupuncture is of no effect. Indeed, placebo analgesia and acupuncture analgesia may use the same opioid mechanism [76]. Conversely, when the mechanisms of placebo and nocebo are made clear, one may like to strengthen the placebo effect and to reduce the nocebo effect, in order to intensify the therapeutic capacity for the good of the patients [76].

Primary Outcome, Secondary Outcome, and Long-Term Effect

Primary outcome of pain alleviation is usually assessed by the visual analog scale. While the immediate analgesic effect is important, the follow-up long-term effect is even more desirable. Compared to oral pills, acupuncture treatment usually takes more time to achieve a visible therapeutic effect. So if the effect of acupuncture is short lasting, the superiority for this treatment modality would be greatly diminished. Likewise, research on the mechanisms of acupuncture effect should also put more emphasis on its long-term effect A good example was made by Harris et al. who used a PET scan to show that one session of acupuncture produced an immediate increase of morphine-binding potential in the brain. This elevation was even stronger when eight sessions of acupuncture were delivered to FM patient in 1 month of time [71]. Long-lasting analgesic effect would naturally induce simultaneous changes in sleep quality, physical activity, quality of life, and sense of well-being. These secondary outcomes are supplementary evidence to support the primary outcome.

Summary and Conclusions

Acupuncture is getting more and more popular in the medical field. This technology can be used for the treatment of distinctive diseases, or an array of conditions such as acute and chronic pain. One of the mechanisms is that it can increase the production and release of opioid peptides [13] and also increase the opioid receptor availability [71] in the discrete regions of the central nervous system. Conversely, acupuncture may just strengthen the homeostasis or activate the self-healing process via modulation of endocrine/immune systems, thereby improving the health status.

While the authentic form of acupuncture is manual needling, the demarcation between manual needling, electroacupuncture (EA), and transcutaneous electric acupoint stimulation (TEAS) is gradually fading. From neurobiological point of view, acupuncture can be regarded as a special form of peripheral stimulation for neuromodulatory effect. For example, during the pharmacological anesthesia for surgical operation, why not make use of the endogenous opioid system to reduce the postoperative pain and nausea/vomiting, simply by putting the skin electrodes on the acupoints prior to chemical anesthesia and leaving the TEAS device kept on for the whole period of surgery. During the treatment of migraine, for example, why not combine the drug intervention with the TEAS, simply by training the patient with the use of the portable TEAS device together with the self-sticky skin electrodes. This way, we can contribute to the global effort of increasing the therapeutic efficiency and, in the meanwhile, lowering the medical cost.

Looking at the future, when the clinical efficacy of acupuncture is made clear and the mechanisms of its action are better elucidated, one would expect that patients, physicians, and insurance providers would show more interest for the use of acupuncture in the clinical practice.

References

1. NIH Consensus Development Conference on Acupuncture. 3–5 Nov 2007. NIH continuing Medical Education. See: Ramsay DJ, Bowman MA, Greenman PE, et al. NIH Consensus Development Panel Acupuncture. JAMA. 1998;280:1518–24.
2. NCCAM, NIH. Get the facts. Acupuncture for pain. Web site: nccam.nih.gov.
3. Nahin RL, Barness PM, Straussman BJ, et al. Costs of complementary and alternative medicine (CAM) and frequency of visits to CAM practitioners: United States, 2007. Natl Health Stat Rep. 2009;18:1–16.
4. Wang SM, Kain ZN, White P. Acupuncture analgesia: I. The Scientific Basis. Pain Med. 2008;106:602–21.
5. Zhao ZQ. Neural mechanisms underlying acupuncture analgesia. Prog Neurobiol. 2008;85(4):355–75.
6. Butler MJ, Sidall PJ. Neurochemical and neurophysiologic effect of needle insertion: clinical implications. In: Cousins J, Carr DB, Horlocker TT, Bridenbaugh PO, editors. Cousins and Bridenbaugh's "neural blockade in clinical anesthesia and pain medicine". 4th ed. Philadelphia: Lippincott, Williams & Wilkins; 2009. p. 763–76.
7. Research Group of Acupuncture Analgesia, Beijing Medical College. The effect of acupuncture on pain threshold of the skin on human volunteers. Chin Med J. 1973;3:151–7.
8. Lu GW, Liang RZ, Xie JQ, et al. Role of peripheral afferent by needling point Zusanli. Sci Sin. 1979;22:680–92.
9. Research Group of Acupuncture Anesthesia. Beijing Medical College: the role of some neurotransmitters of brain in acupuncture analgesia. Sci Sin. 1974;17:112–30.
10. Han JS, Chou PH, Lu CH, et al. The role of central 5-HT in acupuncture analgesia. Sci Sin. 1979;22:91–104.
11. Xie CW, Tang J, Han JS. Central norepinephrine in acupuncture analgesia. Differential effects in brain and spinal cord. In: Takagi H, Simon EJ, editors. Advances in endogenous and exogenous opioids. Tokyo: Kodansha; 1981. p. 288–90.
12. Mayer DJ, Price DD, Raffi A. Antagonism of acupuncture analgesia in man by narcotic antagonist naloxone. Brain Res. 1977; 121:368–72.
13. Han JS. Acupuncture: neuropeptide release produced by electrical stimulation of different frequencies. Trends Neurosci. 2003; 26:17–22.
14. Huang L, Ren MF, Lu JH, et al. Mutual potentiation of the analgesic effects of met-enkephalin, dynorphin A(1–13) and morphine in the spinal cord of the rat. Acta Physiol Sinica. 1987;39:454–46.
15. Sutters KA, Miaskowski C, Taiwo YO, et al. Analgesic synergy and improved motor function produced by combinations of μ-δ- and μ-κ-opioids. Brain Res. 1990;530:290–4.
16. Han JS, Li SJ, Tang J. Tolerance to electroacupuncture and its cross tolerance to morphine. Neuropharmacology. 1981;20:593–6.
17. Tang NM, Dong HW, Wang XM, et al. Cholecystokinin antisense RNA increases the analgesic effect induced by electroacupuncture or low dose morphine: conversion of low responder rats into high responders. Pain. 1997;71(71):81.
18. Han JS. Opioid and anti-opioid peptides: a model of Yin-Yang balance in acupuncture mechanisms of pain modulation. In: Stux G, Hammerschlag R, editors. Clinical acupuncture, scientific basis. Berlin/Heidelberg: Springer; 2001. p. 51–68.
19. Han JS, Wang Q. Mobilization of specific neuropeptides by peripheral stimulation of identified frequencies. News Physiol Sci. 1992;7:176–80.

20. You HJ, Tjolsen A, Arent-Nielson L. High frequency conditioning stimulation evokes supraspinal independent long-term depression but not long term potentiation of the spinal withdrawal reflex in rats. Brain Res. 2006;1090:116–22.

21. Xing GG, Liu FY, Qu XX, et al. Long term synaptic plasticity in the dorsal horn neuron and its modulation by electroacupuncture in rats with neuropathic pain. Exp Neurol. 2007;208:323–32.

22. Zhang WT, Jin Z, Cui GH, et al. Relations between brain network activation and analgesic effect induced by low versus high frequency electrical acupoint stimulation in different subjects: a functional magnetic resonance imaging study. Brain Res. 2003; 982:168–78.

23. Wang L, Fei XY, Zhu B. Chaos analysis of the electrical signal time series evoked by acupuncture. Chaos Solition Fractals. 2007; 33:901–7.

24. Sun RQ, Wang HC, Wan Y, et al. Suppression of neuropathic pain by peripheral electrical stimulation in rats: mu opioid receptor and NMDA receptor implicated. Exp Neurol. 2004;187:23–9.

25. Wang JZ, Zhou HJ, Liu GL, et al. Han's acupoint nerve stimulator for the treatment of spinal cord injury induced muscle spasticity. Chin J Pain Med. 6:217–24.

26. Dong HW, Wang LH, Zhang M, et al. Decreased dynorphin A (1–17) in the spinal cord of spastic rats after the compressive injury. Brain Res Bull. 2005;67:189–95.

27. Liu HX, Tian JB, Luo F, et al. Repeated 100 Hz TENS for the treatment of chronic inflammatory hyperalgesia and suppression of spinal release of substance P in monoarthritic rats. Evid based Complement Alternat Med. 2006;3:101–16.

28. Wang Q, Mao LM, Han JS. Comparison of the antinociceptive effects induced by electroacupuncture and transcutaneous electrical nerve stimulation in the rat. Int J Neurosci. 1992;65:117–29.

29. Ahmed HE, Craig WF, White PF, et al. Percutaneous electrical nerve stimulation: an alternative to antiviral drugs for acute herpes zoster. Anesth Analg. 1998;87:911–4.

30. Cumming M. Percutaneous electrical nerve stimulation – electroacupuncture by another name? A comparative review. Acupunct Med. 2001;19:32–5.

31. Wang BG, Wang EZ, Chen XZ, et al. Acupuncture anesthesia combined with enflurane for cranial operations. Integr Chin West Med China. 1994;14:10–3 (In Chinese).

32. Billota F, Rosa G. "Anesthesia" for awake neurosurgery. Curr Opin Anaesthesiol. 2009;22:560–5.

33. Qu GL, Zhuang XL, Xu GH, et al. Clinical study on kidney transplantation under complex acupuncture and drug anesthesia. Acupunct Res. 1997;4:275–9.

34. Sim CK, Xu PC, Pua HL, et al. Effects of electroacupuncture on intraoperative and postoperative analgesic requirement. Acupunct Med. 2002;20:56–65.

35. Morioka N, Akca O, Doufas AG, et al. Electroacupuncture at the Zusali, Yanlinquan and Kunlun points does not reduce anesthetic requirement. Anesth Analg. 2002;95:98–102.

36. Wang BG, Tang J, White PF, et al. Effect of the intensity of transcutaneous acupoint electrical stimulation on the postoperative analgesic requirement. Anesth Analg. 1997;85:406–13.

37. Chen L, Tang J, White PF, et al. The effect of location of transcutaneous electrical nerve stimulation: acupoint versus nonacupoint stimulation. Anesth Analg. 1998;87:1129–34.

38. Lin ZG, Lo MW, Hsieh CL, et al. The effect of high and low frequency electroacupuncture in pain after lower abdominal surgery. Pain. 2002;99:509–14.

39. White PF, Hamza MA, Recart A, et al. Optimal timing of acustimulation for antiemetic prophylaxis as an adjunct to ondansetron in patients undergoing plastic surgery. Anesth Analg. 2005;100:367–72.

40. Grube T, Uhlemann C, Weiss T, et al. Influence of acupuncture on postoperative pain, nausea and vomiting after cisceral surgery: a prospective, randomized comparative study of metamizole and standard treatment. Schmerz. 2009;23(4):370–6.

41. Korinenko Y, Vincent A, Cutshall SM, et al. Efficacy of acupuncture in prevention of postoperative nausea in cardiac surgery patients. Ann Thorac Surg. 2009;88:637–42.

42. Zarate E, Mingus M, White PF, et al. The use of transcutaneous Acupoint electrical stimulation for preventing nausea and vomiting after laparoscopic surgery. Anesth Analg. 2001;92:629–35.

43. White PF. Use of alternative medical therapies in the perioperative period: is it time to get on board? Anesth Analg. 2007;104:251–4.

44. Shafer SL. Did our brains fall out? Anesth Analg. 2007;104:247–8.

45. Ghoname EA, et al. Percutaneous electrical nerve stimulation for low back pain: a randomized crossover study. J Am Med Assoc. 1999;281:818–23.

46. Ghoname EA, Craig WF, White PF, et al. The effect of stimulus frequency on the analgesic response to percutaneous electrical nerve stimulation in patients with chronic low back pain. Anesth Analg. 1999;88:841–6.

47. Chen XH, Guo SF, Chang CG, Han JS. Optimal conditions for eliciting maximal electroacupuncture analgesia with dense-and-disperse mode stimulation. Am J Acupunct. 1994;22:47–53.

48. Sator-Katzenschager SM, Scharbert G, Kozek-Langenecker SA, et al. The short and long-term benefit in chronic low back pain through adjuvant electrical versus manual auricular acupuncture. Pain Med. 2004;98:1359–64.

49. Gadsby JG, Flowerdew MW. Transcutaneous electrical stimulation and acupuncture-like transcutaneous electrical nerve stimulation for chronic low back pain. Cochrane Database Syst Rev. 2006;(1): CD000210.

50. White PF, Craig WF, Vakharia AS, et al. Percutaneous neuromodulation therapy: does the location of electrical stimulation effect the acute analgesic response? Anesth Analg. 2000;91:949–54.

51. Ernst E, White A. Acupuncture for back pain: a meta-analysis of randomized controlled trials. Arch Intern Med. 1998;158: 2235–41.

52. Yokoyama M, Sun XH, Oku S, et al. Comparison of percutaneous electrical nerve stimulation with transcutaneous electrical nerve stimulation for long-term pain relief in patients with chronic low back pain. Anesth Analg. 2004;98:1552–6.

53. Berman BM, Lao LX, Langenberg P, et al. Effectiveness of acupuncture as adjunctive therapy in osteoarthritis of the knee. Ann Intern Med. 2004;141:901–10.

54. Scharf HP, Mansmann U, Stretberger K, et al. Acupuncture and knee osteoarthritis. A tree-armed randomized trial. Ann Intern Med. 2006;145:12–20.

55. Ahsin S, Saleem S, Bhatti AM. Clinical and endocrinological changes after electroacupuncture treatment in patients with osteoarthritis of the knee. Pain. 2009;147(1-3):60–6.

56. Zhang W, Moslowitz RW, Nuki G, et al. OARSI recommendations for the management of hip and knee osteoarthritis, Part II: OARSI evidence-based, expert consensus guidelines. Osteoarthritis Cartilage. 2008;16(2):137–62.

57. Conaghan PG, Dickson J, Grant RL. Guideline Development Group. Care and management of osteoarthritis in adults: summary of NICE guidance. BMJ. 2008;336(7642):502–3.

58. White A. NICE guideline on osteoarthritis: is it fair to acupuncture? No. Acupunct Med. 2009;27:70–2.

59. Latimer N. NICE guideline on osteoarthritis: is it fair to acupuncture? Yes. Acupunct Med. 2009;27:72–5.

60. Abuaisha BB, Costanzi JB, Boulton AJM. Acupuncture for the treatment of chronic painful peripheral diabetic neuropathy: a long term study. Diabetic Res Clin Pract. 1998;39:115–21.

61. Hamza MA, Proctor TJ, White PF, et al. Percutaneous electrical nerve stimulation: a novel analgesic therapy for diabetic neuropathic pain. Diabetes Care. 2000;23:365–70.

62. Endres HG, Diener HC, Molsberger A. Role of acupuncture in the treatment of migraine. Expert Rev Neurother. 2007;7:1121–34.

63. Li Y, Liang F, Yang X, et al. Acupuncture for treating acute attacks of migraine: a randomized controlled trial. Headache. 2009;49:805–16.

64. Facco E, Liguori A, Petti F, et al. Traditional acupuncture in migraine: a controlled randomized study. Headache. 2008. doi:10.1111/j.1526-4610.2007.00916.x.

65. Jena S, Will CM, Brinkhaus B, et al. Acupuncture in patients with headache. Cephalalgia. 2008;28:969–79.

66. Diener HC. Migraine: is acupuncture clinically viable for treating acute migraine? Nat Rev Neurol. 2009;5:469–70.

67. Spinal Cord Injury Information Network. Updated 2009.

68. Wang JZ, Zhou HJ, Liu GL, et al. Post-traumatic spinal spasticity treated with Han's Acupoint Nerve Stimulator (NASS). Chin J Pain Med. 2000;6:217–24.

69. Martin DP, Sletten CD, Williams BA, et al. Improvement in fibromyalgia symptom with acupuncture: results of a randomized controlled trial. Mayo Clin Proc. 2006;81:749–57.

70. Harris RE, Clauw DJ, Scott DJ, et al. Decreased central mu-opioid availability in fibromyalgia. J Neurosci. 2007;27:10000–6.

71. Harris RE, Zubieta JK, Scott DJ, et al. Traditional Chinese acupuncture ad placebo (sham) acupuncture are differentiated by their effect on mu-opioid receptors (MORs). Neuroimage. 2009;47:1077–85.

72. Streitberger K, Kleinhenz J. Introducing a placebo needle into acupuncture research. Lancet. 1998;352:364–5.

73. Lund I, Naslund J, Lundeberg T. Minimal acupuncture is not a valid placebo control in randomized controlled trials of acupuncture: a physiologist's perspective. Chin Med. 2009;4:1–9.

74. Lambert C, Berlin I, Lee TL, et al. A Standardized transcutaneous electric acupoint stimulation for relieving tobacco urges in dependent smokers. eCAM. 2008;1093:1–9.

75. Dhond R, Kettner N, Napadow V. Do the neural correlates of acupuncture and placebo effects differ? Pain. 2007;128:8–12.

76. Enck P, Benedetti F, Schedlowski M. New insights into the placebo and nocebo response. Neuron. 2008;59:195–206.

77. Research Group of Ear Acupuncture, Jiangsu College of New Medicine. The effect of ear acupuncture on the pain threshold of the skin at thoracic and abdominal region. In: Theoretical study on acupuncture anesthesia. Shanghai: Shanghai People's Press; 1973. p. 27–32.

Manual Therapies

John F. Barnes, Albert L. Ray, and Rhonwyn Ullmann

Key Points

- Manual therapies are an essential part of functional restoration and pain treatment in people with persistent pain.
- Several therapeutic techniques can help with neuroplastic positive changes in brain function (retraining the brain).
- The most critical element in improving function is to find a technique that "fits" the patient best since they all have common elements for brain change.
- The common feature of successful long-term improvement via manual therapies seems to be simultaneous multiple inputs to the brain; some of which incorporate mindful focused attention coupled with sensory and/or motor activities.
- The therapeutic improvements from the manual therapies discussed in this chapter demonstrate long-term effectiveness, unless the person is retraumatized in body, mind, or both.

J.F. Barnes, PT, LMT, NCTMP (✉)
Myofascial Release Treatment Centers and Seminar,
222 West Lancaster Avenue, Suite 100, Paoli, PA, 19301, USA
e-mail: paoli@myofascialrelease.com

A.L. Ray, M.D.
The LITE Center, 5901 SW 74 St, Suite 201,
South Miami, FL 33143, USA

University of Miami Miller School of Medicine,
Miami, FL, USA
e-mail: aray@thelitecenter.org

R. Ullmann, BS, M.S.
The LITE Center, 5901 SW 74 St, Suite 201,
South Miami, FL 33143, USA
e-mail: bearrab@aol.com

Introduction

Manual therapy is an essential and critical part of interdisciplinary functional restoration and pain treatment. There are multiple types of manual therapies. This chapter will present a select few, all of which have clinically shown themselves to be effective for such treatment. Some of these techniques have been in existence for centuries, while others are more recent. However, all of them have evolved over time and experience of the main therapists behind their names and styles, based on what has been the most effective for those suffering from chronic pain. They all have experience and time-testing behind them. Some of the literature is scant in terms of modern "evidence-based" studies for various reasons: some were started and developed long before double-blind randomized controlled trials were considered necessary; some have evolved by therapists who have reported techniques that they find work and were meant to be shared with other practitioners as practical and useful ways to improve function without intending to "prove" their worthiness to a scientific community; some have simply evolved because patients respond to them; and, especially in today's economic climate, research funding to create and implement double-blind randomized trials of these techniques is rare, if available at all. There is, however, crucial and critical thinking behind all of the techniques that will be presented in this chapter. The purpose of this chapter is to present an overview of various manual therapy techniques in order to raise awareness on the part of our readers as to what is available, and we submit that there is much more specific information, as well as courses, available to all who desire a more involved learning of these topics or wish to be able to practice these various techniques.

There is no one particular manual therapy technique that is, by development, superior to others. Different patients respond differently, and whichever technique a person is able to utilize to help themselves is the important discriminator. However, in these authors' experience, those techniques which include more than one "brain input" at a time

T.R. Deer et al. (eds.), *Comprehensive Treatment of Chronic Pain by Medical, Interventional, and Integrative Approaches*,
DOI 10.1007/978-1-4614-1560-2_80, © American Academy of Pain Medicine 2013

seem to be the techniques that offer the most effective opportunities to alter neuroplastic patterns in the brain, and that is why this list of therapies have been chosen for discussion. This mind-body connection "release" via multiple simultaneous brain "inputs" also seems to be one characteristic which makes these techniques more effective than single-modality "traditional" physical therapy for those suffering from persistent pain.

We will now turn to specific manual therapies and begin with the John Barnes technique. Within this section is a more detailed discussion related to the fascia and the mind-body connection within this "connective" tissue system. The principles related to fascial characteristics, however, are applicable to the other therapeutic techniques that follow as well.

John F. Barnes Myofascial Release

Myofascial release is a whole body, hands-on approach for the evaluation and treatment of the human structure. Its focus is the fascial system. Pain associated with physical trauma, an inflammatory or infection process, surgical procedures, or structural imbalance from dental malocclusion, osseous restriction, leg-length discrepancy, and pelvic rotation may all create inappropriate fascial strain.

Trauma and inflammatory responses create myofascial restrictions that can produce tensile pressures of approximately 2,000 lb/in.^{2} on pain-sensitive structures that do not show up in any of the standard tests (x-rays, myelograms, CT scans, electromyography, etc.).

This enormous pressure acts like a "straightjacket" on muscles, nerves, blood vessels, and osseous structures producing the symptoms of pain, headaches, and restriction of motion. Myofascial release allows the chronic inflammatory response to resolve and eradicate the enormous pressure of myofascial restrictions exerted on pain-sensitive structures to alleviate symptoms and to allow the body's natural healing capacity to function properly.

Fascia, an embryologic tissue, reorganizes along the lines of tension (called tensegrity) imposed on the body, adding support to misalignment and contracting to protect the individual from further trauma (real or imagined). This has the potential to alter organ and tissue physiology significantly. Fascial strains can slowly tighten, causing the body to lose its physiologic adaptive capacity. Flexibility and spontaneity of movement are lost, setting the body up for more trauma, pain, and limitation of movement. These powerful fascial restrictions begin to pull the body out of its three-dimensional alignment.

Janet Travell's [1] detailed description of the myofascial element indicates that there is a smooth fascial sheath which surrounds every muscle of the body, so that every muscular fascicle is surrounded by fascia, every fibril is surrounded by fascia, and every microfibril down to the cellular level is surrounded by fascia. Therefore, it is the fascia that ultimately determines the length and function of its muscular component, and muscle becomes an inseparable component of fascia. Because fascia covers the muscle, bones, nerves, organs, and vessels down to the cellular level, malfunction of the system due to trauma, surgery, poor posture, or inflammation can bind down the fascia, resulting in abnormal pressure on any or all of these body components.

As Travell [1] has explained, restrictions of the fascia can create pain or malfunction throughout the body, sometimes with bizarre side effects and seemingly unrelated symptoms that do not always follow dermatome zones. An extremely high percentage of people suffering with pain, loss of motion, or both may have fascial restriction problems.

John F. Barnes Myofascial Release (JFBMFR), along with therapeutic exercise and movement therapy, improves the vertical alignment and lengthens the body, providing more space and less pressure for the proper functioning of osseous structures, neuromatrix system, blood vessels, and organs.

Thus, for example, with an injury to the lumbosacral area, patients have been known to experience distant symptoms such as occipital headaches, upper cervical pain and dysfunction, feelings of tightness around the thoracic area, lumbosacral pain, and tightness and lack of flexibility in the posterior aspect of the lower extremity. During trauma, or with development of a structural imbalance, a proprioceptive memory pattern of pain is established in the central nervous system. Beyond the localized pain from injured nerves, these reflex patterns remain to perpetuate the pain during and beyond healing of the injured tissue, similar to the experience of phantom limb pain.

Once fascia has tightened and is creating symptoms distant from the injury, appropriate traditional localized treatments may produce temporary results; however, they do not treat the "straightjacket" of pressure that is causing the symptoms. Myofascial release (JFBMFR) techniques are performed in conjunction with specific systematic treatment. The gentle tractioning forces applied to the fascial restrictions will elicit heat from a vasomotor response which increases blood flow to the affected area, enhancing lymphatic drainage of toxic metabolic wastes, realignment of fascial planes, and, most importantly, reset the soft tissue proprioceptive sensory mechanism. The activity seems to reprogram the central nervous system, enabling the patient to perform a normal, functional range of motion without eliciting the previous pain patterns [2].

The goal of this form of myofascial release is to remove fascial restrictions and restore the body's equilibrium. When the structure has been returned to a balanced state, it is realigned with gravity. When these aims have been accomplished, the body's inherent ability to self-correct returns, thus restoring optimum function and performance with the least amount of energy expenditure [3]. A more ideal environment

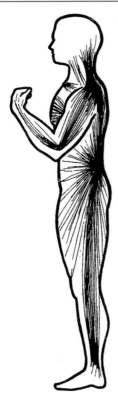

Fig. 80.1 Fascia man (Courtesy of John Barnes)

to enhance the effectiveness of concomitant systematic work therapy is also created (Fig. 80.1).

The trained JFBMFR therapist finds the cause of symptoms by evaluating the fascial system. The technique requires continuous reevaluation during treatment, including observation of vasomotor responses and their location as they occur after a particular restriction has been released.

When the location of the fascial restriction is determined, gentle pressure is applied in its direction. It is hypothesized that this has the effect of pulling the elastocollagenous fibers straight. When hand or palm pressure is first applied to the elastocollagenous complex, the elastic component is engaged, resulting in a "springy" feel. The elastic component is slowly stretched until hands stop at what feels like a firm barrier. This is the collagenous component. This barrier cannot be forced; it is too strong. Instead, the therapist continues to apply gentle sustained pressure, and soon, the firm barrier will yield to the previous melting or springy feel as it stretches further. This yielding phenomenon is related to viscous flow; that is, a low load (gentle pressure) applied slowly will allow a viscous medium to flow to a greater extent than a high load (quickly applied) pressure [4, 5]. The viscosity of the ground substance has an effect on the ground collagen since it is believed that the viscous medium that makes up the ground substance controls the ease with which collagen fibers rearrange themselves (Jenkins DHR). As this rearranging occurs, the collagenous barrier releases, producing a change in tissue length [4].

JFBMFR techniques and myofascial unwinding seem to allow for the complete communication of mind with body and body with mind, which is necessary for healing. The body remembers everything that ever happened to it, and Hameroff's research [6] indicates that the theory of "quantum coherence" points toward the storing of meaningful memory in the microtubules, cylindrical protein polymers that we find in the fascia of cells. Mind-body awareness and healing are often linked to the concept of "state-dependent" memory, learning, and behavior [7, 8]. For example, a certain smell or the sound of a particular piece of music may create a flashback phenomenon, a visual, sensorimotor replay of a past event or an important episode in our lives with such vividness that it is as if it were happening at that moment. Work based on the writings of and expanded upon by Barnes, Hameroff, and colleagues [6] includes position-dependent memory, learning, and behavior, with the structural position being the missing component in Selye's state-dependent theory as it is currently described [7, 8].

During periods of trauma, people form subconscious indelible imprints of the experience that have high levels of emotional content and which could not be processed at the time of occurrence. The body can hold information below the conscious level, as a protective mechanism, so that memories tend to become dissociated, or amnesiac, called memory dissociation, or reversible amnesia. Subconscious holding patterns eventually form for specific muscular tone or tension patterns, and the fascial component then tightens into these habitual positions of strain as a compensation to support misalignment that results (tensegrity effect). Therefore, the repeated postural insults of a lifetime, combined with the tensions of emotional and psychological origin, seem to result in tense, contracted, bunched, and fatigued fibrous tissue. A combination of mental and physical stresses may alter the neuromyofascial and skeletal structure, creating a visible, identifiable physical change which, itself, generates further stress, such as pain, joint restrictions, general discomfort, and fatigue. A chronic stress pattern produces long-term muscular contraction which, if prolonged, can cause energy loss, mechanical inefficiency, pain, cardiovascular pathology, and hypertension [9]. Memories are state (or position) dependent and can therefore be retrieved when the person later repeats that particular state (or position). This information is not available in the normal conscious state, and the body's protective mechanisms keep us away from the positions that our mind-body awareness construes as painful or traumatic.

It has been demonstrated consistently that when a myofascial release technique takes the tissue to a significant position, or when myofascial unwinding allows a body part to assume a significant position three-dimensionally in space, the tissue not only changes and improves, but memories, associated emotional states, and belief systems rise to the conscious level. This awareness, through the positional reproduction of a past event or trauma, allows the individual to grasp the previously hidden information that may be creating or maintaining symptoms or behavior that deter improvement. With the repressed and stored information now at the conscious level, the individual is in a position to learn which holding or bracing patterns have been impeding progress and why. The release of the tissue with its stored emotions and hidden information creates an environment for change. As such, no longer do patients habitually find themselves holding or stiffening to protect themselves from future pain or trauma. Release of fear and emotion takes place simultaneously with physical fascial release and physiologic release of the associated stress hormones.

Fascia and New Explanatory Paradigms

Clinical evidence has demonstrated that restrictions in the fascial system are of considerable importance in relieving pain and restoring function [10]. Myofascial release becomes vitally important when we realize that these restrictions can exert tremendous tensile forces on the neuromuscular-skeletal systems and other pain-sensitive structures, creating the very symptoms that we have been trying to eliminate [11].

An important component of the theory behind the mind-body connection is the ability for people to transmit natural bioelectrical currents along the endogenous electromagnetic fields of the three-dimensional network of the fascial system of another person [4]. Medical applications of exogenous bioelectromagnetics (like x-ray) are very common. Endogenous bioelectromagnetic field, natural within all living beings, has only more recently been studied [4, 12].

Increasingly, medical researchers and experienced health professionals are beginning to view the body as a self-correcting mechanism with bioelectric healing systems. According to Cowley [13], some scientists are starting to explore the body's sensitivity to electromagnetic energy. Electromagnetic fields "trigger the release of stress hormones… [and] can affect such processes as bone growth, communication among brain cells, and even the activity of white cells" [13].

Copper wire is a well-known conductor of electricity. If copper wire becomes twisted or crushed, it loses its ability to conduct energy properly. It is thought that fascia may act like copper wire when it becomes restricted through trauma, inflammatory processes, or poor posture over time. Then, its ability to conduct the body's bioelectricity seems to be diminished, setting up structural compensations and, ultimately, symptoms or restrictions of motion [4]. Just like untwisting a copper wire, myofascial release techniques seem to restore the fascia's ability to conduct bioelectricity, thus creating the environment for enhanced healing. Release

techniques can also structurally eliminate the enormous pressures that fascial restrictions exert on nerves, blood vessels, and muscles [4].

Fascial "Memory"

It appears that not only the myofascial element but also every cell of the body has a consciousness that stores memories and emotions [4, 14]. Research findings suggest that the mind and body act on each other in often remarkable ways. With the help of sophisticated new laboratory tools, investigators are demonstrating that emotional states can translate into altered responses in the immune system, the complex array of organs, glands, and cells that comprises the body's principal mechanism for repelling invaders. The implications of this loop are unsettling. To experts in the field of psychoneuroimmunology, the immune system seems to behave almost as if it had a brain of its own. This is creating a revolution in medicine in the way we view physiology. More than that, it is raising profound and tantalizing questions about the nature of behavior, about the essence of what we are [15].

Fascia is not accessed by traditional mechanical methods such as point mobilization modalities or traditional stretching methods. Fascia, instead, responds to the combination of the intentional application of endogenous bioelectromagnetic energy fields and the sustained mechanical pressure at the myofascial barrier from within the therapist. Through the palms and fingers of the therapist's hands, this gentle, sustained mechanical pressure seems to open memories and experiences in restricted fascia, for upon the release of restrictions, patients commonly become transported back to an injurious experience and with similar emotion, relating the experience in three-dimensional detail [4]. Once the trauma is completely experienced and fascial restrictions have given way, healing can commence. We have yet to learn the cellular mechanism of the healing process, it is believed that as restrictions are removed from fascia, body energy, blood, lymph, neurotransmitters, neuropeptides, and steroids are free to flow, restoring balance, homeostasis, and overall health to the system [4].

Myofascial release is not offered to replace traditional physical therapy techniques, but rather to supplement and enhance them as a complementary approach in evaluating and treating patients with pain, restriction of motion, and structural symptoms.

Yoga

Yoga historically evolved from a Hindu spiritual and ascetic discipline which utilizes specific body postures (asana) along with breath control (prana) and simple meditation to achieve unity of body and mind. Asana is the Sanskrit term for the physical postures of yoga. (Interestingly, many "traditional" Western physical therapy stretches and exercises are based in yoga tradition, but they do not incorporate the mindful focus in addition.) However, asana is only one of eight "limbs" of yoga, the majority of which are more concerned with mental and spiritual well-being rather than the physical. This technique is about creating balance in the body through development of strength and flexibility, including stretching. One style, vinyasa, utilizes the poses quickly in succession to create body heat through movement, while other styles go more slowly to focus on increasing stamina and perfect alignment of the pose.

Yoga has been found to be effective in the treatment of low back pain. In looking at randomized trials of yoga in low back pain with pain level as a mandated outcome measure, five RCTs suggested yoga significantly reduced low back pain compared to usual care, education, or conventional therapeutic exercises [16]. An 8-week yoga program demonstrated reduced pain, reduced catastrophizing, increased acceptance and mindfulness, and increased cortisol levels in women with fibromyalgia [17]. Positive results are shown in primary dysmenorrhea in reducing the pain intensity and duration [18]. In children with functional abdominal pain and irritable bowel syndrome, yoga has reduced pain and frequency, especially in children between 8 and 11 years old [19]. In a yogic prana (breathing) energization technique (YPET) study of fresh simple fractures of extra-articular long and short bones, patients within the yoga treatment showed significant improvement over controls in pain reduction, tenderness reduction, swelling, and increased fracture time density and number of cortices united [20].

Feldenkrais Method or Awareness Through Movement®

Feldenkrais Method is a form of somatic education developed by Dr. Moshe Feldenkrais, a physicist, judo expert, mechanical engineer, and educator who utilized this knowledge base to design a method of gentle movement and directed attention to improve movement and enhance human functioning. Another name for this treatment method is Awareness Through Movement®. It is based on the principles of physics, biomechanics, and an empirical understanding of learning. It has been successfully utilized in all age groups in both physically challenged and physically fit groups, including professional athletes. It is claimed to be useful for helping those with chronic pain, those wishing to improve their self-awareness and self-image, and in central nervous conditions such as multiple sclerosis, cerebral palsy, and stroke.

Literature is scarce for treatment of chronic pain with Feldenkrais Method, but one study of 14 women with nonspecific neck and shoulder pain in a self-report study model demonstrated significant improvement and found the technique "wholesome, but difficult." Additionally, they reported positive changes in posture, balance, a feeling of release, and increased self-confidence, and these positive effects remained after 4–6-month follow-up [21]. In a study comparing Body Awareness Therapy (BAT), Feldenkrais Method (FM), and conventional physiotherapy in patients with nonspecific musculoskeletal disorders, both the BAT and FM groups improved over conventional therapy in pain and quality of life, and they remained stable over time, while the conventional therapy group deteriorated at 1-year follow-up [22].

Pilates

Pilates exercises were developed by Joseph Pilates in the 1920s. There are six principles to Pilates exercises which emphasize precision of movement over quantity of exercise, and these include centering, control, flow, breath, precision, and concentration. Core muscle strength is the foundation of this technique, and these include the deep muscles of the abdomen and back. Pilates exercises are done either on a mat or on specialized equipment that utilizes pulleys and the patient's own body weight for resistance.

Literature review for Pilates-based treatment of chronic pain produced mixed results. One 4-week study for treatment of nonspecific chronic low back pain looked at pain reduction and functional disability, and demonstrated a significant decrease in pain and disability which continued at 12-month follow-up, compared to a control group receiving usual care [23]. Another study compared Pilates training in people with fibromyalgia with a home exercise program of stretching/relaxation found significant improvement in both pain and FIQ (Fibromyalgia Impact Questionnaire) at 12 weeks, but only in FIQ at 24 weeks in the Pilates group [24]. Multiple studies did literature reviews of RCTs including nonspecific low back pain with varied results. In a systematic review and meta-analysis, Lim concluded that Pilates-based exercises are superior to minimal intervention for pain relief, but not superior to other forms of exercise to reduce pain and disability [25]. The La Touche [24] review also found positive effects for reducing pain in nonspecific chronic low back pain but cautions that no studies have identified which specific parameters are to be applied when prescribing Pilates exercises [26]. However, Posadzki's literature review found "some evidence" supporting effectiveness of Pilates in management of low back pain, they point out that no definite conclusions could be drawn, and further research is needed due to the sample sizes, heterogeneity of inclusion/exclusion criteria, etc. [27]. On the contrary, one literature review found no improvement in pain or functionality in low back pain patients when compared to control and lumbar stabilization exercise groups. However, the Pilates group was no worse either [28].

Alexander Technique

The Alexander technique is focused on movement and release of tension in the body. It is designed to improve the ease and freedom of movement, balance, support, and coordination. This technique improves the efficiency with which we move and decreases the energy and effort required. It is more a reeducation of the mind and body, rather than an exercise program, but it is a useful manual therapy. Like Feldenkrais Method, Alexander technique is based on tension patterns in our movement that develop from about age 3–4 years on, and both techniques are designed to reinstate better movement, more "childlike" to make improvement. Both utilize awareness as a major part of change, and both are based on learning philosophies. The Alexander technique is utilized in painful conditions based on the body tensions, usually out of our awareness, involved in painful conditions.

The medical literature regarding treatment of pain with Alexander technique provides supportive evidence for this treatment. One study found Alexander technique alone superior to either massage or massage combined with Alexander technique for chronic back pain [29]. In fact, those patients reported being able to manage their back pain better utilizing Alexander teachings without the excuses made for difficulty in standard exercising, because it "made sense" and they could perform it while carrying out everyday activities or relaxing [30]. Two studies found Alexander lessons effective for chronic pain at 1-year follow-up [31, 32]. A literature review by Ernst found two good studies that demonstrated Alexander technique to be useful in reducing disability in patients suffering from Parkinson's disease and improving pain behavior and disability in patients with back pain. They recommend further study of this technique, as the evidence was not "convincing" [33].

Aquatic Therapy

Water is an excellent medium for recovery from minor to major injuries and chronic pain. It addresses muscle imbalances and postural problems and is also less threatening to patients who are afraid of exercise, pain, and/or reinjury. By creating a safe environment, one in which the patient can feel more in control and one that may not increase pain, can be a stepping-stone to changing the patients perception of pain and of movement.

The properties of water make it ideal for achieving therapeutic goals in a safe and effective environment [34, 35]:

- Buoyancy. Buoyancy is the upward pressure exerted by the fluid in which the body is immersed. Buoyancy opposes the force of gravity, allowing the body to move more freely and easily than on land.
- Decreased compressive forces. This is due to the effects of buoyancy. The deeper one is in water, the greater the decrease in the compressive or weight-bearing forces on all joints, as well as the discs of the spine.
- Even hydrostatic pressure on submerged body parts. There is equal pressure from the water on the body that increases with depth. This is helpful for swelling around the joints or circulatory problems because the static fluid around the joints is forced upward toward the heart by hydrostatic pressure.
- Temperature. Aquatic therapy can be affected in any comfortable water temperature, but heated water (89–91 °F) has been found to be demonstrably more effective, especially for persons with arthritic conditions.

Many patients who are unable or not emotionally or psychologically ready to exercise in a conventional clinic setting can successfully participate in water exercise programs. In addition to the physical benefits (below), the safe environment builds confidence and trust in their ability to move and to exercise:

- Safety. One of the attractions to water as a therapeutic modality is the safety. Water is supportive through its buoyancy, resistive in nature, and equal in hydrostatic pressure on the submerged body part.
- Flexibility/range of motion. Due to the decrease of gravitational forces in water, the body moves freely, and overall weight is diminished so that a body part can be lifted and stretched without as much pain.
- Strengthening. The body in water is working against resistance, yet the patient feels supported and safe in this environment. As strength and endurance improve, resistive devices are available that enable the person to "turn up" the intensity of the exercise, further increasing cardiovascular strength and endurance aspects of reconditioning.
- Muscle reeducation. When movement patterns have been altered due to injury and/or pain, reeducating the whole body as well as the brain can be accomplished effectively in water.
- Balance. The environment in water is ever-changing, and the patient is constantly challenged.

Functional Movement/Restoration

What is "functional movement" and how does it differ from "traditional" physical therapy?

Functional movement is a "functional approach" to exercise and restoration, meaning that it is designed to address "real-world" movements and mimics the broad range of daily movements one might normally do. It teaches the body how to actually move, use, and increase available strength utilizing everyday movement patterns [36, 37]. Basically, it is directed toward the way a patient works, plays, and lives. Its goal is to get the patient back to work, play, and normalized life.

Once an injury and/or pain begins (particularly if it began quite a while ago), the way a patient moves changes due to compensation and fear of pain. This puts stress on more than just the injured area. Changes and pain begin to be noticed in other areas of their body as well. Treating just the injured area, as is often done, does not treat the patient. As patients begin to feel pain in other areas, it frequently affects not just their body, but their mind and their spirit. Treating only the injured area is often not the answer. Integration of mind, body, and spirit simultaneously restores functionality and retrains the brain by creating new and/or restoring normal movement patterns that can help return patients back to life.

Summary

In this chapter, we have reviewed some of the most important manual therapy techniques that are utilized for reducing pain and restoring functionally improved mechanical abilities and mindful peacefulness. The utilization of touch should be apparent in all of these techniques, some of which allow for direct touching as a way to transfer information and energy between the pain sufferer and the therapist helping them, while others do it with indirect touching and "self-touching" of energy (as in yoga). The most important common denominator that we have found among all of these manual techniques is the useful application of mindful focus coupled with simultaneous sensory and/or motor involvement. This double stimulation of the brain seems to us to be the link that alters the brain in a positive way in either depotentiating the long-term potentiation that occurred by sensitization of the pain pathways or those that "clogged" the information transfer ability of the body's connective tissue system, especially the fascia. Once these problems are reversed, our mind-body connections are able to optimize their functions, and we see improvement that not only helps the person feel and function better but is permanent unless new problems develop. This is the important part of the manual therapies presented here, and why they become significantly important adjuncts to more traditional type physical therapies, which do not seem to make the same permanent improvements in persons with persistent pain. Traditional physical therapies are much more effective in treating the type of eudynia where pain is still a symptom of an underlying mechanical problem such as an acute injury, postsurgical problems, or flare-ups of arthritic conditions. Once maldynia develops, the manual therapies reviewed in this chapter become much more useful, because they are effective in changing the neuroplastic dysfunctional brain

states that have developed and in "clearing out" long-standing dysfunctional conditions within the soft tissue, especially, as mentioned, the fascia.

References

1. Travell J. Myofascial pain and dysfunction. Baltimore: Williams & Wilkins; 1983.
2. Barnes J. Myofascial release: the search for excellence. In: Davis C, editor. Complementary therapies in rehabilitation. Thorofare: Slack Inc; 2004. p. 60.
3. Barnes JF, Smith G. The body is a self-correcting mechanism. Phys Ther Forum. July 1987;27.
4. Oschman JL. Energy medicine: the science basis. New York: Churchill Livingstone; 2000.
5. Jenkins DHR. Ligament injuries and their treatment. Rockville: Aspen Publications; 1985.
6. Hameroff SR. Quantum coherence in microtubules: a neural basis for emergent consciousness. J Conscious Stud. 1994;1(1):91–118.
7. Selye H. History and present status of the stress concept. In: Goldberger L, Breznitz S, editors. Handbook of stress. New York: Macmillan; 1982. p. 7–20.
8. Selye H. The stress of life. New York: McGraw-Hill; 1976.
9. Chaitow L. Neuro-muscular technique – a practitioner's guide to soft tissue mobilization. New York: Thorsons; 1985. p. 13–5.
10. Barnes JF. The significance of touch. Phys Ther Forum. 1988; 7:10.
11. Popper KR, Eccles JC. The self and its brain. Berlin: Springer; 1977.
12. National Institutes of Health (U.S.). Alternative medicine: expanding medical horizons. Report to the NIH on alternative medical systems of practices in the United States. Pittsburgh: US Government Printing Office, Superintendent of Documents; 1992. p. 48–50.
13. Cowley G. An electromagnetic storm. Newsweek. 1989;114(2): p. 77.
14. Pert CB. Molecules of emotion: the science behind mind-body medicine. New York: Touchstone; 1997.
15. Kurtz R. Body centered psychotherapy: the Hakomi therapy. Ashland: The Hakomi Institute; 1988.
16. Posadski P, Ernst E. Yoga for low back pain: a systematic review of randomized clinical trials. Clin Rheumatol. 2011;30(9):1257–62.
17. Curtis K, Osadchuk A, Katz J. An eight-week yoga intervention is associated with improvements in pain, psychological functioning and mindfulness, and changes in cortisol levels in women with fibromyalgia. J Pain Res. 2011;4:189–201.
18. Rakhshaee Z. Effect of three yoga poses (cobra, cat and fish poses) in women with primary dysmenorrheal: a randomized clinical trial. J Pediatr Adolesc Gynecol. 2011;24(4):192–6.
19. Brands MM, Purperhart H, Deckers-Kocken JM. A pilot study of yoga treatment in children with functional abdominal pain and irritable bowel syndrome. Complement Ther Med. 2011;19(3): 109–14.
20. Oswal P, et al. The effect of add-on yoga prana energization technique (YPET) on healing of fresh fractures: a randomized control study. J Altern Complement Med. 2011;17(3):253–8.
21. Ohman A, Aström L, Malmgren-Olsson EB. Feldenkrais® therapy as group treatment for chronic pain – a qualitative evaluation. J Bodyw Mov Ther. 2011;15(2):153–61.
22. Malmgren-Olsson EB, Bränholm IB. A comparison between three physiotherapy approaches with regard to health-related factors in patients with non-specific musculoskeletal disorders. Disabil Rehabil. 2002;24(6):308–17.
23. Rydeard R, Leger A, Smith D. Pilates-based therapeutic exercise: effect on subjects with nonspecific chronic low back pain and functional disability: a randomized controlled trial. J Orthop Sports Phys Ther. 2006;36(7):472–84.

24. Altan L, et al. Effect of pilates training on people with fibromyalgia syndrome: a pilot study. Arch Phys Med Rehabil. 2009;90(12): 1983–8.

25. Lim EC, et al. Effects of Pilates-based exercises on pain and disability in individuals with persistent nonspecific low back pain: a systematic review with meta-analysis. J Orthop Sports Phys Ther. 2011;41(2):70–80.

26. La Touche R, Escalante K, Linares MT. Treating non-specific chronic low back pain through the Pilates Method. J Bodyw Mov Ther. 2008;12(4):364–70.

27. Posadski P, Lizis P, Hagner-Derengowska M. Pilates for low back pain: a systematic review. Complement Ther Clin Pract. 2011; 17(2):85–9.

28. Pereira LM, et al. Comparing the Pilates method with no exercise or lumbar stabilization for pain and functionality in patients with chronic low back pain: systematic review and meta-analysis. Clin Rehabil. 2012;26(1):10–20. Epub 2011 Aug 19.

29. Beattie A. Participating in and delivering the ATEAM (Alexander technique lessons, exercise, and massage) interventions for chronic back pain: a qualitative study of professional perspectives. Complement Ther Med. 2010;18(3–4):119–27.

30. Yardley L, et al. Patients' views of receiving lessons in the Alexander technique and an exercise prescription for managing back pain in the ATEAM trial. Fam Pract. 2010;27(2):198–204.

31. Ehrlich GE. Alexander technique lessons were effective for chronic or recurrent back pain at 1 year. Evid Based Med. 2009;14(1):13.

32. Little P, et al. Randomised controlled trial of Alexander technique lessons, exercise, and massage (ATEAM) for chronic and recurrent back pain. Br J Sports Med. 2008;42(12):965–8.

33. Ernst E, Canter PH. The Alexander technique: a systematic review of controlled clinical trials. Forsch Komplementarmed Klass Naturheilkd. 2003;10(6):325–9.

34. Suomi R, Collier D. Effects of arthritis exercise programs on functional fitness and perceived ADL measures in older adults with arthritis. Arch Phys Med Rehabil. 2003;84(11):1589–94.

35. Hinman R, Haywood S, Day A. Aquatic PT for hip and knee OA: results of a single blind randomized control trial. J Am Phys Ther Assoc. 2007;87:32–42.

36. Chek P. Functional exercises from the inside out in "Live with Paul Chek" series. New York: C.H.E.K. Institute; 2003.

37. Santana JC. Functional training: an old concept with a new name. Boca Raton: The Institute of Human Performance (IHP); 2009.

Treatment of Chronic Painful Musculoskeletal Injuries and Diseases with Regenerative Injection Therapy (RIT): Regenerative Injection Therapy Principles and Practice

81

Felix S. Linetsky, Hakan Alfredson, David Crane, and Christopher J. Centeno

Key Points

- Focuses on treatment of pain related to pathology of the connective tissue
- Provides detail explanation of mechanism of action
- Emphasizes neurolytic properties of chemical injectates
- Describes biologic injectates in details
- Compares and explains the significant resemblance of pain maps derived from the interspinous ligaments with those from the spinal and pelvic synovial joints
- Provides a step by step approach to differential diagnosis and treatment
- Describes future directions for regenerative injection therapy

F.S. Linetsky, M.D. (✉)
Department of Osteopathic Principles and Practice,
Nova Southeastern University of Osteopathic Medicine,
Clearwater, FL, USA
e-mail: linetskyom@gmail.com

H. Alfredson, M.D., Ph.D.
Sports Medicine Unit, University of Umea,
Gosta Skoglunds Vag 3, Umea 90738, Sweden
e-mail: hakan.alfredson@idrott.umu.se

D. Crane, M.D.
Regenerative Medicine, Crane Clinic Sports Medicine,
219 Chesterfield Towne Center,
Chesterfield, MO 63005, USA
e-mail: dcranemd@earthlink.net

C.J. Centeno, M.D.
Physical Medicine and Rehabilitation and Pain Medicine,
Regenerative Medicine, Centeno-Schultz Clinic,
403 Summit Blvd, Broomfield, CO 80021, USA
e-mail: centenooffice@centenoclinic.com

Introduction

Regenerative injection therapy (RIT), also known as prolotherapy or sclerotherapy, is a treatment for chronic musculoskeletal pain caused by connective tissue diathesis utilizing chemical or biologic substances [1]. Steroidal and nonsteroidal anti-inflammatory medications are useful in degenerative disease processes with concomitant inflammatory changes or fibrosis which tethers adjacent structures such as nerves or tendons. In such instances, hydrodissection with injectates containing corticosteroid may also prove useful. RIT is a viable, type-specific treatment for chronic conditions that involve collagen destruction or degeneration. Multiple controlled and uncontrolled studies indicated effectiveness of RIT in treating painful degenerative musculoskeletal conditions. Advances in imaging technology such as MRI and diagnostic ultrasound made it possible to visualize soft tissue pathology in the muscles, ligaments, and tendons. Tendinosis is frequently present in the appendicular and axial tendons. The diagnosis of tendinosis requires therapeutic interventions different from corticosteroids. There is literally an army of capable doctors who need biologically active substances to repair or regenerate degenerative pathologic changes. Old and newer injectates used for RIT such as polidocanol, platelet-rich plasma, and stem cells meet these requirements and are rendering impressive results.

The published pain patterns from ligaments, muscles, intervertebral discs, and synovial joints in the cervical thoracic and lumbar regions overlap significantly (Figs. 81.1, 81.2, 81.3, 81.4, 81.5, and 81.6) [2–4, 10–16]. Nonetheless, ligaments and tendons of these regions are rarely included in differential diagnosis. This chapter is addressing the diagnostic and therapeutic approaches to chronic musculoskeletal pain related to the pathology of fibrous collagenous connective tissue that could benefit from RIT.

T.R. Deer et al. (eds.), *Comprehensive Treatment of Chronic Pain by Medical, Interventional, and Integrative Approaches*,
DOI 10.1007/978-1-4614-1560-2_81, © American Academy of Pain Medicine 2013

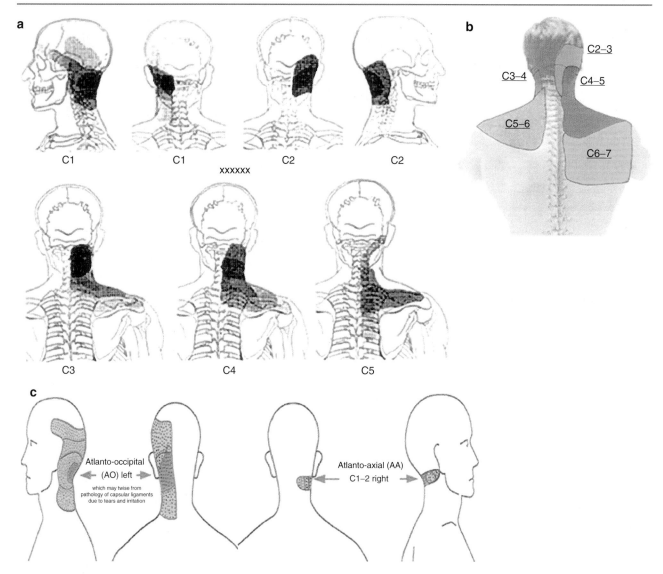

Fig. 81.1 Modified comparative composition of pain distribution in the cervical region provoked by injections of hypertonic saline in to the interspinous ligaments (**a**) Feinstein et al. [2]. Synovial joints: (**b**) (**c**) Significant overlap of these pain maps is due to the fact that injected structures are innervated by the cervical dorsal rami specifically the medial branches (MBDR). Similar relations exist in the thoracic, lumbar, and sacral regions (With permission from Dwyer et al. [3]; and Dreyfuss et al. [4])

Evolution of Terminology

Prior to 1930s, this treatment was called "injection treatment" with addition of a pathologic descriptor such as of injection treatment of varicose veins or injection treatment of hydroceles [17]. Biegeleisen coined the term "sclerotherapy" in 1936 [18].

Concluding that sclerotherapy implied scar formation, Hackett coined the term prolotherapy as "the rehabilitation of an incompetent structure by the generation of new cellular tissue." Hackett's supposition that "… prolotherapy is a treatment to permanently strengthen the 'weld' of disabled ligaments and tendons to bone" led to treatment with injections at the fibro-osseous junctions [11]. More recent work found significant amount of degenerative changes in the midsubstance of the ligaments and tendons as well as ruptures at the fibro-muscular interfaces, and intersubstance changes.

Further, current understanding of the basic science is such that regeneration and repair extend beyond the proliferative stage which is only a short phase of the healing process. More so, proliferation is an integral part of a malignant unsuppressed growth as well as degenerative changes which are present in the bones, synovium, intervertebral discs, ligaments, tendons, and fascial connective tissues. Regenerative injection therapy was coined by Dr. Linetsky because it is a more appropriate nomenclature for the treatment modality which promotes natural healing [1, 19–22].

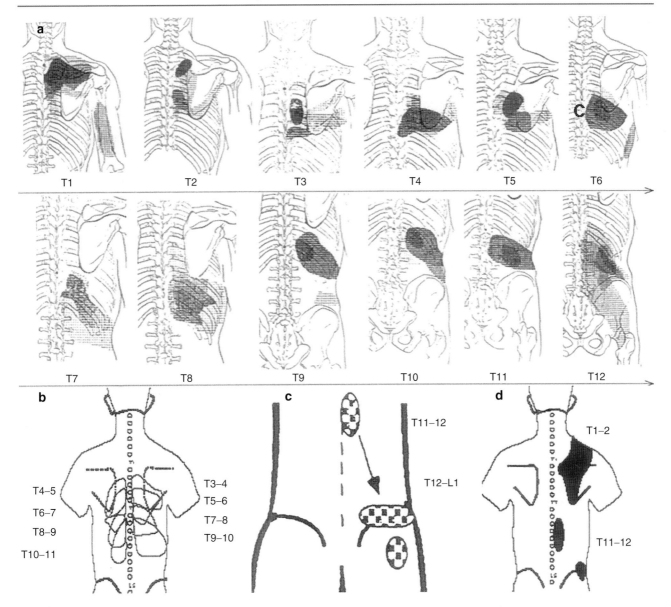

Fig. 81.2 A modified, comparative composition of pain distribution in the thoracic region provoked by injections of hypertonic saline into the interspinous ligaments by Feinstein et al. [2] (Upper two rows – **a**) and thoracic Z-joints (**b**) by Dreyfuss et al. [4], (**c**) by Dussault and Kaplan [5], and (**d**) by Fukui et al. [6]. Significant resemblance of the pain patterns and their overlaps is due to the fact that injected structures receive the same segmental innervated by the thoracic dorsal rami specifically the medial branches (MBDR)

Local Anesthetics in the Diagnosis of Musculoskeletal Pain

Differential diagnosis of musculoskeletal pain based on infiltration of procaine at the fibro-osseous junctions was pioneered in the 1930s by Leriche [16, 19, 22]. Steindler and Luck described that posterior primary rami provide sensory supply to muscles, tendons, thoracolumbar fascia, ligaments, and aponeuroses and their origins and insertions; therefore, no definite diagnosis could be made based on clinical presentation alone. They established the following criteria to prove a causal relationship between the structure and pain symptoms: reproduction of local and referral pain by needle contact, suppression of local tenderness, and referral/radiating pain by procaine infiltration [23]. Haldeman and Soto-Hall [24] infiltrated procaine in to posterior sacroiliac and interspinous ligaments, zygapophyseal joint capsules producing a field block with a marked relaxation of spastic musculature facilitating a routine use of sacroiliac and facet joint manipulations. They have introduced manipulation of axial joints under local anesthesia [24].

The same basic principles have been employed over all of the anatomic areas since the inception of RIT. Local anesthetic diagnostic blocks are still the best available objective confirmation of the precise source of pain in clinical diagnosis [3, 4, 11–17, 22–25].

Fig. 81.3 Modified comparative composition of pain distribution in the lumbar region provoked by injections of hypertonic saline into the (**a**) lumbar interspinous ligaments dots in the midline from Kellgren et al. [7], from lumbar Z-joints, Mooney and Robertson [8] (**b**), and from asymptomatic subjects (**c**) of symptomatic patients (*paravertebral dots*); significant resemblance of the pain patterns and their overlaps is due to the fact that injected structures receive the same segmental innervated by the lumbar dorsal rami specifically the medial branches (MBDR)

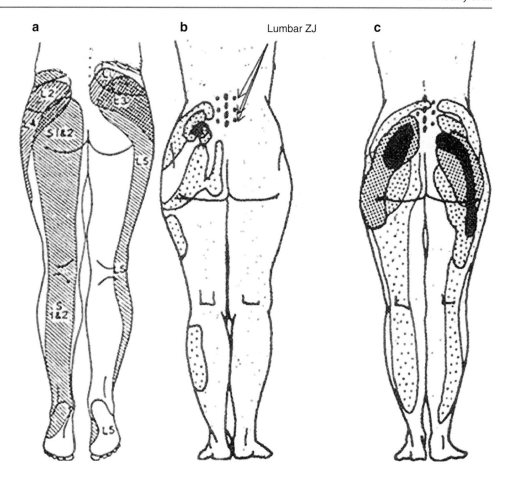

Anatomic Biomechanical and Pathologic Considerations

Ligaments are dull white, dense connective tissue structures that connect adjacent bones. They may be intra-articular, extra-articular, or capsular. Collagen fibers in ligaments may be parallel, oblique, or spiral, each of these orientations contains specific cross-linking formations. Such orientations represent adaptation to specific directions in restriction of joint displacements. Under a light microscope, ligaments have a crimped, wavelike appearance which unfolds during initial loading of collagen [22, 26–28]. When elongated up to 4 % of original length, ligaments and tendons return to their original crimped wave appearance. Beyond 4 % of elongation, they lose elasticity and become permanently laxed, causing joint hypermobility. In degenerated ligaments, subfailure was reported at earlier stages of elongation. At its best, natural healing may restore connective tissue to their pre-injury length, but only 50–75 % of its pre-injury tensile strength [22, 27–30].

There are three types of nerve terminals in posterior spinal ligaments: free nerve endings and the Pacini and the Ruffini corpuscles. A sharp increase in the quantity of free nerve endings at the tips of lumbar spinous processes was documented (Fig. 81.7) [29].

Collagenous tissues are deleteriously affected by nonsteroidal anti-inflammatory drugs (NSAIDs), steroid admin-

istrations, inactivity, and denervation. A single corticosteroid injection into a ligament or tendon has been reported to have debilitating effects on the strength of collagen contained therein [27].

In the presence of repetitive microtrauma with insufficient time for recovery, use of NSAIDs and steroids, tissue hypoxia, metabolic abnormalities, and other less defined causes, connective tissues lose their homeostasis and cycle toward an accelerated degenerative pathway [17, 22, 27, 30, 32–34]. Therefore, a cautious use of anti-inflammatory therapy continues to be a useful, but an adjunctive, therapy [32]. It should be noted that unless homeostasis is reestablished in a joint which the ligament protects, further progressive degenerative changes occur with time when continued laxity is present. A well-known example of this is the development of osteoarthrosis in the knee joint following ACL injury with associated laxity of the joint capsule.

As opposed to ligaments, tendons are glistening whitish collagenous bands interposed between muscle and bone that transmit tensile forces during muscle contraction. There are considerable variations in shape and structure of fibro-osseous attachments and myotendinous junctions. A normal tendon with a cross section of 10 mm in diameter can support a load of 600–1,000 kg [22, 26, 33].

Collagenous tissue response to trauma is inflammatory/regenerative/reparative in nature and varies with the degree

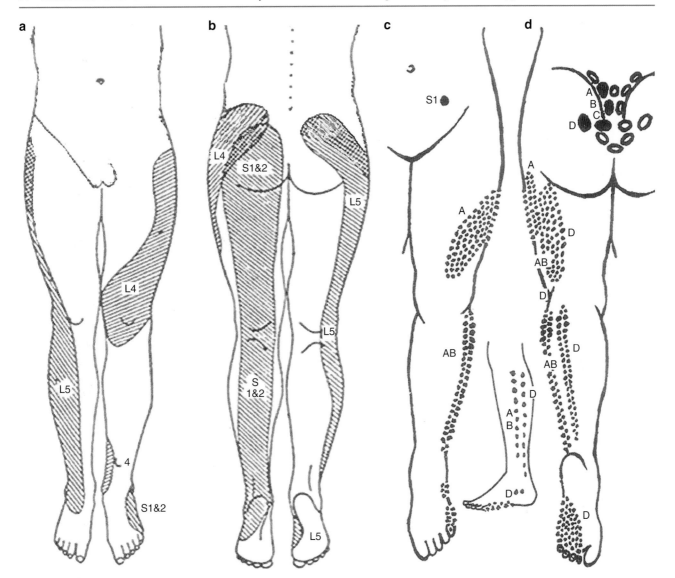

Fig. 81.4 Modified comparative composition of pain distribution from lumbosacral region provoked by injections of hypertonic saline into the (**a**, **b**) interspinous ligaments from L4–5 to S1–2 from Kellgren et al. [7]. (**c**, **d**) Referred pain maps from posterior sacroiliac ligament enthesopathies and sacroiliac joint instability (*AB* from the upper fibers, *CD* lower fibers ileum and sacrum) (Reproduced from Hackett [9]).

Hackett published these maps after abolishing pain with local anesthetic infiltration in more than 7,000 injections over 17 years. Significant resemblance of the pain patterns and their overlaps is due to the fact that injected structures receive the same segmental innervated by the lumbar dorsal rami (Prepared for publication by Felix Linetsky M.D.)

of injury. In the presence of cellular damage, regenerative pathway takes place; in the case of extracellular matrix damage, a combined regenerative/reparative pathway takes place. Both are controlled by hormones, chemical, and growth factors [17, 22, 27, 30, 32–34]. Central denervation, such as in quadriplegia, paraplegia, or hemiplegia, leads to a statistically high, accelerated tendon degeneration [33]. Radiofrequency procedures may not be an exception. Corticosteroids do not arrest or slow the course of degenerative process. Neoneurogenesis and neovasculogenesis are also integral components of degeneration.

The presence of vascular and neural ingrowth into degenerated intervertebral discs, posterior spinal ligaments, the

hard niduses of fibromyalgia, and tennis elbow tendinopathies have been known for some time. Presence of neuropeptides in the facet joint capsules and articular and periarticular tissue of the sacroiliac joints with the absence of inflammatory markers are also well established, rendering the aforementioned structures nociceptive; nonetheless, corticosteroid injections are still the advocated therapeutic interventions [35–39].

More recently, research dedicated to sports medicine shed light on degenerative changes in tendinosis and tendinopathy as a distinct pathologic and clinical entity [40]. The neurovascular ingrowth was studied extensively in Achilles, patellar, and supraspinatus tendinosis. Intratendinous microdialysis

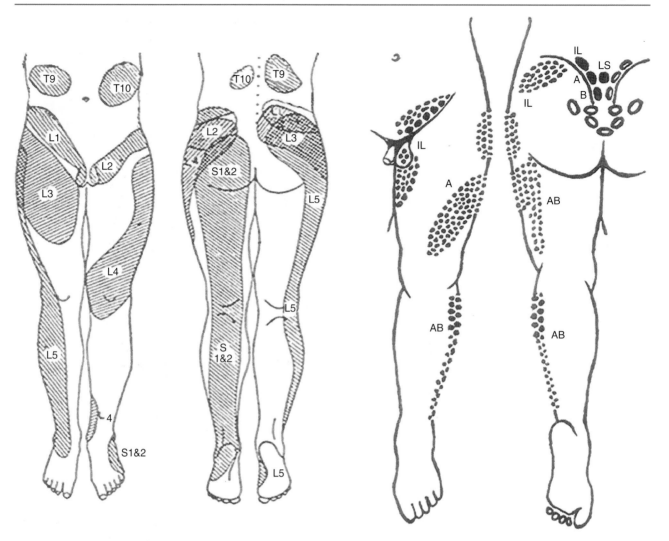

Fig. 81.5 Modified comparative composition of pain distribution from lumbosacral region provoked by injections of hypertonic saline into the (**a, b**) interspinous ligaments from L1–2 to S1–2 from Kellgren et al. [7]. (**c, d**) Trigger areas and referred pain from iliolumbar (*IL*) and posterior sacroiliac (upper *AB*) ligaments (lumbosacral (*LS*) and sacroiliac joint instability). Hackett published these maps after abolishing pain with

local anesthetic infiltration in more than 7,000 injections over 17 years. Significant resemblance of the pain patterns and their overlaps is due to the fact that injected structures are innervated by the same segmental lumbar dorsal rami (From Hackett [9]. Prepared for publication by Felix Linetsky M.D.)

of these tendons found normal prostaglandin E_2 (PGE_2) levels in chronic painful tendinosis. Analyses of biopsies showed no upregulation of pro-inflammatory cytokines. The neurotransmitter glutamate, a potent modulator of pain in the central nervous system, was found in tendinosis. Microdialysis demonstrated significantly higher glutamate levels in chronic painful tendinosis in comparison with pain-free control tendons [41–44]. Significantly, higher lactate levels were found in chronic painful tendinosis in comparison with pain-free normal tendons, implicating either hypoxia or a higher metabolic rate in pathophysiology of tendinosis [45].

Biopsies from the areas with tendinosis and neovascularization followed by immunohistochemical analyses of specimens showed substance P (SP) in the nerves juxtapositioned to the vessels and in the nervi vasorum together with calcitonin gene-related peptide (CGRP) juxtapositioned to the vascular walls [46, 47]. The neurokinin-1 receptor (NK-1R), that is known to have a high affinity for SPP, has been found in the vascular wall [48]. The findings of neuropeptides indicate the presence of a so-called neurogenic inflammation mediated by (SP) – like neuropeptides. The use of diagnostic ultrasound is very helpful in evaluation of tendinosis and

Fig. 81.6 Trigger areas and needle positions for diagnosis and treatment of cervical enthesopathies with small fiber neuropathies and neuralgias with their respective referral pain maps from ligaments and tendons. (*A–C*) Between superior and inferior nuchal lines. *ART* ZJ articular ligaments and periarticular tendons, *IS* Interspinous ligaments (From Hackett [9])

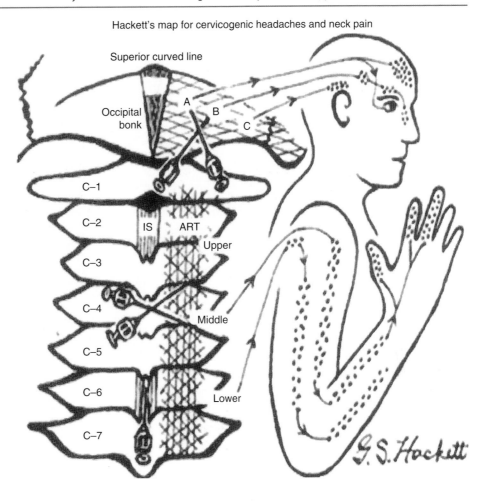

Hackett's map for cervicogenic headaches and neck pain

other musculoskeletal pathology and will be described under radiologic evaluation.

Rationale

The rationale for RIT in chronic painful pathology of ligaments and tendons evolved from clinical, experimental, and histological research performed for injection treatment of hydroceles and hernia. In hydroceles, hypertrophied subserous connective tissue layer reinforced capillary walls and prevented further exudate formation. The same principle is employed in the treatment of chronic bursitis. Conversely in hernias, proliferation and subsequent regenerative/reparative response lead to a fibrotic closure of the defect [17–22].

A similar ability to induce a proliferative regenerative repetitive response in ligaments and tendons was demonstrated in experimental and clinical studies, with a 65 % increased diameter of collagen fibers [18, 49–51]. Multiple recent studies

demonstrated that injecting polidocanol in to the neovascularity proximal to Achilles, patellar, and supraspinatus tendinosis under color Doppler (CD) ultrasound guidance produced an ultrasound-documented resolution of tendinosis and neovascularity, allowing patients return to a full painless activities. Thus, the sclerosing agent acting directly on neovessels is capable of restoring connective tissue homeostasis by modulation of local hemodynamic [52–55].

Clinical Anatomy in Relation to RIT

The shape of a human body is irregularly tubular. This shape, cross-sectionally and longitudinally, is maintained by continuous compartmentalized fascial stacking that incorporates, interconnects, and supports various ligaments, tendons, muscles, neurovascular, and osseous structures. Collagenous connective tissues, despite slightly different biochemical content, blend at their boundaries and at the osseous

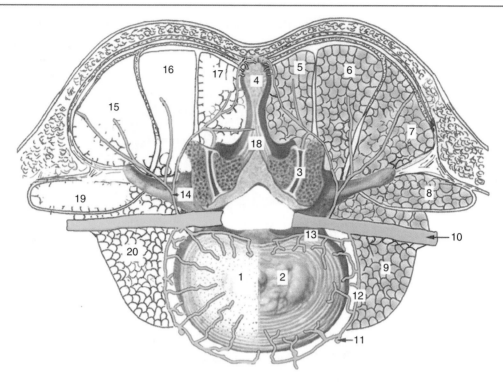

Fig. 81.7 Cross-sectional semi-schematic drawing of lumbar area illustrates *1* vertebral body, *2* intervertebral disc, *3* zygapophyseal joint (*ZJ*), *4* spinous process, *5* multifidus, *6* longissimus thoracis, *7* iliocostalis lumborum, *8* quadratus lumborum, *9* psoas major, *10* ventral ramus, *11* sympathetic trunk, *12* gray ramus communicant, *13* sinuvertebral nerve, *14* dorsal ramus, *15* lateral branch of the dorsal ramus (*LBDR*) in longissimus thoracis compartment, *16* intermediate branch of the dorsal ramus (*IBDR*) in iliocostalis lumborum compartment, *17* medial brunch of the dorsal ramus (*MBDR*) in multifidus compartment, *18* interspinous ligament, *19* quadratus lumborum compartment, and *20* psoas major compartment. MBDR innervates ZJ, multifidi, and interspinous ligaments and forms a several fold increase of the free unmyelinated nerve fibers at the tips of the spinous processes (Modified from Sinelnikov [31]. Modified and prepared for publication by Tracey James. All rights reserved. No part of this picture may be reproduced or transmitted in any form or by any means without written permission from Felix Linetsky M.D.)

structures, functioning as a single unit. This arrangement provides bracing and a hydraulic amplification effect to the muscles, increasing contraction strength up to 30 % (Fig. 81.7) [22, 26, 56–62].

Movements of the extremities, spine, and cranium are achieved through various well-innervated articulations, which are syndesmotic, synovial, and symphysial. For the ease of radiologic evaluation, spinal joints were allocated to the anterior, middle, and posterior columns. Syndesmotic joints are anterior and posterior longitudinal ligaments, anterior and posterior atlantooccipital membranes (ALL and PLL), supraspinous and interspinous ligaments (SSL and ISL), and ligamentum flavum (LF).

Symphysial joints are the intervertebral discs (IVD), which are absent at the cranio-cervical and sacral segments, but present from the sacrococcygeal segments caudally.

Spinal synovial joints are the atlantoaxial (AA), atlantooccipital (AO), zygapophyseal (ZJ), costotransverse (CTJ), and costovertebral (CVJ); sacroiliac (SI) joint is a combined synovial–syndesmotic joint [22, 26, 56, 57].

Differential diagnosis is based on understanding of the regional and segmental anatomy, pathology, as well as segmental, multisegmental, and intersegmental innervation of the compartments and their contents around the spine; this is provided by ventral rami (VR), dorsal rami (DR), gray rami communicants (GRC), sinuvertebral nerves (SVN), and the sympathetic chain (SC) (Fig. 81.7) [22, 26, 56, 57].

Lumbar interspinous ligaments receive innervation from the medial branches of the dorsal rami (MBDR). Three types of nerve terminals in posterior spinal ligaments have been confirmed microscopically. They are the free nerve endings and the Pacini and Ruffini corpuscles. These nerve endings arise from lumbar MB [29]. A sharp increase in the quantity of free nerve endings at the lumbar spinous processes attachments (enthesis) was documented, rendering them putatively nociceptive (Fig. 81.7) [29]. Experimental and empiric observations suggest that a similar arrangement exists at the cervical and thoracic spinous processes, especially at the C2, C7, and T1, rendering them putatively nociceptive (Fig. 81.8) [2, 10, 28, 56]. Willard demonstrated that cervical, thoracic,

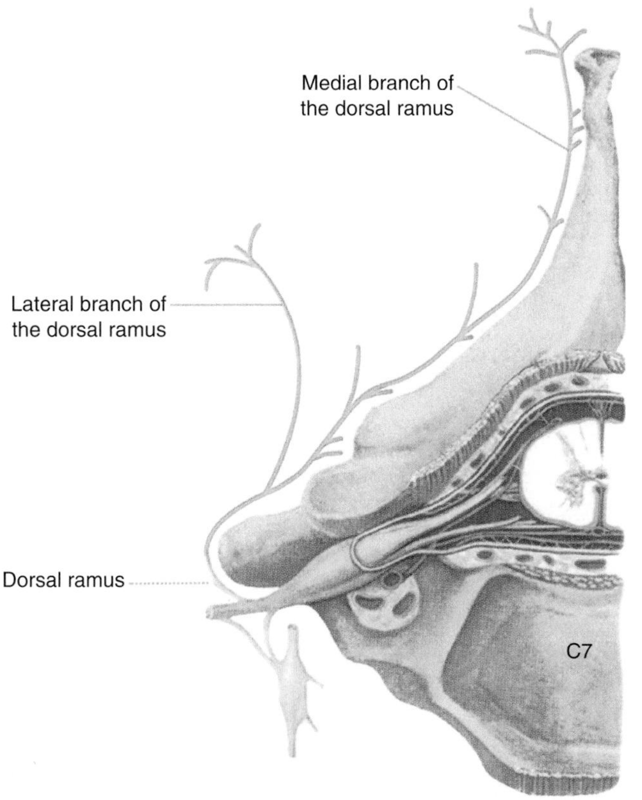

Fig. 81.8 The course of the dorsal ramus proper and its lateral (LBDR) and medial branches (MBDR) represented semi-schematically at the level of C7 (Modified from Sinelnikov [31]. Modified and prepared for publication by Tracey James. All rights reserved. No part of this picture may be reproduced or transmitted in any form or by any means without written permission from Felix Linetsky M.D.)

and lumbar MBs on their distal course are located very close to the bone descending to the very apex of the spinous process, innervating the multifidus and cervical interspinales muscles [28, 56]. A formal recent anatomic study by Zhang et al. reconfirmed these observations in the cervical region [62]. Proximal to the origin, cervical MB is located in the gutter formed by the neighboring ZJ capsules under the semispinalis capitis (SSCa) tendon and supplies twigs to ZJ capsules. Thereafter, MB continues dorsomedially supplying on its course the semispinalis cervices (SSCe) and SSCa. At the mid-lamina level, MB innervates the multifidi and continues adjacent to every spinous process bilaterally below C2 to become a

Thus, MBs do not exclusively supply innervation to the cervical, thoracic, and lumbar ZJ but also to the structures that have enthesis at the spinous processes. This explains the similarity of clinical presentations and the significant overlap of the known pain patterns (Figs. 81.1, 81.2, 81.3, 81.4, 81.5, 81.6, 81.7, and 81.8) [2–4, 10–13, 28, 56, 62].

Current prevailing trends in diagnostic efforts address discogenic, facetogenic, and neurocompressive components of spinal pain. The therapy is directed toward neuromodulation or neuroablation with radiofrequency generators or corticosteroid injections [25]. Example, cervical ZJ is responsible for 54 % of chronic neck pain after whiplash injury; the prevalence may be as high as 65 % [58]. In patients with headaches after whiplash, more than 50 % of the headaches stem from the C2 to C3 z-joint [25, 58]. Intra-articular corticosteroid injections are ineffective in relieving chronic cervical z-joint pain [59]. These statistical data strongly suggest the presence of nociceptors other than ZJ and IVD [22, 25, 58, 59].

Spondyloarthropathies with enthesopathies and muscular, ligamentous, and tendinous pain are rarely, if ever, included in the differential diagnosis or therapeutic plan. The unspoken reasons for this are economical. Major insurance carriers identify the MBDR block as a ZJ block. Any other injections are considered trigger point or ligament injections, and only two ligament or tendon injections or a maximum of three trigger point injections with corticosteroids are reimbursed during the same office visit at a very low rate. The fact that there may be several nociceptors in the same area in the same patient at the same time is disregarded.

The other reason can be explained by the spinal uncertainty principle. In a simple example of two motion segments, the disc, facets, and musculotendinous compartments are each considered as one putative nociceptive unit, the total number of clinically indistinguishable combinations rises to 63 possibilities. It is practically impossible to address such a magnitude of possibilities under fluoroscopic guidance.

In the majority of cases, RIT can be done without radiologic guidance, taking innervation into account. Therefore, it can afford evaluation of many putative nociceptors from the variety of pain presentations and offers a practical advantage that can be accomplished during the same procedure (Fig. 81.9). The syndromes and conditions treated with RIT are listed in Table 81.1 [11, 17–22, 39, 52–55, 57, 60–84].

Clinical Presentation and Evaluation

The list of syndromes and conditions gives the reader the idea that there is a wide variety of presenting complaints including headaches, neck pain, low back pain, pain between the shoulders, mid-scapular pain, pain mimicking pleurisy or various radiculopathies, thoracolumbar area pain, occipital and suboccipital pain, low back and hip pain, neck and shoulder pain, sharp pain with difficulty breathing, tail bone pain with difficulty seating, and any combination of these symptoms. The intensity, duration, and quality of pain are variable, and the onset may be sudden or gradual. The evaluation may reveal postural abnormalities, functional asymmetries, and combinations of kyphoscoliosis, flattening of cervical

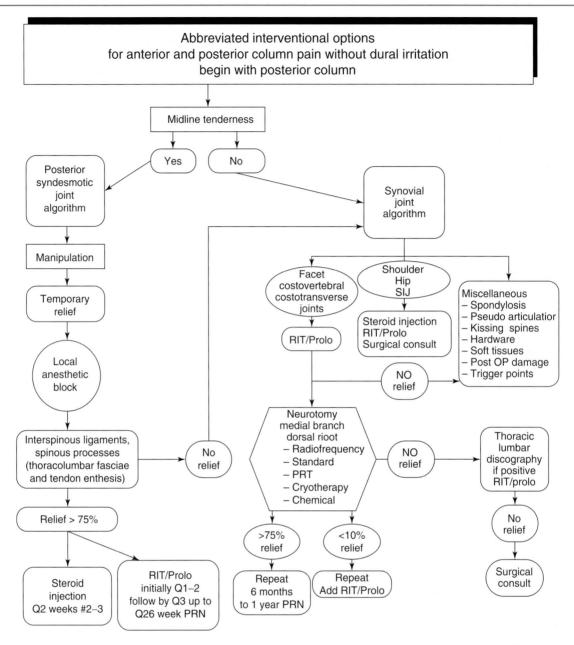

Fig. 81.9 Self-explanatory, modified, abbreviated excerpt from interventional options for spinal and paravertebral pain without dural irritation including large synovial joints (From Linetsky et al. [57])

and lumbar lordosis, and arm or leg length discrepancies. A wide range of increased or restricted passive and active range of motions as well as frank deformities of axial or peripheral joints may be present.

Contractions against resistance usually denote a tendon-related pain, whereas passive attempts to bring a joint to the anatomic range indicate a ligament-related pain. The most reliable, objective clinical finding is tenderness which may be present at the fibro-osseous junction (enthesis) or at the midsubstance of a muscle, ligament, or tendon. Such areas of tenderness are identified and marked and become the sub-

ject of ultrasound investigation and eventually needle probing "needling" and local anesthetic block. The needle placement at the areas of maximum tenderness usually reproduces the pain that becomes temporarily worse during infiltration of local anesthetic and usually subsides within 10–15 s after infiltration. Such diagnostic blocks may be performed with or without fluoroscopic or ultrasound guidance. Abolishment or persistence of tenderness and or local or referred pain concludes the clinical examination and becomes the basis for clinical diagnosis (Figs. 81.9 and 81.10) [11, 22, 57, 63–65].

Table 81.1 The syndromes and conditions treated with RIT

Barre–Lieou syndrome	Acromioclavicular sprain/arthrosis
Cervicocranial syndrome (cervicogenic headaches)	Scapulothoracic crepitus
Temporomandibular pain and dysfunction syndrome	Rotator cuff syndrome: supraspinatus, infraspinatus, subscapularis tendinosis, or impingement
Whiplash injury syndrome, spasmodic torticollis	Proximal and distal biceps tendinosis
Cervical and cervicothoracic spinal pain of "unknown" origin	Tennis and golfer's elbow
Cervicobrachial syndrome (shoulder/neck pain)	Baastrup's disease – kissing spine
Snapping scapulae syndrome or scapulothoracic crepitus	Recurrent shoulder dislocations
Hyperextension/hyperflexion injury whiplash syndromes	Myofascial pain syndrome
Cervical, thoracic, and lumbar facet syndromes	Ehlers–Danlos syndrome
Cervical, thoracic, and lumbar sprain/strain	Marie–Strumpell disease
Cervical, thoracic, and lumbar disc syndrome	Internal disc derangement
Slipping rib syndrome	Failed back surgery syndrome
Costotransverse and costovertebral joint arthrosis pain and subluxations	Low back pain syndrome
Sternoclavicular arthrosis and repetitive sprain and subluxations	Iliac crest syndrome
Acromioclavicular arthrosis and instability	Friction rib syndrome
Repetitive thoracic segmental dysfunction	Sacroiliac joint sprain/strain and instability
Costosternal arthrosis/arthritis	Groin pull/sprain/strain
Tietze's syndrome/costochondritis/chondrosis	Coccydynia syndrome
Interchondral arthrosis	Groin sprains
Xiphoidalgia syndrome	Snapping hip syndrome
	Gluteus minimus and medius tendinosis
	Trochanteric tendinosis
	Patellar tendinosis
	Osgood Schlatter disease
	Achilles tendinosis

Radiologic Evaluation Relevant to RIT

Plain Radiographs

Plain radiographs are of limited diagnostic value in painful pathology of the connective tissue, but may indirectly suggest the presence of such pathology by detecting structural or positional osseous abnormalities, like anterior or posterior listhesis on flexion/extension lateral views and degenerative changes in general with deformities of the osseous and articular components such as osteophyte formations in various parts of the skeleton, ectopic calcifications, and improperly healed fractures [66].

Magnetic Resonance Imaging (MRI)

MRI may detect the pathology of intervertebral disc, ligamentous injury, interspinous bursitis, enthesopathy, ZJ disease, SIJ pathology, neural foramina pathology, bone contusion, infection, fracture, or neoplasia. Magnetic resonance imaging may exclude or confirm spinal cord disease and pathology related to extramedullary, intradural, and epidural spaces. MRI detects cartilage abnormality, degenerative

tendon and ligament pathology, tendinosis, joint effusions, bursitis, soft tissue edema, hematoma, ligament tendon and muscle rupture, and vascular abnormalities [66, 67].

Computed Tomography Scans (CT)

CT scan may detect small avulsion fractures of facets, laminar fracture, fracture of vertebral bodies and pedicles, and neoplastic or degenerative changes in the axial or appendicular skeleton [66].

Bone Scan

Bone scans are useful in assessing entire skeleton to evaluate for metabolically active disease processes [66].

Diagnostic Ultrasound

Gray scale (GS) ultrasound can detect in real time joint effusions, bursitis, cystic formations, synovial hypertrophy, cartilage abnormality, muscle atrophy, attenuation or partial

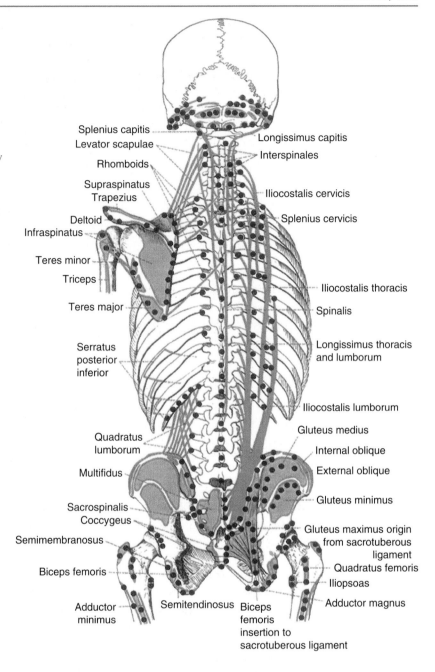

Fig. 81.10 Schematic drawing demonstrating sites of tendon origins and insertions (enthesis) of the paravertebral musculature in the cervical, thoracic, lumbar, and pelvic regions with parts of the upper and lower extremities. Clinically significant enthesopathies with small fiber neuropathies and neuralgias are common at the locations identified by *dots*. *Dots* also represent most common locations of needle insertion and RIT injections (Note: Not all of the locations are treated in each patient) (Modified from Sinelnikov [31]. Modified and prepared for publication by Tracey James. All rights reserved. No part of this picture may be reproduced or transmitted in any form or by any means without written permission from Felix Linetsky M.D.)

disruptions of ligaments, tendons or muscles, ectopic calcifications, tendon enlargement, inhomogeneity in tendinosis, and nerve hypertrophy like in carpal tunnel syndrome. Nerve and tendon subluxations or impingements are evaluated with dynamic ultrasound. GS ultrasound provides real-time needle guidance during various diagnostic or therapeutic injections including aspirations, nerve blocks, and percutaneous needle tenotomy. Ultrasound is becoming a more useful tool in the assessment of myofascial and osseous pain sources because it allows a dynamic pattern recognition as well as direct evaluation and patterning in superficial collagenous structures. Ultrasound is now a preferred method to evaluate rotator cuff pathology in the office setting and is

gaining popularity in knee joint evaluation prior to arthroscopy.

The color Doppler (CD) ultrasound can detect neovascularities to be injected, when present, in tendinosis or synovitis and delineate positions of large vessels and nerves to be avoided during injections [52–55, 68, 69]. Unless the practitioner is very experienced in MSK, ultrasound correlations with plain radiographs, MRI, CT scans, and palpation are highly advisable. There are a multitude of weekend courses in musculoskeletal ultrasound; the industry is promoting the methodology, but the high quality hands on supervised training is not yet available at the academic institutions for the practicing physicians. Gaining a supervised high-quality experience takes time.

Solutions for Injections

Local anesthetics are an important component of the solutions used for RIT and were described under the heading of *Local Anesthetics in the Diagnosis of Musculoskeletal Pain*. When contemporary local anesthetics are combined with hyperosmolar injectates, they provide long-lasting diagnostic/therapeutic blocks, and the reasons for this scientifically proven effect will be described below.

Five types of injectates are used for RIT, and they are:

1. Osmotic shock agents such as hypertonic dextrose, glycerin, or distilled water
2. Chemical irritants such as phenol
3. Chemotactic sclerosing agents such as sodium morrhuate, Sotradecol, or polidocanol
4. Particulates such as pumice suspension
5. Biologic agents such as whole blood, platelet-rich plasma (PRP), autologous conditioned serum (ACS), platelet-poor plasma (PPP), adipose-derived and bone marrow aspirate concentrates with their mesenchymal and hematopoietic biocellular components, and isolated and cultured mesenchymal stem cells

The injectates in groups 1–4 have been used as a single agent in various concentrations or in various combinations with other chemical agents, and their concentrations are mixed with local anesthetics, by the virtue of being injected into connective tissue, all of them become irritants [57, 60, 61, 63–65, 71–74]. Injectates in group 5 are also used as a single injectate agent in various concentrations or in various combinations of the agents and their concentrations.

Experimental studies demonstrated that any solution with osmolality greater than a 1,000 mOsm/l is *neurolytic*, causing separation of the myelin lamellae in myelinated nerve fibers and total destruction in unmyelinated fibers, after soaking for 1 h in solutions with osmolality greater than 1,000 mOsm/l or a distilled water. Hypoosmolar solutions produce a reversible conduction block of rabbit vagus nerve and potentiate the local anesthetics. C fibers showed evidence of axonal damage characterized by accumulation of macrophages and proliferation of Schwann cells. Osmotic fragility of axons is similar to that of erythrocytes after exposure to 0.4 and 0.5 dilutions of normal saline. When administered intrathecally, local anesthetics are more effective in hypobaric solution than in hyperbaric solution [85–88]. In humans, intrathecal hypertonic saline produced good results in chronic intractable pain and is currently used in epidurolysis of adhesions [17, 89–91]. Hypertonic/hyperosmolar dextrose has been successfully used for treatment of enthesopathies with small fiber neuropathies, spondyloarthropathies, and internal disc derangements [1, 11, 17, 19–22, 57, 73, 74].

Pharmacologic *properties of phenol, glycerin, and hypertonic dextrose are both neurolytic and inflammatory*. Various concentrations of water- and glycerin-based phenol solutions have been used to treat pain. The literature suggests that perineural phenol glycerin combinations produce a better regenerative/reparative response; these experimental findings support the use of phenol glycerin or phenol glycerin dextrose solutions in treatment of axial and peripheral enthesopathies with small fiber neuropathies and neuralgias [92–102].

Neurolytic intra-articular injections of a 10 % aqueous phenol, diluted to 5 % with omnipaque or omniscan contrast and local anesthetic, are used in the Pain Management Department of Mayo Clinic to facilitate nursing care in severely debilitated patients [103].

Diluted 5 % phenol in 50 % glycerin solution is used for the treatment of spinal enthesopathies and injections at donor harvest sites of the iliac crest for neurolytic and regenerative/reparative responses. Prior to injection, 1 ml of this solution is mixed with 4 ml of local anesthetic 1,086 mOsm/l [63, 64]. The most common solutions contain lidocaine/dextrose mixtures in various concentrations. Lidocaine is available in 0.5–2 %; dextrose is available in a 50 % concentration.

To achieve a 10 % dextrose concentration, dilution is made with lidocaine in 4:1 proportions (i.e., 4 ml of 1 % lidocaine is mixed with 1 ml of 50 % dextrose) and will produce a 0.8 % lidocaine with osmolality of 555 mOsm/l (*hyperosmolar block*).

To achieve a 12.5 % dextrose concentration, dilution is made with lidocaine in 3:1 proportions (i.e., 3 ml of 1 % lidocaine mixed with 1 ml of 50 % dextrose) and will produce a 0.75 % lidocaine with osmolality of 694 mOsm/l (*hyperosmolar block*).

To achieve a 20 % dextrose concentration, dilution is made with lidocaine in 3:2 proportion (i.e., 3 ml of 1 % lidocaine mixed with 2 ml of 50 % dextrose) and will produce a 0.6 % lidocaine with osmolality of 1,110 mOsm/l (*hyperosmolar neurolytic block*). In two studies, this solution produced a 50 % reduction in low back pain lasting for 2 years.

A 1:1 dilution makes a 25 % dextrose concentration with 0.5 lidocaine solution with osmolality of 1,388 mOsm/l (*hyperosmolar neurolytic block*). In two studies, this solution was used for intradiscal injections.

Dextrose/phenol/glycerin (DPG) solution is referred to as DPG or P2G and contains dextrose and glycerin in equal 25 % amounts, 2.5 % phenol and water. Prior to injection, DPG is diluted in concentrations of 1:2=1,368 mOsm/l, 1:1=2,052 mOsm/l, or 2:3=1,641 mOsm/l with a local anesthetic.

When dextrose-containing solutions are not controlling pain and dysfunction, progression to stronger solutions such as sodium morrhuate, Sotradecol, or polidocanol has been used in various dilutions up to a full strength.

Five percent sodium morrhuate is a mixture of sodium salts of saturated and unsaturated fatty acids of cod liver oil and 2 % benzyl alcohol (chemically very similar to phenol), which acts as both a local anesthetic and a preservative.

This is very well tolerated in selective patients with rheumatoid arthritis or ankylosing spondyloarthropathies, personal observation of the senior author.

Sotradecol® (sodium tetradecyl sulfate injection) is a sterile nonpyrogenic solution for intravenous use as a sclerosing agent. Three percent (30 mg/ml) with 2 % benzyl alcohol: Each mL contains sodium tetradecyl sulfate 30 mg and benzyl alcohol 20 mg. It can be used interchangeably with sodium morrhuate; clinical results are similar, but there is a lesser possibility of allergic reactions.

Polidocanol is a nonionic detergent, containing a polar hydrophilic (dodecyl alcohol) and an apolar hydrophobic (polyethylene oxide) chain as active ingredients. On March 31, 2010, the US Food and Drug Administration (FDA) approved polidocanol injection for the treatment of small varicose veins. Polidocanol is a local anesthetic and antipruritic component of ointments and bath additives. The substance is also used as a sclerosant, an irritant injected to treat varicose veins. Professor Alfredson has extensively used 1 % polidocanol in 1–2 ml increments for the treatment of tendinosis [52–55].

Pumice suspension: Pumice is a substance of volcanic origin consisting chiefly of complex silicates of aluminum, potassium, and sodium. Pumice is insoluble in water and is not attacked by acids or alkali solutions. It is used in this preparation as a material irritant to stimulate the fibrosing process. Extra fine grade is defined as one that passes a 325 mesh sieve at 84 % or more, and only a trace is retained by a 200 mesh sieve:

- Pumice (extra fine grade) – 1.0 g.
- Glycerin – 5.0 ml.
- Polysorbate 80–0.09 ml (2 standard drops).
- Preservatives q.s.
- Lidocaine 1–2 % q.s. ad 100 cc.
- Place in a multidose bottle, sterilize, and shake well before use.

Two to three milliliter of this suspension is drawn in a 10-ml syringe mixed with dextrose formula of a choice or alone. Drawing in to the syringe should be done through the same gage needle that will be used for injection. Suspension was developed by Dr. Gedney for injections of sacroiliac ligaments to stabilize SI and lumbosacral joints [19–22].

Biocellular autografts include whole blood, platelet-rich plasma (PRP), autologous conditioned serum (ACS), platelet-poor plasma (PPP), and adipose- and bone marrow-derived aspirate concentrates with mesenchymal and hematopoietic components [104–109]. Widely popularized and accepted in recent years, these autografts are composed of three ingredients used separately or together:

1. PRP or ACS provides platelet concentrates with cytokines and growth factors.
2. Autologous fat cells provide a living collagen bioscaffold with its intrinsic stromal vascular tissue transferred in the form of a graft or a lyophilized collagen in the form of an injectate which may be utilized as a cellular bioscaffold matrix.

3. Lipoaspirates or adipose tissue plus/minus bone marrow aspirate concentrate provides stromal vascular fraction with supporting mesenchymal stem cells.

PRP is a platelet concentrate of four- to eight-fold above baseline levels that contain signal proteins, platelet-derived growth factors, chemokines, and cytokines that control inflammatory cascade. Autologous conditioned serum (ACS or ACP) contains platelet concentrations of two to three-fold baseline levels, and whole blood contains platelet levels at baseline. It remains a point of debate in the literature which autograft provides a superior collagen growth. It may depend on the structure to be regenerated which level of chemokine and cytokine concentration or MSC concentration or pure scaffold regeneration proves most helpful.

PRP is a reach source of important signal proteins (cytokines) and a variety of growth factors (GF) critical to initiation and maintenance of the entire inflammatory cascade in vivo. Many studies have shown the effectiveness of these GFs in healing.

Bone marrows concentrate with or without supporting matrix releases chemokines and cytokines. Growth factors are known to be a major player in vascular remodeling. The platelets in a bone marrow concentrate upon activation secrete stromal-derived factor (SDF-1). This supports primary adhesion and migration of progenitor cells to the site of injury. Bone marrow stroma contains plastic adherent cells (colony-forming unit fibroblast, CFU-F) that can give rise to a broad spectrum of fully differentiated connective tissues [105–107].

Adipose-derived mesenchymal stem cells (AD-MSCs) also contribute to the growth factor load through direct secretion of growth factors (autocrine amplification system), such as vascular endothelial growth factor (VEGF), insulin-like growth factor 1 (IGF-1), IGF-2, and hepatocyte growth factor. Additional benefits of adipose tissue comparing to bone marrow are greater concentration of mesenchymal stem cells, ready availability, ease and rapidity of harvesting, lower morbidity, and diminished cost. In addition, adipose tissues possess properties which serve as an ideal living bioscaffold or matrix [106, 107].

PRP concentrates are obtained by venous blood draw of 20–120 cc. Centrifugation produces the buffy coat fraction. Various manufacturers utilize proprietary techniques to remove the neutrophils with the intent of maintaining the monocyte fraction along with the platelet fraction of spun cells. The amount of cytotoxicity of neutrophils in vivo is currently a point of contention in the literature. It is therefore up to the practitioner to decide if they wish to manufacture platelet concentrates via a two spin centrifugation technique or utilize a proprietary solution on the market [108, 109].

Bone marrow aspirates are obtained via 12-ga. multiport aspiration needle with a stylet placed within the iliac crest or other appropriate marrow cavity, and 60–120 cc of marrow is aspirated in small aliquots obtained from multiple positions within the marrow cavity. This gives variable numbers of

CD34+ cells in a matrix of total nucleated cells. The total number of cells is based on the aspiration and centrifugation technique. Manufacturer and independent tests are available to measure cell counts [105].

Lipoaspirates, or autologous fat grafting (AFG), are used extensively in aesthetic and reconstructive surgery over the past 20 years. A closed syringe system (Tulip Medical) and cell-friendly microcannulas allow a safe and effective harvest of volumes ranging from 10 to 20 cc. Combined with thrombin-activated PRP, this injectate is accurately placed by guided ultrasonography into damaged muscular, tenoligamentous, and cartilaginous tissue [107].

Practical note: The physician should examine the state and federal laws of their respective practice location to determine what level of cellular processing is permissible under current law.

Isolated and Expanded Stem Cells

Mesenchymal stem cells (MSCs), also known as marrow stromal cells, derive from mesodermal tissues and are pluripotent adult stem cells with therapeutic potential in regenerative medicine [110–116]. It has been shown recently that MSCs are a heterogeneous population of similar cells rather than one distinct cell type [117]. As a result, outside of the ability to select cells via adhesion culture and a handful of hallmark surface markers, there is still no uniformly accepted definition of an MSC [118].

As stated above, MSCs can be easily isolated from many different tissues, including a whole bone marrow aspirate, marrow mobilized whole blood, muscle biopsy, adipose liposuction aspirate, and other tissues [110]. As a rule, the closer the graft source to the treated tissue, the more efficient are the MSCs to differentiate into to the treated tissue type. For example, Vidal compared equine MSCs derived from the bone marrow to ones derived from adipose tissue for their chondrogenic potential and found that bone marrow MSCs produced a more hyaline-like matrix and had improved glycosaminoglycan production [119]. Animal studies demonstrated that bone marrow MSC produced better repair of a tibial osteochondral defect when compared to adipose MSCs [120]. Yoshimura determined that MSCs derived from the synovial tissue of the knee (closest to the target tissue of cartilage defect) produced a better chondrogenesis than bone marrow MSCs [121].

MSC Culture Expansion

A limited amount of cells can be obtained from any tissue. In many instances, the number that can be harvested from the source tissue is less than the quantity of cells needed for tissue repair. One method to obtain larger numbers of cells is to culture them. A delicate balance exists between length of time in culture (which produces more cells) and adverse consequences to the cells (such as genetic transformation).

MSCs are usually expanded in a culture via monolayer. MSCs are placed into a specialized flask and allowed to attach to a plastic surface and fed with a nutrient broth. Because MSCs are contact inhibited, they will grow on this surface until they become confluent at which point they abruptly stop growing. To keep MSCs proliferating in culture, when the colonies are near confluence, the nonadherent cells in the media are discarded and an enzyme is used to detach the MSCs from the plastic surface. The MSCs are then replated in a similar flask, and fresh media is added. Most MSCs are grown in culture for 11–17 days, because some studies have shown decreased differentiation if MSCs are grown for prolonged periods in culture with a higher chance of genetic mutation [122–125].

How Do the MSCs Affect Tissue Repair?

Animal studies have demonstrated the multipotency of MSCs and their ability to differentiate into muscle, bone, cartilage, tendon, and various cells of internal organs. However, these cells also act via paracrine mechanisms to assist in tissue repair. In this context, paracrine is defined as the production of certain growth factors and cytokines by the MSCs which can assist in tissue repair [126].

Donor Versus Autologous MSC Sources

Obviously, autologous stem cells do not have the risk of communicable disease transmission as donor allogeneic cells. However, there are reasons why donor cells are attractive. For example, some studies have shown a decreased differentiation potential for MSCs obtained from older patients [127]. In addition, somatic genetic variants (i.e., trisomy V and VII) have been demonstrated in the MSCs and osteoprogenitors of some patients with osteoarthritis [128].

Use of MSC in Musculoskeltal Diathesis

MSCs have been used in animal and early clinical studies to repair meniscal tissue, cartilage, and intervertebral discs. Izuta et al. demonstrated meniscus repair after MSCs transplant on a fibrin matrix [129]. Horie reported that synovial-derived MSCs after injection into massive rat meniscus tears were able to differentiate and repair meniscal tissue [130]. Yamasaki et al. repopulated devitalized meniscus with MSCs and demonstrated biomechanical properties approximating the normal meniscus [131].

The earliest models of cartilage repair used autologous, cultured chondrocytes [132]; others used MSCs because MSCs have shown innate cartilage repair properties through both differentiation and paracrine signaling [133]. In these studies, an osteochondral defect (OCD) was created, and the MSCs were implanted into the lesion, often in a hydrogel or other carrier or at times through local adherence [134–137]. Partial to robust healing of the OCD takes place over weeks to months [110]. The cartilage produced by these cells was very much like native hyaline cartilage, but subtle differences have been observed [138].

Traditional spinal surgery on degenerated intervertebral discs (IVDs) continues to show disappointing results [139–141]. Conversely, animal studies have shown robust repair of acutely injured IVDs [142–148]. For example, Sakai et al. have published animal models whereby MSCs are combined with atelocollagen and achieved disc repair with improvements in hydration, height, and disc morphology demonstrated on MRI [149]. Richardson et al. and Risbud et al. investigating the coculturing of MSCs with cells from the nucleus pulposus (NP) demonstrated that this technique can produce partially differentiated cells that are capable of repopulating the NP in an animal model [150, 151]. Finally, Miyamoto et al. recently demonstrated that intra-discal transplantation of synovial-derived MSCs prevented disc degeneration through suppression of catabolic genes and perhaps proteoglycan production [152].

Biocellular injectates such as whole blood and PRP are extremely irritating immediately upon injection. Regional pain blocks have therefore become an important adjunct in the treatment paradigm with biocellular autografts. If used with inadequate or improperly placed local anesthesia, even under US guidance, these agents produce overwhelming non-localized deep somatic pain lasting for up to 10 min which subsides to a tolerable level after about 30 min and which follows a typical primary, secondary, and tertiary curve for collagen maturation with the pain levels inherent therein. Thus, pain subsides over the secondary cellular maturation time frame of 6–8 weeks resulting in a pain-free state. Intra-articular hip injections of PRP with or without bioscaffold, in the presence of significant degenerative changes, when used with local anesthesia under US guidance produce a significant pain that subsides to a preinjection level in about 2 weeks.

Clinical Effectiveness

Multiple publications on RIT include randomized trials [63, 72, 75–77, 153], non-randomized publications, and prospective and retrospective clinical studies as well as case reports [65, 78] and systematic reviews [78]. In one of the systematic reviews of prolotherapy injections for chronic low back pain, Yelland et al. [78] included four randomized high-quality

trials with a total of 344 patients. Two of these four studies [72, 76] demonstrated significant differences between the treatment and control group. However, Yelland et al. [78] could not pooled their results because in the study of Ongley et al. [76], manipulation allegedly confounded independent evaluation of results. And in the other study by Kline et al., there was no significant difference in mean pain and disability scores between the groups [72]. The third study was demonstrated no improvement in either group [77]. The fourth study was the earlier one of Yelland et al. reporting only mean pain and disability scores of 40 patients in each group [75] showed no difference between groups. But in each group, there was more than 50 % improvement maintained for more than 2 years. Therefore, Yelland et al.'s [75] study clearly demonstrated that relatively large volumes of normal saline injected in the low back ligaments are therapeutic and are not a placebo. The conclusions of this systematic review were confusing and unrealistic such as that there was conflicting evidence regarding the efficacy of prolotherapy injections in reducing pain and disability in patients with chronic low back pain or that in the presence of co-interventions, prolotherapy injections were more effective than controlled injections, more so when both injections and co-interventions were controlled concurrently.

Another controlled trial is eliminated from the systematic review because it could not be pooled by Wilkinson [63] who demonstrated that when specific diagnosis is applied, the positive results approach 89 %. There is substantial evidence from non-randomized prospective and retrospective studies as well as case reports that cannot be discussed here due to a limited size of this publication [17–22, 65]. Similar results were demonstrated by Alfredson et al. in peripheral tendinosis [52–55] and Topol et al. in groin strains [79–83].

The growing use of biologic agents deserves a special attention. The clinical translation of MSCs from the lab to the bedside is already taking place; Centeno et al. published early case studies in which positive MRI changes were observed in knees and hip joints after MSC injections [143–145]. They have also noted that the complication rate of expanded MSC injection procedures is no greater than other needle-based interventional techniques [146]. Their submitted publication data on 339 patients demonstrated a safety profile better than surgical techniques such as total knee arthroplasty. They have recently submitted for publication a large case series of 250 knee and hip osteoarthritis patients treated with percutaneous injection of MSCs. Prior to MSC injections, two-thirds of the knee patients were total knee arthroplasty (TKA) candidates, only 6 % of the patients opted for TKA after the injections; additionally, both treated groups reported better relief than an untreated comparative group.

Other authors have described similar safety profiles using more invasive surgical implant techniques. Wakatani published an 11-year prospective study of 45 knees (in 41 patients) treated with autologous bone marrow-derived MSCs, with results indicating both safety and efficacy [147]. Nejadnik recently described a comparison between surgically implanted chondrocytes versus MSCs placed by needle in 72 knees [153]. The MSC-treated knees demonstrated good safety, less donor site morbidity, and better efficacy when compared with an autologous chondrocyte implantation procedure. Haleem has noted that autologous, cultured bone marrow MSCs reimplanted into articular cartilage defects in platelet-rich fibrin demonstrated evidence of healed cartilage in some patients [148].

While very little has been published on intervertebral disc repair in humans, some clinical data is available. Yoshikawa recently published on two patients who were treated with surgically implanted MSCs that showed less vacuum phenomenon on follow-up imaging [142]. The only other human data of which we are aware is produced by Centeno's group from 2005 to 2010, under IRB supervision and now being prepared for publication (unpublished data). Replicating the Sakai study [149] wherein cultured MSCs were placed into the disc produced little measureable results, their experience was similar. However, a third case series performed with changes in culture, injection technique, and diagnostic criteria (changed from degenerative disc disease DDD to chronic disc bulge with lumbar radiculopathy). The last model showed encouraging clinical and imaging results. Presented literature, especially newer publications, does offer convincing evidence of RIT efficacy in carefully selected patients, when specific diagnostic entities are treated and strict diagnostic criteria and injection techniques are applied [52–55, 63, 78–84, 142–148].

neovascularities ventral to Achilles tendon, restoration of normal longitudinal microcirculation was documented by power Doppler. Chemomodulation of collagen through inflammatory, proliferative, and regenerative/reparative response is induced by the chemical and pharmacologic properties of all injectates and mediated by cytokines and multiple growth factors.

A relatively large volume of osmotically inert or active injectate assumes the role of a space-occupying lesion in a relatively tight, slowly equilibrating, extracellular compartment of the connective tissue. Inert injectates are also used to disrupt adhesions that have been created by the original inflammatory attempts to heal the injury or for hydrodissection of fibrotic bands.

Temporary repetitive stabilization of the painful hypermobile joints, induced by inflammatory response to the injectates, provides a better environment for regeneration and repair of the affected ligaments and tendons.

Compression of cells by relatively large extracellular volume as well as cell expansion or constriction due to osmotic properties of injectate stimulates the release of intracellular growth factors. Cellular and extracellular matrix damage induced by mechanical transection with the needle stimulates inflammatory cascade, governing release of growth factors [11, 12, 17–22, 49–55, 57, 63–65, 71–104].

Indications for regenerative injection therapy are listed in Table 81.2. General contraindications are those that are applicable to all of the injection techniques. A list of general contraindications is presented in Table 81.3.

Mechanism of Action of Chemical Injectates

Based on literature review [11, 12, 17–22, 49–55, 57, 63–65, 71–104] and the above described pharmacologic properties of the injectates, current understanding of the mechanism of action is complex and multifaceted. Obviously, *phenol- and glycerin*-containing solutions, depending on concentration, produce *temporary neurolysis or neuromodulation* of peripheral nociceptors and provide modulation of antidromic, orthodromic, sympathetic, and axon reflex transmissions. Modulation of sympathetic transmission via nervi vasorum leads to modulation of local hemodynamics in tendons, ligaments, and bone; this in turn decreases blood pressure which leads to pain reduction. Hyper-/hypoosmolar injectates provide the same initial action; purple discoloration of the skin is frequently observed after injection of several adjacent interspinous ligaments.

Conversely, sclerosants act initially on modulation of hemodynamics with subsequent regression of neoneurogenesis. When sclerosant was deposited into pathologic

Vertebral and Paravertebral Injection Sites and Techniques

Any innervated structure is a potential pain generator. The same nerve usually supplies several structures; therefore, there is a significant overlap of all known pain maps (Figs. 81.1, 81.2, 81.3, 81.4, 81.5, and 81.6). The main question is, "How to navigate in this sea of unknown?" For the purpose of RIT, the following step by step approach is implemented. Patients' "pain and tenderness" is accepted for face value without dismissal or allocation to a distant "proven" source. The *knowledge of clinical anatomy, pain patterns, and pathology guiding the clinical investigation* is based on clinical experiments of many researchers over decades. Diagnostic ultrasound may reveal tendinosis and neovascularities in the tender areas.

Tenderness over posterior column structures is an objective finding, especially in the midline, as is the rebound tenderness in any abdominal quadrant [17, 22, 57, 63–65, 104]. The tender areas are identified by palpation and marked.

Table 81.2 Indications for regenerative injection therapy

Cervicogenic headaches	Osteoarthritis, osteoarthrosis/arthritis, spondylolysis, osteochondrosis and spondylolisthesis
Unhealed fractures, pseudoarthrosis	Rheumatoid arthritis with osteoarthritis
Chronic enthesopathies, tendinosis or ligamentosis with small fiber neuropathies and neuralgias after sprains/strains or overuse occupational and postural conditions known as repetitive motion disorders (RMD)	Peripheral nerve and tendon entrapments
Small unhealed painful intersubstance ruptures of muscles ligaments and tendons	Osgood Schlatter disease
Internal disc derangement (cervical, thoracic, lumbar)	Postsurgical cervical, thoracic, and low back pain (with or without instrumentation)
Painful hypermobility and instability of the axial and peripheral joints due to capsular laxity	Other posterior column sources of nociception refractory to steroid injections, nonsteroidal anti-inflammatory therapy (NSAID), and radiofrequency procedures
Vertebral compression fractures exerting stress on adjacent joints and soft tissue	Enhancement of manipulative treatment and physiotherapy

Table 81.3 Contraindications for regenerative injection therapy

General contraindications	Specific contraindications
Allergy to anesthetic solutions	Acute arthritis (septic, gout, rheumatoid, or posttraumatic with hemarthrosis)
Bacterial infection, systemic or localized to the region to be injected	Acute bursitis or tendonitis
Bleeding diathesis secondary to disease or anticoagulants	Acute non-reduced subluxations, dislocations, or fractures
Fear of the procedure or needle phobia	Allergy to injectable solutions or their ingredients such as dextrose (corn), sodium morrhuate (fish), or phenol
Neoplastic lesions involving the musculature and osseous structures	
Recent onset of a progressive neurological deficit including but not limited to severe intractable cephalgia, unilaterally dilated pupil, bladder dysfunction, bowel incontinence, etc.	
Requests for large quantity of sedation and/or narcotics before and after treatment	
Severe exacerbation of pain or lack of improvement after local anesthetic blocks	

Confirmation is obtained by needle tapping the bone and local anesthetic block of the tissue at the enthesis keeping the innervation in perspective.

Using palpable landmarks for guidance, experienced practitioners have been safely injecting, with or without fluoroscopic guidance, the following posterior column elements innervated by the dorsal rami: tendons and ligaments enthesis at the spinous process, lamina, posterior ZJ capsule, and thoracolumbar fascia insertions at the transverse process.

Theoretically, 0.5 % lidocaine solution is an effective, initial diagnostic option for pain arising from posterior column elements when utilized in increments of 0.5–1.0 ml injected after each bone contact; in practice, hyperosmolar lidocaine/dextrose in 4:2 or 3:2 dilution is used initially blocking the structures innervated by terminal filaments of the MB with the sequence as follows:

Step A: In the presence of midline pain and tenderness, enthesis of ligaments and tendons at the spinous process are blocked initially in the midline at the previously marked level(s).

Step B: The blocked area is reexamined about 1 min after each injection for tenderness and movements that provoked pain.

If tenderness remains at the lateral aspects of the spinous processes, injections are carried out to the lateral aspects of their apices, thus continuing on the course of medial branches or dorsal rami. Step B is repeated.

Persistence of paramedial pain is calling for investigative blocks of ZJ capsules (cervical, thoracic, and lumbar) and costotransverse joints. Step B is repeated.

Perseverance of lateral tenderness dictates investigation of the structures innervated by the lateral branches of the dorsal rami, such as the enthesis of iliocostalis or serratus posterior superior/inferior at the ribs, the ventral sheath of thoracolumbar fascia at the lateral aspects of the lumbar transverse processes, or at the iliac crests. Step B is repeated. In this fashion, all potential nociceptors on the course of MB and LB are investigated from their periphery toward their origins. Thus, the differential diagnosis of pain arising from vertebral and paravertebral structures innervated by MB and LB is made based on the results of the

Fig. 81.11 Drawing demonstrating sites of tendon origins and insertions (enthesis) of the paravertebral musculature in the cervical, thoracic, lumbar, and pelvic regions with parts of the upper and lower extremities. Clinically significant enthesopathies with small fiber neuropathies and neuralgias are common at the locations identified by *dots. Dots* also represent most common locations of needle insertion and RIT injections (Note: Not all of the locations are treated in each patient) (Modified from Sinelnikov [31]. Modified and prepared for publication by Tracey James. All rights reserved. No part of this picture may be reproduced or transmitted in any form or by any means without written permission from Felix Linetsky M.D.)

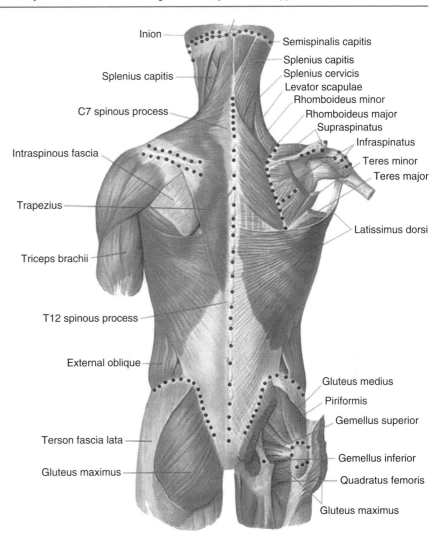

blocks (Figs. 81.9, 81.10, and 81.11). Manipulation under local anesthesia can be performed after anesthetic has taken effect, and the musculature is sufficiently relaxed [154]. Pain from the upper cervical synovial joints presents a diagnostic and a therapeutic challenge; therefore, it is a diagnosis of exclusion.

The possibility of serious complications dictates that all intra-articular injections of the axial synovial joints, specifically atlantoaxial and atlantooccipital, ZJ, costovertebral, and intervertebral discs, should be performed only under fluoroscopic guidance by an experienced practitioner [3, 4, 14–16, 25, 58–61, 73, 74]. Conversely, the intra-articular injections of SJ joint are grossly overemphasized [39, 51, 57, 63, 64, 72]. This was recently proven again by Murakami et al. [155].

Most commonly injected sites of painful spinal enthesopathies of the posterior column are innervated by the medial (MB) and lateral (LB) branches of the dorsal rami:
- Enthesis of ligaments and tendons at the superior, inferior, and lateral surfaces especially at the apex of the spinous processes
- Enthesis at the occipital bone at and between inferior and superior nuchal lines

- Enthesis at the thoracic and lumbar transverse processes
- Capsular ligaments and periarticular enthesis at the cervical thoracic and lumbar ZJs
- Costotransverse joints and capsules
- Tendons and ligaments at the posteromedial, superior, inferior, and lateral surfaces of the iliac crests and spines
- Posterior tubercles and angles of the ribs
  Multiple other common peripheral enthesopathies are depicted in Figs. 81.10 and 81.11 and described below:
- Proximal and distal portions of the clavicle specifically superior acromioclavicular (AC) ligament and AC joint, sternoclavicular (SC) ligament and joint, etc.
- Greater and lesser humeral tuberosities and medial and lateral epicondyles
- Sternum, xiphoid, and anterior ribs
- Pubic tubercles, superior and inferior rami, and ischial spines, tuberosities, and rami
- Greater and lesser femoral trochanters and medial and lateral femoral epicondyles

Side Effects and Complications of RIT

Several types of statistically rare complications occur with regenerative injection therapy [156]. The most recent statistical data on complications came from a survey of 171 physicians providing RIT in 2006 [157].

Responders to the survey had been providing this treatment for a median of 10 years and described treating a median of 500 patients each, giving a median of 2,000 injections each.

The following complications were reported: 164 spinal headaches, 123 pneumothoraxes, 73 temporary systemic reactions, and 54 temporary nerve damage. Sixty-nine adverse events required hospitalization, among them 46 patients with a pneumothorax and none with the spinal headache. Five cases of permanent nerve damage were reported. Only three surveyors included information on the specific injury: one case of mild to moderate leg pain, one case of persistent numbness in a small area of the gluteal region, and one case of persistent numbness in the quadriceps region [157]. These findings were similar to an earlier survey by Dorman of 450 physicians performing RIT/prolotherapy [158]. At that time, 120 respondents revealed that 495,000 patients received injections. Among them, 29 instances of pneumothorax were reported, two of them requiring chest tube placement. Also, 24 of non-life-threatening allergic reactions were reported [158].

Stipulating that each patient had at least three visits and during each visit received at least ten injections, the occurrence of pneumothorax requiring a chest tube was 1 per 247,500 injections. Thus, self-limited pneumothoraxes were 1 per 18,333, and allergic reactions were 1 per 20,625 injections [158].

In the 1960s, five cases of postinjection arachnoiditis were reported [159]. Two were fatal; one was a direct sequence of arachnoiditis and another was a sequence of incompetent shunt and persistent hydrocephalus with increased intracranial pressure. Of the other three cases, the first one with mild paraparesis recovered after a ventriculo-jugular shunt. The second recovered spontaneously with a mild neurological deficit, and the third patient remained paraplegic.

Three other cases of intrathecal injections known to the first author have not been reported in the literature because of medicolegal issues. Two of them resulted in paraplegia. The first occurred after injection at the thoracic level and the second after a lumbar injection. The third case was performed by an untrained person who injected zinc sulfate solution, which is hardly used in today's practice, at the cranio-cervical level, resulting in immediate onset of severe neurologic deficit, quadriplegia, and subsequent hydrocephalus. One case of self-limiting sterile meningitis after lumbosacral sclerosing injections was reported in 1994. Adjacent endplate fractures associated with intradiscal dextrose injections were recently reported [160].

Postspinal puncture headaches have been reported after lumbosacral injections. Two such cases occurred in the first author's practice during the past 20 years. Both patients recovered after 1 week with bed rest and fluids.

Overall, pneumothorax is the most commonly reported complication. Injections of anterior thoracic synovial joints, such as sternoclavicular, costosternal, and interchondral, may also result in pneumothorax.

Conclusions

Double-blind, placebo-controlled, and retrospective studies clearly indicate the effectiveness of RIT in painful degenerative posttraumatic conditions of fibrous connective tissue.

Literature suggests that degenerative cascade is a multietiologic disease process. NSAIDs and steroid preparations have limited use in chronic painful overuse conditions and degenerative painful conditions of ligaments and tendons. Microinterventional regenerative techniques and proper rehabilitation up to 1 year supported with mild opioid analgesics are more appropriate.

Cervical thoracic and lumbar discogenic pain continues to be a therapeutic challenge. Encouraging positive results were published after regenerative injections for lumbar discogenic pain with dextrose-based solutions, methylene blue, and mesenchymal stem cells. The work in this direction continues. It appears that cervical and thoracic discogenic pain may be addressed similarly in the near future.

The future is such that, instead of indirect stimulation of growth factors through inflammatory cascade, specific growth factors or their combinations may be available. The challenge will continue to determining which specific growth factors should be used. The other viable possibility is injection of engineered, type-specific tissue derived from stem-cell research [83, 84, 154]. Some variations of nanotechnology will be also added.

As stated by the late Professor Mooney, "The ideas of regeneration and controlled proliferation are slowly moving from the fringe to the frontier of medical care" [161]. A physician versatile in diagnostic and therapeutic injection techniques may have ample opportunity to implement RIT in the treatment of chronic musculoskeletal pain. More information regarding RIT can be found on linetskymd.com and aarom.org. Full texts of many original articles text books and chapters are available on these websites. The individual training with CME credits is available by the American Academy of Regenerative Orthopedic Medicine (AAROM) at Drs. Linetsky, Centeno, Crane, and Hirsch offices.

Acknowledgments The authors would like to extend their special thanks to Jacqueline Ferreira for invaluable help in the preparation of this manuscript and Tracey James for preparation of the illustrations.

References

1. Linetsky F, Willard F. Use of regenerative injection therapy for low back pain. Pain Clin. 1999;1:27–31.

2. Feinstein B, Langton J, Jameson R, et al. Experiments on pain referred from deep somatic tissues. J Bone Joint Surg Am. 1954;36A:981–96.

3. Dwyer A, Aprill C, Bogduk N. Cervical zygapophyseal joint pain patterns: a clinical evaluation. Spine. 1990;15:458–61.

4. Dreyfuss P, Michaelsen M, Fletcher D. Atlanto-occipital and lateral atlanto-axial joint pain patterns. Spine. 1994;19:1125–31.

5. Dussault RG, Kaplan PA. Facet joint injection: diagnosis and therapy. Appl Radiol. 1994;23:35–39.

6. Fukui S, Ohseto K, Shiotani M. Patterns of pain induced by distending the thoracic zygapophyseal joints. Reg Anesth Pain Med. 1997;22(4):332–336. http://dx.doi.org/10.1016/S1098-7339(97)80007-7

7. Kellgren JH. Observations on referred pain arising from muscle. Clin Sci. 1939;4:35–46.

8. Mooney V, Robertson J. The facet syndrome. Clin Orthop Relat Res. 1976;115:149–156.

9. Hackett G. Ligament and tendon relaxation treated by prolotherapy. 3rd ed. Springfield: Charles C. Thomas; 1958.

10. Kellgren J. On the distribution of pain arising from deep somatic structures with charts of segmental pain areas. Somatic Pain. 1939;4:35–46.

11. Hackett G, Hemwall G, Montgomery G. Ligament and tendon relaxation: treated by prolotherapy. 5th ed. Springfield: Charles C. Thomas; 1991.

12. Simons DG, Travell JG, Simons LS. Myofascial pain and dysfunction: the trigger point manual, vol. 1. Baltimore: Williams & Wilkins; 1991.

13. Bonica J, Loeser J, Chapman C, et al. The management of pain. vol I, 2nd ed. Malvern: Lea & Febiger; 1990; 7:136–139.

14. Dreyfuss P, Tibiletti C, Dreyer S. Thoracic zygapophyseal joint pain patterns: a study in normal volunteers. Spine. 1994;19:807–11.

15. Dussault RG, Kaplan PA, Anderson MW. Fluoroscopy-guided sacroiliac joint injections. Radiology. 2000;214(1):273–7.

16. O'Neill C, Kurgansky M, Derby R, et al. Disc stimulation and patterns of referred pain. Spine. 2002;27:2776–81.

17. Linetsky F, Trescot A, Manchikanti L. Regenerative injection therapy. In: Manchikanti L, Singh V, editors. Interventional techniques in chronic non-spinal pain. Paducah: ASIPP Publishing; 2009. p. 87–98.

18. Biegeleisen H. Varicose veins, related diseases, and sclerotherapy: a guide for practitioners. Fountain Valley: Eden Press; 1994.

19. Linetsky F, Mikulinsky A, Gorfine L. Regenerative injection therapy: history of application in pain management: part I 1930s–1950s. Pain Clin. 2000;2:8–13.

20. Linetsky F, Botwin K, Gorfine L, et al. Position paper of the Florida Academy of Pain Medicine on regenerative injection therapy: effectiveness and appropriate usage. Pain Clin. 2002;4:38–45.

21. Linetsky F, Saberski L, Miguel R, et al. A history of the applications of regenerative injection therapy in pain management: part II 1960s–1980s. Pain Clin. 2001;3:32–6.

22. Linetsky F, Derby R, Saberski L, et al. Pain management with regenerative injection therapy (RIT). In: Boswell M, Cole E, editors. Weiner's Pain management: a practical guide for clinicians. 7th ed. Boca Raton: CRC Press; 2006. p. 939–66.

23. Steindler A, Luck J. Differential diagnosis of pain low in the back: allocation of the source of pain by the procaine hydrochloride method. JAMA. 1938;110:106–13.

24. Haldeman K, Soto-Hall R. The diagnosis and treatment of sacroiliac conditions by the injection of procaine (Novocain). J Bone Joint Surg Am. 1938;3:675–85.

25. Bogduk N. Post-traumatic cervical and lumbar spine zygapophyseal joint pain. In: Evans RW, editor. Neurology and trauma. Philadelphia: WB Saunders; 1996. p. 363–75.

26. Williams P. Gray's anatomy, 38th British edition. Philadelphia: Churchill Livingston, Pearson Professional Limited; 1995.

27. Best T. Basic science of soft tissue. In: Delee J, Drez D, editors. Orthopedic sports medicine principles and practice, vol. 1. Philadelphia: WB Saunders; 1994.

28. Willard F. Gross anatomy of the cervical and thoracic regions: understanding connective tissue stockings and their contents. Presented at the 20th American Association of Orthopedic Medicine annual conference and scientific seminar; a common sense approach to "hidden" pain generators, Orlando, 2003.

29. Yahia H, Newman N. A light and electron microscopic study of spinal ligament innervation. Z Mikrosk Anat Forsch. 1989; 102:664–74.

30. Leadbetter W. Cell-matrix response in tendon injury. Clin Sports Med. 1992;11:533–78.

31. Sinelnikov RD. Atlas of anatomy, vol. 1. Moscow: Meditsina; 1972.

32. Leadbetter W. Anti-inflammatory therapy and sport injury: the role of non-steroidal drugs and corticosteroid injections. Clin Sports Med. 1995;14:353–410.

33. Jozsa L, Kannus P. Human tendons, anatomy, physiology, and pathology. Champaign: Human Kinetics; 1997.

34. Cotran R, Vinay K, Collins T, et al. Robbins pathologic basis of disease. Philadelphia: WB Saunders; 1999.

35. Freemont A. Nerve ingrowth into diseased intervertebral disc in chronic back pain. Lancet. 1997;350:178–81.

36. Ashton I, Ashton B, Gibson S, et al. Morphological basis for back pain: the demonstration of nerve fibers and neuropeptides in the lumbar facet joint capsule but not in the ligamentum flavum. J Orthop Res. 1992;10:72–8.

37. Tuzlukov P, Skuba N, Gorbatovskaya N. The morphological characteristics of fibromyalgia syndrome. Arkh Patol. 1993;4:47–50.

38. Nirschl R, Pettrone F. Tennis elbow. The surgical treatment of lateral epicondylitis. J Bone Joint Surg Am. 1979;61(6A):832–9.

39. Fortin J, Vilensky J, Merkel GJ. Can the sacroiliac joint cause sciatica? Pain Physician. 2003;6(3):269–71.

40. Khan KM, Cook JL, Taunton JE, Bonar F. Overuse tendinosis, not tendinitis part 1: a new paradigm for a difficult clinical problem. Phys Sportsmed. 2000;28(5):38–48.

41. Alfredson H, Thorsen K, Lorentzon R. In situ microdialysis in tendon tissue: high levels of glutamate, but not prostaglandin E2 in chronic Achilles tendon pain. Knee Surg Sports Traumatol Arthrosc. 1999;7:378–81.

42. Alfredson H, Ljung BO, Thorsen K, Lorentzon R. In vivo investigation of ECRB tendons with microdialysis technique: no signs of inflammation but high amounts of glutamate in tennis elbow. Acta Orthop Scand. 2000;71(5):475–9.

43. Alfredson H, Forsgren S, Thorsen K, Lorentzon R. In vivo microdialysis and immunohistochemical analyses of tendon tissue demonstrated high amounts of free glutamate and glutamate NMDAR1 receptors, but no signs of inflammation, in Jumper's knee. J Orthop Res. 2001;19:881–6.

44. Alfredson H, Forsgren S, Thorsen K, Fahlström M, Johansson H, Lorentzon R. Glutamate NMDAR1 receptors localised to nerves in human Achilles tendons. Implications for treatment? Knee Surg Sports Traumatol Arthrosc. 2000;9:123–6.

45. Alfredson H, Bjur D, Thorsen K, Lorentzon R. High intratendinous lactate levels in painful chronic Achilles tendinosis. An investigation using microdialysis technique. J Orthop Res. 2002; 20:934–8.

46. Bjur D, Alfredson H, Forsgren S. The innervation pattern of the human Achilles tendon: studies of the normal and tendinosis tendon with markers for general and sensory innervation. Cell Tissue Res. 2005;320(1):201–6. Epub 2005 Feb 9.

47. Ljung BO, Forsgren S, Fridén J. Substance-P and Calcitonin gene-related peptide expression at the extensor carpi radialis brevis muscle origin: implications for the aetiology of tennis elbow? J Orthop Res. 1999;17(4):554–9.

48. Ljung BO, Alfredson H, Forsgren S. Neurokinin 1-receptors and sensory neuropeptides in tendon insertions at the medial and lateral epicondyles of the humerus. Studies on tennis elbow and medial epicodylalgia. J Orthop Res. 2004;22:321–7.

49. Liu Y, Tipton C, Matthes R, et al. An in situ study of the influence of a sclerosing solution in rabbit medial collateral ligaments and its junction strength. Connect Tissue Res. 1983;11:95–102.

50. Maynard J, Pedrini V, Pedrini-Mille A, et al. Morphological and biochemical effects of sodium morrhuate on tendons. J Orthop Res. 1985;3:234–48.

51. Klein R, Dorman T, Johnson C. Proliferant injections for low back pain: histologic changes of injected ligaments and objective measurements of lumbar spine mobility before and after treatment. J Neurol Ortho Med Surg. 1989;10:2.

52. Öhberg L, Alfredson H. Ultrasound guided sclerosis of neovessels in painful chronic Achilles tendinosis: pilot study of a new treatment. Br J Sports Med. 2002;36:173–7.

53. Alfredson H, Ohberg L. Neovascularisation in chronic painful patellar tendinosis – promising results after sclerosing neovessels outside the tendon challenge the need for surgery. Knee Surg Sports Traumatol Arthrosc. 2005;13(2):74–80. Epub 2004 Nov 26.

54. Alfredson H, Öhberg L. Sclerosing injections to areas of neovascularisation reduce pain in chronic Achilles tendinopathy: a double-blind randomized controlled trial. Knee Surg Sports Traumatol Arthrosc. 2005;13(4):338–44. Epub 2005 Feb 2. PMID:15688235.

55. Alfredson H, Harstad H, Haugen S, Ohberg L. Sclerosing polidocanol injections to treat chronic painful shoulder impingement syndrome-results of a two-centre collaborative pilot study. Knee Surg Sports Traumatol Arthrosc. 2006;14(12):1321–6. Epub 2006 Oct 7.

56. Willard F. The muscular, ligamentous and neural structure of the low back and its relation to back pain. In: Vleeming A et al., editors. Movement stability and low back pain. New York: Churchill Livingston; 1997. p. 1–35.

57. Linetsky F, Parris W, et al. Regenerative injection therapy. In: Manchikanti L, editor. Low back pain. Paducah: ASIPP Publishing; 2002. p. 519–20.

58. Lord S. Chronic cervical zygapophyseal joint pain after whiplash: a placebo-controlled prevalence study. Spine. 1996;21:1737–45.

59. Barnsley L, Lord S, Walis B, et al. Lack of effect of intra-articular corticosteroids for chronic pain in the cervical zygapophyseal joints. N Engl J Med. 1994;330:1047–50.

60. O'Neill C. Intra-articular dextrose/glucosamine injections for cervical facet syndrome, atlanto-occipital and atlanto-axial joint pain, combined ISIS AAOM approach. Presented at the 20th AAOM annual conference and scientific seminar, Orlando, April 30–May 3, 2003.

61. Stanton-Hicks M. Cervicocranial syndrome: treatment of atlanto-occipital and atlanto-axial joint pain with phenol/glycerin injections. Presented at the 20th AAOM annual conference and scientific seminar, Orlando, April 30–May 3, 2003.

62. Zhang J, Tsuzuki N, Hirabayashi S, et al. Surgical anatomy of the nerves and muscles in the posterior cervical spine. A guide for avoiding inadvertent nerve injuries during the posterior approach. Spine. 2003;28:1379–84.

63. Wilkinson H. Injection therapy for enthesopathies causing axial spine pain and the "failed back syndrome": a single blinded, randomized and cross-over study. Pain Physician. 2005;8:167–74.

64. Wilkinson H. The failed back syndrome etiology and therapy. 2nd ed. New York: Springer; 1992.

65. Kayfetz D, Blumenthal L, Hackett G, et al. Whiplash injury and other ligamentous headache: its management with prolotherapy. Headache. 1963;3:1.

66. Resnick D. Diagnosis of bone and joint disorders, volumes 1–6. 3rd ed. Philadelphia: WB Saunders; 1995.

67. Stark D, Bradley W. Magnetic resonance imaging, volumes 1 and 2. 3rd ed. St. Louis: Mosby; 1999.

68. European Society of Musculoskeletal Radiology. http://www.south-staffordshirepct.nhs.uk/policies/clinical/Clin55_DiagnosticUltrasoundProcedures.pdf. Approved 27 Apr 2009. http://www.essr.org/html/img/pool/shoulder.pdf; http://www.essr.org/html/img/pool/elbow.pdf; http://radiology.rsna.org/content/252/1/157.full.pdf.

69. McNally E. Ultrasound of the small joints of the hands and feet: current status. Skeletal Radiol. 2008;37(2):99–113. Epub 2007 Aug 22.

70. Linetsky F, Stanton Hicks M, O'Neil C. Prolotherapy. In: Wallace M, Staats P, editors. Pain medicine & management – just the facts. New York: McGraw-Hill; 2004. p. 318–24.

71. Linetsky F, Saberski L, Dubin J, et al. Letter to the editor. Re: Yelland MJ, Glasziou PP, Bogduk N, et al. Prolotherapy injections, saline injections, and exercises for chronic low-back pain: a randomized study. Spine, 2003; 29:9–16. Spine. Spine. 2004;29(16):1840–1; author reply 1842–3.

72. Klein R, DeLong W, Mooney V, et al. A randomized, double-blind trial of dextrose-glycerin-phenol injections for chronic, low back pain. J Spinal Disord. 1993;6:23–33.

73. Miller M. Treatment of painful advanced internal lumbar disc derangement with intradiscal injection of hypertonic dextrose. Pain Physician. 2006;9(2):115–21.

74. Klein R, O'Neill C, Mooney V, et al. Biochemical injection treatment for discogenic low back pain: a pilot study. Spine J. 2003; 3(3):220–6.

75. Yelland M, Glasziou P, Bogduk N, et al. Prolotherapy injections, saline injections, and exercises for chronic low-back pain: a randomized trial. Spine. 2004;29:9–16.

76. Ongley M, Klein R, Dorman T, et al. A new approach to the treatment of chronic low back pain. Lancet. 1987;2:143–6.

77. Dechow E, Davies R, Carr A, et al. A randomized, double-blind, placebo controlled trial of sclerosing injections in patients with chronic low back pain. Rheumatology. 1999;38:1255–9.

78. Yelland M, Yeo M, Schluter P. Prolotherapy injections for chronic low back pain – results of a pilot comparative study. Australas Musculoskelet Med. 2000;5:20–3.

79. Yelland M, et al. Prolotherapy injections for chronic low back pain: a systematic review. Spine. 2004;19:2126–33.

80. Kon E. Platelet-rich plasma: intra-articular knee injections produced favorable results on degenerative cartilage lesions. Knee Surg Sports Traumatol Arthrosc. 2010;18(4):472–9.

81. Mishra A, et al. Platelet-rich plasma compared with corticosteroid injection for chronic lateral elbow tendinosis. P M R. 2009;1(4):366–70.

82. Topol G, et al. Efficacy of dextrose prolotherapy in elite make kicking-sport athletes with chronic groin pain. Arch Phys Med Rehabil. 2005;86(4):697–702.

83. Topol G, Reeves K. Regenerative injection of elite athletes with career-altering chronic groin pain who fail conservative treatment: a consecutive case series. Am J Phys Med Rehabil. 2008;87:890–902.

84. Kon E, et al. Platelet-rich plasma: new clinical application: a pilot study for treatment of jumper's knee. Injury. 2009;40(6):598–603.

85. Robertson J. Structural alterations in nerve fibers produced by hypotonic and hypertonic solutions. J Biophys Biochem Cytol. 1958;4:349–64.

86. Jewett D, Kind J. Conduction block of monkey dorsal rootlets by water and hypertonic saline solutions. Exp Neurol. 1971;33:225.

87. Barsa et al. Functional and structural changes in the rabbit vagus nerve in vivo following exposure to various hypoosmotic solutions. Anesth Analg. 1982;61(11):912–6.

88. Fink et al. Osmotic swelling effects on neural conduction. Anesthesiology. 1979;51(5):418–23.

89. Hitchcock E, Prandini MN. Hypertonic saline in management of intractable pain. Lancet. 1973;1(7798):310–2.

90. Racz GB, Heavner JE, Trescot A. Percutaneous lysis of epidural adhesions – evidence for safety and efficacy. Pain Pract. 2008; 8(4):277–86. Epub 2008 May 23.

91. Westerlund T, et al. The endoneurial response to neurolytic agents is highly dependent on the mode of application. Reg Anesth Pain Med. 1999;24(4):294–302.

92. Westerlund T, Vuorinen V, Roytta M. The effect of combined neurolytic blocking agent 5 % phenol -glycerol in rat sciatic nerve. Acta Neuropathol (Berl). 2003;106:261–70.

93. Bodine-Fowler SC, Allsing S, Botte MJ. Time course of muscle atrophy and recovery following a phenol-induced nerve block. Muscle Nerve. 1996;19:497–504.

94. Birch M, Strong N, Brittain P, et al. Retrobulbar phenol injection in blind painful eyes. Ann Ophthalmol. 1993;257:267–70.

95. Garland DE, Lilling M, Keenan MA. Percutaneous phenol blocks to motor points of spastic forearm muscles in head-injured adults. Arch Phys Med Rehabil. 1984;65:243–5.

96. Viel E, Pellas F, Ripart J, et al. Peripheral neurolytic blocks and spasticity. Ann Fr Anesth Reanim. 2005;24:667–72.

97. Raj P. Practical management of pain. 3rd ed. St. Louis: Mosby Inc.; 2000.

98. Zafonte RD, Munin MC. Phenol and alcohol blocks for the treatment of spasticity. Phys Med Rehabil Clin N Am. 2001;12:817–32.

99. Kirvela O, Nieminen S. Treatment of painful neuromas with neurolytic blockade. Pain. 1990;41:161–5.

100. Wilkinson HA. Trigeminal nerve peripheral branch phenol/glycerol injections for tic douloureux. J Neurosurg. 1999;90:828–32.

101. Robertson D. Transsacral neurolytic nerve block. An alternative approach to intractable perineal pain. Br J Anaesth. 1983;559:873–5.

102. Trescot A. HansenH. Neurolytic agents: pharmacology and clinical applications. In: Manchikanti L, Singh V, editors. Interventional techniques in chronic non-spinal pain. Paducah: ASIPP Publishing; 2009. p. 53–8.

103. Lamer T. Neurolytic peripheral joint injections in severely debilitated patients. Presented at the annual meeting of the Florida Academy of Pain Medicine, Orlando, 30 July 2005.

104. Broadhurst N, Wilk V. Vertebral mid-line pain: pain arising from the interspinous spaces. J Orthop Med. 1996;18:2–4.

105. Kevy S, Jacobson M. Point of care concentration and clinical application of autologous bone marrow derived stem cells. Presented at the Orthopedic Research Society, 52nd annual meeting. 19–22 March 2006.

106. Aust L, Devlin B, Foster S. Yield of human adipose-derived adult stem cells from lipoaspirates. Cytotherapy. 2004;6:7–14.

107. Alexander R. Use of PRP in autologous fat grafting. In: Shiffman M, editor. Autologous fat grafting. Berlin: Springer; 2010. p. 140–67.

108. Crane D, Everts P. Platelet rich plasma matrix grafts. Pract Pain Manag. 2008;8:12–26. http://www.prolotherapy.com/PPM_JanFeb2008_Crane_PRP.pdf

109. Everts P, Knape J, Weibrich G, et al. Platelet-rich plasma and platelet gel: a review. J Extra Corpor Technol. 2006;38:174–87.

110. Alhadlaq A, Mao JJ. Mesenchymal stem cells: isolation and therapeutics. Stem Cells Dev. 2004;13(4):436–48.

111. Barry FP. Mesenchymal stem cell therapy in joint disease. Novartis Found Symp. 2003;249:86–96; discussion 96–102, 170–4, 239–41.

112. Bruder SP, Fink DJ, Caplan AI. Mesenchymal stem cells in bone development, bone repair, and skeletal regeneration therapy. J Cell Biochem. 1994;56(3):283–94.

113. Cha J, Falanga V. Stem cells in cutaneous wound healing. Clin Dermatol. 2007;25(1):73–8.

114. Gangji V, Toungouz M, Hauzeur JP. Stem cell therapy for osteonecrosis of the femoral head. Expert Opin Biol Ther. 2005;5(4):437–42.

115. Becker AJ, Mc CE, Till JE. Cytological demonstration of the clonal nature of spleen colonies derived from transplanted mouse marrow cells. Nature. 1963;197:452–4.

116. Friedenstein AJ, et al. Precursors for fibroblasts in different populations of hematopoietic cells as detected by the in vitro colony assay method. Exp Hematol. 1974;2(2):83–92.

117. Zhou Z, et al. Comparative study on various subpopulations in mesenchymal stem cells of adult bone marrow. Zhongguo Shi Yan Xue Ye Xue Za Zhi. 2005;13(1):54–8.

118. Schauwer CD, et al. Markers of stemness in equine mesenchymal stem cells: a plea for uniformity. Theriogenology. 2011;75(8):1431–43. Epub 2010 Dec 31.

119. Vidal MA, et al. Comparison of chondrogenic potential in equine mesenchymal stromal cells derived from adipose tissue and bone marrow. Vet Surg. 2008;37(8):713–24.

120. Niemeyer P, et al. Comparison of mesenchymal stem cells from bone marrow and adipose tissue for bone regeneration in a critical size defect of the sheep tibia and the influence of platelet-rich plasma. Biomaterials. 2010;31(13):3572–9.

121. Yoshimura H, et al. Comparison of rat mesenchymal stem cells derived from bone marrow, synovium, periosteum, adipose tissue, and muscle. Cell Tissue Res. 2007;327(3):449–62.

122. Frisbie DD, et al. Evaluation of adipose-derived stromal vascular fraction or bone marrow-derived mesenchymal stem cells for treatment of osteoarthritis. J Orthop Res. 2009;27(12):1675–80.

123. Banfi A, et al. Proliferation kinetics and differentiation potential of ex vivo expanded human bone marrow stromal cells: Implications for their use in cell therapy. Exp Hematol. 2000;28(6): 707–15.

124. Crisostomo PR, et al. High passage number of stem cells adversely affects stem cell activation and myocardial protection. Shock. 2006;26(6):575–80.

125. Izadpanah R, et al. Long-term in vitro expansion alters the biology of adult mesenchymal stem cells. Cancer Res. 2008;68(11): 4229–38.

126. Ladage D, et al. Mesenchymal stem cells induce endothelial activation via paracine mechanisms. Endothelium. 2007;14(2): 53–63.

127. Zhou S, et al. Age-related intrinsic changes in human bone-marrow-derived mesenchymal stem cells and their differentiation to osteoblasts. Aging Cell. 2008;7(3):335–43.

128. Broberg K, et al. Polyclonal expansion of cells with trisomy 7 in synovia from patients with osteoarthritis. Cytogenet Cell Genet. 1998;83(1–2):30–4.

129. Izuta Y, et al. Meniscal repair using bone marrow-derived mesenchymal stem cells: experimental study using green fluorescent protein transgenic rats. Knee. 2005;12(3):217–23.

130. Horie M, et al. Intra-articular Injected synovial stem cells differentiate into meniscal cells directly and promote meniscal regeneration without mobilization to distant organs in rat massive meniscal defect. Stem Cells. 2009;27(4):878–87.

131. Yamasaki T, et al. Meniscal regeneration using tissue engineering with a scaffold derived from a rat meniscus and mesenchymal stromal cells derived from rat bone marrow. J Biomed Mater Res A. 2005;75(1):23–30.

132. Brittberg M, et al. Treatment of deep cartilage defects in the knee with autologous chondrocyte transplantation. N Engl J Med. 1994;331(14):889–95.

133. Caplan AI. Mesenchymal stem cells. J Orthop Res. 1991; 9(5):641–50.

134. Angele P, et al. Engineering of osteochondral tissue with bone marrow mesenchymal progenitor cells in a derivatized hyaluronan-gelatin composite sponge. Tissue Eng. 1999;5(6):545–54.

135. Buckwalter JA, Mankin HJ. Articular cartilage: degeneration and osteoarthritis, repair, regeneration, and transplantation. Instr Course Lect. 1998;47:487–504.

136. Johnstone B, Yoo JU. Autologous mesenchymal progenitor cells in articular cartilage repair. Clin Orthop Relat Res. 1999; 367(Suppl):S156–62.

137. Minas T, Nehrer S. Current concepts in the treatment of articular cartilage defects. Orthopedics. 1997;20(6):525–38.

138. Katakai D. Compressive properties of cartilage-like tissues repaired in vivo with scaffold-free, tissue engineered constructs. Clin Biomech (Bristol, Avon). 2009;24(1):110–6.

139. Fritzell P, Hagg O, Nordwall A. Complications in lumbar fusion surgery for chronic low back pain: comparison of three surgical techniques used in a prospective randomized study. A report from the Swedish Lumbar Spine Study Group. Eur Spine J. 2003; 12(2):178–89.

140. Deyo RA. Lumbar spinal fusion. A cohort study of complications, reoperations, and resource use in the Medicare population. Spine. 1993;18(11):463–70.

141. Elias WJ, et al. Complications of posterior lumbar interbody fusion when using a titanium threaded cage device. J Neurosurg. 2000;93(1 Suppl):45–52.

142. Yoshikawa T. Disc regeneration therapy using marrow mesenchymal cell transplantation: a report of two case studies. Spine (Phila Pa 1976). 2010;35(11):E475–80.

143. Centeno CJ, et al. Regeneration of meniscus cartilage in a knee treated with percutaneously implanted autologous mesenchymal stem cells. Med Hypotheses. 2008;71(6):900–8.

144. Centeno CJ, et al. Increased knee cartilage volume in degenerative joint disease using percutaneously implanted, autologous mesenchymal stem cells. Pain Physician. 2008;11(3):343–53.

145. Centeno CJ, et al. Partial regeneration of the human hip via autologous bone marrow nucleated cell transfer: a case study. Pain Physician. 2006;9(3):253–6.

146. Centeno CJ, et al. Safety and complications reporting on the reimplantation of culture-expanded mesenchymal stem cells using autologous platelet lysate technique. Curr Stem Cell Res Ther. 2010;5(1):81–93.

147. Wakitani S, et al. Safety of autologous bone marrow-derived mesenchymal stem cell transplantation for cartilage repair in 41 patients with 45 joints followed for up to 11 years and 5 months. J Tissue Eng Regen Med. 2011;5(2):146–50.

148. Haleem AM, et al. The clinical use of human culture-expanded autologous bone marrow mesenchymal stem cells transplanted on platelet-rich fibrin glue in the treatment of articular cartilage defects: a pilot study and preliminary results. Cartilage. 2010;1(4):253–61.

149. Sakai D, et al. Transplantation of mesenchymal stem cells embedded in Atelocollagen gel to the intervertebral disc: a potential therapeutic model for disc degeneration. Biomaterials. 2003;24(20):3531–41.

150. Richardson SM, et al. Intervertebral disc cell mediated mesenchymal stem cell differentiation. Stem Cells. 2006;24(3):707–16.

151. Risbud MV, et al. Differentiation of mesenchymal stem cells towards a nucleus pulposus-like phenotype in vitro: implications for cell-based transplantation therapy. Spine. 2004;29(23): 2627–32.

152. Miyamoto T, et al. Intradiscal transplantation of synovial mesenchymal stem cells prevents intervertebral disc degeneration through suppression of matrix metalloproteinase-related genes in nucleus pulposus cells in rabbits. Arthritis Res Ther. 2010; 12(6):R206.

153. Nejadnik H, et al. Autologous bone marrow-derived mesenchymal stem cells versus autologous chondrocyte implantation: an observational cohort study. Am J Sports Med. 2010;38(6): 1110–6.

154. Dreyfuss P, Michaelsen M, Horne M. MUJA: manipulation under joint anesthesia/analgesia: a treatment approach for recalcitrant low back pain of synovial joint origin. J Manipulative Physiol Ther. 1995;18:537–46.

155. Murakami E, et al. Effect of periarticular and intraarticular lidocaine injections for sacroiliac joint pain: prospective comparative study. J Orthop Sci. 2007;12(3):274–80.

156. Peng B, Pang X, Wu Y, et al. A randomized placebo-controlled trial of intradiscal ethylene blue injection for the treatment of chronic discogenic low back pain. Pain. 2010;149(1):124–9.

157. Dagenais S, Ogunseitan O, Haldeman S, et al. Side effects and adverse events related to intraligamentous injections of sclerosing solutions (prolotherapy) for back and neck pain: a survey of practitioners. Arch Phys Med Rehabil. 2006;87:909–13.

158. Dorman T. Prolotherapy: a survey. J Orthop Med. 1993;15: 49–50.

159. Keplinger J, Bucy P. Paraplegia from treatment with sclerosing agents. JAMA. 1960;173:1333–5.

160. Whitworth M. Endplate fracture associated with intradiscal dextrose injection. Pain Physician. 2002;5:379–84.

161. Mooney V. Prolotherapy at the fringe of medical care, or is it the frontier? Spine J. 2003;3:253–4.

Interdisciplinary Functional Restoration and Pain Programs

Steven D. Feinberg, Robert J. Gatchel, Steven Stanos, Rachel Feinberg, and Valerie Johnson-Montieth

Key Points

- An interdisciplinary functional restoration approach to pain management has been empirically shown to be therapeutically and cost-effective.
- The biopsychosocial model of diagnosis and treatment operates on the idea that illness and disability is the result of, and influences, diverse areas of an individual's life, including the biological, psycho-
logical, social, environmental, and cultural components of their existence.
- It is important to identify those individuals at risk for delayed recovery and transitioning from an acute pain episode to a chronic pain condition.
- Functional restoration programs emphasize a biopsychosocial approach including different disciplines and anticipating an individual's gradual progression to a normal lifestyle.
- Treatment approaches include medication optimization, normalization of function, education, physical reactivation, cognitive-behavioral therapy, various mind-body techniques to manage chronic pain, and return of new functional activities.

S.D. Feinberg, M.D. (✉)
Feinberg Medical Group,
825 El Camino Real, Palo Alto, CA 94301, USA

Stanford University School of Medicine,
Stanford, CA, USA

American Pain Solutions,
San Diego, CA USA
e-mail: stevenfeinberg@hotmail.com

R.J. Gatchel, Ph.D., ABPP
Department of Psychology, College of Science,
The University of Texas at Arlington,
313 Life Science Building, Arlington, TX 76019, USA
e-mail: gatchel@vta.edu

S. Stanos, DO
Department of Physical Medicine and Rehabilitation,
Center for Pain Management, Rehabilitation Institute of Chicago,
980 N. Michigan Ave, Suite 800, Chicago, IL 60611, USA

Northwestern University Medical School,
Feinberg School of Medicine,
Chicago, IL, USA
e-mail: sstanos@ric.org

R. Feinberg, PT, DPT
Feinberg Medical Group,
825 El Camino Real, Palo Alto, CA 94301, USA
e-mail: rfeinberg14@gmail.com

V. Johnson-Montieth, B.A., M.A., Ph.D. Candidate
Department of Psychology, University of Texas at Arlington,
Arlington, TX, USA
e-mail: valerie.johnston@mavs.uta.edu

Overview: Pain Rehabilitation and the Restoration of Function

The major purpose of the present chapter is to provide a review of the currently most therapeutically effective method for managing chronic pain—functional restoration (FR). Before doing so, a brief overview of the rehabilitation process will be provided. Indeed, throughout history, the treatment of chronic pain conditions has been difficult, time consuming, expensive, and, all too often, unsuccessful. Many modes of treatment, both invasive (injections, procedures, surgery, etc.) and noninvasive methods (medications, physical therapy, counseling, applications of heat, ice, transcutaneous electrical stimulation, and many others), have been used by the health-care profession in an attempt to eliminate pain and return these patients to a productive, fulfilling life. All too frequently, though, these attempts resulted in failure. Recently, however, an interdisciplinary FR approach to pain management has been empirically shown to be therapeutically and cost-effective. As will be discussed, the FR approach is based on a fundamental understanding of the individual's unique condition as it relates to impairment, disability, and functional limitation.

It should be noted that the *AMA Guides to the Evaluation of Permanent Impairment*, 5th Edition [1], defines impairment as "a loss, loss of use, or derangement of any body part, organ system, or organ function." The 6th Edition [2] defines impairment as "a significant deviation, loss, or loss of use of any body structure or body function in an individual with a health condition, disorder, or disease." One such impairment can involve the loss or abnormality psychologically, physiologically, or functionally at the level of the organs and body systems. Examples of physiologic impairments include muscle weakness, range-of-motion loss, and restriction or lack of ability to perform activities due to related impairments. These impairments can cause inabilities to function in specific vocations including those of being a worker, spouse, student, or parent. Disability is defined by the AMA Guides 5th Edition as "An alteration of an individual's capacity to meet personal, social, or occupational demands because of an impairment." The AMA Guides 6th Edition defines disability as "activity limitations and/or participation restrictions in an individual with a health condition, disorder, or disease." Finally, the American Physical Therapy Association in the Guide to Physical Therapist Practice, Second Edition [3], describes functioning as an umbrella term for body functions, body structures, activities, and participation, denoting a positive interaction between the individual or patient and contextual factors (i.e., background of the individual's life and current situation). Functional limitation is a deviation from normal behavior involved in performing the activities of daily living (ADLs) and may include problems with transfers, standing, ambulation, running, and stair climbing. A formal model proposed by the International Classification of Functioning, Disability and Health (ICF) [4] integrates the individual components into a biopsychosocial-based model where the term "health condition" is exchanged for "chronic pain" (see Fig. 82.1). Chronic pain is affected by body function, activities, and participation as well as influences from the environment and personal factors.

The World Health Organization (WHO) developed a comprehensive model of disablement, the International Classification of Functioning, Disability and Health (ICF) 2009; this classification is depicted in Table 82.1. The ICF framework is intended to describe and measure health and disability at both the individual and population levels and consists of three key components:

1. Body functions and body structures: physiological functions and body parts, respectively; these can vary from the normal state, in terms of loss or deviations, which are referred to as impairments.
2. Activity: task executions by the individual and activity limitations are difficulties the individual may experience while carrying out such activities.
3. Participation: involvement in life situations and participation restrictions are barriers to experiencing such involve-

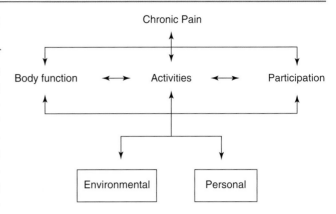

Fig. 82.1 A formal model proposed by the International Classification of Functioning, Disability and Health (ICF) [4] integrates the individual components into a biopsychosocial-based model (Adapted from International Classification of Functioning, Disability and Health (ICF) [4])

Table 82.1 Pain rehabilitation goals

1. Functional improvement
2. Improvement in activities of daily living
3. Relevant psychosocial improvement
4. Rational pharmacologic management (analgesia, mood, and sleep)
5. Return to leisure, sport, work, or other productive activity

From World Health Organization, http://www.who.int/classifications/icf/en/

ment. These components comprise functioning and disability in the model. In turn, they are related interactively to an individual with a given health condition, disorder, or disease and to environmental factors and personal factors of each specific case.

A patient-centered, "whole-person" approach is necessary to effectively address these important individual concepts. A team-centered treatment approach is utilized, focusing on helping patients achieve individual goals, which enable them to improve physical and psychosocial function, decrease pain, and improve quality of life. By working together, the chronic pain rehabilitation team helps patients achieve better outcomes than those achieved by an individual practitioner or interventions (i.e., surgeries, injections, pharmacotherapy, and psychological therapies) in isolation. Basic treatment goals of early and chronic pain rehabilitation programs focus on functional improvement, improved abilities in performing activities of daily living (ADLs), returning to leisure, sport, and vocational activities and improved pharmacologic management of pain and related affective distress (see Table 82.1).

History of Pain Rehabilitation

Early evidence of a rehabilitation approach to the injured person or worker dates back to the Egyptians under Ramses II, in 1,500 B.C. [5]. Further advances in treating pain seemed to be delayed until many years later, with the birth of the field of anesthesia in the 1840s, the isolation and synthesis of morphine by Serturner in 1806, and the discovery of salicylates in willow bark in the late 1800s [6]. Modern advancements in understanding health and health psychology in the 1950s also shaped a more comprehensive view of the complexities of an individual's pain experience. This led to the view that the experience of pain is a complex phenomenon and multiple models have evolved over time to explain it. Traditionally, the biomedical model explains pain through etiologic factors (e.g., injury) or disease whose pathophysiology results in pain. Over time, it became clear this classic biomedical approach to understanding and treating pain was incomplete. Its exclusive application often resulted in unrealistic expectations on the part of the physician and patient, inadequate pain relief, and excessive disability in those with pain that persists well after the original injury has healed.

George Engel [7] developed a novel theory of health care in which the various areas impacting an individual's disease process are taken into consideration. When developing a health-care plan, Engel posited that there were several factors affecting each individual and his/her disease processes. These factors include (1) biological, (2) sociological, (3) environmental, (4) cultural, and (5) psychological. This became known as the biopsychosocial model [8]. This biopsychosocial model was subsequently successfully applied to the assessment and treatment of chronic pain [9, 10]. In contradiction to the biomedical model, this model recognizes pain is ultimately the result of the pathophysiology, plus the psychological state, cultural background/belief system, and relationship/interactions individuals have with their environment (workplace, home, disability system, and health-care providers). To put it more simply, to treat the pain and the illness, the whole person needs attention.

The modern rehabilitation model evolved after World Wars I and II, with the founding of the fields of physical and occupational therapy as a method to rehabilitate returning soldiers who had been injured in performance of service to their country [11]. The practice of pain rehabilitation increasingly developed during the twentieth century by evolving medical specialties of physical medicine and rehabilitation, anesthesia, psychiatry, and occupational medicine. John Bonica, one of the fathers of pain medicine, championed a more comprehensive biopsychosocial multidisciplinary approach in the United States in 1947. This approach expanded to include a team of clinicians at the University of Washington in the 1960s [12]. Bonica's collaboration with Wilbert Fordyce, a psychologist, incorporated operant conditioning and other behavioral approaches with more specialized, structured, and inpatient multi-week programs. In the 1980s, John Loeser formalized a more at structured program the University of Washington. This 3-week long, daily program became a model for interdisciplinary treatment.

An increasingly biopsychosocial approach to pain rehabilitation, facilitated by the merging of behavioral and cognitive fields and subsequent cognitive-behavioral approaches

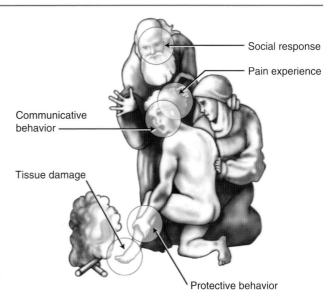

Fig. 82.2 Biopsychomotor response (Modified from Sullivan [15])

to the assessment and treatment of pain, developed in the 1980s and 1990s [13]. A proliferation of pain treatment facilities was seen between 1980 and 1995. These facilities included the advancement of interventional procedures as treatment for chronic pain [14]. A more recent conceptualization by Sullivan [15], the biopsychomotor model, focuses on behaviors within the pain system incorporating three independent behavioral subsystems: (1) communicative, (2) protective, and (3) social response behaviors. In this model, a pain system is assumed to be only adaptive. The sensory component of the pain system is accompanied by behaviors designed to act on the source, or cause of injury or illness. This may help to explain the wide variability observed in pain behaviors seen across different patients, despite relatively similar levels of reported pain intensity and objective tissue pathology. In this model, a more sensory-based model of pain extends to include behavioral factors: communicative behaviors (i.e., grimacing), protective behaviors (i.e., withdrawing a body part from fire), and social responses (i.e., empathy and solicitous behavior from others). This model, as in the biopsychosocial model, emphasizes dysfunction developing in behavioral systems separate from pain sensation. Subsequent treatments targeting pain behavior likely lead to better clinical outcomes and provide a more pragmatic and inclusive model for the spectrum of pain rehabilitation (see Fig. 82.2).

Applying a Biopsychosocial Model to Pain Rehabilitation

The biopsychosocial model of diagnosis and treatment operates on the idea that illness and disability is the result of, and influences, diverse areas of an individual's life, including the biological, psychological, social, environmental, and cultural components of their existence. In individuals with chronic pain conditions, the pain continues past the time the initial injury has healed. There are numerous challenges and issues that the patient faces and that must be addressed. These include guarding of the injured area, fear of movement and reinjury, adoption of the sick role along with cultural beliefs about pain, the loss of productivity, a decrease in beneficial leisure activities, the loss of income, and change in the role and responsibilities within the family and the community at large.

There are several factors identifying those individuals at risk for transitioning from an acute pain episode to a chronic pain condition. These factors are (1) unresponsiveness to traditional therapies normally effective for that particular diagnosis, (2) considerable psychosocial factors which negatively influence recovery, (3) unemployment or lengthy absence from work, (4) history of prior delayed recovery or rehabilitation, (5) the employer is not supportive or accommodative of the needs of the individual, and (6) history of childhood abuse: verbal, physical, or mental. Of the previous factors, lost time from work is most predictive of those at risk of encountering delayed recovery [16].

Chronic pain usually starts with an acute pain episode although, in some cases, there is no acute event, but rather the recognition of a pain problem. When a delayed recovery is recognized, the diagnosis and treatment approach should be reconsidered. At this time, psychosocial risk factors should be identified and the patient either treated by the attending physician or specialist using a biopsychosocial approach, or when appropriate, referred to an FR chronic pain program. A treatment plan addressing the presenting symptoms and attendant risk factors delaying recovery can then be developed and implemented. With a diagnosis of delayed recovery, a program focusing on the individual's biomedical condition, not addressing the complex requirements inherent in delayed recovery, will not be efficacious [9].

Individuals at risk of developing chronic pain conditions, as evidenced by lack of progress toward healing and a return to normalcy, are benefited by a multidisciplinary FR program. Physical and psychological interventions can be employed before disability becomes chronic. Early intervention minimizes long-term treatment costs and the negative physical, psychological, and sociological effects of disability, restoring the individual to an optimal level of functioning [16]. Many times, a purely biomedical model continues to be applied, with a narrow focus on reversing or eliminating nociception, or the "pain generator," and is more focused on a cure than on effective management. The biomedical model ignores or minimizes psychosocial factors, as well as the more complex central changes in the nervous system (i.e., sensitization of tissue, pathways, and neurochemical changes related to affective distress),that, not surprisingly, results in treatment failure (see Table 82.2).

Table 82.2 The biomedical versus the biopsychosocial model of pain

Biomedical model	Biopsychosocial model
Suitable for acute pain management	Suitable for chronic pain management
Concentrates on physical disease mechanisms	Illness behaviors incur[prating cognitive and emotional responses to pain are acknowledged
Accentuates peripheral perception of pain (nociception)	Understands the role central physiological mechanisms play in the modulation of peripheral nociception or the generation of pain experience in the absence of nociception
Approach to understanding/ treating pain is reductionistic	Understanding and treating pain is approached with a multidisciplinary systems perspective
Relies on medical management approaches	Utilizes self-management approaches

History of Functional Restoration and Work Rehabilitation

Historically, FR is a term that was initially used for a variety of pain rehabilitation programs characterized by objective measure of physical function, intensive graded exercise, and multimodal pain/disability management, with both psychosocial and case management features. The concept of functional restoration was first described in the mid-1980s. Functional restoration programs for chronic pain have strong support in the medical literature going back to the early 1990s. The term "functional restoration" has in recent years become increasing popular with evidence-based medicine support, and it has been adopted as the treatment paradigm of choice for chronic conditions and particularly chronic pain states. Indeed, the effectiveness of functional restoration programs has been independently replicated throughout the world [17]. For patients with more complex or refractory problems, a comprehensive multidisciplinary approach to pain management that is individualized, functionally oriented (not pain-oriented), and goal specific has been found to be the most effective treatment approach [10, 18, 19].

Functional restoration (FR) programs, which are based on a return to work model, evolved along with advancements in occupational medicine, beginning in the 1970s. Prior to this, in the 1920s, programs of habit training, focused on restoring workers affected by disease or injury and later, in 1923, by the incorporation of vocational rehabilitation, were mandated at the federal level by the Vocational Rehabilitation Act. In the 1950s, more objective measures were used to track progress and measure outcomes and served as the starting point for more formal work conditioning and work hardening programs. These innovative programs were championed by Lillian Wegg and Florence Cromwell [20]. Subsequently, in the 1970s, work hardening emerged as a formal industrial management service [21], adopting a similar multidisciplinary approach that was used in the management of chronic pain and disability. Standardized work simulation equipment, assessment, and treatment protocols were incorporated into standard practice in the 1980s, leading to formal accreditation by the Commission on Accreditation of Rehabilitation Facilities (CARF) in the late 1980s and early 1990s.

Recent evidence-based guidelines strongly support the use of interdisciplinary functional restoration-based programs for the treatment of chronic pain, including low back pain [19]. For the treatment of chronic nonradicular low back pain, interdisciplinary functional restoration treatment, including cognitive-behavioral interventions, is supported by high-quality evidence. Within these same evidence-based guidelines, shared decision making for potential surgical intervention for low back pain should include a discussion of interdisciplinary treatment, since interdisciplinary therapy was found to be equally effective in long-term outcome studies [22].

Applying Functional Restoration Approach: Multi- and Interdisciplinary Treatment

Functional restoration is an evidence-based, empirically proven component of multi- and interdisciplinary pain management programs, emphasizing physical activity and psychosocial therapy and anticipating an individual's gradual progression to a normal lifestyle. FR programs emphasize a multidisciplinary, biopsychosocial approach in which physicians, psychologists, occupational and physical therapists, and therapists specializing in other relaxation techniques all work in concert with each other. The ultimate goal is the development and implementation of treatment plans individualized to fit each patient's unique needs. These programs are regarded as the treatment of choice for chronic conditions, particularly chronic pain conditions [23]. Such programs are both therapeutically and cost-effective in treating chronic pain conditions and restoring a patient to a productive lifestyle. Moreover, while FR programs are effective for chronic pain conditions, many believe this type of program would be both cost-effective and efficacious for other chronic conditions as well [24].

Gatchel et al. [25] have delineated the described critical elements of a functional restoration approach, which serves as the foundation for most multi- and interdisciplinary rehabilitation-based programs. These elements include quantification of physical deficits on an ongoing basis; psychosocial and socioeconomic assessment used to individualize and monitor progress; an emphasis on reconditioning of the injured area or body part; generic simulation of work or activity; disability management with cognitive-behavioral approaches; psychopharmacologic management focusing on improving

analgesia, sleep, and affective distress; and, in some cases, detoxifying patients from medications (i.e., opioids or benzodiazepines). Individually tailored, these programs initially emphasize moderate physical interventions (i.e., stretching, strengthening, conditioning) and gradually progressing to more active, strenuous therapies with the goal of obtaining maximum rehabilitation and normalization in all facets of a person's lifestyle. This includes return to work, improved socioeconomic factors and self-esteem, and cognitive behavior therapy (CBT) addressing beliefs about pain, the resulting dysfunction, and environmental and socioeconomic factors. Research shows that a chronic pain patient's treatment needs are best addressed by such a multidisciplinary treatment program [26]. However, a biopsychosocial model of health care is not only efficacious in the treatment of chronic pain. Patients presenting with other disease processes are likely to benefit from this type of treatment concept.

Major Components of Functional Restoration

Some confusion has developed with the mixing of terms such as multi- and interdisciplinary models [10]. In the multidisciplinary model, patient care is planned and managed by a team leader, usually a pain specialist (anesthesiologist, physiatrist, neurologist, psychiatrist, or primary care provider), or a psychologist, and often hierarchical, with one or two individuals directing the services of a range of team members, many with individual goals. Treatment may be delivered at different facilities or centers where individual patient progress is not regularly shared between distinct disciplines. In contrast, the more collaborative interdisciplinary model involves team members working together "under one roof" toward a common goal. Team members are able to communicate and consult with other team members on an ongoing basis, facilitated by regular, face-to-face meetings. The interdisciplinary model provides practical strategies for assessing and treating pain-related deconditioning, psychosocial distress, and socioeconomic factors related to disability. An interdisciplinary team model is characterized by team members working together for a common goal, making collective therapeutic decisions, having face-to-face meetings and patient team conferences, and facilitating communication and consultation. Interdisciplinary teams may be led by a physician (medical director), psychologist, or nurse, and it includes comprehensive assessment incorporating pain medicine, pain psychology, physical functional restoration, and vocational rehabilitation. Physical and occupational therapy assessments are also included in the formal assessment. Interdisciplinary programs are usually housed in one facility, with group goal setting, periodic interdisciplinary team meetings assessing and adjusting treatment progress, program coordination, and discharge planning. The physical aspects of these programs focus primarily on restoring joint mobility, muscle strength, endurance, conditioning, and cardiovascular fitness. The psychological aspects focus on cognitive behavioral strategies for pain management. The coordination of vocational and therapeutic recreation services is an important aspect of care, focusing on aiding patients in their return to work, improving behavioral factors (i.e., coping, catastrophizing, and problem solving) in the workplace, clarifying return to work level of functioning, and, in many cases, providing individual therapy.

In general, formal interdisciplinary programs usually last 3–8 weeks, 4–8 h/day, with tailored group and individual therapies provided in an outpatient setting. Program schedules include individual and group-based therapies. Most importantly, regularly scheduled team conferences help to facilitate progress, troubleshoot patient problems, build consensus, improve communication regarding progress (i.e., complete conference notes and communicate to case managers and referring physicians), adjust goals of therapy, and plan for discharge. Long-term follow-up studies of interdisciplinary treatment programs demonstrate improved return to work rates, pain reduction, and quality of life. In special situations, inpatient functional restoration programs may be indicated. Inpatient pain rehabilitation programs typically consist of more intensive functional rehabilitation and medical care than their outpatient counterparts. They may be appropriate for patients who (1) do not have the minimal functional capacity to participate effectively in an outpatient program, (2) have medical conditions that require more intensive oversight, (3) are receiving large amounts of medications necessitating medication weaning or detoxification, or (4) have complex medical or psychosocial diagnoses that benefit from more intensive observation and/or additional consultation during the rehabilitation process. As with outpatient pain rehabilitation programs, the most effective programs combine intensive, daily biopsychosocial rehabilitation with a functional restoration approach. To again summarize, the fundamental elements of a functional restoration approach include assessment of the person's dynamic physical, functional, cultural, and psychosocial status. This includes assessment of strength, sensation, range of motion, aerobic capacity, and endurance, as well as measures of what the individual can and cannot do in terms of general activities of daily living, recreational, and work-related activities. Psychosocial strengths and stressors are assessed, including an analysis of the individual's support system, any history of childhood dysfunction or abuse, evidence of mood disorders or psychiatric comorbidity, assessment of education and skills, medication use, any history of substance abuse, presence of litigation, and work incapacity [24]. We will now review the various issues addressed in a comprehensive FR program.

Normalization of Function

Normalization of function is described as the reestablishment of independence and function, while understanding that some physical limitations may be unavoidable. Functional restoration empowers the individual to achieve maximal functional independence, the capacity to regain or maximize activities of daily living, and return to vocational and avocational activities. Depending on the current functional level of the patient, reaching their maximum level of function may take as long as 6 months to a year as they incorporate both a progressive exercise program and active pain management skills into their lifestyle. For physical limitations that are unavoidable, patients should be instructed on assistive devices and modifications for the home, and/or the workplace to allow them to achieve the highest level of function possible.

Education

At the beginning of any treatment, the patient's understanding and belief system of his or her prognosis and treatment must be ascertained. Information from multiple providers can often be misunderstood. Patients are often informed that nothing else can be done for them. Some are given lifting restrictions of no lifting or carrying greater than 10 lb postsurgically, and they continue to adhere to these restrictions for years after the necessity has lapsed. The treating physician and/or physical or occupational therapists, treating in an acute care model, may have informed the patient not to use the body part if it were painful. All of these can leave the patient with incorrect directions on how to best manage chronic pain.

Before the patient considers participating in a functional restoration program, he or she should be informed regarding the differences between functional restoration and other treatment methods. It is not uncommon for the patient to have seen multiple doctors and therapists without any benefit or with a worsening of symptoms. The patient may have little confidence that a functional restoration approach will be more effective than any of the other treatments that they have tried. Therefore, education about diagnosis, prognosis, and expectations concerning treatment and outcome should begin as soon as possible. Explanation of the changes to the patient's body, his or her personal experience, and how this translates to the symptoms they are experiencing is a connection that the provider must make for the patient. The patient must be provided with a confirmation that variability of symptoms and emotions are normal to their condition. The expectations concerning patient effort in the restoration process are emphasized. The active participation of the patient in the setting of treatment goals, his or her personal control of the process, and the success of the treatment are all important aspects contributing to the likelihood of successful completion of the restoration and a return to normalcy.

The patient must understand that treatment will provoke discomfort and may be perceived as painful, that they will receive help with managing these symptoms, and that the outcome will be significant improvement in their overall functional level. Education regarding goals based on function, not only pain changes, is important to assist the patient in feeling successful and attaining their goals, as many patients believe that the focus of treatment is to simply reduce their pain level. Finally, the patient must be educated about the negative consequences of inactivity and resting. A significant loss of flexibility, strength, and secondary injury from guarding and abnormal movement are all possible, harmful consequences if the patient does not remain active after functional restoration therapy is complete.

Fear of Reinjury or Movement

Kinesiophobia (the fear of movement and reinjury) commonly obstructs the individual's return to work, a normal home life, and leisure activities after an injury has occurred. Fear related to pain, and subsequent avoidance of activities, has been empirically validated as an important factor in determining the patient's activity levels at 6–12 month post-injury [27]. Typically, patients will push themselves to increase social and physical activities in an attempt to confront and overcome the pain and disability of an injury. This may increase the pain, which increases the fear that an as-yet undiagnosed injury or illness is present. This fear may lead to a maladaptive avoidance response, which leads to lack of exercise and a physical deconditioning; this, in turn, leads to lack of muscle strength and flexibility and an increase in pain and infirmity. The patient must then be reexposed to previously avoided activities and assume a participatory role in the recovery process. Crombez et al. [28] found that "over prediction of pain," a construct closely related to fear-avoidance, was reduced by a gradual, paced, and repeated exposure to the activity individualized to the patient's own fear. Studies have suggested that back pain disability for some patients may be determined more by the fear of pain rather than intensity or other biomedical factors [29]. Treatment to overcome fear-avoidance includes patient education, repeated exposure to activities that have been avoided, and taking responsibility in an active role to recovery. Patients are educated on how their beliefs and behaviors can lead to a vicious cycle involving catastrophic thoughts, fear, avoidance, disability, and pain. The patient learns the difference between pain and damage, safe positioning, safe activity, and slow progression of exercise. The activity program consists of the fearful activities initially introduced at low levels and then progressed on an individual basis.

Exposure therapy is a type of cognitive behavioral therapy (CBT – see below) and is used to expose an individual to fear-provoking stimuli. The bioinformational theory of fear states that activation of fear association, followed by the availability of new information refuting the fear expectations, is an intrinsic part of fear memory reduction [30]. A therapy used to develop a hierarchy of fear-producing stimuli uses a photograph series of daily activities, using the upper extremities (PHODA-UE), and a series of daily activities involving the lower extremities (PHODA-LE) [31]. In this therapy, patients judge the threat value of the various activities. The therapist then develops individually tailored practice tasks. The patient begins to perform the tasks, beginning with the least fear-inducing tasks, gradually advancing through the hierarchy to the most fear-inducing tasks [24].

Flare-up Management

Flare-ups, the seemingly uncontrolled, overwhelming symptoms of chronic pain, can feel unmanageable. The physical reactions to these flare-ups can include holding the breath, muscle tightening, tightening of chest and stomach muscles, and nausea. Psychological reactions can include fear, anxiety, worry, feelings of being overwhelmed, and anger. As these reactions take place, the pain level increases, incurring further flare-ups. Flare-up management education gives the patient active tools with which to control these symptoms. In the acute model, passive tools such as ice, heat, massage, TENS, rest, and medications are used for pain control. These passive tools are not as effective with chronic pain and often leave the patient dependent on medical providers. Active tools allow for more independence and a feeling of control. Education on ways to prevent flare-ups, and managing current flare-ups, provides the patient with different ways to control his or her pain.

The patient is educated on a variety of tools from all different aspects, including physical, emotional/behavioral, social, cognitive, spiritual, and environmental [32]. Teaching patients how to perform diaphragmatic breathing through pain, using light stretching or exercise, and ways to pace their activity (including setting limits), relaxation techniques, distraction, and visual imagery are some examples of useful tools. The patient is allowed to take multiple breaks during activities, which allows for control of any intensifying symptoms of anxiety, fear, or any other unconstructive response. These breaks are used for deep breathing, relaxation, stretching, and/or CBT to help the patients to become calm and relaxed, at which time they are able to resume their activities.

Pacing

Pacing is a tool allowing the patient to change the way they perform, or complete an exercise or activity, successfully increasing strength, tolerance, and function, while managing pain levels. The purpose of pacing and goal setting is regulating daily activities and structuring an increase in tolerance by gradually increasing activity. Pacing activity requires the person to break an activity into active and rest periods.

Rest periods are taken before significant increases in pain level occur. It provides structure to the overall activity level, guiding the individual to build an optimum schedule, minimizing pain, and maximizing productivity during the day. Pacing also brings about structure to the day, giving the person a sense of control.

Psychosocial Approaches

Many behavioral and psychosocial variables intensify and aggravate the pain and disability related to chronic pain conditions [26]. These behavioral and psychological variables help maintain the chronic pain condition in some patients. An interdisciplinary approach addresses these variables in an attempt to effectively manage the negative aspects associated with chronic pain. Anxiety, stress, communication skills, ideas about pain, and coping methods are all associated with a patient's ability to successfully or unsuccessfully cope with pain. If patients have negative ideas about themselves and their chronic pain condition, these destructive feelings can spread to their home and families, and they may, in turn, lose the ability to enjoy constructive activities. This reinforces initial negative feelings and causes the patient to become apathetic, depressed, and anxious. The family relationships are negatively modified, responsibility and productivity decrease, and the pain cycle increases with the assimilation of the "sick role." The financial burden that accompanies the loss of productivity and the negative psychosocial and behavioral aspects of the chronic pain condition all contribute to a downward spiral affecting all aspects of a patient's existence [33]. A functional restoration program is designed to recognize all the factors that contribute to an individual's chronic pain experience and to educate and support the patient to manage and alter those factors successfully. Often, the family is included in some sessions to provide them with a perspective of important pain management techniques that they can help with at home with the patient, as well as to modify any solicitous behaviors they may be providing (as discussed above). The group setting of a functional restoration program increases the feelings of companionship and solidarity with others who are experiencing similar changes. In addition, the use of psychological intervention approaches, such as cognitive behavioral therapy (CBT), and mind-body techniques including biofeedback-assisted relaxation training, hypnosis, deep breathing, and coping skills training can all bring about positive change in a patient's existence [34].

Cognitive Behavioral Therapy (CBT)

Cognitive behavioral therapy (CBT), developed by Aaron Beck, is a form of therapy that combines features of both cognitive therapy and behavioral therapy that assists patients in recognizing, confronting, and changing irrational thoughts (Table 82.3). This type of therapy emphasizes the important role of thoughts and how automatic, but inaccurate thoughts or beliefs in certain situations lead to negative moods, unhealthy

Table 82.3 Pain team shared primary objectives of a cognitive behavioral approach for pain patients

Combat demoralization by assisting patients to change their view of their pain from overwhelming to manageable
Teach patients the coping strategies and techniques to help them to adapt and respond to pain and the resultant problems
Assist patients to reconceptualize themselves as active, resourceful, and competent
Learn the associations between thoughts, feelings, and behaviors, subsequently identify and alter automatic, maladaptive patterns
Utilize more adaptive ways of thinking, feeling, and behaving
Bolster self-confidence and patient's attribution of successful outcomes to their own efforts
Help patients anticipate problems proactively and generate solutions, thereby facilitating maintenance and generalization

Adapted from Sullivan [15]

behaviors, and attitudes detrimental to the patient and his progression toward a constructive and adaptive lifestyle.

CBT teaches the patients to recognize and replace maladaptive behaviors with healthy, adaptive behaviors. This form of therapy is frequently used on patients with chronic pain and is especially helpful for those who suffer with comorbid psychosocial illnesses, such as depression, anxiety, or somatoform disorders. CBT encompasses a wide variety of treatments, including relaxation, biofeedback, guided imagery, and acquisition of other adaptive coping mechanisms. The treatment plan is easily adapted to the needs of the individual patient. CBT is an important therapeutic component of a multidisciplinary pain clinic program. CBT is an efficacious, cost-effective therapy for chronic pain conditions; however, it does not treat the physiological mechanisms of the pain itself. It does improve the patient's perception of the pain experience, the appraisal of the pain experience, and the subsequent coping mechanisms, as well as the ability to negate the "sick role" that often is adopted by chronic pain patients and the individual's daily functioning [34].

Mind-Body Techniques for Chronic Pain

The mind-body connection uses the power of thoughts and emotions to train the mind to control the body. The techniques include biofeedback and relaxation therapy which commonly includes diaphragmatic breathing, meditation, imagery, and autogenic training.

Biofeedback

A technique in which people are trained to learn how to control certain internal bodily processes, normally occurring involuntarily, such as heart rate, blood pressure, muscle tension, and skin temperature. The results of biofeedback are measured by electromyography (EMG) which measures muscle tension, surface electrodes which measure the galvanic skin response, thermal biofeedback which measures skin temperature, and an electrocardiograph (ECG) which measures heart rate or an electroencephalograph (EEG) which measures brain-wave activity. The patient is taught to use this information to gain control over these involuntary activities. Such biofeedback is used in pain management, assisting the patient in recognizing and controlling factors that aggravate pain. This technique helps the patient learn the connections between emotions and health, improving a patient's awareness toward his or her own body. Through the use of specific instrumentation and computers, physiologic responses are brought closer to conscious awareness and control by their conversion into auditory or visual feedback. With biofeedback, patients are commonly taught to recognize and release tension in their muscles, decrease stress response, control anxiety, slow breathing and heart rate, and raise their skin temperature. Regardless of the specific technique utilized, successful incorporation of relaxation techniques into a patient's treatment plan offers the patient more active self-management tools. The techniques are applicable to daily self-management of chronic pain, as well as during more problematic periods of flare-ups. Formal relaxation training is usually performed by certified relaxation therapist or other allied health professionals, including licensed psychologists, physical, occupational, and/ or recreational therapists.

Relaxation Therapy

The numerous clinical approaches described for biofeedback training apply equally to relaxation therapy and commonly include diaphragmatic breathing, imagery, and autogenic training. The two chief relaxation methods utilized may also be characterized as deep or brief. Deep methods include autogenic training, meditation, and progressive muscle relaxation; brief methods include paced respiration and self-control relaxation. Autogenic training is a common deep method of relaxation therapy in which the patient imagines being in a peaceful place with pleasant body sensations. Breathing is centered and the pulse is regulated. The patient focuses on his or her body and attempts to make differing parts of the body feel heavy, warm, or cool. Elevated muscle tension has been shown to contribute to chronic musculoskeletal pain [35, 36]. Elevated muscle responses and prolonged muscle tension have also been demonstrated during physical work and stressful situations [37, 38]. A common deep method of relaxation is progressive muscle relaxation. During progressive muscle relaxation training, the patient focuses on contracting and relaxing each of the major muscle groups in attempt to better understand the feeling of tension which can then facilitate subsequent relaxation.

Breathing Techniques: People with chronic pain typically have a dysfunctional breathing pattern, due to living with anxiety, tension, stress, and pain. Abnormal breathing patterns can cause headaches, neck pain, shoulder pain, chest pain, and upper back pain. The body, breath, and mind are linked, and if there are abnormal breath patterns, they are partly due to irregularities in the mind or body. Therefore, if irregularities are eliminated from the physical breath, it has an extremely beneficial effect on the mind as well. When the breath becomes smooth, continuous, slow, and quiet, the mind comes along, also becoming calm and peaceful. The body follows, relaxing much more easily. Diaphragmatic breathing techniques are used in all parts of a functional restoration program to educate and instruct the patient on an effective and active pain management skill. Brief methods are also utilized when the patient senses an acute increase in stress or anxiety. Techniques include self-control meditation (a shortened form of progressive muscle relaxation), paced respiration (the patient breathes slowly and deliberately for a specific time period), and deep breathing (the patient takes a deep breath, holds it for 3–5 s, then slowly releases it). The sequences may be repeated several times to achieve a more relaxed state.

Meditation

Some practitioners consider meditation to be a deep method of relaxation therapy. The ultimate goal is mind-body relaxation and the passive removal of harmful thought processes. Although various forms of meditation are practiced, common forms include mindfulness meditation, transcendental meditation, yoga, and walking meditation. Mindfulness meditation involves the concentration on body sensations and thoughts that occur in the moment. The patient learns to observe these sensations and thoughts without judging them. Yoga and walking meditation are both derived from Zen Buddhism and use controlled breathing and slow, deliberate movements and postures to focus the body and mind. Transcendental meditation involves focusing on a sound or thought and the repetition of a word, mantra, or sound. As with relaxation therapies, meditation may be performed on a daily basis by patients with chronic pain to help maintain a basal level of pain control. It can also be useful in the management of acute and chronic pain "flare-ups."

Guided Imagery

Guided imagery involves the generation-specific mental images with the goal of evoking a general psychophysiological state of relaxation or other specific outcome. The visualizations are initially directed by a practitioner, with the goal of eventual self-guidance. Guided imagery is an essential part of a multi- and interdisciplinary chronic pain management programs. Persistent pain patients typically utilize guided imagery on a daily basis and may need to increase the number of sessions during acute pain "flare-ups."

Physical Medicine Treatments

Physical medicine approaches incorporated into an interdisciplinary program include interventional therapies, passive modalities (i.e., ultrasound, heat, cold), and more active physical therapy interventions including formal physical therapy-directed exercise, aerobic conditioning, strengthening, and stretching. However, the ultimate goal is to teach the patient self-management techniques to decrease and eventually eliminate the reliance upon medical intervention with the ultimate goal of a successful return to work and productivity [24].

Physical Fitness: Aerobic Conditioning, Strengthening, and Stretching

Physical fitness is defined by the American Physical Therapy Association as:

> A dynamic physical state comprising cardiovascular/pulmonary endurance; muscle strength, power, endurance and flexibility; relaxation; and body composition that allows optimal and efficient performance of daily and leisure activities.

Physical activity increases health and fitness, not only to injured body parts, but to the entire person. Exercise has been reported to improve the immune system, cardiovascular system, and digestive functioning; decrease stress levels; improve sleep patterns; and enhance mood. These physically reactivating activities have the benefit of being adaptable to both home and group settings. Physical conditioning encourages socialization in group settings such as health clubs and walking tracks. These activities can also be modified to each individual's physical activity tolerance level. Aerobic activities decrease pain, possibly through endorphin release. These activities also promote increased blood flow to the musculoskeletal system, warming muscle tissue, decreasing stiffness through joint lubrication, increasing circulation, and improving muscle tissue health. Aerobic conditioning and encouraging physical activity has been shown to reduce disability [39], and it was found that high fear-avoiders, randomized to an exercise class, were over three times more likely at 1 year to report reduced disability, compared to those patients randomized to usual general care (in which patients took part in a back to fitness program which included 8, 1-h sessions over a 4-week period which included low-impact aerobic exercises, strengthening, and stretching) [40].

Stretching exercises allow the individual to successfully learn an important pain management tool and a way for the patient to relearn relaxed, not guarded, movement. Although research on the benefit for stretching for prevention of injury in a healthy individual varies [41], this appears to play an important role in pain management. It is important that the patient learn proper stretching techniques, combined with breathing exercises, to allow for benefit and not pain flares. Patients often report increased pain with stretching due to pushing too hard into muscle resistance and other ROM restrictions. With simple modifications and relaxation techniques, stretching can be a useful and helpful tool. Strengthening and stabilization exercises provide increased muscle tone, muscle strength gains, and normalization of demands placed on the body. Strength and stabilization gains allow decreased mechanical stress on passive structures and a shift toward correct muscle usage patterns. Initially, the strengthening program must focus on exercising in a normal movement pattern and not encouraging a learned abnormal pattern. An exercise program begins at a level that the patient can tolerate with only minimal and sometimes moderate pain flares. The exercise program is carefully balanced, as to avoid excessively aggravating activities involving the affected area, causing a prolonged worsening of symptoms rather than an improvement. This is a challenge to the therapist and the patient, as one must distinguish between fear-avoidance and true harm with activity. The approach is often to find a "happy medium," where activity and exercise (while possibly uncomfortable) are not harmful but helpful. Flare management skills, especially pacing, are used to give the patient the pain control to continue with the program.

The program is then expanded and advanced slowly, in order to allow individuals to successfully complete the activities, encouraging their progression to more strength gains. Some examples of strengthening and stabilization tools include balance exercises, use of a physioball, foam roll, and functional exercise in all three planes of motion. Unlike machine-based exercises, functional exercises and exercises focused on stabilization challenge the patient's body to allow development of the necessary strength to negotiate daily activities. More specialized PT-directed therapy for low back pain treatment may include directional preference assessment (i.e., McKenzie therapy) and neuromobilization. For those with compromised joint function, and comorbid conditions that prevent weight-bearing exercise, aquatic therapy shows benefits in edema control and decrease in stress on affected joints while increasing aerobic capacity, muscle strength, and flexibility [24]. Active therapeutic exercise should be individually assessed and adjusted with an emphasis on ensuring compliance and independence with an agreed upon home program after completion of formal therapy. Other treatments used include Tai Chi, yoga, Feldenkrais, and gait training. Typically, a comprehensive program using a combination of all of these techniques to seek the "best fit" for each patient's needs and physical level is encouraged.

Postural Training

Maintaining correct posture is more than just "standing up straight." It requires finding a balance between the head, trunk, pelvis, and lower extremity, as well as engaging the correct musculature, and maintaining this balance throughout different activities. Factors associated with postural issues include a long history of poor posture leading to an imbalance of muscle length and tone, compensatory postures, disuse syndromes, and prolonged bed rest. Suffering from chronic pain can lead to inactivity, increased down time, and prolonged bed rest, which may lead to loss of muscle strength in the postural and lower extremity musculature. Weak and compromised muscles and muscle groups are common areas of compensatory myofascial pain. Therapy can be directed at these specific areas of impairment. Determining and maintaining the correct posture, with both static and dynamic activities, requires extensive external verbal and tactile cueing, an increased sense of body awareness, and an exercise program focused on correcting the muscular imbalance.

Functional Activities

A functional restoration program focuses on supporting and promoting a patient's ability to return to being a productive member of the community, the ability to enjoy leisure activities, and successfully returning to family responsibilities. Functional activities, such as lifting, carrying, pushing/pulling, hand use and the activities performed in daily living, and leisure activities, are practiced. Treatment begins by helping the individual in assessing their current level of physical abilities in different areas. The patient then performs repetitive functional tasks, while being educated on abnormal or guarding physical movement patterns and correct body mechanics. Flare-up management, appropriate pacing, and gradual development of ability are emphasized. Often, patients are fearful of the specific activities that caused their injury, and overcoming this fear requires extensive education and instruction. Concurrent education on anatomy, physiology, mechanical stress on the affected structures with different tasks, and that pain does not always signal damage assists the patient in working through their fear. As the patient improves, they are encouraged to assimilate these practices into their home environment, including recreational activities which also increase socialization, exercise, and the utilization of free time [24].

Wellness Therapies

Wellness is defined by the American Physical Therapy Association as "A multidimensional state of being describing the existence of positive health in an individual as exemplified by quality of life and a sense of well-being." Wellness therapies play a significant role in pain management and functional restoration. These techniques are used as flare management techniques, movement therapies, stress management skills, and coping tools. Wellness therapies

include a variety of physical and mind-based techniques. Indeed, there are many different forms of mind-body relaxation approaches for pain management, but they all have the underlying purpose of connecting the mind and body through breath, allowing the person to reach a higher state of relaxation. Some techniques commonly used include imagery meditation, mindfulness-based stress reduction, breathing exercises, and progressive muscle relaxation. Movement-based wellness therapies, including Tai Chi and Qigong, provide a way to integrate relaxation into movement. Living with chronic pain can lead to guarding, muscle tension, and abnormal movement patterns. In Tai Chi and Qigong, movements are performed slowly, with deliberate and smooth movement. The focus is on breathing and creating inner stillness—quieting the mind and relaxing the body. This allows the patient to relearn how to move without guarding and tension.

Nutrition Education

As we know, proper nutrition is vital to multiple systems in the body including bone health, reducing the risk of heart disease, and controlling obesity. Diet and nutrition can also play an important role in the management of chronic pain. Certain foods such as those high in fat, sugar, and/or caffeine can intensify the pain response. In addition, some foods act as triggers for certain pain conditions, such as migraine headaches. Nutritional education not only includes the basics of nutrition, foods with anti-inflammatory properties, and the role of supplements but also topics on making smarter choices when dining out, label reading, and easy meals to prepare at home.

Treatment of Secondary Conditions

The potential for individuals suffering from a chronic pain condition to develop secondary conditions is great. Disuse syndromes, abnormal compensatory movement patterns, medications, and depression can cause weight gain and secondary myofascial disorders. These disorders are amenable to treatment. Identification of a compensatory movement pattern during the physical therapy evaluation is important. Initial treatment must focus on renormalizing movement, before strength gains or functional activity increases. It is not uncommon for patients to either show minimal gains or a decrease in current physical function, as they learn how to move in the correct pattern with normal muscle function. Nutrition counseling and education is helpful to combat the weight gain from secondary conditions. Drug, tobacco, and alcohol use are addressed as individuals adapt and adopt a healthier lifestyle. Evaluation of any sexual difficulties, sleep disturbances, or any other difficulties arising from depression, medication use, or the chronic pain syndrome should be addressed and treated [24].

Changes to the Environment

Properly adapting a patient's home and work environment and focusing on ergonomic issues and adaptive equipment in the home and in the workplace can lessen the pain and disability suffered by the chronic pain patient. Although the condition that the individual endures may not change, it is of vital importance that we treat the environment to reduce the dysfunction to a minimum. This is done in order to assure the patient's ability to function successfully, thus ensuring their best possible emotional well-being [24].

Functional Restoration Versus Other Similar Approaches (Continuum of Care)

FR with the biopsychosocial model as its basis has been proven to be the most cost-efficient therapy addressing chronic pain conditions in individuals. Because of the success of these interdisciplinary programs in treating these patients in returning them to home and work activities, there are many "programs" which call themselves interdisciplinary, but are not. These treatment programs are much less effective at treating the myriad of biological, psychological, and societal issues facing the chronic pain patient. It should not be necessary to emphasize that the reputation and outcome data from any treatment program are of vital importance.

Overview of Continuum: Parallel to Integrative Unidisciplinary Programs

Unidisciplinary programs, while incorporating treatment by physicians, psychologists, occupational, and physical therapists, may not be as effective as multidisciplinary programs [42]. Unidisciplinary programs require minimal contact within the treatment providers, usually restricted to progress reports or case histories. This kind of program is minimally effective and only as the initial treatment for patients who have been recently injured, presenting with low levels of disability and no simultaneous existing psychiatric disorders.

Work Conditioning and Work Hardening

These programs are intended for patients who, because of physical limitations, are not yet able to return to work. The American Physical Therapy Association defines "work conditioning" as a rigorous, goal-directed, work-oriented conditioning program intended to recondition musculoskeletal systems (i.e., joint integrity and mobility, muscle functioning). This includes strength and endurance, range of motion, and cardiopulmonary function. The intent of work conditioning is to increase the client's physical ability with the object of returning the individual to work. "Work hardening" is used to restore injured workers suffering from long-term injuries and disabilities, to be able to perform employment activities safely. Work hardening programs use actual or simulated work activities in a highly structured, goal-oriented individualized multidisciplinary program, intended to restore the individual's physical, behavioral, and vocational performance. These programs are geared toward increasing productivity, physical tolerance, and worker behaviors; in addition, ergonomics, job coaching, and transitional work development are also addressed. Such programs are most effective when detailed knowledge of the individual's job requirements is available, along with an in-depth understanding of the patient's physical abilities and specific deficits between his or her abilities and capabilities. An individual focus during therapy allows the gap between the end of physical therapy and the return to the workplace to be successfully bridged [24].

Early Intervention Programs

Early identification and suitable management of patients exhibiting signs of delayed recovery is believed to be an effective method of decreasing the likelihood the patient will develop a chronic pain condition. A restricted but intense early prevention program of physical rehabilitation and education allows a patient to distinguish various obstructions to healing and the eventual return to work. These early intervention programs are helpful for those who show signs of an impeded or delayed recovery and the need for instruction and psychological evaluation and intercession. The early intervention functional restoration programs are similar to the full-time FR programs, but at a lower utilization, duration, and cost than the full-time FR treatment programs. They have been found to be both therapeutically and cost-effective, relative to standard care, for low back pain patients. However, one of the difficulties found with early intervention programs is the fact that insurance companies are reluctant to authorize payment for treatment, in spite of the cost-effectiveness of early functional restoration intervention. However, there is a trend toward the identification of risk factors and early intervention by pain specialists and the willingness of insurers to pay for services [14].

Table 82.4 Strategies applied by the rehabilitation team to overcome barriers to collaboration

Stakeholders	Strategies applied
Worker	Pain management
	Relaxation
	Education
	Confrontation
	Rational polypharmacy (analgesia, mood, sleep)
Employer	Education
	Asking employers onion on TRW (therapeutic return to work) setting
	Sensitize employer to the support role in relation to the worker
	Asking insurer to use its authority to exert influence on the employer
Insurer	Education
	Sensitize to the issues involved in intervention
	Clarification of the roles and objectives
	Meeting with insurer's case worker before meeting worker or employer to ensure consistency in information delivered
	Acting without interfering
	Choosing convincing information
	Asking for the case worker's support for the intervention
Physician	Inform the physician about the rehabilitation process
	Convincing him/her to take action to facilitate return to work

Adapted from Loisel et al. [43]

Applying Team Values

Values underlying team decision making in pain rehabilitation has been found to incorporate common decision values shared by team members, workers, and stakeholders. Loisel et al. [43] describes "general values" shared by all that stress the construct that work is therapeutic, pain is multidimensional, and intervention should be graded. These values should, in turn, be shared by team members, the workers, and stakeholders. These values are facilitated by reassurance and the delivering of a single message as a way of more successfully returning a patient to work or previous level of function. These same values can be applied to many barriers presented to the individual patient and stakeholders.

The interdisciplinary team must have a broader view of the disability problem than is typically evidenced in the medical community. Communication between team members and other patient stakeholders (i.e., case manager, adjustor, family members, referring physician) may have some similar, as well as divergent or conflicting, goals. Success of the team may be determined by team values and the decision-making process (see Table 82.4). Curtis initially identified four values important to the rehabilitation team, including

Table 82.5 Team-related values for IPC

Team-related values	Comments
Team unity, credibility	Key factors in taking appropriate action and enhancing worker trust
Collaboration with stakeholders	Effective for coordination of care, constraining if it hinders team decisions
Worker's internal motivation	Demonstrated by autonomy and assertiveness
Workers adherence to the program	Worker and team acting as "allies"
Worker's reactivation	Overcome fear of movement and reinjury
Single message	Regarding patient condition, goals, and action of the team
Patient and team member reassurance	While playing down distressing, less helpful information
Graded intervention	Psychological and *physical* progression in order for patient to restore confidence
Pain is multidimensional	Must also be actively controlled
Work is therapeutic	Expose patient/worker to workplace obstacles, positive relationship between worker and employer, and preparing patient for work hardening and conditioning

Adapted from Loisel et al. [43]

altruism, choice, empowerment, equality, and individualism [44]. Subsequently, important values underlying any team decision-making process have been more recently been delineated [43]. Ten common decision values were identified in an observational study of an interdisciplinary team treating injured workers. The ten identified values were divided into four categories: (1) team-related values, (2) stakeholder-related values, (3) worker-related values, and (4) general values influencing the intervention (see Table 82.5).

References

1. Andersson GBJ, Cocchiarella L, editors. The AMA guides to the evaluation of permanent impairment. 5th ed. Chicago: American Medical Association; 2000.
2. The AMA guides to the evaluation of permanent impairment. 6th ed. Chicago: American Medical Association; 2007.
3. The American Physical Therapy Association. Guide to physical therapist practice. Second edition. American Physical Therapy Association. Phys Ther. 2001;81(1):729–38.
4. International Classification of Functioning, Disability and Health (ICF). http://www.who.int/classifications/icf/en/.
5. Foley BS, Buschbacher RM. Occupational rehabilitation. In: Braddom RL, editor. Physical medicine and rehabilitation. 3rd ed. Philadelphia: Saunders/Elsevier; 2007. p. 1047–54.
6. Zimmerman M. The history of pain concepts and treatment before IASP. In: Merskey H, Loeser J, Dubner R, editors. The paths of pain. Seattle: IASP Press; 1975–2005.
7. Engle GL. The need for a new medical model: a challenge for biomedicine. Science (New Series). 1977;196(4286):129–36.
8. Engel GL. Psychogenic pain and pain-prone patient. Am J Med. 1959;26:899–918.

9. Turk DC, Monarch ES. Biopsychosocial perspective on chronic pain. In: Turk DC, Gatchel RJ, editors. Psychological approaches to pain management: a practitioner's handbook. 2nd ed. New York: Guilford; 2002. p. 3–29.

10. Gatchel RJ, Bruga D. Multi- and interdisciplinary intervention for injured workers with chronic low back pain: invited review. SpineLine. 2005. http://www.spine.org/Pages/Publications/SpineLine/PreviousIssues/2005/sle05sepoct.aspx.

11. Murphy WB, editor. Healing the generations: a history of physical therapy and the American Physical Therapy Association. Alexandria: American Physical Therapy Association; 1995.

12. Bonica JJ. Organization and function of a pain clinic. Northwest Med. 1950;49:593–6.

13. Turk DC. Biopsychosocial perspective on chronic pain. In: Gatchel RJ, Turk DC, editors. Psychological approaches to pain management: a practitioner's handbook. New York: Guilford Press; 1996. p. 33–52.

14. Brena SF. Pain control facilities: patterns of operation and problems of organization in the USA. Clin Anesth. 1985;3:183–95.

15. Sullivan MJ. Toward a biopsychomotor conceptualization of pain. Clin J Pain. 2008;24:281–90.

16. Gatchel RJ, Polatin PB, Noe CE, Gardea MA, Pulliam C, Thompson J. Treatment and cost-effectiveness of early intervention for acute low back pain patients: a one-year prospective study. J Occup Rehabil. 2003;13:1–9.

17. Gatchel R, Okifiji A. Evidence-based scientific data documenting the treatment and cost-effectiveness of comprehensive pain programs for chronic nonmalignant pain. Pain. 2006;7(11):779–93.

18. Flor H, Fyfrich T, Turk DC. Efficacy of multidisciplinary pain treatment centers: a meta-analytic review. Pain. 1992;49(2):221–30.

19. Guzman E. Multidisciplinary rehabilitation for chronic low back pain: systematic review. BMJ. 2001;322:1511–6.

20. Curry R. Understanding patients with chronic pain in work hardening programs. Work programs special interest section newsletter (American Occupational Therapy Association). 1989;3:3.

21. Wegg L. Essentials of work evaluation. Am J Occup Ther. 1960;14:65–9.

22. Chou R, Loeser JD, Owens DK, Rosenquist RW, Atlas SJ, Baisden J, Carragee EJ, Grabois M, Murphy DR, Resnick DK, Stanos SP, Shaffer WO, Wall EM, American Pain Society Low Back Pain Guideline Panel. Interventional therapies, surgery, and interdisciplinary rehabilitation for low back pain: an evidence-based clinical practice guideline from the American Pain Society. Spine. 2009;34(10):1066–77. doi:10.1097/BRS.0b013e3181a1390d.

23. American College of Occupational and Environmental Medicine. Occupational medicine practice guidelines, chronic pain chapter update. Beverly Farms: Occupational and Environmental Medicine Press; 2008.

24. Feinberg SD, Feinberg RM, Gatchel RJ. Functional restoration and chronic pain management. Crit Rev Phys Rehabil Med. 2008;20(3):221–35. doi:10.1615/CritRevPhysRehabilMed.v20.i3.30.

25. Gatchel RG, Mayer TG, Hazard RG, et al. Editorial: functional restoration. Pitfalls in evaluating efficacy. Spine. 1992;17:988–94.

26. Turks DC, Swanson K. Efficacy and cost effectiveness treatment of chronic pain: AN analysis and evidence –based synthesis. In: Schatman MF, Campbell A, editors. Chronic pain management guidelines for multidisciplinary program development. New York: Informa Healthcare; 2007. p. 15–38.

27. Siddall PJ, Cousins MJ. Persistent pain: a disease entity. J Pain Manag. 2007;33 suppl 2:s4–10.

28. Crombez G, Vlaeyen W, Heuts P, et al. Pain related fear is more disabling than pain itself: evidence on the role of pain-related fear in chronic back pain disability. Pain. 2005;80:329–39.

29. Vlaeyen J, Linton S. Fear-avoidance and its consequences in chronic musculoskeletal pain: a state of the art. Pain. 2000;85:17–32.

30. de Jong JR, Johan WS, Vlayen JWS, Onghena P, Goossens MEJB, Geilen M, Mulder H. Fear of movement/ (re)injury in chronic back pain education or exposure in vivo as mediator to fear reduction? Clin J Pain. 2005;21:9–17.

31. Jelinek S, Germes D, Leyckes N. The Photograph series of Daily Activities (PHODA); lower extremities [CD-ROM]. The Netherlands: Hogeschool Zuyd, University Maastricht and Institute for Rehabilitation Research; 2003 (iRv).

32. Harden N, Cohen M. Unmet needs in the management of neuropathic pain. J Pain Symptom Manage. 2003;25(5 Suppl 1):s12–7.

33. Bruel S, Chung OY. Psychological and behavioral aspects of complex regional pain syndrome management. Clin J Pain. 2006;22(5):430–7.

34. Gatchel R, Rollings K. Evidence-informed management of chronic low back pain with cognitive behavioral therapy. Spine J. 2008;8:40–5.

35. McBerth J, Macfarlane G, Bejnamin S, et al. The association between tender points, psychological distress, and adverse childhood experiences: a community-based study. Arthritis Rheum. 1999;42:1397–404.

36. Wheeler A. Myofascial pain disorders: theory to therapy. Drugs. 2004;64:45–62.

37. Sanjsjo I, Melin B, Rissen D, et al. Trapezius muscle activity, neck, and shoulder pain, and subjective experiences during monotonous work in women. Eur J Appl Physiol. 2000;83:235–8.

38. Mork P, Westergaard R. Low-amplitude trapezius activity in work and leisure and the relation to shoulder and neck pain. J Appl Physiol. 2006;100:1142–9.

39. Linton S, van Tulder M. Preventive interventions for back and neck pain problems. Spine. 2001;26:775–87.

40. Klaber J, Carr J, Howarth E. High fear-avoiders of physical activity benefit from an exercise program for patients with back pain. Spine. 2004;29:1167–73.

41. Shrier I. Stretching before exercise; an evidence based approach. Br J Sports Med. 2000;34:324–5.

42. Gatchel RJ, Noe C, Gajarj N, Vakharia A, Polatin PB, Deschner M, Pulliam C. The negative impact on an interdisciplinary pain management program of insurance "treatment carve out" practices. J Workmans Compens. 2001;10:50–63.

43. Loisel P, Falardeau M, Baril R. The values underlying team decision making in work rehabilitation for musculoskeletal disorders. Disabil Rehabil. 2005;27:561–9.

44. Curtis RS. Values and valuing in rehabilitation. J Rehabil. 1998;64:42–7.

Pain and Spirituality

83

Allen R. Dyer and Richard L. Stieg

Key Points

- Pain is a physical symptom, but it is also more than a physical symptom.
- Spirituality (or religion) can be an important source of support and solace in times of difficulty such as facing chronic illness or pain.
- Pain may be seen as a test of faith or endurance.
- Pain and suffering may, for many people, sharpen their sense of meaning and what is important in life.
- Spirituality can be important in the life of physicians as well as in patients.

No one knows where we come from or where we go, but most of us have an intuition that there is a greater dimension that we participate in beyond our present work-----the soul's work
– David Whyte

Introduction

Teaching in the field of pain medicine seems to be dominated by emphasis on pain as a symptom. This is a natural response to the scientism that dominates our medical training, thinking, and practice. The topic of pain and spirituality affords us the opportunity to refocus our attention on the multidimensional aspects of the pain experience, as many have so eloquently done before [1–3]. We introduce our topic by posing several questions: How important is spirituality in the lives

A.R. Dyer, M.D., Ph.D. (✉)
International Medical Corps, 1313 L. Street NW, Suite 220, Washington, DC 20005, USA
e-mail: adyer@internationalmedicalcorps.org

R.L. Stieg, M.D., MHS,
1020 15th St., STE 30N, Denver, CO, 80202, USA
e-mail: rstieg01@aol.com

of patients? How important is the spirituality in the lives of physicians?

What role does spirituality play in health/wellness, recovery from illness, and relief from suffering? How can physicians attend to patients spiritual needs? Can we understand some concepts of spiritual experience in neurophysiological terms? Can such understanding help bridge the gap between the scientific and the spiritual?

Pain and Spirituality

Pain and spirituality are terms that everyone understands, but everyone understands them uniquely. The same words may convey different meanings to different people. "Pain" and "spirituality" are laden with meaning and with ambiguity. In many ways, they are beyond the ability of words to describe. Yet it is language we must use to communicate life's innermost and most personal experiences and their close, ineffable relationship. In order to create a shared understanding that will be important to physicians, no less than patients, we will explore the layers of nuance in pain and spirituality. Especially, the conversation physicians must be prepared to have with their patients depends on some level of mutual understanding and empathy. What is pain? What is spirituality? How do we communicate our experiences of these to others? How do we understand what others intend when they try to communicate their experience to us? Pain is a universal human experience, which in the modern (or postmodern) era may be understood to be either physical or mental/emotion. The dictionary definition reflects this cultural dualism. It tells us that pain is either physical suffering or discomfort (in a particular part of the body) caused by illness or injury or that pain is mental suffering or distress (New Oxford American Dictionary). Body or mind. Either/or. It was not always this way. Aristotle thought of pain as an emotion, like joy. Descartes, who ushered in the idea of a mind-body split, considered pain a sensation. Is physical pain a different experience to emotional pain or different aspects of the same experience? There is an obvious difference between a tooth-ache and heartache, but does it make sense to think of unpleasant experience as issuing from separate realms? We might be tempted to say from a medical point of view that pain is a symptom, a problem, something to be treated or eliminated. And often it is. But we would not wish for a world without sensation. We would not wish to eliminate the warning pains that teach a child to pull its hand away from a fire. We would not wish for a world without emotions, the joys that put our sorrows in perspective or vice versa. These are the experiences that make us human, that give life meaning. It is not always fun. It cannot be.

The question of meaning, what we might call the hermeneutics of pain, leads us to the relationship of pain and spirituality. Spirituality, like pain, is richly laden with meaning and ambiguity. For many people, spirituality can be equated with religion. For many people, their faith, their religion, provides a source of meaning and comfort and understanding. It makes life bearable. It may alleviate pain and suffering. In this sense, religion (or spirituality) becomes medically interesting. But for others, religion may be problematic, a source of dogma, discomfort, or divisiveness. So we are led to make distinctions. We look for the clear and distinct idea that so inspired Descartes, but we communicate with languages rich in nuance and ambiguity, that evoke meanings, rather than truncate them.

Religious or Spiritual?

In the latter part of the twentieth century, there has been a trend to distinguish between religion and spirituality. Older (pre-1960s) definitions of "religion" and "spirituality" typically saw the two as interpenetrating, often interchangeable concepts. Most frequently, spirituality was viewed as the intensely internalized aspects of one's espoused religion. Religion has its times of general spiritual intensification. Spirituality was often considered a path or discipline for incorporating religious precepts into one's personal living and consciousness. Spirituality's connection to religion with its theological and ritual dimensions overseen by a priesthood of some kind was considered essential to keep spirituality "within rational bounds" and not spinning out of control. Beginning with the 1970s, articles related to religion and spirituality began to appear with increasing frequency in the psychotherapy literature. Those articles that defined religion and spirituality in mutually exclusive terms tended to value spirituality and be dismissive of religion. Definitions that saw them as overlapping tended to value both [4–6].

In the current phase of intensified interest in spirituality and religion, the option of regarding oneself as "spiritual" but not necessarily "religious" has increased dramatically. "Religion" in many instances is more closely aligned with the political than with the spiritual, while spirituality retains the sense of a personal concern with meaning and transcendence. These concerns may or may not be grounded in institutional beliefs and practices. Whether this concern for the transcendent necessarily involves the sacred is a matter of personal consideration. Being captivated by a sunset, a sports team, or a political campaign is not intrinsically a spiritual experience simply because one feels connected to something larger than oneself. However, if these experiences are imbued with a sense of connection with the sacred, or ultimate reality, or things as they really are, then that would represent a spiritually significant experience. The ordinary activities of everyday life can thus become invested with spiritual meaning as is the case for a Buddhist focusing mindfully on sweeping the steps or eating a raisin, a Jew reciting a prayer while washing his hands, or a Catholic who views preparing a meal as a sacrament. In this sense, both religiousness and spirituality are seen as reflecting "the feelings, thoughts, experiences, and behaviors that arise from a search for the sacred" [4].

What might spirituality be, then, if not an approximate synonym for religious? Spirituality derives from spirits, ghosts, and the rituals that primitive cultures have developed to help cope with the feelings of lost loved ones. We now say more respectfully "traditional cultures," but our euphemism belies the connection with an unrefined, unenlightened, unscientific struggle to make sense and find meaning of a world beyond our control.

Pain and Evil

Evil stands as the antithesis of good, that which is valued. Evil is bad, and pain is disvalued, hence bad, hence evil. Evil is sometimes divided into natural evil, events beyond human control such as tsunamis and earthquakes, and man-made (human-made) evil, the bad things that people do, assaults, murders, and perhaps wars, the activities of sociopaths who act outside the bounds of conscience and civil responsibility. Illness (and pain) defies such classification. While disvalued, they are not necessarily caused unless one believes in an omnipotent being who causes everything. Such a belief challenges faith. Why would an omnipotent being cause suffering? If not as a deserved punishment, it would clearly be an injustice. This apparent contradiction is called theodicy, the vindication of divine goodness and providence in view of the existence of evil. Why would bad things happen to good people? The question is important not only for those who consider themselves religious, but for anyone who experiences suffering and tries to make sense of their experience. It is a conversation doctors should be having with patients, whose insights about their pain experiences offer clues for ways to help relieve their suffering.

The Case of Job

The Hebrew Bible (Old Testament) poses this question is the Book of Job in the context of man's relationship to God. The Hebrew Bible tells the story of a very pious and prosperous man named Job. He had seven sons and three daughters and many possessions. He constantly feared that his sons may have sinned and cursed God in their hearts, so he offered burnt offerings as a pardon for their sins. God asks Satan his opinion of Job, and Satan suggests that he is only pious because he is prosperous. God gives Satan permission to destroy Job's family and his possessions. In spite of these losses, Job remains faithful. "YHVH has given and YHVH has taken away" (Genesis 31:9). Job does not curse God, but he does question him. Satan asks for permission to afflict Job's body as well and causes Job to break out in boils. Still, he does not curse God, even when his wife urges him to do so. Job's three friends, Eliphaz, Bildad, and Zophar, believe that Job must have sinned to incite God's punishment. They believe Job must deserve his suffering because God always rewards good and punishes evil. Job's fourth friend Elihu takes a different view. He argues that Job may not have committed a specific sin for which he is being punished, but that the he is not perfect, and God as creator is such that his motives cannot be questioned by man. Elihu stresses that real repentance entails renouncing moral authority (the knowledge of good and evil), which is God alone. Elihu therefore underscores the inherent arrogance in Job's desire to "make his case" before God, which presupposes that Job possesses a superior moral standard that can be prevailed upon God. Job prays for forgiveness (for himself and his friends), realizing that he cannot understand the ways of God. His wealth is restored twofold; he is given seven more sons and three more daughters and lives to see the fourth generation.

This kind of introspection lies at the heart of one of the most successful disciplines in the treatment of addiction disorders, the 12-Step Programs of Alcoholics Anonymous and related community organizations such as Narcotics Anonymous. Although not widely used, it may have direct applicability to those suffering with chronic pain and other chronic illnesses [7].

Pain and Suffering

David Morris, in his far reaching analysis of pain in our culture, *The Culture of Pain*, has probably gone farther than anyone else in highlighting the tension and contradictions in our modern understanding of pain [8]. He observes that "The secular, scientific spirit of modern medicine has so eclipsed other systems of thought as almost to erase the memory that pain—far from registering its presence mostly in meaningless mental circuits or in some sterile, living death of hysterical numbness – once possessed redemptive and visionary powers. We need to recover this understanding partly because it shows so clearly how pain inhabits a social realm that sprawls well outside the domain of medicine." Suffering is a passive experience. Something bad or unpleasant, like pain or illness, befalls the person. What Morris is suggesting is that the interpretation of that experience may be redemptive in some way, as with the 12-step programs. Understanding this may put suffering into a different context that allows an individual to overcome it, at least conceptually, by active mastery. That taking control may be religious or spiritual or even political in some self-chosen way, a way that modern medicine may have forgotten or dismissed.

The Case of Ivan Ilych

Ivan Ilych was an ordinary man, Tolstoy tells us in his famous story, *The Death of Ivan Ilych*. He had noble qualities. He was cheerful, good-natured, and industrious. After he graduated from law school, his successes led him from one position to another, marriage, children, a nice house, and a life many might find enviable.

It was while decorating his house that he fell from a ladder, a downfall as it were, hurting his side. Pain entered his life, but it subsided. But it was followed by other sensations, a bad taste in his mouth, a pressure in his side where the pain had been. He became worried and preoccupied. He became irritable and withdrew from social activities. He stopped playing cards with his friends. He saw doctors, got prescriptions, more doctors, and more prescriptions. His pain in his side became a constant ache, which consumed his attention. His appearance changed, and this bothered him. It occurred to him that he might be dying, but his family continued to deny this possibility. He doubted his life, the reality of his accomplishments. When he realized that his life had been unalterably changed, he began to scream and he screamed for days. When death finally came, it was anticlimactic. Ivan Ilych, as he was once known, had already been dead for a long time.

Ivan Ilych's pain takes over his life so gradually that it is almost imperceptible. It is only by contrasting what he was with what he became that we appreciate how dramatic the change was. Tolstoy does not tell us exactly what was wrong with poor Ilych. He suggests that it was related temporally to the fall from the ladder, but that it might have been something different. Was it in his mind or his body or should he try to make that distinction? Tolstoy's story presents us with a distinction between the death of a person as a whole and the death of the whole person long before we began to worry about brain death.

The Role of Spirituality in the Lives of Our Patients

Larry Dossey, MD, has reviewed the world literature (more than 2,000 studies) on the role of spirituality and compassion on health stating that roughly half have shown positive statistical significance [9] and that spirituality/religious involvement correlates with decreased health problems and morbidity. He suggests that healing may be more likely to occur only in the hands of dedicated "healing experts." He discusses the famous Harvard study about intercessory prayer [10], noting while the effects of prayer in this study were statistically positive, the study could not be duplicated elsewhere. Dr. Dossey suggests that the difference was the "expertise" and good intentions of those offering the prayer in the Harvard study versus a more scientific experimental design utilizing people with less experience.

For a period of 2 years, thanks to the generosity of the owners of a private rehabilitation center where I carried out my work (RLS), we had as a regular member of the staff an ordained minister who offered both formal and informal spiritual guidance to our patients. Although a Christian minister, she was very much attuned to the spiritual needs of non-Christians and nonpracticing Christians. In addition to receiving voluntary counseling, the patients were given homework and reading assignments to help them get more in touch with their spiritual sides. Those with addiction disorders were also encouraged to actively participate in 12-step community programs. As one of my duties at this center, I conducted exit interviews on hundreds of patients who had completed this multidisciplinary pain treatment. One of my questions was a general one, "What things

meant the most to you in your time here at the clinic and what was the least helpful?" Almost invariably, somewhat to my surprise, was the answer that the "minister" had by far been the most helpful. When asked why, responses like "learning to cope" and "experiencing less suffering" were common answers.

Peter Levine, author of *Waking the Tiger*, *Healing Trauma*, notes the emergence in many patients of spiritual epiphanies as they successfully master significant physical and emotional trauma and suggests a common physiology if healing trauma is done gradually so that suppressed "survival energy" does not emerge rapidly and overwhelm the individual. Gradual therapeutic movement in this direction provides a vital resource for helping people reengage into life after the devastation of trauma. This is a feeling experience, similar to that experienced in virtually every religious tradition, where suffering is understood as a doorway to awakening [11, 12].

The Role of Spirituality in the Working Lives of Physicians

Recent surveys and papers reflect a growing interest among physicians about spiritual issues, including mindfulness, belonging to an organized religion and formal spiritual techniques such as prayer and meditation [13–15]. In order to address those issues, many healthcare professionals have relegated the job to spiritual counselors such as hospital chaplains. We suggest, however, that the spiritual dimension of patient's lives is too important for the physician to ignore. For many pain medicine practitioners that might call for a significant paradigm shift and we would offer a new medical model of treatment to accomplish that. George Engel identified the need for "a new medical model" in 1977 [16]. The model he proposed was a biopsychosocial model intended to expand the bio-reductionistic model then in force. The bio-reductionistic model held that everything you need to know about medicine could be explained by reducing illness to its biological components. That model was extremely successful up to a point. There had been many advances in biomedicine that supported the treat-the-body-as-a-machine approach. Even organs could be replaced intact like the worn out parts of an old automobile. Now, three decades after the publication of Engel's article, we appreciate that the biological model did not explain enough. We realize how mind (and stress) affect the body-machine and how so many of the illnesses people suffer stem from behavioral causes with physiological correlates.

In defense of Engel's originality and insight, I think it could be said that spirituality is implicit in his consideration of the psychosocial. But it must also be recognized that the discussion of spirituality in modern Western thought is strained and uncomfortable. We think it could also be said that a failure to distinguish the spiritual from the religious has impeded a broader consideration of the spiritual.

In opening up the possibility of a conversation about the role of spirituality in health care, we are aware that we would need to consider everything from the array of organized religions to the most unique forms of New Age individualism. And that is precisely the point. Each patient, each person comes to medicine with his or her own unique experience and outlook and needs. And they may find their own unique path to healing. The doctor and healthcare team do not need to share the same experience, but they need to understand the uniqueness of each person's psychosocial and spiritual needs, as well as their own. The team needs to be aware of the impact their own spiritual belief systems have on their interactions with their patients.

Rachel Naomi Remen, MD, has developed a curriculum that is now used in over 30 medical schools in the United States on the subject of medical practice and spirituality [17]. She also offers ongoing retreats for doctors on this same subject who either wish to teach the subject or who have become in some way dispirited themselves and are in need of refreshing [18]. At one of these weeklong seminars, one of the authors (RLS) was introduced to the simple practice of starting each day with yoga and meditation and "remembering to dedicate oneself each day in practice to our patients." In the course of doing this, one becomes more mindful of patients' needs and a better listener. I would submit that this is an informal spiritual practice that, sadly, many healthcare practitioners have abandoned or never even thought about. Indeed, in a series of focus groups held 10 years ago by the National Pain Foundation patient's suffering with chronic pain repeatedly stated that among their greatest needs were healthcare professionals who would listen to them and validate their pain and suffering; something they felt had been sorely missing in their lives. In addition to starting my workday in the manner above, I have also gotten into the habit of setting a quiet place in my office to talk with patients. We both have an easy chair in between which sits a lamp table with a lighted scented candle (which is quickly extinguished for my migraine and chemically sensitive patients), creating a sense of peacefulness and calmness which the patients very much seem to appreciate.

But what of our strong scientific training background? As a society, we value what we can count. We value scientific proof that something is of benefit before it's socially acceptable. Patients, too (even those who consider themselves on a spiritual pathway), may draw strength by having their subjective experiences validated by the tools of science [19].

Is There a Neurophysiologic Basis for Spiritual Experience?

Andrew Newberg, MD, Associate Professor of Radiology and Psychiatry, University of Pennsylvania, discusses the difficulty in matching subjective experiences (which are so variable among individuals and cultures) and objective measures [20]. Neurophysiological changes such as can be measured with functional MRI (fMRI) only capture some of the picture but show that a vast network of brain structures get involved with such practices as prayer and meditation. For example, parietal lobe structures deactivate as practitioners experience a sense of losing themselves while at the same time limbic areas such as the amygdala and hippocampus become active with intense spiritual/emotional experiences. So, too, are there measurable levels in hormones during such experiences.

James Austin, MD, Clinical Professor of Neurology at the University of Missouri-Columbia, is an academic neurologist. Dr. Austin has studied in Delhi, India, and Kyoto, Japan. His highly technical and intellectual discussion in the book *Measuring the Immeasurable* [21] offers the reader more in-depth discussion of the complexities of the science behind our subject. However, all of our growing understanding of the neurophysiology associated with spiritual experience still begs the question of why humans were given this gift of transformative mind.

Putting Spirituality into Everyday Practice

Death, loss suffering, and pain are all part of the human condition. Though we may lament, rail, and complain, we as human beings cannot escape their inevitability. Our challenge is what to do and how to understand in the face of a fate that is almost unbearable and unacceptable. Physicians and healers attending to those who suffer must be mindful of what their patients suffer. As technicians, it would be nice to be able to remove afflictions, and sometimes, this is possible, but more often, it is the task of the healer to help the patient bear what cannot be removed. For each of us, part of the task is coming to comprehend how to live a life that might be less than what we would hope for. That struggle takes time and has been articulated in a number of ways, some of which are illustrated in Table 83.1 [22, 23].

The notion that when faced with a loss or diagnosed with a serious illness, people go through a series of "stages" has become widespread in lay and professional circles [24]. There are no invariant rules, and several nomenclatures illustrate the process. Immediately, people tend to experience some sense of shock, denial, or at least disbelief that such a thing could happen. Almost all descriptors convey some

Table 83.1 Stages of faith and child development [22, 23]

Age group	Fowler's stages of faith	Developmental stages (Erikson and Piaget)	Key attributes
Infancy	Undifferentiated faith	Trust vs. mistrust (Erikson)	Development of basic trust through relationship with parents or primary caregivers; attachment sets the stage for future relationships
		Sensorimotor (Piaget)	Consistency and dependability of caregiving responses and rituals counter feelings of anxiety and mistrust
			Experiences mediated through senses and physical exploration
Early childhood	Intuitive-projective faith	Autonomy vs. shame *followed by* initiative vs. guilt (Erikson)	Literal and concrete thinking
		Preoperational (Piaget)	Imitative, reflects religious beliefs and behaviors of parents/caregivers
			Beginning to develop a sense of right and wrong, drawn to clear-cut representations of good and evil
			May judge things, experiences, or self according to outcome – e.g., viewing illness as a punishment; poor understanding of cause and effect
			Concerned about security, safety, and the power of caregivers to protect
School years	Mythic-literal faith	Industry vs. inferiority (Erikson)	Fairness is an important construct in understanding the world
		Concrete operations (Piaget)	Beginning to take on the stories, beliefs, and observances that symbolize belonging to one's community
			Superstition and magical thinking may be evident, but symbols and concepts remain concrete and literal
			Fuller understanding of cause and effect
			Increasing ability to separate own perspective from that of others
			Beginning to recognize that rewards and punishments do not necessarily correlate to actions ("bad things happen to good people")
Adolescence into young adulthood	Synthetic-conventional faith *followed by* individuative-reflective faith	Identity vs. role confusion (Erikson)	Development of abstract thinking, flexibility of perspective taking
		Formal operations (Piaget)	Sense of identity and "inferiority" are utmost concerns
			Ability to integrate diverse and even contradictory elements into self-identity
			Attachment to beliefs and personal expression of significant people in their lives
			Dependence on others for validation of and clarity about one's identity
			Experience of the world extends beyond the family to school, work, peers, "street society," the media
			Search for identity may include questioning beliefs and practices of family
			Toward end of this stage, critical reflection leads to intentional choices and renewed clarity about personal ideology and belief systems

sense of anger, which may be one of the most problematic emotions and difficult to deal with, especially if it is displaced, as it often may be, on the person trying to be helpful and responsive. It may be one of the most difficult things for physicians to deal with. Some sort of sadness, depression, and self-pity may follow, especially if open communication of feelings is not encouraged or tolerated. Eventually, one may come to some sort of acceptance, which does not necessarily mean that everything is alright, but rather that the inevitable reality is acknowledged. For physicians and health

Table 83.2   Stages of grief (words for feelings)

Denial	Denial	*Unglaube* (disbelief)
Anger	Anger	*Zorn* (anger)
Bargaining	Accusatory	*Selbstmitleid* (self-pity)
Depression	Self-accusatory	*Traurigkeit* (sadness)
		Gott flehend (pleading with God)
Acceptance	Acceptance	*Anerkennung* (Acknowledgment)

From Kubler-Ross [24]

Table 83.3   The FICA Spiritual History Tool

"How would you like me, your healthcare provider, to address these issues in your healthcare?"

The FICA Spiritual History Tool

F – Faith and Belief

"Do you consider yourself spiritual or religious?" or "Do you have spiritual beliefs that help you cope with stress?" If the patient responds "No," the healthcare provider might ask, "What gives your life meaning?" Sometimes patients respond with answers such as family, career, or nature.

I – Importance

"What importance does your faith or belief have in our life? Have your beliefs influenced how you take care of yourself in this illness? What role do your beliefs play in regaining your health?"

C – Community

"Are you part of a spiritual or religious community? Is this of support to you and how? Is there a group of people you really love or who are important to you?" Communities such as churches, temples, and mosques, or a group of like-minded friends can serve as strong support systems for some patients.

A – Address in Care

The FICA Spiritual History Tool [25]

professionals, the task faced is how to attend to such suffering. How should one enter into conversation with patients? Are there questions to be asked? Comments to be made? A general rule would be to start with open-ended questions, and LISTEN. Let the person narrate his or her own experience. Avoid judging or being prescriptive. These are challenging and sensitive areas because the basis for empathy is our experience even as we realize that others may experience and understand things differently, especially in spiritual matters.

Table 83.1 offers a developmental approach, which places Fowler's stages of faith alongside stages of psychological (and physical) development. Table 83.2, stages of grief (words for feelings), indicates some of the feelings people often report in the weeks or months after experiencing a loss or health diagnosis. Table 83.3, the FICA Spiritual History Tool, could be adopted for office use and suggests some widely used approaches to thinking of human development [25]. The stages offer the practitioner self-discipline to minimize assumptions about how someone should behave or respond. Developmental and stage theories help expand the assess-

ment of the patient as an empathic aid to understanding what their world might be like. For example, to say that someone is being "childish" can be harsh and judgmental. To realize that in the face of a threatening illness, even an adult may struggle, and to approach their suffering in a sympathetic and helpful manner may be the best that one can offer.

Ethics, Pain, and Spirituality

Religion and spirituality are for many a main source for ethical values, reasoned and understood. For the health professional, shared ethical norms orient healing activities in a way that patients, clients, or consumers can depend on the person from whom they seek help. The principle of beneficence, respect for autonomy and self-determination, informed consent, confidentiality, and competence are all norms which have governed professional behavior at least since the time of Hippocrates.

One ethical principle demands special attention in the area of religion and spirituality: the respect for boundaries. This is most basically seen in the proscription against sexual activity with patients. Also, it is the basis for the prohibition against entering into a business relationship or other dual relationship. It stems from the recognition that the patient is a different person, not an extension of the professional and not available for the gratification or exploitation of the professional. This can be problematic in the area of dependency relationships, where in fact the patient does need the expertise of the professional. It is ethically incumbent on the professional to recognize that need and not exploit it.

Another boundary that is important for the professional to recognize is the spiritual boundary. If the professional has strong religious beliefs, he or she must be careful not to attempt to impose them – even subtly – on the patient, realizing that we are not in a position to understand the mysteries of the ultimate.

Summary

We hope the preceding discussion will encourage a significant paradigm shift in the world of pain medicine today. Pain is much more than a medical problem, and medical attempts to eliminate or alleviate pain must also account for the complexities of human suffering. Medicine alone does not solve the problem of pain. Our scientific quest to conquer pain only underscores the reality of its complexity and heightens its mystery. The founders of the American Academy of Pain Medicine (formerly the American Academy of Algology) understood and emphasized the multidimensional nature of pain and the strong need for multidisciplinary approaches to its evaluation and treatment. There have been many scientific advances in the subsequent decades since most of which have shifted the focus of attention once again to pain as a symptom, subject to potential eradication by the wonders of our technology and pharmacologic prowess. These advances need to be coupled with a reawakening about the other important dimensions of pain, including the spiritual. There are many roadblocks to doing so [26]. The training of the postmodern twenty-first century pain medicine physician should reemphasize the importance of psychosocial and spiritual treatment if we are to achieve our goal as a truly unique medical specialty.

References

1. Chapman CR, Turner J. Psychological and psychosocial aspects of acute pain. In: Bonica JJ, Loeser JD, Chapman CR, Fordyce WE, editors. The management of pain. 2nd ed. Philadelphia: Lea & Febiger; 1990. p. 122–33.
2. Turk D, Stieg A. Chronic pain: the necessity of interdisciplinary communication. Clin J Pain. 1987;3:163–7.
3. Stieg RL, Williams RC. Chronic pain as a biosociocultural phenomenon, implications for treatment. Semin Neurol. 1983;3:370.
4. Grosch W. Reflections on cancer and spirituality. South Med J. 2011;104(4):249–305.
5. Newberg A, editor. Why God won't go away: brain science and biology of belief. New York: Ballantine Publishing Group; 2001.
6. Rippentrop EA, Altmaier EM, Chen JJ, Found EM, Keffala VJ. The relationship between religion/spirituality and physical health, mental health and pain in a chronic pain population. Pain. 2005;1(16):311–21.
7. Cleveland M, editor. Chronic illness and the 12 steps. A practical approach to spiritual resilience. Center City: Hazelden Publishing; 1999.
8. Morris D, editor. The culture of pain. Berkeley: University of California Press; 1991.
9. Dossey L. Compassion and healing. In: Goldman D, Small G, editors. Measuring the immeasurable. The scientific case for spirituality. Boulder: Sounds True, Inc.; 2008. p. 47–60.
10. Chibnall JT, Jeral JM, Cerullo MA. Experiments in distant intercessory prayer: God, science, and the lesson of Massah. Arch Intern Med. 2001;161:2529–36.
11. Levine P. Trauma and spirituality. In: Goldman D, Small G, editors. Measuring the immeasurable. The scientific case for spirituality. Boulder: Sounds True, Inc.; 2008. p. 85–100.
12. Levine P. Waking the tiger, healing trauma. Berkeley: North Atlantic Press; 1996.
13. Fung G, Fung C. What do prayer studies prove? Christ Today. 2009;53(5):43–4.
14. Büssing A, Michalsen A, Balzat HJ, Grünther RA, Ostermann T, Neugebauer EA, Matthiessen PF. Are spirituality and religiosity resources for patients with chronic pain conditions? Pain Med. 2009;10:327–39.
15. Büssing A, et al. Spirituality, therapeutic self-efficacy and interest in patients. J Explore Sci and Heal. 2009;5(3):150–1.
16. Engel GL. The need for a new medical model: a challenge for biomedicine. Science. 1977;96(4286):129–36.
17. Remen RN, O'Donnell J, Rabow MW. The Healer's art: education in meaning and service. J Cancer Educ. 2008;23:65–7.
18. Remen R. Graduate physician CME curriculum: detoxifying death. The institute for the study of health and illness at Commonweal. http://www.commonwealhealth.org/?s=detoxifying+death
19. Simon T. An introduction to the scientific case for spirituality. In: Goldman D, Small G, editors. Measuring the immeasurable. The scientific case for spirituality. Boulder: Sounds True, Inc; 2008. p. IX–XI.
20. Newberg A. Spirituality, the brain and health. In: Goldman D, Small G, editors. Measuring the immeasurable. The scientific case for spirituality. Boulder: Sounds True, Inc.; 2008. p. 349–72.
21. Austin J. Selfless insight – wisdom: a thalamic meaning. In: Goldman D, Small G, editors. Measuring the immeasurable. The scientific case for spirituality. Boulder: Sounds True, Inc.; 2008. p. 211–30.
22. Erikson EH. Childhood and society. New York: Triad Paladin Press; 1977.
23. Fowler JW, Dell ML. Stages of faith and identity: birth to teens. Child Adolesc Psychiatr Clin N Am. 2004;13(1):17–33.
24. Kubler-Ross E, Kessler D. On grief and grieving: finding the meaning of grief through the 5 stages of loss. New York: Simon and Schuster; 2005.
25. The FICA Spiritual History Tool. The George Washington University Institute for Spirituality and Health. 2012. www.gwish.org. Accessed 23 Jan 2012.
26. Dubois M, et al. Pain medicine position paper. Pain Med. 2009; 10(6):972–1000.

September Williams

Key Points

- Pain and other health and health-care disparities are related.
- Pain disparity refers to both unequal distribution of increased pain and decreased effective pain care.
- Pain disparity assessment modifies the standard pain assessment to improve pain care.
- Traditional medicine provides a guide to culturally relevant patient-centered pain management.

Introduction

Millions of people in the world have acute and chronic pain because of (1) ignorance of clinicians, (2) lack of a standardized scientific approach, (3) failure to facilitate adequate treatment of pain by legitimate use of opiates, (4) inadequate balance between use of controlled substances for medical purposes and the prevention of their abuse, and (5) lack of appropriate use of the new non-opiate pharmaceuticals and integrative medicine armamentaria which has expanded over the past decade [1, 2]. Of ten developed countries, World Health Organization (WHO) has estimated that 37 % of adults in these populations have constant pain conditions [3]. Pain is a public health concern because of its prevalence and increasing incidence. In 2010, in the United States, adults with constant pain were conservatively estimated at 16 million [4].

S. Williams, M.D.
Clinical Medical Ethics, Palliative Care and Film,
Ninth Month Consults, 401 Pine Street, Unit D, Mill Valley,
CA 94941, USA
e-mail: september.ninthmonth@gmail.com

Pain Disparity

Pain disparity refers to both increased pain and decreased effective pain care. Risk of poor pain care is proportional to the presence of pain itself, particularly when chronic. Pain is an arena of health and health-care disparity because its presence and inadequate management disproportionately affect subgroups of the US and world population (Table 84.1). When groups of people are compared, it may not be possible to clarify causal pathways directly causing differences in health. However, it is well documented that Black and Hispanic peoples are more disadvantaged by health disparities specifically through the mechanism of racism [5]. Racism, how an individual is defined by appearance, is an independent determinant for the quality of health, healthcare, and by corollary pain care [6]. Through racism, ethnic peoples of color are more disadvantaged by health disparities.

Pain Disparity: Oriented Pain Assessment

A given health-care disparity is most easily identified when there is a clear reference point for what is appropriate and reasonable to expect [7]. Palliative medicine literature establishes that it is appropriate and reasonable to expect that most pain can be brought under control by using basic principles of pain management [8]. The best current practice standard of pain medicine is appropriate to expect. However, current best practice pain assessment may not be sufficient for quality care where pain is combined with maximum vulnerability for other unequal health and healthcare.

Controlled chronic pain can be demonstrated by improved patient function, physiologic, emotional, and social comfort. Pain management, falling short of what is reasonable to expect when best practice standards are applied, leads to suspect pain disparity. The pain disparity assessment modifies the standard pain assessment by considering communication,

Table 84.1 Groups at risk for pain disparity

These vulnerable subgroups include those:
Having English as a second language
Being among ethnic peoples of color
With low income or poor education
Being women or transgender
Old or young
Disabled
Living in the inner city or rural areas
Being veterans from the United States Military

Adapted from Blyth [4]

Table 84.2 Effects of palliative care consultation

Sense of well-being and dignity
Information exchange and communication with the clinician
Respect for the patient treatment preferences
Emotional and spiritual support of patients and their families
Management of distressing symptoms
Choice of care
Access to outpatient, benefits, and services

Adapted from Casarrette et al. [9, pp. 368–381]

poverty, health literacy, shared decisional capacity, informed consent, patient concerns about addiction, and unaddressed biopsychosocial needs.

Communication

Pain disparity may be lessened through palliative care consultation. Palliative care consultation enhances communication. The family assessment of treatment at end of life (FATE) was used to compare palliative care consultation with other clinicians managing pain. In one study, care was perceived best with palliative care consults for a variety of reasons (Table 84.2). Effects of palliative care consultation were not race or ethnically related. Improved communication, even for those dying, decreases the negative effect of health-care and health disparities on pain and distressing symptom management across race and ethnic subgroups [9].

Experience and education aside, palliative care consultants may compensate for a key institutional shortcoming of most health-care systems, lost focus on clinician-patient communication under duress of time. Consultants frequently have more dedicated individual time per patient encounter than primary care clinicians. A pain assessment requires patient or proxy interviews exploring loss of function, other distressing symptoms, and pain's relation to them. Emotional, social, psychological, and economic burdens need be explored at the initial evaluation and then re-explored in subsequent encounters. Ultimately, it is the primary care physician who has the long view of a person's chronic pain management failures and successes [10]. Pain consultants assist in prioritizing associated concerns.

Rigorous initial pain assessment should be visible to patients. This, along with continuity of approach in subsequent assessments, provides a shared shorthand for communicating about pain. Pain assessment, like the physical examination, demonstrates to the patient due diligence, a caring and believing clinician. Relevant to communication, the pain assessment can cultivate a working relationship and language between clinician and patient cultures.

Clinician deficit perspectives, associated with deficits in cross cultural or language of communication, may drive poor pain assessment. Patients uncomfortable in the medical culture may present with apparent stoicism, excited expression, or historically appropriate distrust. Observing and responding to these presentations appropriately improve communication.

Poverty

Risk of poverty corresponds with being a person of color in the United States. An analysis of poverty finds nearly a 1:4 ratio of poverty for African Americans, "nonwhite" Hispanic Americans, and Native Americans. This rate is roughly 25 % of the respective populations. In comparison, 13 % of all Americans live in poverty. The highest rates of US poverty are among those living in inner city and rural areas [11]. All ethnic peoples of color are not poor. Nonetheless, most ethnic peoples of color have a disproportionately high risk for chronic pain and pain disparity.

Poorly managed acute pain often leads to persistent pain. Persistent pain can cause loss of function associated with poor employment, decreased educational capacity, and cross generational illiteracy. Clinicians will see pain disparity next to fiscal stress. Pain clinicians need to know that level of fiscal stress relates to medication access, transportation to appointments, basic utilities like telephones, and child care needs while participating in pain therapies. Appropriate social services referrals can diminish some poverty-related effects on poor pain management.

Health Literacy

Limited health literacy is prevalent and associated with low socioeconomic status and poor access to healthcare. Health literacy is defined as the degree to which individuals have the capacity to obtain, process, and understand basic health information and services needed to make appropriate health decisions [12]. Low health literacy is an independent risk factor for health disparities, particularly in older people, who are also disproportionately affected by pain [13]. A pain disparity assessment clarifies a patient's educational level, numerical and reading literacy. Verbal English literacy may mask variable capacity to read and write; particularly in inner-city communities, the elderly and those whose home language is not English. Pain rating scales can serve as an equalizing tool. Commonly, a numerical scale from 1 to 10 is used [14]. Unfortunately, numerical pain scales may be difficult for those with low mathematical, language, and health literacy.

If a patient seems unable to learn the 1–10 scale the clinician should explore that this may herald low health literacy. With this recognition of low health literacy appropriate selection of pain scale can be determined. A common adjustment is to convert the register of the scale to 1–5. The altered scale is multiplied by the clinician to reflect the 1–10 scale. This should be done with notation in the chart. Care should be taken so that other clinicians do not misinterpret a patient report of 5 as moderate pain associated with 5/10, instead of severe pain of 5/5. Each subsequent clinician should follow the same pain assessment scale. Simultaneous notation should be made about patient numerical health literacy.

The numerical pain scale can be substituted with a picture scale in low literacy, cognitive impairment, and children [15]. Picture scale efficacy does not seem as good as the numeric scale. Pictures must be appropriately interpreted in a cultural or age context. For persons with advanced dementia, without speech, or in vegetative states, a pain score can be calculated based on subtle observations of physical distress. Pain interpretation of distress in this population is often best in the hands of caregivers, family, or certified nurse assistants, not the clinician. Whatever pain scale used and therapy anticipated, the pain rating is translated into the language of mild, moderate, or severe pain. This facilitates appropriate initial management, choice of integrative therapies, dose of medication, and procedures.

Shared Decisional Capacity and Informed Consent

Where appropriate, a formal contract should be establish for pain management with patients. When a patient is asked to enter into a pain management contract, there is an extra burden placed on clinicians to assess decisional capacity. Where risk is high, stringency of consent is also high. The two-tiered model of shared decisional capacity may be helpful to gage patient clinician understanding of specific therapies [16]. This tiered approach discloses the risks and benefits of the therapy and considers barriers to explore when understanding of disclosure is blocked. Some of these barriers may be reversible if the clinician and the patient understand their existence (Table 84.3).

The WHO stepwise escalation of drug therapy for pain is based on the pain rating scale [18]. Understanding the value

Table 84.3 Two-tiered assessment of shared decisional capacity

Tier one: disclosure	Tier two: barriers to disclosure
Patient/proxy is able to express	Clinician considers
Medical indication	Physiological states (anoxia, dementia, aphasia)
Expected outcome with therapy	Drugs (prescription/illicit)
Expected outcome without therapy	Pain
Alternative therapies	Stages of death, dying, or grief
Voluntary acceptance of proposed therapy	Educational differences (language, literacy, integrative medicine integration toward complimentary therapies)
	Institutional chauvinisms (ageism, sexism, genderism, classism, professionalism, colonialism, racism)

Modified from Dula and Williams [16], Emanuel [17]

of a patient's previous attempts at pain management, integrative or not, determines the validity of stepwise pain recommendations. Beginning at the lowest level of opiate may not be appropriate, often true for cancer pain and those with established reasons for opiate tolerance or addiction. Use of opiates may be precluded by previous pain management history.

Regardless of the therapy, once pain is being treated, there needs to be a follow-up at relatively close interval [19]. This is particularly for those in health-care undeserved settings using opiates as part of therapy as time between clinic appointments may be prolonged. Telephone or email is being increasingly used for initial follow-up. Pain left unmanaged pushes the neurological response toward constant pain. Follow-up pain assessment and documentation (PAD) is best when including the four domains: analgesia, activity or function, [20] adverse effects (constipation, respiratory depression, sedation, myoclonus, delirium, urinary retention, drowsiness), and aberrant behaviors [21]. Drug-related aberrant behaviors include drug seeking because of pseudo addiction insufficient analgesia resulting in clock watching, tolerance cycle, or addiction.

Addiction Concerns

The National Institute of Drug Abuse (NIDA), of the National Institutes of Health, recommends assessment of addition potential by screening for cigarettes, alcohol, and illicit drug abuse. The screening involves the ask, advise, assess, assist, and arrange (addiction specialist) approach [22]. Each racial, ethnic, age, and gender group has been explored by NIDA for prevalence of addictive behavior by substance abused. For instance, in the United States, African Americans and Americans of European descent have the same prevalence of 6 % addictive behavior and illicit drug abuse. NIDA believes, as an example, racial profiling results in statistical over representation of African Americans in the prison system related to drug abuse.

For those with pain and present addiction or risks, an honest plan needs to be made for pain management. The plan requires knowing the person's base opiate use, efficacy of previous therapies, treatment contracts, and commitment by clinicians to arrange substance abuse treatment. Community resources or state medical board opiate monitoring systems should be used to learn the truest history of prescribed opiates. If methadone maintenance for addiction is in place, it should continue at the same dosage and received at the outpatient facility assigned. The usual dose of methadone should not be changed, baring high side effect profile. Additional opiates of choice may be added to the methadone for pain management.

Refusal of appropriate therapy by those without addiction potential may accentuate pain disparity. Pain left unmanaged often results in a persistent pain cycle. In intact communities of color, there seems a burden of responsible people to not want to leave a legacy of weakness by the use of opiates or to avoid tainting the body with drugs.

Pain and Diseases of Health Disparities

Many diseases of health-care disparities have pain as a fellow traveler. Acute pain is related to discrete events, better localized and so is less evasive. The specialty of emergency medicine has been aggressive about research on acute care pain disparity [23]. Advances in pain science may shift a disease's pain category. An example of such a shift is changing the pain classification of rheumatoid arthritis from the chronic pain category to the more accurate recurrent.

Persistent pain is referred to as chronic pain. Persistent pain is more indolent with a source less easily defined than acute pain. Chronic malignant pain includes cancer, HIV/AIDS, amyotrophic lateral sclerosis (ALS), multiple sclerosis, end-stage organ failure, advanced chronic obstructive pulmonary disease, advanced congestive heart failure, and Parkinsonism. Chronic nonmalignant pain encompasses chronic musculoskeletal pain such as spinal pain or low back pain, chronic degenerative arthritis, osteoarthritis, rheumatoid arthritis, myofascial, chronic headache, migraine, and bone pain. Significantly, this group also tends to be frequently ambiguously reported because it has a neuropathic component associated with nerve compression and visceral pain [24].

Persistent pain occurs more frequently in those with health and health-care disparities. When pain is ascribed to an underlying disease, it tends to be more accepted as "real"

by a scientifically based medicine system. An example is the validation of pain in HIV/AIDS leading to the realization that pain is the second most reported symptom, just behind fever, in AIDS. For many ethnic peoples of color, the scientific basis for pain is less meaningful than the nonphysical suffering pain causes. The health-care community should be aware that its response to undefined pain ranges from care and compassion to judgmental, sometimes devolving into blaming or inappropriate personalization of responsibility [25].

Choice of Pain Therapies

Clinicians caring for people with persistent pain should carefully review and educate themselves about pain relevant reimbursement coding systems. The complexity of the biopsychosocial issues of pain disparity require more diagnostic and treatment time in individuals with multiple health disparities. Clinical pharmacy specialist, social workers, nurses, and behavioral medicine consultants may need clinician support to access indicated medications and therapies. There is a growing understanding that medications alone are frequently inadequate to decrease persistent pain disparity.

Research supports the effectiveness of self-management programs in pain care. A meta-analysis of 17 self-management education programs for arthritis found that they achieved small but statistically significant reductions in pain ratings and reports of disability [26]. Self-Management occurs with or without clinician involvement through emotional, social, and media influences. Formal clinical assistance likely provides better targeted outcomes. Programs have combined pain self-management with therapy for depression, in cancer pain patients [27]. Convenience of schedule, location, and frequency of programs significantly improves participation rates. An individual's reinforced belief that they can control their own pain is a strong determiner for successful pain management [28].

Emotion and pain are closely tied. Harnessing positive emotions shows improvement in pain. Pain, [29] anxiety, depression, and fear form a vicious cycle one entity feeding on the other [30]. Anger is prominent for those in pain. Anger is often directed at health-care providers, significant others, and insurance companies. Of great concern is that studies show anger more manifest as self-loathing than directed at others [31]. Therapies which improve emotional competency, like cognitive behavioral or group therapy, are important adjuncts in pain management. Expressed emotion is a window to pain perception. Cultural transparency in emotional expression between clinicians and patients is required before appropriate psychological support can be provided.

Traditional Medicine and Patient-Centered Care

Increasingly, pain is considered a disease and not simply a distressing symptom. Disease prevention and management are profoundly influenced by community engagement [32]. Community engagement requires culturally relevant care; those who have the problem may have the solution. Traditional medicine provides a guide to culturally relevant, patient-centered care. Among those at highest risk for health-care disparities are Native, Hispanic, African, and monolingual non-English-speaking Asian Americans.

The majority of the world's people use traditional medicine as their primary care. Traditional medicine is "the health practices, approaches, knowledge and beliefs incorporating plant, animal and mineral-based medicines, spiritual therapies, manual techniques and exercises, applied singularly or in combination to treat, diagnose, and prevent illnesses or maintain well-being" [33]. When traditional medicine is used by medical systems outside of the culture of its origin, it is called complimentary or alternative medicine. When the former is used in conjunction with allopathic medicine, it is called integrative medicine. Traditional medicine is based on nonscientific systems and knowledge which have evolved over thousands of years. The cultural practitioner of traditional medicine operates from a shamanistic base, traversing both the physical and the spiritual world. Traditional medicine seeks to create care that incorporates whole patient principles and is closely allied with patient-centered care [34]. In traditional medicine, the healing dialog often exists in the arena of spirituality.

Culture is how a group of individuals define themselves. A person's expression, tolerance, and understanding of the meaning of pain are related to culture [35]. Culture tells people how to behave in relationship to pain [36]. Exploration of cultural touchstones provides a means of initiating a cross-cultural exchange between clinicians and patients about pain. A mnemonic for cultural touchstones is family, spirituality, struggles, and icons of culture (FaSSI).

There is rarely a separation between traditional medicine and spirituality. Consciousness raising therapies like meditation, prayer, and yoga are used in all traditional medicine systems. Spiritual assessment tools can clarify personal cultural values and probable acceptance of traditional medicine by a patient [37]. Among these tools is HOPE: what gives hope, organized religion, preferred response to spirituality, effects of spirituality on illness, pain, and suffering. Another similar spiritual assessment is FICA: faith and beliefs, importance of spirituality to life, community of spiritual support, addressing of spirituality by the clinician. More general cultural familiarity can be found through exploring a cultural or individual resonance with screen narratives, books, and arts [38, 39].

There are specific current and historical struggles affecting communities of health disparities. Some of these struggles deteriorate the biopsychosocial-spiritual axis in a way described as a cultural posttraumatic syndrome [40]. This deterioration, when manifest by escalating nonresponse to allopathic pain management, should prompt consideration of traditional or integrative medicine therapy. Cultural icons and associated rituals provide a shorthand for recognizing a person's identification with a culture. The significance of icons to an individual provides a gentle entree to cross culture exchange between patients and clinicians.

Applying FaSSI allows review of Native American, Hispanic, African, and Asian American traditional medicine. The goal is to provide examples of cross-cultural information about traditional medicine important to pain clinicians during epidemic pain disparity.

Native American Traditional Medicine

In the United States, Native Americans include Alaskan Natives. Applying FaSSI allows review of Native American traditional medicine in relationship to Hispanic, African, and Asian Americans. Though in the US Native Americans include Alaskan Natives, it is the people of the lower 48 states who underscore the historic, cultural, and genetic intersections of those most burdened by health disparities.

Family: Extended family is a crucial factor in the life of Native Americans. Kinships are increased through marriage and adoption rituals. Most American Indian households, until recently, consisted of at least three-generation families. This means that a Native American baby boomer was likely in direct contact with elders born at the turn of the last century. Elder generations frequently are more deeply tied to core cultural practices and values. Family is essential in helping people recover from illness, ameliorating pain and suffering. Family extends to ancestors and clan relationships. It is considered important to have family close at hand when one is hospitalized. Strength is drawn from having support of significant individuals to reaffirm identity. Reflection of the role of family in settling suffering and its cousin, grief, is seen in some ancient Native American practices of burying babies in the home of their bereaved parents. Now, modern parents keep the spirits of their babies from wandering too far by making photographs [41].

Spirituality: A medicine man or woman guides the ailing person to approaches which allow rebalancing between self, nature, and the supernatural. Native religion believes that the

Great Spirit is manifested by the natural environment and kinship relationships. Symptoms of illness, like pain, are brought to the attention of a medicine person after trying customary local folk remedies, herbs and procedures. These initial treatments usually derive from the natural environment. If symptoms do not resolve, the person needs both natural and supernatural assistance. The medicine people provide this combined level of care, being both priest and physician. The medicine person uses rituals to communicate with the Great Spirit, through nature or supernatural intermediaries [42]. There are many spiritual healing forms in Native American culture including the medicine wheel, which is a 10,000-year-old tool. Each Native American tribe has a variation. The medicine wheel of the Lakota people is an example.

The Lakota originates from the lands now occupied largely by the Dakota states. The home geography influences the interpretation of the medicine wheel. The medicine wheel is a circle divided into four equal quarters. The spokes of the wheel each represents direction: north, south, east, and west. The center of the wheel represents "self, balance, harmony, and learning." The quarters of the wheel represent parts of the self's natural, spiritual, and emotional universe. It also describes races of people. Each quadrant has a color. The colors of the quadrants are white, yellow, black, and red. Red symbolizes the South, red people, heart, and emotion. Yellow symbolizes yellow people, the East, sun, spiritual, and values. Black represents black people, the West (where the sun sets), the earth, the physical, and the action. White stands for the North, white people, snow, wind, brain, mental, and decisions [43].

The medicine wheel clarifies the direction of imbalance and how to change when in pain or suffering. The medicine man (woman) interprets the map of the wheel. The symptomatic person may be told to shift toward, for instance, the black, which is also toward the physical. This may be the case if one is too ethereal, spiritual, or yellow, bringing the person back down to earth. The imbalance of illness is thought to be physical, emotional, and related to others in the human and spiritual environment. This complicated calculus of the medicine wheel combines observation of the ill person, with treatments prescribed by the medicine person.

Struggle: Diaspora, being separated from homeland and culture, is a common theme of struggle. Loss of the integrity of Native American traditional medicine preceded damage to the psychosocial cultural system of Native Americans. With the formation of the Indian Health Services, traditional medicine was supplanted. Infectious disease incidence went down, rates of disparity states like alcoholism,

cirrhosis, suicide, homicide, hypertension, cigarette smoking, and diabetes became disproportionately identified with Native communities.

The Trail of Tears, a major struggle in Native American history, underscores the strength of strong cultures and their healing traditions to survive against the odds. Native Americans were forced from their homelands in the southeastern states by federal troops and driven westward to Oklahoma beginning in 1831. The legal justification for this march was the Indian Relocation Act. Seventeen thousand Choctaw people were among the first relocated, 6,000 of who died before reaching the Oklahoma territory. Members of five major Native Nations of the southeast were in the march. The lands, its sustenance, customs, and families were also disrupted and killed in the process of this march [44].

A Native American baby boomer, in pain, could easily has shared a home with a grandparent who personally knew a family member who marched the Trail of Tears. Three-generational knowledge is easily culturally accessible and lays in the base of the current generation's identity. The Indian Freedom of Religion Act, enabling Native Americans to practice traditional spirituality, was only passed by both houses of congress in 1978. The United Nations Declaration of Rights of Indigenous Peoples was passed in 2007 [45, 46].

Icons and Rituals: There is no stronger icon or sets of healing practices in Native American traditional medicine than the "medicine wheel". Replicas of medicine wheels are seen in many places as adornments on fancy dance costumes, braid ties, painted, or as in tradition, laid out with stone and pigments. Other icons include medicine hoops, smudging, sand painting, replicas of spirit animals, and medicine bags. Jewelry is often considered to carry the blessings of those from whom it was received. The amount of jewelry worn is not simply for adornment but for protection.

Notes for Pain Clinicians: Those caring for Native American people should ascertain the level of a patient identification with traditional culture and traditional medicine. Icons and language style provide clues. A formal spiritual assessment (see HOPE and FICA above) provides an entry point for reviewing cultural beliefs. Consultation with traditional Native American healers may be an appropriate care enhancement particularly in refractory pain and in death and dying. During clinical critical points, care should be taken to not remove cultural icons from a person's body if possible. Maintaining identity is important to healing when in allopathic settings [44]. Clinics serving larger numbers of Native American people may have within the clinic community access to traditional healers with whom a practice relationship can be cultivated.

Mexican Traditional Medicine

Family: Family members, including extended family, are responsible for the health of their loved ones. Family contacts the appropriate traditional practitioner on behalf of the symptomatic person. In Mexican traditional medicine, this person is a curandero (a) or a yerbera (o). The family chooses which practitioners to consult first. It is the family that sees that other routine herbs and activities have not helped prior to consultations. Often, the curandero (a) will not ask the ill person about the problem but will refer questions to the family members of the ill person. The idea of autonomy of the patient, without family inclusion, is anathema. The family is responsible for carrying out the instructions that will facilitate cure [47].

Mexican folk medicine divides illness between hot and cold categories. Like Native American medicine, the goal is to keep the symptomatic person in a balance between the two. Heat from fever and respiratory phloem is treated with heat—to draw the heat from the body. A poultice of stewed tomatoes might be applied. Key family members are taught to prepare and apply the poultice. Many herbs have medicinal functions in Latino cultural medicine. These therapies are often found in the family kitchen. Garlic for anorexia, oregano for dry cough, rose water for fever, linseed for constipation, and aloe vera for burns. Many of these have a scientific basis but that is not what drives people to use traditional healers. The curandero prescribes and teaches family to use these therapies.

Family members are charged by the curandero with specific chants or prayers to be said to God for the patient. There are therapeutic and preventive instructions called remedios (remedies). These are preventive teachings using words or parables that instruct and remind the person to use certain preventive practices. An example is the phrase "consejos sobre la regla, which reminds a woman to not eat spicy foods while menstruating." Menstruating is considered to be hot. Spicy foods are also hot, both together would give a profound imbalance in equilibrium. These are verbal sayings which the culture spreads generation by generation for prevention of illness.

Struggle: In 2006, Hispanic people of the United States were estimated to be 44.3 million. In 2000, the same communities were estimated at 35.6 million [48]. Hispanic is a US government term differentiating those Spanish-speaking people born in the Americas from those European born. Fifty percent of the Hispanic peoples in the United States have linage from Mexico. Before the arrival of Spanish colonialist in the 1500s, Mexican people were the indigenous Native peoples of the southern part of North America, including the land in the lower portion of the United States. In the early 1800s, Mexican people fought for their independence from Spain and won. In the mid-1800s after the United States-Mexico War, the USA seized lands previously owned by Mexico. Mexicans living in the United States, who could not repatriate to Mexico for fiscal reasons, suffered the diasporas effect as many immigrant laborers experience today.

The US-Mexico War, ended in proximity to the Emancipation Proclamation. Work previously done by the exploitation of African slave labor was left undone. This period resulted in economic depression of the United States. In the period from the late 1800s until the 1930s, Mexican workers first became essential to the US infrastructure: building railroads, working in foundries, agriculture, and mining [1]. Having known one another in the Mexican-Spanish colonial period, Mexican Americans again met African Americans in the workplace. From 1880 to 1930, the rate of Mexican American lynching in the United States was 27.4 per 100,000 of population. This statistic is second only to that of the African American community during the same period, an average of 37.1 per 100,000 population [49].

Spiritualism: Mexican traditional medicine, heavily influenced by indigenous Native American medicine, strives for balance and harmony. Spiritualism is used in healing and is the basis for a patient's understanding, not scientific principles. Spiritualism in Hispanic culture is a mixture of Catholicism, indigenous/Native Mexican culture, and African influences. The body and the mind are healed at the same time as the spirit. Prayers and chants are said to appeal to God. They are said by the curandero, the patient, and the family. The prayers are also to provide comfort to the patient and decrease fear and anxiety.

Curanderos direct the symptomatic person's own inner energies toward healing. A curandero may transfer energy to the ill person, for example, by laying on of hands. This exchange supports the ill person until they garner their own energies. The curandero may be exhausted (siento debil) or drained by the exercise while the ailing person will be more at ease. The energy is delivered to the curandero through communication with supernatural intermediaries to God. This approach is mostly used when the illness is thought to be supernatural, in combination with specific physical therapies prescribed by the curandero. The curandero uses ancient spiritual practices and references (Mayan, Aztec, origin) and Catholic rituals and practices (Virgin of Guadeloupe, saints with key domains of influence). Mexican traditional medicine presumes that the body and spirit are always connected. Unnatural agents such as pharmaceuticals or drugs are discouraged. The body and blood must be clean as well as the thoughts pure if the ill person is to heal [50].

Icons: Many instruments in healing ceremonies are associated with Catholicism. They are also used to prevent harm to a person while weakened with illness or in daily life. Amulets, medals, holy water, and blessed herbs may be worn by the sick person. These are reminiscent of the medicine bags often found around the neck of Native American people. Prayers are placed in sacramental urns in front of candles, usually written on paper or tree bark. Statues of the Virgin Mary, the Virgin of Guadeloupe, saints, and crucifixes are icons of respect conferring protection seen in jewelry, homes, and vehicles.

Notes for Pain Clinicians: Asking the question, "Has a curandero's assistance been sought?" may open a field of dialog between a clinician and a Latino patient. Demonstrating a respect for a nonscientific basis for healing may resonate with a patient's core values. Both traditional Mexican and allopathic medicine are often used simultaneously, people know when immediate life threatening illness requires one or the other. Use of a curandero may evidence that a patient's belief system significantly includes the supernatural realm. Clinicians who see people presenting with icons of their culture may want to ask, "What does this mean to you?" Expressing interest in the meaning of icons demonstrates respect for a person's beliefs, important because respect may be under siege for those with persistent pain. Pain clinician awareness of the curandero's treatment, prevention, and education plan may be referenced and incorporated in the clinician's therapeutic approach.

African American Traditional Medicine

Family: It is difficult to separate family and struggle in African American history or in response to pain. At slave ports in the United States, Africans were forbidden to use their language, customs, traditions, and healing practices. Families and tribes were dispersed and sold away from one another, fracturing culture and family. Slave owners often allowed traditional African medicine healers to retain skills as means of maintaining the slave work force; sick slaves could not work. Slave doctors and midwives acting as both healers and spiritual guides became key parts of maintaining the extended families created in the slave quarters [51]. These African-born slave healers hid slave illness from owners. This practice of hiding illness and pain protected members of slave extended families from being sold away from one another, experimented on, or made eunuch [52, 53].

The doctor serving African Americans is at best advantage when considered a member of the extended family. Such clinicians demonstrate more "cool" than other clinicians. That is, they absorb heat, stress, and emotional charge related to illness [54]. The responsibility of family to protect, as in Native American and Mexican communities, is paramount. For African Americans, there is historically safety in numbers. The skills, education, icons, and appearance of African American family members are heterogeneous. Capacity to understand and manipulate complex medical systems is generally thought better with more family participants.

Struggle: For Americans of African descent, there are multiple diaspora, the first being the uprooting from Africa. The second being the profound negative effect of slavery on African American family and cultural retention. The third diaspora relates to African American unity with Native Americans and Mexicans. In the Maroon movement, escaped slaves, again separated from their people, preserved some of the traditional base of African medicine. The basis of African traditional medicine, shared reverence for the earth, similar worship styles, and capacity to move agilely over land, formed relationships between the Maroon and Native Americans. African slaves and Native Americans combined families. The March of Tears included 10–18 % of the five nations uprooted from the southeast USA to Oklahoma in the early 1800s [55].

Some African slaves were welcomed into Mexico at the time of the March of Tears to avoid their recapture. By 1810, Mexican slavery was abolished by Mexico's second president, who was of African and indigenous Mexican origin. African slaves originally brought to Mexico by Spanish colonialist became principle fighters for Mexican independence [56].

Spirituality: Because of the multiple diaspora, the African origin of African American traditional medicine is less clear than that of Native, Hispanic, or Chinese Americans. Much of the medical knowledge of African American slaves evolved from Yoruba medicine. Traditional Yoruba medicine began with the migration of the East African Yoruba across the trans-African route leading from the mid-Nile river area to the mid-Niger, West African region [57]. Yoruba medicine traditions incorporated and influenced many other African healing traditions en route to the Atlantic. These traditions included Egyptian medicine which became the source of western medicine disseminated through the Mediterranean to the East (Greece) by the Phoenicians. African cultural healing traditions included medicine men who acted as priest and physicians, similar to the Native American and the Mexican traditions.

Yoruba medicine also sees health as harmony with nature and the supernatural. Disease is considered to reflect disharmony [58]. Evidence of the link between spirit and body is reflected in the persistence of medicine dolls use in the Caribbean. The medicine dolls come from Yoruba tradition. Pins are stuck in the doll replicas of the patient. The pins guide supernatural forces to the points of illness. These African healers were trained to use roots, minerals, and plants for solutions drunk or applied to the body. Therapies had a direct relationship to Yoruba gods or forces. The god forces being Okydnare (the self-existent being of one source), Orisha (good forces), and Ashe (nature). Additionally, in Yoruba medicine, the human physical form has a dual potential through the evolution of the human spirit to supernatural.

This duality of the natural and supernatural is not unlike the Christ story reflected in Christianity. Yoruba spirituality likely helped African American culture become tightly linked to Christianity. It has been said that the key feature of African American Christianity is, "African Americans want to be saved and saved by Jesus Christ" [59]. Suffering is related to sharing kindredness with the suffering of Christ before resurrection. Pain is sometimes thought to be a punishment or originating from hard times endured by previous generations [60].

The therapies used in African traditional medicine are similar to those in Native, Mexican, and Chinese medicine. In Yoruba medicine, the natural world is linked to the spiritual world through the seven major Orisha or good forces. Each Orisha has different capacities corresponding to places on the body and their illnesses. Specific combinations of herbs serve specific Orisha. The African Orisha herbs were replaced by other flora in the Americas with the assistance of Native Americans. African folk medicine remnants are common for self medication of discomfort distressing symptoms include chamomile or ginger for abdominal cramping and garlic, rose hips, lemon, and honey for cough. These therapies originate from distant knowledge of the Orisha.

Okydnare, the self-existent being of one source or life force, may be transferred through the laying on of hands, prayer, and speaking in tongues to a person to relieve pain [61]. Use of drugs alone will likely be less effective among those African Americans with pain disparity inclined to embrace folk or integrative medicine practices. In this case, touch therapies like massage may improve acceptance and effectiveness of medication therapies.

Icons: African Americans may wear symbols of African heritage. It is common for African American college graduates to wear kente cloth sashes with their graduation gowns. Kente cloth is a multicolored silk and cotton woven cloth which originated in eleventh century, West Africa. Different colors and patterns have different meanings. Those used at graduations, mean new beginnings, often have touching pyramid point shapes symbolizing keys. The neck sash itself is a sign of dignity and was original worn by African chiefs.

Styles of hair and clothing often derive from the duo African and African American origin. Children are named to demonstrate African roots. People shake hands with handshakes which communicate kindredness to Africa and a belonging to one another. Frequently the same handshake is recognized by African born, African Americans, and others close to both.

Notes for Pain Clinicians: Intact African American culture is a culture of relationships [62]. As many family members as can fit into the room may be invited by a patient or proxy when clinical information is exchanged. "Dress up" for clinic visits is a sign of the patient's self-worth and respect for the clinician.

"Dress up" may mask, or even improve, the level of discomfort a person is feeling while at clinic. Family confirmation of effective pain management while at home should be sought.

Negative side effect experience may cause patient resistance to pain management. These may be patients more comfortable with self-management programs and integrative medicine. In clinical practice, stoicism may present as a result from spiritual beliefs but also from distrust. Formal spiritual assessment (HOPE or FICA) should be done by the pain clinician. Especially for African Americans, the spiritual assessment is an essential part of the pain disparity assessment. Acknowledging the history of previous medical abuses of African Americans can forge an alliance with the patient to try to do better.

Chinese Traditional Medicine

Family: The traditional Chinese household is three generational: parents, the eldest son and his wife, their children, and unmarried sisters of the eldest son. Commonly, the oldest male in the house will control all the family affairs. It is often seen with older Chinese American women, will defer to oldest man in the family in clinical settings. The first born boy is historically considered the most important child in the household. This practice originated because girl children marry and leave the family. When the oldest man in the family dies, it is the oldest son who will replace him. The traditional family structure is still often maintained in rural modern China, Hong Kong, and Taiwan and frequently in some form in Chinese American families. In families observing this hierarchy, clinicians may find themselves conferring with relatively young men about their elders [63]. A savvy translator of the appropriate Chinese language and the region from which the family has come may be needed for pain assessment, informed consent, and pain contracts.

Struggle: Indentured laborers in the Americas increased in direct response to the end of African slavery in the Americas. The best understanding of the contact between Chinese, African slaves, Native American, and Mexican people in the Americas is in chronicles of indentured Chinese laborers' interactions in the Caribbean and especially in Cuba [64]. This forced diaspora continued from the mid-1800s into the 1900s. During the economic depression following the United States Civil War and WWI, Asian indentured workers like Mexican workers was used as scapegoats for lack of jobs. Chinese workers built railroads, farmed, and mined. Chinese Americans were lynched as were African Americans and Mexican Americans.

The Chinese Exclusion Act specifically targeted Chinese immigrants to the United States. Many Chinese people were forced to return to China in the midst of major Chinese upheaval at the rise of World War II. Of the estimated

20 million people that died in Asia as a result of that war, half were estimated to have been killed in China [65]. The battle of Shanghai in the beginning of World War II is embedded in the memory of many American Chinese elders. From 1910 to 1940, Angel Island in the San Francisco Bay was one of the notorious processing and detention centers. Nearly 60,000 Asian people were detained there. The conditions at the detention center lacked sanitation. Infectious disease was rampant. The barracks burned on the island, aiding the movement to repeal the Chinese Exclusion Act.

Spirituality: Confucianism, Taoism, and Buddhism are historically the three major religions of Chinese people. Confucianism is more a way of thinking about the world than a religion. There are many Christian Chinese as well. Chinese Christianity may be an admixture of values from the major religions and the old Chinese religions predating the three majors.

Spiritual understanding is tightly linked to Chinese medicine. Chinese medicine is estimated to be approximately 5,000 years old. It is significant to many Asian cultures because of the patterns of Chinese migration and integration throughout Asia. The Yellow Emperor Huang Ti took a specific interest in Chinese medicine and learned it in a series of dialogs with practitioners. These dialogs were scribed, the exchanges becoming the written text of Chinese medicine, rare in other traditional medicines [66]. Chinese medicine particularly reflects many refined ideas of Taoism.

Taoism is about the balanced relationship between human beings and nature. The law of Tao deals with the opposites of human beings, ideas, and objects. Opposing energies are kept in check by the Yin and Yang. Yin is described as negative, dark, cold, and feminine. Yang is positive, light warm, and masculine. Persistent imbalance results in illness. These opposite pairs exist on the condition of each other. Chinese medicine also places primary emphasis on the balance of Qi (Chi), or vital energy. Opening blocks in these energies utilizing 12 meridians of the body is the basis of acupuncture. Most conditions of disease are believed caused by an imbalance in energy manifested by wrong diet or strong displays of emotional feelings (drama). Harmony can be restored by self-restraint and herbs. Man is also subject to the universal laws of nature manifested as fire, earth, metal, water, and wood [67]. Each of these properties is ascribed to different organs of the body. The body and the mind are always integrated, for better or worse. Every organ also is considered to encompass properties of taste, emotion, sound, odor, season, climate, power, and fortification of other structures of the body.

Dietary therapeutic manipulations are also controlled by the balance of Yin and Yang or Hot and Cold. Hot disease is treated with herbs or foods that are cold and vice versa to restore the balance. Other procedures in Chinese traditional medicine include meditation, martial arts, (Tai Chi chuan and Kung fu), acumassage, acupressure, and moxibustion (burning of artemisia vulgaris or moxa). Moxibustion works somewhat like sage in Native American healing, the latter being significant in cleansing and the Chinese being opening meridians [68]. The choice of type of therapy is dependent on the physical exam of pulses and ways in which the meridians may be altered.

Icons: Closely related to pain issues are rituals and icons around death. The next life can be altered by disrupting the spirit in its transition through drama. The moment of death, like life, must be calm and balanced. Transition of the spirit is facilitated by the icon of Xi Bo during funerals [69]. Xi Bo yellow and silver squares of paper are folded to resemble ancient coins, then floated on water, and lit on fire at the time of a person's funeral. Xi Bo symbolizes money being offered to a person who has died so that they can go on their journey with the protection of wealth. There are restrictions on who may handle Xi Bo. Pregnant women, or those menstruating, cannot touch Xi Bo. These women are thought to have a power to stop the Xi Bo ability to help the dead in crossing into the next life by consumption of the Xi Bo. Use of Xi Bo paper is so common that they are found in Chinese grocery stores.

The most powerful icon in Chinese culture is the mythical dragon. The dragon is made of the parts of other animals: birds, lizards, and so on. The dragon's power derives from the ability to move from one life form to those whose body parts it shares without dying [70].

Notes for Pain Clinicians: Apparent stoicism or restraint in pain expression may result from patient perception of generations of hardship endured as immigrants. In the setting of family and friends, stoicism is not always a pattern; there are cultural reasons why clinicians may have difficulty "seeing" pain expression in Asian patients. Excess dramatic expression is seen to disrupt balance. Showing weakness is culturally unacceptable for many Asian cultures including Chinese. A Chinese patient may refuse an initial pain medication to avoid showing weakness or because of fears of imbalance; subsequent offers may be accepted after sufficient strength is demonstrated through initial refusals [71]. Wholeness is important in life and death. Clinicians should strive to have all the person's physical parts present for the funeral and transition to the next life.

Conclusion

July of 2011, the Academy of Science, through the Institute of Medicine, issued its extensive report, *Relieving Pain in America: A blueprint for transforming Prevention, Care, Education and Research* [72]. This report affirms the importance of emerging pain science validating a basis for the observed effectiveness of some integrative therapies on pain perception and neuroplasticity [73]. It also identifies pain as an overarching disparity related to most other health-care disparities. Pain disparity oriented additions to the standard pain assessment support integrative medicine.

Pain clinicians committed to expanding their cross-cultural knowledge are better able to address pain disparity. Traditional medicine provides a model for culturally relevant patient-centered approaches to pain care. One third of people in the United States are estimated to use complimentary or alternative medicine [1]. Ethnic peoples of color are disproportionately affected by epidemic pain disparity. The same people rarely are able to access services related to their own cultural traditional medicines: complimentary, alternative, and integrative medicine. Given broader access, integrative medicine with its already firm hand on traditional medicine, is positioned to decrease pain disparity through culturally relevant patient-centered pain care.

References

1. WHO normative guidelines on pain management. 2011. http://www.who.int/medicines/areas/quality_safety/delphi_study_pain_guidelines.pdf. Accessed 5 June 2011.
2. International Association for the Study of pain declaration of Montreal.2011.http://www.iasp-pain.org/Content/NavigationMenu/Advocacy/DeclarationofMontr233al/default.htm. Accessed 10 Aug 2011.
3. Tsang A, Von Korff S, Lee J, et al. Common chronic pain conditions in developed and developing countries: gender and age differences and comorbidity with depression-anxiety disorders.J Pain. 2008;9:883–9.
4. Blyth FM. The demography of chronic pain: an overview. In: Croft P, Blyth FM, van der Windt D, editors. Chronic pain epidemiology: from aetiology to public health. Oxford: Oxford University Press; 2010. p. 19–27.
5. Bonham V. Race, thnicity and pain treatment: striving to understand the causes and solutions to the disparities in pain treatment. J Law Med Ethics. 2001;29:52–68.
6. Whittle J, et al. Racial differences in the use of invasive cardiovascular procedures in the Department of Veterans Affairs medical system. N Engl J Med. 1993;329:621–7.
7. National healthcare disparities report, 2003 summary AHRQ 2002. 2011. http://www.ahrq.gov/qual/nhdr03/nhdrsum03.htm. Accessed 24 June 2011.
8. Bial A, Levine S. UNIPAC three: assessment and treatment of physical pain associated with life limiting illness. In: Storey CP, Levine S, Shega JW, editors. Hospice and palliative care training for physicians: a self study program: a self study program (UNIPAC). Glenview: American Academy of Hospice and Palliative Medicine; 2008.
9. Casarette D, Pickard A, Baily F, et al. Do palliative consultations improve outcome? In: Meier D, Issacs S, Hughes R, editors. Palliative care: transforming the care of serious illness. San Francisco: Jossey-Bass; 2010. p. 369–81.
10. Bodenheimer T, Grumback K, Berenson R. A lifeline for primary care. N Engl J Med. 2009;360(26):2693–6.
11. DeNavas-Walt C, Proctor D, Smith J. Income poverty and health insurance coverage in the united states. In: US census bureau current population reports 2007. Washington, DC: U.S. Government Printing Office; 2008. p. 235.
12. Nielsen-Bohlman L, Panzer A, Kindig A. What is health literacy. In: Committee on Health Literacy, Institute of Medicine, editor. Health literacy: a prescription to end confusion. Washington, DC: National Academic Press; 2004. p. 31–58.
13. Sadore R, Meta K, Simon E. Limited literacy in older people and disparities in health and health care access. J Am Geriatr Soc. 2006;54:770–6.
14. Quill T, Holloway R, Shah M, et al. Pain management. In: Quill T, editor. Primer of palliative care. 5th ed. Glenview: American Academy of Hospice and Palliative Care; 2010. p. 11–2.
15. Huckenberry MJ, Wilson D. Wong-baker faces pain rating scale. In: Wong's essentials of pediatric nursing. 8th ed. St Louis: Mosby; 2008. p. 12–80.
16. Dula A, Williams S. When race matters. Clin Geri Med. 2005; 21:239–53.
17. Emanuel L, editor. Palliative care II: improving care. Philadelphia: Saunders; 2005.
18. WHO Expert Committee. Cancer pain relief and palliative care: report of a WHO expert committee. Geneva: World Health Organization; 1990. p. 7–21.
19. Osteoarthritis pain relief "only a phone call away?". 2011. http://www.niams.nih.gov/Recovery/chronicles/osteoarthritis_phone_call.asp. Accessed 3 July 2011.
20. Karnofsky and ECOG scores. http://www.aboutcancer.com/karnofsky.htm. Accessed 10 Aug 2011.
21. Emanuel LL, Ferris FD, von Gunten CF, Von Roenn J. EPEC-O: Education in Palliative and End-of-life Care for Oncology. Module 2 © The EPEC Project,™ Chicago, IL, 2005. p.12–14.
22. Passik S, Kirsh K, Whitcomb L, et al. A new tool to assess and document pain outcomes in chronic pain patients receiving opioid therapy. Clin Ther. 2009;26(4):552–6.
23. Screening for drug use in general medical settings resource guide. http://www.nida.nih.gov/nidamed/resguide/resourceguide.pdf. Accessed 3 July 2011.
24. Todd KH. Ethnicity and analgesic practice. Ann Emerg Med. 2000; 35:11–6.
25. WHO normative guidelines on pain management. 2011. http://www.who.int/medicines/areas/quality_safety/delphi_study_pain_guidelines.pdf. Accessed 5 June 2011.
26. Pizzo P, Clark M. Summary. In: Institute of Medicine, editor. Reliving pain in America: a blueprint for transforming prevention, care, education and research. Washington, DC: National Academy of Science; 2011. p. S1–16.
27. Warsi A, LaValley MP, Wang PS, Avorn J, Solomon DH. Arthritis self-management education programs. Arthritis Rheumatol. 2003; 48:2207–13.
28. Kroenke K, Spitzer RL, Williams JBW, Löwe B. An ultra-brief screening scale for anxiety and depression: the PHQ-4. Psychosomatic. 2009;50:613–21.
29. Bruce B, Lorig K, Laurent D. Participation in patient self-management programs. Arthritis Care Res. 2007;57(5):851–4.
30. Park S, Sonty N. Positive affect mediates the relationship between pain-related coping efficacy and interference in social functioning. J Pain. 2010;11(12):1267–73.
31. Bair MJ, Wu J, Damush TM, Sutherland JM, Kroenke K. Association of depression and anxiety alone and in combination with chronic musculoskeletal pain in primary care patients. Psychosomataic Med. 2008;70(8):890–7.
32. Okifuji A, Turk D, Curran S. Anger in chronic pain: investigations of anger targets and intensity. J Psychosom Res. 1999;47(1):1–12.
33. Community engagement: definitions and organizing concepts from the literature. In: Principles of community engagement. 2011. http://www.cdc.gov/phppo/pce/. 27 July 2011.
34. World Health Organization. WHO fact sheet no. 134: traditional medicine. 2011. http://www.who.int/mediacentre/factsheets/fs134/en/2008-12-01. Accessed 5 July 2011.
35. Integrative Medicine and Patient-Centered Care. Commissioned for the IOM summit on integrative medicine and the health of the public. 2011. http://www.iom.edu/~/media/Files/Activity%20Files/Quality/IntegrativeMed/Integrative%20Medicine%20and%20Patient%20Centered%20Care.pdf. Accessed 14 July 2011.
36. Wenger AF. Cultural meaning of symptoms. Holist Nurs Pract. 1993;7:22–35.
37. Zborowski M. People in pain. San Francisco: Jossey-Bass; 1969. p. 30–2.
38. Puchalaski CM, Carlson DB. Developing curricula in spirituality in medicine. Acad Med. 1997;73(9):970–4.

39. Colt H, Quadrelli S, Friedman L. Picture of health: medical ethics and the movies. New York: Oxford University Press; 2011. p. 1–560.

40. Azul La Luz W. Hispanios in the valley of death: street-level trauma, cultural-PTSD, overdoses, and suicides in north central New Mexico. 2011. http://repository.unm.edu/handle/1928/10352. Accessed 18 Aug 2011.

41. Defrain J, et al. Stukkbirb: the invisible death. In: Bertman S, editor. Grief and the healing arts. Amityville: Baywood Publishing Company Inc; 1999. p. 427.

42. Joe J, Galerita J, Pino C. Cultural health traditions: American Indian perspective. In: Paxton PP, Branch MF, editors. Safe nursing care for ethnic peoples of color. New York: Appleton-Century-Crofts; 1976. p. 81–98.

43. Vickers J. Medicine wheels: a mystery in stone. Alberta Past. 1992;8(3):6–7, Winter; 93–4.

44. Katz LK. Liberty among the Indians. In: Black women of the old west. New York: Atheneum; 1995. p. 3–6.

45. The American Indian Religious Freedom Act, Public Law No. 95-341, 92 Stat. 469. 2011. http://www.nativeamericanchurch.net/Native_American_Church/LS-AmericanIndianReligiousFreedom Act.html. Accessed 2 July 2011.

46. Canby JC. American Indian law in a nutshell. New York: West Publishing Company; 1988. p. 339, 340.

47. Rodriquez-Dorsey P. Cultural health traditions: Latino/Chicano perspectives. In: Paxton PP, Branch MF, editors. Providing safe nursing care for ethnic peoples of color by Marie Foster Branch and Phyllis Perry Paxton. New York: Appleton-Century-Crofts; 1976. p. 272.

48. U.S. Census Bureau, population estimates July 1, internet release date February 08, 2008. 2011. http://www.census.gov/population/www/socdemo/hispanic/hispanic_pop_presentation.html. 5 July 2011.

49. Shaw R. Beyond the fields: Cesar Chavez, the UFW, and the struggle for justice in the 21st century. Los Angeles: University of California Press; 2008. p. 1–253.

50. The lynching of persons of Mexican origin or descent in the United States, 1848 to 1928. 2011. http://findarticles.com/p/articles/mi_m2005/is_2_37/ai_111897839/pg_9/. Accessed 1 July 2011.

51. Roman OI. Carrrismatic medicine, folk healing and folk sainthood. Anthropology. 1965;75:1152.

52. Jacques G. Cultural health traditions: a black perspective. In: Paxton PP, Branch MF, editors. Safe nursing care for ethnic peoples of color. New York: Appleton-Century-Crofts; 1976. p. 115–44.

53. Hatch J, Holmes A. Rural and small town African American populations and human rights post industrial society. In: Secundy MG, Dula A, Willimas S, editors. Bioethics research concerns and directions for African Americans. Tuskegee: Tuskegee University, National Center for Bioethics in Research and Health Care; 2000. p. 68–80.

54. Dula A. The need for a dialogue with African Americans. In: Dula A, Goering S, Secund M, Williams S, editors. It just ain't fair: westport. Conn: Praeger; 1994. p. 1–315.

55. Thompson RS. Esthetic of the cool. Afr Art. 1973;2(1):40–67.

56. Katz LK. Black women of the old west. New York: Atheneum; 1995. p. 1–79.

57. Gonzales P, Rodriquez R. African roots stretch deep into Mexico. 1996. http://www.mexconnect.com/articles/1935-african-roots-stretch-deep-into-mexico. 4 July 2011.

58. Karade BI. The handbook of Yoruba religious concepts. York Beech: Samuel Weiser, Inc; 1994. p. 1–23.

59. Lipson GJ, Dibble ST, editors. Culture and clinical care. San Francisco: UCSF Nursing Press; 2005. p. 1–14.

60. When we are asked: spirituality (VHS/DVD). Directed by September Williams. USA 2004. USA. Ninth Month Productions/APPEALproject.RWJ. 98 mins. 2011. http://divinity.duke.edu/initiatives-centers/iceol/resources/appeal#details. 25 July 2011.

61. Cultural diversity: pain beliefs and treatment among Mexican-Americans, African-Americans, Chinese-Americans and Japanese-Americans Alvarado, Anthony pain reliefCultural Diversity: Al. 2011. http://commons.emich.edu/cgi/viewcontent.cgi?article=1126&context=honors. Accessed 1 July 2011.

62. Cultural diversity: pain beliefs and treatment among Mexican-Americans, African-Americans, Chinese-Americans and Japanese-Americans Alvarado, Anthony pain reliefCultural Diversity: Al. 2011. http://commons.emich.edu/cgi/viewcontent.cgi?article=1126&context=honors. Accessed 25 June 2011.

63. When we are asked: race, class, culture (VHS/DVD). Directed by September Williams. USA 2004. USA. Ninth Month Productions/APPEALproject.RWJ. 98 mins. 2011. http://divinity.duke.edu/initiatives-centers/iceol/resources/appeal#details. 25 July 2011.

64. Chinese family life. 2011. http://www.mitchellteachers.org/WorldHistory/AncientChinaCurriculum/ModernChineseFamilyLife. Accessed 5 July 2011.

65. Yun L. The coolie speaks: Chinese indentured laborers and African slaves in Cuba. Philadelphia: Temple University Press; 2008. p. 1–336.

66. Japanese occupation of China. 2011. http://factsanddetails.com/china.php?itemid=59. Accessed 20 July 2011.

67. Veith I. The yellow Emperor's classic of internal medicine, 1949. Berkeley: University of California Press; 1970.

68. Lawson-Wood D, Lawson-Wood J. Five elements of acupuncture and Chinese massage. Health Science Press, Wellingborough: UK; 1973.

69. Chow E. Cultural health traditions: Asian perspectives. In: Paxton PP, Branch MF, editors. Safe nursing care for ethnic peoples of color. New York: Appleton-Century-Crofts; 1976. p. 99–115.

70. A Chinese funeral. 2011. http://www.bearspage.info/h/tra/ch/fun.html. Accessed 20 July 2011.

71. Cultural China traditions, myths and legends. Shanghai News and Press Bureau. http://traditions.cultural-china.com/en/13Traditions991.html. 20 July 2011.

72. Cultural diversity: pain beliefs and treatment among Mexican-Americans, African-Americans, Chinese-Americans and Japanese-Americans Alvarado, Anthony pain reliefCultural Diversity: Al. 2011. http://commons.emich.edu/cgi/viewcontent.cgi?article=1126&context=honors. Accessed 70–79. Accessed 1 July 2011.

73. IOM (Institute of Medicine). Relieving pain in America: a blueprint for transforming prevention, care, education, and research. Washington, DC: The National Academies Press; 2011.

Sleep and Chronic Pain

Nicole K.Y. Tang, Claire E. Goodchild,
and Lynn R. Webster

Key Points

- Sleep is essential for well-being, and the lack of it compromises both physical and mental health.
- Complaints of sleep disturbance have been documented in a variety of individuals reporting pain symptoms.
- Common sleep disorders detected in patients reporting pain symptoms include insomnia, periodic limb movement disorder/restless leg syndrome, and obstructive and central sleep apnea.
- Experimental studies have produced evidence indicating a possible reciprocal relationship between pain and sleep, such that pain worsens sleep and sleep deprivation/fragmentation increases pain perception. These findings highlight the importance of addressing sleep disturbance in patients presenting with pain symptoms.

- Pain-related sleep disturbance can be effectively managed using pharmacotherapy (e.g., NSAIDs, opioids, anticonvulsants, antidepressants, hypnotics) and/or psychological therapy (e.g., cognitive behavioral therapy for primary insomnia, pain management program based on cognitive behavioral principles).
- Clinicians should carefully assess the sleep complaints presented by patients with pain symptoms and use the information obtained to devise appropriate treatment plans.

Introduction

Chronic pain can be unrelenting. Unlike acute pain for which therapies could provide relief, chronic pain can seldom be cured. Persistent pain often impairs functioning [1–3]. It may be surprising but chronic pain patients' quality of life has been found to be lower than those of patients with chronic illnesses (e.g., chronic obstructive pulmonary disease) or life-threatening diseases (e.g., HIV/AIDS) [4]. While some individuals manage to live fulfilling lives despite pain, others suffer both physically and mentally and go on to develop anxiety, depression, and even increased suicidal ideation and behavior [5]. One plausible reason is that, to many chronic pain patients, pain is not the only source of distress and disability. Among the many other concomitant health and emotional problems, sleep (or the lack of it) is a particular area with which most chronic pain patients want help.

Increasingly, chronic pain patients have voiced their concerns over their interrupted sleep. Aside from pain reduction, these patients have repeatedly identified better sleep as one of the most important outcomes desired from new forms of treatment [2, 6]. This is a justified request because we now know that the vast majority of chronic pain patients report problems sleeping and more than half of them have insomnia of a severity that warrants clinical attention [7–9]. We also

N.K.Y. Tang, D. Phil. (Oxon) (✉)
Arthritis Research UK Primary Care Centre, Keele University,
Staffordshire, ST5 5BG, UK
e-mail: n.k.y.tang@cphc.keele.ac.uk

C.E. Goodchild, B.Sc., M.Sc., Ph.D.
Department of Psychology,
Institute of Psychiatry, King's College London,
De Crespigny Park, Denmark Hill, London SE5 7UB, UK
e-mail: claire.goodchild@kcl.ac.uk

L.R. Webster, M.D.
Lifetree Clinical Research and Pain Clinic,
3838 South 700 East, Suite 200, Salt Lake City, UT 84106, USA
e-mail: lrwebstermd@gmail.com

T.R. Deer et al. (eds.), *Comprehensive Treatment of Chronic Pain by Medical, Interventional, and Integrative Approaches*,
DOI 10.1007/978-1-4614-1560-2_85, © American Academy of Pain Medicine 2013

know that persistent insomnia is linked to many negative consequences, including reduced daytime functioning (e.g., tiredness, poor concentration, memory, and alertness) and increased mood disturbance (e.g., irritability, lethargy) [10]. Consistently, chronic pain patients with sleep complaints tend to experience greater levels of physical and psychosocial disability than those who do not report any difficulty sleeping [11, 12]. Leaders in the field are now recommending that treatments be diversified, such that the focus is not only on reducing/managing pain but also on improving physical and emotional functioning [13, 14]. Given this context, greater understanding of sleep disturbance in chronic pain and the available treatment options will give clinicians the competitive edge to offer services that truly address the patient's needs.

In this chapter, we will briefly review the basics of sleep, revisiting the importance and structure of sleep and describing the types/patterns of sleep disturbance commonly observed in patients with chronic pain. We will then examine the interplay between pain and sleep and provide a brief road map for sleep assessment. Finally, we will review the recent advances in both pharmacological and psychological treatments for insomnia occurring with chronic pain. The advantages and disadvantages of the existing treatment options will be considered, and avenues for future research and treatment development highlighted.

Background: Sleep Basics

Importance of Sleep

Sleep is essential for well-being, and the lack of it compromises both physical and mental health. The exact role of sleep is unknown, but it is believed to be necessary for homeostasis and to impact protein synthesis, cellular growth and proliferation, metabolism, and immune function among other biological processes. The importance of sleep has been demonstrated in animals: serious pathologies and death resulted when sleep in rats was disrupted via mild physical stimulus, perhaps because of interference with thermoregulation [15].

One possible benefit of sleep is that when cerebral energy output is reduced, cell resources engage in protein synthesis, helping to preserve brain structure and function. Studies in rats showed that sleep deprivation causes a reduction in the proliferation of cells [16]. Another possible vital role for sleep is that of providing a needed period of energy conservation [17], perhaps helping to combat the accumulation of free radicals. Sleep deprivation has been linked to oxidative stress, and recovery sleep has been shown to assist in restoring antioxidant balance [18].

Sleep's association with the immune system is apparent in the need for more sleep when one is sick. Animals with infection increase levels of sleep [19], and infection levels increase when they are deprived of sleep [20]. Sleep deprivation also leads to elevated levels of immunity-related, inflammatory cytokines in rats [21]. It is believed that the dysregulation of the immune system wrought by sleep disorders worsens chronic inflammatory conditions such as rheumatoid arthritis (RA) and fibromyalgia (FM) [22].

In humans, cardinal sequelae of sleeplessness include difficulty concentrating, memory lapses, irritability, fatigue, lethargy, and emotional instability. Insomnia is associated with an elevated risk of road and work accidents [23], and longitudinal studies indicate that insomnia heightens the risk of developing depression, anxiety, and substance-related problems [24–32].

Sleep Architecture

Humans experience two main types of sleep: rapid-eye-movement (REM) sleep and non-rapid-eye-movement (NREM) sleep. NREM sleep can be subdivided into four stages: N1 through N4 sleep (Fig. 85.1) [33, 34]. During a typical night's sleep, the sleeper may cycle through these stages four to six times per night with each cycle lasting, on average, 60–90 min [35]. With each subsequent cycle, REM sleep tends to lengthen while the time spent in deep sleep lessens. The light sleep of stage N1 lasts for 5–10 min, progressing to N2, during which body temperature and heart rate decrease. These sleep stages are followed by the deep sleep – or slow wave sleep (SWS) – phases of N3 and N4. During N3 sleep, delta waves alternate with faster waves, while N4 is marked by delta waves almost exclusively. During stage N4 sleep, the sleeper can only be aroused with vigorous stimulation and, if awakened, does not report dreaming. The SWS phases are followed by the REM period, during which dreams usually occur, breathing is rapid and shallow, heart rate and blood pressure rise, the eyes jerk rapidly, and the brain waves return to the levels observed during the wakened state (Fig. 85.1).

The amount of sleep required varies between individuals, and the amount of sleep obtained is influenced by age, environmental demands, and many other biological, psychological, and social factors. There is no clear consensus what constitutes "normal" sleep, but conventionally, sleep is considered disturbed if it is characterized by a long sleep onset latency (SOL; ≥30 min), long duration of awakening after sleep onset (WASO; ≥30 min), short total sleep time (TST; ≤6.5 h), low-quality/nonrefreshing sleep, or a sleep efficiency (SE; the proportion of time in bed asleep) of 85 % or below (Table 85.1).

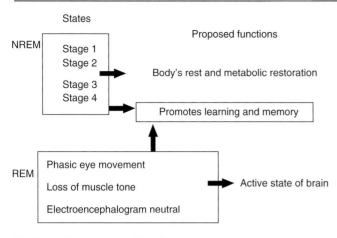

Fig. 85.1 Sleep stages and function

Table 85.1 Abbreviations of sleep architecture

Sleep architecture	
NREM	*Non-rapid-eye-movement sleep* composed of four distinct stages: N1 and N2 are characterized by lighter sleep, while N3 and N4 are regarded as deeper stages of sleep
REM	*Rapid-eye-movement sleep* follows stage N4 sleep, and dreams usually occur during this period. This phase is characterized by rapid, shallow breathing, raised heart rate and blood pressure, jerky eye movement, and brain wave patterns similar to wakefulness. Also known as paradoxical sleep
SWS	*Slow wave sleep:* stages N3 and N4 of NREM; N4 consists almost entirely of SWS
SOL	*Sleep onset latency:* time taken to fall asleep
WASO	*Wake after sleep onset:* time awake following initial onset of sleep
TWT	*Total wake time:* cumulative amount of time awake
TST	*Total sleep time:* cumulative amount of time sleeping
SE	*Sleep efficiency* expressed as a percentage of time in bed asleep: (total sleep time/total time in bed) $\times$ 100 %
SQ	*Sleep quality:* a subjective rating of quality of sleep

Scientific Relevance to Pain Care

Prevalence and Pattern of Sleep Disruption in Chronic Pain

Complaints of sleep disturbance have been documented in a variety of individuals reporting pain symptoms. A large-scale community-based survey investigating the prevalence of sleeping difficulties in multiple European countries found that 23.3 % of participants who reported experiencing pain also reported difficulties sleeping, while only 7.4 % of participants reporting impaired sleep were without pain [36]. In a prospective postal survey of adults in the UK, pain reported at baseline was a significant risk factor for developing insomnia symptoms 1 year later [37]. These findings are consistent with those obtained from the Sleep in America Survey

conducted in 2003, indicating that the presence of bodily pain increased the odds of insomnia by approximately two-fold in older adults [38].

Sleep disturbance is a common consequence of acute pain; estimates of sleep disturbance experienced during hospitalization postsurgery range between 22 and 61 % [39–41]. In these patients, polysomnography (PSG; an instrument to measure sleep) has indicated frequent awakenings, shorter TST and SE, as well as more frequent transitions between the sleep stages with longer duration of N1 sleep, and reduced SWS and REM sleep [40, 42]. This disturbance is generally short-term, and TST returns to preoperative levels within 1 week of hospitalization for the majority of patients [39–41]. Similarly, nighttime pain in patients hospitalized for burn injuries is associated with frequent awakenings and reduced sleep quality and TST. Sleep disturbance was reported by 75 % of patients on at least one night during the 5-day study period [43].

Sleep disturbance is also a common problem in cancer and a number of chronic pain conditions, such as RA, osteoarthritis (OA), FM, headache, and musculoskeletal pain conditions. In a review of cancer-related insomnia, the prevalence of sleep disturbance in this population was estimated between 30 and 50 % post-diagnosis [44]. The insomnia rate only dropped slightly (estimated between 24 and 44 %) when assessed 2–5 years after treatment [44] suggesting insomnia itself is a chronic problem for this population, although cancer pain specifically increases difficulties initiating sleep and frequent awakenings [45].

Confining the focus to chronic noncancer pain, as many as 90 % of the patients attending tertiary pain clinics have complaints with their sleep [7, 8, 11, 46, 47], and approximately 53 % of these patients have insomnia of a severity that warrants clinical attention [9]. Apparently, the pattern of sleep disturbance in these chronic pain patients is largely comparable to that of patients with primary insomnia [48]. Common problems cited by chronic pain patients are initiating sleep and frequent awakenings [7, 8]. Studies using PSG have indicated that chronic pain patients have more microarousals, more body movements during sleep, more frequent transitions between the sleep stages with increased N1 and N2 sleep and reduced N3 and N4, frequent awakenings, and lower SE, compared to healthy volunteers [49, 50]. Sleep disruption experienced by these patients is also characterized by reduced spindle activity at N2 sleep [51], an increase in the rate of cyclic alternating pattern (CAP); [52] a lack of heart rate variability reduction [53] and an intrusion of electroencephalographic (EEG) activity in the alpha range (8–13 cps) during NREM sleep [54]. Although alpha-delta sleep was once thought to be a signature of pain-related sleep disturbance [55], there is now conflicting evidence suggesting otherwise

[56–59]. It remains open as to whether or not there is a neuro-physiological marker of sleep complaints exclusive to the pain population.

Primary Sleep Disorders Other than Insomnia in Chronic Pain

Sleep disorders other than insomnia, including periodic limb movement (PLMD) and sleep apnea, have a heightened prevalence among patients with chronic pain [60, 61]. PLMD and restless leg syndrome (RLS) are closely related movement disorders that often disturb sleep onset and maintenance. PLMD occurs during sleep with spontaneous movement of the lower extremities. RLS occurs during the day or night and is associated with an unpleasant sensation in the lower extremities somewhat relieved with movement. There is always a strong urge to move with RLS, and it can be the genesis of movement and pain at night. Approximately 80 % of patients with RLS have PLMD [62]. The etiology of PLMD and RLS is not well understood, but some forms appear to be due to a dopaminergic dysfunction. Secondary PLMD and RLS have been associated with iron deficiency, folate deficiency, chronic renal failure, OA, and small-sensory-fiber disease [63]. Pain from OA and dysesthesias from small sensory nerve disease are factors that contribute to sleep disturbances with patients who have PLMD and RLS [64].

Chronic headaches appear to be strongly associated with obstructive sleep apnea (OSA); OSA sufferers are seven times more likely to experience chronic headaches (defined as occurring 15 or more times per month) than people in the general population [65]. The severity of the headaches, which tend to occur in the morning, is directly related to the severity of OSA [66]. A strong association also appears to exist between FM and sleep apnea. The prevalence of FM in a study of 50 patients with sleep apnea was tenfold higher than in the general population [67]. Patients with FM often experience OSA [60], and it is possible that OSA plays an etiologic role in some cases of FM. In one case study, a woman with FM and OSA saw great improvement of her FM symptoms after being treated for OSA with nasal continuous positive airway pressure (CPAP) [68]. However, the current research on the link between primary sleep disorders and chronic pain is thin; the rate and variety of comorbid sleep disorders may have been underdetected and/or underreported.

Sleep-Pain Interaction

We have seen that disturbed sleep and chronic pain frequently go together and that the relationship is often assumed to be bidirectional. There are studies showing that the introduction of nociceptive stimuli during sleep can produce cortical arousal [69–71] and that deprivation of sleep – in particular, REM sleep and SWS – can heighten pain intensity [72–74]. However, as more experimental data accrue, the relationship between sleep and pain emerges to be more complex than originally thought.

On the effect of sleep disturbance on pain, there are confusing findings regarding the relative importance of REM sleep and SWS disruption in pain responses. For example, in one study of healthy pain-free sleepers, the loss of 4 h of sleep associated with REM sleep disruption had a greater hyperalgesic effect than the loss of an equal amount of sleep that was associated with NREM sleep interruption [75]. In another study [72], recovery sleep following SWS interruption, but not REM interruption, increased pain thresholds. Contrary to the previous study [75], this finding suggests that SWS plays a more important role than REM sleep in determining the pain tolerance levels . Further, in an elegant study designed to tease apart the effect of sleep deprivation from sleep fragmentation, healthy controls who were in the sleep fragmentation condition demonstrated a significant loss of pain inhibition and an increase in spontaneous pain, while sleep deprivation did not produce any effect on pain thresholds. This interesting finding indicates that the lack of sleep continuity, rather than simple sleep restriction, impairs endogenous pain-inhibitory function and increases spontaneous pain [76].

Pain is frequently cited by patients as the cause of their sleep disturbance [8], and consistently, pain intensity ratings have been found to predict sleep disturbance [47, 77]. However, not all studies identify a significant relationship between pain severity and sleep [78], and certainly not every pain patient has problems sleeping. A subset of individuals with high pain intensity manage to have normal sleep or even regard themselves as "good sleepers" [7, 9, 47, 78]. Although there are clinical studies noting pain to be predictive of subsequent poor sleep, the amount of within-subject variance in sleep explained by pain was rather small and often became nonsignificant when other psychological variables (e.g., pain attention, presleep cognitive arousal) were statistically controlled for [79, 80]. In fact, evidence is accruing to suggest that cognitive behavioral factors common in primary insomnia (such as rumination, worry, health- and sleep-related anxiety, poor stimulus control, pre-sleep arousal, and dysfunctional sleep beliefs) may be better predictors of insomnia severity than pain intensity per se [9, 81, 82, 151].

Clinical Practice

Sleep Assessment

When a pain patient is complaining of insomnia, there are various ways to assess the complaint, such that both the subjective distress of the complaint and the objective characteristics of the sleep disturbance are captured. Although there are sophisticated tests and equipment available for the measurement of sleep, most cases of insomnia are primarily diagnosed by clinical evaluation.

A *detailed clinical interview* should include a careful evaluation of the patient's sleep history, medical and psychiatric history, current and past use of substances, and history of treatment for the sleep problem. When asking the patient about the sleep history, it is important to gather information about the (1) typical sleep-wake schedule; (2) past diagnosis of and treatment for sleep/psychiatric disorder(s); (3) nature and onset of the current sleep complaint; (4) frequency, severity, and duration of the sleep problem; and (5) whether or not the sleep problem has daytime consequences or is causing significant distress. This should provide information to establish if the patient meets the basic diagnostic criteria for insomnia – the three most commonly used classification systems are DSM-IV-TR [83], ICD-10 [84], and ICSD-2 [85]. Moreover, it would be helpful for the clinician to ask questions about the following: the patient's occupation (e.g., doing shift work or jobs requiring frequent long haul travel), general lifestyle (e.g., leading a sedentary lifestyle; napping often; consuming excessive alcohol, drugs, caffeine, and/or other stimulants), current and past life stresses that could cause anxiety and depression (e.g., pain, bereavement, divorce, job loss), bedroom environment (e.g., too hot/cold/ bright/noisy, having a bed partner who snores), general beliefs about sleep (e.g., "I must have 8 h of sleep a night!"), sleep practices (e.g., having a pre-sleep wind-down routine; if woken up, staying in bed for hours to try and go back to sleep), and their typical response to a poor night's sleep (e.g., feeling annoyed and frustrated; worried about losing control over sleep; cutting daytime appointments for fear of not being able to function well; going to bed early to catch up on sleep, even when not sleepy). This should help establish the psychophysiological factors precipitating and perpetuating the sleep problems. There are structured interview schedules available to guide and assist the assessment of insomnia and sleep disorders. Examples of these include the structured interview for sleep disorders according to DSM-III-R [86] and the Duke Structured Interview Schedule for the diagnoses of DSM-IV-TR and International Classification of Sleep Disorder, second edition (ICSD-2) [87]. The use of these instruments, however, requires training and practice.

While a thorough clinical interview should form the core of the evaluation, a combination of self-report questionnaires and a sleep diary (with or without actigraphy) can be used to aid the assessment. *Self-report questionnaires* such as the Insomnia Severity Index [88], the Pittsburgh Sleep Quality Index (PSQI) [89], the Mini-Sleep Questionnaire [90], the Uppsala Sleep Inventory [91], the Medical Outcome Study Sleep Questionnaire [92], and the Dysfunctional Beliefs and Attitudes About Sleep Scale [93, 94] have been used to assess sleep difficulties in chronic pain conditions. However, it must be emphasized that most of these questionnaires are designed to measure sleep quality rather than for diagnostic purposes. As such, their scores should be interpreted with caution as they are neither sufficient to establish a differential diagnosis nor to guide the planning of treatment. Moreover, retrospective responses to these sleep questionnaires are often obscured by recall bias and mood state of the individual at the time of assessment [95].

It is good practice to prescribe 2 weeks of *sleep diaries* to obtain a more stable picture of the sleep pattern [10]. Each diary entry is essentially a short questionnaire to be completed immediately after waking to provide information concerning the previous night for sleep onset latency (SOL), frequency and total duration of wake time after sleep onset (WASO), total sleep time (TST), and sleep efficiency (SE). Depending on the nature of the sleep complaint, sleep diaries may also include reports of sleep quality (SQ), pain, use of medication and substances, daytime sleepiness, and fatigue to provide additional information for assessment and case formulation. Although sleep diaries are generally easy to use and there have been clinical reports suggesting therapeutic benefits associated with regular sleep monitoring, care must be taken to explain to the patient the rationale and procedure of the sleep monitoring so as to enhance adherence.

If appropriate, the use of a sleep diary can be complemented by the use of an *actigraph* (also known as an accelerometer), which is a wristwatch-like device to be worn on the nondominant wrist to measure and record the intensity and duration of physical motion. The rationale behind the use of this technology in sleep research is that frequent and intense movement during the night is indicative of wakefulness. With the aid of an algorithm, data extracted from the actigraph can be used to provide objective estimates of basic sleep parameters, such as SOL, WASO, and TST. The actigraphic measurements of TST, WASO, and SE compare well ($r=0.49$–0.98) with corresponding sleep parameters recorded by polysomnography [96]. Actigraphy has shown modest agreement ($r=0.34$–0.44) when compared with subjective reports of sleep given by people with musculoskeletal pain [77]. Actigraphy has also demonstrated a high degree of stability across nights ($r=0.4$–0.81) [77, 97]. A strong relationship ($r=0.64$) has also been observed between the actigraph measure of TST and the perceived sleep quality reported by women with FM [98]. However, it should be noted that actigraphy is recommended to establish the sleep-wake pattern over time rather than to generate estimates of sleep parameters as this technology may underestimate SOL and overestimate TST in individuals who manage to lie still over long periods. Kushida et al. [99] recommend that sleep diaries and actigraphy should be used simultaneously to provide more detailed information regarding sleep.

Although *polysomnography (PSG)* is considered the gold standard of sleep measurement [10, 99], it is not recommended for routine sleep assessment. PSG can provide information about the architecture of sleep (see "Sleep Architecture") via three measures: electroencephalography (EEG: measurement of brain waves/electrical activity), electrooculography (EOG: measurement of eye movement), and electromyography (EMG: measurement of facial muscle tension) [100]. Coupled with other electrophysiological measures (e.g., EKG, electrocardiograms, nasal/oral air flow, oxygen desaturation, leg movement), the clinician could extract useful information for the diagnosis of sleep disorders such as sleep apnea, PLMD, and RLS (which are described in "Primary Sleep Disorders Other than Insomnia in Chronic Pain"). However, the use of PSG can be intrusive to the patient's sleep, expensive to conduct, and laborious for the clinician to set up and score the results. These limitations are some of the reasons why PSG is often less accessible to the general public and the duration of sleep study is usually restricted to a short period of time (less than three nights). PSG is not indicated unless the pain patient is suspected of having primary sleep disorders. A sleep study is recommended, however, when a patient is on high-dose opioids (>150 mg), considering the strong association between daily opioid dosage and sleep apnea [101]. A home study is less expensive than in-lab PSGs and, in most cases, is sufficient to diagnose sleep-disordered breathing and to differentiate central sleep apnea from OSA. Patients with sleep apnea must be treated accordingly or have their daily opioid dose decreased, after which a repeat sleep study is recommended.

Managing Sleep Disturbance in Patients with Chronic Pain

Sleep disturbance co-occurring with chronic pain can be managed using pharmacotherapy and/or psychological therapy. The sections below describe these treatment approaches, and Table 85.2 provides a summary of their respective mechanisms, advantages, and disadvantages with a view to informing clinical decisions (Table 85.2).

Pharmacological Treatment

A number of pharmacological treatments are available for patients' sleep disturbances and pain; however, adverse effects are frequent, and patients should be monitored closely for medication-related effects on sleep pathology and pain sensitivity. Pharmacologic treatment options to manage pain include nonsteroidal anti-inflammatory drugs, opioids (morphine, oxycodone, methadone, codeine, fentanyl, buprenorphine, hydromorphone, dextropropoxyphene, and pentazocine), tricyclic antidepressants (amitriptyline), and selective norepinephrine reuptake inhibitors (duloxetine). Options to manage sleep disturbances include hypnotics and related drugs, such as benzodiazepines (BZDs-clonazepam) and nonbenzodiazepines (zolpidem, zaleplon, and eszopiclone) [122, 123]. Patients treated with opioids and BZDs should be cautioned not to take more medication than directed, even if pain is

uncontrolled, because unauthorized escalation of doses could be lethal. Opioids and BZD doses should be reduced by approximately 20 % if the patient develops a flu or severe respiratory infection. For nocturnal pain, off-label use of anticonvulsants and antidepressants is less likely than opioids to depress respiration.

Some pharmacologic treatments can impact sleep architecture, sleep restoration, and pain threshold levels. Morphine, for example, has reduced SWS (by 75 %) and REM sleep, while increasing N2 sleep, [124] and in a separate study, morphine and methadone increased N2 sleep and significantly decreased N3 and N4 sleep ($p < 0.001$) [125]. In contrast, patients with chronic pain from OA showed significantly lower pain scores from baseline following morphine sulfate as well as increases in TST and SE [126]. Some newer anticonvulsants have been found to have negligible impacts on sleep architecture, and some may even improve it. For instance, gabapentin and pregabalin were found to promote modest increases in SWS without affecting REM sleep in healthy adults [103, 104, 127, 128].

Additional adverse effects must be considered when treating patients pharmacologically. For example, opioids, particularly methadone, have been associated with a high rate (75 %) of sleep-disordered breathing in patients with chronic pain [129]. Concomitant BZD administration was shown to have a significant additive effect on methadone-related central sleep apnea. In another study, the prevalence of central sleep apnea was found to be 30 % in patients undergoing methadone maintenance treatment [130].

Methadone is not the only opioid associated with alarming levels of sleep apnea. There appears to be a dose relationship of all opioids to central sleep apnea. A linear relationship of opioid dose to central sleep apnea has been reported with immediate release and sustained release formulations. Doses of 150 mg morphine equivalence have approximately a 70 % probability of central sleep apnea [101]. Hypoxia due to hypoventilation has also been observed in patients on chronic opioid therapy even without evidence of sleep apnea (Lynn Webster, personal communication).

Tricyclic antidepressants (TCAs), commonly administered for neuropathic pain, concurrently address symptoms of insomnia and depression. A meta-analysis of 61 clinical trials found that TCAs have demonstrated effectiveness for treatment of diabetic neuralgia and postherpetic neuralgia and to some extent for central pain, atypical facial pain, and postoperative pain after breast cancer treatments [131]. Possible adverse effects of TCAs include drowsiness, dry mouth, blurred vision, constipation, urinary retention, and more serious heart-related conditions [131]. Tricyclic antidepressants have been linked to increased risk of suicide attempts [107, 108] and may reduce seizure thresholds in vulnerable individuals [132]. The newer SNRI formulations (e.g., duloxetine, milnacipran, desvenlafaxine) are reported to have much fewer

Table 85.2 Mechanisms, advantages, and disadvantages of the mainstream pharmacological agents and psychological treatments for chronic pain patients with concomitant insomnia

Treatment	Mechanism	Advantages	Disadvantages
Analgesics (e.g., NSAIDs, opioids)	NSAIDs reduce inflammation and algesia by inhibiting arachidonic acid but have no sedative effect. Inhibition of prostaglandin biosynthesis is through inhibition of COX-1 and COX-2 enzymes. COX-1 activation leads to production of prostacyclin which is cytoprotective. COX-2 is induced in inflammatory cells. The ratio of COX-1 to COX-2 determines the likelihood of adverse effects. Opioids bind to mu, delta, and kappa receptors; effect is to decrease presynaptic calcium flux, which decreases neurotransmitter release. Opioids also increase postsynaptic K+ flux, resulting in hyperpolarization of the neuron, decreasing conductance and transmission. The analgesic and sedative effects of opioids arise from the inhibition of cholinergic, adenosinergic, and GABAergic transmission	The analgesic effects of NSAIDs may reduce nighttime arousal The sedative effects of opioids hasten sleep onset.	Analgesics may increase awakening and alter sleep architecture, suppressing SWS and REM sleep Other side effects include nausea, vomiting, diarrhea, constipation, skin complaints, dry mouth, dizziness, headaches, blurred vision, and fluid retention. The more severe complications are stomach ulcers and kidney/liver failure There is also the risk of addiction with prolonged use of opioids [102]
Anticonvulsants (e.g., gabapentin, pregabalin)	Mechanism is not known but appears to involve activation of the alpha2-delta protein subunit, which decreases Ca+ flux and slows depolarization of neuronal activity of postsynaptic neurons.	Demonstrated efficacy in improving pain and functional measures, including sleep [103] Increase SWS without detrimenting REM sleep [104] Effective in the treatment of RLS and PLMD [105] Pregabalin is thought to be less of a risk for dependence/abuse than other classes of medication [106]	Pain relief happens when optimal dose is achieved. Optimal doses of these drugs vary from individual to individual; careful monitoring and patient titration are required Some patients cannot tolerate these drugs well, particularly those who are on high doses, causing premature drug withdrawals Common adverse effects include dizziness, peripheral edema, somnolence, confusion, headache, dry mouth, and constipation
Tricyclic antidepressants (e.g., amitriptyline, nortriptyline)	Inhibit neuronal uptake of norepinephrine and serotonin into the presynaptic nerve terminals by inhibiting the serotonin and norepinephrine transporters at an approximately 1:8 ratio. They also block postsynaptic sodium, calcium, and potassium channels	Some evidence of pain relief Hasten sleep onset Beneficial for pain patients with concomitant mood problems	Off-label use only; none of the TCAs has been approved by the FDA for treatment of DPNP or any type of pain TCAs alter sleep architecture. Possible side effects include daytime drowsiness, dry mouth, blurred vision, constipation, urinary retention, and heart conditions TCAs may increase the risk of suicide attempt [107, 108] Amitriptyline is a relative contraindication for older patients and patients with any cardiovascular disease [109]

(continued)

Table 85.2 (continued)

Treatment	Mechanism	Advantages	Disadvantages
Selective reuptake inhibitors (e.g., duloxetine, venlafaxine, milnacipran, desvenlafaxine)	Prevent serotonin and norepinephrine form being reabsorbed into the presynaptic terminals. Duloxetine differs from venlafaxine in that it is comparatively more noradrenergic. Venlafaxine has a 30-fold higher affinity for serotonin than for norepinephrine, while duloxetine has a tenfold selectivity for serotonin [110]. Approximate potency ratios (5-HT:NE) are 1:10 for duloxetine and 1:30 for venlafaxine	Lack most of the side effects of tricyclic antidepressants and monoamine oxidase inhibitors; Duloxetine is approved for the management of neuropathic pain associated with diabetic peripheral neuropathy and FM	Nausea is the most common side effect for most drugs in this class; This class of drug is also associated with increased blood pressure and insomnia [110–112]; Cytochrome P450 isoenzymes inducers and inhibitors can affect drug levels
Hypnotics (e.g., clonazepam, zolpidem)	Facilitate GABAergic transmission. BZDs and other hypnotics (non-BZDs) bind to the gamma subunit of the GABA-A receptor, which increases chloride ion conductance and inhibition of the action potentials	Established efficacy for both BZDs and non-BZDs for acute and short-term management; Fast-acting	Potential side effects include daytime drowsiness, dizziness, impaired memory, concentration, and psychomotor performance; There is the risk of tolerance and dependence with extended use, and rebound insomnia may occur after discontinuation [113]
Pain management programs (multidisciplinary programs in the US)	Treatment delivered by multidisciplinary team. Program content varies but generally includes psychoeducation on pain, relaxation techniques, physical exercises, CT for pain, and behavioral pain and stress management strategies; many programs also offer sleep hygiene education	Moderate treatment effects have been achieved for improved coping and self-efficacy regarding pain [114]; The group format encourages social support and facilitates behavioral change [115]	Treatment effects are generally small for reducing pain severity [114]; Focus of treatment is largely on rehabilitation. Not enough individual therapy time for complex cases that present with other comorbid anxiety, mood, and sleep problems; Limited coverage on sleep: only minimal improvements on sleep are detected in graduates of PMPs [116]; Remission rates in a range of pain and functional outcome measures are between 18 and 33 %, with 1–2 % of the patients reliably deteriorate during the period of treatment [117]

| CBT for insomnia | Treatment delivered both individually or in groups by trained psychologists or behavioral sleep medicine specialists. Content varies but generally include psychoeducation on sleep, sleep hygiene, relaxation training, CT for sleep, sleep restriction, stimulus control, paradoxical intention, biofeedback, and imagery training | Highly efficacious and cost-effective; recommended for chronic insomnia [118]
Durable treatment has been achieved in core sleep parameters when CBT-I is directly applied to treat pain-related insomnia [119, 120] | Improved sleep does not necessarily bring about a reduction in pain [119–121]
Remission rates in individuals with pain-related insomnia are between 16 and 57 % [119–121]
Further refinement is required to address sleep-interfering processes specific to chronic pain patients [48]
The initial stage of CBT-I involves cutting down time resting in bed and the introduction of mild sleep deprivation. This may aggravate pain/discomfort for some individuals
The use of sleep restriction therapy involves getting out of bed and going to another room when woken from sleep. This may be difficult for patients who have restricted mobility |

NSAIDs nonsteroidal anti-inflammatory drugs, *COX* cyclooxygenase enzyme, *K+* potassium cation, *GABA* gamma aminobutyric acid, *SWS* slow wave sleep, *REM* rapid eye movement, *Ca+* calcium cation, *RLS* restless leg syndrome, *PLMD* periodic limb movement disorder, *TCAs* tricyclic antidepressants, *FDA* food and drug administration, *DPNP* diabetic peripheral neuropathic pain, *BZDs* benzodiazepines, *CT* cognitive therapy, *PMPs* pain management programs, *CBT-I* cognitive behavioral therapy for insomnia side effects and increased tolerability. This is particularly important to elderly patients who tend to be more sensitive to the side effect profile of many medications.

Benzodiazepines (BZDs) are frequently used to treat sleep disorders, but their efficacy for sleep disturbances complicated by pain is unclear, and more research is needed. Some studies show improved sleep outcomes, including decreased SOL and WASO and increased TST; however, many other studies demonstrate either no effect or heightened levels of pain compared to controls [123]. It should be noted that prolonged use of BZDs has been associated with increased risk of hip fractures in the elderly [133], although some research shows that prior risk factors such as depression and antidepressant use often precede a new BZD prescription in older adults [134]. It appears that newer BZDs and the non-BZDs may offer enhanced safety and greater efficacy as related to sleep outcomes, but data are limited with relation to pain management [123, 135].

Nonpharmacological Treatment

Although pharmacological management of insomnia is commonly used as the first-line treatment for pain-related sleep disturbance, clinical experience tells us that many patients prefer not to have another tablet for sleep, not only because of the adverse effects mentioned above but also for fears of potential drug interaction, tolerance, and dependence. While pharmacotherapy can have a favorable risk-benefit profile in many individuals, evidence in support of its efficacy and safety beyond 6–12 months is currently thin [113]. Long-term hypnotic medication is usually not indicated for the type of insomnia experienced by chronic pain patients, which often is as chronic as the pain itself and requires a different approach of management.

While most cases of insomnia in chronic pain were precipitated by the onset of pain, the relative importance of pain as a maintaining factor decreases as the insomnia persists. Factors perpetuating the insomnia proliferate as the patient develops compensatory strategies to cope with the pain (e.g., resting in pain, inactivity, ruminating about the pain) and the sleep loss (e.g., extending bedtime, daytime naps, drinking large amounts of tea and coffee to stay alert during the day). Similar to what is happening in primary insomnia, these perpetuating factors tend to be cognitive behavioral in nature and are often amenable to psychological treatments grounded on the cognitive behavioral principles. Multidisciplinary pain programs, which are sometimes called pain management programs (PMP), and cognitive behavioral therapy for primary insomnia (CBT-I) are obvious alternatives to pharmacological treatments. These two forms of treatment will be reviewed in this section with a particular focus on their effectiveness for pain-related insomnia.

Pain management programs (PMPs) – frequently referred to as multidisciplinary pain programs in the United States – are usually delivered to groups of patients and cover three main areas. Patients are taught about the physiology, psychology, and function of pain and shown how to utilize relaxation techniques and coping skills. Components of PMPs typically have a strong behavioral focus, encouraging patients to get back in action, pace their activities, set goals, and direct their activities towards achieving those goals. Some PMPs also include cognitive treatment components that focus on identifying and challenging negative thoughts and beliefs about pain and on managing the psychological effects of pain and stress. Although sleep is often discussed in the form of sleep hygiene education in many standard PMPs, it is not normally included as an outcome measure in treatment studies [136]. There are, however, some notable exceptions that have investigated the effect of PMPs on sleep.

A randomized, controlled trial (RCT) conducted by Redondo et al. [137] compared cognitive behavioral therapy (CBT) versus a physical exercise program in 40 women with FM. The CBT comprised eight sessions, each 2.5 h long and 1 week apart, providing information about FM, teaching behavioral techniques for pain management, and advising on sleep and resting. Despite success in improving patients' ability to cope with pain and their daily functioning, sleep did not improve when rated posttreatment or at the 6-month and 1-year follow-up. Similarly, there was no significant improvement in sleep in patients assigned to the physical exercise program.

Gustavsson and von Koch [138] led an RCT comparing a group program of pain and stress management against individual physiotherapy in 37 patients seeking treatment for chronic neck pain. The pain and stress management program involved 7 weekly sessions, each lasting 1.5 h, which taught anatomy, etiology, and physiology concerning neck pain and developing strategies for managing pain and stress, including applied relaxation training. It should be noted that relaxation training is also commonly incorporated in CBT-I; although not specifically instructed to do so, participants in Gustavsson and von Koch's study could have used the relaxation techniques to reduce sleep-interfering somatic and cognitive tension at night. However, those who completed the treatment ($n=29$; 78 %) reported no significant improvement in their sleep after completing the treatment or at the 20-week follow-up [138].

Becker et al. [139] randomly assigned 189 patients seeking treatment for chronic pain to one of three groups: treatment at a multidisciplinary pain center, treatment from a general practitioner (GP), or a 6-month wait-list group. After 6 months, those patients treated by the multidisciplinary pain team reported a small improvement in their sleep as well as reduced pain intensity and improved psychological well-being. However, the clinical significance of the improvement in sleep was not discussed.

Ashworth et al. [116] investigated the within-group effect of a PMP on unhelpful sleep beliefs as well as sleep quality in 42 chronic pain patients. The PMP was delivered in a group format and consisted of 12 weekly sessions. The Pittsburgh Sleep Quality Index (PSQI) [89] and the Dysfunctional Beliefs and Attitudes about Sleep Questionnaire (DBAS) [93, 94] were administered to evaluate improvements in sleep. No improvements were reported for self-reported TST, estimated SE, or dysfunctional beliefs about sleep. However, patients did report shorter SOL and improved satisfaction with sleep quality, and reduced use of medication and daytime dysfunction. There was no control group in this study, and thus the reported benefits in sleep might have been inflated.

Although these studies can be commended for including sleep as an outcome measure, they (with the exception of Ashworth et al. [116]) mostly relied upon single-item ratings of sleep, and none used more detailed sleep diaries or objective measures of sleep, which are more reliable measures of sleep improvement and are commonplace in sleep research. Based on the findings reported above, it appears that only minimal improvements can be obtained in sleep when the focus of the treatment is on better managing pain. One possible explanation for this is that the insomnia experienced by these pain patients, though triggered by pain, is predominantly perpetuated by factors that are not addressed by individual pain clinicians or multidisciplinary programs.

With the growing understanding of pain-related insomnia as a problem in its own right, colleagues in the field have progressed to use CBT-I to specifically address sleep problems in chronic pain. CBT-I involves teaching patients about the science of sleep and the factors that affect it, collaborating with the patient to improve sleep efficiency using strategies such as sleep restriction (reducing time spent in bed to increase physiological sleep pressure) and stimulus control (reestablishing the association between the bed/bedroom and sleep). Cognitive elements of the therapy address sleep-specific worries and beliefs, especially those that instigate sleep-related anxiety (e.g., "if I can't sleep I won't be able to function tomorrow"), and safety-seeking behaviors (e.g., spending excessive time in bed and napping during the day to make up sleep) that further aggravate the sleep problem.

There is an emerging body of research investigating the effectiveness of *CBT-I for treating pain-related insomnia*, and four RCTs have been published during the past decade involving patients with chronic nonmalignant pain.

Currie et al. [119] conducted the first RCT to examine the effectiveness of CBT-I to treat pain-related insomnia. Sixty patients with chronic musculoskeletal pain were randomly

allocated to either CBT-I ($n=32$) or wait-list control. The CBT-I consisted of 7 weekly 2-h sessions delivered in a group format by six psychology doctorial students/interns with previous training in CBT interventions. The content of the treatment included psychoeducation about sleep and good sleep hygiene, relaxation training, cognitive therapy, sleep restriction therapy, and stimulus control. Sleep, pain, and mood were assessed at baseline, posttreatment, and after 3 months using 2-week sleep diaries, actigraphy, PSQI [89], Multidimensional Pain Inventory Pain Severity Scale (MPI-PS) [140], and Beck Depression Inventory (BDI) [141], respectively. Participants receiving CBT-I reported significantly improved SOL, WASO, and SE as measured by the sleep diaries and greater sleep quality measured by the PSQI posttreatment compared to the control group. Within-group analysis also indicated a significant reduction in movement monitored by actigraphy posttreatment compared to the baseline assessment. These improvements were maintained 3 months posttreatment with 16 % of patients achieving improvements that were clinically as well as statistically significant (SOL and WASO <30 min, SE>85 %, and PSQI<6). CBT-I, however, had no significant impact upon pain severity or mood.

Edinger et al. [120] compared CBT-I ($n=18$) with basic sleep hygiene education ($n=18$) and usual care ($n=11$) for treating patients with FM. The CBT-I was delivered by experienced clinical psychologists to patients following an individual format in 6 weekly sessions, the duration of which varied between 15 min and 1 h. The CBT-I consisted of psychoeducation about sleep, sleep restriction therapy, and stimulus control. Sleep was assessed using sleep diaries, actigraphy, and Insomnia Symptom Questionnaire (ISQ) [142]. Pain was assessed using the McGill Pain Questionnaire (MPQ) [143] and the Brief Pain Inventory (BPI) [144] while mood was assessed using the Profile of Mood States (POMS) [145] and the mental health composite score of the Medical Outcomes Survey 36-Item Short-Form Health Survey (SF-36) [146]. Posttreatment patients who received CBT-I reported shorter SOL, longer TST and SE, shorter SOL recorded by actigraphy, and lower ratings on the ISQ (indicating improved sleep) compared to patients receiving usual care, and these differences remained at 6-month follow-up. These improvements in sleep were considered by Edinger et al. [120] to be clinically significant for 57 % of the CBT-I group (TST≥6.5 h, TWT<60 min, and SE≥85 %, which is consistent with that defined in the CBT-I literature). Significant improvements were also observed in mood but not in pain.

Jungquist et al. [121] evaluated the impact of CBT-I on sleep disturbance and pain severity and pain interference. Nineteen patients with chronic neck or back pain individually received 8 weekly sessions of CBT-I from a CBT-trained nurse. The sessions lasted between 30 and 60 min and included sleep hygiene education, cognitive therapy, stimulus control, and sleep restriction. Sleep was measured using sleep diaries and the Insomnia Severity Index (ISI) [88]; pain was assessed using the MPI-PS, [140] the Pain Disability Index (PDI) [147], and a daily pain rating; mood was measured using the BDI [141]. Posttreatment patients reported significant improvements compared with controls in their self-reported SOL, WASO, SE, and overall ISI score. These improvements reached clinical significance for 42 % of the group according to the criteria (SOL and WASO< 15 min) of Jungquist and colleagues [121]. However, the improvements in sleep did not translate to significant improvements in pain and mood.

Vitello et al. [148] evaluated the efficacy of CBT-I on sleep disturbance and pain in 23 older adults with OA. The study follows their parent RCT [149], which compared CBT-I with an attention control condition in older adults with insomnia comorbid with a variety of chronic illnesses and found significant group differences posttreatment for sleep (CBT-I showed greater improvements) but not pain, as measured with MPQ [143]. This is a secondary analysis focusing on the within-group effect in a subgroup of OA patients to examine the durability of sleep improvements and to gauge the extent to which improved sleep can reduce pain.

The CBT-I consisted of 8 weekly sessions delivered in a group format by two clinical psychologists, each session lasting 2 h. The sessions involved teaching good sleep hygiene practice, relaxation training, cognitive therapy, stimulus control, and sleep restriction. Outcome measures included 2-week sleep diaries, short-form MPQ [143], and bodily pain subscale of the SF-36 [146], which were taken at baseline, posttreatment, and 1-year posttreatment. Patients who received CBT-I reported improved SOL (effect size=0.55), WASO (effect size=0.72), and increased SE (effect size=0.88) posttreatment compared to baseline. At 1-year follow-up, all improvements in sleep were maintained, and TST had also increased significantly (effect size=0.46). Although the focus of the study was to examine the efficacy of CBT-I for reducing pain, only a small improvement was reported on the SF-36 measure (effect size=0.31) and was not confirmed when measured with the SF-MPQ. Further, the gain on the SF-36 was not maintained when assessed 1-year posttreatment.

It appears that CBT-I originally developed for the treatment of primary insomnia can be successfully applied to treat pain-related insomnia. The pre-posttreatment effects for sleep are encouraging, ranging from 0.55 to 2.15 for SOL, 0.72–1.45 for WASO, 0.21–0.99 for TST, 0.88–2.01 for SE, and 0.76–3.25 for SQ [119–121, 148]. In terms of clinical significance, between 16 and 57 % of the patients achieved remission at posttreatment, and it appears that those treatments that adopted the individual format produced a higher remission rate than those that adopted the group format.

The knowledge that sleep deprivation/fragmentation increases pain perception has raised the hope that improvements in sleep could result in a significant improvement in pain. Unfortunately, the reciprocal relationship between sleep and pain is not as apparent in the therapeutic context as in the experimental setting. The results from the above-reviewed RCTs indicate that sleep improvement does not necessarily bring about a therapeutic effect on mood and pain [119–121]. The only RCT where an improvement in pain was observed reported inconsistent results from the SF-36 pain items and the SF-MPQ, and the result was obtained from a secondary analysis that specifically looked at the within-group change that will provide larger effect sizes than between-group comparisons [150]. Although it is encouraging to know that CBT-I, if well designed and executed, could have some positive impact on a patient's pain complaint, CBT-I per se is not sufficient to provide meaningful pain relief for patients suffering from chronic pain.

Taken together, PMPs incorporating just the sleep hygiene component of CBT-I typically do not produce any major benefit to pain patient's sleep. Although CBT-I directly applied to treat insomnia is efficacious in alleviating sleep disturbance, its therapeutic effect is not strong enough to prompt a discernable reduction in pain intensity or pain-related interference. The respective limitations of PMPs and CBT-I have led us to think that a hybrid form of psychological treatment that combines the most potent treatment components of PMPs and CBT-I to simultaneously address sleep and pain may be able to produce better outcomes. Given the intractable nature of chronic pain and the demonstrated inconsistent relationship between sleep and pain, the focus of such treatment should not be on using sleep to achieve pain reduction. Instead, we think that using better sleep as a means to improve the patient's daytime functioning, activity level, and overall quality of life may be more a meaningful goal.

Future Directions

We have only just begun to understand more about the impact of acute and chronic pain on sleep and the reverse impact of sleep disturbance on pain perception and tolerance. There are still many basic and clinically relevant questions to be answered. More effort will be required to delineate the mechanisms through which sleep and pain interact, both at the physiological and psychological levels. We know from experimental studies that the presentation of painful stimuli could have an arousal effect on healthy volunteers. However, scant evidence suggests that an increase in pain has the same effects on individuals who have already been experiencing pain for some time. As such, it would be important for future research to further examine these pain-sleep interaction pathways using clinical pain patient samples. In characterizing the impact of sleep disturbances on pain responses, recent additions to the literature indicate that the suppression of SWS and REM sleep may have differential effects on pain perception and that it may be sleep disruption, rather than sleep deprivation, that is contributing to the increased pain complaints. Developing an experimental model of sleep fragmentation that closely approximates the intermittent sleep pattern seen in patients with acute or chronic pain may allow future research to better study the impact of sleep disruption in different contexts. And of course, more research is required to understand the elevated rates of several sleep disorders (e.g., RSL, PLMS, OSA) in subgroups of pain patients.

Currently, there are a number of methods available to manage sleep disturbances concomitant to chronic pain. Each has its own advantages and disadvantages, and clinicians need to weigh the risks and benefits of each approach when planning treatment for their patients. Although both pharmacotherapy and nonpharmacotherapy have demonstrated efficacy in reducing insomnia symptoms, neither has consistently demonstrated that improved sleep is associated with a significant reduction in pain. Perhaps, the relationship between sleep and pain is not completely reciprocal in a therapeutic context. Most RCTs investigating the effect of CBT-I on sleep and pain complaints only had a short follow-up duration. Future RCTs with longer follow-up periods should provide an answer if time is what is needed for the effect of improved sleep on pain to be seen. Also, it is unclear what neuromechanisms underpin the transition from acute to persistent insomnia in chronic pain. It would be interesting to see whether the application of CBT-I could reverse some of these biological changes after treatment. Well-designed, longitudinal imaging studies may shed new light on the neuroplasticity of the brain.

Hybrid treatment that incorporates the most potent components of existing pain and sleep treatments to simultaneously address pain and insomnia may be the way forward if the therapy goal is to achieve significant improvement in both pain and sleep domains. Hybrid treatment could be an integration of psychological treatments of different focus (e.g., PMPs + CBT-I) or a combination of both pharmacological and nonpharmacological treatments (e.g., pregabalin plus CBT-I). More research will be needed to inform the design, structure, format, sequence, and duration of such treatment.

Summary and Conclusion

Chronic pain and insomnia are two of the most common forms of health problems in today's society. Each of them is a debilitating health condition in its own right. When both are presented in the same patient, pain and sleep interact to produce a condition that is even more challenging for the patient to self-manage and for healthcare professionals to treat. Existing evidence indicates that the standard unidimensional approach of treatment is insufficient. Research and clinical efforts are now focusing on better understanding the pain-sleep interaction and developing more effective strategies to deal with both pain and insomnia symptoms simultaneously. A more integrative treatment approach with diverse clinical targets is likely to be the model of effective pain management in the future.

References

1. Becker N, Bondegaard TA, Olsen AK, et al. Pain epidemiology and health related quality of life in chronic non-malignant pain patients referred to a Danish multidisciplinary pain center. Pain. 1997;73:393–400.
2. Casarett D, Karlawish J, Sankar P, et al. Designing pain research from the patient's perspective: what trial end points are important to patients with chronic pain? Pain Med. 2001;2:309–16.
3. Smith BH, Torrance N, Bennett MI, et al. Health and quality of life associated with chronic pain of predominantly neuropathic origin in the community. Clin J Pain. 2007;23:143–9.
4. Smith MT, Carmody TP, Smith MS. Quality of well-being scale and chronic low back pain. J Clin Psychol Med S. 2000;7:175–84.
5. Tang NKY, Crane C. Suicidality in chronic pain: a review of the prevalence, risk factors and psychological links. Psychol Med. 2006;36:575–86.
6. Turk DC, Dworkin RH, Revicki D, et al. Identifying important outcome domains for chronic pain clinical trials: an IMMPACT survey of people with pain. Pain. 2008;137:276–85.
7. Morin C, Gibson D, Wade J. Self-reported sleep and mood disturbance in chronic pain patients. Clin J Pain. 1998;14:311–4.
8. Smith M, Perlis M, Smith M, et al. Sleep quality and presleep arousal in chronic pain. J Behav Med. 2000;23:1–13.
9. Tang NKY, Wright KJ, Salkovskis PM. Prevalence and correlates of clinical insomnia co-occurring with chronic low back pain. J Sleep Res. 2007;16:85–95.
10. Morin CM, Espie CA. Insomnia: a clinical guide to assessment and treatment. New York: Springer; 2004.
11. McCracken LM, Iverson GL. Disrupted sleep patterns and daily functioning in patients with chronic pain. Pain Res Manag. 2002;7:75–9.
12. Theadom A, Cropley M, Humphrey K. Exploring the role of sleep and coping in quality of life in fibromyalgia. J Psychosom Res. 2007;62:145–51.
13. Dworkin RH, Turk DC, Farrar JT, et al. Core outcome measures for chronic pain clinical trials: IMMPACT recommendations. Pain. 2005;113:9–19.
14. Turk DC, Dworkin RH, McDermott MP, et al. Analyzing multiple endpoints in clinical trials of pain treatments: IMMPACT recommendations. Pain. 2008;139:485–93.
15. Rechtschaffen A, Bergmann B, Everson C, et al. Sleep deprivation in the rat: X integration and discussion of the findings. Sleep. 1989;25:68–87.
16. Guzman-Marýn R, Suntsova N, Stewart D, et al. Sleep deprivation reduces proliferation of cells in the dentate gyrus of the hippocampus in rats. J Physiol. 2003;549:563–71.
17. Schmidek W, Zachariassen K, Hammel H. Total calorimetric measurements in the rat: influences of the sleep-wakefulness cycle and of the environmental temperature. Brain Res. 1983;288:261–71.

18. Everson C, Laatsch C, Hogg N. Antioxidant defense responses to sleep loss and sleep recovery. Am J Physiol Regul Integr Comp Physiol. 2005;288:R374–83.

19. Toth L. Sleep, sleep deprivation and infectious disease: studies in animals. Adv Neuroimmunol. 1995;5:79–92.

20. Everson C. Sustained sleep deprivation impairs host defense. Am J Physiol. 1993;265:R1148–54.

21. Everson C. Clinical assessment of blood leukocytes, serum cytokines, and serum immunoglobulins as responses to sleep deprivation in laboratory rats. Am J Physiol Regul Integr Comp Physiol. 2005;289:R1054–63.

22. Ranjbaran Z, Keefer L, Stepanski E, et al. The relevance of sleep abnormalities to chronic inflammatory conditions. Inflamm Res. 2007;56:51–7.

23. Ohayon MM, Caulet M, Philip P, et al. How sleep and mental disorders are related to complaints of daytime sleepiness. Arch Intern Med. 1997;157:2645–52.

24. Becker PM, Brown WD, Jamieson AO. Impact of insomnia: assessment with the sickness impact profile. Sleep Res. 1991;20:206.

25. Breslau N, Roth T, Rosenthal L, et al. Daytime sleepiness: an epidemiological study of young adults. Am J Public Health. 1997; 87:1649–53.

26. Chang PP, Ford DE, Mead LA, et al. Insomnia in young men and subsequent depression. The Johns Hopkins study. Am J Epidemiol. 1997;146:105–14.

27. Ford DE, Kamerow DB. Epidemiologic study of sleep disturbances and psychiatric disorders. An opportunity for prevention? JAMA. 1989;262:1479–84.

28. Mellinger GD, Balter MB, Uhlenhuth EH. Insomnia and its treatment. Prevalence and correlates. Arch Gen Psychiatry. 1985;42:225–32.

29. Neckelmann D, Mykletun A, Dahl AA. Chronic insomnia as a risk factor for developing anxiety and depression. Sleep. 2007;30: 873–80.

30. Simon GE, VonKorff M. Prevalence, burden, and treatment of insomnia in primary care. Am J Psychiatry. 1997;154:1417–23.

31. Vollrath M, Wicki W, Angst J. The Zurich study. VIII. Insomnia: association with depression, anxiety, somatic syndromes, and course of insomnia. Eur Arch Psychiatry Neurol Sci. 1989;239:113–24.

32. Weissman MM, Greenwald S, Nino-Murcia G, et al. The morbidity of insomnia uncomplicated by psychiatric disorders. Gen Hosp Psychiatry. 1997;19:245–50.

33. Stickgold R, James L, Hobson J. Visual discrimination learning requires sleep after training. Nat Neurosci. 2000;3:1237–8.

34. Stickgold R, Whidbee D, Schirmer B, et al. Visual discrimination task improvement: a multi-step process occurring during sleep. J Cogn Neurosci. 2000;12:246–54.

35. McCarley R. Neurobiology of REM and NREM sleep. Sleep Med. 2007;8:302–30.

36. Ohayon MM. Relationship between chronic painful physical condition and insomnia. J Psychiatr Res. 2005;39:151–9.

37. Morphy H, Dunn KM, Lewis M, et al. Epidemiology of insomnia: a longitudinal study in a UK population. Sleep. 2007;30:274–80.

38. Foley D, Ancoli-Israel S, Britz P, et al. Sleep disturbances and chronic disease in older adults: results of the 2003 National Sleep Foundation Sleep in America Survey. J Psychosom Res. 2004; 56:497–502.

39. Gabor JY, Cooper AB, Hanly PJ. Sleep disruption in the intensive care unit. Curr Opin Crit Care. 2001;7:21–7.

40. Redeker NS. Sleep in acute care settings: an integrative review. J Nurs Scholarsh. 2000;32:31–8.

41. Rosenberg-Adamsen S, Kehlet H, Dodds C, et al. Postoperative sleep disturbances: mechanisms and clinical implications. Br J Anaesth. 1996;76:552–9.

42. Redeker NS, Hedges C. Sleep during hospitalization and recovery after cardiac surgery. J Cardiovasc Nurs. 2002;17:56–68.

43. Raymond I, Nielsen TA, Lavigne G, et al. Quality of sleep and its daily relationship to pain intensity in hospitalized adult burn patients. Pain. 2001;92:381–8.

44. Savard J, Morin CM. Insomnia in the context of cancer: a review of a neglected problem. J Clin Oncol. 2001;19:895–908.

45. Dorrepaal KL, Aaronson NK, van Dam FS. Pain experience and pain management among hospitalized cancer patients. A clinical study. Cancer. 1989;63:593–8.

46. Atkinson JH, Ancoli-Israel S, Slater MA, et al. Subjective sleep disturbance in chronic back pain. Clin J Pain. 1988;4:225–32.

47. Pilowsky I, Crettenden I, Townley M. Sleep disturbance in pain clinic patients. Pain. 1985;23:27–33.

48. Tang NKY, Goodchild CE, Hester J, Salkovskis PM. Pain-related insomnia: A comparision study of sleep pattern, psychological characteristics and cognitive-behavioural processes. Clinical journal of pain. 2012;428–436.

49. Wittig R, Zorick F, Blumer D, et al. Disturbed sleep in patients complaining of chronic pain. J Nerv Ment Dis. 1982;170:429–31.

50. Hirsch M, Carlander B, Vergé M, et al. Objective and subjective sleep disturbances in patients with rheumatoid arthritis. A reappraisal. Arthritis Rheum. 1994;37:41–9.

51. Landis C, Lentz M, Rothermel J, et al. Decreased sleep spindles and spindle activity in midlife women with fibromyalgia and pain. Sleep. 2004;27:741–50.

52. Rizzi M, Sarzi-Puttini P, Atzeni F, et al. Cyclic alternating pattern: a new marker of sleep alteration in patients with fibromyalgia? J Rheumatol. 2004;31:1193–9.

53. Martinez-Lavin M, Hermosillo AG, Rosas M, et al. Circadian studies of autonomic nervous balance in patients with fibromyalgia: a heart rate variability analysis. Arthritis Rheum. 1998;41:1966–71.

54. Moldofsky H, Scarisbrick P, England R, et al. Musculoskeletal symptoms and non-REM sleep disturbance in patients with "fibrositis syndrome" and healthy subjects. Psychosom Med. 1975;37:341–51.

55. Moldofsky H, Lue F. The relationship of alpha and delta EEG frequencies to pain and mood in 'fibrositis' patients treated with chlorpromazine and L-tryptophan. Electroencephalogr Clin Neurophysiol. 1980;50:71–80.

56. Horne JA, Shackell BS. Alpha-like EEG activity in non-REM sleep and the fibromyalgia (fibrositis) syndrome. Electroencephalogr Clin Neurophysiol. 1991;79:271–6.

57. Pivik RT, Harman K. A reconceptualization of EEG alpha activity as an index of arousal during sleep: all alpha activity is not equal. J Sleep Res. 1995;4:131–7.

58. Rains J, Penzien D. Sleep and chronic pain: challenges to the alpha-EEG sleep pattern as a pain specific sleep anomaly. J Psychosom Res. 2003;54:77–83.

59. Schneider-Helmert D, Whitehouse I, Kumar A, et al. Insomnia and alpha sleep in chronic non-organic pain as compared to primary insomnia. Neuropsychobiology. 2001;43:54–8.

60. Dauvilliers Y, Touchon J. Sleep in fibromyalgia: review of clinical and polysomnographic data. Neurophysiol Clin. 2001;31:18–33.

61. Moldofsky H, Tullis C, Lue F. Sleep related myoclonus in rheumatic pain modulation disorder (fibrositis syndrome). J Rheumatol. 1986;13:614–7.

62. Montplaisir J, Boucher S, Poirier G, et al. Clinical, polysomnographic, and genetic characteristics of restless legs syndrome: a study of 133 patients diagnosed with new standard criteria. Mov Disord. 1997;12:61–5.

63. Sun ER, Chen CA, Ho G, et al. Iron and the restless legs syndrome. Sleep. 1998;21:371–7.

64. Polydefkis M, Allen RP, Hauer P, et al. Subclinical sensory neuropathy in late-onset restless legs syndrome. Neurology. 2000; 55:1115–21.

65. Sand T, Hagen K, Schrader H. Sleep apnea and chronic headache. Cephalalgia. 2003;23:90–5.

66. Loh N, Dinner D, Foldvary N, et al. Do patients with obstructive sleep apnea wake up with headaches? Arch Intern Med. 1999;159:1765–8.
67. Germanowicz D, Lumertz MS, Martinez D, et al. Sleep disordered breathing concomitant with fibromyalgia syndrome. J Bras Pneumol. 2006;32:333–8.
68. Sepici V, Tosun A, Köktürk O. Obstructive sleep apnea syndrome as an uncommon cause of fibromyalgia: a case report. Rheumatol Int. 2007;28:69–71.
69. Drewes AM, Nielsen KD, Arendt-Nielsen L, et al. The effect of cutaneous and deep pain on the electroencephalogram during sleep – an experimental study. Sleep. 1997;20:632–40.
70. Lavigne G, Zucconi M, Castronovo C, et al. Sleep arousal response to experimental thermal stimulation during sleep in human subjects free of pain and sleep problems. Pain. 2000;84:283–90.
71. Lavigne G, Brousseau M, Kato T, et al. Experimental pain perception remains equally active over all sleep stages. Pain. 2004;110: 646–55.
72. Onen S, Alloui A, Gross A, et al. The effects of total sleep deprivation, selective sleep interruption and sleep recovery on pain tolerance thresholds in healthy subjects. J Sleep Res. 2001;10:35–42.
73. Moldofsky H, Scarisbrick P. Induction of neurasthenic musculoskeletal pain syndrome by selective sleep stage deprivation. Psychosom Med. 1976;38:35–44.
74. Lentz MJ, Landis CA, Rothermel J, et al. Effects of selective slow wave sleep disruption on musculoskeletal pain and fatigue in middle aged women. J Rheumatol. 1999;26:1586–92.
75. Roehrs T, Hyde M, Blaisdell B, et al. Sleep loss and REM sleep loss are hyperalgesic. Sleep. 2006;29:145–51.
76. Smith MT, Edwards RR, McCann UD, et al. The effects of sleep deprivation on pain inhibition and spontaneous pain in women. Sleep. 2007;30:494–505.
77. Wilson KG, Watson ST, Currie SR. Daily diary and ambulatory activity monitoring of sleep in patients with insomnia associated with chronic musculoskeletal pain. Pain. 1998;75:75–84.
78. Chapman JB, Lehman CL, Elliott J, et al. Sleep quality and the role of sleep medications for veterans with chronic pain. Pain Med. 2006;7:105–14.
79. Affleck G, Urrows S, Tennen H, et al. Sequential daily relations of sleep, pain intensity, and attention to pain among women with fibromyalgia. Pain. 1996;68:363–8.
80. Nicassio PM, Moxham EG, Schuman CE, et al. The contribution of pain, reported sleep quality, and depressive symptoms to fatigue in fibromyalgia. Pain. 2002;100:271–9.
81. Theadom A, Cropley M. Dysfunctional beliefs, stress and sleep disturbance in fibromyalgia. Sleep Med. 2008;9:376–81.
82. Smith MT, Perlis ML, Carmody TP, et al. Presleep cognitions in patients with insomnia secondary to chronic pain. J Behav Med. 2001;24:93–114.
83. American Psychiatric Association. Diagnostic and statistical manual of mental disorders. Text Revision edition. 4th ed. Washington, DC: American Psychiatric Association; 2000.
84. World Health Organization. International statistical classification of diseases and related health problems 10th revision. 2007. http://apps.who.int/classifications/apps/icd/icd10online/. Accessed 16 Sep 2009.
85. American Academy of Sleep Medicine. International classification of sleep disorders: diagnostic and coding manual. 2nd ed. Westchester: American Academy of Sleep Medicine; 2005.
86. Schramm E, Hohagen F, Grasshoff U, et al. Test-retest reliability and validity of the structured interview for sleep disorders according to DSM-III-R. Am J Psychiat. 1993;150:867–72.
87. Edinger JD, Kirby AC, Lineberger MD, et al. DUKE structured interview schedule for DSM-IV-TR and international classification of sleep disorders, second edition (ICSD-2) sleep disorder diagnoses. Durham: Veterans Affairs and Duke University Medical Centers; 2006.

88. Bastien C, Vallières A, Morin CM. Validation of the insomnia severity index as a clinical outcome measure for insomnia research. Sleep Med. 2001;2:297–307.
89. Buysse DJ, Reynolds III CF, Monk TH, et al. The Pittsburgh sleep quality index: a new instrument for psychiatric practice and research. Psychiatry Res. 1989;28:193–213.
90. Zomer J, Peled R, Rubin AHE, et al. Mini sleep questionnaire for screening large populations for excessive daytime sleepiness complaints. In: Koella W, Ruther E, Schulz U, editors. Sleep 1984. Stuttgart: Gustav Fisher Verlag; 1985. p. 467–70.
91. Hetta J, Almqvist M, Agren H, et al. Prevalence of sleep disturbances and related symptoms in a middle-aged Swedish population. In: Koella W, Ruther E, Schulz U, editors. Sleep 1984. Stuttgart: Gustav Fischer Verlag; 1985. p. 373–6.
92. Hays RD, Martin SA, Sesti AM, et al. Psychometric properties of the medical outcomes study sleep measure. Sleep Med. 2005; 6:41–4.
93. Morin CM. Insomnia: psychological assessment and management. New York: Guilford Press; 1993.
94. Morin CM. Dysfunctional beliefs and attitudes about sleep: preliminary scale development and description. Behav Ther. 1994; 17:163–4.
95. Espie CA. The psychological treatment of insomnia. Chichester: Wiley; 1991.
96. Tyron W. Issues of validity in actigraphic sleep assessment. Sleep. 2004;27:158–65.
97. Lavie P, Epstein R, Tzischinsky O, et al. Actigraphic measurements of sleep in rheumatoid arthritis: comparison of patients with low back pain and healthy controls. J Rheumatol. 1992;19: 362–5.
98. Landis CA, Frey CA, Lentz MJ, et al. Self-reported sleep quality and fatigue correlates with actigraphy in midlife women with fibromyalgia. Nurs Res. 2003;52:140–7.
99. Kushida CA, Chang A, Gadkary C, et al. Comparison of actigraphic, polysomnographic, and subjective assessment of sleep parameters in sleep-disordered patients. Sleep Med. 2001;2:389–96.
100. Lichstein KL, Riedel BW. Behavioral assessment and treatment of insomnia: a review with an emphasis on clinical application. Behav Ther. 1994;25:659–88.
101. Walker J, Farney R, Rhondeau S, et al. Chronic opioid use is a risk factor for the development of central sleep apnea and ataxic breathing. J Clin Sleep Med. 2007;3:455–61.
102. Ballantyne JC, Mao J. Opioid therapy for chronic pain. N Engl J Med. 2003;349:1943–53.
103. Gilron I. Gabapentin and pregabalin for chronic neuropathic and early postsurgical pain: current evidence and future directions. Curr Opin Anaesthesiol. 2007;20:456–72.
104. Legros B, Bazil C. Effects of antiepileptic drugs on sleep architecture: a pilot study. Sleep Med. 2003;4:51–5.
105. Garcia-Borreguero D, Larrosa O, de la Llave Y, et al. Treatment of restless legs syndrome with gabapentin: a double-blind, crossover study. Neurology. 2002;59:1573–9.
106. Drug Enforcement Administration DoJ. Schedules of controlled substances: placement of pregabalin into schedule V. Final rule. Fed Regist. 2005;70:43633–5.
107. Tiihonen J, Lonnqvist J, Wahlbeck K, et al. Antidepressants and the risk of suicide, attempted suicide, and overall mortality in a nationwide cohort. Arch Gen Psychiatry. 2006;63:1358–67.
108. Perroud N, Uher R, Marusic A, et al. Suicidal ideation during treatment of depression with escitalopram and nortriptyline in genome-based therapeutic drugs for depression (GENDEP): a clinical trial. BMC Med. 2009;7:60.
109. Berger A, Dukes EM, Edelsberg J, et al. Use of tricyclic antidepressants in older patients with painful neuropathies. Eur J Clin Pharmacol. 2006;62:757–64.

110. Bymaster F, Dreshfield-Ahmad L, Threlkeld P, et al. Comparative affinity of duloxetine and venlafaxine for serotonin and norepinephrine transporters in vitro and in vivo, human serotonin receptor subtypes, and other neuronal receptors. Neuropsychopharmacology. 2001;25:871–80.

111. Fava M, Mulroy R, Alpert J, et al. Emergence of adverse events following discontinuation of treatment with extended-release venlafaxine. Am J Psychiatry. 1997;154:1760–2.

112. Thase M. Effects of venlafaxine on blood pressure: a meta-analysis of original data from 3744 depressed patients. J Clin Psychiatry. 1998;59:502–8.

113. Krystal AD. A compendium of placebo-controlled trials of the risks/benefits of pharmacological treatments for insomnia: the empirical basis for U.S. clinical practice. Sleep Med Rev. 2009;13: 265–74.

114. Smith MT, Haythornthwaite JA. Cognitive-behavioral treatment for insomnia and pain. In: Lavigne G, Sessle B, Choiniere M, Soja P, editors. Sleep and pain. Seattle: ISAP; 2007. p. 439–57.

115. British Pain Society. Recommended guidelines for pain management programmes for adults. London: British Pain Society; 2007.

116. Ashworth PCH, Burke BL, McCracken L. Does a pain management programme help you sleep better? Clin Psychol Forum. 2008;184:35–40.

117. Morley S, Williams A, Hussain S. Estimating the clinical effectiveness of cognitive behavioural therapy in the clinic: evaluation of a CBT informed pain management programme. Pain. 2008;137: 670–80.

118. Lichstein KL, Wilson NM, Johnson CT. Psychological treatment of secondary insomnia. Psychol Aging. 2000;15:232–40.

119. Currie SR, Wilson KG, Pontefract AJ, et al. Cognitive-behavioral treatment of insomnia secondary to chronic pain. J Consult Clin Psychol. 2000;68:407–16.

120. Edinger JD, Wohlgemuth WK, Krystal AD, et al. Behavioral insomnia therapy for fibromyalgia patients: a randomized clinical trial. Arch Intern Med. 2005;165:2527–35.

121. Jungquist CR, O'Brien C, Matteson-Rusby S, et al. The efficacy of cognitive behavioral therapy for insomnia in patients with chronic pain. Sleep Med. 2010;11:302–9.

122. Nikolaus T, Zeyfang A. Pharmacological treatments for persistent non-malignant pain in older persons. Drugs Aging. 2004;21:19–41.

123. Menefee LA, Cohen MJ, Anderson WR, et al. Sleep disturbance and nonmalignant chronic pain: a comprehensive review of the literature. Pain Med. 2000;1:156–72.

124. Shaw I, Lavigne G, Mayer P, et al. Acute intravenous administration of morphine perturbs sleep architecture in healthy pain-free young adults: a preliminary study. Sleep. 2005;28:677–82.

125. Dimsdale J, Norman D, Dejardin D, et al. The effect of opioids on sleep architecture. J Clin Sleep Med. 2007;3:33–6.

126. Rosenthal M, Moore P, Groves E, et al. Sleep improves when patients with chronic OA pain are managed with morning dosing of once a day extended-release morphine sulfate (AVINZA): findings from a pilot study. J Opioid Manag. 2007;3:145–54.

127. Foldvary-Schaefer N, De Leon Sanchez I, Karafa M, et al. Gabapentin increases slow-wave sleep in normal adults. Epilepsia. 2002;43:1493–7.

128. Hindmarch I, Dawson J, Stanley N. A double-blind study in healthy volunteers to assess the effects on sleep of pregabalin compared with alprazolam and placebo. Sleep. 2005;28:187–93.

129. Webster L, Choi Y, Desai H, et al. Sleep-disordered breathing and chronic opioid therapy. Pain Med. 2008;9:425–32.

130. Wang D, Teichtahl H, Drummer O, et al. Central sleep apnea in stable methadone maintenance treatment patients. Chest. 2005; 128:1348–56.

131. Saarto T, Wiffen P. Antidepressants for neuropathic pain. Cochrane Database Syst Rev. 2007;CD005454.

132. Haddad PM, Dursun SM. Neurological complications of psychiatric drugs: clinical features and management. Hum Psychopharmacol. 2008;23 Suppl 1:15–26.

133. Chang C, Wu E, Chang I, et al. Benzodiazepine and risk of hip fractures in older people: a nested case-control study in Taiwan. Am J Geriatr Psychiatry. 2008;16:686–92.

134. Bartlett G, Abrahamowicz M, Grad R, et al. Association between risk factors for injurious falls and new benzodiazepine prescribing in elderly persons. BMC Fam Pract. 2009;10:1.

135. Roehrs T, Roth T. Sleep and pain: interaction of two vital functions. Semin Neurol. 2005;25:106–16.

136. Morley S, Eccleston C, Williams A. Systematic review and meta-analysis of randomized controlled trials of cognitive behaviour therapy and behaviour therapy for chronic pain in adults, excluding headache. Pain. 1999;80:1–13.

137. Redondo JR, Justo CM, Moraleda FV, et al. Long-term efficacy of therapy in patients with fibromyalgia: a physical exercise-based program and a cognitive-behavioral approach. Arthritis Rheum. 2004;51:184–92.

138. Gustavsson C, von Koch L. Applied relaxation in the treatment of long-lasting neck pain: a randomized controlled pilot study. J Rehabil Med. 2006;38:100–7.

139. Becker N, Sjogren P, Bech P, et al. Treatment outcome of chronic non-malignant pain patients managed in a Danish multidisciplinary pain centre compared to general practice: a randomised controlled trial. Pain. 2000;84:203–11.

140. Kerns RD, Turk DC, Rudy TE. The West Haven-Yale multidimensional pain inventory (WHYMPI). Pain. 1985;23:345–56.

141. Beck AT, Ward CH, Mendelson MM, et al. An inventory for measuring depression. Arch Gen Psych. 1961;4:561–71.

142. Spielman AJ, Saskin P, Thorpy MJ. Treatment of chronic insomnia by restriction of time in bed. Sleep. 1987;10:45–55.

143. Melzack R. The short-form McGill pain questionnaire. Pain. 1987;30:191–7.

144. Cleeland CS. Measurement of pain by subjective report. In: Chapman CR, Loeser JD, editors. Advances in pain research and therapy, volume 12: issues in pain measurement. New York: Raven; 1989. p. 391–403.

145. McNair DM, Lorr M, Droppleman LF. EDITS manual for the profile of mood states. San Diego: EDITS; 1971.

146. Ware JE, Snow KK, Kosinski M, et al. SF-36 health survey: manual and interpretation guide. Boston: The Health Institute, New England Medical Center; 1993.

147. Tait RC, Pollard CA, Margolis RB, et al. The pain disability index: psychometric and validity data. Arch Phys Med Rehabil. 1987;68:438–41.

148. Vitello MV, Rybarczyk B, Von Korff M, et al. Cognitive behavioral therapy for insomnia improves sleep and decreases pain in older adults with co-morbid insomnia and osteoarthritis. J Clin Sleep Med. 2009;5:355–62.

149. Rybarczyk B, Stepanski E, Fogg L, et al. A placebo-controlled test of CBT for co-morbid insomnia in older adults. J Consult Clin Psychol. 2005;73:1164–74.

150. Haynes PL. Is CBT-I effective for pain? J Clin Sleep Med. 2009;5:363–4.

151. Tang NKY, Goodchild CE, Sanborn AN, Howard J, Salkovskis PM. Deciphering the temporal link between sleep and pain in a heterogeneous chronic pain patient sample: A multilevel daily process study. Sleep. 2012;5(35):675–68.

Empowerment: A Pain Caregiver's Perspective

86

Julia Hallisy

Key Points

- Witnessing a loved one in pain is a significant source of fear and anxiety for caregivers, even if they seem to be coping well.
- Caregivers are often expected to assume complicated medical duties without proper training or emotional support.
- There are many reputable sources of information and support for patients and caregivers, and they need to be made aware of appropriate networks.
- The siblings of an ill child may have an especially difficult time adjusting to the changes in their lives, and their unique situation needs to be acknowledged and addressed.
- Caregivers often experience extreme exhaustion and feelings of isolation, and their own interpersonal relationships may suffer – including their relationship with the patient.
- Many caregivers experience a significant loss of control when the patient enters the hospital, and their knowledge and expertise may not be recognized or utilized.

Introduction

Managing a loved one's pain is one of the most difficult and anxiety-provoking responsibilities facing caregivers. Pain management by caregivers requires information, skills, support, and compassion. Too often, caregivers find that they are overwhelmed by this formidable responsibility and unsure of where to turn for help.

J. Hallisy, B.S., DDS
595 Buckingham Way # 305,
San Francisco 94132, CA, USA
e-mail: julia@empoweredpatientcoalition.org

In my own case, my late daughter Katherine Hallisy was diagnosed at 5 months of age with bilateral retinoblastoma and faced five recurrences of her cancer before her death in February 2000 at the age of ten. Kate's cancer was aggressive and accompanied by episodes of chronic pain. An above-the-knee amputation led to both physical and unrelenting "phantom" pain. Radiation years earlier to Kate's right orbital area eventually led to a non-operable tumor in her skull and proved to be one of our most formidable pain management challenges. I learned that while each pain experience is personal and subjective, in many ways, it is shared by the entire family and each caregiver.

Pain and Patients

The fear of pain is a major concern for cancer patients [1] and for any individual facing a serious or prolonged illness. It is not just the physical burdens of pain that are problematic. The nonphysical manifestations of pain including anxiety, personality changes, feelings of helplessness, a sense of frustration, sudden anger, and guilt can be devastating for the patient's sense of well-being and for their relationships with those around them.

Patients and their advocates and caregivers are given numerous details about a diagnosis and proposed treatment plan, but may receive little information early on about the "pain control plan." Those facing serious illness and their caregivers need to feel confident that they have been given enough information to assess pain levels, training in how to competently manage pain, and assurances that they will have access to the best resources and pain specialists. Those who are taught to view pain as a normal and often inevitable process will not be blindsided and unprepared if pain becomes a challenging issue. I have had many caregivers express their deep-rooted fear that the patient will experience pain that becomes impossible to control and patients often fear untreatable pain more than death itself. These feelings may be impossible to avoid, but addressing them openly and early in the course of treatment may alleviate a great deal of anxiety for both patients and caregivers.

Pain and Caregivers

Pain is ever changing, difficult to manage, and physically and mentally debilitating for both patients and their caregivers. Acting as a caregiver for a patient with severe or chronic pain is one of the most stressful and demanding roles a person can accept. Research studies confirm that caregivers of cancer patients who are in pain have significantly higher levels of depression and anxiety [2]. Aside from the obvious and understandable levels of fear, being a caregiver thrusts people into physically demanding roles that they are often not trained for or emotionally prepared to handle.

Caregivers are often asked to assume intricate medical duties such as assessing pain levels accurately, administering and monitoring powerful medications, and communicating with teams of highly trained medical personnel including oncologists, pharmacists, and nurse practitioners. In my personal situation, I was given a brief tutorial on drawing blood from Kate's central line, flushing the line with heparin, and changing the dressing around the central line, and then I was expected to assume these duties at home on my own. I was also responsible for watching for signs of infection and blood clots. Even as a health-care professional, I was overwhelmed and fearful that I would make a critical mistake that could jeopardize my daughter's health.

Managing my daughter's central line often meant that I was the one causing her physical and emotional pain. We both knew that the line went directly into a vessel near her heart, and we felt the stress associated with changing the dressing or tugging on the skin. It was impossible to have a dressing change that was painless and that did not cause moments of intense stress. It is even more difficult to deal with the patient's pain when it is your actions that are causing the distress. No matter how many times you tell yourself that you are only doing what must be done, this is a predicament that caregivers are not prepared for and often face alone.

Caregivers may not fully comprehend the true scope of their responsibilities, especially when they lead to emotional dilemmas. Health-care professionals need to provide caregivers specific information about the requirements of their duties, but they must also prepare people for the many psychological components that are a part of tending to the ill.

Seeking Information and Support

When my daughter was diagnosed with cancer in 1989, there were few resources available to find current information about retinoblastoma. I was not familiar with the Internet or medical information search companies, so I went to our local medical school bookstore and looked at pediatric textbooks that contained data and statistics that were outdated and frightening.

Fortunately, patients and their advocates now have access to cutting-edge resources for facts and support when facing illness. There are an ever-growing number of people who are willing to take the time and expend the effort to learn about their symptoms, diagnosis, tests, and medications. There are some physicians who discourage their patients from doing their own research and admonish them to "stay off the Internet." Once a patient shows any interest in seeking their own facts, it would be helpful for professionals to be supportive of these efforts and to guide people to reputable sources of information.

The government offers many sites appropriate for the public, including Healthfinder.gov, MedlinePlus, Agency for Healthcare Research and Quality (AHRQ), and the Centers for Disease Control and Prevention (CDC). Patients can be advised to look for web sites that contain the HONcode which guarantees that the site abides by standards for reliable health information.

Another excellent resource is Planetree Health Resource Centers for information and support. Planetree offers "health links" which is a list of the best sites for health information, and some Planetree centers will conduct a literature search and assemble an information packet on a specific illness for a reasonable fee. This is a good resource for people who do not want to spend time doing research or who aren't savvy with computers. Some Planetree centers offer lecture series and links to online support groups as well.

Choosing a Doctor/Changing Doctors

What I look for in a physician has evolved over the last two decades. When Kate was first diagnosed, her pediatrician gave us a referral to an oncologist, which we accepted without question. I didn't know how to research his background, to ask for any other referrals or second opinions, or to set up a brief meeting to see if he seemed to be a "good fit" for our daughter and our family. I have learned over the years that thought and research is needed before establishing relationship with a physician. Extra care should go into choosing a doctor with whom patients are likely to have a long-term relationship such as internists, oncologists, or pain specialists.

I have now set the bar high, and my requirements for a good doctor-patient relationship must include excellent communication and access, a sense of warmth and compassion, absolute truth and transparency, and a feeling of trust. If any of these are lacking, I know I need to make a change. We had the experience of realizing that we needed to leave the care of Kate's oncologist after 8 years of working together, so I have lived through the thought process and the emotional aspects of changing doctors during a complicated treatment plan.

In 1998, we came to the unexpected and immediate conclusion that we needed to find a new oncologist for Kate. Kate had a bad reaction to one of her three chemotherapy drugs, and the decision was made by all to discontinue the medication. We hoped to continue her regimen with the remaining two drugs, knowing that it was less than ideal. Even though all the tests had shown no cancer anywhere in Kate's body at the time, the tumor board and our oncologist decided to invoke a "futile care" policy and stop all chemotherapy. Our oncologist called me at the end of my work day with no advance warning to inform me that the hospital would be stopping treatment because the cancer "will undoubtedly come back." I was supposed to be comforted by his comment "Don't worry – we will be sure you have lots of pain medicine." I was alone, stunned, and panic stricken, and I had to drive home and break the news to my husband. I had never felt so abandoned by a physician or another human being in my life.

There had been times along the way that we weren't happy with this doctor's level of communication or his demeanor, but we made the mistake of brushing these intuitive feelings aside. Now in my work as a patient advocate, I routinely advise people to heed these internal warning signals and to search for a provider who includes them in thought processes, rationales, and the decision-making process. Patients may come to their physicians with misgivings about a specialist or other provider, and I suggest that doctors listen carefully to the patient's concerns and encourage them to find a new practitioner if they are unhappy in any way.

Pain and Family Caregivers, Including Siblings

Many patients suffering from illness and chronic pain are cared for at home by relatives. While family members may seem like the logical choice to be caregivers, they often face unique challenges and stresses. The services of outside caregivers may be a financial burden, and families often want their loved ones to be cared for in their own familiar home environment.

Children caring for parents have their own families, careers, and other responsibilities in addition to the many hours spent providing care for loved ones. Vacations, hobbies, relationships, and travel plans may all have to be altered or abandoned to make time for the patient. Many caregivers are elderly spouses who may have their own health issues and physical limitations. Many family members are so emotionally involved in the situation that it can become difficult to notice subtle changes in the patient's condition. Certainly, fatigue and worry can impair a family member's ability to assess pain levels and to deliver quality care on a consistent basis.

Other family members are impacted by the experiences of the caregiver, including spouses, friends, coworkers, and siblings who may all notice a decline in the caregiver's attitude, health, and demeanor. Children of caregivers may be adversely affected by the stressful situation their parent is facing, and siblings of an ill child may have an especially difficult time adjusting to the changes and the disruption in their household.

I have had the unfortunate and life-altering experience of being a sibling of a critically ill child and the parent of a daughter facing a life-threatening illness. I watched my parents become consumed with making complex medical treatment decisions when my late sister was diagnosed with a congenital cardiac defect that necessitated a complicated open heart surgery. At 7 years old, I desperately wanted to understand what was happening and I sensed that the problem with her heart posed a risk to her life. When I asked my mother point-blank if my sister could die, she broke down in tears and couldn't form an answer. I wanted to know the truth about the situation, but I immediately knew that I had asked the wrong question.

Siblings see their lives change overnight, and they may feel that they are losing touch with their parents both physically and emotionally. Siblings need and want to know the truth, but they want to ease their parent's burden even more, so they internalize their fears and their questions remain unanswered. Siblings often tell me that they felt removed from their sibling's illness and that they had to find their own ways of dealing with the stress of seeing their brother or sister in pain. Ten years after their sister's death, my own two sons react very differently to the memory of Kate's experience with cancer. My younger son who was six at the time remembers more of Kate's exuberant personality and the fun things they did together like playing games on her bed. My older son who was twelve at the time says he "prefers not to think about" the doctors, hospitals, and the episodes of extreme pain he witnessed. His sister's illness and the resulting consequences still make him angry and frustrated. He was just old enough to have the memory of the suffering leave a permanent imprint on his psyche. Editor's note: I would highly recommend eye movement desensitization and reprocessing (EMDR) for the caregiver's older son, even this far removed in time. This process clears out long-term potentiation in the brain and is the most potent and very fast treatment for PTSD symptoms. It is a good tool, but also requires a good therapist to do it successfully. There is an EMDR Guild which lists all certified practitioners in her area.

My sons did not assume medical duties, but they ministered to their sister by being her legs when she was healing from her amputation, watching movies and playing games at her bedside and sharing stories about school and friends to keep her updated on the outside world. Brothers and sisters often play important roles in the life of their sibling, but may do so with the great burden of mystery and worry. Parents naturally want to protect their other children from the hardships of illness which is why it is important for professionals to be prepared to offer guidance or referrals long before siblings have sequestered their emotions or are struggling to cope with a new and stressful family dynamic.

Challenges to Caregivers' Relationships

The stresses to interpersonal relationships often begin so subtly that it can be difficult to realize that they are happening. Friendships, marriages, parental roles, and coworker relationships can all suffer when a person takes on caregiving responsibilities. Being a care provider often demands every free moment and can leave people with little or no time for maintaining or sustaining relationships.

The stress-filled environment of pain control duties can make a person short-tempered, lonely, and defensive. It becomes too easy for the caregiver to feel isolated and overwhelmed and to think that "no one understands" [3]. Caregivers often stop allocating time for themselves and their relationships and may even come to view them as unnecessary intrusions into their duties. Again, medical professionals can caution people about this phenomenon right from the beginning and encourage people to nourish their personal relationships. The reality is that small steps may be in order and caregivers may need to choose one or two people that they will work at staying in contact with. Caregivers can also ask a few people to commit to reaching out and making regular contact with them, which takes the responsibility off their shoulders.

Caregivers need to realize that they will experience an ever-changing range of emotions and communicate to their loved ones that they should expect a wide variance in their demeanor. Conversations with friends or relatives can run the gamut from stoic and forced to prolonged venting sessions about the challenges facing the caregiver. Naturally, some friends will find these conversations difficult, and they will struggle to find the right words of support. In time, the calls and visits may dwindle. Professionals can encourage caregivers to be open and honest about their feelings and to tell people right up front that they are having a bad day or that they just need someone to listen when they want to talk about their problems. Some friends and family will be better at certain roles than others, so caregivers should try to establish a small group of "go-to" people who can help them through these ups and downs.

It's important for caregivers to be reminded to take the time to nurture their relationship with the patient. Caregivers who are feeling isolated and exhausted will not be able to hide these emotions from the patient, who will share in the deleterious effects on their relationship and worry that they are pushing their loved one to the breaking point. It is important for caregivers to remember what their relationship with the patient was like before illness intervened and to try to have moments every day when they set their role as a caregiver aside and interact with the patient as simply a friend, spouse, or child.

Professionals should have current information available for caregivers about new social networking and communication models such as CarePages.com, CaringBridge.org, or LotsaHelpingHands.com. Caregivers and patients can provide online updates for friends and family to stay informed about the patient's condition and about any ways that they may be able to contribute and assist. These sites have the capability to set up meal delivery schedules, blogs, photos, message boards, and monetary donations. These sites are powerful tools for caregivers to stay connected to their supporters and to feel like they are keeping people updated without taking precious time away from the patient.

Caregivers must be told up front that they need to work at becoming accustomed to asking for help from those around them and that a strong and capable caregiver recognizes that they will occasionally need assistance. We must update the definition of a good caregiver from someone who takes on a superhuman role all on their own to someone who is strong enough to realize that they cannot possibly be 100% every hour of every day.

Caring for the Caregiver

Just as each illness has a unique progression and path, each caregiver faces challenges that can be difficult and life-altering. Caregivers may routinely face ongoing stress, sleep deprivation, lack of exercise, compromised nutrition, and insomnia. On a much more serious level, caregivers may struggle with debilitating depression, alcohol or substance abuse, impaired job performance, fears about financial issues, a sense of isolation, and posttraumatic stress disorder.

Caregivers may comprehend that they have to take care of themselves, but making this a reality can feel next to impossible. We were told that many marriages do not survive the serious illness of a child. Apparently, even our marriage was hanging in a life-or-death balance, which was another concern to add to our ever-growing list. While I appreciated the admonishment to take care of my marriage (and still value it to this day), I would like to see caregivers receive specific ideas for keeping their relationships on the right track. Simple suggestions such as taking 15 min each day to talk or simply be alone together, keeping a notebook or journal to share thoughts, sending text messages, or choosing an upbeat song as your inspiration and listening to it together can make a big difference. I would like to see providers consult with therapists to compile lists of small steps to maintain friendships and marriages to distribute to caregivers and then follow up at visits to see if they are taking time away from their duties to care for themselves.

Providers should ask if the caregiver has formed a "caregiving plan" to help cope with the realities and the responsibilities of the situation. The doctor should remind the caregiver that providing care to the patient could go on much longer than anticipated and that additional caregivers may be needed at some point. Caregivers need to find out if any friends or family members are able to help, how any costs will be managed, and if any public or private resources or assistance are available to them.

I would advise caregiver's right from the beginning to think about their "support team" and to choose one or two small things they will do for themselves each day. Professionals can weave this thought process into the initial conversations to stress the importance of caring for the caregiver. A support team can help provide nutritious meals or make trips to the grocery store, they can sit with a loved one while the caregiver walks around the block for 15 min, and they can watch for signs of fatigue and depression that the care provider may not recognize.

It can quickly become difficult to respond to every inquiry or to thank every person who shows kindness. It quickly becomes a time management challenge and yet another source of stress. In time, it just seems easier to have calls go straight to voice mail or to ignore requests for updates. The evolution of Internet updates and patient information web sites is important because friends and family can be updated regularly by one entry, and patients and caregivers can feel good about their ability to communicate and stay connected to others. The above mentioned CarePages, CaringBridge, or LotsaHelpingHands are excellent resources for sharing information with others. In addition, social media such as Facebook and Twitter are excellent means of disseminating and sharing information on a large scale.

Caring for a person experiencing symptoms of pain may lead to feelings of loneliness and isolation. Some friends and visitors will not be able to sustain a relationship in the face of such basic human suffering. It is often just as distressing for visitors to see the toll the disease is taking on the patient as it is for the caregiver. Caregivers may unconsciously begin to isolate themselves from outsiders if they become overwhelmed by the time and energy required to provide constant updates on the patient's condition, if they fear assessment of their skills, or if they feel that others, including their doctors, are making judgments about their decisions.

The Power of Human Touch

It is common for the home environment to develop an institutional feel because it can function like a mini hospital. And just like what happens in a hospital, the caregiver may be in and out of the patient's room dozens of times a day to check on the person, to bring meals, or to administer medications. The caregiver may be so busy with duties that they do not recognize the physical disconnect that is developing between them and the patient.

Studies have shown that the human touch can relieve stress and may even diminish the perception of pain [4].

Touching, hugging, stroking, and even massage therapy send a powerful message to the patient that they are not "damaged" or frightening to others. Humans crave touch – especially as a means of comfort and solace. Studies also show that interacting with and petting animals can lower a patient's blood pressure and relieve stress simply from the beneficial effects of touch [5]. Caregivers should be reminded to utilize massage, acupressure, holding hands, stroking the forehead, or spending time with pets as a means of relieving stress for both themselves and the patient and as a potentially powerful tool to alleviate pain.

Assessing Pain Levels

Evaluating and responding to the patient's pain is a formidable task. In reality, only the patient truly knows what level their pain is at, but caregivers are always on alert and watching for the subtle signals that the patient is uncomfortable. The patient's tone of voice, anxiety level, facial expressions, sighing, and restlessness can all be signs of escalating pain. It is important that caregivers realize that pain is now considered the "fifth vital sign" and that it is just as important to monitor and treat pain symptoms as it is fever or high blood pressure.

If the patient is able, it is always a good idea to involve the individual in assessing the amount of pain. Instead of announcing "I'm going to give you more pain medication," the caregiver can say "I'm noticing that you are frowning and you seem restless. Are you having any pain?" This way, the patient will not receive a dose of pain medication that they may not need, and they will retain a sense of control over their pain management.

When pain medication is being given through a pain pump, caregivers face additional challenges. Caregivers are always instructed not to press the button for the patient, but sometimes by the time a patient wakes up from a narcotic-induced sleep, they are already in significant pain. Should the caregiver press the button? Not press the button? These are the types of real-life dilemmas that caregivers face many times a day and ones that take their toll on their confidence and challenge their sense of morality. Practitioners can help by acknowledging that caregivers may run into ambiguous situations and that they should feel comfortable bringing up these conflicts and asking for help. It will help caregivers to be reminded that each person and each situation is unique and that commonly accepted rules may need to be adjusted.

Caregivers should be informed that when possible, they should include the patient in assessing pain levels and watch for trends or patterns in the signs that precede an episode of pain. The patient will feel less helpless, and the caregiver will become more skilled at recognizing the sometimes subtle indicators of distress. Caregivers need to know that sometimes the rules may need to be changed along the way and that they should never feel that they are doing something wrong or feel the need to be secretive or to hide their pain control decisions from providers.

Administering Pain Medications

Caregivers develop a respect and appreciation for the power of narcotic drugs to relieve pain, but at the same time they have a deep sense of fear and anxiety associated with these powerful medications. When you are administering pain medications, the sense of total responsibility and accountability can be overwhelming. Caregivers routinely fear noxious side effects, oversedation, reduced respirations, and addiction.

What caregivers may fear even more is running low on pain medications (especially on weekends or over holidays), the phenomenon of "breakthrough" pain, and pain control in the middle of the night when they feel particularly alone and vulnerable. Establishing procedures to address these valid concerns will make the task of administering medications much easier for caregivers. Caregivers need to establish a written system or log to monitor pain medication amounts so that they don't run low. Caregivers need to know that breakthrough pain is a common occurrence and that a plan for handling this special pain situation must be in place long before it happens. Caregivers must have an efficient and reliable method to contact a professional during the day, nights, weekends, and holidays if they encounter a problem.

All caregivers should be advised to have a medication log that they use to keep a record of all medications, dosages, times given, and any side effects or other observations. Caregivers need to be instructed to document potentially important observations. Was there breakthrough pain and additional medication needed? Was the patient overly anxious at any time? Were there any new side effects? Is the patient having regular bowel movements and are they being noted? Medication administration records are a vital tool in hospitals, and we need to reinforce this procedure to caregivers. A written record will reduce the stress of trying to rely on memory and worries about overdosage of medication and will facilitate communication with physicians and other providers. Caregivers need to know that administering medications for pain control is an important job and that written notes will make this task easier for them.

Caregivers must be encouraged to keep these logs, and professionals can underscore their importance by asking that they bring them to office visits or have them available during phone consultations. The most efficient system would involve professionals dispensing these forms in their offices or via computer download. Examples of Internet sites that can be of assistance in this effort are www.mymedicineschedule.com and www.PartnersAgainstPain.com. MyMedicineSchedule.com is a free web site that allows patients to "build personalized medication schedules," and the site can even send e-mail reminders to refill prescriptions. PartnersAgainstPain.com offers "pain diary" forms, medication schedules, and pain assessment charts. This type of computer technology is an efficient means of helping caregivers manage medication delivery schedules.

Record keeping is a proven method for reducing errors, monitoring patient progress, and communicating effectively. I would like to see patients and caregivers benefit from these advantages and feel a sense of control and empowerment when managing complex drug regimens at home.

Side Effects and the Fear of Addiction

The side effects of strong pain medications are alarming for caregivers. Nausea, vomiting, loss of appetite, weakness, weight loss, constipation, changes in personality, delirium, night terrors, and oversedation cause caregivers great concern on a daily basis. It can seem like a full-time job to entice a person who has no appetite to eat enough food to keep themselves nourished. Nausea and vomiting are uncomfortable and lead to an almost immediate loss of appetite, weight loss, and weakness. Constipation can be an extremely challenging problem and always carries a risk of infection and bowel obstruction. Bad dreams, a complete change in personality, delirium, and sedation can change the patient into someone who is almost unrecognizable to the caregiver. Caregivers discover quickly how much is at stake and realize how little room there is for error.

The fear of the patient becoming addicted to narcotics is a common and ongoing worry for caregivers. The fact is that many chronic pain patients will become addicted to narcotics at some point in their course of treatment [6]. When I expressed my concerns about my daughter's reliance on narcotics, I was told by our first oncologist "Don't worry about it." Telling a patient or a concerned caregiver not to worry is pointless and ineffective. In hindsight, I would have preferred to hear "Of course dependence is always a concern, but for right now our primary goal is to manage the pain. Addiction, if it happens, can be dealt with later."

This response acknowledges the fear and focuses on the task at hand. Simply telling a caregiver not to worry will only compound the anxiety because the message they will hear is "Your loved one is desperately ill and will likely never come off of narcotics." Even if this is the reality and even if the caregiver is fully aware of the poor prognosis, they will continue to experience stress about addiction. Providers need to educate caregivers about the phenomenon of tolerance and explain that it is normal to experience an increase in the amounts of pain medication over time. When a caregiver is stressed about an increase in dose, they should be reminded of the fact that those experiencing real and ongoing pain will likely need more medication over time [7].

It is important for providers to address side effects, tolerance, and addiction early in the treatment plan and to assure caregivers that they are valid concerns. Ideally, the patient or caregiver express a fear or concern, they are encouraged to voice their questions, the provider answers inquiries both truthfully and with compassion, any fears are acknowledged, and a clear plan is formed to assist the caregiver in dealing with their immediate challenges.

When Pain Escalates

It may be an inevitable part of disease progression to have steadily increasing pain levels. Escalating pain is worrisome to the caregiver, frightening for the patient, and more difficult to manage. Increasing the dose of pain medicine may be medically indicated, but it often causes great angst for both patients and caregivers.

Changing the amount of pain medication mandates a discussion with the physician and patients, and caregivers may have an underlying fear that they are giving the impression that they are giving up or are becoming resigned to the inevitable. Care providers are always concerned that the patient may not be completely honest about escalating pain levels because they don't want to worry the caregiver. Patients may not want to experience more sedation or other side effects.

As patients sense that their prognosis is becoming more guarded, they often want to "be in the moment" and alert enough to interact with loved ones.

Physicians may become frustrated by or question the patient's or the caregiver's resistance to using more medications, but when you take the above fears into account, it becomes easy to understand conflict at this stage. Doctors must be prepared to address these fears and to have the potentially difficult conversations with both patients and caregivers. This is a time for compassionate truth and honesty. I always appreciated our oncologist's candor when he told us that my daughter's escalating pain concerned him and that he was going to order a scan or a blood test to check for disease progression. My fear was acknowledged and out in the open, and I was actively taking steps to address the underlying cause.

A doctor who senses reticence to pain medications can simply confront the issue head on and ask "Does increasing the pain medication make you worry that the illness is progressing?" or "Tell me what worries you about the pain medications we are using." This will address the issue directly and take the pressure off the patient and the caregiver who may be struggling to voice their concerns. Doctors should acknowledge that escalating pain levels cause real fear, that it is a fear that the doctor sees in many patients, and that it could indeed be an indication that the patient has moved into a new phase of their illness. Facing and sharing fears diffuse their ability to run rampant and cause feelings of helplessness. It has been my experience that patients have more fear about the topics their doctors leave unspoken.

Losing Control in the Hospital

Pain management in the hospital setting can be more challenging and anxiety-provoking. The caregiver is no longer at the helm of the ship and may feel a profound loss of control. Patients are rarely as comfortable or relaxed in the hospital as they are at home, and levels of pain medications may need to be increased as an inpatient. Both patients and caregivers will experience disruptions in their daily routine, sleep deprivation, and increased stress levels while hospitalized.

When my daughter was hospitalized, we continued to utilize her regular programmable pain pump, but I no longer had the ability to administer immediate "bolus" injections like I did at home. Kate would have to ask for additional medication, the nurse would have to find a second nurse to confirm the dose, and then the key to unlock the narcotics drawer had to be tracked down in order to retrieve the medication. Often, there would only be one nurse on the floor, especially during meal times. The delivery of much-needed pain medication was delayed by many minutes, which allowed Kate's pain to escalate to a point that the additional dose was not always adequate to completely eliminate her pain. This was a problem we completely avoided at home, but the policies and procedures of a hospital can be a hindrance to efficient and timely pain relief. It seemed surreal to have to watch my child needlessly suffer when we were in a major medical center surrounded by staff and medications.

It was always much more effective to have a pharmacist available to consult at the bedside and to have access to staff members who were trained in pain relief. It is vital for someone to keep a close watch on the dosing schedule and to anticipate the need for additional medications. Providers should take the time to ask the patient and the caregiver what their normal schedule and routine is like and, hopefully, a medication log is being used at home that can be shared with the hospital staff. The caregiver needs to be involved because they are the expert on the patient's daily needs, and the staff should let caregivers know that they need their input and assistance. I would like to see doctors and hospitals routinely acknowledge the efforts and their expertise of caregivers and use this resource for everyone's benefit.

End-of-Life Pain Issues

Once a patient's medical condition progresses to the point that active treatment is not indicated, the need for excellent pain relief is more essential than ever. Caregivers are just as dedicated and focused on providing pain control at the end of life, but it may cause an increased amount of fear and anxiety.

If hospice care is initiated, the caregiver may experience a loss of control and they may feel that they are losing touch with the patient's regular physician. The hospice team members will be making decisions and guiding pain control methods which may make the caregiver feel confused and even abandoned by the doctor. It would be ideal for the patient and the caregiver to know that they can call on the original doctor for support and brief consultations. Caregivers will feel much more comforted by a person that they know, and the physician can reinforce the hospice pain management plan.

Another pressing concern will be the issue of respiratory depression and overdose. The end of life may require greater amounts of pain control medications [8]. The patient's pain may not only be due to the progression of their illness, but from bed sores, weight loss, dehydration, or agitation. Caregivers experience great anxiety about administering a potentially lethal amount of medication. It is a stressful conundrum – you want to see a loved one out of pain, but you don't want to feel responsible for hastening their death.

These moments are the ones that can leave a family in peace or cause regrets and angst for years.

When a physician is informed that one of his or her patients has passed, it would be ideal to send a card or a note to express their condolences about the patient's death and to acknowledge the hard work and dedication of the caregiver.

Conclusion

Pain control issues are only one of the many challenges facing caregivers, but they are often the most difficult. Practitioners play a major role in assisting and supporting caregivers, and they have the power to transform the caregiving experience with information, education, and compassion. Perhaps the most important goal is to acknowledge that caregiving is a difficult job each and every day, but that it is also one of the most rewarding and selfless actions a person can take.

I never heard a doctor or nurse simply state that caring for a terminally ill child was an excruciatingly difficult task, but that it is also a calling to which I had been chosen. It would have made a remarkable difference for Kate's providers to tell me that they had all the confidence in the world in my abilities and that we were doing a wonderful job as a family caring for our daughter and sister. Caregivers need to hear the words.

References

1. Miaskowski C, Kragness L, Dibble S, Wallhagen M. Differences in mood states, health status, and caregiver strain between family caregivers of oncology outpatients with cancer-related pain. J Pain Symptom Manage. 1997;13(3):138–47.
2. Porter LS, Keefe FJ, McBride CM, Pollack K, Fish L, Garst J. Perceptions of patients' self-efficacy for managing pain and lung cancer symptoms: correspondence between patients and family caregivers. Pain. 2002;98:169–78.
3. http://www.thefamilycaregiver.org/connecting_caregivers/the_caregiver_story_project.cfm . Accessed 1 Sep 2009.
4. Carlson K, Eisenstat SA, Ziporyn T. The new Harvard guide to women's health. Cambridge: Belknap Press (Harvard University Press); 2004. 27.
5. Barker SB. Therapeutic aspects of the human-companion animal interaction. Psychiatr Times. 1999;16(2):45.
6. Streltzer J, Johansen L. Prescription drug dependence and evolving beliefs about chronic pain management. Am J Psychiatry. 2006; 163:594–8.
7. Kissin I, Bright CA, Bradley Jr EL. Can Inflammatory pain prevent the development of acute tolerance to alfentanil? Anesth Analg. 2001;92:1296–300.
8. Ward SE, Berry PE, Misiewicz H. Concerns about analgesics among patients and family caregivers in a hospice setting. Res Nurs Health. 1996;19:205–11.

Patient and Caregiver's Perspective

Heidi J. Stokes

Key Points

- Each patient is unique and multidimensional. Chronic pain invades all areas of our lives—physical, emotional, spiritual, and financial.
- Pain is abstract. No words, symbols, or a smiley face chart can begin to explain it.
- Living with chronic pain is a "life"—but not the life anyone dreamed of or desires.
- Patients living with chronic pain have trouble discerning "emergency pain" from chronic pain.
- Doctors excel at providing heroic medicine, but often get bored and frustrated when dealing with patients with chronic pain.
- Americans are led to believe that there is a pill or procedure to fix everything.
- A compassionate, competent, doctor is a rich blessing to patients and to the world.

Introduction

When Dr. Albert Ray asked if I would be willing to write a textbook chapter about pain from a patient's perspective, I said "Yes" without hesitation. While I have no degree in medicine, I have been a lifelong academic in the study of chronic pain.

My scholarship began at the age of 17 when a baffling series of health crises led to a diagnosis of systemic lupus erythematosus in my senior year of high school. It marked the beginning of intense, personal research into my disease and the world of pain it brought along with it. While it was never the field of study I would have voluntarily chosen, it has been a rich education, nonetheless.

Dr. Ray and I met through the *National Pain Foundation.* I had been honored by that organization at their *Triumph Dinner* in San Francisco where I received the 2008 *Triumph Award,* given to an individual living with pain who has made a significant difference in the lives of others. It was a wonderful honor, a Cinderella moment in my life, and I believe such a dinner and award marked a sea change in the way chronic pain is acknowledged and addressed.

First, it indicates a general consensus that chronic pain is real, even though it can't be captured, photographed, or pinned down. And it shows that we are seeing chronic pain as its own category, not treating it as something that tags along with rheumatoid arthritis, lupus, Temporomandibular Joint Dysfunction (TMJ) and Physician Assistant (PA), neurological disorders, and the rest. Chronic pain can stand on its own, regardless of its origins.

The *Triumph Award* says to me that we are not just physical beings, not just systems. That we are complex individuals and attention must be paid not just to our bodies but also our minds, spirit, and emotions. Our illness is not our identity. Its failure to leave the body isn't a failure on the part of the "patient," doctor, or medical community.

The award also recognized that as a person living with chronic pain, you can look at the life you have today and accept it, even embrace it. You can refuse to give in. You can abandon your fear, cherish the moment, and embrace your life. Of course, it is not the life you wanted, but it is life nonetheless. I owe a huge debt of gratitude to the doctors and everyone in the medical community who pulled me through and saved my life.

I love a challenge, and I certainly got one. Sometimes, that challenge is getting up in the morning. But with pain and fatigue, you have to manage. You go to work, you cook dinner for your family, you may run a company (as I do with my husband), you hang onto your integrity, and you do the best you can. And then you do more.

I believe the *Triumph Award* legitimized living with chronic pain.

H.J. Stokes
3504 44th Ave South, Minneapolis, MN, 55406, USA
e-mail: heidi@aaronstokes.com

T.R. Deer et al. (eds.), *Comprehensive Treatment of Chronic Pain by Medical, Interventional, and Integrative Approaches,*
DOI 10.1007/978-1-4614-1560-2_87, © American Academy of Pain Medicine 2013

I'm saying this because the reality of pain is not sharable. There is no Vulcan mind meld. I can tell you my pain, but you can't measure it, and you may not even believe me. You may think I'm there for the drugs. You may think I am a big baby. It happens all the time.

Smiley Faces Pain Chart

We seem stuck in preschool when dealing with pain. In doctor's offices right now, we are still pointing at numbered emoticons—round smiley faces that turn to frowns and then tears—to rate our pain level. You don't know how badly I wanted to have a pain tolerance test—hook my skull up to electrodes and put my hand in a vice—so we could both know what my pain tolerance is and what my pain level means. So I will be believed, perhaps even respected, for what I am battling daily.

My pain began as result of a rampaging immune system that attacked my blood, liver, brain, heart, lungs, and kidneys: systemic lupus erythematosus. A teenager alone in a hospital room far away from family and friends, I asked a doctor how long I had to live. He said if the disease continued to progress—4 years. I believed him. My own godmother lost her daughter at age 14 to lupus. Back in 1977, lupus patients with blood, heart, liver, brain, muscle, and joint involvement didn't live long after their initial diagnosis. Perhaps the fact that it took most patients-years to get an accurate diagnosis contributed to that high mortality. In fact, my doctors had to do an about-face from searching for an infectious agent or parasite, to looking at lupus.

Lupus is like a roller coaster. In the first year, I kept track of the times I was in the hospital—seven. After that, it wasn't quite as important. I've had joint pain and swelling, fever, enlarged spleen, hepatitis, encephalitis, pleurisy, pericarditis, myocarditis, nephritis, and gastritis—a long, long list. At this point, I haven't been in a hospital in years.

A New Source of Pain

But if the crushing fatigue and body aches and pains of lupus were not enough, a rare reaction to the drug Compozine took things to a much higher number on the smiley face chart.

While hospitalized at age 22, this time for gastritis, an injection of Compozine triggered violent spasms in my jaw, face, and mouth. My eyebrows froze in a freakish look of surprise. I couldn't speak, and my tongue became ridged and pointy. Then my jaw started sliding back and forth with such force that it dislocated. I was terrified. When the nurse came into my room, she took one look at me and ran out of the room yelling. Looking at myself in the mirror, I thought, hey, maybe I'm actually *possessed*. Maybe that's what this has been about from the beginning!

The nurse came back with a doctor, not a priest, and gave me a shot of Benadryl. The news spread across the hospital about my reaction, and in moments my room was crowded with nurses, doctors, and orderlies all wanting to take a peek at the spectacle. They had heard of this reaction, but no one had witnessed it firsthand. I felt like I was in the zoo. After the shot, the nurse did tell me what was going on. She said I had a rare drug reaction and I would get better. About 8 h later, the whole ordeal repeated. My jaw started to skate back and forth, and this time I heard snaps and pops. After more Benadryl brought things back to normal, my jaw remained permanently locked shut. I now drank my meals through a straw, and suffered agonizing headaches, before eventually receiving bilateral jaw implants.

The good news was the surgery was successful. After 2 weeks, I could open my mouth, and after about 6 months I could even eat pizza! While I could not move my jaw from side to side, I could finally open and close my mouth. The bad news was that the surgery triggered a severe lupus flare leaving me so ill that for a time, I was dependent on a walker. Things went very well with the implants, until they were recalled by the FDA. They were discovered to be causing severe bone erosion. The FDA ordered the removal of all implants, with no alternatives waiting in the wings. I had the implants for 9 years, and after the first year adjustment period, I was satisfied with them. Then they pulled them out, leaving me with my current bone-on-bone arrangement. I can open my mouth wide enough for a White Castle slider, but not a hotdog. I haven't bitten into an apple in 25 years. The headaches are horrible. On the smiley face chart, the face would be wrinkled and cursing. A visit to the dentist is a torture—let's not even go there.

In those early years of disease and pain, I was a novelty. Lupus wasn't that common, and I was visited, poked, and prodded by many physicians. My case was unique and interesting. Doctors love the heroic aspects of their profession: saving a life, pulling you away from death's grip, and placing you back, once again, into the living.

I found doctors were extremely attentive when the bells and beeps were going off and organs and body systems were compromised. But after the heroics are over, and you are no longer sick enough to be in the hospital (but not well enough to really participate in your own life), you, as a patient, become less important, perhaps even dull. Pretty soon, it's just "hang on and I'll see you in 6 weeks."

Eventually, I realized there is no magic wand, no heroic trek to find the source for healing. Life isn't a television drama where the mysterious disease process that has you by the throat is discovered and pounced on by a genius team of attractive experts with a diagnosis and cure found within the hour, even accounting for commercials. This was a hard lesson to learn as an optimistic Midwestern American who grew up (with television) in the most technologically advanced and wealthy country in the world.

In the first years, I honestly believed the doctors were holding out on me that they did not care that I was living in a deeply compromised and often hopeless state. Or maybe they didn't believe the fact that I was suffering? It was a strange time. Well-meaning people suggested diets, vitamins, coffee enemas, and such. I had a religious person suggest that I must have unrepented sin in my life. This almost-dying thing, this pain, was my fault. I was being punished, and I needed to atone, or confess . . ., something. I remember asking this person why she was wearing glasses. Perhaps, it was only a minor sin. I did, however, play it safe that night and prayed an extra long prayer listing anything and everything I could think of that might have played a role.

But my faith has been a strong lifeline for me. Even though I have a wonderful husband, son, parents, sister, and dear friends, faith has kept me centered. "Faith is something that we hope for and certain of what we do not see." One day I will be well, if not in this world, the next.

But now, back to Earth. Let me tell you a little more about how a person reacts to being ill and in chronic pain.

This Can't Be Happening

I decided at some point in this lingering three-way relationship between me, pain, and my doctor that the problem must be in a failure to fully communicate with my doctor. I believed the problem was a lack of clarity. I would go to my appointment with a detailed list of questions and carefully detailed symptoms. I expected that one day, soon my doctor would comprehend my situation, slap his forehead, and say, "Yes! But of course! You need to take *this* medication! It is all too clear!"

Then would follow the perfect prescription for a pain-free life.

But during the visit, I would realize this wasn't going to happen. I would feel the golf ball-sized lump in my throat, and I would blink very carefully so the tears wouldn't flow down my cheeks. If the doctor was male, as he often was, I also needed to be very careful not to make him think I was some sort of out-of-control emotional woman, a lingering stereotype.

I would leave the doctor's office devastated—without hope.

How can I live this way? How am I going to get back into my life and complete my plans? How on Earth can anyone live like this? But I did, and years continued to pass. Holding out for hope of a cure or relief was difficult. The very doctor that changed my life pulled me out of the woods and kept me out of the hospital—ultimately became unhelpful. At one time, I wanted to kiss his feet; now I wanted to kick him in the shin. I was too upset and too controlled to have a heart to heart with him. I hoped and believed he would help me—that he would understand—and the blood tests would reveal something new. Perhaps, I would be placed on some sort of new treatment.

Of course that didn't happen. I waited, and waited, and I felt myself putting my life on hold. My real identity had nothing to do with illness or pain. I was an extrovert, an athlete, a musician (percussionist), an artist, a friend, a daughter, and a sister. I was Annie Oakley in my high school production of *Annie Get Your Gun.* "Anything you can do, I can do better!"

Lupus made my life, that "real life," stop. My high school friends didn't know how to relate to me because we no longer had anything in common. They were in school with dances and homecoming, and I was being tutored at home in my pj's, my face a huge moon from prednisone, my hair falling out. Besides a concoction to make the pain and fatigue manageable, I needed a book, a manual, some sort of leg up on this situation.

Pain and illness are such great disappointments, both to you and those around you. You want so much to go back to that lovely "old you." That healthy 16-year-old with her whole life ahead of her. Her future? Limitless. You are waiting, waiting for it as the years go by, and then you realize, this is it. I must give her up. I must redefine my life. I must even redefine joy.

Sometimes, I just sit in my office with an ice pack on my head and a heating pad on my neck, and everyone knows I do. I just make sure I take the ice pack off before I see clients. And I have to be aware that pain is often conveyed in my voice and is interpreted as irritation. I must make a special effort in maintaining my voice and carriage. I can be abrupt without knowing it. I become annoyed with people who can't immediately get to the point.

If I can't control my pain or manage it, everything, and I mean everything, becomes compromised. I'm more prone to mistakes. Concentration can be difficult. When you wake up in the morning really achy and sore, you don't feel you can just pop out of bed and start moving. It feels like it's going to kill you. You may panic knowing you have a full day ahead and you can hardly crawl out of bed. You can always think of tomorrow, like the song in *Annie.* It will be better tomorrow.

So, I wake up every day to some level of chronic pain and fatigue. It is part of my life, and I know now there is no perfect prescription. The doctors have only so many weapons at their disposal. You break a bone, you get a cast. You come down with strep throat, you get penicillin. But chronic pain and fatigue are still murky and not particularly intellectually stimulating for either the doctor or patient.

Yes, there are a host of drugs out there, but none of them can totally erase discomfort and all have their side effects. Opiates work to ease pain and bring sleep and can give you a few hours of reprieve, but they begin to lose their effectiveness, and doctors are increasingly fearful of prescribing them.

Today, I treat pain with a combination of ice packs, heat, breathing, stretching, and water exercise with deep muscle Botox injections—which are godsend—muscle relaxants and drugs used to treat diabetic neuropathy. I have a fairly wide range of other medications to manage lupus. It is a long and boring list.

Different Types of Pain

But there is still a lesson that I have had trouble absorbing during this education, one that began after I had been living with pain for years. Just when I thought I was managing my illness very well—that I really knew what I was doing—I found I had more learning to do.

It was because I had become so used to pain that I found myself in serious trouble. The lesson involved the difference between acute pain, get to the doctor pain, and chronic pain. As an example, one day at work, I felt something wet trickling down my neck, it was blood. After a hasty urgent care visit, it was determined I had ruptured my eardrum. I was referred to an ear, nose, and throat specialist who read me the riot act.

"Didn't it hurt?"

"Yes, it hurt like heck."

"Why didn't you come in? You could have damaged hearing in that ear!"

"I just thought it was jaw pain."

He sent me to a new age counselor who talked about how we need to be in touch with our bodies. Whatever, I supposed I did learn a few tips.

It was a little more serious when I was giving birth to my son. Labor had been going on for hours, and I had entered a new pain level. Agony.

"I've never been in this kind of pain in my life," I told the nurse flatly.

"Yes," she said.

Only when the fetal monitor showed my son's heart stuttering and stopping did I get an immediate C-section. Things were not going well in the natural birth department.

"Why didn't you say anything?!" the nurse asked me the following day.

I said, "I did! I told you I had never had that kind of pain before".

She said, "Yes, you told me. However, you were articulate, and should have been screaming!"

"Not being a baby" could have cost me my baby. Even today, I don't regard myself as an expert on distinguishing acute pain from chronic pain. This is one of my husband's greatest fears. He is sure that one day I will have a heart attack or stroke and I will not know it is an emergency. I will think it is just a new addition to the same old, same old world of chronic pain. I agree it is a concern.

My Prescription for Doctors

During the years that it took me to become an award-winning "scholar" of pain, I have had the opportunity to observe many, many doctors. Today, I am able to distill those countless hours and conversations to help you know how your patients see you and what they need from you. Here it goes.

Even before you enter the exam room, stop, read the chart, and collect your thoughts. When you step in, take the time to make eye contact and maybe smile (it's zero on Wong-Baker chart if you need a reference). I honestly find that a simple smile has a major effect on reducing anxiety.

The appointment is only 15 min in your back-to-back schedule, but it holds an entirely different level of importance for us. We have been waiting weeks for these few minutes. We have taken time off work, battled traffic, searched for a parking place, and waited, reading old magazines, in your waiting room. Then we sit in a little exam room all by ourselves, maybe in a less than flattering robe, waiting for your entrance and eventual verdict.

We have come prepared, maybe we've even rehearsed what we would like to say to you, but when you come in and smile, actually see us and acknowledge the situation, angst can dissolve, and a real connection can take place.

Like it or not you've become a major figure in our lives, and our contact with you sometimes feels like our lifeline—it all comes down to those few minutes. There we are, something is wrong with us, and we feel miserably vulnerable. It's awful!

When I talk to you, for goodness' sakes look at me. I know you are rushed and the pressure is extreme, but we need you to be attentive. I want to know that you comprehend my situation and recognize the compromised life I have to live. I don't want sympathy, but a little compassion can go a long way. Be honest and open, and don't be afraid to say, "I am not sure," or "I don't know." Do say, "I am willing to do my best to help you out."

Discuss possible treatments; let us know that there are other approaches or options, even if it is something we might not like. Sometimes simple things are lifesavers. For years, I didn't know ice took down inflammation. I just thought it numbed the pain, and I don't like to be cold. Once, when I was getting a cortisone shot in my shoulder, the PA told me what movements to avoid and what movements would be easy and helpful. It was a surprise, like the ice, and so simple. I wish I had known years before.

There are a lot of resources out there online and a lot of goofy ranters. If you know of a book, a web site, or a support group that you respect, please write it down for us. And if we are taking too much of your time that day, see if you can arrange a follow-up visit or let the nurse know that we need to schedule a longer visit next time.

In my years of study, I have seen arrogant doctors that have no business working with patients. I have also seen doctors who began the healing process as soon as they came through the door, simply through their very presence.

You are in a healing profession. You are giving service. Remember the oath you took to do no harm. Poor interactions can seriously jeopardize the therapeutic relationship that we need to get better, or even just stay the course.

If you are the go-to doctor for my disease, but you don't listen to me or extend any hope, you are going to be giving me only half of what I need. If you can't make headway with a patient, please suggest another doctor for a second opinion. I understand there are difficult, irate, and demanding patients. But you have the home court advantage when they are sitting in your office, possibly in a flimsy hospital gown, wondering if their backside is showing.

Believe me, these people are feeling helpless and isolated. They probably don't know the terminology. They are in your world, not theirs, and everything is new. It's not just the patient that needs you; our families, employers, and friends all depend on you to help patch us together, so we can participate in life and community again. A good, kind, competent doctor is one of the richest, deepest, life-changing blessings a patient can have. Wow, what a gift you can be to this world.

Take a Vacation?

And last, here is something you might not think about. Your patient is likely under financial stress. It costs a fortune to have a chronic illness. Relaxing vacations? Not likely. Help with the housework? I wish. Weekly massage? Forget it.

I don't even want to see a parking meter or a pay ramp when I come to see you.

As for taking time off work, that's the source of our health insurance. No work, no insurance. We may have taken off a day without pay to see you or used another vacation day for our illness. The inconvenience is extraordinary.

Note that the burdens of chronic pain are also financial. Your patients have mortgage payments, car payments, and staggering medical bills. They live with the same stresses you and others have, but must perform under constant duress, and often with frightening uncertainty about their futures. For instance, I have to run a business AND be a wife and mother. That's at least two full-time jobs while living with chronic pain.

I hope this story, from a nonacademic is helpful in your work with patients. If revealing my life with pain helps a new generation of doctors empathize and better treat tomorrow's patients, then my struggle is worth something.

It's been 33 years since those first terrifying and lonely days of early diagnosis—I'm still here! I have learned, and grown, and taken responsibility for my new life. I have found excellent doctors, and we have developed ways to understand and productively work with each other. We are even starting to adequately rate pain by not only viewing its level, but also measuring how it affects our day-to-day life.

It has been quite an education, and I am honored to be able to pass along what I have learned.

I will always be grateful to those doctors who have stuck by me through thick and thin and problem-solved my various needs with diligence, care, expertise, and sometimes even a sense of humor. You are a gift to my family and me: Dr. James Reinersten, Dr. Eric Schned, Dr. John Schousboe, Dr. James Swift, and Dr. Tom Hainlen.

Pain Medicine in Older Adults: How Should It Differ?

88

Debra K. Weiner, Jordan F. Karp, Cheryl D. Bernstein, and Natalia E. Morone

Key Points

- Degenerative skeletal disease is a normal part of aging; imaging should not be used to guide care in the majority of older adults with chronic pain.
- Pain is common, but it is not a normal part of aging; the majority of older adults are motivated to get better, and their pain and associated disability should be treated as aggressively as in younger patients.
- The older adult with chronic pain should not be treated as a chronologically older version of a younger patient with chronic pain; they should be treated as an older adult first and a patient with pain second.
- Successful pain management for the older adult requires differentiating the patient's weak link(s) from their treatment target(s).
- Non-pharmacological pain management strategies should be prioritized for older adults in an effort to limit medication-associated toxicities that are more common and dangerous than those experienced by younger patients.
- All older adults should undergo formal screening of their cognitive function; the older adult with dementia requires an approach to pain evaluation and management that is distinct from that used for cognitively intact patients.
- Primum non nocere: Opioid analgesics and pain itself can both cause harm (e.g., falls, cognitive dysfunction); the potential risks associated with treatment must be weighed against the risks of no treatment.

D.K. Weiner, M.D. (✉)
Geriatric Research, Education and Clinical Center, VA Pittsburgh Healthcare System, Pittsburgh PA, USA

University of Pittsburgh School of Medicine, 3471 Fifth Ave., Suite 500, Pittsburgh, PA 15213, USA

Department of Medicine, Psychiatry and Anesthesiology, University of Pittsburgh School of Medicine, 3471 Fifth Ave., Suite 500, Pittsburgh, PA 15213, USA
e-mail: dweiner@pitt.edu

J.F. Karp, M.D.
University of Pittsburgh School of Medicine, Pittsburgh, PA USA

Department of Psychiatry, University of Pittsburgh Medical Center, 3811 O'Hara Street, Pittsburgh, PA 15213, USA
e-mail: karpjf@upmc.edu

C.D. Bernstein, M.D.
Department of Anesthesiology, University of Pittsburgh School of Medicine, Pittsburgh, PA 15213, USA

5750 Centre Avenue, Suite 400, Pittsburgh, PA 15206, USA
e-mail: berncd@upmc.edu

N.E. Morone, M.D., M.S.
Department of Medicine, University of Pittsburgh School of Medicine, 230 McKee Place, Suite 600, Pittsburgh, PA 15213, USA

Geriatric Research Education and Clinical Center, VA Pittsburgh Healthcare System, Pittsburgh, PA, USA
e-mail: moronene@upmc.edu

Introduction

Older adults (commonly defined as those ≥ age 65) are not simply a chronologically older version of younger patients. Homeostenosis, that is, progressive restriction of an aging organism's capacity to respond to stress because of diminution of its biological, psychological, and social reserves, underlies the distinction of old from young [1]. As pain is a stressor that commonly accompanies aging, the provision of safe, clinically effective, and cost-effective pain care to older adults requires awareness of these specific aging-related changes [2]. The main goals of this chapter are to (1) educate the pain practitioner in basic principles of aging needed to guide the evaluation and treatment of older adults, (2) provide clinical case examples to illustrate the advantages of treatment that is guided by these principles as compared with traditional pain care and why traditional pain care may actually harm these patients, and

T.R. Deer et al. (eds.), *Comprehensive Treatment of Chronic Pain by Medical, Interventional, and Integrative Approaches,*
DOI 10.1007/978-1-4614-1560-2_88, © American Academy of Pain Medicine 2013

(3) offer specific therapeutic guidelines for the treatment of nociceptive, neuropathic, and widespread pain in older patients.

Background

America is aging at a rapid pace. In 2000, approximately 35 million people (12.4 % of the total population) were ≥ age 65, and in 2050, this number is anticipated to rise to an estimated 86.7 million (20.6 % of the total population) [3]. Those ≥ age 85 represent the most rapidly growing segment of the population. Of all chronic health conditions that limit activity and heighten the risk of disability in older adults (e.g., dementia, diabetes mellitus, cardiovascular disease), painful musculoskeletal disorders such as arthritis and low back pain are the most common [4]. Pain practitioners are, therefore, ideally positioned to impact the lives of older adults in a profound way.

Scientific Foundation

The purpose of this section is to present scientific data that negate commonly held beliefs about older adults that have lead to the undertreatment of pain in this vulnerable population.

Myth #1
Pain is a normal part of aging.

Reality #1
Although degenerative skeletal disease is a normal part of aging, chronic pain is not. Additionally, chronic pain can lead to serious health consequences for older adults.

Discussion: While pain is common in older adults, it is not normal. A key principle of aging is as follows: *Many findings that are abnormal in younger patients are common in older people and may not be responsible for a particular symptom* [5]. Using low back pain (LBP) as an example, data demonstrate clearly that degenerative disease of the lumbar spine is nearly ubiquitous in those age 65 and older [6–8] and that magnetic resonance imaging (MRI) evidence of moderate to severe lumbar spinal stenosis occurs not uncommonly in those who are asymptomatic [9]. Although large epidemiological studies that focus exclusively on older adults are lacking, existing data suggest that fewer than half of these individuals experience LBP and an estimated 14 % experience associated functional decline [10]. Degenerative disease

of the appendicular skeleton also is common. For example, asymptomatic hip osteoarthritis occurs in over half of older women [11].

Further, older adults with chronic noncancer pain may experience numerous adverse consequences such as impaired physical function, depression and anxiety, social isolation, sleep and appetite disturbance, impaired neuropsychological performance, an increased burden of medical comorbidity, and excessive utilization of health care resources [10, 12–23]. Community-dwelling older adults with chronic pain also have significantly worse self-rated health (a powerful predictor of morbidity and mortality) than those without pain [24], suggesting that unrelieved pain may be associated with enhanced mortality.

Myth #2
Older adults do not feel pain as much as younger patients; thus, conditions associated with pain in younger patients may not be associated with pain in older adults. Thus, pain treatment does not need to be aggressive in these individuals.

Reality #2
Laboratory data do not support diminished ability of older adults to perceive pain. Some data point to their diminished ability to regulate (through top-down inhibition) peripheral nociceptive stimuli, and this suggests that practitioners may need to provide even more aggressive analgesia to older adults.

Discussion: Histopathological and biochemical studies indicate decreased density of myelinated and unmyelinated peripheral nerve fibers [25–27], and an increased number of degenerated fibers are associated with aging [28]. Selective age-related impairment of myelinated nociceptive fiber function also has been demonstrated [29, 30].

Additional evidence points to age-associated central changes in significant neurotransmitters. In the dorsal horn of the rat, progressive age-related loss of serotonergic and noradrenergic neurons has been demonstrated [31, 32]. There is a decline in the concentration and turnover of catecholamines, gamma-aminobutyric acid (GABA), and opioid receptors [33–35] in the limbic system and a lower density of serotonin receptors [36]. Aging-associated biochemical changes are also evident in the cerebral cortex in general [37–44] and in the prefrontal cortex in particular [45]. Thus, older adults may have an inadequate quantity of key pain-modulating neurochemicals.

Laboratory studies of pain threshold and tolerance have been performed exclusively on healthy individuals. The application of these data to patients in pain is unknown.

Somatosensory thresholds for non-noxious stimuli in healthy older adults increase with age, while results associated with noxious stimuli have been variable and dependent upon the type of stimulus applied [30]. One of the most carefully designed studies comparing pain threshold and tolerance to pressure, heat, and ischemic stimuli in young and old humans demonstrated no significant age-associated differences in response to heat or pressure and significantly lower tolerance and threshold to ischemic stimuli in old versus young [46].

Age differences in temporal summation (i.e., enhancement of perceived pain intensity when noxious stimuli are delivered repetitively above a critical rate), a correlate of wind up in animals, also have been examined in the laboratory, with findings summarized as follows: (1) Older adults appear to have enhanced temporal summation to heat but not pressure as compared with younger individuals [47]. (2) Older adults have enhanced temporal summation in response to electrical stimulation compared to younger adults [48]. These findings suggest that older adults may have reduced capacity to downregulate their nervous system response to pain after an initial period of sensitization [49].

Myth #3

As with younger chronic pain patients, treatment of psychological dysfunction (e.g., depression, anxiety, poor coping skills) is the most important aspect of chronic pain treatment for older adults.

Reality #3

For the majority of older adults with chronic pain, identifying and treating the numerous physical pain contributors (i.e., the appropriate treatment targets) holds the key to optimizing symptomatic relief. The law of parsimony (Occam's razor) *should not* guide treatment, and the "weakest link" may not be the treatment target.

Discussion: Although older adults with chronic pain tend to have more physical limitations than younger patients, in general, they are more psychologically robust, with better coping skills and mental health, less fear avoidance, and a greater sense of life control [50]. While large population-based studies have not been performed, preliminary data indicate an estimated one in three older adults with chronic nonmalignant pain seen in a tertiary referral center's interdisciplinary pain clinic has a high burden of psychological dysfunction [17]. For these individuals, the practitioner should consider prescribing interdisciplinary pain rehabilitation that includes psychological treatment. Two-thirds of the older adults in this sample did not have high levels of psychologi-

cal dysfunction and would not, therefore, require such treatment.

Our research and clinical experience suggests that for the majority of older adults with chronic pain who do not have significant psychological dysfunction, ascertaining the numerous biological/physical contributors to the patient's pain syndrome and their pain-associated functional limitations holds the key to prescribing effective treatment. More often than not, the older adult with chronic pain has numerous contributors to pain, even when the patient reports pain at a single site. A related key principle of aging is as follows: *Because many homeostatic mechanisms are often compromised concurrently, there are usually multiple abnormalities amenable to treatment and small improvements in each may yield dramatic benefits overall* [5]. We recently published a case series of older adults with postherpetic pain and comorbid myofascial pain [51]. These patients had been treated with numerous neuropathic pain medications that resulted in side effects and/or suboptimal pain relief. Significant symptomatic improvement occurred only after the myofascial component of their pain was treated.

Another example of multiple pathologic contributors to single-site pain is chronic low back pain. We have demonstrated that 82% of older adults with chronic low back pain have multiple potential sources of pain including myofascial pain (95.5 %), sacroiliac joint pain (83.6 %), hip disease (24 %), and fibromyalgia syndrome (19.3 %) [52]. Further, while 25 % of these individuals reported neurogenic claudication, 50 % of them also had other spinal/leg pathology that might have accounted for their low back and leg pain.

These data should be considered in the context of studies that have demonstrated substantial rates of failed back surgery syndrome in those who undergo decompressive laminectomy for the treatment of lumbar spinal stenosis [53, 54]. The effect on low back/leg pain is unknown of addressing associated pathology (e.g., fibromyalgia, hip joint arthritis) instead of or in addition to surgically treating the degenerative lumbar disease. Until the answer to this question is ascertained, the most clinically effective and cost-effective treatment(s) for these patients will remain elusive.

A related key principle of aging is as follows: *Presentation of a new disease depends on the organ system made most vulnerable by previous changes, and because the most vulnerable organ system ("weakest link") often differs from the one newly diseased, presentation is often atypical* [5]. Consider, for example, the hospitalized older adult who develops acute confusion (i.e., delirium). The most common causes of delirium in hospitalized older adults are adverse drug reactions and infections [55]. Rational evaluation and treatment of these patients is guided by a search for potentially offensive medications and/or infections such as a urinary tract infection or pneumonia. Unless there are focal neurological findings, brain imaging is not indicated because while the brain is the "weakest link," it is not the treatment target. Similarly, for older adults with low back pain, the lumbar spine may be the weakest link and successful treatment might lie in identifying and treating conditions outside of the spine itself. An illustrative case is presented later in this chapter (Case 1 below).

Myth #4
Treating pain in older adults will reduce the risk of disability.

Reality #4
While quality of life can be improved by treating pain in older adults, effective strategies to reduce the risk of disability are elusive. Preliminary data indicate that brain-targeted as opposed to body-targeted treatment may represent the "missing link." Additional research in this area is needed.

Discussion: While treating pain is essential for improving quality of life and diminishing its interference with performance of daily activities [23], treating pain as a physical symptom does not appear to reduce the risk of future dependent living status, that is, disability. Large studies examining the efficacy of physical therapy for the treatment of chronic low back pain (CLBP) in older adults have not been performed. Preliminary evidence suggests that lumbar spine-focused physical therapy for these patients does not improve pain or physical function [56, 57]. Those who undergo decompressive laminectomy for lumbar spinal stenosis experience less pain, but not significantly improved function [58].

We have gathered several sets of data that support the potential role of the brain in generating pain-related disability in older adults with CLBP. Specifically, evidence supports the following: (1) Neuropsychological performance mediates the relationship between pain and physical function [13]. We have shown in older adults with CLBP that the modest relationship between pain severity and disability is no longer significant when neuropsychological performance (NP) is statistically controlled (i.e., after NP is removed from the relationship). This implies either that NP mediates the relationship between pain and disability or that NP and disability share common pathways in the brain. (2) Older adults with CLBP, as compared with older adults who are pain-free, have structural brain changes in the middle corpus callosum, middle cingulate white matter, and gray matter of the posterior parietal cortex as well as impaired attention and mental flexibility [59]. (3) Older adults with CLBP that is self-reported as being disabling have more severe changes in brain morphology than older

adults with CLBP that is not disabling, and the duration of chronic pain is associated with the severity of changes in brain morphology [60]. The exact cause of the brain changes and the extent to which these changes are reversible or modifiable is not known. (4) Mindfulness meditation, a treatment directed at altering the brain's perception of/reaction to pain, reduces pain's interference with performing daily activities [61]. Additional research in this area may be at the cutting edge of developing treatments that not only reduce pain but reduce the risk of disability for older adults with CLBP. Given the suboptimal outcomes associated with lumbar spine-focused treatments, such research is critically needed.

Myth #5
Opioids should be used with extreme caution if at all in older adults.

Reality #5
Opioids and pain itself are associated with multiple potential deleterious effects. If opioids are prescribed, the adage "start low and go slow" should guide treatment. Meticulous, ongoing follow-up is the only way to answer, "Do the benefits of opioids outweigh their risks?"

Discussion: As with all medications, risks and benefits must be balanced. Opioids may result in a number of deleterious side effects in older patients. As noted in the introduction to this chapter, as people age, there is progressive restriction in their physiological reserve capacity (i.e., homeostenosis). This can take many forms that include decline in neuropsychological performance [62], sarcopenia and reduced mobility [63, 64], changes in analgesic pharmacokinetics and pharmacodynamics [65], and social isolation. When opioids are used, therefore, the practitioner must be vigilant for side effects for which older adults may be at increased risk such as falls, hip fracture, and delirium. And because older adults have enhanced pharmacodynamic sensitivity to opioids [66, 67], the patient and his caregiver must be educated about these risks, even when low doses are prescribed.

That being said, risks associated with opioids must be balanced with the risks associated with pain itself. As summarized in Table 88.1, many of the deleterious effects associated with opioids are identical to those associated with pain. Older adults with chronic low back pain have more impaired balance [68] and, therefore, a greater risk of falls than those who are pain-free. While delirium is a potential side effect of opioids, it is also a potential side effect of pain,

Table 88.1 Opioids in older adults: balancing risks and benefits

Symptom/side effect	Associated with opioids	Associated with pain	Management/monitoring approach
Depression	X	X	Consider treating depression as first step and observe effect on pain
Anxiety	X	X	Consider treating anxiety as first step and observe effect on pain
Agitation	X	X	Consider referral to psychiatry to determine cause and most appropriate treatment of agitation
Mobility difficulty/falls	X	X	Falls risk should always be screened in the older adult with chronic pain. If balance impairment is evident, an assistive device should be recommended along with referral to physical therapy for instruction in proper use. If opioids are considered, education regarding the risk of falls is essential for all older adults. If opioids are considered for the older adult with baseline mobility impairment, the practitioner must refer to physical therapy in an effort to optimize balance *prior* to prescribing opioids
Delirium	X	X	Patients with dementia have a heightened risk of delirium with opioids and with pain. A cognitive function screen should be considered an essential vital sign for older adults
Constipation	X		Discussion about starting a stimulant laxative at the first sign of constipation should occur at the time that the opioid is prescribed
Urinary retention	X		Especially important to educate the older male with benign prostatic hypertrophy and baseline voiding symptoms about this risk
Respiratory depression	X		More common in high doses
Sleep disturbance	X	X	Although nocturnal pain may prompt prescription of an opioid at bedtime, patients should be educated about their potential deleterious impact on sleep
Diminished appetite	X	X	As with other symptoms, the patient should ascertain the relative risks and benefits
Increased utilization of health care resources	?	X	Our clinical experience suggests that drug-seeking behavior is unusual in older adults in the absence of poorly treated pain

especially for hospitalized older adults or those in nursing homes. A study of 541 older adults who underwent hip fracture repair demonstrated that better pain control on higher doses of intravenous morphine was associated with a lower risk of postoperative delirium [69]. Others have shown that cancer patients who require long-term opioids may experience improved neuropsychological performance as a result of more effective pain management [70, 71].

Myth #6

Treatment of pain in older adults with dementia should be guided by the same basic principles as for those who are cognitively intact.

Reality #6

Older adults with dementia are not simply a cognitively impaired version of those who are cognitively intact. An evidence base to guide treatment of pain in older adults with dementia is lacking; there is no substitute for thoughtful implementation and critical observation of empirical interventions.

Discussion: Just as aging is associated with extreme heterogeneity in the deterioration of biological, psychological, and social reserves as well as physical function, so too is

dementia a heterogeneous process. The most common form of dementia is Alzheimer's disease (AD) and the vast majority of data regarding pain, and dementia applies to this condition.

A number of studies that have been done with pain-free older adults in the laboratory highlight that those with Alzheimer's disease have altered pain processing as compared with cognitively intact individuals. Functional brain imaging suggests that those with AD experience enhanced attention to painful stimuli as compared to those without AD [72]. Others have demonstrated that AD patients self-report pain intensity of acute stimuli (e.g., pressure, venipuncture) similar to that of cognitively intact individuals, but that their facial expressions associated with these stimuli are more exaggerated and nonspecific [73, 74]. Data also suggest that other behavioral manifestations of pain, such as guarding, bracing, and rubbing, also may be nonspecific in those with AD [75], that is, these "pain" behaviors may be an expression of the disordered movement that occurs in association with dementia, even in the absence of pain. Additional research in this area is clearly needed so that pain can be accurately detected in patients who have dementia and others with communication impairment.

Evidence also suggests that older adults with dementia may have blunted treatment expectancy [76]. It has been well-established in the pain literature that treatment expectancy is synergistic with pharmacodynamic analgesic efficacy

[77, 78]. That is, the absence of belief in treatment efficacy negatively impacts treatment outcomes, even in those who are cognitively intact. If, in fact, patients with dementia have reduced treatment expectancy, these individuals may require larger analgesic doses to achieve desirable treatment outcomes. The reader should be aware that controlled studies of this hypothesis have never been undertaken and are needed. Until scientific evidence exists, the practitioner should be aware of the differences in pain processing between older adults with and without dementia and approach treatment prescribing accordingly.

Application to Clinical Practice

The key to optimizing treatment outcomes for older adults with chronic pain is to start with comprehensive assessment. The purpose of this assessment is threefold: (1) to identify all treatment targets, (2) to establish the patient's unique pain signature that should be used to determine the efficacy of treatment, and (3) to identify key comorbidities that could constrain various treatment options. Table 88.2 outlines the essential components of a comprehensive history [79] and physical examination for the older adult with chronic pain that is designed to address each of these three goals.

Below is a series of real cases that actualize how to integrate principles of aging into the practice of pain medicine and illustrate how to comprehensively identify treatment targets, establish the older adult's pain signature (i.e., the way(s) that the patient manifests pain such as reduced appetite, difficulty walking, and confusion) [79], and identify potentially limiting comorbidities.

Case 1

An 82-year-old woman presented with low back pain for many years that had started insidiously and had lead to increasing functional limitations. She reported 7–8/10 sharp/burning daily pain that she experienced bilaterally, below the waist, and was worsened by standing, lifting, walking, and bending. There were no red flags. She had undergone numerous treatments without benefit including acupuncture, chiropractic, traction, physical therapy, aqua therapy, multiple epidural corticosteroid injections, and inpatient pain rehabilitation. She took prn naproxen for pain relief. Musculoskeletal examination revealed mild kyphoscoliosis, tenderness to palpation of both sacroiliac regions, and bilateral piriformis taut bands and trigger points. Neurological examination revealed symmetrical reflexes, 5/5 strength throughout, shortened stride length, and an anxious affect. The initial working diagnoses were (1) sacroiliac joint syndrome, (2) myofascial pain, and (3) anxiety

for which physical therapy, sacroiliac joint injections, and gabapentin were prescribed.

One month later, she had experienced no pain reduction or functional improvement. A more detailed history uncovered the development over the past year of change in her voice (softening), handwriting (smaller), posture (increased forward flexion), and facial expression (less animated). A more detailed physical examination uncovered mild cogwheeling of her right arm. A neurology consultation was obtained to address the possibility of Parkinson's disease. The consultant felt that there were "no full-blown Parkinsonian signs or symptoms," but the presence of her masked facies, diminished blink, minimal asymmetrical cogwheeling, Myerson's sign, and tendency to retropulse prompted a trial of levodopa/carbidopa 25/100 bid.

One month later, the patient reported average 4/10 pain (~50 % reduction from baseline), improved posture, and balance as well as walking capacity and flexibility.

Discussion: The synthesis of this case is presented in Fig. 88.1. The treatment targets for this patient were her Parkinson's disease and her myofascial pain. Her pain signature was comprised primarily of decreased physical function. Her impaired gait was also the primary comorbidity of concern. This placed her at heightened risk of falls. Had opioids been prescribed, the practitioner would have had to be especially vigilant for worsening mobility. Prior to prescribing such medications, the patient would have had to be educated about the risk of falls and hip fracture.

This case highlights the fact that PD is not infrequently associated with pain. Forty to fifty percent of patients with PD have pain that is not explained by other obviously painful disorders [80, 81]. Fifteen percent have pain as their presenting symptom (e.g., unilateral shoulder pain) [82]. Twenty-five percent have pain that precedes motor symptoms [83]. Patients may report muscle cramps or tightness, typically in the neck, paraspinal, or calf muscles; painful dystonias; joint pain; neuropathic pain; or less commonly, generalized pain [84]. Oral and genital pain syndromes that are similar to symptoms occurring in patients with tardive dystonia and akathisia from neuroleptics also have been described in patients with PD [85, 86]. The underlying pathogenesis of pain in PD can be central, peripheral, or mixed. Sensory thresholds to experimentally delivered painful stimuli are reduced in PD [87]. Unlike peripherally generated pain, such as that experienced by our patient, central PD pain that is associated with abnormal nociceptive input processing is not affected by dopamine administration [88].

Perhaps most importantly, this case illustrates that successful treatment of the older adult with low back pain requires identifying the proper treatment targets (Parkinson's disease [PD]) rather than simply treating the weak link (axial spondylosis). Had this patient elected to go forward with spinal surgery, the likely outcome, as compared with the actual

Table 88.2 History and physical examination for the older adult with persistent pain: the essentials

History [79]
Answers to the following questions will help to ascertain the older adult's pain signature and, therefore, key treatment outcomes.
1. How strong is your pain (right now, worst/average over past week)?
2. How many days over the past week have you been unable to do what you would like to do because of your pain?
3. Over the past week, how often has pain interfered with your ability to take care of yourself, for example, with bathing, eating, dressing, and going to the toilet?
4. Over the past week, how often has pain interfered with your ability to take care of your home-related chores such as going grocery shopping, preparing meals, paying bills, and driving?
5. How often do you participate in pleasurable activities such as hobbies, socializing with friends, and travel? Over the past week, how often has pain interfered with these activities?
6. How often do you do some type of exercise? Over the past week, how often has pain interfered with your ability to exercise?
7. Does pain interfere with your ability to think clearly?
8. Does pain interfere with your appetite? Have you lost weight?
9. Does pain interfere with your sleep? How often over the past week?
10. Has pain interfered with your energy, mood, personality, or relationships with other people?
11. Over the past week, how often have you taken pain medications?
12. How would you rate your health at the present time? Excellent, good, fair, poor, or bad?
Past history/review of systems: This portion of the history will identify key medical, psychological, and social comorbidities that may impact treatment response.

Medical comorbidities	Relationship to treatment
Constipation	If present at baseline, a stimulant laxative should be prescribed (e.g., senna) at the same time that an opioid is started
Lower extremity edema	May be exacerbated by a nonsteroidal anti-inflammatory drug
Hypertension	Gabapentin and pregabalin can contribute to lower extremity edema
Congestive heart failure Peptic ulcer disease Renal insufficiency	Renal insufficiency should be kept in mind when dosing various analgesics (see Tables 88.4 and 88.5)
Obesity	Some medications may contribute to weight gain, such as gabapentin, pregabalin, and tricyclic antidepressants
Sleep disturbance	While pain may disrupt sleep, opioids are also associated with disruption in sleep architecture
Difficulty walking/falls	While pain itself can contribute to weakness, difficulty walking, and falls, older adults can have mobility difficulty independent of pain. In these individuals, care must be taken to avoid medications that can themselves contribute to mobility impairment, for example, opioids, pregabalin, gabapentin, and tricyclic antidepressants
Memory loss	As noted in the text, pain itself can cause decrements in multiple domains of neuropsychological performance. With effective pain treatment, memory may improve. Practitioners must be aware, however, that many pain medications may contribute to confusion, for example, opioids, pregabalin, gabapentin, tricyclic antidepressants, and others (see Tables 88.4 and 88.5)
Psychological factors	
Depression Anxiety	Untreated depression and/or anxiety can impair top-down inhibition; thus, the older adult with comorbid depression and/or anxiety must be treated for these disorders as part of pain treatment
Coping skills	Poor coping skills (e.g., tendency to catastrophize) can inhibit the efficacy of pain treatment. While most cognitively intact older adults seem to cope well with chronic pain, the minority who do not should be referred for cognitive behavioral therapy as a part of pain treatment
Self-efficacy Confidence in mobility Fear of movement	Physical therapy reduces fear avoidance beliefs (i.e., fear of moving because of concerns about exacerbating pain) in older adults [57]. Older adults with a history of falls may exhibit fear of falling, may have low confidence in mobility, and may have low self-efficacy (i.e., lack of confidence in their ability to engage in certain behaviors to affect desired outcomes). For these individuals, referral to a pain psychologist and physical therapist should be part of pain treatment
Treatment expectancy	Treatment expectancy must be established at the outset of pain evaluation. Patients who believe that treatment will work will likely improve (i.e., placebo effect). Those who believe that treatment will not work will likely not improve (i.e., nocebo effect)

(continued)

Table 88.2 (continued)

Social factors	
Social/caregiver support	Social isolation can interfere with the older adult's ability to distract themselves from their pain and, therefore, intensify their pain experience. This may be especially problematic for the older adult with dementia.
Financial status	The practitioner should always consider the older adult's financial resources when prescribing treatments.

Physical examination
1. Vital signs
(a) Cognitive function
Mini-Cog [92, 93]: Examiner gives the patient three unrelated words to remember. Then, she/he gives the patient a blank piece of paper and asks them to draw a clock with the hands pointing to a specific time. Then, the patient is asked to recall the three words. Patients who are able to recall all three words have a low likelihood of dementia. Those who recall zero words have a high likelihood of dementia. For those who recall 1–2 words, the examiner should assess the accuracy of the clock-drawing test. If there are gross errors, the patient should be referred for evaluation of possible dementia.
(b) Mobility
(c) Traditional vital signs
2. Functional performance
(a) Balance
Modified postural stress test ([94]; see Fig. 88.4): Examiner stands behind the patient with hands on sides of pelvis and states, "I am going to pull you backwards gently and try to throw you off balance…Do not let me…Are you ready?" Then, the examiner pulls the patient toward himself gently. If the patient is able to resist easily, try pulling a little more forcefully and observe response. The older adult whose balance is easily perturbed has decreased postural control and may be at heightened risk for falls.
(b) Basic functional tasks – chair rise, ability to pick up object from floor, ability to place hands behind neck and waist (movements needed for dressing), and manual dexterity (e.g., ability to button and unbutton clothing, tie shoes)
3. Comprehensive identification of pain comorbidities
(a) Knee/hip arthritis in patients with low back pain
(b) Shoulder disease in those with neck/upper back pain
(c) Myofascial pain in all patients, including those with neuropathic pain [51]
4. Comprehensive routine physical examination

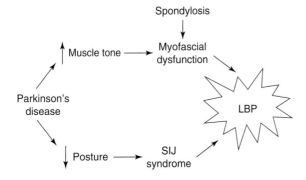

Fig. 88.1 Synthesis of Case 1. For details, see text. *LBP* low back pain, *SIJ* sacroiliac joint

outcome, is depicted in Fig. 88.2. In this figure, the "existing approach" represents common practice and the "proposed approach" is what we recommend.

Case 2

An 82-year-old woman presented with low back pain and right leg pain for two years with documented central canal stenosis on MRI. She had worked full time in a dress shop and was forced to retire 2 years ago because the company was downsizing. She said that her pain started at that time and had gotten progressively more severe. Her pain was made worse by prolonged standing or walking, and she was having increasing difficulty performing heavy housework. Her pain was made better with rest and heat application. She denied fever, chills, weight loss, and change in her bowels or bladder function. She reported poor balance and multiple near falls at home. She lived alone. She was becoming increasingly fearful of leaving her home. Medications at the time of presentation, all of which had been prescribed to treat her pain and pain-associated anxiety, included gabapentin, oxycodone CR, celecoxib, tramadol/acetaminophen, olanzapine, escitalopram, and lorazepam. Physical examination revealed poor balance, dementia (memory problems and very impaired clock-drawing test) [89], kyphoscoliosis, and tenderness of the right sacroiliac joint/lumbar paraspinal musculature/tensor fasciae latae/iliotibial band. Because of extreme guarding behavior, strength testing was invalid.

Because of polypharmacy, high falls risk, and social isolation, the patient was admitted to a nursing home for detoxification. All of her medications were discontinued with the exception of regularly scheduled acetaminophen and prn tramadol. She reported minimal pain and her balance improved markedly. It was recommended that her family strongly consider placing her in an assisted living facility. They chose to seek other opinions from pain practitioners. Immediately following discharge, the patient's pain complaints escalated and multiple other pain regimens were attempted including a morphine pump trial, all of which failed. She was eventually placed in an assisted living facility where she did well.

Discussion: The synthesis of this case is presented in Fig. 88.3. As noted earlier in this chapter, to prescribe effective treatment, the practitioner must differentiate the weak link from the treatment target(s). In this case, chronic pain

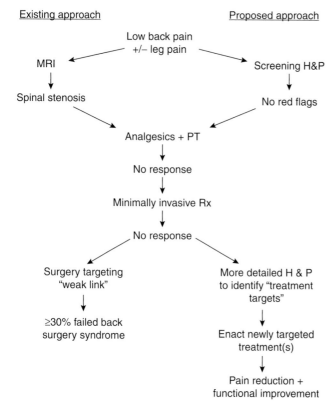

Fig. 88.2 A comparison of two approaches for the management of older adults with low back +/– leg pain. The approach commonly used (existing approach) focuses on imaging to direct treatment. Because the predictive value of abnormal imaging has not been critically examined in older adults and because abnormalities occur commonly, with or without pain, this approach frequently results in failed treatment. The proposed approach relies on a comprehensive history and physical examination to guide treatment that often targets multiple pain contributors. *H&P* history and physical examination, *MRI* magnetic resonance imaging, *PT* physical therapy

was the weak link and fear/social isolation the treatment targets. Her pain signature consisted of pain perseveration and significant utilization of health care resources. The main potentially treatment-limiting comorbidities were her dementia and balance frailty.

One of the first discussions that we have with patients in chronic pain revolves around treatment expectations. Specifically, patients with chronic pain need to understand that it is realistic to expect partial but not complete pain relief. Treatment of the older adult with dementia is complicated by the fact that information provided in treatment counseling sessions may not be remembered and ongoing reinforcement may be necessary. Such reinforcement is often successful when the patient has an involved and supportive caregiver (and one who does not catastrophize about the patient's pain) and health care providers who are willing to communicate a consistent message. In this patient's case, inconsistent messages were delivered (i.e., although it was clear that the patient's fear and social isolation in the setting of dementia were primarily responsible for her suffering, the patient's family insisted that her pain was responsible and more aggressive pain treatment was sought).

While many patients with dementia can report pain reliably [90, 91], the meaning of these reports must be ascertained in order to prescribe effective treatment. Is the patient's pain reporting a manifestation of perseveration (that occurs not uncommonly in patients with dementia)? Or, is the patient's pain reporting a more general signal of distress? Or, is the patient's pain reporting an indication of pain-related suffering? If there is pain-related suffering, then pain-specific treatment must be implemented. In the case of our patient, her pain reporting appeared to be a manifestation of both perseveration and a more general signal of distress (i.e., anxiety surrounding social isolation and dementia). Thus, while treatment did involve analgesics, providing a supportive environment was the primary therapeutic element.

This case highlights the need to screen for dementia at the time of the initial history and physical examination. One of the most efficient and effective screening tools is the Mini-Cog, described in Table 88.2 [92, 93]. It takes no more than 2–3 min to perform. If this testing uncovers the possibility of dementia, the patient should be referred to a geriatrician for further evaluation. Older adults with and without dementia often have mobility difficulty and a risk of falling; thus, a

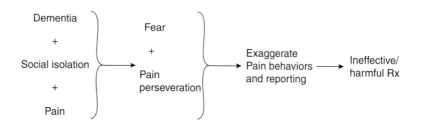

Fig. 88.3 Synthesis of Case 2. For details, see text

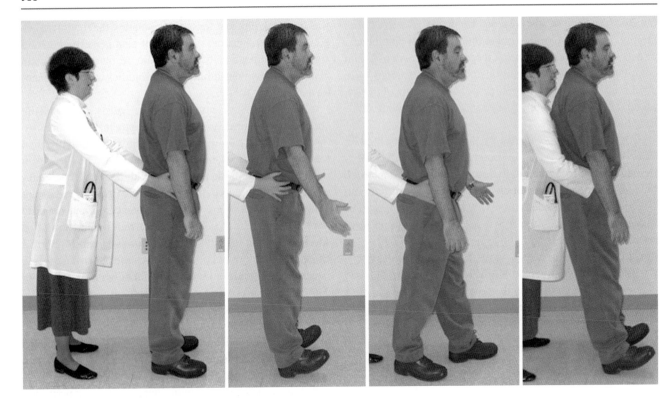

Fig. 88.4 Modified postural stress test. The highest level postural response (i.e., associated with the best balance) is shown on the far left, where there is no obvious movement in response to attempted perturbation. The lowest level "timber response" is shown on the right, where the patient makes no effort to recover upright stance. This response is highly unusual and typically indicates severe supratentorial dysfunction. The middle two photographs depict intermediary responses.

balance screen should also be included as part of the baseline assessment. A modified postural stress test [94] can readily be done in the office and is described in Table 88.2 and shown in Fig. 88.4. If this test reveals poor balance, a referral to physical therapy should precede any intervention that could further impair balance (e.g., opioid prescription).

Case 3

An 85-year-old man with advanced Alzheimer's disease presented, along with his wife of 60 years and their daughter, for treatment recommendations to address "persistent reporting of pain" in his lower back. His primary care provider was concerned because the patient's pain ratings had not changed despite numerous analgesic prescriptions. Most recently, he had been prescribed fentanyl that had been titrated to a dosage of 100 mcg/72 h and resulted in hospitalization because the patient became semicomatose. When the dosage was decreased to 50 mcg/72 h, his mental status returned to baseline and he continued to report pain so a pain clinic consult was requested.

At the time of the evaluation, he was sitting in a wheelchair, appeared very comfortable, smiled throughout most of the interview, and had no pain complaints. His history was unreliable because of advanced dementia. His wife reported that the patient had low back pain for many years. She was asked, "Do you think your husband is suffering from his pain, or is he just talking about it?" Without hesitation, she replied, "Oh…he's just talking about it." Together, we decided that the most appropriate treatment would include tapering him off the fentanyl and have him participate in a local day care program for socialization and distraction. His family was educated about the fact that patients with chronic low back pain cannot be made pain-free and that the main goal of treatment is preservation and/or improvement in function to the extent possible. She understood and fully supported the plan.

Discussion: The synthesis of this case is presented in Fig. 88.5 and reinforces the complexities of pain evaluation and management in older adults with dementia. In this patient, chronic pain was the weak link and pain perseveration the treatment target. Pain perseveration was also the major component of his pain signature. The main potentially treatment-limiting comorbidity was his dementia (i.e., increased risk of falls and/or delirium with opioids). As opposed to the patient in *Case 2* whose pain reporting reflected pain perseveration as a general signal of distress, this patient's pain reporting was a simple representation of pain perseveration that was treated with distraction. Often, this type of perseveration behavior in older adults with

Fig. 88.5 Synthesis of Case 3. For details, see text

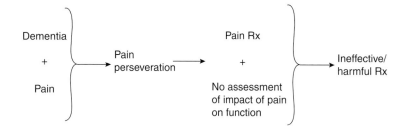

dementia is more a problem for the caregiver (i.e., it is stressful to observe the perceived suffering of a loved one, contributing to caregiver burden) than for the patient, and treatment strategies should keep this in mind.

This case also highlights the importance of patient-centered or patient/caregiver-centered decision making. In busy office practices, it may be difficult to take the extra time required to engage in these discussions. Not doing so, however, may lead to unnecessary morbidity, as was the case with this patient.

Case 4

A 67-year-old man presented with low back and left leg pain for 10 months. He had injured his back nearly 50 years earlier associated with heavy lifting. He was treated conservatively and his pain abated within 1–2 months. Ten months ago, he experienced the insidious onset of sharp/burning pain in his left lower back with occasional radiation to the left leg (lateral aspect) that was getting progressively more severe. He reported occasional weakness and numbness of the left leg and progressively more restricted walking tolerance. At the time of presentation, he ambulated with a walking stick and could go one-half block before he had to stop because of pain. He reported multiple falls because his leg "gave way." His pain was worsened by lying prone and trying to straighten his leg while lying supine. It was made better by lying on his side and assuming a fetal position. He denied fever, chills, or change in his bowels/bladder.

A lumbar MRI performed 2 months following the onset of his pain revealed diffuse lumbar spondylosis and moderate central canal stenosis. Treatment had included (1) physical therapy for lumbar spinal stenosis that resulted in no improvement in his pain or function; (2) tramadol that was ineffective; (3) gabapentin that caused nausea, vomiting, and a 15-lb weight loss; and (4) hydrocodone/acetaminophen that was associated with moderate pain relief. Spinal surgery was recommended, but he declined. His only significant medical comorbidity was hypertension.

Notable on physical examination was blood pressure 178/96, ¾ in. leg length discrepancy, mild scoliosis, mild left piriformis tenderness, and an antalgic gait with favoring of the left leg. His gait was slow but steady when performed

with his walking stick. Examination of the left hip revealed <15° painful internal rotation. Right hip exam was normal. Neurological exam revealed symmetrical lower extremity reflexes and 5/5 strength throughout with the exception of the left hip flexors and left quadriceps that were 4/5. When the patient was lying supine and asked to raise his left leg, he did so by picking it up with his hands. Hip x-rays revealed marked joint space narrowing of the superior and inferior aspects on the left and no abnormalities on the right. Based on these findings, he was instructed to continue regularly scheduled hydrocodone/acetaminophen and he was referred to physical therapy specifically directed toward the left hip. If these strategies are ineffective, he will be referred for intra-articular hip injection. If he is refractory to all noninvasive and minimally invasive treatments, he will be referred for consideration of a total hip replacement.

Discussion: The synthesis of this case is shown in Fig. 88.6. The treatment target was his hip osteoarthritis. His pain signature consisted of severe self-reported pain and difficulty walking. His significant comorbidities included hypertension and difficulty walking/falls. Because his symptoms were initially attributed to the lumbar spine, he underwent an unnecessary lumbar MRI and was prescribed medications that resulted in significant adverse events, physical therapy that was ineffective, and a referral for spinal surgery that would likely not have relieved the "pain generator."

This case is presented to highlight the important contribution of hip osteoarthritis to low back pain. The hip-spine syndrome was first described in 1983 and refers to symptoms that exist in the setting of concurrent degenerative pathology in the hip and spine [95]. Three types of hip-spine syndrome were postulated: (1) *simple,* when history and physical examination clearly indicate whether the hip or the spine is the primary source of pain; (2) *complex,* when both the hip and the spine are responsible for pain; these cases are said to require ancillary investigations such as nerve root infiltration and intra-articular blocks of the hip joint to disentangle the primary source of pain; and (3) *secondary,* when altered hip function (e.g., flexion deformity with advanced OA) directly changes spinal biomechanics that cause low back pain. The contribution of hip OA to CLBP also is supported by more recent data. Specifically, total hip replacement surgery for patients with severe hip pain and advanced OA on x-ray

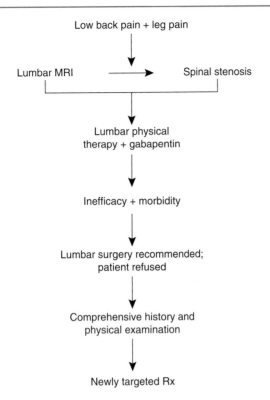

Low back pain + leg pain

↓

Lumbar MRI ⟶ **Spinal stenosis**

↓

Lumbar physical therapy + gabapentin

↓

Inefficacy + morbidity

↓

Lumbar surgery recommended; patient refused

↓

Comprehensive history and physical examination

↓

Newly targeted Rx

Fig. 88.6 Synthesis of Case 4. For details, see text. *MRI* magnetic resonance imaging

reduces low back pain and improves overall spine function [96]. In patients with low back pain, diminished hip range of motion predicts poor outcomes following spinal manipulation [97] and after lumbar percutaneous electrical nerve stimulation (unpublished data). Preliminary data suggest that patients with self-reported hip OA respond less favorably to decompressive laminectomy for the treatment of lumbar spinal stenosis (LSS) than those without hip OA [98].

It is likely that many older adults have hip-spine syndrome that is both complex and secondary in which both the hip and spine are pain generators, but altered hip function causes abnormal spinal biomechanics and low back pain, that is, altered hip function adds insult to injury. Although severe hip flexion deformity may be absent, we hypothesize that underlying lumbar spondylosis makes the lower back vulnerable and, therefore, more modest alterations in hip function may be needed to cause low back pain. So, the lumbar spine is the weak link and the hip is the treatment target. Well-controlled studies are needed to test this hypothesis. Until definitive answers are available, practitioners must approach the older adult with low back and/or leg pain using a broad perspective to avoid unnecessary "diagnostics" and misguided/potentially harmful treatments. Table 88.3 highlights key history and physical examination differences between pain generated by lumbosacral degeneration and that associated with hip OA. It should be noted that hip x-rays alone

cannot be used to make a diagnosis of clinically meaningful hip OA. Fewer than 50 % of patients with radiographic evidence of hip OA report pain [11]. A definitive diagnosis of hip OA should be based on a combination of clinical examination and x-ray findings [99, 100]. Thus, careful examination of the hip should be a routine part of evaluating all older adults who present with low back and/or leg pain.

Treatment Guidelines

The overarching goal of treatment for the older adult with chronic pain is to optimize function and quality of life while minimizing the potential for adverse effects associated with treatment. To accomplish this goal, an integrative stepped-care approach that combines non-pharmacological and pharmacological modalities is recommended. Specific recommendations for treating older adults with nociceptive pain, neuropathic pain, and widespread pain are provided below.

Nociceptive Pain

Figure 88.7 depicts an integrative stepped-care approach for the treatment of nociceptive pain. Topical preparations, cognitive behavioral therapy, interdisciplinary pain treatment, and complementary and alternative modalities (CAM) may be used at any step, either alone or in combination. The individual steps shown in Fig. 88.7 are arranged from treatments associated with relatively low risk (step 1) to those associated with high risk (step 7).

At the foundation of treatment are education, weight loss, exercise, and other physical therapy approaches (including assistive devices). Sometimes, these approaches are alone sufficient to accomplish desired outcomes. For the older adult with fibromyalgia who is capable of participating in aerobic exercise, no further treatment may be needed. For the patient with kyphosis related to vertebral compression fractures and associated lumbar strain, a four-wheeled walker often is very effective for reducing pain and improving mobility. Education should be targeted at ensuring realistic treatment expectations (i.e., pain reduction but not elimination and improved function despite the persistence of pain) and quelling any pain-associated fears (e.g., becoming crippled and/or losing independence because of pain, having cancer associated with pain).

To avoid risks associated with systemic medication, injections should be considered for the older adult with pain in one or two joints, for example, knee osteoarthritis (OA). Trigger point injections can be an effective adjunct for treating myofascial pain syndromes [101]. There is no strong evidence to guide the prescription of spinal injections for older adults with chronic low back pain (CLBP). In general, injection

Table 88.3 Differentiation of lumbosacral from hip-generated low back/leg pain

Feature	Lumbosacral	Hip	Comments
Pain location	Above pelvis; if comorbid spinal stenosis, pain may involve buttocks and/or legs	Most common referral patterns are buttocks, groin, and thigh	If sacroiliac joint syndrome (SIJS) complicates hip disease, SI pain can coexist with buttocks/groin/thigh pain
Leg pain	Present if comorbid spinal stenosis or knee/hip disease	Often	Radiculopathy pain typically extends the entire leg. Although hip pain can be referred to the lower leg and/or foot, most commonly it involves the buttocks, groin, and thigh
Groin pain	Absent	Often	SI pain can be referred to the groin, so if SIJS complicates lumbosacral pathology, groin pain can occur
Movements that aggravate pain	Spinal extension	Leg extension / Hip internal rotation	If comorbid SIJS, side lying and/or flexion may worsen pain
Movements that alleviate pain	Spinal flexion	Hip flexion / Hip external rotation	If spine and hip disease co-occur, response to movement patterns may be atypical
Posture	Spinal flexion	Leans forward, with flexion at the hip	When spine or hip disease is mild, there may be no obvious postural abnormalities
Associated symptoms	Paresthesias, radiculopathic pain, lower extremity weakness	Lower extremity weakness	If spine and hip disease co-occur, symptoms can overlap
X-ray findings	Poor predictive validity for pain	Poor predictive validity for pain	Degenerative disease of the lumbar spine exists in >90 % of older adults without low back pain [8], and spinal stenosis is not uncommon in older adults [9]
			53 % of women with radiographic hip OA report no pain [11]. A definitive diagnosis of hip osteoarthritis should be based on ACR criteria [99]

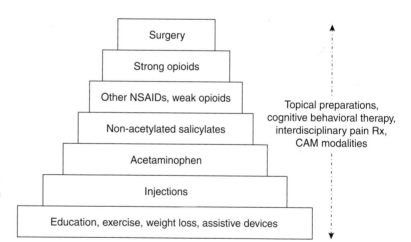

Fig. 88.7 Stepped-care approach for the treatment of nociceptive pain. *CAM* complementary and alternative medicine, *NSAIDs* nonsteroidal anti-inflammatory drugs (Reprinted from: Weiner and Cayea [178], with permission from Debra Weiner and IASP Press)

therapies should be viewed as a tool to enhance compliance with rehabilitation efforts, which represent the mainstay of nociceptive pain treatment. For older adults with diabetes mellitus, patients should be instructed to monitor their blood sugar carefully following corticosteroid injections.

Systemic pharmacologic treatment of mild to moderate nociceptive pain should start with regularly scheduled acetaminophen because of its relatively safe side effect profile and few drug-drug or drug-disease interactions. Acetaminophen exerts its analgesic effect by weak, reversible, nonspecific cyclooxygenase inhibition, and, therefore, prostaglandin synthesis. It has no anti-inflammatory or antiplatelet effect and uncommonly causes gastrointestinal (GI) bleeding or nephrotoxicity [65]. An overdose of 10 g can cause liver failure and death. Hepatic injury can occur with lower doses when the patient drinks alcohol heavily or is taking hepatic enzyme inducing medications (e.g., rifampin, carbamazepine, phenytoin, phenobarbital). Preexisting liver disease, malnourishment, fasting, or dehydration can also increase the risk of liver injury. Table 88.4 provides dosing guidelines, pharmacokinetics, key drug-drug and drug-disease interactions, and important adverse effects associated with acetaminophen and other medications used for nociceptive pain. To avoid breakthrough pain, it is important to dose analgesics around the clock [102].

When acetaminophen does not provide adequate analgesia or when an anti-inflammatory effect is needed, a nonacetylated salicylate such as salicylsalicylic acid should be considered [103]. As with all nonsteroidal anti-inflammatory drugs (NSAIDs), these drugs primarily promote analgesia via reversible inhibition of cyclooxygenase-2 that in turn blocks prostaglandin-associated sensitization of peripheral nociceptors [104]. Nonacetylated salicylates have a superior safety profile compared with other NSAIDs. They rarely cause GI bleeding. This is of particular clinical importance as adults over the age of 60 have a 3–4 % risk of bleeding while taking NSAIDs as compared to 1 % of the general population [65]. The nonacetylated salicylates also do not interfere with platelet function. Since many older adults are taking a daily aspirin for underlying diabetes or coronary artery disease, this latter benefit is also clinically relevant. These drugs can be combined with opioids if needed.

If a nonacetylated salicylate fails to relieve pain adequately, traditional NSAIDs or weak opioids can be considered. Because of the serious adverse events associated with NSAIDs, we advise that they be used only for brief periods in the setting of inflammatory disorders (e.g., a 7-day course of ibuprofen for an acute flare of gout or pseudogout). NSAIDs cause gastrointestinal bleeding, ulceration, and perforation. Additionally, because of renal prostaglandin inhibition with associated renal artery vasodilatation, NSAIDs promote fluid retention and may worsen or precipitate congestive heart failure, hypertension, and renal injury; cognitive dysfunction also may occur [65]. Although an NSAID can be combined with misoprostol or a proton-pump inhibitor to reduce the risk of gastrointestinal bleeding, we avoid the chronic use of NSAIDs in older adults whenever possible.

Recommended weak opioids include codeine and hydrocodone. The latter is more potent than codeine (10 mg of hydrocodone is equivalent to 60–80 mg of codeine). Like all opioids, they work by binding to mu receptors in the central nervous system. Their half-life is prolonged in patients with chronic kidney disease. Generally, older adults have an increased pharmacodynamic sensitivity to opioids [66, 105] and are more likely to experience the adverse effects of constipation, sedation, nausea, urinary retention, and cognitive impairment [106]. They are also more at risk for falling, especially if they have preexisting mobility impairment

[107]. Because constipation with chronic opioid use is very common, practitioners should anticipate this and advise use of a stimulant laxative such as senna to patients at the first sign of constipation (e.g., 2–3 days without a bowel movement).

While opioids may be required at night, sleep quality may be affected by their nighttime use. Opioids both suppress rapid eye movement (REM) sleep and reduce total time spent in stage 4 (e.g., slow wave or "deep") sleep [108–110]. If sedation or daytime fatigue develops, initiation of methylphenidate (usually at starting doses of 2.5 mg daily or twice daily) can be considered, although large, well-controlled trials are lacking. The novel wake-promoting agents – modafinil and armodafinil – are treatment options for fatigue associated with chronic pain and the sedation commonly encountered with opioid pharmacotherapy. These agents may have safer side effect profiles than central nervous system stimulants, but care must be taken when prescribing for older adults because of potential cardiovascular and elimination concerns. Our recommendations, based on clinical experience, are to initiate treatment with half the recommended starting dose (50 mg/day for modafinil; 25–50 mg/day for armodafinil). Close attention should be paid to increases in blood pressure and heart rate with all of these agents.

Opioids also can cause hypogonadism because they bind to hypothalamic receptors and limit the production of gonadotropin-releasing hormones [111–117]. Estrogen and testosterone production is secondarily reduced resulting in hypogonadism [118–124]. While opioid-induced hypogonadism occurs in both sexes, it is more commonly recognized in men. The symptoms of hypogonadism in older adults include impotence in men and diminished libido in both men and women. Symptomatic improvement is seen after hormone supplementation [125]. Rat studies indicate that low testosterone is associated with increased pain sensitivity [126]. Preliminary evidence also suggests that hypogonadism may limit the antinociceptive properties of opioids [127]. At this time, there are no human studies demonstrating the effect of hypogonadism on pain sensitivity.

Tramadol is a weak mu opioid receptor agonist and blocks the reuptake of norepinephrine and serotonin. It has a similar side effect profile as the typical opioids. Tramadol should be used cautiously or not at all in patients taking other serotonergic medications because of its potential to contribute to serotonin syndrome. Typically used in neuropathic pain, this drug is described in more detail below.

If weak opioids are ineffective, a strong opioid should be considered. Among older adults, oxycodone, the combination of oxycodone/acetaminophen, and morphine are all used commonly. Long-acting preparations of oxycodone and morphine are appropriate in equianalgesic doses for long-term use. Alternative agents such as hydromorphone and

Table 88.4 Oral analgesics for nociceptive pain

Medication class	Medication	Recommended dosing	Pharmacokinetics	Key drug–drug interactions	Key drug–disease interactions	Important adverse effects
Other analgesic	Acetaminophen	325–1,000 mg q 4–6 h Maximum daily dose 4,000 mg	Metabolized via glucuronidation Clearance may be reduced in frail older adults	Hepatic injury can occur with modest doses when concomitant use of hepatic enzyme inducing medications (e.g., rifampin, carbamazepine, phenytoin, phenobarbital).	None	Hepatic necrosis with acute 10 g ingestion or chronic use of >4 g/day. Increased toxicity from chronic use occurs with heavy alcohol use, malnourishment, pre-exiting liver disease – decrease maximum daily dose to 2 g Nephrotoxicity (dose dependent)
Non-acetylated salicylates	Salsalate	500–750 mg bid Maximum dose 3,000 mg/day	Metabolized by hydrolysis to salicylate; also metabolized via glucuronidation	No significant drug–drug interactions	See other NSAIDs below	Does not interfere with platelet function; GI bleeding rare
Other NSAIDs	Ibuprofen Naproxen	400 mg tid-qid 250–500 mg bid	CYP2C9/19 CYP2C9 and CYP1A2; clearance significantly reduced with advanced age	Concomitant use of NSAIDs with diuretics and antihypertensives may decrease their effectiveness. Use with corticosteroids and/or warfarin increases the risk of peptic ulcer disease. Increases concentration of lithium and methotrexate	Use NSAIDs with caution in patients with chronic renal failure, heart failure, hypertension, and peptic ulcer disease history	Risk of GI bleeding increased in persons ≥60 years. Cognitive impairment possible with higher doses. These NSAIDs should be reserved for short-term use in the older adult.
Cyclooxygenase (COX-2) inhibitor	Celecoxib	100 mg bid	CYP2C9/19	Same as NSAIDs above	Same as NSAIDs above	Because of relatively long half-life, naproxen should not be first choice for older adults. COX-2 inhibitor has less GI toxicity, but similar renal toxicity to other NSAIDS. Given long half-life and perhaps greater cardiac toxicity make it not a preferred agent for older adults.
Weak opioids	Codeine Hydrocodone	15–30 mg q 4–6 h 5–10 mg q 4–6 h (alone or in combination with acetaminophen)	Prodrug metabolized by CYP2D6 CYP2D6;not studied in older adults	Few clinically significant drug-drug interactions. Quinidine can inhibit the analgesic effect of codeine.	For all opioids, increased risk of falls in patients with dysmobility. May worsen or precipitate urinary retention when BPH present. Increased risk of delirium in those with dementia. Codeine has active renal metabolites that can accumulate with advancing age and renal insufficiency.	Because of increased sensitivity to opioids older adults at greater risk for sedation, nausea, vomiting, constipation, urinary retention, respiratory depression, and cognitive impairment.

(continued)

Table 88.4 (continued)

		Dosing	Metabolism	Drug interactions	Seizure/renal considerations	Side effects/comments
Opiate receptor agonist/SNRI	Tramadol	Initiate at 25 mg qd. Increase by 25–50 mg daily in divided doses every 3–7 days as tolerated to max dose of 100 mg Four times a day (QID). Renal dosing 100 mg Twice a day (BID).	Prodrug metabolized by CYP2D4, 2B6 and 2D6.	Sedative medications and other opioids. Risk of serotonin syndrome in combination with SSRI and triptans. Seizure risk with MAOI. Rare reports of interaction with warfarin and digoxin. Quinidine can inhibit the analgesic effect.	Seizure disorder (avoid if history of seizures). Adjust dose with renal insufficiency; maximum dose 100 mg bid.	Seizures and orthostatic hypotension. Other side effects similar to traditional opioids including sedation, confusion, respiratory depression.
Strong opioids	Oxycodone (short and long-acting)	Start with 5 mg (short acting) q 4–6 h; after 7 days, determine dose requirements, then convert to long acting.	CYP2D6	As above	As above. Oxycodone and morphine have active renal metabolites that can accumulate with advancing age and renal insufficiency.	As above. Stong opioids to avoid in older adults: pentazocine, meperidine.
	Morphine (short and long-acting)	Start with 2.5 mg q 4 h and titrate by 2.5 mg increments q 7 days. Convert to long acting after dosing requirements determined.	Large first pass effect and high hepatic extraction ratio results in higher serum levels and decreased clearance; glucuronidation to active renally cleared metabolites.			
	Hydromorphone	Start with 2 mg q 4 h. Increase after 7 days if needed.	Glucuronidation; not studied in older adults			Dose of opioid required (for weak, strong, and tramadol) can be reduced by combining with a non-opioid agent such as acetaminophen.
	Fentanyl transdermal	Start with 12 mcg patch q 72 h. If ineffective after 1 week, increase to 25 mcg. 48 h dosing interval may be required.	CYP3A4			Constipation is very common with all opioids, but not universal; a stimulant laxative (e.g., senna) should be prescribed if needed.
	Methadone	Start with 1 mg q 12–24 h (po, buccal, sc). Titrate ≥q 7d.	CYP3A4; not studied in older adults	Phentyoin can increase clearance		Fentanyl patch, methadone and other sustained-release opioids should be avoided in those who are opioid-naïve. EKG should be obtained and monitored in those on methadone, as may be associated with prolonged QT interval.

fentanyl also can be considered. Although methadone has a long and variable half-life, it can be a very effective analgesic [128]. Meperidine and pentazocine should not be prescribed in the older adult because of enhanced toxicity. For the patient who benefits from opioids but has limiting side effects, an intrathecal opioid pump might be considered.

While many complementary and alternative modalities are not covered by third-party payers, the evidence base for their efficacy in older adults is growing. Data indicate that lumbar percutaneous electrical nerve stimulation is effective for the treatment of chronic low back pain (CLBP), although the minimally effective dose of electrical stimulation has not been determined [56, 57]. Preliminary data indicate that mindfulness meditation reduces pain interference with daily activities in older adults with CLBP [61]. Periosteal stimulation has short-term benefits in reducing pain and improving function in older adults with chronic knee pain and advanced osteoarthritis [129]. Tai Chi and hypnosis may help improve osteoarthritis-associated pain and functional limitations [130, 131]. Given the toxicities associated with pharmacological management of chronic pain in older adults, additional research is needed to expand the scope of proven complementary and alternative modalities that have a favorable risk profile [132].

Practitioners should be aware that vitamin D deficiency is not uncommon in older adults and can contribute to pain, wasting, weakness, and gait instability/falls [133, 134]. Over the years, the recommended serum vitamin D level has varied. Recent studies suggest that 25-OH vitamin D levels between 30–32 ng/mL are optimal to prevent fractures and secondary hyperparathyroidism [135–140]. For patients with vitamin D levels below 20 ng/mL, we recommend supplementation with 50,000 IU once weekly for 3 months and then serum levels should be rechecked. If the level is normal, the patient should be placed on 1,000 IU daily for maintenance. If the vitamin D level is between 20 and 30 ng/mL, patients may be supplemented with 1,000 IU daily. Other studies recommend more aggressive vitamin D supplementation with 50,000 IU biweekly for 3 months in patients with levels below 10 ng/mL. Supplementation with 50,000 IU once weekly for 3 months is recommended for those with levels between 10 and 32 ng/mL [135].

Vitamin D supplementation is well tolerated in older adults and may have considerable benefits. Vitamin D and calcium supplementation may reduce hip and non-vertebral fractures and fall risk [141–143]. A recent study of statin-associated myalgia demonstrated symptomatic improvement after vitamin D supplementation in deficient patients [144]. Other studies have demonstrated improvement of nonspecific muscle pain after vitamin D supplementation in deficient patients [145]. In one case series, chronic back pain and failed back surgery syndrome improved after vitamin D supplementation [146], although studies have had conflicting results. Despite contradictory data on the relationship between vitamin D levels and fibromyalgia pain [147], we routinely measure vitamin D levels in these patients and supplement if insufficient levels are found.

Neuropathic Pain

An algorithmic approach to the treatment of neuropathic pain is depicted in Fig. 88.8. Monotherapy with an antidepressant or anticonvulsant is the standard-of-care first-line approach for generalized neuropathic pain. For severe pain, an opioid alone or combined with another drug may be necessary. Topical preparations and peripheral nerve blockade are effective for localized symptoms and may be combined with systemic treatments. Those with intractable symptoms may benefit from interventional treatments such as spinal cord and peripheral nerve stimulation.

Table 88.5 contains guidelines for dosing, pharmacokinetics, key drug-drug and drug-disease interactions, and important adverse effects associated with medications used to treat neuropathic pain. Gabapentin and pregabalin have no significant end-organ toxicities and are safe for long-term use in older adults. When initiating and/or titrating these medications, practitioners must be vigilant for the development of sedation, confusion, and/or gait unsteadiness. Starting with a low dose and titrating, these medications slowly can help to avoid these side effects. Weight gain and peripheral edema also occur not uncommonly.

Secondary tricyclic antidepressants (TCAs) are well studied for the treatment of neuropathic pain and provide effective analgesia at approximately 30–50 % of the antidepressant dose [148]. In general, caution should be exercised when prescribing this class of medications for older adults. Amitriptyline has the greatest anticholinergic potential and is contraindicated in older adults. If the practitioner wishes to prescribe a TCA, desipramine and nortriptyline are preferred agents. TCAs in general are contraindicated in patients with a history of myocardial infarction, QT prolongation, and/or bundle branch block, and a screening EKG should always be obtained prior to initiating them in older adults [149]. They also are contraindicated in patients with untreated narrow-angle glaucoma because of their potential to exacerbate this condition. Other commonly encountered anticholinergic side effects include sedation, confusion, dizziness, xerostomia, constipation, gait unsteadiness/falls, and urinary retention [107, 150]. For older adults with medical comorbidities that themselves contribute to these symptoms (e.g., urinary hesitancy in the older male with prostatism, poor cognitive function in the patient with dementia, gait unsteadiness typically related to multiple factors), an alternative to TCAs should be considered.

The newer serotonin and norepinephrine reuptake inhibitor (SNRI) antidepressants, duloxetine and venlafaxine, and

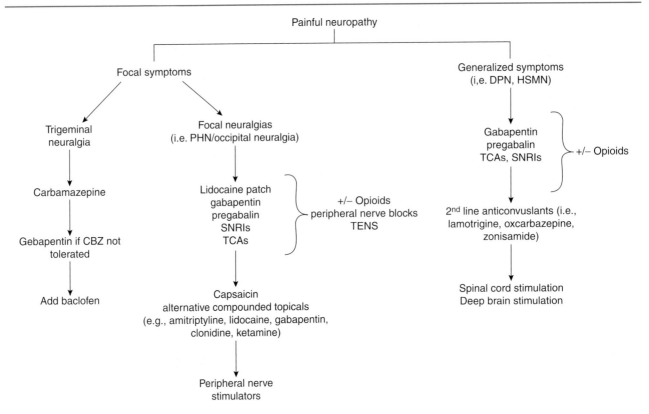

Fig. 88.8 Algorithmic approach for the treatment of painful neuropathy. *CBZ* carbamazepine, *DPN* diabetic peripheral neuropathy, *HSMN* hereditary sensory/motor neuropathy, *PHN* postherpetic neuralgia, *SNRI* serotonin/norepinephrine reuptake inhibitor, *TENS* transcutaneous electrical nerve stimulation, *TCA* tricyclic antidepressant

o-desmethylvenlafaxine are effective for neuropathic pain and have fewer side effects than the TCAs [151, 152]. Duloxetine is Food and Drug Administration (FDA) approved for painful diabetic neuropathy. It is contraindicated for patients with uncontrolled narrow-angle glaucoma and should ordinarily not be prescribed to patients with substantial alcohol use or evidence of chronic liver disease. Nausea (especially during induction or dose escalations) and orthostatic hypotension are not uncommon adverse drug reactions. Venlafaxine, o-desmethylvenlafaxine, and duloxetine, in addition to causing orthostatic hypotension [153], can cause sustained elevations in blood pressure, may lower seizure threshold in patients with a history of seizure, and increase the risk of abnormal bleeding, especially when co-prescribed with NSAIDs, aspirin, or other drugs that affect coagulation.

If monotherapy with a first-line anticonvulsant or antidepressant provides suboptimal analgesia, these medications may be combined. Combining modest doses of gabapentin and morphine is more effective than larger doses of either drug alone [154]. Second-line anticonvulsants, lamotrigine, oxcarbazepine, and zonisamide, are effective for some types of neuropathic pain including painful diabetic polyneuropathy [155, 156].

Opioid analgesics are first-line options for moderate to severe nerve pain [157]. Traditional opioids as well as methadone, a long-acting opioid and N-Methyl-D-aspartic acid (NMDA) antagonist, are effective. Tramadol, a weak mu-receptor agonist with serotonin and norepinephrine reuptake blockade, also is effective for neuropathic pain [158, 159]. Serotonin syndrome may occur when tramadol is combined with other serotonergic medications (e.g., triptans, various antidepressants). Tramadol also lowers the seizure threshold and increases the risk of seizure in patients taking serotonin reuptake inhibitors, tricyclic antidepressants and other tricyclic compounds (e.g., cyclobenzaprine), and other opioids. At therapeutic doses, tramadol has no effect on heart rate, left-ventricular function, or cardiac index, although orthostatic hypotension has been observed.

While tramadol is currently approved for the treatment of moderate to moderately severe chronic pain in adults, a newer compound, tapentadol, is approved for the treatment of moderate to severe acute pain in adults [160]. The analgesic efficacy of tapentadol is thought to occur via mu-receptor agonism and norepinephrine reuptake blockade. The side effect profile of tapentadol is similar to tramadol, but given its recent release, it has not been as extensively used with

Table 88.5 Oral analgesics for neuropathic pain

Medication class	Medication	Recommended dosing	Pharmacokinetics	Key drug-drug interactions	Key drug-disease interactions	Important adverse effects
Anticonvulsants	Gabapentin	Initiate at 100 mg nightly. Increase by 100 mg weekly. Renal dosing: CLcr 30–59 mg/min, titrate to 600 mg bid; CLcr 15–29 mg/min, titrate to 300 mg bid; CLcr <15 mg/min, titrate to 300 mg qd. Supplemental dosing after dialysis	Renal elimination. Nonlinear pharmacokinetics. Plasma concentration increases disproportionately to dose	Other CNS/sedative medications	Dementia, ataxia	Confusion, dizziness, somnolence, peripheral edema, weight gain. Withdrawal syndrome with abrupt discontinuation
	Pregabalin	Initiate at 25–50 mg nightly. Increase by 25–50 mg weekly up to 100 mg BID. Max dose 300 mg Once a day (QD). Renal dosing: CLcr 30–60 mg/min adjust dose to 150–300 mg QD. CLcr 15–30 mg/min adjust dose to 75–150 mg QD. CLcr <15 mg/min adjust dose to 25–50 QD. Supplement dose after dialysis	Renal elimination. Linear pharmacokinetics (plasma concentration is dose proportionate)	Other CNS/sedative medications	Dementia, ataxia	Confusion, dizziness, somnolence, peripheral edema, weight gain
	Carbamazepine	Initiate at 50 mg nightly. Increase by 50 mg every week up to 100 mg BID. Target dose 200–600 mg QD. Max dose 1,200 mg QD. Adjust dose for serum levels (4–12 mg/L). Patients on multiple CNS medications may have toxicity at lower serum levels.	Metabolized by CYP450 3A4; induces CYP450	CYP3A4 inhibitors increase serum CBZ levels. CYP3A4 inducers decrease serum CBZ levels. CBZ induces hepatic activity and can lower concentration of numerous drugs		Slurred speech, gait instability, poor coordination; Syndrome of Inappropriate Antidiuretic Hormone Secretion (SIADH); rare severe reactions: Stevens-Johnson syndrome, aplastic anemia, hepatotoxicity, drug-induced lupus. Monitor LFTs, CBC, and serum sodium after initiation and during treatment.
TCAs	Nortriptyline Desipramine	10 mg at night. Increase by 10 mg weekly. Max dose 50 mg at night	Metabolized by CYP2D6	CYP2D6 inhibitors increase serum levels. CYP2D6 inducers decrease serum levels. Other CNS/sedative medications	Myocardial infarction and bundle branch block; seizures, narrow-angle glaucoma, prostatic hypertrophy; dementia, falls	Arrhythmia, prolongation of QT interval and conduction block. Severe cases may lead to torsades de pointes. EKG prior to use in older adults. Orthostatic hypotension, sedation, confusion, constipation, urinary retention, SIADH

(continued)

Table 88.5 (continued)

Medication class	Medication	Recommended dosing	Pharmacokinetics	Key drug-drug interactions	Key drug-disease interactions	Important adverse effects
Dual reuptake inhibitors (SNRIs)	Venlafaxine	Initiate at 37.5 mg daily. Increase by 37.5 mg weekly up to 150 mg daily. Max dose 225 mg daily	Metabolized by CYP2D6	Contraindicated within 14 days of MAOI use. May precipitate serotonin syndrome when combined with triptans, tramadol, and other antidepressants.	HTN and uncontrolled narrow-angle glaucoma. Precipitation of mania in bipolar disorder	Sedation/falls, insomnia, nausea, xerostomia, and constipation. Abrupt discontinuation may result in withdrawal syndrome.
	Duloxetine	Initiate at 20–30 mg daily. Increase to 60 mg after 1 week. Max dose 60 mg. Not recommended in ESRD or with CLcr<30 mL/min.	Metabolized by CYP1A2 and CYP2D6	CYP2D6 inhibitors; contraindicated within 14 days of MAOI use. May precipitate serotonin syndrome when combined with triptans, tramadol, and other antidepressants.	HTN, uncontrolled narrow-angle glaucoma, and seizure disorder. Precipitation of mania in patients with bipolar disorder	Nausea, dry mouth, sedation/falls, urinary retention, and constipation. Abrupt discontinuation may result in withdrawal syndrome and low risk of hepatotoxicity, but contraindicated with hepatic disease and heavy alcohol
Topical agents	Lidocaine patch 5 %	1–3 patches topically 12 h on 12 h off. Only 3 ± 2 % of lidocaine patch absorbed. 95 % lidocaine remains in patch form	Hepatically metabolized Unknown if lidocaine is metabolized in the skin. Negligible serum metabolite levels after topical application, that is, minimal systemic absorption	Use with caution in patients taking class I antiarrhythmics (tocainamide and mexiletine).	Severe hepatic disease and non-intact skin	Site reactions. Symptoms of lidocaine toxicity are rare and include nausea, nervousness, tinnitus, metallic taste, confusion, and tremor. Toxicity seen with serum lidocaine levels of >5 mcg/mL. Serum levels with lidocaine patch typically 0.13 mcg/mL
	Capsaicin	Apply thin layer to affected area QID	Cutaneous action. Maximum effect noted after 4–6 weeks of use	None known	Irritation on non-intact skin	Skin reactions and burning. Avoid contact with eyes and sensitive skin areas. Respiratory irritation/cough if inhaled
Muscle relaxants	Baclofen	Initiate at 5 mg nightly. Increase by 5 mg every week as tolerated. Max dose 10 mg TID. Dose adjustment with renal insufficiency	Minimal metabolism; 85 % excreted unchanged in liver and feces	CNS depressants	Ataxia, renal disease, dementia, and seizures	Not recommended for older adults. Confusion, nausea, and sedation Abrupt withdrawal syndrome with hallucinations, seizures, muscle rigidity, and high fever. If severe, may lead to rhabdomyolysis, multi-organ system failure, and death
Opioid analgesics	See Table 88.4					

CBC complete blood count, *CBZ* Carbamazepine, *CLcr* creatinine clearance, *CNS* central nervous system, *CYP* Cytochrome P450, *EKG* electrocardiogram, *ESRD* end-stage renal disease, *HTN* hypertension, *LFTs* liver function tests, *MAOI* monoamine oxidase inhibitor, *NSAID* nonsteroidal anti-inflammatory drug older adults. The potential side effects associated with opioids are numerous and described earlier in this chapter.

Focal nerve pain is often amenable to treatment with peripheral nerve blockade, topical treatments, and transcutaneous electrical stimulation. Depending on the older adult's risk profile, these treatments may be chosen as first line for those with localized pain. Peripheral nerve blocks with local anesthetics and steroid are used to treat ilioinguinal, occipital, and postherpetic neuralgia. Complications from these interventions are rare and include bleeding and infection. The lidocaine patch and other compounded topical medications (e.g., gabapentin, clonidine, amitriptyline, ketamine either alone or combined) may be beneficial. Capsaicin relieves painful symptoms but may itself be painful and requires 4–6 weeks of use before taking effect.

As noted earlier in this chapter, treatment of comorbid myofascial pain (MP) in older adults with focal nerve pain may result in dramatic pain reduction, as evidenced by our clinical experience with a number of older adults who presented with refractory postherpetic neuralgia [51]. In these patients, pain reduction related to successful non-pharmacological treatment of MP afforded significant dose reduction or complete discontinuation of opioids.

Neuropathic pain secondary to trigeminal neuralgia (TN) is unique and may respond to treatment with carbamazepine (CBZ). Compared to other anticonvulsants, however, CBZ may be less well tolerated [161]. The risk of serious dermatologic reactions (e.g., Stevens-Johnson syndrome), aplastic anemia and agranulocytosis, and hyponatremia must be weighed prior to initiating treatment with CBZ. Gabapentin, while less effective for TN, is a reasonable alternative for those older adults who do not tolerate CBZ. Baclofen, a muscle relaxant, is effective for TN and may be combined with CBZ or gabapentin [162], but muscle relaxants generally should be avoided in older adults as highlighted in the 2012 [163].

Multidisciplinary pain treatment combining physical therapy, occupational therapy, and psychology may be beneficial for those with refractory symptoms. As for patients with nociceptive pain, those with neuropathic pain who benefit from opioids but have limiting side effects, an intrathecal opioid pump might be considered. Spinal cord or peripheral nerve stimulation is a final resort for those who fail systemic, topical, and other non-pharmacological treatments [164, 165]. Motor cortex stimulation may treat severe neuropathic pain involving the face or as a result of intracerebral pathology (i.e., stroke) [166]. A psychological evaluation is required prior to these invasive procedures.

Widespread Pain

Fibromyalgia (FMS) syndrome, the classical condition defined by widespread musculoskeletal pain from which older adults suffer, affects 7 % of community-dwelling women aged 60–79 [167]. Diagnosis requires a history of pain in at least three of four body quadrants lasting at least 3 months and pain with palpation (using 4 kgf) at 11 or more of 18 specific points on the body [168]. Morning stiffness, fatigue, nonrestorative sleep, neuropsychiatric disturbances (e.g., impaired memory, depression), paresthesias, and irritable bowel and bladder symptoms commonly accompany FMS. Depression and/or anxiety should be screened routinely, given their common co-occurrence in FMS and their potential for interfering with analgesic efficacy and treatment adherence.

The first step in treating the older adult with FMS is education. This is especially relevant for older adults and their caregivers who may be puzzled and frightened by the presence of widespread pain; it may be interpreted as a life-threatening condition. A patient-centered care model should be adopted so that the patient, physician, and caregiver collaborate in developing a personalized treatment plan. After providing education, evidence-based non-pharmacological and pharmacological treatments should be implemented.

To date, there have been no non-pharmacological or pharmacological treatment studies of FMS restricted to older adults. Although pharmacological approaches are an important mode of treatment, there is no evidence to support long-term benefit and they should never be used without proven non-pharmacological approaches such as cognitive behavioral therapy and aerobic exercise [169]. When depression or anxiety is comorbid, an antidepressant should be utilized. Low-dose tricyclic antidepressants such as nortriptyline or desipramine improve both sleep quality and symptoms on the global assessment scale and lead to improvement in tender point score, pain, and fatigue [170]. Because of the anticholinergic and cardiac side effects noted above, it may be difficult to increase the dose of tricyclics to a level with antidepressant efficacy. Fluoxetine alone or in combination with amitriptyline also has beneficial effects [171]. We do not, however, recommend the use of either fluoxetine or amitriptyline in older adults. Fluoxetine has a long half-life, and as noted earlier in this chapter, amitriptyline is more sedating than other tricyclics and has the highest anticholinergic burden. Symptom improvement was not observed in a randomized, double-blind, placebo-controlled study of citalopram [172].

If depression or anxiety is comorbid with FMS and nortriptyline or desipramine is contraindicated, a serotonin norepinephrine reuptake inhibitor such as duloxetine or milnacipran would be suitable. In a 3-month study, compared to placebo, treatment with duloxetine (60 mg twice daily) resulted in more improvement on the Fibromyalgia Impact Questionnaire (FIQ) and a number of other outcomes, independent of its effect on mood [173]. Milnacipran, twice daily, improved pain and other outcome measures in 125 patients with FMS over 12 weeks [174]. Duloxetine is not recommended for patients with end-stage renal disease (ESRD) or severe renal impairment (estimated creatinine clearance <30 mL/min). Milnacipran should not be used in patients with ESRD, and in those with creatinine clearance of 5–29 mL/min, the dose should be reduced by 50 %.

Pregabalin, discussed in the section on neuropathic pain, is one of three FDA-approved medications (duloxetine and milnacipran are the other two) for the treatment of FMS. Because of its anxiolytic properties, if symptoms or anxiety are prominent (and depression is not present), pregabalin may be a good first-line medication. Its molecular precursor, gabapentin, has proven efficacious in the treatment of FMS in mixed age adults [175].

Tramadol, discussed in the section on nociceptive pain, has efficacy in FMS for reducing pain and improving physical function [176]. Tramadol also has been found to be effective in treating the pain of osteoarthritis [177], a disorder that frequently coexists with FMS in older adults.

Cyclobenzaprine has strong efficacy evidence for reducing pain in FMS [169], but because of its strong anticholinergic potential, decreased clearance in older adults, and potential to disrupt cardiac conduction, it should be used cautiously [178].

Future Directions

The field of pain and aging is in its infancy, having originated because of an obvious societal need rather than a distinct body of knowledge. To optimize the treatment of the burgeoning population of older adults, numerous questions must be answered: (1) What drives functional decline in older adults with chronic pain? How should future treatment be targeted to most effectively ameliorate this decline? (2) What is the efficacy and safety of pharmacological and non-pharmacological treatments for older adults? Studies must be designed that include adequate numbers of older adults to provide a meaningful answer to this question. (3) How should our health care resources be funneled to optimize benefits and decrease risks? Until health care policy changes, how can we improve the training of students and health care providers to evaluate and manage pain in older adults in a clinically effective and cost-effective way?

Summary/Conclusions

Older adults with chronic pain should be thought of and cared for as older adults first and as pain patients second. Their management often requires the cooperation of an interdisciplinary team rather than a pain physician in isolation. Until an adequate evidence base exists to direct the treatment of these patients, care should proceed carefully and comprehensively.

References

1. Becker PM, Cohen HJ. The functional approach to the care of the elderly: a conceptual framework. J Am Geriatr Soc. 1984; 32:923.
2. Karp JF, Shega JW, Morone NE, Weiner DK. Advances in understanding the mechanisms and management of persistent pain in older adults. Br J Anaesth. 2008;101(1):111–20.
3. US Bureau of the Census. 1997. Aging in the United States – past, present, and future. http://www.census.gov/ipc/prod/97agewc.pdf. Accessed on 1st Jan 2010.
4. Centers for Disease Control and Prevention. 2008. Health, United States, 2008. http://www.cdc.gov/nchs/data/hus/hus08.pdf. Accessed on 1st Jan 2010.
5. Resnick NM, Marcantonio ER. How should clinical care of the aged differ? Lancet. 1997;350:1157–8.
6. Boden SD, Davis DO, Dina TS, Patronas NJ, Wiesel SW. Abnormal magnetic-resonance scans of the lumbar spine in asymptomatic subjects – a prospective investigation. J Bone Joint Surg Am. 1990;72(3):403–8.
7. Weiner DK, Distell B, Studenski S, Martinez S, Lomasney L, Bongiorni D. Does radiographic osteoarthritis correlate with flexibility of the lumbar spine? J Am Geriatr Soc. 1994;42:257–63.
8. Hicks GE, Morone N, Weiner DK. Degenerative lumbar disc and facet disease in older adults: prevalence and clinical correlates. Spine. 2009;34(12):1301–6.
9. Jarvik JJ, Hollingworth W, Heagerty P, Haynor DR, Deyo RA. The longitudinal assessment of imaging and disability of the back (LAIDBack) study: baseline data. Spine. 2001;26(10):1158–66.
10. Reid MC, Williams CS, Gill TM. Back pain and decline in lower extremity physical function among community-dwelling older persons. J Gerontol Med Sci. 2005;60A(6):793–7.
11. Lane NE, Nevitt MC, Hochberg MC, Hung Y-Y, Palermo L. Progression of radiographic hip osteoarthritis over eight years in a community sample of elderly white women. Arthritis Rheum. 2004;50(5):1477–86.
12. Bosley BN, Weiner DK, Rudy TE, Granieri E. Is chronic nonmalignant pain associated with decreased appetite in older adults? Preliminary evidence. J Am Geriatr Soc. 2004;52:247–51.
13. Weiner DK, Rudy TE, Morrow L, Slaboda J, Lieber SJ. The relationship between pain, neuropsychological performance, and physical function in community-dwelling older adults with chronic low back pain. Pain Med. 2006;7(1):60–70.
14. Karp JF, Reynolds CF, Butters MA, Dew MA, Mazumdar S, Begley AE, et al. The relationship between pain and mental flexibility in older adult pain clinic patients. Pain Med. 2006;7:444–52.
15. Rudy TE, Weiner DK, Lieber SJ, Slaboda J, Boston JR. The impact of chronic low back pain on older adults: a comparative study of patients and controls. Pain. 2007;13:293–301.
16. Carey TS, Evans A, Hadler N, Kalsbeek W, McLaughlin C, Fryer J. Care-seeking among individuals with chronic low back pain. Spine. 1995;20(3):312–7.
17. Weiner DK, Rudy TE, Gaur S. Are all older adults with persistent pain created equal? Preliminary evidence for a multiaxial taxonomy. Pain Res Manag. 2001;6(3):133–41.
18. Williamson GM, Schulz R. Pain, activity restriction, and symptoms of depression among community-residing adults. J Gerontol. 1992;47:367–72.

19. Williams AK, Schulz R. Association of pain and physical dependency with depression in physically ill middle-aged and elderly. Phys Ther. 1988;68(8):1226–30.

20. Casten RJ, Parmelee PA, Kleban MH, Lawton MP, Katz IR. The relationships among anxiety, depression, and pain in a geriatric institutionalized sample. Pain. 1995;61:271–6.

21. Gentili A, Weiner DK, Kuchibhatla M, Edinger JD. Factors that disturb sleep in nursing home residents. Aging Clin Exp Res. 1997;9:207–13.

22. Wilson KG, Watson ST, Currie SR. Daily diary and ambulatory activity monitoring of sleep in patients with insomnia associated with chronic musculoskeletal pain. Pain. 1998;75:75–84.

23. Weiner DK, Haggerty CL, Kritchevsky SB, Harris T, Simonsick EM, Nevitt M, et al. How does low back pain impact physical function in independent, well-functioning older adults? Evidence from the Health ABC cohort and implications for the future. Pain Med. 2003;4(4):311–20.

24. Reyes-Gibby CC, Aday L, Cleeland C. Impact of pain on self-rated health in the community-dwelling older adults. Pain. 2002;95(1–2):75–82.

25. O'Sullivan DJ, Swallow M. The fibre size and content of the radial and sural nerves. J Neurol Neurosurg Psychiatry. 1968;31:464–70.

26. Ochoa J, Mair WG. The normal sural nerve in man. II. Changes in the axons and Schwann cells due to aging. Acta Neuropathol. 1969;13:217–39.

27. Rafalowska J, Drac H, Rosinska K. Histological and electrophysiological changes of the lower motor neuron with aging. Pol Med Sci Hist Bull. 1976;15:271–80.

28. Drac H, Babiuch M, Wisniewska W. Morphological and biochemical changes in peripheral nerves with aging. Neuropatol Pol. 1991;29:49–67.

29. Chakour MC, Gibson SJ, Bradbeer M, Helme RD. The effect of age on A delta- and C-fibre thermal pain perception. Pain. 1996;64:143–52.

30. Gibson SJ, Farrell M. A review of age differences in the neurophysiology of nociception and the perceptual experience of pain. Clin J Pain. 2004;20:227–39.

31. Iwata K, Fukuoka T, Kondo E, et al. Plastic changes in nociceptive transmission of the rat spinal cord with advancing age. J Neurophysiol. 2002;87:1086–93.

32. Ko ML, King MA, Gordon TL, Crisp T. The effects of aging on spinal neurochemistry in the rat. Brain Res Bull. 1997;42:95–8.

33. Amenta F, Zaccheo D, Collier WL. Neurotransmitters, neuroreceptors and aging. Mech Ageing Dev. 1991;61:249–73.

34. Barili P, De Carolis G, Zaccheo D, Amenta F. Sensitivity to ageing of the limbic dopaminergic system: a review. Mech Ageing Dev. 1998;106:57–92.

35. Spokes EG. An analysis of factors influencing measurements of dopamine, noradrenaline, glutamate decarboxylase and choline acetylase in human post-mortem brain tissue. Brain. 1979;102:333–46.

36. Kakiuchi T, Nishiyama S, Sato K, Ohba H, Nakanishi S, Tsukada H. Age-related reduction of [11C]MDL100,907 binding to central 5-HT(2A) receptors: PET study in the conscious monkey brain. Brain Res. 2000;883:135–42.

37. DeKosky ST, Scheff SW, Markesbery WR. Laminar organization of cholinergic circuits in human frontal cortex in Alzheimer's disease and aging. Neurology. 1985;35:1425–31.

38. Grote SS, Moses SG, Robins E, Hudgens RW, Croninger AB. A study of selected catecholamine metabolizing enzymes: a comparison of depressive suicides and alcoholic suicides with controls. J Neurochem. 1974;23:791–802.

39. McGeer E, McGeer P. Neurotransmitter metabolism in the ageing brain. In: Terry R, Gershon S, editors. Neurobiology of aging. New York: Raven; 1976. p. 389–401.

40. Robinson D. Changes in MAO and monoamines with human development. Fed Proc. 1975;34:103–7.

41. Rogers J, Bloom F. Neurotransmitter metabolism and function in the aging nervous system. In: Finch CE, Schneider EL, editors. Handbook of the biology of aging. New York: Van Nostrand Reinhold; 1985. p. 645–62.

42. White P, Hiley CR, Goodhardt MJ, et al. Neocortical cholinergic neurons in elderly people. Lancet. 1977;1:668–71.

43. Wong DF, Wagner HNJ, Dannals RF, et al. Effects of age on dopamine and serotonin receptors measured by positron tomography in the living human brain. Science. 1984;226:1393–6.

44. Marcusson JO, Morgan DG, Winblad B, Finch CE. Serotonin-2 binding sites in human frontal cortex and hippocampus. Selective loss of S-2A sites with age. Brain Res. 1984;311:51–6.

45. Grachev ID, Swarnkar A, Szeverenyi NM, Ramachandran TS, Apkarian AV. Aging alters the multichemical networking profile of the human brain: an in vivo (l)H-MRS study of young versus middle-aged subjects. J Neurochem. 2001;77:292–303.

46. Edwards RR, Fillingim RB. Age-associated differences in responses to noxious stimuli. J Gerontol A Biol Sci Med Sci. 2001;56:M180–5.

47. Lautenbacher S, Kunz M, Strate P, Nielsen J, Arendt-Nielsen L. Age effects on pain thresholds, temporal summation and spatial summation of heat and pressure pain. Pain. 2005;115:410–8.

48. Farrell M, Gibson S. Age interacts with stimulus frequency in the temporal summation of pain. Pain Med. 2007;8:514–20.

49. Gagliese L. What do experimental pain models tell us about aging and clinical pain? Pain Med. 2007;8:475–7.

50. Wittink HM, Rogers WH, Lipman AG, McCarberg BH, Ashburn MA, Oderda GM, et al. Older and younger adults in pain management programs in the United States: differences and similarities. Pain Med. 2006;7(2):151–63.

51. Weiner DK, Schmader KE. Postherpetic pain: more than sensory neuralgia? Pain Med. 2006;7:243–9.

52. Weiner DK, Sakamoto S, Perera S, Breuer P. Chronic low back pain in older adults: prevalence, reliability, and validity of physical examination findings. J Am Geriatr Soc. 2006;54:11–20.

53. Ciol MA, Deyo RA, Howell E, Kreif S. An assessment of surgery for spinal stenosis: time trends, geographic variations, complications, and reoperations. J Am Geriatr Soc. 1996;44:285–90.

54. Cloyd JM, Acosta FLJ, Ames CP. Complications and outcomes of lumbar spine surgery in elderly people: a review of the literature. J Am Geriatr Soc. 2008;56:1318–27.

55. Inouye SK. Delirium in older persons. N Engl J Med. 2006;354(11):1157–65.

56. Weiner DK, Rudy TE, Glick RM, Boston JR, Lieber SJ, Morrow L, et al. Efficacy of percutaneous electrical nerve stimulation (PENS) for the treatment of chronic low back pain in older adults. J Am Geriatr Soc. 2003;51:599–608.

57. Weiner DK, Perera S, Rudy TE, Glick RM, Shenoy S, Delitto A. Efficacy of percutaneous electrical nerve stimulation and therapeutic exercise for older adults with chronic low back pain: a randomized controlled trial. Pain. 2008;140:344–57.

58. Weinstein JN, Tosteson TD, Lurie JD, Tosteson ANA, Blood E, Hanscom B, et al. Surgical versus nonsurgical therapy for lumbar spinal stenosis. N Engl J Med. 2008;358:794–810.

59. Buckalew N, Haut M, Morrow LA, Weiner DK. Chronic pain is associated with brain volume loss in older adults: preliminary evidence. Pain Med. 2008;9(2):240–8.

60. Buckalew N, Haut MW, Morrow L, Perera S, Weiner D. Brain morphology differences in older adults with disabling chronic low back pain. J Am Geriatr Soc. 2009;57(4):S58.

61. Morone NE, Greco CM, Weiner DK. Mindfulness meditation for the treatment of chronic low back pain in older adults: a randomized controlled pilot study. Pain. 2008;134:310–9.

62. Ratcliff G, Dodge H, Birzescu M, Ganguli M. Tracking cognitive function over time: ten-year longitudinal data from a community-based study. Appl Neuropsychol. 2003;10(2):76–88.

63. Rolland Y, Czerwinski S, AbellanvanKan G, Morley JE, Cesari M, Onder G, et al. Sarcopenia: its assessment, etiology, pathogenesis, consequences and future perspectives. J Nutr Health Aging. 2008;12:433–50.

64. Ferrucci L, Guralnik JM, Simonsick E, Salive ME, Corti C, Langlois J. Progressive versus catastrophic disability: a longitudinal view of the disablement process. J Gerontol Ser A Biol Sci Med Sci. 1996;51(3):M123–30.

65. Hanlon JT, Guay DRP, Ives TJ. Oral analgesics: efficacy, mechanism of action, pharmacokinetics, adverse effects, drug interactions and practical recommendations for use in older adults. In: Gibson SJ, Weiner DK, editors. Pain in older persons, progress in pain research and management. Seattle: IASP Press; 2005.

66. Kaiko RF. Age and morphine analgesia in cancer patients with postoperative pain. Clin Pharmacol Ther. 1980;28:823–6.

67. Kaiko RF, Wallenstein SL, Rogers AG, et al. Narcotics in the elderly. Med Clin North Am. 1982;66:1079–89.

68. Hicks GE, Simonsick EM, Harris TB, Newman AB, Weiner DK, Nevitt MA, et al. Cross-sectional associations between trunk muscle composition, back pain and physical function in the Health ABC study. J Gerontol Med Sci. 2005;60A(7):882–7.

69. Morrison RS, Magaziner J, Gilbert M, Koval KJ, McLaughlin MA, Orosz G, et al. Relationship between pain and opioid analgesics on the development of delirium following hip fracture. J Gerontol Med Sci. 2003;58(1):76–81.

70. Tassain V, Attal N, Fletcher D, Brasseur L, Degieux P, Chauvin M, et al. Long term effects of oral sustained release morphine on neuropsychological performance in patients with chronic non-cancer pain. Pain. 2003;104:389–400.

71. Jamison RN, Schein JR, Vallow S, Ascher S, Vorsanger GJ, Katz NP. Neuropsychological effects of long-term opioid use in chronic pain patients. J Pain Symptom Manage. 2003;26(4): 913–21.

72. Cole LJ, Farrell MJ, Duff EP, Barber JB, Egan GF, Gibson SJ. Pain sensitivity and fMRI pain-related brain activity in Alzheimer's disease. Brain. 2006;129:2957–65.

73. Porter FL, Malhotra KM, Wolf CM, Morris JC, Smith MC. Dementia and response to pain in the elderly. Pain. 1996;68:413–21.

74. Kunz M, Scharmann S, Hemmeter U, Schepelmann K, Lautenbacher S. The facial expression of pain in patients with dementia. Pain. 2007;133:221–8.

75. Shega JW, Rudy T, Keefe FJ, Perri LC, Mengin OT, Weiner DK. Validity of pain behaviors in persons with mild to moderate cognitive impairment. J Am Geriatr Soc. 2008;56:1631–7.

76. Benedetti F, Arduino C, Costa S, Vighetti S, Tarenzi L, Rainero I, et al. Loss of expectancy-related mechanisms in Alzheimer's disease makes analgesic therapies less effective. Pain. 2006;121: 133–44.

77. Benedetti F. What do you expect from this treatment? Changing our mind about clinical trials. Pain. 2007;128:193–4.

78. Finiss DG, Benedetti F. Mechanisms of the placebo response and their impact on clinical trials and clinical practice. Pain. 2005;114:3–6.

79. Weiner DK, Herr K. Comprehensive assessment & interdisciplinary treatment planning: an integrative overview. In: Weiner DK, Herr K, Rudy TE, editors. Persistent pain in older adults: an interdisciplinary guide for treatment. New York: Springer Publishing Company; 2002. p. 18–57.

80. Goetz CG, Tanner CM, Levy M, Wilson RS, Garron DC. Pain in Parkinson's disease. Mov Disord. 1986;1(1):45–9.

81. Witjas T, Kaphan E, Azulay JP, Blin O, Ceccaldi M, Pouget J, et al. Nonmotor fluctuations in Parkinson's disease – frequent and disabling. Neurology. 2002;59:408–13.

82. O'Sullivan SS, Williams DR, Gallagher DA, Massey LA, Silveira-Moriyama L, Lees AJ. Nonmotor symptoms as presenting complaints in Parkinson's disease: a clinicopathological study. Mov Disord. 2008;1(1):101–6.

83. Wolters EC. Variability in the clinical expression of Parkinson's disease. J Neurol Sci. 2008;266:197–203.

84. Truong DD, Bhidayasiri R, Wolters E. Management of non-motor symptoms in advanced Parkinson's disease. J Neurol Sci. 2008;266:216–28.

85. Ford B, Greene P, Fahn S. Oral and genital tardive pain syndromes. Neurology. 1994;44:2115–9.

86. Ford B, Louis ED, Greene P, Fahn S. Oral and genital pain syndromes in Parkinson's disease. Mov Disord. 1996;11:421–6.

87. Djaldetti R, Shifrin A, Rogowski Z, Sprecher E, Melamed E, Yarnitsky D. Quantitative measurement of pain sensation in patients with Parkinson disease. Neurology. 2004;62:2171–5.

88. Tinazzi M, Del Vesco C, Defazio G, Fincati E, Smania N, Moretto G, et al. Abnormal processing of the nociceptive input in Parkinson's disease: a study with CO_2 laser evoked potentials. Pain. 2008;136:117–24.

89. Tuokko H, Hadjistavropoulos T, Miller JA, Beattie BL. The clock test: a sensitive measure to differentiate normal elderly from those with Alzheimer disease. J Am Geriatr Soc. 1992;40:579–84.

90. Weiner DK, Peterson B, Logue P, Keefe FJ. Predictors of pain self-report in nursing home residents. Aging Clin Exp Res. 1998;10:411–20.

91. Chibnall J, Tait R. Pain assessment in cognitively impaired and unimpaired older adults: a comparison of four scales. Pain. 2001;92:173–86.

92. Borson S, Scanlan J, Brush M, Vitaliano P, Dokmak A. The Mini-Cog: a cognitive vital signs measure for dementia screening in multi-lingual elderly. Int J Geriatr Psychiatry. 2000;15:1021–7.

93. Scanlan J, Borson S. The Mini-Cog: receiver operating characteristics with expert and naïve raters. Int J Geriatr Psychiatry. 2001;16:216–22.

94. Wolfson LI, Whipple R, Amerman P, Kleinberg A. Stressing the postural response. A quantitative method for testing balance. J Am Geriatr Soc. 1986;34:845–50.

95. Offierski CM, Macnab MB. Hip-spine syndrome. Spine. 1983;8(3):316–21.

96. Ben-Galim P, Ben-Galim T, Rand N, Haim A, Hipp J, Dekel S, et al. Hip-Spine syndrome: the effect of total hip replacement surgery on low back pain in severe osteoarthritis of the hip. Spine. 2007;32(19):2099–102.

97. Fritz JM, Whitman JM, Flynn TW, Wainner RS, Childs JD. Factors related to the inability of individuals with low back pain to improve with a spinal manipulation. Phys Ther. 2004;84(2):173–90.

98. Airaksinen O, Herno A, Turunen V, Saari T, Suomlainen O. Surgical outcome of 438 patient treated surgically for lumbar spinal stenosis. Spine. 1997;22(19):2278–82.

99. Altman R, Alarcon G, Appelrouth D, et al. The American College of Rheumatology criteria for the classification and reporting of osteoarthritis of the hip. Arthritis Rheum. 1991;34(5):505–14.

100. Lane NE. Osteoarthritis of the hip. N Engl J Med. 2007;357: 1413–21.

101. Borg-Stein J. Treatment of fibromyalgia, myofascial pain, and related disorders. Phys Med Rehabil Clin N Am. 2006;17:491–510.

102. Weiner DK. Office management of chronic pain in the elderly. Am J Med. 2007;120(4):306–15.

103. AGS Panel on Persistent Pain in Older Persons. The management of persistent pain in older persons. J Am Geriatr Soc. 2002;50(6 suppl):S205–24104.

104. Nikolaus T, Zeyfang A. Pharmacological treatments for persistent non-malignant pain in older persons. Drugs Aging. 2004;21:19–41.

105. Bellville JW, Forrest Jr WH, Miller E, Brown Jr BW. Influence of age on pain relief from analgesics. A study of postoperative patients. JAMA. 1971;217(13):1835–41.

106. Weiner DK, Hanlon JT. Pain in nursing home residents – management strategies. Drugs Aging. 2001;18(1):13–29.

107. Weiner DK, Hanlon JT, Studenski SA. Effects of central nervous system polypharmacy on falls liability in community-dwelling elderly. Gerontology. 1998;44:217–21.

108. Kay DC, Pickworth WB, Neider GL. Morphine-like insomnia from heroin in nondependent human addicts. Br J Clin Pharmacol. 1981;11(2):159–69.

109. Shaw IR, et al. Acute intravenous administration of morphine perturbs sleep architecture in healthy pain-free adults: a preliminary study. Sleep. 2005;28(6):677–82.

110. Walder B, Tramer MR, Blois R. The effects of two single doses of tramadol on sleep: a randomized, cross-over trial in healthy volunteers. Eur J Anaesthesiol. 2001;18(1):36–42.

111. Katz N, Mazer NA. The impact of opioids on the endocrine system. Clin J Pain. 2009;25:170–5.

112. Cicero T. Effects of exogenous and endogenous opiates on the hypothalamic-pituitary-gonadal axis in the male. Fed Proc. 1980;39:2551–4.

113. Drolet G, Dumont EC, Gosselin I, et al. Role of endogenous opioid system in the regulation of the stress response. Prog Neuropsychopharmacol Biol Psychiatry. 2001;25:729–41.

114. Genazzani AR, Genazzani AD, Volpogni C, et al. Opioid control of gonadotropin secretion in humans. Hum Reprod. 1993;8:151–3.

115. Grossman A, Moult PJ, Gaillard RC, et al. The opioid control of LH and FSH release: effects of a met-enkephalin analogue and naloxone. Clin Endocrinol. 1981;14:41–7.

116. Jordan D, Tafini JAM, Ries C, et al. Evidence for multiple opioid receptors in the human posterior pituitary. J Neuroendocrinol. 1996;8:883–7.

117. Veldhuis JD, Rogol AD, Samojlik E, et al. Role of endogenous opiates in the expression of negative feedback actions of androgen and estrogen on pulsatile properties of luteinizing hormone secretion in man. J Clin Invest. 1984;74:47–55.

118. Cicero TJ, Bell RD, Wiest WG, et al. Function of the male sex organs in heroin and methadone users. N Engl J Med. 1975;292:882–7.

119. Abs R, Verhelst J, Maeyaert J, et al. Endocrine consequences of long-term intrathecal administration of opioids. J Clin Endocrinol Metab. 2000;85:2215–22.

120. Finch PM, Roberts LJ, Price L, et al. Hypogonadism in patients treated with intrathecal morphine. Clin J Pain. 2000;16:251–4.

121. Paice JA, Penn RD. Amenorrhea associated with intraspinal morphine. J Pain Symptom Manage. 1995;10:582–3.

122. Winkelmuller M, Winkelmuller W. Long-term effects of continuous intrathecal opioid treatment in chronic pain of nonmalignant etiology. J Neurosurg. 1996;85:458–67.

123. Daniell HW. DHEAS deficiency during consumption of sustained-action prescribed opioids: evidence for opioid-induced inhibition of adrenal androgen production. J Pain. 2006;7:901–7.

124. Daniell HW. Hypogonadism in men consuming sustained-action oral opioids. J Pain. 2002;3:377–84.

125. Daniell HW, Lentz R, Mazer NA. Open-label pilot study of testosterone patch therapy in men with opioid induced androgen deficiency (OPIAD). J Pain. 2006;7:200–10.

126. Forman LJ, Tingle V, Estilow S, et al. The response to analgesia testing is affected by gonadal steroids in the rat. Life Sci. 1989;45:447–54.

127. Stoffel EC, Ulibarri CM, Folk JE, et al. Gonadal hormone modulation of mu, kappa, and delta opioid antinociception in male and female rats. J Pain. 2005;6(4):261–74.

128. Gallagher R. Methadone: an effective, safe drug of first choice for pain management in frail older adults. Pain Med. 2009;10(2):319–26.

129. Weiner DK, Rudy TE, Morone N, Glick R, Kwoh CK. Efficacy of periosteal stimulation therapy for the treatment of osteoarthritis-associated chronic knee pain: an initial controlled clinical trial. J Am Geriatr Soc. 2007;55:1541–7.

130. Gay MC, Philippot P, Luminet O. Differential effectiveness of psychological interventions for reducing osteoarthritis pain: a comparison of Erickson hypnosis and Jacobson relaxation. Eur J Pain. 2002;6:1–16.

131. Song R, Lee E, Lam P, Bae S. Effects of tai chi exercise on pain, balance, muscle strength, and perceived difficulties in physical functioning in older women with osteoarthritis: a randomized clinical trial. J Rheumatol. 2003;30:2039–44.

132. Morone NE, Greco CM. Mind-body interventions for chronic pain in older adults: a structured review. Pain Med. 2007;8(4):359–75.

133. Holick MF. Vitamin D deficiency. N Engl J Med. 2007;357: 266–81.

134. van der Wielen RP, Lowik MR, van den Berg H, et al. Serum vitamin D concentrations among elderly people in Europe. Lancet. 1995;346:207–10.

135. Khazai N, Judd SE, Tangpricha V. Calcium and vitamin D skeletal and extraskeletal health. Curr Rheumatol Rep. 2008;10:110–7.

136. Heaney RP, Dowell MS, Hale CA, et al. Calcium absorption varies within the reference range for serum 25-hydroxyvitamin D. J Am Coll Nutr. 2003;22:142–6.

137. Chapuy MC, Arlot ME, Duboeuf F, et al. Vitamin D3 and calcium to prevent hip fractures in elderly women. N Engl J Med. 1992;327:1637–42.

138. Chapuy MC, Pamphile R, Paris E, et al. Combined calcium and vitamin D3 supplementation in elderly women: confirmation of reversal of secondary hypoparathyroidism and hip fracture risk: the Decalyos II study. Osteoporos Int. 2002;13:257–64.

139. Trivedi DP, Doll R, Khaw KT. Effect of four monthly oral vitamin D3 (cholecalciferol) supplementation on fractures and mortality in men and women living in the community: randomised double blind controlled trial. Br Med J. 2003;326:469.

140. Dawson-Hughes B, Harris SS, Krall EA, et al. Effect of calcium and vitamin D supplementation on bone density in men and women 65 years of age or older. N Engl J Med. 1997;337: 670–6.

141. Bischoff-Ferrari HA, Dawson-Hughes B, Willett WC, et al. Effect of vitamin D on falls: a meta-analysis. JAMA. 2004;291:1999–2006.

142. Bischoff-Ferrari HA, Dietrich T, Orav EJ, et al. Higher 25-hydroxyvitamin D concentrations are associated with better lower-extremity function in both active and inactive persons aged > or =60y. Am J Clin Nutr. 2004;80:752–8.

143. Boonen S, Lips P, Bouillon R, et al. Need for additional calcium to reduce the risk of hip fracture with vitamin D supplementation: evidence from a comparative meta-analysis of randomized controlled trials. J Clin Endocrinol Metab. 2007;92: 1415–23.

144. Ahmed W, Khan N, Glueck CJ, et al. Low serum 25 (OH) vitamin D levels (<32ng/ml) are associated with reversible myositis-myalgia in statin-treated patients. Transl Res. 2009;153:11–6.

145. Badsha H, Daher M, Ooi Kong K. Myalgias or non-specific muscle pain in Arab or Indo-Pakistani patients may indicate vitamin D deficiency. Clin Rheumatol. 2009;28:971–3.

146. Schwalfenberg G. Improvement of chronic back pain or failed back surgery with vitamin D repletion: a case series. J Am Board Fam Med. 2009;22:69–74.

147. Tandeter H, Grynbaum M, Zuili I, et al. Serum 25-OH vitamin D levels in patients with fibromyalgia. Isr Med Assoc J. 2009;11:339–42.

148. Collins SL, Moore RA, McQuay HJ, et al. Antidepressants and anticonvulsants for diabetic neuropathy and postherpetic neuralgia: a quantitative systematic review. J Pain Symptom Manage. 2000;47:449–58.

149. Roose SP, Laghrissi-Thode F, Kennedy JS, et al. Comparison of paroxetine and nortriptyline in depressed patients with ischemic heart disease. J Am Med Assoc. 1998;279:287–91.

150. Dworkin RH, Backonja M, Rowbotham MC, et al. Advances in neuropathic pain: diagnosis, mechanisms, and treatment recommendations. Arch Neurol. 2003;60:1524–34.

151. Goldstein DJ, Lu Y, Detke MJ, Lee TC, Iyengar S. Duloxetine vs. placebo in patients with painful diabetic neuropathy. Pain. 2005;116(1–2):109–18.

152. Sindrup SH, Bach FW, Madsen C, Gram LF, Jensen TS. Venlafaxine versus imipramine in painful polyneuropathy: a randomized, controlled trial. Neurology. 2003;60:1284–9.

153. Johnson EM, et al. Cardiovascular changes associated with venlafaxine in the treatment of late-life depression. Am J Geriatr Psychiatry. 2006;14(9):796–802.

154. Gilron I, Bailey JM, Tu D, Holden RR, Weaver DF, Houlden RL. Morphine, gabapentin, or their combination for neuropathic pain. N Engl J Med. 2005;352:1324–34.

155. Guay DR. Oxcarbazepine, topiramate, zonisamide, and levetiracetam: potential use in neuropathic pain. Am J Geriatr Pharmacother. 2003;1:18–37.

156. Eisenberg E, Lurie Y, Braker C, et al. Lamotrigine reduces painful diabetic neuropathy: a randomized, controlled study. Neurology. 2003;60:1508–14.

157. Eisenberg E, McNicol ED, Carr DB. Efficacy and safety of opioid agonists in the treatment of neuropathic pain of nonmalignant origin. J Am Med Assoc. 2005;293:3043–52.

158. Sindrup SH, Andersen G, Madsen C, et al. Tramadol relieves pain and allodynia in polyneuropathy: a randomised, double-blind, controlled trial. Pain. 1999;83:85–90.

159. Boureau F, Legallicier P, Kabir-Ahmadi M. Tramadol in postherpetic neuralgia: a randomized, double-blind, placebo-controlled trial. Pain. 2003;104:323–31.

160. Hartrick C, et al. Efficacy and tolerability of tapentadol immediate release and oxycodone HCl immediate release in patients awaiting primary joint replacement surgery for end-stage joint disease: a 10-day, phase III, randomized double-blind, active- and placebo-controlled study. Clin Ther. 2009;31(2):260–71.

161. Rowan AJ, et al. New onset geriatric epilepsy: a randomized study of gabapentin, lamotrigine, and carbamazepine. Neurology. 2005;64(11):1868–73.

162. He L, Wu B, Zhou M. Non-antiepileptic drugs for trigeminal neuralgia. Cochrane Database Syst Rev. 2006;3:(CD004029).

163. The American Geriatrics Society 2012 Beers Criteria Update Expert Panel. American Geriatrics Society updated Beers criteria for potentially inappropriate medication use in older adults. J Am Geriatr Soc 2012;60:616–631.

164. North RB, Wetzel FT. Spinal cord stimulation for chronic pain of spinal origin - a valuable long-term solution. Spine. 2002;27:2584–91.

165. Stajanovic MP. Stimulation methods for neuropathic pain. Curr Pain Headache Rep. 2001;5:130–7.

166. Saitoh Y, Yoshimine T. Stimulation of primary motor cortex for intractable deafferentation pain. Acta Neurochir Suppl. 2007;97:51–6.

167. Wolfe F, Ross K, Anderson J, Russell IJ, Hebert L. The prevalence and characteristics of fibromyalgia in the general population. Arthritis Rheum. 1995;38:19–28.

168. Wolfe F, Smythe HA, Yunus MB, Bennett RM, Bombardier C, Goldenberg DL, et al. The American College of Rheumatology 1990 criteria for the classification of fibromyalgia-report of the multicenter criteria committee. Arthritis Rheum. 1990;33:160–72.

169. Goldenberg DL, Burckhardt C, Crofford L. Management of fibromyalgia syndrome. J Am Med Assoc. 2004;292(19):2388–95.

170. Carette S, McCain GA, Bell DA, Fam AG. Evaluation of amitriptyline in primary fibrositis. A double-blind, placebo-controlled study. Arthritis Rheum. 1986;29(5):655–9.

171. Goldenberg D, Mayskiy M, Mossey C, et al. A randomized, double-blind crossover trial of fluoxetine and amitriptyline in the treatment of fibromyalgia. Arthritis Rheum. 1996;39(11):1852–9.

172. Norregaard J, Volkmann H, Danneskiold-Samsoe B. A randomized controlled trial of citalopram in the treatment of fibromyalgia. Pain. 1995;61(3):445–9.

173. Arnold LM, Lu Y, Crofford LJ, Wohlreich M, Detke MJ, Iyengar S, et al. A double-blind, multicenter trial comparing duloxetine with placebo in the treatment of fibromyalgia patients with or without major depressive disorder. Arthritis Rheum. 2004;50(9):2974–84.

174. Gendreau R, Mease P, Rao S, Kranzler J, Clauw D. Milnacipran: a potential new treatment of fibromyalgia. Arthritis Rheum. 2003;48:S616.

175. Arnold L, Goldenberg D, Stanford S, Lalonde J, Sandhu H, Keck P, et al. Gabapentin in the treatment of fibromyalgia: a randomized, double-blind, placebo-controlled, multicenter trial. Arthritis Rheum. 2007;56(4):1336–44.

176. Bennett RM, Kamin M, Karim R, Rosenthal N. Tramadol and acetaminophen combination tablets in the treatment of fibromyalgia pain: a double-blind, randomized, placebo-controlled study. Am J Med. 2003;114(7):537–45.

177. Katz W. Pharmacology and clinical experience with tramadol in osteoarthritis. Drugs. 1996;52(3):39–47.

178. Weiner DK, Cayea D. Low back pain and its contributors in older adults: a practical approach to evaluation and treatment. In: Pain in older persons, progress in pain research and management, vol. 35. Seattle: IASP Press; 2005. p. 332.

Pain Medicine and Primary Care: The Evolution of a Population-Based Approach to Chronic Pain as a Public Health Problem

Rollin M. Gallagher

Key Points

- The concept of pain as a major public health problem has been gaining traction, fueled by societal awareness of three intersecting health crises: *first*, pain's contribution to rising health-care costs affecting the competiveness of American business; *second*, hundreds of thousands of American troops returning home with chronic pain and comorbidities such as PTSD (post-traumatic stress disorder); TBI (traumatic brain injury); CARF [no expansion needed]; JCAHO (Joint Commission for the Accreditation of Health Care Organizations); ACGME (Accreditation Council for Graduate Medical Education); VHA (Veterans Health Administration); TENS (transcutaneous electrical nerve stimulation) substance abuse, and suicide risk; and *third*, a growing epidemic of prescription analgesic drug abuse.
- "The pain medicine and primary care community rehabilitation model" (PMPCCRM) is proposed as a performance-based system of integrated, biopsychosocial, interdisciplinary, patient-centered team care in primary care offices closely supported by interdisciplinary pain medicine specialty clinics.
- The PMPCCRM is adopted as the stepped care model in two major capitated health-care systems that rely on cost-effective outcomes, the Department of Veteran Affairs and Department of Defense;

however, the goals of PMPCCRM will only be achieved with adequate training to an appropriate level of competency for all clinicians in the system, including both primary care providers and pain medicine specialists.

Introduction

This chapter outlines our progress in establishing chronic pain as a public health problem and in developing a population-based approach to pain management that relies heavily on an informed and skilled primary care sector in the medical home model. Other AAPM book chapters deal with the causes and complexities of different pain conditions and their treatments. This chapter will focus on gains that have been made in structuring models of care that improve primary care treatment and elevate the critically important role that primary care providers play in managing chronic pain.

In 1999, I wrote the following "Conclusion" in a paper for the *Medical Clinics of North America*: "Primary care and pain medicine: A community solution to the public health problem of chronic pain" [1]:

This paper presents commonly accepted evidence that defines chronic pain as a public health problem crying out for a re-organization of the manner in which our health care system manages pain. I have endeavored to present some of the conceptual, administrative and communication factors that may contribute to sustaining the present system of ineffective care. I have described several different but common models of care and why they have been ineffective. Finally, I have introduced the rationale for a new model of care that would remediate some of these problems. This model emphasizes the critical role of two new players in the specialized medical care of pain who relate closely to the functional restoration roles of physical therapists and behavioral specialists. The two new players are the informed *primary care physician* in a community practice, and the *pain medicine specialist* (Fig. 89.1).

Informed *community primary care physicians* contribute their expertise in longitudinal, comprehensive management combined with their more intimate knowledge of health, family and other psychosocial factors and community resources that

R.M. Gallagher, M.D., MPH
Department of Psychiatry, Anesthesiology and Critical Care, University of Pennsylvania Perelman School of Medicine, Philadelphia, PA, USA

Pain Policy Research and Primary Care, Penn Pain Medicine Center, Philadelphia, PA, USA

Pain Management, Philadelphia Veterans Health System, Philadelphia, PA, USA
e-mail: rgallagh@mail.med.upenn.edu

Fig. 89.1 The pain medicine and primary care community rehabilitation model (PMPCCR)

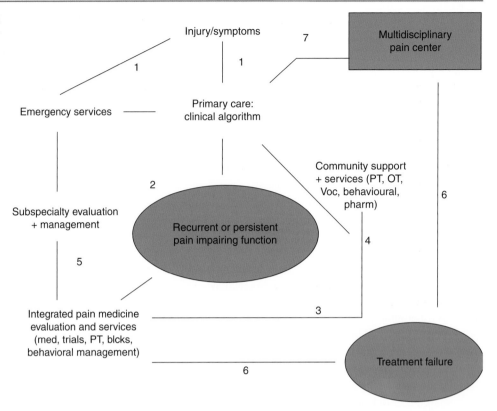

might importantly influence the outcome of pain treatment. *Pain medicine specialists* may have initial training and practice experience in a traditional specialty (e.g., anesthesiologist, psychiatrist, neurologist, neurosurgeon, physiatrist) but are now defined by having been board certified by credentialing and examination in the new specialty of pain medicine. The pain medicine specialist provides consultative support to the network of primary care physicians, physical therapists, and behavioral clinicians in the community centers, introduces new cost-effective technology rapidly into the system, and organizes and monitors the cost-effective and timely functioning of a complimentary network of needed sub-specialty services in the tertiary setting.

This model can be built gradually by selective practice collaborations with like-minded practitioners over time and will be supported by the insurance industry who already recognize the need for such a system, by health care system administrators who recognize the competitive advantages of such a system, and by regulators and certifying bodies, such as CARF, that recognize the value of such a system of care. Critical to success will be access to consistent information about the performance of the system, specifically the outcomes of patients as measured most importantly by function and costs, and the professionals' adherence to the processes enhancing quality care that is cost-effective. To demonstrate cost-effectiveness, the system will need to utilize uniform measures of outcomes used nationally to establish performance against accepted benchmarks of quality and cost-effectiveness. Support for such a model can be solicited from health industry constituents such as insurers, managed care companies, and state and federal agencies, and from health care systems such as hospital networks, particularly those with capitated risk. The challenge for these entities will be to identify and support key leaders and practitioners possibly outside traditional specialty structures, who have the necessary commitment to developing such a model.

My editorial in *Clinical Journal of Pain*, then the official journal of the American Academy of Pain Medicine, fol-

lowed shortly: "The pain medicine and primary care community rehabilitation model: Monitored care for pain disorders in multiple settings" [2]. Both of these papers called for a population-based approach to pain management.

This chapter will review our progress in adopting this population-based approach. I will particularly emphasize some of the structural changes in medicine that are encouraging, even in some cases mandating, the pain medicine and primary care community rehabilitation model and the centrality of a well-trained and rewarded primary care sector for the chronic disease management of pain. I will also marshal some of the emerging evidence that is accumulating to support these changes.

The Decade of Pain Control and Research

Where have we come since 1999? Over the ensuing decade, progress was slow. Our health-care system continued to expand in costs and size without any indication that quality was improving and with considerable data demonstrating deterioration in many sectors and a widening of disparities in health care. Much was written about chronic pain's role in the health economy and its contribution to its costs and disparities. Although certain sectors of American health care (e.g., the Veterans Health System followed by JCAHO) promoted evaluating pain systematically, and the United States Congress declared the "Decade of Pain Control and Research," 2001–2010 [3, 4], the medical establishment made little progress in addressing the deficits in research funding and training and the organizational factors in the health system that perpetuated the public health problem of pain [5, 6].

During the early part of the decade, concerted efforts by the American Pain Foundation joined by the Pain Care Coalition (American Academy of Pain Medicine, American Pain Society, American Headache Association) led to a bill (the so-called Rogers Bill named after its sponsor in Congress, Rep. Bill Rogers from Michigan) to establish a Pain Institute at NIH and more funding for research. Congressional support for this bill was tepid however. The AAPM and American Board of Pain Medicine made applications to the ACGME to establish expanded training for pain medicine specialists but was turned down on two occasions by a negative vote by ABMS members of the review committee – although other non-ABMS members voted for expanding training. Finally, beginning in 2008, the concept of pain as a major public health problem began gaining traction in a wider sector of American society, fueled by three intersecting societal crises. *First*, pain was demonstrated to contribute to the problem of rising health-care costs and its effects on the competiveness of American business and America's economy [7]. *Second*, hundreds of thousands of American troops were returning home from Iraq and Afghanistan for care in the military and veteran health systems with chronic pain, many with comorbidities such as PTSD and post-concussive syndrome, and as substance abuse and suicide rates rose in this population, pain was discovered to be a driving factor [8–10]. *Third,* emerging data demonstrating a growing epidemic of prescription analgesic drug abuse [11, 12] was brought to American consciousness by the national press. Meanwhile, the American Pain Foundation led the development of the Pain Forum, a consortium of professional, patient-centered, and industry organizations, and the Pain Care Coalition expanded to include a powerful partner, the American Society of Anesthesiology. Together, these groups successfully helped marshal three bills through congress: the Veterans Pain Care Act (2008) [13], the Military Pain Care Act (2009) [14], and the inclusion of the provisions of the original NIH Rogers Bill in the national health-care bill for health-care reform (2011) [15]. With the passage of these bills, which require a yearly progress report to congress, rapid transformative changes are occurring in pain management and research in the veterans and military health systems and in NIH. The former two systems, which are capitated and deliver care to a population of patients under a fixed budget, are most relevant to a discussion of the immediate changes that are needed in the health-care system. The NIH, which has long overlooked funding for the naturalistic, health systems, and combination trials demanded by the public health problem of pain [16], much less the development of new treatments, is most relevant in the long run for promoting research that improves the evidence basis for pain management.

Evolving Models of Primary Care for Pain

The *VA Health Administration* (VHS) has instituted a progression of activities, consistent with the PMPCCR model, leading to the publication and dissemination of a Directive, written by this author and Robert Kerns, National Program Director for Pain Management. The Directive outlines a new standard of care for pain for the entire VA [17], Stepped Pain Care [18] Rosenberger et al. Federal Practitioner (2011), which directs that a biopsychosocial model of patient-centered chronic pain care be provided seamlessly and collaboratively in primary care, secondary care, and tertiary care with movement between sectors depending on complexity, treatment refractoriness, comorbidities, and risk. The model is consistent with the medical home model in the national health act in that it emphasizes routine primary care screening for pain and comprehensive assessment, case management by interdisciplinary teams, shared decision-making with patients and their families, and patient self-management. System support for primary care is provided by pharmacy through medication and opioid management, by behavioral health with screening and management of mental health comorbidities, and by evidence-based guidelines and clinical algorithms, as in Fig. 89.2. The evidence basis for this model is emerging from clinical trials and cohort studies in primary care systems, most notably in the VHA, in which specific primary care enhancements improve outcomes in primary care practices managing pain [19–25].

To promote this transformation in all 153 VHA medical facilities and their related outpatient clinics, the VHA's national pain management office is supported by the National Pain Management Strategy Coordinating Committee (NPMSCC), consisting of representatives from several other program offices (e.g., anesthesia, education, mental health, neurology, nursing, primary care, PM&R, research, and quality improvement), and a National Pain Leadership Group consisting of VISN (regional) and facility "points-of-contact," which discuss implementation progress in monthly meetings. National and regional workshops for "pain champions" in each primary care setting are being held in conjunction with transformation of VA care to primary care Pain Aligned Care Teams (PACT) in the medical home model. National workgroups have identified core "competencies" for VHA primary care providers in pain management, as listed in Table 89.1. To provide for the needs of the huge population requiring pain management, these competencies will necessarily be extended considerably to encompass many office-based procedures and interventions as improved training proceeds in primary care, both in postgraduate medical education and continuing education.

One innovative contribution of the academic and private sector to post-training continuing education is academic detailing, as established by the University of New Mexico's

Fig. 89.2 Stepped model of care, Veterans Health System

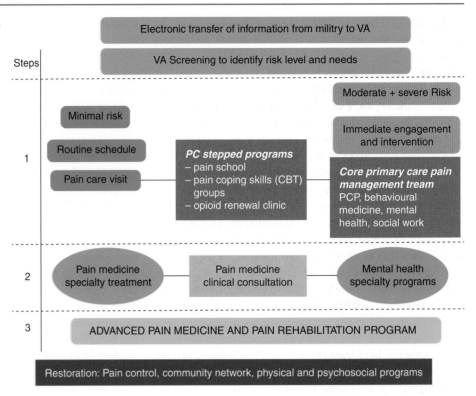

Table 89.1 Topics of the First National Pain Medicine Summit, American Medical Association (AMA), November 2009

1. What should all physicians know about pain medicine (i.e., where is the line drawn between primary care pain medicine competency and specialty pain medicine competency)?
2. How should pain medicine be taught?
3. What are the parameters that define the field of pain medicine?
4. What mechanisms do we need to establish the competency of a physician who wishes to practice pain medicine?
5. What are the barriers that prevent patients from receiving adequate pain care, other than the absence of competent pain medicine physicians?

ECHO model of using videoconferencing technology to train providers while they care for patients with complex chronic pain that is beyond the scope of their initial training. In the model of a resident case conference, interdisciplinary teams of clinicians (pain medicine specialists, psychologists, psychiatrists, social workers, and physical therapists) use videoconferencing links to supervise simultaneously several providers whose patients have difficulty accessing specialty pain care due to one or more factors such as distance, transportation, and illness severity. Evaluation of the impact of this model on the outcomes of patients with hepatitis C has shown outcomes equivalent to direct specialty care [26]. Although patient outcomes for pain specialty supervision are not yet published, supervised providers exhibit high satisfaction, confidence in pain care, and the growing capacity to manage chronic pain complexity independently of the specialty team.

Providers must attend weekly 2-h conferences for a year and present to and follow with the pain team at least ten cases over that year before sufficient knowledge and skill transfer is achieved so they can approximate pain medicine practice at a specialist level. The ECHO concept has been adopted for trial in six different regions of the VHA in what is now called the Specialty Care Access Network or SCAN-ECHO, and each site is now actively providing such telehealth supervision with plans to link to direct telehealth patient care. The end result will be primary care providers with direct pain management training in a preceptorship model similar to residency training. To support such a successful postgraduate medical education intervention, credentialing organizations are now challenged to find an acceptable way to test and credentialing such providers in primary care pain medicine.

The Department of Defense (DoD), led by the Army Surgeon General and guided by the Defense and Veterans Pain Management Initiative (DVPMI), in 2009 chartered the Army Pain Task Force, including pain experts from the VA, Navy, and Air Force. The task force intensively studied the problem of pain management in the military over a 6-month period, making dozens of site visits to "best practices" as well as holding three retreats, and published a 163-page report [27] which thoroughly outlined the deficiencies in care and made over 100 recommendations for transforming pain care in the military. Key among the recommendations was adoption of the stepped care model for providing uniform standards for pain care in the military and in the VA. Subsequently, the VA-DoD Health Executive Council (HEC), codirected by the Under Secretaries for Health of both the VA and the DoD, chartered a Pain Management Working Group (PMWG). The PMWG, cochaired by this author, is charged with helping establish a single system of continuous, collaborative, and effective pain care, research, and education for the VA and DoD. The Defense and Veterans Center for Integrated Pain Management (DVCIPM) is a newly functional office chartered under the lead of the army to help operationalize the work of the HEC-PMWG. Projects underway include PASTOR, a standardized pain assessment to be used in all chronic pain encounters, no matter the setting but particularly in primary care, to assist providers in real-time clinical decision-making. The assessments will generate both cross-sectional reports for primary care providers at time of initial assessment as well as longitudinal reports on clinical outcomes. All data will be entered in a data registry and used to establish the benchmarks needed for health-care administrators to address planning and policy, consistent with the PMPCCR model as outlined in the beginning of this chapter. The HEC-PMWG hopes to coordinate DoD and VHA activities in at least two rapidly developing programs, the assessment and data registry project, PASTOR, and the SCAN-ECHO postgraduate training project.

Changes in the "Medical Establishment"

Finally, led by the American Medical Association (AMA), other organizations outside the VA and military have called for changes based on wide recognition of pain medicine training deficiencies for all physicians, particularly primary on who fall the largest burden of care [28–30]. Through the concerted efforts of the AMA's Pain and Palliative Medicine Specialty Section Council (PPMSSC), under the direction of its chairman, Philipp M. Lippe, MD, FACS, the AMA hosted the first national summit on Pain Medicine in 2009. The entire process and its outcomes are described in a 2010 paper in *Pain Medicine* [31]. The process began with the adoption of Resolution 321 (A-08) at an AMA Annual House of Delegates meeting in June 2008. Resolution 321 (A-08) states, in part, that "....the AMA encourages relevant specialties to collaborate in studying: (1) the scope and practice and body of knowledge encompassed by the field of Pain Medicine; (2) the adequacy of undergraduate, graduate, and post graduate education in the principles and practices of the field of Pain Medicine, considering the current and anticipated medical need for the delivery of quality pain care; and (3) appropriate training and credentialing criteria for this multi-disciplinary field of medical practice." Over several months, representatives from all clinical specialties in the AMA convened in a modified Delphi process with representatives of the VA, the military, and major pain organizations. Their task was to identify the most

Table 89.2 Pain management core competencies, primary care

1. Conduct comprehensive pain assessment
2. Negotiate behaviorally specific and feasible goals
3. Know/use common metrics for measuring function
4. Optimize patient communication
  (a) How to provide reassurance
  (b) How to foster pain self-management
5. Conduct routine physical/neurological examinations
6. Judiciously use diagnostic tests/procedures and secondary consultation
7. Assess psychiatric/behavioral comorbidities
8. Know accepted clinical practice guidelines
9. Use rational, algorithmic-based polypharmacy
10. Manage opioids safely and effectively
Additional competencies
11. Provide office-based procedures (potentially guided by ultrasound)
  Trigger point injections
  Joint injections
  Peripheral nerve blocks
12. Provide brief or sustaining psychotherapeutic enhancements
  Cognitive reframing
  Motivational interviewing
  Problem-solving
  Supportive patient and family counseling
  Goal-oriented, patient-centered pain management planning
  Relaxation training and meditation
  Weight and food management
13. Supervise/prescribe physical therapies
  Exercise regimens (McKenzie; Krause)
  Ice and stretch
  Neuromodulation (TENS, inferential stimulator)

pressing issues affecting the care of pain. The top five issues that emerged from this process are outlined in Tables 89.1 and 89.2.

A retreat was held the day prior to the annual midyear meeting of the AMA in Houston, Texas, in November 2009. Participants thoroughly considered the problem in an open, transparent forum. For the most part, they did not defending turf or position but honestly attempted to understand the problem and agree on the best approach for the benefit of medicine and the population. For the first time, pain medicine specialists, surgeons, internists, family physicians, psychiatrists, and others, most in leadership positions in medical schools, the AMA, community practice, and various large organizations, contributed their ideas openly and constructively. The meeting imparted a general sense of a medical community of interest and intent. Regarding education of primary care providers, one of the workgroups, charged with answering the Delphi process-generated question, "What should all physicians know about Pain Medicine (i.e., where is the line drawn between primary care Pain Medicine competency and specialty Pain Medicine competency)?" recommended the following five "next steps" [32]: (1) The AAPM should collaborate with the Association of American Medical Colleges about standards for undergraduate education. (2) Each medical specialty should establish specific pain medicine competencies through ACGME. (3) The American Board of Medical Specialties should recognize pain medicine as a primary specialty to ensure adequacy and consistency of pain medicine specialty training/certification nationally and to assure uniform and reliable education for students in medical schools. (4) The Council on Medical Education of the AMA should resolve to develop a specific educational package on competencies for pain medicine. (5) Gaps in pain care in the ACGME programs should be filled by surveying the Association Program Specialty Directors of ACGME to determine what is currently being taught and what needs to be taught about pain medicine in their programs. The survey could be developed from core competency standards for primary care, perhaps adopting the VA's competencies, as outlined in Table 89.1. Efforts for a follow-up summit to assess progress are underway.

Passage of the National Health Reform Act of 2010 that included the language of the original Rogers Bill required that the NIH attends to pain research and education and charter an Institute of Medicine (IOM) Committee to study and make recommendations for a widespread societal approach to addressing the problem of chronic pain. Since then, NIH has established several working groups to address deficiencies in education and research in pain management [33]. The IOM recently convened the recommended committee and completed a report, "Relieving Pain in America: A Blueprint for Transforming Prevention, Care, Education, and Research," that comprehensively reviewed the public health burden of pain, collated and summarized the literature outlining clinical deficits and needs, and commented on the relevant needed research [34]. The IOM report cogently compiled and summarized an incredible breadth and depth of information supporting the need for a population approach such as presented by the PMPCCR model and the education and training required to establish such a model. However, strikingly absent from the report were specific suggestions for reform of education and training of physicians, which presents the most salient challenge if society is to effectively address the public health problem of pain as the IOM report outlined in such detail. The AMA report went much further. A demand for AAMC-mandated reform of medical student education, ACGME-mandated reform of primary care residency and pain fellowship training as outlined in the AMA Summit Report, would drive the system toward a PMPCCR model and real system change. Causes of this reluctance may reflect the membership of the IOM Committee, which largely represented traditional specialty, research, and patient advocacy interests. Tellingly, there was no representation on the panel from internal medicine or family practice, the specialties that bear the largest burden of pain, whereas there were three psychologists, two ethicists, and one writer.

The Future

The management of pain can no longer be put on medicine's back burner. Society now demands change. Medicine's guild-like structures support the tribal identities that perpetuate fragmented pain care. Doctors would like to continue lucrative practices that focus on technically difficult procedures that are highly reimbursed. These identities and structures are threatened by a new model of integrated and patient-centric team care based in primary care offices and closely supported by the well-trained pain medicine specialist. Thoughtful, biopsychosocial chronic disease management is professionally rewarding if a provider is sufficiently trained and supported because it is effective. There is no greater pleasure than relieving suffering and restoring meaningful life. However, if one has to close practice because reimbursement favors only procedures completed, not outcomes, then change will not occur. Society must make the changes – medicine will not.

How different care will be allocated among primary care and specialty care remains to be determined. There will be two polarities in this determination; either may evolve, or some combination depending on circumstances. Both scenarios emphasize the importance of the primary care provider. In the first scenario, pain medicine specialists will acquire much more specialty training in biopsychosocial pain medicine, encompassing all the training needed for managing complex chronic pain. Primary care providers will continue to enlarge the scope of their practices in pain management but leave complexity and risk management cases to the specialists. In the second scenario, primary care physicians will become subspecialists in pain medicine, with an extra year or more of training much like they do in palliative care, cardiology, and pulmonology, and will care for the vast majority of patients with chronic pain at both the primary and secondary levels of care. They will adopt many of the roles and techniques now practiced in pain medicine specialty care. Pain medicine specialists will manage only the technically complex case requiring special, expensive equipment and training and practiced in tertiary care centers. The collaborative models of care that evolve in these two scenarios will be determined by a complex interaction of health economics, medical politics, and medical science. Hopefully, the patient's and society's mutual best interests will be served by measurement based choices in health care that will drive the ultimate model that emerges.

Several specific self-care and primary care enhancement models have already been examined. Davies, Quintner, and colleagues describe how a state in Australia implemented a

Fig. 89.3 Disease management in a population of patients in pain [6]

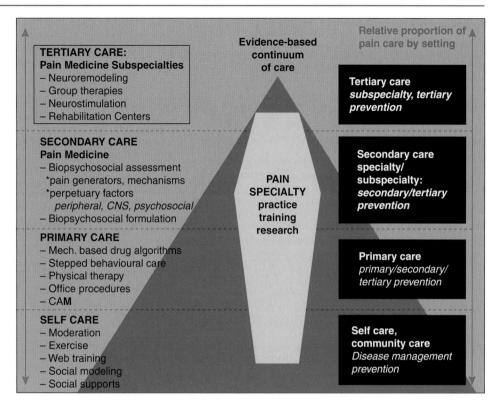

publicly funded self-management program that greatly reduced the need for primary care and pain specialty care visits and reduced wait times for specialty pain care [35]. Wiedemer et al. describe how a structured opioid management program run by pharmacists in a veterans hospital's primary care clinic reduced aberrant behavior and identified patients with substance use disorders needing referral to addiction treatment [23]. Dobscha and colleagues, in a controlled clinical trial, showed that enhancing primary care of pain with telephone-assisted consultation and support for emotional responses to pain, such as depression, improved patient outcomes and costs over "treatment as usual" condition [36]. Kroenke, Bair, and colleagues implemented a stepped care approach in primary care that demonstrated clinical efficacy for chronic pain with comorbid depression [37].

Who knows whether the primary care subspecialty model, pain medicine specialty model, or some hybrid, depending on local/regional conditions, will dominate the future of pain management. Society and its inevitable reinforcement of efficiency will assure that the PMPCCR model will prevail ultimately. In any case, the optimal result will be the engagement of patient and provider within a seamless continuum of pain management within a health system and society that maximizes pain control, function, and overall quality of life. The widespread use of e-health supported by interactive technologies will engage patient in active, positive, neuromodulatory behavioral and emotional self-management strategies. These strategies will be culturally socialized within a supportive family, workplace, and community milieu that provides for self-actualization and productivity that enhances self-esteem, rather than destroying it. These strategies will be a foundation of a person-in-pain's biopsychosocial medical pain management, rather than an adjunct to a series of procedures, medications, and other biomedical interventions or outside the clinical milieu altogether. Patients will learn new coping skills that are transferable to other challenges and settings in their life course.

When entering the health system, access to an evidence-based stepped model of care will marshal resources appropriate to the level of need to achieve shared patient-centered goals. A population-based allocation of resources will achieve efficiencies and effectiveness unheard of in today's confusing, inefficient medical environment. Figure 89.3 depicts such a population-based system of care, with the majority of care being self-care using evidence-based methods of primary prevention such as weight control and exercise – much like cardiovascular care relies on self-management of diet and exercise to reduce risk of CV disease. Once pain symptoms ensue, then a seamless stepped model, relying on a healthy foundation of self-management, will begin in primary care. Biopsychosocial outcomes will be continuously monitored so that there are no barriers to pain specialty treatment and "chronification" does not progress to "maldynia" and its attendant costs to patient, family, and society [38].

References

1. Gallagher RM. Pain medicine and primary care: a community solution to pain as a public health problem. Med Clin North Am. 1999;83(5):555–85.

2. Gallagher RM. The pain medicine and primary care community rehabilitation model: monitored care for pain disorders in multiple settings. Clin J Pain. 1999;15(1):1–3.

3. Lippe PM. The decade of pain control and research. Pain Med. 2000;1(4):286.

4. Loeser J. The decade of pain control and research. APS Bull. 2003;13(3). http://www.ampainsoc.org/library/bulletin/may03/article1.htm. Accessed 29 Aug 2011.

5. Gallagher RM. The AMA in health care reform: a "flexner report" to improve pain medicine training and practice. Pain Med. 2010;11(10):1437–9.

6. Dubois M, Gallagher RM, Lippe P. Pain medicine position paper. Pain Med. 2009;10(6):972–1000.

7. Stewart WF, Ricci JA, Chee E, Morganstein D, Lipton R. Lost productive time and cost due to common pain conditions in the US workforce. JAMA. 2003;290(18):2443–54.

8. Gironda RJ, Clark ME, Massengale JP, Walker RL. Pain among veterans of operations enduring freedom and Iraqi freedom. Pain Med. 2006;7(4):339–43.

9. Kerns RD, Dobscha SK. Pain among veterans returning from deployment in Iraq and Afghanistan: update on the Veterans Health Administration Pain Research Program. Pain Med. 2009;10(7):1161–4.

10. Lew HL, Otis JD, Tun C, Kerns RD, Clark ME, Cifu DX. Prevalence of chronic pain, posttraumatic stress disorder, and persistent postconcussive symptoms in OIF/OEF Veterans: polytrauma clinical triad. J Rehabil Res Dev. 2009;46(6):697–702.

11. Gilson AM, Kreis PG. The burden of the nonmedical use of prescription opioid analgesics. Pain Med. 2009;10(S2):S89–100.

12. Birnbaum HG, White AG, Schiller M, Waldman T, Cleveland JM, Roland CL. Societal costs of prescription opioid abuse, dependence, and misuse in the United States. Pain Med. 2011;12(4):657–67.

13. Section 501 of Veterans' Mental Health and Other Care Improvements Act of 2008, Public Law 110-387. 2008. http://www.gpo.gov/fdsys/pkg/PLAW-110publ387/pdf/PLAW-110publ387.pdf. Accessed 10 Oct 2008.

14. Section 711 of National Defense Authorization Act for FY 2010, Public Law 111-84. 2009. http://www.gpo.gov/fdsys/pkg/PLAW-111publ84/pdf/PLAW-111publ84.pdf.Accessed 28 Oct 2009.

15. Section 4305 of Patient Protection and Affordable Care Act, Public law 111-148. 2010. http://www.gpo.gov/fdsys/pkg/PLAW-111publ148/pdf/PLAW-111publ148.pdf. Accessed 23 Mar 2010.

16. Rathmell JP, Carr DB. The scientific method, evidence-based medicine, and rational use of interventional pain treatments. [editorial] (Comment on Merrill DG. Hoffman's glasses: evidence-based medicine and the search for quality in the literature of interventional pain medicine. Reg Anesth Pain Med. 2003;28:547–580) Reg Anesth Pain Med. 2003;28:498–501.

17. VHA DIRECTIVE 2009-053, Pain management. 2011. http://www1.va.gov/vhapublications/viewpublication.asp?Pub_ID=2238. Accessed 23 Aug 2011.

18. Rosenberger PH, Philip EJ, Lee A, Kerns RD. The VHA's national pain management strategy: implementing the stepped care model. Fed Pract. 2011;28(8):39–42.

19. Dobscha SK, Corson K, Perrin NA, Hanson GC, Leibowitz RQ, Doak MN, Dickinson KC, Sullivan MD, Gerrity MS. Collaborative care for chronic pain in primary care: a cluster-randomized trial. JAMA. 2009;301(12):1242–52.

20. Kroenke K, Bair MJ, Damush TM, Wu J, Hoke S, Sutherland J, Tu W. Optimized antidepressant therapy and pain self-management in primary care patients with depression and musculoskeletal pain: a

randomized controlled trial. J Am Med Assoc. 2009;301(20):2099–110.

21. Lin EHB, Katon W, Von Korff M, et al. Effect of improving depression care on pain and functional outcomes among older adults with arthritis: a randomized controlled trial. JAMA. 2003;290(18):2428–9.

22. Ahles TA, Wasson JH, Seville JL, et al. A controlled trial of methods for managing pain in primary care patients with or without co-occurring psychosocial problems. Ann Fam Med. 2006;4(4):341–50.

23. Wiedemer N, Harden P, Arndt R, Gallagher RM. The opioid renewal clinic, a primary care, managed approach to opioid therapy in chronic pain patients at risk for substance. Pain Med. 2007;8(7):573–84.

24. Trafton J, Martine S, Michel M, Lewis E, Wang D, Combs A, Scales N, Tu S, Goldstein MK. Evaluation of the acceptability and usability of a decision support system to encourage safe and effective use of opioid therapy for chronic, noncancer pain by primary care providers. Pain Med. 2010;11(4):575–85.

25. Bair M. Overcoming fears, frustrations, and competing demands: an effective integration of pain medicine and primary care to treat complex pain patients. Pain Med. 2007;8(7):544–5.

26. Arora S, Thornton K, Murata G, Derning P, et al. Outcomes of treatment for hepatitis C virus infection by primary care providers. N Engl J Med. 2011;364:2199–207.

27. Office of the Army Surgeon General, Pain Management Task Force Final report: providing a standardized DoD and VHA vision and approach to pain management to optimize the care for warriors and their families. http://www.armymedicine.army.mil/prr/pain_management.html. Accessed 29 Aug 2011.

28. Gallagher R. Physician variability in pain management: are the JCAHO standards enough? Pain Med. 2003;4(1):1–3.

29. Corrigan C, Desnick L, Marshall S, Bentov N, Rosenblatt RA. What can we learn from first-year medical students' perceptions of pain in the primary care setting? Pain Med. 2011;12(8):1216–22.

30. Norris TE. Chronic pain, medical students, and primary care commentary on "what can we learn from first-year medical students' perception of pain in the primary care setting". Pain Med. 2011;12(8):1137–8.

31. Lippe PM, Brock C, David J, Crossno R, Gitlow S. The first national pain medicine summit – final summary report. Pain Med. 2010;11:1447–68.

32. Gallagher R. What should all physicians know about pain medicine? Workgroup report. The first national pain medicine summit – final summary report. Pain Med. 2010;11:1450–2.

33. Reid MC, Bennett DA, Chen WG, et al. Improving the pharmacologic management of pain in older adults: identifying the research gaps and methods to address them. Pain Med. 2011;12(9):1336–57. doi:10.1111/j.1526-4637.2011.01211.x. Epub 2011 Aug 11.

34. Institute of Medicine. Relieving pain in America: a blueprint for transforming prevention, care, education, and research. 2011. http://www.iom.edu/Reports/2011/Relieving-Pain-in-America-A-Blueprint-for-Transforming-Prevention-Care-Education-Research.aspx. Accessed 29 Aug 2011.

35. Davies S, Quinter J, Parsons R, Parkitny L, Knight P, Forrester E, Roberts M, Graham C, Visser E, Antill T, Packer T, Schug SA. Preclinic group education sessions reduce waiting times and costs at public pain medicine units. Pain Med. 2011;12(1):59–71.

36. Dobscha SK, Corson K, Flores JA, Tansill EC, Gerrity MS. Veterans affairs primary care clinicians' attitudes toward chronic pain and correlates of opioid prescribing rates. Pain Med. 2008;9(5):564–71.

37. Kroenke K, Bair MJ, Damush TM, Wu J, Hoke S, Sutherland J, Tu W. Optimized antidepressant therapy and pain self-management in primary care patients with depression and musculoskeletal pain: a randomized controlled trial. JAMA. 2009;301(20):2099–110.

38. Gallagher RM. Chronification to maldynia: biopsychosocial failure of pain homeostasis. Pain Med. 2011;12(7):993–5.

Pain Care Beyond the Medical Practice Office: Utilizing Patient Advocacy, Education, and Support Organizations

William Rowe

Key Points

- There are numerous, credible pain patient education, support, and advocacy organizations.
- The medical practitioner has little time or experience to provide some of the critical assistance elements for their patients.
- Pain patient education, support, and advocacy organizations can provide helpful support and education for pain patients that make a critical difference in their ability to successfully manage their pain.
- Medical practitioners should include referrals to these organizations as standard treatment recommendations.

Why Utilize Patient Education and Advocacy Organizations?

Living with chronic pain is a total-person experience. Chronic pain affects all aspects of an individual's life. The physical effects are clear—pain, sleep deprivation, and curtailed capacity to function. The emotional effects should also be clear—in most cases depression, sense of loss, fear and anxiety, frustration, and diminished hope and confidence. The social effects should also be clear—diminished social activities and contacts, strained marital, family and work relationships, and withdrawal. The effects on work and career should also be obvious—diminished capacity to perform, diminished ability to achieve career goals, possible loss, or end of work life.

W. Rowe, M.A.
American Pain Foundation,
201 N. Charles Street, Suite 710,
Baltimore 21201, MD, USA
e-mail: wrowe@painfoundation.org

These effects in turn contribute to spiraling the individual into a mixed state of pain, fear, withdrawal, anger, anxiety, frustration, hopelessness, and defeat. How does the medical practitioner deal with all of that in the 10, 15, or 20 min of the periodic office visit? Most people living with chronic pain need a great deal more than what can be provided in the typical office visit. The days and weeks are long when living with pain, and the need for information and support is continuous beyond the medical office visit. The physical-psychosocial impact of pain is well documented [1].

In addition referring to other practitioners who offer complementary therapies, one resource, often not utilized by medical practitioners, is encouraging patients to check out and connect to the multitude of helpful, credible patient education and support organizations. There are many organizations that provide comprehensive information and various support services. Some are defined by a particular pain disease, and some are general about pain in all of its forms. Most have comprehensive websites with information and resources that can assist the person with pain to manage their pain. They all also serve the very important function of connecting the person with pain to others who are living with pain. A common experience of people living with pain is isolation and a sense of being alone and the only person living this pain experience. These patient support sites offer a community of people and an inventory of information and resources to ameliorate the isolation.

There are many potential benefits for people with pain who consult and utilize patient education and support organizations. A short list would include:

- Access to comprehensive, helpful information about their pain condition and treatment options for their pain
- Access to credible, practical, and tested tools for improving your well-being and reducing pain
- Breaking the sense of isolation and connecting individuals to others who immediately understand their challenges
- Presenting links to a multitude of organizations and resources that can be specific to an individual's needs

- Presenting information about key pain advocacy issues and offering instruction and ways to become better personal advocates and advocates for improved pain policy
- Presenting credible and useful information to help people with pain to better communicate with their health-care providers, with family members, and with one's social and work networks
- Presenting information about the latest and future treatment options for pain
- Presenting a general message of hope and confidence that people are listening and working to improve pain care

These benefits are tangible, measurable benefits for people living with pain. Promoting patients to connect to credible patient advocacy, education, and support organizations offers the practitioner an active and helpful complement to the medical services that take place in the office and relieves the practitioner from the challenging and time-consuming burden of being the only source of expertise and consolation. Investigating these resources presents opportunities for patients to take charge of their pain, to become informed, connected, and empowered to take actions to improve their lives.

Patient Organizations and Resources

There are many patient organizations that provide credible information and helpful resources and services for people living with pain. Some focus on specific diseases, and some are about pain and its variety of causes and manifestations. The leading national organizations providing information and support for people with pain are the *American Pain Foundation* (*APF*) (www.painfoundation.org) and the *American Chronic Pain Association* (www.theacpa.org). Each offers a variety of resources that are web-based and some print and personal resources. In 2010, a third national pain organization, the *National Pain Foundation*, gifted its web and program resources to the American Pain Foundation enhancing the breadth of content of the APF.

A short list of organizations that focus on a particular pain condition includes the *Reflex Sympathetic Dystrophy Syndrome Association* (www.rsdsa.org) which focuses on what is now referred to as complex regional pain syndrome, *TNA The Facial Pain Association* (www.fpa-support.org) which focuses on facial pain conditions such as trigeminal neuralgia, *Lupus Foundation of America* (www.lupus.org), *The Neuropathy Association* (www.neuropathy.org), the *National Vulvodynia Association* (www.nva.org), *Ehlers-Danlos National Foundation* (www.ednf.org), the *Interstitial Cystitis Association* (www.ichelp.org), the *National Headache Foundation* (www.headaches.org), and the *National Fibromyalgia and Chronic Pain Association* (www.fmcpaware.org).

In order to illustrate how a national pain patient organization might be helpful to a person with pain and a helpful supplement to the practitioner's work, consider a scenario where Jane Doe has just visited her doctor with complaints of debilitating low back pain and a long-term, persistent, generalized pain in her shoulders, neck, and upper back. She explains that her shoulder and neck pains have been preventing her from engaging in many of her usual activities and cutting her off from friends. After a thorough history and exam, her doctor diagnosed severe muscle strain in her lower back and possibly a fibromyalgia condition. He recommends customary treatment choices for both conditions and that she consult the resources about back pain and fibromyalgia at the APF website, www.painfoundation.org. He explains in a few minutes his diagnoses offering basic information about muscular strain and fibromyalgia and encourages her to "read-up" on these conditions on the website.

That evening Jane opens up the website of the APF and sees the homepage:

Jane notices a couple of paths to follow: (a) Click on the "Learn About Pain" button; (b) Click on the "PainAid—Support" button. She starts her search with "Learn About Pain" and sees that there is section on "Pain Conditions" where "Fibromyalgia" and "Back Pain" are listed. A search on each of these paths uncovers pages and pages of information about these conditions including Tip Sheets, Fact Sheets, Handbooks, archived webinars, treatment information and self-help resources, interviews with experts, FAQs and links to professionally moderated chat rooms on fibromyalgia and back pain, patient stories, and comprehensive lists of resources including books, websites, and articles. Following the PainAid path, she discovers a list of regularly scheduled professionally moderated Live Chats and a large list of Discussion Boards including a topic section on Fibromyalgia and another on Back Pain.

Jane's first visit to the APF site is more exploratory where she finds topics, skim reads various sections, and makes mental notes for her return. Her initial impressions include a major sense of relief after reading descriptions of "fibromyalgia" and "muscle strain back pain" that provide her a strong sense that the diagnoses were correct. She also was immediately gratified to read the words of others who are experiencing similar pains and limitations confirming that she was not imagining her pains and not "crazy or weak" because she felt those pains. The words she read from others were exact descriptions of what she was experiencing. The quick read of information about treatments also confirmed that the recommendations from her physician were appropriate and standard for the pains she experienced.

After several days of exploring, reading deeper, and viewing webinars on the subjects, Jane felt very informed and equipped to take charge of her pains. She followed her doctor's instructions with confidence and added some treatment activities including gentle stretching and guided relaxation techniques to her self-care. She participated in chats and discussion boards and shared her experiences and learned from the experiences of others. In a brief time, her low back muscle pain ended, and she learned to manage her fibromyalgia pain. After a few months Jane engaged in some of the advocacy opportunities outlined on the website and felt encouraged that her advocacy was contributing to better care for others who might be in the early stages of addressing their chronic pain.

The information and support that Jane received was vital to her understanding her pain, vital to her commitment to her treatment regimen, vital to her confidence and optimism, and a major contributor to the successful management of her pain. This story is representative of many who utilize the assistance of patient information and support organizations. The list presented earlier is only a small representation of the type and number of organizations available for pain patient support. Patient information, support, and advocacy organizations are a useful supplement to the advice and medical decision making that goes on in the medical office.

Reference

1. Fine PG. Long term consequences of chronic pain: mounting evidence for pain as a neurological disease and parallels with other chronic disease states. Pain Med. 2011;12:996–1004.

Neonatal Pain

Celeste Johnston, Marsha Campbell-Yeo, Ananda
Fernandes, and Manon Ranger

Key Points

- Excessive exposure to painful invasive procedures is part of the experience of hospitalized neonates.
- Pain is not treated in more than half of invasive procedures in neonates.
- Assessment of pain in neonates requires a multidimensional approach that also accounts for gestational age
- Although effective for postoperative pain, analgesics, including opiates, topical agents, and nonsteroidal anti-inflammatory agents, are not appropriate for minor procedural pain in neonates.
- Non-pharmacological approaches to pain management have proven to be effective for minor procedural pain.

Introduction

Pain in infants was essentially ignored up until the 1980s. The few reports that did exist were small observational studies [1–4]. In 1987, the first randomized trial on pain in neonates was published in the *Lancet,* in which it was reported that the standard for anesthesia for neonates undergoing repair of pat-

C. Johnston, R.N., D.E. (✉) • M. Ranger, R.N., Ph.D.
School of Nursing, McGill University,
3506 University Street, Wilson Hall, Montreal,
QC H3A 2A7, Canada
e-mail: dceleste.johnston@mcgill.ca

M. Campbell-Yeo, R.N., M.N., Ph.D.
Department of Maternal Newborn Program, IWK Health Care,
5850/5980 University Ave., P.O. Box 9700,
Halifax, NS B3K 6R8, Canada

A. Fernandes, M.S.N., Ph.D.
Coimbra School of Nursing,
Coimbra, Lisbon, Portugal

ent ductus arteriosus was inadequate and that infants who received an opiate-based anesthetic over the usual nitrous oxide had fewer postoperative complications [5]. At the time that article appeared, there was an increased interest in the issue of pain in infants, but there were several challenges in order to proceed. The first challenge was how to assess pain in a uniformly nonverbal population, especially given that most definitions of pain included self-report [6]. The second challenge was to determine which analgesics were effective for which conditions with considerations for safety in this vulnerable population. As will be reported below, there was a need for alternate non-pharmacological approaches to pain control, and thus, studies were required to test which ones were effective for pain, particularly procedural pain.

Infants undergoing surgery now typically receive adequate anesthesia and analgesia due to the pioneering study mentioned above [5] as well as subsequent studies on the effects of surgical pain on neonates [7, 8]. Guidelines on the treatment of surgical pain in neonates suggest opiates for major surgery, and this is usually followed [9, 10]. Now, attention has moved to common procedural pain management [11].

Infants who are hospitalized in neonatal intensive care units are subjected to numerous procedures as part of necessary monitoring and therapeutic interventions. Many of these procedures involve tissue damage, such as heel lance, intravenous line insertions, lumbar punctures, or have been considered to be painful although typically not tissue damaging per se, such as endotracheal intubation or suctioning of in situ endotracheal tubes. Estimates of procedural pain range from 10 per day to 5 per week, with approximately half receiving no pain management strategies [9, 10, 12, 13]. This high exposure to untreated procedural pain at a time of increased developmental plasticity is not inconsequential [14–16]. There is peripheral hypersensitivity [17], behavioral blunting [18, 19], altered cortisol response [20], and altered thermal sensitivity into childhood [21–24].

The challenges of measuring pain in this population, of using pharmacological interventions and of alternate interventions, are being met to some extent. The current state of knowledge on these topics will be presented in this chapter with a conclusion regarding the remaining unmet challenges.

Pain Assessment

An accurate pain evaluation is an essential step to its management. Although it is well recognized, researched, and has been incorporated into best practice clinical guidelines, this task remains challenging in critically ill infants. Through the recognition that preterm infants feel pain, tremendous advancements in this field have been made and have prompted the development of various unidimensional and multidimensional pain assessment measures [25, 26]. Behaviors identified as being reliable proxy indicators for pain evaluation, such as facial expressions and cry, are not without their limits. As critically ill preterm and term neonates may have limited neurological development and energy to construct a proper observable response to pain, it is not uncommon for these fragile babies to not display any detectable cues of such suffering [27, 28]. With the fast progress of neuroimaging techniques, research focus has shifted to measurement of cortical activity related to noxious events, perhaps providing clinical researchers opportunities to explore the use of associated signals to identify and better understand the pain process. Nonetheless, to date, behavioral displays caused by pain remain the best available means to evaluate the infantile forms of self-report and should be used as "surrogate" measures in clinical practice [6].

Behavioral and Physiological Responses

For National Institute for the Humanities (NICU) practitioners, decoding the subtle infantile expressions of pain remains challenging. This critical task requires a certain level of experience, skill in pain evaluation, and adequate time and patience to regularly observe for expressions of pain. The complex nature of this subjective experience does not aid this matter. To aid clinicians, numerous behavioral or composite pain assessment instruments have been developed, some with more solid psychometric properties than others. These scales predominantly include (1) behavioral signs: facial actions, cry, and body motions; and (2) physiological indicators: heart rate, respiratory rate, arterial oxygen saturation, and blood pressure [29]. Among these, facial expressions have been recognized to be the most stable, sensitive, and reliable proxy measures of pain [4, 13, 30]. Out of the ten facial actions first described in the important work by Grunau and Craig [i.e., Neonatal Facial Coding System (NFCS)] [31], three most frequent and typical expressions have been identified: brow bulge, eye squeeze, and nasolabial furrow [29, 32]. These facial displays have been included in many observational pain scales used to assess infant's pain.

According to neurological developmental principles, "excitability" precedes the capacity of the infant to self-regulate a response, and a vigorous behavioral reaction to a stimulus may reflect neurological maturity [33]. Thus, the absence of observational reactions to a noxious stimulus in a preterm neonate is an indicator of immaturity rather than no pain perception [34]. Moreover, in response to a noxious stimulation, a complex disposition at the spinal or brainstem level is required to enable an infant to display a visible facial expression; this requiring a coordinated motor neuron activity27. Reports of blunted behavioral cues of pain in preterm infants despite cerebral hemodynamic changes have stressed the importance of relying on other means of pain assessment indicators in populations with limited observable behavioral displays [28, 35, 36]. Slater et al. [28] described facial expression latency following a heel-lance procedure in preterm infants and reported that only 64 % of their sample displayed observable facial expression. Moreover, a significant effect of postmenstrual age upon the latency of pain behavior was shown.

Even though more than 40 pain assessment tools are available, no single instrument has demonstrated superiority over the others for use across varied painful conditions or clinical situations. Thus, no specific measure has been set as the "gold standard" for pain assessment of infants in research and clinical practice [37].

Of all of the pain measures developed for use in preterm and term neonates, the Premature Infant Pain Profile (PIPP) is perhaps the most well-known and clinically used multidimensional assessment instrument [38]. As such, it has been reported as being one of the most valid and reliable infant acute pain measure available. In a recent review evaluating their instrument, 13 years after its initial development, the authors were able to index 62 studies that reported having used the PIPP, thus contributing to its validation over the years [32]. Aside from being well established and having solid psychometric features, the particularity of the PIPP is that it includes two contextual variables, behavioral state and gestational age (GA), which have been shown to contribute to the pain response [30, 31, 39, 40]. Other examples of scales that take into account one of these factors are the multidimensional Neonatal Pain, Agitation, and Sedation Scale (N-PASS) [41] and the behavioral Neonatal Infant Pain Scale (NIPS) [42]. As mentioned previously, many acute pain assessment instruments have been developed with varying levels of psychometric testing; some having gone through only very basic testing. Following is a list of those that have published data, two are multidimensional (1, 2) and three behavioral (3–5) instruments: (1) Crying, Requires Increased oxygen, Increased vital signs, Expression, Sleeplessness (CRIES) [43]; (2) *Douleur aiguë du nouveau-né* (DAN) [44]; (3) Scale for Use in Newborn (SUN) [45]; (4) Pain Assessment

Table 91.1 Summary of neonatal pain scales

Type/context pain	Measurement scale	Validated age group
Procedural pain	CRIES	32 weeks–2 months
	DAN	Preterm–3 months
	PIPP	28 weeks–1 months
	NIPS	Premature–6 weeks
	N-PASS	Premature–3 months
	PAIN	26–47 weeks
	SUN	24–40 weeks
	BIIP	23–32 weeks
	DSVNI	37–40 weeks
Postoperative pain	CRIES	As above
	PIPP	
	N-PASS	
Prolonged pain	EDIN	Preterm–9 months

in Neonates scale (PAIN) [46]; and (5) Behavioral of Indicators of Infant Pain (BIIP) which includes two hand actions [47]. The multidimensional tool Distress Scale for Ventilated Newborn Infants (DSVNI) [48] is the first of its kind to focus specifically on ventilated newborn infants. The only scale developed to evaluate prolonged pain in preterm and term neonates until age of 6 to 9 months is the *Échelle de douleur et d'inconfort du nouveau-né* (EDIN) [49]. For a more comprehensive review of the various pain assessment tools developed for use in preterm and term infants, refer to review manuscripts (Table 91.1) [26, 50, 51].

To evaluate pain in critically ill infants, health-care professionals often rely upon unstable and nonspecific physiological indicators such as heart rate, arterial oxygen saturation, respiratory rate, and blood pressure. These parameters could be viewed as more "objective" or quantifiable than other more qualitative behavioral indicators. However, relying on physiological markers can lead to misinterpretation of pain intensity since they have been shown to decrease the internal consistency of many multidimensional pain assessment instruments, are not well correlated to behavioral indicators, and are not specific to the pain response [30, 52, 53]. Other physiological indicators lacking specificity that have been studied to assess stress and pain in neonates are cortisol level from saliva samples [54], skin conductance (palmar sweating) [55–58], and biomarkers such as analysis of heart rate variability [59].

In a sample of 149 infants undergoing an acute painful procedure, Stevens and others examined the factor structure of 19 pain indicators, both physiological and behavioral [29]. Facial actions accounted for a greater proportion of the variance (close to 40 %) with oxygen saturation, heart rate, cry, and heart rate variability accounting for lesser, but important, contributions of 8–26 % of the additional explained variance. As many physiological cues and some behavioral cues, such as crying, are not specific to pain, researchers and clinicians

are faced with the difficult task of discriminating between these to decide whether they are truly indicative of pain and not of other similarly manifested states, such as agitation, distress, anxiety, stress, or hunger.

Cortical Responses

As discussed previously, in addition to manifesting related states (i.e., stress, hunger, agitation, etc.) that can be difficult to distinguish from pain expressions, the fragile and immature condition of critically ill infants may lessen their capability to organize and exhibit perceived pain as a recognizable response. Consequently, clinical researchers have explored the use of associated signals to identify pain. The search for a more objective, specific, and sensitive means of measuring pain in this population is inspiring researchers to develop clinically applicable tools. Neuroimaging techniques are becoming more common in pain research; understanding the strengths and limitations of these approaches is important for professionals considering their application for the study and clinical management of pain in neonates. Although we may be far from clinically applicable instruments, promising results have been reported for the use of noninvasive electroencephalography (EEG) [36, 60, 61] and neuroimaging techniques to measure sensory input processing, such as in studies of somatosensory cortical activation [62]. As such, these novel approaches to measuring pain are beginning to provide validation for observational methods [27].

It has been demonstrated with near-infrared spectroscopy (NIRS) that cerebral hemodynamic changes (presumably due to cortical activation) occur in response to stressful and/or painful stimuli in term and preterm newborn infants [63–65]. NIRS is a noninvasive technique that detects subtle changes in the brain (or tissue) concentration of oxygenated and deoxygenated hemoglobin, which are inferred to reflect changes in cerebral metabolism and perfusion. An additional feature of NIRS, as compared to magnetic resonance imaging (MRI) and positron-emission tomography (PET) devices, is its portability directly to the bedside of these fragile patients which allows for continuous signal recording capable of capturing responses to intermittent stimuli.

The study of hemodynamic changes to assess the functional activation in the brain is based on the assumption that a given stimulus will induce a neuronal response which in turn triggers local vasodilation with an increase in cerebral blood volume (CBV) and cerebral blood flow (CBF) [66]. There have been significant advances in this field in the last decade; however, understanding of how blood flow, metabolism, and neuronal activity interact to affect the NIRS signals remains incomplete. Establishing validity of the NIRS measures has also proven difficult because few alternative technologies exist to serve as a gold standard 67. NIRS technology is sensitive to various factors that may confound results. Conditions related to critical illness that may result in metabolic somatosensory changes could confound pain-related activation measurement using NIRS. Patient movement can cause artifacts and disruptions in data collection. Although NIRS has excellent temporal resolution, it has poor spatial resolution when compared to other functional and structural imaging techniques such as MRI [67]. Therefore, it remains difficult to accurately identify the exact region that is sampled by the NIR light [68]. However, conducting multichannel functional NIRS trials allows for a more accurate mapping of cortical areas and improved discrimination [69] but remains difficult in preterm and term neonates to conduct due to their extremely small heads.

Although our understanding of the multidimensional experience of pain has advanced over the last century, many avenues remain unexplored. NIRS has potential as a noninvasive portable technique for assessing pain evoked cerebral activation in critically ill infants. However, given the complexity of NIRS technology, the paucity of research supporting its use in pain measurement in critically ill infants, and the need for tight control of many confounding factors as well as artifacts, more studies are clearly needed. At this stage, it is perhaps best to consider this neurodiagnostic technique, as well as others previously enumerated, solely as research tools that will improve our understanding of pain perception, increase the psychometric features of currently available pain assessment instruments, and perhaps assess the efficacy of pharmacological and non-pharmacological treatments.

Pharmacological Treatment of Procedural Pain

The most common drugs used to treat neonatal pain include topical and local anesthetics, acetaminophen, and opiates [70]. There are several difficulties with providing pharmacological treatments for procedural pain including safety concerns, insufficient data on specific neonatal pharmacokinetic and pharmacodynamics, difficulty in pain assessment, and lack of long-term neurodevelopmental follow-up. In addition, large variation in reported efficacy for procedural pain attenuation has limited their use in this population.

Topical Anesthetics

Topical anesthetics have been reasonably well researched in this population primarily related to several assumed benefits including noninvasive method of administration, lack of systemic effects, and potential for effectiveness. In an early review paper, Taddio and colleagues [71] evaluated the use

of lidocaine–prilocaine cream (EMLA®, Astra Pharma) compared to placebo in treating pain from heel lance, venipuncture, arterial puncture, lumbar puncture, percutaneous venous catheter placement, and circumcision in preterm and term infants. Nine randomized controlled trials (RCTs) were included. Unfortunately, for the most commonly performed procedure in the NICU, heel lance for blood procurement, EMLA was not shown to be beneficial. Similarly, in two later studies examining the effect of tetracaine 4 % gel (Ametop®, Smith & Nephew), on the pain of heel lance in both preterm and term newborns, no reduction in pain scores or duration of crying was noted between the groups [72, 73]. It has been postulated that variation in perfusion and skin thickness of an infant's heel may contribute to this ineffectiveness [74].

Similarly, the use of topical anesthetic has not been shown to be effective in diminishing pain associated with the insertion of intravenous lines or peripherally inserted central catheters (PICC) [75–77]. Some evidence was provided for the use of EMLA in relieving pain during venipuncture; however, results remain inconclusive. There have been five clinical trials examining the effect of topical anesthetic (EMLA and tetracaine 4 %) for pain associated with venipuncture [76, 78–81]. Results show that the application of local anesthetic could decrease the duration of cry but increase the procedure time [79], as well as being dose (0.5 vs. 1 ml) [78] and application time dependent (30 vs. 60 min) [76, 80].

There are no known contradictions to using preemptive local or topical anesthetics for lumbar puncture in neonates, and their use has been associated with increased success in obtaining cerebral spinal fluid (CFS) [82] and potential benefits related to a reduction in pain score and physiological stability [83]. In a randomized trial comparing the effect of lidocaine–prilocaine (EMLA) (1 g over 60–90 min) compared to placebo for 60 infants undergoing a lumbar puncture, infant in the intervention group had lower mean HR at needle insertion ($P = 0.001$) and needle withdrawal ($P < 0.001$) and lower total behavioral score again at insertion ($P < 0.004$) and needle withdrawal ($P < 0.001$) [84].

Currently, the most widely utilized local anesthetic for injection is lidocaine hydrochloride 1 %. It is effective as an adjuvant pain relieving strategy for lumbar puncture, chest tube insertion, and circumcision [85–89].

The use of EMLA to relieve pain caused by a frequently performed procedure in neonates, circumcision, has been shown to be more effective than placebo, as indicated by changes in physiological and behavioral pain indicators [86], and these findings were similar to a later Cochrane systematic review [71]. In another Cochrane review regarding pain relief for circumcision that included 35 trials involving 1,997 full-term and preterm infants, when compared to placebo, dorsal penile nerve block (DPNB), EMLA, and sweet taste all reduced pain response [90]. Of the six trials ($n = 190$) specifically examining EMLA compared to placebo, infants receiving EMLA demonstrated significantly lower facial action scores, decreased time crying, and lower heart rate. However, when EMLA and sweet taste were compared with DPNB, crying and elevation in heart rate were lowest in the DPNB group. Despite the large number of trials, small sample sizes, lack of blinding, large variations in practice, and little use of age appropriate validated pain tools limited the author's ability to make concise recommendations. The authors concluded that topical anesthetic in conjunction with DPNB as well as other pain relieving strategies could be safely implemented as part of routine practice related to circumcision.

Acetaminophen

Acetaminophen is one of the most commonly used analgesics for both mild ongoing pain and intermittent medical procedures [91]. Interestingly, despite its widespread use, there is limited evidence regarding its efficacy related to procedural pain alleviation in newborns [92–95]. Even at very high oral doses (40 mg/kg), it did not diminish the pain associated with heel lance [96]. The widespread use of prophylactic acetaminophen prior to immunization has been recently refuted, although its administration for local pain or swelling postinjections is still supported [97, 98].

The efficacy of intravenous acetaminophen has been better studied, and it appears to be beneficial for the relief of postoperative pain and act as an opioid sparing agent [99–101]. Its use for intermittent procedure pain has not been reported.

Opioids

Although opioids continue to be the mainstay in the neonatal intensive care unit (NICU) for the treatment of ongoing painful conditions such as necrotizing enterocolitis, operative procedures, and postoperative care, their use for more common single procedures performed in the NICU has been less promising [91]. Systemic administered drugs, specifically opioids, are highly sensitive to development [102, 103] and have significantly slower clearance in neonates [104–108]. Morphine and fentanyl are the predominate opioids used in hospitalized newborns with morphine being the most studied.

There have been conflicting reports regarding the efficacy and safety of intermittent and continuous intravenous infusions morphine for routine medical procedures and the stress associated with mechanical ventilation. Morphine does not appear to be beneficial for some of the commonly performed procedures in the NICU such as tracheal suctioning [109] or heel lance [110]. Validated pain scores were not significantly

different for 42 preterm infants, mean GA at birth of 27 weeks, randomized to receive a loading dose, and continuous infusion of morphine or placebo during heel lance over three time points [110]. Conversely, in an earlier study conducted by Anand [111], procedural pain (endotracheal suctioning) response was found to be much lower in the infants receiving morphine compared to placebo. Similarly in a much larger trial, pain scores in response to endotracheal suctioning were lower with morphine [112]. However, the incidence of longer duration of mechanical ventilation, hypotension, and severe intraventricular hemorrhage was higher in infants receiving more frequent intermittent doses of morphine regardless of assigned group.

In a systematic review of 13 RCTs examining the effectiveness of opioid analgesia in reducing the pain experienced from mechanical ventilation, the authors concluded that there was insufficient data to support the routine use of opioids in mechanically ventilated newborns [113]. The broad range of opioid dose and variation in type of analgesia in the trials also contributed to the findings. Of note, pain scores were significantly lower in four of the trials, and the authors did recommend that opioids should be used cautiously and in combination with well-validated pain scoring measures to evaluate their effectiveness. The authors also reported a higher incidence of hypotension and poorer neurodevelopmental outcome associated with midazolam compared to morphine. Therefore, if sedation is required, morphine appears to be a safer choice than midazolam.

There do appear to be some acutely painful conditions that warrant the use of morphine. Intravenous morphine was found to be more advantageous than topical application of tetracaine for the management of pain associated with insertion of a central venous catheter in neonates [75]. Remifentanil, a fast-acting opioid, has also been found to be analgesic for the insertion of a PICC. When compared to placebo, a 0.03 mcg/kg infusion of remifentanil significantly lowered the pain score of very preterm neonates undergoing insertion of a PICC. Mean pain scores [NIPS and PIPP] at skin preparation T1 and needle insertion T2 were significantly different to baseline T0 and recovery T3. No improvement was noted with respect to the number of attempts needed to successfully perform the procedure [114].

There is increasing consensus that opioids with rapid onset in combination with anticholinergics and muscle relaxants should be used for all infants undergoing elective intubation [115, 116]. In a review of nine trials, Shah [117] reported that the use of premedication was associated with a reduction in physiological pain indicators and intubation times. The most common and preferred agents reported were fentanyl, atropine, and rocuronium, although differences in medication and dosages were common across sites [118]. Morphine's slower onset of peak effect could contribute to its lack of efficacy [119]. Results from studies examining two synthetic agents, alfentanil and remifentanil, are promising [120, 121]. Ongoing research to determine the optimal dosage, administration route, and combination of medications as well as the long-term neurodevelopmental effects are warranted [118].

Alternate Strategies for the Treatment of Procedural Pain

Given the frequency of painful procedures in neonatal intensive care units and the difficulties with pharmacological management, the use of alternate or non-pharmacological strategies alone or as adjuvant management is highly recommended.

Alternate and non-pharmacological interventions that have been studied to relieve procedural pain in infants may be categorized in two main groups according to their nature. The earliest group of interventions studied focused on offering pleasant sensorial stimuli or manipulation of the infant's environmental boundaries such as oro-tactile stimulation as in the case of nonnutritive sucking (NNS), oro-gustatory stimulation by sweet solutions, containment and facilitated tucking, and vestibular stimulation, while investigation of the second group of interventions centered on maternal proximity such as breastfeeding and skin-to-skin (SSC) contact came later.

The exact mechanisms underlying the comforting effect of these interventions remains unclear, but it has been postulated that they involve both opioid and non-opioid-mediated systems, namely, the oxytocinergic system. Although there are scant data in neonates regarding endogenous descending, inhibitory mechanisms, the engagement of mechanisms that release endorphins is well established in adults [122, 123] There is a suggestion from the animal literature that the endogenous system is not well developed prior to 32 weeks postconception, but it is likely that it is well developed enough in neonates after 32 weeks, and possibly earlier, to provide some comfort [15, 124].

Oro-Tactile Stimulation by NNS

Sucking movements start in uterus around 12–14 weeks postconceptional age (PCA) [125], the sucking reflex develops around the 17th week postconception, and regular sucking activity is found in fetuses of 27–28 weeks PCA. NNS is stimulated in neonates by placing a pacifier in the infant's mouth.

Based on its effect in reducing fussing and crying in preterm infants in neonatal care [126], several studies have looked at NNS, comparing it to other interventions or no intervention in order to determine whether it decreases the responses of neonates to painful procedures. NNS has been found to reduce the increase in heart rate [127]; reduce crying time in term and preterm neonates [127–132], even in those who are intubated and ventilated [133]; and reduce pain scores [129, 131, 134–139].

Compared to swaddling, NNS after heel lance interrupted crying earlier (23.2 s vs. 58.7) and promoted a faster decline in heart rate although infants spent more time in an alert state (59 % of the time vs. 22 %, $P<0.01$) [140]. Compared to rocking, heart rate was also significantly reduced by NNS, but these infants slept more in the rocking group [128]. Compared to sucrose, glucose, and sucrose with pacifier, the median pain scores of term infants who received NNS for venipuncture was significantly lower (2) than that of infants who received sweet solutions (5). Although the scores with sucrose and pacifier (1) were the lowest, they were not significantly different from NNS alone ($P=0.06$) [136].

Adding other interventions to NNS appears to be beneficial. In a crossover trial, pacifier alone was compared to pacifier plus music therapy, music therapy alone, and no intervention during and after heel lance [139]. All three interventions improved the pain response, compared to no intervention, but NNS combined with music was associated with the lowest NIPS scores and the highest transcutaneous oxygen saturation ($TcPaO_2$) levels, while music therapy alone produced the lowest heart rate. Regarding the synergistic effect of simultaneously using NNS and sweet solutions, while adding a pacifier to sucrose or glucose seems to enhance the effect of sweet solutions used alone [130, 131], adding sucrose or glucose to a pacifier seems to provide no additional benefit than using a pacifier alone [134–138].

Including pacifier with glucose in a combined intervention named sensorial saturation (SS) that includes, besides taste, sight, touch, voice, and smell has shown to be more efficacious than glucose with pacifier in reducing the pain scores of term newborns during heel lance [137].

Oro-Gustatory Stimulation by Sweet Taste

The capacity of infants to distinguish between flavors, namely, sucrose, quinine, and corn oil has been demonstrated [141], and the calming effects of sweet taste have been known for a long time. Animal studies reinforce the evidence from studies in human infants that sucrose, glucose, and fructose but not lactose have a calming and pain-reducing effect, increasing the latency to withdraw from a heated surface in rat pups [142]. A recently updated Cochrane systematic review including 44 studies concluded that sucrose is efficacious and safe to use in single and repeated heel lances and should be considered for venipuncture since it significantly reduces pain behaviors and composite measures [143]. The authors of this review state that for other procedures such as eye examination for retinopathy of prematurity, bladder catheterization, nasogastric tube insertion, circumcision, and subcutaneous injections, further studies are required due to conflicting evidence and that the use of sucrose in extremely low birth weight and unstable and/or ventilated neonates needs to be addressed.

The recommended dose is a small volume of 0.05–0.5 ml of a 24 % sucrose solution for preterm neonates and 1–2 ml, administered 2 min prior to the painful procedure, for term neonates [143]. Concentrations of sucrose have varied from 12 to 50 %, but a ceiling effect seems to be reached at 25 % [144]. The most common method of administration is via syringe or dropper placing the solution on the anterior surface of the infants' tongue, but a pacifier dipped in a sucrose solution may also be used and is estimated to deliver approximately 0.1 ml [134]. The repeated use of sucrose for heel lance seems to not reduce its efficacy [144, 145]. Regarding concerns about long-term effects, one study has found a poorer neurobehavioral development in neonates younger than 31 weeks PCA [146]. However, a secondary analysis of the same data showed that increased risk occurred in neonates who had more than ten doses of sucrose in 24 h [147]. A subsequent study has found that infants who had procedural pain consistently managed by sucrose and pacifier in the first 28 days of life had no difference in adverse events or clinical outcomes such as intraventricular hemorrhage compared to infants who received no sucrose [148].

Glucose is another well-studied source of sweet taste. Its efficacy in a volume range of 0.3–2 ml of a 30 % solution has been shown for heel lance [149] and venipuncture [136, 150, 151], both in term [149, 150] and preterm [151] infants, as well as for subcutaneous injections in very preterm neonates (25–32 weeks GA) [152].

Comparisons between similar volumes and concentrations of sucrose and glucose show similar effects in reducing pain scores [126, 153–155], and both sucrose [156] and glucose [157] compare favorably to a topical anesthetic cream for venipuncture in full-term newborns.

Favoring Behavioral Organization Through Swaddling or Containment

Wrapping young infants in a cloth is part of the traditional way of care in many cultures [158]. An extensive systematic review of 78 studies evaluating the effects of swaddling, four of which examining pain control, concluded that it reduces crying, physiologic distress, and motor activity; increases sleep; and improves neuromuscular development in preterm infants [158]. Regarding pain control during heel lance, neonates over 30 weeks PCA returned to their baseline facial activity, heart rate, and arterial oxygen saturation levels more quickly [158]. A meta-analysis of four unpublished studies conducted in Thailand also supported the

efficacy of swaddling, with moderate to large mean effect sizes in full-term babies during heel lance [159].

Containment or facilitated tucking by holding the infant in a side lying position, arms and legs flexed near the trunk [160], also has been shown to reduce behavioral signs of distress of very low birth weight infants during heel lance [161], endotracheal suctioning [162], and pharyngeal suctioning [163]. Facilitated tucking seems to be more efficacious than water or oxycodone in reducing pain scores during pharyngeal suctioning and heel lance in very low birth weight infants and was equivalent to 0.2 ml of 24 % glucose but presents less short-term adverse effects, such as desaturation and/or bradycardia, than oral glucose [164]. In addition, in two studies, facilitated tucking was performed by parents, offering them an opportunity to participate in alleviating their infants' distress [163, 164].

Vestibular Stimulation

Rocking has also been a traditional way to calm infants and promote sleep. When compared to the use of a pacifier after heel lance in term infants, while both interventions reduced crying and can therefore be considered efficacious, rocking promoted arousal levels more than pacifiers, which promoted sleep [128]. A more recent trial compared rocking, expressed breast milk, 20 % sucrose, water, NNS, and massage in term, stable neonates [165]. Neonates were rocked by lifting the baby's head off the cot on the palm of the hand but not the body and making rocking movements in a gentle, rhythmic manner during and up till 2 min after heel lance. Like infants in the NNS group, infants who received rocking cried less and had lower pain scores at 2 and 4 min after the painful procedure, while infants in the sucrose group had a reduced pain score only at 30 sec [165]. Another trial in preterm infants during heel lance compared simulated rocking (infants in supine or side lying position on an oscillating air mattress), sucrose, usual incubator care with no intervention, and a combination of simulated rocking and sucrose [166, 167]. Simulated rocking combined with sucrose decreased facial expression by 40 % and so did sucrose alone, while simulated rocking was no better than incubator care, suggesting that the pain-reducing effect was related to the sucrose administration.

Auditory Stimulation

Human fetuses' capacity of perceiving sound at different frequencies and responding to them develops from 19 weeks of GA to term [167]. Their ability to learn and remember auditory stimuli from the intrauterine environment as early as 22 weeks GA has been put into evidence by conditioning studies [168].

It was demonstrated that infants as young as 3 days preferred their mothers' voice to the voice of another female [169], and exposure to familiar sounds has been associated to improved physiological stability [170]. The soothing effects of familiar sounds during painful procedures have been evaluated in a few trials. Maternal heart rate, Japanese drum with identical rhythm, and no sound were offered to 131 full-term infants who underwent heel lance [171]. Infants exposed to maternal heart beat had reduced facial response and crying, as well as lower levels of salivary cortisol. Following an identical rationale, 20 preterm infants 32–36 weeks were exposed to recorded and filtered maternal "singsong" voice or to no voice during a heel-lance procedure in a randomized crossover design [172]. No significant differences were found in pain scores between conditions, and the authors conclude that maternal voice alone, without other components of maternal presence, may not be enough to reduce pain response.

The effects of music to reduce pain have also been examined. A recent systematic review of RCTs of music for medical indications in the neonatal period found six studies that looked at painful procedures, three for circumcision and three for heel lance [173]. Only one of the studies on circumcision [174] had high-methodological quality and showed a lower pain score, lower heart rate increase, and higher arterial oxygen saturation levels, while the other two studies found no significant differences between groups. For heel lance, three trials were included but considered to have poor methodological quality [173]. One crossover trial with 27 infants 28 weeks GA or more found a significant decrease in heart rate and pain scores and an improvement in arterial oxygen saturation levels with music but also with music combined with NNS and with NNS alone [139]. Another crossover trial including 14 infants of 29–36 weeks PCA found a significant effect on heart rate, behavioral state, and pain scores only in infants over 31 weeks [175].

Auditory stimulation may be administered through different types of sounds, from music to direct or recorded maternal voice, or filtered voice and heart beat that would resemble the sound heard in the womb. Significant changes during the maturation process occurring in the last trimester of pregnancy with implication on the frequencies and levels of intensity that can be perceived by neonates of different GAs pose an important challenge when designing appropriate auditory interventions and methodologically sound studies.

Olfactory Stimulation

During their prenatal experience, human fetuses are exposed to the numerous compounds of the amniotic fluid, which play an active role in shaping the development of chemosensory sensitivity and preferences [176]. It has been demonstrated that newborns are able to discriminate odors and have

head-orientation behavior toward their own amniotic fluid, showing their preference for a familiar versus non familiar odor [177]. In preterm infants, responses elicited by odorants are weak and irregular at 24 weeks PCA but reliable by week 28 [176]. Given the soothing effect of the smell of amniotic fluid in term neonates separated from their mothers following birth [177], the effect of olfactory stimulation for painful procedures has gained increasing interest.

To determine the soothing effect of familiar and unfamiliar odor in full-term infants undergoing a routine heel lance, 44 breast-fed newborns were randomized to 4 groups [178]: (1) infants naturally familiarized with their mother's milk odor (2), infants previously familiarized with vanilla odor (3), infants not previously exposed to vanilla odor, and (4) infants who received no intervention. Results showed that the neonates in group 1 and 2 who received the odors during and after heel lance showed less distress during the recovery phase compared with the heel lance phase. Furthermore, the infants who were not exposed previously to the vanilla odor and those in the control group showed no difference in grimacing and cry during and after the heel lance. Babies who smelled their mother's milk exhibited significantly less motor agitation during the heel lance compared with the other groups. Whether familiarization to the odor was obtained through the mother or without the mother did not make a difference as shown in a replication of the previous study, in which the calming effects of familiar odor were visible during the heel-lance phase [179]. In healthy preterm newborns, a familiar odor compared to unfamiliar or no odor also reduced crying and grimacing [180]. A comparison between mother's milk, non-mother's milk, and formula milk given to healthy full-term neonates showed that crying, grimacing, and motor activity during heel lance were decreased only by exposure of the infant's own mother's milk [180].

Olfactory stimulation has been used in full-term and preterm infants during heel lance as a component of SS, an intervention that combines visual stimulation (looking the baby in the face to attract his attention), auditory stimulation (speaking to the infant gently but firmly), tactile stimulation (massaging the infant's face and back), and gustatory stimulation (glucose with pacifier) [137, 138, 181]. Within the original concept of SS, olfactory stimulation was provided by letting the infant smell the fragrance of baby oil on the therapist's hands [138], but a modified version without perfume has also shown to be effective in reducing pain scores of full-term healthy neonates [181]. Moreover, the modified intervention was shown to be more effective on a cry scale [182] than 1 ml of 30 % glucose with pacifier, raising questions regarding the importance of the olfactory component of SS.

The mechanism underlying the comforting effect of intrauterine, maternal, and familiarized smell remains unclear but it has been postulated that it is an opioid-mediated system. This hypothesis derives, on one hand, from knowledge that the taste system and the olfactory system are linked and that the antinociceptive effect of sweet taste is opioid mediated [183]. Conversely, animal studies indicated that the opioid system modulates olfactory learning and odor preferences [184].

Maternal Proximity

Breast Milk and Breastfeeding

The mother–infant dyad has an innate mutual bond that is key to survival. Infants actively mediate this bond by eliciting distress cues when separated from their mother that in turn heightens a mothers' instinctive need to protect and comfort their young. Therefore, it is not surprising that researchers returned to this basic human premise to investigate whether maternal presence could diminish the effects of repeated procedural pain exposure during prolonged hospitalization. The first studies followed the oro-gustatory research and focused on the use of breast milk or breastfeeding to attenuate the pain associated with common newborn procedures such as heel lance, venipuncture, and intramuscular injection. In a systematic review of eleven clinical trials, six examining the effectiveness of supplemental breast milk and five examining breastfeeding, breast milk giving orally by syringe was no different than water and significantly less beneficial than sweet taste in both full-term and preterm infants undergoing routine procedural pain from heel lance and venipuncture [185]. In contrast, breastfeeding when compared to placebo was shown to provide analgesia. In addition, when comparing to sweet taste, breastfeeding has been shown to be equivocal [186] and may even be superior [187]. Healthy term neonates (37–42 weeks of gestation at least 60 h old) undergoing heel lance for metabolic screening had lower median PIPP scores in the breastfeeding group (3.0) than those infants receiving 1 ml sucrose solution (8.5). The benefits of glucose and breastfeeding may be cumulative when provided simultaneously [188]. The efficacy of breastfeeding to diminish the painful effects of immunization appears to continue to at least 1 year of age. Consistent findings have been reported in three studies. Breast-fed infants when compared to controls experienced significantly shorter duration of crying, 35.85 vs. 76.24 s, $P=0.001$ [189] and 20.0 s (0–120) vs. 150.0 (0–180), $P=0.001$ [190] and 125.33 vs. 148.66 [191]. NIPS scores were also significantly reduced when infants were breast-feed, B 3.0 (0–6) vs. 6.0 (0–7), $P = 0.001$ [190].

Maternal contact is likely to be the mediating factor why breastfeeding when compared to supplemental breast milk alone is effective. During heel lance, infants being held by mother and breast-fed or being held by mother with pacifier cried significantly less (33 and 45 %) compared to being held by non-mother with pacifier (66 %, $P<0.01$ and $P=0.03$) [192].

SCC Contact

SSC between an infant and mother is also referred to as kangaroo mother care (KMC) due to its similarity to marsupial maternal care [193]. During KMC, a diaper-clad infant is held upright, at an angle of approximately 60°, between the mother's breasts, providing maximal skin-to-skin contact between baby and parent. Full skin contact and maternal presence have been shown to be beneficial for both term and preterm infants. Advantages for the infant are numerous: stable heart and respiratory rates, balanced thermoregulation, decreased apnea and periodic breathing, improved weight gain, accelerated maturation of the autonomic and circadian systems, and analgesia to painful therapeutic procedures [194–197]. KMC was originally implemented as an alternative to the incubator to maintain preterm infants' body temperature and increase survival rate in South America where incubators were in short supply [193]. During this time, it was serendipitously noted that infants spent more time in quiet sleep state [197, 199]. Since quiet state is associated with decreased pain response [31, 200], the idea developed to use KMC for procedural pain. In addition, it appeared that holding with skin-to-skin contact provided more comfort than holding with clothed body-to-skin contact [201]. The difference in skin-to-skin contact comfort may be related to inborn tactile receptor response and regulation of opiates, oxytocin, beta endorphins, and vagal tone [202, 203].

Initially studied in full-term neonates, 10–15 min of KMC prior to heel lance reduced crying by 82 %, grimacing by 65 %, and elevation in heart rate (8–10 vs. 36–38) compared to infants who stayed in a cot [204]. Later in the first study to examine the effects of KMC in preterm neonates, pain scores (PIPP) [32, 38], as well as the individual components of decreased facial action, heart rate acceleration, and increased arterial oxygen saturation changes, were reported as lower for the neonates who received KMC compared to those remaining in an incubator during heel lance [196]. Following these studies, numerous trials followed.

In a Cochrane review on skin-to-skin contact for procedural pain in infants, 13 studies that meet the inclusion criteria all show positive results [205]. KMC during heel lance significantly reduced pain scores in full- and in preterm neonates as young as 28 weeks GA [196, 206–210], as well as venipuncture [206] and intramuscular injection [211, 212]. KMC during heel lance has also been associated with a shortened duration of crying [213, 214], more robust heart rate variability [215], and better regulated neurobehavioral response assessed by the Newborn Individualized

Developmental Care and Assessment Program (NIDCAP) [216]. Of interest, two of those studies [210, 211] showed that KMC was more effective than sweet taste.

Summary

Pain in neonates is an important issue in particular as neonates are a vulnerable population due both to their helplessness, their inability to report verbally, and their highly developing nervous system. Although they cannot self-report, there are validated ways to measure their pain, and new techniques hold promise for further specificity. There is a need to search for safe analgesics for this population. Such searches should begin with infants and not extrapolate down from other populations. Endogenous mechanisms show somewhat surprising effectiveness for procedural pain. Being inexpensive and easily implemented, the use of these strategies should be implemented [116].

References

1. McGraw MB. Neural maturation as exemplified in the changing reactions of the infant to pin prick. Child Dev. 1941;12:31–42.
2. Owens ME. Pain in infancy: conceptual and methodological issues. Pain (Amsterdam). 1984;20:213–30.
3. Owens ME. Assessment of infant pain in clinical settings. J Pain Symptom Manag. 1986;1:29–31.
4. Johnston CC, Strada ME. Acute pain responses in infants: a multidimensional description. Pain (Amsterdam). 1986;24:373–82.
5. Anand KJ, Sippell WG, Aynsley-Green A. Randomised trial of fentanyl anaesthesia in preterm babies undergoing surgery: effects on the stress response. Lancet. 1987;1(8524):62–6.
6. Anand KJS, Craig KD. New perspectives on the definition of pain. Pain (Amsterdam). 1996;67:3–6.
7. Anand KJ, Hickey PR. Halothane-morphine compared with high-dose sufentanil for anesthesia and postoperative analgesia in neonatal cardiac surgery. N Engl J Med. 1992;326(1):1–9.
8. Anand KJS, Aynsley-Green A. Measuring severity of surgical stress in newborn infants. J Pediatr Surg. 1988;23:297–305.
9. Carbajal R, Rousset A, Danan C, et al. Epidemiology and treatment of painful procedures in neonates in intensive care units. JAMA. 2008;300(1):60–70.
10. Johnston CC, Barrington K, Taddio A, Carbajal R, Filion F. Pain in Canadian NICU's: have we improved over the past 12 years? Clin J Pain. 2010;27(3):225–32.
11. American Academy of P, Committee on F, Newborn, Canadian Paediatric S, Fetus, Newborn C. Prevention and management of pain in the neonate. [An update reprint of Pediatrics. 2006;118(5):2231–41; PMID: 17079598]. Adv Neonatal Care. 2007;7(3):151–160.
12. Simons SH, van Dijk M, Anand KS, Roofthooft D, van Lingen RA, Tibboel D. Do we still hurt newborn babies? A prospective study of procedural pain and analgesia in neonates. Arch Pediatr Adolesc Med. 2003;157(11):1058–64.
13. Stevens B, McGrath P, Gibbins S, et al. Procedural pain in newborns at risk for neurologic impairment. Pain (Amsterdam). 2003;105(1–2):27–35.
14. Fitzgerald M, Beggs S. The neurobiology of pain: developmental aspects. [Review] [120 refs]. Neuroscientist. 2001;7(3):246–57.
15. Fitzgerald M, Walker SM. Infant pain management: a developmental neurobiological approach. Nat Clin Pract Neurol. 2009; 5(1):35–50.
16. Grunau RE, Thanh Tu M. Long-term consequences of pain in human neonates. Anand KJS, Stevens BJ, McGrath PJ (ed.), 3rd editions, Pain Neonates and Infants: Elsevier 2007;3.
17. Fitzgerald M, Millard C, McIntosh N. Cutaneous hypersensitivity following peripheral tissue damage in newborn infants and its reversal with topical anaesthesia. Pain (Amsterdam). 1989;39: 31–6.
18. Johnston CC, Stevens BJ. Experience in a neonatal intensive care unit affects pain response. Pediatrics (Evanston IL). 1996;98(5): 925–30.
19. Grunau RE, Oberlander TF, Whitfield MF, Fitzgerald C, Lee SK. Demographic and therapeutic determinants of pain reactivity in very low birth weight neonates at 32 weeks' postconceptional age. Pediatrics (Evanston IL). 2001;107(1):105–12.
20. Grunau RE, Haley DW, Whitfield MF, Weinberg J, Yu W, Thiessen P. Altered basal cortisol levels at 3, 6, 8 and 18 months in infants born at extremely low gestational age. J Pediatr. 2007;150(2): 151–6.
21. Walker SM, Franck LS, Fitzgerald M, Myles J, Stocks J, Marlow N. Long-term impact of neonatal intensive care and surgery on somatosensory perception in children born extremely preterm. Pain. 2009;141(1–2):79–87.
22. Hermann C, Hohmeister J, Demirakca S, Zohsel K, Flor H. Long-term alteration of pain sensitivity in school-aged children with early pain experiences. Pain (Amsterdam). 2006;125(3): 278–85.
23. Hohmeister J, Demirakca S, Zohsel K, Flor H, Hermann C. Responses to pain in school-aged children with experience in a neonatal intensive care unit: cognitive aspects and maternal influences. Eur J Pain. 2009;13(1):94–101.
24. Goffaux P, Lafrenaye S, Morin M, Patural H, Demers G, Marchand S. Preterm births: can neonatal pain alter the development of endogenous gating systems? Eur J Pain. 2008;12(7):945–51.
25. Anand KJS, Hickey PR. Pain and its effects in the human neonate and fetus. N Engl J Med. 1987;19:1321–9.
26. Ranger M, Johnston CC, Anand KJ. Current controversies regarding pain assessment in neonates. Semin Perinatol. 2007;31(5): 283–8.
27. Slater R, Cantarella A, Franck L, Meek J, Fitzgerald M. How well do clinical pain assessment tools reflect pain in neonates? PLoS Med. 2008;5(6e129):0928–33.
28. Slater R, Cantarella A, Yoxen J, et al. Latency to facial expression change following noxious stimulation in infants is dependent on postmenstrual age. Pain. 2009;146(1–2):177–82.
29. Stevens B, Franck L, Gibbins S, et al. Determining the structure of acute pain responses in vulnerable neonates. Can J Nurs Res. 2007;39(2):32–47.
30. Craig KD, Whitfield MF, Grunau RV, Linton J, Hadjistavropoulos HD. Pain in the preterm neonate: behavioural and physiological indices. Pain (Amsterdam). 1993;52:287–99.
31. Grunau RVE, Craig KD. Pain expression in neonates: facial action and cry. Pain (Amsterdam). 1987;28:395–410.
32. Stevens B, Johnston C, Gibbins S, Taddio A, Yamada J. The premature infant pain profile (PIPP): evaluation 13 years after development. Clin J Pain. 2010;26(9):813–30.
33. Als H. Towards a synactive theory of development: promise for the assessment of infant individuality. Infant Ment Health J. 1982; 3:229–43.
34. Gibbins S, Stevens B, Beyene J, Chan PC, Bagg M, Asztalos E. Pain behaviours in extremely low gestational age infants. Early Hum Dev. 2008;84(7):451–8.
35. Slater R, Cantarella A, Gallella S, et al. Cortical pain responses in human infants. J Neurosci. 2006;26(14):3662–6.

36. Slater R, Fabrizi L, Worley A, Meek J, Boyd S, Fitzgerald M. Premature infants display increased noxious-evoked neuronal activity in the brain compared to healthy age-matched term-born infants. Neuroimage. 2010;52(2):583–9.

37. Anand KJ. Pain assessment in preterm neonates. Pediatrics (Evanston IL). 2007;119(3):605–7.

38. Stevens B, Johnston C, Petryshen P, Taddio A. Premature infant pain profile: development and initial validation. Clin J Pain. 1996;12(1):13–22.

39. Johnston CC, Stevens B, Craig KD, Grunau RV. Developmental changes in pain expression in premature, full-term, two- and four-month-old infants. Pain. 1993;52(2):201–8.

40. Stevens BJ, Johnston CC, Horton L. Factors that influence the behavioral pain responses of premature infants. Pain (Amsterdam). 1994;59(1):101–9.

41. Hummel P, Puchalski M, Creech SD, Weiss MG. Clinical reliability and validity of the N-PASS: neonatal pain, agitation and sedation scale with prolonged pain. J Perinatol. 2008;28(1):55–60.

42. Lawerence J, Alcock D, McGrath PJ, Kay J, MacMurray SB, Dulberg C. The development of a tool to assess neonatal pain. Neonatal Netw. 1993;12:59–66.

43. Krechel SW, Bildner J. CRIES: a new neonatal postoperative pain measurement score. Initial testing of validity and reliability. Paediatr Anaesth. 1995;5:53–61.

44. Carbajal R, Paupe A, Hoenn E, Lenclen R, Olivier M. APN: evaluation behavioral scale of acute pain in newborn infants. [French]. Arch Pediatr. 1997;4(7):623–8.

45. Blauer T, Gerstmann D. A simultaneous comparison of three neonatal pain scales during common NICU procedures. Clin J Pain. 1998;14(1):39–47.

46. Hudson-Barr D, Capper-Michel B, Lambert S, Palermo TM, Morbeto K, Lombardo S. Validation of the Pain Assessment in Neonates (PAIN) scale with the Neonatal Infant Pain Scale (NIPS). Neonatal Netw. 2002;21(6):15–21.

47. Holsti L, Grunau RE. Initial validation of the behavioral indicators of infant pain (BIIP). Pain (Amsterdam). 2007;132(3):264–72.

48. Sparshott M. The development of a clinical distress scale for ventilated newborn infants: identification of pain and distress based on validated behavioural scores. J Neonatal Nurs. 1996;2:5–11.

49. Debillon T, Zupan V, Ravault N, Magny JF, Dehan M. Development and initial validation of the EDIN scale, a new tool for assessing prolonged pain in preterm infants. Arch Dis Child Fetal Neonatal Ed. 2001;85(1):F36–41.

50. Stevens BJ, Pillai Riddell R, Oberlander TE, Gibbins S, Anand KJS, McGrath PJ. Assessment of pain in neonates and infants, Pain in neonates and infants, vol. 3. Toronto: Elsevier; 2007. p. 67–90.

51. Duhn LJ, Medves JM. A systematic integrative review of infant pain assessment tools. [Review] [71 refs]. Adv Neonatal Care. 2004;4(3):126–40.

52. Johnston CC, Stevens BJ, Yang F, Horton L. Differential response to pain by very premature neonates. Pain. 1995;61(3):471–9.

53. Sweet SD, McGrath PJ. Physiological measures of pain. In: Finley GA, McGrath PJ, editors. Measurement of pain in infants and children. Seattle: IASP Press; 1998. p. 59–81.

54. Grunau RE, Holsti L, Haley DW, et al. Neonatal procedural pain exposure predicts lower cortisol and behavioral reactivity in preterm infants in the NICU. Pain. 2005;113(3):293–300.

55. Harrison D, Boyce S, Loughnan P, Dargaville P, Storm H, Johnston L. Skin conductance as a measure of pain and stress in hospitalised infants. Early Hum Dev. 2006;82(9):603–8.

56. Hellerud BC, Storm H. Skin conductance and behaviour during sensory stimulation of preterm and term infants. Early Hum Dev. 2002;70(1–2):35–46.

57. Storm H. Development of emotional sweating in preterms measured by skin conductance changes. Early Hum Dev. 2001;62(2):149–58.

58. Eriksson M, Storm H, Fremming A, Schollin J. Skin conductance compared to a combined behavioural and physiological pain measure in newborn infants. Acta Paediatr. 2008;97(1):27–30.

59. Oberlander T, Saul JP. Methodological considerations for the use of heart rate variability as a measure of pain reactivity in vulnerable infants. Clin Perinatol. 2002;29(3):427–43.

60. Slater R, Worley A, Fabrizi L, et al. Evoked potentials generated by noxious stimulation in the human infant brain. Eur J Pain. 2009;14(3):321–6.

61. Slater R, Cornelissen L, Fabrizi L, et al. Oral sucrose as an analgesic drug for procedural pain in newborn infants: a randomised controlled trial. Lancet. 2010;376(9748):1225–32.

62. Lagercrantz H. The birth of consciousness. Early Hum Dev. 2009;85(10 Suppl):S57–8.

63. Slater R, Boyd S, Meek J, Fitzgerald M. Cortical pain responses in the infant brain. Pain. 2006;123(3):332–4.

64. Bartocci M, Bergqvist LL, Lagercrantz H, Anand KJ. Pain activates cortical areas in the preterm newborn brain. Pain (Amsterdam). 2006;122(1–2):109–17.

65. Limperopoulos C, Gauvreau K, O'Leary H, Bassan H, Eichenwald EC, Ringer S. Cerebral hemodynamic changes during intensive care of premature infants. Pediatrics (Evanston IL). 2008;122(5):e1006–13.

66. Soul JS, du Plessis AJ. New technologies in pediatric neurology. Near-infrared spectroscopy. [Review] [53 refs]. Semin Pediatr Neurol. 1999;6(2):101–10.

67. Wolfberg AJ, du Plessis AJ. Near-infrared spectroscopy in the fetus and neonate. [Review] [110 refs]. Clin Perinatol. 2006;33(3):707–28.

68. Hoshi Y. Functional near-infrared optical imaging: utility and limitations in human brain mapping. Psychophysiology. 2003;40(4):511–20.

69. Becerra L, Harris W, Joseph D, Huppert T, Boas DA, Borsook D. Diffuse optical tomography of pain and tactile stimulation: activation in cortical sensory and emotional systems. Neuroimage. 2008;41(2):252–9.

70. Hall RW, Shbarou RM. Drugs of choice for sedation and analgesia in the neonatal ICU. Clin Perinatol. 2009;36(1):15–26.

71. Taddio A, Ohlsson A, Einarson TR, Stevens B, Koren G. A systematic review of lidocaine-prilocaine cream (EMLA) in the treatment of acute pain in neonates. Pediatrics. 1998;101(2):E1.

72. Jain A, Rutter N. Local anaesthetic effect of topical amethocaine gel in neonates: randomised controlled trial. Arch Dis Child Fetal Neonatal Ed. 2000;82(1):F42–5.

73. Larsson BA, Jylli L, Lagercrantz H, Olsson GL. Does a local anaesthetic cream (EMLA) alleviate pain from heel-lancing in neonates? Acta Anaesthesiol Scand. 1995;39(8):1028–31.

74. Larsson BA, Norman M, Bjerring P, Egekvist H, Lagercrantz H, Olsson GL. Regional variations in skin perfusion and skin thickness may contribute to varying efficacy of topical, local anaesthetics in neonates. Paediatr Anaesth. 1996;6:107–10.

75. Taddio A, Lee C, Yip A, Parvez B, McNamara PJ, Shah V. Intravenous morphine and topical tetracaine for treatment of pain in [corrected] neonates undergoing central line placement. [Erratum appears in JAMA. 2006;295(13):1518]. J Am Med Assoc. 2006;295(7):793–800.

76. Lemyre B, Hogan DL, Gaboury I, Sherlock R, Blanchard C, Moher D. How effective is tetracaine 4% gel, before a venipuncture, in reducing procedural pain in infants: a randomized double-blind placebo controlled trial. BMC Pediatr. 2007;7:7.

77. Ballantyne M, McNair C, Ung E, Gibbins S, Stevens B. A randomized controlled trial evaluating the efficacy of tetracaine gel for pain relief from peripherally inserted central catheters in infants. Adv Neonatal Care. 2003;3(6):297–307.

78. Lindh V, Wiklund U, Hakansson S. Assessment of the effect of EMLA during venipuncture in the newborn by analysis of heart rate variability. Pain. 2000;86(3):247–54.

79. Larsson BA, Tannfeldt G, Lagercrantz H, Olsson GL. Venipuncture is more effective and less painful than heel lancing for blood tests in neonates. Pediatrics (Evanston IL). 1998;101(5):882–6.

80. Jain A, Rutter N. Does topical amethocaine gel reduce the pain of venipuncture in newborn infants? A randomised double blind controlled trial. Arch Dis Child Fetal Neonatal Ed. 2000;83(3): F207–10.

81. Acharya AB, Bustani PC, Phillips JD, Taub NA, Beattie RM. Randomised controlled trial of eutectic mixture of local anaesthetics cream for venipuncture in healthy preterm infants. Arch Dis Child Fetal Neonatal Ed. 1998;78(2):F138–42.

82. Quinn M, Carraccio C, Sacchetti A. Pain, punctures, and pediatricians. Pediatr Emerg Care. 1993;9:12–4.

83. Pinheiro JM, Furdon S, Ochoa LF. Role of local anesthesia during lumbar puncture in neonates. Pediatrics. 1993;91(2):379–82.

84. Kaur G, Gupta P, Kumar A. A randomized trial of eutectic mixture of local anesthetics during lumbar puncture in newborns. Arch Pediatr Adolesc Med. 2003;157(11):1065–70.

85. Brady-Fryer B, Wiebe N, Lander JA. Pain relief for neonatal circumcision. [Review] [99 refs]. Cochrane Database Syst Rev. 2004;4:CD004217..

86. Benini F, Johnston CC, Faucher DJ, Aranda JV. Topical anesthesia during circumcision in newborn infants. J Am Med Assoc. 1993;270:850–3.

87. Taddio A, Stevens B, Craig K, et al. Efficacy and safety of lidocaine-prilocaine cream for pain during circumcision. N Engl J Med. 1997;336(17):1197–201.

88. Lehr VT, Taddio A. Topical anesthesia in neonates: clinical practices and practical considerations. Semin Perinatol. 2007;31(5): 323–9.

89. Yamada J, Stinson J, Lamba J, Dickson A, McGrath PJ, Stevens B. A review of systematic reviews on pain interventions in hospitalized infants. Pain Res Manag. 2008;13(5):413–20.

90. Brady-Fryer B, Wiebe N, Lander JA. Pain relief for neonatal circumcision. Cochrane Database Syst Rev. 2008;1.

91. Anand KJ, Johnston CC, Oberlander TF, Taddio A, Lehr VT, Walco GA. Analgesia and local anesthesia during invasive procedures in the neonate. Clin Ther. 2005;27(6):844–76.

92. Shah V, Taddio A, Ohlsson A. Randomised controlled trial of paracetamol for heel prick pain in neonates. Arch Dis Child Fetal Neonatal Ed. 1998;79(3):F209–11.

93. Macke JK. Analgesia for circumcision: effects on newborn behavior and mother/infant interaction. J Obstet Gynecol Neonatal Nurs. 2001;30(5):507–14.

94. Howard CR, Howard FM, Weitzman ML. Acetaminophen analgesia in neonatal circumcision: the effect on pain. Pediatrics (Evanston IL). 1994;4:641–6.

95. Taddio A, Manley J, Potash L, Ipp M, Sgro M, Shah V. Routine immunization practices: use of topical anesthetics and oral analgesics. Pediatrics (Evanston IL). 2007;120(3):e637–43.

96. Badiee Z, Torcan N. Effects of high dose orally administered paracetamol for heel prick pain in premature infants. Saudi Med J. 2009;30(11):1450–3.

97. Manley J, Taddio A. Acetaminophen and ibuprofen for prevention of adverse reactions associated with childhood immunization. [Review] [16 refs]. Ann Pharmacother. 2007;41(7):1227–32.

98. Prymula R, Siegrist CA, Chlibek R, et al. Effect of prophylactic paracetamol administration at time of vaccination on febrile reactions and antibody responses in children: two open-label, randomised controlled trials. Lancet. 2009;374(9698):1339–50.

99. Agrawal S, Fitzsimons JJ, Horn V, Petros A. Intravenous paracetamol for postoperative analgesia in a 4-day-old term neonate. Paediatr Anaesth. 2007;17(1):70–1.

100. Prins SA, Van Dijk M, Van Leeuwen P, et al. Pharmacokinetics and analgesic effects of intravenous propacetamol vs rectal paracetamol in children after major craniofacial surgery. Paediatr Anaesth. 2008;18(7):582–92.

101. Wilson-Smith EM, Morton NS. Survey of i.v. paracetamol (acetaminophen) use in neonates and infants under 1 year of age by UK anesthetists. Paediatr Anaesth. 2009;19(4):329–37.

102. Nandi R, Beacham D, Middleton J, Koltzenburg M, Howard RF, Fitzgerald M. The functional expression of mu opioid receptors on sensory neurons is developmentally regulated; morphine analgesia is less selective in the neonate. Pain. 2004;111(1–2):38–50.

103. Nandi R, Fitzgerald M. Opioid analgesia in the newborn. Euro J Pain: EJP. 2005;9(2):105–8.

104. Allegaert K, Simons SH, Vanhole C, Tibboel D. Developmental pharmacokinetics of opioids in neonates. [Review] [31 refs]. J Opioid Manag. 2007;3(1):59–64.

105. Bouwmeester NJ, Anderson BJ, Tibboel D, Holford NH. Developmental pharmacokinetics of morphine and its metabolites in neonates, infants and young children. Br J Anaesth. 2004;92(2): 208–17.

106. Lynn AM, Slattery JT. Morphine pharmacokinetics in early infancy. Anaesthesia. 1987;66:136–9.

107. Zuppa AF, Mondick JT, Davis L, Cohen D. Population pharmacokinetics of ketorolac in neonates and young infants. Am J Ther. 2009;16(2):143–6.

108. Koren G. Postoperative morphine infusion in newborn infants: assessment of disposition. J Pediatr. 1985;107:963–7.

109. Simons SH, van Dijk M, van Lingen RA, et al. Routine morphine infusion in preterm newborns who received ventilatory support: a randomized controlled trial. JAMA. 2003;290(18):2419–27.

110. Carbajal R, Lenclen R, Jugie M, Paupe A, Barton BA, Anand KJ. Morphine does not provide adequate analgesia for acute procedural pain among preterm neonates. Pediatrics. 2005;115(6): 1494–500.

111. Anand KJ, Barton BA, McIntosh N, et al. Analgesia and sedation in preterm neonates who require ventilatory support: results from the NOPAIN trial. Neonatal Outcome and Prolonged Analgesia in Neonates [Published erratum appears in Arch Pediatr Adolesc Med. 1999;153(8):895]. Arch Pediatr Adolesc Med. 1999;153(4): 331–338.

112. Anand KJ, Hall RW, Desai N, et al. Effects of morphine analgesia in ventilated preterm neonates: primary outcomes from the NEOPAIN randomised trial. Lancet. 2004;363(9422): 1673–82.

113. Bellu R, de Waal KA, Zanini R. Opioids for neonates receiving mechanical ventilation. Cochrane Database Syst Rev. 2005;1: CD004212.

114. Lago P, Tiozzo C, Boccuzzo G, Allegro A, Zacchello F. Remifentanil for percutaneous intravenous central catheter placement in preterm infant: a randomized controlled trial. Paediatr Anaesth. 2008;18(8):736–44.

115. Lago P, Garetti E, Merazzi D, et al. Guidelines for procedural pain in the newborn. Acta Paediatr. 2009;98(6):932–9.

116. American Academy of Pediatrics Committee on F, Newborn, American Academy of Pediatrics Section on S, et al. Prevention and management of pain in the neonate: an update. Pediatrics (Evanston IL). 2006;118(5):2231–41.

117. Shah V, Ohlsson A. The effectiveness of premedication for endotracheal intubation in mechanically ventilated neonates. A systematic review. Clinics Perinatol. 2002;29(3):535–54.

118. Kumar P, Denson SE, Mancuso TJ. Premedication for nonemergency endotracheal intubation in the neonate. Pediatrics. 2010; 125(3):608–15.

119. Lemyre B, Doucette J, Kalyn A, Gray S, Marrin ML. Morphine for elective endotracheal intubation in neonates: a randomized trial [ISRCTN43546373]. BMC Pediatr. 2004;4(1):20.

120. Choong K, AlFaleh K, Doucette J, et al. Remifentanil for endotracheal intubation in neonates: a randomised controlled trial. Arch Dis Child Fetal Neonatal Ed. 2010;95(2):F80–4.

121. Pereira e Silva Y, Gomez RS, Marcatto Jde O, Maximo TA, Barbosa RF, Silva AC Simoes e. Morphine versus remifentanil for intubating preterm neonates. Arch Dis Child Fetal Neonatal Ed. 2007;92(4):F293–4.

122. Melzack R, Wall P. Pain mechanisms: new theory. Science (Washington DC). 1965;150:971–9.

123. Benedetti F. Placebo and endogenous mechanisms of analgesia. Handb Exp Pharmacol. 2007;177:393–413.

124. Fitzgerald M, Millard C, MacIntosh N. Hyperalgesia in premature infants. Lancet (London). 1988;1(8580):292.

125. de Vries JIP, Visser GH, Prechtl HF. The emergence of fetal behaviour. I. Qualitative aspects. Early Hum Dev. 1982;7(4):301–22.

126. Pinelli J, Symington A. Non-nutritive sucking for promoting physiologic stability and nutrition in preterm infants [Systematic Review]. Cochrane Database Syst Rev 2007;1.

127. Corbo MG, Mansi G, Stagni A, et al. Nonnutritive sucking during heelstick procedures decreases behavioral distress in the newborn infant. Biol Neonate. 2000;77(3):162–7.

128. Campos RG. Rocking and pacifiers: two comforting interventions for heelstick pain. Res Nurs Health. 1994;17(5):321–31.

129. Elserafy FA, Alsaedi SA, Louwrens J, Mersal AY, Bin Sadiq B. Oral sucrose and a pacifier for pain relief during simple procedures in preterm infants: a randomized controlled trial. Ann Saudi Med. 2009;29(3):184–8.

130. Curtis SJ, Jou H, Ali S, Vandermeer B, Klassen T. A randomized controlled trial of sucrose and/or pacifier as analgesia for infants receiving venipuncture in a pediatric emergency department. BMC Pediatr. 2007;7:27.

131. Akman I, Ozek E, Bilgen H, Ozdogan T, Cebeci D. Sweet solutions and pacifiers for pain relief in newborn infants. J Pain. 2002;3(3):199–202.

132. Field T, Goldson E. Pacifying effects of nonnutritive sucking on term and preterm neonates during heelstick procedures. Pediatrics (Evanston IL). 1984;74:1012–5.

133. Miller HD, Anderson GC. Nonnutritive sucking: effects on crying and heart rate in intubated infants requiring assisted mechanical ventilation. Neonatal Intensive Care. 1994;46–48.

134. Stevens B, Johnston C, Franck L, Petryshen P, Jack A, Foster G. The efficacy of developmentally sensitive interventions and sucrose for relieving procedural pain in very low birth weight neonates. Nurs Res. 1999;48(1):35–43.

135. Boyle EM, Freer Y, Khan-Orakzai Z, et al. Sucrose and non-nutritive sucking for the relief of pain in screening for retinopathy of prematurity: a randomised controlled trial. Arch Dis Child Fetal Neonatal Ed. 2006;91(3):F166–8.

136. Carbajal R, Chauvet X, Couderc S, Olivier-Martin M. Randomised trial of analgesic effects of sucrose, glucose, and pacifiers in term neonates [see comments]. Br Med J. 1999;319(7222):1393–7.

137. Bellieni CV, Bagnoli F, Perrone S, et al. Effect of multisensory stimulation on analgesia in term neonates: a randomized controlled trial. Pediatr Res. 2002;51(4):460–3.

138. Bellieni CV, Buonocore G, Nenci A, Franci N, Cordelli DM, Bagnoli F. Sensorial saturation: an effective analgesic tool for heel-prick in preterm infants: a prospective randomized trial. Biol Neonate. 2001;80(1):15–8.

139. Bo LK, Callaghan P. Soothing pain-elicited distress in Chinese neonates. Pediatrics (Evanston IL). 2000;105(4):E49.

140. Campos RG. Soothing pain elicited distress in infants with swaddling and pacifiers. Child Dev. 1989;60:781–92.

141. Graillon A, Barr RG, Young SN, Wright JH, Hendricks LA. Differential response to intraoral sucrose, quinine and corn oil in crying human newborns. Physiol Behav. 1997;62(2):317–25.

142. Blass EM, Ciaramitaro V. A new look at some old mechanisms in human newborns: taste and tactile determinants of state, affect, and action. Monogr Soc Res Child Dev. 1994;59:1–80.

143. Stevens B, Yamada J, Ohlsson A. Sucrose for analgesia in newborn infants undergoing painful procedures. Cochrane Database Syst Rev. 2010;1:CD001069.

144. Gaspardo CM, Miyase CI, Chimello JT, Martinez FE, Martins Linhares MB. Is pain relief equally efficacious and free of side effects with repeated doses of oral sucrose in preterm neonates? Pain. 2008;137(1):16–25.

145. Harrison D, Loughnan P, Manias E, Gordon I, Johnston L. Repeated doses of sucrose in infants continue to reduce procedural pain during prolonged hospitalizations. Nurs Res. 2009;58(6):427–34.

146. Johnston CC, Filion F, Snider L, et al. Routine sucrose analgesia during the first week of life in neonates younger than 31 weeks' postconceptional age. Pediatrics. 2002;110(3):523–8.

147. Johnston CC, Filion F, Snider L, et al. How much sucrose is too much sucrose? Pediatrics (Evanston IL). 2007;119(1):226.

148. Stevens B, Yamada J, Beyene J, et al. Consistent management of repeated procedural pain with sucrose in preterm neonates: is it effective and safe for repeated use over time? Clin J Pain. 2005;21(6):543–8.

149. Akcam M, Ormeci AR. Oral hypertonic glucose spray: a practical alternative for analgesia in the newborn. Acta Paediatr. 2004;93(10):1330–3.

150. Eriksson M, Gradin M, Schollin J. Oral glucose and venipuncture reduce blood sampling pain in newborns. Early Hum Dev. 1999;55(3):211–8.

151. Deshmukh LS, Udani RH. Analgesic effect of oral glucose in preterm infants during venipuncture–a double-blind, randomized, controlled trial. J Trop Pediatr. 2002;48(3):138–41.

152. Carbajal R, Lenclen R, Gajdos V, Jugie M, Paupe A. Crossover trial of analgesic efficacy of glucose and pacifier in very preterm neonates during subcutaneous injections. Pediatrics. 2002;110(2 Pt 1):389–93.

153. Okan F, Coban A, Ince Z, Yapici Z, Can G. Analgesia in preterm newborns: the comparative effects of sucrose and glucose. Eur J Pediatr. 2007;166(10):1017–24.

154. Guala A. Glucose or sucrose as an analgesic for newborns: a randomised controlled blind trial. Minerva Pediatr. 2001;53(4):271–4.

155. Isik U. Comparison of oral glucose and sucrose solutions on pain response in neonates. J Pain. 2000;1(4):275–8.

156. Abad F, Diaz-Gomez NM, Domenech E, Gonzalez D, Robayna M, Feria M. Oral sucrose compares favourably with lidocaine-prilocaine cream for pain relief during venipuncture in neonates. Acta Paediatr. 2001;90(2):160–5.

157. Gradin M, Eriksson M, Holmqvist G, Holstein A, Schollin J. Pain reduction at venipuncture in newborns: oral glucose compared with local anesthetic cream. Pediatrics. 2002;110(6):1053–7.

158. van Sleuwen BE, Engelberts AC, Boere-Boonekamp MM, Kuis W, Schulpen TW, L'Hoir MP. Swaddling: a systematic review. [Review] [82 refs]. Pediatrics (Evanston IL). 2007;120(4):e1097–106.

159. Prasopkittikun T, Tilokskulchai F. Management of pain from heel stick in neonates: an analysis of research conducted in Thailand. J Perinat Neonatal Nurs. 2003;17(4):304–12.

160. Huang CM, Tung WS, Kuo LL, Ying-Ju C. Comparison of pain responses of premature infants to the heelstick between containment and swaddling. J Nurs Res. 2004;12(1):31–40.

161. Corff KE, Seideman R, Venkataraman PS, Lutes L, Yates B. Facilitated tucking: a nonpharmacologic comfort measure for pain in preterm neonates. J Obstet Gynecol Neonatal Nurs. 1995;24(2):143–7.

162. Ward-Larson C, Horn RA, Gosnell F. The efficacy of facilitated tucking for relieving procedural pain of endotracheal suctioning in very low birthweight infants. MCN Am J Matern Child Nurs. 2004;29(3):151–6. quiz 157–158.

163. Axelin A, Salantera S, Lehtonen L. 'Facilitated tucking by parents' in pain management of preterm infants-a randomized crossover trial. Early Hum Dev. 2006;82(4):241–7.

164. Axelin A, Salantera S, Kirjavainen J, Lehtonen L. Oral glucose and parental holding preferable to opioid in pain management in preterm infants. Clin J Pain. 2009;25(2):138–45.

165. Mathai S, Natrajan N, Rajalakshmi NR. A comparative study of nonpharmacological methods to reduce pain in neonates. Indian Pediatr. 2006;43(12):1070–5.

166. Johnston CC, Stremler RL, Stevens BJ, Horton LJ. Effectiveness of oral sucrose and simulated rocking on pain response in preterm neonates. Pain. 1997;72(1–2):193–9.

167. Hepper PG, Shahidullah BS. Development of fetal hearing. Arch Dis Child. 1994;71(2):F81–7.

168. Hepper PG. Fetal memory: does it exist? What does it do? [Review] [59 refs]. Acta Paediatr Suppl. 1996;416:16–20.

169. DeCasper AJ, Fifer WP. Of human bonding: newborns prefer their mothers voices. Science (Washington DC). 1980;208:1174–6.

170. Standley JM, Moore RS. Therapeutic effects of music and mother's voice on premature infants. Pediatr Nurs. 1995;21(6):509–12. 574.

171. Kurihara H, Chiba H, Shimizu Y, et al. Behavioral and adrenocortical responses to stress in neonates and the stabilizing effects of maternal heartbeat on them. Early Hum Dev. 1996;46(1–2):117–27.

172. Johnston CC, Filion F, Nuyt AM. Recorded maternal voice for preterm neonates undergoing heel lance. Adv Neonatal Care. 2007;7(5):258–66.

173. Hartling L, Shaik MS, Tjosvold L, Leicht R, Liang Y, Kumar M. Music for medical indications in the neonatal period: a systematic review of randomised controlled trials. Arch Dis Child Fetal Neonatal Ed. 2009;94(5):F349–54.

174. Joyce BA, Keck JF, Gerkensmeyer J. Evaluation of pain management interventions for neonatal circumcision pain. J Pediatr Health Care. 2001;15(3):105–14.

175. Butt ML, Kisilevsky BS. Music modulates behaviour of premature infants following heel lance. Can J Nurs Res. 2000;31(4):17–39.

176. Schaal B, Marlier L, Soussignan R. Olfactory function in the human fetus: evidence from selective neonatal responsiveness to the odor of amniotic fluid. Behav Neurosci. 1998;112(6):1438–49.

177. Varendi H, Christensson K, Porter RH, Winberg J. Soothing effect of amniotic fluid smell in newborn infants. Early Hum Dev. 1998;51(1):47–55.

178. Rattaz C, Goubet N, Bullinger A. The calming effect of a familiar odor on full-term newborns. J Dev Behav Pediatr. 2005;26(2):86–92.

179. Goubet N, Strasbaugh K, Chesney J. Familiarity breeds content? Soothing effect of a familiar odor on full-term newborns. J Dev Behav Pediatr. 2007;28(3):189–94.

180. Goubet N, Rattaz C, Pierrat V, Bullinger A, Lequien P. Olfactory experience mediates response to pain in preterm newborns. Dev Psychobiol. 2003;42(2):171–80.

181. Bellieni CV, Cordelli DM, Marchi S, et al. Sensorial saturation for neonatal analgesia. Clin J Pain. 2007;23(3):219–21.

182. Bellieni C, Maffei M, Ancora G, et al. Is the ABC pain scale reliable for premature babies? Acta Paediatr. 2007;96(7):1008–10.

183. Gibbins S, Stevens B. Mechanisms of sucrose and non-nutritive sucking in procedural pain management in infants. Pain Res Manag. 2001;6(1):21–8.

184. Jahangeer AC, Mellier D, Caston J. Influence of olfactory stimulation on nociceptive behavior in mice. Physiol Behav. 1997;62(2):359–66.

185. Shah PS, Aliwalas LL, Shah V. Breastfeeding or breast milk for procedural pain in neonates. Cochrane Database Syst Rev. 2008;1.

186. Carbajal R, Veerapen S, Couderc S. Breastfeeding as an analgesic for term newborns during venipunctures. Proc Acad Pediatr Soc. 2002;2105

187. Codipietro L, Ceccarelli M, Ponzone A. Breastfeeding or oral sucrose solution in term neonates receiving heel lance: a randomized, controlled trial. Pediatrics (Evanston IL). 2008;122(3):e716–21.

188. Gradin M, Finnstrom O, Schollin J. Feeding and oral glucose–additive effects on pain reduction in newborns. Early Hum Dev. 2004;77(1–2):57–65.

189. Efe E, Ozer ZC. The use of breast-feeding for pain relief during neonatal immunization injections. Appl Nurs Res. 2007;20(1):10–6.

190. Dilli DK, Küçük IG, Dallar Y. Interventions to reduce pain during vaccination in infancy. J Pediatr. 2009;154(3):385–90.

191. Abdel Razek A, Az El-Dein N. Effect of breast-feeding on pain relief during infant immunization injections. Int J Nurs Pract. 2009;15(2):99–104.

192. Phillips RM, Chantry CJ, Gallagher MP. Analgesic effects of breast-feeding or pacifier use with maternal holding in term infants. Ambul Pediatr. 2005;5(6):359–64.

193. Charpak N, Ruiz-Pelaez JG, Charpak Y. Rey-Martinez kangaroo mother program: an alternative way of caring for low birth weight infants? One year mortality in a two cohort study. Pediatrics (Evanston IL). 1994;94(6:Pt 1):t-10.

194. Conde-Agudelo A, Diaz-Rossello JL, Belizan JM. Kangaroo mother care to reduce morbidity and mortality in low birthweight infants. [update of Cochrane Database Syst Rev. 2000;(4):CD002771; PMID: 11034759]. [Review] [21 refs]. Cochrane Database of Syst Rev. 2003;(2):CD002771.

195. Engler AJ, Ludington-Hoe SM, Cusson RM, et al. Kangaroo care: national survey of practice, knowledge, barriers, and perceptions. MCN, Am J Matern Child Nurs. 2002;27(3):146–53.

196. Feldman R, Eidelman AI. Skin-to-skin contact (Kangaroo Care) accelerates autonomic and neurobehavioural maturation in preterm infants. Dev Med Child Neurol. 2003;45(4):274–81.

197. Johnston CC, Stevens B, Pinelli J, et al. Kangaroo care is effective in diminishing pain response in preterm neonates. Arch Pediatr Adolesc Med. 2003;157(11):1084–8.

198. Moore ER, Anderson GC, Bergman N. Early skin-to-skin contact for mothers and their healthy newborn infants. Cochrane Database Syst Rev. 2007;4.

199. Acolet D, Sleath K, Whitelaw A. Oxygenation, heart rate, and temperature in very low birthweight infants during skin-to-skin contact with their mothers. Acta Paediatr Scand. 1989;78:189–93.

200. Bohnhorst B, Heyne T, Peter CS, Poets CF. Skin-to-skin (kangaroo) care, respiratory control, and thermoregulation. J Pediatr. 2001;138(2):193–7.

201. Stevens BJ, Johnston C, Petryshen P, Taddio A. Premature infant pain profile: development and initial validation. Clin J Pain. 1996;12(1):13–22.

202. Arditi H, Feldman R, Eidelman AI. Effects of human contact and vagal regulation on pain reactivity and visual attention in newborns. Dev Psychobiol. 2006;48(7):561–73.

203. Mooncey S, Giannakoulopoulos X, Glover V, Acolet D, Modi N. The effect of mother-infant skin-to-skin contact on plasma cortisol and beta-endorphin concentrations in preterm newborns. Infant Behav Dev. 1997;20(4):553–7.

204. Michelsson K, Christensson K, Rothganger H, Winberg J. Crying in separated and non-separated newborns: sound spectrographic analysis. Acta Paediatr. 1996;85(4):471–5.

205. Gray L, Watt L, Blass EM. Skin-to-skin contact is analgesic in healthy newborns. Pediatrics (Evanston IL). 2000;105(1):e14.

206. Johnston C, Campbell-Yeo M, Fernandes A, Inglis D, Streiner D, Zee R. Skin-to-skin care for procedural pain in neonates (Protocol). Cochrane Database Syst Rev. 2010;(3):Art. No.: CD008435. DOI: 008410.001002/14651858.CD14008435.

207. Akcan E, Yigit R, Atici A. The effect of kangaroo care on pain in premature infants during invasive procedures. Turk J Pediatr. 2009;51(1):14–8.

208. Johnston CC, Filion F, Campbell-Yeo M, et al. Enhanced kangaroo mother care for heel lance in preterm neonates: a crossover trial. J Perinatol. 2009;29(1):51–6.

209. Johnston CC, Filion F, Campbell-Yeo M, et al. Kangaroo mother care diminishes pain from heel lance in very preterm neonates: a crossover trial. BMC Pediatr. 2008;8:13.

210. Castral TC, Warnock F, Leite AM, Haas VJ, Scochi CG. The effects of skin-to-skin contact during acute pain in preterm newborns. Euro J Pain: EJP. 2008;12(4):464–71.

211. de Sousa Freire NjB, Santos Garcia JoB, Carvalho Lamy Z. Evaluation of analgesic effect of skin-to-skin contact compared to oral glucose in preterm neonates. Pain (Amsterdam). 2008;139(1):28–33.

212. Chermont AG, Falcao LF, de Souza Silva EH, de Cassia Xavier Balda R, Guinsburg R. Skin-to-skin contact and/or oral 25% dextrose for procedural pain relief for term newborn infants. Pediatrics. 2009;124(6):e1101–7.

213. Kashaninia Z, Sajedi F, Rahgozar M, Noghabi FA. The effect of kangaroo care on behavioral responses to pain of an intramuscular injection in neonates. J Spec Pediatr Nurs. 2008;13(4): 275–80.

214. Kostandy RR, Ludington-Hoe SM, Cong X, et al. Kangaroo care (skin contact) reduces crying response to pain in preterm neonates: pilot results. Pain Manag Nurs. 2008;9(2):55–65.

215. Ludington-Hoe SM, Hosseini R, Torowizc DL. Skin-to-skin contact (kangaroo care) analgesia for preterm infant heelstick. AACN Clin Issues. 2005;16(3):373–87.

216. Cong X, Ludington-Hoe SM, McCain G, Fu P. Kangaroo care modifies preterm infant heart rate variability in response to heel stick pain: pilot study. Early Hum Dev. 2009;85(9):561–7.

217. Ferber SG, Makhoul IR. The effect of skin-to-skin contact (kangaroo care) shortly after birth on the neurobehavioral responses of the term newborn: a randomized, controlled trial. Pediatrics (Evanston IL). 2004;113(4):858–65.

Assessing Disability in the Pain Patient

Steven D. Feinberg and Christopher R. Brigham

Key Points

- Assessing disability in the pain patient is often difficult due to both administrative and clinical issues, yet this assessment is essential.
- Clinically, quantifying pain remains problematic as chronic pain is a subjective phenomenon, often associated with confounding behavioral, characterological, personality, and psychological issues.
- Typically, the physician does not define "disability"; rather, the physician defines clinical issues, functional deficits, and, when requested, impairment. Disability is most often an administrative determination.
- The assessment of disability associated with chronic pain is complex, and the evaluator must approach the clinical evaluation with recognition of the many factors associated with the experience of pain and disability.

- The treating physician who has a doctor–patient relationship with the claimant may have a different perspective than the "independent" disability evaluator.
- While an independent medical evaluation has some similarities to a comprehensive medical consultation, there are significant differences.

Introduction

Assessing disability in the pain patient is often difficult due to both administrative and clinical issues, yet this assessment is essential. Administratively, it is complicated by numerous states, federal, and private systems and policies with different definitions and benefit systems. Clinically, quantifying pain remains problematic as chronic pain is a subjective phenomenon, often associated with confounding behavioral, characterological, personality, and psychological issues. Additionally, the terms impairment and disability are often misunderstood. Furthermore, underlying personality structure and motivation are often determinates for disability. Chronic-pain complaints may be linked with significant disability [1]. Typically, the physician does not define "disability"; rather, the physician defines clinical issues, functional deficits, and, when requested, impairment. Disability is most often an administrative determination.

Pain is the most common cause of disability, with chronic low back pain alone accounting for more disability than any other condition [2]. Disability related to back pain has increased, although there is no significant change in back injuries or pain [3, 4]. Headache disorders are frequently associated with work loss [5]. Despite advances in physiologic understanding and interventions, challenges associated with chronic pain and disability increase.

The pain associated with specific recognized physical conditions needs to be distinguished from somatoform pain disorder. The essential feature of somatoform pain

S.D. Feinberg, M.D. (✉)
Feinberg Medical Group,
825 El Camino Real, Palo Alto, CA 94301, USA

Stanford University School of Medicine,
Stanford, CA, USA

American Pain Solutions,
San Diego, CA, USA
e-mail: stevenfeinberg@hotmail.com

C.R. Brigham, M.D.
Brigham and Associates, Inc,
N. Kalaheo Avenue, Suite C-312, Kailua, HI 96734, USA

American Medical Association,
Chicago, IL, USA
e-mail: cbrigham@cbrigham.com

T.R. Deer et al. (eds.), *Comprehensive Treatment of Chronic Pain by Medical, Interventional, and Integrative Approaches*,
DOI 10.1007/978-1-4614-1560-2_92, © American Academy of Pain Medicine 2013

disorder in DSM-IV [6] is preoccupation with pain in the absence of physical findings that adequately account for the pain and its intensity, as well as the presence of psychological factors that are judged to have a major role. Somatization is defined as a person's conscious or unconscious use of the body or bodily symptoms for psychological purposes or psychological gain [7, 8]. Somatization is characterized by the propensity to experience and report somatic symptoms that have no pathophysiologic explanation, to misattribute them to disease, and to seek medical attention for them. Somatization can be acute or chronic and may be associated with medical comorbidity, an underlying psychiatric syndrome, a coexistent personality disorder, or a significant psychosocial stressor [9]. Somatoform disorders, factitious disorders, and malingering represent various degrees of illness behavior characterized by the process of somatization.

It is important to recognize that in chronic-pain states, physical and psychological factors typically are both present and overlap and that a quality physical examination is critical before dismissing the problem as being purely psychological.

The *biopsychosocial* approach is currently viewed as the most appropriate perspective to the understanding, assessment, and treatment of chronic-pain disorders and disability [2–4, 10, 11]. Chronic pain reflects a complex and dynamic interaction among biological, psychological, and social factors.

Pain, impairment, and disability may coexist, or be independent [5]. Pain is a subjective experience defined by the International Association for the Study of Pain as "an unpleasant sensory and emotional experience associated with actual or potential tissue damage or described in terms of such damage" [12]. Impairment is defined in the AMA *Guides to the Evaluation of Permanent Impairment* (AMA *Guides*) [13] as "a significant deviation, loss, or loss of use of any body system or function in an individual with a health condition, disorder, or disease." Typically, the AMA *Guides* determines impairment on the basis of specific objective findings, rather than on subjective complaints. The AMA *Guides* defines disability as "an umbrella term for activity limitations and/or participation restrictions in an individual with a health condition, disorder or disease." Waddell notes that pain is a symptom, not a clinical sign, or a diagnosis, or a disease, whereas disability is restricted activity [14]. Managing pain does not guarantee that the disability will lessen or resolve. There is not a direct relationship between pain and disability.

Although it is appealing to define disability on the basis of objective as opposed to subjective factors, this is not always the case. The Institute of Medicine Committee on Pain and Disability and Chronic Illness Behavior concluded that "the notion that all impairments should be verifiable by objective evidence is administratively necessary for an entitlement program. Yet this notion is fundamentally at odds with a realistic understanding of how disease and injury operate to incapacitate people. Except for a very few conditions, such as the loss of a limb, blindness, deafness, paralysis, or coma, most diseases and injuries do not prevent people from working by mechanical failure. Rather, people are incapacitated by a variety of unbearable sensations when they try to work" [15].

Assessing disability in the pain patient is thus a challenging endeavor. While some individuals present with a clear and direct connection between pathology and loss of function, it is problematic to measure loss of functional ability in the individual whose behavior and perception of disability and functional loss is significant, sometimes far exceeding that which would be expected from the physical pathology. Some people with chronic pain seek the designation of being "disabled" because of perceived incapacity associated with their portrayed pain and physical dysfunction. For some, seeking such designation is a logical extension of suffering a loss of capacity and utilizing an available benefit system. Others may portray being disability as a reflection of anger, dissatisfaction, or a sense of entitlement.

For some, the designation of being disabled is more complex and may involve seeking attention and/or other benefits that for some observers may seem excessive, unreasonable, and unnecessary. The request for assistance or insurance benefits may take various forms such as a disability parking permit, avoiding waiting lines, housing assistance, help with household chores, and benefits such as monetary payments or subsidies. The individual may claim incapacity (including from work) and request disability benefits under various private, state, or federal programs.

The physician performing a clinical evaluation that will be used to determine disability should perform a biopsychosocial assessment, recognizing the array of factors that relate to the experience of pain and disability. From a physical perspective, it is necessary to clarify the physical pathology. Some pathology cannot be directly measured (headache, neuropathic pain, etc.), and other pathology may have been missed (tumor, herniated disk, complex regional pain syndrome). Secondary to problems with chronic pain, there may be other problems, such as physical deconditioning and secondary psychological issues. Two individuals with similar injuries and resulting pathological changes may present with distinctly different experiences and perceptions. The first may have little or no complaints or perceived disability, while the second individual may present with significant pain behavior and dysfunction.

There may be other nonphysical (psychosocial, behavioral, and cultural) ramifications that may help explain the second individual's pain presentation and assertion of functional loss despite physical findings that do not support the reported disability. Assuming the individual is presenting in an honest and credible manner, the physician then must opine on impairment or functional issues considering physical and these other nonphysical factors. If requested, the physician may also opine on disability. Opining on disability requires an understanding of specific definitions of disability and often specific occupational functional requirements.

Symptom magnification, i.e., illness behavior, is common, particularly in the context of subjective experiences such as chronic pain or litigation. When the individual is not credible or there is purposeful misrepresentation, such as malingering, it may not be possible to accurately define any disability.

The assessment of disability associated with chronic pain is complex, and the evaluator must approach the clinical evaluation with recognition of the many factors associated with the experience of pain and disability.

Symptom Magnification and Malingering

Symptom magnification, inappropriate illness behavior, and embellishment are not uncommon (malingering is less common but occurs and should be considered), particularly in medicolegal circumstances and entitlement programs. Therefore, evaluators need to consider whether the presenting complaints are congruent with recognized conditions and known pathophysiology and have been consistent over time. The evaluator should also determine if there is inappropriate illness behavior.

Pain behaviors (i.e., facial grimacing, holding or supporting affected body part or area, limping or distorted gait, shifting, extremely slow movements, rigidity, moaning, or inappropriate use of a cane) may indicate symptom magnification.

Nonorganic findings, i.e., findings that are not explained by physical pathology, may also support a conclusion of symptom magnification. Nonorganic findings have been described dating back to the early part of the twentieth century [16]. Since that time, a number of nonorganic signs have been defined [17]. In an effort to maximize information from the evaluation, physicians routinely test for nonorganic physical signs. Gordon Waddell, M.D., described five signs to assist in determining the contribution of psychological factors to patients' low back pain [18]. He was specifically interested in developing screening tests to determine the likelihood a patient would have a good outcome from surgery. The physician must perform all five Waddell tests—evaluation for excessive tenderness, regional weakness, overreaction, distraction, and simulation. Isolated positive signs have no clinical or predictive value, and only a score of three or more positive signs is considered clinically significant. These tests were not designed to detect malingering.

Malingering is defined in the *Diagnostic and Statistical Manual for Mental Disorders, Fourth Edition-Text Revised (DSM-IV-TR)* [19] as the "intentional production of false or grossly exaggerated physical or psychological symptoms, motivated by external incentives such as avoiding military duty, avoiding work, obtaining financial compensation, evading criminal prosecution, or obtaining drugs." The DSM-IV-TR states:

Malingering should be suspected if any combination of the following is noted:

1. Medicolegal context of presentation (e.g., the person is referred by an attorney to the clinician for examination)
2. Marked discrepancy between the person's claimed stress or disability and the objective findings
3. Lack of cooperation during the diagnostic evaluation and in complying with the prescribed treatment regimen
4. The presence of antisocial personality disorder

Malingering occurs along a spectrum—from embellishment to symptom magnification to blatant misrepresentation. The possibility of obtaining disability benefits or financial rewards or being relieved from other responsibilities, such as work, increases the likelihood of malingering. Patients may unconsciously or consciously exaggerate their symptoms. With malingering, the intent is purposeful. Ill-defined complaints occur in a circumscribed group, perhaps in a setting of poor morale or conflict, also may be viewed with suspicion. If there are suggestions of significant illness behavior or malingering, a careful investigation including a multidisciplinary evaluation and psychological testing may be required [20, 21].

Treating Physician Versus Independent Medical Evaluation

The treating physician who has a doctor–patient relationship with the claimant may have a different perspective than the "independent" disability evaluator. The treating physician often takes a patient-advocate role and may have little desire or experience to comment on disability, nor will that physician be able to define disability in an independent manner [22].

Frequently, conflict and distrust develops between claimants and the independent evaluating physicians who evaluate them and the claims examiners handling their claim. Patients often report that their problem is being discounting, while physician disability evaluators and claims representatives may express doubt and skepticism about claimants' chronic-pain complaints and reported loss of functional capacity.

The physician has the predicament of viewing the subjective reports in relationship with the objective evidence of tissue damage or organ pathology to come up with some final assessment about the extent to which the patient really is disabled from functional activities. It is not difficult to see how the treating physician advocating for the patient will have a different perspective than the "independent" physician evaluating a claimant for disability.

The "independent" medical evaluator (IME) is also not without his or her biases, and in some jurisdictions, only plaintiff and defense IMEs are the norm. The true IME is used by both sides and in some settings is referred to as the "agreed" medical evaluator (AME).

When the physician provides treatment, the doctor–patient relationship is one of trust. The physician is acting as an agent for the patient. When performing a disability evaluation, the physician is acting as agent for the state or agency requesting the evaluation. In 1992, Sullivan and Loeser recommended that physicians refuse to do disability evaluation on patients they are treating [23].

The problem with this is that adverse consequences may ensue for the patient who may be cut off from benefits absent a signed disability form.

Disability Versus Impairment

The two main terms when discussing disability are impairment and disability. The following definitions are from the AMA *Guides,* the World Health Organization (WHO), and from various state and federal programs.

The AMA *Guides to the Evaluation of Permanent Impairment*, Sixth Edition (hereafter referred to as the *Guides*), defines disability as "an umbrella term for activity limitations and/or participation restrictions in an individual with a health condition, disorder or disease." The AMA *Guides* defines *impairment* as "a significant deviation, loss, or loss of use of any body system or function in an individual with a health condition, disorder, or disease." The sixth edition, published in December 2007, introduces new approaches to rating impairment. The leadership for this edition was provided by Robert Rondinelli, M.D., an experienced physical medicine and rehabilitation physician; therefore, this edition reflects principles of this specialty. An innovative methodology is used to enhance the relevancy of impairment ratings, improve internal consistency, promote greater precision, and simplify the rating process. The approach is based on a modification of the conceptual framework of the International Classification of Functioning, Disability, and Health (ICF), although the fundamental principles underlying the *Guides* remain unchanged.

The World Health Organization (WHO) defines impairment as "any loss or abnormality of psychological, physiological or anatomical structure or function." Problems in body function or structure involve a significant deviation or loss. Impairments of structure can involve an anomaly, defect, loss, or other significant deviation in body structures.

The *International Classification of Functioning, Disability, and Health* (ICF) [24] changes the emphasis from the word "disability" to *activity* and *activity limitation* (WHO 2000). ICF defines activity as "something a person does, ranging from very basic elementary or simple to complex." Activity limitation is "a difficulty in the performance, accomplishment, or completion of an activity. Difficulties in performing activities occur when there is a qualitative or quantitative alteration in the way in which activities are carried out. Difficulty encompasses all the ways in which the doing of the activity may be affected."

Federal and state agencies generally use a definition that is specific to a particular program or service. To be found disabled for purposes of Social Security disability benefits, individuals must have a severe disability (or combination of disabilities) that has lasted, or is expected to last, at least 12 months or result in death and which prevents working at a "substantial gainful activity" level (1). Impairment is described as an anatomical, physiological, or psychological abnormality that can be shown by medically acceptable clinical and laboratory diagnostic techniques.

The Americans with Disabilities Act (ADA) has a three-part definition of *disability*. Under ADA, an individual with a disability is a person who (1) has a physical or mental impairment that substantially limits one or more major life activities, or (2) has a record of such an impairment, or (3) is regarded as having such an impairment. A *physical impairment* is defined by ADA as "any physiological disorder or condition, cosmetic disfigurement, or anatomical loss affecting one or more of the following body systems: neurological, musculoskeletal, special sense organs, respiratory (including speech organs), cardiovascular, reproductive, digestive, genitourinary, hemic and lymphatic, skin, and endocrine."

Regardless of the system, the term impairment defines a measurable change (any loss or abnormality psychological, physiological, or anatomical structure or function) and is consistent and measurable across different systems and programs. On the other hand, disability is a social construct in that each program or system defines it differently and assigns different weights and benefits to those definitions. One can be "disabled" in one system of benefits and not in another despite the same impairment. Disability usually results from an impairment that results in a functional loss of ability to perform an activity.

It is imperative to distinguish the difference between impairment and disability. One individual can be impaired significantly and have no disability, while another individual can be quite disabled with only limited impairment.

For example, a person with a below-knee amputation may be working full time quite successfully as a pianist and, therefore, would not meet the Social Security Administration (SSA's) definition of being disabled. On the other hand, this same pianist might have a relatively minor injury to a digital nerve that severely limits his/her ability to perform basic work activities such as playing a difficult piano concerto. In some disability systems, a person in this situation might meet the definition of partial disabled, even though he/she can do other work.

Perhaps, another way to distinguish the terms disability and impairment is as follows: Some diseases cause a negative change at the molecular, cellular, or tissue level which leads to a structural or functional change at the organ level, a measurable impairment. At the level of the person, there is a deficit in daily activities and this is the disability.

Because of this difference between impairment and disability, and despite the fact that many disability systems are work-injury-loss related, the widely used AMA *Guides* has stated that impairment ratings are not intended for use as direct determinants of work disability. The impairment rating is rather based on universal factors present in all individuals, the level of impact of the condition on performance of activities of daily living, rather than on performance of work-related tasks. The sixth edition of the AMA *Guides* states on p. 6 that "the relationship between impairment and disability remains both complex and difficult, if not impossible, to predict."

While it is true that the AMA *Guides* is a widely used source (the vast majority of state workers' compensation systems require some use of the different editions of the AMA *Guides*) for assessing and rating an individual's permanent impairments, there are a number of states and the federal government's SSA disability program that do not recognize the AMA *Guides* for rating impairment. In addition, the Veterans Administration has its own unique set of disability rating criteria. There is clearly no consensus on a universal system to measure impairment.

Depending upon the system, impairment is necessary for disability, but other factors are considered. Different disability programs attempt to combine medical information and the associated impairment with nonmedical factors that bear on the individual's ability to compete in the open labor market. Other considerations include age, educational level, and past work experience. Physicians typically provide the data regarding the medical condition and impairment, while nonmedical issues are the purview of disability adjudicators.

The AMA Guides and Chronic Pain

The *Guides* provides a discussion of the assessment of pain in Chapter 3—Pain-Related Impairment. The AMA *Guides* states that subjective complaints are included in the provided impairment ratings, and up to 3% whole person permanent impairment may be provided in only unusual circumstances, including that there is no other basis to rate impairment.

Pain specialist physicians may feel that the AMA *Guides* method of impairment rating do not adequately address the

"disability" and functional loss caused by some chronic-pain states. Since the *Guides* limits itself for the most part to describing measurable objective changes or impairment, chronic-pain states, despite causing significant functional losses, are not provided significant impairment ratings.

The American Academy of Pain Medicine has characterized pain with updated terminology, namely, *eudynia* for nociceptive pain and *maldynia* for neuropathic pain. Eudynia (nociceptive pain) is a normal physiologic response to noxious events and injury to somatic or visceral tissue. It can be beneficial and serves as an early warning mechanism. Eudynia often is acute, but can also be persistent (e.g., cancer pain). Eudynia usually is correlated directly with the resultant impairment. In this scenario, pain would appropriately be incorporated into the organ system impairment rating. Maldynia or neuropathic pain often results in significant dysfunction. Whatever pathology exists, it is not well measured with our current testing abilities and the clinician often has difficulty correlating the pathology with the level of reported dysfunction.

The AMA Guides and Maximal Medical Improvement (MMI)

The AMA *Guides* states that an impairment rating can only be done when the individual has reached maximal medical improvement (MMI), i.e., "the point at which a condition has stabilized and is unlikely to change (improve or worsen) substantially in the next year, with or without treatment." It is necessary to determine that the patient is stable and that no further restoration of function is probable. If the examinee shows up and is in the middle of a flare-up or has had a new injury that interferes with the examination, it is premature to do an impairment rating. In other words, the examinee must be stabilized medically for the physician to fairly assess the impairment rating. If the condition is changing or likely to improve substantially with medical treatment, the impairment is not permanent and should not be rated.

The AMA Guides and Activities of Daily Living (ADL)

The AMA *Guides* reflects the severity of the medical condition and the degree to which the impairment decreases an individual's ability to perform common activities of daily living (ADL), *excluding* work.

Throughout the fifth edition of the AMA *Guides*, the examiner is given the opportunity to adjust the impairment rating based on the extent of any activities of daily living (ADL) deficits (5th Ed). The fifth edition of the AMA *Guides* describes typical ADLs as:

- Self-care and personal hygiene (urinating, defecating, brushing teeth, combing hair, bathing, dressing oneself, eating)
- Communication (writing, typing, seeing, hearing, speaking)
- Physical activity (standing, sitting, reclining, walking, climbing stairs)
- Sensory function (hearing, seeing, tactile feeling, tasting, smelling)
- Nonspecialized hand activities (grasping, lifting, tactile discrimination)
- Travel (riding, driving, flying)
- Sexual function (orgasm, ejaculation, lubrication, erection)
- Sleep (restful, nocturnal sleep pattern)

In the sixth edition, a distinction is made between ADLs, basic activities (such as feeding, bathing, hygiene), and instrumented ADLs, complex activities (such as financial management and medications). This edition also distinguishes between activity "execution of a task or action by an individual" and participation "involvement in a life situation" and between activity limitations "difficulties an individual may have in executing activities" and participation restrictions "problems an individual may experience in involvement in life situations."

AMA Guides Impairment Rating Percentages

A 0% whole person impairment (WPI) rating is assigned to an individual with an impairment if the impairment has no significant organ or body system functional consequences and does not limit the performance of the common activities of daily living. A 90–100% WP impairment indicates a very severe organ or body system impairment requiring the individual to be fully dependent on others for self-care, approaching death. The *Guides* impairment ratings reflect the severity and limitations of the organ/body system impairment and resulting functional limitations.

The AMA *Guides* provides weighted percentages for various body parts, but since the total impairment cannot exceed 100%, the Guides provides a combined values chart to enable the physician to account for the effects of multiple impairments with a summary value. Subjective concerns, including fatigue, difficulty in concentrating, and pain, when not accompanied by demonstrable clinical signs or other independent, measurable abnormalities, are generally not given separate impairment ratings. Impairment ratings in the Guides already have accounted for commonly associated pain, including that which may be experienced in areas distant to the specific site of pathology.

The Guides does not deny the existence or importance of these subjective complaints to the individual or their functional impact but notes that there has not yet identified an accepted method within the scientific literature to ascertain how these concerns consistently affect organ or body system functioning. The physician is encouraged to discuss these concerns and symptoms in the impairment evaluation.

The AMA Guides and Work Disability

Impairment assessment is provided by the *Guides*; however, the *Guides* does not define disability. An individual can have a disability in performing a specific work activity but not have a disability in any other social role. An impairment evaluation by a physician is only one aspect of disability determination. A disability determination also includes information about the individual's skills, education, job history, adaptability, age, and environment requirements and modifications. Assessing these factors can provide a more realistic picture of the effects of the impairment on the ability to perform complex work and social activities. If adaptations can be made to the environment, the individual may not be disabled from performing that activity (in this scenario though, the impairment is still present).

The *Guides* is not intended to be used for direct estimates of loss of work capacity (disability). Impairment percentages derived according to the Guides criteria do not measure work disability. Therefore, it is inappropriate to use the *Guides'* criteria or ratings to make direct estimates of work disability.

Independent Medical Evaluation (IME)

While an independent medical evaluation has some similarities to a comprehensive medical consultation, there are significant differences. An independent medical evaluation involves an examination by a health care professional at the request of a third party in which no medical care is provided.

The terminology for these evaluations varies in different areas of the country and includes terms like independent medical evaluation or examination (IME), or in California, an agreed medical evaluation (AME) or qualified medical evaluation or examination (QME). The AME serves both sides of a dispute at the same time and, in a sense, serves as the "medical judge." These evaluations otherwise are typically at the request of one side or the other (defense or plaintiff/applicant).

Medicine and law have different approaches. The practice of law is based on the advocacy system and is contentious and argumentative in nature by design. It is a system that allows different and conflicting points of view to be heard with resolution achieved by way of a jury, judge, or through arbitration. The practice of medicine is focused on diagnosing and treating patients to the best of the physician's ability to help them regain and maintain good health.

Physicians providing either a one-time consultation or ongoing medical care are accustomed to having their advice sought and followed by a usually grateful patient. Whereas in the legal system, physicians can expect to have their opinions challenged vigorously and in detail by skilled attorneys. In some cases, physicians may have their credentials and ability to testify as an expert questioned in a harsh and demeaning manner. While the attack may seem personal, in fact, it is only a method used by attorneys to discredit physicians' testimony to either have it thrown out or its value minimized. A skilled attorney will ask questions that are often difficult to answer, and physicians may find that the opportunity for explanation may be limited.

Possible Versus Probable

The gold standard for a medical opinion is "beyond a reasonable degree of medical probability." Physicians do not have to be 100% certain, but they must form opinions that are medically probably or greater than a 50% chance of being correct. Anything less than this is termed "possible." Anything is possible, but to be accepted as medically reasonable, with a causal relationship, the term probable must be used. It is actually wise to keep away from using specific percentages, as this is hard to substantiate.

Evaluation Process

An independent medical evaluation involves an examination by a health care professional at the request of a third party in which no medical care is provided or suggested. The physician is not involved in the medical care of the examinee (there is no physician/patient relationship or privilege with some exceptions—please see liability issues below) and serves to provide a medical opinion to clarify issues associated with the case. The disability evaluation report is not necessarily to facilitate the well-being of the patient. Medical expertise is assumed for a disability evaluation, as is impartiality and objectivity, but such is not always the case. Unlike a medical consultation, the disability evaluation is not confidential and, further, should be easily read and understood by nonmedical personnel. Standards for independent medical evaluations have been published [25].

Referral Sources

Disability evaluations are an integral part of case management and are utilized widely by insurers and attorneys in a variety of arenas, including workers' compensation, personal injury, and long-term disability.

Workers' compensation systems are no fault, but litigation issues often center around causation, the extent and duration of medical care needs, the length of temporary disability, the extent and cost of permanent impairment and/or disability, and issues of apportionment to nonindustrial causation. An insurance carrier or third-party administrator typically handles claims. Some employers are partially or fully self-insured.

Personal injury litigation including malpractice cases involves primarily the cause and extent of injuries and the level of associated disability. Once a lawsuit is filed, the defendant is generally allowed one IME. In these cases, the defendant is counting on the IME to be unusually thorough as the case may hinge on the examination findings and report conclusions.

Long-term disability cases range from Social Security benefits for persons expected to be totally disabled for at least 12 months to individuals who have purchased or been provided by their employer private disability insurance policies.

Report Quality Issues

While the quality of the physician's testimony at a deposition, arbitration, or trial may be critical, the initial-typed report is typically most important. This report is relied upon in any settlement negotiation and often becomes part of the evidence. The disability evaluation report should be valid, defensible, and readable. A well-written report will assist the physician during cross-examination and may even discourage the opposing attorney from calling the physician to testify. The report itself may lead to early case settlement or resolution. Most often, the physician will be judged by the quality of the written report.

A quality evaluation report is responsive to the specific questions asked by the referral source. The report should be understandable by nonmedical individuals. Often, a verbal report is provided prior to submission of a written report, thus giving the referrer the opportunity to further direct specific questions or concerns or to even defer on receiving a written report. The physician should always maintain integrity but should remember that there is no traditional doctor–patient relationship and the payer is the client.

Report Writing Technique

Evaluation reports should be without spelling errors and should be grammatically correct. The report structure should include appropriate formatting with headings and categories. Bold lettering, italics, underlining, numbering, and bullet points can be used for clarity and emphasis. All material and records reviewed should be listed. Paragraphs should be kept relatively short, and separate ideas should be put in distinct categories. Unnecessary repetition should be avoided. It is of critical importance to use unambiguous language that can be easily understood by the referral source.

Pre-evaluation Issues

Prior to examining the claimant, the physician's office will receive a request for a disability evaluation by the referral source. A chart should be made up and all verbal and written correspondence noted in the record. It is important to provide documentation regarding charges, and usually a curriculum vita will be requested. Some physicians insist on a prepayment advance prior to reviewing records, providing an examination report, or attending a deposition, arbitration, or trial. Charges should include costs for late cancellations, records review, the actual examination, report writing, research, meeting time with the referral source, deposition, arbitration, and trial testimony time. It is important to identify who will be notifying the examinee of the appointment date and time. It is appropriate to review records in advance to assure that all historical items are reviewed with the examinee.

Interactions with the Examinee

If the evaluation is being accomplished at the request of the examinee's attorney or as an agreed medical examiner, there is an implied understanding that the physician is serving in that individual's best interest. When examining for the defense (the "other side"), it is not uncommon to find an examinee who is, at a minimum, suspicious and maybe even hostile.

Depending on the jurisdiction, the claimant's attorney or representative and sometimes even a court reporter may attend the evaluation. This may or not be permissible, dependent on the setting. Any other individual attending the appointment should remain silent and not provide information except for significant others. The claimant may request to tape record the examination; however, whether this is permissible is dependent on the jurisdiction.

It is important in any scenario to carefully explain your role including the fact that the disability evaluation is not meant to be a comprehensive medical evaluation covering all possible problems and that no doctor–patient relationship is implied. Risk is reduced by having the examinee signed an informed consent form. There is usually no confidentiality. Typically, the disability evaluation physician's opinions and any recommendations are not discussed with the examinee unless such is specifically requested by the referral source.

It is recommended that the examinee be told to not perform any maneuver that her or she feels will be harmful to them. Adequate gown coverage is important and a chaperone is recommended.

Evaluation Report Writing

Introduction

Physicians are well aware of the usual details covered in a standard history and physical examination. The disability evaluation report goes into much greater detail in certain areas as compared to a medical consultation since often other factors contribute to the issues of portrayed pain and disability.

The examinee's pre-injury status is carefully detailed. It is very important to determine if there was any disability predating the injury. The history of the injury, subsequent events, and medical care up to the present time are carefully ascertained.

Any inconsistency between the individual's report and information found in the medical record is noted. It is important to remember that individuals often have selective memories and, sometimes, what they remember is not accurate. The medical record is of critical importance; however, it is possible that the health care professional left something out or misunderstood the examinee. Therefore, just because something is not reported in the medical record does not mean that it did not happen as described by the examinee.

A quality disability evaluation report takes all of these factors into consideration. The disability evaluation physician is neither a magician nor fortune-teller, but must assess all the information available and provide a medically reasonable explanation. All the disability evaluation physician can do is to give a sincere and honest opinion and state what is medically probable.

Identifying Information

The report starts out with the identifying information consisting of the date of the report, the name of address of the referral source(s), the name of the examinee, the claim or other identifying numbers (like the date of injury), and the date of the exam if different than the report date. For workers' compensation cases, the employer's name is often listed as well.

Purpose of the Examination

The report should be addressed directly to the referral source. The first report paragraph typically notes the purpose of the exam and any other specific questions asked or reasons for the evaluation. You may add a paragraph noting that the report is based upon the personal interview and examination of the examinee, combined with review of available medical records and radiographs and other submitted information. A list of all records reviewed is either listed in the body of the report or attached as an addendum. You may choose to ask to see examinee picture identification such as a driver's license. You should identify if the examinee was accompanied by an interpreter or any other person (significant other, friend, relative, lawyer, nurse, etc.) and whether the examinee tape recorded the examination. Document that the examinee was informed the purposes of the examination and that there was no doctor–patient relationship and that the examinee should not perform any maneuvers that the individual would consider harmful or injurious.

Examinee Introduction

The next paragraph lists the examinee's age, handedness, and marital status. In the workers' compensation arena, the employer, years on the job, and current work status can be listed.

Pertinent History

For most evaluations, there is a point in time when problems surfaced either due to a specific injury or illness or on a cumulative trauma basis, and this should be identified. You may identify that prior to some identified point in time, the examinee described being in good health without ongoing disability, or that second, the examinee had a pre-injury (or illness) history of pertinence. You should describe any *relevant* prior history of injuries or illness (this might include auto accidents, illnesses, prior work or other injuries, surgeries, etc.) and document a history from the examinee regarding the injury/illness itself and subsequent symptoms and medical care (including medications prescribed and tests/procedures accomplished). You should assess whether the history is consistent with the records, recognizing that examinees do not always recollect their medical history correctly nor are medical records always correct.

Current Symptoms

The current symptoms are carefully documented. A pain diagram can be useful. The examinee is given the opportunity to detail all symptoms and complaints. Any loss of function (activities of daily living) or loss of pre-injury capacity is described. Body parts involved include location and radiation of symptoms and referral patterns along with spatial characteristics, duration periodicity, and intensity/severity.

Pain complaints associated with disability are often described with two components: the character of the pain

(i.e., continuous, non-fluctuating; continuous fluctuating; episodic; paroxysmal, etc.) and the quality of the pain (e.g., burning; freezing; sharp; pins and needles; aching; dull; hot; cold; numbing; and electrical).

Additional descriptors should be listed (tingling, numbness, weakness, swelling, color change, temperature change, sweating, skin or hair growth changes, etc.). Provocative or aggravating factors that worsen the pain and palliative factors that alleviate the symptoms should be detailed. The current intensity of the pain is described on a 10-point scale, where "0" represents no pain and "10" represents the worst pain imaginable. Any bowel, bladder, sexual, or sleep dysfunction should be described.

The presence of any examinee-perceived emotional (anxiety, depression, etc.) or cognitive dysfunction should be noted. Additional relevant information may be obtained from significant others.

Assess

1. What is the *cause of the pain* (the examinee's perspective of what tissue abnormalities are causing the current problem)?
2. The *meaning of the pain* (what is and is not causing further tissue damage, and what is the meaning of the complaint is, i.e., whether there is progression, sinister illness, and/or concern present).
3. The *impact of the pain* on the examinee's life including interference in vocational, social, recreational activities, etc. We recommend a listing of an average day and daily activities.
4. Note the examinee's *perception of appropriate treatment*. An individual who is directed toward a passive treatment approach will have little interest in an active, functional restoration approach.
5. Note the examinee's *goals* to be achieved with further treatment.

Functional History

Obtain information regarding activities of daily living (ADLs—feeding, grooming, bathing, dressing, and toileting) and physical functional activities during an average day (exercise, outdoor activities, shopping, recreation, household chores, etc.). A description of the examinee's daily routine and changes from pre-injury status are documented.

Current and Past Medications

Obtain a list of past and current medications. We find it helpful to request that the examinee brings all current medications to the examination. The examiner should assess medication effectiveness, side effects, and any evidence of misuse or abuse.

Review of Systems

Consider constitutional, head and neck, cardiovascular, respiratory, genitourinary, gastrointestinal, neurological, psychiatric, and musculoskeletal symptoms in the review.

Past Medical and Surgical History

The examiner should especially note relevant injuries and illnesses including accidents (auto and other). There should be a review of all past significant or similar medical diagnoses, treatments, allergies, previous hospitalizations, and surgical procedures plus any history of psychiatric disorders/treatments/hospitalizations. Note potentially significant other medical problems like diabetes, cardiovascular or pulmonary disease, hypertension, arthritis, gout, etc.

Family History

The examinee should be questioned about relevant family history issues especially any alcoholism, substance abuse, major injuries, disability, pain, etc. Disability, illness, or death in the family may affect how the individual responds to his or her own medical problems. A family history of certain diseases may explain symptoms in the examinee that have not previously been well explained.

Personal History

Information in this section can be of critical importance, and areas of concern include the following:

- Childhood, i.e., was the examinee's childhood normal, dysfunctional, or abusive (sexual/verbal/physical)?
- Education, i.e., years of formal education, military service, and any legal history (litigation or incarceration).
- Marital status, i.e., has the examinee ever been married, how many times, and for how long? Was there any associated abuse history?
- Children, i.e., if there are children, what ages and how many? Is there a significant other and is that person working or disabled?
- Current living situation.
- Illicit substance use or abuse? If positive, provide previous and current usage level.
- Tobacco, caffeine, and alcohol usage.
- Current income source, if any (family members, workers' compensation, pension, long-term disability, state disability, Social Security, etc.).

- Work history: The occupational history should include not only the titles, types, and physical intensity of previous jobs but also continuity and length of previous positions. Attitudes about work (work "ethic") can be of considerable importance.

Physical Examination

The physical examination is similar for the disability evaluation as it is for a medical consultation, but it is important to document negative, positive, and nonorganic findings. If you are performing an impairment evaluation, perform the assessment according to specific examination requirements in the AMA *Guides*. When giving testimony, an opposing attorney can make the disability evaluating physician feel quite uncomfortable when parts of the examination are not documented.

The examination integrates information obtained from physical findings to support or refute diagnoses suggested during the history taking. The examination may uncover physical findings not readily apparent from the history or even known to the patient.

The physical examination is not limited to but is directed to the concerned body parts, and when a change or abnormality is identified, the appropriate regional examination is expanded.

The *general observation* of the examinee includes a behavioral examination including such issues as cooperation and attentiveness, along with any pain behaviors or unusual activities. The individual's sitting and standing tolerance is noted and all measurements recorded. Nonphysiologic findings are also noted.

Patient descriptors can include the patient as a good, poor, or fair historian and, when appropriate, can include such terms as pleasant and cooperative (vs. unpleasant and uncooperative), angry or hostile, and/or garrulous or loquacious.

Any *pain behavior* should be noted (verbal—sighing, moaning, groaning and nonverbal—grimacing, guarding, splinting, clutching, bizarre gait).

Constitutional findings refer to the examinee's general appearance (e.g., body habitus, deformities, development, nutrition, and attention to grooming) and vital signs (e.g., height, weight, temperature, blood pressure, pulse, respirations). Any adaptive aids such as braces/splints and walking aids/wheelchair are noted including whether such is appropriate or inappropriate.

Other physical examination findings, dependent on the context of the evaluation, may include:

- *Head, eyes, and ears*—General appearance, deformities, assistive devices (e.g., hearing aids, glasses), and visual/auditory acuity.

- *Mouth, throat, and nose*—General appearance, general dental condition, and patency of airway.
- *Neck*—General appearance, vascular distension, auscultation for bruits, active range of motion (AROM) and passive range of motion (PROM), and lymph nodes.
- *Cardiovascular*—Auscultation of the heart, examination of peripheral pulses, inspection of vascular refilling, varicosities, swelling, and edema.
- *Respiratory and chest*—General appearance of the chest, breasts for masses or tenderness, auscultation of lungs and upper airways, observation of breathing pattern, and examination for peripheral clubbing or cyanosis.
- *Gastrointestinal/genitourinary*—Inspection of abdomen and pelvis, auscultation of bowels, palpation of abdominal organs, and rectal examination.
- *Genitourinary*—Directed as appropriate.
- *Integumentary*—Inspection and palpation of skin and subcutaneous tissues for color, mottling, sweating, temperature changes, atrophy, tattoos, lesions, scars, rashes, ulcers, and surgical incisions.
- *Musculoskeletal*—Inspection, percussion, and palpation of joints, bones, and muscles/tendons noting any deformity, effusion, misalignment, laxity, crepitation, masses, or tenderness; assessment of AROM and PROM and stability of joints; inspection of muscle mass, spinal alignment, and symmetry; and assessment of muscle strength and tone.
- *Provocative tests*—Maneuvers for thoracic outlet syndrome, Phalen's and Tinel's for carpal tunnel, foraminal compression for cervical radiculopathy, straight leg raising for sciatica, etc.
- *Neurologic*—Assessment of level of consciousness (alert, lethargic, stuporous, comatose) and mental status (e.g., orientation, memory, attention and concentration, thought processes and content, speech and communication/language and naming, fund of knowledge, insights into current condition) and assessment of cranial nerves. The neurologic examination also includes assessment of (1) sensation to pinprick, two-point discrimination, sensibility, vibration, and proprioception; (2) assessment of sphincter tone and reflexes (e.g., bulbocavernosus); (3) assessment of deep tendon reflexes (DTR) in the upper and lower extremities, including pathologic reflexes (e.g., Babinski, Hoffman, palmomental, etc.); (4) assessment of coordination (e.g., finger/nose, heel/shin, rapid alternating movements) and tandem gait; and (5) functional mobility including gait and station.
- *Nonphysiologic behaviors*—assessed such as Waddell signs (e.g., superficial skin tenderness, stimulation of back pain by axial loading or trunk rotation, differences in straight leg raising response between supine and sitting positions, regional nonanatomic weakness or numbness, and overreaction/disproportionate pain responses).

Impression

List the diagnostic categories and/or the differential diagnoses.

Discussion

We recommend a succinct summary of the history and physical examination followed by opinions (when requested) on the specific issues requested by the client.

Causation and apportionment are often critical issues to be discussed along with prognosis. The evaluator must be able to determine whether the problem or disability was pre-existing or caused by an event or occurrence, which is not a subject of the claim. If there is a basis for causation for the claim in question, is it fully or partially responsible?

The evaluator must be able to distinguish between an *aggravation and an exacerbation*. An aggravation results from a new event or injury causing a worsening, hastening, or deterioration of a preexisting condition. An exacerbation is a temporary increase in the symptomatology of a preexisting condition.

The issue of whether and when the examinee has reached *maximal medical improvement* (MMI) may also be addressed. The disability evaluator may also be asked to discuss the *prognosis and future medical care* needs of the condition and other costs as part of a life-care plan.

Lastly, the *face-to-face time* spent with the examinee should be listed (some physicians also document records review, research, and report preparation time as well) followed with the examiner's name and signature. Copies of the report to the appropriate parties should be noted.

Functional Capacity Evaluation

The disability evaluator may be asked to address the examinee's functional ability or work capacity. The opinion is based on a review of medical records, the historical and physical examination, test results, and the examinee's functional capacity. The evaluation is made difficult when the individual demonstrates pain behaviors and a suboptimal effort on examination and testing.

The report should include the number of hours to be worked per day, sitting, standing, and walking tolerance, as well as lifting and carrying capabilities. For the upper extremities, the ability to perform forceful and repetitive activities should be discussed. Other factors to be considered are reaching, pushing, pulling, grasping or gripping, bending, crouching, squatting, climbing, balancing, working on uneven terrain, and working at heights. For difficult cases, a formal functional capacity evaluation (FCE) may be helpful.

A physical or functional capacity evaluation (FCE) is a systematic process of assessing an individual's physical capacities and functional abilities. Testing, lasting one-half day to several days, is usually carried out by a physical or occupational therapist with special training and expertise in this area.

The FCE matches human performance levels to the demands of a specific job or work activity or occupation. The FCE establishes the physical level of work an individual can perform. The FCE is useful in determining job placement, job accommodation, or return to work after injury or illness. An FCE can provide objective information regarding functional work ability in the determination of occupational disability status.

The FCE is a tool that can be used to make objective and reliable assessments of the individual's condition. Its precise data format provides information that can be used in various contexts. The FCE may be used (1) to determine the individual's ability to safely return to work full time or on modified duty; (2) to determine if work restrictions, job modifications, or reasonable accommodations are necessary to prevent further injury; (3) to determine the extent to which impairments exist, or the degree of physical disability for compensation purposes; and (4) to predict the potential ability to perform work following acute rehabilitation or a work-hardening/work-conditioning program.

A physical or functional capacity evaluation (FCE) provides additional information beyond what can be determined by the physician-directed disability evaluation, but the FCE does have its limitations as well. The functional capacity of the examinee who does not provide a full effort cannot be accurately assessed. Further, while providing a greater depth of testing than the physician physical examination, the FCE can only measure capacity in a controlled environment over a short period of time and does not necessarily equate with full-time, real-world, everyday life and job tasks.

Reason for the Opinion

The evaluation physician cannot base opinions solely on only the basis of "education, training, and experience." Rather, the disability evaluator must provide a clear description of why a conclusion has been reached. What are the facts in the case that cause you to formulate that opinion? It is important to discuss unusual or abnormal findings.

Post-evaluation Issues

Disability evaluation reports should be completed and sent with appropriate billing to the referral source. The examinee and the treating physician are not provided copies of the disability evaluation report unless requested by the referral source although this is uncommon. Depending upon the particular situation, the referral source should be contacted by phone so the disability evaluator can discuss any opinions or recommendations. In some cases, a written report may not be required or desired at that time. This is particularly true when the opinion generated is not deemed to be in the best interest of the referral source's case.

Testimony

The disability evaluator should be prepared to be deposed and to attend an arbitration hearing or trial. Depositions are usually requested by the opposing counsel to gauge the potential effectiveness of the physician as a witness. Should the case go forward to arbitration or trial, the effectiveness of the disability evaluation physician goes beyond medical knowledge, but also involves the individual's presentation and demeanor in front of a judge and/or jury.

Credibility is always increased through the observer's perception of the physician's honesty and integrity. It is always best to be honest and not appear to be trying to "help" the case of the referral source. Any potential negative information or opinions should have been discussed previously with the referring attorney or claims person as to how to deal with it in the least damaging manner. While honesty and integrity are essential, there is no need to volunteer information that might be damaging to your referral source. It is ultimately the job of the disability evaluation physician to be an expert witness, not to "make" the case for the referral source. It is never appropriate to demean or demonize the claimant or treating physicians.

Physician Disability Evaluation Liability Issues

The claimant may not be pleased with the disability evaluator's opinions. In recent years, medical malpractice lawsuits against physicians who conduct disability evaluations have become more common. Despite the absence of a traditional physician–patient relationship, physicians who conduct disability evaluations still have various legal duties to the examinee, although this issue is in flux and ever changing [26]. Examinees generally can successfully sue IME physicians for negligently causing physical injury during the examination, failing to take reasonable steps to disclose significant medical findings to the patient, and disclosing confidential medical information to third parties without authorization, but they *cannot* successfully sue for inaccurate or missed diagnoses.

Summary

The evaluation of pain and disability is complex and multi-faceted. The evaluating physician must approach such an evaluation from a biopsychosocial perspective. Often, these evaluations are performed in the context of an independent medical evaluation, i.e., an examination by a health care professional at the request of a third party in which no medical care is provided. The evaluation results in a report that must reflect a thorough evaluation, answer the specific issues requested by the client, and be easily understandable by non-medical individuals. These evaluations are part of the legal or advocacy system that may be contentious and argumentative. The skilled independent medical examiner must always maintain impartiality and provide conclusions that are supportable. A thoughtful and thorough evaluation is of considerable value to all involved.

References

1. Aronoff GM. Chronic pain and the disability epidemic. Clin J Pain. 1991;7:330–8.
2. Gatchel RJ, Okifuji A. Evidence-based scientific data documenting the treatment- and cost-effectiveness of comprehensive pain programs for chronic nonmalignant pain. J Pain. 2006;7:779–93.
3. Turk DC, Gatchel RJ, editors. Psychological approaches to pain management: a practitioner's handbook. 2nd ed. New York: Guilford; 2002.
4. Turk DC, Monarch ES. Biopsychosocial perspective on chronic pain. In: Turk DC, Gatchel RJ, editors. Psychological approaches to pain management: a practitioner's handbook. 2nd ed. New York: Guilford; 2002.
5. Robinson JP, Turk DC, Loeser JD. Pain, impairment, and disability in the AMA guides. Guides newsletter. Nov/Dec 2004.
6. American Psychiatric Association. Committee on nomenclature and statistics. Diagnostic and statistical manual of mental disorders. Rev. 3rd ed. Washington, DC: American Psychiatric Association; 1987. Diagnostic and statistical manual of mental disorders. 4th ed. Washington, DC: American Psychiatric Association; 1994.
7. Ensalada LH, Brigham C. Somatization. Guides newsletter. July–Aug 2000.
8. Lipowski ZJ. Somatization: the concept and its clinical application. Am J Psychiatry. 1988;145:1358–68.
9. Lipowski ZJ. Somatization and depression. Psychosomatics. 1990;31:13–21.
10. Gatchel RJ. Comorbidity of chronic mental and physical health disorders: the biopsychosocial perspective. Am Psychol. 2004;59:792–805.
11. Gatchel RJ. Clinical essentials of pain management. Washington, DC: American Psychological Association; 2005.
12. Merskey H, Bogduk N. Classification of chronic pain: descriptions of chronic pain syndromes and definitions of pain terms. 2nd ed. Seattle: IASP Press; 1994.
13. Rondinelli R, editor. AMA guides to the evaluation of permanent impairment. 6th ed. Chicago: AMA Press; 2007.
14. Waddell G. The back pain revolution. 2nd ed. Edinburgh: Churchill Livingstone; 2004.
15. Institute of Medicine Committee on Pain, Disability, and Chronic Illness Behavior (Osterweis M, Kleinman A, Mechanic D, eds.). Pain and disability: clinical, behavioral, and public policy perspectives. Washington, DC: National Academies Press; 1987. p. 28.
16. Collie J. Malingering and feigned sickness. London: Edward Arnold Ltd; 1913.
17. Brigham C, Ensalada LH. Nonorganic findings. Guides newsletter, Sept–Oct 2005.
18. Waddell G, McCulloch JA, Kummel E, Venner R. Nonorganic physical signs in low-back pain. Spine. 1980;5:117–25.
19. American Psychiatric Association. Diagnostic and statistical manual of mental disorders. Text revision. 4th ed. Washington, DC: American Psychiatric Association; 2000.
20. Rogers R, editor. Clinical assessment of malingering and deception. 2nd ed. New York: Guilford Publications; 1997.
21. Meyerson A. Malingering. In: Kaplan H, Sadock B, editors. Textbook of psychiatry. 7th ed. New York: Williams & Wilkins; 2000.
22. Barth RJ, Brigham CR. Who is in the better position to evaluate, the treating physician or an independent examiner? Guides newsletter, 8, Sept–Oct 2005.
23. Sullivan MD, Loeser JD. The diagnosis of disability. Arch Intern Med. 1992;152:1829–35.
24. WHO. International classification of functioning, disability and health: ICF. Geneva: World Health Organization; 2001.
25. Nierenberg C, Brigham C, Direnfeld LK, Burket C. Standards for independent medical examinations. Guides newsletter. Nov/Dec 2005
26. Baum K. Independent medical examinations: an expanding source of physician liability, offer insights and suggestions for limiting physician liability in these situations. Ann Intern Med. 2005;142:974–8.

The Double Effect: In Theory and in Practice

Lynn R. Webster

Key Points

- The principle of double effect has roots in the Hippocratic Oath and moral teachings of the Catholic Church as outlined by Thomas Aquinas.
- The double effect allows serious harm to a person as a secondary effect resulting from a primary action that is good. To satisfy double effect, only the primary good action must be intended, the good outcome must not be produced by means of the bad effect, and the good must outweigh the harm caused.
- The principle has clinical relevance whenever an intervention performed to benefit a patient has the potential or certitude of also causing harm, such as when opioids are administered during end-of-life care.
- Everyday clinical decisions raise questions that involve the difficulty of determining clinician intent, disagreements regarding the limits of patient autonomy, the tension between proponents of compassionate pragmatism vs. moral absolutism, and interpreting the laws that govern the ending of human life.
- Opioids given as therapy for chronic, nonmalignant pain can also cause detriment as well as benefit to individuals and to society and may be considered in light of double effect.
- The question of whether double effect continues as a valuable clinical guide given recent technological advances and the current state of medical ethics remains unresolved.

L.R. Webster, M.D.
Clinical Research,
3838 South 700 East, Suite 200, Salt Lake City, UT 84106, USA
e-mail: lynnw@lifetreepain.com

Introduction

It is not always possible to perform clinical interventions that benefit a patient without also triggering some degree of harm. The double effect (DE) is both a moral and pragmatic principle to determine whether the good outcome resulting from an action outweighs any detrimental secondary effects. The principle's underpinnings are lodged in medieval, theological thought, and the continuing clinical significance of DE to a diverse, technological society is the subject of much debate among scientists and philosophers. In the scientific literature, DE is most often invoked to address questions of what is moral and ethical in end-of-life care.

The following discussion will trace the principle's beginnings, its usual clinical applications, and the areas where DE is most subject to differing interpretations. Reaching beyond the end-of-life debate, the analysis will turn to decisions that must be made while caring for patients who suffer chronic, nonmalignant pain. The question remains open as to whether the arguments raised serve to nullify, modify, or only reinforce the strictures of DE principle, in part or in whole.

The History and Specifics of Double Effect (DE)

The DE has been described variously as a rule, a principle, and a doctrine. The word "doctrine" connotes religious observance in keeping with DE's beginnings in the moral teachings of the Catholic Church as outlined by Thomas Aquinas [1]. In the *Summa Theologica* (II-II, Qu. 64, Art.7), Aquinas reasons, "Nothing hinders one act from having two effects, only one of which is intended, while the other is beside the intention" [2]. Reaching back further still, DE's emphasis on the physician's responsibility to safeguard the total life and well-being of a patient can be traced to the ancient Greek principle of non-maleficence encoded in the Hippocratic Oath.

T.R. Deer et al. (eds.), *Comprehensive Treatment of Chronic Pain by Medical, Interventional, and Integrative Approaches,*
DOI 10.1007/978-1-4614-1560-2_93, © American Academy of Pain Medicine 2013

As interpreted today, DE principle allows bad effects to occur as the result of good action as long as four essential components are satisfied:

1. The primary act in itself must be morally good or at least indifferent.
2. Only the good effect must be intended and not the bad effect.
3. The good effect must not be produced by means of the bad effect.
4. The good achieved must sufficiently outweigh in proportion the harm caused.

The most typical clinical application cited to illustrate DE is the giving of opioids to ease end-of-life pain even when doing so may hasten death. Direct killing through the administration of a lethal drug such as KCl is forbidden. The giving of high-dose opioids, however, has pain relief as its aim and is permissible under DE.

A look at each DE criterion will show how this judgment follows:

- The No. 1 component, which says the primary action must not be morally wrong, appears to be satisfied here: Opioids are not in themselves evil agents, despite their somewhat checkered reputation among laypeople and even some physicians.
- The second component is met because the primary aim is pain control, while death is a potential but unintended secondary evil.
- The third requirement also appears to be met as death is a possible side effect but not the primary means of pain control.
- Most clinicians who treat terminally ill patients, the patients themselves, and their families assign a degree of benefit to a peaceful, pain-free death. They would agree that the fourth component of proportionality is satisfied when a patient who is already close to death and who would otherwise suffer excruciating, escalating pain is relieved of that suffering – even if to do so hastens the inevitable.

The reasoning behind this classic end-of-life scenario appears unimpeachable but is, in fact, anything but controversy free. The biggest areas of contention concern the difficulty of determining clinician intent, the arguments for and against limitations on patient autonomy, and the sometimes unshared view that the ultimate good lies in prolonging life. Furthermore, end-of-life care is only one area in which clinical interventions invoke DE; indeed, anytime an action is performed that raises the possibility of harm to the patient, DE questions are raised.

Intended or Only Foreseen Outcomes

An important distinction occurs between secondary bad outcomes that are "foreseen" and those that are "intended." Many are the examples where an outcome can be reasonably predicted considering the clinical action taken, yet the outcome is not intended (and may even be dreaded) by the physician. For instance, a clinician gives a needed medication that is likely to cause the side effect of nausea. The nausea is certainly not intended, although it is foreseen; thus, steps are taken to minimize the patient's discomfort.

Yet, intention may be difficult to discern. Some critics argue that it is no different to foresee an outcome when one reasonably expects it will occur than to intend that outcome. Take, for example, the clinician who administers a dose of opioids that reasonably could be expected to hasten a death. The question is whether the person performing that action intends a quicker death as a means of ending suffering. This would violate DE, which states that a harm that would be acceptable as a side effect must not occur as a primary means.

Others contend these are very different matters indeed. Sulmasy argues that a clinician who expects, desires, and even prays for a gravely ill patient's death still does not intend the death as a primary aim [3]. This type of reasoning comes from supporters of DE's clinical relevance, who argue that the ambiguities of intent need not render DE impracticable.

Some ethicists make a further distinction between outcomes that *may* occur as opposed to those that certainly will. The question is, for example, whether palliative care involving large doses of opioids is permitted when death is certain or when it is only possible.

Proportionality: How Much Harm Is Too Much?

The fourth rule of proportionality is very important in applying DE principle. It is not enough that bad effects merely be unintended and not the primary action – they must also fail to outweigh the good achieved.

One can see a continuum of proportional harm where the harm rendered is most grave at either end. At one end of the continuum, physicians, perhaps fearing regulatory or other sanctions, administer doses of opioids too weak to relieve pain. At the other end, physicians administer doses larger than needed for pain control that prove lethal. One can see that the proportionality of harm applies not just to doses that may hasten death but to the harm of allowing patients to suffer pain needlessly. In between the two poles lies the therapeutic window.

Applications of Good and "Evil"

In Catholic doctrine, DE differentiates between casts of evil from a religious point of view. No good outcomes must be achieved through evil acts performed with intent. Today, although most Americans are religious, dissent arises as to what constitutes "evil," raising the possibility that words like "detriment" and "harm," which are less fraught with theological judgment, could serve as pragmatic alternatives. Even commonly used terms like "compassion" and "morality" are open to interpretation. Analysts are obliged to wrestle with universal applications of this type of terminology and also with whether the intent behind a given action matters more than its result.

Moral Absolutism Versus Pragmatism

Moral absolutists take the view that the killing of innocents as a primary aim is never justified. A vivid example is that of the pregnant woman who must be rid of a fetus in order to live. The particulars could include eclampsia or malignant hypertension that would kill both the woman and the fetus unless action is taken. To the absolutist, to abort a fetus to save the life of the mother violates DE by perpetrating a primary evil; however, no violation occurs when one performs an operation to remove the uterus (a primary good), though the fetus dies as a result (a secondary evil). Although the operation goes against the argument of some ethicists who would insist that death should be only a possibility – never a certainty – in general, the action is permissible even by the precepts of moral absolutism as represented by Catholic theology: Removal of the uterus whereby the fetus *will* die is (morally) lawful; abortion is not.

Proponents of a viewpoint that could be termed *compassionate pragmatism* reject this solution as being tainted by circular logic and ask, "Why subject the mother to a needless operation?" They argue against the capacity of DE to resolve questions raised by euthanasia and abortion [3]. Why, for example, subject a woman with an ectopic pregnancy to an unnecessary operation – removal of the fallopian tube – to satisfy the requirement that a fetus death must be a side effect, not a means of treatment? Instead, pragmatists argue, why not administer an intramuscular injection of methotrexate to kill the fetus? could be administered. Again, in this example, the fetus will die anyway, and the woman, under the strictest DE interpretation, must undergo an operation to remove organs, thus enduring an unnecessary harm, the pragmatic argument goes [3].

The pragmatist is particularly concerned with apparent inconsistencies in the limits placed on patient autonomy by DE principle. For instance, Shaw points out that killing a person directly is forbidden, although sex changes – which would be seen as horrific mutilation under different circumstances – are allowed. The question raised is why patient autonomy reigns supreme in one instance but not the other:

> The prohibition of euthanasia must derive from a belief that direct killing of the innocent is supremely and always wrong in a way that dreadful mutilations are not. That belief may or may not be true. The patient should decide for himself. [4]

Despite the pragmatist's rejection of moral absolutism, questions of patient autonomy and clinician intent can complicate pragmatic decisions. For example, palliative care advocates who argue passionately for a dying patient's right to pain control often see physician-assisted suicide as an unacceptable overextension of the concept of patient autonomy, a contradiction of a physician's role as healer and an invitation to abuse the practice.

Reconciling the Terminology

Ethics and *morals* are two terms that describe the individual's responsibility to do right and not wrong in relation to one's fellow man. The two somewhat synonymous terms carry different connotations for many people. *Ethics*, with roots in the teachings of Aristotle, describes universal standards of upright character, while *morals* (from the Latin "mores") are more often invoked relative to the standards of a particular social group.

Yet ethics are created in an ongoing fashion and are often defined as the situation dictates. Such *situational ethics* are frequent in DE examples utilizing warfare where many types of gain to the aggressor are deemed "good" sufficient to outweigh the proportion of evil suffered by adversaries.

Cultural relativity also plays a role in what constitutes unallowable harm to a patient. Eastern cultures, for example, may not stress individual autonomy. In addition, some other modern societies do not share equally the United States' uneasiness with physician-assisted suicide; in the Netherlands, for example, acceptance of the practice is far broader [5], though some point to the Dutch as evidence of a "slippery slope" toward involuntary euthanasia.

One could also ask what is meant by "compassion" today. Physicians are expected to do more than present choices and informed consent to patients. They must also listen and empathize, understand the cultural and social significance of certain decisions to the patient, and help patients cope with stress, anxiety, and physical pain [6].

Whenever we apply relative terminology to medical practice, we are responsible for achieving results that are not only theoretically satisfying but also clinically beneficial. One must take special care not to utilize the concept of pragmatism to describe that which is merely convenient to the clinician. When ethics become too situational, the fourth DE component of proportionality may be given too much weight. This occurs when an achieved benefit such as mere clinical expediency is deemed sufficient to outweigh deleterious effects.

Fresh Thinking and Revised Criteria

Western society places great value on individual autonomy. To safeguard this principle, Quill, Dresser, and Brock have offered revised criteria that they believe mesh better with today's medical realities and that help mitigate some of the ethical ambiguities unforeseen by crafters of DE absolutism. They suggest medical decision making be guided by:

- The patient's informed consent
- The patient's degree of suffering
- The absence of less harmful treatment alternatives [7]

In this view, the patient's autonomy and the rule of proportionality are weighted more heavily than the inexact science of ascertaining a clinician's intent or the absolute prohibition against purposefully causing death.

Traditional Clinical Applications (Mostly End of Life)

The impact of DE on medicine is most clearly seen in cases of terminal illness. The application of DE to end-of-life care is contained in the following summation given by the *International Consensus Conference in Critical Care*:

> The patient must be given sufficient analgesia to alleviate pain and distress; if such analgesia hastens death, this "double effect" should not detract from the primary aim to ensure comfort. [8]

DE says death is not a medical treatment and cannot be utilized as a primary aim. Prohibitions would include physician-assisted suicide, euthanasia (voluntary or involuntary) and – in the strictest interpretation – even the withholding of life-sustaining treatment in some instances.

One can see physician actions as a descending ladder organized from the greatest to the least degree of intervention (Fig. 93.1).

Before addressing the different categories of physician action using medical ethics or personal conscience, it is first advisable to understand what the law says about DE.

Double Effect and the Law

The fear that DE opens the door to legalized euthanasia is a prime motivator behind the precepts that get codified into law. The principle has in the past come into conflict with laws forbidding acts or omissions that hasten death. Australian law, for example, clarifies that acting to kill or allowing a person to kill oneself is unacceptable. Palliative care must be "reasonable" and "in good faith" and is never to be confused with euthanasia [9].

In the United States, recent federal focus has been on forbidding clinicians to help people die. The Pain Relief Promotion Act (PRPA) (H.R.2260), which would have imposed stiff penalties on clinicians for assisting the suicide of a patient, was passed by the House of Representatives in 2000 only to stall in committee, never becoming law. The proposal was alternately praised and damned by physicians. The American Medical Association (AMA) hailed the act for acknowledging that death may be hastened by appropriate,

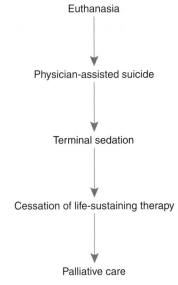

Fig. 93.1 Descending ladder of physician action in end-of-life care

Euthanasia

↓

Physician-assisted suicide

↓

Terminal sedation

↓

Cessation of life-sustaining therapy

↓

Palliative care

aggressive palliative care. But critics decried the attempt to override state law, putting federal authorities in charge of medical determinations such as how high a dose indicates "intent" to assist suicide rather than to relieve pain [10].

The failure of the PRPA was followed by a challenge from the US Attorney General to Oregon's physician-assisted suicide law attempting to outlaw the prescribing of medications to assist with a suicide on the grounds that to do so does not serve "a legitimate medical purpose" under the federal Controlled Substances Act. In the end, the US Supreme Court refuted the challenge, specifying that Congress has not granted medical decision-making power to the attorney general, though it is possible such power could still be granted in the future [11, 12].

The Supreme Court has affirmed that patients have a right to palliative care and also upholds states' rights to pass their own laws regarding physician-assisted suicide; a majority of states have passed laws forbidding the assisting of suicide [13, 14].

US criminal law forbids causing death but protects posing a risk to life if the risk is justified by expected benefits. US law also says a physician is to stop treatment when a competent patient requests, even with the foreknowledge of death. When palliative care does not bring adequate relief, "there is a growing consensus [in the United States] that sedation to the point of comfortable sleep is permissible" [15]. Thus, the law and common medical practice stand against DE, which says the cause of death cannot be intentional.

In general, US law recognizes the right to discontinue life-sustaining therapy but stops short of endowing a patient with the right to die. Some supporters of a patient's right to die find the distinction counterintuitive, asking why the refusal of life-supporting therapy is protected, but the choice to ask a physician for assistance in ending one's life is not [16].

The argument for the patient's right to die is offset by the belief that laws allowing assisted suicide are based on a "cynical argument ... that killing pain and deliberately killing patients are essentially similar, that neither laws nor doctors can effectively distinguish them, that therefore we must allow *both* if we allow either" [17]. So the argument continues unabated.

Is the DE Argument Based on a "Myth?"

Opioids confer enormous benefits for the dying, including the relief of pain and dyspnea. Their side effects include:
- Sedation
- Respiratory depression
- Hypotension
- Vomiting
- Myoclonus
- Delirium
- Anxiety
- Agitation

Do they also hasten death? Some experts in pain and palliative care say no and would render moot DE's relevance to questions of high-dose opioids administered to the dying. Several researchers argue that little evidence supports the precipitation of death so often associated with the giving of opioids at the end of life [18, 19]. Fohr performed an exhaustive literature review, concluding that the belief that opioids hasten death via respiratory depression is "more myth than fact" and further posits that a false belief in DE leads to the undertreatment of pain because physicians fear to hasten death [19]. The American Academy of Pain Medicine (AAPM) and the American Pain Society (APS) uphold the principle that patients on opioid therapy develop tolerance quickly to the risk of respiratory depression and that pain itself antagonizes the effect, further reducing the risk [20].

It is argued that opioids given to dying patients may appear to hasten a death that is instead the result of the disease process and also that benzodiazepines and barbiturates are more likely to induce a sedation that could lead to death than are opioids. However, other literature supports the potential of opioids for hastening death – particularly in patients with sleep apnea – [21–23] and warns against counting on tolerance to confer complete protection to respiratory depression. Research has found that development of tolerance to respiratory depression is highly variable and may lag behind tolerance to other effects, never becoming complete even for long-term opioid users [24, 25].

Categories of Clinician Action

Clinical actions in the treatment of terminal patients throw into sharp relief society's views on patient autonomy and clinician intent. Many commentators take pains to differentiate

the DE-supported use of opioids that may hasten death from the practice of euthanasia. Though some argue for euthanasia or physician-assisted suicide as humane practices, the prohibitions of law and of many individual consciences would disagree. Therefore, the largest gray areas in DE application exist in the categories of terminal sedation and the cessation of life-sustaining therapy, both of which do occur commonly in medical practice.

"Foreseen" and "intended" consequences can be in the eye of the beholder, depending on whether one believes the action achieved is good in proportion to the bad. Research does support the assertion that clinicians, particularly non-specialists, fear to hasten death [26]. The danger exists that, hamstrung by ambiguities, clinicians may refuse to give adequate pain control.

Euthanasia

Euthanasia is the intentional administering of medication or other interventions to cause a patient's death. This can be either voluntary at the request of a competent patient who has received informed consent or involuntary, lacking the request of a competent patient. In DE terms, the intention (to relieve pain) may be laudable, but the primary action (voluntary killing) is impermissible.

The following experience, the memory of a then 26-year-old intern illustrates the daily experiences of clinicians who work with dying patients:

> I will never forget this patient because the experience was terribly painful. He was over 90 and in the VA hospital waiting to die. He did not have a terminal illness – he was just old. He could walk only with tremendous pain. He could perform no other meaningful activities. He was half blind, had partial hearing, couldn't sleep, and was tormented with bowel and bladder problems. He hurt all over, and he had no family. This man did not want to live. Every time I passed his bed, he would grab at me, cry and plead for me to help him die. He suffered physically and emotionally as much as anyone can suffer. His only hope was to escape. I was obliged to observe him being tortured by his own existence. I had nightmares of hearing him scream. Obviously I couldn't comply with his request. My own personal conscience tells me I couldn't have done it then, and I couldn't do it now. But that doesn't mean I don't believe someone could.

The intern who chronicled that memory is the first author of this chapter, now many years removed. The question at stake is whether the preservation of life is always the ultimate value. DE forbids causing a grave harm as an end in itself, but could the law of proportionality sometimes support the belief that allowing a person to suffer excruciating pain with no hope of relief is itself an unjustifiable harm?

Those who argue that active euthanasia – not just acts of omission and "letting die" – can be a compassionate, clinical act are buoyed by the belief that consequences, such as a pain-free death, matter as much or more than absolute prohibitions against deliberate killing [27].

The absolutist would disagree sharply, lobbying for limitations on patient autonomy and the need to scrutinize the clinician's intent as opposed to the clinical outcome. One worry is that a clinician, endowed with too much decision-making power, could succumb to skewed intentions and – overfocused on ending pain – begin euthanizing without consent. Some experts argue it is relatively easy to prove intent by reviewing the medical record of drugs given and actions taken; but this supposition depends mightily on the qualifications of the person doing the looking.

Physician-Assisted Suicide

Physician-assisted suicide refers to the providing of medications or other interventions to a patient who intends to use them to end his or her life [7]. In general, it is assumed that the physician knows what the patient intends. The value assigned to patient autonomy is thus brought directly into conflict with the DE prohibition against intending a patient's death.

Distinctions of intention may be unclear: How, for example, can a physician know for certain what a patient will do with medications sufficient to either relieve pain or to cause death (if taken in high enough quantities)? Is it sufficient to violate DE if a physician knows a death will result from his action, even if it is the patient's own final action that brings the death about?

In addition to the prohibitions enforced by law, a fair number of medical professionals and associations oppose physician-assisted suicide, believing it reflects a failure to provide adequate palliative care and psychological support to the dying. The American Medical Association (AMA) has announced its firm opposition to physician-assisted suicide as a contradiction of the physician's role as healer. The familiar arguments that pit the right to a pain-free death and patient autonomy against the need to safeguard life and guard against a "slippery slope" of suspect clinician intent also apply here.

Terminal Sedation

Terminal sedation refers to the administration of a dose larger than is needed for analgesia with the goal of sedating the patient to the point of unconsciousness to relieve untreatable pain. This action often occurs in tandem with the cessation of life-sustaining therapies. The intentionality of causing death is incompatible with DE, although many physicians perform this action, which is supported by current medical ethical standards and allowed by law. The practice is not meant to provide mere clinical expediency and should be driven only by the patient's symptoms. It requires informed consent from the patient or the permission of a surrogate. Critics complain that terminal sedation is comparable to slow euthanasia and could be easily abused by clinicians.

Cessation of Life-Sustaining Therapy

Cessation of life-sustaining therapy involves the withholding or withdrawing of life-sustaining medical treatments from the patient to let him or her die. This is where DE conflicts most strongly with commonly accepted medical ethics and clinical reality. A survey showed that 39 % of physicians who had sedated patients while stopping life-sustaining treatment had not just foreseen but had intended to hasten the death of the patient [7].

Fear of violating the absolute prohibition against intentionally causing death may lead some physicians to refuse to withdraw nonbeneficial, life-sustaining treatment, even when such a refusal clearly violates the wishes of the patient and the patient's family. The nitty-gritty of the debate is summarized thus "Many persons and groups reject the position that death should never be intentionally hastened when unrelievable suffering is extreme and death is desired by the patient" [7]. Here, pragmatic compassion butts heads with moral absolutism.

Palliative Care

Palliative care concentrates on improving quality of life for terminal patients. It involves the administering of opioids or other medications to relieve pain with the potential incidental consequence of causing respiratory depression sufficient to result in the patient's death. Courts have upheld a patient's right to palliative care as long as the primary purpose is to relieve pain, not to hasten death.

For some commentators and clinicians in the field, it is sometimes difficult to distinguish between the dose of medication that relieves suffering and the dose of medication that ends a life in order to bring about the same aim: the relief of suffering. In particular, it may be difficult to distinguish between euthanasia and palliative care when death is not just a potential but a known outcome of interventions.

Some clarification can be found in the knowledge that morphine and other opioids are pain-relieving aids, not mere agents of death as would be carbon monoxide. Some also insist that a lag is needed between pain relief and death, meaning doses that instantly kill a patient constitute euthanasia rather than palliative care [9].

In some cases, the confusion causes needless suffering. It has been estimated that greater than 90 % of pain associated with severe illness is relievable if established guidelines are followed [15]. Yet the literature contains examples of physicians and nurses refusing to administer "as needed" doses of opioids – even to patients who are close to death and suffering excruciating pain from advanced malignancies – for fear of "causing" a patient's death [15].

In the matter of palliative care, the line between the dose that kills and the dose that relieves pain grows narrower as the patient reaches the end. In practice, healthcare providers in hospice and palliative care accept hastened death as the price of giving optimal treatment to patients who are dying. Some admit they have hastened a death to end unendurable pain, then ponder whether they have crossed a line where their "intent" was to administer death rather than symptom relief.

The fact remains that if the disease process were not present, the need to end suffering would not be either. Yet neither is the DE component of proportionality to be forgotten:

> After all, physicians are not permitted to relieve the pain of kidney stones with potentially lethal doses of opiates simply because they foresee but do not intend the hastening of death! A variety of substantive medical and ethical judgments provide the justificatory context: the patient is terminally ill, there is an urgent need to relieve pain and suffering, death is imminent, and the patient or the patient's proxy consents. [28]

Impact of the Technology on DE Debate

Current techniques sometimes provide alternatives that manage pain without hastening death. In this way, advances in technology change the DE conversation. Many proponents of palliative care who campaign strenuously for better pain control for the dying believe that those who plead for allowing patients to die may be motivated by an unwillingness or inability to provide adequate interventions. A call to increase the skills and training of those who care for the dying appeared in the letters column of the *New England Journal of Medicine*: "It is sad that our care of the dying has lagged behind other forms of medical care, justifying the fear of many persons that they will not be able to die with dignity and comfort" [29].

A patient's comfort as he or she nears death may well depend as heavily on the absence of psychological and emotional agony as it does on the relief of physical pain. In general, using sedation to relieve a patient's psychic symptoms courts greater controversy than using the same dose to address physical symptoms.

Technology is important to this distinction. The advent of spinal opioid treatment, which delivers opioid analgesia without triggering psychic effects, is one advance in pain treatment that reframes the question of what constitutes adequate relief of suffering at the end of life. The following cases presented at the 2002 *American Pain Society* meeting illustrate the point:

Two of three patients, all of whom suffered advanced malignancies, intractable pain, and unacceptable side effects such as mental clouding, were implanted with an intrathecal pump to deliver analgesia. Both patients attained greater than 50 percent pain relief and increased cognitive function. However, this latter benefit came at a price: an increase in anxiety, depression, and difficult issues that presented conflicts with family members [30].

When pain can be relieved at the end of life without significant psychic side effects, who is there to help patients deal with the extraordinary psychological burden presented by their situation? Palliative care *must* seek to answer this question.

DE Applications to a Nonterminal, Chronic-Pain Population

The precepts of DE apply outside the realm of terminal illness, encompassing any clinical intervention that measures harm against benefit. Physicians and other clinicians who specialize in the care of patients suffering from chronic, nonmalignant pain are accustomed to weighing the benefit against the harm, from clinical and regulatory standpoints, even if they have never thought of the process in terms of DE. One can see DE applications in microcosm and macrocosm, pertaining to the individual and the relative good of society as a whole.

The giving of opioids to manage chronic, nonmalignant pain can be considered a primary good, thus satisfying the first component of DE. However, what if opioids are being given knowingly to someone who is not gaining adequate pain relief from opioids and who suffers from an active addiction? The intent might be to help that person forestall the agony of withdrawal symptoms, so ostensibly the goal is to ease suffering. However, the clinician should consider that any benefit gained is likely to be short term and that to continue to provide opioids to people with addiction may tip the balance.

On a macro level, overdose deaths involving pain medications are increasing [31]. Based on historical data, a small percentage of patients with chronic, nonmalignant pain who are prescribed opioids could die, either by intentional or unintentional overdose. Some may also die from suicide if pain is not treated. The secondary evil occurs as a result of the good intent and primary action: the giving of opioids to relieve pain and improve physical function and quality of life for the majority of patients. Thus, the fourth component of proportionality is important in determining how much good is achieved at the risk of ill effect.

Assume a few patients in a pain practice may inject, distribute, or otherwise misuse opioids prescribed for pain. The intended good effect is pain relief, and the detrimental effect is drug abuse or addiction from overdose. Opioid prescribing for chronic pain is based on the belief that the large numbers of patients who use their medications as directed derive substantial benefit, outweighing the harm caused by a smaller number of patients who misuse them. However, if a clinician's prescribing becomes careless, resulting in a larger number of patients harmed than helped by opioids, at that point, the prescribing clinician's action would not meet the rule of proportionality.

Summary

DE has been described as a means of explaining exceptions to the absolute prohibition to purposefully ending human life [28]. Supporters maintain its value as a moral compass and clinical aid. However, DE principle is frequently challenged as containing too much ambiguity to serve as a truly useful clinical guide, and modifications through compassionate pragmatism are intended to bring DE in line with current medical ethics.

Whatever a clinician's personal convictions, it is imperative to clarify the wishes of patients or their surrogates and to give whatever treatments provide the greatest comfort and cause the least harm. While supporting patient autonomy, one should try to ensure that a patient's expressed desire to die does not stem from inadequate, though available, pain control or lack of psychological support. DE is one guide for a clinician to consult, along with relevant laws and accepted medical practices, when in the view of the patient, the benefit of living no longer outweighs the pain endured in meeting the inevitable end.

Acknowledgment   Beth Dove of Dove Medical Communications, Salt Lake City, Utah, contributed technical writing and manuscript review. (Note: Please note the spelling of Dove – not Dover – Medical Communications).

References

1. Mangan J. An historical analysis of the principle of double effect. Theol Stud. 1949;10:41–61.
2. Aquinas T. (13th c). Summa Theologica II-II, Q. 64, art. 7, "Of Killing". In: Baumgarth WP, Richard J, Regan SJ, editors. On law, morality, and politics. Indianapolis/Cambridge: Hackett Publishing Co; 1988. p. 226–7.
3. Sulmasy DP. Killing and allowing to die: another look. J Law Med Ethics. 1998;26(1):55–64.
4. Shaw AB. Two challenges to the double effect doctrine: euthanasia and abortion. J Med Ethics. 2002;28(2):102–4.
5. Purdy L. Ending life [book review]. JAMA. 2006;295(7):830–1.
6. Tauber AI. Patient autonomy and the ethics of responsibility. Cambridge: MIT Press; 2005.
7. Quill TE, Dresser R, Brock DW. The rule of double effect – a critique of its role in end-of-life decision making. N Engl J Med. 1997;337(24):1768–71.
8. Carlet J, Thijs LG, Antonelli M, et al. Challenges in end-of-life care in the ICU. Statement of the 5th International Consensus Conference in Critical Care: Brussels, Belgium, April 2003. Intensive Care Med. 2004;30(5):770–84. Epub 2004 Apr 20.
9. McGee A. Double effect in the criminal code 1899 (QLD): a critical appraisal. QUT Law Just J. 2004;4(1):46–57.
10. Orentlicher D, Caplan A. The pain relief promotion Act of 1999: a serious threat to palliative care. JAMA. 2000;283(2):255–8.
11. Annas GJ. Congress, controlled substances, and physician-assisted suicide – elephants in mouseholes. N Engl J Med. 2006;354(10):1079–84.
12. Kapp MB. The U.S. Supreme court decision on assisted suicide and the prescription of pain medication: limit the celebration. J Opioid Manag. 2006;2(2):73–4.
13. Vacco v. Quill, 117 S.Ct. 2293. 1997.
14. Washington v. Glucksberg, 117 S.Ct. 2258. 1997.
15. Quill TE, Meier DE. The big chill – inserting the DEA into end-of-life care. N Engl J Med. 2006;354(1):1–3.
16. Canick SM. Constitutional aspects of physician-assisted suicide after Lee v. Oregon. Am J Law Med. 1997;23(1):69–96.
17. Reality check on the pain relief promotion act. Secretariat for Pro-Life Activities, United States Conference of Catholic Bishops, 3211 4th Street, N.E., Washington, DC 20017–1194 (202) 541–3070. http://www.nccbuscc.org/prolife/issues/euthanas/reality2.htm. Accessed 17 Aug 2006.
18. Sykes N, Thorns A. The use of opioids and sedatives at the end of life. Lancet Oncol. 2003;4(5):312–8.
19. Fohr SA. The double effect of pain medication: separating myth from reality. J Palliat Med. 1998;1(4):315–28.
20. The use of opioids for the treatment of chronic pain: a consensus statement from American Academy of Pain Medicine and American Pain Society. Approved by the AAPM Board of Directors on 29 June 1996. Approved by the APS Executive Committee on 20 Aug 1996. http://www.ampainsoc.org/advocacy/opioids.htm. Accessed 19 July 2005. Under review.
21. Farney RJ, Walker JM, Cloward TV, Rhondeau S. Sleep-disordered breathing associated with long-term opioid therapy. Chest. 2003;123(2):632–9.
22. Wang D, Teichtahl H, Drummer O, Goodman C, Cherry G, Cunnington D, Kronborg I. Central sleep apnea in stable methadone maintenance treatment patients. Chest. 2005;128(3):1348–56.
23. Webster LR, Grant BJB, Choi Y. Sleep apnea associated with methadone and benzodiazepine therapy [abstract]. Poster presented at the 22nd annual meeting of the American Academy of Pain Medicine (AAPM), San Diego, 2006.
24. White JM, Irvine RJ. Mechanisms of fatal opioid overdose. Addiction. 1999;94(7):961–72.
25. Santiago TV, Pugliese AC, Edelman NH. Control of breathing during methadone addiction. Am J Med. 1977;62(3):347–54.
26. Schwartz JK. The rule of double effect and its role in facilitating good end-of-life palliative care: a help or a hindrance? J Hosp Palliat Nurs. 2004;6(2):125–33.
27. Snelling PC. Consequences count: against absolutism at the end of life. J Adv Nurs. 2004;46(4):350–7.
28. McIntyre A. Doctrine of double effect. In: Edward NZ, editors. The stanford encyclopedia of philosophy. Summer 2006 ed. 2006. http://plato.stanford.edu/archives/sum2006/entries/double-effect/. Accessed August 20, 2012.
29. Patterson JR, Hodges MO. The rule of double effect [letter]. N Engl J Med. 1998;338(19):1389.
30. Cahana A. Is optimal pain relief always optimal? Bioethical considerations of interventional pain management at the end of life. Am Pain Soc Bull. 2002;12(3):1–4.
31. Webster LR. Methadone-related deaths. J Opioid Manag. 2005;1(4):211–7.

Failure to Treat Pain

Kenneth L. Kirsh, Steven D. Passik, and Ben A. Rich

Key Points

- Despite issues of misuse and abuse with opioid analgesics, pain continues to be undertreated and many barriers exist to proper access to pain care.
- In place of a pure disease model, there is a need to get back to incorporating issues of palliation into medicine in order to live up to the calling to reduce suffering.
- While there has been a trend towards under-prescribing controlled medications for pain out of fear of regulatory sanction, several cases have shown that undertreatment of pain can also be a cause for civil liability.
- The failure to treat pain is fundamentally a failure of empathy and prescribers need to acknowledge their own strengths and weaknesses in this area in an open and honest fashion.
- In addition to issues of empathy, prescribers need to be aware of social psychological phenomenon such as observer-subject bias and the psychoanalytic notion of projective identification when assessing and treating patients with chronic pain issues.

K.L. Kirsh, Ph.D. (✉)
Department of Behavioral Medicine,
The Pain Treatment Center of the Bluegrass,
2416 Regency Rd, Lexington, KY 40503, USA
e-mail: doctorken@windstream.net

S.D. Passik, Ph.D.
Department of Psychology and Behavioral Sciences,
Memorial Sloan-Kettering Cancer Center,
641 Lexington Avenue, 7th Floor, New York, NY 10022, USA
e-mail: passiks@mskcc.org

B.A. Rich, JD, Ph.D.
School of Medicine Alumni Association Endowed Chair of Bioethics,
University of California, Davis School of Medicine,
4150 V Street, Suite 2500, Sacramento, CA 95817, USA
e-mail: barich@ucdavis.edu

Introduction

Simply stated, there is an epidemic of undertreated pain, and it has been recognized as a major public health problem [1]. The question that begs to be answered, candidly and definitively, is how such a state of affairs could have developed at the very time when advances in medical science and technology offer a wide variety of pharmacological and non-pharmacological measures for the management of pain. The problem of undertreated pain is complex, and therefore, so too must be any plausible explanation of it.

Barriers to Effective Pain Management

The barriers to pain management are so well recognized by now that they might, somewhat pejoratively, be characterized as "the usual suspects" (see Table 94.1). With the advent of managed care, a barrier that has increased in significance is the lack of adequate reimbursement by third party payers for pain management [2]. There are also patient-centered barriers that, to a significant degree, mirror the clinician-related problems of ignorance and fear concerning the use of opioids in pain management [3]. Until recently, one might reasonably anticipate that patients would share such knowledge deficits since what they did know about pain management would be largely dependent upon what their clinicians could impart to them. However, with the rise of the internet, many patients now have access to a wealth of information on pain management that may or may not be within the working knowledge of the clinicians whom they encounter.

An elucidation of these barriers actually raises more questions than it answers. During a time when the ethical and legal debate over physician-assisted suicide came to a head in the 1990s, national health-care organizations (representing physicians, nurses, and other types of health-care professionals) insisted that the role of their professions was to treat disease and relieve suffering, not cause or hasten a patient's death [4]. Yet, just as the health professions were reaffirming

Table 94.1 Barriers to effective pain management

Inadequate clinical and continuing education on the assessment and management of pain
Insufficient understanding of the adverse clinical and psychological impact of undertreated pain on patients and their families, and consequently, a failure to make pain relief a priority in patient care
The virtual absence of monitoring of pain management by clinicians or accountability for demonstrable deficiencies in clinician knowledge, skills, and attitudes with regard to the assessment and management of pain
A regulatory environment that has historically been, and to a significant extent continues to be, hostile to appropriately aggressive pain management practices

Table 94.2 Comparison of the curative versus palliative model

Curative model	Palliative model
Analytic and rational	Humanistic and personal
Clinical puzzle solving	Patient as person
Mind-body dualism	Mind-body unity
Disvalues subjectivity	Privileges subjectivity
Biomedical model	Biocultural model
Discounts idiosyncrasy	Privileges idiosyncrasy
Death = failure	Unnecessary suffering = failure

their clinical priority and professional responsibility to relieve suffering, the clinical literature was documenting their manifest failure to do so [5]. This failure was not merely a phenomenon of rural, outpatient settings where a lack of state-of-the-art pain management strategies might be anticipated but in the citadels of the most prestigious academic medical centers [6]. Clearly, a major disconnect between the goals and aspirations of the health professions on the one hand, and the real life experience of patients on the other had been revealed. If, as the opponents of physician-assisted suicide maintained, virtually all pain can be safely and effectively managed, and doing so is one of the primary professional responsibilities of clinicians, then how could the previously identified barriers to effective pain management have produced this epidemic of undertreated pain?

The Culture of Medicine and the Culture of Pain

One response is that the prescriber's purported duty to relieve pain and suffering is much more rhetoric than a reflection of a genuinely felt sense of professional responsibility [7]. Twenty-five years ago, in a seminal article on the subject, Cassell wrote that the major goal of medicine is to reduce or relieve suffering [8]. Nearly 10 years later, he elaborated on this issue, stating that modern medicine largely fails to relieve suffering adequately [9].

A major issue involves the biomedical model of disease and the curative model of medical practice, which causes the prescriber to focus on the pathophysiology of disease rather than the patient's experience of illness. Unless and until clinicians can focus on the patient as person, rather than the body as the locus of a disease process, they cannot begin to address pain and suffering. The major problem posed by the curative model of medical practice is that its essential features stand in stark contrast, indeed, diametric opposition to those of the palliative model (see Table 94.2) [10].

In the curative paradigm, pain is a symptom of an underlying medical condition. Patient reports of pain constitute information that facilitates the diagnosis of the underlying

condition and the formulation of a treatment plan. From this perspective, measures intended to reduce or possibly even eliminate the pain would be counterproductive, as they would (theoretically) deprive the clinician of potentially important information. This propensity to categorize pain as a clinical datum to be processed rather than a personal experience calling for a compassionate response by the clinician can itself exacerbate the problem by causing the patient to feel abandoned.

The Cultivation of Ignorance

The barrier of knowledge deficits on the part of clinicians in the assessment and management of pain has been documented in the clinical literature for decades [11]. These deficits can be directly linked to the virtual absence of pain management in the medical school curriculum [12]. This curricular void has produced not just knowledge deficits that clinicians themselves recognize but also myths and misinformation about the risks (especially addiction to opioid analgesics) and potential side effects of opioids that are perpetuated in the informal medical curriculum from one generation of physicians to another [13]. A clinician in the full grip of these pervasive myths and misinformation could, and commonly did, invoke the ancient medical maxim of primum non nocere as the moral basis for withholding opioid analgesics from patients who required them for pain relief.

The Proliferation of Fear

Surveys of physicians consistently reveal a high level of anxiety concerning regulatory oversight of their prescribing of opioid analgesics [14]. The primary fear factor has been a well-established pattern and practice of state medical boards of charging physicians with "overprescribing" pain medications, particularly opioid analgesics for patients with chronic nonmalignant pain [15]. More recently, physicians who treat large numbers of chronic nonmalignant pain patients have been increasingly made the targets of DEA (Drug Enforcement Administration) investigations and federal criminal prosecutions for "drug trafficking" [16]. In a host of guidelines and policy statements, physicians are admonished to balance a patient's need for opioid analgesics with their purported responsibility as prescribers to prevent drug abuse, diversion, and trafficking [17]. The combination of these factors perpetuated what one commentator has characterized as an "ethic of underprescribing" in the medical community [18]. Such an ethic, of course, runs counter to the ancient and core value of the medical profession concerning the relief of suffering.

The fear factor was significantly complicated when a few health-care institutions and professionals were held liable for substantial damages in civil actions alleging a failure to manage pain. The first such case was brought against a skilled nursing facility in North Carolina. The crux of the complaint was that a nursing administrator had discontinued a pain management regimen for an elderly patient with metastatic prostate cancer because she considered it to be excessive. A jury found the facility that employed her guilty of gross negligence and assessed compensatory and punitive damages in the amount of $15 million [19]. Ten years later, a California jury awarded damages of $1.5 million to the family of an elderly patient who died of lung cancer. The basis for the award was that the patient's pain had been ineffectively managed by the physician who had been responsible for his care during a 5-day hospitalization prior to his death [20]. This case achieved substantial national notoriety for a number of important reasons. First, because tort reform legislation in California precluded the recovery of damages in a medical malpractice suit for pain and suffering following the death of the patient, the civil action against the physician and hospital was brought under the state elder abuse statute, which allowed such a postmortem award. Second, prior to the litigation, the Medical Board of California had investigated a complaint against the physician by the patient's family. Its reviewing expert had found the physician's pain management to be inadequate, yet the board declined to take any disciplinary action. The stark contrast between how the board saw the case and how the jury saw the case seemed to epitomize the disparity noted much earlier by Cassell.

Such cases established what was, but should not have been, an entirely new precedent (i.e., liability of health-care institutions and professionals for undertreating pain). The underlying premise of these civil actions was quite straightforward – pain management is like any other aspect of patient care in that if it is done negligently or otherwise inappropriately; it can give rise to professional liability and the award of substantial monetary damages [21]. Such jury verdicts indicate that lay jurors take the clinician's responsibility to relieve pain and suffering very seriously. Similarly, state medical boards began to recognize that failure to properly manage a patient's pain might constitute unprofessional practice and thereby justify disciplinary action against a prescriber who had, in effect, subjected a patient to unnecessary pain or suffering. In 1999, Oregon became the first state to impose sanctions on a physician solely and exclusively for failure to properly manage the pain of several of his patients who were gravely ill or dying [22]. Subsequently, in 2003, the Medical Board of California pursued disciplinary action against a physician for failing to demonstrate in his care of an elderly patient dying of mesothelioma that he understood the nature and properties of some of the analgesics he prescribed for the patient [23]. Given the failure of the California Board to take any action in the case just 2 years earlier, this suggests a remarkable shift in attitude and approach to allegations of substandard pain management practice.

The Emerging Paradigm

Failure to appropriately assess and treat pain is now generally recognized as a form of substandard care and unprofessional practice. Many state medical board policies, and the model policy of the Federation of State Medical Licensing Boards, admonish physicians that effective pain management is an essential feature of quality patient care. Failure to provide such care, or to refer a patient to a clinician who can provide it, can constitute the basis for disciplinary action and/or malpractice liability. Organizations such as the American Academy of Pain Medicine and the American Pain Society, among others, have promulgated clinical practice guidelines to assist clinicians in fulfilling their responsibilities to all patients with pain. However, it would be presumptuous and overly simplistic to conclude that simply promulgating guidelines and promoting continuing professional education will magically remove the barriers to pain relief [24]. There are attitudes and ways of thinking in the culture of medicine and the health professions that contribute significantly to the problem of undertreated pain.

The Role of Empathy

The failure to treat pain is fundamentally a failure of empathy. From a clinical and psychological perspective, there are multiple pragmatic and psychological factors that argue against the ability of the health-care provider and the patient to relate to one another. If they could, it is hard to argue that the problem of undertreated pain would be of the magnitude that it has been, even when we take the previously mentioned barriers into account. Perhaps those involved in patient care will ultimately be better served if they simply learn to accept the fact that they are unable to rely solely on their empathy. While they may be, at their core, good caring people, this is not sufficient to make them competent or effective in the treatment of pain. Ultimately, the use of rating scales and aids that facilitate the objective measure of pain, and thereby communication about it, are the only hope in allowing for better, more empathic pain care. Ultimately, the souring of the regulatory and legal climates surrounding pain management creates fear, and fear widens the gulf between doctor and patient [25].

When students begin health-care training, it is easy to elicit from them expressions that their primary motivation for doing so is the desire to help people. What aspect of intervening in the care of another human being meets this criterion more readily than treating pain? When young medical trainees first enter their clinical rotations, they are psychologically very close to patients. A study of the content of the nightmares experienced by trainees revealed that residents at the beginning of training often find themselves in the patient role in a nightmare, such as being operated on without anesthesia [26]. It is important to make a marked distinction between this early form of sympathy, wherein a trainee overidentifies with the patient and the more appropriate level and skill of empathy, which entails putting oneself objectively in the viewpoint of another without taking on their emotional investment in the situation. Medical education provides the necessary distance to allow for empathy and perspective taking, as opposed to actually feeling the pain of the patient. This distance is probably necessary to allow physicians to do what they must do to other human beings in situations where, if there were too much emotional investment, perhaps it would be impossible to perform painful procedures. Thus, distance begins to develop, and by the end of training, residents' nightmares more commonly put them in the physician role. But is this distance good or bad thing when they are called upon to treat pain?

When we hear that older, non-white females have the highest likelihood of being undertreated for their cancer pain or that Hispanics are half as likely to receive pain medications in emergency rooms when they have the same long bone fractures as whites, are we to believe that medicine is ageist, racist, and sexist [27–29]? Or that in AIDS patients, being uneducated is a risk factor for poor pain care (along with a history of a substance abuse)? [30] Or is it possible – that in fields historically dominated by younger, educated, white men – that being different from your physician works against you somehow and drives the likelihood of their ability to empathize with your suffering even further underground?

These issues have perhaps been best studied in cancer. That the undertreatment of pain is a problem in oncology only reinforces the fact that the problem of undertreatment is even more profound in nonmalignant pain. In cancer clinics, studies have been done to examine how well oncologists and oncology nurses can intuit their patients' suffering. In studies of the agreement of patients' self report with reports given by their professional caregivers about their estimations of the patients' pain, depression, and overall quality of life, agreement tends to occur for the lowest intensity of the symptom [31–34]. Thus, as long as the patients say that they are not in a lot of pain or are not too depressed or that there are no major problems in quality of life, their physicians and nurses agree with them. But when problems become more intense, the agreement falls off dramatically, leading to a marked tendency to underestimate the suffering of patients in many different facets.

Pragmatic Factors

There are many pragmatic considerations that detract from the experience of empathy for people in pain. They can be roughly categorized into system-related, patient-related, and professional-related barriers. The first, system-related barriers, includes time pressures created by the very brief time in which the physician and patient are in the room together and reimbursement issues that fail to adequately compensate the physician for treating pain and thereby lower attention to and interest in pain management [25, 35–38]. Second, patient-related barriers include the multiple fears patients harbor that inhibit them from aggressively and accurately reporting pain and suffering to their physicians – from the fear of addiction to fears of being a bad patient and fears of distracting the physician from the treatment of their primary disease to not wanting to acknowledge pain for fear that it may represent progression of disease [39]. These barriers lead to inhibited communication about pain, which in turn fails to provide the physician with the building blocks for empathy and concern. Beliefs such as "no news is good news" and "don't ask, don't tell" are quite common among patients. Finally, there are physician-related barriers, such as the failure to acquire adequate knowledge of pain assessment and management and the fear of regulatory oversight.

Unconscious Processes: The Mechanics of (Unempathic) Judgment

Cognitive and social psychologists have described numerous unconscious aspects of how humans make judgments that are out of awareness and have referred to these as the "mechanics of judgment" [40–44]. For example, when four items are randomly placed in four different positions, the item in the third position is preferred and chosen an inordinate number of times. This is not something people are generally aware of, yet it colors the perceptions of quality and preference. This use of subtle preferences and prototypes goes on out of conscious awareness. To what extent do physicians' judgments of pain and suffering in their patient, so important to the ability to empathize, fall victim to such mechanical aspects of the way humans think and make judgments?

Are patients thought to be in pain or not, to require attention or not, because of processes that go on out of awareness for the person making the assessment? When one hears that there is a consistent inability to match the patient's assessment of their pain, depression, or quality of life, one might come to believe that the physician might be using a prototype of "what an outpatient with cancer feels" than what the individual patient sitting in front of them actually feels. This would be a fruitful avenue for further research.

Social psychologists have identified one such unconscious process that would seem most relevant to this discussion, namely, the observer-subject bias [45]. When one person looks at another's behavior and is asked to make a judgment about why that person is acting the way that they are, the observer is likely to posit a *characterological* explanation for the behavior (often termed the fundamental attribution error). On the other hand, when one is asked why they themselves are behaving in the way that they are, they tend to posit *situational* explanations (often termed the self-serving bias).

Unconscious Content

Is there unconscious sadism and hostility towards people in pain harbored by practitioners of medical and related disciplines that impede pain management? In classic papers on the undertreatment of pain, the insightful and brutally honest Sam Perry believed this to be the case [46, 47]. Are the pain patients who are nonresponsive to our ministrations actually thwarting our desires to help? Does this lead to engendering anger and sadistic impulses? Are patients who are seen to be "bringing their problems onto themselves," such as addicts and obese people, deserving of our scorn? If not, how do we explain the callous treatment they sometimes receive (i.e., carrying out painful procedures without the provision of adequate analgesia)? In a classic paper "Hate in the Counter-Transference," Winnicott [48] examines how patients who are depressed and self-destructive (like so many people in chronic pain) engender unconscious hate in their caregivers that can drive the patient into despair. Do people who have been the victims of abuse and neglect (like so many people in chronic pain) manage to unconsciously and unwittingly engage us in faulty caregiver scenarios that perpetuate more of the same? This process has been called projective identification by the psychoanalysts and is as germane to the care of people with pain as they are to psychoanalytic treatments of non-pain patients [49–51]. Yet psychoanalysts continually involve themselves in introspection and their own psychotherapy and supervision to examine themselves for such tendencies. Would all of us who treat patients benefit from doing the same?

Summary

The problem of undertreated pain can be solved. To do so, we need to address the medical and legal climates and the realities of a clinical situation that detract from empathic care. These realms are intricately tied to one another. In the end, professionals will need to accept the fact that, while they are caring people, there are too many barriers to the treatment of pain and the provision of empathic care that they simply cannot be overcome flying by the seats of our collective pants. We will have to accept our limitations and then work to overcome them with technologic and educational initiatives that promote communication and empathy such as screening tools and other aids.

References

1. Brenna SF, editor. Chronic pain: America's hidden epidemic. New York: Atheneum/SMI; 1978.
2. Hoffman DE. Pain management and palliative care in the era of managed care: issues for health insurers. J Law Med Ethics. 1998;26:267–89.
3. Bostrom M. Summary of the mayday fund survey: public attitudes about pain and analgesics. J Pain Symptom Manage. 1997;13:166–8.
4. Quill TE, Lo B, Brock DW. Palliative options of last resort. JAMA. 1997;278:2099–104.
5. Cleeland CS, Gonin R, Hatfield AK, et al. Pain and it's treatment in outpatients with metastatic cancer. N Engl J Med. 1994;330:592–6.
6. The SUPPORT Principal Investigators. A controlled trial to improve care for seriously ill hospitalized patients. JAMA. 1995;274:1591–8.
7. Foley KM. Pain relief into practice: rhetoric or reform? J Clin Oncol. 1995;13:2149–51.
8. Cassell EJ. The nature of suffering and the goals of medicine. N Engl J Med. 1982;306:639–45.
9. Cassell EJ. The nature of suffering and the goals of medicine. New York: Oxford University Press; 1991.
10. Fox E. Prominence of the curative model care, a residual problem. JAMA. 1997;278:761–3.
11. Von Roenn JH, et al. Physician attitudes and practice in cancer pain management. Ann Intern Med. 1993;119(2):121–6.
12. Weiner RS. An interview with John J. Boncia, M.D. Pain Pract. 1989;1:2.
13. Hill CS. When will adequate pain treatment be the norm? JAMA. 1995;274:1881–2.
14. Skelly FJ. Fear of sanctions limits prescribing pain drugs. Am Med News. 1994;15:19.
15. Hoover v. Agency for Health Care Administration, 676 So. 2d 1380 (Fla. Dist. Ct. App. 1996).
16. Brushwood DB. The chilling effect is no myth. Available at http://www.doctordeluca.com/Library/WOD/ChillingEffectNoMyth04.htm. Accessed on 13th July 2012.
17. Suthers JW. Professional Standards Committee of the Colorado Prescription Drug Abuse Task Force. Colorado Guidelines of Professional Practice for Controlled Substances. Denver, CO: Colorado Prescription Drug Abuse Task Force; 3rd ed. 1999.

18. Martino AM. In search of a new ethic for treating patients with chronic pain: what can medical boards do? J Law Med Ethics. 1998;26:332–49.

19. Estate of Henry James v. Hillhaven Corp., 89 CVS 64 (Super. Ct. Hertford Co., N.C. 1991).

20. Bergman v. Chin, M.D. No. H205732-1 (Cal. App. Dept. Super. Ct. Feb. 16, 1999).

21. Rich BA. A prescription for the pain: the emerging standard of care for pain management. William Mitchell Law Rev. 2000;26:1–91.

22. In the Matter of Paul A. Bilder, M.D. Stipulated Order. Oregon Board of Medical Examiners; 1999. Available at: http://www.drug-policy.org/docUploads/Bilder_v_Oregon_Stipulated_Order.pdf. Accessed on 13th July 2012.

23. Accusation of Eugene Whitney, M.D. Medical Board of California. Case No. 12-2002-133376. 2003.

24. Max MB. Improving outcomes of analgesic treatment: is education enough? Ann Intern Med. 1990;113(11):885–9.

25. Passik SD, Kirsh KL. Fear and loathing in the pain clinic. Pain Med. 2006;7(4):363–4.

26. Marcus ER. Medical student dreams about medical school: the unconscious developmental process of becoming a physician. Int J Psychoanal. 2003;84(Pt 2):367–86.

27. Cleeland CS. Undertreatment of cancer pain in elderly patients. JAMA. 1998;279(23):1914–5.

28. Cleeland CS, Gonin R, Baez L, Loehrer P, Pandya KJ. Pain and treatment of pain in minority patients with cancer. The Eastern Cooperative Oncology Group Minority Outpatient Pain Study. Ann Intern Med. 1997;127(9):813–6.

29. Todd KH, Samaroo N, Hoffman JR. Ethnicity as a risk factor for inadequate emergency department analgesia. JAMA. 1993;269(12):1537–9.

30. Breitbart W, Passik S, McDonald MV, Rosenfeld B, Smith M, Kaim M, Funesti-Esch J. Patient-related barriers to pain management in ambulatory AIDS patients. Pain. 1998;76(1–2):9–16.

31. Grossman SA, Sheidler VR, Swedeen K, Mucenski J, Piantadosi S. Correlation of patient and caregiver ratings of cancer pain. J Pain Symptom Manage. 1991;6(2):53–7.

32. Passik SD, McDonald M, Dugan W, Theobald D. Oncologists' recognition of depression in their patients with cancer. J Clin Oncol. 1998;16(4):1594–600.

33. McDonald M, Passik SD, Dugan W, Rosenfeld B, Theobald D, Edgerton S. Nurses' recognition of depression in their patients with cancer. Oncol Nurs Forum. 1999;26(3):593–9.

34. Fisch MJ, Titzer ML, Kristeller JL, Shen J, Loehrer PJ, Jung SH, Passik SD, Einhorn LH. Assessment of quality of life in outpatients with advanced cancer: the accuracy of clinician estimations and the relevance of spiritual well-being – a Hoosier Oncology Group Study. J Clin Oncol. 2003;21(14):2754–9.

35. Mechanic D, McAlpine DD, Rosenthal M. Are patients' office visits with physicians getting shorter? N Engl J Med. 2001;344(3):198–204.

36. Ohtaki S, Ohtaki T, Fetters MD. Doctor-patient communication: a comparison of the USA and Japan. Fam Pract. 2003;20(3):276–82.

37. Balkrishnan R, Hall MA, Mehrabi D, Chen GJ, Feldman SR, Fleischer Jr AB. Capitation payment, length of visit, and preventive services: evidence from a national sample of outpatient physicians. Am J Manag Care. 2002;8(4):332–40.

38. Joranson DE. Are health-care reimbursement policies a barrier to acute and cancer pain management? J Pain Symptom Manage. 1994;9(4):244–53.

39. Ward SE, Goldberg N, Miller-McCauley V, Mueller C, Nolan A, Pawlik-Plank D, Robbins A, Stormoen D, Weissman DE. Patient-related barriers to management of cancer pain. Pain. 1993;52(3):319–24.

40. Gati I, Tversky A. Weighting common and distinctive features in perceptual and conceptual judgments. Cognit Psychol. 1984;16(3):341–70.

41. Kahneman D. A perspective on judgment and choice: mapping bounded rationality. Am Psychol. 2003;58(9):697–720.

42. Kahneman D, Tversky A. On the reality of cognitive illusions. Psychol Rev. 1996;103(3):582–91; discussion 592–6.

43. Johnson-Laird PN, Girotto V, Legrenzi P. Reasoning from inconsistency to consistency. Psychol Rev. 2004;111(3):640–61.

44. Redelmeier DA, Koehler DJ, Liberman V, Tversky A. Probability judgement in medicine: discounting unspecified possibilities. Med Decis Making. 1995;15(3):227–30.

45. Haro JM, Kontodimas S, Negrin MA, Ratcliffe M, Suarez D, Windmeijer F. Methodological aspects in the assessment of treatment effects in observational health outcomes studies. Appl Health Econ Health Policy. 2006;5(1):11–25.

46. Perry SW. Irrational attitudes toward addicts and narcotics. Bull N Y Acad Med. 1985;61(8):706–27.

47. Perry SW. Undermedication for pain on a burn unit. Gen Hosp Psychiatry. 1984;6(4):308–16.

48. Winnicott DW. Counter-transference. III. Br J Med Psychol. 1960;33:17–21.

49. Rizq R. Ripley's Game: projective identification, emotional engagement, and the counselling psychologist. Psychol Psychother. 2005;78(Pt 4):449–64.

50. Waska R. Addictions and the quest to control the object. Am J Psychoanal. 2006;66(1):43–62.

51. Yahav R, Oz S. The relevance of psychodynamic psychotherapy to understanding therapist-patient sexual abuse and treatment of survivors. J Am Acad Psychoanal Dyn Psychiatry. 2006;34(2):303–31.

Index

T.R. Deer et al. (eds.), *Comprehensive Treatment of Chronic Pain by Medical, Interventional, and Integrative Approaches*,
DOI 10.1007/978-1-4614-1560-2, © American Academy of Pain Medicine 2013

Printed in the United States of America